Shnider and Levinson's
Anesthesia for Obstetrics

Shnider and Levinson's Anesthesia for Obstetrics

Fourth Edition

Edited by

Samuel C. Hughes, M.D.
Professor of Anesthesia and Perioperative Care
University of California San Francisco
Director, Obstetrical Anesthesia
San Francisco General Hospital
San Francisco, California

Gershon Levinson, M.D.
Staff Anesthesiologist
California Pacific Medical Center
San Francisco, California

Mark A. Rosen, M.D.
Professor and Vice Chairman of Anesthesia and Perioperative Care
Professor of Obstetrics, Gynecology & Reproductive Sciences
Director, Anesthesia Residency Training Program
University of California San Francisco
Director, Obstetrical Anesthesia
Moffitt-Long Hospital (UCSF Medical Center)
San Francisco, California

LIPPINCOTT WILLIAMS & WILKINS
A **Wolters Kluwer** Company
Philadelphia • Baltimore • New York • London
Buenos Aires • Hong Kong • Sydney • Tokyo

Acquisitions Editor: Craig Percy
Developmental Editor: Tanya Lazar
Production Editor: W. Christopher Granville
Manufacturing Manager: Colin Warnock
Cover Designer: Mark Lerner
Compositor: TechBooks
Printer: Courier Westford
Cover Illustration: Mother and Child, Eskimo Sculpture by Peter Anoutak

© 2002 by LIPPINCOTT WILLIAMS & WILKINS
530 Walnut Street
Philadelphia, PA 19106 USA
LWW.com

Printed in the USA

Library of Congress Cataloging-in-Publication Data

Shnider and Levinson's anesthesia for obstetrics / edited by Samuel C. Hughes, Gershon Levinson, Mark A. Rosen.—4th ed.
    p. ; cm.
    Rev. ed. of: Anesthesia for obstetrics. 3rd ed. c1993.
    Includes bibliographical references and index.
    ISBN 0-683-30665-0
    1. Anesthesia in obstetrics. I. Title: Anesthesia for obstetrics. II. Hughes, Samuel C.
III. Levinson, Gershon, 1943– IV. Rosen, Mark A. V. Shnider, Sol M., 1929–
    [DNLM: 1. Anesthesia, Obstetrical. WO 450 S5586 2001]
RG732 .A553 2001
617.9′682—dc21   200103831

Care has been taken to confirm the accuracy of the information presented and to describe generally accepted practices. However, the authors, editors, and publisher are not responsible for errors or omissions or for any consequences from application of the information in this book and make no warranty, expressed or implied, with respect to the currency, completeness, or accuracy of the contents of the publication. Application of this information in a particular situation remains the professional responsibility of the practitioner.

The authors, editors, and publisher have exerted every effort to ensure that drug selection and dosage set forth in this text are in accordance with current recommendations and practice at the time of publication. However, in view of ongoing research, changes in government regulations, and the constant flow of information relating to drug therapy and drug reactions, the reader is urged to check the package insert for each drug for any change in indications and dosage and for added warnings and precautions. This is particularly important when the recommended agent is a new or infrequently employed drug.

Some drugs and medical devices presented in this publication have Food and Drug Administration (FDA) clearance for limited use in restricted research settings. It is the responsibility of the health care provider to ascertain the FDA status of each drug or device planned for use in their clinical practice.

10 9 8 7 6 5 4 3 2 1

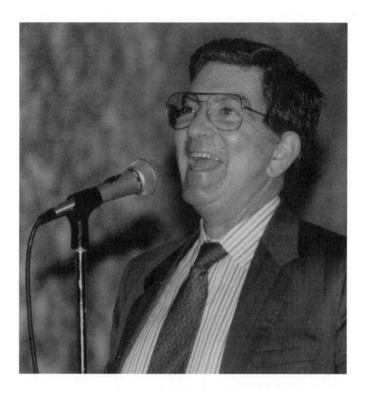

Sol M. Shnider, M.D. (1929–1994)

Born in Yorktown, Saskatchewan, Canada, Dr. Shnider received his
medical degree from the University of Manitoba and undertook
residency training in anesthesia at Columbia University in New York.
He spent most of his professional life dedicated to teaching
and research in the field of obstetrical anesthesia at the
University of California San Francisco. Dr. Shnider was a founding
member of the Society for Obstetric Anesthesia and Perinatology,
recipient of numerous awards and honors, and the first editor of this
book. Indeed, he was one of the pioneers of modern obstetrical
anesthesia. He is remembered by many around the world for his
contributions and impact as a great physician, educator, investigator,
and mentor. He died prematurely at the peak of his illustrious
career. We dedicate this book to our teacher, mentor and friend,
Sol M. Shnider, M.D.

PREFACE

Anesthesia for Obstetrics in its previous editions taught obstetric anesthesia to the majority of today's practitioners. Since the publication of the first edition in 1979, this book has become the international standard in the field, with translations in Spanish, French, Portuguese, German, and Japanese. This textbook has served as a valuable clinical guide and reference source for more than a generation of students and clinicians. Most of the currently prominent obstetric anesthesiologists "grew-up" on this now classic textbook.

The field of obstetric anesthesia has grown dramatically over the years. This is demonstrated by the growth of obstetric anesthesia subspecialty societies around the world such as the Society for Obstetric Anesthesia and Perinatology (SOAP), the Obstetric Anaesthetists Association (OAA), Club Italiano Anestesisti Obstetrici (CIAO), Club d'Anesthésie-Réanimation en Obstétrique (CARO), and the Norsk Interesse gruppe for Obstetrisk Interesserte Anestesileger.

The third edition was published in 1993 and since then, significant changes and advances in the field of obstetric anesthesia have occurred. For example, the introduction of combined spinal epidural anesthesia in the late 1980s is now used for 80% of parturients receiving regional analgesia in some centers. Controversies and new research continue to require alterations and additions to the text. The chapter on the effects of anesthesia and uterine activity in labor has undergone a major revision because of the heated controversy and extensive research in this area. Some chapters are completely new to this edition, others were totally rewritten, and the rest were significantly revised. For example, the chapters on anesthesia for cesarean section and regional anesthesia for labor and delivery have undergone major revisions prompted by a large body of research and changing clinical practice. The chapter on intraspinal opioids has undergone considerable updating, with a new introduction on mechanisms of pain. Chapters on neurosurgery and amniotic fluid embolism have been completely rewritten. The exciting and emerging field of fetal surgery has been highlighted in this revision, and this chapter remains the original and classic source of information in this field. There is a new chapter on airway management, a critical factor in avoiding maternal mortality and morbidity. We trust the reader will discover many other important, practical, and clinically useful changes throughout the text.

We wrote this book to facilitate learning and to serve as a guide to clinical care for the pregnant patient and delivery room care for the newborn. We are particularly grateful to our 48 contributors, including 25 new authors, who represent the next generation of leaders in the field. These new authors bring a fresh outlook to this text. Many of the authors are nationally and internationally recognized as authorities in anesthesiology, perinatology, and the law. The book has grown with the field of obstetric anesthesia over the years. This is reflected by the number of contributors: 17 in the first edition and now 48 in this fourth edition. We trust this edition will serve as an even more valuable standard reference textbook, focused for the clinician, continuing the quality of the previous three editions.

This text was written as a foundation and clinical reference for students and clinicians to learn the challenging field and undertake the rewarding practice of obstetric anesthesia. We have tried to present the classic information in an organized and accessible manner, as well as to discuss the many controversies and less well-established practice issues and concerns. Our focus however remains the clinical practice and the practical aspects of obstetrical anesthesia. While we have included extensive references in each chapter to help guide the practitioner, we also present clear outlines of clinical practice with suggested techniques. The most basic aspects of clinical practice are clearly outlined so that the reader can quickly answer routine clinical questions and form a management plan.

This book is dedicated to the late Sol M. Shnider, M.D., our teacher, mentor and friend, who was an inspiration in our professional careers. The book was initially, and remains, inspired by the hundreds of residents we have trained at the University of California San Francisco over the years, and whom we have had the privilege of teaching. They are the energy and light that have made this book possible. It is our hope that they and the many students in other programs around the world will continue to find this book useful, not only in training but also in practice. We hope they will continue to learn and ultimately expand upon this knowledge.

No book of this scope is published without the strong support of colleagues, family, and friends. We are extremely thankful to contributors for their valuable time and effort which make this book possible. We wish to acknowledge the patience of our families and friends during the preparation of this book: Donald, Dana, Shelley, Jim, Sandy (SCH); Jean, Charles, Jonathan (GL); and Fonda, Sasha, Kayla (MAR). We are also very grateful to Judy Johnson and Russell Brent whose editorial professionalism and talented abilities made major contributions to the quality of this book. Judy Johnson has worked with Sol and us for many years; she worked on the previous three editions of this book and provided invaluable continuity, friendship, an abiding dedication and enthusiasm, as well as tireless effort. Although new to this project, Russell Brent proved masterful in his assistance, particularly in graphics preparation, skilled efficiency in organizing and managing the numerous manuscript versions and their references, and timely rationing of his sagacious wit, which added much joy in the preparation of this book.

Samuel C. Hughes, M.D.
Gershon Levinson, M.D.
Mark A. Rosen, M.D.

CONTRIBUTING AUTHORS

Deborah L. Anderson, C.N.M.
Assistant Clinical Professor
Department of Obstetrics, Gynecology
    and Reproductive Science
University of California San Francisco
San Francisco General Hospital
San Francisco, California

Valerie A. Arkoosh, M.D.
Chair,
Department of Anesthesiology
Professor of Anesthesiology,
    Obstetrics and Gynecology
MCP Hahnemann University
Philadelphia, Pennsylvania

Rhonda K. Arnette, M.D.
Research Fellow, Obstetrical Anesthesia
Department of Anesthesia and
    Perioperative Care
University of California San Francisco
San Francisco, California

Cedric R. Bainton, M.D.
Professor of Anesthesia
    and Perioperative Care (Emeritus)
University of California San Francisco
San Francisco, California

Gerard M. Bassell, M.B., B.S.
Professor of Anesthesiology,
    Obstetrics and Gynecology
University of Kansas School of Medicine
Wichita, Kansas

Diane R. Biehl, M.D.
Professor
Department of Anesthesia
University of Manitoba
Section Head
Obstetrical Anesthesia
St. Boniface General Hospital
Winnipeg, Manitoba, Canada

Philip R. Bromage, M.B.B.S., F.R.C.A., F.R.C.P.C.
Professor of Anaesthesia (Emeritus)
McGill University
Montreal, Quebec, Canada

William R. Camann, M.D.
Associate Professor of Anesthesia
Harvard Medical School
Director of Obstetric Anesthesia
Brigham and Women's Hospital
Boston, Massachusetts

A. Sue Carlisle, Ph.D., M.D.
Professor of Anesthesia and Perioperative Care
University of California San Francisco
Chief, Anesthesia and Peroperative Care
San Francisco General Hospital
San Francisco, California

H.S. Chadwick, M.D.
Associate Professor of Anesthesiology
Director, Obstetric Anesthesia
University of Washington
Seattle, Washington

Theodore G. Cheek, M.D.
Associate Professor of Anesthesia and
    Obstetrics and Gynecology
Associate Director of Obstetric Anesthesia
University of Pennsylvania
Philadelphia, Pennsylvania

Sheila E. Cohen, M.B., Ch.B., F.R.C.A.
Professor of Anesthesia and Obstetrics
    and Gynecology (by courtesy)
Stanford University School of Medicine
Director of Obstetric Anesthesia
Lucile Salter Packard Children's Hospital
Stanford, California

Patricia A. Dailey, M.D.
Staff Anesthesiologist
Mills Peninsula Health Services
Burlingame, California

Sanjay Datta, M.D., F.F.A.R.C.S. (Eng)
Professor of Anesthesia
Harvard Medical School
Senior Staff Anesthesiologist
Brigham and Women's Hospital
Boston, Massachusetts

Richard E. Dodge, Esq. (*Deceased*)
Attorneys-at-Law
McNamara, Houston, Dodge, McClure,
    and Ney Corporation
Walnut Creek, California

Barbara A. Dodson, M.A., M.D.
Professor of Anesthesia and Perioperative Care
University of California San Francisco
San Francisco, California

M. Joanne Douglas M.A., M.D., F.R.C.P.C.
Clinical Professor of Anesthesia
Head, Division of Obstetric Anaesthesia
University of British Columbia Faculty of Medicine
Head, Department of Anesthesia
British Columbia Women's Hospital and Health Center
Vancouver, British Columbia, Canada

Kenneth Drasner, M.D.
Professor of Anesthesia
 and Perioperative Care
University of California San Francisco
Director, Postoperative Pain Service
San Francisco General Hospital
San Francisco, California

James C. Eisenach, M.D.
Francis M. James III Professor
 of Anesthesiology
Wake Forest University School of Medicine
Winston-Salem, North Carolina

Mieczyslaw Finster, M.D.
Professor of Anesthesia,
 Obstetrics and Gynecology
College of Physicians and Surgeons
 of Columbia University
Attending Anesthesiologist New York
 Presbyterian Hospital
New York, New York

Robert R. Gaiser, M.D.
Associate Professor of Anesthesiology
Director, Obstetric Anesthesia
Associate Professor of Pharmacology
University of Pennsylvania
Philadelphia, Pennsylvania

George A. Gregory, M.D.
Professor of Anesthesia and Pediatrics
Department of Anesthesia and
 Perioperative Care
University of California San Francisco
San Francisco, California

Holly C. Gunn, M.D.
Staff Anesthesiologist
Capitol Anesthesiology Association
Austin, Texas

Brett B. Gutsche, M.D.
Professor of Anesthesiology,
 Obstetrics and Gynecology
University of Pennsylvania
Philadelphia, Pennsylvania

Stephen Halpern, M.D., MSc, F.R.C.P.C.
Associate Professor of Anaesthesia
 Obstetrics and Gynaeology
University of Toronto
Director of Obstetrical Anaesthesia
Sunnybrook and Women's
 Health Sciences Centre
Toronto, Ontario, Canada

Joy L. Hawkins, M.D.
Professor of Anesthesiology
Director of Obstetric Anesthesia
University of Colorado School of Medicine
Denver, Colorado

Samuel C. Hughes, M.D.
Professor of Anesthesia and
 Perioperative Care
University of California San Francisco
Director, Obstetrical Anesthesia
San Francisco General Hospital
San Francisco, California

Charlize Kessin, M.D.
Staff Anesthesiologist
Department of Cardiac Surgery
Hospital Nove de Julho
Assistant in Anesthesia
Department of Surgery
Hospital das Clinicas
Universidade de Sao Paulo
Sao Paulo, Brazil

Sarah J. Kilpatrick, M.D., Ph.D.
Professor of Obstetrics and Gynecology
Director, Division of Maternal-Fetal Medicine
University of Illinois at Chicago
Chicago, Illinois

Tekoa L. King, C.N.M., M.P.H.
Associate Professor
Department of Obstetrics, Gynecology
 and Reproductive Sciences
University of California San Francisco
San Francisco, California

Russell K. Laros, Jr., M.D.
Professor of Obstetrics, Gynecology &
 Reproductive Sciences
University of California San Francisco
San Francisco, California

Gershon Levinson, M.D.
Staff Anesthesiologist
Department of Anesthesia
California Pacific Medical Center
San Francisco, California

Andrew M. Malinow, M.D.
Professor of Anesthesiology
 and Obstetrics,
 Gynecology & Reproductive Sciences
University of Maryland School
 of Medicine
Chief, Obstetric Anesthesiology
University of Maryland Hospital
Baltimore, Maryland

Susan R. Gorman Maloney, M.D.
Staff Anesthesiologist
California Pacific Medical Center
Assistant Professor of Anesthesia
University of California San Francisco
San Francisco, California

Dennis T. Mangano, Ph.D., M.D.
Chairman of the Board
Chief Scientific Officer
The Ischemia Research
    and Education Foundation
San Francisco, California

Gertie F. Marx, M.D.
Professor of Anesthesiology (Emeritus)
Albert Einstein College of Medicine
Bronx, New York

Anthony C. Miller, M.D.
Commander, Medical Corps, United States Navy
Assistant Head
Department of Anesthesia
Director of Obstetric Anesthesia
Naval Medical Center
Portsmouth, Virginia

Pamela J. Morgan, M.D., C.C.F.P., F.R.C.P.C.
Associate Professor of Anesthesiology
University of Toronto
Staff Anesthesiologist
Sunnybrook & Women's College Health Sciences Centre
Toronto, Ontario, Canada

Julian T. Parer, M.D., Ph.D.
Professor of Obstetrics, Gynecology
    and Reproductive Sciences
Director, Perinatal Medicine and Genetics
Director, Maternal-Fetal Medicine
    Fellowship Training Program
University of California San Francisco
San Francisco, California

Stephen H. Rolbin, M.D., C.M., F.R.C.P. (C)
Assistant Professor of Anaesthesiology
University of Toronto
Staff Anesthesiologist
Sunnybrook & Women's College Health Sciences Centre
Toronto, Ontario, Canada

Mark A. Rosen, M.D.
Professor and Vice Chairman of Anesthesia
    and Perioperative Care
Professor of Obstetrics, Gynecology
    and Reproductive Sciences
Director, Anesthesia Training Program
University of California San Francisco
Director, Obstetrical Anesthesia
Moffitt-Long Hospital (UCSF Medical Center)
San Francisco, California

Alan C. Santos, M.D., M.P.H.
Associate Director of Anesthesiology
St. Luke's – Roosevelt Hospital Center
New York, New York

Susan H. Sniderman, M.D.
Professor of Clinical Pediatrics
University of California San Francisco
San Francisco General Hospital
San Francisco, California

Margaret Srebrnjak, M.D., F.R.C.P.C.
Lecturer, Department of Anaesthesia
University of Toronto
Director of Obstetrical Anaesthesia
St. Michael's Hospital
Toronto, Ontario, Canada

Robin A. Stackhouse, M.D.
Associate Professor of Anesthesia and Perioperative Care
University of California San Francisco
San Francisco General Hospital
San Francisco, California

Steve M. Yentis, M.D., M.B.B.S., F.R.C.A.
Consultant Anaesthetist
Chelsea & Westminster Hospital
Honorary Senior Lecturer
Imperial College School of Medicine
London, United Kingdom

CONTENTS

I OBSTETRIC PHYSIOLOGY AND PHARMACOLOGY

1 Maternal Physiologic Alterations
During Pregnancy   3
Theodore G. Cheek and Brett B. Gutsche

2 Uteroplacental Circulation and Respiratory
Gas Exchange   19
Julian T. Parer, Mark A. Rosen, and
Gershon Levinson

3 Effects of Anesthesia on Uterine Activity
and Labor   41
Anthony C. Miller

4 Perinatal Pharmacology   61
Alan C. Santos and Mieczyslaw Finster

II ANESTHESIA FOR VAGINAL DELIVERY

5 Choice of Local Anesthetics in Obstetrics   73
Kenneth Drasner and Philip R. Bromage

6 Nonpharmacologic Methods
of Pain Relief During Labor   95
Deborah L. Anderson and Samuel C. Hughes

7 Systemic Medication for Labor
and Delivery   105
M. Joanne Douglas and Gershon Levinson

8 Regional Anesthesia for Labor
and Delivery   123
Mark A. Rosen, Samuel C. Hughes, and
Gershon Levinson

9 Intraspinal Analgesia in Obstetrics   149

   Part I *Opioids and Other
           Non—local Anesthetics*   149
           James C. Eisenach

   Part II *Clinical Applications*   155
           Samuel C. Hughes

10 Inhalation Analgesia and Anesthesia for
Labor and Vaginal Delivery   189
Steve M. Yentis and Sheila E. Cohen

III OBSTETRIC COMPLICATIONS

11 Anesthesia for Cesarean Section   201
Samuel C. Hughes, Gershon Levinson, and
Mark A. Rosen

12 Anesthesia for Postpartum Sterilization   237
Stephen H. Rolbin and Pamela J. Morgan

13 Anesthesia for Surgery During Pregnancy   249
Gershon Levinson

14 Anesthesia for Fetal Procedures
and Surgery   267
Mark A. Rosen

15 Anesthesia for Abnormal Positions and
Presentations, Shoulder Dystocia, and
Multiple Births   287
Susan R. Gorman Maloney and Gershon Levinson

16 Anesthetic Considerations for the Hypertensive
Disorders of Pregnancy   297
Robert R. Gaiser, Brett B. Gutsche, and
Theodore G. Cheek

17 Anesthesia for Preterm Labor
and Delivery   323
Andrew M. Malinow and Patricia A. Dailey

18 Coagulation Disorders and Hemoglobinopathies
in the Obstetric and Surgical Patient   345
Russell K. Laros, Jr.

19 Amniotic Fluid Embolism   355
Valerie A. Arkoosh

20 Antepartum and
Postpartum Hemorrhage   361
William R. Camann and Diane R. Biehl

IV ANESTHETIC COMPLICATIONS

21 Difficult Airway Management   375
Robin A. Stackhouse and Cedric R. Bainton

22 Pulmonary Aspiration
of Gastric Contents   391
Theodore G. Cheek and Brett B. Gutsche

23 Neurologic Complications of Regional
Anesthesia for Obstetrics   409
Philip R. Bromage

24 Anesthesia-Related Maternal Mortality   429
Joy L. Hawkins, Gerard M. Bassell, and
Gertie F. Marx

25 Obstetric Anesthesia and Lawsuits   441

    Part I *General Considerations
            and Recommendations*   441
            Richard E. Dodge

    Part II *Review of Obstetric Anesthesia
             Closed Claims*   446
             H.S. Chadwick and Holly C. Gunn

V   NONOBSTETRIC DISORDERS
    DURING PREGNANCY

26 Anesthesia for the Pregnant
    Cardiac Patient   455
    Dennis T. Mangano

27 Perioperative Management of the
    Pregnant Patient with Asthma   487
    A. Sue Carlisle

28 Anesthesia for the Pregnant
    Diabetic Patient   497
    Sanjay Datta

29 Anesthesia for Neurosurgery
    During Pregnancy   509
    Barbara A. Dodson and Mark A. Rosen

30 Anesthesia for the Pregnant Patient
    with Neuromuscular Disorders   529
    Samuel C. Hughes

31 Anesthesia for the Morbidly Obese
    Pregnant Patient   545
    Sheila E. Cohen

32 Anesthesia for the Pregnant Patient
    with Immunologic Disorders   559
    Margaret Srebrnjak and Stephen Halpern

33 Human Immunodeficiency Virus in the
    Delivery Suite   583
    Samuel C. Hughes and Patricia A. Dailey

VI FETUS AND NEWBORN

34 Anesthesia and the
    Drug-Addicted Mother   599
    Samuel C. Hughes and Charlize Kessin

35 Fetal Evaluation: Routine and
    Indicated Tests   613
    Sarah J. Kilpatrick and Russell K. Laros, Jr.

36 Electronic Fetal Monitoring and Diagnosis
    of Fetal Asphyxia   623
    Julian T. Parer and Tekoa L. King

37 Evaluation of the Neonate   639
    Gershon Levinson, Samuel C. Hughes,
    and Mark A. Rosen

38 Resuscitation of the Newborn   657
    Susan H. Sniderman, Gershon Levinson, and
    George A. Gregory

APPENDIX A: Guidelines for Regional
    Anesthesia in Obstetrics   671

APPENDIX B: Practice Guidelines for
    Obstetrical Anesthesia   673

APPENDIX C: Optimal Goals for
    Anesthesia Care in Obstetrics   679

APPENDIX D: Fetal and Neonatal Effects
    of Maternally Administered Drugs   681
    Rhonda K. Arnette

Index   691

Shnider and Levinson's
Anesthesia for Obstetrics

ONE

OBSTETRIC PHYSIOLOGY AND PHARMACOLOGY

Shnider and Levinson's Anesthesia for Obstetrics,
edited by Samuel C. Hughes, et al.
Lippincott Williams & Wilkins,
Philadelphia, © 2001.

CHAPTER 1

MATERNAL PHYSIOLOGIC ALTERATIONS DURING PREGNANCY

THEODORE G. CHEEK, M. D. AND BRETT B. GUTSCHE, M. D.

Pregnancy, labor, and delivery profoundly alter maternal physiology and the response to anesthesia. Pregnancy has been described as the only normal physiologic state in which most physiologic parameters are altered. These changes are seen in the common physical complaints of pregnancy. Breathlessness and frequent upper respiratory tract infections reflect increased respiratory drive and airway swelling. Ankle edema, leg varices, and hemorrhoids indicate lower extremity venous engorgement and stasis. Heartburn, nausea, and vomiting imply decreased gastric emptying, increased gastric acidity, and decreased gastroesophageal junction tone. Back pain accompanies increased lumbar vertebral lordosis and weight-bearing strain. Urinary frequency and infection is evidence of the decreased capacity of the bladder. Early in pregnancy, rising levels of progesterone, estrogen, human chorionic gonadotropin, and prostaglandin play a primary role in the anatomic and physiologic changes of pregnancy. As pregnancy progresses, the enlarging uterus assumes a more important role in the alteration of respiratory, circulatory, gastrointestinal, renal, and skeletal functions. This chapter reviews these physiologic changes and discusses their implications for anesthesia care of the parturient. Familiarity with this subject will contribute to the best possible anesthetic outcome. Detailed reviews on maternal physiologic changes are available for further study (1–5).

RESPIRATORY CHANGES DURING PREGNANCY

The respiratory changes that occur during pregnancy are of special significance to the anesthetist (Tables 1.1 and 1.2). Ventilation increases during and after the first trimester of pregnancy, and shortness of breath may occur during the latter months of pregnancy. Capillary engorgement of the mucosa throughout the respiratory tract causes swelling of the nasal and oral pharynx, larynx, and trachea. As a result, the parturient frequently appears to have symptoms of upper respiratory tract infection and laryngitis, with nasal congestion and voice change (6). These changes may be markedly exacerbated by a mild upper respiratory tract infection, fluid overload, or the edema associated with pregnancy-induced hypertension, which occasionally leads to a severely compromised airway (7). The effects of labor on the oropharynx are reported to change the Mallampati examination score (8).

Manipulation of the upper airway requires special care. Suctioning, the placement of airways, and careless laryngoscopy may result in trauma and bleeding. Manipulation of the nasal airway is often associated with brisk epistaxis. Upper airway obstruction may occur early in anesthetic induction. When endotracheal intubation is performed, a 6- to 7-mm cuffed endotracheal tube is recommended because swelling of the false vocal cords often decreases the area of the glottic opening. Attempts to intubate the parturient's trachea with an 8-mm cuffed tube, suitable for the nonpregnant adult

woman, may result in trauma and an inability to pass the endotracheal tube. Breast engorgement can interfere with laryngoscopy, making the use of a short-handled blade necessary (9).

Minute ventilation is increased by 30% at the seventh week of pregnancy and about 50% at term primarily as a result of an increased tidal volume with little change (or at most a slight increase) in respiratory rate (10–12). This is likely caused by either progesterone-induced increased sensitivity to carbon dioxide or a direct progesterone stimulus (5, 13). Hyperventilation precedes maternal increased metabolic rate (5).

As a result of this increased alveolar ventilation at term, maternal $Paco_2$ is usually decreased to about 32 mm Hg, but little maternal alkalosis occurs because of a compensatory renal excretion of serum bicarbonate of about 4 mEq/L (i.e., from 26 to 22 mEq/L). During labor, particularly in the latter first stage and second stage as pain becomes severe, maternal minute ventilation may be increased by as much as 300% compared with the nonpregnant state, with the development of marked maternal hypocarbia ($Paco_2$ 20 mm Hg or less) and alkalemia (pH greater than 7.55) (Fig. 1.1) (14). This marked respiratory alkalosis may cause loss of consciousness and hypoventilation between painful contractions (Fig. 1.2) and a leftward shift of the oxyhemoglobin curve, causing oxygen to be more tightly bound to maternal hemoglobin and thus compromising its availability to the fetus (15, 16). It has been demonstrated that effective epidural analgesia alone can markedly diminish maternal hyperventilation and oxygen consumption, as well as attenuate the hypoxic episodes associated with painful labor (Fig. 1.3) (14, 17–21).

Lung volumes and lung capacities are not greatly changed by pregnancy. Changes are primarily limited to the functional residual capacity (FRC), which is decreased 15% to 20% in the gravida at term (Fig. 1.4). It has been shown that most of this decrease is caused by a reduction in the expiratory reserve volume secondary to an increase in tidal volume. Vital capacity, taken in the upright position, remains essentially unchanged throughout pregnancy according to most studies because of an increase in inspiratory reserve. A measurable decrease in vital capacity during pregnancy occurs in obese women (22) or may indicate pulmonary or cardiovascular dysfunction (1). Earlier data (23) have indicated that total lung capacity at term is decreased about 5% as a result of a 4-cm elevation of the diaphragm caused by the gravid uterus. A later study disputes these findings and indicates there is a 5- to 7-cm increase in chest circumference that compensates for the elevation of the diaphragm (24). Contrary to some reports, the diaphragm is not splinted at term but moves freely (25). Radiographs taken during normal pregnancy show increased central lung markings that may simulate mild pulmonary edema (26). A recent study of Qs/Qt (pulmonary shunt) in the third trimester found normal values of 12.8% to 15.3% compared with 2% to 5% in normal nonpregnant women (27). These findings were observed in all maternal positions (not just supine) and

Table 1.1. CHANGES IN THE RESPIRATORY SYSTEM AT TERM

Variable	Direction of Change	Average Change
Minute ventilation	⇑	+50%
Alveolar ventilation	⇑	+70%
Tidal volume	⇑	+40%
Respiratory rate	⇑	+15%
Arterial PO_2	⇑	+10 mm Hg
Inspiratory lung capacity	⇑	+5–15%
Oxygen consumption	⇑	+20%
Dead space (anat)	⇔	No change
Lung compliance (alone)	⇔	No change
Arterial pH	⇔	No change
Vital capacity	⇔	No change
FEV 1	⇔	No change
PEF (peak exp flow)	⇔	No change; decrease postpartum
Diffusing capacity	⇔	No change
Maximum breathing capacity	⇔	No change
Closing volume	⇔ or ⇓	No change
Alveolar dead space	⇔ or ⇓	None or −5%
Airway resistance	⇓	−36%
Total pulmonary resistance	⇓	−50%
Total compliance	⇓	−30%
Chest wall compliance (alone)	⇓	−45%
Arterial PCO_2	⇓	−10 mm Hg
Serum bicarbonate	⇓	−4 mEq/L
Total lung capacity	⇓	−0–5%
Functional residual capacity	⇓	−15–20%
Expiratory reserve volume	⇓	−20%
Residual volume	⇓	−20%

Adapted from references 10–12, 17, 23, 24, 28–34, 43, 44, and Brancazio LR, Laifer SA, Schwartz T. Peak expiratory flow rate in normal pregnancy. *Obstet Gynecol* 1997;89:383–386.

may further explain why pregnant women feel breathless near term.

The supine position markedly impairs respiratory function in late pregnancy. Measurements of closing volume (lung volume during expiration at which airways begin to close in the dependent zones of the lungs) have shown that, in one third to one half of supine pregnant women, closing capacity will exceed FRC. This means that in the supine position the mother is at risk of hypoxemia, as well as impaired organ perfusion (28, 29). One would also expect the pregnant woman to be more susceptible to atelectasis and to develop an increased oxygen alveolar-arterial (A-a) gradient more readily. Although this concept has been challenged (30), most studies in normal parturients demonstrate a wide variability in A-a gradient and dead space—to—tidal-volume ratio (31, 32), which highlights the risk of the supine position. In the upright position, measurements of

Table 1.2. BLOOD GASES IN PREGNANCY

Normal (Sea Level)		1388 m (650 mm Hg)
pH:	7.40–7.47 (arterial)	7.46
pH:	7.38 (venous)	
PaO_2:	85–103 mm Hg	88 mm Hg
$PaCO_2$:	27–33.5 mm Hg	26.6 mm Hg
HCO_3:	21–27 mEq/L	18.2 mEq/L
BE:	−2 to −4	

Adapted from Hankins GD, Clark SL, Harvey CJ, Uckan EM, Cotton D, Van Hook JW. Third-trimester arterial blood gas and acid base values in normal pregnancy at moderate altitude. *Obstet Gynecol* 1996;88:347–350.

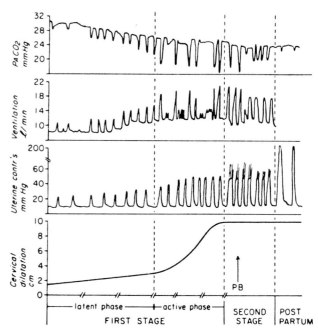

Figure 1.1. The progressive hyperventilation and hypocapnia experienced by the unmedicated woman during successive stages of labor is caused by increasing intensity of painful uterine contractions. Painful expulsion efforts during the second stage result in ventilation nearly double that of early labor, which can be partially relieved by pudendal block. (Reprinted by permission from Bonica JJ, ed. *Obstetric Analgesia and Anesthesia.* Amsterdam: World Federation of Societies of Anaesthesiologists; 1980.)

small airway function (closing volume and flow-volume loops) are similar to nonpregnant values.

Oxygen uptake in pregnancy is markedly increased both at rest (about 20%) and during exercise (33, 34) at term compared with the nonpregnant state. This increase is due to an elevated maternal metabolism and the increased work required in breathing. Longitudinal sleep studies after 35 weeks of gestation

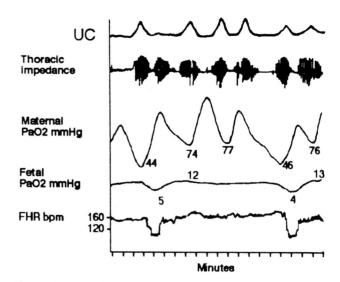

Figure 1.2. Maternal and fetal hypoxia during hypoventilation between contractions is caused by excessive maternal hyperventilation. (Reprinted by permission from Bonica JJ. Labour pain. In: Wall PD, Melzack R, eds. *Textbook of Pain.* Edinburgh: Churchill Livingstone; 1984; as redrawn from Huch A, Huch R, Schneider H, Rooth G. Continuous transcutaneous monitoring of fetal oxygen tension during labour. *Br J Obstet Gynaecol* 1977;84[suppl]:1–39.)

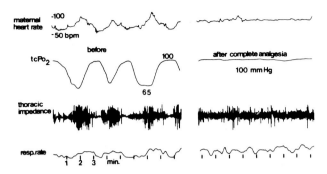

Figure 1.3. Maternal hyperventilation during painful uterine contractions results in hypoventilation between contractions with a corresponding decrease in transcutaneous oxygen pressure (tcPo$_2$) to 65 to 70 mm Hg. After effective epidural analgesia tcPo$_2$ is maintained at a stable 100 mm Hg. (Reprinted by permission from Huch R, Huch A, Lubbers DW, eds. In: *Transcutaneous Po$_2$*. New York: Thieme-Stratton; 1981:139.)

have shown maternal Spo$_2$ to normally range from 91% to 98% (mean 95.2%) at night (35). Some women may experience Spo$_2$ below 90% up to 20% of the time. Oxygen consumption is increased by an additional 63% with painful uterine contractions. Regional analgesia during the first and second stage of labor eliminates this additional increase in oxygen consumption (20). Flow-volume loops, timed-forced expiratory volume, and other flow characteristics during pregnancy are little changed from the nonpregnant state (30). In the immediate postpartum period, most maternal respiratory mechanics remain unchanged. However, maximum expiratory pressure, which is a measure of cough strength, is mildly to moderately reduced until ≈4 hours postpartum (36).

Changes of respiratory function during pregnancy are important to the anesthetist. The decrease in FRC combined with the increased minute ventilation increases the rapidity of induction with inhalation anesthetics. The decrease in FRC will increase the uptake of the more insoluble inhalation drugs, whereas the increased minute ventilation hastens the uptake of

the more soluble inhalation drugs. In addition, the minimum alveolar concentration (MAC) of potent inhalation drugs has been found to decrease during pregnancy by 24% to 40% in animal studies (37, 38) and 28% in a human study (39). The above factors combine to increase the parturient's sensitivity to inhalation anesthetic agents. Low concentrations of inhalation gases administered for analgesia may produce general anesthesia with loss of protective airway reflexes. Higher doses, which are safe in the nonpregnant patient, may produce overdosage with cardiopulmonary depression in the parturient.

Decreased FRC combined with increased oxygen consumption and increased A-a gradient lower the maternal oxygen reserve and make the pregnant patient in labor more vulnerable to hypoxia. This justifies an increased fraction of inspired oxygen in high-risk parturients either in labor or under general anesthesia. Induction of anesthesia with endotracheal intubation in the parturient breathing 100% oxygen, in contrast to the nonparturient, is associated with a much faster decrease in Pao$_2$ after 1 minute of apnea (Fig. 1.5). Time to desaturation (100% to 95%) is 173 seconds and 243 seconds in pregnant and nonpregnant females, respectively (40). The tendency for rapid development of hypoxia is aggravated by increased oxygen consumption during labor. The risk of hypoxia on induction can be decreased with 2 to 3 minutes of 100% oxygen by mask (41) or by several deep breaths of 100% oxygen before induction of general anesthesia (42). End tidal carbon dioxide in pregnancy closely mirrors arterial carbon dioxide in contrast to the gradient seen in the nonpregnant patient. This could be caused by decreased physiologic dead space, a change in the dynamics of alveolar emptying, increased cardiac output, and hemodilution (43, 44). High thoracic regional block, routinely performed for cesarean section, does not alter resting Paco$_2$ or minute ventilation (45). In contrast, thoracic regional block decreases coughing force and further decreases FRC (46). These findings support the use of supplementary oxygen and attention to the mother's ability to clear the airway during cesarean section. The anesthetic implications of the respiratory changes in pregnancy are summarized in Table 1.3.

In our opinion, the anatomic changes of the airway and the more rapid desaturation during apnea are strongly linked to the

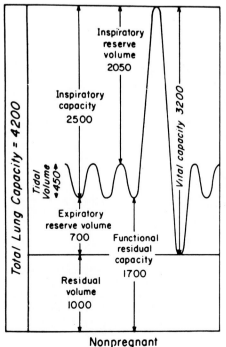

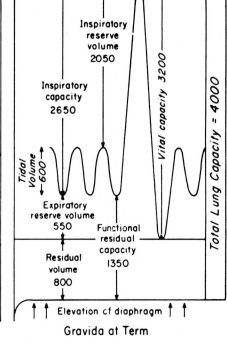

Figure 1.4. Pulmonary volumes and capacities during pregnancy, labor, and postpartum period. (Reprinted by permission from Bonica JJ, ed. In: *Principles and Practice of Obstetric Analgesia and Anesthesia*. Philadelphia: Davis; 1967:24.)

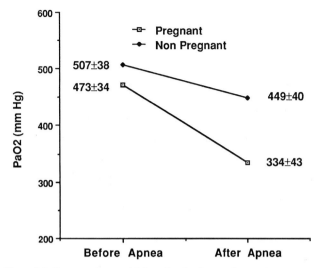

Figure 1.5. Decrease in arterial Po$_2$ after 1 minute of apnea in pregnant and nonpregnant patients. (Graph developed from data in Archer GW Jr, Marx GF. Arterial oxygen tension during apnea in parturient women. *Br J Anaesth* 1974;46:358–360.)

Table 1.3. RESPIRATORY CHANGES: ANESTHETIC SIGNIFICANCE

A. Airway management is more challenging
  1. Weight gain and breast engorgement hinder laryngoscopy
  2. Swollen mucosa bleeds easily; avoid intranasal manipulation
  3. Use smaller endotracheal tube (6–7 mm)
B. Response to anesthetics
  1. MAC decreased
  2. Decreased FRC results in faster induction with insoluble agents
  3. Increased VE speeds induction with soluble agents
  4. Rapid overdose with loss of airway reflexes
C. Greater risk of hypoxemia
  1. Decreased FRC means less oxygen reserve
  2. Increased oxygen consumption
  3. Rapid airway obstruction
D. Excessive mechanical hyperventilation (P$_{ET CO_2}$ < 24) may reduce maternal cardiac output and uterine blood flow
E. Maternal and fetal hypoxemia is associated with pain-induced hyper- and hypoventilation; can be avoided with effective analgesia

Table 1.4. CHANGES IN CARDIOVASCULAR SYSTEM

Variable	Direction of Change	Average Change
Blood volume	⇑	+35
Plasma volume	⇑	+45%
Red blood cell volume	⇑	+20%
Cardiac output	⇑	+40–50%
Stroke volume	⇑	+30%
Heart rate	⇑	+15–20%
Femoral (uterine?) venous pressure	⇑	+15 mm Hg
Total peripheral resistance	⇓	−15%
Mean arterial blood pressure	⇓	−15 mm Hg
Systolic blood pressure	⇓	−0–15 mm Hg
Diastolic blood pressure	⇓	−10–20 mm Hg
Central venous pressure	⇔	No change

Adapted from references 50–66.

increased maternal risks of morbidity and mortality associated with emergency general anesthesia discussed later in Chapter 24. This is particularly true when accompanied by maternal problems such as obesity, airway abnormalities, pregnancy-induced hypertension, and prolonged difficult labor.

CARDIOVASCULAR CHANGES DURING PREGNANCY

During pregnancy, numerous changes occur in the cardiovascular system that provide for the needs of the fetus and prepare the mother for delivery (Table 1.4). The diaphragmatic rise shifts the position of the heart leftward and may cause an enlarged appearance on radiographic examination (Fig. 1.6). Doppler and M-mode echocardiography in pregnant women at 38 weeks of gestation indicate an increase in end-diastolic chamber size compared with that of nonpregnant women (4.86 cm vs. 4.67 cm) and an increase in total left ventricular wall thickness (2.01 cm vs. 1.69 cm) (47). Asymptomatic pericardial effusion has been reported in some parturients by echocardiographic examination (48). An innocent grade I to II systolic heart murmur caused by increased blood flow and tricuspid annulus dilation may be heard. A third heart sound and occasionally a fourth may be heard in late pregnancy (49). The electrocardiogram may show an increase in benign dysrhythmia; reversible ST, T,

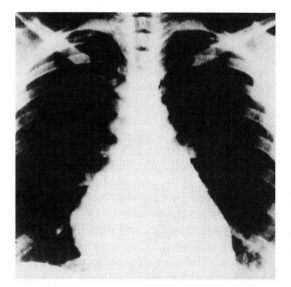
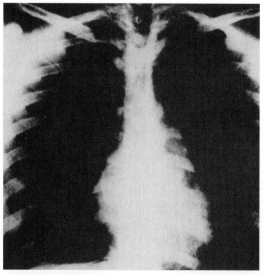

Figure 1.6. Chest radiograph of a woman during pregnancy (*left*) and postpartum (*right*). (Reprinted by permission from Burwell CS, McAnulty JH, Ueland K, eds. *Heart Disease in Pregnancy: Physiology and Management.* Boston: Little, Brown; 1986:60–63.)

Table 1.5. DISTRIBUTION OF WEIGHT GAIN DURING PREGNANCY

	Increase in Weight in Grams (and Pounds) up to:			
Tissue Fluid	*10 wk*	*20 wk*	*30 wk*	*40 wk*
Fetus	5 (0.01)	300 (0.7)	1500 (3.3)	3400 (7.5)
Placenta	20 (0.04)	170 (0.4)	430 (0.9)	650 (1.4)
Amniotic fluid	30 (0.07)	350 (0.8)	750 (1.7)	800 (1.8)
Uterus	140 (0.3)	320 (0.7)	600 (1.3)	700 (2.1)
Breasts	45 (0.1)	180 (0.4)	360 (0.8)	405 (0.9)
Blood	100 (0.2)	600 (1.3)	1300 (2.9)	1250 (2.8)
Extracellular extravascular fluid (no edema present)	0 (0)	30 (0.06)	80 (0.2)	1680 (3.7)
Subtotal	340 (0.7)	1950 (4.3)	5020 (11.1)	9115 (20.2)
Maternal reserves	310 (0.7)	2050 (4.5)	3480 (7.7)	3345 (7.4)
Total weight gain	650 (1.4)	4000 (8.8)	8500 (18.7)	12,500 (27)

Reprinted with permission from Hytten F, Chamberlain G. *Clinical Physiology in Obstetrics.* Oxford: Blackwell Scientific; 1980:217.

and Q wave changes; and some left axis deviation. These normal findings must be differentiated from those indicating heart disease, which include (a) systolic murmur greater than grade III, (b) any diastolic murmur, (c) severe arrhythmias, and (d) unequivocal cardiac enlargement on radiographic examination (26, 50).

Much of the average 12.5 kg weight gain in pregnancy is attributed to the increase in intravascular and extravascular fluid (Table 1.5). Maternal blood volume markedly increases during pregnancy (Fig. 1.7) (51–53). Plasma volume increases from 40 to 70 mL/kg, and red blood cell volume from 25 to 30 mL/kg. The plasma volume increase may be mediated by a resetting of the osmotic threshold for thirst and vasopressin secretion (54). Progesterone stimulates aldosterone production. Estrogen enhances renin activity, which modulates water absorption. The increase in maternal blood volume begins in the first trimester, has its maximum rate of increase in the second trimester, and continues to increase at a slower rate early in the third trimester. Contrary to earlier studies conducted with subjects in the supine position, maternal blood volume decreases only slightly, if at all, late in the third trimester (52). Near term there is about a 35% to 40% expansion of the blood volume by 1000 to 1500 mL compared with the nonpregnant state. Much of this increased

blood volume perfuses the gravid uterus, and with contractions 300 to 500 mL may be forced from the uterus into the maternal vascular system (53, 55). An average blood loss of less than 500 mL occurs in a normal vaginal delivery. With the uncomplicated vaginal delivery of twins or with cesarean section, maternal blood loss exceeding 1000 mL is rare. The normal nonpregnant blood volume is not reached until 7 to 14 days postpartum (53).

Erythropoietin, which rises by 8 weeks of gestation, stimulates red blood cell mass production (56). Hemoglobin increases at a slower rate than plasma volume, which accounts for the relative anemia of pregnancy (51). Nevertheless, a hemoglobin of less than 11 g or a hematocrit of 33% at any time during pregnancy represents maternal anemia, usually secondary to iron deficiency.

The normal parturient is well prepared to lose considerable blood at the time of delivery and rarely will require transfusion unless blood loss exceeds 1500 mL. The parturient has an increased blood volume and, at the time of delivery, the uterus contracts, essentially providing an autotransfusion in excess of 500 mL of blood (55). The contracted uterus also effectively decreases the vascular space by the same volume. However, the gravida with hypertension, whether essential or pregnancy-induced, usually has a diminished blood volume at term that may be less than that of her normal nonpregnant counterpart (see Chapter 16) (57). Blood loss in these patients is not well tolerated, especially by the fetus before delivery.

During the first trimester of pregnancy, cardiac output is increased by approximately 30% to 40%. An additional increase occurs during the second trimester. Earlier studies indicate that cardiac output then decreases toward nonpregnant values during the third trimester. These earlier studies, however, were done with the gravid patient supine. Lees et al. (58, 59) and Ueland et al. (60) showed that the pronounced decrease in cardiac output after 28 weeks that occurs in the supine position was due primarily to obstruction of the inferior vena cava. They also found a decrease in cardiac output in the sitting and lateral position as the patient approached term, but this decrease was of a much smaller magnitude than that seen in the supine position (Fig. 1.8). Invasive and echo human studies agree with these results (Fig. 1.9) (61–64).

During labor, cardiac output increases with uterine contractions 15% during the latent phase, 30% during the active phase, and 45% during the expulsive stage compared with prelabor values (65). This increase in cardiac output is due to an increase in both heart rate and stroke volume (64, 65). Each uterine contraction increases cardiac output by an additional 10% to 25% (66). The greatest increase occurs immediately after delivery, when the cardiac output is an average of 80% above prelabor values (67); this increase is attributed to autotransfusion and the increased venous return associated with uterine involution.

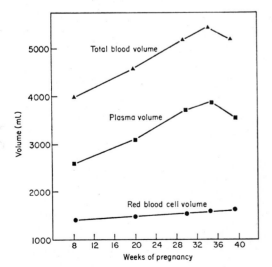

Figure 1.7. Changes in total blood volume, plasma volume, and red blood cell volume in normal pregnancy. Note the continued increase in red blood cell volume and plasma volume late in the third trimester. (Reprinted by permission from Moir DD, Carty MJ. In: Moir DD (ed) *Obstetric Anesthesia and Analgesia.* Baltimore: Williams & Wilkins; 1977.)

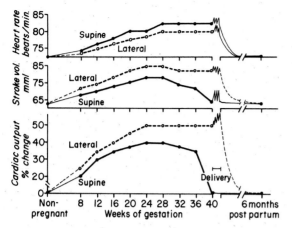

Figure 1.8. Changes in maternal heart rate, stroke volume, and cardiac output during pregnancy with the gravida in the supine and lateral position. These curves are based on data derived from several studies by Ueland (52, 60, 65, 66, 67). (Reprinted by permission from Bonica JJ, ed. *Obstetric Analgesia and Anesthesia.* Amsterdam: World Federation of Societies of Anaesthesiologists; 1980.)

Cardiac output then gradually declines (67, 68) to nonpregnant levels by 2 weeks after delivery. Although an increase in myocardial contractility in pregnancy has been suggested in the past (47), recently this has been disputed (69). Detailed reviews of the relationship between cardiac output, blood volume, and endocrinologic influences are available (69, 70, 70a).

Despite the increase in cardiac output, blood pressure (BP) is not increased during normal pregnancy, in part because of a 21% and 34% decrease in systemic and pulmonary vascular resistance, respectively (69), and an increase in aortic compliance (70b). The decreased systemic vascular resistance results in part from the blood flow through the developing low resistance vascular bed of the uterine intervillous space. This flow is about 10% of maternal cardiac output at term gestation. Many researchers attribute the decrease in vessel tone to α- and β-receptor down-regulation and prostacyclin changes that result in increased renal, uterine, and extremity blood flow (71–74).

This may also explain the decreased maternal chronotropic response after the administration of test doses of epinephrine and isoproterenol (75, 76). Other investigators argue that the effect of pregnancy on autonomic receptor number and function is small (77, 78). If autonomic receptor down-regulation occurs, it helps to explain the improved oxygen delivery and dissipation of heat generated by increased maternal and fetoplacental metabolism. Despite a general decrease in vascular tone, there is a greater maternal dependence on vasomotor response to maintain hemodynamic stability (79). This may explain in part the 50% decrease in maternal BP observed in older studies of complete sympathectomy (80). Some investigators suggest that an even greater decrease in vagal tone in pregnancy may allow for relatively normal sympathetic function (81, 82). This may explain why few women become severely bradycardic despite high sympathectomy commonly seen at cesarean section. These observations also underscore the importance of fluid administration before regional block in pregnancy–a subject that is discussed in greater detail in Chapter 11. Normal ambulatory BP by gestational age can be seen in Table 1.6 (83). During labor, each uterine contraction is associated with a 5% to 20% increase in BP (Fig. 1.10) (55).

Measurement of Blood Pressure in Pregnancy

Much has been published recently over the proper measurement of BP. It appears that automatic oscillometric BP monitors underestimate diastolic BP by about 10 mm Hg and overestimate systolic BP by about 10 mm Hg in laboring women when compared to auscultatory methods (84, 85). Diastolic BP may be better estimated in pregnancy from phase V (disappearance) and not phase IV (muffling) of Korotkoff sounds (86, 87). BP obtained from the dependent left arm in the left decubitus position agrees closely with or approximates supine or sitting BP (88–90).

Aortocaval Compression

Up to 15% of pregnant patients near term develop signs of shock—including hypotension, pallor, sweating, nausea, vomiting, and changes in cerebration—when they assume the supine

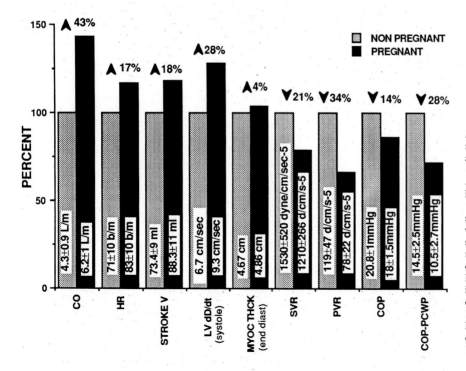

Figure 1.9. Hemodynamic changes of pregnancy from echocardiographic and pulmonary artery catheter monitors in healthy women. *CO* indicates cardiac output; *HR*, heart rate; *STROKE V*, stroke volume; *LV dD/dt (systole)*, left ventricle change (diameter/time); *MYOC THCK (end diast)*, myocardial thickness; *SVR*, systemic vascular resistance; *PVR*, pulmonary vascular resistance; *COP*, colloid oncotic pressure; *COP—PCWP*, colloid oncotic pressure minus pulmonary capillary wedge pressure. (Data extracted from Robson SC, Hunter S, Moore M, Dunlop W. Haemodynamic changes during the puerperium: A Doppler and M-mode echocardiographic study. *Br J Obstet Gynaecol* 1987;94:1028–1039; and Clark SL, Cotton DB, Lee W, et al. Central hemodynamic assessment of normal term pregnancy. *Am J Obstet Gynecol* 1989;161:1439–1442.)

Table 1.6. TWENTY-FOUR–HOUR AMBULATORY BLOOD PRESSURE MONITORING VALUES ACCORDING TO GESTATIONAL AGE

Gestational Age	Mean mm Hg	SD	Range mm Hg	Upper mm Hg
Normal				
9–17 wk (n = 9)				
SBP	111	5	101–118	121
DBP	65	4	60–71	73
MAP	80	4	73–86	88
18–22 wk (n = 83)				
SBP	112	7	96–127	126
DBP	66	5	56–78	76
MAP	81	5	71–93	91
26–30 wk (n = 140)				
SBP	114	7	97–133	128
DBP	68	5	56–84	78
MAP	83	5	69–101	93
31–40 wk (n = 44)				
SBP	115	8	103–136	131
DBP	70	6	57–85	82
MAP	85	6	75–100	97

Reprinted with permission from Brown MA, Robinson A, Bowyer L, et al. Ambulatory blood pressure monitoring in pregnancy: What is normal? *Am J Obstet Gynecol* 1998;178:836–842.

position. Howard et al. (91) described the syndrome and named it the "supine-hypotension syndrome." By injection of radiopaque dye in a femoral vein, Kerr et al. (92) showed that the inferior vena cava was totally obstructed by the gravid uterus in the supine position in 10 of 12 women. In part, blood from below the obstructed inferior vena cava returned to the heart via the paravertebral (epidural) veins emptying into the

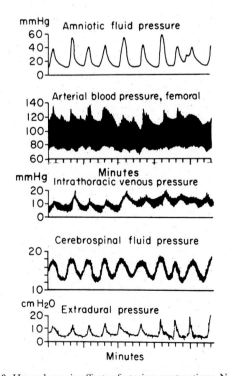

Figure 1.10. Hemodynamic effects of uterine contractions. Note the increase in arterial blood pressure and central venous pressure, which is reflected in cerebrospinal fluid and extradural pressures. (Reprinted by permission from Bonica JJ, ed. *Obstetric Analgesia and Anesthesia.* Amsterdam: World Federation of Societies of Anaesthesiologists; 1980; as drawn from Hendricks CH. Hemodynamics of a uterine contraction. *Am J Obstet Gynecol* 1958;76:968–982.)

azygos system. Turning the gravid patient on her side partially relieved the obstruction of the vena cava. The maternal symptoms of supine hypotension were attributed to lack of venous return to the heart. Compression of the inferior vena cava is most common late in pregnancy before the presenting fetal part becomes fixed in the pelvis. This compression produces pooling of venous blood and increased venous pressure in the lower torso and lower extremities, which may explain the tendency toward phlebitis and the development of venous varicosities in pregnancy. The increase in uterine venous pressure may affect the well being of the fetus through a resultant decrease in uterine blood flow. Blood flow to the uterus is directly related to the perfusion pressure, that is, uterine artery minus venous pressure. In the supine position, even without arterial hypotension, uterine perfusion pressure decreases as a result of the increased uterine venous pressure.

Bieniarz et al. (93) produced serial radiographs of the aorta in 70 subjects after injection of radiopaque dye in the femoral arteries and found the aorta to be partially occluded when the gravid subject was supine. Compression of the aorta is not associated with maternal symptoms but causes arterial hypotension in the lower extremities and uterine arteries, which can further decrease uterine blood flow and result in fetal hypoxia/asphyxia (94). Hence, even with normal upper extremity maternal BP, uteroplacental perfusion may decrease in the supine position. Kauppila et al. (95) found that turning the mother at term from the left lateral to the supine position decreased the intervillous blood flow by 20%. Similarly, Huch et al. (15) demonstrated a 40% decrease in transcutaneous fetal oxygen tension when the mother was turned from the lateral to the supine position (Fig. 1.11). Subsequently, Abitbol (96), Marx et al. (97), and Aldrich et al. (98), using scalp pH, Doppler flow, and infrared spectroscopy, have provided further evidence of decreased fetal cerebral oxygenation when the mother assumes the supine position (Fig 1.12).

It is imperative that anesthesiologists appreciate the importance of the syndrome now called *aortocaval compression* and realize that anesthesia may augment its signs and symptoms. The ill effects of aortocaval compression on the mother and fetus may manifest as early as the 20th week of gestation. Drugs causing vasodilation, such as halothane and thiopental, or techniques causing sympathetic blockade, such as subarachnoid or epidural block, will further decrease venous return to the heart in the presence of vena caval obstruction. Sympathetic block impairs the parturient's ability to compensate for the decreased venous return by vasoconstriction. Thus, arterial hypotension is much more common and severe during anesthesia in pregnancy compared with the nonpregnant state (80).

Prevention of aortocaval compression is preferred to treatment. The gravida at term should never be allowed to assume

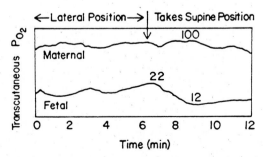

Figure 1.11. Continuous monitoring of maternal and fetal transcutaneous P_{O_2} during labor. Fetal P_{O_2} was monitored using a fetal scalp transcutaneous oxygen electrode. When mother turned from the lateral to the supine position, fetal P_{O_2} promptly decreased. (Modified from Huch A, Huch R, Schneider H, Rooth G. Continuous transcutaneous monitoring of fetal oxygen tension during labour. *Br J Obstet Gynaecol* 1977;84[suppl]:1–39.)

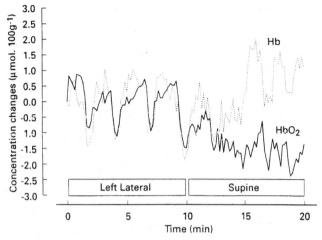

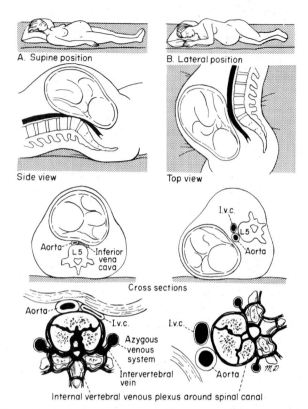

Figure 1.12. Representative changes from baseline in cerebral oxyhemoglobin (*solid line*) and deoxyhemoglobin (*dotted line*) concentrations in a term fetus with mother moving from left lateral to supine position. (Reprinted by permission from Aldrich CJ, D'Antona D, Spencer JA, et al. The effect of maternal posture on fetal cerebral oxygenation during labour. *Br J Obstet Gynaecol* 1995;102:14–19.)

Figure 1.13. Lateral and cross-sectional views of uterine aortocaval compression in the supine position and its resolution by lateral positioning of the pregnant woman. (Reprinted by permission from Bonica JJ, ed. *Obstetric Analgesia and Anesthesia.* Amsterdam: World Federation of Societies of Anaesthesiologists; 1980.)

the supine position (Figs. 1.13, 1.14). Left to their own devices, 98% of women beyond 30 weeks of gestation naturally avoid the supine position at night (99). Physicians would do well to heed this natural protective instinct. Nonreassuring fetal heart rate patterns are more often observed in parturients placed in the supine position or partially wedged position, particularly in the presence of major conduction or general anesthesia (100). Prevention of aortocaval compression consists of left uterine displacement (LUD), which can be accomplished by manual displacement of the uterus in which the uterus is lifted and displaced to the left. Alternatively, the patient may be positioned on her left side either by tipping the operating or delivery table 15 degrees to the left or by using sheets, a foam rubber wedge, or an inflatable bag to elevate the right buttock and back 10 to 15 cm. Stationary left uterine displacers such as the one designed by Colon-Morales (101), which is placed under the patient's right hip, are effective. In about 10% of women, right uterine displacement is more effective than LUD. This is demonstrated if maternal vital signs or the fetal heart rate pattern is more favorable in the right uterine displaced position. Complete lateral position after activating an epidural block is not associated with an increase in failed or lopsided block. Indeed, this position is associated with a lower incidence of nonreassuring fetal heart rate patterns (100). Placing the patient in the Trendelenburg posi-

tion without LUD is an inappropriate means of prophylaxis and may actually worsen the condition by shifting the uterus further back onto the vena cava and aorta. An unusually large uterus, such as that seen with twins or polyhydramnios, may require as much as 30 degrees of uterine displacement to avoid aortocaval compression (102). Intense bearing down during the second stage of labor has also been shown to cause aortocaval compression (103). During cesarean section, neonates from mothers with uterine displacement had less frequent and less severe depression by Apgar score and less acidosis than neonates from mothers in the supine position (104). If hypotension develops in the gravid patient near term, one should immediately suspect inferior vena cava occlusion and displace the uterus to the left or turn the mother to the complete lateral position without delay.

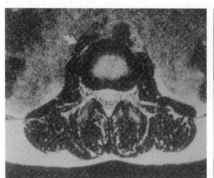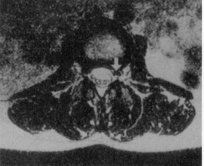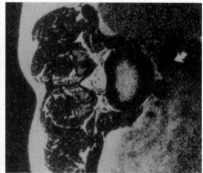

Figure 1.14. Magnetic resonance imaging of the same subject at L2 to L3 intervertebral disc. *A* = nonpregnant; *B* = pregnant supine; *C* = pregnant lateral. Vena cava can be seen (*curved arrows*) in the nonpregnant supine and the pregnant lateral positions but not in the pregnant supine position. Engorgement of intervertebral veins can be seen in the pregnant supine position. (Reprinted by permission from Hirabayashi Y, Shimizu R, Fukuda H, Saitoh K, Igarashi T. Effects of the pregnant uterus on the extradural venous plexus on the supine and lateral positions as determined by magnetic resonance imaging. *Br J Anaesth* 1997:78:317–319.)

Table 1.7. COAGULATION FACTORS AND INHIBITORS DURING NORMAL PREGNANCY

Factor	Nonpregnant	Late Pregnancy
Factor I (fibrinogen)	200–450 mg/dL	400–650 mg/dL
Factor II (prothrombin)	75–125%	100–125%
Factor V	75–125%	100–150%
Factor VII	75–125%	100–250%
Factor VIII	75–150%	200–500%
Factor IX	75–125%	100–150%
Factor X	75–125%	150–250%
Factor XI	5–125%	50–100%
Factor XII	75–125%	100–200%
Factor XIII	75–125%	35–75%
Antithrombin III	85–110%	75–100%
Antifactor Xa	85–110%	75–100%
Platelet count	$\Longleftrightarrow$ or $\Downarrow$	
PT	$\Downarrow$ 20%	
PTT	$\Downarrow$ 20%	
Fibrin split products	$\Uparrow$	

Adapted with permission from Hathaway WE, Bonnar J., eds. Coagulation in pregnancy. In: *Perinatal Coagulation*. New York: Grune & Stratton; 1978.

Oxygen transport during pregnancy is increased. Although a lower hematocrit decreases oxygen-carrying capacity from 19.5 to 16.0 vol/100 mL, this is overcome by other compensatory changes. Increased ventilation in pregnancy results in arterial oxygen tensions averaging 103 mm Hg. Increased cardiac output, vasodilation of the uterus and kidneys, and hemodilution increase blood flow to important target organs. Kambam et al. (105) have shown that the maternal oxyhemoglobin dissociation P50 is shifted to the right from 26.7 to 30.2 mm Hg at term. This increases the available oxygen at the tissue level.

There is a 14% decline in plasma colloid oncotic pressure (COP) (20.8 ± 1 mm Hg to 18 ± 1.5 mm Hg) that may favor mild edema formation in late pregnancy (71). A reported 28% decline in plasma COP to pulmonary capillary wedge pressure gradient (14.5 ± 2.5 to 10.5 ± 2.7) (Fig. 1.9) implies a tendency to develop pulmonary edema in the presence of altered pulmonary capillary permeability or markedly increased cardiac preload (61). After delivery, COP often decreases further. Combined with sustained high cardiac output, women with severe preeclampsia or who have recently received β-agonist therapy are at particular risk of pulmonary edema in the postpartum period. In a recent series, radiolabelled interstitial lung water increased in 7 of 20 normal pregnant women. This was not associated with an increased incidence of pulmonary edema (106). Increased lymphatic flow, not easily measured in humans, may explain why more parturients do not experience pulmonary edema.

In general, the clotting factor substrate increases with gestational age. Thus, the pregnant woman takes on a compensated hypercoagulable state as gestation progresses. This, combined with rapid myometrial contraction during placental separation, help to prevent excessive maternal blood loss at delivery. These changes in clotting substrate also place the pregnant woman at greater risk of deep vein thrombosis. Factors VII, VIII, and X and especially plasma fibrinogen are markedly increased after the third month of gestation (Table 1.7). A 20% decline in the platelet count seen at term does not influence bleeding time (107). Platelet function is increased in response to epinephrine, arachidonic acid, collagen, and adenosine. It is not unusual to see platelet counts of 150,000 (See Chapter 23, Fig. 23.7). Clotting measured with thromboelastography tends to be more rapid (108). Fibrinolysis, formerly thought to be depressed in pregnancy, has been shown to be normal. Levels of plasminogen are increased, but plasminogen activator is depressed as a result of sequestration at sites of fibrin deposition (109).

Table 1.8. CARDIOVASCULAR CHANGES: ANESTHETIC SIGNIFICANCE

A. Venodilation may increase the incidence of accidental epidural vein puncture.
B. Healthy parturient will tolerate up to 1500 mL blood loss; transfusion rarely required (hemorrhage at delivery remains an important risk).
C. Oxytocin with a free water IV infusion may lead to fluid overload.
D. High hemoglobin level (> 14) indicates low-volume state caused by preeclamsia, hypertension, or inappropriate diuretics.
E. Cardiac output remains high in first few hours postpartum; women with cardiac or pulmonary disease remain at risk after delivery.
F. Epidural block reduces cardiac work during labor and may be beneficial in some cardiac disease states.
G. Maternal blood pressure of < 90 to 95 mm Hg during regional block should be of concern because it may be associated with a proportional decrease in uterine blood flow.
H. ALWAYS AVOID AORTOCAVAL COMPRESSION: 70–80% of supine parturients with a T4 sympathectomy develop significant hypotension.

Leukocyte levels increase during pregnancy to a high of 12,000 to 21,000/mL during the third trimester; this has been attributed to increases in plasma-free cortisol and estrogen levels (107). Leukocyte chemotaxis and antigen adherence is impaired (110, 111). The anesthetic significance of the cardiovascular changes is summarized in Table 1.8.

NERVOUS SYSTEM CHANGES DURING PREGNANCY

Anesthetic requirement (MAC) for inhalation agents is decreased by up to 40% during pregnancy, as measured in animals (37, 38, 112) and by 28% for isoflurane in humans (113). Thus, concentrations of inhalation agents that would not produce loss of consciousness in the surgical patient may cause unconsciousness in the parturient, thereby subjecting her to the dangers of airway obstruction, vomiting, and aspiration. The thiopental requirement for hypnosis in human pregnancy is reportedly decreased by 17% (114). The mechanism for the decrease in MAC is uncertain, but hormonal, serotonergic, and endogenous opiate changes during pregnancy may be responsible. Progesterone, the plasma and cerebrospinal fluid (CSF) levels of which increase 10- to 20-fold (Fig. 1.15) during late pregnancy (115–118), has a sedative activity (119) and in large doses induces loss of consciousness in humans (120). Metabolites of

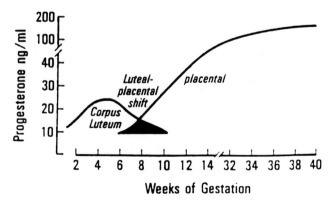

Figure 1.15. A shift of progesterone production from the corpus luteum to the placenta occures at approximately the eight to ninth week of gestation. The black area represents the estimated duration for this functional transition. (Reprinted by permission from Yen SCC. Endocrine and other evaluations of the fetal environment. In: Creasy RK, Resnik R, eds. *Maternal-Fetal Medicine: Principles and Practice.* 2nd ed. Philadelphia: WB Saunders; 1989:376.)

progesterone are also reported to produce unconsciousness (121). Anesthetic requirements for inhalation drugs in the postpartum period return to normal in 3 to 5 days (122, 123). These changes correlate with decreased progesterone levels but not with β-endorphins. Progesterone has also been associated with the cerebral vasodilation seen in pregnancy (124).

The role of endorphins in pregnancy is not fully understood. Maternal β-endorphin blood levels increase during gestation (125–127). They also increase significantly in most parturients during labor and delivery; the increase is proportional to the frequency and duration of uterine contractions, reflecting the stress of labor (127–129). Cesarean section performed with the patient under general anesthesia is associated with a marked increase of β-endorphin levels (130). Lumbar epidural analgesia itself is not associated with an increase in β-endorphins and blocks their elevation in labor, vaginal delivery, and cesarean section. This indicates that major conduction analgesia decreases the stress of labor. The effects of physiologic increases in β-endorphins on the subjective responses to the pain of parturition or MAC are unclear (128, 129, 131).

During pregnancy in rats, Gintzler found that a progressive increase in pain tolerance was abolished by an administration of an opioid antagonist (131). Steinbrook et al. found that, whereas plasma β-endorphin levels increased in pregnancy and during labor, CSF levels remained unchanged (127). Guistino et al. (132) reported that women who exercised during pregnancy, when compared with controls, had 34% higher plasma β-endorphin levels at the end of labor (≈59 pg vs. ≈44 pg) and lower visual analog pain scores (60 vs. 85). Although this difference was statistically significant, there was no clinical difference in terms of discomfort levels. Intrathecal administration of β-endorphin in higher than physiologic concentrations produces effective analgesia during labor (133). Thus, a pregnancy-induced activation of the endorphin system may contribute to a decreased anesthetic requirement. A norepinephrine-acetylcholine mediated antinociceptive pathway in humans has also been proposed and studied (134).

Density of CSF decreases in pregnancy to 1.00030 ± 0.00004 g/mL (nonpregnant = 1.00049 ± 0.00004 g/mL) (135). Theoretically, this change would increase the possibility of some intrathecal drugs acting in a hyperbaric manner. In fact, most non—dextrose-containing local anesthetic and opioid combinations in use are mildly hypobaric in pregnancy.

Circulatory changes within the vertebral column have important effects on subarachnoid and epidural techniques of regional analgesia. As a result of increased intraabdominal pressure, epidural veins become engorged, making accidental intravascular injection during lumbar epidural or caudal epidural block common. Baseline extradural pressures are higher ($+ 1$ cm H_2O) in full-term parturients than in nonpregnant women ($- 1$ cm H_2O). As labor progresses, this pressure increases steadily to reach 4 to 10 cm H_2O at the conclusion of the first stage of labor (Fig. 1.10). Second-stage bearing-down efforts can raise the extradural pressure to 60 cm H_2O (136) as a result of progressive venous engorgement and the muscle activity of bearing down. CSF pressures in the second stage of labor may reach 70 cm H_2O during contractions and bearing-down efforts. The use of the hanging-drop technique to identify the epidural space and entering the space during a contraction may increase the hazard of dural puncture. Although injection of local anesthetics into the epidural space during a contraction in the first stage of labor has been shown to have no effect on the resulting level of anesthetic block (137), such injections in the subarachnoid space during contractions may produce increased upward spread of the block, especially if the mother strains.

The gravid patient requires less local anesthetic to produce the same level of spinal or epidural block than does her nonpregnant counterpart (138–141). Some authors suggest that the epidural volume dose for patients during cesarean section is no different than for nonpregnant surgery patients (142, 143).

However, in one study (142), the nonpregnant group was unusually obese and not a valid control. Close inspection of the second study (141) shows a small but evident decrease in epidural dose requirements for cesarean section.

The approximately 30% reduction of local anesthetic required to produce a similar level of subarachnoid block in the gravid patient may be explained by a number of mechanisms: (a) swelling of the epidural veins, which decreases the volume of CSF in the vertebral column; (b) labor-induced increases in CSF pressure (144); and (c) increased neurosensitivity to local anesthetics. In the past, this decrease in local anesthesia requirement was explained completely by the engorgement of epidural veins, which decreased the volume of the subarachnoid and epidural spaces and prevented loss of local anesthetic solution through the intervertebral foramina (145, 146). This theory has received recent support from Carpenter et al., who showed with lumbosacral magnetic resonance imaging that CSF volume was a primary determinant of block spread (147), and Igarashi et al., who demonstrated engorgement of epidural vessels and the progressive narrowing of the epidural space during pregnancy with epiduroscopy (147a). Others have suggested that acid-base changes in CSF (139, 148) and/or hormonal changes such as elevated progesterone levels may increase nerve sensitivity to local anesthetics (149–151). Datta et al. have shown an increase in human CSF progesterone levels in pregnant (122 ± 8 ng) compared with nonpregnant women (61 ± 2.3 ng) (152). Lidocaine blockade of the median nerve was faster in pregnant (4 minutes) compared with nonpregnant (11.5 minutes) women (153). However, progesterone applied directly to nerve-conduction preparations does not affect local anesthesia conduction blockade (154). It is suggested that the increased sensitivity to conduction blockade seen with chronic progesterone treatment in animals (150) is an indirect effect that requires some time to develop. Some of the possible progesterone mechanisms include (a) alteration of receptor activity, (b) modulation of sodium channels, or (c) altered permeability of the nerve membrane (155). Others have disputed the effect of pregnancy and progesterone on spinal root local anesthetic susceptibility (156).

Although CSF protein binding of local anesthetics does not appear to be altered in pregnancy, the increased lumbar lordosis of pregnancy may enhance cephalad spread of local anesthetic solutions placed in the CSF. Several authors suggest that the duration and maximal level of block obtained with both epidural and subarachnoid analgesia begin to decline in the first 3 days postpartum (157, 158).

Data published in 1942 by Gibbs and Reid stated that the electroencephalogram (EEG) at the end of pregnancy showed "a slowing of the cortical activity . . . and an absence of high voltage fast records." Keunen et al. have recently shown that there is no change in EEG during pregnancy and that any changes during pregnancy should be considered abnormal (159).

GASTROINTESTINAL CHANGES DURING PREGNANCY

Pregnancy is associated with a shift in the position of the stomach caused by the gravid uterus, which changes the angle of the gastroesophageal junction (160). This frequently results in incompetence of the gastroesophageal pinchcock mechanism (high pressure zone), which allows gastric reflux and production of esophagitis and heartburn in 45% to 70% of pregnant women (161, 162). The presence of this condition makes the parturient prone to silent regurgitation, active vomiting, and aspiration during general anesthesia or impaired consciousness from any cause.

Although gastric motility and emptying time in pregnancy have been debated in recent years (see Table 3, Chapter 22) (163), there is general agreement that stomach emptying time

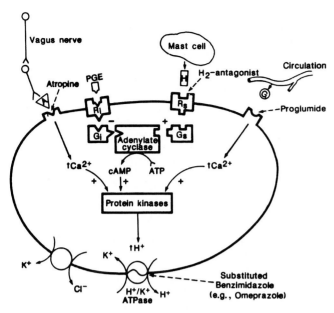

Figure 1.16. Cartoon of parietal (oxyntic) cell showing pathways that stimulate hydrogen ion secretion. *Dashed arrows* show sites of action of various antisecretory agents. (Reprinted by permission from Wolfe MM, Soll AH. The physiology of gastric acid secretion. *N Engl J Med* 1988;319:1707–1715.

can be prolonged in pregnancy and is certainly delayed in labor (164, 165). The enlarged uterus displaces the pylorus upward and backward and may also retard gastric emptying. The hormone gastrin produced by the placenta raises the acid, chloride, volume, and enzyme content of the stomach to levels above normal (166). Even if the gastric volume and pH of nonlaboring gravidae were the same as the nonpregnant population, greater risk would still surround the pregnant laboring patient because of changes in esophageal sphincter tone (167), along with other factors such as pregnancy-and labor-related nausea, pain, fear, ketosis, drugs, disease states, obesity, and recent food ingestion, and loss of airway reflexes due to any cause may act singly or in combination to increase the chance of gastric material entering the airway.

The stomach is lined by glands containing chief cells, which produce pepsinogen and oxyntic (parietal) cells, which in turn produce hydrochloric acid. Acid output can range from 5 mmol/h to 38 mmol/h, while gastric fluid production averages 1500 mL/24 h (168, 169). Proton pump blockers such as omeprazole decrease acid production by blocking the cellular hydrogen ion pump (170). Histamine greatly amplifies acid production through intracellular cyclic adenosine monophosphate release. This effect can be inhibited with H_2-blocking agents such as cimetidine and ranitidine (Fig. 1.16).

Intragastric pressure is increased during the last weeks of pregnancy and may reach levels exceeding 40 cm H_2O in cases of obesity, multiple gestation, and hydramnios (171). Epidural analgesia has minimal effects on gastric emptying (172). Opioids delay stomach-emptying time (173), and opioids and anticholinergics decrease lower gastroesophageal tone (174–177).

All parturients must be considered at risk of pulmonary aspiration of both acid material, causing the acid aspiration syndrome of Mendelson, and solid material, associated with atelectasis, lung abscess, and mechanical obstruction. The magnitude and prevention of this problem are considered in Chapter 22.

RENAL CHANGES DURING PREGNANCY

Renal plasma flow (RPF) increases by 40% to 90% and glomerular filtration rate (GFR) increases rapidly by 50% to 60% above nonpregnant values by the fourth month of gestation (178–180). Increased aldosterone levels contribute to increased total body water and sodium (181). The threshold for antidiuretic hormone secretion may be reset, which contributes to decreased plasma osmolality and slightly lower plasma sodium levels. During the third trimester, RPF and GFR gradually return toward normal levels. Compression of the aorta caused by the gravid uterus in the supine patient may decrease renal blood flow to levels below those preceding pregnancy. The high RPF and GFR result in an increase in creatinine clearance. The upper limits of normal for blood urea nitrogen (BUN) and serum creatinine values are reduced by 40% in the pregnant woman, BUN to 6 to 9 mg/dL and creatinine to 0.4 to 0.6 mg/dL during normal pregnancy (182, 183). Creatinine may rise slightly by the 3rd trimester, but clearance does not change. There is evidence that GFR is stimulated by more than one mechanism (184, 185). Tubular reabsorption of electrolytes and water increases in proportion to the GFR. During pregnancy, the body takes on between 500 and 800 mEq sodium and 300 mEq potassium (183, 186, 187). Plasma renin activity is increased, as is the renin substrate angiotensin, to which the normal gravid patient has decreased sensitivity (188, 189). Glucosuria of 1 to 10 g/d (190) and proteinuria of up to 300 mg/d are common and may not be associated with any pathologic condition (191).

Renal calyces, pelves, and ureters dilate after the third month of gestation. Early dilation is due to progesterone production, which induces atony of the calyces and ureters (192–194). Later, the ureters are compressed at the pelvic brim by the enlarging uterus, further contributing to this dilation. The resulting urinary stasis contributes to the frequency of urinary tract infections during pregnancy.

HEPATIC AND ENDOCRINE CHANGES DURING PREGNANCY

Liver size, histology, and blood flow do not undergo much change in pregnancy (195, 196). Microsomal activity increases (197), as does RNA content. Increased serum glutamic-oxaloacetic transaminase, lactic dehydrogenase, alkaline phosphatase, and cholesterol levels are common during pregnancy and labor, with 80% of parturients having an abnormal bromsulfophthalein excretion test result (198, 199). Transferases (AST and ALT) and gamma glutamyl transpeptidase (GGT) activity and production increase (200). These abnormal liver function test results do not necessarily indicate hepatic disease. Serum bilirubin is unaltered. Both total protein and the albumin-to-globulin ratio are decreased in pregnancy (201). Decreased serum albumin levels may result in higher free blood levels of some substances that are highly protein bound. Hepatic synthesis of corticosteroid-binding globulin doubles in pregnancy. Unbound plasma cortisol in term pregnancy is approximately 2.5 times that of nonpregnant women (202).

Average serum cholinesterase activity is reduced by 24% before delivery and by 33% at 3 days postpartum, returning to normal by 2 to 6 weeks postpartum (203, 204). Despite these lower levels of activity, prolonged respiratory impairment rarely occurs following appropriate doses of succinylcholine. This may be due to a larger volume of distribution for serum cholinesterase at term and agrees with the prolonged succinylcholine block seen in the first postpartum days as this volume rapidly contracts (205). Prolonged neuromuscular impairment, rarely lasting more than 20 minutes, has been reported in 2% to 6% of parturients having genotypically normal but often low levels of serum pseudocholinesterase. Dehydration, acidosis, diabetes mellitus, electrolyte abnormalities, and magnesium, trimethaphan, and cholinesterase inhibitors may depress or interact with serum cholinesterase activity (204, 206). These conditions have been associated with prolonged recovery from succinylcholine. Monitoring muscle twitch with a nerve stimulator when succinylcholine is used in the gravid patient is useful in preventing prolonged muscle weakness (207). The hydrolysis of 2-chloroprocaine, which requires serum pseudocholinesterase, appears normal in the parturient (208). Although pregnancy is associated with mild thyroid gland hypertrophy and bound T3 and T4 increase by 50%, free thyroxine and triiodothyronine levels remain normal (209). Profound alterations in gestational hormones are thoroughly reviewed by Cunningham et al. (210).

Calcium-dependent nitric oxide synthase activity is increased 2- to 4-fold by pregnancy. Nitric oxide synthase plays a role in smooth muscle adaptations of pregnancy (211, 212).

Decrease in plasma concentrations of atrial natriuretic peptide (ANP) is one of the mechanisms whereby blood volume is increased and maintained during pregnancy. The competitive relationship between ANP and the renin-aldosterone system in regulating sodium balance and fluid volume is preserved during pregnancy (213).

Insulin sensitivity is decreased in the last half of pregnancy, in part due to placental insulinase production. Resting glucose is lower and postprandial blood glucose levels are higher in pregnancy. This so-called "diabetogenic" profile of pregnancy is discussed in greater detail in Chapter 28.

UTERINE BLOOD FLOW IN PREGNANCY

During pregnancy, the uterus undergoes substantial changes in size and blood flow, particularly the blood flow to the placental intervillous space to allow fetal gas, nutrient, and waste exchange between the mother and fetus. The physiologic changes, mechanisms of exchange across the placenta, uterine blood flow, and impact of various anesthetic agents and techniques are described in Chapter 2.

REFERENCES

1. Chamberlain G, Broughton-Pipkin F. *Clinical Physiology in Obstetrics*. 3rd ed. Oxford: Blackwell Scientific Publications; 1998.
2. Metcalfe J, Stock MK, Barron DH. Maternal physiology during gestation. In: Knobil K, Neill JD, eds. *The Physiology of Reproduction*. 2nd ed. New York: Raven Press; 1994.
3. Lapinsky SE. Alterations in cardiopulmonary physiology during pregnancy. *Semin Respir Crit Care Med* 1998;19:201–208.
4. Lockitch G. Clinical biochemistry of pregnancy. *Crit Rev Clin Lab Sci* 1997;34:67–139.
5. Weinberger SE, Weiss ST, Cohen WR, Weiss JW, Johnson TS. Pregnancy and the lung. *Am Rev Respir Dis* 1980;121:559–581.
6. Mackenzie AI. Laryngeal oedema complicating obstetric anaesthesia. *Anaesthesia* 1978;33:271.
7. Heller PJ, Scheider EP, Marx GF. Pharyngolaryngeal edema as a presenting symptom in pre-eclampsia. *Obstet Gynecol* 1983;62:523–527.
8. Farcon EL, Kim MH, Marx GF. Changing Mallampati score during labour. *Can J Anaesth* 1994;41:50–51.
9. Datta S, Briwa J. Modified laryngoscope for endotracheal intubation of obese patients. *Anesth Analg* 1981;60:120–122.
10. Prowse CM, Gaensler EA. Respiratory acid base changes during pregnancy. *Anesthesiology* 1965;26:381–392.
11. Pernoll ML, Metcalf J, Kovach PA, Wachtel R, Dunham MJ. Ventilation during rest and exercise in pregnancy and postpartum. *Respir Physiol* 1975;25:295–310.
12. Clapp JF II, Seaward BL, Sleamaker RH, Hiser J. Maternal physiologic adaptations to early human pregnancy. *Am J Obstet Gynecol* 1988;159:1456–1460.
13. Lyons HA, Antonio R. The sensitivity of the respiratory center in pregnancy and after the administration of progesterone. *Trans Assoc Am Phys* 1959;72:173–180.
14. Bonica JJ. Labour pain. In: Wall PD, Melzack R, eds. *Textbook of Pain*. Edinburgh: Churchill Livingstone; 1984:377–392.
15. Huch A, Huch R, Schneider H, Rooth G. Continuous transcutaneous monitoring of fetal oxygen tension during labour. *Br J Obstet Gynaecol* 1977;84 (suppl):1–39.
16. Burden RJ, Janke EL, Brighouse D. Hyperventilation-induced unconsciousness during labour. *Br J Anaesth* 1994;73:838–839.
17. Fisher A, Prys-Roberts C. Maternal pulmonary gas exchange: A study during normal labor and extradural blockade. *Anaesthesia* 1968;23:350–356.
18. Peabody JL. Transcutaneous oxygen measurement to evaluate drug effects. *Clin Perinatol* 1979;6:109–121.
19. Sangoul F, Fox GS, Houle GL. Effect of regional analgesia on maternal oxygen consumption during the first stage of labor. *Am J Obstet Gynecol* 1975;121:1080–1083.
20. Hagerdal M, Morgan CW, Sumner AE, Gutsche BB. Minute ventilation and oxygen consumption during labor with epidural analgesia. *Anesthesiology* 1983;59:425–427.
21. Griffin RP, Reynolds F. Maternal hypoxaemia during labour and delivery: The influence of analgesia and effect on neonatal outcome. *Anaesthesia* 1995;50:151–156.
22. Eng M, Butler J, Bonica JJ. Respiratory function in pregnant obese women. *Am J Obstet Gynecol* 1975;123:241.
23. Cugell DW, Frank NR, Gaensler EA. Pulmonary function in pregnancy. I. Serial observations in normal women. *Am Rev Tuberc* 1953;67:568–599.
24. Leontic EA. Respiratory disease in pregnancy. *Med Clin North Am* 1977;61:111–128.
25. McGinty AP. The comparative effects of pregnancy and phrenic nerve interruption on the diaphragm and their relation to pulmonary tuberculosis. *Am J Obstet Gynecol* 1938;35:237–248.
26. Metcalfe J, McAnulty JH, Ueland K. *Burwell and Metcalfe's Heart Disease and Pregnancy: Physiology and Management*. 2nd ed. Boston: Little, Brown; 1986:25.
27. Hankins GDV, Harvey CJ, Clark EM, Uckan EM, VanHook JW. The effects of maternal position and cardiac output on intrapulmonary shunt in normal third-trimester pregnant women. *Obstet Gynecol* 1996;88:327–330.
28. Bevan DR, Holdcroft A, Loh L, MacGregor WG, O'Sullivan JC. Closing volume and pregnancy. *Br Med J* 1974;1:13–15.
29. Russell IF, Chambers WA. Closing volume in normal pregnancy. *Br J Anaesth* 1981;53:1043–1047.
30. Baldwin GR, Moorthi DS, Whelton JA, MacDonnell K. New lung functions and pregnancy. *Am J Obstet Gynecol* 1977;127:235–239.
31. Awe RJ, Nicotra MB, Newsom TD, Viles R. Arterial oxygenation and alveolar-arterial gradients in term pregnancy. *Obstet Gynecol* 1979;53:182–186.
32. Lyons G, Tunstall GL. Maternal blood gas tensions (PAO2-PAO2) physiological shunt and VD/VT during general anaesthesia for caesarean section. *Br J Anaesth* 1979;51:1059–1062.
33. Clapp JF, III. Oxygen consumption during treadmill exercise before, during and after pregnancy. *Am J Obstet Gynecol* 1989;161:1458–1464.
34. McMurray RG, Katz VL, Berry MJ, Cefalo RC. The effect of pregnancy on metabolic responses during rest, immersion, and aerobic exercise in the water. *Am J Obstet Gynecol* 1988;158:481–486.
35. Bourne T, Ogilvy AJ, Williamson K. Nocturnal hypoxaemia in late pregnancy. *Br J Anaesth* 1995;75:678–682.
36. Gupta A, Johnson A, Johansson A, Berg G, Lennmarken C. Maternal respiratory function following normal vaginal delivery. *Int J Obstet Anesth* 1993;2:129–133.
37. Palahniuk RJ, Shnider SM, Eger EI II. Pregnancy decreases the requirements for inhaled anesthetic agents. *Anesthesiology* 1974;41:82–83.
38. Datta S, Migliozzi RP, Flanagan HL, Krieger NR. Chronically administered progesterone decreases halothane requirements in rabbits. *Anesth Analg* 1989;68:46–50.
39. Gin T, Chan MTV. Decreased minimum alveolar concerntratin of isoflurane in pregnant humans. *Anesthesiology* 1994;81:829–832.
40. Baraka AS, Hanna MT, Jabbour SI, et al. Preoxygenation of pregnant and nonpregnant women in the head-up versus supine position. *Anesth Analg* 1992;75:757–759.
41. Byrne F, Oduro-Dominah A, Kipling R. The effect of pregnancy on pulmonary nitrogen washout. *Anaesthesia* 1987;42:148–150.
42. Norris MC, Kirkland MR, Torjman MC, Goldberg ME. Denitrogenation in pregnancy. *Can J Anaesth* 1989;36:523–525.
43. Shankar KB, Moseley H, Vemula V, Kumar Y. Physiological dead space during general anaesthesia for Caesarean section. *Can J Anaesth* 1987;34:373–376.
44. Shankar KB, Mushlin PS. Arterial to end-tidal gradients in pregnant subjects [letter; comment]. *Anesthesiology* 1997;87:1596–1598.
45. Moya F, Smith B. Spinal anesthesia for cesarean section. Clinical and biochemical studies of effects on maternal physiology. *JAMA* 1962;179:609–614.

46. Askrog VF Smith TC, Eckenhoff JE. Changes in pulmonary ventilation during spinal anesthesia. *Surg Gynecol Obstet* 1964;119:563–567.

47. Robson SC, Hunter S, Moore M, Dunlop W. Haemodynamic changes during the puerperium: A Doppler and M-mode echocardiographic study. *Br J Obstet Gynaecol* 1987;94:1028–1039.

48. Enein M, Zina AA, Kassem M, el-Tabbakh G. Echocardiography of the pericardium in pregnancy. *Obstet Gynecol* 1987;69:851–853.

49. Cutforth R, MacDonald CB. Heart sounds and murmurs in pregnancy. *Am Heart J* 1966;71:741–747.

50. Elkayam U, Gleicher N. Hemodynamics and cardiac function during normal pregnancy and the puerperium. In: Elkayam U, Gleicher N, eds. *Cardiac Problems in Pregnancy.* New York: Alan R. Liss; 1990:5–24.

51. Assali NS, Brinkman CR III. Disorders of maternal circulatory and respiratory adjustments. In: Assali NS, Brinkman CR III, eds. *Pathophysiology of Gestation: Maternal Disorders*, vol 1. New York: Academic Press; 1972:278–285.

52. Ueland K. Maternal cardiovascular dynamics. VII. Intrapartum blood volume changes. *Am J Obstet Gynecol* 1976;126:671–677.

53. Pritchard JA. Changes in blood volume during pregnancy and delivery. *Anesthesiology* 1965;26:393–399.

54. Lindheimer MD, Barron WM, Durr J, Davison JM. Water homeostasis and vasopressin release during rodent and human gestation. *Am J Kidney Dis* 1987;9:270–275.

55. Hendricks CH. Hemodynamics of a uterine contraction. *Am J Obstet Gynecol* 1958;76:968–982.

56. Cotes PM, Canning CE, Lind T. Changes in serum immunoreactive erythropoietin during the menstrual cycle and normal pregnancy. *Br J Obstet Gynaecol* 1983;90:304–311.

57. Goodlin RC, Dobry CA, Anderson JC, Woods RE, Quaile M. Clinical signs of normal volume expansion during pregnancy. *Am J Obstet Gynecol* 1983;145:1001–1009.

58. Lees MM, Taylor SH, Scott DB. A study of cardiac output at rest throughout pregnancy. *J Obstet Gynaecol Br Commonw* 1967;74:319–328.

59. Lees MM, Scott DB, Kerr MG. The circulatory effects of recumbent postural change in late pregnancy. *Clin Sci* 1967;32:453–465.

60. Ueland K, Novy MJ, Peterson EN. Maternal cardiovascular dynamics. IV. The influence of gestational age on the maternal cardiovascular response to posture and exercise. *Am J Obstet Gynecol* 1969;104:856–864.

61. Clark SL, Cotton DB, Lee W, et al. Central hemodynamic assessment of normal term pregnancy. *Am J Obstet Gynecol* 1989;161:1439–1442.

62. Mabie WC, DiSessa TG, Crocker LG, Sibai BM, Arheart KL. A longitudinal study of cardiac output in normal human pregnancy. *Am J Obstet Gynecol* 1994;170:849–856.

63. Sadaniantz A, Saint Laurent L, Parisi AF. Long-term effects of multiple pregnancies on cardiac dimensions and systolic and diastolic function. *Am J Obstet Gynecol* 1996;174:1061–1064.

64. Warner MH, Fairhead AC, Rawles J, MacLennan FM. An investigation of the changes in aortic diameter and an evaluation of their effect on Doppler measurement of cardiac output in pregnancy. *Int J Obstet Anesth* 1996;5:73–78.

65. Ueland K, Hansen JM. Maternal cardiovascular dynamics. III. Labor and delivery under local and caudal analgesia. *Am J Obstet Gynecol* 1969;103:8–18.

66. Ueland K, Hansen JM. Maternal cardiovascular dynamics. II. Posture and uterine contractions. *Am J Obstet Gynecol* 1969;103:1–7.

67. Hansen JM, Ueland K. The influence of caudal analgesia on cardiovascular dynamics during labour and delivery. *Acta Anaesthesiol Scand* 1966;23 (suppl):449–452.

68. Walters WAW, McGregor WG, Hills M. Cardiac output at rest, during pregnancy and the puerperium. *Clin Sci* 1966;30:1–11.

69. Poppas A, Shroff SG, Korcarz CE, et al. Serial assessment of the cardiovascular system in normal pregnancy. Role of arterial compliance and pulsatile arterial load. *Circulation* 1997;95:2407–2415.

70. Longo LD. Maternal blood volume and cardiac output during pregnancy: A hypothesis of endocrinologic control. *Am J Physiol* 1983;245:R720–R729.

70a. Clapp JF III, Capeless E. Cardiovascular function before, during, and after the first and subsequent pregnancies. *Am J Cardiol* 1997;80:1469–1473.

70b. Hart MV, Morton MJ, Hosenpud JD, Metcalfe J. Aortic function during normal human pregnancy. *Am J Obstet Gynecol* 1986;154:887–891.

71. Oian P, Maltau JM, Noddeland H, Fadnes HO. Oedema: Preventing mechanisms in subcutaneous tissue of normal pregnant women. *Br J Obstet Gynaecol* 1985;92:1113–1119.

72. Goodman RP, Killom AP, Brash AR, Branch RA. Prostacyclin production during pregnancy: Comparison of production during normal pregnancy and pregnancy complicated by hypertension. *Am J Obstet Gynecol* 1982;142:817–822.

73. Ylikorkala O, Jouppila P, Kirkinen P, Viinikka L. Maternal prostacyclin, thromboxane, and placental blood flow. *Am J Obstet Gynecol* 1983;145:730–732.

74. Clark KE, Austin JE, Seeds AE. Effect of bisenoic prostaglandins and arachidonic acid on the uterine vasculature of pregnant sheep. *Am J Obstet Gynecol* 1982;142:261–268.

75. DeSimone CA, Leighton BL, Norris MC, Chayen B, Menduke H. The chronotropic effect of isoproterenol is reduced in term pregnant women. *Anesthesiology* 1988;69:626–628.

76. Paller MS. Decreased pressor responsiveness in pregnancy: Studies in experimental animals. *Am J Kidney Dis* 1987;9:308–311.

77. Pantuck CB, Smiley RM. Longitudinal study of beta and alpha adrenergic receptor properties during human pregnancy. *Am J Obstet Gynecol* 1997;177:234–242.

78. Ramsay MM, Pipkin FB, Rubin PC. Pressor, heart rate and plasma catecholamine responses to noradrenaline in pregnant and nonpregnant women. *Br J Obstet Gynaecol* 1993;100:170–176.

79. Goodlin RC. Venous reactivity and pregnancy abnormalities. *Acta Obstet Gynecol Scand* 1986;65:345–348.

80. Assali NS, Prystowsky H. Studies on autonomic blockade. I. Comparison between the effects of tetraethyl ammonium chloride (TEAC) and high selective spinal anesthesia on the blood pressure of normal and toxemic pregnancy. *J Clin Invest* 1950;29:1354–1366.

81. Ekholm EM, Piha SJ, Antila KJ, Erkkola RU. Cardiovascular autonomic reflexes in mid-pregnancy. *Br J Obstet Gynaecol* 1993;100:177–182.

82. Kuo CD, Chen GY, Yang MJ, Tsai YS. The effect of position on autonomic nervous activity in late pregnancy. *Anaesthesia* 1997;52:1161–1165.

83. Brown MA, Robinson A, Bowyer L, et al. Ambulatory blood pressure monitoring in pregnancy: What is normal? *Am J Obstet Gynecol* 1998;178:836–842.

84. Marx GF, Schwalbe SS, Cho E, Whitty JE. Automated blood pressure measurements in laboring women: Are they reliable? *Am J Obstet Gynecol* 1993;168:796–798.

85. Hasan MA, Thomas TA, Pryse-Roberts C. Comparison of automatic oscillometric arterial pressure measurement with conventional auscultatory measurement on the labour ward. *Br J Anaesth* 1993;70:141–144.

86. Shennan A, Gupta M, Halligan DJ, Taylor DJ, deSwiet M. Lack of reproducibility in pregnancy of Korotkoff phase IV as measured by mercury sphygmomanometry. *Lancet* 1996;347:139–142.

87. Brown MA, Reiter L, Smith B, Buddle ML, Morris R, Whitworth JA. Measuring blood pressure in pregnant women: A comparison of direct and indirect methods. *Am J Obstet Gynecol* 1994;171:661–667.

88. Kinsella SM, Black AMS. Reporting of "hypotension" after epidural analgesia during labour. Effect of choice of arm and timing of baseline readings. *Anaesthesia* 1998;53:131–135.

89. Clark SL, Cotton DB, Pivarnik JM, et al. Position change and central hemodynamic profile during normal third-trimester pregnancy and post partum. *Am J Obstet Gynecol* 1991;164:883–887.

90. Kinsella SM. Blood pressure measurement in pregnant women in the left lateral recumbent position (letter/reply). *Am J Obstet Gynecol* 1998;179:867–868.

91. Howard BK, Goodson JH, Mengert WF. Supine hypotension syndrome in late pregnancy. *Obstet Gynecol* 1953;1:371–377.

92. Kerr MG, Scott DB, Samuel E. Studies of the inferior vena cava in late pregnancy. *Br Med J* 1964;1:532–533.

93. Bieniarz I, Crottogini JJ, Curachet E. Aortocaval compression by the uterus in late human pregnancy. *Am J Obstet Gynecol* 1968;100:203–217.

94. Marx GF. Aortocaval compression: Incidence and prevention. *Bull NY Acad Med* 1974;50:443–446.

95. Kauppila A, Kokinen M, Puolakka J, Tuimala R, Kuikka J. Decreased intervillous and unchanged myometrial blood flow in supine recumbency. *Obstet Gynecol* 1980;55:203–205.

96. Abitbol MM. Supine position in labor and associated fetal heart rate changes. *Obstet Gynecol* 1985;65:481–486.

97. Marx GF, Patel S, Berman JA, Farmakides G, Schulman H. Umbilical blood flow velocity waveforms in different maternal positions and with epidural analgesia. *Obstet Gynecol* 1986;68:61–64.

98. Aldrich CJ, D'Antona D, Spencer JA, et al. The effect of maternal posture on fetal cerebral oxygenation during labour. *Br J Obstet Gynaecol* 1995;102:14–19.

99. Mills GH, Chaffe AG. Sleeping position adopted by pregnant women of more than 30 weeks gestation. *Anaesthesia* 1994;49:249–250.

100. Preston R. Crosby ET, Kotarba H, Dudas H, Elliott RD. Maternal positioning affects fetal heart rate changes after epidural analgesia for labour. *Can J Anaesth* 1993;40:1136–1141.

101. Colon-Morales MA. A self-supporting device for continuous left uterine displacement during cesarean section. *Anesth Analg* 1970;49:223–224.

102. Kim YI, Chandra P, Marx GF. Successful management of severe aortocaval compression in twin pregnancy. *Obstet Gynecol* 1975;46:362–364.

103. Bassell GM, Humayun SG, Marx GF. Maternal bearing down efforts–another fetal risk? *Obstet Gynecol* 1980;56:39–41.

104. Crawford JS. Anesthesia for section: Further refinements of a technique. *Br J Anaesth* 1973;45:726–731.

105. Kambam JR, Handte RE, Brown WU Jr, Smith BE. Effect of normal and preeclamptic pregnancies on the oxyhemoglobin dissociation curve. *Anesthesiology* 1986;65:426–427.

106. MacLennan FM, MacDonald AF, Campbell DM. Lung water during the puerperium. *Anaesthesia* 1987;42:141–147.

107. Pitkin RM, Witte DL. Platelet and leukocyte counts in pregnancy. *JAMA* 1979;242:2696–2698.

108. Sharma SK, Philip J, Wiley J. Thromboelastographic changes in healthy parturients and postpartum women. *Anesth Analg* 1997;85:94–98.

109. Fletcher AP, Alkjaersig NK, Burstein R. The influence of pregnancy upon blood coagulation and plasma fibrinolytic function. *Am J Obstet Gynecol* 1979;134:743–751.

110. Krause PJ, Ingardia CJ, Pontius LT, Malech HL, LoBello TM, Maderazo EG. Host defense during pregnancy: neutrophil chemotaxis and adherence. *Am J Obstet Gynecol* 1987;157:274–280.

111. Taylor RN. Immunobiology of human pregnancy. *Curr Probl Obstet Gynecol Fertil* 1998;21:5–23.

112. Thomas BA, Anzalone TA, Rosinia FA. Progesterone decreases the MAC of desflurane in the nonpregnant ewe. *Anesthesiology* 1995;83:A952.

113. Gin T, Chan MTV. Decreased minimum alveolar concentration of isoflurane in pregnant humans. *Anesthesiology* 1994;81:829–832.

114. Gin T, Mainland P, Chan MTV, Short TG. Decreased thiopental requirement in early pregnancy. *Anesthesiology* 1997;86:73–78.

115. Lurie AO, Weiss JB. Progesterone in cerebrospinal fluid during human pregnancy. *Nature* 1967;215:1178.

116. Yannone ME, McCurcy JR, Goldfein A. Plasma progesterone levels in normal pregnancy, labor and the puerperium. II. Clinical data. *Am J Obstet Gynecol* 1968;101:1058–1061.

117. Datta S, Hurley RJ, Naulty SJ, et al. Plasma and cerebrospinal fluid progesterone levels in pregnant and nonpregnant women. *Anesth Analg* 1986;65:950–954.

118. Hirabayashi Y, Shimizu R, Saitoh K, Fukuda H. Cerebrospinal fluid progesterone in pregnant women. *Br J Anaesth* 1995;75:683–687.

119. Selye H. Studies concerning the anesthetic action of steroid hormones. *J Pharmacol Exp Ther* 1941;73:127–141.

120. Merryman W. Progesterone "anesthesia" in human subjects. *J Clin Endocrinol Metab* 1954;14:1567–1569.

121. Mok WM, Herschkowitz S, Krieger NR. In vivo studies identify 5 alpha-pregnan-3 alpha-ol-20-one as an active anesthetic agent. *J Neurochem* 1991;57:1296–1301.

122. Zhou HH, Norman P, DeLima LG, Mehta M, Bass D. The minimum alveolar concentration of isoflurane in patients undergoing bilateral tubal ligation in the postpartum period. *Anesthesiology* 1995;82:1364–1368.

123. Chan MTV, Gin T. Postpartum changes in minimum alveolar concentration of isoflurane. *Anesthesiology* 1995;82:1360–1363.

124. Lu GP, Cho E, Marx GF, Gibson J. Cerebral hemodynamic response to female sex hormones in the rat. *Microvasc Res* 1996;51:393–395.

125. Houck JC, Kimball C, Chang C, Pedigo NW, Yamamura HI. Placental beta-endorphin-like peptides. *Science* 1980;207:78–80.

126. Csontos K, Rust M, Halt V, Mahr W, Kromer W, Teschemacher HJ. Elevated plasma beta-endorphin levels in pregnant women and their neonates. *Life Sci* 1979;25:835–844.

127. Steinbrook RA, Carr DB, Datta S, Naulty JS, Lee C, Fisher J. Dissociation of plasma and cerebrospinal fluid beta-endorphin immunoreactivity levels during pregnancy and parturition. *Anesth Analg* 1982;61:893–897.

128. Pilkington JW, Nemeroff CB, Mason GA, Prange AJ. Increase in plasma beta-endorphin like immunoreactivity at parturition in normal women. *Am J Obstet Gynecol* 1983;145:111–113.

129. Thomas TA, Fletcher JE, Hill RG. Influence of medication, pain and progress in labour on plasma beta-endorphin-like immunoreactivity. *Br J Anaesth* 1982;54:401–408.

130. Abboud TK, Noueihid R, Khoo S, et al. Effect of induction of general and regional anesthesia for cesarean section and maternal plasma beta-endorphin levels. *Am J Obstet Gynecol* 1983;146:927–930.

131. Gintzler AR. Endorphin-mediated increases in pain threshold during pregnancy. *Science* 1980;210:193–195.

132. Guistino V, Bazzano C, Edwards WT. Effects of physical activity on maternal plasma beta-endorphin levels and perception of labor pain. *Am J Obstet Gynecol* 1989;160:707–712.

133. Oyama T, Akitoma M, Takeo T, Ling N, Guillemin R. Beta-endorphin in obstetric analgesia. *Am J Obstet Gynecol* 1980;137:613–616.

134. Eisenach JC, Detweiler DJ, Tong C, D'Angelo R, Hood DD. Cerebrospinal fluid norepinephrine and acetylcholine concentrations during acute pain. *Anesth Analg* 1996;82:621–626.

135. Richardson MG, Wissler RN. Density of lumbar cerebrospinal fluid in pregnant and nonpregnant humans. *Anesthesiology* 1996;85:326–330.

136. Galbert MW, Marx GF. Extradural pressures in the parturient patient. *Anesthesiology* 1974;40:499–502.

137. Sivakumaran C, Ramanathan S, Chalon J, Turndorf H. Uterine contractions and the spread of local anesthetics in the epidural space. *Anesth Analg* 1982;61:127–129.

138. Bonica JJ. Maternal physiologic and psychologic alterations. In: Cosmi E, ed. *Obstetric Anesthesia and Perinatology*. New York: Appleton-Century-Crofts; 1981:28–29.

139. Fagraeus L, Urban B, Bromage P. Spread of epidural analgesia in early pregnancy. *Anesthesiology* 1983;58:184–187.

140. Bromage P. Physiology and pharmacology of epidural analgesia. *Anesthesiology* 1967;28:592–622.

141. James KS, McGrady E, Patrick A. Combined spinal-extradural anaesthesia for preterm and term cesarean section: Is there a difference in local anesthetic requirements? *Br J Anaesth* 1997;78:498–501.

142. Grundy EM, Zamora AM, Winnie AP. Comparison of spread of epidural anesthesia in pregnant and nonpregnant women. *Anesth Analg* 1978;57:544–546.

143. Sharrock NE, Greenidge J. Epidural dose responses in pregnant and nonpregnant patients. *Anesthesiology* 1978;51:S298.

144. Marx GF, Oka Y, Orkin LR. Cerebrospinal fluid pressures during labor. *Am J Obstet Gynecol* 1967;84:213–219.

145. Bromage PR. Continuous lumbar epidural analgesia for obstetrics. *Can Med Assoc J* 1961;85:1136–1140.

146. Marx GF, Bassell GM. Physiologic considerations of the mother. In: Marx GF, Bassell GM, eds. *Obstetric Analgesia and Anaesthesia*. New York: Elsevier Publications; 1980:35.

147. Carpenter RL, Hogan QH, Liu SS, Crane B, Moore J. Lumbosacral cerebrospinal fluid volume is the primary determinant of sensory block extent and duration during spinal anesthesia. *Anesthesiology* 1998;89:24–29.

147a. Igarashi T, Hirabayashi Y, Shimizu R, Saitoh K, Fukuda H, Suzuki H. The fiberscopic findings of the epidural space in pregnant women. *Anesthesiology* 2000;92:1631–1636.

148. Dautenhahn DL, Fagraeus L. Acid-base changes of spinal fluid during pregnancy. *Anesth Analg* 1984;63:204.

149. Datta S, Lambert DH, Gregus J, Gissen AJ, Covino BG. Differential sensitivities of mammalian nerve fibers during pregnancy. *Anesth Analg* 1983;62:1070–1072.

150. Flanagan HL, Datta S, Lambert DH, Gissen AJ, Covino B. Effect of pregnancy on bupivacaine-induced conduction blockade in the isolated rabbit vagus nerve. *Anesth Analg* 1987;66:123–126.

151. Sevarino FB, Gilbertson LI, Gugino LD, Courtney MA, Datta S. The effect of pregnancy on the nervous system response to sensory stimulation. *Anesthesiology* 1988;69:A695.

152. Datta S, Hurley R, Naulty SJ, et al. Plasma and cerebrospinal fluid progesterone concentrations in pregnant and nonpregnant women. *Anesth Analg* 1986;65:950–954.

153. Butterworth JF, Walker FO, Lyzak SZ. Pregnancy increases median nerve susceptibility to lidocaine. *Anesthesiology* 1990;72:962–965.

154. Bader AM, Datta S, Moller B, Covino BG. Acute progesterone treatment has no effect on bupivacaine-induced conduction blockade in the isolated rabbit vagus nerve. *Anesth Analg* 1990;71:541–544.

155. Datta S. Comment. *Obstet Anesth Digest* 1994;14:175–176.

156. Dietz FB, Jaffe RA. Pregnancy does not increase susceptibility to bupivacaine in spinal root axons. *Anesthesiology* 1997;87:610–616.

157. Abouleish EI. Postpartum tubal ligation requires more bupivacaine for spinal anesthesia than does cesarean section. *Anesth Analg* 1986;65:897–900.

158. Marx GF. Regional analgesia in obstetrics. *Anaesthesia* 1972;21:84–91.

159. Keunen RWM, Vliegen JHR, van der Pol DAE, Gerretsen G, Stam CJ. The electroencephalogram during normal third trimester pregnancy and six months post-partum. *Br J Obstet Gynaecol* 1997;104:256–258.

160. Vanner RG. Mechanisms of regurgitation and its prevention with cricoid pressure. *Int J Obstet Anesth* 1993;2:207–215.

161. Hart DM. Heartburn in pregnancy. *J Int Med Res* 1978;6(suppl):1–5.

162. Marrero JM, Goggin PM, de Caestecker JS, Pearce JM, Maxwell JD. Determinants of pregnancy heartburn. *Br J Obstet Gynaecol* 1992;99:731–734.

163. O'Sullivan GM, Sutton AJ, Thompson SA, Carrie LE, Bullingham MB. Noninvasive measurement of gastric emptying in obstetric patients. *Anesth Analg* 1987;66:505–511.

164. Christofides ND, Ghatei MA, Bloom SR, Borberg C, Gillmer MD. Decreased plasma motilin concentration in pregnancy. *Br Med J* 1982;285:1453–1454.

165. Davison JS, Davison MC, Hay DM. Gastric emptying time in late pregnancy and labour. *J Obstet Gynaecol Br Commonw* 1970;77:37–41.

166. Attia RR, Ebeid AM, Fischer JE, Goudsouzian NG. Maternal-fetal and placental gastrin concentrations. *Anaesthesia* 1982;37:18–21.

167. Fisher RS, Roberts GS, Grabowski CJ, Cohen S. Altered lower esophageal sphincter function during early pregnancy. *Gastroenterology* 1978;74:1233–1237.

168. Brook FP. Physiology of the stomach. In: Berk JE, ed. *Gastroenterology*. Philadelphia: WB Saunders; 1985:874–940.

169. Feldman M, Richardson CT. Total 24 hour gastric acid secretion in patients with duodenal ulcer: Comparison with normal subjects and the effects of cimetidine and parietal cell vagotomy. *Gastroenterology* 1986;90:540–544.

170. Ewart MC, Yau G, Gin T, Kotur CF, Oh TE. A comparison of the effects of omeprazole and ranitidine on gastric secretion in women undergoing elective caesarean section. *Anaesthesia* 1990;45:527–530.

171. Spence AA, Moir DD, Finlay WEI. Observations on intragastric pressure. *Anaesthesia* 1967;22:249–256.

172. Wilson J. Gastric emptying in labor: Some recent findings and their clinical significance. *J Int Med Res* 1978;6(suppl):54–62.

173. Nimmo WS, Wilson J, Prescott LF. Narcotic analgesics and delayed gastric emptying in labour. *Lancet* 1975;1:890–893.

174. Hall AW, Moosa AR, Clark J, Cooley GR, Skinner DB. The effect of premedication drugs on the lower esophageal high pressure zone and reflux status in rhesus monkeys and man. *Gut* 1975;16:347–352.

175. Brock-Utne JG, Rubin J, Downing JW, Dimopoulos GE, Mishal MG, Naicker M. The administration of metoclopramide with atropine. *Anaesthesia* 1976;31:1186–1190.

176. Brock-Utne JG, Rubin J, Welmas S, Dimopoulos GE, Mishal MG, Downing JW. The action of commonly used anti-emetics on the lower esophageal sphincter. *Br J Anaesth* 1978;50:295–298.

177. Brock-Utne JG, Rubin J, Welman S, Dimopoulos GE, Mishal MG, Downing JW. The effect of glycopyrrolate (Robinul) on the lower esophageal sphincter. *Can Anaesth Soc J* 1978;2:144–146.

178. Dafnis E, Sabatini S. The effect of pregnancy on renal function–physiology and pathophysiology. *Am J Med Sci* 1992;303:184–205.

179. Dignam WJ, Titus P, Assali NS. Renal function in human pregnancy. I. Changes in glomerular filtration rate and renal plasma flow. *Proc Soc Exp Biol Med* 1958;97:512–514.

180. Davison JM, Dunlop W. Renal hemodynamics and tubular function normal human pregnancy. *Kidney Int* 1980;18:152–161.

181. Brown MA, Sinosich MJ, Saunders DM, Gallery ED. Potassium regulation and progesterone-aldosterone interrelationships in human pregnancy: a prospective study. *Am J Obstet Gynecol* 1986;155:349–353.

182. Berman LB. The pregnant kidney. *JAMA* 1974;230:111–112.

183. Lindheimer MD, Katz AI. Pregnancy and the kidney. *J Reprod Med* 1973;11:14–18.

184. Gaboury CL, Woods LL. Renal reserve in pregnancy. *Semin Nephrol* 1995;15:449–453.

185. Sturgiss SN, Wilkinson R, Davison JM. Renal reserve during human pregnancy. *Am J Physiol* 1996;271:F16–20.

186. Katz AI, Lindheimer MD. Renal handling of acute sodium loads in pregnancy. *Am J Physiol* 1973;225:696–699.

187. Lindheimer MD, Richardson DA, Ehrlich EN, Katz AI. Potassium homeostasis in pregnancy. *J Reprod Med* 1987;32:517–522.

188. Sundsfjord JA, Aakvaag A. Plasma renin activity, plasma renin substrate and urinary aldosterone excretion in the menstrual cycle in relation to the concentration of progesterone and oestrogens in the plasma. *Acta Endocrinol* 1972;71:519–529.

189. Talledo OE, Chesley LC, Zuspan FP. Renin-angiotensin system in normal and toxemic pregnancies. III. Differential sensitivity to angiotensin II and norepinephrine in toxemia at pregnancy. *Am J Obstet Gynecol* 1968;100:218–221.

190. Davison JM, Dunlop W. Renal hemodynamics and tubular function normal human pregnancy. *Kidney Int* 1980;18:152–161.

191. Toback FG, Hall PW, Lindheimer MD. Effect of posture on urinary protein patterns in nonpregnant, pregnant and toxemic women. *Obstet Gynecol* 1970;35:765–768.

192. Van Wagenen G, Jenkins RH. An experimental examination of factors causing ureteral dilation of pregnancy. *J Urol* 1939;42:1010–1020.

193. Bailey RR, Rolleston GL. Kidney length and ureteric dilatation in the puerperium. *J Obstet Gynaecol Br Commonw* 1971;78:55–61.

194. Hertzberg BS, Carroll BA, Bowie JD, et al. Doppler US assessment of maternal kidneys: analysis of intrarenal resistivity indexes in normal pregnancy and physiologic pelvicaliectasis. *Radiology* 1993;186:689–692.

195. Duke J. Pregnancy and cirrhosis: management of hematemesis by Warren shunt during third trimester gestation. *Int J Obstet Anesth* 1994;3:97–102.

196. Reynolds F. Pharmacokinetics. In: Chamberlain G, Broughton Pipkin F, eds. *Clinical Physiology in Obstetrics*. 3rd ed. Oxford: Blackwell Scientific Publications; 1998:243.

197. Corke BC. Drugs and obstetric anesthesia. In: Wood M, Wood AJJ, eds. *Drugs and Anesthesia: Pharmacology for the Anesthetist*. Baltimore: Williams & Wilkins; 1990:347.

198. Smith BE, Moya F, Shnider SM. The effects of anesthesia on liver function during labor. *Anesth Analg* 1962;41:24–31.

199. Yip DM, Baker AL. Liver diseases in pregnancy. *Clin Perinatol* 1985;12:683–694.

200. Walker FB IV, Hoblit DL, Cunningham FG, Combes B. Gamma glutamyl transpeptidase in normal pregnancy. *Obstet Gynecol* 1974;43:745–749.

201. McNair RD, Jaynes RV. Alterations in liver function during normal pregnancy. *Am J Obstet Gynecol* 1960;80:500–505.

202. Rosenthal HE, Slaunwhite WR Jr, Sandberg AA. Transcortin: a corticosteroid-binding protein of plasma. X. Cortisol and progesterone interplay and unbound levels of these steroids in pregnancy. *J Clin Endocrinol Metab* 1969;29:352–367.

203. Shnider SM. Serum cholinesterase activity during pregnancy, labor and puerperium. *Anesthesiology* 1965;26:335–339.

204. Weissman DB, Ehrenwerth J. Prolonged neuromuscular blockade in a parturient associated with succinylcholine. *Anesth Analg* 1983;62:444–446.

205. Leighton BL, Cheek TG, Gross JB, et al. Succinylcholine pharmacodynamics in peripartum patients. *Anesthesiology* 1986;64:202–205.

206. Ravindran RS, Cummins DF, Pantazis KL, Strausberg BJ, Baenziger JC. Unusual aspects of low levels of pseudo-cholinesterase in a pregnant patient. *Anesth Analg* 1982;61:953–955.

207. Viegas O. Guest discussion: Correlation of plasma cholinesterase activity and duration of action of succinylcholine during pregnancy. *Anesth Analg* 1977;56:81–82.

208. O'Brien J, Abbey V, Hinsvark O, Perel J, Finster M. Metabolism and measurement of chloroprocaine: An ester type local anesthetic. *J Pharm Sci* 1979;68:75–78.

209. Harada A, Hershman JM, Reed AW, et al. Comparison of thyroid stimulators and thyroid hormone concentrations in the sera of pregnant women. *J Clin Endocrinol Metab* 1979;48:793–7.

210. Cunningham FG, MacDonald PC, Gant NF (eds). Human pregnancy: Overview, organization and diagnosis. In: *Williams Obstetrics*. 20th ed. Norwalk CT: McGraw-Hill; 1996: Chapter 1.

211. Weiner CP, Knowles RG, Moncada S. Induction of nitric oxide synthases early in pregnancy. *Am J Obstet Gynecol* 1994;171:838–843.

212. Boulanger H, Berkane N, Pruna A. Role of nitric oxide (NO) in pregnancy and in preeclampsia. *Nephrologie* 1997;18:81–90.

213. Thomsen JK, Foghanderson N, Jaszczak P, Giese J. Atrial-natriuretic-peptide (ANP) decrease during normal pregnancy as related to hemodynamic changes and volume regulation. *Acta Obstet Gynecol Scand* 1993;72:103–110.

Shnider and Levinson's Anesthesia for Obstetrics,
edited by Samuel C. Hughes, et al.
Lippincott Williams & Wilkins,
Philadelphia, © 2001.

CHAPTER 2

UTEROPLACENTAL CIRCULATION AND RESPIRATORY GAS EXCHANGE

JULIAN T. PARER, M.D., Ph.D., MARK A. ROSEN, M.D., AND
GERSHON LEVINSON, M.D.

The placenta is a union of maternal and fetal tissues for purposes of physiologic exchange. Because many stillbirths and depressed fetuses are the result of intrauterine asphyxia, the factors responsible for adequacy of placental function, particularly respiratory gas exchange, assume great importance.

PLACENTAL ANATOMY AND CIRCULATION

The human placenta is described as a villous hemochorial type. The villi are projections of fetal tissue surrounded by chorion that are exposed to circulating maternal blood. The chorion is the outermost fetal tissue layer. At term, the human placenta weighs about 500 g and is disc shaped, with a diameter of approximately 20 cm and a thickness of 3 cm. The normal fetal–to–placental-weight ratio is approximately 6:1 at term. Before this, the placenta is relatively heavier and the ratio is less (e.g., 3:1 at 30 weeks of gestation).

Circulation of blood through the placenta is illustrated in Figure 2.1. The maternal blood is carried initially in the uterine arteries, and these ultimately divide into spiral arteries in the basal plate. Blood is spurted, probably under arterial pressure, from these arteries into the intervillous space. It traverses upward toward the chorionic plate, passing fetal villi, and finally drains back to veins in the basal plate. It is likely that, throughout this passage past the villi, the maternal blood is exchanging substances with fetal blood within the villi.

The fetal circulation within the placenta is quite different. Blood is carried into the placenta by two umbilical arteries that successively divide into smaller vessels within the fetal villi. Ultimately, capillaries traverse the tips of the fetal villi, and it is at this point that exchange occurs with maternal blood within the intervillous space. The blood is finally collected into a single umbilical vein in the umbilical cord, and this carries the nutrient-rich and waste-poor blood to the fetus.

Fetal and maternal blood are separated by three microscopic tissue layers in the human placenta. The first layer is the fetal trophoblast, which consists of cytotrophoblast and syncytiotrophoblast. The syncytiotrophoblast is the metabolically active part of the placenta, where much of the endocrine function of the placenta occurs. The other tissue layers are fetal connective tissue, which serves to support the villi, and the endothelium of fetal capillaries (Fig. 2.2).

The quantitative relationship of fetal and maternal blood flow and relative concentrations of substances at any one point in the human placenta are quite complex. The relative rates of blood flow in various areas of the placenta are also quite variable, and there is a continually-changing concentration of nutrients

and waste materials in various areas of the placenta as exchange occurs (1).

MECHANISMS OF EXCHANGE

Substances are exchanged across the placental membrane by five mechanisms (Fig. 2.3) (2).

1. Diffusion

This is a physicochemical process in which no energy is required and substances pass from one area to another on the basis of a concentration gradient. The respiratory gases, oxygen and carbon dioxide, the fatty acids, and the smaller ions (e.g., Na^+ and Cl^-) are transported by this mechanism (2).

Facilitated diffusion describes the mechanism of passage of glucose and some other carbohydrates. With this mechanism, substances still pass down a concentration gradient, but the rate of passage is greater than can be explained by the gradient alone. Possibly, carrier molecules are involved, and there may be need for energy expenditure.

Glucose crosses the placenta via facilitated-diffusion carriers inserted in both microvillous and basal membranes. In this mode of transport, the movement of glucose down its concentration gradient to the fetus is dependent on blood flow and plasma concentrations, and also on cellular energy supply. Changes in glucose transport have been postulated for several placental pathophysiologies including intrauterine growth restriction (IUGR), diabetes, and preeclampsia.

2. Active Transport

This mechanism allows for the passage of substances in a direction against the concentration gradient. Energy is required; carrier molecules are involved; and active transport is subject to inhibition by certain metabolites. The amino acids, water-soluble vitamins, and some of the larger ions (e.g., Ca^{++} and Fe^{++}) are transported by this mechanism.

a) *Primary active transport*: Movement of a substance takes place against its concentration (i.e., uphill) via a specific protein carrier, which uses the energy in adenosine triphosphate (ATP) to drive transport.

b) *Secondary active transport*: Movement of one transport substrate down its gradient (e.g., sodium entry into cells) via a protein carrier provides the energy for movement of a coupled transport substrate via carrier.

Amino acids are transported by a series of transporters with multiple substrate specificities. They can be divided into two types, those co-transported with sodium (secondary active transport) and those independent of sodium. Amino acids are transported uphill from the maternal circulation into the fetal

19

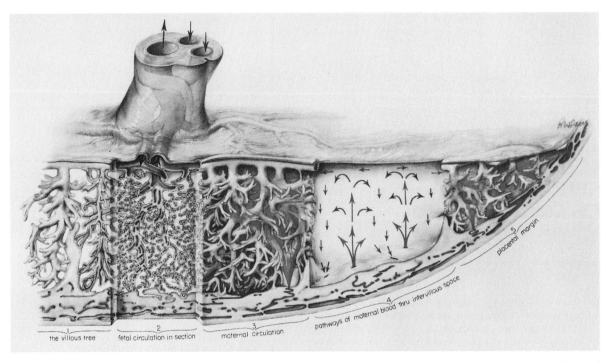

Figure 2.1. Composite drawing of the placenta showing its structure and circulation. *1,* villus tree; *2,* cross section of the fetal circulation; *3* and *4,* hemodynamics of maternal circulation according to the concepts of Ramsey et al. (From Ramsey EM, and the Carnegie Institution of Washington. In: Greenhill JP. *Obstetrics.* 13th ed. Philedelphia: WB Saunders Co; 1965.)

circulation; however, the intracellular placental concentrations of most amino acids are higher than the fetal plasma concentrations. For most amino acids therefore, the major energy-requiring step is that which transports them from the maternal circulation into the placenta.

Alterations in amino acid transport have been postulated in a number of placental pathophysiologies. Animal and human studies have shown clear deficits in certain classes of amino acids in intrauterine growth restriction (IUGR). Studies on placental amino acid transporters from term and preterm human tissues have shown a greater than 5-fold increase in transport capacity between 10 and 40 weeks of gestation and decreases in amino acid transport capacity in both IUGR and macrosomic diabetes.

3. Bulk Flow

This describes the passage of substances resulting from a hydrostatic or osmotic gradient. Water is transported by this

mechanism and may also carry some solutes with it under the influence of this mechanism.

Water diffuses rapidly across the placenta in both directions, but since there is no "concentration" difference, this mechanism does not drive fetal uptake. Fetal water acquisition (bulk flow) results from the maternal/fetal movement of water in response to an osmotic gradient. An osmotic gradient of less than 1 mOsm is sufficient to drive fetal water acquisition at term. The movement of water is dependent on the pumping on NaCl and thus on ATP and may therefore be sensitive to conditions that produce reductions in cellular energy supply, such as hypoxia. There are several conditions of pregnancy in which water permeabilities

Figure 2.2. Drawing from an electron micrograph of cross-section through parts of two fetal villi, showing tissue layers that separate fetal and maternal blood in the human placenta. The cytotrophoblastic layer is much less distinct in the third trimester than is depicted here. (Reprinted by courtesy of Berkeley Bio-Engineering, Inc., Berkeley, CA.)

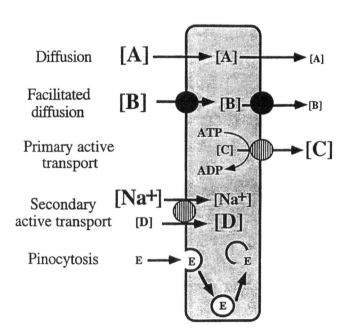

Figure 2.3. Modes of transport of molecules across the placenta.

or the forces driving water movement may be altered. These include polyhydramnios, oligohydramnios, and nonimmune fetal hydrops.

4. Pinocytosis

Some large molecules such as the immune globulins are transported by being enclosed in small vesicles consisting of cell membranes.

The cellular uptake of proteins (by endocytosis) involves binding of the protein to a specific receptor on the cell surface followed by the pinching off of a plasma membrane vesicle, which moves in the interior of the cell. Acidification of the endocytic vesicles releases the protein and the vesicle recycles to the cell surface. Efflux, or exocytosis, reverses this process. Sequestration of the specific protein into vesicles takes place followed by transfer of the vesicle to the cell surface, fusion with the plasma membrane, and release of the protein.

Iron circulates into an iron-binding protein, transferrin. Iron-bound transferrin binds specifically to transferrin receptors on the syncytiotrophoblast microvillous surface. These receptors are internalized in a plasma membrane (endocytic) vesicle and the iron is then released to the cell, while the iron-free transferrin, still bound to its receptor, is recycled back to the microvillous surface, along with the plasma membrane fragment.

5. Breaks

The delicate, filmy villi may at times break off within the intervillous space, and the contents may be extruded into the maternal circulation. It is also thought that maternal intravascular contents may be taken up by the fetal circulation at times. The most important result of this is seen when fetal Rh-positive red blood cells are deposited in the vascular system of an Rh-negative mother, resulting in alloimmunization and subsequent erythroblastosis fetalis.

DIFFUSION

When limitations of placental transfer occur in the human, they usually are first recognized as limitations of those substances that are exchanged by diffusion. For example, an acute decrease in placental function limits passage of oxygen to and carbon dioxide from the fetus, resulting in fetal asphyxia. A more chronic decrease in placental function may result in limitation of substances necessary for growth (e.g., carbohydrates), thus giving rise to a fetus that is growth restricted. Hence, the process of diffusion is examined in some detail.

Fick's diffusion equation describes the physicochemical process:

$$\text{Rate of transfer} = \text{concentration gradient} \times \text{area} \times \text{permeability}/\text{membrane thickness}$$

Each of the factors determining rate of passage of substances by diffusion is considered in turn.

Concentration Gradient

The concentration gradient of a substance across the placenta is equal to the difference between the mean maternal blood concentration and the mean fetal blood concentration within each of the exchanging areas. As noted above, however, it is most unlikely that this gradient is constant throughout the placenta because of the placenta's peculiar circulatory anatomy. It probably varies from place to place and also from time to time in any particular area. However, by considering a simplified exchanging membrane with blood flowing in from each side, each of the factors that would affect the concentration gradient can be conceptually discussed (Fig. 2.4). These factors are

1. Concentration of substance in maternal arterial blood
2. Concentration of substance in fetal arterial blood
3. Maternal intervillous space blood flow
4. Fetal-placental blood flow

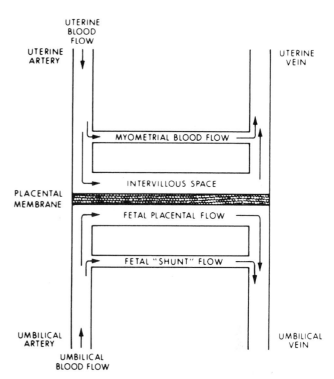

Figure 2.4. Simplified diagram of pattern of circulation through the placenta. (Reprinted by courtesy of Berkeley Bio-Engineering, Inc., Berkeley, CA.)

5. Diffusing capacity of the placenta for the substance
6. Ratio of maternal to fetal blood flow in exchanging areas

This is analogous to ventilation-to-perfusion ratios as applied to the lung. Inequalities in the ratio give rise to decreased efficiency of transfer. Exchange of substances is optimal if the flows are evenly matched.

7. Binding of substances to molecules and dissociation rates

Depending on the rate of dissociation, this reaction time could limit the transfer of a substance. This does not appear to be limiting with regard to the dissociation of oxygen and hemoglobin.

8. Geometry of exchanging surfaces with respect to blood flow

If the blood flows are traveling in the same direction during exchange, the system is called concurrent. If the blood flows are traveling in opposite directions, the system is called countercurrent. This latter system is the most efficient from the exchange point of view. As can be seen in Figure 2.1, in the human placenta it is unlikely that either of these simplified concepts holds. The human pattern has been described as the multivillous stream system (1). The evaluation of the mean concentration gradient of any nutrient in this system becomes extremely complex.

9. The metabolism of the substance

If a substance is consumed within the placenta, its rate of passage across the placenta will not be reflected by the concentration gradient. For example, oxygen is consumed in considerable quantities by the trophoblast and the rate of passage appears to be relatively inefficient when based on oxygen tension gradients alone.

Area of the Placenta

The villous surface area of the human term placenta (3) is approximately 11 m^2. In comparison, the lung has an alveolar surface area of 70 m^2. The area of actual exchange, the vasculosyncytial membrane—that is, the area where fetal capillaries approach closely enough to the surface to exchange materials with maternal blood—is 1.8 m^2.

Placental area is decreased in a number of clinical situations. An acute decrease occurs with abruptio placentae. With part of the placenta separated, the fetus does not necessarily expire through asphyxia. Its ability to survive depends on the placental reserve that existed before the episode of abruption. Some placentas, particularly those in cases of maternal hypertension or those that have infarcted fibrotic areas, have a reduced area available for exchange and, hence, lowered reserve. Thus, the placenta of a mother with long-term hypertension is likely to be smaller than expected, as is the fetus. The infarctions are thought to be caused by maternal arteriolar deficiencies giving rise to devitalization of certain cotyledonary areas, resulting in fibrosis of the villi. Additionally, in certain cases of intrauterine infection or congenital defects, the placentas are decreased in size and area. Large placentas are found in certain diabetics and in erythroblastosis fetalis. In the former case, it is not certain whether the increased area improves the transfer of nutrients to the fetus. In the latter case, most of the increased placental mass is thought to be hydropic in origin and, hence, is unlikely to improve the exchange characteristics of the placenta.

Permeability of the Placental Membrane

The permeability of a membrane to a substance depends on characteristics of both the membrane and the substance that is being exchanged. The units for permeability can be found by a transposition of Fick's diffusion equation. There are three major determinants of permeability:

1. Molecular size. A molecular weight of 1000 is a rough dividing line between those substances that cross the placenta by diffusion and those that are relatively impermeable by diffusion. Below a molecular weight of 1000, the rate of passage of the molecule is related to its weight unless other properties (see below) prevent or hasten rate of passage. A common clinical example is found in cases in which it is necessary to anticoagulate a pregnant woman. If one uses heparin, with a molecular weight above 6000, one does not concomitantly heparinize the fetus. However, with the use of warfarin (Coumadin), with a molecular weight of 330, the fetus will also be anticoagulated. This is considered undesirable, particularly in the intrapartum period when fetal bleeding may occur. Also, warfarin may have some teratogenic effects in the first trimester.

2. Lipid solubility. A lipid-soluble substance traverses the placenta more rapidly than one that is not lipid soluble.

3. Electrical charge. This deters the passage of a substance across the placenta. For example, succinylcholine, commonly used during balanced anesthesia, is highly ionized and is poorly diffusible across the placenta despite its molecular weight of 361. Thiopental, with a molecular weight of 264, is lipid soluble, relatively unionized, and moves very rapidly into the fetal circulation.

Substances are classified into those in which the rate of passage is either "permeability limited" or "flow limited" (4). A substance that has poor permeability is limited in its rate of passage across the placenta by permeability and not by rates of blood flow. Hence, increasing the rate of blood flow will not improve its rate of passage by much. The majority of biologic molecules are limited in their rate of passage across the placenta by resistance of diffusion. However, substances that are highly permeable are limited by the rate of blood flow. Oxygen and carbon dioxide are examples of this. Decreasing the rate of blood flow decreases the rate of exchange considerably.

Diffusion Distance

The average distance for diffusion across the placenta (3) has been measured as approximately 3.5 μ. This contrasts with the much smaller distance from alveolus to pulmonary capillary in the lung (0.5 μ). The diffusion distance decreases as the placenta matures, but it is not clear whether this improves the placenta's characteristics for exchange. The distance is increased in

several conditions, such as erythroblastosis fetalis and congenital syphilis. This increased distance probably is due to villous edema and presumably decreases the organ's efficiency for exchange. Fibrous or calcific deposits in the placental vasculature, such as are found in diabetes mellitus or preeclampsia, presumably increase diffusion distance.

UTERINE BLOOD FLOW

Because uterine blood flow is one of the prime determinants of passage of a number of critical substances across the placenta, its characteristics, the factors affecting it, and the effects of anesthesia on uterine blood flow are discussed in the latter portion of this chapter.

Uterine blood flow rises progressively throughout pregnancy and in the term fetus is approximately 700 mL/min (Fig. 2.5). This represents about 10% of the cardiac output. Approximately 70% to 90% of the uterine blood flow passes through the intervillous space, and the remainder largely supplies the myometrium.

The uterine vascular bed is thought to be almost maximally dilated under normal conditions, with little capacity to dilate further (5). It is not autoregulated, so flow is proportional to the mean perfusion pressure. However, it is capable of marked vasoconstriction by α-adrenergic action. It is not responsive to changes in respiratory gas tensions. The uterine blood flow is determined by the following relationship:

Uterine blood flow

= uterine arterial pressure − uterine venous pressure/ uterine vascular resistance

Hence, any factor affecting either of the three values on the right side of the above relationship will alter uterine blood flow. A number of causes of decreased uterine blood flow are shown in Table 2.1.

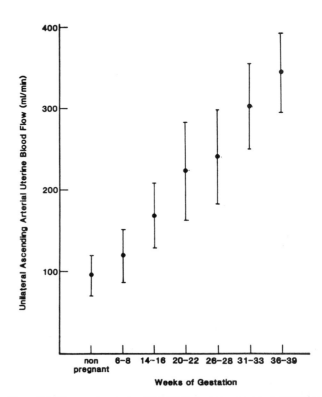

Figure 2.5. Changes in uterine blood flow during pregnancy. Assuming equal flow in both uterine arteries, total uterine blood flow as measured by a transvaginal duplex Doppler ultrasound would be about 700 mL/min. (Reprinted by permission from Thaler I, Manor D, Itskovitz J, et al. Changes in uterine blood flow during human pregnancy. *Am J Obstet Gynecol* 1990;162:121–125.)

Table 2.1. FACTORS CAUSING DECREASED UTERINE BLOOD FLOW

Uterine contractions
Hypertonus
   Abruptio placentae
   Tetanic contraction
   Overstimulation with oxytocin
Hypotension
   Sympathetic block
   Hypovolemic shock
   Supine hypotensive syndrome
Hypertension
   Essential
   Preeclamptic
Vasoconstriction, endogenous
   Sympathetic discharge
   Adrenal medullary activity
Vasoconstrictors, exogenous
   Most sympathomimetics (α-adrenergic effects)
   Exception is ephedrine (primarily β-adrenergic effect)

Uterine contractions decrease uterine blood flow as a result of increased uterine venous pressure brought about by increased intramural pressure of the uterus. There may also be a decrease in uterine arterial pressure with contractions. Uterine hypertonus causes a decreased uterine blood flow through the same mechanism.

In sheep, it has been shown that, if uterine arterial perfusion pressure is altered without changing the resistance of the uterine vascular bed, there is a direct relationship between uterine blood flow and the pressure (5). Hence, hypotension through any of the mechanisms noted in Table 2.1 will cause a decrease in blood flow.

In the case of maternal arterial hypertension, it is likely that there is a concomitant increased vascular resistance that is shared by the uterine vascular bed. This therefore results in a decrease in uterine blood flow. Either endogenous or exogenous vasoconstriction results in decreased blood flow because of increased uterine vascular resistance.

There are few useful means of increasing uterine blood flow when it is known to be suboptimal. The most important clinical considerations are the avoidance or correction of factors responsible for an acute decrease in blood flow (e.g., excessive uterine activity or maternal hypotension).

Some of the β-mimetic agents that are used as uterine relaxants for preterm labor may increase uterine blood flow, but this effect, if it occurs, is small and may only be a result of decreased uterine tonus. There are a number of experimental means of increasing uterine blood flow, sometimes transiently, but these have no real clinical use. Examples of such treatments include estrogens, acetylcholine, nitroglycerin, cyanide, ischemia, and mild hypoxia, the latter either acute or chronic (6).

Clinically, it has been known for many years that maternal bed rest may improve the outcome in suspected fetal growth restriction. There is some evidence that bed rest does improve fetal growth, as evidenced by increasing estriol excretion (7).

UMBILICAL BLOOD FLOW

The umbilical blood flow in the undisturbed fetus at term is about 120 mL/kg/min or 360 mL/min. Such measurements have been obtained by noninvasive methods using ultrasound techniques (8). This is somewhat higher than values obtained immediately after birth, but the latter are probably affected by cord manipulation during the birth process. The measurements have not yet found clinical applicability, but the same technique can be used to calculate the peak systolic-to-diastolic (S/D) ratio, which is a reflection of vascular resistance distal to the point of measurement.

The umbilical blood flow in the human is considerably less than that of the sheep, where it is approximately 200 mL/kg/min (9). The differences may be explained by the somewhat higher metabolic rate of the sheep (body temperature 39°C) and differences in hemoglobin concentrations (sheep, 10 g/dL vs. human, 15 g/dL). It is important to recognize this species difference because the bulk of our information regarding fetal circulatory physiology comes from the chronically instrumented sheep fetus. In sheep, the umbilical blood flow is approximately 45% of the combined ventricular output (9), and about 20% of this blood flow is "shunted," that is, it does not exchange with maternal blood (1). It either is carried through actual vascular shunts within the fetal side of the placenta or else it does not approach closely enough to maternal blood for exchange with it.

Umbilical blood flow is unaffected by acute moderate hypoxia but is decreased by severe hypoxia (10). Whether the umbilical cord is innervated is still in question; however, umbilical blood flow decreases with the administration of catecholamines. It is also decreased by acute cord occlusion. There are no known means of increasing umbilical flow in patients in whom it is thought to be decreased chronically. However, certain fetal heart rate patterns (i.e., variable decelerations) have been ascribed to transient umbilical cord compression in the fetus during labor. Manipulation of maternal position either to the lateral or Trendelenburg position can sometimes abolish these patterns, the implication being that cord compression has been relieved.

Blood Flow Studies in the Human Fetus

Blood Velocity Wave Forms. Real-time directed Doppler ultrasound has been used to investigate human fetal, placental, and uterine blood flows (11). Doppler ultrasound allows for measurement of velocity waveforms of red blood cells traveling in vessels. The velocity data can be used to make inferences about blood flow, vascular resistance, and myocardial contractility. Blood flow velocity waveforms have a characteristic appearance that varies from vessel to vessel (see Fig. 2.10). The observed waveform shape is affected by the pumping ability of the heart, the heart rate, the elasticity of the vessel wall, the outflow impedance, and the blood viscosity. Waveforms in arteries supplying low-resistance vascular beds have a characteristically high forward velocity during diastole, whereas absent or reverse diastolic flow is seen in arteries supplying high-resistance vascular beds. These observations prompted the definition of indices of flow that could be related to the vascular resistance of a downstream vascular bed. The most commonly used indices are:

$$\text{Pulsatility Index: PI} = V_{max} - V_{min}/V_{mean}$$
$$\text{Pourcelot Ratio: PR} = V_{max} - V_{min}/V_{max}$$
$$\text{AB (S/D) Ratio: AB} = V_{max}/V_{min}$$

where V_{max} = Point of maximal blood flow velocity/cardiac cycle
         V_{min} = Point of minimal blood flow velocity/cardiac cycle
         V_{mean} = Mean blood flow velocity/cardiac cycle

Blood Flow. Doppler ultrasound permits the estimation of blood flows in the human fetus. Blood flow is calculated using the formula:

$$Q = (V \times A)/\text{Cos }\theta$$

where V = mean velocity as averaged over many cardiac cycles (cm/s)
        A = estimated cross-sectional area of the vessel (cm^2)
        θ = angle between the Doppler beam and the direction of flow of the blood

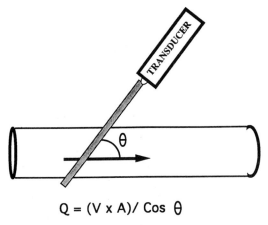

$$Q = (V \times A)/ Cos\ \theta$$

Figure 2.6. The blood flow (Q) through a vessel is quantitated as the product of mean velocity (V) of red blood cells and cross-sectional area (A) of the vessel, divided by the cosine of the angle of insonation of the vessel ($Cos\ \theta$). (Modified from Copel JA, Grannum PA, Hobbins JC, Cunningham FG, eds. Doppler ultrasound in obstetrics. In: *Williams Obstetrics*. 16th ed. Norwalk, CT: Appleton & Lange; 1988.)

This calculation (Fig. 2.6) is complicated by the variation in the velocity of blood cells across a vascular lumen. Cells flow faster in the center of the vessel and slower near the vessel wall. The overall flow in a vessel is the sum of the different flows across the lumen. For this reason, satisfactory volume flow measurements can best be made on large vessels (4 to 10 mm in diameter) with appropriate Doppler angles (30 to 60 degrees). The two-dimensional echo Doppler provides a means of estimating fetal cardiac output by quantifying blood flow volume at the atrioventricular valve orifices. The estimated cardiac output of the human fetus ($553\ mL^{-1} \cdot kg^{-1} \cdot min^{-1}$) is higher than that of the sheep ($450\ mL^{-1} \cdot kg^{-1} \cdot min^{-1}$). In addition, the right and left ventricular outputs are more similar in the human, as compared with the sheep. The ratio of right-to-left ventricular outputs decreases with advancing gestation, from 1.3 at 15 weeks to 1.1 at 40 weeks. In normal pregnancy, high forward velocity levels in the umbilical artery are maintained throughout diastole. A lowered diastolic flow, as seen in severe intrauterine growth restriction, may reflect raised placental resistance (12). Marx et al. used Doppler ultrasound waveform analysis to demonstrate a significant reduction in umbilical artery vascular resistance (S/D ratio) with epidural analgesia in healthy laboring women (13). Youngstrom et al. (14) investigated the effect of more extensive epidural anesthesia (and maternal sympathetic blockade) on umbilical artery flow velocity waveforms in healthy, nonlaboring women undergoing elective cesarean section. They found no statistically significant change in umbilical artery resistance (S/D ratio).

OXYGEN TRANSFER TO THE FETUS

As mentioned previously, it is likely that most stillbirths and cases of fetal depression are the result of inadequate exchange of the respiratory gases. Oxygen has the lowest storage-to-utilization ratio of all nutrients in the fetus. From animal experimentation, it can be calculated that in a term fetus the quantity of oxygen is approximately 42 mL and the normal oxygen consumption is approximately 21 mL/min (10). This means that, in theory, the fetus has a 2-minute supply of oxygen. However, fetuses do not consume the total quantity of oxygen in their body within 2 minutes, nor do they expire after this time. In fact, irreversible brain damage does not occur until about 10 minutes have elapsed (15). This is because the fetus has a number of important compensatory mechanisms that enable it to survive on a lesser quantity of oxygen for longer periods. Clinical situations in which there is total cessation of oxygen delivery are

rare. These include sudden total abruption of the placenta or complete umbilical cord compression, generally after prolapse of the cord.

It is known from animal experimentation that the compensations that occur in the hypoxic fetus are (a) redistribution of blood flow to vital organs, including heart, brain, and placenta; (b) decreased total oxygen consumption (e.g., with moderate hypoxia, the fetal oxygen consumption drops to 50% of the normal level); and (c) dependence of certain vascular beds on anaerobic metabolism. These compensatory mechanisms appear to be initiated with mild hypoxia and result in the maintenance of oxygen supply to vital organs during times of oxygen limitation (10).

It is of value to examine the factors that determine oxygen transfer from mother to fetus (Table 2.2). Because the transfer of oxygen to the fetus depends on rates of blood flow and not limitations to diffusion, the respective blood flow on each side of the placenta assumes major importance for maintenance of fetal oxygenation. Animal work suggests that in the normal placenta there is a "safety factor" of approximately 50% in the uterine blood flow. That is, the uterine blood flow will drop to half its normal value before severe fetal acidosis becomes evident (16) and oxygen uptake declines (17). This applies only to the normal situation with normal placental reserve and is unlikely to be the case in pathologic situations, such as in the infant of a hypertensive mother. In such situations, the placental function may be adequate for oxygenation but not for fetal growth, and a growth-restricted infant may result from such a pregnancy. Furthermore, with superimposition of uterine contractions on such a fetus, there may be transient inadequacy of uterine blood flow during the uterine contractions; this may be recognized by responses of the fetal heart rate (i.e., late decelerations).

Additional important determinants of fetal oxygenation include oxygen tension in maternal arterial and fetal arterial blood. In general, maternal arterial oxygen tension depends on adequate ventilation and pulmonary integrity. Disruptions of this function are relatively rare in obstetrics, although they can occur with pulmonary diseases such as asthma, with congestive heart failure, or in mothers with congenital cardiac defects. The oxygen affinity and oxygen capacity of maternal and fetal blood are also important determinants of fetal oxygen transfer. At a given oxygen tension, the quantity of oxygen carried by blood depends on the oxygen capacity, which depends on the hemoglobin concentration, and on the oxygen affinity. The oxygen affinity of fetal blood is greater than that of maternal blood (Fig. 2.7). That is, the oxygen dissociation curve of the fetus is to the left of that of the mother. In addition, the hemoglobin concentration of fetal blood is approximately 15 g/100 mL in the term fetus, whereas that of the mother is approximately 12 g/100 mL. Both of these factors, an increased oxygen affinity and higher oxygen capacity, confer advantages to the fetus for

Table 2.2. FACTORS AFFECTING OXYGEN TRANSFER FROM MOTHER TO FETUS

Intervillous blood flow
Fetal-placental blood flow
Oxygen tension in maternal arterial blood
Oxygen tension in fetal arterial blood
Oxygen affinity of maternal blood
Oxygen affinity of fetal blood
Hemoglobin concentration or oxygen capacity of maternal blood
Hemoglobin concentration or oxygen capacity of fetal blood
Maternal and fetal blood pH and P_{CO_2} (Bohr effect)
Placental diffusing capacity
Placental vascular geometry
Ratio of maternal to fetal blood flow in exchanging areas
Shunting around exchange sites
Placental oxygen consumption

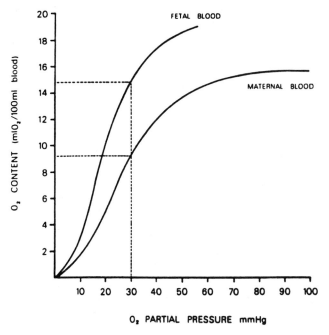

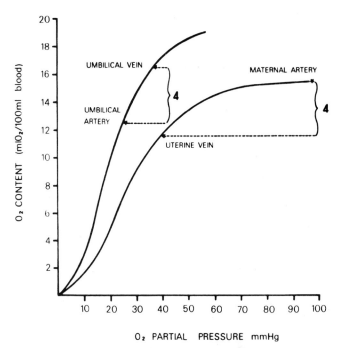

Figure 2.7. Oxygen dissociation curves of maternal and fetal blood. *Vertical broken line* illustrates the higher oxygen affinity of fetal blood— fetal blood is more highly saturated with oxygen than is maternal blood at the same oxygen partial pressure. (Reprinted by permission from Parer JT, ed. Uteroplacental physiology and exchange. In: *Handbook of Fetal Heart Rate Monitoring*. Philadelphia: WB Saunders; 1997:40.)

Figure 2.9. Oxygen contents and tensions, and arteriovenous oxygen concentration differences (*brackets*), on fetal and maternal side of the placenta. These are probable values in the undisturbed human, although use has been made of data from many sources, including experimental animals.

oxygen uptake across the placenta (Fig. 2.8). Probable values of the oxygen content and oxygen tension in umbilical vessels and maternal uterine artery and vein are illustrated in Figure 2.9.

Because most measurements have been made in the human fetus during or after labor, the values of oxygen saturation, oxygen tension, and pH are generally depressed compared with those of the mother. In fact, investigations on chronically-instrumented animals have shown that the oxygen saturation and content of fetal blood and acid-base status is very close to that of maternal blood; only the P_{O2} is lower. The arterio-venous oxygen differences across each side of the placenta are also illustrated in Figure 2.9. Notice that the quantity of oxygen delivered or taken up by each 100 mL of circulating blood in the placenta is approximately equal in the mother and fetus. This further suggests approximate equality of blood flows on each side of the placenta. A number of additional miscellaneous factors determine the rate of oxygen transfer across the placenta; they are listed in Table 2.2 as the last six determinants. They appear to be relatively minor compared with the major factors already outlined.

CARBON DIOXIDE AND ACID-BASE BALANCE

Carbon dioxide crosses the placenta even more readily than does oxygen. In general, the determinants for oxygen transfer also apply to carbon dioxide transfer across the placenta. It is limited by rate of blood flow and not by resistance to diffusion. The carbon dioxide tension in fetal blood in the undisturbed state is close to 40 mm Hg (1). It is well known that the maternal arterial carbon dioxide tension is approximately 34 mm Hg, and the mother is in a state of compensated respiratory alkalosis. The pH of fetal blood under undisturbed conditions is probably close to 7.4, and the bicarbonate concentration is close to that of maternal blood.

Bicarbonate and the fixed acids cross the placenta much more slowly than does carbon dioxide; that is, equilibration takes a matter of hours rather than seconds. There is a situation analogous to "respiratory acidosis" that occurs in the fetus when blood flow, either uterine or umbilical, is acutely compromised. In such cases, the pH drops and carbon dioxide tension is elevated, but the metabolic acid-base status remains unchanged. This occurs during severe or profound fetal decelerations (called variable decelerations) in association with certain uterine contractions, especially during the second stage of labor. These acid-base

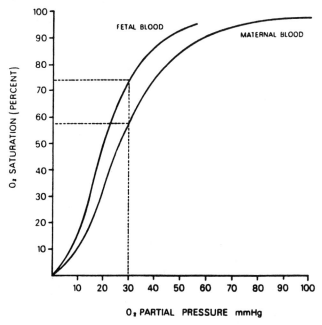

Figure 2.8. Oxygen dissociation curves relating oxygen content of blood to oxygen partial pressure in maternal and fetal blood. This relationship illustrates the even greater oxygen content of fetal blood when the greater hemoglobin content of fetal blood is taken into account. (Reprinted by permission from Parer JT. Uteroplacental physiology and exchange. In: *Handbook of Fetal Heart Rate Monitoring*. Philadelphia: WB Saunders; 1997:41.)

changes are generally rapidly resolved with cessation of the contraction and the bradycardia. However, as noted earlier, if there is a significant oxygen lack that is unrelieved, the fetus will decrease its oxygen consumption, redistribute blood flow, and depend partly on anaerobic metabolism to supply its energy needs, albeit with decreased efficiency. Under these conditions, lactate (an end product of anaerobic metabolism) is produced, resulting in a metabolic acidosis. The acidosis may also be aggravated by a combined respiratory acidosis because of retained carbon dioxide. Unlike carbon dioxide, lactate is lost slowly from the fetus.

Lactate is transported by specific, pH-dependent carriers, while protons pass to the maternal circulation via channels, lipid diffusion, co-transport, and specific proton-pumping ATPases.

CLINICAL IMPLICATIONS

Fetal compromise results from a disruption of normal placental exchange mechanisms. With a knowledge of the components involved in exchange of nutrients and waste materials across the placenta, potential problems can be recognized and corrections made.

The most important components of placental exchange are the rates of blood flow on each side of the placenta and the area available for exchange. Uterine blood flow will decline in the presence of factors causing decreased perfusion pressure or increased uterine vascular resistance. Common clinical occurrences are hypotension, hypertension, endogenous or exogenous vasoconstriction, and possibly severe psychologic stress. The uterine vascular bed, as previously noted, is not autoregulated and has little capacity to dilate further. During labor, it is most likely that the rate of uterine blood flow is the limiting factor in cases of fetal compromise because of the intermittent decline in uterine blood flow with each uterine contraction. In addition, transient or persistent umbilical cord compression may cause fetal asphyxia.

OBSTETRIC ANESTHESIA AND UTERINE BLOOD FLOW

Obstetric anesthesia and analgesia may directly affect uterine blood flow or may alter the response of the uteroplacental circulation to noxious stimuli and to various pharmacologic agents (Table 2.3). Uterine blood flow varies directly with the perfusion pressure (i.e., uterine arterial minus uterine venous pressure) and inversely with uterine vascular resistance. Obstetric anesthesia may affect uterine blood flow by (a) changing the perfusion pressure, that is, altering the uterine arterial or venous pressure; or (b) changing uterine vascular resistance either directly through changes in vascular tone or indirectly by altering uterine contractions or uterine muscle tone.

Direct measurement of human uterine blood flow is not easy because of the relative inaccessibility of the human uteroplacental circulation. Clinically, changes in uterine blood flow are presumed from assessment of fetal and neonatal acid-base and heart rate status. In the late 1970s, a group of Finnish investigators developed a quantitative, highly reproducible method for measuring both the intervillous and myometrial components of human uterine blood flow based on the clearance of xenon-133 given intravenously (18, 19).

Currently, the most popular technique for assessing uteroplacental circulation is Doppler ultrasound. Actual measurements of blood flow require precise measurement of the cross-sectional areas of the vessel. An additional problem in converting velocity measurements to actual flows is the difficulty in precisely measuring the angle between the ultrasound beam and the vessel. Describing the relationship between the Doppler waveform during systole and diastole—that is, the S/D ratio—allows one to study relative changes without actually measuring absolute flow.

Doppler arterial waveforms in most vessels show high systolic velocity and little or no diastolic velocity. During pregnancy, maternal uteroplacental vessels show continuous diastolic flow (Fig. 2.10). Any decrease, absence, or reversal of end-diastolic flow velocity is considered abnormal. The use of a true mean velocity measurement that is more accurate has improved the quality of this technique, but it is effective only in the hands of experts (20).

The vast majority of information on the effects of anesthesia on uteroplacental circulation has been derived mainly from animal experiments. The development of chronic maternal-fetal animal preparations has allowed precise measurement of changes in uterine and placental blood flow and of the effect of these changes on fetal cardiovascular and acid-base status (Fig. 2.11) using various techniques (21–23). The following section reviews the effects of commonly used anesthetic agents, techniques, and adjuvants, and of anesthetic complications on uterine blood flow.

INTRAVENOUS INDUCTION AGENTS

Barbiturates

Ultra short-acting barbiturates are most commonly used for induction of anesthesia and are usually followed by endotracheal intubation and nitrous oxide maintenance. Palahniuk and Cumming (24) studied this sequence and reported that uterine blood flow decreased by 20% after induction of anesthesia without a significant decrease in maternal arterial blood pressure. Fetal oxygen saturation and pH also decreased. They postulated that the increase in uterine vascular resistance was due to maternal catecholamine release during light anesthesia.

Shnider et al (25). reported that, in sheep, intravenous induction of anesthesia with thiopental and succinylcholine followed by direct laryngoscopy and endotracheal intubation resulted in an increase in arterial plasma norepinephrine of 89% from control. Blood pressure rose by 65%, uterine vascular resistance rose by 42%, and uterine blood flow fell by 24%. These acute cardiovascular changes quickly diminished with the termination of airway manipulation. Alon et al (26), also studying pregnant sheep, reported that uterine blood flow decreased by about 40% during thiopental induction and endotracheal intubation, then rapidly increased significantly to a point approximately 28% ± 27% above baseline values during anesthetic maintenance with isoflurane (Fig. 2.12). Jouppila et al. (27), using the radioactive xenon technique, corroborated these findings in humans. During the induction of general anesthesia for cesarean section, they found a marked decrease in placental blood flow with a mean reduction of 35%.

Propofol

In contrast to thiopental, uterine blood flow demonstrated no change during induction of anesthesia with propofol (2 mg/kg) despite a significant increase in mean arterial blood pressure. Unlike the uterine blood flow response during maintenance of anesthesia with isoflurane, maintenance of anesthesia with infusions of propofol at either 150, 300, or 450 $\mu g^{-1} \cdot kg^{-1} \cdot min^{-1}$ (26) did not change uterine blood flow from preinduction baseline values, and it remained stable throughout anesthesia (Fig. 2.13).

Diazepam

In pregnant sheep, diazepam in doses as high as 0.5 mg/kg did not alter maternal or fetal cardiovascular function or uteroplacental blood flow (28). However, larger doses produced an 8% to 12% decrease in arterial pressure with an equivalent decrease in uterine blood flow. Fetal oxygenation was not affected. Cosmi (29) also observed that the bolus injection of diazepam to the ewe in doses of 0.18 mg/kg had no deleterious effects on maternal or fetal blood pressure or acid-base status.

Table 2.3. DRUG EFFECTS ON UTERINE/PLACENTAL BLOOD FLOW*

Drug	Model and Technique	Dosage/Blood Level	Effect	Reference
Induction Agents				
Thiopental	Microsphere-ewe	Standard	40% initial decrease UBF	26
Thiopental	Xenon-human	Standard	Marked decrease placental BF	27
Propofol	Microsphere-ewe	≤450 mg/kg/min	No change UBF from baseline	26
Diazepam	Sheep gravid	0.5 mg/kg	No change utero/placental flow	28
Ketamine	Sheep gravid	0.7 mg/kg	UBF constant	34
Ketamine	Sheep gravid	≤5 mg/kg	Dose-related decrease UBF, increase uterine tone	35
Ketamine	Human recommendations	0.25–1 mg/kg	No adverse effect	37–40
Inhalation Drugs				
Halothane	Sheep gravid	Up to 1.5%	No effect or slight increase UBF	51
Halothane	Monkey and sheep	>2 MAC	Dose-related decrease UBF	51, 53
Isoflurane	Sheep gravid	1%	25% increase UBF	51
Desflurane	No UBF studies			
Sevoflurane	No UBF studies			
Local Anesthetics				
Lidocaine	Uterine artery (human)	400 μg/mL	Vasoconstriction (supraclinical dose)	54
Lidocaine	Sheep gravid	2–4 μg/mL Blood level	No change UBF	60
2 CP	Guinea pigs	2 mg/kg	No change UBF	61
Bupivacaine	Human/ultrasound	≈140 mg epidural	No change UBF	63
Ropivacaine	Human/ultrasound	≈140 mg epidural	No change UBF	63
Cocaine	Sheep gravid	0.5–2.8 mg/kg	Dose-related decrease UBF	66
Epidural Block				
Uncomplicated by hypotension			No change UBF	69, 77–80
Catecholamines				
Epinephrine 1:200K	Human/xenon	10 mL w 2CP epidural	No change intervillous BF	87
Epinephrine	Sheep gravid	20 μg IV	Decrease UBF 40% for 60 sec	82
Epinephrine	Guinea pig	0.2–1 μg/kg	Dose-related decrease UBF	83
Isoproterenol	Pregnant ewe	4, 16, 80 μg IV	Dose-related transient decrease UBF	182
Stress	Monkey/flow probe	Severe stress	Marked reduction UBF	91
	Human	Very anxious	Higher catechols and abnormal FHT	93
Vasopressors				
Ephedrine	Monkey/flow probe	10–15 mg IV	Restores UBF better than other pressors	99
Ephedrine	Gravid sheep	5–10 mg IV	Restores UBF after SAB	98
Ephedrine	Xenon-human	25 mg IV	No decrease IVBF	74
Phenylephrine	Human clinical outcome	20–100 μg IV	Restored maternal BP and possibly UBF	101, 183, 184
Dopamine	Sheep gravid	Doses to correct BP	Decrease UBF	105, 106
Ritodrine	Sheep gravid	Therapeutic doses	Decrease UBF	83, 110
Terbutaline	Sheep gravid	Therapeutic doses	Decrease UBF	111
Antihypertensives				
Hydralazine	Hypertensive sheep	Dose to normalize BP	Increase UBF while decreasing BP	112
Hydralazine	Human hypertension/xenon	125 μg/min	Increase umbilical BF, no change IVBF	115
Nitroglycerin	Hypertensive sheep	Infusion	Increase UBF while decreasing BP	116
Nitroprusside	Hypertensive sheep	Infusion	Decrease UBF, restrict to induction use	113, 185
Labetalol	Human/PEC/xenon/US	1 mg/kg	No change in IVBF or fetal BF	127
Calcium Channel Blockers				
Verapamil	Pregnant ewe	0.2 mg/kg	25% decrease UBF 2 min	130
Nicardipine	Pregnant rabbit	Low and high dose	Dose-related decrease UBF	131
Nifedipine	Pregnant ewe	5–10 μg/kg 90 min	UBF decrease transient, fetal hypoxia	186
Magnesium sulfate	Pregnant ewe	4 gm load, 2–4 gm/h	Initial decrease UBF, then normalization	143
Epidural opioids				
MS, Fentanyl, Sufentanil	Pregnant ewe	Clinical doses	No effect UBF	146–148
Clonidine	Pregnant ewe	300 μg epidural	No significant change UBF	187
Clonidine	Pregnant ewe	300 μg IV	Significant decrease UBF, fetal hypoxia	187
Dantrolene	Pregnant ewe	1.2–2.4 mg/kg	No change UBF	166
Respiratory gases				
Hypocapnia	Pregnant ewe	Mechanical hyperventilation	Decrease UBF 25%	171
Hypercapnia	Pregnant ewe	Art P_{CO_2} > 60 mm Hg	Decrease UBF	169

*Table prepared by Dr. T. Cheek.

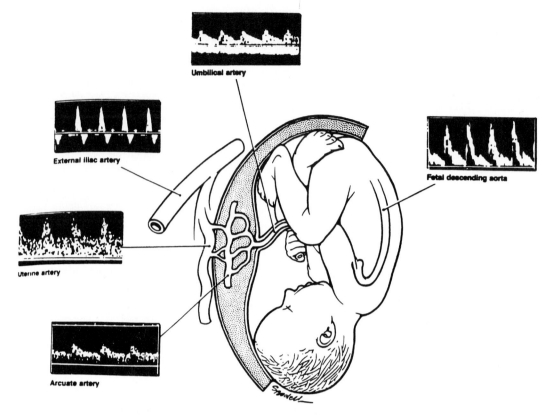

Figure 2.10. Doppler waveforms from normal pregnancy. Shown clockwise are normal waveforms from the maternal arcuate, uterine, and external iliac arteries and from the fetal umbilical artery and descending aorta. Reversed end-diastolic flow velocity is apparent in the external iliac artery, whereas continuous diastolic flow characterizes the uterine and arcuate vessels. Finally, note the greatly diminished end-diastolic flow in the fetal descending aorta. (Modified from Copel JA, Grannum PA, Hobbins JC, Cunningham FG, eds. Doppler ultrasound in obstetrics. In: *Williams Obstetrics.* 16th ed. Norwalk, CT: Appleton & Lange; 1988.)

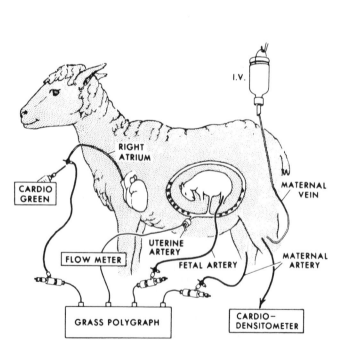

Figure 2.11. Diagram of sheep experimental preparation with chronically implanted maternal and fetal intravascular catheters and an electromagnetic flow probe around a branch of uterine artery. (Reprinted by permission from Ralston DH, Shnider SM, deLorimier AA. Effects of equipotent ephedrine, metaraminol, mephentermine and methoxamine on uterine blood flow in the pregnant ewe. *Anesthesiology* 1974; 40:354–370.)

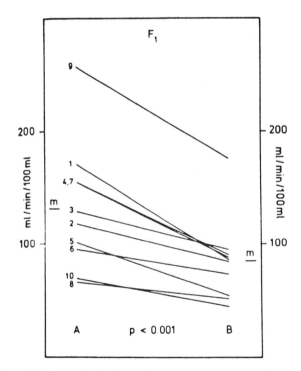

Figure 2.12. The individual intervillous flow changes: A = before anesthesia; B = immediately following induction of anesthesia with 4 mg/kg thiopental and 1 mg/kg succinylcholine; m = mean value. (Reprinted by permission from Jouppila P, Kuikka J, Jouppila R, Hollmén A. Effect of induction of general anesthesia for cesarean section on intervillous blood flow. *Acta Obstet Gynecol Scand* 1979;58:249–253.)

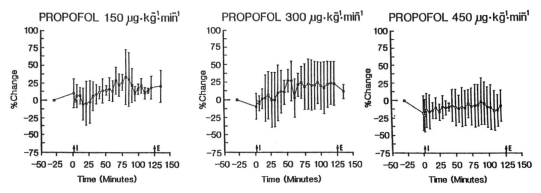

Figure 2.13. Changes in uterine blood flow following induction with 2 mg/kg propofol, 1.5 mg/kg succinylcholine, endotracheal intubation, and infusion of varying doses of propofol with 50% (inspired concentration) N_2O in oxygen. I = intubation; E = extubation. (Reprinted by permission from Alon E, Bell RH, Gillie MH, Parer JT, Rosen MA, Shnider SM. Effects of propofol and thiopental on maternal and cardiovascular and acid-base variables in the pregnant ewe. *Anesthesiology* 1993;78:562–576.)

Ketamine

Ketamine usually increases arterial blood pressure. Greiss and Van Wilkes (30) and Ralston et al. (31) demonstrated that drugs that increase maternal arterial blood pressure as a result of vasoconstriction may lead to a decrease in uterine blood flow with consequent fetal hypoxia and acidosis. Levinson et al. (32) administered 5 mg/kg of ketamine to a group of pregnant ewes near term. They found a 15% increase in mean maternal blood pressure and a 10% increase in uterine blood flow. Eng et al. (33) reported similar results in monkeys. Craft et al. (34) administered 0.7 mg/kg ketamine to pregnant sheep and noted similar results. Maternal effects consisted of a slight increase in blood pressure and cardiac output (up to 16%) and a moderate increase in uterine resting tone, whereas uterine blood flow remained relatively constant.

Cosmi (35) evaluated the effects of ketamine in pregnant sheep not in labor and during labor. In the ewes not in labor (condition resembling that of elective cesarean section), the drug was administered intravenously in doses of 1.8 to 2.2 mg/kg. Anesthesia was maintained with nitrous oxide and oxygen, and ventilation was controlled. Under these conditions, ketamine produced increases in mean maternal blood pressure and heart rate and in uterine blood flow without significant changes in fetal cardiovascular and acid-base status. However, when ketamine in doses of 0.9 to 5 mg/kg was given to the ewes in labor, Cosmi observed a marked increase of maternal ventilation, as well as increases in uterine tone and frequency and intensity of uterine contractions, and a slight decrease of uterine blood flow. These changes were dose related and accompanied by fetal tachycardia and acidosis. Similarly, Galloon (36) reported a dose-related increase in uterine muscle tone after ketamine administration in patients undergoing therapeutic abortion during the second trimester.

Therefore, there appears to be some variability in the maternal circulatory response to ketamine related in part to the presence or absence of labor, the dosage, and the stage of gestation. It would appear, however, that ketamine in the usual clinical doses (0.25 to 1 mg/kg) does not adversely affect uterine blood flow. Several studies report normal neonatal clinical and acid-base conditions after the administration of ketamine in doses up to 1 mg/kg for vaginal and abdominal delivery (35, 37–40).

HALOGENATED INHALATION AGENTS

The effect of inhalation analgesia-anesthesia on the uteroplacental circulation and on the fetus is still a controversial matter. Some authors (41–44) report fetal asphyxia, whereas others (32, 33) indicate that well-conducted inhalation anesthesia produces no effects on the fetus or the uteroplacental circulation.

Halogenated agents have a unique and specific place in obstetric anesthesia because of their potent uterine relaxant properties. Hence, they are the agent of choice when uterine relaxation is required—for example, for version and extraction, breech delivery, retained placenta, tetanic contractions, and surgical manipulations (45–47). Attempts to improve fetal oxygenation by increasing maternal inspired oxygen concentration (48) stimulated interest in the use of halothane with lower concentrations of nitrous oxide for cesarean section (49). In addition, its use has also been recommended to improve fetal oxygenation in case of fetal distress caused by uterine tetany (50).

Several investigators have studied the effect of halothane on uterine blood flow. Palahniuk and Shnider (51) found that in the pregnant ewe during light and moderately deep anesthesia (1 and 1.5 minimum alveolar concentration [MAC]), maternal blood pressure was slightly depressed (less than 20% from control), but uterine vasodilation occurred and uteroplacental blood flow was maintained. Neither fetal hypoxemia nor metabolic acidosis occurred. Deep levels of anesthesia (2 MAC) produced greater reductions in maternal blood pressure and cardiac output. Despite uterine vasodilation, uterine blood flow decreased and the fetuses became hypoxic and acidotic. Similar results have been reported by Carenza and Cosmi (52) in pregnant sheep and by Eng et al. (53) in pregnant monkeys. Furthermore, Cosmi and Marx (41) reported that in humans, light-to-moderate planes of halothane anesthesia (i.e., 0.5 to 1 vol/100 mL) did not alter either maternal cardiovascular function or fetal acid-base status. In contrast, deep planes (i.e., 1.5 vol/100 mL or greater) produced maternal hypotension and fetal acidosis.

Shnider et al. (25) studied the effects in pregnant ewes of halothane 0.5% inspired combined with 50% nitrous oxide and oxygen. They reported a 22% increase in uterine blood flow during the 1-hour administration period. Thus, it seems that low concentrations of halothane do not adversely affect uteroplacental circulation and, in fact, produce uterine vasodilation. Increasing concentrations produce progressive decreases in the uterine blood flow due to maternal hypotension.

Studies by Palahniuk and Shnider (51) indicate that isoflurane is essentially indistinguishable from halothane in its effects on maternal and fetal cardiovascular and acid-base status. Light planes of anesthesia do not decrease uterine blood flow, but deep planes do. Similarly, Alon et al. (26) reported that, in pregnant ewes, light anesthesia produced by inhalation of isoflurane 1% combined with 50% nitrous oxide and oxygen produced a 25% increase in uterine blood flow (Fig. 2.14).

Available data suggest equipotent doses of enflurane, desflurane, and sevoflurane act similarly to halothane and isoflurane with respect to their effects on uterine tone, uterine vasculature, and perfusion. All inhalation agents have dose-dependent

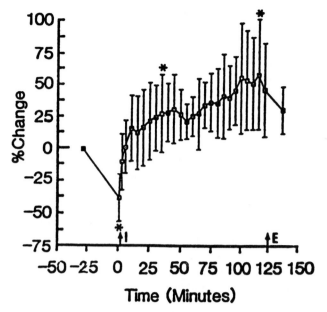

Figure 2.14. Changes in uterine blood flow following induction with 5 mg/kg thiopental, 1.5 mg/kg succinylcholine, endotracheal intubation, and maintenance with 1% isoflurane and 50% (inspired concentration) N_2O in oxygen. I = intubation; E = extubation; *asterisk* = statistically significant differences from control values ($P < .05$). (Reprinted by permission from Alon E, Bell RH, Gillie MH, Parer JT, Rosen MA, Shnider SM. Effects of propofol and thiopental on maternal and cardiovascular and acid-base variables in the pregnant ewe. *Anesthesiology* 1993;78:562–576.)

effects on uterine tone. In clinical situations when uterine tone is increased (e.g., uterine hyperstimulation, tetanic contraction), halogenated agents will decrease uterine tone, and if maternal blood pressure is maintained, result in improved uteroplacental perfusion.

LOCAL ANESTHETICS

Gibbs and Noel (54) and Cibils (55) demonstrated a vasoconstricting effect of both lidocaine and mepivacaine using an *in vitro* preparation of human uterine artery segments obtained from cesarean hysterectomy specimens. The concentrations of

local anesthetics ranged from 400 to 1000 $\mu g/mL$, concentrations well above levels achieved during clinical use. Uterine vasoconstriction was not seen with lower concentrations or in uterine arteries taken from nonpregnant hysterectomy specimens, indicating that the response was dose related and occurred only during pregnancy. Pretreatment of the strips with phenoxybenzamine (an α-adrenergic blocker) did not abolish the vasoconstrictive response.

Greiss et al. (56), injecting 20, 40, and 80 mg boluses of either lidocaine or mepivacaine into the dorsal aorta of eight anesthetized pregnant ewes, found a dose-related, transient (2 to 3 minutes) decrease in uterine blood flow and a simultaneous increase in intrauterine pressure (Fig. 2.15). Uterine arterial blood levels were not measured. These investigators also infused lidocaine, mepivacaine, bupivacaine, and procaine directly into the uterine artery of nonpregnant ewes. The following uterine arterial concentrations reduced mean uterine blood flow by 40%: bupivacaine 5 $\mu g/mL$, mepivacaine 40 $\mu g/mL$, procaine 40 $\mu g/mL$, and lidocaine 200 $\mu g/mL$. Such enormously high concentrations could not occur during epidural anesthesia in the absence of an intravenous injection.

Subsequent studies in the pregnant ewe by Fishburne et al. (57) and Pue et al. (58) produced similar findings of uterine vasoconstriction occurring only at very high blood levels, which might be found in the uterine vasculature during paracervical blocks (close proximity of the injected drugs to the uterine arteries) or during systemic toxic reactions. Morishima et al. (59) found that during lidocaine-induced maternal convulsions in the pregnant ewe, uterine blood flow was reduced by 55% to 71% of control values. The lack of uterine vasoconstriction with low blood levels of lidocaine was demonstrated by Biehl et al. (60). These investigators infused the local anesthetic intravenously to produce blood levels (2 to 4 $\mu g/mL$) in the pregnant ewe comparable to those usually found in the human parturient undergoing epidural anesthesia during the first and second stages of labor. They found that a 2-hour exposure to these low concentrations of lidocaine did not significantly decrease uterine blood flow or increase intraamniotic pressure. Similarly, lidocaine in a dose of 0.4 mg/kg or 2-chloroprocaine in doses up to 2 mg/kg administered intravenously to guinea pigs did not significantly decrease uterine blood flow velocity (61, 62).

In a clinical study of women undergoing cesarean section with epidural anesthesia, Alahuhta et al. demonstrated that 115 to

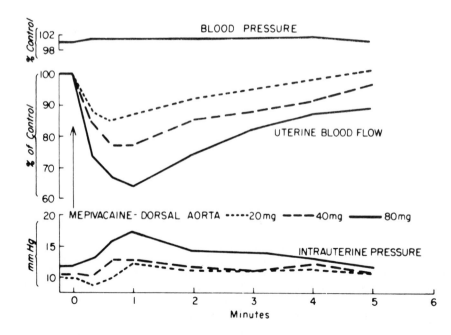

Figure 2.15. Effects of increasing intraaortic doses of mepivacaine on uterine blood flow and intrauterine pressure in pregnant ewes near term. Note the progressive decrease in uterine blood flow with similar inverse changes in intrauterine pressure. (Reprinted by permission from Greiss FC Jr, Still JG, Anderson SG. Effects of local anesthetic agents on the uterine vasculatures and myometrium. *Am J Obstet Gynecol* 1976;124:889–899.)

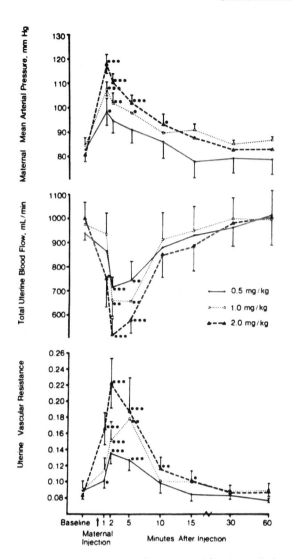

Figure 2.16. Responses of maternal mean arterial pressure (*top*), total uterine blood flow (*middle*), and uterine vascular resistance (*bottom*) to maternal administrations of cocaine. *Single asterisks* indicate $P < .001$. (Reprinted by permission from Woods JR Jr, Plessinger MA, Clark KE. Effect of cocaine on uterine blood flow and fetal oxygenation. *JAMA* 1987;257:957–961.)

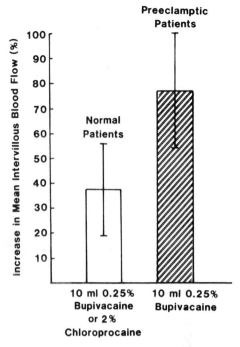

Figure 2.17. Percentage increase in mean intervillous blood flow values ($\pm$SE) after epidural anesthesia for labor in normal and preeclamptic patients. (Redrawn by permission from Hollmén A, Jouppila R, Jouppila P, Koivula A, Vierola H. Effect of extradural analgesia using bupivacaine and 2-chloroprocaine on intervillous blood flow during normal labour. *Br J Anaesth* 1982;54:837–842; and Jouppila P, Jouppila R, Hollmén A, Koivula A. Lumbar epidural analgesia to improve intervillous blood flow during labor in severe preeclampsia. *Obstet Gynecol* 1982;59:158–161.)

140 mg 0.5% ropivacaine had no effect on uterine blood flow (63).

Cocaine is a potent local anesthetic with unique vasoconstrictive properties. Studies on the effect of intravenous cocaine on uterine blood flow have shown that cocaine at doses between 0.5 mg/kg and 2.8 mg/kg produced a dose-related reduction in uterine blood flow (Fig. 2.16) (64–66). Cocaine may significantly decrease uterine blood flow and thus should be avoided or administered cautiously and sparingly to human parturients.

REGIONAL ANESTHESIA

The most frequent complication of spinal, lumbar epidural, and caudal anesthesia is systemic hypotension. The decrease in mean arterial blood pressure reduces uterine blood flow proportionately (67, 68). However, epidural anesthesia uncomplicated by arterial hypotension is associated with no alterations in uterine blood flow (69, 70).

Jouppila et al. (19, 71, 72) and Hollmén et al. (73, 74) extensively studied the effect of regional anesthesia for labor or cesarean section on uteroplacental perfusion. Studies in healthy women not in labor undergoing cesarean section indicated that

neither epidural (19) nor spinal (75) anesthesia uncomplicated by hypotension is associated with changes in intervillous blood flow. However, women with preeclampsia showed an improvement in intervillous blood flow following initiation of the block.

Healthy women in labor showed a 35% increase in intervillous blood flow following the administration of 10 mL of either 0.25% bupivacaine or 2% chloroprocaine (Fig. 2.17) (73). In patients with pregnancy-induced hypertension, the epidural injection of 10 mL 0.25% bupivacaine resulted in a much more significant improvement in intervillous blood flow; the increase amounted to 77% (72). These investigators (71, 73), using smaller volumes of drug (e.g., 4 mL 0.5% bupivacaine with or without epinephrine 1:200,000), found no improvement in placental blood flow. The authors postulated that the more widespread sympathectomy obtained with larger volumes, together with the relief of pain and anxiety, tends to restore uterine blood flow to its normal-nonstressed basal condition.

Studies using Doppler ultrasound to measure uteroplacental arterial flow velocity waveforms have confirmed, with rare exception (76), the lack of deleterious effects of epidural anesthesia on uterine blood flow (77–80). These studies involved women receiving epidural blocks to T3 to T5 dermatome levels for elective cesarean sections. These women were prehydrated with 1 to 2 L balanced salt solution, positioned with left uterine tilt, and received either lidocaine 2% or bupivacaine 0.5%, both with and without epinephrine 1:200,000.

CATECHOLAMINES AND STRESS

Adrenergic stimulation produced by either exogenous or endogenous catecholamines can constrict uterine vessels and reduce uterine blood flow. Exogenous catecholamines (primarily epinephrine) are administered with local anesthetics to produce vasoconstriction at the site of injection. Endogenous catecholamines (both epinephrine and norepinephrine) are released during anxiety and pain. Vasopressors are frequently used to prevent or treat spinal or epidural hypotension.

Epinephrine

Epinephrine has significant effects on both α- and β-adrenergic receptors. High epinephrine blood levels achieved by accidental intravascular injection of epinephrine-containing local anesthetics produce α-adrenergic effects, including hypertension, increased total peripheral resistance, uterine vasoconstriction, increased uterine activity, and decreased uterine blood flow. In ewes given 0.10 to 1 $\mu g^{-1} \cdot kg^{-1} \cdot min^{-1}$ epinephrine, maternal pressure rose 65% above control and uterine blood flow fell by 55% to 75% (81). Injection of epinephrine 20 μg in pregnant ewes decreased uterine blood flow by 40% for about 60 seconds (82). Similarly, injections of 0.2 to 1 $\mu g/kg$ epinephrine in the pregnant guinea pig produced transient dose-related decreases in uterine artery blood flow velocities (61, 83).

Low blood levels of epinephrine, such as occur from systemic absorption during caudal or epidural block, have been shown to produce a generalized β-adrenergic response that becomes maximal 15 minutes after epidural injection (84). A number of studies of the β-adrenergic effects of epinephrine on the uterine vessels have produced conflicting results.

Rosenfeld et al. (85) infused 50 to 100 μg epinephrine intravenously over a 5-minute period into pregnant ewes and produced a generalized β-adrenergic effect with tachycardia and increased cardiac output and blood flow to skeletal muscles. However, although blood pressure did not change, uterine blood flow decreased by almost 50%. These investigators postulated that the uterine artery in the pregnant ewe may be more sensitive to the α-adrenergic effects of epinephrine, while vasculature of skeletal muscle, adipose tissue, and other visceral organs may be more sensitive to the β-adrenergic effects. In contrast, deRosayro et al. (86) studied the effects of epidural epinephrine (100 μg) without local anesthetic drugs on the cardiovascular system of anesthetized pregnant ewes. Except for slight tachycardia, there were no significant cardiovascular changes. Uterine blood flow remained stable. Wallis et al. (69) did find a transient 14% reduction in uterine blood flow in pregnant ewes that received epidural epinephrine (60 to 80 μg) combined with 1.5% chloroprocaine. These ewes had decreases in total peripheral resistance and increases in cardiac output, although blood pressure did not change. Because uterine blood flow did not change in animals that received only chloroprocaine, the decrease in uterine blood flow was possibly due to the combination of epinephrine absorbed from the epidural space and sympathectomy produced by the local anesthetic.

Albright et al. (87) did not corroborate these latter findings. These investigators reported that 10 mL epidural chloroprocaine with 1:200,000 epinephrine did not alter *human* intervillous blood flow during epidural anesthesia for labor despite a reduction in mean blood pressure of 11 mm Hg. Levinson et al. (88) compared 2% lidocaine alone to 2% lidocaine with 1:200,000 epinephrine administered for epidural anesthesia for cesarean section. They found no adverse effects of epinephrine on the mother or neonate as ascertained by the incidence of hypotension, low Apgar scores, or abnormal fetal acid-base status.

In summary, there may be transient fluctuations in uterine blood flow after epidural anesthesia with epinephrine-containing solutions. However, these have little effect on the healthy fetus.

Stress

Myers (89) reported that maternal stress and anxiety in the pregnant rhesus monkey produced fetal asphyxia, likely due to uterine vasoconstriction as a consequence of maternal catecholamine release. Shnider et al.(90) found that stress sufficient to produce maternal hypertension resulted in a precipitous fall in uterine blood flow and an increase in plasma norepinephrine in pregnant ewes. Similarly, Martin and Gingerick (91) found a marked reduction in uterine blood flow in response to severe stress in the pregnant rhesus monkey.

Lederman et al. (92, 93) reported that both primiparous and multiparous parturients who were very anxious during labor had increased circulating epinephrine blood levels and a higher incidence of abnormal fetal heart rate patterns compared with those who were less anxious. Again, we presume that these findings are due to uterine hypoperfusion.

Vasopressors

Vasopressors with predominant α-adrenergic activity reduce uterine blood flow and may adversely affect the fetus (94, 95). Methoxamine, phenylephrine, angiotensin, or norepinephrine treatment of spinal hypotension in animals diminishes uterine blood flow and leads to fetal asphyxia (95–97). Ephedrine, mephentermine, and metaraminol restore uterine blood flow toward normal (Fig. 2.18) (98–100).

Studies of treatment of spinal or epidural hypotension using either low-dose phenylephrine (20 to 100 μg), or ephedrine (10 to 15 mg) in elective cesarean sections have not confirmed the animal data (101, 102). Using an impedance cardiograph to measure stroke volume, ejection fraction, and end-diastolic volume, Ramanathan and Grant (101) showed that both ephedrine and phenylephrine produce venoconstriction to a greater degree than arterial constriction, improve venous return (cardiac preload), increase cardiac output, and likely restore uterine perfusion. Ephedrine may have a more selective constriction of systemic vessels during pregnancy, and therefore preserve uterine perfusion (103). The beneficial effects of ephedrine compared with phenylephrine have been shown in Doppler ultrasound studies by Alahuhta et al., in which phenylephrine, not ephedrine, increased uterine vascular resistance (104).

Drugs such as ephedrine, which support maternal blood pressure by augmenting venous return and by central adrenergic stimulation (positive inotropic and chronotropic activity), have minimal effects on uterine blood flow in the normotensive mother and restore uterine blood flow when used to treat spinal or epidural hypotension (Fig. 2.19). Human studies suggest that carefully titrated doses of phenylephrine may also produce beneficial hemodynamic effects without adversely affecting the fetus and may be useful in selected patients. For the overwhelming majority of patients, ephedrine remains the vasopressor of choice.

Dopamine, a catecholamine that stimulates dopaminergic and α- and β-adrenergic receptors, has been studied in normotensive and hypotensive pregnant sheep. In normotensive animals, Callender et al. (105) reported that doses that increase maternal blood pressure and cardiac output decrease uterine blood flow. Rolbin et al. (106) reported that dopamine, when used to treat spinal hypotension, corrected maternal blood pressure but resulted in a further decrease in uterine blood flow. This was due to a significant increase in uterine vascular resistance despite minimal changes in total peripheral resistance. Conflicting results were reported by Cabalum et al. (107), who found that dopamine infusion in doses similar to those used by Rolbin restored uterine blood flow with the correction of hypotension. A possible explanation for the differences found in these studies is that Cabalum et al. did not place the flow probe around a branch of the uterine artery but rather the internal iliac artery, and thus their flow signal may not reflect that of the uterine circulation (108). A vasoconstrictive effect on uterine blood vessels has been reported with β-adrenergic drugs such as isoxsuprine (109), ritodrine (82, 110), and terbutaline (111). The effects of dopamine on the uterine vessels likely represent an increased sensitivity of these vessels to dopamine's α-adrenergic stimulation.

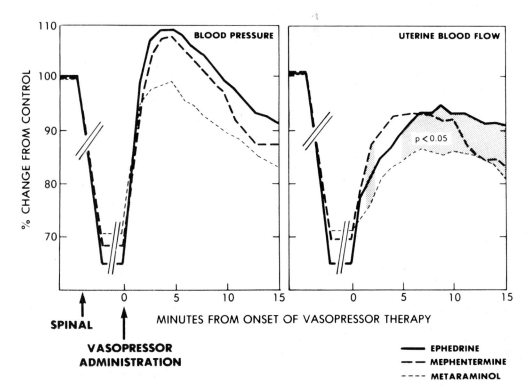

Figure 2.18. Average response patterns to ephedrine and slow infusions of mephentermine and metaraminol after hypotension induced by spinal anesthesia. After 4 minutes, uterine blood flow was significantly higher with ephedrine and mephentermine than with metaraminol therapy. (Reprinted by permission from James FM III, Greiss FC Jr, Kemp RA. An evaluation of vasopressor therapy for maternal hypotension during spinal anesthesia. *Anesthesiology* 1970;33:25–34.)

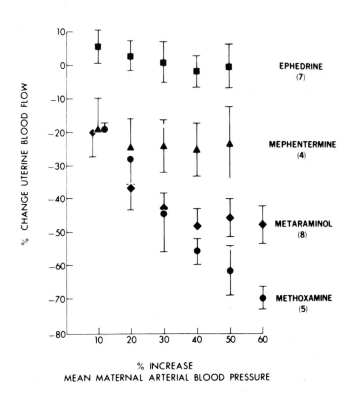

Figure 2.19. Mean changes in uterine blood flow at equal elevations of mean arterial blood pressure after vasopressor administration. (Reprinted by permission from Ralston DH, Shnider SM, deLorimier AA. Effects of equipotent ephedrine, metaraminol, mephentermine and methoxamine on uterine blood flow in the pregnant ewe. *Anesthesiology* 1974;40:354–370.)

ANTIHYPERTENSIVE AGENTS

Hypertensive disorders of pregnancy frequently require therapy. Ideally, drugs used to treat maternal hypertension should reduce blood pressure and uterine vascular resistance so that uterine blood flow is either unchanged or increased.

Hydralazine

Hydralazine, a slow-acting antihypertensive drug, is used widely in the treatment of gestational hypertension. The effects of hydralazine on uterine blood flow in the hypertensive pregnant ewe have been studied by Brinkman and Assali (112). These investigators induced severe hypertension and reduction in uterine blood flow by placing a modified Goldblatt clamp around one renal artery and removing the contralateral kidney. Hydralazine, in this preparation, reduced blood pressure while increasing uterine blood flow. Similarly, in a study by Ring et al. (113) on phenylephrine-induced hypertension, hydralazine slowly lowered the blood pressure while significantly increasing uterine blood flow, although uterine blood flow did not return to normal (Fig. 2.20). During cocaine-induced hypertension in the pregnant ewe, hydralazine did not restore uterine blood flow as maternal blood pressure returned to normal (Fig. 2.21) (114). In humans the effects of intravenously infused hydralazine (incremental doses up to 125 μg/min during 60 minutes) were studied by Jouppila et al. (115) in 10 women with acute or superimposed severe preeclampsia. The intervillous and umbilical vein blood flows were measured before and during hydralazine infusion with the xenon-133 method and with a combination of real-time and Doppler ultrasound equipment, respectively. Maternal blood pressure decreased and pulse rate increased during the infusion. Hydralazine did not change the intervillous blood flow but increased the blood flow in the umbilical vein. The results indicated that hydralazine affected the placental and fetal circulations differently.

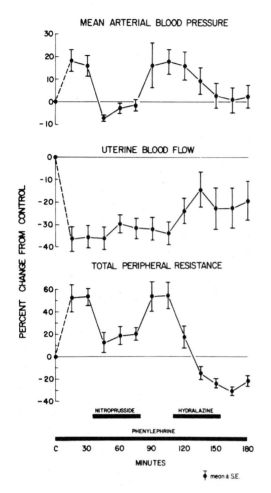

Figure 2.20. Percentage change from control of maternal arterial blood pressure, uterine blood flow, and total peripheral resistance during phenylephrine-induced hypertension and correction of hypertension with nitroprusside and hydralazine. Hydralazine, but not nitroprusside, resulted in a significant increase in uterine blood flow ($P < .05$). (Reprinted by permission from Ring G, Krames E, Shnider SM, Wallis KL, Levinson G. Comparison of nitroprusside and hydralazine in hypertensive pregnant ewes. *Obstet Gynecol* 1977;50:598–602.)

Nitroglycerin

Craft et al. (116) found that a nitroglycerin infusion administered to pregnant ewes during phenylephrine-induced hypertension resulted in a reduction in blood pressure associated with improved uterine blood flow. Sublingual nitroglycerin has been used to relax the uterus in patients with uterine hyperstimulation and fetal heart rate decelerations (117). Intravenous nitroglycerin may also prove useful when managing fetal bradycardia reported in conjunction with intrathecal opioids. Nitroglycerin appears to bring about a decrease in uterine tone and likely increases uterine blood flow in this clinical situation. With acute cocaine intoxication in sheep, nitroglycerin has been shown to decrease maternal blood pressure, but did not significantly improve uterine blood flow (Chapter 34, Fig. 34.8) (118). Intravenous nitroglycerin has been used to facilitate uterine relaxation and preserve uterine blood flow during fetal surgery (see Chapter 14).

Nitroprusside

Nitroprusside, a rapidly-acting antihypertensive agent, is popular in the management of nonobstetric-hypertensive emergencies. Similar to hydralazine, the drug causes a decrease in total

peripheral resistance and an increase in coronary and mesenteric blood flow (119–121). Ring et al. (113) reported that, although nitroprusside decreased total peripheral resistance, it failed to correct the fall in uterine blood flow (Fig. 2.20). In contrast, using isolated uterine arteries from pregnant patients (obtained during cesarean-hysterectomy), Nelson and Suresh (122) demonstrated that, although both nitroprusside and hydralazine inhibited norepinephrine-induced uterine artery contraction, nitroprusside had a greater potency compared to hydralazine in producing direct vasodilation of the uterine arteries from pregnant humans.

Labetalol

Labetalol is a combined α- and β-adrenergic blocking agent. It is used orally to decrease blood pressure in preeclamptic women (123–125). It is also used intravenously to rapidly decrease blood pressure in severely preeclamptic women and to attenuate the hemodynamic response to tracheal intubation (126). Intravenously administered, labetalol does not alter uterine blood flow in preeclamptic women at rest (127), nor does it alter placental perfusion in pregnant hypertensive rats (128). In the near-term pregnant ewe, intravenous-bolus administration of labetalol ameliorated the effects of increased circulating norepinephrine on maternal arterial pressure and uterine blood flow and produced less adrenergic blockade in the fetus than in the mother (129).

CALCIUM CHANNEL BLOCKING DRUGS

Calcium channel blocking drugs are potentially useful in obstetrics. They produce arteriolar vasodilation and may be effective agents in the management of preeclampsia. They slow atrioventricular conduction and may have a role in maternal and fetal supraventricular tachyarrhythmias. Additionally, they inhibit uterine contractility and thus may be useful in the treatment of preterm labor.

Murad et al. (130) studied the hemodynamic effects of *verapamil* in the awake pregnant ewe. Verapamil (0.2 mg/kg) administered intravenously over 3 minutes resulted in a variety of maternal cardiovascular changes: a transient (2 to 5 minutes) decrease in systolic, diastolic, and mean blood pressures; and increase in central venous, mean pulmonary artery, and pulmonary capillary wedge pressures. These results are consistent with the negative inotropic and peripheral vasodilating effects of verapamil. Cardiac output, systemic peripheral vascular resistance, and pulmonary vascular resistance were unaffected. Uterine blood flow decreased by 25% at 2 minutes, then remained slightly below control levels for 30 minutes after drug injection. Thus, the effects of verapamil on uterine blood flow suggest that the drug should be used with caution in cases of uteroplacental insufficiency.

Studies of *nicardipine* in rabbits (131) and monkeys (132) and *nifedipine* in sheep (133) have shown that these drugs decrease uteroplacental blood flow. On the other hand, studies in humans using Doppler ultrasound have shown that short-term *oral* administration does not significantly alter uteroplacental circulation (134, 135). Nifedipine has been increasingly used for management of preterm labor (136–140).

MAGNESIUM SULFATE

Since its first use in obstetrics reported in 1925 by Lazard (141) and Dorsett (142), magnesium sulfate has been used parenterally as an adjunct in the management of certain hypertensive diseases of pregnancy, especially preeclampsia and eclampsia. Its effects on the central and peripheral nervous systems and on neuromuscular transmission are discussed in Chapters 16 and 17. Its action on the maternal and fetal cardiovascular

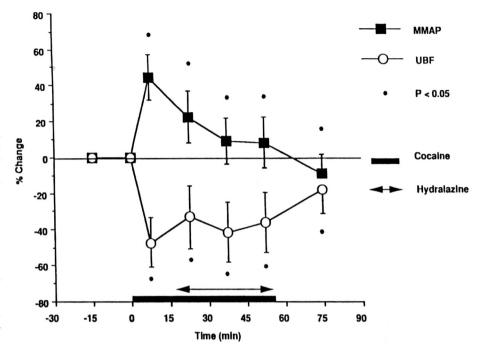

Figure 2.21. Effect of hydralazine therapy on cocaine-induced maternal hypertension. Percentage change in maternal mean arterial pressure (*MMAP*) and uterine blood flow (*UBF*) during cocaine administration and hydralazine therapy (n = 10). The *arrow* represents the time of hydralazine treatment. Both drugs were discontinued at 55 minutes. Values are expressed as ± SD. Changes are compared to baseline values with significance noted (*asterisk* = P < .05). (Reprinted by permission from Vertommen JD, Hughes SC, Rosen MA, et al. Hydralazine does not restore uterine blood flow during cocaine-induced hypertension in the pregnant ewe. *Anesthesiology* 1992;76:580–587.)

systems and uteroplacental circulation has been investigated in pregnant normotensive and hypertensive ewes (143, 144).

Magnesium sulfate was administered to the mother in amounts sufficient to produce a constant serum concentration of 5 to 12 mEq/L in a study by Dandavino et al. (143) and 5 to 7 mEq/L in a study by Krames et al. (144). Dandavino et al. found that magnesium sulfate produced a fall in the systemic arterial blood pressure in both hypertensive and normotensive animals. However, this effect was transient, lasting less than 10 minutes. The uteroplacental blood flow increased by about 10%. Administration of high doses of magnesium sulfate (a 4-g bolus injection followed by a 2-to 4-g/h infusion) produced an initial and transitory decrease of maternal arterial pressure that was greater in the hypertensive than in the normotensive animals. However, 5 to 10 minutes after the start of the infusion, the mean arterial pressure in both groups had returned to control values. The uteroplacental blood flow increased by an average of 13.5% in the normotensive and 7.7% in the hypertensive animals. Krames et al. found that magnesium sulfate produced a decrease in mean arterial blood pressure of 7% with a 7% rise in uterine vascular conductance, thereby resulting in no change in uterine blood flow.

The results of these studies suggest that magnesium sulfate has only a mild and transient effect on maternal arterial pressure and uterine blood flow.

INTRASPINAL OPIOIDS

Epidural opioids are widely used for the treatment of labor pain. Studying pregnant ewes near term, Rosen et al. (145) administered 20 mg morphine into the epidural space. These investigators found no significant changes in uterine blood flow nor, indeed, in any maternal or fetal cardiovascular or acid-base variable during a 2-hour study period. Craft et al. (146) confirmed these findings. They found no significant deleterious effects on uterine blood flow or maternal or fetal hemodynamic or acid-base parameters following administration to the awake pregnant ewe of 50, 75, or 100 μg fentanyl (146–148) or 10 or 20 μg sufentanil (Craft JB Jr, unpublished data). However, intrathecal opioids may cause acute hypotension in 10% to 15% of parturients and this could decrease uterine blood flow if untreated (see Chapter 9).

CLONIDINE

Clonidine is used orally as an antihypertensive agent, intravenously to rapidly control hypertensive emergencies, and epidurally to produce analgesia by an opiate-independent mechanism. It acts primarily by stimulation of α_2-adrenergic receptors, although in high concentrations it will stimulate other receptor subtypes. It causes constriction of human uterine arteries *in vitro* by a mixed α_1- and α_2-adrenergic mechanism (149).

The effects on uterine blood flow of orally-administered clonidine have not been studied, but it has been used safely for many years without apparent adverse maternal, fetal, or neonatal effects (150–153). In normotensive pregnant ewes, intravenous clonidine increases intraamniotic pressure and decreases uterine blood flow without altering maternal or fetal blood pressure (154). The effect on uterine blood flow of intravenous clonidine in a hypertensive animal model has not been studied.

Intravenously administered α_2-adrenergic agonists such as clonidine have also been shown to have other adverse effects. These include rapid placental transfer (153, 154), maternal and fetal hypoxemia (155, 156), hyperglycemia (157), and decreased heart rate. The mechanism of the hypoxemia is not well understood since it is not a result of respiratory or cardiovascular depression or pulmonary vasoconstriction (156). The hyperglycemia is the result of inhibition of insulin release (157).

DANTROLENE

Dantrolene is currently indispensable in the treatment of malignant hyperthermia, although infrequent malignant hyperthermia has been reported during labor and delivery (158–163). Pretreatment of susceptible patients with oral dantrolene before induction of labor or a cesarean section is controversial. Recommended regimens include dantrolene 25 mg orally 4 times a day for 5 days before delivery, then for 3 days after delivery in progressively decreasing doses (day 1, 25 mg 3 times; day 2, 25 mg twice; day 3, 25 mg once) (164). Dantrolene crosses the placenta with a fetal-to-maternal ratio of 0.18 to 0.4 and no apparent adverse effects in the infants (164, 165). Craft et al. (166) studied 1.2 mg/kg and 2.4 mg/kg dantrolene administered intravenously to awake pregnant ewes and demonstrated the drug's maternal and fetal safety. Maternal blood pressure

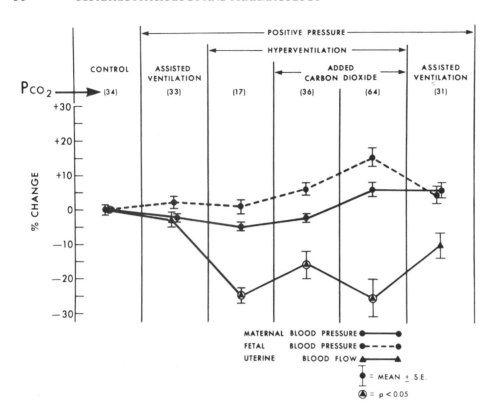

Figure 2.22. Changes from control values in mean maternal and fetal arterial blood pressure and uterine blood flow during five periods of positive pressure ventilation. Mean maternal Pa_{CO_2} during each period is indicated at the *top* of the figure. (Reprinted by permission from Levinson G, Shnider SM, deLorimier AA, Steffenson JL. Effects of maternal hyperventilation on uterine blood flow and fetal oxygenation and acid-base status. *Anesthesiology* 1974;40:340–347.)

and cardiac output increased slightly, but no significant changes were observed in maternal heart rate, central venous pressure, or uterine blood flow. Fetal heart rate decreased by 25% at 3 minutes but had returned to normal at 10 minutes. No clinically significant changes in maternal or fetal acid-base status were noted.

RESPIRATORY GASES

Contrary to earlier beliefs, *moderate* hypoxia, hypercapnia, and hypocapnia do not affect uteroplacental blood flow (167, 168). On the other hand, marked changes in respiratory gases decrease placental perfusion. Dilts et al. (169) measured uterine blood flow in pregnant sheep during severe maternal hypoxia induced by ventilating the lungs with 6% or 12% oxygen gas mixtures. When the lungs were ventilated with a gas mixture containing 6% oxygen, there was an increase in cardiac output and a decrease in maternal systemic vascular resistance. Uteroplacental vascular resistance increased, and uterine blood flow decreased markedly. Milder hypoxia induced with 12% oxygen produced changes that were qualitatively smaller. These investigators attributed these hemodynamic changes to the enhanced output of catecholamines induced by hypoxia. When the mother was made hypoxic by reducing arterial P_{O_2} to 40 mm Hg, the fetus also became hypoxic.

Effects of maternal *hypercapnia* on the uteroplacental circulation are variable. An increase (170), decrease (171), and no change (172, 173) have been reported. Walker et al. (174), using chronic unanesthetized sheep preparations, found that by increasing the arterial P_{CO_2} to 60 mm Hg, uterine blood flow increased. Mean arterial pressure rose, while uterine vascular resistance was unchanged. However, at Pa_{CO_2} levels above 60 mm Hg, uterine vascular resistance increased progressively and uterine blood flow fell despite further increases in mean arterial pressure.

Maternal *hypocapnia* is a frequent phenomenon in pregnant women. It may occur spontaneously as a result of painful uterine contractions, anxiety, and apprehension during labor, or improperly performed Lamaze technique. Controlled ventilation

during anesthesia may also accidentally produce severe maternal alkalemia. Controversy still exists regarding its effects on the fetus and the uteroplacental circulation. Some investigators have reported that marked hyperventilation (Pa_{CO_2} of 17 mm Hg or less) causes uteroplacental vasoconstriction, decreases uteroplacental blood flow, and induces fetal hypoxia, acidosis, and neonatal depression (175, 176). Others have denied that maternal hyperventilation, even of marked degree, is harmful to the fetus. These investigators found minimal changes in the acid-base status of the fetus and no significant effect on uteroplacental blood flow (177, 178). Levinson et al. (171) studied changes in uterine blood flow and fetal oxygenation in unanesthetized pregnant ewes during mechanical hyperventilation. In order to evaluate separately the effects of maternal hypocapnia and positive-pressure ventilation, carbon dioxide was added to the inspired air during mechanical hyperventilation to produce normocapnia and hypercapnia. Uterine blood flow decreased by approximately 25% during all hyperventilation periods (Fig. 2.22). Because the reduction in uterine blood flow was unrelated to changes in maternal Pa_{CO_2} (range 17 to 64 mm Hg) or pH (range 7.74 to 7.24), the decrease probably was caused by the mechanical effect of positive pressure ventilation.

Metabolic alkalosis may also be detrimental to the fetus as a result of decreased uteroplacental blood flow and displacement of the maternal oxygen-hemoglobin dissociation curve to the left, resulting in increased affinity of maternal hemoglobin for oxygen and decreased release at the placenta (176, 179–181). In the pregnant ewe, Cosmi (29) found that maternal metabolic alkalosis induced by intravenous infusion of trihydroxymethylaminomethane caused maternal bradycardia and hypotension, decreased uterine blood flow, and induced fetal hypoxia and acidosis. Ralston et al. (180) produced maternal alkalemia with the infusion of sodium bicarbonate in normal pregnant ewes and found a 16% reduction in uterine blood flow with a concomitant decrease in fetal oxygenation and pH. In contrast, in Cosmi's study (29), the infusion of small doses of sodium bicarbonate (e.g., 100 mEq over 12 minutes) to the acidotic ewe did not alter uterine blood flow.

SUMMARY

Intravenous induction agents, inhalation and local anesthetics, endogenous and exogenous catecholamines and vasopressors, antihypertensive agents and magnesium sulfate, respiratory gases, and metabolic alkalosis can all alter uterine blood flow. Their net effect on uterine blood flow ultimately depends on how these agents alter uterine perfusion pressure relative to uterine vascular resistance. The effects of anesthetic drugs are summarized in Table 2.3.

REFERENCES

1. Metcalfe J, Bartels H, Moll W. Gas exchange in the pregnant uterus. *Physiol Rev* 1967;47:782–838.
2. Longo LD. Placental transfer mechanisms: An overview. In: Wynn RM, ed. *Obstetrics and Gynecology Annual.* New York: Appleton-Century-Crofts; 1972:103–138.
3. Aherne W, Dunnill MS. Morphometry of the human placenta. *Br Med Bull* 1966;22:5–8.
4. Meschia G. Physiology of transplacental diffusion. In: Wynn RM, ed. *Obstetrics and Gynecology Annual.* New York: Appleton-Century-Crofts; 1976:21–38.
5. Assali NS, Brinkman CR III. The uterine circulation and its control. In: Longo LD, Bartels H, eds. *Respiratory Gas Exchange and Blood Flow in the Placenta.* Washington, DC: US Department of Health, Education and Welfare; 1972:121–141.
6. Greiss F Jr. Concepts of uterine blood flow. In: Wynn RM, ed. *Obstetrics and Gynecology Annual.* New York: Appleton-Century-Crofts; 1973:55–83.
7. Beischer NA, Drew JH, Kenny JM, O'Sullivan EF. The effect of rest and intravenous infusion of hypertonic dextrose on subnormal estriol excretion in pregnancy. In: Milunsky A, ed. *Clinics in Perinatology.* Philadelphia: WB Saunders; 1974:253–272.
8. Gill RW, Trudinger BJ, Garrett WJ, Kossoff G, Warren PS. Fetal umbilical venous flow measured in utero by pulsed Doppler and B-mode ultrasound. *Am J Obstet Gynecol* 1981;139:720–725.
9. Heymann MA. Fetal cardiovascular physiology. In: Creasy RK, Resnik R, eds. *Maternal-Fetal Medicine: Principles and Practice.* Philadelphia: WB Saunders; 1984:259–273.
10. Court DJ, Parer JT. Experimental studies in fetal asphyxia and fetal heart rate interpretation. In: Nathanielsz PW, Parer JT, eds. *Research in Perinatal Medicine,* vol 1. Ithaca, NY: Perinatology Press; 1985:114–164.
11. Trudinger BJ, Giles WB, Cook CM. Flow velocity wave-forms in the maternal uteroplacental and fetal placental circulation. *Am J Obstet Gynecol* 1985;152:155–163.
12. Fleischer A, Schulman H, Farmakides G, Bracero L, Blattner P, Randolph G. Umbilical velocity wave ratios in intrauterine growth retardation. *Am J Obstet Gynecol* 1985;151:502–505.
13. Marx GF, Patel S, Berman JA, Farmakides G, Schulman H. Umbilical blood flow velocity waveforms in different maternal positions and with epidural analgesia. *Obstet Gynecol* 1986;68:61–64.
14. Youngstrom P, Veille JC, Kanaan C, Wilson B. Umbilical artery flow velocity waveforms before and during epidural anesthesia for cesarean section. *Anesthesiology* 1988;69:A704.
15. Myers RE. Two patterns of perinatal brain damage and their conditions of occurrence. *Am J Obstet Gynecol* 1972;112:246–276.
16. Parer JT, Behrman RE. The influence of uterine blood flow on the acid-base status of the rhesus monkey. *Am J Obstet Gynecol* 1970;107:1241–1249.
17. Wilkening RB, Meschia G. Fetal oxygen uptake, oxygenation and acid-base balance as a function of uterine blood flow. *Am J Physiol* 1983;24:H749–H755.
18. Rekonen A, Luotola H, Pitkanen M, Kuikka J, Pyorala T. Measurement of intervillous and myometrial blood flow by an intravenous ^{133}Xe method. *Br J Obstet Gynaecol* 1976;83:723–728.
19. Jouppila R, Jouppila P, Kuikka J, Hollmén A. Placental blood flow during caesarean section under lumbar extradural analgesia. *Br J Anaesth* 1988;50:275–278.
20. Palmer SK, Zamudio S, Coffin C, Parker S, Stamm E, Moore LG. Quantitative estimation of human artery blood blow redistribution in pregnancy. *Obstet Gynecol* 1992;80:1000–1006.
21. McParland P, Pearce JM. Doppler blood flow in pregnancy: review article. *Placenta* 1988;9:427–450.
22. Trudinger BJ, Giles WB, Cook CM. Uteroplacental blood flow velocity: Time waveforms in normal and complicated pregnancy. *Br J Obstet Gynaecol* 1985;92:39–45.
23. Copel JA, Grannum PA, Hobbins JC, Cunningham FG, eds. Doppler ultrasound in obstetrics. In: *Williams' Obstetrics.* 16th ed. Norwalk, CT: Appleton & Lange; 1988.
24. Palahniuk RJ, Cumming M. Foetal deterioration following thiopentone-nitrous oxide anaesthesia in the pregnant ewe. *Can Anaesth Soc J* 1977;24:361–370.
25. Shnider SM, Wright RG, Levinson G, et al. Plasma norepinephrine and uterine blood flow changes during endotracheal intubation and general anesthesia in the pregnant ewe. In: *Abstracts of Scientific Papers.* Chicago: American Society of Anesthesiologists; 1978:115.
26. Alon E, Ball RH, Gillie MH, Parer JT, Rosen MA, Shnider SM. Effects of propofol and thiopental on maternal and fetal cardiovascular and acid-base variables in the pregnant ewe. *Anesthesiology* 1993;78:562–576.
27. Jouppila P, Kuikka J, Jouppila R, Hollmén A. Effect of induction of general anesthesia for cesarean section on intervillous blood flow. *Acta Obstet Gynecol Scand* 1979;58:249–253.
28. Mofid M, Brinkman CR III, Assali NS. Effects of diazepam on uteroplacental and fetal hemodynamics and metabolism. *Obstet Gynecol* 1973;41:364–368.
29. Cosmi EV. Fetal homeostasis. In: Scarpelli EM, Auld PAM, eds. *Pulmonary Physiology of the Fetus, Newborn and Child.* Philadelphia: Lea & Febiger; 1975:61.
30. Greiss FC Jr, Van Wilkes D. Effects of sympathomimetic drugs and angiotensin on the uterine vascular bed. *Obstet Gynecol* 1964;23:925–930.
31. Ralston DH, Shnider SM, deLorimier AA. Effects of equipotent ephedrine, metaraminol, mephentermine and methoxamine on uterine blood flow in the pregnant ewe. *Anesthesiology* 1974;40:354–370.
32. Levinson G, Shnider SM, Gildea JE, deLorimier AA. Maternal and foetal cardiovascular and acid-base changes during ketamine anaesthesia in pregnant ewes. *Br J Anaesth* 1973;45:1111–1115.
33. Eng M, Berges PU, Bonica JJ: The effects of ketamine on uterine blood flow in the monkey. In: *Abstracts of Scientific Papers.* Atlanta: Society for Gynecological Investigation; 1973:48.
34. Craft JB Jr, Coaldrake LA, Yonekura JL, et al. Ketamine, catecholamines, and uterine tone in pregnant ewes. *Am J Obstet Gynecol* 1983;146:429–434.
35. Cosmi EV. Effetti della ketamina sulla madre e sul feto. Studio sperimentale e clinico. *Minerva Anestesiol* 1977;43:379.
36. Galloon S. Ketamine for obstetric delivery. *Anesthesiology* 1976;44:522–524.
37. Chodoff P, Stella JG. Use of Cl-581-A phencyclidine derivative for obstetrical anesthesia. *Anesth Analg* 1966;45:527–530.
38. Meer FM, Downing JW, Coleman AJ. An intravenous method of anesthesia for caesarean section. II. Ketamine. *Br J Anaesth* 1973;45:191–196.
39. Akamatsu TJ, Bonica JJ, Rehmet R, Eng M, Ueland K. Experiences with the use of ketamine for parturition. I. Primary anesthetic for vaginal delivery. *Anesth Analg* 1974;53:284–287.
40. Hodgkinson R, Marx GF, Kim SS, Miclat NM. Neonatal neurobehavioral tests following vaginal delivery under ketamine, thiopental and extradural anesthesia. *Anesth Analg* 1977;56:548–553.
41. Cosmi EV, Marx GF. The effect of anesthesia on the acid-base status of the fetus. *Anesthesiology* 1969;30:238–242.
42. Brann AW Jr, Myers RE, DiGiacomo R. The effect of halothane-induced maternal hypotension in the fetus. In: *Medical Primatology 1970.* Proceedings of the 2nd Conference on Experimental Medicine and Surgery in Primates, New York, 1969. S Karger, Basel; 1971:637.
43. Moir DD. Anaesthesia for caesarean section. An evaluation of a method using low concentrations of halothane and 50 per cent of oxygen. *Br J Anaesth* 1970;42:136–142.
44. Bonica JJ. Halothane in obstetrics. In: Shnider SM, Moya F, eds. *The Anesthesiologist, Mother and Newborn.* Baltimore: Williams & Wilkins; 1974:114–121.
45. Allard E, Guimond C. L'halothane en obstetrique. *Can Anaesth Soc J* 1964;11:38–87.
46. Stoelting VK. Fluothane in obstetric anesthesia. *Anesth Analg* 1964;43:243–246.
47. Crawford JS. The place of halothane in obstetrics. *Br J Anaesth* 1962;34:386–390.

48. Marx GF, Mateo CV. Effects of different oxygen concentrations during general anesthesia for elective cesarean section. *Can Anaesth Soc J* 1971;18:587–593.

49. Galbert MW, Gardner AE. Use of halothane in a balanced technique for cesarean section. *Anesth Analg* 1972;51:701–704.

50. Phillips JM, Evans JA. Acute anesthetic and obstetric management of patients with severe abruptio-placenta. *Anesth Analg* 1970;49:998–1004.

51. Palahniuk RJ, Shnider SM. Maternal and fetal cardiovascular and acid-base changes during halothane and isoflurane anesthesia in the pregnant ewe. *Anesthesiology* 1974;41:462–472.

52. Carenza L, Cosmi EV. Analgo-anetesia in travaglio e nel parto: Valutazione des metodi e dei farmaci. In: *58th Congress of the Italian Society of Obstetrics and Gynecology*. Fidenza, Italy: Mattioli Publ; 1977:286.

53. Eng M, Bonica JJ, Akamatsu TJ, Berges PU, Der Yuen D, Ueland K. Maternal and fetal responses to halothane in pregnant monkeys. *Acta Anaesthesiol Scand* 1975;19:154–158.

54. Gibbs CP, Noel SC. Human uterine artery responses to lidocaine. *Am J Obstet Gynecol* 1976;126:313–315.

55. Cibils LA. Response of human uterine arteries to local anesthetics. *Am J Obstet Gynecol* 1976;126:202–210.

56. Greiss FC Jr, Still JG, Anderson SG. Effects of local anesthetic agents on the uterine vasculatures and myometrium. *Am J Obstet Gynecol* 1976;124:889–899.

57. Fishburne JI, Hopkinson RB, Greiss FC Jr. Responses of gravid uterine vasculature to arterial levels of local anesthetic agents. In: *Abstracts of Scientific Papers*. Seattle: Society for Obstetric Anesthesia and Perinatology; 1977:37.

58. Pue AF, Plumer MH, Resnik R, Brink GW. Effects of local anesthetics on uterine blood flow in pregnant sheep. In: *Abstracts of Scientific Papers*. Seattle: Society for Obstetric Anesthesia and Perinatology; 1977:47.

59. Morishima HO, Gutsche BB, Keenaghan JB, Barkus BS, Covino BG. The effect of lidocaine-induced maternal convulsions on the fetal lamb. In: *Abstracts of Scientific Papers*. New Orleans: American Society of Anesthesiologists; 1977:293.

60. Biehl D, Shnider SM, Levinson G, Callender K. The direct effects of circulating lidocaine on uterine blood flow and foetal well-being in the pregnant ewe. *Can Anaesth Soc J* 1977;24:445–451.

61. Chestnut DH, Weiner CP, Martin JG, Herrig JE, Wang JP. Effect of intravenous epinephrine on uterine artery blood flow velocity in the pregnant guinea pig. *Anesthesiology* 1986;65:633–636.

62. Chestnut DH, Weiner CP, Herrig JE. The effect of intravenously administered 2-chloroprocaine upon uterine artery blood flow velocity in gravid guinea pigs. *Anesthesiology* 1989;70:305–308.

63. Alahuhta S, Rasanen J, Jouppila P, et al. The effects of epidural ropivacaine and bupivacaine for cesarean section on uteroplacental and fetal circulation. *Anesthesiology* 1995;83:23–32.

64. Foutz SE, Kotelko DM, Shnider SM, et al. Placental transfer and effects of cocaine on uterine blood flow and the fetus. *Anesthesiology* 1983;59:A422.

65. Moore TR, Sorg J, Key TC, Resnik R. Effects of intravenous cocaine on uterine blood flow and cardiovascular parameters in the pregnant ewe. In: *Abstracts of Scientific Papers*. Phoenix: Society for Gynecological Investigation; 1985:175.

66. Woods JR Jr, Plessinger MA, Clark KE. Effect of cocaine on uterine blood flow and fetal oxygenation. *JAMA* 1987;257:957–961.

67. Greiss FC Jr, Crandell DL. Therapy for hypotension induced by spinal anesthesia during pregnancy. *JAMA* 1965;191:793–796.

68. Greiss FC Jr. Pressure-flow relationship in the gravid uterine vascular bed. *Am J Obstet Gynecol* 1966;96:41–47.

69. Wallis KL, Shnider SM, Hicks JS, Spivey HT. Epidural anesthesia in the normotensive pregnant ewe: Effects on uterine blood flow and fetal acid-base status. *Anesthesiology* 1976;44:481–487.

70. Brotanek V, Vasicka A, Santiago A, Brotanek JD. The influence of epidural anesthesia on uterine blood flow. *Obstet Gynecol* 1973;42:276–282.

71. Jouppila R, Jouppila P, Hollmén A, Kuikka J. Effects of segmental extradural analgesia on placental blood flow during normal labour. *Br J Anaesth* 1978;50:563–567.

72. Jouppila P, Jouppila R, Hollmén A, Koivula A. Lumbar epidural analgesia to improve intervillous blood flow during labor in severe preeclampsia. *Obstet Gynecol* 1982;59:158–161.

73. Hollmén A, Jouppila R, Jouppila P, Koivula A, Vierola H. Effect of extradural analgesia using bupivacaine and 2-chloroprocaine on intervillous blood flow during normal labour. *Br J Anaesth* 1982;54:837–842.

74. Hollmén AI, Jouppila R, Albright GA, Jouppila P, Vierola H, Koivula A. Intervillous blood flow during caesarean section with prophylactic ephedrine and epidural anaesthesia. *Acta Anaesthesiol Scand* 1984;28:396–400.

75. Jouppila P, Jouppila R, Barinoff T, Koivula A. Placental blood flow during caesarean section performed under subarachnoid blockade. *Br J Anaesth* 1984;56:1379–1382.

76. Baumann H, Alon E, Atanassoff P, Pasch TH, Huch A, Huch R. Effect of epidural anesthesia for cesarean delivery on maternal femoral arterial and venous, uteroplacental, and umbilical blood flow velocities and waveforms. *Obstet Gynecol* 1990;75:194–198.

77. Giles W, Lah F, Trudinger B. The effect of epidural anaesthesia for caesarean section on maternal uterine and fetal umbilical artery blood flow velocity waveforms. *Br J Obstet Gynaecol* 1987;94:55–59.

78. Petrikovsky B, Cohen M, Tancer M. Uterine and umbilical blood flow during caesarean section under epidural anaesthesia. *Acta Obstet Gynecol Scand* 1988;67:737–739.

79. Morrow RJ, Rolbin SH, Ritchie JWK, Haley S. Epidural anaesthesia and blood flow velocity in mother and fetus. *Can J Anaesth* 1989;36:519–522.

80. Turner GA, Newnham JP, Johnson C, Westmore M. Effects of extradural anaesthesia on umbilical and uteroplacental arterial flow velocity waveforms. *Br J Anaesth* 1991;67:306–309.

81. Barton MD, Kilam AP, Meschia G. Response of ovine uterine blood flow to epinephrine and norepinephrine. *Proc Soc Exp Biol Med* 1974;145:996–1003.

82. Hood DD, Dewan DM, James FM II. Maternal and fetal effects of epinephrine in gravid ewes. *Anesthesiology* 1986;64:610–613.

83. Chestnut DH, Ostman LG, Weiner CP, Hdez MJ, Wang JP. The effect of vasopressor agents upon uterine artery blood flow velocity in the gravid guinea pig subjected to ritodrine infusion. *Anesthesiology* 1988;68:363–366.

84. Bonica JJ, Akamatsu TJ, Berges PU, Morikawa K, Kennedy WF Jr. Circulatory effects of peridural block. II. Effects of epinephrine. *Anesthesiology* 1972;34:514–522.

85. Rosenfeld CR, Barton MD, Meschia G. Effects of epinephrine on distribution of blood flow in the pregnant ewe. *Am J Obstet Gynecol* 1976;124:156–163.

86. deRosayro AM, Nahrwold ML, Hill AB. Cardiovascular effects of epidural epinephrine in the pregnant sheep. *Reg Anesth* 1981;6:4.

87. Albright GA, Jouppila R, Hollmén AI, Jouppila P, Vierola H, Koivula A. Epinephrine does not alter human intervillous blood flow during epidural anesthesia. *Anesthesiology* 1981;54:131–135.

88. Levinson G, Shnider SM, Krames E, Ring G. Epidural anesthesia for cesarean section: Effects of epinephrine in the local anesthetic solution. In: *Abstracts of Scientific Papers*. Chicago: American Society of Anesthesiologists; 1975:285.

89. Myers RE. Maternal psychological stress and fetal asphyxia: A study in the monkey. *Am J Obstet Gynecol* 1975;122:47–59.

90. Shnider SM, Wright RG, Levinson G, et al. Uterine blood flow and plasma norepinephrine changes during maternal stress in the pregnant ewe. *Anesthesiology* 1979;50:524–527, 1979.

91. Martin CB Jr, Gingerick B. Uteroplacental physiology. *J Obstet Gynecol Neonatal Nurs* 1976;5(suppl):16–25.

92. Lederman RP, Lederman E, Work BA Jr, McCann DS. The relationship of maternal anxiety, plasma catecholamines and plasma cortisol to progress in labor. *Am J Obstet Gynecol* 1978;132:495–500.

93. Lederman RP, Lederman E, Work B, McCann DS. Anxiety and epinephrine in multiparous labor: Relationship to duration of labor and fetal heart rate pattern. *Am J Obstet Gynecol* 1985;153:870–877.

94. Adamsons K, Mueller-Heubach E, Myers RE. Production of fetal asphyxia in the rhesus monkey by administration of catecholamines to the mother. *Am J Obstet Gynecol* 1971;109:248–262.

95. Eng M, Berges PU, Ueland K, Bonica JJ, Parer JT. The effects of methoxamine and ephedrine in normotensive pregnant primates. *Anesthesiology* 1971;35:354–360.

96. Shnider SM, deLorimier AA, Asling JH, Morishima HO. Vasopressors in obstetrics. II. Fetal hazards of methoxamine administration during obstetric spinal anesthesia. *Am J Obstet Gynecol* 1970;106:680–686.

97. Greiss FC Jr, Gobble FL Jr. Effect of sympathetic nerve stimulation on the uterine vascular bed. *Am J Obstet Gynecol* 1967;97:962–967.

98. James FM III, Greiss FC Jr, Kemp RA. An evaluation of vasopressor therapy for maternal hypotension during spinal anesthesia. *Anesthesiology* 1970;33:25–34.

99. Eng M, Berges PU, Parer JT, Bonica JJ, Ueland K. Spinal anesthesia and ephedrine in pregnant monkeys. *Am J Obstet Gynecol* 1973;115:1095–1099.

100. Shnider SM, deLorimier AA, Steffenson JL. Vasopressors in obstetrics. III. Fetal effects of metaraminol infusion during obstetric spinal hypotension. *Am J Obstet Gynecol* 1970;108:1017–1022.

101. Ramanathan S, Grant GJ. Vasopressor therapy for hypotension due to epidural anesthesia for cesarean section. *Acta Anaesthesiol Scand* 1988;32:559–565.

102. Moran DH, Perillo M, Bader AM, Datta S. Phenylephrine in treating maternal hypotension secondary to spinal anesthesia. *Anesthesiology* 1989;71:A857.

103. Tong C, Eisenach JC. The vascular mechanism of ephedrine's beneficial effect on uterine perfusion during pregnancy. *Anesthesiology* 1992;76:792–798.

104. Alahuhta S, Rasanen J, Jouppila P, et al. Ephedrine and phenylephrine for avoiding maternal hypotension due to spinal anesthesia for cesarean section: Effects on uteroplacental and foetal haemodynamics. *Int J Obstet Anesth* 1992;1:129–134.

105. Callender K, Levinson G, Shnider SM, Feduska N, Biehl DR, Ring G. Dopamine administration in the normotensive pregnant ewe. *Obstet Gynecol* 1978;51:586–589.

106. Rolbin SH, Levinson G, Shnider SM, Biehl DR, Wright R. Dopamine treatment of spinal hypotension decreases uterine blood flow in the pregnant ewe. *Anesthesiology* 1978;51:36–40.

107. Cabalum T, Zugaib M, Lieb S, Nuwayhid B, Brinkman CR III, Assali NS. Effect of dopamine on hypotension induced by spinal anesthesia. *Am J Obstet Gynecol* 133:630–634, 1979.

108. Tabsh K, Nuwayhid B, Erkkola R, et al. Hemodynamic responses of the pelvic vascular bed to vasoactive stimuli in pregnant sheep. *Biol Neonate* 1981;39:52–60.

109. Ehrenkranz RA, Hamilton LA, Bennan SC, Oakes GK, Walker AM, Chez RA. Effects of salbutamol and isoxsuprine on uterine and umbilical blood flow in pregnant sheep. *Am J Obstet Gynecol* 1977;128:287–293.

110. Enrenkranz RA, Walker AM, Oakes GK, McLaughlin MK, Chez RA. Effect of ritodrine infusion on uterine and umbilical blood flow in pregnant sheep. *Am J Obstet Gynecol* 1976;126:343–349.

111. Chestnut DH, Weiner CP, Wang JP, Herrig JE, Martin JG. The effect of ephedrine upon uterine artery blood flow velocity in the pregnant guinea pig subjected to terbutaline infusion and acute hemorrhage. *Anesthesiology* 1987;66:508–512.

112. Brinkman CR III, Assali NS. Uteroplacental hemodynamic response to antihypertensive drugs in hypertensive pregnant sheep. In: Lindhimer MD, Katz AL, Zuspan FP, eds. *Hypertension in Pregnancy*. New York: John Wiley; 1976:363–375.

113. Ring G, Krames E, Shnider SM, Wallis KL, Levinson G. Comparison of nitroprusside and hydralazine in hypertensive pregnant ewes. *Obstet Gynecol* 1977;50:598–602.

114. Vertommen JD, Hughes SC, Rosen MA, et al. Hydralazine does not restore uterine blood flow during cocaine-induced hypertension in the pregnant ewe. *Anesthesiology* 1992;76:580–587.

115. Jouppila P, Kirkinen P, Koivula A, Ylikorkala O. Effects of dihydralazine infusion on the fetoplacental blood flow and maternal prostanoids. *Obstet Gynecol* 1985;65:115–118.

116. Craft JB Jr, Co EG, Yonekura ML, Gilman RM. Nitroglycerin therapy for phenylephrine-induced hypertension in pregnant ewes. *Anesth Analg* 1980;59:494–499.

117. Bell E. Nitroglycerin and uterine relaxation (letter). *Anesthesiology* 1996;85:683.

118. Kessin C, Hughes SC, Rosen MA, Johnson JL, Parer JT, Kan R. Nitroglycerin improves decreased uterine blood flow in the pregnant ewe with cocaine-induced hypertension. *Anesthesiology* 1995;83:A937.

119. Schlant RC, Tsagaris TS, Robertson RJ Jr. Studies on the acute cardiovascular effects of intravenous sodium nitroprusside. *Am J Cardiol* 1972;9:51–59.

120. Styles MB, Coleman AJ, Leary WP. Some hemodynamic effects of sodium nitroprusside. *Anesthesiology* 1973;38:173–176.

121. Ross G, Cole PV. Cardiovascular actions of sodium nitroprusside in dogs. *Anaesthesia* 1973;28:400–406.

122. Nelson SH, Suresh MS. Comparison of nitroprusside and hydralazine in isolated uterine arteries from pregnant and nonpregnant patients. *Anesthesiology* 1988;68:541–547.

123. Mabie WC, Gonzalez AR, Sibai BM, Amon E. Comparative trial of labetalol and hydralazine in the acute management of severe hypertension complicating pregnancy. *Obstet Gynecol* 1987;70:328–333.

124. Pickles CJ, Symonds EM, Pipkin FB. The fetal outcome in a randomized double-blind controlled trial of labetalol versus placebo in pregnancy-induced hypertension. *Br J Obstet Gynaecol* 1989;96:38–43.

125. Plouin P-F, Breart G, Maillard F, Papiernik E, Relier J-P. Comparison of antihypertensive efficacy and perinatal safety of labetalol and methyldopa in the treatment of hypertension in pregnancy: A randomized controlled trial. *Br J Obstet Gynaecol* 1988;95:868–876.

126. Ramanathan J, Sibai BM, Mabie WC, Chauhan D, Ruiz AG: The use of labetalol for attenuation of the hypertensive response to endotracheal intubation in preeclampsia. *Am J Obstet Gynecol* 1988;159:650–654.

127. Joupilla P, Kirkinen P, Koivula A, Ylikorkala O. Labetalol does not alter the placental and fetal blood flow or maternal prostanoids in pre-eclampsia. *Br J Obstet Gynaecol* 1986;93:543–547.

128. Ahokas RA, Mabie WC, Sibai BM, Anderson GD. Labetalol does not decrease placental perfusion in the hypertensive term-pregnant rat. *Am J Obstet Gynecol* 1989;160:480–484.

129. Eisenach JC, Mandell G, Dewan DM. Maternal and fetal effects of labetalol in pregnant ewes. *Anesthesiology* 1991;74:292–297.

130. Murad SHN, Tabsh KMA, Shilyanski G, et al. Effects of verapamil on uterine blood flow and maternal cardiovascular function in the awake pregnant ewe. *Anesth Analg* 1985;64:7–10.

131. Lirette M, Holbrook RH, Katz M. Cardiovascular and uterine blood flow changes during nicardipine HCI tocolysis in the rabbit. *Obstet Gynecol* 1987;69:79–82.

132. Ducsay CA, Thompson JS, Wu AT, Novy MJ. Effects of calcium entry blocker (nicardipine) tocolysis in rhesus macaques: Fetal plasma concentrations and cardiorespiratory changes. *Am J Obstet Gynecol* 1987;157:1482–1486.

133. Harake B, Gilbert RD, Ashwal S, Power GG. Nifedipine: Effects on fetal and maternal hemodynamics in pregnant sheep. *Am J Obstet Gynecol* 1987;157:1003–1008.

134. Mari G, Kirshon B, Moise KJ, Lee W, Cotton DB. Doppler assessment of the fetal and uteroplacental circulation during nifedipine therapy for preterm labor. *Am J Obstet Gynecol* 1989;161:1514–1518.

135. Pirhonen JP, Erkkola RU, Erblad UU, Nyman L. Single dose of nifedipine in normotensive pregnancy: Nifedipine concentrations, hemodynamic responses, and uterine and fetal flow velocity waveforms. *Obstet Gynecol* 1990;76:807–811.

136. Papatsonis DN, Kok JH, van Geijn HP, Bleker OP, Ader HJ, Dekker GA. Neonatal effects of nifedipine and ritodrine for preterm labor. *Obstet Gynecol* 2000;95:477–481.

137. Neri I, Valensise H, Facchinetti F, Menghini S, Romanini C, Volpe A. 24-hour ambulatory blood pressure monitoring: a comparison between transdermal glyceryl-trinitrate and oral nifedipine. *Hypertens Pregnancy* 1999;18:107–113.

138. Gyetvai K, Hannah ME, Hodnett ED, Ohlsson A. Tocolytics for preterm labor: a systematic review. *Obstet Gynecol* 1999;94:869–877.

139. Carr DB, Clark AL, Kernek K, Spinnato JA. Maintenance oral nifedipine for preterm labor: a randomized clinical trial. *Am J Obstet Gynecol* 1999;181:822–827.

140. Scardo JA, Vermillion ST, Newman RB, Chauhan SP, Hogg BB. A randomized, double-blind, hemodynamic evaluation of nifedipine and labetalol in preeclamptic hypertensive emergencies. *Am J Obstet Gynecol* 1999;181:862–866.

141. Lazard EM. A preliminary report on the intravenous use of magnesium sulfate in puerperial eclampsia. *Am J Obstet Gynecol* 1925;9:178–188.

142. Dorsett L. The intramuscular injection of magnesium sulfate for the control of convulsions in eclampsia. *Am J Obstet Gynecol* 1926;11:227–231.

143. Dandavino A, Woods JR Jr, Murayama L, Brinkman CR III, Assali NS. Circulatory effects of magnesium sulfate in normotensive and renal hypertensive pregnant sheep. *Am J Obstet Gynecol* 1977;127:769–774.

144. Krames E, Ring G, Wallis KL, Levinson G, Shnider SM. The effect of magnesium sulfate on uterine blood flow and fetal well-being in the pregnant ewe. In: *Abstracts of Scientific Papers*. Chicago: American Society of Anesthesiologists; 1975:287.

145. Rosen MA, Hughes SC, Curtis JD, Norton M, Levinson G, Shnider SM. Effects of epidural morphine on uterine blood flow and acid-base status in the pregnant ewe. *Anesthesiology* 1982;57:A383.

146. Craft JB Jr, Bolan JC, Coaldrake LA, et al. The maternal and fetal cardiovascular effects of epidural morphine in the sheep model. *Am J Obstet Gynecol* 1982;142:835–839.

147. Craft JB Jr, Robichaux AG, Kim HS, et al. The maternal and fetal cardiovascular effects of epidural fentanyl in the sheep model. *Am J Obstet Gynecol* 1984;148:1089–1104.

148. Craft JB Jr, Coaldrake LA, Bolan JC, et al. Placental passage and uterine effects of fentanyl. *Anesth Analg* 1983;62:894–898.

149. Ribeiro CAF, Macedo TA. Pharmacological characterization of the postsynaptic alpha-adrenoceptors in human uterine artery. *J Pharm Pharmacol* 1986;38:600–605.

150. Horvath JS, Phippard A, Korda A, Henderson-Smart DJ, Child A, Tiller J. Clonidine hydrochloride: A safe and effective antihypertensive agent in pregnancy. *Obstet Gynecol* 1985;66:634–638.

151. Hartikaninen-Sorri A-L, Heikkinen JE, Koivisto M. Pharmacokinetics of clonidine during pregnancy and nursing. *Obstet Gynecol* 1987;69:598–600.

152. Tuimala R, Punnonen R, Kauppila E. Clonidine in the treatment of hypertension during pregnancy. *Ann Chir Gynaecol* 1985;74(suppl):47–50.

153. Huisjes HJ, Hadders-Algra M, Touwen BCL. Is clonidine a behavioral teratogen in the human? *Early Hum Dev* 1986;14:43–48.

154. Eisenach JC, Castro MI, Dewan DM, Rose JC, Grice SC. Intravenous clonidine hydrochloride toxicity in pregnant ewes. *Am J Obstet Gynecol* 1988;160:471–476.

155. Jansen CAM, Lowe KC, Nathanielsz PW. The effects of xylazine on uterine activity, fetal and maternal oxygenation, cardiovascular function, and fetal breathing. *Am J Obstet Gynecol* 1984;148:386–390.

156. Eisenach JC. Intravenous clonidine produces hypoxemia by a peripheral alpha$_2$-adrenergic mechanism. *J Pharmacol Exp Ther* 1988;244:247–252.

157. Metz SA, Halter JB, Robertson RP. Induction of defective insulin secretion and impaired glucose tolerance by clonidine: Selective stimulation of metabolic alpha-adrenergic pathways. *Diabetes* 1978;27:554–562.

158. Wadhwa RK. Obstetric anesthesia for a patient with malignant hyperthermia susceptibility. *Anesthesiology* 1977;46:63–64.

159. Willatts SM. Malignant hyperthermia susceptibility: Management during pregnancy and labour. *Anaesthesia* 1979;34:41–46.

160. Lips FJ, Newland M, Dutton G. Malignant hyperthermia triggered by cyclopropane during cesarean section. *Anesthesiology* 1982;56:144–146.

161. Cupryn JP, Kennedy A, Byrick RJ. Malignant hyperthermia in pregnancy. *Am J Obstet Gynecol* 1984;150:327–328.

162. Gibbs JM. Unexplained hyperpyrexia during labor (letter). *Anaesth Intensive Care* 1984;12:375.

163. Doublas MJ, McMorland GH. The anaesthetic management of the malignant hyperthermia susceptible parturient. *Can Anaesth Soc J* 1986;33:371–378.

164. Shime J, Gare D, Andrews J, Britt B. Dantrolene in pregnancy: Lack of adverse effects on the fetus and newborn infant. *Am J Obstet Gynecol* 1988;159:831–834.

165. Morison DH. Placental transfer of dantrolene (letter). *Anesthesiology* 1983;59:265.

166. Craft JB Jr, Goldberg NH, Lim M, et al. Cardiovascular effects and placental passage of dantrolene in the maternal-fetal sheep model. *Anesthesiology* 1988;68:68–72.

167. Greiss FC Jr, Anderson SG, King LC. Uterine vascular bed: Effects of acute hypoxia. *Am J Obstet Gynecol* 1972;113:1057–1064.

168. Makowski EL, Hertz RH, Meschia G. Effect of acute maternal hypoxia and hyperoxia on the blood flow to the pregnant uterus. *Am J Obstet Gynecol* 1973;115:624–629.

169. Dilts PV Jr, Brinkman CR III, Kirschbaum TH, Assali NS. Uterine and systemic hemodynamic interrelationships and their response to hypoxia. *Am J Obstet Gynecol* 1969;103:138–157.

170. Assali NS, Holm LW, Sehgal N. Hemodynamic changes in fetal lambs in utero in response to asphyxia, hypoxia and hypercapnia. *Circ Res* 1962;11:423–430.

171. Levinson G, Shnider SM, deLorimier AA, Steffenson JL. Effects of maternal hyperventilation on uterine blood flow and fetal oxygenation and acid-base status. *Anesthesiology* 1974;40:340–347.

172. Huckabee WE. Uterine blood flow. *Am J Obstet Gynecol* 1962;84:1623–1633.

173. Wolkoff AS, McGee JA, Flowers CE, Bawden JW. Alterations in uterine blood flow in the pregnant ewe. I. Associated changes in blood gases. *Obstet Gynecol* 1964;23:636–637.

174. Walker AM, Oakes GK, Ehrenkranz R, McLaughlin M, Chez RA. Effects of hypercapnia on uterine and umbilical circulation in conscious pregnant sheep. *J Appl Physiol* 1976;41:727–733.

175. Morishima HO, Daniel SS, Adamsons K Jr, James LS. Effects of positive pressure ventilation of the mother upon the acid-base state of the fetus. *Am J Obstet Gynecol* 1965;93:269–273.

176. Motoyama EK, Rivard G, Acheson F, Cook CD. Adverse effect of maternal hyperventilation on the foetus. *Lancet* 1966;1:286–288.

177. Lumley J, Renou P, Newman W, Wood C. Hyperventilation in obstetrics. *Am J Obstet Gynecol* 1969;103:847–855.

178. Parer JT, Eng M, Aoba H, Ueland K. Uterine blood flow and oxygen uptake during maternal hyperventilation in monkeys at cesarean section. *Anesthesiology* 1970;32:130–135.

179. Johnson GH, Brinkman CR III, Assali NS. Effects of acid and base infusion on umbilical hemodynamics. *Am J Obstet Gynecol* 1972;112:1122–1128.

180. Ralston DH, Shnider SM, deLorimier AA. Uterine blood flow and fetal acid-base changes after bicarbonate administration to the pregnant ewe. *Anesthesiology* 1974;40:348–353.

181. Buss DD, Bisgard EG, Rawlings CA, Rankin JHG. Uteroplacental blood flow during alkalosis in the sheep. *Am J Physiol* 1975;228:1497–1500.

182. Norris MC, Arkoosh VA, Knobler R. Maternal and fetal effects of isoproterenol in the gravid ewe. *Anesth Analg* 1997;85:389–394.

183. Thomas DG, Robson SC, Redfern N, Hughes D, Boys RJ. Randomized trial of bolus phenylephrine or ephedrine for maintenance of arterial pressure during spinal anaesthesia for caesarean section. *Br J Anaesth* 1996;76:61–65.

184. Moran DH, Perillo M, LaPorta RF, Bader AM, Datta S. Phenylephrine in the prevention of hypotension following spinal anesthesia for cesarean delivery. *J Clin Anesth* 1991;3:301–305.

185. Ellis SC, Wheeler AS, James FM III, et al. Fetal and maternal effects of sodium nitroprusside used to counteract hypertension in gravid ewes. *Am J Obstet Gynecol* 1982;143:766–770.

186. Blea CW, Barnard JM, Magness RR, Phernetton TM, Hendricks SK. Effect of nifedipine on fetal and maternal hemodynamics and blood gases in the pregnant ewe. *Am J Obstet Gynecol* 1997;176:922–930.

187. Castro MI, Eisenach JC. Pharmacokinetics and dynamics of intravenous, intrathecal, and epidural clonidine in sheep. *Anesthesiology* 1989;71:418–425.

Shnider and Levinson's Anesthesia for Obstetrics,
edited by Samuel C. Hughes, et al.
Lippincott Williams & Wilkins,
Philadelphia, © 2001.

CHAPTER 3

EFFECTS OF ANESTHESIA ON UTERINE ACTIVITY AND LABOR

ANTHONY C. MILLER*, M.D.

The course of labor significantly influences the choices and management of analgesia and anesthesia for the parturient. Similarly, anesthesia and analgesia may affect the progress of labor and method of delivery. This chapter will review the effects of anesthesia on labor.

DEFINITIONS

The frequency of uterine contractions and the pressure they generate define uterine activity. It is monitored indirectly by a tocodynamometer applied to the maternal abdomen or directly by an intrauterine pressure catheter (IUPC) inserted into the uterine cavity. The tocodynamometer responds to the changing shape of the lower abdomen caused by a uterine contraction and measures only the frequency of contractions, not the pressure generated. The IUPC measures contraction pressure, resting tone, and frequency of uterine contractions.

Several systems have been devised for describing uterine activity. One of the earliest, yet still commonly used, was developed by Caldeyro-Barcia and Alvarez (1). The pressures generated by the uterine contractions (peak minus resting pressure in mm Hg) in a 10-minute period are summed and the result is expressed in Montevideo units (named after the location of the authors). Thus, if in 10 minutes there were three contractions, each peaking 50 mm Hg above baseline, the uterine activity would be equivalent to 150 Montevideo units. Another system calculates the area under the uterine pressure curve and yields a result that is expressed in torr-minutes or uterine activity units (2). Alternatively, only the number of contractions in a given period is measured (3). All of these methods have been used in assessing the effect of drugs on uterine activity.

As originally described by Friedman (Fig. 3.1 and 3.2) (4), progress of labor refers to increasing cervical dilation and effacement combined with the descent of the presenting fetal part in the pelvis. The first stage of labor extends from the beginning of cervical dilation and effacement (onset of regular, painful contractions) to complete cervical dilation (commonly referred to as being "10 cm"). The first stage is divided into the latent and active phases, which are distinguished by the rate of cervical dilation. Although an arbitrary cervical dilation is often used to divide these two phases, the transition is unique to each labor and can often be determined only in retrospect. The second stage of labor extends from complete cervical dilation until delivery of the infant, and the third stage, from then until the placenta is delivered (5).

Dystocia, or abnormal progress of labor (long or difficult labor), results from abnormalities of any one or more of the following: (a) expulsive forces (either uterine contraction or voluntary muscle effort in the second stage); (b) fetal presentation, position, or development; (c) the maternal bony pelvis; or (d) the birth canal (6). The abnormal patterns that comprise dystocia

are presented in Table 3.1. Diagnosis and treatment of abnormal labor are crucial because it is the most common indication for primary cesarean section in the United States, and it may be associated with increased perinatal morbidity and mortality (6, 7).

Uterine relaxation refers to a diminution in contraction amplitude or resting uterine tone. Tocolysis is the production of relaxation by a pharmacologic agent (the tocolytic).

Active Management of Labor (AML) is an obstetric management technique used by some to shorten labor and reduce the frequency of cesarean section for dystocia (3). Although the definition is not standardized, AML usually comprises four elements: (a) admitting to the labor ward only those women whose contractions are associated with cervical change or rupture of membranes, (b) early amniotomy, (c) frequent examinations to detect dystocia, and (d) aggressive use of oxytocin to treat dystocia. Studies conflict regarding the success of AML in reducing cesarean section rates (8–10).

INHALATION AGENTS

Halothane, enflurane, and isoflurane produce a dose-dependent reduction in uterine tone (Fig. 3.3) (11–14). Studies of isoflurane demonstrate that halogenated agents reduce both the frequency of contractions and the interval between them (15). Whereas analgesic concentrations of these agents diminish uterine activity, anesthetic amounts nearly eliminate it (15, 16). There is no clinically relevant difference in the profound relaxation produced by all three agents (14). In contrast to the volatile anesthetics, nitrous oxide has little or no effect on the uterus (12, 14, 16).

The ability of volatile agents to cause rapid and profound uterine relaxation can be used to dissipate a tetanic contraction or facilitate intrauterine manipulations. To avoid postpartum hemorrhage, the concentration must be rapidly reduced after delivery. At lower concentrations (less than 0.5% halothane, 1% enflurane, or 1.5% isoflurane), the uterine response to oxytocin is preserved (15, 17). Furthermore, inhalation agents in low concentrations do not increase the blood loss from cesarean section (18–20). Inhalation analgesia for vaginal delivery with very low doses of enflurane or isoflurane (such as 0.2 minimal alveolar concentration [MAC]) appears to have minimal effect on uterine activity, duration of labor, and postpartum blood loss.

Little has been written about the effects of the newer anesthetic agents, desflurane and sevoflurane, on uterine activity. However, given that they are halogenated ethers similar in structure to other agents in use, one would expect their effects on the uterus to be similar. One study confirmed that sevoflurane does suppress uterine activity but to a lesser extent than halothane or isoflurane (21). Two studies have shown that maternal blood loss after cesarean section does not differ among groups receiving sevoflurane vs. isoflurane or desflurane vs. enflurane (22, 23). In the usual clinical concentrations, there do not appear to be significant differences among the halogenated agents in their effect on uterine tone.

*The views expressed in this article are those of the author and do not necessarily reflect the official policy or position of the Department of the Navy, Department of Defense, or the U.S. Government.

Table 3.1. PROLONGED LABOR: DIAGNOSTIC FEATURES

	Prolonged Latent Phase	Protracted Dilation (Slow Slope Active Phase)	Arrested Dilation (Active Phase Arrest)	Protracted Descent of Fetus	Arrest of Descent
Nulliparas	> 20 h	< 1.2 cm/h	No cervical dilation for > 2 h	< 1.2 cm/h	No descent for > 1 h
Multiparas	> 14 h	< 1.5 cm/h		< 1.5 cm/h	

Based upon information from Committee on Technical Bulletins of the American College of Obstetricians and Gynecologists. *Dystocia and the Augmentation of Labor.* ACOG Technical Bulletin No. 218; December 1995.

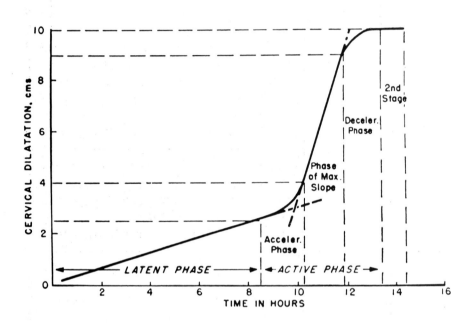

Figure 3.1. The average nulliparous labor curve (cervical dilation vs. time) based on a study of 500 primigravidas. (Reprinted by permission from Friedman EA. Primigravid labor. A graphicostatistical analysis. *Obstet Gynecol* 1955;6:567–589.)

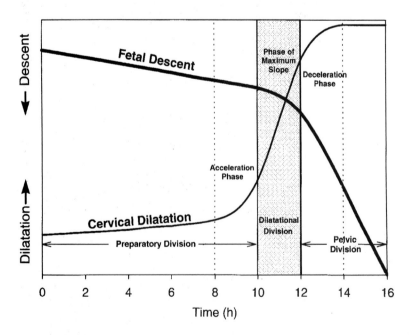

Figure 3.2. Labor course depicting the expected evolution of the dilation and descent curves. It is divided functionally into (1) a preparatory division that includes the latent and acceleration phases; (2) a dilational division equivalent to the phase of maximum slope; and (3) a pelvic division that encompasses both the deceleration phase and the second stage. (Illustration courtesy of Dr. L. Casey, redrawn from Friedman EA, 1978.) (Reprinted by permission from Cunningham FG, MacDonald PC, Gant NF, Leveno KJ, Gilstrap LC, eds. Normal labor and delivery: Parturition. In: *Williams Obstetrics.* 20th ed. Norwalk, CT: Appleton & Lange; 1997:269.)

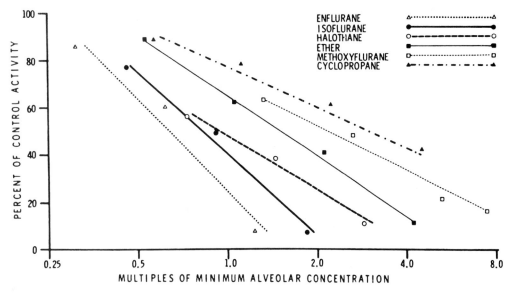

Figure 3.3. The effect of inhaled anesthetics on isolated human gravid uterine muscle. (Reprinted by permission from Tjeuw MTB, Yao F, Poznak A. Depressant effects of anesthetics on isolated human gravid and nongravid uterine muscle. *Chin Med J* 1986;9:235–242.)

PARENTERAL AGENTS

One study concluded that 100 mg intravenous (IV) meperidine administered during the active phase of labor produced either no change or an increase in uterine activity (24). However, there was no control group, and many labors were augmented. Another investigation reported increases in uterine activity after meperidine, pentazocine, or low spinal anesthesia (25). Both studies concluded that analgesia might lower circulating maternal epinephrine concentrations and improve contractility via a decrease in β-adrenergic stimulation.

However, Petrie et al. reported that, in the absence of analgesia, total uterine activity increases throughout labor (26). They studied several IV analgesics and hypnotics by comparing the slope of uterine activity vs. time in the pre- and postinjection periods (Fig. 3.4). They reported that meperidine, morphine, hydroxyzine, and promethazine did not change uterine activity significantly, but the postinjection uterine activity slope changed from the expected positive to negative. This finding implies that

these agents could slow parturition, although the authors did not include direct measurements of labor progress.

Friedman suggested that the inhibitory effects of parenteral opioids on uterine contractility might occur only during the latent phase (27). Furthermore, he determined that, while barbiturates caused dose-related inhibition of uterine contractility, the benzodiazepine-diazepam has no such effect (27).

Rayburn et al. compared IV fentanyl (50 to 100 $\mu g/h$) and meperidine (25 to 50 mg/2 to 3 hours) in a randomized, non-blinded study (28). There was no difference between the groups with respect to efficacy of the analgesics, duration of labor, or mode of delivery. While opioids remain the most frequently prescribed alternative to epidural analgesia, they often fail to provide adequate analgesia for labor.

With respect to ketamine, one study concluded that 2 mg/kg administered during second trimester abortions caused an increase in intrauterine pressure, whereas at cesarean section the same dose caused no change (see Chapter 13, Figs. 13.19 and

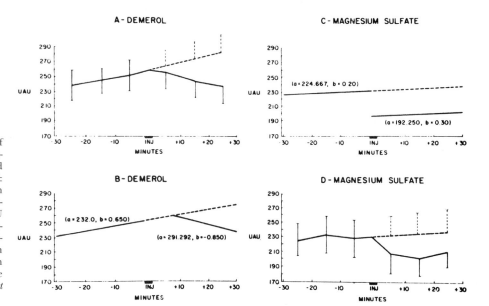

Figure 3.4. Effect on uterine activity of the administration of meperidine (Demerol) and magnesium sulfate. *A* and *D*, mean uterine activity units (*UAU* ± SE) per 10-minute segment of labor in the preinjection and postinjection periods contrasted with the expected UAU (– – –) for that period. *B* and *C*, regression line for the preinjection period contrasted with the observed postinjection values. (Reprinted by permission from Petrie RH, Wu R, Miller FC, et al. The effect of drugs on uterine activity. *Obstet Gynecol* 1976;48:431–435.)

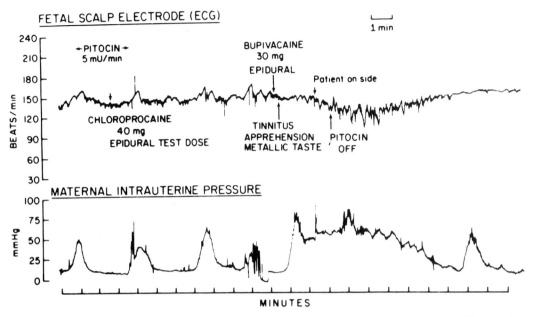

Figure 3.5. Tetanic uterine contraction occurring after inadvertent intravenous injection of bupivacaine. (Reprinted by permission from Greiss FC, Still JG, Anderson SG. Effects of local anesthetic agents on the uterine vasculatures and myometrium. *Am J Obstet Gynecol* 1976;124:889–899.)

13.20) (29). In a study using postpartum uterine pressures conducted by Marx et al., ketamine increased uterine activity briefly but did not affect uterine tone (30).

In summary, parenteral opioids and tranquilizers have little effect on uterine contractility. However, any heavy sedation caused by these drugs might prolong the latent phase. Barbiturates do inhibit uterine contractions in a dose-dependent fashion but are rarely used in current obstetric practice.

REGIONAL ANALGESIA

Epidural Analgesia

The effects of regional analgesia on the progress and outcome of labor are controversial. Although many studies demonstrate differences in the labors of women receiving epidural analgesia, firm conclusions about causality are difficult to draw because the group of patients that receives epidural analgesia is different from the group that does not (31). For example, the epidural group comes to the hospital at an earlier stage of labor, and many in the group already have prolonged labors before the block has begun (32–34). They are also more likely to have induction or augmentation of their labors (34, 35). Women receiving conduction analgesia have often found other methods of analgesia inadequate earlier in labor (36, 37). Melzack et al. reported that labor pain (such as that leading to a request for epidural analgesia) correlates with physical factors such as the ratio of the woman's usual weight to her height (38), and Hess et al. suggested that severe pain in labor predicts cesarean delivery (39). Using radiographic pelvimetry, Floberg et al. showed that patients who request epidural analgesia are more likely to have small pelvic outlet capacity (40). All of these differences create selection bias when comparing patients who received epidural analgesia with those who did not.

Furthermore, it can be very difficult to determine precisely when a given labor started. One must either rely on the parturient's perception of when her contractions became painful and regular or use an arbitrary event such as the time of admission to the hospital (6). Therefore, it is very difficult to make meaningful comparisons concerning the length of labor between women who do and do not request epidural analgesia.

While all of these confounding variables make it nearly impossible to discern the precise effects of epidural analgesia per se, local anesthetics themselves can have a direct effect on the uterus. The high concentrations that might be achieved with an accidental intravascular injection or paracervical block can increase uterine tone (41), and very high concentrations can lead to tetanic contractions (Fig. 3.5). In vitro studies of uterine muscle strips demonstrate that local anesthetics increase tone but decrease the rate and strength of contractions (42).

More important, though, are the effects of local anesthetic concentrations usually achieved clinically. To examine these effects, it is easiest to consider the stages of labor separately, although such a division is somewhat artificial.

First Stage of Labor

It has generally been believed that regional anesthesia administered in the latent phase will significantly prolong labor, whereas the same technique applied when labor is well established will have less effect. This idea first appeared as an aside in two early series evaluating caudal anesthesia for labor (43, 44). Friedman and Sachtleben studied the effects of caudal anesthesia on the first stage of labor and concluded that, if begun in the latent phase, it will lengthen labor substantially (45, 46). However, in the first study, the authors themselves admitted that their own data did not support such a conclusion (45). In the second study, the authors compared women who were experiencing prolongation of the latent phase with normal controls, yet, as stated above, this was subject to selection bias (46). Most subsequent studies have not specifically examined the effect of epidural analgesia on the length of the latent phase. In fact, the normal length of the latent phase is poorly defined and the effects of regional analgesia on it are difficult to evaluate. However, while not directly reporting data regarding the latent phase, a randomized trial by Clark et al. comparing epidural analgesia to IV opioids suggests that the latent phase is not prolonged by the regional block (47). Controversy persists regarding an association between early regional analgesia administration and subsequent operative delivery; this issue is discussed below in **Second Stage of Labor and Mode of Delivery**.

With regard to the active phase of the first stage, several nonrandomized studies suggest that epidural analgesia has a

Table 3.2. LENGTHS OF THE FIRST AND SECOND STAGES OF LABOR

Group	No Regional Anesthesia		Regional Anesthesia	
	First Stage (h)	*Second Stage (min)*	*First Stage (h)*	*Second Stage (min)*
Nulliparous				
Mean ± SD	8.1 ± 4.3	54 ± 39	10.2 ± 4.4	79 ± 53
Multiparous				
Mean ± SD	5.7 ± 3.4	19 ± 21	7.4 ± 3.8	45 ± 43

All means are significantly different ($P < .0001$).
Data from University of California San Francisco.
Modification from Kilpatrick SJ, Laros RK. Characteristics of normal labor. *Obstet Gynecol* 1989;74:85–87.

minimal effect on duration. In a retrospective study, Crawford noted no difference in the duration of the first stage of labor regardless of parity or use of oxytocin (48). Jouppila et al. matched women receiving epidural analgesia with controls for parity and spontaneous or induced labor (49). They determined that, although the total length of the first stage was greater in nulliparas receiving epidural analgesia, once the analgesia was begun the remainder of the first stage was the same duration as that for the controls with equivalent cervical dilation. In multiparas, no difference in the first-stage duration was detected. Studd et al. found that women in unaugmented labor who were given epidural blocks had longer first stages than those not receiving blocks (32). However, the rate of cervical dilation was no different between the groups; the epidural group merely had been admitted at a lesser cervical dilation. Women whose labors were augmented exhibited no effects of epidural analgesia on the duration of the first stage. Moir and Willocks found that the rate of cervical dilation was increased in 70% and unchanged in another 18.6% of women when epidural analgesia was established (50). Other clinicians have reported enhanced and more effective uterine contractility following epidural anesthesia (51–53), and some have recommended conduction analgesia for parturients with incoordinate uterine activity (50, 53–56), multiple gestation (57), or breech presentation (58, 59).

On the other hand, some studies have indicated that the first stage of labor is longer in women who receive epidural analgesics. In a retrospective study, Schussman et al. found longer first stages in low-risk parturients who had received epidural analgesia, even when those who required induction of labor were excluded (35). Kilpatrick and Laros reviewed the records of 6,991 women who did not require induction or augmentation of labor and concluded that the use of conduction anesthesia is associated with a longer first stage (Table 3.2) (60). Read et al. (61) and Willdeck-Lund et al. (62) also reported decreased uterine activity and cervical dilation rate after commencement of epidural analgesia. In a nonrandomized study of primiparas whose labors were managed actively, Carli et al. found that epidural analgesia was associated with a longer first stage compared to a variety of other analgesic options (63). Newton et al. observed that epidural analgesia did not cause a change in myometrial contractility but was associated with slower cervical dilation (64). However, in that study parturients in the epidural group already had slower cervical dilation rates before receiving analgesia. It is difficult to draw meaningful conclusions from these nonrandomized, retrospective studies. For example, Kilpatrick and Laros included in their regional anesthesia group spinal anesthetics during the second stage administered most commonly for operative delivery, presumably after prolonged or difficult labors without regional analgesia. The study by Willdeck-Lund concerned changes in uterine tone that occurred 30 minutes after establishment of an epidural block, which is probably not meaningful for the long-term outcome of labor.

In an effort to resolve the discrepancies in the nonrandomized studies, seven prospective investigations randomized parturients to either epidural analgesia or parenteral opioids (Table 3.3) (47, 65–70) Robinson et al. (69) and Philipsen and Jensen (67) randomized parturients to receive either intramuscular meperidine or intermittent boluses of bupivacaine. In both studies, duration of the first stage was the same in both groups, and the analgesia was significantly better in the epidural group.

Thorp et al. (70) and Ramin et al. (68) compared epidural bupivacaine infusions and IV meperidine-promethazine. Both studies found that epidural analgesia was associated with longer labors (only Thorp reported the first stage separately), increased use of oxytocin augmentation, and superior analgesia. The authors of the latter study repeated the investigation with the modification that the control group received IV meperidine by patient-controlled analgesia to make its pain relief more comparable to the epidural group (66). They did not report the duration of labor for the entire cohort, but for the two thirds of patients who were treated as randomized, those receiving epidural analgesia had longer first stages. Unfortunately, by analyzing such a subgroup, the authors may have introduced selection bias.

In their randomized trial, Clark et al. compared epidural bupivacaine and fentanyl with IV meperidine (47). There was no difference in the length of the first stage as a whole or in the active phase between groups, whether analyzed by intention-to-treat or protocol-compliance.

Recently, Bofill et al. compared an infusion of epidural bupivacaine and fentanyl with IV butorphanol in a randomized study (65). Despite superior analgesia at all times, the epidural group did not have a longer average first stage. A metaanalysis of prospective studies comparing epidural analgesia and parenteral opioids concluded that epidural analgesia prolongs the first stage and provides superior pain relief (71). All of these prospective studies are examined in more depth in **Epidural Analgesia and Increased Cesarean Section rate** (see below).

Other Considerations

Studies have been divided regarding whether the choice of local anesthetic affects length of the first stage. While some investigators have suggested that lidocaine might be associated with a depression of uterine activity (72–74), others have found no difference among bupivacaine, ropivacaine, S(−)-bupivacaine (levobupivacaine), lidocaine, and chloroprocaine (75–83). Conversely, two studies comparing identical concentrations of ropivacaine and bupivacaine suggest that ropivacaine reduces operative vaginal deliveries (84, 85). However, recent studies have shown that ropivacaine is less potent than bupivacaine (86, 87). Thus, the difference in mode of delivery might relate more to the lesser potency of ropivacaine than any intrinsic difference between the drugs.

Many studies have detected a transient decrease in uterine activity after the establishment of an epidural block. However, perhaps it is not the block itself that is responsible for

Table 3.3. SUMMARY OF PROSPECTIVE STUDIES COMPARING EPIDURAL ANALGESIA AND PARENTERAL OPIOIDS

Study	Epidural Analgesia	Opioid	First Stage (1)	Second Stage (1)	Instrumental Delivery (1)	Cesarean Section (1)	Quality of Analgesia (1)	Comments
Robinson et al. (1980)[69]	0.5% bupiv boluses	IM meper+ perphenazine	0	↑	↑	(2)	↑	
Philipsen et al. (1989)[67]	0.375% bupiv boluses	IM meper + IA	0	0	0	0	↑	No second stage analgesia provided
Thorp et al. (1993)[70]	0.25% bupiv bolus and 0.125% bupiv infusion	IV meper + promethazine	↑	↑	0	↑	↑	Criticized for study design
Ramin et al. (1995)[68]	0.25% bupiv bolus and 0.125% bupiv + 2 μg/mL fent infusion	IV meper + promethazine	↑ (3)	↑ (3)	↑	↑	↑	Over one third of subjects crossed to other treatment
Sharma et al. (1997)[66]	0.25% bupiv bolus and 0.125% bupiv + 2 μg/mL fent infusion	IV meper by PCA	↑(4)	0(4)	0(5)	0	↑	Nearly one third of subjects crossed to other treatment
Bofill et al. (1997)[65]	0.25% bupiv + 50–100 μg fent bolus and 0.125% bupiv + 1.5 μg/mL fent infusion	IV butor	0	0	↑ (6)	0	↑	
Clark et al. (1998)[47]	0.25% bupiv + 50 μg fent bolus and 0.125% bupiv + 1 μg/mL fent infusion	IV meper	0(5)	0(5)	0(7)	0(7)	(8)	52% of opioid group crossed to epidural
Halpern et al. (1998)[71]	(9)	(9)	↑	↑	↑	0	↑	Meta-analysis
Zhang et al. (1999)[178]	(9)	(9)	0/↑ (10)	↑	0/↑ (10)	0	(11)	Meta-analysis and quantitative review from NICHHD (12)

1. Study result with respect to effect of epidural analgesia on variable.
2. No cesarean sections occurred in this study.
3. First and second stages were not reported separately.
4. Labor duration was reported only for the protocol-compliant cohort.
5. From the intention-to-treat analysis.
6. Half of the forceps deliveries were for "resident training."
7. From the intention-to-treat and protocol-compliant analyses.
8. Not reported, but high crossover rate suggests superiority of epidural analgesia.
9. Meta-analysis of prospective studies.
10. Minimal increase, if any.
11. Not reported.
12. Epidemiologists from the National Institute of Child Health and Human Development.
0 = no change; ↑ = increased in epidural analgesia group; bupiv = bupivacaine; butor = butorphanol; fent = fentanyl; IA = inhalation analgesia; IM = intramuscular; IV = intravenous; meper = meperidine; PCA = patient-controlled analgesia.

this phenomenon. Cheek et al. showed that women who received a 1000 mL IV fluid bolus exhibited a decrease in uterine activity for 20 minutes, yet those who received a 500 mL bolus or maintenance fluid only did not demonstrate any change in activity (88). The establishment of an epidural block did not affect uterine contractions in any of the groups, and the overall duration of labor was the same in all three groups. This phenomenon, which could be related to inhibited release of oxytocin or atrial natriuretic peptide, may partially explain the transient decrease in uterine contractility commonly associated with epidural analgesia. Nevertheless, the effect should not dissuade the anesthesiologist from administering a clinically indicated fluid bolus before epidural analgesia. Scull et al. demonstrated that, although plasma β-endorphin and cortisol levels decrease after the establishment of epidural analgesia at a cervical dilation of 5 cm or less, oxytocin concentrations and the frequency of uterine contractions are unchanged (89).

Craft et al. demonstrated that the decreased uterine activity associated with epidural analgesia did not occur when the patient was in the lateral position (90). By analyzing uterine activity before and after top-up doses of bupivacaine during epidural block, Schellenberg also concluded that aortocaval compression, not local anesthetic administration, was the apparent reason for decreased uterine activity (91). These investigations suggest that decreased uterine perfusion can occur in the absence of demonstrable hypotension.

Epinephrine is sometimes added to local anesthetics to augment analgesia, prolong duration, and decrease blood concentration, effects that are mediated by α-adrenergic receptors. However, β-agonism could depress uterine activity. Older studies with large doses of epinephrine (100 to 125 μg) during caudal anesthesia suggested that it prolonged the first stage (92, 93). However, several other studies using concentrations of epinephrine ranging from 1:200,000 to 1:1,000,000 combined with lidocaine, bupivacaine, and chloroprocaine concluded that it does not prolong the first stage (74, 90, 94–99).

A common side effect of regional anesthesia is hypotension, and occasionally vasopressors must be used to restore maternal

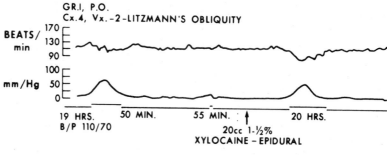

Figure 3.6. Three mg methoxamine were administered to treat maternal hypotension following epidural anesthesia. The upper tracing (*fetal heart rate*) shows a severe fetal bradycardia; the lower tracing (*intraamniotic pressure*) shows the tetanic uterine contraction that resulted from methoxamine. (Reprinted by permission from Vasicka A, Hutchinson HT, Eng M, Allen CR. Spinal and epidural anesthesia, fetal and uterine response to acute hypotension and hypertension. *Am J Obstet Gynecol* 1964;90:800–810.)

blood pressure. These drugs may have direct effects on uterine muscle. There are both α- and β-adrenergic receptors in uterine muscle. α-adrenergic vasopressors such as Phenylephrine (Neo-Synephrine) and methoxamine (Vasoxyl) may cause an increase in uterine tone and tetanic contractions (Fig. 3.6). Ephedrine has little effect on uterine activity.

Other aspects of the epidural technique—such as intermittent bolus injection vs. continuous infusion (100–103); the addition of fentanyl (104–107), alfentanil (108), or sufentanil (109–110); and the administration of pain relief by patient-controlled epidural analgesia (PCEA) (111–114) have generally been shown not to affect the duration of the first stage of labor. A single study, however, suggested that reducing the dose of bupivacaine and adding fentanyl to a continuous infusion increased the time from epidural insertion to full dilation, although the length of the first stage of labor was the same (115). Reducing the concentration of ropivacaine from 0.2% to 0.125% when administered by PCEA (116) or of bupivacaine from 0.25% to 0.1% by intermittent bolus (117) did not affect the duration of the first stage, nor did reducing the concentration of bupivacaine from 0.25% to 0.0625% (with sufentanil) by continuous infusion (99). Another investigation reported an overall shorter duration of labor after analgesia was begun in the PCEA group vs. the conventional epidural group, but the authors did not report the stages of labor separately (118).

Second Stage of Labor and Mode of Delivery

Some studies (32, 119) have indicated that patients receiving epidural analgesia have longer second stages, yet others (120–123) have failed to establish a difference. Epidural block has been reported to affect not only the duration of the second stage of labor, but also the frequency of instrumental (forceps and vacuum) and cesarean delivery. Investigators report an incredible range in frequency of operative vaginal deliveries in association with conduction block. Jouppila et al. (49) reported no vacuum deliveries in multiparas who received epidural analgesia. However, Browne and Catton (124) found an operative vaginal delivery rate of 84.2% in parturients who had received epidural blockade. A recent retrospective study of over 7,300 deliveries reported far more forceps (30.7% vs. 4.0%) and vacuum (3.5% vs. 0.7%) deliveries in the epidural group but no increase in cesarean section (125). Similarly, epidural analgesia has been reported to have no effect on the risk of cesarean birth (65, 66) and, conversely, to increase the risk of cesarean birth by up to nearly 12-fold (70) (Table 3.3) summarize these studies.

How Epidural Analgesia Might Affect the Second Stage

There are several reasons why conduction analgesia could affect the length of the second stage and the mode of delivery: (a) interference with oxytocin release, (b) impairment of maternal expulsive efforts, (c) increase in fetal malposition, (d) effects of second-stage analgesia per se, and (e) accentuation of the difficulties associated with nulliparity. Each of these factors is considered below.

Release of Oxytocin

Some authorities have proposed that distention of the lower vagina by the fetal presenting part leads to an increase in the release of oxytocin, and that this *Ferguson reflex* might be interrupted by epidural blockade. However, it is not clear that such a reflex exists in humans, because a correlation cannot be demonstrated between a rise in the plasma concentration of oxytocin and spontaneous delivery (127). Furthermore, tremendous variation exists among parturients in the serum concentration of oxytocin necessary to produce adequate uterine contractility (128), and an increase in oxytocin receptors may be more important than the plasma concentration (129). Two prospective, randomized, double-blind studies reached conflicting conclusions with regard to the effects of an oxytocin infusion for women receiving epidural analgesia with respect to the duration of labor and operative delivery (130, 131).

Maternal Expulsive Effort

Epidural blockade can affect the adequacy of the maternal expulsive effort. Nearly 50% of patients given 0.25% bupivacaine by bolus injections lose the urge to bear down, and this can be associated with instrumental delivery (48). Motor block and loss of the bearing-down reflex are associated with increasing concentration of bupivacaine (0.5% vs. 0.25%) but not with increasing volume of injection (33, 132, 132a). On the other hand, the quality of analgesia is related more to the volume injected than the concentration of bupivacaine (132, 133). The use of more dilute local anesthetics has gained popularity.

Fetal Malposition

Several retrospective and prospective nonrandomized studies have reported an increase in fetal malposition (persistent occiput posterior or transverse position) and the use of rotational forceps in patients who received epidural analgesia (32, 134, 135). These studies suggest that the malposition might result from relaxation of the pelvic muscles caused by the conduction block, while other prospective studies do not attribute an increase in malposition to epidural analgesia. In their nonrandomized investigation of over 1,000 parturients, Thornburn and Moir noted that, although malposition did occur more often in the epidural group, it was not necessarily related to the degree of motor weakness (33). They further speculated that the abnormality of labor resulting in malposition might also have caused the severe pain that led to the mother's choice of epidural analgesia. A randomized trial of nulliparas showed that patients for whom epidural analgesia was withheld once the fetal head reached the ischial spines were more likely to deliver from the occiput posterior or transverse position than women who received analgesia until delivery (136). Floberg et al. demonstrated in a study of more than 1,400 women that small pelvic outlet capacity is associated with both persistent occiput posterior position and the use of epidural analgesia, but epidural blockade is not independently associated with malposition (40).

Second Stage Analgesia

Some investigators have suggested that the high rate of forceps deliveries, especially rotational forceps, associated with epidural analgesia might be decreased if longer second stages were accepted (32, 137). Because it had been noted that neonatal mortality was associated with longer labor (138), older obstetric teaching dictated operative delivery if the second stage persisted beyond 1 (139) or 2 (118, 140) hours. Thus, many of the labors in the early studies may have been terminated by forceps delivery because an arbitrary amount of time had elapsed. However, it may not be necessary to intervene at any particular time as long as the fetal heart rate pattern is reassuring (140–142). The American College of Obstetricians and Gynecologists (ACOG) recommends that, as long as fetal monitoring is reassuring, the second stage should not be considered prolonged in the presence of epidural analgesia until 3 hours have passed for nulliparas or 2 hours for parous women (Table 3.4) (126). Arbitrary use of forceps for teaching purposes or convenience certainly increases the forceps delivery rate.

Four studies have shown that, for parturients receiving epidural analgesia, delaying maternal expulsive effort until the fetal head is below the level of the ischial spines (136), visible at the introitus (139, 143), 1 or 2 hours have passed since attainment of complete cervical dilation (127, 143), or the mother feels an irresistible urge to push (143) reduces the incidence of forceps delivery. Two other investigations demonstrated no increase in spontaneous deliveries in such parturients who delayed pushing (144, 145).

Other areas of investigation concern whether the continuation of epidural analgesia throughout the second stage or the provision of a "perineal dose" increases the duration of the second stage and the incidence of operative delivery. (A "perineal dose" is a bolus of local anesthetic intended to block the sacral roots, and it is given with the patient in the sitting position.) Hoult et al. suggested that allowing the analgesia to wear off during the expulsive effort might improve the chance of spontaneous delivery (134). Similarly, Walton and Reynolds indicated that the use of sitting top-up doses in the first stage increases the

likelihood of operative vaginal delivery (146). However, a study by Phillips and Thomas contradicts this conclusion (136). Patients whose epidural analgesia was continued until delivery did not have longer second stages or higher rates of instrumental delivery than parturients whose analgesia was allowed to dissipate. In fact, for women older than 25 years, those given epidural blocks were less likely to be delivered instrumentally.

Chestnut et al. conducted three prospective, randomized, double-blind studies in which women were randomized to have epidural infusions either continued or converted to saline during the second stage (119, 121, 122). When 0.75% lidocaine was used, there was no difference in the length of the second stage or in the incidence of instrumental delivery (121). However, analgesia was not significantly different, either. When the local anesthetic was 0.125% bupivacaine, the group whose infusions were continued had significantly more low forceps and midpelvis vacuum deliveries, longer second stages, and more motor block (119). The analgesia was significantly better for these women. Parturients who had continuous infusions of 0.0625% bupivacaine plus 2 μg/mL fentanyl maintained until delivery had better analgesia than those whose infusions were changed to saline, and there was no difference between groups in duration of the second stage or rate of instrumental deliveries (122). However, the analgesia was "only marginally better" in the group whose bupivacaine-fentanyl infusions were continued (147). In all three studies, there was no difference in cesarean section among groups.

Three other prospective trials have also examined this issue. In a randomized trial of 200 nulliparas, Johnsrud et al. showed that a continuous infusion of 0.25% bupivacaine during the second stage did not affect its duration or the incidence of operative vaginal delivery if routine IV oxytocin infusions were employed (148). Luxman et al. randomized women to have intermittent boluses of 0.25% bupivacaine stopped at 8 cm dilation or continued until delivery, and they reported no difference in oxytocin augmentation, length of the second stage, or instrumental or cesarean delivery (149). In a nonrandomized study, Gal et al. compared 3% chloroprocaine epidurally to local perineal infiltration of 1% lidocaine for patients who had received epidural bupivacaine in the first stage (77). There was no difference in the length of the second stage, but the epidural group had six times more low forceps deliveries.

Parity

Most studies regarding parity have shown that, among those receiving epidural analgesia, nulliparas are more likely than multiparas to have an instrumental delivery (32, 34, 48, 49, 120, 132, 146, 150–157). However, one study has indicated the reverse (158), and another has suggested no difference (159).

Prevalence Studies

Because women who receive epidural analgesia can be so different from other parturients, it may be inappropriate to presume that the high rates of operative delivery observed for these patients are a result of the analgesia. Several studies have attempted to resolve this issue by examining the impact of a change in the prevalence of epidural analgesia on the overall percentage of operative delivery in an obstetric department, and most report no change when conduction analgesia became available (160–165).

Palmer et al. reported that a 28.8% increase in regional analgesia for labor was associated with a 25.5% decrease in cesarean section rate over the same 7-year period (166). Similarly, Poma found that a more than doubling in the use of regional analgesia over a 7-year period (to a total prevalence of 30.4%) was associated with a fall in cesarean section rate from 25.5% to 15.5% (167). Forceps deliveries also decreased in the study period, while vacuum extractions increased.

Examining the phenomenon from another perspective, Johnson and Rosenfeld studied the effects of a sudden decrease in

---

Table 3.4. ACOG DEFINITIONS FOR PROLONGED SECOND STAGE OF LABOR

Nullipara
More than 2 h without regional analgesia
More than 3 h with regional analgesia

Multipara
More than 1 h without regional analgesia
More than 2 h with regional analgesia

Based upon information from Committee on Technical Bulletins of the American College of Obstetricians and Gynecologists. *Operative Vaginal Delivery.* ACOG Technical Bulletin No. 196; August 1994.

epidural use after a change in reimbursement (168). Although the epidural rate fell from 71% to 27%, there was no change in cesarean section rates, yet there was a decrease in the average length of the second stage and in forceps deliveries.

Prospective Randomized Studies

Several prospective randomized comparisons between epidural analgesia and parenteral opioids have been reported (Table 3.3) (71). Two older studies by Philipsen et al. (67) and Robinson et al. (69) randomized women of mixed parity to receive epidural block or intramuscular meperidine once they requested analgesia. The former investigation reported no difference in the duration of the second stage or the rate of instrumental or cesarean delivery (67). However, no epidural injections were given during the second stage, and only 44% of patients received more than one dose. The latter study compared 0.5% bupivacaine (a concentration rarely used for analgesia today) with meperidine and promethazine combined with inhalation analgesia (69). The investigators found that the patients who received epidural analgesia had longer second stages and more forceps deliveries. (There were no cesarean deliveries.) In both studies, the epidural block provided superior analgesia.

Epidural Analgesia and Increased Cesarean Section Rate

As a result of several recent retrospective studies (135, 169–171), suggesting that epidural analgesia is associated with increased risk of cesarean section for dystocia, several newer prospective studies have been published (47, 65, 66, 68, 69). Because of the potential selection bias in their retrospective studies (170, 171), Thorp et al. conducted a prospective, randomized, unblinded investigation of 93 nulliparas in spontaneous labor who received epidural analgesia or IV meperidine plus promethazine (70). The epidural patients received an initial bolus of 0.25% bupivacaine followed by an infusion of 0.125% bupivacaine. The control group received IV meperidine 75 mg plus promethazine 25 mg every 90 minutes as needed. The authors concluded that epidural analgesia is associated with (a) a slowing of cervical dilation, (b) an increase in the duration of the first and second stages, (c) a greater likelihood of oxytocin augmentation, (d) an increase in fetal malposition (persistent occiput transverse or posterior), and (e) cesarean section for dystocia. There was no difference between the groups with regard to instrumental delivery, and the quality of analgesia was superior at all times in the epidural group. The authors further concluded that there is little or no increased risk of cesarean section if epidural analgesia is delayed until at least 5 cm cervical dilation. However, this investigation has been extensively criticized for methodological problems (172–176).

Ramin et al. recently reported another prospective, randomized, unblinded comparison of epidural analgesia with parenteral opioids (68). Women of mixed parity (n = 1,330) in spontaneous labor with cervical dilation of 3 to 5 cm were randomized to receive epidural bupivacaine 0.25% followed by infusion of bupivacaine 0.125% plus fentanyl 2 μg/mL or up to four doses of IV meperidine 50 mg plus promethazine 50 mg. Epidural analgesia was associated with better analgesia, longer labors (the first and second stages were not reported separately), second stages lasting more than 2 hours, more use of oxytocin, and more low forceps and cesarean deliveries for dystocia, especially in parous women. This study was criticized because over one third of the patients did not receive the analgesia to which they were randomized and because of the analytic methods used (172). As a result, the same group conducted another investigation comparing the same type of epidural analgesia with meperidine by patient-controlled IV analgesia (PCIA) in 358 women of mixed parity (66). The authors hoped that the use of PCIA would reduce the crossover between groups. Using an intention-to-treat analysis (analyzing groups by original randomization as opposed to protocol-compliance), the authors concluded that there was no difference between groups in instrumental delivery or cesarean section for all indications (Table 3.5). Analgesia was superior in the epidural group, and more infants of mothers receiving PCIA required naloxone. Again, nearly one third of the parturients in each group were not compliant with the protocol. The same authors recently reported similar preliminary results from an investigation of the same design involving parturients with preeclampsia (177).

Bofill et al. randomized 100 nulliparas who had reached at least 4 cm cervical dilation to receive epidural infusion of bupivacaine 0.125% plus fentanyl 1.5 μg/mL or IV butorphanol (1 to 2 mg IV/1 to 2 hours as needed) (65). There were no differences in the length of the first or second stages, oxytocin use, or cesarean sections for dystocia. More operative vaginal deliveries occurred in the epidural group, but the authors stated that most were for resident training. As in all of the prospective studies, the analgesia provided by the epidural technique was significantly better than that for the opioid group.

Table 3.5. METHOD OF DELIVERY BASED UPON INTENT-TO-TREAT ANALYSIS ACCORDING TO RANDOMIZATION

Method of Delivery	Epidural Analgesia (%) (n = 358)	Intravenous Meperidine Analgesia (%) (n = 357)
Spontaneous*	89	91
Instrumental vaginal*		
Total	7	4
Low forceps[†]	6	3
Outlet forceps[‡]	1	1
Cesarean delivery*		
Total	4	5
Dystocia	3	3
Nonreasurring FHR tracing	1	2
Overall operative delivery*	11	9

FHR = fetal heart rate.
*There were no significant differences between the two groups.
[†]Low forceps: +2 cm to +4 cm below the ischeal spines.
[‡]Outlet forceps: fetal head at the perineum.
From Sharma SK, Sidawi JE, Ramin SM, Lucas MJ, Leveno KJ, Cunningham G. Cesarean delivery;
A randomized trial of epidural versus patient-controlled meperidine analgesia during labor.
Anesthesiology 1997;87:487–494.

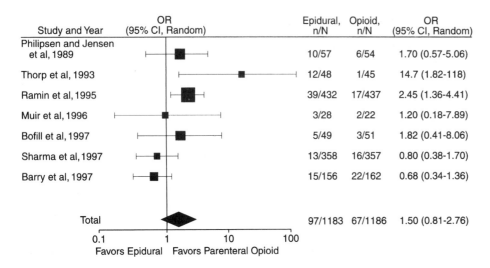

Study and Year	OR (95% CI, Random)	Epidural, n/N	Opioid, n/N	OR (95% CI, Random)
Philipsen and Jensen et al, 1989		10/57	6/54	1.70 (0.57-5.06)
Thorp et al, 1993		12/48	1/45	14.7 (1.82-118)
Ramin et al, 1995		39/432	17/437	2.45 (1.36-4.41)
Muir et al, 1996		3/28	2/22	1.20 (0.18-7.89)
Bofill et al, 1997		5/49	3/51	1.82 (0.41-8.06)
Sharma et al, 1997		13/358	16/357	0.80 (0.38-1.70)
Barry et al, 1997		15/156	22/162	0.68 (0.34-1.36)
Total		97/1183	67/1186	1.50 (0.81-2.76)

0.1   1   10   100
Favors Epidural   Favors Parenteral Opioid

Figure 3.7. Total rate of cesarean delivery did not differ significantly between patients receiving epidural anesthesia (8.2% [97/1183]) vs. parenteral opioids (5.6% [67/1186]) for labor. (Reprinted by permission from Halpern SH, Leighton BCL, Ohlsson A, Barrett JFR, Rice A. Effect of epidural vs. parenteral opioid analgesia on the progress of labor; Ameteanalysis. *JAMA* 1998;280:2105–2110.)

In their randomized trial of nulliparas, Clark et al. compared 156 women assigned to receive an epidural infusion of bupivacaine 0.125% plus fentanyl 1 μg/mL (after a bolus of 0.25% bupivacaine and 50 μg fentanyl) with 162 assigned to IV meperidine 50 to 75 mg every 90 minutes as needed (47). There were no differences between groups with respect to oxytocin use, length of second stage, spontaneous delivery, use of forceps or vacuum extractor, cesarean section for any indication, or cesarean section for dystocia. The conclusions regarding operative delivery are even more remarkable, given that they were true whether the data were analyzed according to intention-to-treat or protocol-compliance. The superior analgesia of the epidural technique is confirmed by the 52% crossover rate from the intravenous to the regional method.

An analysis of 10 prospective comparisons of epidural analgesia and parenteral opioids concluded that epidural analgesia does not cause an increase in overall cesarean section rate or section for dystocia among nulliparas or multiparas (Fig. 3.7) (71). Epidural blocks were associated with longer first and second stages, increased oxytocin use, increased instrumental delivery (overall, but not for dystocia) better analgesia and satisfaction, and better neonatal outcome (Table 3.6).

Zhang et al., a group of epidemiologists from the National Institute of Child Health and Human Development, presented a "quantitative summary" of seven randomized trials and five observational studies (178). In addition to a thorough review of the results, strengths, and weaknesses of the various papers, the authors conducted a metaanalysis of the randomized trials. After considering all of the data, they came to the following conclusion: Epidural analgesia increases the requirement for oxytocin augmentation, slightly increases the likelihood of instrumental delivery, and might prolong the duration of labor; however, it does not increase the risk of cesarean delivery.

Timing of Analgesia

In an attempt to resolve some of the contradictions in the literature, many studies have examined the contributions of various aspects of epidural analgesia technique. For example, in response to Thorp's findings (70, 171), Chestnut et al. investigated whether the timing of the initiation of epidural analgesia affected the outcome of labor in nulliparas (179, 180). Both studies had the same basic design: the authors enrolled parturients who requested epidural analgesia while at a cervical dilation of 3 or 4 cm. At that time, the women were randomized either to begin epidural analgesia immediately (early group) or to wait until a cervical dilation of 5 cm (late group). The early group received intermittent boluses of 0.25% bupivacaine until they reached 5 cm dilation when an infusion of 0.125% bupivacaine was begun. The late group received up to two doses

of IV nalbuphine 10 mg until reaching a cervical dilation of 5 cm, at which point they received the same epidural analgesia as the early group. The first study examined nulliparas already receiving IV oxytocin at the time of randomization (179), and the second, nulliparas in spontaneous labor at the time of randomization (180). Both studies found no difference between the early and late groups with respect to length of the first stage after randomization, length of the second stage, incidence of malposition, frequency of instrumental deliveries, or cesarean section for all indications. Initial analgesia and maternal satisfaction were better in the early group.

Rogers et al. reported that, among women who deliver vaginally, epidural placement at 4 cm or less is associated with shorter labor as opposed to later placement (181). Two other studies, one retrospective (182) and one prospective (183), suggest that it makes no difference to the outcome of labor whether epidural analgesia is commenced before or after 3 or 4 cm dilation.

Choice of Local Anesthetic

Study results are conflicting on whether the choice and concentration of local anesthetic affect the second stage of labor and mode of delivery. Abboud et al. concluded that patients receiving 0.125% bupivacaine infusions are less likely to have spontaneous deliveries than those receiving 0.75% chloroprocaine or 0.75% lidocaine infusions (76), whereas Feiss et al. detected no difference in the incidence of forceps deliveries between women receiving 0.25% bupivacaine or 2% chloroprocaine (184). With respect to the effects resulting from decreasing the concentration of bupivacaine by adding an opioid, some studies report a decrease in instrumental and cesarean deliveries (185, 186), while others report no change (99, 115, 174, 175). Whereas most studies comparing ropivacaine to bupivacaine for labor epidural analgesia report no difference in length of the second stage or mode of delivery (78, 79, 176, 187–191), two investigations suggest that ropivacaine may increase the likelihood of spontaneous delivery (80, 192). Therefore, ropivacaine and bupivacaine may need further evaluation after their relative potencies have been better evaluated (86, 87, 193, 194).

Infusion vs. Intermittent Bolus

Studies comparing continuous epidural infusions with intermittent bolus injections have yielded conflicting results. Smedstad and Morison showed that there was no difference in the length of the second stage or in the quality of analgesia between groups of women who received 0.25% bupivacaine by bolus or infusion (195). However, the infusion group had significantly more outlet forceps deliveries. Li et al. compared 0.25% bupivacaine bolus injections with infusions of 0.0625% or 0.125% bupivacaine at various rates and found no difference in duration of the

Table 3.6.

Outcome	Epidural n/N	Opioid n/N	OR or WMD (95% CI)	P Value
Instrumented delivery*	179/1155	104/1164	2.19 (1.32–7.78)	.02
Instrumented delivery for dystocia*	13/106	18/105	0.68 (0.31–1.49)	.25
Labor length, 1st stage, min[†]	524	555	42 (17–68)	.02
Labor length, 2nd stage, min[†]	581	609	14 (5–23)	.003
Oxytocin after analgesia*	218/487	165/514	1.80 (1.01–3.21)	.04
Fever (>38.0°C)*	156/675	37/696	5.35 (3.67–7.80)	<.001
Hypotension*	312/839	1/845	74.2 (4.0–1375)	<.001
Pain, 1st stage, mm[†,‡]	N = 1017	N = 1014	−40 (−38 to −42)	<.001
Pain, 2nd stage, mm[†,‡]	N = 536	N = 526	−29 (−21 to −38)	<.001
Dissatisfaction*	117/781	324/800	0.25 (0.20–0.32)	<.001
Apgar score <7 at 1 min*	39/1004	68/1011	0.54 (0.35–0.82)	.001
Apgar score <7 at 5 min*	9/1089	25/1087	0.38 (0.18–0.81)	.003
Need for naloxone in the newborn*	3/407	14/408	0.24 (0.07–0.77)	<.001

An odds ratio (OR) of less than 1 favors epidural analgesia; n indicates the number of events; N, the total number of patients in the analysis.
*Dichotomous data are shown as OR and 95% confidence interval (CI) using a random effects model.
[†]Continuous data are shown as weighted mean difference (WMD) and 95% CI using a random effects model; negative numbers favor epidural analgesia; N indicates the total number of patients in the analysis.
[‡]Visual analog pain scores use a 100-mm scale.
Adapted from Halpern SH, Leighton BL, Ohlsson A, Barrett JFR, Rice A. Effect of epidural vs parenteral opioid analgesia on the progress of labor; A meta-analysis. *JAMA* 1998;280;2105–2110.

second stage, motor block, mode of delivery, or quality of analgesia (103). Similarly, Boutros et al. found no difference using bupivacaine plus sufentanil (196). In an investigation comparing boluses and infusions of bupivacaine with fentanyl, D'Athis et al. found better analgesia in the infusion group but no difference in the mode of delivery (101). Bogod et al. compared 0.5% bupivacaine injections with infusions of the 0.125% concentration and reported no difference in mode of delivery or maternal satisfaction (100). When comparing intermittent boluses of 0.25% bupivacaine with an infusion of 0.125%, Lamont et al. detected no difference in duration of the second stage, length of expulsive effort, mode of delivery, or neonatal outcome (102). The analgesia was superior and there was a lower frequency of hypotension in the infusion group. In a retrospective study of epidural bupivacaine-fentanyl boluses vs. infusions, Driver et al. concluded that the infusion group was less likely to require cesarean section (197). The use of dilute continuous infusions may lead to better patient satisfaction and lower doses of local anesthetic, but the effect upon operative deliveries is hard to predict given the many variables involved.

Patient-Controlled Epidural Analgesia

Several studies have compared continuous epidural infusions with PCEA and found no difference in the length or outcome of labor (112–114, 196, 198). Viscomi and Eisenach found no effect on the mode of delivery, but they reported a shorter duration of labor in the PCEA group (118). In a study comparing PCEA solutions, Paech reported fewer spontaneous deliveries in women receiving 0.25% bupivacaine compared to more dilute concentrations plus fentanyl (199). However, there were more nulliparas in the 0.25% bupivacaine group. A similar investigation comparing 0.2% and 0.125% ropivacaine by PCEA reported no difference in length of second stage or mode of delivery (116).

Effect of Technique

Naulty et al. examined the effect of a change in the technique of epidural analgesia upon operative delivery (200). Instead of using intermittent boluses of a high concentration of lidocaine during the first stage of labor and no analgesia during the

second stage, the investigators administered low concentrations of bupivacaine with fentanyl by continuous infusion until delivery. Although the fraction of patients receiving epidural analgesia increased, the overall number of operative vaginal deliveries and cesarean sections decreased. Olofsson et al. compared 0.25% bupivacaine plus epinephrine with 0.125% bupivacaine plus sufentanil 10 μg by intermittent bolus. 201). The lower concentration of local anesthetic plus opioid was associated with less use of oxytocin and fewer instrumental and abdominal deliveries. A similar study found that, when compared for use in bolus administration, 0.125% bupivacaine plus fentanyl is associated with a shorter second stage and fewer forceps deliveries than plain 0.25% bupivacaine (117). However, another study found no difference in second stage duration or mode of delivery among groups receiving bupivacaine 0.25%, 0.625% with sufentanil, or 0.625% with sufentanil and epinephrine (99).

Adjuvants

Many investigations have compared a variety of epidural analgesia recipes using the *opioids* fentanyl, sufentanil, alfentanil, and butorphanol added to bupivacaine, and most show no effect on the duration of the second stage or mode of delivery (104–106, 108, 109, 201, 211). However, two prospective, randomized, double-blind studies have suggested that the addition of sufentanil to intermittent epidural bolus injections of bupivacaine might increase the frequency of spontaneous delivery (110, 208).

Abboud et al. reported that the addition of *epinephrine* 1:300,000 to 0.5% bupivacaine and 1.5% lidocaine or epinephrine 1:200,000 to 2% chloroprocaine did not affect the duration of the second stage or the mode of delivery (94–96). Similarly, epinephrine 1:1,000,000 added to bupivacaine improved analgesia but did not affect second stage or delivery mode in a study by Dahl et al. (99). Additionally, Zador and Nilsson demonstrated that adding epinephrine to lidocaine administered by continuous infusion had no effect upon the duration of the second stage (74).

It is unclear whether the addition of *clonidine* to epidural analgesia will be advantageous, because of its associated side effects (209, 210). However, prospective investigations have demonstrated no difference in duration of labor when clonidine was added to bupivacaine-epinephrine-sufentanil (211), bupivacaine-sufentanil (212), bupivacaine-fentanyl (213), or bupivacaine-fentanyl-neostigmine (213). One of the studies also showed no difference in mode of delivery (211). (Mode of delivery was not reported in the others.)

Obstetric Management

Many studies have examined the effects of epidural analgesia as though it were the most influential variable in labor. However, other factors beyond analgesia, especially obstetric management, exert at least as great an effect upon the rate of operative delivery. At the National Maternity Hospital in Dublin, where AML originated, the use of epidural analgesia has increased nearly 6-fold without a concomitant rise in instrumental or cesarean deliveries (214). Four studies demonstrated that encouraging an attempt at vaginal birth after prior cesarean section combined with staff education and the use of management protocols for treating dystocia can decrease the rate of cesarean section by up to 50% (215–218). In all of the investigations, the use of epidural analgesia increased over the period of the study. The frequency with which an obstetrician's patients receive epidural analgesia is not associated with his or her cesarean rate for dystocia (219). Rogers et al. concluded that active management shortens labor for women who receive epidural analgesia (181).

Other studies have demonstrated the extent to which factors other than analgesia affect cesarean section rate. All of the following are associated with variations in abdominal delivery rates: maternal age (for nulliparas) (220), physician age (221), group vs. solo practice (221), private vs. clinic patient (222, 223), private nonteaching hospital vs. public or private teaching hospital (224), insurance coverage (225), surgeon's malpractice premium (226), obstetric case mix (227), midwife vs. obstetrician management (228), family physician vs. obstetrician management (229), availability of perinatologists (230), the choice of labor nurse (231), department policies (232), and the patient's subjective rating of pain during the latent phase (233). Parrish et al. suggested that increases in primiparity, maternal age, and birth weight account for 25% of the increase in primary cesarean section rate in the United States (234). Using multivariate analysis, Piper et al. demonstrated that the use of epidural analgesia, active phase duration, parity, patient height, birth weight, and station at complete cervical dilation together account for less than 25% of the

variance in second stage duration (235). The remaining variance is unexplained.

INTRATHECAL AND COMBINED SPINAL-EPIDURAL ANALGESIA

There has recently been a resurgence of interest in intrathecal analgesia for labor, especially using the combined spinal-epidural (CSE) technique (Chapter 9) (236). Spinal analgesia provides excellent pain relief with minimal to no motor block. This facilitates maternal ambulation, perhaps even better than very dilute epidural solutions, although the effect of walking on the progress of labor may be minimal (Table 3.7) (237). Two hundred and twenty-nine women who received a combined spinal-epidural block for labor were randomly allocated to stay in bed or spend at least 20 minutes of every hour out of bed during labor; there was no significant difference in duration of labor (Fig. 3.8), analgesia requirements, mode of delivery, or condition of the baby at birth (238).

Honet et al. demonstrated that there is no difference among intrathecal fentanyl, sufentanil, and meperidine with respect to the duration and outcome of labor (239). The addition of epinephrine does not appear to affect the progress of labor (240–242).

Several studies have compared CSE to conventional bupivacaine epidural analgesia. Abouleish et al. reported that the subarachnoid injection of 0.2 mg morphine prolongs the first stage of labor but does not affect mode of delivery (243). Other studies with intrathecal sufentanil (244), fentanyl-bupivacaine (245–247), or sufentanil-bupivacaine-epinephrine (248) compared to epidural bupivacaine with or without adjuvants demonstrated no effect on the duration or outcome of labor. A single investigation comparing spinal to epidural administration of sufentanil found no difference with respect to labor progress (249). After randomizing nulliparas to CSE with bupivacaine 2.5 mg plus sufentanil 10 μg or epidural bupivacaine 0.25%, Tsen et al. determined that cervical dilation and first stage were more rapid in the CSE group, while there were no differences in second stage or mode of delivery (250). In a prospective trial, Nageotte et al. randomized nulliparas to receive 10 μg intrathecal sufentanil followed by an epidural infusion of 0.0625% bupivacaine plus fentanyl 2 μg/mL or an epidural bolus of 0.25% bupivacaine plus 50 μg fentanyl followed by an infusion of 0.125% bupivacaine plus 2 μg/mL fentanyl (251). The CSE group had a lower incidence of operative vaginal delivery. However, there

Table 3.7. COMPARISON OF THE EFFECT OF WALKING ON SELECTED LABOR AND DELIVERY OUTCOMES IN NULLIPAROUS AND PAROUS WOMEN*

Outcome	Nulliparous Women			Parous Women		
	Walking Group (n = 272)	Usual-Care Group (n = 272)	P Value	Walking Group (n = 264)	Usual-Care Group (n = 259)	P Value
Labor—hour						
First stage	7.6 ± 3.9	7.3 ± 3.9	.47	4.6 ± 2.4	4.7 ± 2.4	.60
Second stage	1.0 ± 0.9	0.9 ± 0.8	.46	0.2 ± 0.3	0.2 ± 0.3	.42
Labor augmentation—No. (%)[†]	95 (35)	99 (36)	.72	27 (10)	38 (15)	.12
Forceps delivery—No. (%)	21 (8)	15 (6)	.30	2 (1)	2 (1)	.99
Cesarean birth—No. (%)	19 (7)	21 (8)	.74	4 (2)	10 (4)	.10

* Values are means ± SD.
[†] Labor augmentation was defined as stimulation of labor with oxytocin because of inadequate uterine contractions.
Data from Bloom SL, McIntire DD, Kelly MA, et al. Lack of effect of walking on labor and delivery. *N Engl J Med* 1998;339:76–79.

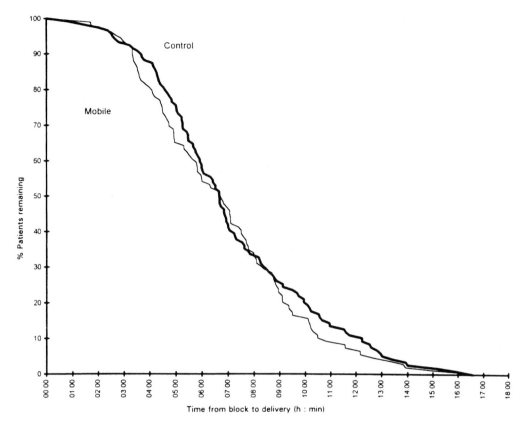

Figure 3.8. Effect of maternal ambulation on labor with low-dose combined spinal-epidural analgesia. There was no difference in the percentage of patients remaining in labor over time(mobile women in labor with combined spinal-epidural [n = 110] vs. patients on bed rest [n = 119]). (Reprinted by permission from Collis RE, Harding SA, Morgan BM. Effect of maternal ambulation on labour with lowdose combined spinal-epidural analgesia. *Anesthesia* 1999;54:535–539.)

were no differences in rate of cesarean section, pain relief, or satisfaction. A similar, smaller study reached the same conclusion regarding mode of delivery when comparing intrathecal sufentanil to epidural bupivacaine when both were followed by epidural bupivacaine-fentanyl by PCEA (252). The intrathecal group had better motor and pain scores. Palmer et al. showed that adding bupivacaine to fentanyl administered intrathecally as part of a CSE technique did not affect the incidence of cesarean vs. vaginal delivery (253).

Gambling et al. randomized parturients to receive CSE or IV meperidine (254). The CSE group received 10 μg intrathecal sufentanil followed later in labor by a bolus of 0.25% bupivacaine and an infusion of 0.125% bupivacaine with fentanyl. The IV group received 50 mg meperidine plus promethazine followed by 50 mg meperidine every hour. An intention-to-treat analysis determined that there was no difference between groups with respect to forceps delivery for dystocia, cesarean section overall, or section for dystocia. CSE was associated with longer first and second stages, more use of oxytocin, more low forceps deliveries for nonreassuring fetal heart rate abnormalities, superior analgesia, and better maternal satisfaction. CSE was also associated with more operative deliveries for profound fetal bradycardia within the first hour after initiation of analgesia, but there was no overall difference in neonatal outcome.

While others have also reported that fetal bradycardia is associated with the administration of intrathecal opioids (255), one prospective study did not find an association between CSE and fetal heart rate abnormalities (256). A retrospective study concluded that CSE is not associated with an increased risk of emergency cesarean section (257) (See Chapter 9).

One investigation suggests no difference in length of labor or mode of delivery among groups receiving various doses of intrathecal clonidine, sufentanil, or a combination of the two (258). However, each group was small. Clonidine has been shown to improve epidural and spinal analgesia (259) for labor and will undergo further evaluation in the future (See Chapter 9).

SUMMARY AND CONCLUSIONS

Although there is controversy regarding the effects of epidural analgesia on labor, it is possible to draw several conclusions.

1) **Epidural analgesia is safe for the fetus** and may improve neonatal outcome.

2) As demonstrated by maternal satisfaction in the prospective studies (Table 3.3) **epidural block provides unparalleled analgesia**. Harrison et al. studied primigravidas who chose epidural analgesia, meperidine-promethazine, Entonox (N_2O-O_2), or transcutaneous electrical nerve stimulation (260). Only epidural analgesia provided complete relief of pain. Furthermore, 46% of parturients who received meperidine-promethazine reported no relief. MacArthur et al. surveyed 11,701 women months to years after delivery (261). Of those who received epidural analgesia, 69% reported full satisfaction—more than twice the percentage for any other method. Therefore, despite its disadvantages, there is no equally-effective substitute for epidural labor analgesia.

3) Provided that uterine displacement is maintained and hypotension avoided, **epidural analgesia probably has little effect on the progress of labor during the first stage**. A transient decrease in uterine activity, possibly related to the IV fluid bolus, may occur after establishment of the block, but normal contractions resume within 30 minutes. **There is no reason to avoid epidural analgesia during the latent phase of the first stage,**

especially since parenteral analgesics have also been suspected of its prolongation (27). It is more important to provide pain relief on request than to deny it until an arbitrary cervical dilation has been attained.

4) **Epidural analgesia can increase the length of the second stage, but using the minimum effective concentration of local anesthetic appears to minimize this problem**. The addition of small amounts of opioid to the epidural solution allows one to reduce the local anesthetic concentration and may improve the chance for spontaneous delivery. In any case, less fetal acidosis develops during a prolonged first or second stage when epidural analgesia is employed (73, 74, 262–265).

5) **The rate of low and outlet instrumental deliveries might be increased in parturients, especially nulliparas, who receive epidural blockade**. However, several studies have demonstrated that such low-station operative vaginal procedures do not increase neonatal morbidity (138, 266–269). Furthermore, a retrospective study of more than 15,000 deliveries showed that epidural analgesia is not associated with increased incidence or severity of birth-canal trauma (270). Epidural analgesia may allow difficult labors to proceed for longer periods with oxytocin augmentation, thereby avoiding a cesarean section, even if an assisted vaginal delivery is ultimately required.

Finally, **epidural analgesia does not increase the likelihood of cesarean section**.

In light of what is known about the effects of epidural analgesia upon labor, what are appropriate goals when managing such a block? First, strive for analgesia, not anesthesia. Totally painless labor and a dense motor block are rarely in the parturient's best interest. Moreover, most women prefer to maintain some sensation, even if it is mildly uncomfortable, rather than receive a dense motor block. Second, reevaluate the block frequently. Labor is a dynamic process, and effective analgesia that facilitates spontaneous delivery requires constant refinement. Finally, **analgesia should be initiated whenever the patient requests it, and it should be maintained until delivery unless there is a strong indication that such a course is not in the patient's or fetus's interest**. If requested to allow a block to subside, before taking such action, consider the following with the obstetrician: Has the women been coached to bear-down properly? Would the use of an oxytocin infusion be helpful? Would decreasing the rate or concentration of the epidural infusion be a better course? Does the patient believe that more sensation would be helpful? When I am asked to discontinue an epidural infusion during the second stage, I ask the obstetrician to discuss the matter with the woman in my presence. Rarely does the patient believe that pain would be helpful. If necessary, one can usually adjust the epidural block to provide more helpful pressure sensation without increasing discomfort.

The course of labor is quite unpredictable because it is influenced by so many factors. Many things, including regional analgesia, affect the progress of labor. Judicious management by both anesthesiologist and obstetrician can result in maternal comfort without unnecessarily prolonging labor or increasing the risk to mother or baby.

REFERENCES

1. Alvarez H, Caldeyro-Barcia R. Contractility of the human uterus recorded by new methods. *Surg Gynecol Obstet* 1950;91:1–13.
2. Hon EH, Paul RH. Quantitation of uterine activity. *Obstet Gynecol* 1973;42:368–370.
3. O'Driscoll K, Meagher D, Boylan P. *Active Management of Labor.* 3rd ed. London: Mosby-Year Book; 1993.
4. Friedman EA. The functional divisions of labor. *Am J Obstet Gynecol* 1971;109:274–280.
5. Cunningham FG, MacDonald PC, Gant NF. Parturition: Biomolecular and physiological processes. In: *Williams Obstetrics.* 18th ed. Norwalk, CT: Appleton & Lange; 1989:213.
6. Cunningham FG, MacDonald PC, Gant NF, et al. Dystocia due to abnormalities of the expulsive forces. In: *Williams Obstetrics.* 19th ed. Norwalk, CT: Appleton and Lange; 1993:475–491.
7. Committee on Technical Bulletins of the American College of Obstetricians and Gynecologists. Dystocia and the augmentation of labor. ACOG Technical Bulletin No. 218; 1995.
8. Rogers R, Gilson GJ, Miller AC, et al. Active management of labor: Does it make a difference? *Am J Obstet Gynecol* 1997;177:599–605.
9. Peaceman AM, Lopez-Zeno JA, Minogue JP, et al. Factors that influence route of delivery–active versus traditional labor management. *Am J Obstet Gynecol* 1993;169:940–944.
10. Frigoletto FD, Lieberman E, Lang JM, et al. A clinical trial of active management of labor. *N Engl J Med* 1995;333:745–750.
11. Naftalin NJ, McKay DM, Phear WPC, et al. The effects of halothane on pregnant and nonpregnant human myometrium. *Anesthesiology* 1977;46:15–19.
12. Munson ES, Maier WR, Caton D. Effects of halothane, cyclopropane and nitrous oxide on isolated human uterine muscle. *J Obstet Gynaecol Br Commonw* 1969;76:27–33.
13. Munson ES, Embro WJ. Enflurane, isoflurane, and halothane and isolated human uterine muscle. *Anesthesiology* 1977;46:11–14.
14. Tjeuw MTB, Yao F, Van Poznak A. Depressant effects of anesthetics on isolated human gravid and non-gravid uterine muscle. *Chin Med J* 1986;9:235–242.
15. Abadir AR, Humayen SG, Calvello D, et al. Effects of isoflurane and oxytocin on gravid human uterus in vitro. *Anesth Analg* 1987;66:S1.
16. Vasicka A, Kretchmer H. Effect of conduction and inhalation anesthesia on uterine contractions: Experimental study of the influence of anesthesia on intra-amniotic pressures. *Am J Obstet Gynecol* 1961;82:600–611.
17. Marx GF, Kim YO, Lin CC, et al. Postpartum uterine pressures under halothane or enflurane anesthesia. *Obstet Gynecol* 1978;51:695–698.
18. Coleman AJ, Downing JW. Enflurane anesthesia for cesarean section. *Anesthesiology* 1975;43:354–357.
19. Galbert MW, Gardner AE. Use of halothane in a balanced technique for cesarean section. *Anesth Analg* 1972;51:701–704.
20. Moir DD. Anaesthesia for caesarean section. *Br J Anaesth* 1970;42:136–142.
21. Yamakage M, Mori T, Tsujiguchi N, et al. Inhibitory effects of halothane, isoflurane, and sevoflurane on contractility and intracellular Ca2+ concentrations of pregnant myometrium in rats [abstract]. *Anesthesiology* 1998;89:A1050.
22. Abboud TK, Zhu J, Richardson M, et al. Desflurane: A new volatile anesthetic for cesarean section. *Acta Anaesthesiol Scand* 1995;39:723–726.
23. Gambling DR, Sharma SK, White PF, et al. Use of sevoflurane during elective cesarean birth: a comparison with isoflurane and spinal anesthesia. *Anesth Analg* 1995;81:90–95.
24. DeVoe SJ, DeVoe KJ, Rigsby WC, et al. Effect of meperidine on uterine contractility. *Am J Obstet Gynecol* 1969;105:1004–1007.
25. Filler WWJ, Hall WC, Filler NW. Analgesia in obstetrics. *Am J Obstet Gynecol* 1967;98:832–846.
26. Petrie RH, Wu R, Miller FC, et al. The effect of drugs on uterine activity. *Obstet Gynecol* 1976;48:431–435.
27. Friedman EA. Effects of drugs on uterine contractility. *Anesthesiology* 1965;26:409–422.
28. Rayburn WF, Smith CV, Parriott JE, et al. Randomized comparison of meperidine and fentanyl during labor. *Obstet Gynecol* 1989;14:604–606.
29. Oats JN, Vasey DP, Waldron BA. Effects of ketamine on the pregnant uterus. *Br J Anaesth* 1979;51:1163–1166.
30. Marx GF, Hwang HS, Chandra P. Postpartum uterine pressures with different doses of ketamine. *Anesthesiology* 1979;50:163–166.
31. Mock PM, Santos-Eggimann B, Clerc Berod A, et al. Are women requiring unplanned intrapartum epidural analgesia different in a low-risk population? *Int J Obstet Anesth* 1999;8:94–100.
32. Studd JW, Crawford JS, Duignan NM, et al. The effect of lumbar epidural analgesia on the rate of cervical dilatation and the outcome of labour of spontaneous onset. *Br J Obstet Gynaecol* 1980;87:1015–1021.
33. Thornburn J, Moir DD. Extradural analgesia: The influence of volume and concentration of bupivacaine on the mode of delivery, analgesic efficacy and motor block. *Br J Anaesth* 1981;53:933–939.
34. Willdeck-Lund G, Lindmark G, Nilsson BA. Effect of segmental epidural block on the course of labour and the condition

of the infant during the neonatal period. *Acta Anaesthesiol Scand* 1979;23:301–311.

35. Schussman LC, Woolley FR, Larsen LC, et al. Epidural anesthesia in low-risk obstetrical patients. *J Fam Pract* 1982;14:851–858.
36. Raabe N, Belfrage P. Lumbar epidural analgesia in labour: A clinical analysis. *Acta Obstet Gynecol Scand* 1976;55:125–129.
37. Moore J, Murnaghan GA, Lewis MA. A clinical evaluation of the maternal effects of lumbar extradural analgesia for labour. *Anaesthesia* 1974;29:537–544.
38. Melzack R, Kinch R, Dobkin P, et al. Severity of labour pain: Influence of physical as well as psychologic variables. *Can Med Assoc J* 1984;130:579–584.
39. Hess PE, Pratt SD, Soni AK, et al. An association between severe labor pain and cesarean delivery. *Anesth Analg* 2000;90:881–886.
40. Floberg J, Belfrage P, Ohlsén H. Influence of the pelvic outlet capacity on fetal head presentation at delivery. *Acta Obstet Gynecol Scand* 1987;66:127–130.
41. Evans JA, Chastain GM, Philips JM. The use of local anesthetic agents in obstetrics. *South Med J* 1969;62:519–524.
42. McCaughey HS Jr, Corey EL, Eastwood D, et al. Effects of synthetic anesthetics on the spontaneous motility of human uterine muscles in vitro. *Obstet Gynecol* 1962;19:233–240.
43. Ritmiller LF, Rippmann ET. Caudal analgesia in obstetrics: Report of thirteen years' experience. *Obstet Gynecol* 1957;9:25–28.
44. Siever JM, Mousel LH. Continuous caudal anesthesia in three hundred unselected obstetric cases. *JAMA* 1943;122:424–426.
45. Friedman EA, Sachtleben MR. Caudal anesthesia. The factors that influence its effect on labor. *Obstet Gynecol* 1959;13:442–450.
46. Friedman EA, Sachtleben MR. Dysfunctional labor. I. Prolonged latent phase in the nullipara. *Obstet Gynecol* 1961;17:135–148.
47. Clark A, Carr D, Loyd G, et al. The influence of epidural analgesia on cesarean delivery rates: A randomized, prospective clinical trial. *Am J Obstet Gynecol* 1998;179:1527–1533.
48. Crawford JS. The second thousand epidural blocks in an obstetric hospital practice. *Br J Anaesth* 1972;44:1277–1286.
49. Jouppila R, Jouppila P, Karinen J-M, et al. Segmental epidural analgesia in labour: Related to the progress of labour, fetal malposition and instrumental delivery. *Acta Obstet Gynecol Scand* 1979;58:135–139.
50. Moir DD, Willocks J. Management of incoordinate uterine action under continuous epidural analgesia. *Br Med J* 1967;2:396–400.
51. Cowles GT. Experiences with lumbar epidural block. *Obstet Gynecol* 1965;26:734–739.
52. Akamatsu TJ. Advances in obstetric anesthesiology during the period 1960–1970. In: Fabian LW, ed. *Clinical Anesthesiology: A Decade of Clinical Progress.* Philadelphia: Davis; 1971:222.
53. Ruppert H. The influence of extradural spinal anesthesia on the motility of the gravid uterus. First World Congress of Anesthesiologists; Minneapolis: Burgess; 1956.
54. Moir DD, Willocks J. Continuous epidural analgesia in incoordinate uterine action. *Acta Anaesthesiol Scand* 1966;23(suppl):144–153.
55. Mercer WH, Simons EG, Philpott RH. The use of lumbar epidural analgesia during the first stage of labour in high risk pregnancies. *South Afr Med J* 1974;48:774–779.
56. Climie GR. The place of continuous lumbar epidural analgesia in the management of abnormally prolonged labour. *Med J Aust* 1964;2:447–450.
57. Crawford JS. An appraisal of lumbar epidural blockade in labour in patients with multiple pregnancy. *Br J Obstet Gynaecol* 1975;82:929–935.
58. Crawford JS. An appraisal of lumbar epidural blockade in patients with a singleton fetus presenting by the breech. *J Obstet Gynaecol Br Commonw* 1974;81:867–872.
59. Donnai P, Nicholas AD. Epidural analgesia, fetal monitoring and the condition of the baby at birth with breech presentation. *Br J Obstet Gynaecol* 1975;82:360–365.
60. Kilpatrick SJ, Laros RK. Characteristics of normal labor. *Obstet Gynecol* 1989;74:85–87.
61. Read MD, Hunt LP, Anderson JM, et al. Epidural block and the progress and outcome of labor. *J Obstet Gynaecol* 1983;4:35–39.
62. Willdeck-Lund G, Lindmark G, Nilsson BA. Effect of segmental epidural analgesia upon the uterine activity with special reference to the use of different local anaesthetic agents. *Acta Anaesthesiol Scand* 1979;23:519–528.
63. Carli F, Creagh-Barry P, Gordon H, et al. Does epidural analgesia influence the mode of delivery in primiparae managed actively?

A preliminary study of 1250 women. *Int J Obstet Anesth* 1993;2:15–20.
64. Newton ER, Schroeder BC, Knape KG, et al. Epidural analgesia and uterine function. *Obstet Gynecol* 1995;85:749–755.
65. Bofill JA, Vincent RD, Ross EL, et al. Nulliparous active labor, epidural analgesia, and cesarean delivery for dystocia. *Am J Obstet Gynecol* 1997;177:1465–1470.
66. Sharma SK, Sidawi JE, Ramin SM, et al. Cesarean delivery: A randomized trial of epidural versus patient-controlled meperidine analgesia during labor. *Anesthesiology* 1997;87:487–494.
67. Philipsen T, Jensen N-H. Epidural block or parenteral pethidine as an analgesic in labour; a randomized study concerning progress in labour and instrumental deliveries. *Eur J Obstet Gynecol Reprod Biol* 1989;30:27–33.
68. Ramin SM, Gambling DR, Lucas MJ, et al. Randomized trial of epidural versus intravenous analgesia during labor. *Obstet Gynecol* 1995;86:783–789.
69. Robinson JO, Rosen M, Evans JM, et al. Maternal opinion about analgesia for labour: A controlled trial between epidural block and intramuscular pethidine combined with inhalation. *Anaesthesia* 1980;35:1173–1181.
70. Thorp JA, Hu DH, Albin RM, et al. The effect of intrapartum epidural analgesia on nulliparous labor: A randomized, controlled, prospective trial. *Am J Obstet Gynecol* 1993;169:851–858.
71. Halpern SH, Leighton BL, Ohlsson A, et al. Effect of epidural vs. parenteral opioid analgesia on the progress of labor: A meta-analysis. *JAMA* 1998;280:2105–2110.
72. Lowensohn RI, Paul R, Fales S, et al. Intrapartum epidural anesthesia: An evaluation of effects on uterine activity. *Obstet Gynecol* 1974;44:388–393.
73. Zador G, Nilsson BA. Low dose intermittent epidural anaesthesia with lidocaine for vaginal delivery. II. Influence on labour and foetal acid-base status. *Acta Obstet Gynecol Scand* 1974;34(suppl):17–30.
74. Zador G, Nilsson BA. Continuous drip lumbar epidural anaesthesia with lidocaine for vaginal delivery. II. Influence on labour and foetal acid-base status. *Acta Obstet Gynecol Scand* 1974;34(suppl):41–49.
75. Abboud TK, Khoo SS, Miller F, et al. Maternal, fetal, and neonatal responses after epidural anesthesia with bupivacaine, 2-chloroprocaine, or lidocaine. *Anesth Analg* 1982;61:638–644.
76. Abboud TK, Afrasiabi A, Sarkis F, et al. Continuous infusion epidural analgesia in parturients receiving bupivacaine, chloroprocaine, or lidocaine: Maternal, fetal, and neonatal effects. *Anesth Analg* 1984;63:421–428.
77. Gal D, Choudhy R, Ung K-A, et al. Segmental epidural analgesia for labor and delivery. *Acta Obstet Gynecol Scand* 1979;58:429–431.
78. Muir HA, Writer D, Douglas J, et al. Double-blind comparison of epidural ropivacaine 0.25% and bupivacaine 0.25%, for the relief of childbirth pain. *Can J Anaesth* 1997;44:599–604.
79. Owen MD, D'Angelo R, Gerancher JC, et al. 0.125% Ropivacaine is similar to 0.125% bupivacaine for labor analgesia using patient-controlled epidural infusion. *Anesth Analg* 1998;86:527–531.
80. Writer WD, Ahlen K, Hedlund C, et al. Ropivacaine compared to bupivacaine for epidural labour analgesia: A prospective meta-analysis [abstract]. *Reg Anesth* 1996;21:385.
81. Gautier P, De Kock M, Van Steenberge A, et al. A double-blind comparison of 0.125% ropivacaine with sufentanil and 0.125% bupivacaine with sufentanil for epidural labor analgesia. *Anesthesiology* 1999;90:772–778.
82. Fischer C, Blanie P, Jaouen E, et al. Ropivacaine, 0.1%, plus sufentanil 0.5 μg/mL, versus bupivacaine, 0.1%, plus sufentanil 0.5 μg/mL, using patient-controlled epidural analgesia for labor: a double-blind comparison. *Anesthesiology* 2000;92:1588–1593.
83. Burke D, Henderson DJ, Simpson AM, et al. Comparison of 0.25% S(−)-bupivacaine with 0.25% RS-bupivacaine for epidural analgesia in labour. *Br J Anaesth* 1999;83:750–755.
84. Writer WDR, Stienstra R, Eddleston JM, et al. Neonatal outcome and mode of delivery after epidural analgesia for labour with ropivacaine and bupivacaine: A prospective meta-analysis. *Br J Anaesth* 1998;81:713–717.
85. Campbell DC, Zwack RM, Crone LL, Yip RW. Ambulatory labor epidural analgesia: Bupivacaine versus ropivacaine. *Anesth Analg* 2000;90:1384–1389.
86. Capogna G, Celleno D, Fusco P, et al. Relative potencies of bupivacaine and ropivacaine for analgesia in labour. *Br J Anaesth* 1999;82:371–373.

87. Polley LS, Columb MO, Naughton NN, et al. Relative analgesic potencies of ropivacaine and bupivacaine for epidural analgesia in labor: Implications for therapeutic indexes. *Anesthesiology* 1999;90:941–943.

88. Cheek TG, Samuels P, Miller F, et al. Normal saline i.v. fluid load decreases uterine activity in labour. *Br J Anaesth* 1996;77:632–635.

89. Scull TJ, Hemmings GT, Franco C, et al. Epidural analgesia in early labour blocks the stress response but uterine contractions remain unchanged. *Can J Anaesth* 1998;45:626–630.

90. Craft JB, Epstein BS, Coakley CS. Effect of lidocaine with epinephrine versus lidocaine (plain) on induced labor. *Anesth Analg* 1972;51:243–246.

91. Schellenberg JS. Uterine activity during lumbar epidural analgesia with bupivacaine. *Am J Obstet Gynecol* 1977;127:26–31.

92. Gunther RE, Bauman J. Obstetrical caudal anesthesia. I. A randomized study comparing 1 per cent lidocaine plus epinephrine. *Anesthesiology* 1969;31:5–19.

93. Gunther RE, Bellville JW. Obstetrical caudal anesthesia. II. A randomized study comparing 1 per cent mepivacaine with 1 per cent mepivacaine plus epinephrine. *Anesthesiology* 1972;37:288–298.

94. Abboud TK, David S, Nagappala S, et al. Maternal, fetal, and neonatal effects of lidocaine with and without epinephrine for epidural anesthesia in obstetrics. *Anesth Analg* 1984;63:973–979.

95. Abboud TK, Shiek-al-Eslam A, Yanagi T, et al. Safety and efficacy of epinephrine added to bupivacaine for lumbar epidural analgesia in obstetrics. *Anesth Analg* 1985;64:585–591.

96. Abboud TK, Der Sakissian L, Terrasi J, et al. Comparative maternal, fetal, and neonatal effects of chloroprocaine with and without epinephrine for epidural anesthesia in obstetrics. *Anesth Analg* 1987;66:71–75.

97. Eisenach J, Grice SC, Dewan DM. Epinephrine enhances analgesia produced by epidural bupivacaine during labor. *Anesth Analg* 1987;66:447–451.

98. Grice SC, Eisenach JC, Dewan DM. Labor analgesia with epidural bupivacaine plus fentanyl: Enhancement with epinephrine and inhibition with 2-chloroprocaine. *Anesthesiology* 1990;72:623–628.

99. Dahl V, Hagen I, Koss KS, et al. Bupivacaine 2.5 mg/mL versus bupivacaine 0.625 mg/mL and sufentanil 1 μg/mL with or without epinephrine 1 μg/mL for epidural analgesia in labour. *Int J Obstet Anesth* 1999;8:155–160.

100. Bogod DG, Rosen M, Rees GAD. Extradural infusion of 0.125% bupivacaine at 10 ml h-1 to women during labour. *Br J Anaesth* 1987;59:325–330.

101. D'Athis F, Machebouef M, Thomas H, et al. Epidural analgesia with a bupivacaine-fentanyl mixture in obstetrics: Comparison of repeated injections and continuous infusion. *Can J Anaesth* 1988;35:116–122.

102. Lamont RF, Pinney D, Rodgers P, et al. Continuous versus intermittent epidural analgesia: A randomised trial to observe obstetric outcome. *Anaesthesia* 1989;44:893–896.

103. Li DF, Rees GAD, Rosen M. Continuous extradural infusion of 0.0625% or 0.125% bupivacaine for pain relief in primigravid labour. *Br J Anaesth* 1985;57:264–270.

104. Celleno D, Capogna G. Epidural fentanyl plus bupivacaine 0.125 per cent for labour: Analgesic effects. *Can J Anaesth* 1988;35:375–378.

105. Chestnut DH, Owen CL, Bates JN, et al. Continuous infusion epidural analgesia during labor: A randomized double-blind comparison of 0.0625% bupivacaine/0.0002% fentanyl versus 0.125% bupivacaine. *Anesthesiology* 1988;68:754–759.

106. Jones G, Paul DL, Elton RA, et al. Comparison of bupivacaine and bupivacaine with fentanyl in continuous extradural analgesia during labour. *Br J Anaesth* 1989;63:254–259.

107. Murphy JD, Henderson K, Bowden MI, et al. Bupivacaine versus bupivacaine plus fentanyl for epidural analgesia: Effect on maternal satisfaction. *Br Med J* 1991;302:564–567.

108. Kavuri S, Janardhan Y, Fernando E, et al. A comparative study of epidural alfentanil and fentanyl for labor pain relief [abstract]. *Anesthesiology* 1989;71:A846.

109. Van Steenberge A, Debroux HC, Noorduin H. Extradural bupivacaine with sufentanil for vaginal delivery—a double-blind trial. *Br J Anaesth* 1987;59:1518–1522.

110. Vertommen JD, Vandermeulen E, Van Aken H, et al. The effects of the addition of sufentanil to 0.125% bupivacaine on the quality of analgesia during labor and on the incidence of instrumental deliveries. *Anesthesiology* 1991;74:809–814.

111. Gambling DR, Yu P, McMorland GH, et al. A comparative study of patient controlled epidural analgesia (PCEA) and continuous infusion epidural analgesia (CIEA) during labour. *Can J Anaesth* 1988;35:249–254.

112. Fontenot RJ, Price RL, Henry A, et al. Double-blind evaluation of patient-controlled epidural analgesia during labor. *Int J Obstet Anesth* 1993;2:73–77.

113. Ferrante FM, Lu L, Jamison SB, et al. Patient-controlled epidural analgesia: Demand dosing. *Anesth Analg* 1991;73:547–552.

114. Lysak SZ, Eisenach JC, Dobson CE. Patient-controlled epidural analgesia during labor: A comparison of three solutions with a continuous infusion control. *Anesthesiology* 1990;72:44–49.

115. Russell R, Quinlan J, Reynolds F. Motor block during epidural infusions for nulliparous women in labour: A randomized double-blind study of plain bupivacaine and low dose bupivacaine with fentanyl. *Int J Obstet Anesth* 1995;4:82–88.

116. Tiong-Heng Sia A, Ruban P, Chong JL, Wong K. Motor blockade is reduced with ropivacaine 0.125% for parturient-controlled epidural analgesia during labour. *Can J Anaesth* 1999;46:1019–1023.

117. James KS, McGrady E, Quasim I, Patrick A. Comparison of epidural bolus administration of 0.25% bupivacaine and 0.1% bupivacaine with 0.0002% fentanyl for analgesia during labour. *Br J Anaesth* 1998;81:507–510.

118. Viscomi C, Eisenach JC. Patient-controlled epidural analgesia during labor. *Obstet Gynecol* 1991;77:348–351.

119. Chestnut DH, Vandewalker GE, Owen CL, et al. The influence of continuous epidural bupivacaine analgesia on the second stage of labor and method of delivery in nulliparous women. *Anesthesiology* 1987;66:774–780.

120. Cox SM, Bost JE, Faro S, et al. Epidural anesthesia during labor and the incidence of forceps delivery. *Tex Med* 1987;83:45–47.

121. Chestnut D, Bates JN, Choi WW. Continuous infusion epidural analgesia with lidocaine: Efficacy and influence during the second stage of labor. *Obstet Gynecol* 1987;69:323–327.

122. Chestnut DH, Laszewski LJ, Pollack KL, et al. Continuous epidural infusion of 0.0625% bupivacaine-0.0002% fentanyl during the second stage of labor. *Anesthesiology* 1990;72:613–618.

123. Niv D, Ber A, Rudick V, et al. Mode of vaginal delivery and epidural analgesia. *Isr J Med Sci* 1988;24:80–83.

124. Browne RA, Catton DV. The use of bupivacaine in labour. *Can Anaesth Soc J* 1971;18:23–32.

125. Ploeckinger B, Ulm MR, Chalubinski K, et al. Epidural anaesthesia in labour: Influence on surgical delivery rates, intrapartum fever and blood loss. *Gynecol Obstet Invest* 1995;39:24–27.

126. Committee on Technical Bulletins of the American College of Obstetricians and Gynecologists. Operative vaginal delivery. ACOG Technical Bulletin No. 196; 1994.

127. Goodfellow CF, Hull MGR, Swaab DF, et al. Oxytocin deficiency at delivery with epidural analgesia. *Br J Obstet Gynaecol* 1983;90:214–219.

128. Amico JA, Seitchik J, Robinson AG. Studies of oxytocin in plasma of women during hypocontractile labor. *J Clin Endocrinol Metab* 1984;58:274–279.

129. Carsten ME, Miller JD. A new look at uterine muscle contraction. *Am J Obstet Gynecol* 1987;157:1303–1315.

130. Saunders NJ St G, Spily H, Gilbert L, et al. Oxytocin infusion during second stage of labour in primiparous women using epidural analgesia: A randomised double blind placebo controlled trial. *Br Med J* 1989;299:1423–1426.

131. Shennan AH, Smith R, Browne D, et al. The elective use of oxytocin infusion during labour in nulliparous women using epidural analgesia. A randomised double-blind placebo-controlled trial. *Int J Obstet Anesth* 1995;4:78–81.

132. Crawford JS. Lumbar epidural block in labour: A clinical analysis. *Br J Anaesth* 1972;44:66–74.

132a. Maloney SR, Johnson JL, Hughes SC, et al. Epidural bupivacaine decreases Pushing Strength (Abstract). In: Abstracts of Scientific papers of the Annual meeting of the Society for Obstetric Anesthesia and Perinatology; San Diego, CA:2001.

133. Christiaens F, Verborgh C, Dierick A, Camu F. Effects of diluent volume of a single dose of epidural bupivacaine in parturients during the first stage of labor. *Reg Anesth Pain Med* 1998;23:134–141.

134. Hoult J, MacLennan AH, Carrie LES. Lumbar epidural analgesia in labour: Relation to fetal malposition and instrumental delivery. *Br Med J* 1977;1:14–16.

135. Lieberman E, Lang JM, Cohen A, et al. Association of epidural analgesia with cesarean delivery in nulliparas. *Obstet Gynecol* 1996;88:993–1000.

136. Phillips KC, Thomas TA. Second stage of labour with or without extradural analgesia. *Anaesthesia* 1983;38:972–976.

137. Belfrage P, Raabe N. Continuous epidural anesthesia with a low frequency of instrumental deliveries [letter]. *Acta Obstet Gynecol Scand* 1976;55:469–470.

138. Niswander KR, Gordon M. Safety of the low-forceps operation. *Am J Obstet Gynecol* 1973;117:619–629.

139. Maresh M, Choong KH, Beard RW. Delayed pushing with lumbar epidural analgesia in labour. *Br J Obstet Gynaecol* 1983;90:623–627.

140. Derham RJ, Crowhurst J, Crowther C. The second stage of labour: Durational dilemmas. *Aust N Z J Obstet Gynaecol* 1991;31:31–36.

141. Cohen WR. Influence of the duration of second stage labor on perinatal outcome and puerperal morbidity. *Obstet Gynecol* 1977;49:266–269.

142. Moon JM, Smith CV, Rayburn WF. Perinatal outcome after a prolonged second stage of labor. *J Reprod Med* 1990;35:229–231.

143. Fraser WD, Marcoux S, Krauss I, et al. Multicenter, randomized, controlled trial of delayed pushing for nulliparous women in the second stage of labor with continuous epidural analgesia. *Am J Obstet Gynecol* 2000;182:1165–1172.

144. Gleeson NC, Griffith AP. The management of the second stage of labour in primiparae with epidural analgesia. *Br J Clin Pract* 1991;45:90–91.

145. Manyonda IT, Shaw DE, Drife JO. The effect of delayed pushing in the second stage of labor with continuous lumbar epidural analgesia. *Acta Obstet Gynecol Scand* 1990;69:291–295.

146. Walton P, Reynolds F. Epidural analgesia and instrumental delivery. *Anaesthesia* 1984;39:218–223.

147. Chestnut DH. Epidural anesthesia and instrumental vaginal delivery [editorial]. *Anesthesiology* 1991;74:805–808.

148. Johnsrud M-L, Dale PO, Lovland B. Benefits of continuous infusion epidural analgesia throughout vaginal delivery. *Acta Obstet Gynecol Scand* 1988;67:355–358.

149. Luxman D, Wolman I, Niv D, et al. Effect of second-stage 0.25% epidural bupivacaine on the outcome of labor. *Gynecol Obstet Invest* 1996;42:167–170.

150. Brown SE, Vass ACR. An extradural service in a district general hospital. *Br J Anaesth* 1977;49:243–246.

151. Hollmén A, Jouppila R, Pihlajaniemi R, et al. Selective lumbar epidural block in labour: A clinical analysis. *Acta Anaesthesiol Scand* 1977;21:174–181.

152. Bleyaert A, Soetens M, Vaes L, et al. Bupivacaine, 0.125 per cent, in obstetric epidural analgesia: Experience in three thousand cases. *Anesthesiology* 1979;51:435–438.

153. Maltau J, Andersen HT. Continuous epidural anaesthesia with a low frequency of instrumental deliveries. *Acta Obstet Gynecol Scand* 1975;54:401–406.

154. Kaminski HM, Stafl A, Aiman J. The effect of epidural analgesia on the frequency of instrumental obstetric delivery. *Obstet Gynecol* 1987;69:770–773.

155. Morgan BM, Rehar S, Lewis PJ. Epidural analgesia for uneventful labour. *Anaesthesia* 1980;35:57–60.

156. James DK, Chiswick ML. Kielland's forceps: Role of antenatal factors in prediction of use. *Br Med J* 1979;1:10–11.

157. Doughty A. Selective epidural analgesia and the forceps rate. *Br J Anaesth* 1969;41:1058–1062.

158. Hawkins JL, Hess KR, Kubicek MA, et al. A reevaluation of the association between instrumental delivery and epidural analgesia. *Reg Anesth* 1995;20:50–56.

159. Youngstrom P, Sedensky M, Frankmann D, et al. Continuous epidural infusion of low-dose bupivacaine-fentanyl for labor analgesia [abstract]. *Anesthesiology* 1988;69:A-686.

160. Bailey PW, Howard FA. Epidural analgesia and forceps delivery: Laying a bogey. *Anaesthesia* 1983;38:282–285.

161. Noble AD, deVere RD. Epidural analgesia in labour [letter]. *Br Med J* 1970;1:296.

162. Lyon DS, Knuckles G, Whitaker E, et al. The effect of instituting an elective labor epidural program on the operative delivery rate. *Obstet Gynecol* 1997;90:135–141.

163. Gribble RK, Meier PR. Effect of epidural analgesia on the primary cesarean rate. *Obstet Gynecol* 1991;78:231–234.

164. Fogel ST, Shyken JM, Leighton BL, et al. Epidural labor analgesia and the incidence of cesarean delivery for dystocia. *Anesth Analg* 1998;87:119–123.

165. Yancey MK, Pierce B, Schweitzer D, Daniels D. Observations on labor epidural analgesia and operative delivery rates. *Am J Obstet Gynecol* 1999;180:353–359.

166. Palmer CM, Van Maren GA, Alves DM. Relation between regional anesthesia for labor and cesarean section rate [abstract]. *Anesthesiology* 1998;89:A-1029.

167. Poma PA. Vanishing forceps delivery. *Am J Perinatol* 1999;16:227–231.

168. Johnson S, Rosenfeld JA. The effect of epidural anesthesia on the length of labor. *J Fam Pract* 1995;40:244–247.

169. Niehaus LS, Chaska BW, Nesse RE. The effects of epidural anesthesia on type of delivery. *J Am Board Fam Pract* 1988;1:238–244.

170. Thorp JA, Parisi VM, Boylan PC, et al. The effect of continuous epidural analgesia on cesarean section for dystocia in nulliparous women. *Am J Obstet Gynecol* 1989;161:670–675.

171. Thorp JA, Eckert LO, Ang MS, et al. Epidural analgesia and cesarean section for dystocia: Risk factors in nulliparas. *Am J Perinatol* 1991;8:402–410.

172. Miller AC. The effects of epidural analgesia on uterine activity and labor. *Int J Obstet Anesth* 1997;6:2–18.

173. Segal S, Datta S. Epidural analgesia and frequency of cesarean section [letter]. *Am J Obstet Gynecol* 1994;171:1396–1397.

174. Camann W. Epidural analgesia and frequency of cesarean section [letter]. *Am J Obstet Gynecol* 1994;171:1399.

175. Chestnut DH. Does epidural analgesia during labor affect the incidence of cesarean delivery? *Reg Anesth* 1997;22:495–499.

176. McGrady EM. Extradural analgesia: Does it affect progress and outcome in labour [editorial]? *Br J Anaesth* 1997;78:115–117.

177. Lucas MJ, Sharma SK, Leveno KJ, et al. A randomized trial of labor epidural analgesia in women with preeclampsia [abstract]. *Anesthesiology* 1998;89:A-1033.

178. Zhang J, Klebanoff MA, DerSimonian R. Epidural analgesia in association with duration of labor and mode of delivery: A quantitative review. *Am J Obstet Gynecol* 1999;180:970–977.

179. Chestnut DH, Vincent RD, McGrath JM, et al. Does early administration of epidural analgesia affect obstetric outcome in nulliparous women who are receiving intravenous oxytocin? *Anesthesiology* 1994;80:1193–1200.

180. Chestnut DH, McGrath JM, Vincent RD, et al. Does early administration of epidural analgesia affect obstetric outcome in nulliparous women who are in spontaneous labor? *Anesthesiology* 1994;80:1201–1208.

181. Rogers R, Gilson G, Kammerer-Doak D. Epidural analgesia and active management of labor: Effects on length of labor and mode of delivery. *Obstet Gynecol* 1999;93:995–998.

182. Ohel G, Harats H. Epidural anesthesia in early compared with advanced labor. *Int J Gynaecol Obstet* 1994;45:217–219.

183. Luxman D, Wolman I, Groutz A, et al. The effect of early epidural block administration on progression and outcome of labor. *Int J Obstet Anesth* 1998;7:161–164.

184. Feiss P, Collet D, Vincelot A. Peridural analgesia in labor. Comparison between bupivacaine and 2-chloroprocaine [in French]. *Cah Anesthesiol* 1986;34:95–98.

185. Pratt SD, Soni AK, Sarna MC, et al. Ultra low dose labor epidural solution affects obstetric outcome but not anesthesiologist work load: A preliminary report of a review of 2511 patients [abstract]. *Anesth Analg* 1997;84:S403.

186. Parker RK. Influence of labor epidural management on outcome in obstetrics [abstract]. *Reg Anesth* 1992;17:31.

187. Russell R, Reynolds F. Epidural infusion of low-dose bupivacaine and opioid in labour: Does reducing motor block increase the spontaneous delivery rate? *Anaesthesia* 1996;51:266–273.

188. Scrutton MJL, Porter JS, O'Sullivan G. Comparison of three different loading doses to establish epidural analgesia in labour. *Int J Obstet Anesth* 1998;7:165–169.

189. McCrae AF, Jozwiak H, McClure JH. Comparison of ropivacaine and bupivacaine in extradural analgesia for the relief of pain in labour. *Br J Anaesth* 1995;74:261–265.

190. McCrae AF, Westerling P, McClure JH. Pharmacokinetic and clinical study of ropivacaine and bupivacaine in women receiving extradural analgesia in labour. *Br J Anaesth* 1997;79:558–562.

191. Stienstra R, Jonker TA, Bourdrez P, et al. Ropivacaine 0.25% versus bupivacaine 0.25% for continuous epidural analgesia in labor: A double-blind comparison. *Anesth Analg* 1995;80:285–289.

192. Eddleston JM, Holland JJ, Griffin RP. A double-blind comparison of 0.25% ropivacaine and 0.25% bupivacaine for extradural analgesia in labour. *Br J Anaesth* 1996;76:66–71.

193. McDonald SB, Liu SS, Kopacz DJ, Stephenson CA. Hyperbaric spinal ropivacaine: a comparison to bupivacaine in volunteers. *Anesthesiology* 1999;90:971–977.

194. Polley LS, Columb MO, Naughton NN, Wagner DS, van de Ven CJM. Relative analgesic potencies of ropivacaine and bupivacaine for epidural analgesia in labor. *Anesthesiology* 1999;90:944–950.

195. Smedstad KG, Morison DH. A comparative study of continuous and intermittent epidural analgesia for labour and delivery. *Can J Anaesth* 1988;35:234–241.

196. Boutros A, Blary S, Bronchard R, Bonnet F. Comparison of intermittent epidural bolus, continuous epidural infusion and patient controlled-epidural analgesia during labor. *Int J Obstet Anesth* 1999;8:236–241.

197. Driver I, Popham P, Glazebrook C, et al. Epidural bupivacaine/fentanyl infusion vs. intermittent top-ups: A retrospective study of the effects on mode of delivery in primiparous women. *Eur J Anaesthesiol* 1996;13:515–520.

198. Sia AT, Chong JL. Epidural 0.2% ropivacaine for labour analgesia: Parturient- controlled or continuous infusion. *Anaesth Int Care* 1999;27:154–158.

199. Paech MJ. Patient controlled epidural analgesia during labour: Choice of solution. *Int J Obstet Anesth* 1993;2:65–72.

200. Naulty JS, Smith R, Ross R. Effect of changes in labor analgesic practice on labor outcome [abstract]. *Anesthesiology* 1988;69:A-660.

201. Olofsson C, Ekblom A, Edman-Ordeberg G, et al. Obstetric outcome following epidural analgesia with bupivacaine-adrenaline 0.25% or bupivacaine 0.125% with sufentanil–a prospective randomized controlled study in 1000 parturients. *Acta Anaesthesiol Scand* 1998;42:284–292.

202. Ahn NN, Karambelkar D, Cannelli G, et al. Epidural alfentanil and bupivacaine for analgesia during labor [abstract]. *Anesthesiology* 1989;71:A-845.

203. Naulty JS, Ross R, Bergen W. Epidural sufentanil-bupivacaine for analgesia during labor and delivery [abstract]. *Anesthesiology* 1989;71:A-842.

204. Carp H, Johnson MD, Bader AM, et al. Continuous epidural infusion of alfentanil and bupivacaine for labor and delivery [abstract]. *Anesthesiology* 1988;69:A-687.

205. Hoyt M, Youngstrom P. Neonatal neurobehavioral effects of continuous epidural infusion of fentanyl/bupivacaine/epinephrine in labor [abstract]. *Anesthesiology* 1990;73:A-984.

206. Hunt CO, Naulty JS, Malinow AM, et al. Epidural butorphanol-bupivacaine for analgesia during labor and delivery. *Anesth Analg* 1989;68:323–327.

207. Cohen S, Amar D, Pantuck CB, et al. Epidural analgesia for labour and delivery: Fentanyl or sufentanil? *Can J Anaesth* 1996;43:341–346.

208. Steinberg RB, Dunn SM, Dixon DE, et al. Comparison of sufentanil, bupivacaine, and their combination for epidural analgesia in obstetrics. *Reg Anesth* 1992;17:131–138.

209. Eisenach JC, Detweiler D, Hood D. Hemodynamic and analgesic actions of epidurally administered clonidine. *Anesthesiology* 1993;78:277–287.

210. Chassard D, Mathon L, Dailler F. Extradural clonidine combined with sufentanil and 0.0625% bupivacaine for analgesia in labour. *Br J Anaesth* 1996;77:458–462.

211. Claes B, Soetens M, Van Zundert A, et al. Clonidine added to bupivacaine- epinephrine-sufentanil improves epidural analgesia during childbirth. *Reg Anesth Pain* Med 1998;23:540–547.

212. D'Angelo R, Evans E, Dean LA, et al. Spinal clonidine prolongs labor analgesia from spinal sufentanil and bupivacaine. *Anesth Analg* 1999;88:573–576.

213. Owen MD, Ozsarac O, Sahin S, et al. Low-dose clonidine and neostigmine prolong the duration of intrathecal bupivacaine-fentanyl for labor analgesia. *Anesthesiology* 2000:92:361–366.

214. Impey L, MacQuillan K, Robson M. Epidural analgesia need not increase operative delivery rates. *Am J Obstet Gynecol* 2000;182:358–363.

215. Iglesias S, Burn R, Saunders LD. Reducing the cesarean section rate in a rural community hospital. *Can Med Assoc J* 1991;145:1459–1464.

216. Socol ML, Garcia PM, Peaceman AM, et al. Reducing cesarean births at a primarily private university hospital. *Am J Obstet Gynecol* 1993;168:1748–1754.

217. Lagrew DC, Morgan MA. Decreasing the cesarean section rate in a private hospital: Success without mandated clinical changes. *Am J Obstet Gynecol* 1996;174:184–191.

218. Lagrew DC, Adashek JA. Lowering the cesarean section rate in a private hospital: Comparison of individual physicians' rates, risk factors, and outcomes. *Am J Obstet Gynecol* 1998;178:1207–1214.

219. Segal S, Blatman R, Doble M, Datta S. The influence of the obstetrician in the relationship between epidural analgesia and cesarean section for dystocia. *Anesthesiology* 1999;91:90–96.

220. Gilbert WM, Nesbitt TS, Danielsen B. Childbearing beyond age 40: Pregnancy outcome in 24,032 cases. *Obstet Gynecol* 1999;93:9–14.

221. Poma PA. Effects of obstetrician characteristics on cesarean delivery rates: A community hospital experience. *Am J Obstet Gynecol* 1999;180:164–1372.

222. Neuhoff D, Burke MS, Porreco RP. Cesarean birth for failed progress in labor. *Obstet Gynecol* 1989;73:915–920.

223. Cary AJ. Intervention rates in spontaneous term labour in low risk nulliparous women. *Aust N Z J Obstet Gynaecol* 1990;30:46–51.

224. Gregory KD, Ramicone E, Chan L, Kahn KL. Cesarean deliveries for Medicaid patients: A comparison in public and private hospitals in Los Angeles County. *Am J Obstet Gynecol* 1999;180:1177–1184.

225. Haas JS, Udvarhelyi S, Epstein AM. The effect of health coverage for uninsured pregnant women on maternal health and the use of cesarean section. *JAMA* 1993;270:61–64.

226. Localio AR, Lawthers AG, Bengtson JM, et al. Relationship between malpractice claims and cesarean delivery. *JAMA* 1993;269:366–373.

227. Lieberman E, Lang JM, Heffner LJ, Cohen A. Assessing the role of case mix in cesarean delivery rates. *Obstet Gynecol* 1998;92:1–7.

228. Butler J, Abrams B, Parker J, et al. Supportive nurse-midwife care is associated with a reduced incidence of cesarean section. *Am J Obstet Gynecol* 1993;168:1407–1413.

229. Hueston WJ, Applegate JA, Mansfield CJ, et al. Practice variations between family physicians and obstetricians in the management of low-risk pregnancies. *J Fam Pract* 1995;40:345–351.

230. Clark SL, Xu W, Porter TF, et al. Institutional influences on the primary cesarean section rate in Utah, 1992–1995. *Am J Obstet Gynecol* 1998;179:841–845.

231. Radin TG, Harmon JS, Hanson DA. Nurses' care during labor: Its effect on the cesarean birth rate of healthy, nulliparous women. *Birth* 1993;20:14–21.

232. Poma PA. Effect of departmental policies on cesarean delivery rates: A community hospital experience. *Obstet Gynecol* 1998;91:1013–1018.

233. Wuitchik M, Bakal D, Lipshitz J. The clinical significance of pain and cognitive activity in latent labor. *Obstet Gynecol* 1989;73:35–42.

234. Parrish KM, Holt VL, Easterling TR, et al. Effect of changes in maternal age, parity, and birth weight distribution on primary cesarean delivery rates. *JAMA* 1994;271:443–447.

235. Piper JM, Bolling DR, Newton ER. The second stage of labor: Factors influencing duration. *Am J Obstet Gynecol* 1991;165:976–979.

236. Rawal N, VanZundert A, Holmstrom B, et al. Combined spinal-epidural technique. *Reg Anesth* 1997;22:406–423.

237. Bloom SL, McIntire DD, Kelly MA, et al. Lack of effect of walking on labor and delivery. *N Engl J Med* 1998;339:76–79.

238. Collis RE, Harding SA, Morgan BM. Effect of maternal ambulation on labour with low-dose combined spinal-epidural analgesia. *Anaesthesia* 1999;54:535–539.

239. Honet JE, Arkoosh VA, Norris MC, et al. Comparison among intrathecal fentanyl, meperidine, and sufentanil for labor analgesia. *Anesth Analg* 1992;75:734–739.

240. Grieco WM, Norris MC, Leighton BL, et al. Intrathecal sufentanil for labor analgesia: The effects of adding morphine or epinephrine. *Anesth Analg* 1993;77:1149–1154.

241. Campbell DC, Banner R, Crone LA, et al. Addition of epinephrine to intrathecal bupivacaine and sufentanil for ambulatory labor analgesia. *Anesthesiology* 1997;86:525–531.

242. Camann WR, Mintzer BH, Denney RA, et al. Intrathecal sufentanil for labor analgesia: Effects of added epinephrine. *Anesthesiology* 1993;78:870–874.

243. Abouleish E, Rawal N, Shaw J, et al. Intrathecal morphine 0.2 mg versus epidural bupivacaine 0.125% or their combination: Effects on parturients. *Anesthesiology* 1991;74:711–716.

244. D'Angelo R, Anderson MT, Philip J, et al. Intrathecal sufentanil compared to epidural bupivacaine for labor analgesia. *Anesthesiology* 1994;80:1209–1215.

245. Collis RE, Davies DWL, Aveling W. Randomised comparison of combined spinal-epidural and standard epidural analgesia in labour. *Lancet* 1995;345:1413–1416.

246. Dresner M, Bamber J, Calow C, et al. Comparison of low-dose epidural with combined spinal-epidural analgesia for labour. *Br J Anaesth* 1999;83:756–760.

247. Price C, Lafreniere L, Brosnan C, Findley I. Regional analgesia in early active labour: Combined spinal epidural vs. epidural. *Anaesthesia* 1998;53:951–955.

248. Kartawiadi L, Vercauteren MP, Van Steenberge AL, et al. Spinal analgesia during labor with low-dose bupivacaine, sufentanil, and epinephrine. A comparison with epidural analgesia. *Reg Anesth* 1996;21:191–196.

249. Dunn SM, Connelly NR, Steinberg RB, et al. Intrathecal sufentanil versus epidural lidocaine with epinephrine and sufentanil for early labor analgesia. *Anesth Analg* 1998;87:331–335.

250. Tsen LC, Thue B, Datta S, Segal S. Is combined spinal-epidural analgesia associated with more rapid cervical dilation in nulliparous patients when compared with conventional epidural analgesia? *Anesthesiology* 1999;91:920–925.

251. Nageotte MP, Larson D, Rumney PJ, et al. Epidural analgesia compared with combined spinal-epidural analgesia during labor in nulliparous women. *N Engl J Med* 1997;337:1715–1719.

252. Rosenfeld DJ, Ackal T, Fournet K, et al. A comparison of epidural bupivacaine and intrathecal sufentanil with PCEA throughout labor [abstract]. *Anesthesiology* 1998;89:A-1025.

253. Palmer CM, Van Maren G, Nogami WM, Alves D. Bupivacaine augments intrathecal fentanyl for labor analgesia. *Anesthesiology* 1999;91:84–89.

254. Gambling DR, Sharma SK, Ramin SM, et al. A randomized study of combined spinal-epidural analgesia versus intravenous meperidine during labor: Impact on cesarean delivery rate. *Anesthesiology* 1998;89:1336–1344.

255. Clarke VT, Smiley RM, Finster M. Uterine hyperactivity after intrathecal injection of fentanyl for analgesia during labor: A cause of fetal bradycardia [letter]? *Anesthesiology* 1994;81:1083.

256. Nielsen PE, Erickson JR, Abouleish EI, et al. Fetal heart rate changes after intrathecal sufentanil or epidural bupivacaine for labor analgesia: Incidence and clinical significance. *Anesth Analg* 1996;83:742–746.

257. Albright GA, Forster RM. Does combined spinal-epidural analgesia with subarachnoid sufentanil increase the incidence of emergency cesarean section? *Reg Anesth* 1997;22:400–405.

258. Gautier PE, De Kock M, Fanard L, et al. Intrathecal clonidine combined with sufentanil for labor analgesia. *Anesthesiology* 1998;88:651–656.

259. Eisenach JC, De Kock M, Klimschaw W. α2-adrenergic agonists for regional anesthesia: A clinical review of clonidine (1984–1995). *Anesthesiology* 1996;85:655–675.

260. Harrison RF, Shore M, Woods T, et al. A comparative study of transcutaneous electrical nerve stimulation (TENS), Entonox, pethidine + promazine and lumbar epidural for pain relief in labor. *Acta Obstet Gynecol Scand* 1987;66:9–14.

261. MacArthur C, Lewis M, Knox EG. Evaluation of obstetric analgesia and anaesthesia: Long-term maternal recollections. *Int J Obstet Gynecol* 1993;2:3–11.

262. Pearson JF, Davies P. The effect of continuous lumbar epidural analgesia on the acid-base status of maternal arterial blood during the first stage of labour. *J Obstet Gynaecol Br Commonw* 1973;80:218–224.

263. Belfrage P, Raabe N, Thalme B, et al. Lumbar epidural analgesia with bupivacaine in labor. Determinations of drug concentration and pH in fetal scalp blood and continuous fetal heart rate monitoring. *Am J Obstet Gynecol* 1975;121:360–365.

264. Thalme B, Belfrage P, Raabe N. Lumbar epidural analgesia in labour. I. Acid-base balance and clinical condition of mother, fetus, and newborn child. *Acta Obstet Gynecol Scand* 1974;53:27–35.

265. Thalme B, Raabe N, Belfrage P. Lumbar epidural analgesia in labour. II. Effects on glucose, lactate, sodium, chloride, total protein, haematocrit and haemoglobin in maternal, fetal and neonatal blood. *Acta Obstet Gynecol Scand* 1974;53:113–119.

266. Livnat EJ, Fejgin M, Scommegna A, et al. Neonatal acid-base balance in spontaneous and instrumental vaginal deliveries. *Obstet Gynecol* 1978;52:549–551.

267. McBride WG, Black BP, Brown CJ, et al. Method of delivery and developmental outcome at five years of age. *Med J Aust* 1979;1:301–304.

268. Gilstrap LC, Hauth JC, Schiano S, et al. Neonatal acidosis and method of delivery. *Obstet Gynecol* 1984;63:681–685.

269. Friedman EA, Sachtleben-Murray MR, Dahrouge D, et al. Long-term effects of labor and delivery on offspring: A matched-pair analysis. *Am J Obstet Gynecol* 1984;150:941–945.

270. Walker MPR, Farine D, Rolbin SH, et al. Epidural anesthesia, episiotomy, and obstetric laceration. *Obstet Gynecol* 1991;77:668–671.

Shnider and Levinson's Anesthesia for Obstetrics,
edited by Samuel C. Hughes, et al.
Lippincott Williams & Wilkins,
Philadelphia, © 2001.

CHAPTER 4

PERINATAL PHARMACOLOGY

ALAN C. SANTOS, M.D., M.P.H. AND MIECZYSLAW
FINSTER, M.D.

Perinatal pharmacology involves the pharmacologic processes of drug absorption, distribution, biotransformation, and excretion, not in one individual but in two: the mother and the fetus. The perinatal period begins with the preimplantation blastocyst and extends to the neonate at 28 days of age. The discovery of vaginal adenosis in young women whose mothers were exposed to diethylstilbestrol during pregnancy (1) demonstrates that drugs administered during the perinatal period are capable of producing long-term effects.

This chapter focuses on the period of parturition and the effect of anesthetic drugs on the fetus and neonate. The basic concepts of placental drug transfer (absorption) (2), fetal and neonatal disposition of anesthetic drugs (distribution, biotransformation, excretion) (3, 4), and the clinical implications of anesthetic drug effects on the newborn (5) are examined. Because local anesthetics are among the most commonly used drugs for obstetric anesthesia, they are used to illustrate many of the important principles of perinatal pharmacology.

DETERMINANTS OF PLACENTAL TRANSFER

To achieve a physiologic effect, a critical concentration of "free" drug (i.e., nonionized and nonprotein bound) must arrive at and react with a given tissue receptor site (Fig. 4.1) (2–4, 6). To reach the fetus, a maternally-administered drug must first traverse the placenta, a process determined by maternal, placental, and fetal factors (Fig. 4.2).

Maternal Factors

Drug delivery to the placental exchange site depends on the fraction of total uterine blood flow that perfuses the intervillous space. Total uterine blood flow in women at term gestation is estimated to be approximately $150 \text{ mL} \cdot \text{kg}^{-1} \cdot \text{min}^{-1}$ of the total weight of the gravid uterus (7) (about 10% of cardiac output). In sheep, total uterine blood flow is 250 to $350 \text{ mL} \cdot \text{kg}^{-1} \cdot \text{min}^{-1}$ (8), and approximately 80% perfuses the intervillous space (Fig. 4.3) (9). A similar distribution probably exists in women.

Little information is available on how changes in maternal hemodynamics alter delivery of a drug to the placenta. To illustrate the complexity of this process, assume that a drug is injected as an intravenous bolus to a woman in active labor. During the peak of a uterine contraction, uterine arterial flow decreases; hence, the drug is unable to reach the placenta, at least during the first maternal circulation time. Indeed, lower concentrations of diazepam have been measured in infants born to mothers given the drug intravenously at the onset of uterine contraction, compared with newborns whose mothers received diazepam during uterine diastole (10). The supine position may cause maternal vena caval and/or aortic compression, which could also alter drug delivery to the placenta. Maternal hypotension or hypertension may also affect delivery of a drug to the

placenta to an unknown extent. Studies of drug transfer across the rabbit placenta, perfused in situ, showed that a decrease in maternal blood pressure of 35% reduced the placental clearance of meperidine, but not bupivacaine (11). Neither did the addition of adrenaline affect the placental clearance of bupivacaine (12). The uterine artery concentration of "free drug" (cm) that arrives at the intervillous space is itself dependent on the following factors (Table 4.1).

Dose

Increasing the total dose of drug, regardless of the route of administration, increases the maternal aretrial blood concentration (13). As a result, fetal drug blood concentration increases as well.

Injection Site

Intravenous administration results in the highest peak concentration of drug. Injection of local anesthetic into the highly vascular caudal epidural space results in higher peak maternal blood levels than occur after lumbar epidural administration (14), whereas maternal concentrations of local anesthetics are similar after injection into the lumbar epidural, pudendal, or paracervical areas (13–15).

Adjuvants

Epinephrine reduces the peak maternal local anesthetic concentration by 30% to 50% with lidocaine or mepivacaine but has little effect on peak levels of bupivacaine or etidocaine (Fig. 4.4) (13–16).

Individual Drug Pharmacokinetics

Maternal metabolism and elimination reduces drug concentrations in blood perfusing the intervillous space. In human volunteers, the elimination half-lives for the commonly-administered local anesthetics range from 1.5 hours for lidocaine to 3.5 hours for bupivacaine (17). Detailed pharmacokinetic studies in pregnant women have not been possible. In one study, the elimination half-life of lidocaine was 60 to 90 minutes after an intravenous bolus injection of 3 mg/kg (15). When bupivacaine is administered epidurally for cesarean section, the drug disappears from maternal blood in two phases, an initial rapid elimination with a half-life of 47 minutes and a slower elimination phase with a half-life of 9 hours (18). The time to achieve maximum serum concentration (about 15 minutes) and the terminal elimination half-life after epidural administration of bupivacaine were similar in pregnant and nonpregnant women (19).

Pregnancy-related conditions, such as preeclampsia, may result in higher maternal blood concentrations of anesthetic drugs due to impaired hepatic metabolism and decreased hepatic blood flow. This is particularly true for drugs having a high hepatic-extraction ratio, such as lidocaine, because their metabolism is sensitive to fluctuations in hepatic blood flow. For instance, in one study, the total clearance of lidocaine was slower

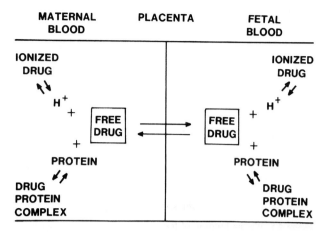

Figure 4.1. Drug in blood or tissue exists in several forms: ionized, protein bound, or nonionized, nonprotein-bound free form. It is this lipid-soluble, free form of the drug that readily passes through biologic membranes such as the placenta.

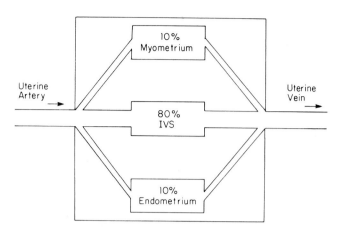

Figure 4.3. The distribution of uterine blood flow in the pregnant sheep. A similar distribution may occur in the human. (Modified from Makowski EL, Meschia G, Droegemueller W, Battaglia FC. Distribution of uterine blood flow in the pregnant sheep. *Am J Obstet Gynecol* 1968;101:409–412.)

and area under the plasma concentration vs. time decay curve greater in preeclamptic compared to normotensive parturients given lidocaine for epidural anesthesia during cesarean delivery (20). Preoperative treatment of parturients with an H₂-receptor antagonist (cimetidine, ranitidine) is often used to reduce the risk of gastric acid pulmonary aspiration. However, these H₂-receptor antagonists may affect pharmacokinetics of concurrently administered drugs by binding to hepatic cytochrome P-450 (CYP) and reducing hepatic blood flow and renal clearance of drug (21–23). Indeed, altered drug disposition has been documented with long-term cimetidine treatment of surgical patients (24). The effects may be less pronounced with ranitidine (21). However, as used clinically in obstetrics for the purpose of acid aspiration prophylaxis, H₂-receptor antagonists do not alter the pharmacokinetics of epidurally-administered local anesthetics (25–28). The potential effects of protein binding on the placental transfer of anesthetic drugs are perhaps the most confusing and least understood. *In vitro* studies using the dually perfused single cotyledon model of the human placenta have demonstrated that a doubling of the albumin concentration in

the maternal perfusate results in a halving of the transfer ratio for two of the commonly used local anesthetics, ropivacaine and bupivacaine (Table 4.2) (29). Thus, it is possible that reductions in the maternal level of plasma proteins, such as can occur with severe preeclampsia, can enhance fetal exposure to anesthetic agents (30). However, the ability to predict the degree of placental transfer for drugs having different protein-binding

Table 4.1. FACTORS THAT DETERMINE THE CONCENTRATION OF FREE DRUG IN UTERINE ARTERIAL BLOOD (C$_m$)

Total dose
Route of administration
Presence of epinephrine in anesthetic solution
Maternal metabolism and excretion
Maternal protein binding
Maternal pH and pK$_a$ of drug

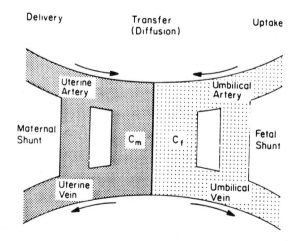

Maternal
A Blood flow to IVS
B Uterine artery concentrations of "free drug" (C$_m$)

Placental
C/t=A(C$_m$-C$_f$)/X

(Fick's Law of Passive Diffusion)

Fetal
A Umbilical blood flow
B Umbilical artery concentration of "free drug" (C$_f$)

Figure 4.2. A schematic diagram of the placental exchange site and the maternal, placental, and fetal factors that influence drug transfer and fetal drug uptake. *IVS*, intervillous space; *C/t*, rate of diffusion; *K*, diffusion constant of drug and membrane; *A*, surface available for transfer; *C$_m$*, drug concentration in maternal blood; *C$_f$*, drug concentration in fetal blood; *X*, thickness of membrane.

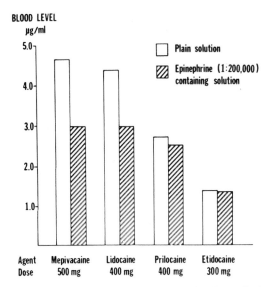

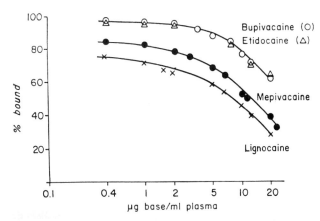

Figure 4.5. Plasma binding of four anilide local anesthetics at plasma concentrations of 0.4 to 20 μg/mL. (Reprinted by permission from Tucker GT, Mather LE. Pharmacokinetics of local anesthetic agents. *Br J Anaesth* 1975;47:213–224.)

Figure 4.4. The peak concentration of various local anesthetics after epidural administration with and without epinephrine. (Reprinted by permission from Covino BG, Vassallo HG. *Local Anesthetics: Mechanisms of Action and Clinical Use.* New York: Grune & Stratton; 1976:104.)

capacities is less certain. Plasma protein binding of local anesthetic varies with the individual drug and its concentration (Fig. 4.5). At the usually encountered clinical concentrations, the percentage of binding for lidocaine and mepivacaine is 50% to 70%, and for bupivacaine and etidocaine it is 95% (17, 31). The higher degree of protein binding with bupivacaine as compared to lidocaine was thought to impede placental transfer by reducing the concentration of free drug available for diffusion (Fig. 4.1). Indeed, lower fetal–to–maternal blood concentration ratios have been reported for bupivacaine as compared to lidocaine (32–35). However, the lower-umbilical vein–to–maternal vein concentration ratio of bupivacaine is caused by the difference in fetal and maternal plasma protein binding (higher in the mother) rather than more restrictive transfer (32, 33). For example, consider a hypothetical situation in which the total maternal plasma concentrations of lidocaine and bupivacaine are 2 mg/mL and their plasma protein binding is 50% and 90%, respectively (Fig. 4.6). The corresponding free concentration of drug will be 1 and 0.2 mg/mL, respectively. At equilibrium, the free-drug concentration will be equal on both sides of the placenta. However, protein binding of lidocaine and bupivacaine in the fetus (25% and 50%, respectively) is lower than in the mother. As a result, the total lidocaine concentration in the fetal plasma is

1.33 mg/mL and the fetal-to-maternal concentration ratio is 0.67. The corresponding values for bupivacaine are 0.4 and 0.2 mg/mL.

Pregnancy may reduce the protein binding of some drugs. For example, plasma protein binding of bupivacaine is reduced during human pregnancy (34). The rate of drug-protein dissociation is also important in assessing the significance of local anesthetic protein binding. Tucker (31) suggested that protein binding of local anesthetic does not significantly impede diffusion of drug across the placenta because the dissociation of drug from protein is essentially instantaneous. This could not be substantiated for bupivacaine but has been documented for fentanyl, an opioid bound to plasma albumin (36).

The pK$_a$ of a drug is the pH at which 50% of the drug is ionized and 50% is nonionized. Because most local anesthetics and opioids are weak bases, with pK$_a$s above maternal pH, a significant quantity of these drugs exists in the lipid-soluble, nonionized form in maternal blood.

Placental Factors

Once a given drug has reached the intervillous space, the quantity transferred per unit time is described by Fick's equation of passive diffusion (Fig. 4.2), expressed mathematically as

$$Q/t = K \cdot A(C_m - C_f / X)$$

where K is a diffusion constant determined by drug physicochemical properties such as molecular weight, lipid solubility, degree of ionization, and spatial configuration. This equation states that the amount of transfer is proportional to the difference in free-drug concentration between maternal and fetal blood, and the surface area available for diffusion is inversely related to the thickness of the membrane. At equilibrium, the concentration of free drug on both sides of the membrane is equal. Therefore, placental drug transfer is facilitated by a high concentration of nonionized, lipid-soluble, nonprotein-bound drug. High molecular weight, poor lipid solubility, and a high degree of ionization will impede but not totally prevent the transfer of a drug across the placenta. Muscle relaxants such as succinylcholine, atracurium, and vecuronium, which are highly ionized, do cross the placenta but only to a negligible extent (37–39). Changes within the placental circulation may also affect the rate of transfer. For instance, maternal hypoxia results in a reduced transfer of lidocaine, presumably due to stagnation of the circulation within the placental unit (40).

It has been proposed that if the blood flow to the fetal side of the placenta can be measured (such as in some animal models), calculating the placental clearance is the more appropriate way

Table 4.2. THE EFFECT OF INCREASING MATERNAL PERFUSATE ALBUMIN CONCENTRATION ON MATERNAL: FETAL CONCENTRATION RATIO (TRANSFER RATIO)

Transfer Ratio	Albumin Concentration	
	2 g/100 mL	*4 g/100 mL*
Ropivacaine	0.82 ± 0.03	0.42 ± 0.07*
Bupivacaine	0.74 ± 0.01	0.40 ± 0.03*

*Significantly lower than maternal perfusate containing 2 g/100 mL albumin.
Mean ± SEM
Adapted from Johnson RF, Cahana A, Olenick M, et al. A comparison of the placental transfer of ropivacaine versus bupivacaine. *Anesth Analg* 1999;89:703–708.

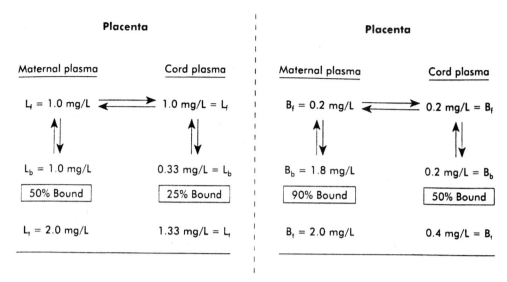

Figure 4.6. Illustration of how distribution of local anesthetics across the placenta can be predicted from differences in drug protein binding in the maternal and fetal plasma. *L*, lidocaine; *B*, bupivacaine; *f*, *b*, *t*, free, bound, and total drug concentration, respectively. Lidocaine umbilical–to–maternal-vein(UV/MV) ratio = 0.67; bupivacaine UV/MV ratio = 0.2. (Reprinted by permission from Tucker GT, Mather LE. Properties, absorption, and disposition of local anesthetic agents. In Cousins MJ, Bridenbaugh PO, eds. *Neural Blockade in Clinical Anesthesia and Management of Pain.* 2nd ed. Philadelphia: Lippincott; 1988:95.)

of expressing drug transfer to the fetus (41). At steady state,

$$Cl = Qu\,(Cuv - Cua)/Cma$$

where   Cl = clearance, in vol/time
     Qu = umbilical blood flow
     Cuv = umbilical vein drug concentration
     Cua = umbilical artery drug concentration
     Cma = maternal arterial drug concentration

Uptake and metabolism of drugs by the placenta would be expected to decrease fetal drug exposure. The placenta has considerable cholinesterase activity and has been shown to metabolize some anesthetic compounds, such as cocaine and paraaminobenzoic acid (42, 43). However, the capacity of the placenta to metabolize clinically-used anesthetic drugs is too limited to be of significance in reducing their transfer to the fetus (41). For example, remifentanil is a new opioid that is rapidly hydrolyzed by serum and tissue cholinesterases, in contrast to other opioid analgesics, like sufentanil, which undergo hepatic metabolism. Remifentanil crosses the placenta readily. Its degradation by placental cholinesterases is negligible as suggested by a umbilical vein (UV)–to maternal-artery (MA) ratio similar to that seen with sufentanil (Table 4.3) (44). Placental absorption of dexmedetomidine and clonidine has been shown to affect fetal blood levels of these drugs (Fig. 4.7) (45).

Fetal Factors

Fetal uptake, distribution, metabolism, and elimination determine drug disposition and physiologic effects once a drug has diffused across the placental exchange site.

FETAL UPTAKE OF DRUGS

Fetal uptake is determined by the solubility of the drug in fetal blood (which includes drug dissolved in plasma water, as well as drug bound to red blood cell and plasma protein components), the quantity and distribution of fetal blood flow to the intervillous space, and the concentration of drug in fetal blood returning to the placenta (Fig. 4.2). In addition, the pH gradient existing between maternal and fetal blood influences the concentration of drug at equilibrium. Local anesthetics are

weak bases, with pK$_a$s ranging from 7.6 for mepivacaine to 8.9 for procaine. At an increased hydrogen ion concentration (or lower pH) more local anesthetic exists in the ionized state. At pH 7.40, lidocaine is 24% nonionized, whereas at pH 7.0, 11% exists in the nonionized form (Fig. 4.8). Thus, a 0.40 pH gradient would cause a 54% increase in the amount of ionized drug. Such a pH gradient may exist between a mother and an asphyxiated fetus. Because the ionized form of the drug does not pass through lipid membranes as readily as the lipid-soluble, nonionized form, a weakly basic drug may accumulate in the more acid fetal blood. Clinical and laboratory evidence suggests that this phenomenon of "ion trapping" may indeed occur. Brown et al. (46) found high UV–to MV concentration ratios of lidocaine and mepivacaine in neonates with umbilical artery pH values of 7.03 to 7.23 at delivery. Biehl et al. (47) induced acidosis in fetal lambs during constant-rate intravenous infusion of lidocaine into the mother. Higher fetal blood lidocaine concentrations were seen with fetal acidosis (pH 6.90 to 7.18) than when fetal pH was normal (7.30 to 7.35). Correction of fetal acidosis with bicarbonate (fetal pH 7.22 to 7.40) resulted in a decrease in fetal blood lidocaine concentration (Fig. 4.9). In a recent study, Johnson et al., using isolated dually perfused human placental cotyledons, demonstrated that increasing maternal drug

Table 4.3. REMIFENTANIL BLOOD CONCENTRATIONS AND PLACENTAL TRANSFER

		Remifentanil
	n	*Mean* ± *SD*
MA (µg/mL)	16	1.32 ± 0.80
UV (µg/mL)	15	0.73 ± 0.27
UA (µg/mL)	10	0.20 ± 0.07
UV/MA	15	0.88 ± 0.78
UA/UV	10	0.29 ± 0.07

MA = maternal artery; UV = umbilical vein; UA = umbilical artery. Reprinted with permission from Kan RE, Hughes, SC, Rosen MA, Kessin C, Preston PG, Lobo EP. Intravenous remifentanil: Placental transfer, maternal and neonatal effects. *Anesthesiology* 1998;88: 1467–1474.

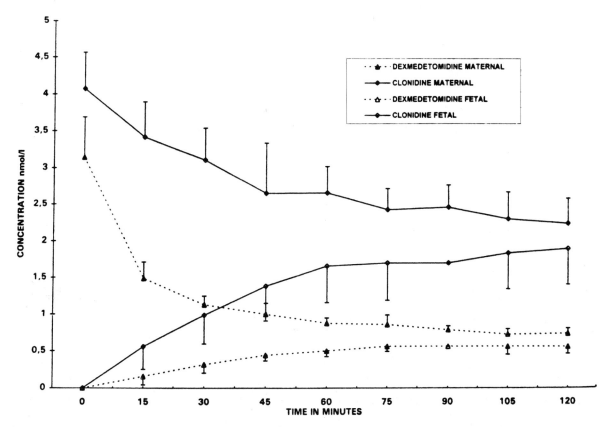

Figure 4.7. Maternal disappearance and fetal appearance of clonidine ($n = 4$) and dexmedetomidine ($n = 4$) after a bolus dose of the drug. A total of 250 ng of the drug (radioactively labeled and unlabeled) was added to the maternal reservoir at the start of the experiment. The mean peak clonidine and dexmedetomidine concentrations measured at 0-time were 4.1 (SD ± 0.49) nmol/L, and 3.1 (SD ± 0.55) nmol/L, respectively. (Reprinted by permission from Ala-Kokko TI, Pienimäki P, Lamela E, Hollmén AI, Pelkonen O, Vähäkangas K. Transfer of clonidine and dexmedetomidine across the isolated perfused human placenta. *Acta Anaesthesiol Scand* 1997;41:313–319.)

binding limited the increase in placental transfer seen with fetal acidosis. If this finding is applicable to parturients, bupivacaine, because of its greater binding to serum proteins, may be a better drug to use in the presence of fetal acidosis than lidocaine (48).

Although ion trapping may account for the higher fetal blood levels of local anesthetics and opioids, reduced fetal clearance of these drugs due to alterations in fetal cardiac output or umbilical or hepatic blood flow, or changes in the blood-to-tissue distribution of these drugs during metabolic acidosis, might also explain the observed findings. For example, the infusion of lidocaine into asphyxiated baboon fetuses resulted in increased drug uptake in the heart, brain, and liver, as compared with nonasphyxiated controls (49).

Fetal umbilical blood flow to the placental exchange site is obviously essential for fetal drug uptake (Fig. 4.10). Fetal-placental flow in the lamb is 200 to 250 mL/min/kg body weight, representing approximately 50% (Fig. 4.11) of the combined ventricular output (8). The fraction of this output perfusing the placenta increases with fetal asphyxia due to uteroplacental insufficiency (50) and may decrease with cord compression.

Local anesthetics transferred across the placenta may adversely affect fetal circulatory adaptations to asphyxia, including

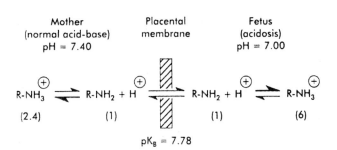

Figure 4.8. Mechanism by which amide local anesthetics accumulate on the fetal side of the placenta with profound fetal acidosis ("ion trapping"). (Reprinted by permission from Brown WU, Bell GC, Alper MH. Acidosis, local anesthetics and the newborn. *Obstet Gynecol* 1976;48:27–30.)

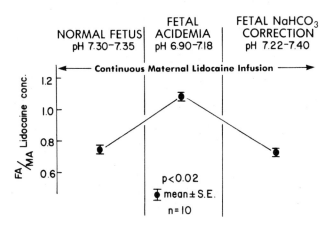

Figure 4.9. Fetal–to–maternal arterial (*FA/MA*) lidocaine ratios were significantly higher during fetal acidemia than during control or during pH correction with bicarbonate. (Reprinted by permission from Biehl D, Shnider SM, Levinson G, Callender K. Placental transfer of lidocaine: Effects of fetal acidosis. *Anesthesiology* 1978;48:409–412.)

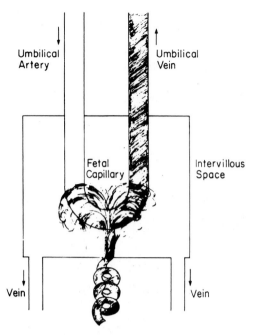

Figure 4.10. Circulatory pathways at the intervillous space. The fetal umbilical artery carries blood to the intervillous space, where exchange of oxygen, carbon dioxide, and drugs occurs. The maternal spinal artery enters at the base, and fountain-like spurts of blood bathe the branching villi, which contain fetal capillaries. Blood returns to the fetus via the umbilical vein, whereas uterine veins drain maternal blood from the intervillous space. Hemodynamic alterations may occur at several sites: umbilical artery or vein (cord compression); intervillous space (fetal capillary compression with increased intrauterine pressure); uterine vein (vena caval obstruction with a parturient in the supine position); or uterine artery (spinal hypotension or α-adrenergic stimulation). How hemodynamic changes influence placental transfer is poorly understood.

increased placental blood flow. In the chronically-instrumented pregnant ewe, lidocaine infusion resulting in clinically-relevant maternal and fetal plasma levels of the drug is well tolerated by the partially asphyxiated mature fetal lamb (51). However, the preterm fetus loses its cardiovascular adaptation to asphyxia and its condition deteriorates further when exposed to lidocaine (52). In contrast, fetal heart rate, blood pressure and acid-base status are maintained in the asphyxiated preterm fetal lamb during bupivacaine exposure, despite a return in organ blood flows from elevated asphyxial levels to baseline (53).

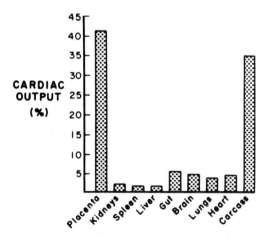

Figure 4.11. Percent distribution of combined ventricular output in fetal lamb near term (measured with radioactive microspheres). (Reprinted by permission from Pang LM, Mellins RB. Neonatal cardiorespiratory physiology. *Anesthesiology* 1975;43:171–196.)

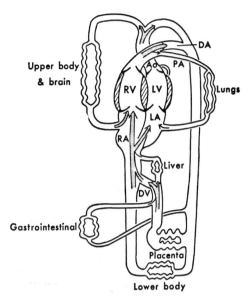

Figure 4.12. The fetal circulation. (Reprinted by permission from Rudolph AM. *Congenital Diseases of the Heart: Clinical Physiologic Considerations in Diagnosis and Management.* Chicago: Year Book Medical Publishers; 1974:2.)

Studies of drug transfer across rabbit placenta, perfused in situ, indicate that a reduction in umbilical blood flow may increase the fetal-to-maternal concentration ratio but reduce the rate of placental transfer of drugs such as bupivacaine, lidocaine, and meperidine (30). Further complicating the contribution of hemodynamic factors to fetal drug uptake is the nonhomogeneity of maternal and fetal blood flow within the placenta (54, 55). Inasmuch as most anesthetic drugs cross the placenta by a process of flow-dependent passive diffusion, changes in the maternal-to-fetal circulation ratios in various parts of the placenta undoubtedly may modulate drug transfer. Little information is available in this area.

FETAL DISTRIBUTION OF DRUGS

The fetal circulation is unique in several ways and can greatly modify drug distribution (Fig. 4.12). A variable proportion of the umbilical venous blood returning from the placenta perfuses the liver; the remainder flows through the ductus venosus (56). Fetal hepatic uptake of drug may protect against rapid attainment of high drug levels on the arterial side of the fetal circulation (Fig. 4.13) (57, 58). Dilution of umbilical venous blood in the fetal right atrium and shunting of blood across the foramen ovale and ductus arteriosus also modify fetal drug distribution.

The concentration of drug returning to the placenta in umbilical arterial blood is determined by the quantity of drug entering the fetal circulation (the input), fetal tissue uptake, fetal pH, protein binding and, possibly, nonplacental routes of fetal drug elimination (Table 4.4). Rapid placental transfer of

---

Table 4.4. FACTORS THAT DETERMINE THE CONCENTRATION OF FREE DRUG IN FETAL UMBILICAL ARTERIAL BLOOD (C_f)

Umbilical venous blood concentration (input)
Fetal pH
Fetal protein binding
Fetal tissue uptake
Nonplacental routes of fetal drug elimination
Fetal hepatic metabolism
Fetal renal excretion

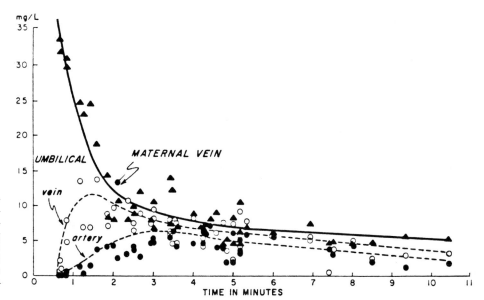

Figure 4.13. Thiopental blood concentrations in the maternal and umbilical veins and umbilical artery following an intravenous injection of the drug (4 gm/kg) to the mother. (Reprinted by permission from Kosaka Y, Takahashi T, Mark LC. Intravenous thiobarbiturate anesthesia for cesarean section. *Anesthesiology* 1969;31:489–506.)

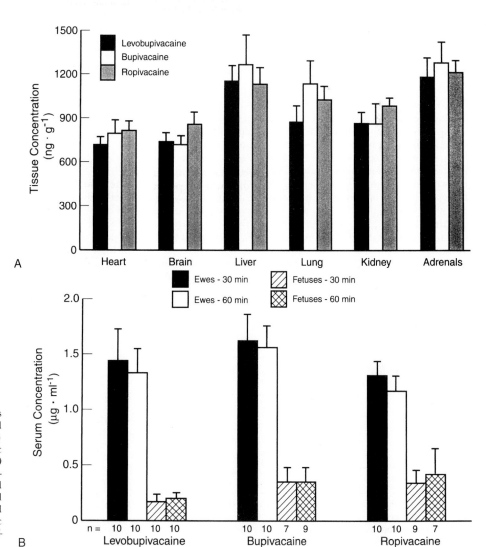

Figure 4.14. Fetal tissue concentrations (ng/g) (*Graph A*) and maternal and fetal serum concentrations (μg/mL) (*Graph B*) of levobupivacaine, racemic bupivacaine, and ropivacaine at 30 (serum only) and 60 minutes of intravenous infusion to the ewe. (Reprinted by permission from Santos AC, Karpel B, Noble G. The placental transfer and fetal effects of levobupivacaine, racemic bupivacaine and ropivacaine. *Anesthesiology* 1999;90:1698–1703.)

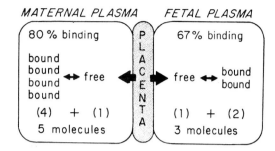

Figure 4.15. Differential protein binding of drug by maternal and fetal blood would account for differences in *total* drug concentrations on both sides of the placenta when free drug concentrations were, in fact, equal. (Reprinted by permission from DeJong RH. *Local Anesthetics.* Springfield, IL: Charles C Thomas; 1976:204.)

anesthetic drugs is paralleled by their rapid distribution to highly perfused fetal organs (57, 58). For instance, after intravenous administration of levobupivacaine, bupivacaine, or ropivacaine to pregnant sheep, the fetal tissue concentrations of all three drugs were considerably greater than the fetal serum concentrations (Fig. 4.14) (59).

Fetal red blood cells and serum proteins bind local anesthetics to a lesser degree than do maternal red blood cells and proteins (60). This may be clinically significant, because at a given total drug concentration more drug would be in the unbound free form, the fraction presumably responsible for physiologic effects (Fig. 4.15) (16).

FETAL METABOLISM AND EXCRETION OF DRUGS

Fetal hepatic enzyme activity is generally less than in adults. Oxidative and conjugative detoxification pathways, both of which are involved in the metabolism of many drugs, are deficient in the fetal or neonatal animal (61). In humans, although fetal metabolism of amide local anesthetics has not been studied, indirect evidence suggests that the human fetus can metabolize these drugs. Although hepatic CYP activity is absent in fetuses of several animal species either early or late in gestation, human fetal liver microsomes have significant CYP levels and NADPH cytochrome C reductase as early as the 14th week of gestation (62, 63). This suggests that even the premature human fetus can metabolize numerous drugs, including most local anesthetics.

A study comparing the pharmacokinetics of lidocaine among adult ewes and fetal and neonatal lambs showed that the metabolic clearance in the newborn was similar to, and renal clearance was greater than, that in the adult (Table 4.5) (64). Nonetheless, the elimination half-life was more prolonged in

the newborn. This was attributed to a greater volume of distribution and tissue uptake of the drug so that, at any given time, the neonate's liver and kidneys were exposed to a smaller fraction of lidocaine accumulated in the body. Similar results were obtained in another study involving administration of lidocaine to human infants in a neonatal intensive care unit (65). Prolonged elimination half-lives in the newborn compared with the adult have been noted for other amide local anesthetics (66).

Table 4.5. PHARMACOKINETICS OF LIDOCAINE IN ADULT SHEEP AND NEWBORN LAMBS

	Adult	Neonatel
Vdβ (I/kg)	1.84	3.94
T1/2α (min)	5	5
T1/2β (min)	31	51
C1 (mL/min/kg)	41	54
Renal Cl (mL/min/kg)	1.0	9.2

Adapted from Morishima HO, Finster M, Pedersen H, et al. Pharmacokinetics of lidocaine in fetal and neonatal lambs and adult sheep. *Anesthesiology* 1979;50:431–436.

REFERENCES

1. Herbst AL, Ulfelder H, Poskanzer DC. Adenocarcinoma of the vagina: Association of maternal stilbestrol therapy with tumor appearance in young women. *N Engl J Med* 1971;284:878–881.
2. Mirkin BL, Singh S. Placental transfer of pharmacologically active molecules. In: Mirkin BL, ed. *Perinatal Pharmacology and Therapeutics.* New York: Academic Press; 1976.
3. Mirkin BL. Drug distribution in pregnancy. In: Boreus L, ed. *Fetal Pharmacology.* New York: Raven Press; 1973:1–26.
4. Mirkin BL. Maternal and fetal distribution of drugs in pregnancy. *Clin Pharmacol Ther* 1973;14:643–647.
5. Levinson G, Shnider SM. Placental transfer of local anesthetics: Clinical implications. In: Marx GF, ed. *Parturition and Perinatology.* Philadelphia: Davis; 1973.
6. Mirkin BL. Perinatal pharmacology: Placental transfer, fetal localization, and neonatal disposition of drugs. *Anesthesiology* 1975;43:156–170.
7. Assali NS, Douglass RA, Baird WM, Nicholson DB, Suyemoto R. Measurement of uterine metabolism. IV. Results in normal pregnancy. *Am J Obstet Gynecol* 1953;66:248–253.
8. Comline RS, Silver M. Placental transfer of blood gases. *Br Med Bull* 1975;31:25–31.
9. Makowski EL, Meschia G, Droegemueller W, Battaglia FC. Distribution of uterine blood flow in the pregnant sheep. *Am J Obstet Gynecol* 1968;101:409–412.
10. Haram K, Bakke OM, Johanessen KH, Lund T. Transplacental passage of diazepam during labor: Influence of uterine contractions. *Clin Pharmacol Ther* 1978;24:590–599.
11. Gaylard DG, Carson RJ, Reynolds F. Effect of umbilical perfusate pH and controlled maternal hypotension on placental drug transfer in the rabbit. *Anesth Analg* 1990;71:42–48.
12. Laishley RS, Carson RJ, Reynolds F. Effect of adrenaline on placental transfer of bupivacaine in the perfused in situ rabbit placenta. *Br J Anaesth* 1989;63:439–443.
13. Covino BG, Vassallo HG. *Local Anesthetics: Mechanisms of Action and Clinical Use.* New York: Grune & Stratton; 1976:100.
14. Lund PC, Bush DF, Covino BG. Determinants of etidocaine concentration in the blood. *Anesthesiology* 1975;42:497–503.
15. Shnider SM, Way EL. The kinetics of transfer of lidocaine (Xylocaine) across the human placenta. *Anesthesiology* 1968;29:944–950.
16. DeJong RH. *Local Anesthetics.* Springfield, IL: Charles C. Thomas; 1977:197.
17. Tucker GT, Mather LE. Pharmacokinetics of local anesthetic agents. *Br J Anaesth* 1975;47:213–224.
18. Magno R, Berlin A, Karlsson K, Kjellmer I. Anesthesia for cesarean section. IV. Placental transfer and neonatal elimination of bupivacaine following epidural analgesia for elective cesarean section. *Acta Anaesthesiol Scand* 1976;20:141–146.
19. Pihlajamäki K, Kanto J, Lindberg R, Karanko M, Kiilholma P. Extradural administration of bupivacaine: Pharmacokinetics and metabolism in pregnant and nonpregnant women. *Br J Anaesth* 1990;64:556–562.
20. Ramanathan J, Botorff M, Jeter JN, et al. The pharmacokinetics and maternal and neonatal effects of epidural lidocaine in preeclampsia. *Anesth Analg* 1986;65:120–126.
21. Abernethy DR, Greenblatt DJ, Eshelman FN, Shader RI. Ranitidine does not impair oxidative or conjugative metabolism: Noninteraction with antipyrine, diazepam, and lorazepam. *Clin Pharmacol Ther* 1984;35:188–192.
22. Reimann IW, Klotz U, Frolich JC. Effects of cimetidine and ranitidine on steady-state propranolol kinetics and dynamics. *Clin Pharmacol Ther* 1982;32:749–757.
23. Wieslaw P, Jague LL, Tepperman BL, et al. Histamine H$_1$ and H$_2$ receptor vasodilation of canine intestinal circulation. *Am J Physiol* 1977;233:E219–224.

24. Feely J, Wilkinson GR, Wood AJJ. Reduction of liver blood flow and propranolol metabolism by cimetidine. *N Engl J Med* 1981;304:692–695.

25. Dailey PA, Hughes SC, Rosen MA, et al. Effect of cimetidine and ranitidine on lidocaine concentrations during epidural anesthesia for cesarean section. *Anesthesiology* 1988;69:1013–1017.

26. Flynn RJ, Moore J, Collier PS, Howard PJ. Single dose oral H_2-antagonists do not affect plasma lidocaine levels in the parturient. *Acta Anaesthesiol Scand* 1989;33:593–596.

27. O'Sullivan GM, Smith M, Morgan B, et al. H_2 antagonists and bupivacaine clearance. *Anaesthesia* 1988;43:93–95.

28. Brashear WT, Zuspan KJ, Lazebnik N, et al. Effect of ranitidine on bupivacaine disposition. *Anesth Analg* 1991;72:369–376.

29. Johnson RF, Cahana A, Olenick M, et al. A comparison of the placental transfer of ropivacaine versus bupivacaine. *Anesth Analg* 1999;89:703–708.

30. Johnson RF, Herman N, Arney TL, Gonzalez H, Johnson HV, Downing JW. Bupivacaine transfer across the human term placenta: A study using the dual perfused placental model. *Anesthesiology* 1995;82:459–468.

31. Tucker GT. Plasma binding and disposition of local anesthetics. *Int Anesthesiol Clin* 1975;13:33–59.

32. Kennedy RL, Miller RP, Bell JU, et al. Uptake and distribution of bupivacaine in fetal lambs. *Anesthesiology* 1986;65:247–253.

33. Kennedy RL, Bell JU, Miller RP, et al. Uptake and distribution of lidocaine in fetal lambs. *Anesthesiology* 1990;72:483–489.

34. Wulf H, Münstedt P, Maier CH. Plasma protein binding of bupivacaine in pregnant women at term. *Acta Anaesthesiol Scand* 1991;35:129–133.

35. Hamshaw-Thomas A, Rogerson N, Reynolds F. Transfer of bupivacaine, lignocaine and pethidine across rabbit placenta: Influence of maternal protein binding and fetal flow. *Placenta* 1984;5:61–70.

36. Vella LM, Knott C, Reynolds F. Transfer of fentanyl across the rabbit placenta. *Br J Anaesth* 1986;8:49–54.

37. Drábková J, Crul JF, van der Kleijn E. Placental transfer of 14C labelled succinylcholine in near-term Macaca mulatta monkeys. *Br J Anaesth* 1973;45:1087–1095.

38. Flynn PJ, Frank M, Hughes R. Use of atracurium in caesarean section. *Br J Anaesth* 1984;56:599–605.

39. Dailey PA, Fisher DM, Shnider SM, et al. Pharmacokinetics, placental transfer and neonatal effects of vecuronium and pancuronium administered during cesarean section. *Anesthesiology* 1984;60:569–574.

40. Waters JJ, Ramanathan S. Placental transfer of lidocaine during maternal hypoxia [abstract]. *Anesthesiology* 1991;75:A-828.

41. Reynolds F, Knott C. Pharmacokinetics in pregnancy and placental drug transfer. In: Milligan SR, ed. *Oxford Reviews of Reproductive Biology.* Vol 11. New York: Oxford University Press; 1989:389.

42. Roe DA, Little BB, Bawdon RE, Gilstrap L. Metabolism of cocaine by human placentas: Implication for fetal exposure. *Am J Obstet Gynecol* 1990;163:715–718.

43. Van Petten GR, Hirsch GH, Cherrington AD. Drug-metabolizing activity of the human placenta. *Can J Biochem* 1968;46:1057–1061.

44. Kan RE, Hughes SC, Rosen MA, Kessin C, Preston PG, Lobo EP. Intravenous remifentanil: Placental transfer, maternal and neonatal effects. *Anesthesiology* 1998;88:1467–1474.

45. Ala-Kokko TI, Pienimäki, Hollmén AI, Pelkonen O, Vähäkangas K. Transfer of clonidine and dexmedetomidine across the isolated perfused human placenta. *Acta Anaesthesiol Scand* 1997;41:313–319.

46. Brown WU Jr, Bell GC, Alper MH. Acidosis, local anesthetics and the newborn. *Obstet Gynecol* 1976;48:27–30.

47. Biehl D, Shnider SM, Levinson G, Callender K. Placental transfer of lidocaine: Effects of fetal acidosis. *Anesthesiology* 1978;48:409–412.

48. Johnson RF, Herman NL, Johnson HV, Arney TL, Paschall RL, Downing JW. Effects of fetal pH on local anesthetic transfer across the human placenta. *Anesthesiology* 1996;85:608–615.

49. Morishima HO, Covino BG. Toxicity and distribution of lidocaine in non-asphyxiated and asphyxiated baboon fetuses. *Anesthesiology* 1996;54:182–186.

50. Rudolph AM. *Congenital Diseases of the Heart: Clinical-Physiologic Considerations in Diagnosis and Management.* Chicago: Year Book Medical Publishers; 1974.

51. Morishima HO, Santos AC, Pedersen H, et al. Effect of lidocaine on the asphyxial responses in the mature fetal lamb. *Anesthesiology* 1987;66:502–507.

52. Morishima HO, Pedersen H, Santos AC, et al. Adverse effects of maternally administered lidocaine on the asphyxiated preterm fetal lamb. *Anesthesiology* 1989;71:110–115.

53. Santos AC, Yun EM, Bobby PD, Noble G, Arthur GR, Finster M. The effects of bupivacaine, L-nitro-L-arginine-methyl-ester and phenylephrine on cardiovascular adaptation to asphyxia in the preterm fetal lamb. *Anesth Analg* 1997;84:1299–1306.

54. Power GG, Hill EP, Longo LD. Analysis of uneven distribution of diffusing capacity and blood flow in placenta. *Am J Physiol* 1972;222:740–746.

55. Power GG, Longo LD, Wagner NN, Kuhl DE, Forster RE II. Uneven distribution of maternal and fetal placental blood flow, as demonstrated using macroaggregates, and its response to hypoxia. *J Clin Invest* 1967;46:2053–2063.

56. Pang LM, Mellins RB. Neonatal cardiorespiratory physiology. *Anesthesiology* 1975;43:171–196.

57. Finster M, Morishima HO, Boyes RN, Covino BG. The placental transfer of lidocaine and its uptake by fetal tissues. *Anesthesiology* 1972;36:159–163.

58. Finster M, Morishima HO, Mark LC, Perel JM, Dayton PG, James LS. Tissue thiopental concentrations in the fetus and newborn. *Anesthesiology* 1972;36:155–158.

59. Santos AC, Karpel B, Noble G. The placental transfer and fetal effects of levobupivacaine, racemic bupivacaine, and ropivacaine. *Anesthesiology* 1999;90:1698–1703.

60. Mather LE, Long G, Thomas J. The binding of bupivacaine to maternal and foetal plasma proteins. *J Pharm Pharmacol* 1971;23:359–365.

61. Dawkins MJ. Biochemical aspects of developing function in newborn mammalian liver. *Br Med Bull* 1966;22:27–33.

62. Waddell WJ, Marlowe GC. Disposition of drugs in the fetus. In: Mirkin BL, ed. *Perinatal Pharmacology and Therapeutics.* New York: Academic Press; 1976:119.

63. Yaffe SJ. Developmental factors influencing interactions of drugs. *Ann NY Acad Sci* 1976;281:90–97.

64. Morishima HO, Finster M, Pedersen H, et al. Pharmacokinetics of lidocaine in fetal and neonatal lambs and adult sheep. *Anesthesiology* 1979;50:431–436.

65. Mihaly GW, Moore RG, Thomas J, Triggs EJ, Thomas D, Shanks CA. The pharmacokinetics and metabolism of the anilide local anaesthetics in neonates. *Eur J Clin Pharmacol* 1978;13:143–152.

66. Brown WU Jr, Bell GC, Lurie AO, Scanlon JW, Alper MH. Newborn blood levels of lidocaine and mepivacaine in the first postnatal day following maternal epidural anesthesia. *Anesthesiology* 1975;42:698–707.

TWO

ANESTHESIA FOR VAGINAL DELIVERY

Shnider and Levinson's Anesthesia for Obstetrics, edited by Samuel C. Hughes, et al. Lippincott Williams & Wilkins, Philadelphia, © 2001.

CHAPTER 5

CHOICE OF LOCAL ANESTHETICS IN OBSTETRICS

KENNETH DRASNER, M.D. AND PHILIP R. BROMAGE, M.B., B.S., F.F.A.R.C., F.R.C.P. (C)

Local anesthetics are used to provide analgesia for labor and anesthesia for instrumented or operative deliveries. Although a broad range of local anesthetics are available for use in obstetrics, only three (lidocaine, chloroprocaine, and bupivacaine) have stood the test of time, while the role of two new agents (ropivacaine, levobupivacaine) has yet to be defined. This chapter will focus on these agents with only brief mention of the rationale underlying the exclusion of others. It sets out to describe the major advantages and disadvantages, and to suggest those drugs and concentrations likely to be best suited for the diverse clinical requirements of obstetric anesthetic practice. Opinions obviously change as fresh data become available in the neverending quest for greater safety and efficacy. However, it is somewhat surprising that complications have been the primary force driving the evolution of obstetric anesthesia during the past 2 decades.

It should be appreciated that one cannot discuss anesthetics independent of technique or specific clinical requirements, and these interrelated factors are considered relative to optimal care of the mother and fetus. Additionally, the use of spinal opioids in conjunction with local anesthetics has moved us closer to the goal of pain relief without motor block, has improved the quality of operative anesthesia, and has changed the landscape of postoperative analgesia. Thus, it will be necessary to touch briefly on some aspects of local anesthetic-opioid mixtures, although the main treatment of spinal opioids is presented in Chapter 9.

DESIDERATA

As with any choice, the question must be asked: What do we really want? All too often, this essential question to the act of selection has not been adequately considered. Fortunately, in the context of obstetric anesthesia, the objectives that underlie rational selection are easily defined and have guided practice over the past 45 years.

Labor Analgesia: Five basic requirements must be met for relief of pain during labor and delivery, as set out in Table 5.1. The drug must obviously provide effective analgesia and be safe for the mother. Additionally, in terms of the three Ps listed in Table 5.1: the expulsive forces of labor must be unaffected; tone should be preserved in the muscles of the birth canal to facilitate rotation of the fetal head; and the fetus must not be intoxicated by placental transfer of potentially depressing drugs nor should the drugs jeopardize fetal gas exchange. With respect to the latter, dosages should be kept to a minimum consistent with efficacy, and every means should be sought to minimize placental transfer. In addition, caution must be exercised when using vasoactive drugs that may diminish uterine blood flow.

Operative Delivery. Anesthetic requirements for cesarean section are clearly very different from analgesic requirements for vaginal delivery. Perhaps less appreciated are the subtle differences between the requirements for cesarean section and most other surgical procedures First, profound muscle relaxation is rarely necessary since the abdominal muscles are well stretched by the enlarged uterus. Second, analgesia must be profound in all lumbosacral segments, including the resistant segments L5 and S1, which carry nociceptive input during manipulation of the uterus and adjacent structures. In contemporary North American obstetric practice, this nociceptive input and the incidence of pain and nausea are heightened by the maneuver of eventrating the uterus for uterine repair (1). In European practice, most repairs are done in situ but, even then, partial rotation of the uterus on its long axis may generate appreciable pain if the L5 and S1 segments are not well anesthetized. Finally, segmental analgesia must extend higher than the sixth thoracic dermatome, which, theoretically, should be sufficient to interrupt all afferent impulses from the lower abdomen. Clinical experience shows that, contrary to theoretic expectations, analgesia is often inadequate unless blockade extends to include T4 or even to the apex of the axilla. Subarachnoid and lumbar epidural blockade are the most favorable anesthetic techniques to achieve these goals. Caudal anesthesia requires excessively large amounts of local anesthetic and is therefore not recommended for cesarean section.

TECHNIQUE-RELATED FACTORS: GENERAL CONSIDERATIONS AND RECENT DEVELOPMENTS

Spinal vs. Epidural Anesthesia. Surveys of anesthetic practice document increased use of spinal anesthesia for cesarean section over the last decade. This trend is likely to continue as recent evidence suggests that a spinal block provides better and more cost-effective anesthesia than an epidural block for uncomplicated, elective cesarean section (2). Furthermore, the recent manufacture of smaller-gauge and "noncutting" spinal needles (i.e., 26- to 29-gauge Quincke and 22- to 27-gauge Whitacre and Sprotte) has reduced the incidence of spinal puncture headaches to 1% to 2% (see Chapters 8, 9, and 11), eliminating one of the principal advantages of epidural anesthesia for cesarean section. Additionally, the safety and efficacy of modest doses of intrathecal opioids have brought spinal anesthesia in line with epidural analgesia with respect to effective postoperative analgesia. Preservative-free morphine in a small dose of 0.1 mg will provide 16 to 24 hours of postoperative analgesia with minimal risk of respiratory depression (3, 4). The quality of intraoperative analgesia can also be augmented by including a short-acting lipophilic agent such as fentanyl (10 to 25 μg) or sufentanil (5 to 10 μg) (5–7).

Subarachnoid block has obvious appeal because intense and extensive analgesia is obtained from a small dose of local anesthetic and blood concentrations never reach a level that could possibly have a depressant effect on the fetus. Moreover, the technique has the virtue of speed. The block can be performed and an anesthetic level to T3 established in 5 to 10 minutes, whereas a carefully titrated epidural anesthetic may

Table 5.1. REQUIREMENTS OF A LOCAL ANESTHETIC AGENT FOR RELIEF OF PAIN IN LABOR AND DELIVERY

Effective and controllable analgesia
Maternal safety
No weakening of maternal *p*owers
No alteration of maternal *p*assages
No depression of the *p*assenger (fetus)

take 20 to 30 minutes to reach the same segmental level. Even then, sensation may still persist in segments L5 and S1. Weighed against the advantage of speed is the unpredictability of segmental analgesic spread: none of the traditional indices of anesthetic dose, such as height, spinal length, body weight, or ponderal index, exerts any degree of statistical power for predicting segmental analgesic spread in parturient patients (8). Furthermore, the rapidity of sympathetic blockade is prone to cause precipitous changes of cardiovascular dynamics. As a result, the incidence of arterial hypotension is high and corrective vasopressor treatment is often needed, even in the presence of adequate hydration and left uterine displacement (9).

Unlike subarachnoid block, epidural analgesia requires dosages of local anesthetic agents large enough to cause appreciable transfer across the placenta, with the resulting possibility of fetal depression. Epidural blockade, however, has a slower onset, and the maternal cardiovascular system is more readily controlled than in the precipitous onset of subarachnoid block. Moreover, when a continuous catheter technique is used, dosage can be titrated to achieve a more precise segmental level, and an inadequate initial level can be raised by injecting a supplementary dose. As with spinal anesthesia for cesarean section, opioids have become standard adjuvants to improve the intraoperative quality of epidural analgesia and to prolong postoperative analgesia. However the opioid doses required by the epidural route are 5 to 10 times greater than when injected directly into the

intrathecal space. Thus, consideration must be given to minimizing maternal vascular uptake and placental transfer to the fetus.

Regardless of which drug is chosen, the key to successful epidural analgesia is time. Between 20 and 30 minutes is required to ensure solid analgesia, especially in segments L5 and S1. In a hurried milieu, a high incidence of intraoperative pain or discomfort must be expected if the operating team does not appreciate and abide by this inherent constraint of epidural blockade.

New Techniques for Labor and Delivery. Two recent developments threaten the distinction between spinal and epidural anesthesia for labor and delivery: combined spinal-epidural anesthesia (CSE) and continuous spinal anesthesia (CSA). The former is discussed in detail in Chapters 8 and 9.

Epidural vs. CSA. In the medicolegal climate of contemporary obstetric practice, cesarean section rates in the United States have climbed to 25% to 30%. Consequently, of all epidural catheters inserted for relief of pain in labor, one fourth to one third will end up providing surgical anesthesia for cesarean section. This change of purpose brings with it a distinct advantage of continuous catheter techniques for labor, a consideration that has traditionally favored the epidural technique. However, the recent development of small-bore intrathecal catheters may overcome this barrier, permitting more expanded use of intrathecal analgesia in this population (10, 11). However, there are no catheters currently approved for this use. Moreover, while experience with this technique in obstetrics is encouraging (12), it is far too limited to assess its safety and efficacy.

LOCAL ANESTHETIC AGENTS: GENERAL CONSIDERATIONS
Ester-Linked Agents

Local anesthetics are divided into two main pharmacologic genera, depending on their molecular structure: those with an ester linkage and those with an amide linkage (Fig. 5.1). The esters,

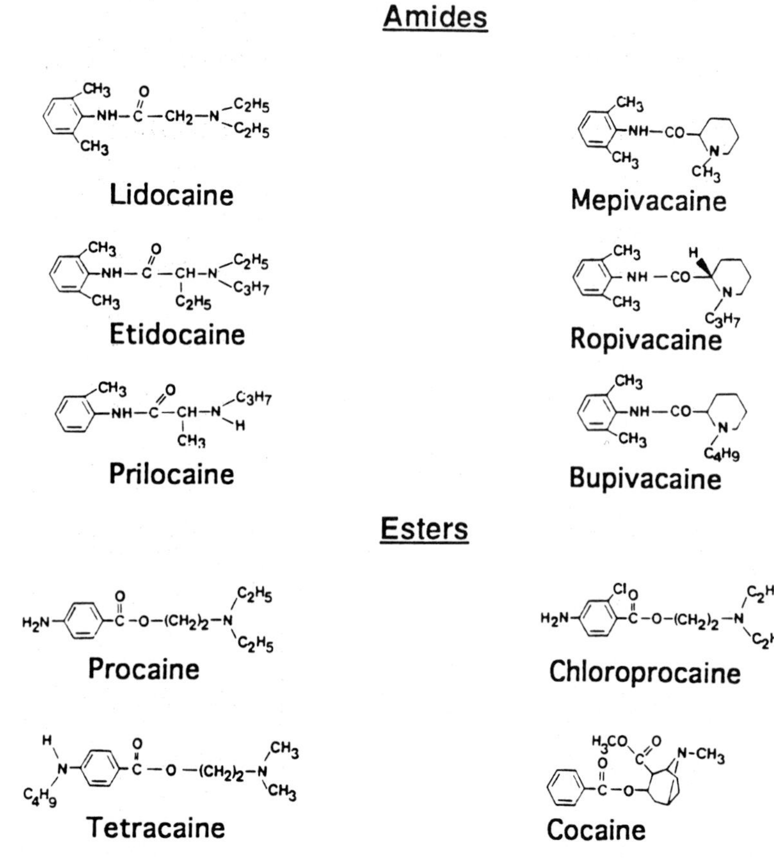

Figure 5.1. Chemical structures of local anesthetics.

Table 5.2. HALF-LIFE OF CHLOROPROCAINE (IN SECONDS)

	Mean ± SD
Mothers (n = 7)	20.9 ± 5.8
Umbilical cords (n = 7)	42.6 ± 11.2
Male controls (n = 6)	20.6 ± 4.1
Female controls (n = 5)	25.2 ± 3.7
Homozygous atypical cholinesterase carriers	106.0 ± 45.0

Reprinted by permission from O'Brien JE, Abbey V, Hinsvark O, Perel J, Finster M. Metabolism and measurement of 2-chloroprocaine, an ester-type anesthetic. *J Pharmacol Sci* 1979;68:75–79.

such as procaine, chloroprocaine, and tetracaine, are metabolized in the bloodstream by plasma pseudocholinesterase at different speeds, with chloroprocaine having the fastest rate of hydrolysis. However, some esters (such as piperocaine) are metabolized more readily by the liver than by plasma pseudocholinesterase. Paraaminobenzoic acid, the end-product of ester cleavage, passes across the placenta freely but does not appear to cause appreciable fetal depression (13). However, it is a known allergen and likely contributes to the higher incidence of reactions to ester-based anesthetics.

Chloroprocaine (Nesacaine)

Overview. Chloroprocaine has many of the attributes of the ideal epidural local anesthetic for obstetrics. It has a very fast onset, produces good quality sensory blockade, and has minimal systemic toxicity due to a rapid rate of hydrolysis. Unfortunately, these major advantages have been offset by significant limitations and complications. Nonetheless, chloroprocaine still has a valuable, if limited, role to play in obstetric anesthesia.

Chloroprocaine is quickly metabolized in the bloodstream in the presence of normal pseudocholinesterase. The *in vitro* plasma half-life is 21 seconds for maternal blood and 43 seconds for umbilical cord blood (14), translating into very low systemic concentrations, minimal drug transfer across the placenta, and continued rapid hydrolysis despite the lower esterase activity of the fetal circulation (Table 5.2 and Fig. 5.2) (15). This rapid metabolism imparts minimal risk of systemic toxicity, making it perhaps the safest agent for use in obstetrics.

A concentration of 1.5% to 2% is adequate for relief of first-stage labor pain, but a 3% solution is required for perineal analgesia and relaxation, or for cesarean section. Although the quality of sensory block is excellent, the duration of action is relatively short, lasting only 35 to 50 minutes with epinephrine added. Consequently, repetitive injection is often necessary even for routine uncomplicated cesarean section, presenting a minor drawback to its use for operative delivery.

A second, and more significant, barrier to its routine use is its effect on the efficacy of other epidural agents. Chloroprocaine, or one of its metabolites (4-amino-2-chlorobenzoic acid), impairs the anesthetic or analgesic action of epidural bupivacaine, fentanyl, and morphine, an effect that appears to occur whether these agents are used concurrently or even sequentially (16–21).

Chloroprocaine Toxicity: A Tale of Two Preservatives?

In addition to the limitations imposed by its short duration of action and its interference with other neuraxial agents, use of chloroprocaine has been associated with significant complications. These complications have arisen, at least in part, from preservatives added to the anesthetic solution to prevent chloroprocaine's oxidative decomposition.

In the recent past, chloroprocaine was suspected to be neurotoxic because of reports of neurologic injury presumed

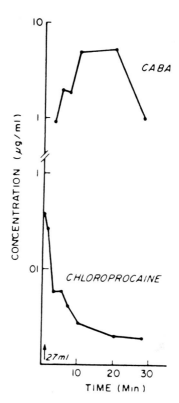

Figure 5.2. Plasma concentrations of chloroprocaine and chloroamino-benzoic acid (*CABA*) in a typical patient following epidural anesthesia (multiple injections) for vaginal delivery. (Reprinted by permission from Kuhnert BR, Kuhnert PM, Porochaska BS, Gross TL. Plasma levels of 2-chloroprocaine in obstetric patients and their neonates after epidural anesthesia. *Anesthesiology* 1980;53:21–25.)

secondary to intrathecal injection of chloroprocaine intended for epidural administration (22–24). However, the circumstances of these cases failed to clearly identify this mechanism of injury, as some did not have definitive evidence for intrathecal injection and several were complicated by significant hypotension. The animal experiments that followed also failed to establish this mechanism of injury, providing instead conflicting evidence regarding chloroprocaine neurotoxicity (25–31). The most widely cited were experiments by Gissen, in which exposure of isolated rabbit vagus nerves to the commercial solution of 3% chloroprocaine containing 0.2% sodium bisulfite and with a pH of approximately 3.0 produced irreversible block, while exposure to the same solution buffered to a pH of 7.3 resulted in complete recovery (26). Additional experiments in this model indicated that irreversible block could result from the combination of bisulfite and a low pH in the absence of anesthetic, suggesting that liberation of sulfur dioxide might be the etiology of injury. Although the prevailing conclusion was that bisulfite was the etiology of injury and that chloroprocaine per se was not neurotoxic, data from various other models did not consistently support these findings (31). More recent *in vivo* studies also call this conclusion into question and, ironically, suggest that bisulfite might actually be neuroprotective (32).

Nonetheless, concern for neurotoxicity induced Astra Pharmaceuticals to introduce a new formulation of chloroprocaine (Nesacaine-MPF), replacing metabisulfite with disodium ethylenediaminetetraacetic acid (EDTA), a chelating agent of heavy metals. Unfortunately, this new preservative brought with it a less serious, but nonetheless distressing, complication. Within 2 years of its introduction, Fibuch et al. reported a 40% incidence of severe back pain when this formulation was administered epidurally to patients undergoing ambulatory surgery (33). The backache was severe, unrelenting, lasting for a period of several hours, and often exceeding the pain from the surgical

Table 5.3. EFFECT OF ANESTHETIC SOLUTION ON BACK PAIN

		% Patients			
		Type 1*		Type 2†	
Group	Solution (Initial Volume/Supplemental Volume)	Immediate‡	24 h‡	Immediate§	24 h‖
1	2% lidocaine HCl (30 mmL/10 mL)	15	30	5	0
2	3% chloroprocaine w/EDTA (15 mL/5 mL)	5	30	10	5
3	3% chloroprocaine w/EDTA (30 mL/10 mL)	25	10	50	60
4	3% chloroprocaine w/o EDTA w/metabisulfite (30 mL/10 mL)	35	35	10	15
5	3% chloroprocaine w/EDTA pH adjusted (30 mL/10 mL)	20	30	25	30

*Type 1 = localized superficial pain confined to the area of neddle insertion.
†Type 2 = deep, aching, or burning pain confined to the lumbar area but diffuse in location.
‡Not statistically significant.
§Group 3 differs significantly from groups 1, 2, and 4 ($P < .0032$).
‖Group 3 differs significantly from groups 1, 2, and 4 ($P < .0001$); group 5 differs significantly from group 1 ($P < .0001$).
EDTA, ethylenediaminetetraacetic acid; w/, with; w/o, without.
Data from Stevens RA, Urmey WF, Urquhart BL, Kao, T. Back pain after epidural anesthesia with chloroprocaine. *Anesthesiology* 1993;78:492–497.

procedure. The authors postulated that binding of calcium reduced local tissue concentrations, inducing hypocalcemic tetany of the paraspinous muscles. Although this theory never gained universal acceptance, the causal relationship between epidural administration of Nesacaine-MPF and severe back pain was undeniable (34–36). During a study investigating thermal regulation, severe back pain was noted in four of five volunteers receiving Nesacaine-MPF, but none of 10 receiving lidocaine, and none of four receiving saline (34). In another study, 10 volunteers receiving three sequential escalating doses of epidural Nesacaine-MPF reported back pain that increased in severity following resolution of each block (35). But the most convincing evidence was derived from a prospective systematic investigation by Stevens et al. (36). These investigators administered five anesthetic solutions (including chloroprocaine with and without EDTA), and divided back pain into two distinct categories: superficial pain limited to the site of needle insertion, and deep and aching pain poorly localized in the lumbar region. The former had a similar incidence among groups, while the latter was significantly greater in incidence and intensity for patients receiving chloroprocaine containing EDTA (Table 5.3). Ultimately, this complication led to the abandonment of EDTA in favor of a formulation devoid of any preservative or antioxidant, and packaged in colored vials to reduce the rate of oxidation. Although removal of all preservatives resolved the frequent occurrence of back pain, continued concerns regarding chloroprocaine's neurotoxicity forbade intrathecal use and warrant heightened vigilance to avoid intrathecal placement during epidural administration.

Current Usage

Epidural. In spite of the rapid potency and very low toxicity of chloroprocaine, the need for repetitive injection and its interference with the analgesic efficacy of other adjuvants have relegated chloroprocaine to a relatively narrow role in obstetric analgesia. However, there are situations in which chloroprocaine can prove quite valuable. First, the onset of analgesia with 3% chloroprocaine is fast enough to substitute for subarachnoid analgesia in many cases where rapid anesthesia is required for instrumented delivery, retained placenta, or urgent cesarean section. A lowlumbar epidural injection of 12 to 15 mL will provide analgesia up to the umbilicus, and 20 mL will provide anesthesia for cesarean section. Obviously, a test dose should be used to exclude inadvertent subarachnoid injection but, as previously noted, the

danger of systemic toxicity is virtually nonexistent because of its rapid hydrolysis by plasma pseudocholinesterase. Second, the "chloroprocaine save" can salvage inadequate epidural anesthetics when it is believed that the catheter is positioned within the epidural space but blockade fails to extend to an adequate segmental level after a maximum safe dose of amide local anesthetic has been administered (37). Supplementary doses of 10 to 20 mL 3% chloroprocaine are generally sufficient to achieve a satisfactory surgical level of anesthesia.

Intrathecal. Concern for potential neurotoxicity prohibits deliberate intrathecal administration of this agent.

Procaine

One of the earliest anesthetics, procaine enjoyed widespread popularity as an intrathecal agent for several decades. It has a relatively short half-life, making it somewhat unsuitable for cesarean sections. For a short period of time, it gained favor as an intrathecal agent combined with tetracaine, procaine being used to facilitate onset. However, clinical comparisons to bupivacaine were unfavorable, the combination producing a higher incidence of hypotension and more prolonged block (38). Recent concerns regarding transient pain and/or dysesthesia with lidocaine have generated a modicum of renewed interest in this anesthetic for short surgical procedures (see **Lidocaine: Minor Toxicity**). However, the limited data are not encouraging with reference to quality of anesthesia, the presence of side effects and a reduced, but still significant, incidence of postoperative buttock/leg pain (39). Additionally, unpublished animal data from the laboratory of one of the co—authors suggests that spinal procaine has a poor therapeutic index with respect to neurotoxicity.

Piperocaine (Metycaine)

Piperocaine enjoyed a period of popularity in the 1940s and 1950s, but its slow hydrolysis rate gave it no advantage in terms of fetal toxicity, and it was discarded in favor of the more effective amide agents such as lidocaine.

Tetracaine (Pontocaine)

Tetracaine has a long duration of action and might seem to be a desirable epidural agent for use in labor. However, epidural tetracaine produces profound motor block with relatively poor analgesia (40). This pattern of dissociated blockade is particularly undesirable in obstetrics, in which sensory analgesia is needed while motor block interferes with the active management of parturition. Although tetracaine remains an effective and popular drug for subarachnoid block, its slow onset, variability, and somewhat excessive duration are ill suited for instrumented or operative delivery, and have led to its near abandonment in obstetrics in favor or lidocaine and bupivacaine.

AMIDE-LINKED AGENTS

The amide-linked agents include the most effective local anesthetics currently available. Unfortunately, these drugs are metabolized in the liver, and their half-lives are long. They have relatively low molecular weights (under 300) and high lipid solubilities, and thus all transfer across the placenta in greater or lesser amounts. The ease of placental transfer is also determined by their degree of ionization at physiologic pH. Transfer is favored by a high proportion of nonionized drug, and this, in turn, is favored by a low dissociation constant, or pK_a. For example, the five agents: lidocaine, etidocaine, mepivacaine, ropivacaine, and bupivacaine can be ranked in order of pK_a and diffusibility. Thus: mepivacaine (pK_a 7.65) > etidocaine (pK_a 7.76) > lidocaine (pK_a 7.85) > ropivacaine (pK_a 8.1) > bupivacaine (pK_a 8.16).

From this scale, it can be seen that mepivacaine is likely to show the greatest degree of placental transfer, and bupivacaine, the least. In the past, it was thought that highly protein-bound local anesthetics such as bupivacaine and etidocaine (41, 42) would not traverse the placenta as easily as less highly protein-bound drugs such as lidocaine. However, Morishima et al. (43) demonstrated that low fetal blood levels do not imply limited placental transfer. Studies in the pregnant guinea pig indicated that the total amount of local anesthetic reaching the fetus was the same for lidocaine and etidocaine. Highly protein-bound and lipid-soluble drugs have greater tissue uptake, and lower blood levels therefore result. The influence of protein binding and lipid solubility on fetal uptake of local anesthetics is discussed more fully in Chapter 4.

Lidocaine (Xylocaine)

Overview

Initially synthesized by Lofgren and Lundqvist in 1943, lidocaine was introduced into clinical practice in the United States in 1948. As an anesthetic agent, lidocaine is well suited for many of the requirements of obstetric practice. It provides excellent sensory block when administered epidurally for labor analgesia, and produces spinal or epidural anesthesia suitable for the time constraints of routine cesarean section. Unfortunately, use of spinal lidocaine has recently been plagued with major and minor complications that impact its use and threaten its viability as an intrathecal agent. Moreover, unlike chloroprocaine, these complications are all clearly linked to the anesthetic and are not attributable to preservatives or other components of the anesthetic solution.

In the early years, lidocaine hydrochloride was the standard agent for epidural analgesia in labor and for operative delivery. At that time, the provision of effective pain relief was the principal aim, and in most units relatively little attention was paid to the maintenance of motor power and the muscle tone of the birth canal. Moreover, infusion devices were primitive and imprecise; thus, intermittent bolus doses of 1% lidocaine were customary (44). After the introduction of bupivacaine into obstetrics, it became clear that bupivacaine provided a more favorable ratio of sensory-to-motor block (45). The advantage claimed for lidocaine was a lower incidence of fetal heart rate disturbances compared with bupivacaine (46), but this was achieved at the

expense of reliable perineal analgesia (47). Additionally, placental transfer of lidocaine was shown to be appreciable, with studies demonstrating that fetal accumulation of the maternal dose was 2.8 times higher for lidocaine than for bupivacaine (48, 49). Although Apgar scores were usually high (50, 51) and the time to sustained respiration short, neurobehavioral studies of the newborn after maternal lidocaine and mepivacaine epidurals indicated the possibility of subtle depression of some reflexes that was not seen after bupivacaine or chloroprocaine (52, 53). Later experience questioned the practical significance of these neurobehavioral changes (54, 55), and the pendulum of opinion swung back in favor of lidocaine's safety. In fact, the utility of neurobehavioral testing recently has been questioned. These issues are discussed in greater detail in Chapter 37.

Major Neurologic Toxicity

Concern that lidocaine might induce neurotoxic damage emerged in 1991, with a report by Rigler et al. of four cases of cauda equina syndrome following continuous spinal anesthesia CSA (56). Three of these cases were associated with the administration of 5% lidocaine delivered through a small-bore catheter specifically marketed for CSA. In all four cases, there was evidence of a restricted sacral block, and to achieve adequate anesthesia a dose of local anesthetic was administered which was greater than that routinely used with a single injection technique. These circumstances led the authors to postulate that the combination of maldistribution combined with repetitive injection produced neurotoxic concentrations of anesthetic within the subarachnoid space (56). This mechanism of injury was consistent with the clinical course of eight additional cases associated with lidocaine reported to the Food and Drug Administration (57). Studies performed with models of the subarachnoid space also support this etiology for injury—administration of hyperbaric local anesthetic through a sacrally—directed catheter produces a restricted distribution (58–60), and high concentrations can be achieved with clinically relevant dosages (Fig. 5.3) (58, 59).

Data from other *in vitro* and *in vivo* investigations provide abundant support for anesthetic toxicity as the mechanism of injury (61–70). Studies using isolated segments of frog or crayfish axon (61, 63, 64) or cell culture (62) demonstrate conduction failure (61–64), loss of membrane potential (62, 63), accumulation of intracellular calcium (62), and cell death (62)

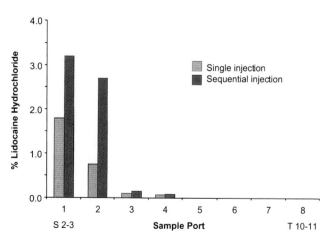

Figure 5.3. Effect of three sequential injections on distribution of lidocaine through a 28-gauge catheter on the model of the subarachnoid space. Two experiments are presented. In the first, 1 mL hyperbaric lidocaine hydrochloride was injected over 60 seconds; in the second, three sequential 1-mL injections (5 minutes apart) were made with the catheter in the same fixed position. (Reprinted by permission from Rigler ML, Drasner K. Distribution of catheter-injected local anesthetic in a model of the subarachnoid space. *Anesthesiology* 1991;75:684–692.)

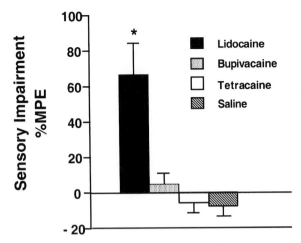

Figure 5.4. Sensory function 4 days after intrathecal administration of 5% lidocaine with 7.5% dextrose; 0.75% bupivacaine with 8.25% dextrose; 5% tetracaine with 5% dextrose; or normal. Tail-flick latency values were calculated as the average of latencies for the proximal, middle, and distal portions of the tail, and are expressed as percent maximum possible effect, where $\%MPE = \{(\text{tail-flick latency} - \text{baseline})/(\text{cut-off} - \text{baseline})\} \times 100$. Data represent mean ±SEM. (Reprinted by permission from Drasner K, Sakura S, Chan V, Bollen A, Ciriales R. Persistent sacral sensory deficit induced by intrathecal local anesthetic infusion in the rat. *Anesthesiology* 1994;80:847–852.)

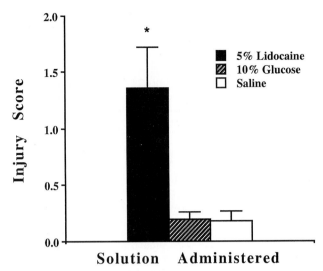

Figure 5.5. Nerve injury score for sections obtained 12 mm caudal to the conus 7 days after an intrathecal infusion of 5% lidocaine, 10% glucose in sterile water, or normal saline. Nerve injury scores were based on all fascicles present in each nerve cross-section. Each fascicle was assigned an injury score of 0–3, where 0 = normal; 1 = mild; 2 = moderate; and 3 = severe. The injury score for each cross-section was calculated as the average score of all fascicles in each section. Data reflect the mean ± SEM. The injury score for 5% lidocaine–treated animals differed significantly from that for 10% glucose–or saline-treated animals. (Reprinted by permission from Hashimoto K, Sakura S, Bollen AW, Ciriales R, Drasner K. Comparative toxicity of glucose and lidocaine administered intrathecally in the rat. *Reg Anesth Pain Med* 1998:23:444–445.)

with clinical concentrations of lidocaine, but not glucose (64). It should be appreciated that the absolute concentration having an effect in an isolated segment of nonmammalian axon or in cell culture must be interpreted with caution. Nonetheless, these results raise concern that concentrations of lidocaine below those achieved in spinal canal models (58, 59) might induce diverse deleterious effects (62–64) and that the neurotoxicity of lidocaine might exceed that of bupivacaine and tetracaine (64).

Studies using chronic indwelling catheters in rats demonstrate that deficits may occur *in vivo* with intrathecal lidocaine at concentrations used for spinal anesthesia. Administration of anesthetic in a restricted pattern can induce functional loss that closely parallels clinical injury and causes histologic damage consistent with impairment (65–70). Additionally, when administered in equal volumes, impairment produced by 5% lidocaine with 7.5% glucose was found to exceed that of 0.75% bupivacaine with 8.25% glucose or 0.5% tetracaine with 5% glucose (Fig. 5.4) (65); glucose alone neither induced injury (Fig. 5.5) (66) nor altered the toxicity of lidocaine (68).

Review of the cases of cauda equina syndrome led Rigler et al. to advocate abandonment of 5% lidocaine in favor of lower concentrations (56, 71), a recommendation adopted four years later by the manufacturer. However, this suggestion was based on limited available data demonstrating concentration-dependent injury derived from in vitro studies (72), peripheral nerve models (73) or experiments that failed to control for anesthetic dose (29). Surprisingly, preliminary *in vivo* data suggest that the toxicity from a fixed dose of lidocaine may be roughly equivalent whether the anesthetic is administered as a 5% or a 2% solution (74). Thus, the extent to which risk of toxicity is reduced by use of a lower, clinically effective, concentration remains to be established. Nonetheless, a 5% solution greatly exceeds the concentration needed for adequate blockade and a higher injectate concentration might pose some additional risk should anesthetic not be diluted by cerebrospinal fluid. (CSF)

Approval for dedicated small-bore catheters (>24 gauge) for continuous spinal anesthesia was ultimately withdrawn, effectively removing these devices from clinical practice in the United States. However, removal of these devices has not eliminated risk. Practitioners remain at liberty to use large-bore (epidural)

catheters for this purpose, and many resort to this technique following inadvertent dural puncture during attempted epidural placement. In fact, there is some evidence to suggest that this strategy might possibly decrease risk of postdural puncture headache comparable to placement of an epidural catheter at an alternative interspace (75). Moreover, ongoing studies evaluating the use of small-bore catheters for obstetric anesthesia show promise (76), and clinicians will likely see these catheters reintroduced into clinical practice. *Avoidance of injury therefore requires an understanding of the factors that contribute to neurotoxicity, and appropriate clinical management* (Table 5.4).

The experience with continuous spinal anesthesia (and with lidocaine) uncovered fundamental issues of toxicity that have proven to have broad relevance to the safe conduct of single-injection spinal anesthesia and continuous epidural anesthesia. As with continuous spinal anesthesia, repeat injection after a "failed" single-injection spinal may confer risk (77). If sensory block is inadequate because of maldistribution, there is the potential (albeit less than with a catheter in fixed position) for

---

Table 5.4. CONTINUOUS SPINAL ANESTHESIA: GUIDELINES FOR ANESTHETIC ADMINISTRATION

1. Insert catheter just far enough to confirm and maintain placement.
2. Use the lowest effective anesthetic concentration.
3. Place a limit on the amount of anesthetic to be used.
4. Administer a test dose and assess the extent of block.
5. If maldistribution is suspected, use maneuvers to increase the spread of local anesthetic (e.g., change the patient's position, alter the lumbosacral curvature, switch to a solution with a different baricity).
6. If well-distributed sensory anesthesia is not achieved before the dose limit is reached, abandon the technique.

Adapted from Rigler ML, Drasner K, Krejcie TC, et al. Cauda equina syndrome after continuous spinal anesthesia. *Anesth Analg* 1991;72:275–281.

Table 5.5. SPINAL ANESTHESIA GUIDELINES FOR ANESTHETIC ADMINISTRATION AFTER A "FAILED SPINAL"

1. Aspiration of CSF should be attempted before and after injection of anesthetic.
2. Sacral dermatomes should always be included in an evaluation of the presence of a spinal block.
3. If CSF is aspirated after anesthetic injection, it should be assumed that the local anesthetic has been delivered into the subarachnoid space; total anesthetic dosage should be limited to the maximum dose a clinician would consider reasonable to administer in a single injection.
4. If an injection is repeated, the technique should be modified to avoid reinforcing the same restricted distribution.
5. If CSF cannot be aspirated after injection, repeat injection of a full dose of local anesthetic should not be considered unless careful sensory examination (conducted after sufficient time for development of sensory anesthesia) reveals no evidence of block.

CSF = cerebrospinal fluid.
Modified from Drasner K, Rigler ML. Repeat injection after a "failed spinal": At times, a potentially unsafe practice. *Anesthesiology* 1991;75:713–714.

repeat injections to distribute in the same restricted pattern, which could result in neurotoxic concentrations of local anesthetic. Accordingly, guidelines for management of a failed spinal have been proposed which include an assessment of the likelihood of technical error (e.g., movement of the needle), and an appropriate adjustment of dosage for the repeat injection (Table 5.5). For example, if CSF can be aspirated immediately following injection of local anesthetic, it should be assumed that the full dose of local anesthetic has been delivered intrathecally—the combined dosage from the two injections should not exceed the maximum a clinician would consider reasonable to administer in a single injection.

There is a third mechanism by which relatively high doses of anesthetic find their way into the subarachnoid space—inadvertent intrathecal injection of a dose intended for epidural administration. As previously discussed, concerns for neurotoxicity with misplaced anesthetic emerged in the 1980s with reports of deficits associated with administration of chloroprocaine. However, appreciation that lidocaine was not completely innocuous removed the conceptual barrier needed for recognition of similar injuries induced by this anesthetic (78, 79). Furthermore, that injuries occurred with a second anesthetic agent suggested a common mechanism, casting further doubt that neural deficits associated with chloroprocaine were due to the antioxidant. These injuries, therefore, underscore the critical importance of the test dose and fractional administration during epidural administration of anesthetic. Additionally, should high doses of an anesthetic be administered through a misplaced catheter, repetitive withdrawal of small volumes of CSF and replacement with saline should be considered regardless of the anesthetic agent.

Taken together, these clinical reports combined with supportive experimental data provided compelling evidence that injury might result if high doses of anesthetic are administered intrathecally. Then, in 1997, two articles appearing in the same issue of *Anesthesiology* raised suspicion that neurologic deficits might occur with administration of lidocaine at a dose recommended for single-injection spinal anesthesia (80, 81). The first was a case report of cauda equina syndrome following a routine spinal performed with 100 mg lidocaine with epinephrine (80). The second was a prospective study of regional anesthesia from France (81). In this database were roughly 40,000 spinal anesthetics with 12 neurologic deficits that could not be explained on the basis of trauma. Of these, nine occurred with lidocaine, including three that were permanent. Although far from conclusive, an analysis of these cases pointed to toxicity as the most likely etiology of injury (82). Accordingly, modifications in technique have been proposed that may decrease risk of injury (Table 5.6). Most critically, it has been suggested that the dose of lidocaine used for single-injection spinal anesthesia not exceed 75 mg.

Minor "Toxicity"

The reports of major toxicity associated with high doses of intrathecal lidocaine served as a catalyst for identification of a syndrome of pain and/or dysesthesia that commonly follows

Table 5.6. LIDOCAINE SPINAL ANESTHESIA: SUGGESTED GUIDELINES

1. Dosage should be limited to 75 mg.
2. Concentration should not exceed 2.0%.
3. Epinephrine should not be used to enhance anesthesia or prolong the duration of block.
4. Consider alternative techniques for outpatients and for patients positioned with stretch on lumbosacral roots, e.g., lithotomy.

Modified from Drasner K. Lidocaine spinal anesthesia: A vanishing therapeutic index? *Anesthesiology* 1995;87:469–472.

spinal anesthesia with standard intrathecal doses of lidocaine. In their initial report of four cases, Schneider et al. suggested that these symptoms represented a transient neurotoxic effect of lidocaine and proposed the term "transient radicular irritation" (TRI) (83). However, uncertainty regarding etiology has led to the abandonment of this term in favor of the less specific term "transient neurologic symptoms" (TNS). Additionally, all four patients were in lithotomy position, leading the authors to also postulate that this produced stretch on the nerve roots of the cauda equina, reducing tissue perfusion, and increasing vulnerability of the nerve fibers (83). A follow-up study performed at the same institution by Hampl et al. documented a remarkably high incidence of symptoms associated with lidocaine (Table 5.7) (84). When questioned by a research nurse blinded to the anesthetic, 44 of 120 patients (37%) reported symptoms while only one of 150 patients receiving bupivacaine was symptomatic. Data from both nonrandomized (85, 86) and randomized (87–89) studies have subsequently confirmed that symptoms are quite common with lidocaine but infrequent with bupivacaine or tetracaine. Although these symptoms appear self-limited, the pain can be quite severe. In one study, 48% of symptomatic patients rated their pain as 4 or greater on a scale from 0 to 10, and 30% rated it as 8 or greater (86). In some cases, pain has been so incapacitating as to require rehospitalization for pain management (90).

Although the etiology and significance of these symptoms remain to be established, the evolving literature has succeeded in

Table 5.7. TRANSIENT NEUROLOGIC SYMPTOMS (TNS) AFTER SPINAL ANESTHESIA

	5% Lidocaine	0.5% Bupivacaine
Total	120	150
Paresthesia	12	9
> 1 Puncture	9	18
Lithotomy	120	93
TNS	44	1

From Hampl K, Schneider M, Ummenhofer W, Drewe J. Transient neurologic symptoms after spinal anesthesia. *Anesth Analg* 1995; 81:1148–1153.

identifying or eliminating other factors that contribute to their occurrence. For example, the high osmolarity of the standard hyperbaric 5% lidocaine solution (>800 mOsm/L) was shown not to be a factor, as the incidence was similar when lidocaine was administered in a solution containing 2.7% glucose (88). Subsequent data suggested that the addition of epinephrine or even the elimination of glucose has no significant effect (86, 89). Unfortunately, studies have also documented that reducing the concentration of lidocaine from 5% to 2% (89, 91) or even lower (92) fails to alter the incidence of TNS. Although these findings may seem counterintuitive, it is critical to appreciate the difference between the anesthetic concentration in the injected solution and bathing the nerve roots in the subarachnoid space. In the absence of extreme maldistribution, it is the dose administered that will determine the concentration in the subarachnoid space.

Data from a multicenter epidemiologic study of 1,863 patients provide strong support for lithotomy enhancing TNS with lidocaine, the relative risk being 2.6 (95% confidence interval [CI], 1.5 to 4.5) compared with other positions (86). Interestingly, patients in another study having knee arthroscopy under lidocaine spinal anesthesia had a 13% incidence of TNS compared with 5% for those undergoing inguinal herniorrhaphy (89). The authors suggested that, as with lithotomy, positioning for arthroscopy with the nonoperative leg flexed at the knee and the operative leg manipulated to facilitate surgery contributed to the development of symptoms by producing stretch of the lumbosacral nerves.

Additional data from the aforementioned epidemiologic study provide information concerning other potential risk factors for TNS (86). In addition to lithotomy position, outpatient status was found to be a significant factor (relative risk [RR], 3.6; 95% CI, 1.9 to 6.8), while obesity was of borderline significance (RR, 1.6; 95% CI, 1.0 to 2.5). The impact of these factors and their interaction can be readily appreciated by reviewing Table 5.8 (86). Equally important, many factors postulated to have an effect did not alter risk, including type and size of spinal needle, level and approach for spinal puncture, blood-tinged CSF, and, most surprisingly, the dose of lidocaine. However, the dose range was relatively narrow, and a more recent study reported a lower incidence of symptoms when a "conventional dose" of lidocaine (50 mg) was replaced with a "minidose" (20 mg) combined with 25 μg fentanyl (93). Whether this effect was due to the dose limitation, the addition of fentanyl, or their interaction remains to be determined.

Although there have been case reports of TNS in parturients (94), obstetric patients may be at lower risk. First, based on the aforementioned data, one might predict that use of lidocaine for cesarean section would not have a low incidence of TNS because of supine positioning and inpatient status. Additionally, in a nonrandomized prospective study, none of 67 parturients receiving lidocaine developed symptoms (95% CI, 0% to 4.5%), including 18 who were in lithotomy position (95). Obviously, it will be necessary to see whether these findings hold up as additional data become available.

There has been considerable speculation that severe deficits following high doses of intrathecal lidocaine and episodes of pain and/or dysesthesia following single-injection spinal anesthesia represent different points on a spectrum of toxicity. The occurrence of more significant dysfunction in the former would be consistent with the greater anesthetic exposure. Whether transient dysfunction and permanent injury are mediated by the same mechanism is of substantial importance. In addition to engendering greater concern, factors affecting transient dysfunction could be investigated using existing animal models of neurotoxicity. The corollary would also prove useful, i.e., TNS could serve as a surrogate clinical end point for more serious injury, providing an invaluable tool for evaluating the safety of anesthetic agents and techniques. However, although the data are far too limited to draw reasonable conclusions, discrepancies between factors affecting TNS and experimental animal data cast doubt on a common mechanism. For example, in contrast to the clinical studies cited above, epinephrine appears to substantially enhance functional impairment and histologic damage induced by intrathecal administration of lidocaine (67). Similarly, prilocaine appears to have a low incidence of TNS (87) yet induce similar injury in an experimental model of neurotoxicity (96). At a minimum, such inconsistencies raise doubt that TNS will be a valuable surrogate marker for major toxicity.

Alternative etiologies for TNS have been proposed, but only one, myofascial pain, has garnered much support. Proponents of this theory point to the association with positioning, the nature of these symptoms, and isolated case reports of relief with trigger-point injection (97–99). However, ascribing these symptoms to a musculoskeletal origin is difficult because of the disproportionally high incidence of TNS observed with lidocaine (84–89). One explanation offered to account for this disparity is that local anesthetics differ with respect to an intervening factor, i.e., motor block, and that the higher incidence with lidocaine is due to more profound musculoskeletal relaxation with this anesthetic. However, differences in motor block among anesthetics do not appear adequate to account for the large discrepancy in symptoms (87, 100). Moreover, in a randomized study comparing spinal and general anesthesia, symptoms consistent with TNS occurred in 8 of 30 patients (27%) given lidocaine but in only one of the 30 patients receiving a general anesthetic with muscle relaxation (101).

Current Usage

Epidural. Lidocaine's quick onset is used to advantage by many for establishing effective pain control for labor. Generally administered as a 1.5% solution containing epinephrine, an initial dose of 3 to 5 mL serves as a reasonable test for intrathecal and intravascular placement. Absence of block or elevated heart rate is often followed by an additional 3 to 8 mL or, alternatively, a similar volume of a low concentration of bupivacaine, levobupivacaine, or ropivacaine. As discussed above, the more favorable experience with bupivacaine has relegated lidocaine to a minor position with respect to infusions for maintenance of analgesia during labor. However, along with chloroprocaine, lidocaine is often used to provide anesthesia for instrumented or assisted delivery, and is particularly favored if there is a high likelihood of requiring cesarean section.

The slow onset and prolonged motor block produced by bupivacaine, as well as its potential cardiac toxicity, have helped to establish lidocaine's dominance as the epidural agent of choice for cesarean section. As such, a total of 18 to 25 mL of a 2% solution in incremental doses is needed to raise the upper segmental level of analgesia to the third or fourth thoracic segments. Epinephrine 1:200,000 should be added to reduce vascular absorption, minimizing the risk of systemic toxicity while increasing effective anesthesia to approximately 75 minutes. This prolongation and enhancement of block may also, in part, be due

---

Table 5.8. FACTORS WHICH MODIFIED RISK OF TNS WITH LIDOCAINE

Lithotomy	Outpatient	TNS
No	No	3.1%
Yes	No	7.7%
No	Yes	9.5%
Yes	Yes	24.3%

From Freedman J, Li D, Drasner K, et al. Transient neurologic symptoms after spinal anesthesia: An epidemiologic study of 1863 patients. *Anesthesiology* 1998;89:633–641.

to epinephrine's α-2 activity. If necessary, repetitive injection is made using a plain solution and a volume approximately half that which was required to establish anesthesia. Segmental analgesic efficacy and maternal comfort, without fetal depression, may also be increased by including a lipid-soluble opioid, such as fentanyl (50 to 100 μg) or sufentanil (30 μg) (102). Following delivery of the infant, epidural morphine (2.5 to 4 mg) may be administered via the epidural catheter for prolonged postoperative analgesia (103, 104).

Although onset of epidural lidocaine is a bit sluggish compared to chloroprocaine, it may be hastened by elevating the pH of the solution. As discussed under the section **Adjuvants** later in this chapter, alkalinization favors the nonprotonated species, facilitating penetration and delivery to the site of action. An alternative approach is to add CO_2, which presumably decreases intracellular pH, leading to diffusion trapping of the cationic form. Carbonated lidocaine has been available in Canada and Europe since 1970, but not in the United States. Initial clinical studies with this agent showed great promise in terms of its faster onset and more intense analgesia, especially in the resistant segments of L5 and S1 (105–107). Later comparisons reported somewhat disappointing findings (108–110), while more recent double-blind comparisons confirmed the significantly faster profiles of sensory and motor block with the carbonated salts (111, 112).

Spinal. As discussed above, issues of major toxicity and TNS have severely impacted the enthusiasm for spinal lidocaine. Nonetheless, lidocaine is still widely used for spinal anesthesia in the parturient. Adherence to a ceiling dose of 75 mg should minimize risk though the effect of pregnancy on susceptibility to toxicity is not known. Because subarachnoid blockade spreads further in obstetric patients than in the normal population, this recommendation poses little limitation as 60 to 75 mg will produce a reliable upper segmental level analgesia in the range of T4 or C8 even when administered in the sitting position at L3 to L4. Recent experimentation with very low doses (20 mg) combined with fentanyl suggests these may be adequate for cerclage or instrumented delivery (93). Use of such low doses should virtually eliminate risk of major toxicity and may minimize the incidence of TNS. Because concentration can be reduced without loss of efficacy, there is little justification to use 5% lidocaine. However, as previously discussed dilution of 5% lidocaine appears to have no effect on the incidence of TNS and the extent to which risk of major toxicity is actually reduced by use of a lower, clinically-relevant, concentration remains to be established.

Prilocaine (Citanest)

Prilocaine was introduced into obstetrics with the hope that its rapid metabolism and low acute toxicity would make it a useful drug in this population. Unfortunately, the phenolic metabolite of prilocaine, α-ortho-toluidine, can cause significant methemoglobinemia (113, 114). Because the fetus is vulnerable to any reduction of oxygen supply, it is generally accepted that the risk of methemoglobinemia is a contraindication to the use of prilocaine as an epidural agent for relief of pain in labor or for cesarean section (115). However, these concerns do not apply to its use as a spinal anesthetic due to the low dose requirement. Consequently, recent issues regarding lidocaine's toxicity may herald expanded use of prilocaine as an intrathecal agent in obstetric anesthesia.

Although never achieving the popularity of lidocaine, prilocaine has been used as an intrathecal agent for more than 30 years (116, 117). It has a duration of action similar to lidocaine, making it more suitable than bupivacaine for short procedures such as cerclage or instrumented deliveries. Most critically, there is evidence suggesting that, in contrast to lidocaine and similar to bupivacaine, spinal administration of prilocaine has a low incidence of TNS. In a survey of over 5,000 spinal anesthetics

performed with prilocaine, Konig did not uncover any cases associated with TNS (118). However, data collection was neither prospective nor blinded, and the incidence of TNS with prilocaine was not directly compared to that of other anesthetics. Lack of comparison with lidocaine is particularly problematic because the reported incidence of TNS is highly variable and, as previously noted, dependent upon factors such as patient positioning. In an effort to overcome these limitations, Hampl et al. performed a prospective double-blind study in women undergoing short gynecologic procedures in lithotomy position, a population at high risk of TNS (87). Patients were randomly assigned to receive a hyperbaric solution of lidocaine, prilocaine, or bupivacaine. TNS occurred in 9 of 30 patients receiving 2% lidocaine, 1 of 30 patients receiving 2% prilocaine, and 0 of 30 patients receiving 0.5% bupivacaine. As expected, times to ambulate and to void with prilocaine were similar to lidocaine and significantly shorter than with bupivacaine. Taken together, these two reports suggest that prilocaine might be a suitable alternative to spinal lidocaine for short obstetric procedures. However, far more data and experience are required to draw reasonable conclusions regarding risk of TNS (or other potential problems) with prilocaine. Moreover, prilocaine is not currently approved for use in the United States, nor is there any formulation available that would be appropriate for intrathecal administration.

Mepivacaine (Carbocaine)

Mepivacaine is an effective amide agent with a slightly longer duration of action than lidocaine, but its long half-life in the neonate (9 hours vs. less than 3 hours for lidocaine) led to a decline in its use as an epidural agent in obstetric practice (52, 119). However, as with prilocaine, the search for alternatives to lidocaine for spinal anesthesia have generated interest in mepivacaine as a short-acting intrathecal agent. Unfortunately, the data concerning TNS with mepivacaine are limited, conflicting, and fairly discouraging (120–124).

In a prospective randomized study of 200 patients, Hiller and Rosenberg reported a 30% incidence of TNS in patients receiving 4% mepivacaine with 9.5% glucose compared with 3% for those receiving 0.5% bupivacaine with 8% glucose (121). In contrast, in a randomized study of ambulatory patients undergoing knee arthroscopy, none of 30 patients receiving 45 mg 1.5% mepivacaine developed TNS compared with 6 of 27 receiving 60 mg 2% lidocaine (120). However, a follow-up dose-ranging study performed at the same institution by Zayas et al. reported a 7.4 % incidence with 30 to 60 mg isobaric 1.5% mepivacaine used for the same surgical procedure (122). To further confuse matters, in a similar dose-ranging study by Pawlowski et al., none of 60 patients receiving 60 to 80 mg isobaric 2% mepivacaine for anterior cruciate ligament by repair reported symptoms consistent with TNS (123). Finally, in a prospective study of 90 patients undergoing mainly urologic procedures, TNS was observed in 6 of 30 patients receiving lidocaine (20%), in 11 of 30 patients receiving mepivacaine (37%), and in 0 of 30 patients (0%) receiving bupivacaine (124).

Bupivacaine (Marcaine, Sensorcaine)

Bupivacaine is a congener of mepivacaine, with three methyl groups added to the piperidine ring of the mepivacaine molecule. This important agent was introduced into clinical practice by Telivuo in 1963 (125). When used as an epidural anesthetic agent for labor, bupivacaine produces high-quality analgesia with minimal motor blockade. These favorable characteristics, along with its minimal effect on the fetus, have established bupivacaine as the most commonly used local anesthetic for epidural analgesia during labor and delivery. As an intrathecal agent, bupivacaine has a relatively unblemished record, and it has become an increasingly popular anesthetic

Table 5.9. PERCENTAGE OF SIGNIFICANT ELECTROCARDIOGRAPHIC RHYTHM ABNORMALITIES, HEMODYNAMIC CHANGES, OR DEATH IN ACIDOTIC SHEEP AFTER INJECTION OF LIDOCAINE OR BUPIVACAINE AT TWO DOSE LEVELS

	Lidocaine (%)		Bupivacaine (%)	
	5.7 mg/Kg (n = 5)	11.4 mg/Kg (n = 6)	2.1 mg/Kg (n = 6)	4.2 mg/Kg (n = 6)
Atrioventricular conduction block	0	0	0	50
Wide QRS complex rhythm	0	0	33	30
Wide QRS complex bradycardia	0	0	50	83
Wide QRS complex tachycardia	0	0	0	17
Electromechanical dissociation	0	0	17	66
Death	0	0	17	100

Modified from data in Rosen MA, Thigpen JW, Shnider SM, Foutz SE, Levinson G, Koike M. Bupivacaine-induced cardiotoxicity in hypoxic and acidotic sheep. *Anesth Analg* 1985;64:1089–1096.

for cesarean section due to recent concerns regarding lidocaine toxicity.

Early studies with epidural bupivacaine for labor and delivery were marred by the use of excessive concentrations for the required task. Solutions of 0.25% to 0.5% provided excellent relief of pain but at the cost of unnecessary maternal motor blockade and immobility. Clinical studies by Van Steenberge et al. in the early 1970s challenged the wisdom of providing such intense segmental blockade throughout labor (126–128). Concentrations of 0.125% bupivacaine with low-dose epinephrine (1:800,000) were shown to provide adequate comfort while retaining muscular tone (126–128). Subsequent studies documented the feasibility of using even lower concentrations when combined with an epidural opioid (0.0625% bupivacaine with fentanyl 2 μg/mL) (129, 130), setting off an empiric search for the optimal mixture to provide maternal comfort with the least depression of the fetus or the muscular powers of parturition. This remains an area of significant clinical investigation (131–134).

Use of epidural bupivacaine has been shown to have little impact on the fetus. Early studies by Scanlon et al. (53) used neurobehavior tests to assess the effect of absorbed bupivacaine on the newborn after maternal epidural analgesia with rather high cumulative maternal doses of bupivacaine. They found that the umbilical vein concentrations of 110 ± 20 ng/mL at delivery were apparently innocuous. Later studies of placental transfer by Kennedy et al. demonstrated the favorable pharmacokinetics of bupivacaine compared with lidocaine (48, 49). Moreover, detectable neurobehavioral effects have been absent even after administration of high volumes of 0.75% bupivacaine for cesarean section (135, 136). (The issue of placental transfer and its effect on the fetus are discussed more thoroughly in Chapters 4 and 37.)

In contrast to its applicability for labor and delivery, epidural bupivacaine is rather unsuitable for cesarean section. If administered as a 0.5% solution, it has a slow onset (40), provides less intense anesthesia than lidocaine 2%, and has a high incidence of prolonged motor block. Faster onset and better surgical conditions can be achieved with a 0.75% concentration, and this formulation enjoyed popularity as a single-shot agent for some years. Unfortunately, tragic cases of refractory cardiac arrest were associated with its use, and 0.75% bupivacaine was withdrawn from obstetric practice. While elimination of this solution reduced the maximum exposure, concern for bupivacaine toxicity reinforced modifications in practice standards that may have had an even greater impact on patient safety. Specifically, these cases underscored the critical importance of the test dose and fractionated administration of anesthetic, particularly when large volumes of concentrated local anesthetics are used for cesarean section.

The cardiotoxicity of bupivacaine has been exhaustively investigated using numerous models, including isolated heart

(137–139) and heart tissue (140, 141), as well as *in vivo* toxicity in mice (142), rabbits (143), rats (144), cats (145), dogs (146–148), sheep (149–151), and monkeys (152). Although some studies failed to demonstrate unique cardiotoxic properties of bupivacaine (146, 147, 152), the weight of evidence clearly suggested that the cardiotoxicity of bupivacaine far exceeds that of lidocaine (Table 5.9 and Fig. 5.6) (137, 138, 140, 145, 148, 150, 151).

The most likely mechanism for bupivacaine's cardiotoxicity relates to the nature of its interaction with cardiac sodium channels (140) (Figs. 5.7 and 5.8 and Table 5.9). Both lidocaine and bupivacaine block voltage-gated sodium channels of nerve and heart. These channels, which open briefly during the upstroke of the action potential, are responsible for fast conduction. Indeed, blockade at the level of the nerve membrane is the primary mechanism of action of local anesthetics. Although blockade of cardiac sodium channels by lidocaine is well tolerated, the same does not hold true for bupivacaine (140). When electrophysiologic differences between lidocaine and bupivacaine were compared using voltage clamp experiments with guinea pig papillary muscle, lidocaine was found to enter the sodium channel quickly and to leave quickly. Recovery from bupivacaine block during diastole was noted to proceed relatively slowly, making it far more potent with respect to depressing V_{max} (conduction) in ventricular muscle. As a result, bupivacaine has been labeled a "fast-in, slow-out" agent (Fig. 5.7 and 5.8) (140). Similar effects were observed in a subsequent study of isolated rabbit Purkinje fiber-ventricular muscle (141). These effects likely set the stage for unidirectional block and reentry, a concept supported by epicardial mapping studies conducted in rabbit heart (139). Additional mechanisms that may play an important role in bupivacaine cardiotoxicity include depression of atrioventricular nodal conduction (153) and myocardial contractility (154), as well as indirect effects mediated via the central nervous system (CNS) (143, 144). More recent studies of cardiotoxicity have centered on comparisons of bupivacaine with two new local anesthetics, ropivacaine and bupivacaine, and are addressed later in this chapter.

Most of the reported cases of bupivacaine cardiotoxicity involved obstetric patients (155). The reason for the apparent higher incidence during pregnancy has never been established. It may have been due to the more frequent use of 0.75% bupivacaine in this population, or that pregnancy made it easier to accidentally puncture a dilated epidural vein. Physiologic changes during pregnancy might also have made the parturient more susceptible or more difficult to resuscitate. Indeed, all of the cases of cardiac arrest occurred in women who were positioned on their backs for resuscitative purposes when toxic convulsions began. Thus, intractable arrest might have been due, in part, to the iatrogenic insult of unrelieved aortic caval compression. Animal studies on the sensitivity to bupivacaine cardiotoxicity

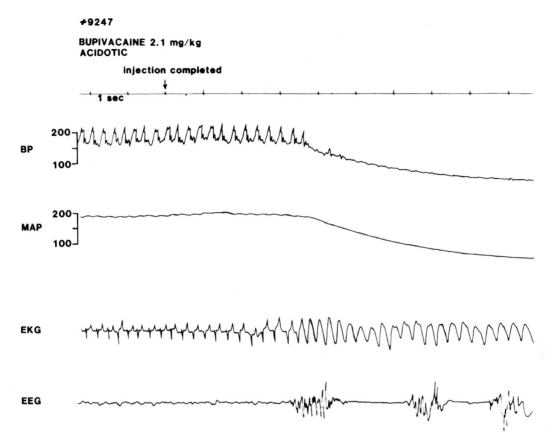

≠9247

BUPIVACAINE 2.1 mg/kg
ACIDOTIC

injection completed

1 sec

BP

MAP

EKG

EEG

Figure 5.6. Hemodynamic effects of rapid intravenous injection (over 10 seconds) of bupivacaine 2.1 mg/kg into a ewe with respiratory acidosis. Within seconds of completion of the injection, convulsant activity is noted on the electroencephalogram (*EEG*). The electrocardiogram (*EKG*) develops a wide QRS complex rhythm, and arterial blood pressure (*BP*) falls precipitously. (Reprinted by permission from Rosen MA, Thigpen JW, Shnider SM, Foutz SE, Levinson G, Koike M. Bupivacaine-induced cardiotoxicity in hypoxic and acidotic sheep. *Anesth Analg* 1985;64:1089–1096.)

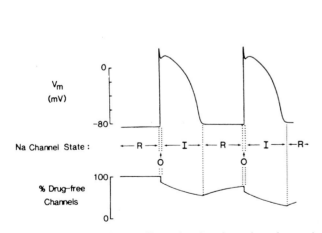

Figure 5.7. Schematic diagram illustrating time-dependent changes in sodium channel states (*middle*) and block of sodium changes (*bottom*) associated with the cardiac action potential (*top*) in the presence of a local anesthetic drug. The top trace shows two simulated ventricular muscular action potentials. *Vm* = transmembrane voltage. The drug binds to sodium channels in open (*O*) and inactivated (*I*) states but has a very low affinity for channels in the rested (*R*) state. Drug association during diastole is time dependent and, with a drug such as bupivacaine, may be incomplete even at normal heart rates. This results in an accumulation of drug-associated (blocked) channels with successive beats. (Reprinted by permission from Clarkson CW, Hondeghem LM. Mechanism for bupivacaine depression of cardiac conduction: Fast block of sodium channels during the action potential with slow recovery from block during diastole. *Anesthesiology* 1985;62:396–405.)

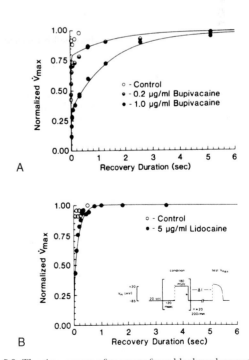

Figure 5.8. The time course of recovery from block under control conditions and in the presence of bupivacaine (*A*) or lidocaine (*B*). The pulse protocol is shown in the inset. (Reprinted by permission from Clarkson CW, Hondeghem LM. Mechanism for bupivacaine depression of cardiac conduction: Fast block of sodium channels during the action potential with slow recovery from block during diastole. *Anesthesiology* 1985;62:396–405.)

during pregnancy also failed to provide clear insight regarding the higher incidence in the parturient, yielding instead conflicting results. For example, Morishima et al. (156) and Kotelko et al. (149) found that pregnant sheep were more susceptible, while Eisler et al. (157) found that the lethal dose for intravenous bupivacaine in rabbits did not change with pregnancy. Similarly, more recent studies by Santos et al. demonstrate that pregnancy does not enhance the systemic toxicity of bupivacaine or ropivacaine in sheep (158). Although one must be cautious in extrapolating from these animal studies to the clinical situation of unintended intravascular injection of a local anesthetic, the weight of evidence suggests lack of unique susceptibility to anesthetic cardiotoxicity during pregnancy.

Fortunately, bupivacaine's potential cardiotoxicity has little relevance to its use as an epidural analgesic for labor, when small volumes or dilute local anesthetics are used, or when used as an intrathecal agent for cesarean section. Concerning the latter, bupivacaine perhaps has the best track record of any available anesthetic with respect to neurotoxicity and, as discussed previously, is associated with a low incidence of TNS (86). Although the duration of block is somewhat prolonged for routine cesarean section performed by an agile surgeon, it is arguably more consistent than that achieved with tetracaine.

Current Usage

Epidural. Bupivacaine is currently the most commonly used epidural anesthetic agent for control of pain during labor. As such, it is often combined with the opioids, fentanyl or sufentanil, and recommendations and opinions regarding optimal concentration and combinations are voluminous. This information is summarized in Chapters 8 and 9. Table 8.3 outlines a common approach to lumbar epidural analgesia for labor with bupivacaine. As discussed above, 0.5% bupivacaine has a slow onset, excessive duration, and, compared to 2% lidocaine, less potency for cesarean section, while 0.75% is proscribed from obstetric practice. Accordingly, use of epidural bupivacaine for cesarean section is not recommended, unless a particularly long surgery is anticipated.

Spinal. Apprehension regarding intrathecal lidocaine has fortified bupivacaine's preeminent status as the intrathecal agent of choice for cesarean section. Excellent surgical conditions and maternal comfort can be achieved with doses of 10 to 15 mg, which can be administered as a hyperbaric or isobaric solution (8, 159–161). Inclusion of a lipid soluble opioid (e.g., 10 to 25 μg fentanyl) can improve maternal comfort and/or reduce anesthetic requirement (5–7), while effective postoperative analgesia can be achieved with a small dose (0.1 mg) of preservative-free morphine (3, 4). Use of intrathecal bupivacaine for cesarean section is discussed in Chapter 11.

THE NEW GENERATION AMIDES: CHIRAL COMPOUNDS

Concern for bupivacaine toxicity and the withdrawal of 0.75% solution created a perceived void in the local anesthetic armamentarium. Clinical development soon centered on the asymmetric carbon adjacent to the amino group of the N-substituted pipecolyl xylidines, bupivacaine and propivacaine. Before proceeding further, a brief review of stereochemistry may prove useful (162). *Isomers* are different compounds that have the same molecular formula. A subset of isomers that have atoms connected by the same sequence of bonds yet differ in their spatial orientation are called *stereoisomers* while the term *Chiral* is drawn from the Greek "Cheir" for "hand", and thus makes reference to anatomical structures that are non-superimposable mirror-images.

Enantiomers are a particular class of stereoisomers that exist as mirror images. Those that have identical physical properties except for the direction of the rotation of the plane of polarized light, which is not surprising since they only differ with respect to symmetry. This forms the basis of one classification scheme, the enantiomer labeled *dextrorotatory* (or +) if the rotation is to the right (clockwise) and *levorotatory* (or −) if to the left (counterclockwise). A *racemic* mixture is a mixture of equal parts of enantiomers and is optically inactive because the rotation caused by the molecules of one isomer is canceled by the opposite rotation of its enantiomer. These compounds can also be classified based on absolute configuration, most frequently designated R (*rectus*) or S (*sinister*) based on the Cahn-Ingold-Prelog system (163). Most critically, despite identical physical properties, enantiomers may differ significantly with respect to their biologic activity.

Ropivacaine (Naropin)

Chemically speaking, ropivacaine is the S(−)-enantiomer of N-propyl pipecolyl xylidine (Fig. 5.1). It is therefore a homolog of mepivacaine and bupivacaine, having a propyl on the pipecolyl ring as opposed to a methyl (mepivacaine) or butyl group (bupivacaine or levobupivacaine), respectively. Interest in this compound stemmed from experimental data that S-enantiomers are less cardiotoxic than their mirror image relatives (164, 165). An added advantage was that S(−)-propivacaine was known to have a longer duration of action than R(+) propivacaine, at least in part, derived from a greater propensity for vasoconstriction (166). Early data offered great promise for clinical practice. In volunteer studies, infusions of ropivacaine were better tolerated than bupivacaine with respect to CNS symptoms or depression of cardiac contractility and conductivity (167), while clinical studies appeared to indicate roughly equivalent sensory anesthesia when administered for brachial plexus block (168, 169) or for epidural anesthesia (170, 171). Additionally, motor effects were less pronounced, which, along with earlier electrophysiologic data suggesting *preferential* C fiber blockade (172), opened up the exciting possibility of a more favorable differential block (i.e., greater sensory block than motor block). This particularly valuable characteristic for obstetric anesthesia achieved some support from studies comparing low concentrations of ropivacaine and bupivacaine for labor analgesia (173–178). Meanwhile, *in vitro* (179) and *in vivo* (151, 180, 181) experimental studies provided data supporting the claim for reduced cardiac toxicity compared with bupivacaine.

Unfortunately, as might be predicted based on the shorter side chain and less lipid solubility (182), recent animal and clinical data suggest that ropivacaine may, in fact, be less potent than bupivacaine. Using tail-flick response in the rat to assess the antinociceptive effects of epidural and intrathecal anesthetic, Kanai et al. found ropivacaine to be less potent than levobupivacaine or bupivacaine (183). More direct evidence for a difference in clinical potency is derived from two recent studies using minimum local analgesic concentration (MLAC) to compare epidural ropivacaine with bupivacaine for labor analgesia (Fig. 5.9) (184, 185). This methodology uses an "up-down" sequential allocation, analogous to determination of volatile anesthetic minimum alveolar concentration, in which the concentration administered is determined by the response of the previous patient in the same treatment group (186). The results of these studies are consistent, both reporting ropivacaine to be approximately 60% as potent as bupivacaine, and neither reporting a difference in motor block. It should be appreciated that this methodology does have limitations, the most critical is the lack of information regarding the *slope* or *shape* of the dose-response curve. (These issues are beyond the scope of this chapter and the interested reader is directed to recent editorials, letters to the editor (187, 188) and an excellent review of enantiomer local anesthetics (189). Nonetheless, these studies

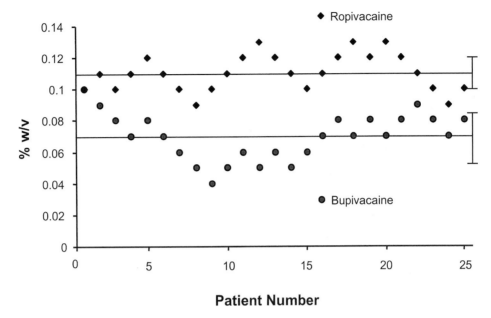

Figure 5.9. The median effective local analgesic concentration of ropivacaine and bupivacaine as determined by the technique of up-down sequential allocation. The minimum local analgesic concentration (*MLAC*) for ropivacaine is 0.111% wt/vol and 0.067% wt/vol for bupivacaine. Error bars represent 95% confidence intervals. The testing interval was 0.01% wt/vol. (Reprinted by permission from Polley LS, Columb MO, Naughton NN, et al. Relative analgesic potencies of ropivacaine and bupivacaine for epidural analgesia in labor. *Anesthesiology* 1999;90:944–950.)

document differences in EC_{50} at relevant end points, providing strong evidence for clinically relevant differences in potency.

Studies comparing ropivacaine to bupivacaine for spinal anesthesia have also found ropivacaine to have lower potency (190–192). In a volunteer study, McDonald et al. administered doses of 4 to 12 mg ropivacaine and bupivacaine using a double-blind, randomized, crossover design (191). Ropivacaine was found to be half as potent, and, equally important, equipotent doses had a similar clinical profile and a higher incidence of back pain. Similarly, in a clinical study of patients undergoing knee arthroscopy, Gautier et al. reported ropivacaine to be roughly two thirds as potent as bupivacaine (192), findings consistent with data reported by Malinovsky et al., in patients undergoing urologic procedures (190). Although neither of these studies reported episodes of TNS with ropivacaine, the data did not suggest any clinical advantage over bupivacaine for short surgical procedures.

The question of potency is obviously central to the potential clinical value of ropivacaine. If more drug must be administered to achieve the desired clinical effect, the perceived benefits with respect to cardiac toxicity, CNS effects, or motor block may be diminished, ablated, or even reversed. At present, the data are inadequate to provide a clear answer, but it is unlikely that use of epidural ropivacaine will confer unique clinical advantage.

The placental transfer and fetal effects of levobupivacaine, bupivacaine, and ropivacaine recently have been evaluated in pregnant sheep (193). The data demonstrated that maternal infusion of equimolar solutions of these three local anesthetics produced no important changes in the pregnant ewe or her fetus. There were no changes in the baseline blood pressure, uterine blood flow, or intraamniotic or central venous pressures at 30 and 60 minutes of infusion with any of the three local anesthetics.

Current Usage

Epidural. Since the release of ropivacaine for clinical use in 1996, numerous studies have evaluated ropivacaine 0.2% and 0.25% for labor, comparing it to the same concentrations of bupivacaine. These studies found similar pain relief and drug consumption (mg/h), as well as similar maternal and fetal safety

(173, 175–178, 194). These studies demonstrated no appreciable differences in the motor block resulting from use of either of these drugs. Current practice in obstetric anesthesia, however, generally involves the use of more dilute local anesthetic solutions. A study by Owen et al., comparing ropivacaine 0.125% with bupivacaine 0.125% using patient-controlled epidural analgesia (PCEA), concluded that "these two drugs are clinically indistinguishable at this concentration." They had demonstrated effective analgesia with both drugs but no difference in the amount of local anesthetics used, sensory levels, motor blockade, duration of labor, or mode of delivery (195). However, in a study comparing ropivacaine 0.125% with sufentanil 7.5 µg (10 mL) and bupivacaine 0.125% with sufentanil 7.5 µg administered by an intermittent bolus technique, it was suggested that less motor blockade resulted from use of ropivacaine (196). A meta-analysis of several earlier studies comparing ropivacaine 0.25% to bupivacaine 0.25% also suggested that the intensity of motor block was lower with ropivacaine (197). Spontaneous deliveries were reported to be more frequent with ropivacaine, and instrumental deliveries occurred less frequently. Although these earlier studies have demonstrated that ropivacaine 0.125% to 0.25% provides effective labor analgesia when administered epidurally, the doses studied in comparison to bupivacaine may not be appropriate.

As described earlier in this chapter, the relative potencies of bupivacaine and ropivacaine for labor analgesia appear not to be equivalent as assumed in most studies of these drugs. Capogna et al. (198) and Polley et al. (199) demonstrated that the MLAC for bupivacaine is 0.067 to 0.093% wt/vol, while the MLAC for ropivacaine is 0.111 to 0.156% wt/vol (Fig. 5.9). Thus, ropivacaine has only 60% of bupivacaine's potency, and most studies have compared equiconcentrations but not equipotent drug concentrations. The decreased motor effects of ropivacaine appear to be purely the result of its being a less potent local anesthetic. It has been suggested that in the study by Gautier et al., for example, the comparisons of ropivacaine 0.125% wt/vol to bupivacaine 0.075% wt/vol would have been more appropriate (200). The MLAC studies also call into question the purported advantages claimed for ropivacaine regarding a greater safety from cardiotoxicity compared to bupivacaine, since equiconcentrations were most often studied (201, 202).

More recent clinical evaluations have focused on dilute concentrations of ropivacaine by either continuous infusion (131) or PCEA administration (132, 133, 203) with fentanyl or sufentanil. It has been demonstrated that epidural fentanyl reduces the local anesthetic requirements by 19% to 31% (204–206). By the addition of opioids to ropivacaine, less local anesthetic (lower concentrations or lower hourly infusion rates) should be required. Meister et al. (132) demonstrated that both ropivacaine and bupivacaine 0.125% with fentanyl 2 μg/mL administered by PCEA (6 mL/h basal rate, 5 mL bolus, 10-minute lockout, 30 mL/h dose limit) provided highly effective analgesia. There were no differences in local anesthetic use, pain scores, or side effects. However, the group that received ropivacaine developed significantly less motor block. In these studies, the hourly local anesthetic use decreased from 19 mL/h (used in their previous study of plain ropivacaine and bupivacaine 0.125%) (195) to approximately 13.7 mL/h with the addition of fentanyl. The authors asserted that there is a threshold dose of local anesthetic required to cause motor block that is exceeded at higher local anesthetic doses. Consequently, administration of ropivacaine 0.125% with fentanyl 2 μg/mL produced effective analgesia at a dose below this threshold, while bupivacaine at the same concentration exceeds this threshold and produces more motor block. While these differences appear directly related to differences in potencies of these two local anesthetics, these authors suggest that women who received ropivacaine would have self-administered more ropivacaine if differences in MLAC between the two agents were true. Similar arguments have been made by Campbell et al., who studied ropivacaine and bupivacaine 0.08% plus fentanyl 2 μg/mL administered by PCEA to women in labor (203). A 20-mL dose of the study solution was first administered in divided doses and then by PCEA pump set for a 5-mL bolus with a 10-minute lockout period with no background infusion or hourly dose limit. They demonstrated less motor blockade with ropivacaine (ability to ambulate, spontaneous micturition, lower incidence of forceps delivery). These authors have also questioned the MLAC values for ropivacaine and bupivacaine, and stated that the use of dilute solutions of local anesthetic administered by PCEA supports the concept that there is lesser motor block with ropivacaine. However others, using ropivacaine 0.1% with sufentanil 0.5 μg/mL, have not found a significant difference in forceps deliveries, for example, compared to bupivacaine at the same concentration (133). Women who received a ropivacaine solution used similar amounts of local anesthetic solutions and had similar visual analog scale (VAS) scores during labor; however, they requested more supplemental boluses to achieve analgesia during the second stage and maternal satisfaction was significantly lower ($P < .0001$). This study seems to support the MLAC findings that ropivacaine is simply a less potent drug compared with bupivacaine. Ropivacaine has a longer half-life than bupivacaine because of the S-enantiomer form and greater vasoconstrictor properties, which may explain subtle differences as more dilute concentrations are administered by PCEA (207). The appropriate clinical dose of ropivacaine and its potency compared to bupivacaine remain under investigation, and further studies to evaluate the ED$_{90}$ or ED$_{95}$ may be needed (134, 208–212).

Ropivacaine is now a widely used local anesthetic, and it provides effective analgesia for labor and delivery in concentrations from 0.08% to 0.25%. It has proven to be safe for both the mother and fetus (213–216). However, it appears to be less potent than bupivacaine and may not have unique pharmacologic properties to warrant its clinical use. In a multicenter study of 0.2% bupivacaine administered at either 4, 6, 8, or 10 mL/h, 6 mL/h appeared to be the lowest effective rate that provided the best combination of effective pain relief, minimal motor block, and least need for rebolusing (217). It seems likely, however, that more dilute solutions (0.0625% to 0.10%) in larger administered volumes (10 to 20 mL) with the addition of an opioid (203, 209) or epinephrine (218) will prove more popular.

Ropivacaine has also been used successfully for cesarean section in both the 0.5% (219–222) and the 0.75% concentrations (223–225). The higher concentration seems unnecessary since the studies to date suggest ropivacaine 0.5% when administered epidurally at a volume of 20 to 25 mL is as effective as bupivacaine 0.5%, although the duration of the motor block may be shorter with ropivacaine (219). In support of the MLAC studies suggesting that ropivacaine is less potent than bupivacaine, however, it has been demonstrated that 0.5% ropivacaine may be associated with insufficient motor blockade for major orthopedic surgeries (226).

Spinal. Intrathecal ropivacaine 0.25 mg, administered as part of the CSE technique for labor has also proved successful but appears to have no unique benefit compared to bupivacaine (227, 228). However, this is an area of ongoing research, and whether there is such an effect–and the appropriate intrathecal dose–has yet to be determined (229, 230).

Levobupivacaine (Chirocaine)

Early work by Aberg et al. had demonstrated the favorable toxicologic properties of the S(−)-enantiomer of bupivacaine (165). However, lack of a perceived need and inadequate methods for large-scale production of single enantiomer compounds would delay its introduction into clinical practice for 3 decades. Although levobupivacaine is similar to ropivacaine, both chemically and historically, the evolving experimental and clinical data highlight two important distinctions: (1) the evidence for levobupivacaine's reduced cardiotoxicity is more compelling, not being entangled in issues of potency; and (2) there is little to suggest selective or more favorable differential block compared with the R(+)-enantiomer or the racemic mixture.

Although the mechanism of death was not explored, Aberg et al. demonstrated that LD$_{50}$ for the S(−)-enantiomer of bupivacaine exceeded that of its antipode, despite comparable *in vitro* and *in vivo* anesthetic activity (165). Interestingly, the difference between the two enantiomers was less pronounced in experiments using subcutaneous rather than intravenous injections, likely reflecting the greater vasoconstrictive properties of the S(−)-enantiomer (231).

Concern for bupivacaine toxicity heightened interest in an alternative long-acting amide and focused study on the comparative cardiovascular effects of racemic bupivacaine and its two enantiomers; almost all have found stereospecificity. For example, the S(−)-enantiomer has been shown to produce less depression of V$_{max}$ and action potential duration than the R(+)-isomer in guinea pig papillary muscle (164); similarly, in isolated rabbit heart, the S(−)-isomer has been found to induce less prolongation of the QRS interval than its antipode (232) or the racemic mixture (233), and is associated with a reduced incidence of potentially fatal arrhythmias (232). *In vivo* studies in conscious sheep (234, 235) and anesthetized swine (236) also demonstrate lower toxicity than racemic bupivacaine as evidenced by less prolongation of the QRS interval (236), significantly fewer and less deleterious arrhythmias (235), and a higher lethal dose (234–236). In one of these studies (235), three animals died after 150 to 200 mg bupivacaine from the sudden onset of ventricular fibrillation, while equivalent doses of levobupivacaine produced nonfatal arrhythmias that automatically returned to sinus rhythm. Although there are studies that have failed to document stereoselective arrhythmogenesis, this failure may reflect the nature of the experimental model (237). Finally, although caution must be exercised in interpreting surrogate end points, a study in volunteers found levobupivacaine to have less significant cardiac depression than racemic bupivacaine with respect to stroke index, acceleration index, and ejection fraction (238).

Unlike ropivacaine, levobupivacaine's reduced toxicity cannot be easily dismissed on the basis of lower potency. Levobupivacaine has been shown to provide similar anesthesia when administered epidurally for cesarean section (239), lower abdominal surgery (240), and lower extremity surgery (241), and when used for supraclavicular brachial plexus block (242) or for local infiltration for inguinal herniorrhaphy (243). When evaluating levobupivacaine 0.5% and bupivacaine 0.5% for cesarean delivery, Bader et al. noted no significant differences between these two drugs in time to onset of motor block, time to offset of sensory and motor block, and quality of analgesia (239). Time to regression to T10 was 329 ± 79 minutes for levobupivacaine and 317 ± 81 minutes for bupivacaine, and time to complete offset was over 425 minutes with both drugs. Concentrations of levobupivacaine between 0.08% and 0.25% administered epidurally for labor analgesia have also produced analgesia equivalent to the same concentrations of bupivacaine (244–246). For example, Burke et al. compared the efficacy of bolus doses of 0.25% levobupivacaine with 0.25% bupivacaine and found no significant differences in analgesia, spread of sensory block, percentage of patients with motor block, or incidence of adverse effects. Perhaps most germane are the findings of an "up-down" sequential allocation study by Lyons et al., which compared the MLAC of levobupivacaine and racemic bupivacaine (247). As previously noted, this is the methodology that has provided the most convincing data suggesting the nonequivalence of ropivacaine. In contrast to the findings with ropivacaine, the MLAC of levobupivacaine was 0.083% wt/vol (95% CI, 0.065 to 0.101), the MLAC of bupivacaine was 0.081% wt/vol (95% CI, 0.055 to 0.108), and the calculated potency ratio of levobupivacaine to bupivacaine was 0.98 (95% CI, 0.67 to 1.41). Of note, in molar terms the ratio was actually 0.87 (95% CI, 0.60 to 1.25), the difference due to the percentage of levobupivacaine used in this study calculated using the free base. Nonetheless, this difference is not statistically significant and the effect size is not likely to impact levobupivacaine's apparently favorable therapeutic index.

Current Usage

Epidural. Relatively limited clinical investigation of levobupivacaine in obstetric anesthesia has been undertaken, and its place in labor analgesia has yet to be established. However, the available data suggest that levobupivacaine is quite similar to racemic bupivacaine and should be highly effective in concentrations of 0.0625% to 0.125%. In a volunteer study of intradermal injections using serial dilutions of bupivacaine enantiomers, it was noted that the S(−)-enantiomer produced greater vasoconstriction and appeared longer acting (248). Thus, when more dilute solutions of levobupivacaine are studied clinically using techniques such as PCEA (as has been done with ropivacaine [132, 133, 203]), subtle differences may emerge (248).

It is unlikely that levobupivacaine will be more useful than bupivacaine for routine cesarean section under epidural anesthesia, owing to the relatively slow onset of action, prolonged duration of anesthesia, and inferior sensory blockade of both drugs at the 0.5% concentration compared with 2% lidocaine. In unique cases where greater surgical time is required and repetitive dosing is not desired, the likely decreased cardiotoxicity of levobupivacaine would make it potentially safer than bupivacaine yet equally efficacious. This characteristic may offer significant advantage for peripheral blocks in the nonobstetric arena.

Spinal. The available experimental (183) and clinical information (249) is inadequate to determine the usefulness of levobupivacaine for spinal anesthesia in obstetrics. Although it has a tendency to produce vasoconstriction at low concentrations, it is unlikely that spinal levobupivacaine will confer clinical advantage over spinal bupivacaine in this population.

ADJUVANTS

Carbon Dioxide, Sodium Bicarbonate: pH Adjustment

Slow onset of epidural analgesia for cesarean section can be a minor drawback or a serious limitation. The onset of analgesia

can be hastened by increasing the proportions of nonionized, lipid-soluble base in the anesthetic solution. Commercially-prepared carbonated lidocaine, as a salt of carbonic acid, has an appreciably faster onset than the orthodox hydrochloride solution, especially in the resistant segments L5 and S1 (107, 112). Although the carbonated formulation of lidocaine has been available in Canada for the past 20 years, it is not approved in the United States, where pH adjustment with freshly added sodium bicarbonate is a workable but more primitive substitute (250). One milliequivalent of sodium bicarbonate (i.e., 1 mL 8.4% sodium bicarbonate solution) added to every 10 mL lidocaine hydrochloride, or 3% chloroprocaine, increases the pH to between 7.08 and 7.51 (251). In spite of the handicap of having to add bicarbonate just before injection, the benefits are worthwhile in terms of the faster onset and more profound analgesia when chloroprocaine or lidocaine is chosen as the primary anesthetic agent. Such is not the case with bupivacaine as alkalinization does not appear to hasten its onset (150). Moreover, the margin between satisfactory alkalinization and complete precipitation of the base is very narrow, and pH adjustment of bupivacaine must therefore be done carefully with one tenth the amount of bicarbonate used for lidocaine (251).

Epinephrine

This vasoconstrictor has a long history as an important adjuvant for subarachnoid and epidural anesthesia. Recently, the use of epinephrine has become controversial, partly because of variables peculiar to the drug itself, partly because of physicochemical differences among the newer local anesthetics and opioid agents to which it is added, and partly due to renewed concerns regarding toxicity when used as an intrathecal agent.

Epidural Administration. The principal reason for using epinephrine is to slow vascular uptake of local anesthetics and opioids, and to so favor their uptake into the lipids of the cord and canal, thereby increasing the intensity and duration of their neural blockade (252–256). At the same time, fetal uptake of local anesthetics and opioids is reduced through slowing of maternal vascular uptake and reduction of placental transfer (257). In addition, epidural epinephrine alone at a concentration of $5\ \mu g/mL$ has been shown to induce a mild degree of segmental analgesia in volunteers, an effect apparently mediated by postsynaptic α-2 agonism (258). Although this effect may add to the cumulative intensity of analgesia provided by local anesthetic-opioid mixtures, the intrinsic epinephrine contribution is likely too small to be distinguished from the vasoactive effects that determine competition for drug uptake between the aqueous and lipid phases within the spinal canal. The outcome of this competition between aqueous and lipid phases depends on the inherent lipid solubility of each local anesthetic or opioid under study; the more lipid-soluble the agent, the less striking is the relatively smaller extra advantage from adding epinephrine. Thus, the sensory and motor-blocking qualities of lidocaine, with a low lipid/water partition coefficient of 2.7, are markedly enhanced by adding epinephrine, whereas epidural bupivacaine with a lipid-solubility coefficient 10 times greater, is less affected, and it is difficult to demonstrate any enhancement of its sensory block from the addition of epinephrine, although intensification of motor block can be seen (259). Similarly, epinephrine intensifies the sensory and side effects of epidural morphine to a greater degree than a more lipid-soluble agent such as sufentanil (256, 258). However, epinephrine does reduce the vascular uptake of the lipid-soluble opioids, so lower maternal blood levels and fetal drug transfer may be expected if epinephrine is added to a bolus injection of epidural fentanyl or sufentanil for cesarean section or to an epidural infusion for relief of pain in labor.

Spinal Administration. Epinephrine is commonly added to anesthetic solutions to enhance the intensity and prolong the duration of spinal anesthesia. This practice has been largely limited in obstetric anesthesia to use with lidocaine because the duration of plain bupivacaine is more than adequate for routine cesarean section. Although fears that intraspinal epinephrine might contribute to spinal cord ischemia have periodically emerged, such concerns have been generally dismissed and have not affected practice. In addition to a vast clinical experience suggesting safety, the limited experimental studies produced reassuring data concerning epinephrine's effect on spinal cord blood flow. Most significantly, studies in animals with radioactive microspheres and with the hydrogen washout technique showed some reduction of flow in the dura mater after intrathecal injection of epinephrine but failed to show any significant reduction of flow in the spinal cord (260–262).

Unfortunately, more recent clinical experience and laboratory data have called into question the safety of adding epinephrine to lidocaine for spinal anesthesia (67, 80). As discussed in a previous section, recent reports of neurologic sequelae suggest that the threshold for toxicity with spinal lidocaine may lie at or close to the upper end of the clinical dose range (80–82). Experimental studies of spinal anesthesia demonstrate that adding epinephrine further compromises this already narrow therapeutic index (Fig. 5.10) (67). These recent experimental data do not actually conflict with earlier findings as epinephrine alone produced neither functional impairment nor histologic damage. While such findings do not exclude epinephrine impacting directly on neural tissue, they are more consistent with an indirect effect likely mediated by epinephrine-induced vasoconstriction. Thus, whereas epinephrine-induced vasoconstriction might be well tolerated, the reduction in blood flow could delay absorption of lidocaine, increasing neuronal exposure to anesthetic and hence toxicity. Regardless of mechanism, these recent findings indicate that recommendations for maximum safe intrathecal dose of lidocaine should consider whether the solution contains epinephrine. However, given the apparently narrow therapeutic index of spinal lidocaine and the availability of viable alternatives (e.g., bupivacaine), the use of lidocaine with epinephrine would best be avoided.

Meperidine

Part opioid, part local anesthetic, this familiar compound was among the first opioid agents to be tested as the sole epidural agent for relief of pain in labor. Initial reports were controversial, mainly as a result of the use of conservative doses of 25 mg (263), but later studies confirmed epidural analgesic efficacy when larger doses of meperidine were used alone or as an adjuvant to a dilute local anesthetic solution (264–266). In contrast to other currently-available opioids, meperidine is capable of producing surgical anesthesia when administered intrathecally in humans (267) and has been used in obstetric anesthesia for labor pain (268), postpartum tubal ligation (268), and cesarean section (269, 270). As such, its use may be associated with a high incidence of nausea (268, 270) and pruritus (271). Of far greater concern, however, is the lack of adequate toxicologic data supporting the safety of administering these relatively high anesthetic doses intrathecally. Recent preliminary data reinforce this concern, suggesting that the potential for sensory impairment and morphologic damage with intrathecal meperidine exceeds that of an equivalent dose of lidocaine (272).

CONCLUSION

The agents available for obstetric regional anesthesia have undergone continuous reevaluation over the past 2 decades, with significant improvements in the safety of analgesia and the management of difficult labor. Indeed, it is interesting that choices that seemed so obvious in the recent past could appear ill-advised in the light of new evidence or experience. With the possible exception of chloroprocaine, co-administration of two or more analgesic agents with widely different target sites has superseded the traditional view that, in obstetric practice, local anesthetics are safest and best when given alone for major spinal blockade; opioid adjuvants have played the major part in this change of outlook. Anesthetic administered by infusion for labor has become the norm, the use of CSE and PCEA is increasing, and the immediate future should see definition of the role of CSA. A number of the older anesthetics are undergoing reevaluation, while the use of two new agents, ropivacaine and levobupivacaine, has yet to be defined. While neither appears poised to significantly alter the clinical practice of obstetric anesthesia, the data are clearly inadequate to completely exclude this possibility.

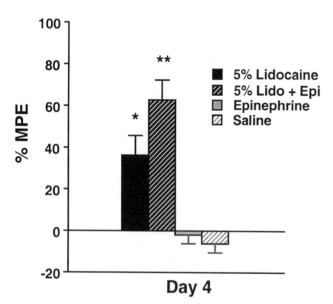

Figure 5.10. Sensory function 4 days after intrathecal administration of 5% lidocaine, 5% lidocaine with epinephrine (0.2 mg/mL), epinephrine (0.2 mg/mL), or saline. Tail-flick latency values were calculated as the average of latencies for the proximal, middle, and distal portions of the tail, and are expressed as percent maximum possible effect, where $\%MPE = \{(\text{tail-flick latency} - \text{baseline})/(\text{cut-off} - \text{baseline})\} \times 100$; $Lido + Epi$ = lidocaine plus epinephrine. Data represent mean ± SEM. $*P < .05$ vs. epinephrine or saline.$** P < .05$ vs. all other groups. (Reprinted by permission from Hashimoto K, Hampl K, Nakamura Y, Bollen A, Feiner J, Drasner K. Epinephrine increases the neurotoxic potential of intrathecally administered lidocaine in the rat. *Anesthesiology.* In press.)

REFERENCES

1. Hershey DW, Quilligan EJ. Extraabdominal uterine exteriorization at cesarean section. *Obstet Gynecol* 1978;52:189–192.
2. Riley ET, Cohen SE, Macario A, Desai JB, Ratner EF. Spinal versus epidural anesthesia for cesarean section: A comparison of time efficiency, costs, charges, and complications. *Anesth Analg* 1995;80:709–712.
3. Abboud TK, Dror A, Mosaad P, et al. Mini-dose intrathecal morphine for the relief of post-cesarean section pain: Safety, efficacy, and ventilatory responses to carbon dioxide. *Anesth Analg* 1988;67:137–143.
4. Palmer CM, Emerson S, Volgoropolous D, Alves D. Dose-response relationship of intrathecal morphine for postcesarean analgesia [published erratum appears in *Anesthesiology* 1999;90:1241]. *Anesthesiology* 1999;90:437–444.
5. Belzarena SD. Clinical effects of intrathecally administered fentanyl in patients undergoing cesarean section. *Anesth Analg* 1992;74:653–657.
6. Choi DH, Ahn HJ, Kim MH. Bupivacaine-sparing effect of fentanyl in spinal anesthesia for cesarean delivery. *Reg Anesth Pain Med* 2000;25:240–245.
7. Shende D, Cooper GM, Bowden MI. The influence of intrathecal fentanyl on the characteristics of subarachnoid block for caesarean section. *Anaesthesia* 1998;53:706–710.

8. Norris MC. Patient variables and the subarachnoid spread of hyperbaric bupivacaine in the term patient. *Anesthesiology* 1990;72:478–482.

9. Kee WD, Khaw KS, Lee BB, Lau TK, Gin T. A dose-response study of prophylactic intravenous ephedrine for the prevention of hypotension during spinal anesthesia for cesarean delivery. *Anesth Analg* 2000;90:1390–1395.

10. Hurley R, Lampert D. Continuous spinal anesthesia with a microcatheter technique: Preliminary experience. *Anesth Analg* 1990;70:97–102.

11. Drasner K, Connolly M, Reece W. Evaluation of a 28-gauge catheter for continuous spinal anesthesia. *Anesth Analg* 1990;70:S88.

12. Arkoosh V, Palmer C, Van Maren G, Yun E, Wissler R. Continuous intrathecal labor analgesia: Safety and efficacy [abstract]. *Anesthesiology* 1998;89:A-1041.

13. Usubiaga JE, La Iuppa M, Moya F, Wikinski JA, Velazco R. Passage of procaine hydrochloride and para-aminobenzoic acid across the human placenta. *Am J Obstet Gynecol* 1968;100:918–923.

14. O'Brien JE, Abbey V, Hinsvark O, Perel J, Finster M. Metabolism and measurement of chloroprocaine, an ester-type local anesthetic. *J Pharm Sci* 1979;68:75–78.

15. Kuhnert BR, Kuhnert PM, Prochaska AL, Gross TL. Plasma levels of 2-chloroprocaine in obstetric patients and their neonates after epidural anesthesia. *Anesthesiology* 1980;53:21–25.

16. Hodgkinson R, Husain FJ, Bluhm C. Reduced effectiveness of bupivacaine 0.5% to relieve labor pain after prior injection of chloroprocaine 2% [abstract]. *Anesthesiology* 1982;57:A-201.

17. Kotelko DM, Thigpen JW, Shnider SM, et al. Postoperative epidural morphine analgesia after various local anesthetics [abstract]. *Anesthesiology* 1983;59:A-413.

18. Grice SC, Eisenach JC, Dewan DM. Labor analgesia with epidural bupivacaine plus fentanyl: Enhancement with epinephrine and inhibition with 2-chloroprocaine. *Anesthesiology* 1990;72:623–628.

19. Camann WR, Hartigan PM, Gilbertson Ll, Johnson M, Datta S. Chloroprocaine antagonism of epidural opioid analgesia: A receptor-specific phenomenon? *Anesthesiology* 1990;73:860–863.

20. Corke BC, Carlson CG, Dettbarn WD. The influence of 2-chloroprocaine on the subsequent analgesic potency of bupivacaine. *Anesthesiology* 1984;60:25–27.

21. Eisenach JC, Schlairet TJ, Dobson CE, Hood DH. Effect of prior anesthetic solution on epidural morphine analgesia. *Anesth Analg* 1991;73:119–123.

22. Moore D, Spierkijk J, van Kleef J, Coleman R, Love G. Chloroprocaine neurotoxicity: Four additional cases. *Anesth Analg* l982;61:155–159.

23. Ravindran R, Bond V, Tasch M, Gupta C, Luerssen T. Prolonged neural blockade following regional anesthesia with 2-chloroprocaine. *Anesth Analg* 1980;59:447–454.

24. Reisner L, Hochman B, Plumer M. Persistent neurologic deficit and adhesive arachnoiditis following intrathecal 2-chloroprocaine injection. *Anesth Analg* 1980;59:452–454.

25. Ravindran R, Turner M, Muller J. Neurologic effects of subarachnoid administration of 2-chloroprocaine-CE, bupivacaine, and low pH normal saline in dogs. *Anesth Analg* 1982;61:279–283.

26. Gissen A, Datta S, Lambert D. The chloroprocaine controversy. II. Is chloroprocaine neurotoxic? *Reg Anesth* 1984;9:135–144.

27. Barsa J, Batra M, Fink B, Sumi S. A comparative in vivo study of local neurotoxicity of lidocaine, bupivacaine, 2-chloroprocaine, and a mixture of 2-chloroprocaine and bupivacaine. *Anesth Analg* 1982;61:961–967.

28. Rosen MA, Baysinger CL, Shnider SM, et al. Evaluation of neurotoxicity after subarachnoid injection of large volumes of local anesthetic solutions. *Anesth Analg* 1983;62:802–808.

29. Ready LB, Plumer MH, Haschke RH, Austin E, Sumi SM. Neurotoxicity of intrathecal local anesthetics in rabbits. *Anesthesiology* 1985;63:364–370.

30. Wang BC, Hillman DE, Spielholz NI, Turndorf H. Chronic neurological deficits and Nesacaine-CE—an effect of the anesthetic, 2-chloroprocaine, or the antioxidant, sodium bisulfite? *Anesth Analg* 1984;63:445–447.

31. Kalichman MW, Powell HC, Reisner LS, Myers RR. The role of 2-chloroprocaine and sodium bisulfite in rat sciatic nerve edema. *J Neuropathol Exp Neurol* 1986;45:566–575.

32. Taniguchi M, Bollen AW, Drasner K. Is sodium bisulfite neurotoxic? [abstract] *Anesthesiology* 2000;93:A838.

33. Fibuch E, Opper S. Back pain following epidurally administered Nesacaine-MPF. *Anesth Analg* 1989;69:113–115.

34. Hynson J, Sessler D, Glosten B. Back pain in volunteers after epidural anesthesia with chloroprocaine. *Anesth Analg* 1991;72:253–256.

35. Levy L, Randel G, Pandit S. Does chloroprocaine (Nesacaine-MPF) for epidural anesthesia increase the incidence of backache [letter]? *Anesthesiology* 1989;71:476.

36. Stevens R, Urmey W, Urquhart B, Kao T. Back pain after epidural anesthesia with chloroprocaine. *Anesthesiology* 1993;78:492–497.

37. Crosby E, Read D. Salvaging inadequate epidural anaesthetics: "The chloro-procaine save". *Can J Anaesth* 1991;38:136–137.

38. Hauch MA, Hartwell BL, Hunt CO, Datta S. Comparative effects of subarachnoid hyperbaric bupivacaine and tetracaine-procaine for cesarean delivery. *Reg Anesth* 1990;15:81–85.

39. Hodgson PS, Liu SS, Batra MS, et al. Procaine compared with lidocaine for incidence of transient neurologic symptoms. *Reg Anesth Pain Med* 2000;25:218–222.

40. Bromage PR. A comparison of bupivacaine and tetracaine in epidural analgesia for surgery. *Can Anaesth Soc J* 1969;16:37–45.

41. Tucker GT, Boyes RN, Bridenbaugh PO, Moore DC. Binding of anilide-type local anesthetics in human plasma. II. Implications in vivo, with special reference to transplacental distribution. *Anesthesiology* 1970;33:304–314.

42. Tucker GT, Boyes RN, Bridenbaugh PO, Moore DC. Binding of anilide-type local anesthetics in human plasma. I. Relationships between binding, physicochemical properties, and anesthetic activity. *Anesthesiology* 1970;33:287–303.

43. Morishima HO, Daniel SS, Finster M, Poppers PJ, James S. Transmission of mepivacaine hydrochloride (Carbocaine) across the human placenta. *Anesthesiology* 1966;27:147–154.

44. Spoerel WE, Thomas A, Gerula GR. Continuous epidural analgesia: Experience with mechanical injection devices. *Can Anaesth Soc J* 1970;17:37–51.

45. Bromage PR. *Epidural Analgesia*. Philadelphia: Saunders; 1978.

46. Abboud TK, Afrasiabi A, Sarkis F, et al. Continuous infusion epidural analgesia in parturients receiving bupivacaine, chloroprocaine, or lidocaine–Maternal, fetal, and neonatal effects. *Anesth Analg* 1984;63:421–428.

47. Chestnut DH, Bates JN, Choi WH. Continuous infusion epidural analgesia with lidocaine: Efficacy and influence during the second stage of labor. *Obstet Gynecol* 1987;69:323–327.

48. Kennedy RL, Bell JU, Miller RP, et al. Uptake and distribution of lidocaine in fetal lambs. *Anesthesiology* 1990;72:483–489.

49. Kennedy RL, Miller RP, Bell JU, et al. Uptake and distribution of bupivacaine in fetal lambs. *Anesthesiology* 1986;65:247–253.

50. Shnider SM, Way EL. Plasma levels of lidocaine (Xylocaine) in mother and newborn following obstetrical conduction anesthesia: Clinical applications. *Anesthesiology* 1968;29:951–958.

51. Fox GS, Houle GL. Transmission of lidocaine hydrochloride across the placenta during cesarean section. *Can Anaesth Soc J* 1969;16:135–143.

52. Scanlon JW, Brown WU, Weiss JB, Alper MH. Neurobehavioral responses of newborn infants after maternal epidural anesthesia. *Anesthesiology* 1974;40:121–128.

53. Scanlon JW, Ostheimer GW, Lurie AO, et al. Neurobehavioral responses and drug concentrations in newborns after maternal epidural anesthesia with bupivacaine. *Anesthesiology* 1976;45:400–405.

54. Kuhnert BR, Harrison MJ, Linn PL, Kuhnert PM. Effect of maternal epidural anesthesia on neonatal behavior. *Anesth Analg* 1984;63:301–308.

55. Brown WU. Neonatal neurobehavioral tests following vaginal delivery under ketamine, thiopental, and extradural anesthesia: Guest discussion. *Anesth Analg* 1977;56:548–553.

56. Rigler M, Drasner K, Krejcie T, et al. Cauda equina syndrome after continuous spinal anesthesia. *Anesth Analg* 1991;72:275–281.

57. Bensons JS. FDA Safety Alert: Cauda equina syndrome associated with the use of small-bore catheters in continuous spinal anesthesia. Rockville, MD: Food and Drug Administration; May 29, 1992.

58. Rigler M, Drasner K. Distribution of catheter-injected local anesthetic in a model of the subarachnoid space. *Anesthesiology* 1991;75:684–692.

59. Ross B, Coda B, Heath C. Local anesthetic distribution in a spinal model: A possible mechanism of neurologic injury after continuous spinal anesthesia. *Reg Anesth* 1992;17:69–77.

60. Robinson R, Stewart S, Meyers M, et al. Distribution of local anesthetic in a model of the subarachnoid space: A digital video image processing technique and its application to catheter-injected anesthetic. *Anesthesiology* 1994;81:1053–1060.

61. Bainton C, Strichartz G. Concentration dependence of lidocaine-induced irreversible conduction loss in frog nerve. *Anesthesiology* 1993;81:657–667.
62. Gold MS, Reichling DB, Hampl KF, Drasner K, Levine JD. Lidocaine toxicity in primary afferent neurons from the rat. *J Pharmacol Exp Ther* 1998;285:413–421.
63. Kanai Y, Katsuki H, Takasaki M. Graded, irreversible changes in crayfish giant axon as manifestations of lidocaine neurotoxicity in vitro. *Anesth Analg* 1998;86:569–573.
64. Lambert L, Lambert D, Strichartz G. Irreversible conduction block in isolated nerve by high concentrations of local anesthetics. *Anesthesiology* 1994;80:1082–1093.
65. Drasner K, Sakura S, Chan V, Bollen A, Ciriales R. Persistent sacral sensory deficit induced by intrathecal local anesthetic infusion in the rat. *Anesthesiology* 1994;80:847–852.
66. Hashimoto K, Bollen A, Ciriales R, Drasner R. Comparative toxicity of glucose and lidocaine administered intrathecally in the rat. *Reg Anesth Pain Med* 1998;23:444–450.
67. Hashimoto K, Hampl K, Nakamura Y, et al. Epinephrine increases the neurotoxic potential of intrathecally administered local anesthetic in the rat. *Anesthesiology*. In press.
68. Sakura S, Chan V, Ciriales R, Drasner K. The addition of 7.5% glucose does not alter the neurotoxicity of 5% lidocaine administered intrathecally in the rat. *Anesthesiology* 1995;82:236–240.
69. Sakura S, Bollen A, Ciriales R, Drasner K. Local anesthetic neurotoxicity does not result from blockade of voltage-gated sodium channels. *Anesth Analg* 1995;81:338–346.
70. Sakura S, Hashimoto K, Bollen A, Ciriales R, Drasner K. Intrathecal catheterization in the rat: An improved technique for morphologic analysis of drug-induced injury. *Anesthesiology* 1996;85:1184–1189.
71. Drasner K, Rigler M, Krejcie T, et al. Catheter spinal anesthesia and cauda equina syndrome: An alternative view. *Anesth Analg* 1991;73:369–370.
72. Byers M, Fink B, Kennedy R, Middaugh M, Hendrickson A. Effects of lidocaine on axonal morphology, microtubules, and rapid transport in rabbit vagus nerve in vitro. *J Neurobiol* 1973;4:125–143.
73. Kalichman M, Powell H, Myers R. Quantitative histologic analysis of local anesthetic-induced injury to rat sciatic nerve. *J Pharmacol Exp Ther* 1989;250:406–413.
74. Sakura S, Chan V, Ciriales R, Drasner K. Intrathecal infusion in the rat results in dose-dependent, but not concentration-dependent, sacral root injury [abstract]. *Anesthesiology* 1993;78:A856.
75. Norris MC, Leighton BL. Continuous spinal anesthesia after unintentional dural puncture in parturients. *Reg Anesth* 1990;15:285–287.
76. Arkoosh VA. Personal communication, October 2000.
77. Drasner K, Rigler M. Repeat injection after a "failed spinal"–At times, a potentially unsafe practice [letter]. *Anesthesiology* 1991;75:713–714.
78. Drasner K, Rigler M, Sessler D, Stoller M. Cauda equina syndrome following intended epidural anesthesia. *Anesthesiology* 1992;77:582–585.
79. Cheng A. Intended epidural anesthesia as possible cause of cauda equina syndrome. *Anesth Analg* 1993;78:157–159.
80. Gerancher J. Cauda equina syndrome following a single spinal administration of 5% hyperbaric lidocaine through a 25-gauge Whitacre needle. *Anesthesiology* 1997;87:687–689.
81. Auroy Y, Narchi P, Messiah A, et al. Serious complications related to regional anesthesia: Results of a prospective survey in France. *Anesthesiology* 1997;87:479–486.
82. Drasner K. Lidocaine spinal anesthesia: A vanishing therapeutic index? *Anesthesiology* 1997;87:469–472.
83. Schneider M, Ettlin T, Kaufmann M, et al. Transient neurologic toxicity after hyperbaric subarachnoid anesthesia with 5% lidocaine. *Anesth Analg* 1993;76:1154–1157.
84. Hampl KF, Schneider MC, Ummenhofer W, Drewe J. Transient neurologic symptoms after spinal anesthesia. *Anesth Analg* 1995;81:1148–1153.
85. Tarkkila P, Huhtala J, Tuominen M. Transient radicular irritation after spinal anaesthesia with hyperbaric 5% lignocaine. *Br J Anaesth* 1995;74:328–329.
86. Freedman J, Li D, Drasner K, et al. Transient neurologic symptoms after spinal anesthesia: An epidemiologic study of 1,863 patients. *Anesthesiology* 1998;89:633–941.
87. Hampl KF, Heinzmann-Wiedmer S, Luginbuehl I, et al. Transient neurologic symptoms after spinal anesthesia: A lower incidence with prilocaine and bupivacaine than with lidocaine. *Anesthesiology* 1998;88:629–633.
88. Hampl KF, Schneider MC, Thorin D, Ummenhofer W, Drewe J. Hyperosmolarity does not contribute to transient radicular irritation after spinal anesthesia with hyperbaric 5% lidocaine. *Reg Anesth* 1995;20:363–368.
89. Pollock JE, Neal JM, Stephenson CA, Wiley CE. Prospective study of the incidence of transient radicular irritation in patients undergoing spinal anesthesia. *Anesthesiology* 1996;84:1361–1367.
90. Fenerty J, Sonner J, Sakura S, Drasner K. Transient radicular pain following spinal anesthesia: Review of the literature and report of a case involving 2% lidocaine. *Int J Obstet Anesth* 1996;5:32–35.
91. Hampl KF, Schneider MC, Pargger H, et al. A similar incidence of transient neurologic symptoms after spinal anesthesia with 2% and 5% lidocaine. *Anesth Analg* 1996;83:1051–1054.
92. Pollock JE, Liu SS, Neal JM, Stephenson CA. Dilution of spinal lidocaine does not alter the incidence of transient neurologic symptoms. *Anesthesiology* 1999;90:445–450.
93. Ben-David B, Maryanovsky M, Gurevitch A, et al. A comparison of minidose lidocaine-fentanyl and conventional-dose lidocaine spinal anesthesia. *Anesth Analg* 2000;91:865–870.
94. Newman L, Iyer N, Tuman K. Transient radicular irritation after hyperbaric lidocaine spinal anesthesia in parturients. *Int J Obstet Anesth* 1997;6:132–134.
95. Wong CA, Slavenas P. The incidence of transient radicular irritation after spinal anesthesia in obstetric patients. *Reg Anesth Pain Med* 1999;24:55–58.
96. Kishimoto T, Ciriales R, Bollen A, Drasner K. Comparison of the neurotoxicity of intrathecal lidocaine and prilocaine in the rat [abstract]. *Anesthesiology* 1998;87:A-1421.
97. Dahlgren N. Transient radicular irritation after spinal anaesthesia [letter]. *Acta Anaesthesiol Scand* 1996;40:865.
98. Hartrick CT. Transient radicular irritation: A misnomer? [letter; comment]. *Anesth Analg* 1997;84:1392–1393.
99. Naveira FA, Copeland S, Anderson M, Speight K, Rauck R. Transient neurologic toxicity after spinal anesthesia, or is it myofascial pain? Two case reports. *Anesthesiology* 1998;88:268–270.
100. Ewart MC, Rubin AP. Subarachnoid block with hyperbaric lignocaine. A comparison with hyperbaric bupivacaine. *Anaesthesia* 1987;42:1183–1187.
101. Hiller A, Karjalainen K, Balk M, Rosenberg P. Transient neurological symptoms after spinal anaesthesia with hyperbaric 5% lidocaine or general anaesthesia. *Br J Anaesth* 1999;82:575–579.
102. Preston PG, Rosen MA, Hughes SC, et al. Epidural anesthesia with fentanyl and lidocaine for cesarean section: Maternal effects and neonatal outcome. *Anesthesiology* 1988;68:938–943.
103. Fuller JG, McMorland GH, Douglas MJ, Palmer L. Epidural morphine for analgesia after caesarean section: A report of 4880 patients. *Can J Anaesth* 1990;37:636–640.
104. Palmer CM, Nogami WM, Van Maren G, Alves DM. Postcesarean epidural morphine: A dose-response study. *Anesth Analg* 2000;90:887–891.
105. Bromage PR. A comparison of the hydrochloride salts of lidocaine and prilocaine for epidural analgesia. *Br J Anaesth* 1965;37:753–761.
106. Bromage PR. Improved conduction blockade in surgery and obstetrics: Carbonated local anaesthetic solutions. *Can Med Assoc J* 1967;97:1377–1384.
107. Bromage PR, Burfoot MF, Crowell DE, Trunant AP. Quality of epidural blockade. III. Carbonated local anaesthetic solutions. *Br J Anaesth* 1967;39:197–209.
108. Morison DH. A double-blind comparison of carbonated lidocaine and lidocaine hydrochloride in epidural anaesthesia. *Can Anaesth Soc J* 1981;28:387–389.
109. Martin R, Lamarche Y, Tetreault L. Comparison of clinical effectiveness of lidocaine hydrocarbonate and lidocaine hydrochloride with and without epinephrine in epidural anaesthesia. *Can Anaesth Soc J* 1981;28:224–227.
110. Cole CP, McMorland GH, Axelson JE. Evaluation of epidural blockade comparing lidocaine hydrocarbonate and lidocaine hydrochloride for caesarean section [abstract]. *Anesthesiology* 1983;59:A-411.
111. Sukani R, Winnie AP. Clinical pharmacokinetics of carbonated local anesthetics. I. Subclavian perivascular brachial block model. *Anesthesiology* 1987;66:739–745.
112. Nickel PM, Bromage PR, Sherrill DL. Comparison of hydrochloride and carbonated salts of lidocaine for epidural analgesia. *Reg Anesth* 1986;11:62–67.
113. Fujimori M, Nishimura K. Methemoglobinemia due to local anesthetics (a preliminary report). *Far East J Anaesth* 1964;4:4.

114. Lund PC, Cwik JC. Propitocaine (Citanest) and methemoglobinemia. *Anesthesiology* 1965;26:569–571.

115. Scott DB. *Citanest and methemoglobinemia: Discussion, Citanest.* Edited by Wiedling S. ed. Copenhagen Universitetsforlaget I Aarhus; 1965:199.

116. Crankshaw TP. Citanest (prilocaine) in spinal analgesia. *Acta Anaesthesiol Scand* 1965;16(suppl):287–290.

117. Menegel O, Linhares S, Spiegel P, Goncalves B. Clinical evaluation of prilocaine in spinal anesthesia. *Rev Bras Anestesiol* 1970;20:327–331.

118. Konig W, Ruzicic D. Absence of transient radicular irritation after 5000 spinal anaesthetics with prilocaine [letter]. *Anaesthesia* 1997;52:182–183.

119. Brown WU Jr, Bell GC, Jurie AO, et al. Newborn blood levels of lidocaine and mepivacaine in the first postnatal day following maternal epidural anesthesia. *Anesthesiology* 1975;42:698–707.

120. Liguori GA, Zayas VM, Chisholm MF. Transient neurologic symptoms after spinal anesthesia with mepivacaine and lidocaine. *Anesthesiology* 1998;88:619–623.

121. Hiller A, Rosenberg P. Transient neurological symptoms after spinal anaesthesia with 4% mepivacaine and 0.5% bupivacaine. *Br J Anaesth* 1997;79:301–305.

122. Zayas VM, Liguori GA, Chisholm MF, Susman MH, Gordon MA. Dose response relationships for isobaric spinal mepivacaine using the combined spinal epidural technique. *Anesth Analg* 1999;89:1167–1171.

123. Pawlowski J, Sukhani R, Pappas AL, et al. The anesthetic and recovery profile of two doses (60 and 80 mg) of plain mepivacaine for ambulatory spinal anesthesia. *Anesth Analg* 2000;91:580–584.

124. Salmela L, Aromaa U. Transient radicular irritation after spinal anesthesia induced with hyperbaric solutions of cerebrospinal fluid-diluted lidocaine 50 mg/ml or mepivacaine 40 mg/ml or bupivacaine 5 mg/ml. *Acta Anaesthesiol Scand* 1998;42:765–769.

125. Telivuo L. A new long-acting local anaesthetic for pain relief after thoracotomy. *Ann Chir Gynaecol Fenn* 1963;52:513.

126. Van Zundert A, Vaes L, Soetens M, et al. Every dose given in epidural analgesia for vaginal delivery can be a test dose. *Anesthesiology* 1987;67:436–440.

127. Geerinckx K, Vanderick G, Van Steenberge AL, Bouche R, De Muylder E. Bupivacaine 0.125% in epidural block analgesia during childbirth: Maternal and foetal plasma concentrations. *Br J Anaesth* 1974;46:937–941.

128. Bleyaert A, Soetens M, Vaes L, Van Steenberge AL, Van Der Donck A. Bupivacaine 0.125% in obstetric epidural analgesia: Experience in three thousand cases. *Anesthesiology* 1979;51:435–438.

129. Chestnut D, Owen C, Bates J, et al. Continuous infusion epidural analgesia during labor: A randomized, double-blind comparison of 0.0625% bupivacaine, 0.0002% fentanyl versus 0.125% bupivacaine. *Anesthesiology* 1988;68:754–759.

130. Chestnut DH, Laszewski LJ, Pollack KL, et al. Continuous epidural infusion of 0.0625% bupivacaine, 0.0002% fentanyl during the second stage of labor. *Anesthesiology* 1990;72:613–618.

131. Finegold H, Mandell G, Ramanathan S. Comparison of ropivacaine 0.1% fentanyl and bupivacaine 0.125%—fentanyl infusions for epidural labour analgesia. *Can J Anaesth* 2000;47:740–745.

132. Meister GC, D'Angelo R, Owen M, Nelson KE, Gaver R. A comparison of epidural analgesia with 0.125% ropivacaine with fentanyl versus 0.125% bupivacaine with fentanyl during labor. *Anesth Analg* 2000;90:632–637.

133. Fischer C, Blanie P, Jaouen E, et al. Ropivacaine, 0.1%, plus sufentanil, 0.5 microg/ml, versus bupivacaine, 0.1%, plus sufentanil, 0.5 microg/ml, using patient-controlled epidural analgesia for labor: A double-blind comparison. *Anesthesiology* 2000;92:1588–1593.

134. Campbell DC, Breen TW, Kronberg JE, Nunn R, Fick G. Comparison of the effects of ropivacaine vs bupivacaine on maternal ambulation and spontaneous micturition [abstract]. *Anesthesiology* 2000;93:A-1044.

135. Magno R, Berlin A, Karlsson K, Kjellmer I. Anesthesia for cesarean section IV: Placental transfer and neonatal elimination of bupivacaine following epidural analgesia for elective cesarean section. *Acta Anaesthesiol Scand* 1976;20:141–146.

136. McGuinness GA, Merkow AJ, Kennedy RL, Erenberg A. Epidural anesthesia with bupivacaine for Cesarean section: Neonatal blood levels and neurobehavioral responses. *Anesthesiology* 1978;49:270–273.

137. Block A, Covino BG. Effect of local anesthetic agents on cardiac conduction and contractility. *Reg Anesth* 1981;6:55–61.

138. Tanz RD, Heskett T, Loehning RW, Fairfax CA. Comparative cardiotoxicity of bupivacaine and lidocaine in the isolated perfused mammalian heart. *Anesth Analg* 1984;63:549–556.

139. de La Coussaye JE, Brugada J, Allessie MA. Electrophysiologic and arrhythmogenic effects of bupivacaine. A study with high-resolution ventricular epicardial mapping in rabbit hearts. *Anesthesiology* 1992;77:132–141.

140. Clarkson CW, Hondeghem LM. Mechanism for bupivacaine depression of cardiac conduction: Fast block of sodium channels during the action potential with slow recovery from block during diastole. *Anesthesiology* 1985;62:396–405.

141. Moller RA, Covino BG. Cardiac electrophysiologic effects of lidocaine and bupivacaine. *Anesth Analg* 1988;67:107–114.

142. de Jong RH, Bonin JD. Deaths from local anesthetic-induced convulsions in mice. *Anesth Analg* 1980;59:401–405.

143. Bernards CM, Artu AA. Hexamethonium and midazolam terminate dysrhythmias and hypertension caused by intracerebroventricular bupivacaine in rabbits. *Anesthesiology* 1991;74:89–96.

144. Thomas RD, Behbehani MM, Coyle DE, Denson DD. Cardiovascular toxicity of local anesthetics: An alternative hypothesis. *Anesth Analg* 1986;65:444–450.

145. de Jong RH, Ronfeld RA, de Rosa RA. Cardiovascular effects of convulsant and supraconvulsant doses of amide local anesthetics. *Anesth Analg* 1982;61:3–9.

146. Liu P, Feldman HS, Covino BM, Giasi R, Covino BG. Acute cardiovascular toxicity of intravenous amide local anesthetics in anesthetized ventilated dogs. *Anesth Analg* 1982;61:317–322.

147. Liu PL, Feldman HS, Giasi R, Patterson MK, Covino BG. Comparative CNS toxicity of lidocaine, etidocaine, bupivacaine, and tetracaine in awake dogs following rapid intravenous administration. *Anesth Analg* 1983;62:375–379.

148. Sage DJ, Feldman HS, Arthur GR, et al. The cardiovascular effects of convulsant doses of lidocaine and bupivacaine in the conscious dog. *Reg Anesth* 1985;10:175–183.

149. Kotelko DM, Shnider SM, Dailey PA, et al. Bupivacaine-induced cardiac arrhythmias in sheep. *Anesthesiology* 1984;60:10–18.

150. Rosen MA, Thigpen JW, Shnider SM, et al. Bupivacaine-induced cardiotoxicity in hypoxic and acidotic sheep. *Anesth Analg* 1985;64:1089–1096.

151. Nancarrow C, Rutten AJ, Runciman WB, et al. Myocardial and cerebral drug concentrations and the mechanisms of death after fatal intravenous doses of lidocaine, bupivacaine, and ropivacaine in the sheep. *Anesth Analg* 1989;69:276–283.

152. Munson ES, Tucker WK, Ausinsch B, Malagodi MH. Etidocaine, bupivacaine, and lidocaine seizure thresholds in monkeys. *Anesthesiology* 1975;42:471–478.

153. Komai H, Rusy BF. Hyperkalemia and bupivacaine block of AV conduction. *Anesthesiology* 1980;53:S210.

154. Courtney KR. Relationship between excitability block and negative inotropic actions of antiarrhythmic drugs. *Proc West Pharmacol Soc* 1984;27:181–184.

155. Albright GA. Cardiac arrest following regional anesthesia with etidocaine or bupivacaine. *Anesthesiology* 1979;51:285–287.

156. Morishima HO, Pedersen H, Finster M, et al. Bupivacaine toxicity in pregnant and nonpregnant ewes. *Anesthesiology* 1985;63:134–139.

157. Eisler EA, Thigpen JW, Shnider SM, et al. Bupivacaine cardiotoxicity in normal and acidotic rabbits [abstract]. *Anesthesiology* 1984;61:A-233.

158. Santos AC, Arthur GR, Wlody D, et al. Comparative systemic toxicity of ropivacaine and bupivacaine in nonpregnant and pregnant ewes. *Anesthesiology* 1995;82:734–740; discussion 27A.

159. Russell IF, Holmqvist EL. Subarachnoid analgesia for caesarean section. A double-blind comparison of plain and hyperbaric 0.5% bupivacaine. *Br J Anaesth* 1987;59:347–353.

160. Richardson MG, Collins HV, Wissler RN. Intrathecal hypobaric versus hyperbaric bupivacaine with morphine for cesarean section. *Anesth Analg* 1998;87:336–340.

161. Norris M. Height, weight, and the spread of subarachnoid hyperbaric bupivacaine in the term parturient. *Anesth Analg* 1988;67:555–558.

162. Sokolov VI. *Introduction to Theoretical Stereochemistry.* New York: Gordon & Breach; 1991.

163. Cahn R, Ingold C, Prelog V. The specification of asymmetric configuration in organic chemistry. *Experientia* 1956;12:81.

164. Vanhoutte F, Vereecke J, Verbeke N, Carmeliet E. Stereoselective effects of the enantiomers of bupivacaine on the electrophysiological

properties of the guinea-pig papillary muscle. *Br J Pharmacol* 1991;103:1275–1281.

165. Aberg G. Toxicological and local anaesthetic effects of optically active isomers of two local anaesthetic compounds. *Acta Pharmacol Toxicol* 1972;31:273–286.

166. Akerman B, Hellberg IB, Trossvik C. Primary evaluation of the local anaesthetic properties of the amino amide agent ropivacaine (LEA 103). *Acta Anaesthesiol Scand* 1988;32:571–578.

167. Scott DB, Lee A, Fagan D, et al. Acute toxicity of ropivacaine compared with that of bupivacaine. *Anesth Analg* 1989;69:563–569.

168. Hickey R, Hoffman J, Ramamurthy S. A comparison of ropivacaine 0.5% and bupivacaine 0.5% for brachial plexus block. *Anesthesiology* 1991;74:639–642.

169. Hickey R, Rowley CL, Candido KD, et al. A comparative study of 0.25% ropivacaine and 0.25% bupivacaine for brachial plexus block. *Anesth Analg* 1992;75:602–606.

170. Brockway MS, Bannister J, McClure JH, McKeown D, Wildsmith JA. Comparison of extradural ropivacaine and bupivacaine. *Br J Anaesth* 1991;66:31–37.

171. Brown DL, Carpenter RL, Thompson GE. Comparison of 0.5% ropivacaine and 0.5% bupivacaine for epidural anesthesia in patients undergoing lower-extremity surgery. Anesthesiology 1990;72:633–636.

172. Bader AM, Datta S, Flanagan H, Covino BG. Comparison of bupivacaine- and ropivacaine-induced conduction blockade in the isolated rabbit vagus nerve. *Anesth Analg* 1989;68:724–727.

173. Stienstra R, Jonker TA, Bourdrez P, et al. Ropivacaine 0.25% versus bupivacaine 0.25% for continuous epidural analgesia in labor: A double-blind comparison. *Anesth Analg* 1995;80:285–289.

174. Eddleston JM, Holland JJ, Griffin RP, et al. A double-blind comparison of 0.25% ropivacaine and 0.25% bupivacaine for extradural analgesia in labour. *Br J Anaesth* 1996;76:66–71.

175. McCrae AF, Jozwiak H, McClure JH. Comparison of ropivacaine and bupivacaine in extradural analgesia for the relief of pain of labour. *Br J Anaesth* 1995;74:261–265.

176. Gaiser RR, Venkateswaren P, Cheek TG, et al. Comparison of 0.25% ropivacaine and bupivacaine for epidural analgesia for labor and vaginal delivery. *J Clin Anesth* 1997;9:564–568.

177. Benhamou D, Hamza J, Eledjam JJ, et al. Continuous extradural infusion of ropivacaine 2 mg ml-1 for pain relief during labour. *Br J Anaesth* 1997;78:748–750.

178. Muir HA, Writer D, Douglas J, Weeks S, Gambling D, Macarthur A. Double-blind comparison of epidural ropivacaine 0.25% and bupivacaine 0.25% for the relief of childbirth pain. *Can J Anaesth* 1997;44:599–604.

179. Moller R, Covino BG. Cardiac electrophysiologic properties of bupivacaine and lidocaine compared with those of ropivacaine, a new amide local anesthetic. *Anesthesiology* 1990;72:322–329.

180. Reiz S, Haggmark S, Johansson G, Nath S. Cardiotoxicity of ropivacaine–a new amide local anaesthetic agent. *Acta Anaesthesiol Scand* 1989;33:93–98.

181. Feldman HS, Arthur GR, Covino BG. Comparative systemic toxicity of convulsant and supraconvulsant doses of intravenous ropivacaine, bupivacaine, and lidocaine in the conscious dog. *Anesth Analg* 1989;69:794–801.

182. Covino BG, Vassallo H. Chemical aspects of local anesthetic agents. In: Covino BG, ed. *Local Anesthetics: Mechanisms of Action and Clinical Use.* New York: Grune & Stratton; 1976:6–11.

183. Kanai Y, Tateyama S, Nakamura T, Kasaba T, Takasaki M. Effects of levobupivacaine, bupivacaine, and ropivacaine on tail-flick response and motor function in rats following epidural or intrathecal administration. *Reg Anesth Pain Med* 1999;24:444–452.

184. Capogna G, Celleno D, Fusco P, Lyons G, Columb M. Relative potencies of bupivacaine and ropivacaine for analgesia in labour. *Br J Anaesth* 1999;82:371–373.

185. Polley LS, Columb MO, Naughton NN, Wagner DS, van de Ven CJ. Relative analgesic potencies of ropivacaine and bupivacaine for epidural analgesia in labor: Implications for therapeutic indexes. *Anesthesiology* 1999;90:944–950.

186. Dixon WJ, Massey FJ. *Introduction to Statistical Analysis.* 4th ed. New York: McGraw-Hill; 1983:428–439.

187. D'Angelo R, James RL. Is ropivacaine less potent than bupivacaine? [editorial; comment]. *Anesthesiology* 1999;90:941–943.

188. Polley LS, Columb MO. Potency, impotency, and importance [letter]! *Anesth Analg* 2000;91:765–766.

189. Reynolds F. Does the left hand know what the right hand is doing? An appraisal of single enantiomer local anesthetics. *Int J Obstet Anesth* 1997;6:257–269.

190. Malinovsky JM, Charles F, Kick O, et al. Intrathecal anesthesia: Ropivacaine versus bupivacaine. *Anesth Analg* 2000;91:1457–1460.

191. McDonald SB, Liu SS, Kopacz DJ, Stephenson CA. Hyperbaric spinal ropivacaine: A comparison to bupivacaine in volunteers. *Anesthesiology* 1999;90:971–977.

192. Gautier PE, De Kock M, Van Steenberge A, et al. Intrathecal ropivacaine for ambulatory surgery. *Anesthesiology* 1999;91:1239–1245.

193. Santos AC, Karpel B, Noble G. The placental transfer and fetal effects of levobupivacaine, racemic bupivacaine, and ropivacaine. *Anesthesiology* 1999;90:1698–1703.

194. Eddleston JM, Holland JJ, Griffin RP, et al. A double-blind comparison of 0.25% ropivacaine and 0.25% bupivacaine for extradural analgesia in labour. *Br J Anaesth* 1996;76:66–71.

195. Owen MD, D'Angelo R, Gerancher JC, et al. 0.125% Ropivacaine is similar to 0.125% bupivacaine for labor analgesia using patient-controlled epidural infusion. *Anesth Analg* 1998;86:527–531.

196. Gautier P, De Kock M, Van Steenberge A, et al. A double-blind comparison of 0.125% ropivacaine with sufentanil and 0.125% bupivacaine with sufentanil for epidural labor analgesia. *Anesthesiology* 1999;90:772–778.

197. Writer WD, Stienstra R, Eddleston JM, et al. Neonatal outcome and mode of delivery after epidural analgesia for labour with ropivacaine and bupivacaine: A prospective meta-analysis. *Br J Anaesth* 1998;81:713–717.

198. Capogna G, Celleno D, Fusco P, Lyons G, Columb M. Relative potencies of bupivacaine and ropivacaine for analgesia in labour. *Br J Anaesth* 1999;82:371–373.

199. Polley LS, Columb MO, Naughton NN, Wagner DS, van de Ven CJ. Relative analgesic potencies of ropivacaine and bupivacaine for epidural analgesia in labor: Implications for therapeutic indexes. *Anesthesiology* 1999;90:944–950.

200. Polley LS, Columb MO. Comparison of epidural ropivacaine and bupivacaine in combination with sufentanil for labor. *Anesthesiology* 2000;92:280–281.

201. Knudsen L, Suurküla MB, Bloomberg S, et al. Central nervous and cardiovascular effects of I.V. infusions of ropivacaine, bupivacaine and placebo in volunteers. *Br J Anaesth* 1997;78:507–514.

202. Scott SB, Lee A, Fagon D, et al. Acute toxicity of ropivacaine compared with that of bupivacaine. *Anesth Analg* 1989;69:563–569.

203. Campbell DC, Zwack RM, Crone LA, Yip RW. Ambulatory labor epidural analgesia: Bupivacaine versus ropivacaine. *Anesth Analg* 2000;90:1384–1389.

204. Lysak SZ, Eisenach JC, Dobson CE. Patient-controlled epidural analgesia during labor: A comparison of three solutions with a continuous infusion control. *Anesthesiology* 1990;72:44–49.

205. D'Angelo R, Gerancher JC, Eisenach JC, Raphael BL. Epidural fentanyl produces labor analgesia by a spinal mechanism. *Anesthesiology* 1998;88:1519–1523.

206. Lyons G, Columb M, Hawbhotne L, Dresner M. Extradural pain relief in labour: Bupivacaine sparing by extradural fentanyl is dose dependent. *Br J Anaesth* 1997;78:493–497.

207. Pinder AJ, Dresner M. Ropivacaine and bupivacaine with fentanyl for labor epidural anesthesia. *Anesth Analg* 2000;91:1310–1311.

208. Breen TW, Campbell DC, Kronberg JE, Nunn RT, Fick GH. The clinically relevant potencies of ropivacaine and bupivacaine: A PCEA study [abstract]. *Anesthesiology* 2000;93:A-1101.

209. Smiley RM, Kim-Lo SH, Goodman SR, Jackson MA, Landau R. Patient-controlled epidural analgesia with 0.0625% ropivacaine versus bupivacaine with fentanyl during labor [abstract]. *Anesthesiology* 2000;93:A1065.

210. Smith T, Thomas JA, Owen MD, Harris LC, D'Angelo R. 0.075% Epidural ropivacaine and bupivacaine produce indistinguishable labor analgesia [abstract]. *Anesthesiology* 2000;93:A1066.

211. Debon R, Allaouichiche B, Duflo F, Boselli E, Chassard D. The analgesic effect of sufentanil combined with ropivacaine 0.2% for labor analgesia: A comparison of three sufentanil doses. *Anesth Analg* 2001;92:180–183.

212. Beilin Y, Galea M, Zahn J, Bodian CA. Epidural ropivacaine for the initiation of labor epidural analgesia: A dose finding study. *Anesth Analg* 1999;88:1340–1345.

213. McClellan KJ, Faulds D. Ropivacaine: An update of its use in regional anaesthesia. *Drugs* 2000;60:1065–1093.
214. Van de Velde M. Analgesia for labor pain with ropivacaine. *Acta Anaesthesiol Belg* 2000;51:131–134.
215. Johnson RF, Cahana A, Olenick M, et al. A comparison of the placental transfer of ropivacaine versus bupivacaine. *Anesth Analg* 1999;89:703–708.
216. Irestedt L, Ekblom A, Olofsson C, Dahlstrom AC, Emanuelsson BM. Pharmacokinetics and clinical effect during continuous epidural infusion with ropivacaine 2.5 mg/ml or bupivacaine 2.5 mg/ml for labour pain relief. *Acta Anaesthesiol Scand* 1998;42:890–896.
217. Cascio MG, Gaiser RR, Camann WR, et al. Comparative evaluation of four different infusion rates of ropivacaine (2 mg/mL) for epidural labor analgesia. *Reg Anesth Pain Med* 1998;23:548–553.
218. Gaiser RR, Lewin SB, Cheek TG, Gutsche BB. Effects of immediately initiating an epidural infusion in the combined spinal and epidural technique in nulliparous parturients. *Reg Anesth Pain Med* 2000;25:223–227.
219. Griffin RP, Reynolds F. Extradural anaesthesia for caesarean section: A double-blind comparison of 0.5% ropivacaine with 0.5% bupivacaine. *Br J Anaesth* 1995;74:512–516.
220. Datta S, Camann W, Bader A, VanderBurgh L. Clinical effects and maternal and fetal plasma concentrations of epidural ropivacaine versus bupivacaine for cesarean section. *Anesthesiology* 1995;82:1346–1352.
221. Alahuhta C, Rasanen J, Jouppila P, et al. The effects of epidural ropivacaine and bupivacaine for cesarean section on uteroplacental and fetal circulation. *Anesthesiology* 1995;83:23–32.
222. Crosby E, Sandler A, Finucane B, et al. Comparison of epidural anaesthesia with ropivacaine 0.5% and bupivacaine 0.5% for caesarean section. *Can J Anaesth* 1998;45:1066–1071.
223. Irestedt L, Emanuelsson BM, Ekblom A, Olofsson C, Reventlid H. Ropivacaine 7.5 mg/ml for elective caesarean section. A clinical and pharmacokinetic comparison of 150 mg and 187.5 mg. *Acta Anaesthesiol Scand* 1997;41:1149–1156.
224. Morton CP, Bloomfield S, Magnusson A, Jozwiak H, McClure JH. Ropivacaine 0.75% for extradural anaesthesia in elective caesarean section: An open clinical and pharmacokinetic study in mother and neonate. *Br J Anaesth* 1997;79:3–8.
225. Bjornestad E, Smedvig JP, Bjerkreim T, et al. Epidural ropivacaine 7.5 mg/ml for elective Caesarean section: a double-blind comparison of efficacy and tolerability with bupivacaine 5 mg/ml. *Acta Anaesthesiol Scand* 1999;43:603–608.
226. Concepcion M, Arthur GR, Steele SM, Bader AM, Covino BG. A new local anesthetic, ropivacaine. Its epidural effects in humans. *Anesth Analg* 1990;70:80–85.
227. Shah MK, Sia AT, Chong JL. The effect of the addition of ropivacaine or bupivacaine upon pruritus induced by intrathecal fentanyl in labour. *Anaesthesia* 2000;55:1008–1013.
228. Levin A, Datta S, Camann WR. Intrathecal ropivacaine for labor analgesia: A comparison with bupivacaine. *Anesth Analg* 1998;87:624–627.
229. Wali A, Mena G, Imiak S, Vadhera R, Suresh M. Determination of the dose response for intrathecal ropivacaine in laboring parturients [abstract]. *Anesthesiology* 2000;93:A-1099.
230. Palmer C, Nogami W, Alves D. Intrathecal ropivacaine and fentanyl for labor analgesia [abstract]. *Anesthesiology* 2000;93:A-1090.
231. Aps C, Reynolds F. An intradermal study of the local anaesthetic and vascular effects of the isomers of bupivacaine. *Br J Clin Pharmacol* 1978;6:63–68.
232. Mazoit JX, Boico O, Samii K. Myocardial uptake of bupivacaine: II. Pharmacokinetics and pharmacodynamics of bupivacaine enantiomers in the isolated perfused rabbit heart. *Anesth Analg* 1993;77:477–482.
233. Mazoit JX, Decaux A, Bouaziz H, Edouard A. Comparative ventricular electrophysiologic effect of racemic bupivacaine, levobupivacaine, and ropivacaine on the isolated rabbit heart. *Anesthesiology* 2000;93:784–792.
234. Chang DH, Ladd LA, Wilson KA, Gelgor L, Mather LE. Tolerability of large-dose intravenous levobupivacaine in sheep. *Anesth Analg* 2000;91:671–679.
235. Huang YF, Pryor ME, Mather LE, Veering BT. Cardiovascular and central nervous system effects of intravenous levobupivacaine and bupivacaine in sheep. *Anesth Analg* 1998;86:797–804.
236. Morrison SG, Dominguez JJ, Frascarolo P, Reiz S. A comparison of the electrocardiographic cardiotoxic effects of racemic bupivacaine, levobupivacaine, and ropivacaine in anesthetized swine. *Anesth Analg* 2000;90:1308–1314.
237. Groban L, Deal DD, Vernon JC, James RL, Butterworth J. Ventricular arrhythmias with or without programmed electrical stimulation after incremental overdosage with lidocaine, bupivacaine, levobupivacaine, and ropivacaine. *Anesth Analg* 2000;91:1103–1111.
238. Bardsley H, Gristwood R, Baker H, Watson N, Nimmo W. A comparison of the cardiovascular effects of levobupivacaine and racbupivacaine following intravenous administration to healthy volunteers. *Br J Clin Pharmacol* 1998;46:245–249.
239. Bader AM, Tsen LC, Camann WR, Nephew E, Datta S. Clinical effects and maternal and fetal plasma concentrations of 0.5% epidural levobupivacaine versus bupivacaine for cesarean delivery. *Anesthesiology* 1999;90:1596–1601.
240. Kopacz DJ, Allen HW, Thompson GE. A comparison of epidural levobupivacaine 0.75% with racemic bupivacaine for lower abdominal surgery. *Anesth Analg* 2000;90:642–648.
241. Cox CR, Faccenda KA, Gilhooly C, Bannister J, Scott NB, Morrison LM. Extradural S(-)-bupivacaine: Comparison with racemic RS-bupivacaine. *Br J Anaesth* 1998;80:289–293.
242. Cox CR, Checketts MR, Mackenzie N, Scott NB, Bannister J. Comparison of S(−)-bupivacaine with racemic (RS)-bupivacaine in supraclavicular brachial plexus block. *Br J Anaesth* 1998;80:594–598.
243. Bay-Nielsen M, Klarskov B, Bech K, Andersen J, Kehlet H. Levobupivacaine vs bupivacaine as infiltration anaesthesia in inguinal herniorrhaphy. *Br J Anaesth* 1999;82:280–282.
244. Lyons G, Columb M, Wilson RC, Johnson RV. Epidural pain relief in labour: Potencies of levobupivacaine and racemic bupivacaine. *Br J Anaesth* 1998;81:899–901.
245. Burke D, Henderson DJ, Simpson AM, et al. Comparison of 0.25% S(-)-bupivacaine with 0.25% RS-bupivacaine for epidural analgesia in labour. *Br J Anaesth* 1999;83:750–755.
246. Donaldson L, Young A, Eldridge J, et al. A comparison of 0.125% levobupivacaine and 0.125% bupivacaine epidural infusions for labor analgesia [abstract]. *Anesthesiology* 1999;90:A-43.
247. Lyons G, Columb M, Wilson RC, Johnson RV. Epidural pain relief in labour: Potencies of levobupivacaine and racemic bupivacaine [published erratum appears in *Br J Anaesth* 1999;82:488]. *Br J Anaesth* 1998;81:899–901.
248. Aps C, Reynolds F. An intradermal study of the local anaesthetic and vascular effects of the isomers of bupivacaine. *Br J Clin Pharmacol* 1978;6:63–68.
249. Burke D, Kennedy S, Bannister J. Spinal anesthesia with 0.5% S(-)-bupivacaine for elective lower limb surgery. *Reg Anesth Pain Med* 1999;24:519–523.
250. DiFazio CA, Carron H, Grosslight KR, et al. Comparison of pH-adjusted lidocaine solutions for epidural anesthesia. *Anesth Analg* 1986;65:760–764.
251. Peterfreund RA, Datta S, Ostheimer GW. pH-adjustment of local anesthetic solutions with sodium bicarbonate: Laboratory evaluation of alkalinization and precipitation. *Reg Anesth* 1989;14:265–270.
252. Bromage PR, Robson JG. Concentrations of lignocaine in the blood after intravenous, intramuscular, epidural and endotracheal administration. *Br J Anaesth* 1961;16:461–478.
253. Burfoot MF, Bromage PR. The effects of epinephrine on mepivacaine absorption from the spinal epidural space. *Anesthesiology* 1971;35:488–492.
254. Burn AGL, Van Kleef JW, Gradines MP, Olthof G, Spierdijk J. Epidural anesthesia with lidocaine and bupivacaine: Effect of epinephrine on the plasma concentration profile. *Anesth Analg* 1986;65:1281–1284.
255. Jamous MA, Hand CW, Moore RA, Teddy PJ, McQuay HJ. Epinephrine reduces systemic absorption of extradural diacetylmorphine. *Anesth Analg* 1986;65:1290–1294.
256. Klepper ID, Sherrill DL, Boetger CL, Bromage PR. Analgesic and respiratory effects of extradural sufentanil in volunteers and the influence of adrenaline as an adjuvant. *Br J Anaesth* 1987;59:1147–1156.
257. Abboud TK, David S, Nagappala S, et al. Maternal, fetal and neonatal effects of lidocaine with and without epinephrine for epidural anesthesia in obstetrics. *Anesth Analg* 1984;63:973–979.
258. Bromage P, Camporesi E, Durant P, Nielsen C. Influence of epinephrine as an adjuvant to epidural morphine. *Anesthesiology* 1983;58:257–262.

259. Bromage PR, El-Faqih S, Husain I, Naguib M. Epinephrine and fentanyl as adjuvants to 0.5% bupivacaine for epidural analgesia. *Reg Anesth* 1989;14:189–194.

260. Dohi S, Takeshima R, Naito H. Spinal cord blood flow in dogs: The effects of tetracaine, epinephrine, acute blood loss and hypercapnia. *Anesth Analg* 1987;66:599–606.

261. Kozody R, Palahniuk RJ, Wade JG, Cumming M. The effect of subarachnoid epinephrine and phenylephrine on spinal cord blood flow. *Can Anaesth Soc J* 1984;31:503–508.

262. Porter SS, Albin MS, Watson WA, Bunegin L, Pantoja G. Spinal cord and cerebral blood flow responses to subarachnoid injection of local anesthetics with and without epinephrine. *Acta Anaesthesiol Scand* 1985;29:330–338.

263. Perris BW. Epidural pethidine in labour: A study of dose requirements. *Anaesthesia* 1980;35:380–382.

264. Husemeyer RP, Davenport HT, Cummings AJ, Rosankiewicz JR. Comparison of epidural and intramuscular pethidine for analgesia in labour. *Br J Obstet Gynaecol* 1981;88:711–717.

265. Brownridge P. Epidural bupivacaine-pethidine mixture chemical experience using a low-dose combination in labour. *Aust N Z J Obstet Gynaecol* 1988;28:17–24.

266. Baraka A, Maktabi M, Noueihid R. Epidural meperidine-bupivacaine for obstetric analgesia. *Anesth Analg* 1982;61:652–656.

267. Framewo CE, Naguib M. Spinal anaesthesia with meperidine as the sole agent. *Can Anaesth Soc J* 1985;32:553–557.

268. Booth JV, Lindsay DR, Olufolabi AJ, et al. Subarachnoid meperidine (Pethidine) causes significant nausea and vomiting during labor. The Duke Women's Anesthesia Research Group. *Anesthesiology* 2000;93:418–421.

269. Kafle SK. Intrathecal meperidine for elective caesarean section: A comparison with lidocaine. *Can J Anaesth* 1993;40:718–721.

270. Nguyen Thi TV, Orliaguet G, Ngu TH, Bonnet F. Spinal anesthesia with meperidine as the sole agent for cesarean delivery. *Reg Anesth* 1994;19:386–389.

271. Norris MC, Honet JE, Leighton BL, Arkoosh VA. A comparison of meperidine and lidocaine for spinal anesthesia for postpartum tubal ligation. *Reg Anesth* 1996;21:84–88.

272. Ibusuki, Fang Z, Bollen A, Drasner K. Comparative neurotoxicity of intrathecal meperidine and lidocaine in the rat [abstract]. *Anesthesiology* 2000;93:A725.

Shnider and Levinson's Anesthesia for Obstetrics,
edited by Samuel C. Hughes, et al.
Lippincott Williams & Wilkins,
Philadelphia, © 2001.

CHAPTER 6

NONPHARMACOLOGIC METHODS OF PAIN RELIEF DURING LABOR

DEBORAH L. ANDERSON, C.N.M. AND SAMUEL C. HUGHES, M.D.

The experience of childbirth ranges from agony to ecstasy. It is a multidimensional experience that includes intense physical, emotional, psychological, developmental, social, cultural, and spiritual components (1–83). It differs in meaning and quality for each laboring woman (Fig. 6.1) and changes as labor progresses (2). In a study examining relative intensity of differing acute and chronic pain conditions, labor pain ranked among the most intense pains recorded (Fig. 6.2) (2). Even though most women rate their labor pain as severe, while few women report little or no pain, satisfaction with the childbirth experience is not always closely related to experiencing less pain (3, 4). Nonpharmacologic methods of pain relief during labor began gaining popularity in the 1930s, during a time when the undesirable effects of ether and twilight sleep (scopolamine and morphine) gave impetus to consumers and health care providers to search for other methods of pain relief. Since then, many nonpharmacologic methods have been used by women in labor. Today, whether a parturient wants analgesia or anesthesia support during labor, no analgesia or anesthesia, or a combination of the different options, nonpharmacologic methods of pain relief during labor may be useful tools in helping women to cope with the pain of labor. Nonpharmacologic methods may be used instead of opioids and epidural analgesia or as an adjunct to these methods, and may benefit mother and baby by decreasing opioid use or delaying epidural placement until the active phase of labor (5).

HYPNOSIS

The word hypnosis derives from the Greek word *hypnos,* which means sleep. The hypnotic state is not, however, a sleep state, but "a focused state of intense concentration, characterized by heightened responsiveness to suggestions, cues, and signals from the surrounding environment (or the hypnotist)" (6).

Suggestibility, a key factor in achieving the hypnotic state, varies from individual to individual and can be tested for. Approximately 15% of the general population is highly suggestible, 70% can enter some degree of hypnosis, and 15% are difficult to hypnotize (6).

Although its use in the United States has not been widespread, hypnosis has been used in obstetrics since the nineteenth century. It has primarily been used as a method to assist women with pain control during labor.

Self-hypnosis and posthypnotic suggestion are two common hypnotic techniques used to alter pain perception during childbirth. Training begins anywhere from the first to the third trimester and usually consists of six individual or group sessions.

Self-hypnosis is taught to the patient so that she may produce hypnoanalgesia for herself during her labor. She may use self-hypnosis to cope with a difficult isolated contraction or to place herself in trance for an extended period of her labor. Common techniques are relaxation, active imagination, distraction, and glove anesthesia. Glove anesthesia is a technique in which the patient creates a numb feeling in her hand through suggestion; she then spreads the numbness to others parts of her body by placing the numb hand on the area she would like affected (7). This training is begun and practiced repeatedly during the antenatal period.

With posthypnotic suggestion, the antenatal patient is prepared for the labor and delivery experience while in the hypnotic state. Under hypnosis childbirth education, suggestion and repetition are used to modify the fear-tension-pain response that childbirth may engender. A conditioned reflex of comfort, control, and confidence with labor is learned wherein the parturient is able to modify the perception and interpretation of and reaction to the pain of labor.

Although numerous studies have been published reporting that the use of hypnosis during labor results in decreased anxiety, lower analgesia use, and lower perceived pain, most studies were not well designed and were subject to bias (8). Only two randomized-controlled studies have been reported in the literature (9, 10). Freeman et al. (9) evaluated the effect of self-hypnosis on pain relief, satisfaction, and analgesic requirements for women in their first labor. Sixty-five primigravidas with normal pregnancies were randomized to a hypnosis group or a control group. All women attended weekly antenatal classes. The hypnosis group additionally was seen weekly after 32 weeks of gestation where, under hypnosis, they received training for relaxation, pain relief, and glove anesthesia. Hypnotic depth was also assessed in the experimental group; 5 subjects were good hypnotic subjects, 19 moderate, and 5 poor. There was no difference in the proportion of women receiving epidural or pethidine between the hypnosis and control groups; however, good or moderate hypnotic subjects had fewer epidurals than did poor hypnotic subjects. There was a trend for labor to be more satisfying for women in the hypnosis group, with a subset of moderate or good hypnotic subjects finding hypnosis to be exceptionally helpful.

In the most comprehensive study to date, Harmon et al. (10) evaluated the effects of hypnosis as an adjunct to childbirth education. Sixty low-risk nulliparous women attending six regular prenatal classes were evaluated for hypnotic susceptibility and then randomized to a hypnosis or control group. Women in the hypnosis group were taught hypnotic induction then given a cassette tape recording of the induction and suggestions for deep relaxation, enjoyment of childbirth, and glove anesthesia. The control group was given a cassette tape of standard relaxation exercises, visualization for distraction, and pushing and breathing techniques to be used during labor. All subjects were instructed to practice with their tapes daily. Compared with the hypnotically-trained group, a significantly larger proportion of the control group received tranquilizers and opioids during labor.

Baram (6) cites the following risks associated with the use of hypnosis: precipitating a psychotic reaction, making an existing disorder worse, masking a significant physical illness, and

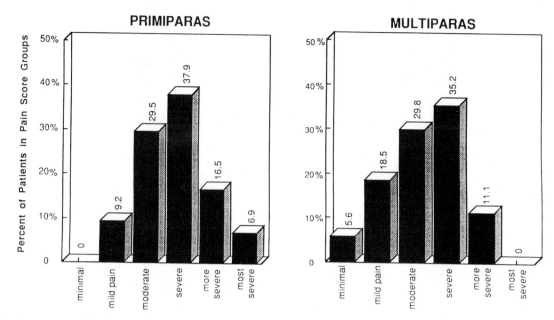

Figure 6.1. Distribution of Pain Rating Index (PRI) scores for primiparas and multiparas in six intervals of the PRI range. There is a wide range of pain scores in both primiparas and multiparas. (Adapted and reprinted by permission from Melzack R, Taenzer P, Feldman P, Kinch RA. Labour is still painful after prepared childbirth training. *Can Med Assoc J* 1981;125:357–363.)

indiscriminately removing neurotic symptoms that have strong psychodynamic meaning.

NATURAL CHILDBIRTH

The term "natural childbirth" was coined by Grantly Dick-Read in the 1930s (11). Dick-Read viewed childbirth as a natural physiologic process and one that is not inherently painful. He believed that labor pain arose from socially induced expectations. He described the "fear-tension-pain syndrome" as the cause of most childbirth pain. He hypothesized that fear produced tension in the lower uterus, which, in turn, resulted in pain perception (12). His training centered around eliminating

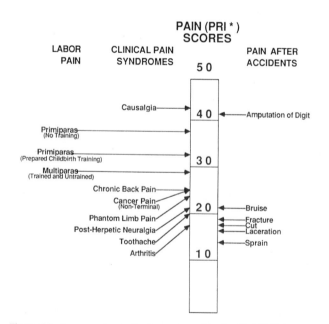

Figure 6.2. A comparison of pain scores using the McGill Pain Questionnaire, comparing labor pain and pain of other patients in a general hospital pain clinic. *McGill Pain Questionnaire Pain Rating Index. (Reprinted by permission from Melzack R. The myth of painless childbirth [The John J. Bonica Lecture]. *Pain* 1984;19:321–337.)

labor pain by educating women about normal labor and delivery processes, correcting faulty expectations regarding parturition pain, teaching progressive muscle relaxation and breathing techniques, and encouraging husband participation (12, 13). Although Dick-Read's method is limited by his assertion that labor is naturally a painless experience, he made substantial contributions to the historical development of the content of contemporary childbirth preparation classes.

PSYCHOPROPHYLAXIS

Dr. Fernand Lamaze, a French obstetrician, introduced the psychoprophylactic method of pain relief to the West after learning about the method during a 1951 visit to Russia (14). Lamaze modified the psychoprophylactic method developed in Russia by Nicolayev, brought it back to Paris, and shortly thereafter the Lamaze method became popular in the United States (13). This technique combines positive conditioning of the mother with education about the process of childbirth, the goal being to lessen fear and provide techniques to cope with labor pain. The basis of psychoprophylaxis is the belief that the pain of labor and delivery can be suppressed by reorganization of cerebral cortical activity. Conditioned pain reflexes associated with uterine contractions and perineal distention can be replaced by newly created "positive" conditioned reflexes. The mother is taught to respond to the beginning of a contraction by immediately taking a deep "cleansing breath," gently exhaling, then breathing in a specific breathing pattern until the contraction ends. She may also focus her eyes on a specific object or location away from herself, concentrate on release of muscle tension, and maintain the proper breathing rhythm with the help and "coaching" of a spouse or friend. The increased concentration required of her by these activities distracts from or inhibits the pain of uterine contraction. Lamaze preparation usually begins 6 weeks before delivery. Instruction includes normal anatomy and physiology of pregnancy, labor, and delivery; training in relaxation and breathing techniques; and providing the mother with knowledge and a greater sense of personal control over her birth experience.

Although there may appear to be some similarity between psychoprophylaxis and hypnosis, proponents of psychoprophylaxis point out that their technique freely engages the mother's conscious and cooperative efforts. When Samko and Schoenfeld investigated the relationship between hypnotic susceptibility and successful Lamaze childbirth, they found no correlation (15).

Over the past 50 years, studies of the effects of psychoprophylaxis and natural childbirth on analgesia and anesthesia use during labor have produced inconsistent results. Some authors (16–19) report a decreased use of analgesia and anesthesia, while others (20–24) report no difference. These inconsistent findings may reflect self-selection bias, variable content of childbirth preparation classes, differing patient populations, methodologic problems, or variations in care received by control groups.

Many contemporary childbirth preparation classes include a combination or modification of the content of both the psychoprophylactic and natural childbirth methodologies (25). In general, current childbirth classes also include analgesia and anesthesia options, a wide variety of nonpharmacologic methods of pain relief, information to improve pregnancy and birth outcomes, preparation about what parents will encounter in the maternity care system, current obstetric technology, and methods to increase self-confidence in the birthing process (26).

ACUPUNCTURE

Acupuncture has been a component of the health care system of China for over 2,500 years. The paradigm of traditional Chinese medicine describes patterns of energy flow (Qi) through the body that are essential to health. An imbalance or disruption of this flow is responsible for pain or disease. It is believed that acupuncture treats illness by correcting imbalances of energy flow (Qi) (27).

Conventional science has produced evidence that demonstrates that opioid peptides are released during acupuncture and that opioid antagonists reverse the analgesic effects of acupuncture (27). Acupuncture has also been documented to produce alterations in immune functions, secretion of neurotransmitters, secretions of neurohormones, and regulation of blood flow. Which of these changes mediates the therapeutic effect of acupuncture is unclear (27).

Acupuncture involves stimulation of anatomical locations on the skin by a variety of techniques. Most commonly, stimulation of acupuncture points is achieved through penetration of the skin with thin, solid, metallic needles, which are then manipulated by hand or by electrical stimulation (27). Acupuncture points selected for treatment vary from practitioner to practitioner. Figure 6.3 illustrates acupuncture points used to provide analgesia during labor (28).

Acupuncture use in the antepartum or intrapartum period has been investigated as a pain relief method during labor. Weekly antepartal acupuncture treatments beginning at 36 weeks of gestation have not been found to reduce the need for labor analgesia or epidural anesthesia use during labor (29–32).

There are few studies in the English language medical literature that examine the efficacy of acupuncture as a labor and delivery analgesic. Small numbers of patients, a wide variation in acupuncture sites, techniques, and length of administration, and biased study designs make it difficult to evaluate variable results.

In a recent, nonrandomized, controlled study from Sweden, Ternov et al. (33) evaluated the analgesic effect of intrapartum acupuncture by comparing the need for other methods of analgesia and anesthesia in women who were or were not given acupuncture. Ninety women in an experimental group who were at least 3 cm dilated received acupuncture intermittently throughout labor and had access to all traditional pain relief methods (epidural, pudendal, meperidine, nitrous oxide, and sterile water blocks). The control group received traditional pain relief methods only. Sixty percent of the women receiving acupuncture requested no additional analgesic during

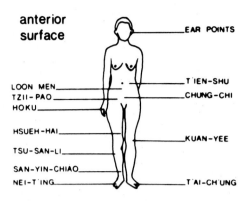

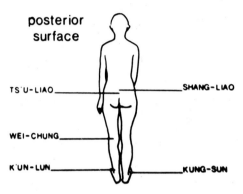

Figure 6.3. Sites of acupuncture points chosen by the acupuncturist to provide analgesia during labor. (Reprinted by permission from Wallis L, Shnider SM, Palahniuk RJ, Spivey HL. An evaluation of acupuncture analgesia in obstetrics. *Anesthesiology* 1974;41:596–601.)

labor compared to 13% in the control group. In addition, of the women who used additional analgesia, significantly fewer women in the acupuncture group used intramuscular meperidine, nitrous oxide, or pudendal nerve block. No adverse effects were noted. Ninety-four percent of the experimental group reported that they would consider acupuncture in future labors.

Further rigorous trials are necessary to understand the role of acupuncture as an obstetric analgesic.

TRANSCUTANEOUS ELECTRICAL NERVE STIMULATION

Transcutaneous electrical nerve stimulation (TENS) is a technique that was introduced as a screening procedure to predict which patients would respond well to indwelling dorsal column stimulators for analgesia (34, 35). Although TENS failed to predict implant outcome, it did produce local analgesia, suggesting other applications of the technique. The use of electricity for analgesia dates from the Greek and Roman use of the torpedo fish, which can emit a 200-V charge (34). Although the use of electricity in modern medicine has been erratic and has not always been safe, developments in the field of electronics and publication of the gate theory of pain in 1965 revived interest in analgesia by electrical stimulation of the afferent nervous system (35).

The gate theory of pain hypothesizes that an area of central nervous system, the substantia gelatinosa in the dorsal horn, acts as a "gate" that, when activated or "closed," inhibits pain sensations from reaching the conscious brain. Theoretically, it is stimulation of large, myelinated A-β nerve fibers that "close the gate," or increase the pain-modulating function of the substantia gelatinosa. Pain sensations or input transmitted by the A-Δ and C nerve fibers may thus be altered or blocked

(36, 37). TENS is thought to affect the A-β fibers similarly, although this hypothesis is controversial (38, 39). Others have suggested that the endogenous opioid system is responsible for the effects of TENS (40, 41), although more recent work refutes this claim (42, 43). Regardless of its mechanism of action, TENS has proved effective in a variety of operative situations (44–46), although not all studies are supportive (46). For obstetrics, TENS offers the possibility of analgesia for labor and delivery produced with minimal intervention and essentially no risk. However, the clinical results to date have been variable.

Technique

The use of this technique is fairly simple. The equipment can be set up in minutes, involving the parturient in the management of her analgesia by allowing her to adjust stimulation as required. Skin electrodes made of a conductive adhesive, 37 × 150 mm (Tenzcare), are applied symmetrically to either side of the T10 to L1 region of the spine. Smaller electrode pads may be added to the sacral area for the second stage of labor, to be used in combination with T10 to L1 stimulation (Fig. 6.4). The electrical current is a biphasic pulse from 30 to 250 μsec in duration, with an amplitude of 0 to 75 mA and a frequency of 40 to 150 Hz. Each manufacturer recommends slightly different limits, and there is some disagreement on the shape of the stimulation waveform. The best results in obstetrics come from a continuous low level of stimulation during labor, with a higher level instituted during contractions. The baseline level of stimulation is usually increased as labor progresses; otherwise, analgesia tends to fade. Some manufacturers offer hand-held devices that allow the mother to adjust (increase) the stimulation with contractions according to need. The mother experiences a tingling sensation in the areas around the electrodes, and the best analgesia is achieved when stimulation is increased until muscle activity around the area is stimulated. The degree of stimulation needed (and tolerated) varies from patient to patient.

The use of this technique seems to be completely safe; its greatest risk is unsatisfactory analgesia. In a European study, measurements of current density in urinary bladders of nonpregnant women using TENS have revealed a current that is below the proposed safety standard of 0.5 μA/mm (48). The stimulators used in the United States have an even lower output and should thus fall within the safety limits.

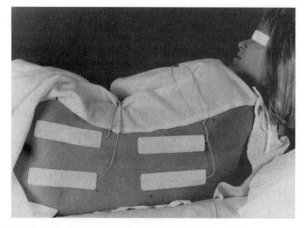

Figure 6.4. Placement of transcutaneous electrical nerve stimulation (TENS) electrodes on a patient's back. Electrodes are easily applied, much like an electrocardiogram pad, and have wires leading to a nerve stimulator. The apparatus is easily operated and can be placed at the bedside or clipped to a patient's gown if she is ambulatory.

In a systematic review of randomized-controlled trials on the effectiveness of TENS in reducing labor pain, Carrol et al. (49) analyzed eight reports involving 352 women receiving TENS and 360 acting as controls. They concluded that the evidence from randomized trials for analgesic benefits from TENS during labor is not compelling. Although no consistent method of measuring pain intensity or relief was found, no study demonstrated any difference in pain scores obtained during labor between TENS and control groups. Significant analgesic benefit with a TENS intervention compared to a sham TENS control group was recorded in only one study where postpartum retrospective questions about pain relief were obtained. The authors additionally concluded that findings were contradictory with regard to need for additional analgesic requirements following TENS use. One study found that a statistically significant number of women would use TENS in future labors. No adverse events were reported.

The effectiveness of TENS as an adjuvant to combined spinal-epidural anesthesia was investigated by Tsen et al. in a randomized double-blind study (50). The authors found that the quality or duration of labor analgesia provided by the spinal portion of combined spinal epidural did not differ with the use of a TENS unit.

In a prospective, randomized, sham-controlled study, TENS decreased postoperative opioid analgesic requirements and opioid-related side effects when utilized as an adjunct to patient-controlled analgesia after lower abdominal gynecologic surgery (e.g., hysterectomy or myomectomy) (51). The authors also concluded that use of TENS at mixed frequencies (2 and 100 Hz) of stimulation produced a greater opioid-sparing effect than low (2 Hz) or high (100 Hz) frequencies. Chen et al. (52) studied the effect of the location of TENS stimulation on postoperative (total abdominal hysterectomy or myomectomy) opioid analgesic requirement. Periincisional dermatomal and Zusanli acupoint (a Chinese acupoint on the lower legs) stimulation were equally effective in decreasing the postoperative opioid analgesic requirement and opioid side effects, and were significantly more effective than sham acupoint stimulation. Whether TENS is effective in reducing postoperative cesarean section pain has yet to be studied.

STERILE WATER BLOCKS

Intracutaneous injections of sterile water in the skin over the sacrum have been shown to relieve first-stage back pain (53–57). This method has also been used to relieve other painful conditions, such as peripheral nerve injury pain, phantom limb pain, shoulder-arm pain, low back pain (58), urolithiasis pain (59), and whiplash pain (60).

Using a 25-gauge needle, four 0.1- to 0.15-mL papules of nonpreserved sterile water are injected into the intracutaneous skin of the sacrum during a contraction. Corresponding to the borders of the sacrum, two of the four injections are placed over the posterior-superior iliac spines and the remaining two are administered 2 cm inferior and 1 cm medial to the first injections (Fig. 6.5). An intense sharp or burning pain results, usually lasting from 20 to 30 seconds. Relief of back pain occurs within 2 minutes and lasts for 45 minutes to 3 hours. The injections may be repeated periodically.

The postulated mechanism of action is that the sterile water injection produces osmotic stimulation from the salt-free water and distention pain in the cutaneous layers, thus stimulating skin nociceptors and inhibiting pain transmission to the dorsal horn (54). The discomfort caused by these injections may additionally raise β-endorphin levels in the cerebrospinal fluid.

Four randomized-controlled studies (53–56) have shown sterile water blocks to be an effective treatment for first-stage labor back pain. Subcutaneous injections of sterile water are as effective as intracutaneous papules (54). Despite good pain

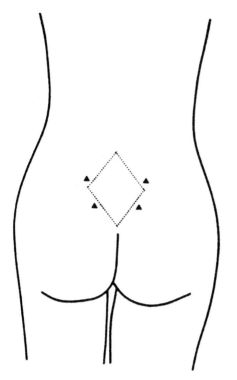

Figure 6.5. Localization of sterile water papules or subcutaneous saline injections in relation to the Michaelis' rhomboid. (Reprinted by permission from Ader L, Hansson B, Wallin G. Parturition pain treated by intracutaneous injections of sterile water. *Pain* 1990;41:133–138.)

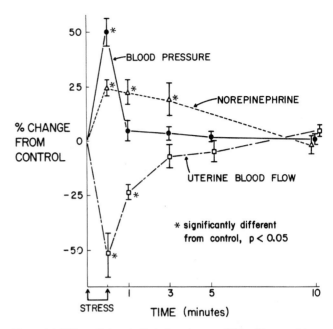

Figure 6.6. Effect of electrically induced stress (30 to 60 seconds) on maternal arterial blood pressure, plasma norepinephrine levels, and uterine blood flow. All values subsequent to control are given as mean percentage change with standard error. (Reprinted by permission from Shnider SM, Wright RG, Levinson G, et al. Uterine blood flow and plasma norepinephrine changes during maternal stress in the pregnant ewe. *Anesthesiology* 1979;50:524–527.)

relief during labor, some women find the temporary pain of sterile water papules to be less acceptable than back pain and would decline the same treatment during future labors (53, 57). Risks of sterile water blocks relate only to possible complications of a needle puncture.

SOCIAL AND PROFESSIONAL SUPPORT OF WOMEN IN LABOR

The provision of a supportive companion during labor is perhaps one of the most successful measures for helping women to cope with the pain of labor. It is welcomed by most parturients and is without adverse side effects. Support can be provided by health care professionals, husbands or partners, friends or family members, childbirth educators, or individuals who are trained and hired specifically to give support during labor (doulas).

Descriptive studies of women's childbirth experiences suggest that continuous emotional support (presence, listening, reassurance, encouragement, assurance that she will not be left alone), advice, information, anticipatory guidance, and tangible assistance in coping with labor (touch and comfort measures) are measures that women find supportive during labor (61, 62).

In a systematic review of 14 randomized-controlled trials, the effects of continuous female support during labor on mothers and babies were assessed (61). Selected labor outcomes in trials involving over 5,000 women who received continuous support during labor from female caregivers were compared to women who received usual care. The caregivers were professionals such as nurses, midwifes, or childbirth educators, or nonprofessionals such as doulas, family, or friends. The authors concluded that continuous support reduced the likelihood of the use of medications for pain relief. In addition, operative vaginal delivery,

cesarean delivery, and a 5-minute Apgar score less than seven were also reduced.

Scott et al. (63) contrasted the effects of intermittent to continuous social support during labor on childbirth outcomes in 11 separate randomized clinical trials by means of meta-analysis. Continuous support when compared to routine care was significantly associated with a decreased need for the use of any analgesia, shorter labors, and a reduced need for oxytocin, forceps, and cesarean sections. Interestingly, intermittent support was not significantly associated with this outcome.

The reason that a supportive companion during labor is associated with these favorable obstetric labor outcomes may be due to a decreased level of anxiety in women who receive support during labor. Animal and human studies have demonstrated that abnormal amounts of stress during labor may result in deleterious effects in mother and fetus. Myers (64) and Morishima (65) demonstrated that monkeys that were frightened or hurt by researchers during labor developed decreased uterine blood flow and subsequent fetal hypoxia and asphyxia. Shnider et al. (66) have demonstrated that in the pregnant ewe psychological and painful physiologic stressors result in increased plasma norepinephrine levels and reduced uterine blood flow (Fig. 6.6). Lederman et al. (67, 68) investigated the relationship of maternal anxiety and catecholamines to progress in labor. They found that women who had higher epinephrine levels during active phase labor had a significantly longer duration of active phase labor than did women with lower epinephrine levels.

Rigorously-controlled investigations are needed to further understand this phenomenon in humans. What is a normal amount of labor stress and what is an excessive and possibly detrimental amount of labor stress have yet to be determined. In any case, minimizing maternal stress during labor is a supportive intervention health care providers can easily provide to their patients.

Currently in the United States, most laboring women are accompanied by their spouses or partners. Although women consistently rate the presence of their husbands in labor and delivery as important and helpful (69), the effect of the partners' presence on labor outcomes has not been adequately studied.

HYDROTHERAPY

Although warm water immersion during labor has been used for relaxation and pain relief for many years, its promotion as a comfort and pain management strategy for parturients began to appear in the obstetric literature in the 1980s (70). Since then, water immersion has become increasingly popular among consumers, and is frequently recommended by consumer advocates. Many hospitals are adding tubs or whirlpools to their labor rooms (71).

According to Nikodem (72), "the bioengineering and physiologic principles underlying hydrotherapy, i.e., buoyancy, hydrostatic pressure, and specific heat, can be applied to labouring women in water." The soothing effect of warm water and its transfer of heat to the body may result in relaxation of muscles and bring about mental relaxation. Physical and mental relaxation may decrease adrenaline and cortisol secretion, which may result in better uterine perfusion and uterine activity (71). When the body is immersed, hydrostatic pressure is the same to all body parts and provides equal resistance to all of the submerged body (71). This creates a relaxing stimulus. Buoyancy may also result in less muscular tension and more pleasant sensations.

Descriptive studies have suggested that hydrotherapy may result in decreased use of pharmacologic pain relief measures (73, 74). Three randomized-controlled trials on water immersion during labor found differing results (71, 75, 76). Rush et al. (75) investigated the effects of water immersion on opioid and epidural requirements in laboring women. Three hundred ninety-three women who used unlimited whirlpool bath during labor were compared to 392 women who received conventional care. The tub group required significantly fewer pharmacologic agents than controls. Two other studies (71, 76) comprising small sample sizes found water immersion did not alter the use of analgesia or anesthesia.

MATERNAL POSITION

Laboring women usually change positions frequently during labor. Through trial and error and their natural tendency to seek comfort, they will find positions that are comparatively more comfortable than others (7). Common positions used during labor include standing, walking, kneeling, leaning, hands and knees, squatting, supine, and lateral.

Several studies have been published addressing maternal position during labor and its effect on pain perception and analgesia use. An upright position during labor has been associated with a reduction in analgesic requirements (77–80) and decreased pain (79, 81, 82). In contrast, Bloom et al. (83) found no difference in analgesia use and no change in pain perception with an upright position.

The reason that an upright position might help women cope with the pain of labor may relate to an increased sense of control, distraction, or stimulation of other body sensations that may compete with painful stimuli (7).

PRENATAL ANESTHESIA VISITS

Some anesthesiologists set up prenatal anesthesia clinics to provide mothers with the opportunity to discuss anesthesia for labor and delivery prior to the onset of labor. During the visit, a medical history is taken, choices of anesthesia are discussed, and the questions and concerns of the mother are addressed.

If individual interviews are impractical, a session during which an anesthesiologist meets with a group of expectant parents to discuss anesthetic alternatives and address questions and concerns should be arranged. The prenatal anesthetic visit can avoid much of the mutual anxiety that often occurs on the labor floor when an anesthesiologist is called to see a parturient in pain about whom he or she knows nothing. Many anesthesia units distribute a brochure to prospective parents, describing pain relief in childbirth.One such brochure prepared by the American Society of Anesthesiologists through the society's Committee on Communications and Committee on Obstetrical Anesthesia is represented in the Appendix of this chapter.

REFERENCES

1. Lowe N. The pain and discomfort of labor and birth. *JOGNN* 1996;25:82–92.
2. Melzack R. The myth of painless childbirth (The John J. Bonica Lecture). *Pain* 1984;19:321–327.
3. Ranta P, Spalding M, Kangas-Saarela T, et al. Maternal expectations and experiences of labour pain–options of 1091 Finnish parturients. *Acta Anaesthesiol Scand* 1995;39:60–66.
4. Morgan BM, Bulpitt CJ, Clifton P, Lewis PJ. Analgesia and satisfaction in childbirth (the Queen Charlotte's 1000 mother survey). *Lancet* 1982;2:808–810.
5. Simkin P. Reducing pain and enhancing progress in labor: A guide to nonpharmacologic methods for maternity caregivers. *Birth* 1995;22:161–171.
6. Baram D. Hypnosis in reproductive health care: A review and case reports.*Birth* 1995;22:37–42.
7. Simkin P. Non-pharmacolocgical methods of pain relief during labour. In: Chalmers I, Enkin M, Kearse M, eds. *Effective Care in Pregnancy and Child Birth.* New York: Oxford University Press; 1989:893–912.
8. Werner W, Schauble P, Knudson M. An argument for the revival of hypnosis in obstetrics. *Am J Clin Hypnosis* 1982;24:149–171.
9. Freeman R, Macaulay A, Eve L, Chamberlain G. Randomised trial of self hypnosis for analgesia in labour. *Br Med J* 1986;292:657–658.
10. Harmon T, Hynan M, Tyre T. Improved obstetric outcomes using hypnotic analgesia and skill mastery combined with childbirth education. *J Consul Clin Psychol* 1990;58:525–530.
11. Dick-Read G. *Childbirth Without Fear.* 2nd ed. New York: Harper & Row; 1959.
12. Beck N, Geden E, Brouder G. Preparation for labor: A historical perspective. *Psychosom Med* 1979;41:243–258.
13. Pitcock C, Clark R. From Fanny to Fernand: The development of consumerism in pain control during the birth process. *Am J Obstet Gynecol* 1992;167:581–587.
14. Lamaze R. *Painless Childbirth: Psychoprophylactic Method.* London: Burke; 1958.
15. Samko MR, Schoenfeld LS. Hypnotic susceptibility and the Lamaze childbirth experience. *Am J Obstet Gynecol* 1975;294:1205–1207.
16. Hetherington SE. A controlled study of the effect of prepared childbirth classes on obstetric outcomes. *Birth* 1990;17:86–90.
17. Charles A, Norr K, Block C, Meyering S, Meyers E. Obstetric and psychological effects of psychoprophylactic preparation for childbirth. *Am J Obstet Gynecol* 1978;131:44–52.
18. Scott JR, Rose NB. Effect of psychoprophylaxis (Lamaze preparation) on labor and delivery in primiparas. *N Engl J Med* 1976; 294:1205–1207.
19. Zax M, Sameroff A, Farnum J. Childbirth education, maternal attitudes, and delivery. *Am J Obstet Gynecol* 1975;123:185–190.
20. Sturrock WA, Johnson JA. The relationship between childbirth education classes and obstetric outcome. *Birth* 1990;17:82–85.
21. Patton LL, English EC, Hambleton JD. Childbirth preparation and outcomes of labor and delivery in primiparous women. *J Fam Pract* 1985;20:375–378.
22. Delke I, Minkoff H, Grunebaum A. Effect of Lamaze childbirth preparation on maternal plasma beta-endorphin immunoreactivity in active labor. *Am J Perinatol* 1985:2:317–319.

23. Brewin C, Bradley C. Perceived control and the experience of childbirth. *Br J Clin Psychol* 1982;21:263–269.

24. Hughey MJ, McElin TW, Young T. Maternal and fetal outcome of Lamaze-prepared patients. *Obstet Gynecol* 1978;51:643–647.

25. Gagnon A. Antenatal education for childbirth/parenthood (protocol for a Cochrane review). In: *The Cochrane Library*. Issue 2. Oxford: Update Software; 2000.

26. Zwelling E, Childbirth education in the 1990s and beyond. *JOGNN* 1996;25:425–432.

27. NIH Consensus Development Panel. Acupuncture: NIH Consensus Development Panel on acupuncture. *JAMA* 1998;280:1518–1524.

28. Wallis L, Shnider S, Palahniuk R, Spivey H. An evaluation of acupuncture analgesia in obstetrics. *Anesthesiology* 1974;41:596–601.

29. Lyrenäs S, Lutsch H, Hetta J, Lindberg B. Acupuncture before delivery: Effect on labor. *Gynecol Obstet Invest* 1987;24:217–224.

30. Lyrenäs S, Lutsch H, Hetta J, Nyberg F, Willdeck-Lundh G, Lindberg B. Acupuncture before delivery: Effect of pain perception and the need for analgesics. *Gynecol Obstet Invest* 1990;29:118–124.

31. Zeisler H, Tempfer C, Mayerhofer K, Barrada M, Husslein P. Influence of acupuncture on duration of labor. *Gynecol Obstet Invest* 1998;46:22–25.

32. Tempfer C, Zeisler H, Heinzl H, Hefler L, Husslein P, Kainz C. Influence of acupuncture on maternal serum levels of interleukin-8, prostaglandin F_2 alpha, and beta-endorphin: A matched pair study. *Obstet Gynecol* 1998;92:245–248.

33. Ternov K, Nilsson M, Löfberg L, Algotsson L, Akeson J. Acupuncture for pain relief during childbirth. *Acupunct Electrother Res* 1998;23:19–26.

34. Tyler E, Caldwell G, Ghia JN. Transcutaneous electrical nerve stimulation: An alternative approach to the management of postoperative pain. *Anesth Analg* 1982;61:449–456.

35. Melzack R, Wall PD. Pain mechanisms: A new theory. *Science* 1965;150:971–979.

36. Shealy CN, Mortimer JT, Reswick JB. Electrical inhibition of pain by stimulation of the dorsal columns: Preliminary clinical report. *Anesth Analg* 1967;46:489–491.

37. Long DM. External electrical stimulation as a treatment of chronic pain. *Minn Med* 1974;57:195–198.

38. Melzack R, Taenzer P, Feldman P, Kinch RA. Labour is still painful after prepared childbirth training. *Can Med Assoc J* 1981;125:357–363.

39. Bundsen P, Peterson L-E, Selstam U. Pain relief in labor by transcutaneous electrical nerve stimulation: A prospective matched study. *Acta Obstet Gynecol Scand* 1981;60:459–468.

40. Woolf CJ, Mitchell D, Barrett GD. Antinociceptive effect of peripheral segmental electrical stimulation in the rat. *Pain* 1980;8:237–252.

41. Solomon RA, Viernstein MC, Long DM. Reduction of postoperative pain and narcotic use by transcutaneous electrical nerve stimulation. *Surgery* 1980;87:142–146.

42. Abram SE, Reynolds AC, Cusick JF. Failure of naloxone to reverse analgesia from transcutaneous electrical stimulation in patients with chronic pain. *Anesth Analg* 1984;60:81–84.

43. Stanley TH, Cazalaa JA, Atinault A, Coeytaux R, Limoge A, Louville Y. Transcutaneous cranial electrical stimulation decreases narcotic requirements during neurolept anesthesia and operation in man. *Anesth Analg* 1982;61:863–866.

44. Rooney S-M, Jain S, Goldiner PL. Effect of transcutaneous nerve stimulation on postoperative pain after thoracotomy. *Anesth Analg* 1983;62:1010–1012.

45. Bourke DL, Smith BAC, Erickson J, Gwartz B, Lessard L. TENS reduces halothane requirements during hand surgery. *Anesthesiology* 1984;61:769–772.

46. McCallum MD, Glynn CJ, Moore RA, Lammer P, Phillips AM. Transcutaneous electrical nerve stimulation in the management of acute postoperative pain. *Br J Anaesth* 1988;61:308–312.

47. Reynolds RA, Glandstone N, Ansari AM. Transcutaneous electrical nerve stimulation for reducing narcotic use after cesarean section. *J Reprod Med* 1987;32:843–846.

48. Bundsen P, Ericson K. Pain relief in labor by transcutaneous electrical nerve stimulation: Safety aspects. *Acta Obstet Gynecol Scand* 1982;61:1–5.

49. Carroll D, Tramèr, M, McQuay H, Nye B, Moore A. Transcutaneous electrical nerve stimulation in labour pain: A systematic review. *Br J Obstet Gynaecol* 1997;104:169–175.

50. Tsen LC, Thomas J, Segal S, Datta S, Bader AM. Transcutaneous electrical nerve stimulation does not augment combined spinal epidural labour analgesia. *Can J Anaesth* 2000;47:38–42.

51. Hamza M, White P, Hesham A, Ghoname E. Effect of the frequency of transcutaneous electrical nerve stimulation on the postoperative opioid analgesic requirement and recovery profile. *Anesthesiology* 1999;91:1232–1238.

52. Chen L, Tang J, White P, et al. The effect of location of transcutaneous electrical nerve stimulation on postoperative opioid analgesic requirement: Acupoint versus nonacupoint stimulation. *Anesth Analg* 1998;87:1129–1134.

53. Labrecque M, Nouwen A, Bergeron M, Rancourt J. A randomized controlled trial of nonpharmacologic approaches for relief of low back pain during labor. *J Fam Pract* 1999;48:259–263.

54. Mårtensson L, Wallin G. Labour pain treated with cutaneous injections of sterile water: A randomized controlled trial. *Br J Obstet Gynaecol* 1999;106:633–637.

55. Trolle B, Moller M, Kronborg H, Thomsen S. The effect of sterile water blocks on low back labor pain. *Am J Obstet Gynecol* 1991;164:1277–1281.

56. Ader L, Hansson B, Wallin G. Parturition pain treated by intracutaneous injections of sterile water. *Pain* 1990;41:133–138.

57. Lytzen T, Cederberg L, Möller-Nielsen J. Relief of low back pain in labor by using intracutaneous nerve stimulation (INS) with sterile water papules. *Acta Obstet Gynecol Scand* 1989;68:341–343.

58. Melzack R. Prolonged relief of pain by brief, intense, transcutaneous somatic stimulation. *Pain* 1975;1:357–373.

59. Bengtsson J, Worning A, Gertz J. Pain due to urolithiasis treated by intracutaneous injection of sterile water. *Ugeskr Laeger* 1981;143:3463–3465.

60. Byrn C, Borenstein P, Linder L. Treatment of neck and shoulder pain in whip-lash syndrome patients with intracutaneous sterile water injections. *Acta Anaesthesiol Scand* 1991;35:52–53.

61. Hodnett ED. Caregiver support for women during childbirth (Cochrane review). In: *The Cochrane Library*. Issue 4. Oxford: Update Software; 1999.

62. Rooks J. *Midwifery and Childbirth in America*. Philadelphia: Temple University Press; 1997.

63. Scott K, Berkowitz G, Klaus M. A comparison of intermittent and continuous support during labor: A meta-analysis. *Am J Obstet Gynecol* 1999;180:1054–1059.

64. Myers R. Maternal psychological stress and fetal asphyxia: A study in the monkey. *Am J Obstet Gynecol* 1975;122:47–59.

65. Morishima H, Pedersen H, Finsler M. The influence of maternal psychological stress on the fetus. *Am J Obstet Gynecol* 1978;131:286–290.

66. Shnider S, Wright R, Levinson G, et al. Uterine blood flow and plasma norepinephrine changes during maternal stress in the pregnant ewe. *Anesthesiology* 1979;50:524–527.

67. Lederman R, Lederman E, Work B, McCann D. The relationship of maternal anxiety, plasma catecholamines, and plasma cortisol to progress in labor. *Am J Obstet Gynecol* 1978;132:495–499.

68. Lederman R, Lederman E, Work B, McCann D. Anxiety and epinephrine in multiparous women in labor: Relationship to duration of labor and fetal heart rate pattern. *Am J Obstet Gynecol* 1985;153:870–877.

69. Keirse M, Enkin M, Lumley J. Social and professional support during labor. In: Chalmers I, Enkin M, Kearse J, eds. *Effective Care in Pregnancy and Child Birth*. New York: Oxford University Press; 1989:805–814.

70. McCandlish R, Renfrea M. Immersion in a tub during labor and birth: The need for evaluation. *Birth* 1993;20:79–85.

71. Schorn M, McAllister J, Blanco J. Water immersion and the effect on labor. *J Nurse Midwifery* 1993;38:336–342.

72. Nikodem V. Immersion in a tub during pregnancy, labour and birth (Cochrane review). In: *The Cochrane Library*. Issue 3. Oxford: Update Software; 1999.

73. Burnes E, Greenish K. Pooling information. *Nurs Times* 1993;89:47–49.

74. Waldenstrom U, Nilsson C. Warm tub bath after spontaneous rupture of the membranes. *Birth* 1992;199:57–63.

75. Rush J, Burlock S, Lambert K, Loosley-Millman M, Huchison B, Enkin M. The effects of whirlpool baths in labor: A randomized, controlled trial. *Birth* 1996;23:136–143.

76. Cammu H, Clasen K, VanWettere L, Derde M. 'To bathe or not to bathe' during the first stage of labor. *Acta Obstet Gynecol Scand* 1994;73:468–472.

77. Albers L, Anderson D, Cragin L, et al. The relationship of ambulation in labor to operative delivery. *J Nurse Midwifery* 1997;42:4–8.

78. MacLennan A, Crowther C, Derham R. Does the option to ambulate during spontaneous labour confer any advantage or disadvantage? *J Matern Fetal Med* 1994;3:43–48.

79. Andrews C, Chrzanowski M. Maternal position, labor and comfort. *Appl Nurs Res* 1990;3:7–13.

80. Fenwick L, Simkin P. Maternal positioning to prevent or alleviate dystocia in labor. *Clin Obstet Gynecol* 1987;30:83–89.

81. Melzack R, Bélanger E, Lacroix R. Labor pain: Effect of maternal position on front and back pain. *J Pain Symptom Manage* 1991;8:476–480.

82. Waldenstroem R, Gottvall K. A randomized trial of birthing stool or conventional semirecumbent position for second-stage labor. *Birth* 1991;18:5–10.

83. Bloom S, McIntire D, Kelly M, et al. Lack of effect of walking on labor and delivery. *N Engl J Med* 1998;339:76–79.

Shnider and Levinson's Anesthesia for Obstetrics,
edited by Samuel C. Hughes, et al.
Lippincott Williams & Wilkins,
Philadelphia, © 2001.

APPENDIX

ANESTHESIA & YOU . . .
PLANNING YOUR
CHILDBIRTH

AMERICAN SOCIETY OF ANESTHESIOLOGISTS*

One of the most thrilling and gratifying experiences in your life will be the birth of your child. This significant event should be made as safe and pleasant as possible for both you and your baby. Your obstetrician, anesthesiologist, and nurses want to help you and your partner reach this goal.

Each woman's labor is unique to her. The amount of labor pain you feel will differ from that felt by other women in labor. It depends on factors such as your level of pain tolerance, the size and position of the baby, strength of uterine contractions and prior birth experiences. Medical decisions regarding control of your labor pain must be made for you specifically.

Some women achieve adequate pain control with the breathing and relaxation techniques learned at childbirth classes. Others may find them inadequate.

Many mothers are reconsidering the idea that childbirth is "natural" only without medication, and they are choosing to have pain relief during labor and delivery to help them experience a more comfortable childbirth.

ANALGESICS AND ANESTHETICS

Analgesia is the full or partial relief of painful sensations. Anesthesia is usually considered to be a more intense blockage of all sensations, including muscle movement. Your wishes and your medical condition are important in selecting the type of pain relief administered to you. Be assured that your physicians will prescribe or administer medications only in the amounts and during those stages of labor that are best for the safety and well-being of your baby. There are several choices for pain relief:

Intravenous "I.V." Medication? Pain-relieving medications that are injected into a vein or muscle will help dull your pain but may not eliminate it completely. These I.V. medications are usually prescribed by your obstetrician. Because they sometimes make both you and your baby sleepy, they are used mainly during early labor.

Local Anesthesia? Other pain-relieving medications may be injected in the vaginal and rectal areas by your obstetrician at the time of delivery. These medications are local anesthetics. They provide a numbness or loss of sensation in a small area. Local anesthesia is often used to ease the pain of delivery or when an episiotomy incision is done to assist the delivery. It does not, however, lessen the pain of contractions.

Regional Blocks? Regional blocks can reduce the discomfort of labor and provide either analgesia or anesthesia. Regional blocks refer to epidural and spinal blocks. They are administered in the lower back, usually by a specialist physician called an anesthesiologist. Local anesthetics and other drugs are used for these procedures to reduce or "block" pain and other sensations over a wider region of the body. Epidural analgesia may be used for labor and vaginal delivery. An epidural block may be used to provide anesthesia for a cesarean section. A spinal block may be used to provide labor analgesia or anesthesia for a cesarean delivery. A combined spinal/epidural block also may be used for labor analgesia and/or anesthesia in certain cases.

REGIONAL BLOCKS FOR LABOR

Regional blocks for labor and delivery have become very popular because of the comfort they provide. The epidural block decreases sensation in the lower areas of your body, yet you remain conscious. The right time to administer the epidural block will vary from patient to patient.

If you request an epidural block, your obstetrician and anesthesiologist will evaluate you and your baby, taking into account your state of health and past anesthetic experiences, the progress of labor, and your baby's responses.

How is the epidural block performed? An epidural block is given in the lower back. You will either be sitting up or lying on your side. The block is administered below the level of the spinal cord. This is called a lumbar epidural block. The block also may be given in the tailbone area. This is called a caudal block.

Before the block is performed, your skin will be cleansed with an antiseptic solution. The anesthesiologist will use local anesthesia to numb an area of your lower back or near the tailbone. A special needle is placed in the epidural space just outside the spinal sac. A tiny flexible tube called an epidural catheter is inserted through this needle. Occasionally, the catheter will touch a nerve, causing a brief tingling sensation down one leg.

Once the catheter is positioned properly, the needle is removed and the catheter is taped in place. Additional medications are given as needed without another needle being inserted. The medication bathes the nerves and blocks out the pain. This produces epidural analgesia.

How soon will the epidural block take effect? Because the medication needs to be absorbed into several nerves, the onset is gradual, not immediate. Pain relief will begin to occur within 10 to 20 minutes after the medication has been injected.

What will I feel after the block takes effect? Although significant pain relief will occur, you still may be aware of pressure or sensations with contractions. You may feel your obstetrician's examinations as labor progresses. Depending on your circumstances and your baby's condition, your anesthesiologist adjusts the degree of numbness for your comfort and to assist labor and delivery. You might notice some degree of temporary numbness, heaviness, or weakness in your legs.

What is a combined spinal/epidural block? A combined spinal/epidural block uses both techniques and can provide pain relief much faster. An injection of medication is made into the spinal sac followed by the placement of the epidural catheter. There may be less numbness with this technique. Some women may be able to walk around after the block is in place. A variation of this technique is sometimes referred to as a "walking epidural."

How long will the block last? The duration of epidural analgesia can be extended usually for as long as you need it. After the epidural catheter is placed, additional medication can be administered through it as needed. Throughout your labor, your comfort and progress will be monitored frequently and medications adjusted accordingly. A nurse may assist your anesthesiologist with this monitoring. After delivery, the epidural catheter will

---

be removed and, within a few hours, sensations will return to normal.

Will the epidural block affect my baby? Considerable research has shown that epidural analgesia and anesthesia can be safe for both mother and baby, with little or no effect on the infant. However, medical judgment, special skills, precautions, and treatments are required. That is why a qualified anesthesiologist should perform this procedure.

Will it slow down my labor? Each mother may respond differently to the various epidural medications. Some may have a brief period of decreased uterine contractions. Many, however, are pleasantly surprised to learn that after the epidural medications have made them more comfortable and relaxed, their labor may actually progress faster.

Can I "push" when needed? Regional analgesia allows you to rest during the longest part of labor, which occurs during cervical dilation. Then, when your cervix is completely dilated and it is time to push, you will have energy in reserve. The regional block can reduce your pain while allowing you to push when needed. Even if you do not have the urge to push, you should be able to do so with instruction.

If the baby's head needs to be guided through the birth canal with forceps or a vacuum instrument, the block can be intensified to provide anesthesia and muscle relaxation.

What are the risks of a regional block? Although not common, complications or side effects can occur, even though you are monitored carefully and your anesthesiologist takes special precautions to avoid them. To help prevent a decrease in blood pressure, fluids will be administered intravenously (into one of your veins). In addition, during your labor, you will be positioned usually on your side. After delivery, you should remain in bed until the block wears off.

Shivering may occur and is a common reaction. Sometimes it happens during labor and delivery, even if you did not receive any anesthetic medications. Keeping you warm often helps it subside.

Although uncommon, a headache may develop following the block procedure. By holding as still as possible while the needle is placed, you help to decrease the likelihood of a headache. The discomfort, sometimes lasting a few days, often can be reduced or eliminated by simple measures such as lying flat, drinking fluids, and taking pain tablets. Occasionally, a patient may need additional treatment if the headache persists.

On rare occasion, the anesthetic medication may affect the chest muscles and make it seem harder to breathe. Oxygen can be given to relieve this feeling and help the breathing.

The veins located in the epidural space become swollen during pregnancy. There is the risk that the anesthetic medication could be injected into one of them. To help avoid unusual reactions stemming from this, your anesthesiologist will first administer a test dose of medication and you may be asked if you notice any dizziness, a funny taste, rapid heart beat, or numbness.

Your anesthesiologist carefully evaluates your condition, makes medical judgments, takes safety precautions and provides special treatment throughout the procedure. You should feel free to talk with your anesthesiologist about your options for pain relief and their possible side effects.

ANESTHESIA FOR CESAREAN BIRTHS

Epidural, spinal, or general anesthesia may be given safely for cesarean section deliveries. Choices depend on several factors, including the medical conditions of you and your baby and, when possible, your preferences.

How is the epidural block given for a cesarean delivery? If you already have a labor epidural catheter in place and then need a cesarean delivery, it is usually possible for your anesthesiologist to inject additional anesthetic medication through the same catheter to enhance pain relief safely. This stronger concentration of medication converts the analgesia to anesthesia. Anesthesia is necessary to numb the entire abdomen completely for the surgical incision. If you prefer to have an epidural block during your cesarean childbirth and you did not have labor epidural analgesia, there usually is enough time to provide epidural anesthesia.

What is spinal anesthesia? Spinal anesthesia is given using a much thinner needle in the same location of the back where an epidural block is placed. The main differences are that a much smaller dose of anesthesia medication is needed for a spinal block, and it is injected into the sac of spinal fluid below the level of the spinal cord. Once the spinal anesthetic medication is injected, the onset of numbness is quite rapid.

When is general anesthesia used? General anesthesia is used when a regional block is not possible or is not the best choice for medical or other reasons. It can be started quickly and causes a rapid loss of consciousness. It is used when an urgent vaginal or cesarean delivery is required, as in rare instances of problems with the baby or vaginal bleeding. In these circumstances, general anesthesia is quite safe for the baby.

One of the most significant concerns during general anesthesia is whether there is food or liquids in the mother stomach. During unconsciousness, "aspiration" could occur, meaning that some stomach contents could come up and then go into the lungs. Here, they could possibly cause pneumonia. Your anesthesiologist, therefore, takes extra precautions to protect your lungs, such as placing a breathing tube into your mouth and windpipe after you are anesthetized. Before your cesarean delivery, you also may be given an antacid to neutralize stomach acid.

It is best to remember, though, that YOU SHOULD NOT EAT OR DRINK ANYTHING AFTER YOUR LABOR PAINS BEGIN, regardless of your plans for delivery or pain control. Sometimes during labor, small sips of water, clear liquids, or ice chips are permissible with your physician's consent.

Will I receive a separate bill from the anesthesiology? Your anesthesiologist is a physician specialist, like your obstetrician or pediatrician, whose medical services have been requested. You likely will receive a bill for your anesthesiologist's professional service as you would from your other physicians. If you have any financial concerns, your anesthesiologist or an office staff member will answer your questions. You will note that your hospital charges separately for medications and equipment used.

Modern anesthesiology offers today's mothers a variety of choices for a more comfortable childbirth. It is the goal of your anesthesiologist to answer your questions, ease your fears, and make your labor and delivery as safe as possible for you and your baby.

Please discuss your anesthesia-related questions or concerns with your obstetrician. A consultation with an anesthesiologist usually can be arranged before your anticipated delivery. The more prepared you are—in other words, the more you "plan your childbirth"—the more comfortable and memorable the birth of your baby will be.

"Anesthesia & You . . . Planning Your Childbirth" has been prepared by the American Society of Anesthesiologists through the cooperative efforts of the Society's Committee on Communications and the Committee on Obstetrical Anesthesia.

Shnider and Levinson's Anesthesia for Obstetrics,
edited by Samuel C. Hughes, et al.
Lippincott Williams & Wilkins,
Philadelphia, © 2001.

CHAPTER 7

SYSTEMIC MEDICATION FOR LABOR AND DELIVERY

M. JOANNE DOUGLAS, M.D., F.R.C.P.C. AND GERSHON LEVINSON, M.D.

Despite the increasing use of regional analgesia during labor, systemic medications are widely used to relieve labor pain and anxiety. There is no ideal, universally applicable analgesic agent for use during childbirth. All systemic medications used for pain relief in labor cross the placenta and may have a depressant effect on the fetus. The amount of depression depends on the dose of the drug, route and time of administration before delivery, and the presence of obstetric complications.

Systemic drugs administered during labor can be classified into four broad categories:

1. *Opioids* are used to relieve pain during the first and second stages of labor.
2. *Sedative-tranquilizers*, either alone or in combination with an opioid, are occasionally used during the first stage of labor.
3. *Dissociative or amnesic drugs*, such as ketamine, are used infrequently. Ketamine in low subanesthetic doses may be used as an analgesic during the second stage of labor or as an adjunct to regional anesthesia for cesarean section. The use of ketamine as an induction agent for cesarean section is discussed in Chapter 11.
4. *Antagonists*, are drugs used to reverse possible adverse effects of the above medications.

OPIOIDS

Opioids are probably the most commonly used medication for labor analgesia. In many facilities where epidural analgesia is unavailable or maternal condition contraindicates its use, opioids remain the analgesics of choice for labor pain. However, for many parturients opioids do not provide adequate analgesia during labor and delivery (Fig. 7.1) in safe doses, that is those that do not result in side effects such as hypoventilation, obtundation of reflexes, postural hypotension or neonatal depression. The escalating nature of labor pain results in administration of larger doses of opioids as labor progresses; as the dose of opioid is increased, the likelihood of undesirable maternal and neonatal side effects increases as well (1). Opioids can provide mild-to-moderate analgesia but cannot be used to completely eliminate pain. Because all opioids in appropriate doses produce comparable pain relief, the choice of drug depends on potential maternal and neonatal side effects and the desired onset and duration of action.

Common maternal side effects from administration of opioids are sedation (Fig. 7.2) (1) and respiratory depression. Porter et al. (2) reported that oxygen desaturation occurred in 29% of women who received analgesia with opioid alone vs. 8% of those who received neither opioids nor sedatives (Table 7.1). Apnea may occur with therapeutic doses of the more potent opioids (3), with potentially serious maternal and fetal

consequences (Fig. 7.3). In equianalgesic doses, most opioids probably produce a comparable shift of the carbon dioxide response curve to the right. Some opioids such as fentanyl (4) may produce a more rapid, transient shift in the response curve. The peak respiratory depression of fentanyl may be of much greater magnitude than equianalgesic doses of other opioids.

Orthostatic hypotension resulting from peripheral vasodilation (5) is another possible side effect of opioid administration. When the usual analgesic doses of opioids are administered to parturients in the wedged, supine position, maternal blood pressure, heart rate, and rhythm are unaffected. However, severe hypotension with maternal and fetal distress may develop if these women ambulate, sit up, or are moved too vigorously.

Opioids produce nausea and vomiting probably by direct stimulation of the chemoreceptor trigger zone in the medulla. The emetic effects are dose related, and equianalgesic doses of the commonly used opioids usually produce equal amounts of nausea and vomiting. However, some patients experience more nausea with one opioid than with others.

Although opioids usually stimulate smooth muscle, they decrease gastric motility and gastric emptying (6). The intramuscular (IM) route of opioid administration has a variable response and may not produce and maintain sufficient blood concentrations to provide analgesia (7). During labor, drug absorption from traditional IM injection sites may be altered with higher maternal plasma levels after deltoid injection than after gluteus injection (Fig. 7.4) (8). Because of this variability in absorption and response, many recommend the intravenous (IV) route. A comparison of IM meperidine 150 mg with self-administered IV meperidine (0.25 mg/kg available at 10-minute intervals) for labor analgesia found that the IV group received less meperidine than the IM group (9). Ratings of pain were nonsignificantly better in the IV group. IV opioids can be administered by the nurse or patient controlled; both techniques have been used effectively during labor (10).

Since opioids rapidly cross the placenta, the fetus and neonate are affected (11–13). During labor, the fetal heart rate (FHR) pattern may show loss of variability (14). In the neonate, respiratory depression is the most serious side effect, but subtle effects on neonatal neurobehavior also occur. With most opioids, the maximum neonatal depression of Apgar scores occurs in newborns delivered 2 to 3 hours after maternal IM administration (15–17), and with a shorter interval after IV administration.

Meperidine

Meperidine is one of the most commonly used opioids in obstetrics, although studies have consistently found that maternal ratings of pain remain high following its administration (18–21). The usual dosage is 50 to 100 mg IM or 25 to 50 mg IV. The peak analgesic effect occurs 40 to 50 minutes after IM and 5 to

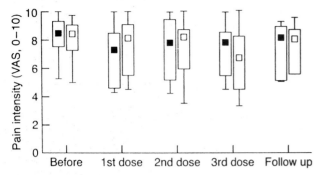

Figure 7.1. Pain intensity before and following morphine (dose 0.05 mg/kg body weight) or meperidine (dose 0.5 mg/kg body weight) given intravenously at iterative doses. Values are presented in box plot with median and interquartile range and total range indicated by vertical whiskers. No significant effect was found after each dose. ■ = morphine; □ = meperidine. (Reprinted by permission from Olofsson Ch, Ekblom A, Ekman-Ordeberg G, Hjelm A, Irestedt L. Lack of analgesic effect of systemically administered morphine or pethidine on labour pain. *Br J Obstet Gynaecol* 1996;103:968–972.)

Table 7.1. INCIDENCE OF DESATURATION IN WOMEN RECEIVING INTRAVENOUS ANALGESICS

Analgesic*	Desaturation Incidents	Total	%	Relative Risk	P Value
None	19	214	8	1[†]	
Meperidine	28	112	25	3.4 (1.8–6.5)	.01
Butorphanol	30	98	31	4.5 (2.5–8.3)	.05
Sedation alone	8	31	26	3.6 (1.5–8.7)	.01
Opioids and sedation	28	107	26	3.6 (2.0–6.7)	.01
Opioids alone	30	103	29	4.2 (2.2–8.0)	.01

* Meperidine denoted exposure to meperidine or meperidine plus promethazine; butorphanol, exposure to butorphanol, butorphanol plus promethazine, or butorphanol plus hydroxyzine; sedation alone, exposure to either promethazine or hydroxyzine; and opioids and sedation, exposure to meperidine plus promethazine or butorphanol plus hydroxyzine.

[†] Reference group.

Reprinted with permission from Porter KB, O'Brien WF, Kiefert V, Knuppel RA. Evaluation of oxygen desaturation events in singleton pregnancies. *J Perinatol* 1992;12:103–106.

10 minutes after IV administration. The duration of action is 3 to 4 hours.

The placental transfer and fetal and neonatal effects of this drug have been studied extensively. Meperidine reaches the fetal circulation within 90 seconds of maternal IV administration, and fetal and maternal concentrations achieve equilibrium within 6 minutes (Fig. 7.5) (22). In most studies, maternal and umbilical cord blood levels are similar at delivery (23, 24). Meperidine is predisposed to "trapping" in the fetus in the presence of fetal compromise (25). The elimination half-life of meperidine in the newborn is reported to be between 13 (26) and 23 hours (27), and the neonate will excrete meperidine for 3 to 6 days. The half-life of normeperidine is 62 hours, and it is present in the neonate for even longer periods than meperidine (28). Normeperidine is a more polar compound than meperidine, and therefore it crosses the placenta more slowly.

The effects of meperidine on the fetus include altered electroencephalogram (29), decreased or arrested respiratory movements (30), decreased fetal movements (31), and decreased beat-to-beat variability (32). In the pregnant ewe, IV meperidine did not affect the fetal blood pressure, heart rate, arterial oxygen, or acid-base status (33). However, in humans, fetal oxygenation measured with a transcutaneous oxygen electrode decreased following maternal IV administration of 50 mg

meperidine (34). This was followed by a decrease in FHR variability (Fig 7.6).

Maternally administered meperidine may affect the neonate by prolonging the time to sustained respiration (35), decreasing Apgar scores (15), lowering oxygen saturation (36), decreasing minute volume (17), and causing respiratory acidosis (37, 38), and abnormal neurobehavioral examinations (39, 40). These effects are related to the dose and to the time interval between maternal administration and delivery of the infant.

Shnider and Moya (15) studied a group of parturients with no medical or obstetric complications. If meperidine (100 mg or less) was given within 1 hour of birth, the incidence of depressed babies was similar to an unmedicated group (Fig. 7.7). There was a significant increase in the percentage of depressed babies born during the second hour after drug administration, even if mothers had received only 50 mg meperidine. Increased doses tended to prolong the period in which significant neonatal depression was observed. The addition of a barbiturate not only prolonged the period but also increased the percentage of neonatal depression (Fig. 7.8). Neonatal depression after meperidine may be prolonged. Oxygen saturation is significantly depressed for at least 30 minutes after birth in full-term babies of mothers who receive 100 mg meperidine 2 to 4 hours before birth (36). Neonatal hypercapnia may persist for up to 5 hours (37).

A recent study examined the effects of a continuous infusion of meperidine during labor on the neonatal breathing pattern during active and quiet sleep (41). The infusion was terminated 5.5 ± 2.1 hours before delivery, and the neonates were compared to infants whose mothers did not receive opioids. During quiet sleep, the investigators found that the respiratory variables were similar, but during active sleep, there were significantly more apneic episodes in the meperidine group than in the control group (37.1 ± 25.1 vs. 11.2 ± 13.9). Additionally, the drug-affected infants spent a greater amount of time with lower oxygen saturation than did the control group (Fig. 7.9).

The reason for the delay in the appearance of neonatal depression after maternal administration of meperidine is unclear. The delay may relate to the quantity of parent drug transferred across the placenta during the first hour after administration. Following maternal IV administration of 50 mg meperidine, Kuhnert et al. (28, 42, 43) measured the concentrations of meperidine and normeperidine in umbilical cord venous and arterial plasma at delivery and in the urine of the neonate for 3 days postpartum. The investigators found that, as the time from administration of the drug to delivery (drug-delivery interval [DDI]) increased, the level of meperidine in both cord

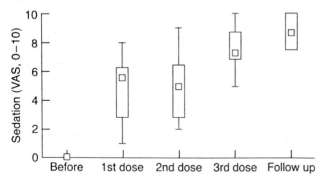

Figure 7.2. Sedation scores before and after successive doses of opioid. There was no significant difference in results between the two opioids, so data for morphine and meperidine have been combined. Box and whisker plots represent median with interquartile range. (Reprinted by permission from Olofsson Ch, Ekblom A, Ekman-Ordeberg G, Hjelm A, Irestedt L. Lack of analgesic effect of systemically administered morphine or pethidine on labor pain. *Br J Obstet Gynaecol* 1996;103:968–972.)

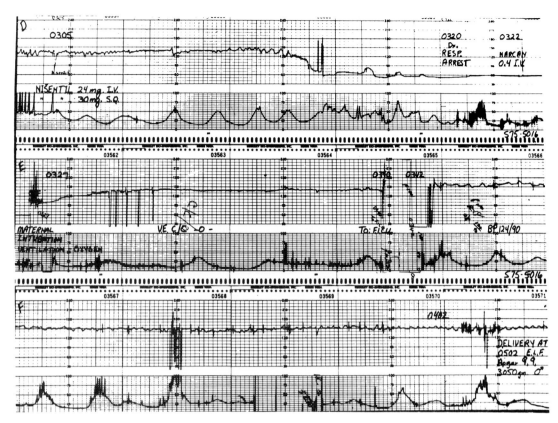

Figure 7.3. Continuous fetal heart rate monitor strip from a patient who received Nisentil intravenously and subcutaneously. Ten minutes after medication, a sustained fetal bradycardia developed, and maternal respiratory arrest was noted shortly thereafter. The mother was treated with Narcan, endotracheal intubation, and controlled ventilation with 100% oxygen. Fetal heart rate rapidly improved, and a vigorous neonate was delivered 2 hours later. (Labor record provided by R.H. Paul M.D., University of Southern California, Los Angeles.)

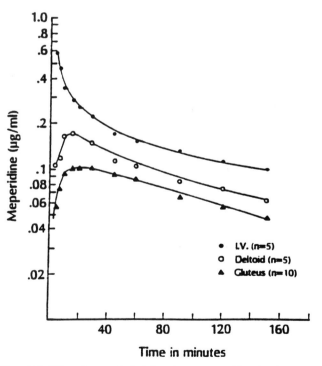

Figure 7.4. Effect of route of administration on meperidine levels during labor. Gluteus vs. intravenous curves are significantly different (F[1.8] = 10.53; $P < .01$). Gluteus vs. deltoid curves are significantly different (F[1.8] = 9.7; $P < .02$). (Reprinted by permission from Lazebnik N, Kuhnert BR, Carr PC, Brashear WT, Syracuse CD, Mann LI. Intravenous, deltoid, or gluteus administration of meperidine during labor? *Am J Obstet Gynecol* 1989;160:1184–1189.)

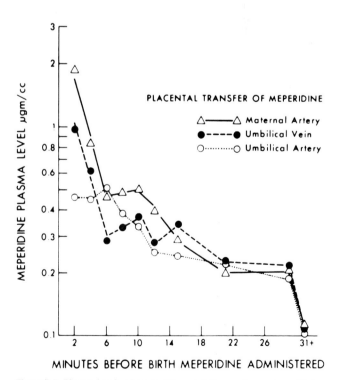

Figure 7.5. Plasma levels of meperidine at delivery after maternal intravenous administration of 50 mg at various intervals from 30 seconds to 4 hours before delivery. (From data in Shnider SM, Way EL, Lord MJ. Rate of appearance and disappearance of meperidine in fetal blood after administration of narcotic to the mother. *Anesthesiology* 1966;27: 227–228.)

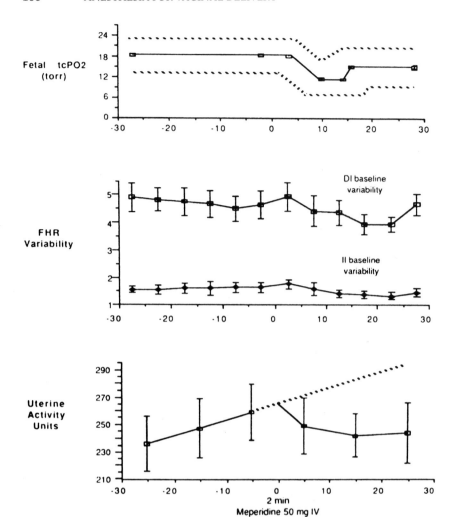

Figure 7.6. Fetal tcPo₂, FHR variability (short-term, DI; long-term, II) and uterine activity (uterine activity units) ± SE following a 2-minute injection of 50 mg meperidine at time 0 minutes. (Reprinted by permission from Baxi LV, Petrie RH, James LS. Human fetal oxygenation (*tcPo₂*), heart rate variability and uterine activity following maternal administration of meperidine. *J Perinat Med* 1988;16:23–29.)

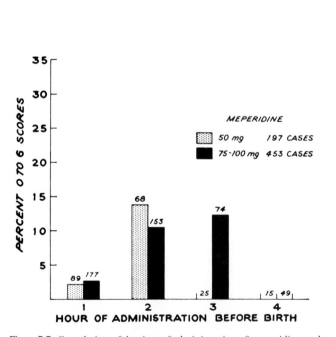

Figure 7.7. Correlation of the time of administration of meperidine and neonatal depression according to Apgar scores. (Reprinted by permission from Shnider SM, Moya F. Effects of meperidine on the newborn infant. *Am J Obstet Gynecol* 1964;89:1009–1015.)

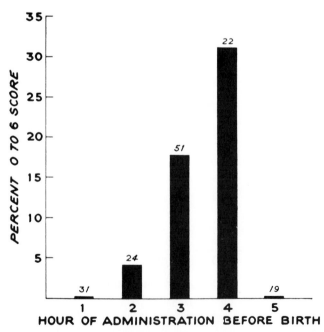

Figure 7.8. Correlation of the time of administration of meperidine-secobarbital and neonatal depression according to Apgar scores. (Reprinted by permission from Shnider SM, Moya F. Effects of meperidine on the newborn infant. *Am J Obstet Gynecol* 1964;89:1009–1015.)

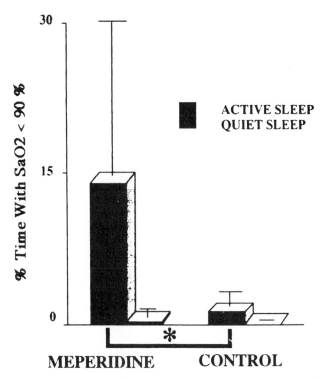

Figure 7.9. Percentage of time with oxygen saturation (SaO$_2$) <90% during sleep states in neonates following a continuous infusion of meperidine. Infants were studied for a total of 240 minutes, starting 60 minutes after delivery. *P < .01 vs. control group. (Reprinted by permission from Hamza J, Benlabed M, Orhant E, Escourrou P, Curzi-Dascalova L, Gaultier C. Neonatal pattern of breathing during active and quiet sleep after maternal administration of meperidine. *Pediatr Res* 1992;32:412–416.)

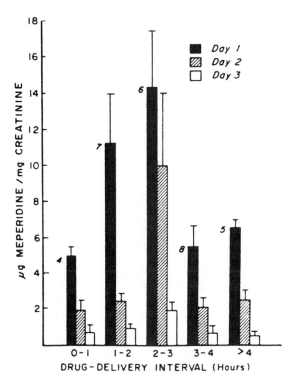

Figure 7.10. Relationship between the drug-delivery interval and the urinary excretion of meperidine by the neonate. (Reprinted by permission from Kuhnert BR, Kuhnert PM, Tu AL, Lin DCK. Meperidine and normeperidine levels following meperidine administration during labor. II. Fetus and neonate. *Am J Obstet Gynecol* 1979;133:909–914.)

vein and artery decreased. With a short DDI, the cord vein levels were higher than cord artery levels, indicating fetal tissue uptake. With longer DDIs, umbilical artery levels equaled or exceeded venous levels, indicating excretion of the drug across the placenta. Measurements of neonatal urine levels of meperidine indicated that fetal exposure to the drug is highest 2 to 3 hours after administration of the opioid to the mother. This agrees with the findings of Belfrage et al. (35). Neonates born to mothers who received meperidine 2 to 3 hours before delivery excreted the greatest amount of drug (Fig. 7.10) (28, 42, 43). Those infants whose mothers had shorter or longer DDIs excreted significantly less drug, indicating that maximal fetal tissue uptake of meperidine occurs 2 to 3 hours following maternal administration.

Another possible reason for the delay in neonatal depression is the continued presence of a pharmacologically active metabolite. Using a nonspecific colorimetric assay, Morrison et al. (44, 45) reported that after IV administration of meperidine to pregnant women, there were three distinct types of metabolic patterns. Neonatal depression was associated with one of these patterns, in which high and prolonged blood levels of unidentified metabolites were found. Of the known metabolites of meperidine, only normeperidine is a central nervous system depressant. Kuhnert et al. (42) reported that normeperidine levels in umbilical cord blood were highest 4 hours or more after administration of a single IV dose of meperidine to the mother. In contrast to meperidine, Kuhnert et al. found that cord normeperidine levels increased with increases in the DDI and that the metabolite reached its highest level when the DDI was the longest (Fig. 7.11). Thus, meperidine reaches a peak in the neonate at a 2- to 3-hour DDI, and normeperidine reaches a peak much later. Others (35, 46) have found a similar pattern.

Kuhnert et al. (47) measured umbilical cord samples and neonatal urine samples for meperidine and normeperidine from 11 neonates whose mothers had received multiple doses of IV meperidine. Blood samples were also collected from 5 of the neonates every 24 hours for 72 hours. The results of the study suggested that administration of multiple doses of meperidine over long-time intervals resulted in maximum accumulation of meperidine and normeperidine in fetal tissues. This could have significant neonatal implications.

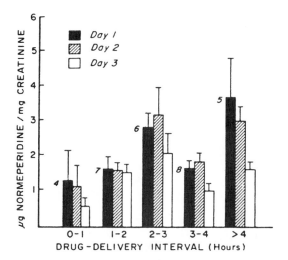

Figure 7.11. Relationship between the drug-delivery interval and the urinary excretion of normeperidine by the neonate. (Reprinted by permission from Kuhnert BR, Kuhnert PM, Tu AL, Lin DCK. Meperidine and normeperidine levels following meperidine administration during labor. II. Fetus and neonate. *Am J Obstet Gynecol* 1979;133:909–914.)

In a study in rhesus monkeys, administration of 2 mg/kg IV meperidine (or two such doses 4 hours apart) during labor produced respiratory depression in three of eight newborns (48). The greatest respiratory depression occurred in newborns with the highest plasma levels of meperidine and normeperidine. In contrast to humans, neonatal plasma normeperidine concentrations in the monkey were more closely associated with respiratory depression than were meperidine concentrations. They also found the normeperidine-to-meperidine ratios in the monkeys were considerably higher than in humans.

In addition to depressant effects seen at birth, meperidine use is associated with subtle effects on neonatal behavior in humans (39, 40, 49, 50) and primates (51). Depression of habituation to an auditory stimulus as well as other subtle neurobehavioral changes are directly proportional to the maternal dose of meperidine (50 to 150 mg) and are present 20 to 60 hours after birth (28, 39, 40). Kuhnert et al. (52) showed that the longer the DDI, the poorer the scores on the Brazelton Neonatal Behavioral Assessment Scale (Fig. 7.12) at 12 hours and 3 days of age. Their findings suggest that the poorer neonatal neurobehavioral test scores are due to normeperidine. Overall, it appears that the acute neonatal effects of maternal administration of meperidine, as manifested by decreased Apgar scores, are due to high tissue levels of meperidine, whereas the more subtle and prolonged effects on neurobehavior are due to normeperidine. It should be emphasized that the statistically significant differences in neurobehavioral examination scores were so slight as to be of doubtful clinical significance, although they are useful in elucidating pharmacologic mechanisms. Administration of IV naloxone to the mother approximately 15 minutes before delivery reverses the neonatal neurobehavioral effects of meperidine for approximately 2 hours after birth, following which the depressant effects are again seen (53).

Longer-term studies involving infant monkeys suggest that later behavior (3 to 12 months) may also be affected (54).

Monkeys exposed to meperidine, through administration to their dams during labor, showed an alteration in the pattern of maturation of spontaneous behaviors.

Meperidine also affects initiation of successful breastfeeding. Righard and Alade (55) observed 72 neonates for 2 hours following birth. Sixteen of 17 unmedicated infants who were in constant skin contact with their mother for at least 1 hour after birth sucked correctly by 2 hours, 1 incorrectly. Twenty-one infants whose mothers had received meperidine during labor were also in continuous contact. Eight of these infants sucked correctly, 3 incorrectly, and 10 were still not sucking at 2 hours. In a separation group (removed from mother's abdomen after approximately 20 minutes), none of the meperidine infants sucked correctly: 4 incorrectly, and 15 were not sucking. Nissen et al. (56) concluded that meperidine affected breastfeeding behavior more if the dose to delivery time interval was short. Higher meperidine concentrations were associated with a poor first breastfeeding performance.

Fentanyl

Because of its rapid onset of action, profound analgesic capabilities, and lack of active metabolites, fentanyl is a popular IV or IM analgesic for labor (57, 58). Fentanyl 100 μg is equianalgesic to morphine 10 mg. The usual IM dose is 50 to 100 μg, and the usual IV dose is 25 to 50 μg. IV fentanyl produces analgesia almost immediately. The peak effect follows within 3 to 5 minutes, and the duration of action is 30 to 60 minutes. After IM administration, analgesia begins in 7 to 8 minutes, peaks at about 30 minutes, and lasts 1 to 2 hours.

As with all opioids, fentanyl rapidly crosses the placenta. It appears in the fetal blood as early as 1 minute, with levels peaking at 5 minutes (59). In maternal blood, approximately 60% to 80% of fentanyl is bound by plasma albumin, thus leaving one third unbound and available for placental transfer. In pregnant sheep, fentanyl had no effect on uterine tone or on uterine blood flow (59).

In a group of neonates similar in age, size, and having a similar surgical procedure, the elimination half-life for fentanyl was highly variable, between 75 and 441 minutes (60). Fentanyl has a lower molecular weight than alfentanil and sufentanil and is highly lipophilic, both factors contributing to its placental transfer, especially where there are fluctuations in maternal blood flow (61). As it is a basic drug, fentanyl will be more ionized in the fetus than in the mother. In cases of fetal acidosis, more drug will be "trapped" in the fetus. The highest concentration of fentanyl in colostrum after a low analgesic dose ($2 \mu g \cdot kg^{-1}$) occurred at 45 minutes with almost no fentanyl detectable at 10 hours (62).

Patient-controlled IV fentanyl for labor analgesia has been utilized. There are few randomized, controlled studies, and most are limited in their conclusions because of the small number of patients studied. Rayburn et al. (63) studied IV fentanyl for labor analgesia in an observational study of 137 laboring women who received 50 or 100 μg IV fentanyl during active labor. The lower dose was usually given initially. The investigators measured maternal and umbilical vein fentanyl levels at delivery and collected information as to the number of requests for the drug and the total dose required. The cumulative dose varied in accordance with maternal needs (mean 140 ± 42 μg; range, 50 to 600 μg); but as seen in Figure 7.13, many women received multiple injections and relatively large cumulative doses. Regardless of the maternal dose, newborn drug levels were low and always less than maternal levels (Fig. 7.14). The newborns were compared with a similar group of consecutively chosen infants whose mothers had required no analgesia during labor. Infants born to the women who received fentanyl had outcome measurements (i.e., Apgar scores, umbilical blood gas values, and neurobehavioral exams) similar to the control groups. The last dose of fentanyl was usually given 2 hours before delivery. Naloxone was

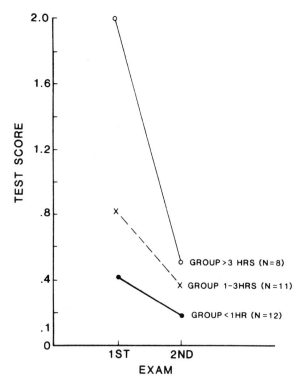

Figure 7.12. The relationship between the drug-delivery interval and the mean number of abnormal reflexes in the meperidine group. (Reprinted by permission from Kuhnert BR, Linn PL, Kennard MJ, Kuhnert PM. Effects of low doses of meperidine on neonatal behavior. *Anesth Analg* 1975;64:335–342.)

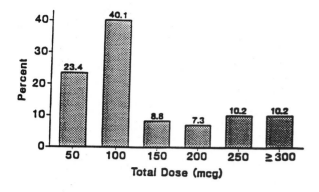

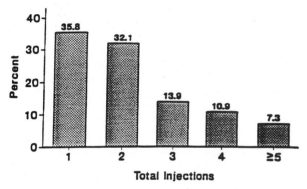

Figure 7.13. Fentanyl citrate use according to the number of injections and total cumulative dose. (Reprinted by permission from Rayburn W, Rathke A, Leuschen P, Chleborad J, Weidner W. Fentanyl citrate analgesia during labor. *Am J Obstet Gynecol* 1989;161:202–206.)

administered to one infant, but there was no other evidence of deleterious effects.

In another study, Rayburn et al. (64) compared the efficacy of IV meperidine and fentanyl in a randomized, unblinded study of 105 parturients. Analgesia was comparable, but there was a lower incidence of side effects, nausea, vomiting, and sedation in the fentanyl group. Neonatal complications (Apgar less than 7, need for ventilatory support, naloxone use) were more common

in the meperidine group. A further study compared patient-controlled and nurse-administered fentanyl for labor analgesia and found both techniques were effective and safe (65).

Smith et al. (66) compared the effects of IV fentanyl (50 μg) on fetal biophysical parameters in 12 women who requested analgesia during labor with 12 parturients who did not require analgesia. Continuous real-time ultrasound imaging was performed by blinded observers on all 24 patients. Information collected included number and duration of fetal body movements during and between contractions, duration and total time of fetal breathing episodes, FHR baseline, and presence of diminished beat-to-beat variability. The single dose of IV fentanyl had no effect on incidence and duration of gross body movement, although the number of movements between contractions and as a percentage of total time was reduced. No breathing episodes were observed during the first 10 minutes after fentanyl, and there was a transient reduction of FHR variability and a regular sine wave-like baseline in the study group. The decrease in FHR variability is common to all opioids.

A randomized, unblinded study comparing IV patient-controlled analgesia with fentanyl to epidural analgesia in 20 patients found that epidural analgesia was more effective and had fewer side effects (67). None of the neonates in either group required naloxone, and all had similar Apgar scores and pH. Respiratory monitoring in the newborns revealed that oxygen saturation was lower in the fentanyl group (Fig. 7.15). It is important to note that IV fentanyl was not used in the second stage of labor.

Lawes et al. (68) studied the use of fentanyl and droperidol supplementation before induction of general anesthesia in a group of severely hypertensive parturients. Fentanyl 200 μg in two divided doses and droperidol 5 mg were administered over a 5-minute period. A standard induction with lidocaine, etomidate, and succinylcholine was given, followed by maintenance of anesthesia with a volatile anesthetic. Most of the mothers had a degree of metabolic acidemia, as did their neonates. The neonates who did not have metabolic acidosis did not appear to be significantly depressed.

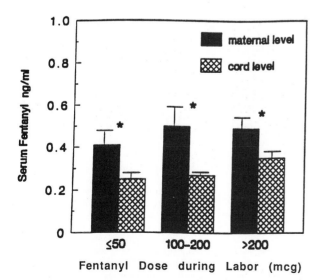

Figure 7.14. Maternal and cord serum fentanyl citrate concentrations at delivery according to maternal dose during labor (*$P < .03$; bars = SEM). (Reprinted by permission from Rayburn W, Rathke A, Leuschen P, Chleborad J, Weidner W. Fentanyl citrate analgesia during labor. *Am J Obstet Gynecol* 1989;161:202–206.)

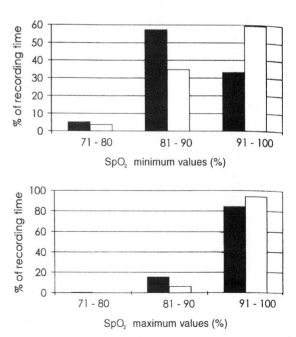

Figure 7.15. Minimum and maximum values of the neonatal arterial oxyhemoglobin saturation (*SPo*₂), percentage of the recording time. ■ = fentanyl group, □ = epidural group. $P < .001$ in both minimum and maximum values. (Reprinted by permission from Nikkola EM, Ekblad UU, Kero PO, Alihanka JJM, Salonen MAO. Intravenous fentanyl PCA during labor. *Can J Anaesth* 1997;44:1248–1255.)

Table 7.2. COMPARISON OF NARCOTIZED (REQUIRED NALOXONE) AND NON—NARCOTIZED NEONATES

	Narcotized Neonates (n = 3)	Non—narcotized Neonates (n = 29)	P Value
PCA duration (min)	279 ± 191	213 ± 160	.489
Total fentanyl dose (μg)	770 ± 233	300 ± 287	.027
Consumption rate (μg·kg^{-1} min^{-1})	0.07 ± 0.07	0.02 ± 0.01	.045

Although the duration of PCA use was similar, the total dose of maternal fentanyl administered and the maternal consumption rate were significantly greater in those neonates who received naloxone than those who did not (Wilcoxon two-sample test. Mean ± SD).
Reprinted with permission from Morley-Forster PK, Weberpals J. Neonatal effects of patient-controlled analgesia using fentanyl in labor. *Int J Obstet Anesth* 1998;7:103–108.

Morley-Forster and Weberpals (69) retrospectively studied the neonatal effects of IV patient-controlled labor analgesia with fentanyl. Thirty-two charts were analyzed for information regarding birth weight, gestational age, Apgar scores, naloxone use, and umbilical venous gases. As this was a retrospective study, fentanyl use was often continued into the second stage of labor. This study found a 44% incidence of 1-minute Apgar scores less than 6, and three infants required naloxone for an Apgar score of 4. A comparison of vigorous (Apgar greater than 6) and depressed (Apgar less than 5) neonates did not reveal any differences in patient-controlled analgesia duration, last dose to delivery time, total fentanyl dose, or consumption rate. The only predictive factor for naloxone use was the total amount of fentanyl received (770 ± 233 μg vs. 300 ± 287 μg), but it is important to remember that the total number of affected infants requiring naloxone was small (Table 7.2).

Sufentanil, Alfentanil, and Remifentanil

The more lipid-soluble opioids sufentanil and alfentanil have not gained popularity for parenteral administration for labor analgesia, as they have little advantage over fentanyl. Sufentanil also crosses the placenta by passive diffusion, with transfer limited by its higher maternal protein binding (70), and increases markedly with fetal acidosis (71). In a study comparing intrathe-

cal, epidural, and IV sufentanil, Camann et al. (72) administered 10 μg sufentanil to 24 laboring parturients. The epidural and IV routes failed to produce satisfactory analgesia (Fig. 7.16).

Alfentanil has a lower lipid solubility and higher protein binding than fentanyl, which may reduce its rate of placental transfer. However, its pK$_a$ of 6.5 would tend to increase placental transfer. Using the human placental lobule model, Zakowski et al. (73) demonstrated that alfentanil crossed the placenta rapidly (less than 5 minutes). Similar to fentanyl and sufentanil, its transfer is maternal blood flow limited (61). Golub et al. (51) reported that alfentanil produced long-term behavioral effects in infant monkeys following maternal administration.

IV alfentanil has been used to ablate the hypertensive response to intubation in parturients with severe preeclampsia. (74) In a study comparing alfentanil with fentanyl in that setting, Rout and Rocke (75) found that alfentanil 10 μg/kg was as effective as fentanyl 2.5 μg/kg in obtunding the pressor response to intubation. There was a lower umbilical arterial PO$_2$ in the alfentanil group.

Remifentanil is a new ultrashort-acting opioid that is unique in that it is hydrolyzed by nonspecific blood and tissue esterases. Kan et al. (76) administered an IV infusion of 0.1 μg·kg^{-1}·min^{-1} remifentanil to 19 parturients having a cesarean section under epidural anesthesia. Maternal arterial, umbilical arterial, and umbilical venous blood samples were obtained at delivery for analysis of drug concentrations of

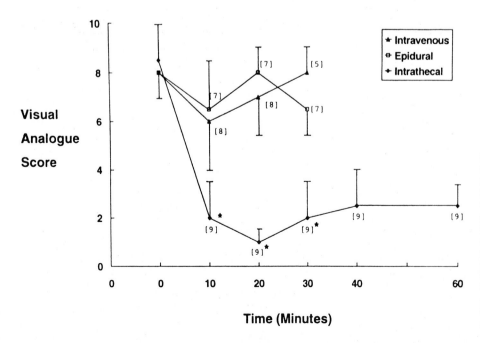

Figure 7.16. Visual analog scale scores (median, interquartile rante) after sufentanil administration. Insufficient numbers of patients precluded data tabulation after 30 minutes in the intravenous and epidural groups. Numbers in brackets indicate number of patients in each group at the time of assessment. *P < .001, intrathecal vs. intravenous and epidural; P < .001 vs. intrathecal baseline visual analog scale score. (Reprinted by permission from Camann WR, Denney RA, Holby ED, Datta S. A comparison of intrathecal, epidural, and intravenous sufentanil for labor analgesia. *Anesthesiology* 1992;77:884–887.)

remifentanil, its metabolite (remifentanil acid), and blood gases. Maternal vital signs and neonatal Apgar scores and neurobehavioral assessments (NACS) were also assessed. These investigators concluded that remifentanil crossed the placenta (mean umbilical-vein–to–maternal-artery ratio 0.88 ± 0.78) but appeared to be rapidly metabolized, redistributed, or both. The newborns were alert despite the presence of maternal sedation. A remifentanil infusion (50 μg/mL at 0.15 μg · kg^{-1} · min^{-1}) has been used to facilitate epidural catheter placement in a parturient (77). The authors report excellent analgesia and suggest that a remifentanil infusion may be advantageous in patients who are unable to remain still during epidural placement. Thurlow and Waterhouse (78) used patient-controlled analgesia with remifentanil (20 μg over 20 seconds with a lockout time of 3 minutes) in two patients with documented platelet abnormalities and reported very good analgesia with no adverse neonatal sequelae. Remifentanil has also proven useful as part of a general anesthetic regimen in patients with cardiac disease (79, 80).

Morphine

Although a few physicians still rely on morphine for labor analgesia, most prefer to use other opioids due to concerns about morphine's neonatal effects. Morphine is usually administered in doses of 5 to 10 mg IM or 2 to 3 mg IV. The peak analgesic effect is 1 to 2 hours after IM administration and 20 minutes after IV administration. The duration of action is 4 to 6 hours.

In equianalgesic doses, morphine may produce more respiratory depression of the newborn than does meperidine. Shute and Davis (16) described a "morphinized baby" as one that, with external stimulation, would inspire once or twice and then lapse into apnea, from which it was difficult to arouse. These investigators suggested that the dosage, the DDI, trauma at delivery, and condition of the infant in utero enhanced the neonatal effects of morphine. In newborns (12 to 60 hours of age), morphine shifts the CO_2 response curve to the right and downward to a greater extent than meperidine (Fig. 7.17) (81). In this study by Way et al., the ratio of meperidine to morphine was 10:1, but the total dose was about one third of that which would be used for analgesia in an adult. The investigators postulated that there was an altered biologic disposition of morphine, i.e., a greater permeability of the infant brain to morphine.

Recently, Gerdin et al. (82) examined the maternal kinetics of morphine in labor. They found that morphine was rapidly

eliminated by the parturient. Although the transplacental transfer was rapid, they suggested that the short maternal elimination half-life would decrease the exposure of the infant to morphine.

Two studies have reevaluated the efficacy of morphine for labor pain relief (1, 83). Other than for back pain, morphine was unsuccessful at relieving pain even at doses that produced heavy maternal sedation. This recent evidence, coupled with the known neonatal effects, does not suggest that there is any clinical advantage to morphine for labor analgesia.

SEDATIVE-TRANQUILIZERS

The amount of anxiety and fear some woman experience during labor and delivery can be minimized by proper psychological preparation and the continuous presence of a supportive person (84). In practice, however, some women significantly benefit from pharmacologic intervention to reduce their anxiety. Furthermore, these drugs promote sleep, and this hypnotic effect may be beneficial in early labor. The phenothiazines, as well as drugs such as hydroxyzine and droperidol, are potent antiemetics and reduce the nausea and vomiting commonly seen during labor or when opioids are used.

Barbiturates

Barbiturates possess no analgesic action and, indeed, may produce an antianalgesic effect (85, 86). In the presence of severe pain, administration of these drugs may result in an excited, disoriented, and unmanageable parturient. With low doses (50 to 100 mg IM pentobarbital) there is no significant respiratory depression (87). In larger doses or with the addition of opioids to smaller doses, barbiturates are associated with respiratory depression and obtundation of protective airway reflexes.

All the barbiturates rapidly cross the placenta, and equilibrium between mother and fetus is achieved in minutes (Fig. 7.18) (88, 89). When used for sedation in the parturient, they have prolonged depressant effects on the neonate. Shnider and Moya (15) showed that the addition of secobarbital (100 mg IM or 200 mg per os) to meperidine (50 to 100 mg IM) increases the incidence of depressed newborns. High doses of barbiturates (600 to 1000 mg) produce neonatal somnolence, flaccidity, hypoventilation, and failure to feed for up to 2 days (90). Even with

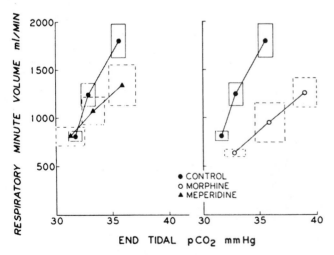

Figure 7.17. Effect of equianalgesic doses of morphine and meperidine on the CO_2 response curve in the newborn. The standard error of the means is indicated by the *rectangles* around each *point*. (Reprinted by permission from Way WL, Costley EC, Way EL. Respiratory sensitivity of the newborn infant to meperidine and morphine. *Clin Pharmacol Ther* 1965;6:454–461.)

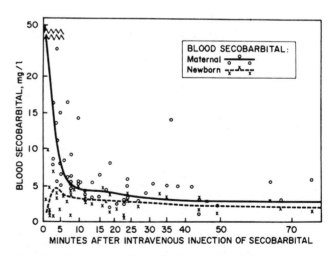

Figure 7.18. Scattergram of blood levels of secobarbital in maternal venous and umbilical cord blood after a single intravenous injection of 250 mg sodium secobarbital from 1 to 75 minutes before delivery. Secobarbital crosses the placenta rapidly, and the neonatal blood level at delivery is approximately 70% of that in the mother. (Reprinted by permission from Root B, Eichner E, Sunshine I. Blood secobarbital levels and their clinical correlation in mothers and newborn infants. *Am J Obstet Gynecol* 1961;81:948–956.)

smaller doses, resulting in no depression of the Apgar score, the newborn's attention span may be decreased for 2 to 4 days (91). For these reasons, most consider barbiturates to be contraindicated in the parturient.

Phenothiazine Derivatives and Hydroxyzine

Promethazine, propiomazine, and hydroxyzine seem to be equally effective in relieving anxiety, reducing opioid requirements, and controlling emesis. Differences between these drugs are relatively minor. Propiomazine has a shorter onset time and duration than promethazine (92). Promethazine is a respiratory stimulant, whereas propiomazine is a mild respiratory depressant. Hydroxyzine has a slight disadvantage in that it cannot be used intravenously.

Despite the rapid placental transfer and decrease in beat-to-beat variability of the FHR, recommended doses of these drugs do not seem to cause neonatal depression. Powe et al. (92) compared three IM analgesic regimens: meperidine 50 mg, meperidine 50 mg plus promethazine 50 mg, and meperidine 50 mg plus propiomazine 20 mg. The addition of either tranquilizer to meperidine did not potentiate analgesia or increase the incidence of depressed newborns but did increase maternal sedation. Similarly, hydroxyzine 50 to 100 mg alone or combined with an opioid produced increased tranquility without increased neonatal depression (93–95).

Benzodiazepines

In obstetrics, benzodiazepines may be used as sedatives, opioid adjuvants, anticonvulsants, and premedicants prior to cesarean section. These drugs possess anxiolytic, hypnotic, anticonvulsant, muscle relaxant, and antegrade amnesic effects. Specific benzodiazepine receptors are found throughout the central nervous system. The pharmacologic effects of benzodiazepines have been attributed to an increase in the quantity or facilitation of the effectiveness of the inhibitory neurotransmitters γ-aminobutyric acid (GABA) and glycine (Fig. 7.19) (96). The glycine-mimetic actions in the spinal cord produce muscle relaxation, while enhanced inhibitory neurotransmitter

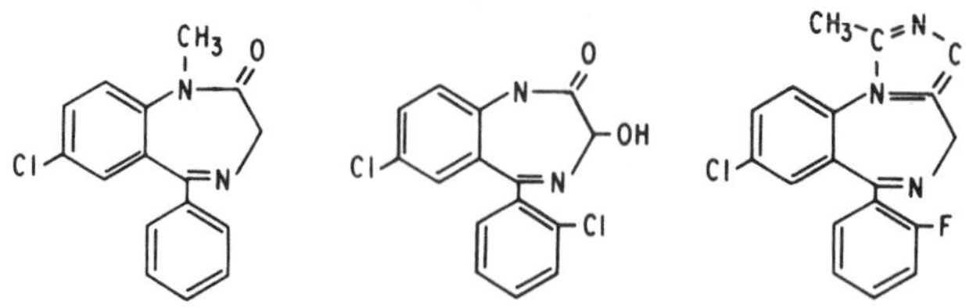

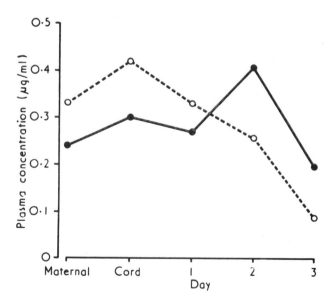

Figure 7.20. Structural formulas of midazolam and two commonly used benzodiazepines, diazepam and lorazepam. Note the fused imidazole ring the distinguishes midazolam from other benzodiazepines. (Reprinted by permission from Reves JG, Fragen RJ, Vinik HR, Greenblatt DJ. Midazolam: Pharmacology and uses. *Anesthesiology* 1985;62:310–324.)

effects of GABA in the brain result in sedation and anticonvulsant activity. The antianxiety effects are likely the result of both glycine- and GABA-mediated inhibition of neuronal pathways in the cortex and brain stem. All benzodiazepines have similar molecular structures, are lipophilic, and rapidly cross the placenta. Diazepam, lorazepam, and midazolam (Fig. 7.20) are the three benzodiazepines clinically used in obstetrics.

Diazepam

Diazepam has been extensively studied in obstetrics, but due to its effects on the neonate it is used only for specific indications, e.g., preeclampsia. Diazepam is metabolized in the liver to a pharmacologically active metabolite, N-desmethyldiazepam, and to hydroxydiazepam. Diazepam has a half-life of 14 to 90 hours; N-desmethyldiazepam has a half-life of 30 to 100 hours and undergoes enterohepatic recirculation, which can cause a return of drowsiness 6 to 8 hours later. The drug rapidly crosses the placenta, and maternal and fetal blood levels are approximately equal within minutes of an IV dose (97). At birth, fetal blood levels may exceed maternal levels (Fig. 7.21) (98–100). The neonate is capable of metabolizing small doses of diazepam. When the total maternal dosage during labor exceeds 30 mg, the drug and its active metabolite persist in pharmacologically active concentrations for at least a week in the neonate (98). When IV diazepam 0.3 mg/kg was used for induction of general

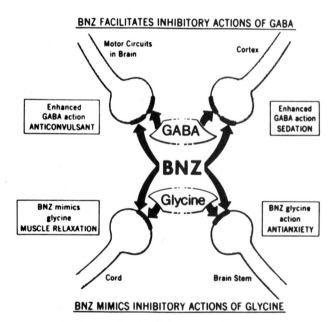

Figure 7.19. Mechanisms and sites of action of benzodiazepines (*BNZ*). (Reprinted by permission from Richter JJ. Current theories about the mechanisms of benzodiaepines and neuroleptic drugs. *Anesthesiology* 1981;54:66–72.)

Figure 7.21. Mean plasma concentration of diazepam and desmethyldiazepam showing crossover in degradation curves. Diazepam (∞); Desmethyldiazepam (••). (Reprinted by permission from Cree JE, Meyer J, Hailey DM. Diazepam in labor: Its metabolism and effect on the clinical condition and thermogenesis of the newborn. *Br Med J* 1973;4:251–255.)

anesthesia for cesarean delivery, the concentration of diazepam in some neonates 2 hours after delivery was in the lower range of plasma levels found in adults taking 15 mg diazepam daily (101). The principal adverse effects of large doses of diazepam on the neonate are hypotonia, lethargy, decreased feeding, and hypothermia (98, 101–104). Apnea may also occur (105–107).

In small doses, there are minimal fetal and neonatal effects (99). Although beat-to-beat variability of the FHR is markedly decreased even with small IV doses (5 to 10 mg) (108), there are no adverse effects on fetal or neonatal acid-base or clinical status (99, 108). Small doses (2.5 to 10 mg) of IV diazepam used for anxiolysis in patients undergoing cesarean section under regional anesthesia (109) did not sedate the newborn—as evidenced by Apgar scores (72% 8—10 without diazepam, 71% with diazepam)—and did not alter umbilical vein or artery oxygen or acid-base status, but did decrease newborn muscle tone. The Scanlon neurobehavioral examination showed decreased tone at 4 hours but not at 24 hours of age.

A theoretical objection to the use of diazepam in obstetrics was raised by the work of Schiff et al. (110). Sodium benzoate, which is used as a buffer in the injectable form of the drug, is a potent bilirubin-albumin uncoupler. The displacement of lipid-soluble bilirubin from its albumin-binding sites could increase the susceptibility of the infant to kernicterus. Schiff et al. advised caution in using injectable diazepam in infants when serum bilirubin levels are increased. Providing only small doses of maternal diazepam are used, subsequent problems with bilirubin binding in the neonate are unlikely (111).

Small IV doses of diazepam (2.5-mg doses to a total of 10 mg) may help allay extreme apprehension and anxiety without producing significant adverse fetal or neonatal effects. When larger doses are used, as in the therapy of preeclampsia or eclampsia, the neonate should be observed carefully for at least 36 hours after delivery as apnea, hypotonia, and hypothermia might occur.

Lorazepam

Lorazepam is five times as potent as the same dose of diazepam (112). In contrast to diazepam, it has a shorter half-life and less than 1% of the drug is transformed to other metabolites. Houghton (113) reported that 0.05 mg · kg^{-1} (approximately 3.5 mg) IM lorazepam 90 minutes before elective cesarean section produced no measurable antianxiety or amnesic effects in the mother but did produce lower neurobehavioral scores on the Brazelton Neonatal Behavioral Assessment Scale in the neonate. In addition, the neonates had increased respiratory rates for up to 7 days. The drug did not adversely affect Apgar scores, neonatal blood gases at 8, 24, and 48 hours after birth, temperature, or feeding patterns. Other studies have demonstrated adverse effects on neonatal feeding after maternal premedication with lorazepam 1 mg per os (114) and neonatal respiratory depression after lorazepam 2 mg per os (115). It would appear that, despite its short half-life and lack of pharmacologically active metabolites, lorazepam does not offer significant advantages over diazepam in obstetric anesthesia.

Midazolam

Midazolam differs from other benzodiazepines in that it is water soluble, has a rapid onset and short duration of action, and can be administered intravenously or intramuscularly without producing pain at the injection site. In common with other benzodiazepines, it has anxiolytic, sedative-hypnotic, amnesic, anticonvulsant, and muscle-relaxant properties. Midazolam is approximately three to four times as potent as diazepam. After IV administration, its onset is immediate and maximum effects occur by 3 minutes. Following IM injection, its onset time is 5 minutes and maximum effects are seen in about 20 minutes. As with other benzodiazepines, clinically useful doses produce minimal cardiovascular or respiratory change (116).

In the pregnant, ewe the drug rapidly crosses the placenta but not to the same extent as does diazepam (117, 118). In humans, 5 mg IV midazolam administered during labor or just prior to cesarean section resulted in lower neonatal Apgar scores (119).

One possible drawback to the use of midazolam is anterograde amnesia. A 5-mg IV dose of midazolam produces approximately 30 minutes of amnesia (120). While usually considered a desirable effect in the surgical patient, it is undesirable in the obstetric patient who wants full awareness and recall of the birth of the baby. Kanto et al. (120) administered 0.075 mg/kg IV midazolam following delivery of the baby in 11 patients having a cesarean section under epidural anesthesia. All patients had profound sedation and remembered the baby being delivered, but most remembered nothing further until moving to the recovery room. This is in contrast to the findings of Camann et al. (121), who described their experience with midazolam (2 to 7 mg) administered during cesarean delivery. Twenty-four to 48 hours postoperatively, the women complained of having no recall of the birth. A similar experience was reported by Heyman and Salem (121a).

AGONIST-ANTAGONIST AGENTS

These drugs are synthetic agonist-antagonist opioid analgesics. The major advantage reputed to these drugs is the ceiling effect for respiratory depression. In nonpregnant patients, analgesic doses of butorphanol (2 mg) and nalbuphine (10 mg) produce respiratory depression equivalent to 10 mg morphine. However, whereas larger doses of morphine produce more respiratory depression, increasing doses of butorphanol and nalbuphine do not (Fig. 7.22) (122, 123). The proposed explanation for this ceiling effect is that they are primarily strong κ- and σ-agonists and weak μ-antagonists. The potential advantage of this ceiling effect on respiratory depression is usually not clinically significant in obstetric practice because of the comparable ceiling effect on analgesia.

Nalbuphine is commonly used for parenteral labor analgesia. It has a rapid onset of action and its plasma half-life is 5 hours. It crosses the placenta rapidly and, because of its agonist-antagonist actions, is used by some instead of meperidine. Nalbuphine is usually considered to be equipotent to morphine

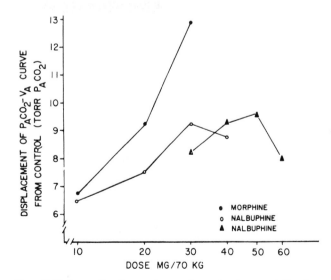

Figure 7.22. Dose-effect for respiratory depression by cumulative doses of morphine (•) and nalbuphine (○) in 8 subjects. Data of larger doses of nalbuphine (▲) were obtained from an additional 10 subjects who did not receive morphine. Abscissa is log scale. (Reprinted by permission from Romagnoli A, Keats AS. Ceiling effect for respiratory depression by nalbuphine. *Clin Pharmacol Ther* 1980;27:478–485.)

on a milligram-per-milligram basis. After IV administration to the mother in labor, measurement of umbilical cord blood nalbuphine concentrations demonstrated that nalbuphine crossed the placenta and entered the fetal circulation (124). Newborn concentrations varied substantially, ranging from one third to six times the simultaneous maternal concentration.

A comparison of meperidine and nalbuphine in a mixed parity group of mothers found that the mean pain scores were higher in the first 2 hours in the meperidine group (125). However, more multiparous patients received meperidine. NACS of the neonates were similar between groups at 6 to 10 hours of age. Patient-controlled IV administration increases patient satisfaction and appears to produce less drowsiness (126). Complications from nalbuphine administration are rare, although a persistent fetal sinusoidal heart pattern appearing after nalbuphine administration has been reported (127), as has bradycardia (128, 129). It is used intramuscularly as well as intravenously.

Analgesia with **butorphanol** is similar to that following meperidine. Maduska and Hajghassemali (130) compared butorphanol (1 or 2 mg IM) with meperidine (40 or 80 mg IM) as analgesics during labor and found them equally effective and safe for the neonate. Placental transfer of butorphanol was equivalent to meperidine, that is, fetal–to–maternal serum drug concentration ratios were approximately the same. Hodgkinson et al. (131) studied the same doses of the drugs but administered them intravenously and also found them to be comparable, including having similar minimal neurobehavioral effects at 4 and 24 hours of age. Quilligan et al. (132), in a similar study, reported that IV butorphanol (1 mg) produced greater analgesia at 30 minutes than meperidine 40 mg. Studies of its use in labor suggest that side effects are less with butorphanol. Neurobehavioral studies on the newborns are similar. A study that evaluated FHR patterns associated with butorphanol administration found that there was a strong association with the appearance of a sinusoidal FHR pattern (133).

Atkinson et al. (134) enrolled 155 parturients in a double-blind randomized trial of butorphanol 1 to 2 mg or fentanyl 50 to 100 μg. Both drugs were administered intravenously every 1 to 2 hours. Fifty-five patients were not evaluated as they did not require analgesia or decided to have epidural analgesia, or delivery occurred within 2 hours after the first dose. Greater temporary pain relief resulted from butorphanol than from fentanyl administration (Fig. 7.23). Neonatal outcomes were similar, but naloxone was required in 28% of fentanyl infants and 16% of butorphanol infants (not significant) (Table 7.3).

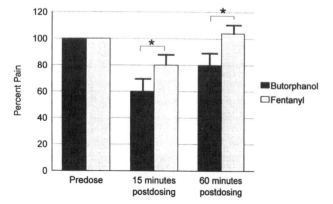

Figure 7.23. Percentage change in pain after first doses of butorphanol and fentanyl. Significant differences between two analgesia groups as indicated: *$P < .05$. (Reprinted by permission from Atkinson BD, Truitt LJ, Rayburn WF, Turnbull GL, Christensen HD, Wlodaver A. Double-blind comparison on intravenous butorphanol (Stadol) and fentanyl (Sublimaze) for analgesia during labor. *Am J Obstet Gynecol* 1994;171:993–998.)

Table 7.3. NEONATAL OUTCOMES: COMPARISON OF INTRAVENOUS BUTORPHANOL AND FENTANYL

	Butorphanol ($n = 50$)	Fentanyl ($n = 50$)
Apgar score ≤ 3		
1 min	4 (8%)	4 (8%)
5 min	1 (2%)	2 (4%)
Apgar score < 7		
1 min	11 (22%)	10 (20%)
5 min	5 (10%)	6 (12%)
Umbilical artery		
pH < 7.20	2 (4%)	4 (8%)
pH	7.30 ± 0.06	7.28 ± 0.08
Po_2 (mm Hg)	24.2 ± 7.6	23.9 ± 8.3
Pco_2 (mm Hg)	45.8 ± 8.7	46.2 ± 7.9
Base deficit (mmol/L)	−3.30 ± 1.8	−3.50 ± 2.3
Ventilatory support	0 (0%)	5 (10%)
Neonatal naloxone	8 (16%)	14 (28%)
Meconium staining	16 (32%)	20 (48%)
Neurobehavioral score		
2–4 h	28.4 ± 4.5	28.4 ± 3.7
24–36 h	32.2 ± 2.8	31.7 ± 2.9

There was no significant difference between the two groups. Reprinted with permission from Atkinson BD, Truitt LJ, Rayburn WF, Turnbull GL, Christensen HD, Wlodaver A. Double-blind comparison of intravenous butorphanol (Stadol) and fentanyl (Sublimaze) for analgesia during labor. *Am J Obstet Gynecol* 1994;171:993–998.

The main side effects associated with both butorphanol and nalbuphine are drowsiness and dizziness. As with other opioids, some patients complain of weakness, nausea, diaphoresis, and a sense of floating. They can cause psychotomimetic effects, but not as severe as with pentazocine. Butorphanol, but not nalbuphine, may increase mean pulmonary artery pressure, pulmonary capillary wedge pressure, mean aortic pressure, pulmonary vascular resistance, and myocardial work (135).

Tramadol

Tramadol is an analgesic that possesses opioid-agonist properties (mainly μ-receptor with minimal effect at Δ or κ-binding sites) and activates monoaminergic spinal inhibition of pain. It is only partially reversed by opioid antagonists (136). It is equipotent with meperidine, one fifth as potent as nalbuphine, and one tenth as potent as morphine (137). Side effects seen with its use include dizziness, nausea, sedation, dry mouth, and sweating (138).

In laboring patients, analgesia from tramadol, morphine, and meperidine was comparable, as was the side-effect profile (139). Approximately 20% of patients experienced no relief from the drug administered. Another study compared tramadol's efficacy with meperidine in nulliparous patients and found that an IM dose of 100 mg tramadol was equivalent in analgesia to 75 mg meperidine but with fewer side effects (140). In this study, the neonates of mothers receiving meperidine had a lower respiratory rate. It is still too early to determine whether tramadol will have a place in the management of labor pain.

DISSOCIATIVE OR AMNESIC DRUGS
Ketamine

IM or IV administration of ketamine produces a state referred to as "dissociative anesthesia," which is characterized by intense analgesia with only superficial sleep. In obstetrics, the drug may be used as an induction agent for general anesthesia (1 mg/kg)

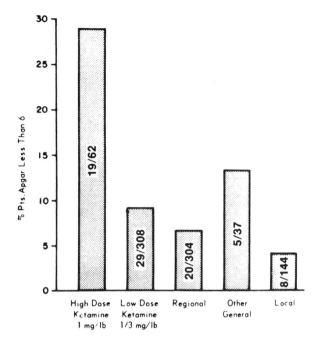

Figure 7.24. Comparison of high-dose and low-dose ketamine anesthesia with regional, local, and other general anesthetics. (Reprinted by permission from Janeczko GF, El-Etr AA, Younes S. Low-dose ketamine anesthesia for obstetrical delivery. *Anesth Analg* 1974;53:828–831.)

or in very small doses (0.25 mg/kg) as a systemic analgesic in the awake parturient.

In both dose ranges, ketamine produces minimal maternal respiratory depression but usually increases arterial blood pressure 10% to 25% (141). Undesirable hypertension may occur, and the drug should not be given to parturients with high blood pressure. In low doses, maternal ketamine does not depress the neonate (Fig. 7.24) (142) but will have some effect on neurobehavior (143).

Ketamine in intermittent IV doses of 10 to 15 mg can be titrated to produce intense maternal analgesia without loss of consciousness. The onset of action is less than 30 seconds, and recovery is rapid (4 minutes), as evidenced by orientation to time, place, and person. Undesirable hallucinations are minimal, especially if the anesthesiologist provides pleasant verbal reassurance and encouragement.

Low-dose ketamine is particularly useful for parturients in whom imminent vaginal delivery of the fetus is expected or for parturients with spotty regional analgesia for either vaginal delivery or cesarean section. After the initial dose, the patient should remain awake and responsive, and the dose may be repeated at intervals of 2 to 5 minutes. The total dose should not exceed 100 mg over a 30-minute period. Amnesia for delivery is common and may be undesirable. A suggested technique is described in Table 7.4.

Table 7.4. LOW-DOSE KETAMINE ANALGESIA: A SUGGESTED TECHNIQUE

1. Administer a nonparticulate antacid, such as sodium citrate 30 mL.
2. Check blood pressure.
3. Administer an initial dose of ketamine (10 to 15 mg), not to exceed 0.25 mg · kg^{-1}.
4. Maintain continuous verbal contact with patient to provide reassurance and monitor her sensorium.
5. If necessary, give additional 10- to 15-mg doses of ketamine every 2 to 5 minutes, up to a maximum total dose of 1 mg · kg^{-1}.

With the recent discovery that the S(+) isomer of ketamine is more potent with fewer side effects than the racemic mixture, there may be a resurgence in its use for obstetric analgesia (144).

Scopolamine (Hyoscine)

Scopolamine, like atropine, is a belladonna derivative with vagolytic action, resulting in decreased salivary secretions and gastric motility (145). Placental transfer is rapid; after IV administration (0.3 to 0.6 mg) fetal tachycardia and loss of beat-to-beat variability are produced within 10 to 25 minutes and last 60 to 90 minutes (146). Unlike atropine, scopolamine crosses the blood-brain barrier and produces profound amnesia and mild sedation, presumably by its anticholinergic actions in the central nervous system (147). Amnesia does not occur until at least 20 minutes after IV administration. Scopolamine does not possess analgesic properties and, like most sedatives, will result in severe agitation, marked excitement, and loss of inhibitions in the presence of severe pain. Hallucinations and delirium are common if a parturient in active labor is given scopolamine without adequate analgesia. "Twilight sleep," once a popular analgesic-amnesic technique, consisted of the administration of a single dose of morphine and scopolamine during labor followed by later injections of scopolamine only. Maternal amnesia for labor and delivery was intense, neonatal opioid depression was common, and the parturient was difficult to manage. Scopolamine per se has no adverse effects on the progress of labor or significant respiratory depressant effects on the neonate (90).

The authors believe that scopolamine has little place as a sedative during labor, because maternal amnesia is no longer desired by most parturients. No good data exist to prove that scopolamine, when used as a premedicant prior to general anesthesia for cesarean section, decreases the incidence of maternal awareness for the operation.

ANTAGONISTS
Physostigmine (Antilirium)

Physostigmine is an anticholinesterase agent that, unlike its analog neostigmine, rapidly crosses the blood-brain barrier and increases central nervous system acetylcholine. It is extremely effective in reversing the delirium and sedation produced by scopolamine and other sedative drugs with anticholinergic activity (148, 149). It is probably a nonspecific central nervous system stimulant. The usual dose is 0.5 to 2 mg intravenously given in 0.5 mg increments. Total doses of 3 to 4 mg are occasionally necessary. The duration of action is 1 to 2 hours. Although bradycardia after physostigmine administration is uncommon, atropine should be readily available.

The drug has been used in obstetrics and found to be a safe and rapidly effective agent for reversing the delirium and somnolence produced by scopolamine. When used prior to delivery, it is not associated with fetal bradycardia. The drug will reverse the decreased beat-to-beat variability produced by atropine and scopolamine (146). The clinical condition of newborns of mothers who have received physostigmine does not seem to be adversely affected (148, 149).

Naloxone

Naloxone is currently the preferred opioid antagonist. Unlike nalorphine (Nalline) and levallorphan (Lorfan), the earlier available opioid antagonists, it has no agonist activity and thus produces no cardiorespiratory or central nervous system depression. Opioid antagonists have been administered in three ways: (a) to the mother with each dose of opioid, (b) to the mother 10 to 15 minutes before delivery, and (c) to the neonate immediately after delivery (150, 151).

The rationale for administering an opioid and opioid antagonist simultaneously is to provide maximum analgesia with minimal respiratory depression. Numerous studies have proved (152) that the antagonists will reverse the analgesia as well as the respiratory depression and therefore offer no advantage, except when used in conjunction with spinal opioids (see Chapter 9).

The rationale for administering naloxone just before delivery is to allow placental transfer and intrauterine reversal of opioid depression in the fetus and neonate. Many consider this approach inadvisable because removal of maternal analgesia immediately before delivery is unfair to the mother, may result in an uncontrollable and difficult delivery, and is usually unnecessary insofar as the neonate is concerned.

The rationale for administering naloxone routinely to all neonates whose mothers have received opioids within 4 hours of delivery is that even apparently vigorous babies will have some central nervous system depression and alteration of neurobehavioral status (40, 150). The objection to this approach is based on the lack of documentation of long-term safety of naloxone. The short-term safety of naloxone is well documented. Even when administered in excessive doses, no adverse effects are seen.

It is apparent that opiate receptors and endogenous opioid substances (enkephalins and endorphins) have a normal physiologic function (153, 154). These compounds may be important neurotransmitters and be involved in hypothalamic-pituitary function and the integration of sensory stimuli. Naloxone acts by displacing opioids from the receptor sites in the central nervous system and blocks the physiologic effects of enkephalins and endorphins; theoretically, it may adversely influence the neonate's response to stress. Indeed, several investigators using animal models have demonstrated that very large doses of naloxone administered directly to the fetus or neonate decreased their ability to respond to asphyxia (155–157). Until further studies are performed, the routine administration of naloxone to all neonates is not recommended.

It should be emphasized that adverse neonatal effects of naloxone have never been demonstrated in humans, and the drug should not be withheld when indicated. Parturients who receive an absolute or relative overdose of opioids, as evidenced by obtundation or hypoventilation, should receive naloxone. Depressed infants who have a high probability of being narcotized and do not respond to routine resuscitation with oxygenation, ventilation, and tactile stimulation should also receive naloxone.

In adults, the usual initial dose is 0.4 mg intravenously. The neonatal dose is 0.1 mg/kg either intravenously or, if perfusion is good, intramuscularly. Effects are seen within minutes and last 1 to 2 hours. Because of the relatively short duration of naloxone, the opioid-overdosed mother or neonate must be observed carefully and repeat doses of the antagonist administered if necessary. Naloxone should not be used in opioid addicts or their neonates because acute withdrawal symptoms may be precipitated.

Flumazenil

Flumazenil is a specific benzodiazepine antagonist (158). Reports of its use in obstetrics are scant. In one report (105), a woman with eclampsia had received 120 mg of diazepam shortly before cesarean section. Her newborn was hypotonic and had persistent apnea that required respiratory support. Following an initial IV bolus of flumazenil, the infant started to breathe spontaneously. He was then treated with a flumazenil infusion, which was continued until the fifth day. In two other cases (106, 107), flumazenil was used in hypotonic, apneic newborns to reverse maternal diazepam administered for severe preeclampsia.

CONCLUSION

In summary, almost all medications administered systemically to the mother rapidly cross the placenta and produce fetal and neonatal effects. Commonly seen are FHR abnormalities that probably are of little consequence. Newborn respiratory depression may have greater consequences if unrecognized and untreated. Neurobehavioral abnormalities are common but their significance is uncertain.

REFERENCES

1. Olofsson Ch, Ekblom A, Ekman-Ordeberg G, Hjelm A, Irestedt L. Lack of analgesic effect of systemically administered morphine or pethidine on labour pain. *Br J Obstet Gynaecol* 1996;103:968–972.
2. Porter KB, O'Brien WF, Kiefert V, Knuppel RA. Evaluation of oxygen desaturation events in singleton pregnancies. *J Perinatol* 1992;12:103–106.
3. Garner EG, Smith CV, Rayburn WF. Maternal respiratory arrest associated with intravenous fentanyl use during labor. A case report. *J Reprod Med* 1994;39:818–820.
4. Downes JJ, Kemp RA, Lambersen CJ. The magnitude and duration of respiratory depression due to fentanyl and meperidine in man. *J Pharmacol Exp Ther* 1967;158:416–420.
5. Eckenhoff JE, Oech SR. The effects of narcotics and antagonists upon respiration and circulation in man. *Clin Pharmacol Ther* 1960;1:483–524.
6. Wilson J. Gastric emptying in labour: Some recent findings and their clinical significance. *J Int Med Res* 1978;6:54–60.
7. Austin KL, Stapleton JV, Mather LE. Multiple intramuscular injections: a major source of variability in analgesic response to meperidine. *Pain* 1980;8:47–62.
8. Lazebnik N, Kuhnert BR, Carr PC, Brashear WT, Syracuse CD, Mann LI. Intravenous, deltoid, or gluteus administration of meperidine during labor? *Am J Obstet Gynecol* 1989;160:1184–1189.
9. Robinson JO, Rosen M, Evans JM, Revill SI, David H, Rees GAD. Self-administered intravenous and intramuscular pethidine. A controlled trial in labor. *Anaesthesia* 1980;35:763–770.
10. Rayburn W, Leuschen P, Earl R, Woods M, Lorkovic M, Gaston-Johansson F. Intravenous meperidine during labor: A randomized comparison between nursing- and patient-controlled administration. *Obstet Gynecol* 1989;74:702–705.
11. Apgar V, Burns JJ, Brodie BB, Papper EM. The transmission of meperidine across the human placenta. *Am J Obstet Gynecol* 1952;64:1368–1370.
12. Moya F, Thorndike V. Passage of drugs across the placenta. *Am J Obstet Gynecol* 1962;84:1778–1798.
13. Moore J, Carson RM, Hunter RJ. A comparison of the effects of pentazocine and pethidine administered during labour. *J Obstet Gynaecol Br Commonw* 1970;77:830–836.
14. Petrie RH, Yeh S-Y, Murata Y, et al. The effect of drugs on fetal heart rate variability. *Am J Obstet Gynecol* 1978;130:294–299.
15. Shnider SM, Moya F. Effects of meperidine on the newborn infant. *Am J Obstet Gynecol* 1964;89:1009–1015.
16. Shute E, Davis M. The effect on the infant of morphine administered in labor. *Surg Gynecol Obstet* 1933;57:727.
17. Roberts H, Kane KM, Percival N, Snow P, Please NW. Effects of some analgesic drugs used in childbirth. *Lancet* 1957;1:128–132.
18. Robinson JO, Rosen M, Evans JM, et al. Maternal opinion about analgesia for labor. A controlled trial between epidural block and intramuscular pethidine combined with inhalation. *Anaesthesia* 1980;35:1173–1181.
19. Isenor L, Penny-MacGillivray T. Intravenous meperidine infusion for obstetric analgesia. *J Obstet Gynecol Neonatal Nurs* 1993;22:349–356.
20. Philipsen T, Jensen N-H. Maternal opinion about analgesia in labor and delivery. A comparison of epidural blockade and intramuscular pethidine. *Eur J Obstet Gynecol Reprod Biol* 1990;34:205–210.
21. Morgan B, Bulpitt CJ, Clifton P, Lewis PJ. Effectiveness of pain relief in labor: Survey of 1000 mothers. *BMJ* 1982;285:689–690.
22. Shnider SM, Way EL, Lord MJ. Rate of appearance and disappearance of meperidine in fetal blood after administration of narcotic to the mother. *Anesthesiology* 1966;27:227–228.

23. Beckett AH, Taylor JF. Blood concentrations of pethidine and pentazocine in mother and infant at time of birth. *J Pharm Pharmacol* 1967;19:50S–52S.

24. Moore J, McNabb TG, Glynn JP. The placental transfer of pentazocine and pethidine. *Br J Anaesth* 1973;45(suppl):798–801.

25. Gaylard DG, Carson RJ, Reyns F. Effect of umbilical perfusate pH and controlled maternal hypotension on placental drug transfer in the rabbit. *Anesth Analg* 1990;71:42–48.

26. Cooper LV, Stephen GW, Aggett PJA. Elimination of pethidine and bupivacaine in the newborn. *Arch Dis Child* 1977;52:638–641.

27. Caldwell J, Wakile LA, Notarianni LJ, et al. Maternal and neonatal disposition of pethidine in childbirth: A study using quantitative gas chromatography-mass spectrometry. *Life Sci* 1978;22:589–596.

28. Kuhnert BR, Kuhnert PM, Prochaska AL, Sokol RJ. Meperidine disposition in mother, neonate, and nonpregnant females. *Clin Pharmacol Ther* 1980;27:486–491.

29. Rosen MG, Scibetta JJ, Hochberg CJ. Human fetal electroencephalogram. III. Pattern changes in presence of fetal heart rate alterations and after use of maternal medications. *Obstet Gynecol* 1970;36:132–140.

30. Boddy K, Dawes GS. Fetal breathing. *Br Med Bull* 1975;31:3–7.

31. Zimmer EZ, Divon MY, Vadasz A. Influence of meperidine on fetal movements and heart rate beat-to-beat variability in the active phase of labor. *Am J Perinatol* 1988;5:197–200.

32. Yeh SY, Forsythe A, Hon EH. Quantification of fetal heart beat-to-beat interval differences. *Obstet Gynecol* 1973;41:355–363.

33. Jenkins VR II, Dilts PV Jr. Some effects of meperidine hydrochloride on maternal and fetal sheep. *Am J Obstet Gynecol* 1971;109:1005–1010.

34. Baxi LV, Petrie RH, James LS. Human fetal oxygenation (tcPo2), heart rate variability and uterine activity following maternal administration of meperidine. *J Perinat Med* 1988;16:23–29.

35. Belfrage P, Boréus LO, Hartvig P, Irestedt L, Raabe N. Neonatal depression after obstetrical analgesia with pethidine. The role of the injection-delivery time interval and of the plasma concentrations of pethidine and norpethidine. *Acta Obstet Gynecol Scand* 1981;60:43–49.

36. Taylor ES, von Fumetti HH, Essig LL, Goodman SN, Walker LC. The effects of demerol and trichloroethylene on arterial oxygen saturation in the newborn. *Am J Obstet Gynecol* 1955;69:348–351.

37. Koch G, Wendel H. The effect of pethidine on the postnatal adjustment of respiration and acid base balance. *Acta Obstet Gynecol Scand* 1968;47:27–37.

38. De Boer FC, Shortland D, Simpson RL, Clifford WA, Catley DM. A comparison of the effects of maternally administered meptazinol and pethidine on neonatal acid-base status. *Br J Obstet Gynaecol* 1987;94:256–261.

39. Brackbill Y, Kane J, Manniello RL, Abramson D. Obstetric meperidine usage and assessment of neonatal status. *Anesthesiology* 1974;40:116–120.

40. Hodgkinson R, Bhatt M, Wang CN. Double-blind comparison of the neurobehavior of neonates following the administration of different doses of meperidine to the mother. *Can Anaesth Soc J* 1978;25:405–411.

41. Hamza J, Benlabed M, Orhant E, Escourrou P, Curzi-Dascalova L, Gaultier C. Neonatal pattern of breathing during active and quiet sleep after maternal administration of meperidine. *Pediatr Res* 1992;32:412–416.

42. Kuhnert BR, Kuhnert PM, Tu AL, Lin DCK. Meperidine and normeperidine levels following meperidine administration during labor. II. Fetus and neonate. *Am J Obstet Gynecol* 1979;133:909–914.

43. Kuhnert BR, Kuhnert PM, Tu AL, Lin DCK, Foltz RL. Meperidine and normeperidine levels following meperidine administration during labor. I. Mother. *Am J Obstet Gynecol* 1979;133:904–908.

44. Morrison JC, Wiser WL, Rosser SI, et al. Metabolites of meperidine related to fetal depression. *Am J Obstet Gynecol* 1973;115:1132–1137.

45. Morrison JC, Whybrew WD, Rosser SI, Bucovaz ET, Wiser WL, Fish SA. Metabolites of meperidine in the fetal and maternal serum. *Am J Obstet Gynecol* 1976;126:997–1002.

46. Freeman DS, Gjika HB, Van Vunakis H. Radioimmunoassay for normeperidine: Studies on the N-dealkylation of meperidine and anileridine. *J Pharmacol Exp Ther* 1977;203:203–212.

47. Kuhnert BR, Kuhnert PM, Philipson EH, Syracuse CD. Disposition of meperidine and normeperidine following multiple doses during labor. II. Fetus and neonate. *Am J Obstet Gynecol* 1985;151:410–415.

48. Golub MS, Eisele JH Jr, Kuhnert BR. Disposition of intrapartum narcotic analgesics in monkeys. *Anesth Analg* 1988;67:637–643.

49. Hodgkinson R, Husain FJ. The duration of effect of maternally administered meperidine on neonatal neurobehavior. *Anesthesiology* 1982;56:51–52.

50. Belsey EM, Rosenblatt DB, Lieberman BA, et al. The influence of maternal analgesia on neonatal behaviour: I. Pethidine. *Br J Obstet Gynaecol* 1981;88:398–406.

51. Golub MS, Eisele JH Jr, Donald JM. Obstetric analgesia and infant outcome in monkeys: Neonatal measures after intrapartum exposure to meperidine or alfentanil. *Am J Obstet Gynecol* 1988;158:1219–1225.

52. Kuhnert BR, Linn PL, Kennard MJ, Kuhnert PM. Effects of low doses of meperidine on neonatal behavior. *Anesth Analg* 1985;64:335–342.

53. Hodgkinson R, Bhatt M, Grewal G, Marx GF. Neonatal neurobehavior in the first 48 hours of life: Effect of the administration of meperidine with and without naloxone in the mother. *Pediatrics* 1978;62:294–298.

54. Golub MS, Donald JM. Effect of intrapartum meperidine on behavior of 3- to 12-month-old infant rhesus monkeys. *Biol Neonate* 1995;67:140–148.

55. Righard L, Alade MO. Effect of delivery room routines on success of first breast-feed. *Lancet* 1990;336:1105–1107.

56. Nissen E, Widström A-M, Lilja G, et al. Effects of routinely given pethidine during labor on infants' developing breastfeeding behaviour. Effects of dose-delivery time interval and various concentrations of pethidine/norpethidine in cord plasma. *Acta Paediatr* 1997;86:201–208.

57. Rosaeg OP, Kitts JB, Koren G, Byford LJ. Maternal and fetal effects of intravenous patient-controlled fentanyl analgesia during labor in a thrombocytopenic parturient. *Can J Anaesth* 1992;39:277–281.

58. Kleiman SJ, Wiesel S, Tessler MJ. Patient-controlled analgesia (PCA) using fentanyl in a parturient with a platelet function abnormality. *Can J Anaesth* 1991;38:489–491.

59. Craft JB Jr, Coaldrake LA, Bolan JC, et al. Placental passage and uterine effects of fentanyl. *Anesth Analg* 1983;62:894–898.

60. Koehntop DE, Rodman JH, Brundage DM, Hegland MG, Buckley JJ. Pharmacokinetics of fentanyl in neonates. *Anesth Analg* 1986;65:227–232.

61. Giroux M, Teixera MG, Dumas JC, Desprats R, Grandjean H, Houin G. Influence of maternal blood flow on the placental transfer of three opioids—fentanyl, alfentanil, sufentanil. *Biol Neonate* 1997;72:133–141.

62. Steer PL, Biddle CJ, Marley WS, Lantz RK, Sulik PL. Concentration of fentanyl in colostrum after an analgesic dose. *Can J Anaesth* 1992;39:231–235 .

63. Rayburn W, Rathke A, Leuschen P, Chleborad J, Weidner W. Fentanyl citrate analgesia during labor. *Am J Obstet Gynecol* 1989;161:202–206.

64. Rayburn WF, Smith CV, Parriott JE, Woods RE. Randomized comparison of meperidine and fentanyl during labor. *Obstet Gynecol* 1989;74:604–606.

65. Rayburn WF, Smith CV, Leuschen MP, Hoffman KA, Flores CS. Comparison of patient-controlled and nurse-administered analgesia using intravenous fentanyl during labor. *Anesthesiol Rev* 1991;18:31–36.

66. Smith CV, Rayburn WF, Allen KV, Bane TM, Livezey GT. Influence of intravenous fentanyl on fetal biophysical parameters during labor. *J Mat Fetal Med* 1996;5:89–92.

67. Nikkola EM, Ekblad UU, Kero PO, Alihanka JJM, Salonen MAO. Intravenous fentanyl PCA during labor. *Can J Anaesth* 1997;44:1248–1255.

68. Lawes EG, Downing JW, Duncan PW, Bland B, Lavies N, Gane GAC. Fentanyl-droperidol supplementation of rapid sequence induction in the presence of severe pregnancy-induced and pregnancy-aggravated hypertension. *Br J Anaesth* 1987;59:1381–1391.

69. Morley-Forster PK, Weberpals J. Neonatal effects of patient-controlled analgesia using fentanyl in labor. *Int J Obstet Anesth* 1998;7:103–107.

70. Johnson RF, Herman N, Arney TL, Johnson HV, Paschall RL, Downing JW. The placental transfer of sufentanil: Effects of fetal pH, protein binding, and sufentanil concentration. *Anesth Analg* 1997;84:1262–1268.

71. Krishna BR, Zakowski MI, Grant GH. Sufentanil transfer in the human placenta during in vitro perfusion. *Can J Anaesth* 1997;44:996–1001.

72. Camann WR, Denney RA, Holby ED, Datta S. A comparison of intrathecal, epidural, and intravenous sufentanil for labor analgesia. *Anesthesiology* 1992;77:884–887.

73. Zakowski MI, Ham AA, Grant GJ. Transfer and uptake of alfentanil in the human placenta during in vitro perfusion. *Anesth Analg* 1994;79:1089–1093.

74. Dann NL, Hutchinson A, Cartwright DP. Maternal and neonatal responses to alfentanil administration before induction of general anaesthesia for Caesarean section. *Br J Anaesth* 1987;59:1392–1396.

75. Rout CC, Rocke DA. Effects of alfentanil and fentanyl on induction of anaesthesia in patients with severe pregnancy-induced hypertension. *Br J Anaesth* 1990;65:468–474.

76. Kan RE, Hughes SC, Rosen MA, Kessin C, Preston PG, Lobo EP. Intravenous remifentanil. Placental transfer, maternal and neonatal effects. *Anesthesiology* 1998;88:1467–1474.

77. Brada SA, Egan TD, Viscomi CM. The use of remifentanil infusion to facilitate epidural catheter placement in a parturient: A case report with pharmacokinetic simulations. *Int J Obstet Anesth* 1998;7:124–127.

78. Thurlow JA, Waterhouse P. Patient-controlled analgesia in labour using remifentanil in two parturients with platelet abnormalities. *Br J Anaesth* 2000;84:411–413.

79. Scott H, Bateman C, Price M. The use of remifentanil in general anesthesia for Caesarean section in a patient with mitral valve disease. *Anaesthesia* 1998;53:695–697.

80. Johnston AJ, Hall JM, Levy DM. Anaesthesia with remifentanil and rocuronium for caesarean section in a patient with long-QT syndrome and an automatic implantable cardioverter-defibrillator. *Int J Obstet Anesth* 2000;9:133–136.

81. Way WL, Costley EC, Way EL. Respiratory sensitivity of the newborn infant to meperidine and morphine. *Clin Pharmacol Ther* 1965;6:454–461.

82. Gerdin E, Salmonson T, Lindberg B, Rane A. Maternal kinetics of morphine during labour. *J Perinat Med* 1990;18:479–487.

83. Olofsson Ch, Ekblom A, Ekman-Ordeberg G, Granström L, Irestedt L. Analgesic efficacy of intravenous morphine in labour pain: A reappraisal. *Int J Obstet Anesth* 1996;5:176–180.

84. Kennell J, Klaus M, McGrath S, Robertson S, Hinkley C. Continuous emotional support during labor in a US hospital. A randomized controlled trial. *JAMA* 1991;265:2197–2201.

85. Clutton-Brock JC. Some pain threshold studies with particular reference to thiopentone. *Anaesthesia* 1960;15:71–72.

86. Dundee JW. Alterations in response to somatic pain associated with anaesthesia. II. The effect of thiopentone and pentobarbitone. *Br J Anaesth* 1960;32:407–414.

87. Keats AS, Kurosu Y. Increased ventilation after pentobarbital in man. *Surv Anesthesiol* 1957;1:473–474.

88. Root B, Eichner E, Sunshine I. Blood secobarbital levels and their clinical correlation in mothers and newborn infants. *Am J Obstet Gynecol* 1961;81:948–956.

89. Kosaka Y, Takahashi T, Mark LC. Intravenous thiobarbiturate anesthesia for cesarean section. *Anesthesiology* 1969;31:489–506.

90. Snyder FF. *Obstetric Analgesia and Anesthesia: Their Effects Upon Labor and the Child.* Philadelphia: WB Saunders; 1949.

91. Irving FC. Advantages and disadvantages of barbiturates in obstetrics. *R I Med J* 1945;28:493.

92. Powe CE, Kiem IM, Fromhagen C, Cavanagh D. Propiomazine hydrochloride in obstetrical analgesia. A controlled study of 520 patients. *JAMA* 1962;181:280–294.

93. Benson C, Benson RC. Hydroxyzine-meperidine analgesia and neonatal response. *Am J Obstet Gynecol* 1962;84:37–43.

94. Brelje MC, Garcia-Bunuel R. Meperidine-hydroxyzine in obstetric analgesia. *Obstet Gynecol* 1966;27:350–354.

95. Zsigmond EK, Patterson RL. Double-blind evaluation of hydroxyzine hydrochloride in obstetric anesthesia. *Anesth Analg* 1967;46:275–280.

96. Richter JJ. Current theories about the mechanisms of benzodiazepines and neuroleptic drugs. *Anesthesiology* 1981;54:66–72.

97. Cavanagh D, Condo CS. Diazepam: A pilot study of drug concentrations in maternal blood, amniotic fluid and cord blood. *Curr Ther Res* 1964;6:122–126.

98. Cree JE, Meyer J, Hailey DM. Diazepam in labor: Its metabolism and effect on the clinical condition and thermogenesis of the newborn. *Br Med J* 1973;4:251–255.

99. Scher J, Hailey DM, Beard RW. The effects of diazepam on the fetus. *J Obstet Gynaecol Br Commonw* 1972;79:635–638.

100. DeSilva JAF, D'Anconte L, Kaplan J. The determination of blood levels and the placental transfer of diazepam in humans. *Curr Ther Res* 1964;6:115–121.

101. Bakke OM, Haram K, Lygre T, Wallem G. Comparison of the placental transfer of thiopental and diazepam in caesarean section. *Eur J Clin Pharmacol* 1981;21:221–227.

102. Flowers CE, Rudolph AJ, Desmond MM. Diazepam (Valium) as an adjunct in obstetric analgesia. *Obstet Gynecol* 1969;34:68–81.

103. Shannon RW, Fraser GP, Aitken RG, Harper JR. Diazepam in preeclamptic toxaemia with special reference to its effect on the newborn infant. *Br J Clin Pract* 1972;26:271–275.

104. Owen JR, Irani SF, Blair AW. Effect of diazepam administered to mothers during labor on temperature regulation of neonate. *Arch Dis Child* 1972;47:107–110.

105. Dixon JC, Speidel BD, Dixon JJ. Neonatal flumazenil therapy reverses maternal diazepam. *Acta Paediatr* 1998;87:225–226.

106. Cone AM, Nadel S, Sweeney B. Flumazenil reverses diazepam-induced neonatal apnoea and hypotonia [letter]. *Eur J Pediatr* 1993;152:458–459.

107. Richard P, Autret E, Bardol J, et al. The use of flumazenil in a neonate. *Clin Toxicol* 1991;29:137–140.

108. Yeh SY, Paul RH, Cordero L, Hon EH. A study of diazepam during labor. *Obstet Gynecol* 1974;43:363–373.

109. Rolbin SH, Wright RG, Shnider SM, et al. Diazepam during cesarean section—Effects on neonatal Apgar scores, acid-base status, neurobehavioral assessment and maternal and fetal plasma norepinephrine levels. In: *Abstracts of Scientific Papers.* New Orleans: American Society of Anesthesiologists; 1977:449.

110. Schiff D, Chan G, Stern L. Fixed drug combinations and the displacement of bilirubin from albumin. *Pediatrics* 1971;48:139–141.

111. Nathenson G, Cohen MI, McNamara H. The effect of Na benzoate on serum bilirubin of the Gun rat. *J Pediatr* 1975;86:799–803.

112. Comer WH, Elliot HW, Nomoff N, Navarro G, Ruelius HW, Knowles JA. Pharmacology of parenterally administered lorazepam in man. *J Int Med Res* 1973;1:216–225.

113. Houghton DJ. Use of lorazepam as a premedicant for caesarean section: An evaluation of its effects on the mother and the neonate. *Br J Anaesth* 1983;55:767–771.

114. Crawford JS. Premedication for elective caesarean section. *Anaesthesia* 1979;34:892–897.

115. McAuley DM, O'Neill MP, Moore J, Dundee JW. Lorazepam premedication for labor. *Br J Obstet Gynaecol* 1982;89:149–154.

116. Reves JG, Fragen RJ, Vinik HR, Greenblatt DJ. Midazolam: Pharmacology and uses. *Anesthesiology* 1985;62:310–324.

117. Conklin KA, Graham CW, Murad S, et al. Midazolam and diazepam: Maternal and fetal effects in the pregnant ewe. *Obstet Gynecol* 1980;56:471–474.

118. Vree TB, Reekers-Ketting JJ, Fragen RJ, Arts THM. Placental transfer of midazolam and its metabolite 1-hydroxymethylmidazolam in the pregnant ewe. *Anesth Analg* 1984;63:31–34.

119. Wilson CM, Dundee JW, Moore J, Howard PJ, Collier PS. A comparison of the early pharmacokinetics of midazolam in pregnant and nonpregnant women. *Anaesthesia* 1987;42:1057–1062.

120. Kanto J, Aaltonen L, Erkkola R, Äärimaa L. Pharmacokinetics and sedative effect of midazolam in connection with caesarean section performed under epidural analgesia. *Acta Anaesthesiol Scand* 1984;28:116–118.

121. Camann W, Cohen MB, Ostheimer GW. Is midazolam desirable for sedation in parturients [letter]? *Anesthesiology* 1986;65:441.

121a. Heyman HJ, Salem MR. FS midazolam desirable for sedation in parturients? Reply [letter] *Anesthesiology* 1987;66:577.

122. Gal TJ, DiFazio CA, Moscicki J. Analgesic and respiratory depressant activity of nalbuphine: A comparison with morphine. *Anesthesiology* 1982;55:367–374.

123. Romagnoli A, Keats AS. Ceiling effect for respiratory depression by nalbuphine. *Clin Pharmacol Ther* 1980;27:478–485.

124. Wilson SJ, Errick JK, Balkon J. Pharmacokinetics of nalbuphine during parturition. *Am J Obstet Gynecol* 1986;155:340–344.

125. Frank M, McAteer EJ, Cattermole R, Loughnan B, Stafford LB, Hitchcock AM. Nalbuphine for obstetric analgesia. A comparison of nalbuphine with pethidine for pain relief in labor when

administered by patient-controlled analgesia (PCA). *Anaesthesia* 1987;42:697–703.

126. Podlas J, Breland BD. Patient-controlled analgesia with nalbuphine during labor. *Obstet Gynecol* 1987;70:202–204.

127. Feinstein SJ, Lodeiro JG, Vintzileos AM, Campbell WA, Montgomery JT, Nochimson DJ. Sinusoidal fetal heart rate pattern after administration of nalbuphine hydrochloride: A case report. *Am J Obstet Gynecol* 1986;154:159–160.

128. Giannina G, Guzman ER, Lai Y-L, Lake MF, Cernadas M, Vintzileos AM. Comparison of the effects of meperidine and nalbuphine on intrapartum fetal heart rate tracings. *Obstet Gynecol* 1995;86:441–445.

129. Roumen FJME, Aardenburg R, da Costa AJ, Maertzdorf WJ. Fetal bradycardia following administration of nalbuphine during labor. *J Matern Fetal Med* 1994;3:27–30.

130. Maduska AL, Hajghassemali M. A double-blind comparison of butorphanol and meperidine in labor: Maternal pain relief and effect on the newborn. *Can Anaesth Soc J* 1978;25:398–404.

131. Hodgkinson R, Huff RW, Hayashi RH, Husain FJ. Double-blind comparison of maternal analgesia and neonatal neurobehaviour following intravenous butorphanol and meperidine. *J Int Med Res* 1979;7:224–230.

132. Quilligan EJ, Keegan KA, Donahue MJ. Double-blind comparison of intravenously injected butorphanol and meperidine in parturients. *Int J Gynaecol Obstet* 1980;18:363–367.

133. Hatjis CG, Meis PJ. Sinusoidal fetal heart rate pattern associated with butorphanol administration. *Obstet Gynecol* 1986;67:377–380.

134. Atkinson BD, Truitt LJ, Rayburn WF, Turnbull GL, Christensen HD, Wlodaver A. Double-blind comparison of intravenous butorphanol (Stadol) and fentanyl (Sublimaze) for analgesia during labor. *Am J Obstet Gynecol* 1994;171:993–998.

135. Popio KA, Jackson DH, Ross AM, Schreiner BF, Yu PN. Hemodynamic and respiratory effects of morphine and butorphanol. *Clin Pharmacol Ther* 1978;23:281–287.

136. Raffa RB, Friderichs E, Reimann W, Shank RP, Codd EE, Vaught JL. Opioid and nonopioid components independently contribute to the mechanism of action of tramadol, an 'atypical' opioid analgesic. *J Pharmacol Exp Ther* 1992;260:275–285.

137. Sinatra RS, Sramcik JL. Tramadol. Its use in pain management. *Anesth Clin North Am* 1998;2:53–69.

138. Lee CR, McTavish D, Sorkin EM. Tramadol. A preliminary review of its pharmacodynamic and pharmacokinetic properties and therapeutic potential in acute and chronic pain states. *Drugs* 1993;46:313–340.

139. Prasertsawat PO, Herabutya Y, Chaturachinda K. Obstetric analgesia: Comparison between tramadol, morphine, and pethidine. *Curr Ther Res* 1986;40:1022–1028.

140. Viegas OAC, Khaw B, Ratnam SS. Tramadol in labor pain in primiparous patients. A prospective comparative clinical trial. *Eur J Obstet Gynecol Reprod Biol* 1993;49:131–135.

141. Akamatsu TJ, Bonica JJ, Rehmet R, Eng M, Ueland K. Experiences with the use of ketamine for parturition. I. Primary anesthetic for vaginal delivery. *Anesth Analg* 1974;53:284–287.

142. Janecszko GF, El-Etr AA, Younes S. Low-dose ketamine anesthesia for obstetrical delivery. *Anesth Analg* 1974;53:828–831.

143. Hodgkinson R, Marx GF, Kim SS, Miclat NM. Neonatal neurobehavioral tests following vaginal delivery under ketamine, thiopental, and extradural anesthesia. *Anesth Analg* 1977;56:548–553.

144. Kohrs R, Durieux ME. Ketamine: Teaching an old drug new tricks. *Anesth Analg* 1998;87:1186–1193.

145. Eger EI II. Atropine, scopolamine, and related compounds. *Anesthesiology* 1962;23:365–383.

146. Boehm FH, Egilmez A, Smith BE. Physostigmine's effect on diminished fetal heart rate variability caused by scopolamine, meperidine and propiomazine. *J Perinat Med* 1977;5:214–222.

147. Safer DJ, Allen RP. The central effects of scopolamine in man. *Biol Psychiatry* 1971;3:347–355.

148. Smiler BG, Bartholomew EG, Sivak BJ, Alexander GD, Brown EM. Physostigmine reversal of scopolamine delirium in obstetric patients. *Am J Obstet Gynecol* 1973;116:326–329.

149. Smith DB, Clark RB, Stephens SR, Sherman RL, Hyde ML. Physostigmine reversal of sedation in parturients. *Anesth Analg* 1976;55:478–480.

150. Telford J, Keats AS. Narcotic-narcotic antagonist mixtures. *Anesthesiology* 1961;22:465–484.

151. Gerhardt T, Bancalari E, Cohen H, Rocha LF. Use of naloxone to reverse narcotic respiratory depression in the newborn infant. *J Pediatr* 1977;90:1009–1012.

152. Wiener PC, Hogg MI, Rosen M. Neonatal respiration, feeding and neurobehavioural state. Effects of intrapartum bupivacaine, pethidine and pethidine reversed by naloxone. *Anaesthesia* 1979;34:996–1004.

153. Snyder SH. Opiate receptors in the brain. *N Engl J Med* 1977;296:266–271.

154. Kosterlitz HW, Hughes J. Possible physiological significance of enkephalin, an endogenous ligand of opiate receptors. *Adv Pain Res Ther* 1976;1:641–645.

155. Goodlin RC. Naloxone administration and newborn rabbit response to asphyxia. *Am J Obstet Gynecol* 1981;140:340–341.

156. LaGamma EF, Itskovitz J, Rudolph AM. Effects of naloxone on fetal circulatory responses to hypoxemia. *Am J Obstet Gynecol* 1982;143:933–940.

157. Young RSK, Hessert TR, Pritchard GA, Yagel SK. Naloxone exacerbates hypoxic-ischemic brain injury in the neonatal rat. *Am J Obstet Gynecol* 1984;150:52–56.

158. Hoffman EJ, Warren EW. Flumazenil: A benzodiazepine antagonist. *Clin Pharm* 1993;12:641–656.

Shnider and Levinson's Anesthesia for Obstetrics,
edited by Samuel C. Hughes, et al.
Lippincott Williams & Wilkins,
Philadelphia, © 2001.

CHAPTER 8

REGIONAL ANESTHESIA FOR LABOR AND DELIVERY

MARK A. ROSEN, M.D., SAMUEL C. HUGHES, M.D., AND
GERSHON LEVINSON, M.D.

Regional anesthetic techniques are very effective for intrapartum analgesia. They are widely promoted and recommended, and are widely accepted by parturients. Properly conducted, they are very safe in current practice. Regional anesthetic techniques provide analgesia while allowing the parturient to remain awake and participate in her labor and delivery, and provide superior analgesia to alternative methods. In contrast to parenteral or general inhalation anesthesia techniques, regional anesthesia decreases the likelihood of fetal drug depression and maternal aspiration pneumonitis, and more reliably reduces the cycle of maternal hyperventilation associated with painful uterine contractions and hypoventilation between contractions. The associated reduction in maternal catecholamines provided by complete analgesia results in improved uteroplacental perfusion, potentially most beneficial for the parturient with pregnancy-induced hypertension. Effective analgesia blunts the hemodynamic effects associated with painful uterine contractions, which may be detrimental to patients with certain medical conditions such as cardiac valvular disease (see Chapter 26) or intracranial vascular disease (see Chapter 29). Further, epidural analgesia can provide assistance with vaginal breech, preterm, or twin delivery (see Chapter 15).

The most common forms of regional anesthesia are lumbar epidural, spinal, combined spinal-epidural, pudendal, and local perineal infiltration. Other techniques include caudal, paracervical, lumbar sympathetic, and paravertebral somatic nerve block. Each technique can be used to block most of the nerves carrying pain impulses during the first or second stage of labor, or both.

PAIN PATHWAYS

The pain of labor arises primarily from nociceptors in uterine and perineal structures. Visceral afferent nerve fibers transmitting pain sensation during the first stage of labor result primarily from uterine contractions and cervical dilation, and travel with sympathetic fibers to enter the neuraxis at the 10th, 11th, and 12th thoracic and 1st lumbar spinal segments (Fig. 8.1). These fibers synapse in and make connections with other ascending and descending fibers in the dorsal horn, particularly in lamina V (Figs. 8.2 and 8.3). In late first-stage and second-stage labor, pain impulses increasingly originate from pain-sensitive areas in the perineum (pelvic floor distention, vagina) and travel via somatic nerve fibers of the pudendal nerve to enter the neuraxis at the 2nd, 3rd, and 4th sacral segments. The afferent sensory component of pain can be largely relieved by blockade of the neural pathways at several anatomic sites. The relevant anatomy of some of these regional obstetric anesthetic techniques is shown in Figures 8.4 and 8.5.

PREPARATION FOR REGIONAL BLOCKADE

Guidelines for safe patient care in regional anesthesia in obstetrics have been put forth by the American Society of Anesthesiologists and are contained in an appendix to this book. Before initiating a regional block, preparation must be made for potential complications, which could include total spinal anesthesia, systemic toxicity from local anesthetics accidentally injected intravenously, and hemodynamic or airway sequelae. Regional anesthesia must be initiated and maintained only in an area in which resuscitation equipment and drugs are immediately available. Necessary equipment includes positive-pressure breathing apparatus for ventilating with 100% oxygen, appropriate suction device, airway equipment (including oral and nasal airways, laryngoscopes, endotracheal tubes, and stylets), and drugs for managing the airway and supporting the circulation to manage procedurally related complications of the regional anesthetic administered. We suggest that a device such as the laryngeal mask airway also be readily available. We recommend that each labor room be equipped with oxygen supply and suction, and a bed that rapidly can be placed in Trendelenburg (head-down) position. The equipment that we suggest be readily available for maternal resuscitation is listed in Table 8.1.

TECHNIQUES OF REGIONAL ANESTHESIA
Lumbar Epidural Anesthesia (Figures 8.6–8.12)

Lumbar epidural analgesic techniques for labor are characterized by numerous variations of drug regimens, including those with and without local anesthetics, opioids, and/or epinephrine, and some that include other, more novel agents such as clonidine. Advocates and rationale for various regimens depend on many factors, including patient expectations, staffing and availability of anesthesiologists, and institutional expectations. Below are described techniques that are commonly used and that have been found satisfactory by the authors.

Once labor has been well established, the patient has requested epidural analgesia for pain relief, has been evaluated, and her consent obtained, and following consultation with her obstetrician, a continuous lumbar epidural block may be administered. The authors believe that epidural analgesia can be appropriate at virtually any time of labor when the parturient experiences painful uterine contractions, providing there are no medical or obstetric contraindications. In the past, epidural analgesia had been withheld until a parturient was in the active phase of labor (4 to 6 cm dilated), or was experiencing strong uterine contractions lasting 1 minute or longer at regular intervals of 3 minutes. As discussed in Chapter 3, this has been the source of considerable controversy, but there is no evidence that administering an epidural analgesic in early labor is harmful. In

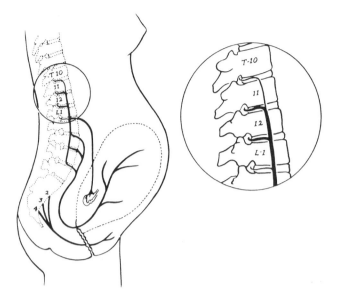

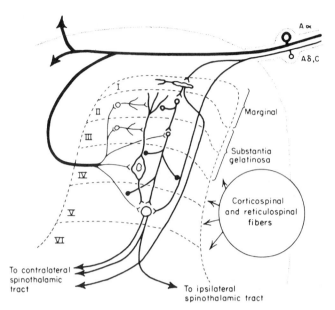

Figure 8.1. Parturition pain pathways. Afferent pain impulses from the cervix and uterus are carried by nerves that accompany sympathetic fibers and enter the neuraxis at T10, T11, T12, and L1 spinal level. Pain pathways from the perineum travel to S2, S3, and S4 via the pudendal nerve. (Reprinted by permission from Bonica JJ. The nature of pain of parturition. *Clin Obstet Gynaecol* 1975;2:511.)

Figure 8.3. A simplified model of the synaptic connections within the six laminae of the dorsal horn. Pain impulses during parturition are transmitted via A-delta and C fibers to the dorsal horn, where multiple synaptic connections are made. Descending corticospinal and reticulospinal fibers carry impulses that may modulate pain information at the dorsal horn, a possible neurophysiologic mechanism for cortical modification of afferent pain stimuli. (Reprinted by permission from Bonica JJ. The nature of pain of parturition. *Clin Obstet Gynaecol* 1975;2:501.)

fact, many parturients do not experience labor as substantially painful until the active phase.

After placement of a needle or plastic catheter in the epidural space, either a specific test dose or testing regimen (see below) must be used to rule out accidental subarachnoid or intravenous (IV) placement (Table 8.2). Analgesia is then established by injecting the local anesthetic or opioid (Table 8.3). The mother is maintained on her side to prevent aortocaval compression. If unilateral analgesia occurs, the patient is turned to the opposite

side and more local anesthetic (5 to 10 mL) is injected. With continuous infusion techniques, sufficient perineal anesthesia is usually achieved by the time of delivery and a perineal dose of local anesthetic is usually not required for spontaneous vaginal delivery. With intermittent injections, segmental anesthesia is provided during labor with repeated injections until perineal

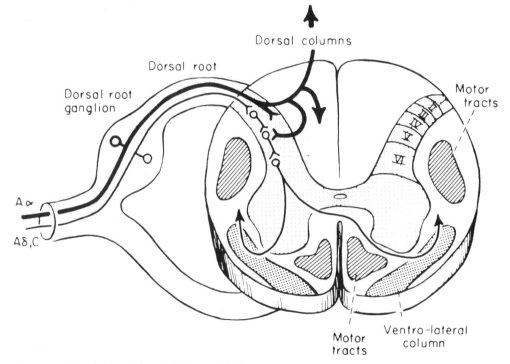

Figure 8.2. Schematic cross section of the spinal cord. A-delta and C fibers make multiple synaptic connections in the dorsal horn. Cell bodies in lamina V send axons to the ipsilateral and contralateral ventral column to make up the spinothalamic system. (Reprinted by permission from Bonica JJ. The nature of pain of parturition. *Clin Obstet Gynaecol* 1975;2:500.)

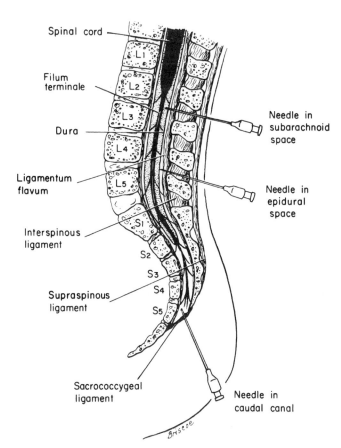

Figure 8.4. Schematic diagram of lumbosacral anatomy showing needle placement for subarachnoid, lumbar epidural, and caudal blocks.

Table 8.1. RESUSCITATION EQUIPMENT

Positive pressure breathing apparatus
Oxygen supply
Laryngoscope and blades
Endotracheal tubes: adult—6.0, 6.5, 7.0, 7.5
Stylets
Oral and nasal airways
Laryngeal mask airways
Suction catheters
Drugs: ephedrine, phenylephrine
      thiopental, propofol,
      succinylcholine
      epinephrine, atropine
      labetalol, hydralazine,
      nitroglycerin (parenteral, sublingual spray)
      calcium
      naloxone
Supplies for venous access and fluid resuscitation
Each labor room should contain an oxygen supply, suction, and bed capable of rapid Trendelenburg position.
Equipment and drugs for cardiopulmonary resuscitation (including a defibrillator) should be readily available.

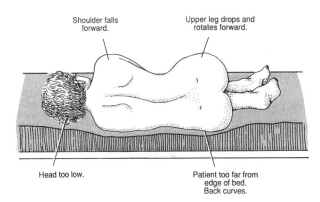

Figure 8.6. Incorrect position for placement of subarachnoid or epidural block. Shoulders have fallen forward, upper leg has rotated forward, and the patient is positioned too far from the edge of the bed so that there is no support from the edge and the back can curve.

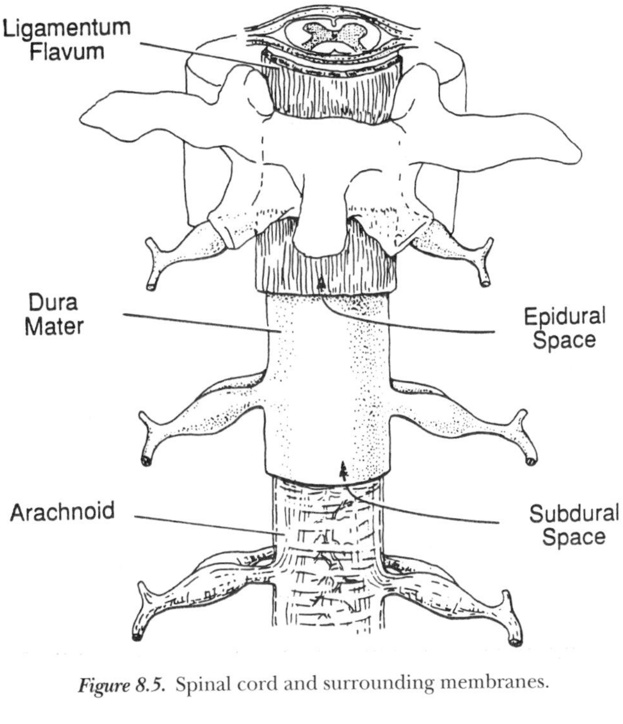

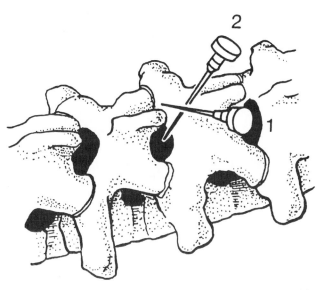

Figure 8.7. Vertebral position with patient in incorrect position. The vertebrae rotate forward, and if the needle is inserted in the usual way (1) the apophyseal joints are encountered. The direction the needle must follow is shown in 2.

Figure 8.5. Spinal cord and surrounding membranes.

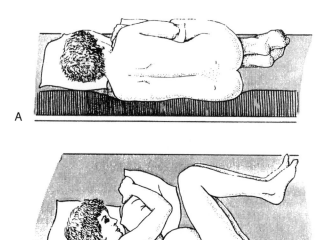

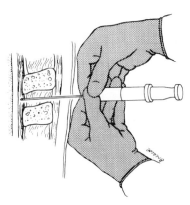

Figure 8.11. Needle is slowly advanced with both hands to prevent too rapid progression and inadvertent dural puncture. Following each incremental advance, intermittent pressure is applied to plunger.

Figure 8.8. Correct position for placement of subarachnoid or epidural block. *A*: The back is straight and vertical, shoulders are square, and the upper leg is prevented from rolling forward. *B*: Correct position viewed from above.

anesthesia is required. With perineal distention by the fetal presenting part, 10 to 15 mL of drug is administered. The authors favor either lidocaine 1.0% to 2.0% or 2-chloroprocaine 2% or 3% to produce rapid onset of profound analgesia and muscle relaxation.

Continuous Infusion Lumbar Epidural Anesthesia (Table 8.4)

Continuous infusion of low concentrations of local anesthetic with or without opioids into the epidural space is commonly used. The technique provides a continuous stable anesthetic level, avoiding the fluctuations in pain relief often found with conventional intermittent epidural injections during labor. A number of studies have suggested significant advantages to this approach (1–16). The total amount of local anesthetic injected is usually less with this technique. Because of the dilute local anesthetic solutions used, the amount of motor block is minimal. This allows the parturient greater mobility in bed. Pelvic muscle tone is maintained, possibly decreasing the incidence of malpositions, and the parturient is better able to make expulsive efforts during the second stage of labor.

There appear to be fewer hypotensive episodes during infusion epidurals (8, 10, 13), possibly due to fewer fluctuations in sympathetic block. The technique also offers advantages to the busy anesthesiologist. Without intermittent injections, there is no need for the time-consuming repeat test doses or the necessary close monitoring of the patient after a reinjection. This

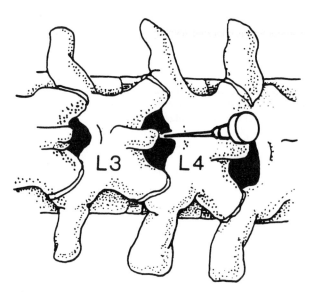

Figure 8.9. Vertebral position with patient correctly positioned.

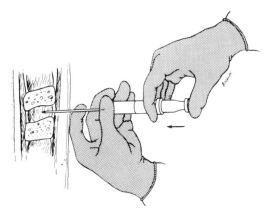

Figure 8.10. Loss-of-resistance technique for identifying epidural space. Needle is placed in interspinous ligament, and resistance to pressure on plunger of syringe is determined. Needle is stabilized with left hand, while thumb of right hand applies intermittent pressure to plunger.

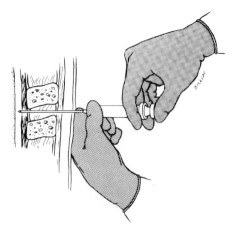

Figure 8.12. When needle passes through ligamentum flavum and enters the epidural space, there will be a sudden loss of resistance.

Table 8.2. LUMBAR EPIDURAL ANESTHESIA FOR LABOR AND VAGINAL DELIVERY: SUGGESTED TECHNIQUE

1. Evaluate patient by the anesthesiologist and obtain consent.
2. Verify that the patient has been examined by an individual qualified in obstetrics, the maternal and fetal status and progress of labor have been evaluated, and a physician is readily available to manage any obstetric complications that arise.
3. Check resuscitation equipment and oxygen-delivery system.
4. Assure adequate venous access (18-gauge plastic indwelling catheter usually sufficient).
5. Apply blood pressure cuff and check baseline pressure.
6. Administer a fluid bolus before starting block (about 500 mL balanced salt solution).
7. Position patient: sitting position (useful in very obese patients) or lateral position. Have nurse available to reassure patient, to help with positioning and monitoring, and to prevent patient movement during placement of the block.
8. Wash back with an appropriate antiseptic solution and drape the lumbar area.
9. Palpate lumbar spinous processes and choose widest interspace below L3.
10. Place an epidural needle (17- to 18-gauge) in the epidural space in the usual manner.
    a. Midline approach is most popular but lateral or paramedian approach is used by some.
    b. Loss-of-resistance technique with saline- (or air-) filled syringe most commonly used.
11. Aspirate for blood or cerebrospinal fluid.
12. Administer 3–5 mL preservative-free saline or dilute local anesthetic to facilitate passage of catheter.
13. Insert catheter and remove needle. Catheter should be threaded 3–4 cm into the epidural space (threading further may increase incidence of one-sided or single dermatome blocks; threading less makes dislodgment from epidural space more common. Note: multiorificed catheters have ports recessed 1 cm from tip). Aspirate catheter for blood or cerebrospinal fluid.
14. Administer a test dose. (See text for discussion.) Use of a 3-mL test dose of local anesthetic containing epinephrine 1:200,000 ($5 \mu g \cdot mL^{-1}$) is most common. Observe for heart rate increase within 60 sec or evidence of spinal blockade within 3–5 min. If test dose is negative, administer additional drug in divided doses as required to obtain desired pain relief.
15. Maintain patient in lateral-tilted (nonsupine) position throughout labor to prevent aortocaval compression.
16. Monitor blood pressure every 1–2 min for the first 10 min after injection of local anesthetic, then every 10–30 min until the block wears off. In some patients, more frequent assessments may be indicated.
17. During the first 20 min after the initial dose, the patient must be monitored and not left unattended. Hypotension or other sequelae may also occur after a top-up dose, and the patient should be appropriately monitored.
18. If hypotension occurs (decrease in systolic blood pressure greater than 20–30% of baseline or below 100 mm Hg), ensure left uterine displacement, infuse intravenous fluids rapidly, and, if necessary, administer ephedrine 5–15 mg IV. If hypotension persists, administer additional vasopressor and oxygen.
19. Monitor fetal heart rate and uterine contractions continuously by electronic means before and after instituting an epidural block.
20. Aspirate catheter for blood or cerebrospinal fluid before each top-up dose. Consider a test dose. Bolus doses should be fractionated.
21. After delivery, remove catheter and ensure the tip of the catheter is removed intact.

Table 8.3. DRUG REGIMENS FOR LUMBAR EPIDURAL ANESTHESIA FOR LABOR AND VAGINAL DELIVERY

1. Epidural catheter is positioned and placement verified as described in Table 8.2.
2. Initial block—options include:
    a. Bupivacaine 0.125–0.25% (10–15 mL)
    b. Bupivacaine 0.125% (10–15 mL) + fentanyl 50–100 μg
    c. Fentanyl 50–100 μg (or sufentanil 10–15 μg) in 10 mL saline (after 3-mL test dose of lidocaine 1.5% + epinephrine 1:200,000)
3. Subsequent analgesia—options include:
    a. Intermittent boluses—repeat as above, as necessary, to maintain maternal comfort
    b. Continuous infusions—10–15 mL/h
       1. Bupivacaine 0.0625–0.125% + fentanyl 1–2 $\mu g \cdot mL^{-1}$ (or sufentanil 0.1–0.3 $\mu g \cdot mL^{-1}$)
       2. Bupivacaine 0.125–0.25% without opioid
       3. Addition of epinephrine 1:400,000 (2.5 $\mu g \cdot mL^{-1}$) to either of the above
    c. PCEA
       1. Initial bolus as in 2a. or 2b. above
       2. Basal infusion—6 mL/h: bupivacaine as in 3b. (continuous infusion) above
       3. Demand bolus dose 3–5 mL: bupivacaine as in 3b. (continuous infusion) above
       4. Lockout interval: 10 min
4. If perineal anesthesia is required, administer 10–15 mL local anesthetic, lidocaine 1.0–2% or chloroprocaine 2–3%.

PCEA = patient-controlled epidural analgesia.
Note: Equipotent doses of local anesthetics, including bupivacaine, chloroprocaine, lidocaine, levobupivacaine, and ropivacaine, can be used interchangeably.

catheter. Between visits, the patient must be closely supervised by trained nurses. Staff experienced in managing possible complications of epidural analgesia must be immediately available.

A variety of infusion devices may be used. However, it is important that the device used have a number of safety features. Flow rate should be adjustable and accurate, with adjustment controls that cannot be changed by accident. The solution reservoir and

Table 8.4. CONTINUOUS INFUSION LUMBAR EPIDURAL FOR LABOR AND VAGINAL DELIVERY: SUGGESTED TECHNIQUE

1. Place epidural catheter in usual manner.
2. Use appropriate test dose regimen to rule out accidental intravascular or subarachnoid injection.
3. Start infusion at appropriate time (depending on agent used for initial block).
4. Check sensory level and adequacy of anesthesia regularly. Adjust infusion rate based on dermatomal level. Increase concentration of local anesthetic or add opioid if block is not adequate.
5. Maintain patient in lateral position throughout labor to prevent aortocaval compression. Patient should turn from side to side regularly to avoid a one-sided block.
6. Monitor blood pressure every 1–2 min for the first 10 min after initial injection of local anesthetic, then every 10–30 min during the infusion and until the block wears off.
7. Ability of the patient to lift legs should be checked regularly to monitor motor block.
8. Careful nursing supervision is mandatory.
9. Diminishing analgesia may indicate intravascular migration. A repeat test dose should be administered before any bolus injections.
10. Development of motor block may indicate subarachnoid migration. Catheter location should be verified by aspiration, careful sensory motor examination, and, if necessary, cautious administration of a test dose.

does not mean, however, that the anesthesiologist can ignore the patient following establishment of the block. To safely achieve optimum analgesia and patient satisfaction, the anesthesiologist should examine and interview the patient at regular intervals. At those times, he or she can make necessary adjustments in the rate of infusion or concentration of local anesthetic, and detect any signs of intravascular or subarachnoid migration of the tubing should be clearly and prominently labeled, and precautions must be taken to eliminate the possibility of injection of other drugs by mistake.

The potential complications of this technique are intravascular or subarachnoid migration of the catheter during the infusion, or the development of progressively higher levels of anesthesia with resulting hypotension and ventilatory difficulties. In reality, it is unlikely that serious complications would occur with the technique as outlined above. Should the epidural catheter migrate into a blood vessel, the only side effect would probably be loss of pain relief. Significant systemic toxicity is avoided because of the very low rate of infusion of local anesthetic. For example, bupivacaine 0.125% infused at 10 mL/h would only inject 12.5 mg of drug per hour–an amount that would not cause systemic toxicity.

Should the epidural catheter accidentally puncture the dura mater, the onset of motor block would be slow and easily diagnosed. During a 30-minute period, 6.25 mg bupivacaine would be infused, an amount that would prevent the patient from raising her legs, thereby alerting the staff to an intrathecal injection. If the infusion rate is too high, the slowly ascending sensory level will be easily recognized. Despite the inherent safety of continuous infusion epidurals for obstetric anesthesia, mishaps may occur if a properly trained and vigilant medical and nursing staff is not in attendance.

Spinal Anesthesia (Table 8.5)

Spinal anesthesia, often called saddle block, is administered immediately before delivery. For a true saddle block, a small dose of hyperbaric local anesthetic (e.g., bupivacaine 4 to 5 mg, lidocaine 15 to 20 mg, or tetracaine 3 mg) is injected into the subarachnoid space with the patient in the sitting position, to accomplish only sacral anesthesia. More commonly, however,

---

Table 8.5. SPINAL ANESTHESIA FOR VAGINAL DELIVERY: SUGGESTED TECHNIQUE

1. Check resuscitation equipment and anesthesia machine prior to block.
2. Assure intravenous access and administer a fluid bolus before starting block
3. Apply blood pressure cuff and check control blood pressure.
4. Position patient: The sitting position is most common. Lateral decubitus with reverse Trendelenburg may be used, especially if there is a preterm infant or a multigravida in whom fetal descent may be very rapid.
5. Prepare and drape lumbar area.
6. Palpate lumbar spinous process and choose widest interspace below L3.
7. Place needle in subarachnoid space in the usual manner. Use small-gauge (22–27), noncutting, pencil-point needle. If cutting tip (Quincke) is used, bevel should be inserted parallel to longitudinal dural fibers.
8. Inject hyperbaric solution of tetracaine, 4 mg; lidocaine, 30 mg; or bupivacaine, 5.0 to 7.5 mg immediately after a uterine contraction when the patient is relaxed and not straining.
9. Maintain patient in sitting or reverse Trendelenburg position for 30 sec, then place supine with legs in stirrups.
10. Monitor blood pressure every 1–2 min for the first 10 min after injection of local anesthetic, then every 5–10 min.
11. If hypotension occurs (decrease in systolic blood pressure greater than 20–30% of baseline or below 100 mm Hg), ensure left uterine displacement, infuse intravenous fluids rapidly, and place patient in 10- to 20-degree Trendelenburg position. If blood pressure is not restored promptly, administer ephedrine 5–15 mg intravenously. If hypotension persists, administer additional vasopressor and oxygen.
12. Following delivery and episiotomy repair, check for hypotension when the patient's legs are taken out of stirrups.

Table 8.6. CONTINUOUS SPINAL ANESTHESIA

1. Lumbar puncture is performed in the usual manner. Any approach to the subarachnoid space may be used. A standard epidural needle is placed. If the use of a microcatheter is planned, a standard 25- or 26-gauge spinal needle or a specially designed needle may be used.
2. The bevel of the epidural needle should be positioned laterally (i.e., parallel to the longitudinal dural fibers) until the dura is pierced, then directed cephalad.
3. The catheter is passed only 2–3 cm beyond the tip of the needle. This distance is sufficient to prevent accidental dislodgement but short enough to prevent curling or passage of the catheter into a dural sleeve. If the catheter cannot be threaded into the subarachnoid space, the needle and the catheter should be withdrawn together and the procedure repeated. A catheter should never be withdrawn through a needle because a portion of it may be sheared off.
4. After the catheter has been inserted, the needle is slowly withdrawn over the catheter, taking care not to simultaneously remove the catheter.
5. Aspiration of cerebrospinal fluid indicates proper placement of the catheter. With a 32-gauge microcatheter, aspiration of cerebrospinal fluid may not be possible.
6. A local anesthetic solution or opioid may be used. Drugs are usually administered in a volume of at least 1.0 mL.
7. Suggested drugs are hyperbaric lidocaine (15–30 mg); bupivacaine (2.5–7.5 mg); sufentanil (2.5–5–10 μg); fentanyl (10–25 μg); or morphine (25–100 μg). Combinations of local anesthetics and opioids are discussed in Chapter 9.

---

a T10 to S5 dermatomal anesthetic distribution is desired and can be accomplished with slightly larger doses of bupivacaine (7.5 mg), lidocaine (30 mg), or tetracaine (4 mg). Small-bore, pencil-point spinal needles will decrease the incidence of postdural puncture headache (PDPH) (17, 18).

Continuous Spinal Anesthesia (Table 8.6)

Passing a catheter into the subarachnoid space has several advantages. Intermittent doses of small amounts of local anesthetic or opioid can be administered until the appropriate level of anesthesia is achieved. This is particularly useful for high-risk patients in whom an unplanned high block may produce serious cardiovascular or respiratory problems. It is also useful in very obese patients in whom placement of an epidural is technically difficult or impossible (19). Following an accidental dural puncture during a planned epidural ("wet tap"), the anesthesiologist may choose to proceed with continuous spinal anesthesia. Routine use of spinal techniques for labor analgesia is discussed in Chapter 9 (20).

Disadvantages of the technique include an increased risk for infection and nerve trauma, although this has not proved to be a significant problem. Concern that the large-bore needle commonly used for continuous techniques would produce an unacceptably high incidence of PDPH also has not been supported by clinical studies (21–23). It has been postulated that the catheter produces an inflammatory reaction, which helps seal the hole in the dura and prevent cerebrospinal fluid (CSF) leakage, thereby reducing the incidence of headache.

Microcatheters that will pass through a standard 25- or 26-gauge spinal needle have been investigated, but experience with microcatheters is still limited. Serious questions of safety in regard to neurologic injury have been raised (24–28), and in June 1992 the U.S. Food and Drug Administration (FDA) recalled these catheters. However, there is ongoing investigation with microcatheters and opioids for labor analgesia under the auspices of the FDA (20), and if technical difficulties with insertion and maintenance of these microcatheters prove surmountable and the question of safety is resolved, the continuous technique may become much more popular.

Combined Spinal-Epidural Analgesia

Combined spinal-epidural (CSE) analgesia in labor has become a popular technique in many obstetric centers, and this approach is discussed extensively in Chapter 9. The technique combines the benefits of a spinal anesthetic, including rapid onset and near certainty of placement (CSF flow) with the benefits of epidural anesthesia, such as the use of a catheter for a continuous, potentially prolonged infusion of local anesthetics of variable concentrations as indicated. There are several sets of unique equipment provided by various manufacturers for CSE. The CSE technique can also be performed by placing a standard epidural needle in the usual manner at L3 to L4 or L4 to L5, and then placing a long spinal needle (24 gauge or smaller and 124 mm or longer) through the epidural needle to enter the subarachnoid space. For labor, an opioid such as fentanyl (10 to 25 μg) or sufentanil (2.5 to 10 μg) may be injected alone or with a local anesthetic such as isobaric bupivacaine (1 to 2.5 mg) (Chapter 9 II: Table 9.3). The administration of intrathecal fentanyl (25 μg) and bupivacaine (2.5 mg) will provide analgesia for approximately 90 minutes (range 20 to 245 minutes) (29).

Intrathecal fentanyl alone is a common choice for CSE. In one study, the median effective dose was 14 μg (confidence interval, 13 to 15 μg), and there was no benefit shown in increasing the dose beyond 25 μg (30). In another study, the mean duration of intrathecal sufentanil (10 μg) for labor analgesia was 102 ± 49.8 minutes (Chapter 9 II, Fig. 9.9) (31). However, a dose of 5.0 μg may be more appropriate. After the intrathecal dose is administered, an epidural catheter is then placed for further administration of local anesthetic for labor analgesia or instrumental or surgical delivery as needed. For labor, an epidural infusion is initiated with a bolus of bupivacaine 0.0625% to 0.125% with 0.0002% fentanyl (2 μg · mL) or an equivalent dose of ropivacaine or levobupivacaine (Chapter 9 II: Table 9.7). The CSE technique has been widely used for labor analgesia and anesthesia for cesarean section and other surgical procedures (32).

When the CSE technique is used for labor, it has the benefit of allowing maternal ambulation, if desired, and is often referred to as a walking epidural. While it is not clear that walking itself offers any real advantage (33, 34), studies suggest that it can be safely done (35–37). However, specific criteria to allow walking must be developed and followed if accidents are to be avoided (Chapter 9 II: Table 9.4) (38). Even if ambulation is not encouraged, establishing analgesia promptly with minimal initial motor blockade is satisfying to the patient and the obstetricians and nurses. The use of this technique remains somewhat controversial, and the side effects, as with any technique, must be carefully considered (Fig. 8.13) (39).

Side Effects of CSE

The side effects of the CSE technique are similar to those encountered with epidural or intrathecal opioids combined with those of spinal anesthesia. They include pruritus, nausea, vomiting, hypotension, respiratory depression, PDPH, urinary retention, and fetal heart rate (FHR) abnormalities (Table 8.7). Although there are numerous potential side effects, the most common is pruritus, which has been reported to occur in 80% of patients receiving intrathecal sufentanil (40); however, few of these patients require treatment. Hypotension occurs in 5% to 10% of patients who receive intrathecal fentanyl or sufentanil (41, 42). The incidence of hypotension is similar to that seen with routine labor epidural (Fig. 8.14) and is treated in the same manner. Nausea and vomiting (2% to 3%), respiratory depression (very rare), and PDPH (1% or less) are not common and can be managed fairly easily (Table 8.7). However, FHR abnormalities are perhaps more common. Fetal bradycardia with the CSE technique was mentioned in early descriptive studies of the technique (41, 43, 44). Three nonrandomized studies have reported that the risk of fetal bradycardia is similar after intrathecal sufentanil or epidural bupivacaine (45–47). In contrast, a greater risk of fetal bradycardia with intrathecal opioids was found compared with epidural analgesia in two other nonrandomized studies (48, 49). Two additional randomized

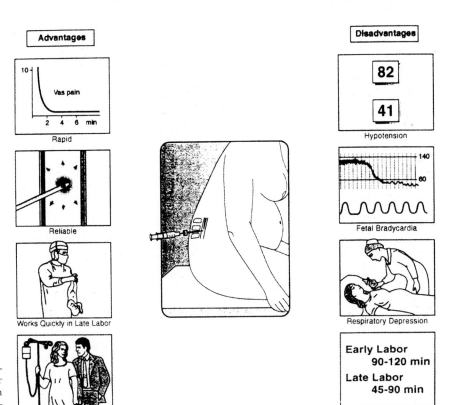

Figure 8.13. The advantages and disadvantages of combined spinal-epidural analgesia for labor. (Reprinted by permission from Eisenach JC. Combined spinal-epidural analgesia in obstetrics. *Anesthesiology* 1999;91:299–302.)

Table 8.7. SIDE EFFECTS OF INTRATHECAL OPIOIDS—COMBINED SPINAL EPIDURAL (CSE)

Problems	Treatments	Comments
Pruritus	• Naloxone 40–100 μg, IV • Nalbuphine 5–10 mg, IV • Diphenhydramine 25 mg, IV • Propofol 10 mg, IV • Droperidol 0.0625 mg (?)	10–25% may need some therapy, but few (< 5%) have severe pruritus; more problematic with intrathecal morphine; treat early if patient is concerned
Hypotension	• IV fluids, maternal positioning (LUD), and ephedrine, as usual	Occurs in 5–10% of laboring women with intrathecal opioids; probably catecholmine mediated but cause unproven
Respiratory depression	• O$_2$ as needed (ventilation rarely necessary) • Naloxone 40–100 μg or more as indicated	Rarely clinically significant but has occurred with sufentanil 10 μg (lower dose [5 μg] may decrease incidence); depression immediately or at 0.5–2 h; more common when previous opioids administered
Nausea and vomiting	• Naloxone 40–100 μg (?) • Metoclopramide 5–10 mg, IV • Droperidol 0.0625 mg, IV(?) • Other agents—ondansetron, dolasetron, propofol (also see Pruritus above)	Often hard to differentiate from obstetric causes; use lowest effective dose of opioid
PDPH	• Postpartum management as needed; epidural blood patch highly effective	Headache uncommon (< 1%); incidence similar to that with use of routine epidural technique
Urinary retention	• Catheterization • Naloxone 400–800 μg may be required for treatment	Catheterization (single time) often provides resolution
FHR abnormalities	• Maintain maternal BP, saturation, LUD • Fluids and ephedrine • Nitroglycerin (50–200 μg IV or 400–800 μg [1–2 puffs] sublingual)	Incidence unclear; mechanism not defined—sudden catecholamine changes and/or increased uterine tone implicated

LUD = left uterine displacement; PDPH = postdural puncture headache. FHR = fetal heart rate; BP = blood pressure; IV = intravenous.

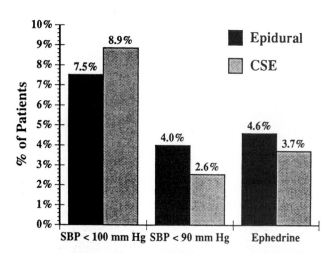

Figure 8.14. Hypotension and use of ephedrine within 60 minutes of induction of epidural or combined spinal-epidural labor analgesia. *SBP* = systolic blood pressure. (Reprinted by permission from Norris MC, Grieco WM, Borkowski M, et al. Complications of labor analgesia: Epidural versus combined spinal epidural techniques. *Anesth Analg* 1994;79:529–537.)

studies have examined this question and found similar incidences of FHR changes with the CSE technique and routine epidural anesthesia (34, 50). FHR abnormalities occur commonly during labor and have been reported to occur with IV meperidine, paracervical blocks, epidural local anesthetics, and intrathecal opioids (51). It has also been suggested that women in severe pain or with induced labor may be at greater risk for FHR changes (47, 49) and that a selection bias may be created by administering CSE to these women. This issue is currently being examined, and the clinician must remain alert to newer research findings (51). However, it is the authors' view that FHR changes are likely similar after CSE and epidural analgesia during labor, and patients must be appropriately monitored and treated. Management of FHR changes might include treatment of maternal hypotension, maternal position change (left uterine displacement [LUD]), supplemental oxygen administration, IV fluid bolus, and treatment of uterine hyperstimulation. Uterine hyperstimulation has been postulated as a possible mechanism for fetal bradycardia associated with the CSE technique (see Chapter 9). Terbutaline (1.25 to 2.5 mg IV or subcutaneously) or nitroglycerin (50 to 200 μg IV or 400 to 800 μg [2 puffs] sublingual) can be useful for treatment of uterine hyperstimulation. FHR abnormalities usually respond to this management, and in a large retrospective review the incidence of emergency cesarean sections was no different in women receiving CSE for labor analgesia compared with either no regional technique or systemic medication (1.3% vs. 1.4%) (52).

Table 8.8. CAUDAL BLOCK FOR LABOR AND VAGINAL DELIVERY

1. Prepare as for epidural block (Table 8.2).
2. Position patient: Lateral is most commonly used, but prone position with bolster under hips is also popular. Have nurse available to reassure patient, to help with positioning, and to prevent movement during placement of the block.
3. Prepare and drape the caudal area.
4. Using the coccyx as a landmark for the midline, palpate the sacral hiatus and the sacrococcygeal ligament.
5. Place a 16- to 18-gauge epidural needle in the caudal canal in the usual manner.
   a. After positioning the needle, remove drapes and perform rectal examination to exclude the possibility of inadvertent puncture of the rectum, cervix, and fetal presenting part, and subsequent anesthetic intoxication of the fetus.
   b. Change gloves, replace drape, and pass catheter through needle.
6. Aspirate for blood or cerebrospinal fluid.
7. Administer local anesthetic as for epidural anesthetic. For a T10 level, a total volume of 15–20 mL local anesthetic is often necessary.

Caudal Anesthesia (Table 8.8)

A caudal block may be administered after labor is established. Caudal blocks are performed with patients positioned either on their side (Fig. 8.15) or prone with a bolster placed under the thighs. Using the coccyx as a landmark for the midline, the sacral cornu and sacrococcygeal ligament are palpated (Fig. 8.16). The needle is then placed in the canal (Figs. 8.17 and 8.18). When a caudal block is performed late in labor, or when the fetal head is in the perineum, some recommend that a maternal rectal examination be performed to exclude the possibility of accidental puncture of the fetal presenting part and subsequent anesthetic intoxication of the fetus (Fig. 8.19) (53). After aspiration, a test dose of local anesthetic is given through the needle and/or catheter, because it is possible to puncture the dural sac that ends at the second vertebra or a dural sleeve of a sacral nerve root and produce spinal anesthesia. This is a highly vascular space as well, and inadvertent IV injection is possible. In a recent review of obstetric epidural analgesia, signs of central nervous system toxicity occurred more frequently with the caudal approach (1 in 600) than with the lumbar route (1 in 3500) (54). The volume of local anesthetic necessary to provide a T10 block usually varies between 15 and 20 mL, with subsequent doses of 15 mL to maintain analgesia. Placing the patient in a head-down position, it may be necessary to achieve a T10 block with smaller volumes of drug. Very large volumes would be needed for a cesarean section, and thus the caudal block technique is an imprudent choice except for labor analgesia.

Insertion of two catheters (double-catheter technique), a lumbar epidural catheter for labor and a caudal catheter for vaginal delivery, was popular many years ago. It permitted one to achieve a segmental block (T10 to L1) early in labor and then, at

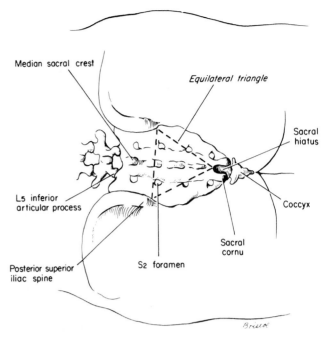

Figure 8.16. Sacrum, showing bony landmarks for identifying sacral cornua and sacral hiatus. Sacral hiatus is usually located 2.5 inches above the tip of coccyx or at the apex of an equilateral triangle formed by posterior—superior iliac spines and sacrococcygeal ligament.

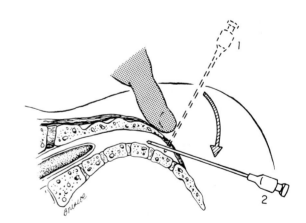

Figure 8.17. Technique of caudal anesthesia. Thumb is placed between sacral cornua at apex of sacral hiatus. Needle is inserted through sacrococcygeal ligament at an angle of approximately 45 degrees (needle position 1). Once the ligament is penetrated, the needle is repositioned as shown and advanced 1 to 2 cm into caudal canal (needle position 2).

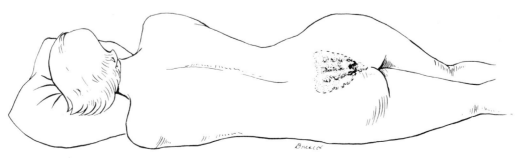

Figure 8.15. Lateral position for caudal block. Note forward tilt of upper hip. For the right-handed physician, the patient should lie on her left side.

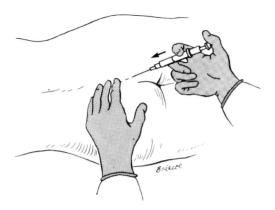

Figure 8.18. Position of needle in caudal canal verified by rapidly injecting a 2- to 3-mL bolus of saline and not palpating an impulse under the fingertips.

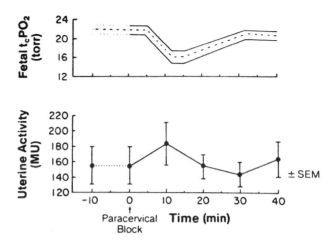

Figure 8.20. Decreased fetal oxygenation in association with fetal bradycardia following paracervical block anesthesia. (Reprinted by permission from Baxi LV, Petrie RH, James LS. Human fetal oxygenation following paracervical block. *Am J Obstet Gynecol* 1979;135:1109–1112.)

the time of delivery, by not injecting the lumbar epidural catheter but instead activating the caudal catheter, the mother would feel contractions, have maximal ability to push, and still have profound perineal analgesia. This technique is now rarely used because similar analgesia can be achieved by other techniques.

Lumbar epidural is preferable to caudal anesthesia for the following reasons: (a) segmental T10 to T12 levels can be achieved in early labor when sacral anesthesia is not required; (b) less drug is needed during labor; (c) pelvic muscles retain their tone, and rotation of the fetal head is more easily accomplished; and (d) even though there is an increased risk of dural puncture, often a lumbar epidural is technically easier for the anesthesiologist to administer and less painful for the patient during the placement of the needle than a caudal anesthetic. Caudal anesthesia administered just before delivery was recommended over lumbar epidural anesthesia in that the onset of perineal anesthesia and muscle relaxation is more rapid. However, use of the CSE technique in this setting allows for the rapid onset of analgesia with epidural catheter placement for potential surgical intervention. Thus, caudal anesthesia is rarely used today for analgesia during labor unless a lumbar epidural is contraindicated or technically difficult.

Paracervical Block Anesthesia

Paracervical block is a relatively simple method used by obstetricians to provide analgesia during labor. Local anesthesia is

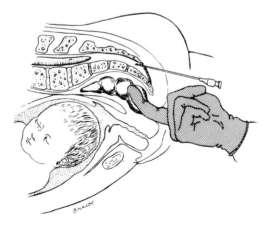

Figure 8.19. Prior to injection of medication or placement of catheter, a rectal examination is performed to rule out inadvertent misplacement of needle with rectal or fetal puncture.

injected submucosally into the fornix of the vagina lateral to the cervix. Frankenhauser's ganglion, containing all the visceral sensory nerve fibers from the uterus, cervix, and upper vagina, is anesthetized. The somatic sensory fibers from the perineum are not blocked; thus, the technique is only effective during the first stage of labor. The major disadvantage of paracervical block anesthesia is the relatively high frequency of fetal bradycardia following the block. This bradycardia is associated with decreased fetal oxygenation (Fig. 8.20), fetal acidosis, and an increased likelihood of neonatal depression. Bradycardia usually develops within 2 to 10 minutes and lasts from 3 to 30 minutes (Fig. 8.21). The etiology of bradycardia is still unclear, but evidence suggests that it is primarily related to decreased uterine blood flow from uterine vasoconstriction induced by the local anesthetic applied in close proximity to the artery (Fig. 8.22) (55, 56).

This possibly may be exacerbated by high fetal blood levels of local anesthetics (57). Fetal drug levels in infants with bradycardia are occasionally higher than simultaneously drawn maternal levels, suggesting that local anesthetics may reach the fetus by a more direct route than maternal systemic absorption. Some investigators have postulated that high concentrations of local anesthetics reach the fetus by diffusion across the uterine arteries.

Although the precise cause of fetal bradycardia may be controversial, the significance is not. Paracervical block bradycardia indicates decreased fetal oxygenation. Increased neonatal morbidity and, indeed, mortality occur when bradycardia follows paracervical block. Because of the potential fetal and neonatal hazards, the authors believe that this technique should not be used when there is known uteroplacental insufficiency or preexisting concern for fetal well-being (e.g., abnormal FHR tracing). There may be exceptions if other anesthetic techniques are contraindicated or pose a greater hazard to the mother or fetus.

When the technique is used, the drug dosage must be kept to a minimum. Safe use of this technique requires that injections are superficial (i.e., just below the mucosa), aspiration is done before injection, and FHR is monitored closely after the injection. The block is performed with the patient in the lithotomy position. A needle is placed through the vaginal mucosa just lateral to the cervix at the 3-o'clock position. After aspiration for blood, 5 to 10 mL low-concentration local anesthetic is injected. FHR is monitored continuously during the next 5 to 10 minutes. If there is no bradycardia, the block is repeated on the other side just lateral to the cervix at the 9- o'clock position with the same volume of drug. FHR and maternal blood pressure

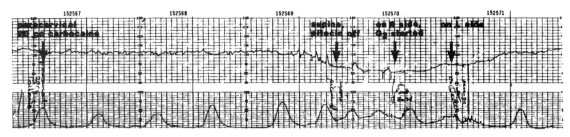

Figure 8.21. Course of fetal bradycardia induced by paracervical block. (Reprinted by permission from Parer JT, ed. *Handbook of Fetal Heart Rate Monitoring.* 2nd ed. Philadelphia: WB Saunders; 1997.)

are monitored closely during the next 10 minutes. This technique will reduce the incidence of fetal bradycardia; however, the occurrence of postblockade fetal bradycardia cannot be entirely eliminated (58). The duration of pain relief will vary from 40 minutes with 1.5% chloroprocaine to 90 minutes with 1% mepivacaine. In the United States, bupivacaine is contraindicated for paracervical block anesthesia in obstetrics. The block may be repeated at intervals depending on the duration of action of the local anesthetic. If the cervix has reached 8 cm of dilation, the block should be used with caution lest an injection into the fetal scalp occur.

Lumbar Sympathetic Block

Bilateral lumbar sympathetic block interrupts the pain impulses from the uterus, cervix, and upper third of the vagina without motor blockade, and may be used to provide analgesia during the first stage of labor. For relief of perineal pain during the second stage, a pudendal nerve block or subarachnoid block must be added.

The lumbar sympathetic block is performed at the level of the second lumbar vertebra. Using a 22-gauge, 10-cm needle, the transverse process is located; the needle is then redirected and advanced an additional 5 cm so that the tip is at the anterolateral surface of the vertebral column just anterior to the medial attachment of the psoas muscle (59). The needle is aspi-

rated in two planes to detect blood or CSF, and then following a test dose a total of 10 mL local anesthetic is injected in fractionated amounts. This volume will allow the anesthetic to spread along the length of the sympathetic chain. The procedure must be performed on both sides. Bupivacaine 0.5% will provide 2 to 3 hours of anesthesia.

Following the block, the patient must be monitored as closely as with a lumbar epidural or caudal anesthetic. Maternal hypotension may occur and is especially common with larger volumes of local anesthetic, which spreads to and anesthetizes the celiac plexus and splanchnic nerves. Systemic toxic reactions from accidental intravascular injection or accidental spinal or epidural injection also can occur. Consequently, prior to performing the block, preparations for those complications must be made. There is some evidence that lumbar sympathetic block accelerates the first stage of labor (60), and it should be used cautiously in the presence of rapidly progressive labor lest tumultuous contractions result (61). Recently, another study confirmed that lumbar sympathetic blocks are associated with an increased speed of labor compared with epidural blocks in nulliparous women whose labor was induced (62, 63).

Compared to continuous lumbar epidural analgesia, lumbar sympathetic block is technically more difficult to perform, involves more painful needle placement, and does not provide second-stage analgesia. Consequently, it is seldom performed in obstetrics. Further, few anesthesiologists have proficiency in performing this block, and the goals of analgesia with minimal motor blockade can be achieved by epidural techniques. However, it may be useful for a parturient with a history of back surgery in which successful epidural analgesia has failed or is precluded.

Pudendal Block and Local Perineal Infiltration Anesthesia

These blocks are usually administered by the obstetrician during the second stage of labor or just before delivery to alleviate the pain from distention of the lower vagina, vulva, and perineum. They are useful for spontaneous vaginal delivery and outlet-forceps and vacuum deliveries, but may not provide sufficient anesthesia for midpelvic instrumental delivery, or procedures such as repair of a cervical or upper-vaginal laceration or manual removal of a retained placenta. Pudendal nerve block also causes motor blockade to the perineal muscles and the external anal sphincter. Pudendal block is most commonly performed transvaginally. With the patient in the lithotomy position, the physician palpates the ischial spine, places a needle guide (Iowa trumpet) under the spine, and introduces a 20-gauge needle through the guide until the point rests on the vaginal mucosa. The needle is advanced approximately 1 cm, piercing the sacrospinous ligament; after aspirating for blood, 10 mL local anesthetic (lidocaine or mepivacaine 1% or chloroprocaine 2%) is injected. The technique is then repeated on the opposite side.

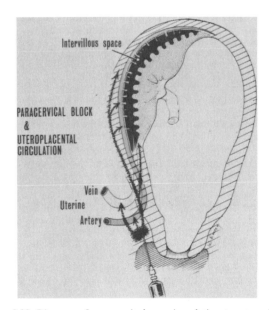

Figure 8.22. Diagram of paracervical area in relation to uteroplacental circulation. (Reprinted by permission from Asling JH, Shnider SM, Margolis AJ, Wilkinson GL, Way EL. Paracervical block anesthesia in obstetrics. II. Etiology of fetal bradycardia following paracervical block anesthesia. *Am J Obstet Gynecol* 1970;107:626–634.)

PREVENTION AND MANAGEMENT OF COMPLICATIONS

Contraindications to Epidural, Caudal, and Spinal Anesthesia

There are relatively few absolute contraindications to major conduction anesthesia. These include (a) patient refusal, (b) infection at site of needle injection, (c) hypovolemic shock, and (d) significant coagulopathies.

A specific platelet count that is predictive of a higher incidence of regional anesthetic complications has not been determined (64, 65). The decision to administer an epidural or spinal anesthetic to a patient receiving low-molecular-weight heparin (LMWH) must be made on an individual basis. The recommendations of a consensus conference of the American Society of Regional Anesthesia (66, 67) include the following: In patients receiving LMWH, needle placement should not occur for at least 10 to 12 hours after the LMWH dose. Patients receiving higher doses of LMWH (e.g., enoxaparin 1 mg · kg^{-1} twice daily) require longer delays (24 hours). If possible, epidural catheters should be removed prior to the initiation of LMWH thromboprophylaxis. If not, catheter removal should be delayed until 10 to 12 hours after a dose of LMWH. Subsequent dosing should not occur for at least 2 hours after catheter removal.

Preexisting neurologic disease of the spinal cord or peripheral nerves is a relative contraindication, but at times regional anesthesia may be in the best interest of the mother and neonate. Each case should be evaluated individually.

Test Dose Regimens

An epidural needle or catheter may be unintentionally placed in either the subarachnoid space or a blood vessel. A variety of regimens have been suggested for testing an epidural to allow the anesthesiologist to recognize this misplacement before a subarachnoid or intravascular injection of an inappropriately large amount of drug. These tests include aspiration, incremental injection of dilute local anesthetics, injection of local anesthetics with epinephrine, or injection of air. The test regimen should be safe, use readily available drugs or equipment, and ideally have a high degree of sensitivity and specificity—that is, few false-positive or -negative findings. Fulfilling these criteria is difficult, and controversy exists regarding which regimen to use.

Aspiration of the needle or catheter is the simplest way to detect intravascular or subarachnoid placement. However, there are numerous case reports of unintentional intravascular or subarachnoid injections occurring after negative aspiration (68–70).

Aspiration does not appear to be reliable with single end-hole epidural catheters (69, 71), but some claim aspiration always detects IV placement of multiple-orifice epidural catheters (72, 73). This claim has not been substantiated, and we believe a review of safety steps in epidural anesthesia correctly concluded that aspiration is not reliable as the sole test; it is specific, but not sensitive (74).

Norris et al (75). studied 1029 laboring women, using multiple-orifice epidural catheters with incremental injections of dilute solutions of local anesthetic agents and opioids. They concluded that aspiration did safeguard against the risks of unintentional IV catheter placement and that an additional test dose was unnecessary. These catheters were also tested with 2 mL plain local anesthetic to identify possible subarachnoid placement. In a subsequent study (76), these investigators again concluded that because aspiration alone detects almost all intravenously placed multiorifice catheters in laboring women, a subsequent epinephrine test dose is unnecessary. However, in their study, at least two and probably three IV catheters were not detected by aspiration alone. With slow infusion of dilute local anesthetic and opioid mixtures, if the catheter were accidentally placed into an epidural vein, regression of analgesia would probably occur before systemic local anesthetic toxicity developed. Presumably, the anesthesiologist would then recognize catheter misplacement. However, delayed recognition of a misplaced epidural catheter delays delivery of adequate analgesia to the parturient. Further, with failed recognition of a catheter in an epidural vein, if an emergency cesarean section were to become necessary, a large IV dose of local anesthetic might be injected. **Careful aspiration followed by an appropriate test dose increases the likelihood that an intravascular catheter will be detected** (77).

Currently, the most commonly used test dose is local anesthetic with 15 to 20 μg epinephrine—that is, 3 to 4 mL of a 1:200,000 solution. Since the function of a test dose is to allow recognition of either an accidental dural or intravascular puncture, a local anesthetic test dose should contain an amount of drug sufficient to rapidly produce a low spinal block if injected into the subarachnoid space and also should provide a reliable indication of an accidental intravascular injection. An accidental subarachnoid block achieved with the test dose should not exceed the upper thoracic dermatomes, and the response to an accidental intravascular injection should not produce serious toxicity to either the mother or the fetus.

Lidocaine appears to be the preferred local anesthetic for use as an epidural test dose. When 3 mL 1.5% hyperbaric lidocaine is injected into the subarachnoid space at the second lumbar level, sensory anesthesia at the S2 dermatome level occurs within 2 minutes (70).

In a study of orthopedic patients receiving either continuous epidural or continuous spinal anesthesia, 3 mL of three different anesthetic solutions were compared: 60 mg lidocaine 2%, 7.5 mg bupivacaine 0.25%, and 15 mg bupivacaine 0.5%. All three solutions contained epinephrine. Variables studied every 2 minutes over the first 10 minutes after injection included (a) presence of a sensory level $\geq$ T12; (b) presence of a motor block; and (c) anesthesia of segments L1, L2, S2, and S5. The administration of 60 mg lidocaine 2% with epinephrine produced a motor block in all patients having an intrathecal catheter 6 minutes after injection, whereas none of the patients receiving the same solution through the epidural catheter presented a motor block. This was not the case for either of the two bupivacaine solutions studied. The authors concluded that lidocaine 2% with epinephrine at a dose of 60 mg is the test dose of choice to detect the intrathecal misplacement of an epidural catheter. The presence of motor block was the most reliable clinical sign (78).

Other studies of subarachnoid isobaric bupivacaine have also shown that owing to variable time of onset and spread with doses of 8 to 15 mg, this drug is unreliable for a test dose (79–82). Similarly, ropivacaine has proven to be an unreliable agent for a test dose (83–86).

Epinephrine is the most commonly used drug for identifying intravascular misplacement of an epidural catheter. The initial study of the use of 15 μg epinephrine with local anesthetic showed that this dose, if injected into a blood vessel, would rapidly produce a transient increase in heart rate of 20 to 30 beats per minute (bpm) and usually a slight increase in blood pressure (87). Although this study tested the IV dose of 15 μg epinephrine in nonobstetric patients, similar changes occur in the parturient when an epidural vein is accidentally cannulated and epinephrine injected (Fig. 8.23) (88–90).

The time of onset to tachycardia is within 60 seconds and the duration is only approximately 60 seconds. Thus, the anesthesiologist must use either an electrocardiogram monitor or a pulse oximeter during the first minute following the test dose to determine whether an accidental intravascular injection has occurred. **In the obstetric patient, the epinephrine test dose should be injected during uterine diastole, preferably soon after a uterine contraction. A sudden and fast acceleration in maternal heart rate (MHR) of at least 10 bpm occurring within 1 minute of injection indicates an IV injection** (89). In the parturient, MHR

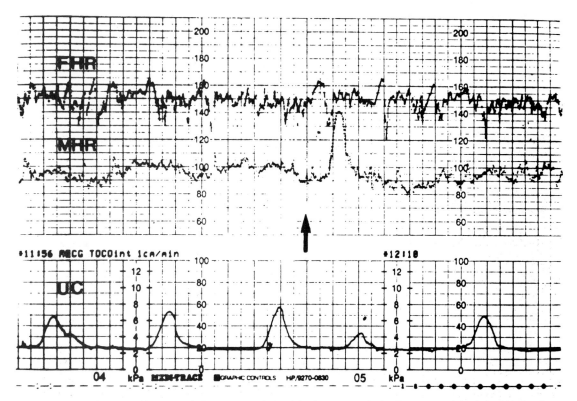

Figure 8.23. A peak increase in maternal heart rate lasting 40 seconds in a laboring woman during intravenous injection of 12.5 mg bupivacaine plus 12.5 μg epinephrine in 10 mL physiologic saline, recorded with the use of a direct electrocardiogram mode of fetal monitoring with dual heart rate capacity. *Arrow* shows start of injection. Thirty seconds is represented between each pair of vertical lines. (Reprinted by permission from Van Zundert AA, Vaes LE, De Wolf AM. ECG monitoring of mother and fetus during epidural anesthesia. *Anesthesiology* 1987;66:584–585.)

response to an IV injection of epinephrine 15 μg has an acceleratory phase of 1.2 bpm (i.e., the rate of increase in MHR is faster than 1.2 bpm for each second), which is different than the 0.69-bpm MHR acceleration induced by labor pain (90).

Although tachycardia and perhaps a modest increase in blood pressure are the two most objective signs, occasionally epinephrine in this dosage may produce other obvious signs such as acute perspiration and tachypnea, or subjective signs such as patient complaints of apprehension or unease. The parturient will often state that she feels "different," that she is apprehensive, possibly short of breath, or has palpitations or a "funny" feeling in her chest.

If uterine activity is being monitored with an intraamniotic catheter, it is not uncommon to find that the subsequent contraction is diminished in amplitude (Fig. 8.23). This occurs because the small dose of epinephrine exerts a β-mimetic effect on uterine activity. This change in uterine activity is not consistent and may be quite subtle, but when present, it is often dramatic. Criticisms of using epinephrine as a test dose to determine accidental intravascular injection in the parturient include a high incidence of false-positive (91) and false-negative (92) results, and possible adverse effects on uterine blood flow and fetal well-being (91, 93). Unlike the nonpregnant woman, the IV injection of 15 μg epinephrine into a pregnant woman produces only a 10-bpm increase in heart rate (89). This is not surprising, as the normal pregnant woman is less sensitive to chronotropic agents (94). However, patients with preeclampsia are **more** sensitive to both the pressor and chronotropic effects of epinephrine (95–97), and some are concerned that epinephrine might produce a serious adverse maternal reaction in the preeclamptic.

Epinephrine (10 to 20 μg) accidentally administered intravenously may produce a significant but very transient decrease in uterine blood flow (Fig. 8.24). This decrease in both degree and duration is similar to that which occurs with a uterine contraction during labor (Fig. 8.25). If a fetus can withstand a uterine

contraction without developing severe distress, the fetus should be able to withstand the transient change in uterine blood flow that might occur with an intravascular injection of a small dose of epinephrine. It should be noted that the decrease in uterine blood flow after epinephrine administration occurs only if the

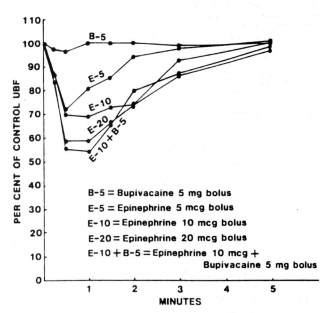

Figure 8.24. Changes in uterine blood flow in the pregnant ewe following intravenous administration of various small amounts of epinephrine and bupivacaine. (Reprinted by permission from Hood DD, Dewan DM, Rose JC, James FM III. Maternal and fetal effects of intravenous epinephrine containing solutions in gravid ewes [abstract]. *Anesthesiology* 1983;59:A393.)

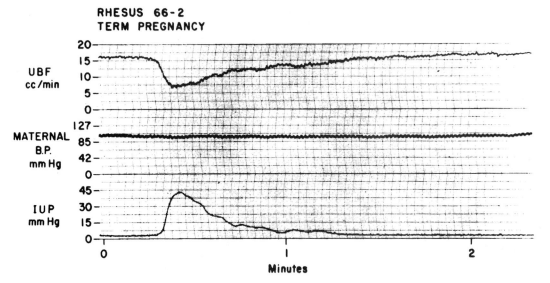

Figure 8.25. Uterine contraction in a pregnant monkey, showing the concomitant "mirror image" decrease in uterine blood flow. This phenomenon probably occurs with every contraction in every woman in labor. *UBF* = uterine blood flow (measured by electromagnetic flow meter); *IUP* = intrauterine pressure. (Reprinted by permission from Greiss F Jr. Uterine blood flow during labor. *Clin Obstet Gynecol* 1968;11:96.)

drug is injected intravenously. It does not occur with an epidural injection.

The incidence of false-positive results can be reduced by repeating the test dose when the response has been equivocal. The incidence of false-negative results is reduced if the test dose is administered between contractions, when MHR is relatively slow and stable, and if the maternal heart is carefully monitored as previously described. There are also potential problems with suggested alternatives to epinephrine. Subconvulsant doses of local anesthetics, such as 100 mg lidocaine (98) or 2-chloroprocaine (99), rely solely on the subjective responses of the mother, which may be unreliable in the anxious parturient. Furthermore, if injected subarachnoid, these doses may produce an unacceptably high block. Alternatives using doses of catecholamines that produce a greater increase in MHR without adverse effects on uterine blood flow, such as isoproterenol 5 μg (94, 100–103), involve the preparation of impractical dilutions of available drugs. The use of isoproterenol also is not recommended in an epidural test dose because insufficient animal neurotoxicology data exist.

An injection of air (1 mL) and the use of the Doppler over the heart have also been suggested (104) but have not achieved widespread popularity. Precordial Doppler monitoring, using standard external heart rate Doppler monitors, can detect air (microbubbles or a 1-mL bolus) injected through intravenously located epidural catheters (71, 104). The Doppler test has a low false-positive rate and a high positive predictive value. Thus far, no patients have developed complications from the air injection. Intrathecal injection of small amounts of air is safe; the radiographic technique of pneumoencephalography requires intrathecal injection of 20 to 30 mL of air. IV injection of air (1 mL) is probably quite safe: there are no reported cases of symptomatic air emboli following identification of the epidural space using the air loss-of- resistance technique, which is associated with a 43% incidence of precordial Doppler heart tone changes (105).

The Doppler test, however, requires a subjective interpretation of Doppler sound changes, requires additional personnel to position and hold the Doppler transducer, cannot be easily performed with the patient on her side, and precludes continuous monitoring of the fetus during injection unless a second external FHR monitor is available. The technique may be useful in selected patients in whom even small amounts of IV epinephrine are contraindicated. *Furthermore, recent studies suggest that this regimen is unreliable with multiorifice catheters* (106).

In summary, using epinephrine in the test dose provides a reasonably reliable indication of accidental intravascular placement of the epidural needle or catheter. The potential benefit outweighs the hazards of a brief decrease in uterine blood flow.

Despite confidence in the correct position of the epidural needle or catheter by a negative test dose response, as well as negative aspiration, it is still prudent to administer the total dose in fractional amounts of perhaps 5 mL, then to wait and observe the patient for at least 30 seconds between each injection.

Hypotension

Hypotension remains the most common side effect of major conduction anesthesia for vaginal delivery (107). Mild-to-moderate reductions in maternal blood pressure that do not adversely affect the mother may have profound effects on uterine blood flow and fetal well-being.

Despite an increased blood volume of 40% above prepregnant levels, the parturient at term is particularly susceptible to hypotension during major conduction anesthesia (108, 109). Partial or complete inferior vena cava and aortic occlusion from compression by the gravid uterus is present in the majority of parturients lying in the supine position (Figs. 8.26 and 8.27) (110–114). Vena caval obstruction not only impedes venous return to the heart, thereby causing hypotension (Fig. 8.28), but also increases uterine venous pressure, further decreasing uterine blood flow. In most parturients, an increase in resting sympathetic tone compensates for the effects of caval compression, and blood pressure is maintained (Fig. 8.29). However, when sympathetic tone is abolished acutely, as with spinal or epidural anesthesia, marked decreases in blood pressure may result. It is believed by many that hypotension occurs less frequently and may be less severe with epidural than with spinal anesthesia. This is likely due, in large part, to the gradual onset of epidural anesthesia, allowing time for compensatory mechanisms to modify the cardiovascular effects produced. The addition of sodium bicarbonate to local anesthetics to increase the speed of onset of epidural blockade has become increasingly popular (115). Associated with this faster onset may be a greater incidence of hypotension (116). **In general, the higher the level of sympathetic blockade, the greater the incidence and severity of hypotension**. Diminished intravascular volume—frequently found with preeclampsia, antepartum bleeding, or dehydration—may further promote maternal hypotension.

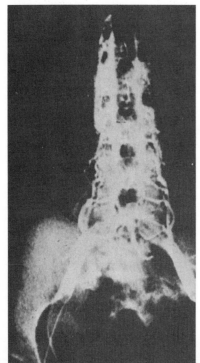

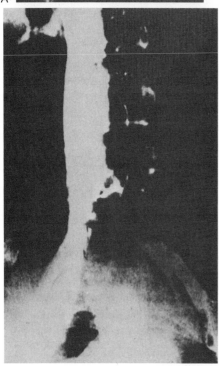

Figure 8.26. A: Venogram in the supine position just before cesarean section. Dye has been injected into both femoral veins but does not reach the inferior vena cava, traversing instead the paravertebral veins. B: Same patient just after cesarean section. The dye now easily reaches the inferior vena cava. (Reprinted by permission from Kerr MG, Scott DB, Samuel E. Studies of the inferior vena cava in late pregnancy. *Br Med J* 1964;1:532–533.)

Most parturients tolerate systolic blood pressures of 80 to 90 mm Hg without ill effects. The fetus, however, is highly sensitive to decreased maternal arterial blood pressure. In contrast to other vital organs, with acute decreases in maternal blood pressure, there is no autoregulation of blood flow to the uterus. With spinal- or epidural-induced hypotension, uterine blood flow decreases linearly with blood pressure (117–119).

The fetal consequences of the reduced uterine blood flow depend on the degree and duration of the fall and the preexisting status of the uteroplacental circulation. When uterine blood flow is inadequate, fetal asphyxia will develop (120–124). The precise degree and duration of hypotension necessary to cause fetal distress seems to be variable. Conduction anesthesia producing a maternal systolic blood pressure of less than 70 mm Hg consistently produced sustained fetal bradycardia (125). When maternal systolic blood pressure was between 70 and 80 mm Hg for 4 minutes or longer, some fetuses developed sustained bradycardia. With maternal systolic blood pressure less than 100 mm Hg for about 5 minutes, abnormal FHR patterns developed (126, 127). A systolic pressure of less than 100 mm Hg for 10 to 15 minutes may lead to fetal acidosis and bradycardia (128). **In all these studies, FHR returned to normal with correction of hypotension.** Moya and Smith (129) reported an increased incidence of low Apgar scores when maternal systolic blood pressure decreased to between 90 and 100 mm Hg for longer than 15 minutes (Fig. 8.30). Women who had even greater decreases in blood pressure, but were promptly treated, delivered vigorous neonates.

Several investigators (130–132) have shown that when the hypotension (defined as a systolic blood pressure lower than 100 mm Hg or a greater than 30% decrease from baseline) associated with regional anesthesia is promptly corrected, it has no effect on the clinical condition of the newborn as assessed by Apgar score at 1 and 5 minutes of age, or the Neurologic Adaptive Capacity Score (NACS) at 15 minutes, 2 hours, and 24 hours of age (132). However, hypotension does appear to be associated with an increase in base deficit and a decrease in pH in umbilical cord blood. These changes are small (pH value change of 0.02 to 0.04 with epidural and slightly greater with spinal hypotension) and thought to be of little clinical significance. In summary, hypotension is best prevented. Systolic blood pressures of less than 100 mm Hg in a previously normotensive parturient are usually treated. In the hypertensive patient, a decrease of 20% to 30% of her control blood pressure probably should be treated.

Several preventive measures can be taken to minimize the incidence and severity of hypotension following conduction anesthesia in obstetrics. For routine spinal or epidural blocks for labor and vaginal delivery, the following measures commonly have been recommended:

1. IV infusion of 500 mL of balanced, non–dextrose-containing solution administered within 30 minutes of a low epidural or saddle block (dermatome level of T10). A modest amount of volume preload does not appear to be harmful and may make significant decreases in maternal blood pressure less likely, less precipitous, or easier to treat with vasopressors. It should be noted that several studies have questioned the value of volume preloading with crystalloid in preventing hypotension (133), even with spinal anesthesia for cesarean section (134, 135). To effectively prevent the hypotension associated with a sympathetic block, IV volume administration must produce a large enough increase in blood volume to result in a significant increase in cardiac output (136). Sufficient amounts of IV crystalloid administered rapidly produce an increase in cardiac filling pressures; however, the intravascular half-life is short and this increase is quickly reversed after the onset of sympathetic blockade (137, 138). It also has been demonstrated that a fluid bolus during labor may produce a transient decrease in the frequency of uterine contractions (139, 140). This transient decrease (about 20 minutes) was found to occur with rapid administration of 1000 mL crystalloid but not with 500 mL. In both of these studies, hydration of 500 or 1000 mL did not further decrease the low incidence of hypotension.

Although dextrose-containing solutions may be useful in reducing maternal ketosis (141), they are undesirable

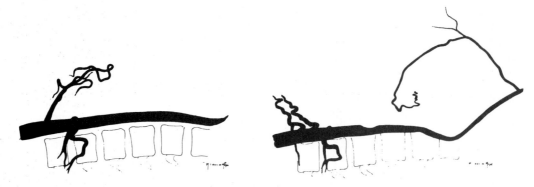

Figure 8.27. Schematic of lateral angiograms obtained from two women lying in the supine position. In the nonpregnant woman (*left*) there is a clear gap between the vertebral column and the aorta. Note the uniform width of the aorta. In the pregnant patient near term (*right*), the aorta is clearly displaced in the dorsal direction, encroaching on the shadow of the spine. The aorta is narrowed at the level of the lumbar lordosis. (Reprinted by permission from Bieniarz J, Crottogini JJ, Curuchet E, et al. Aortocaval compression by the uterus in late human pregnancy. *Am J Obstet Gynecol* 1978;100:203–217.)

in the large volumes required for acute IV loading prior to regional anesthesia. Adverse effects include maternal hyperglycemia (often associated with an osmotic diuresis), fetal hyperglycemia, and subsequent neonatal hyperinsulinemia and hypoglycemia (142–144). Evidence indicating hyperglycemia increases the brain's susceptibility to anoxic injury is further cause for avoiding hyperglycemia during labor and delivery (145).

2. Vasopressor prophylaxis is not recommended for epidural or spinal analgesia for labor. The frequency of hypotension is not great, and when it does occur, it is usually mild and easily treated. Furthermore, placental transfer

of ephedrine may increase FHR and variability, making interpretation of the FHR tracing during labor more difficult (Figs. 8.31 and 8.32) (146).

3. Continuous LUD should be applied to minimize aortocaval compression. Aortocaval compression results in changes in uteroplacental blood flow, which can be deleterious to the fetus. During labor, fetal oxygen saturation can rapidly decrease when a mother assumes the supine position, even in the absence of maternal hypotension or hypoxemia (147). During the second stage of labor, a time-related decrease in fetal pH has been reported when the mother is delivered in the supine lithotomy position.

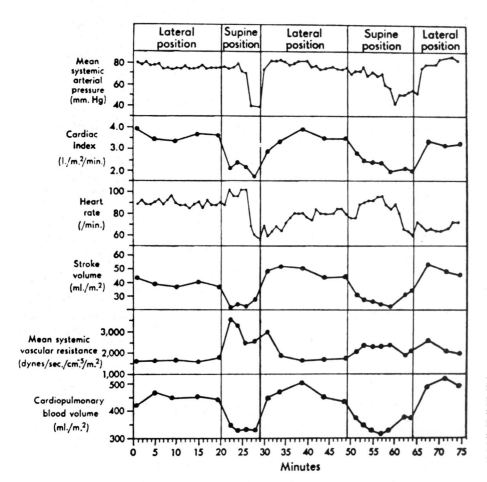

Figure 8.28. Serial hemodynamic studies in a patient who exhibited supine hypotension. After the patient was lying supine for 6 minutes, a profound fall in arterial pressure and pulse rate was seen. (Reprinted by permission from Kerr MG. Cardiovascular dynamics in pregnancy and labour. *Br Med Bull* 1968;24:19–24.)

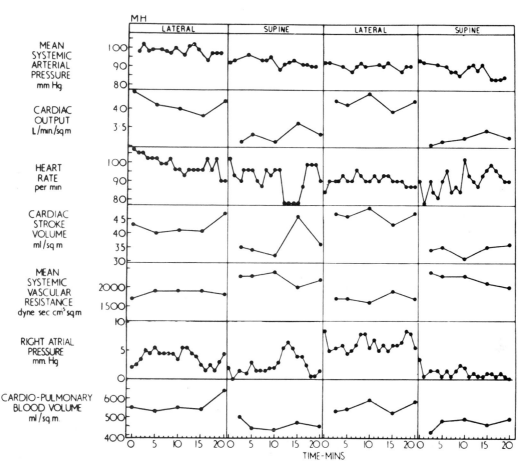

Figure 8.29. Hemodynamic parameters in a patient during late pregnancy who developed a reduced cardiac output in the supine position. The patient was asymptomatic. Note that the changes could be reproduced by turning the patient a second time. (Reprinted by permission from Scott DB. Inferior vena caval occlusion in late pregnancy. In: Marx GF, ed. *Parturition and Perinatology.* Philadelphia: Davis; 1973:42.)

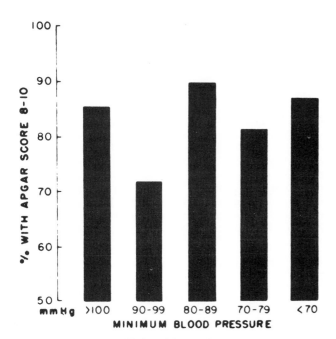

Figure 8.30. In a series of babies delivered by cesarean section under spinal anesthesia, maternal systolic blood pressures below 90 mm Hg were treated immediately. Mothers with systolic blood pressures between 90 and 99 mm Hg were not considered to be hypotensive and were not treated. Note that even this mild degree of hypotension, when uncorrected, resulted in neonatal depression. (Reprinted by permission from Lichtiger M, Moya F. In: Lichtiger M, ed. *Introduction to the Practice of Anesthesia.* Hagerstown, MD: Harper & Row; 1974:313.)

This fetal acidosis is not seen if the mother is tilted to the left (148). Laboring patients should remain in the lateral or semilateral position.

4. Frequent monitoring of arterial blood pressure is mandatory after institution of epidural or spinal analgesia for labor. This will allow early recognition and prompt therapy of hypotension.

Therapy for epidural or spinal hypotension includes more LUD, rapid fluid infusion, the Trendelenburg position to increase venous return, IV ephedrine, and oxygen administration. Administration of oxygen to the mother may not necessarily raise the fetal Pao$_2$ until the hypotension is corrected. After spinal hypotension in pregnant ewes, fetal Pao$_2$ returned to normal only after maternal arterial blood pressure was restored (Fig. 8.33) (149).

In general, it appears that vasopressors with a mixture of both α- and β-adrenergic activity exert as much, if not more, effect on venous capacitance as arteriolar resistance. As a result, they restore blood pressure to a large extent by increasing venous return to the heart (cardiac preload) and cardiac output. Pure α-adrenergic agents, on the other hand, work mostly on the arterioles and, when used to treat spinal hypotension, will not return cardiac output or vital organ blood flow to preanesthetic values (150). Studies in pregnant sheep made hypotensive with spinal anesthesia show that ephedrine, mephentermine, and metaraminol–vasopressors with mixed α-and β-adrenergic activity–returned uterine blood flow toward control while restoring maternal arterial blood pressure (149, 151). Fetal deterioration was, in fact, arrested and often reversed (149). In sheep, vasopressors with primarily peripheral

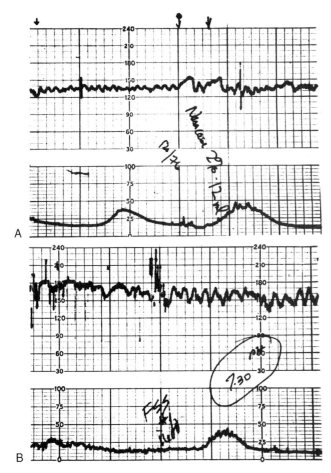

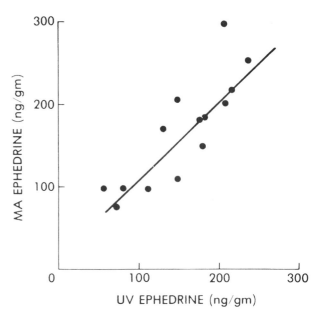

Figure 8.32. The plot of ephedrine levels in maternal arterial blood (*MA*) against levels in umbilical-cord venous blood (*UV*) in ng/g plasma. The R value is 0.73. The equation for the regression line is: y = 30.9 + 0.73x. (Reprinted by permission from Hughes SC, Ward MG, Levinson G, et al. Placental transfer of ephedrine does not affect neonatal outcome. *Anesthesiology* 1985;63:217–219.

Figure 8.31. *A*: Epidural administration of 240 mg chloroprocaine (Nesacaine). Baseline fetal heart rate is approximately 135 beats per minute. *B*: Fetal tachycardia and marked increase in heart rate variability (saltatory pattern) in the same patient as in *A*. The tracing was obtained approximately 1 hour after ephedrine therapy (10 mg intravenous, 25 mg intramuscular) for mild epidural hypotension. The fetal scalp blood pH at this time was 7.3. (Reprinted by permission from Wright RG, Shnider SM, Levinson G, Rolbin SH, Parer JT. The effect of maternal administration of ephedrine on fetal heart rate and variability. *Obstet Gynecol* 1981;57:734–738.)

α-adrenergic action (such as methoxamine or phenylephrine) were harmful to the fetus because they produced further uterine vasoconstriction (152, 153).

Despite numerous animal studies demonstrating adverse effects of α-adrenergic agents in obstetrics, several investigators (154–158) have compared the safety and efficacy of ephedrine and phenylephrine in the treatment of maternal hypotension associated with regional anesthesia for cesarean section. Healthy women undergoing elective cesarean section under either epidural or spinal anesthesia were prehydrated with IV crystalloid. Decreases in blood pressure were promptly treated with small IV doses of either ephedrine or phenylephrine. Phenylephrine produced no adverse neonatal effects as assessed by umbilical cord blood gases or Apgar scores. In one study, mean umbilical artery pH was higher in the phenylephrine group than in the ephedrine group (158). Uterine blood flow was not measured in these studies. However, maternal stroke volume and end-diastolic volume did not differ following ephedrine or phenylephrine therapy, indicating that for these conditions and drug dosages, both ephedrine and phenylephrine worked by augmenting venous return (Fig. 8.34).

Despite these studies, we believe that ephedrine is the vasopressor of choice for the treatment of anesthesia-induced hypotension in obstetrics. It is clearly superior in most animal studies and has a long record of safety in clinical obstetrics. Even if excessive doses are administered, it appears to be safe. In a study of the prophylactic administration of vasopressors in pregnant ewes (159), ephedrine or mephentermine in doses sufficient to raise the mean arterial blood pressure 40% to 50% above control values had no significant effects on uterine blood flow (Chapter 2: Fig. 2.18). Although ephedrine may cross the placenta and has been reported to increase FHR and beat-to-beat variability, no adverse fetal or neonatal effects have been noted (146, 160).

Nevertheless, in clinical situations in which the parturient may not tolerate ephedrine's potential β-mimetic effects or when ephedrine is ineffective, phenylephrine is an acceptable alternative.

In a classic study published in 1969, Marx et al (161). found better fetal biochemical and neonatal clinical conditions when spinal hypotension was prevented rather than treated. However, direct application of these results to today's practice should be made with caution because preventive measures for and treatment of hypotension have changed significantly since that time. Other investigators (130–132, 162) have demonstrated no significant difference in Apgar scores or blood gases between neonates of mothers who become hypotensive and those who do not, provided hypotension is detected early and treated quickly.

Local Anesthetic Convulsions

Central nervous system toxicity occurs when a critical brain tissue concentration of local anesthetic is exceeded. These excessive brain tissue concentrations are almost invariably associated with high blood levels that result from accidental intravascular injection, accumulation of local anesthetic during repeated injections over a prolonged period of time, or rapid systemic absorption of local anesthetic from a highly vascular area. The rate of administration, the total dose of drug, and the physical status of the patient affect tolerance to local anesthetics (163). Accidental intravascular injection may occur with any regional anesthetic technique, including paracervical and pudendal blocks (164). Therefore, when a needle or catheter is placed, a test

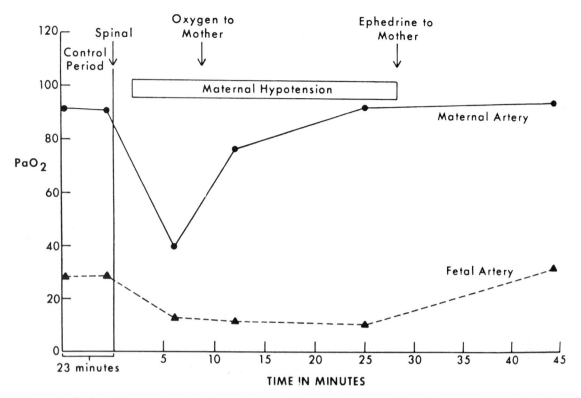

Figure 8.33. Changes in fetal arterial oxygen tension after maternal spinal hypotension, maternal hypoxia, oxygen administration, then ephedrine administration to the mother. (Reprinted by permission from Shnider SM, deLorimier AA, Holl JW, Chapler FK, Morishima HO. Vasopressors in obstetrics. I. Correction of fetal acidosis with ephedrine during spinal hypotension. *Am J Obstet Gynecol* 1968;102:911–919.)

regimen should be used (described earlier) to include aspiration of the catheter to determine whether a blood vessel has been entered before drug injection (76). When local anesthetics are injected, particularly large volumes of concentrated local anesthetics (e.g., for cesarean section), they should be administered in divided (fractionated) doses while observing for signs of systemic toxicity and the onset of spinal anesthesia.

The elimination half-life of amide local anesthetics is 2 to 3 hours. Therefore, systemic accumulation of amide local anesthetics to near-toxic levels may occur with large doses repeated at frequent intervals. During properly conducted regional anesthesia, toxic concentrations of local anesthetics resulting from absorption are rarely seen (54, 163, 165). The current use of more dilute local anesthetics for labor analgesia further reduces this risk.

The reported incidence of convulsions during obstetric regional anesthesia varies widely from 0% to 0.5% (54, 166–172). In more recent reports, convulsions due to local anesthetic tox-

icity have become increasingly rare, with an incidence of 1 in 5000 to 9000 (173–175). A prospective review of 10,995 epidural blocks placed either for labor analgesia (n = 7648) or cesarean section (n = 3311) revealed no convulsions but four cases of minor central nervous system toxicity (tinnitus, visual disturbance, slurred speech, altered conscious state) (54). Three of these cases occurred following injection via a lumbar epidural (1 in 3500; 0.03%), and the other followed a caudal anesthetic (1 in 600; 0.17%). Thus, the caudal approach may confer a higher risk of toxicity.

While careful technique, including regimens to test epidural catheter placement, has reduced the incidence of convulsions, in a review of the American Society of Anesthesiology's Closed Claims Project database, convulsions were the primary damaging event in the obstetric anesthesia files. Convulsions were associated with epidural anesthesia in 85% of the cases reviewed (i.e., those cases that resulted in legal action), and 76% of these appeared to be due to local anesthetic toxicity. In the

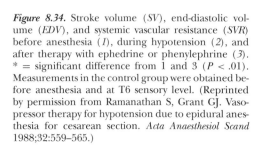

Figure 8.34. Stroke volume (*SV*), end-diastolic volume (*EDV*), and systemic vascular resistance (*SVR*) before anesthesia (*1*), during hypotension (*2*), and after therapy with ephedrine or phenylephrine (*3*). * = significant difference from 1 and 3 (*P* < .01). Measurements in the control group were obtained before anesthesia and at T6 sensory level. (Reprinted by permission from Ramanathan S, Grant GJ. Vasopressor therapy for hypotension due to epidural anesthesia for cesarean section. *Acta Anaesthesiol Scand* 1988;32:559–565.)

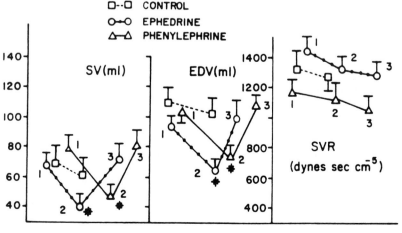

Table 8.9. SIGNS AND SYMPTOMS OF LOCAL ANESTHETIC–INDUCED SYSTEMIC TOXICITY

Central nervous system
  Cerebral cortex
    Stimulation—restlessness, nervousness, incoherent speech, metallic taste, dizziness, blurred vision, tremors, and convulsions
    Depression—unconsciousness
  Medulla
    Stimulation—increased blood pressure, heart and respiratory rate, nausea, and vomiting
    Depression—hypotension, apnea, and asystole
Cardiovascular
  Heart—bradycardia, ventricular tachycardia and fibrillation, decreased contractility
  Blood vessels—vasodilation and hypotension
Uterus
  Uterine vasoconstriction and uterine hypertonus resulting in fetal distress

cases reviewed for which convulsion was listed as the primary damaging event, the outcome was neurologic injury or death to the mother, newborn, or both in 74% of the cases (176). In all probability, in most clinical circumstances of convulsions associated with obstetric regional anesthesia, prompt recognition and treatment usually results in full recovery of the mother and fetus. While the number of claims involving convulsions in the United States has decreased since 1984 (176) and the incidence of convulsions was reported as 0% recently in a prospective review from Australia (54), this remains a significant potential complication. The toxicity of local anesthetics, including the cardiotoxicity of bupivacaine, is discussed in Chapter 5. A summary of the signs and symptoms of local anesthetic toxic reactions is shown in Table 8.9.

Treatment involves:

Early recognition of the reaction. By constant observation of the patient and her vital signs and by talking to her, it is possible to become aware of the impending toxic reaction and to take steps to prevent it from becoming serious.

Prevention of progression of the reaction. Small doses of barbiturates given intravenously may prevent convulsions. The depressant effect of the barbiturate may intensify the depression that results from the local anesthetic, but small doses of thiopental (Pentothal®50 to 100 mg), diazepam (Valium®5 mg), or midazolam (Versed®1 to 2 mg), repeated as needed, are probably safe. At the same time, oxygen should be given by a mask so that the patient is well oxygenated should a convulsion occur.

Maintenance of oxygenation despite convulsions and/or vomiting. Convulsions are not lethal, but the anoxia and acidosis that they produce may be. The airway should be cleared of foreign material and the patient ventilated with 100% oxygen with a positive-pressure breathing apparatus. At times, ventilating the unparalyzed—convulsing patient may be difficult and it may be necessary to paralyze her with succinylcholine (80 to 100 mg). Tracheal intubation with a cuffed endotracheal tube to facilitate ventilation and/or protect the airway from aspiration may also be necessary.

Support of the circulation. Elevation of the legs, displacement of the uterus off the vena cava and aorta, and rapid administration of IV fluids and vasopressors (ephedrine, initially) may be needed to support the depressed circulation.

Treatment of cardiac arrest. Cardiac arrest should be treated using standard advanced cardiac life-support (ACLS) protocols. Appropriate equipment and medication should be immediately available in the labor and delivery unit (64). LUD should be maintained if possible. Delivery of the fetus, by relieving vena caval obstruction, may facilitate cardiopulmonary resuscitation (CPR) (177). The American Heart Association has stated: "Several authors now recommend that the decision to perform a peripartum cesarean section should be made rapidly with

delivery effected within 4 to 5 minutes of the arrest" (178). While an emergency cesarean section has the best chance of improving the outcome for the mother and newborn, this decision must be considered carefully, to include (a) the differential diagnosis of cardiac arrest, (b) the age of the fetus, and (c) the availability of equipment and supplies (179).

Consideration of the fetus. As soon as possible after the convulsion, the condition of the fetus should be assessed to decide the subsequent course of delivery. Prompt maternal resuscitation will usually restore uterine blood flow and fetal oxygenation, allow fetal excretion of local anesthetic to the mother via the placenta, and obviate the need for emergent cesarean section (180).

Total Spinal

Total spinal anesthesia may occur from an excessive spread of local anesthetic administered intrathecally, extradurally, or subdurally (potential space between dura mater and arachnoid mater). Dural perforation by an epidural catheter may occur when the catheter is initially inserted or during the course of a previously uneventful, continuous epidural anesthetic by migration of the catheter (174, 181). A total or high spinal may lead to profound hypotension, dyspnea, inability to speak, and ultimately a loss of consciousness. The subdural space has been referred to as the "third space to go astray" and also can lead to a total spinal (182). Acute, life-threatening respiratory depression has been reported after an opioid was injected through an epidural catheter placed and initially used successfully as part of a CSE for cesarean section (183). The catheter appears to have migrated subdurally in the postoperative period. While placement of an epidural catheter during the CSE technique seems extremely safe, accidental intrathecal insertion of an epidural catheter is possible, as well as migration of a catheter, and thus the catheter must always be tested to rule out this rare but real possibility (184). Paech et al. reported eight unexpectedly high blocks in 10,995 epidurals in obstetric patients (1 in 1400; 0.07%), only two of which required tracheal intubation (1 in 5500; 0.02%) (54).

Subdural injection of a local anesthetic leads to an unexpectedly high but patchy block (182, 185). A subdural block has a variable spread that ultimately is quite extensive for the volume of local anesthetic injected. It is often a patchy block, has a delayed onset, and has a relatively mild motor block (186). The subdural space is the potential space between the dura mater and the arachnoid mater and extends intracranially so that the cranial nerves may be involved. A retrospective review in nonobstetric patients suggested that the incidence of subdural injection may be as high as 0.82%. However, this has not been the authors' experience (187).

Although infrequent, the possibility of total spinal anesthesia necessitates the immediate presence of personnel who can promptly diagnose and treat this complication, with immediate availability of necessary equipment. Treatment consists of establishing an airway, ventilation with oxygen, and provision of cardiovascular support. Tracheal intubation should be performed as soon as possible to protect the airway from aspiration. A total spinal block will not necessarily produce relaxation of the jaw muscles, and succinylcholine may be required for intubation. The Trendelenburg position and LUD should be used to increase venous return to the heart. Fluids and ephedrine should be administered as necessary to maintain blood pressure. If a large dose of local anesthetic accidentally has been injected intrathecally following management of the patient's airway, ventilation and circulation consideration should be given to performing another lumbar puncture and draining CSF.

Severe bradycardia progressing to cardiac asystole has been reported in young healthy patients not premedicated with atropine (188–190). Decreases in heart rate to less than 60 bpm should be promptly treated by increasing venous return and, if necessary, by promptly administering atropine and/or

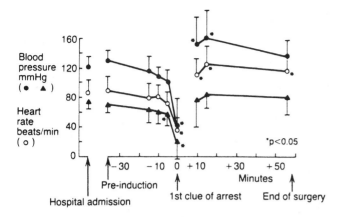

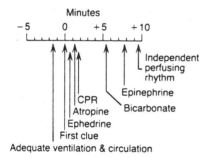

Figure 8.35. Composite display of vital signs (*upper graph*) and key events (*lower graph*) in 14 cases of cardiac arrest during spinal anesthesia. Events are shown in relation to the first clue of impending cardiac arrest (located at 0 minutes on the time scale). The values for systolic blood pressure (*closed circles*), diastolic blood pressure (*closed triangles*), and heart rate (*open circles*) are mean ± SD. *P < .05 vs. hospital admission values. (Reprinted by permission from Caplan RA, Ward RJ, Posner K, Cheney FW. Unexpected cardiac arrest during spinal anesthesia: A closed claims analysis of predisposing factors. *Anesthesiology* 1988;68:5–11.)

ephedrine. If conventional doses of atropine or ephedrine are not effective, IV epinephrine should be administered (190).

In cases of **cardiac arrest** associated with high spinal anesthesia, poor neurologic outcome has been reported with routine (basic) CPR (190). Of the 14 healthy patients who suffered cardiac arrest during spinal anesthesia, bradycardia was the first sign in 7 (50%). While all patients were resuscitated after cardiac arrest, six suffered neurologic injury and died in the hospital. Of the eight survivors, only one recovered to perform routine daily self-care. It is believed that a high sympathetic blockade allows increased peripheral blood flow during CPR and prevents the usual preferential perfusion of the brain. In the cases cited by Caplan, epinephrine was not administered for about 8 minutes (average) after the onset of asystole. Epinephrine should be given "early" in the management of sudden bradycardia (Fig. 8.35). It is speculated that early administration of epinephrine may improve cerebral perfusion during CPR and decrease the high incidence of neurologic damage that occurs in these circumstances. It is recommended that a full resuscitation dose of epinephrine be given immediately upon recognition of cardiac arrest during a spinal or epidural anesthetic (190, 191).

Underlying, undiagnosed medical problems also must be considered in these circumstances. In a case report of cardiac arrest that occurred during spinal anesthesia for cesarean section, a cardiomyopathy was ultimately diagnosed (192). Prompt endotracheal intubation, delivery of the infant, CPR that included epinephrine (1 mg IV) and atropine, as well as an epinephrine infusion and intensive care management, led to a good recovery of the mother and newborn in this case. Thus, concomitant medical problems also must be considered, as well as a differential diagnosis that includes anaphylactic shock, eclampsia,

amniotic fluid, air or thromboembolism, and total caval compression.

Vasopressor-Induced Hypertension

The interaction of vasoactive drugs and ergot derivatives may lead to severe maternal hypertension and possible cerebrovascular accidents (193). Particularly dangerous is the combination of a purely α-adrenergic agent, such as methoxamine, and the ergot derivatives ergonovine and methylergonovine. Ergot derivatives, when used alone, also may be associated with postpartum hypertension (165). However, these drugs may be life-saving in the face of maternal hemorrhage (see Chapter 20). Prophylactic vasopressors or ergot derivatives should be used with caution in parturients with hypertension. If acute postpartum hypertension occurs, treatment might include (a) labetalol 10 to 20 mg intravenously, repeated every 5 minutes up to 1 mg · kg^{-1}; (b) nitroprusside (Nipride) infusion 50 mg in 500 mL; (c) nitroglycerin infusion 50 mg in 500 mL, or sublingual spray 0.4 to 0.8 mg; (d) hydralazine 10 to 20 mg intravenously, which can be repeated every 15 minutes, or other agents such as phentolamine (Regitine) or trimethaphan (Afronad).

Backache

Local tenderness at the site of epidural or spinal placement and transient backache are relatively common, particularly if placement of the block was difficult. This usually clears within several days to 3 weeks and may be related to superficial irritation of the skin or periosteal irritation or damage. However, postpartum backache that persists several months or longer has been reported (194, 195). Although these reports received a great deal of attention, postpartum backache is common, with or without regional anesthesia. Postpartum backache may be related to hormonal changes, softening of maternal ligaments, and mechanical changes (e.g., exaggerated lumbar lordosis and maternal weight gain). In the studies by MacArthur et al., the data were obtained from a mailed questionnaire to 11,701 women who had delivered 1 to 9 years earlier. They found back pain was more common in those who delivered vaginally using epidural analgesia than in those who delivered vaginally without epidural analgesia (18.9% vs. 10.5%). However, this study has been questioned for a number of reasons, including the degree of recall accuracy and the possible bias of recall information (196). Prospective studies of postpartum backache have not supported the data obtained from retrospective surveys. In a prospective study of 1042 parturients, Breen et al. found the incidence of back pain 1 to 2 months after delivery was 44% in women who received epidural anesthesia and 45% in those who did not (197). These results were supported by Russell et al., who found that about 33% of women reported backache that lasted for at least 3 months postpartum, whether they received epidural analgesia or not (198). The chief link to backache within the first 3 months postpartum appears to be antenatal backache (197, 198). Weight gain during the pregnancy also may be a factor (197). Although postpartum back pain is common, it does not appear related to the use of regional analgesia or a particular epidural technique (198–200).

Dense or Prolonged Epidural Block

The goal of epidural analgesia for labor is to achieve pain relief; motor blockade is usually not needed or desired. Thus, increasingly dilute epidural solutions, as well as the CSE technique, have become popular (see Chapter 9) (16). However, more concentrated local anesthetics (bupivacaine 0.125% to 0.25%) are sometimes required for incomplete analgesia or top-up doses. After long-continuous infusions or repeated bolus dosing, significant motor block can develop and may be bothersome to the patient and the nursing staff (201). This may also make voluntary maternal expulsive efforts more difficult during the second stage of labor and lead to prolonged epidural blocks in the postpartum period, particularly if epinephrine is added to the anesthetic solution. A dense block during the course of labor epidural analgesia can be easily managed by decreasing the epidural infusion rate or decreasing the concentration of the local anesthetic. If a dense block is bothersome, discontinuing the infusion for 30 minutes may be helpful, followed by restarting the infusion with a more dilute local anesthetic solution. An unexpectedly prolonged block is most often related to the prolonged administration of a concentrated local anesthetic with epinephrine. This occurred more often with etidocaine, which is no longer commonly used (202–205). Neurologic complications of both labor and delivery itself, as well as regional analgesia, must be considered (see Chapter 23) (206). While an epidural hematoma is often considered in this situation, it is extremely unlikely without a coagulation abnormality or the administration of an anticoagulant. The reported incidence of epidural hematomas is 0.2 to 3.7 per 100,000 epidural blocks for obstetric patients (206). A block that slowly regresses and does not progress would argue against an epidural hematoma. A dense, one-sided block would also make this diagnosis unlikely. However, consultation with a neurologist is appropriate if more routine causes of a prolonged block do not explain the clinical findings. The increasing use of dilute local anesthetic solutions for labor should decrease the incidence of this problem.

Urinary Retention

Urinary retention during labor is not uncommon but appears to be more likely with regional analgesia. However, a recent study of women receiving dilute epidural local anesthetic solutions with opioids demonstrated that women were able to void in most cases (16). In an older study, it was noted that 14.2% of women had bladder dysfunction after a normal vaginal delivery compared with 37.5% of women who had an instrumental vaginal delivery. None of these women had regional anesthesia (207). More recent examination of this problem found a much lower overall incidence. Among women who received epidural analgesia, the incidence was 2.7% compared with 0.1% in women without regional anesthesia (208). Although it has been demonstrated that epidural opioids likely cause urinary retention by their direct sacral spinal action and effect on the detrusor muscle (Chapter 9 II, Fig. 9.25) (209), this seems unlikely in routine practice with dilute local anesthetic and opioid infusions for labor.

Urinary retention during labor and postpartum is no doubt affected by numerous obstetric factors, including perineal trauma, edema, lengthy labor, prolonged second stage, instrumental delivery, and pain. Patients in labor and postpartum should be observed for possible bladder distention and urinary bladder catheterization performed as indicated.

Inadequate or Failed Blocks

Epidural techniques for labor analgesia are extremely effective in skilled hands. However, a failure rate as high as 2% to 5% may occur with incomplete pain relief in 10% to 15% of patients (210). Failed or inadequate blocks typically result from failure to identify the epidural space or from malposition of the catheter. The higher failure rates may be related to inexperience of the practitioner (particularly those in training) or rapid progression of labor. In some instances, for example, there is not time to repeat the placement of a failed epidural catheter.

When there is a question concerning the correct placement of an epidural catheter in labor, the clinician might inject 10 to 15 mL of a more concentrated local anesthetic (1.5% lidocaine; 2% to 3% 2-chloroprocaine) in divided doses to verify placement. If this does not promptly provide significant analgesia, the epidural catheter should be replaced without prolonged attempts to verify placement.

A unilateral epidural block in labor is not uncommon and can occur despite the use of a good technique. In a prospective analysis (n = 10,995), Paech et al. noted that 1.3% of epidural catheters placed for labor or cesarean section needed to be replaced for unilateral or asymmetric blocks (54). While this problem has been attributed to obstruction in the epidural space (dorsomedian connective tissue) (211), anatomical causes are less likely than patient position (prolonged time on one side) or excessive catheter length in the epidural space. Withdrawal of the catheter by 1 to 2 cm and injection with a larger volume of dilute local anesthetic usually solves the problem. In prospective studies, the ideal length for a multiorifice catheter insertion in the epidural space has been determined to be 4 to 6 cm (212, 213).

In the obese parturient, epidural block is typically placed with the patient in the sitting position. The catheter should not be fixed with tape until the patient has returned to her side or lateral position since the magnitude of catheter movement with position change can be more than 4 cm in the obese parturient (214). The patient in labor often experiences a great deal of movement compared to a patient undergoing a cesarean section, for example, and catheters can become dislodged despite careful placement. Therefore, catheters may need to be replaced on occasion, particularly during prolonged labor or in the obese parturient. In a review of anesthesia outcome in the morbidly obese parturient, it was noted that 94% of these patients ultimately obtained successful epidural anesthesia despite the technical difficulties. However, the epidural catheters needed to be replaced once in 46% of the patients and two or more times in 21% of the patients (19).

When surgery is contemplated in a parturient with a "questionable" epidural catheter, a spinal anesthetic may be preferable to use of the epidural catheter. However, high spinal anesthesia has been reported when spinal anesthesia follows a failed ("spotty") epidural anesthetic, and caution is indicated (215–218).

When an epidural anesthetic is used for a cesarean section and anesthesia is found to be incomplete *after* the incision is made, several choices are possible to remedy the situation. Often, simply waiting for the epidural block to take effect will be successful, particularly if bupivacaine or ropivacaine has been used. Other choices include administration of additional local anesthetic to reinforce the block (5 to 10 mL), administration of small IV doses of an analgesic (50 to 100 μg fentanyl), or IV ketamine (0.25 mg·kg^{-1}). One or two doses of ketamine may provide adequate analgesia until the onset of a "slow" but otherwise successful epidural. Alternatively, the surgical team might infiltrate locally in the surgical field with a local anesthetic if it appears there is a missed segment. Finally, low-dose inhalation analgesia with nitrous oxide may be helpful. The risk of aspiration must be kept in mind with use of supplemental IV and/or inhalation agents. The technique must be conscious (not unconscious) sedation. Regardless of the approach, adequate anesthesia must be provided, and the use of general anesthesia may be necessary in some cases, particularly if surgery is urgent or an incision has been made and the patient is in pain. Conversion of an epidural anesthetic to a general anesthetic for cesarean section was necessary in 54 of 4624 cases (1.2%) in a training center in Australia (54).

Although epidural analgesia for labor is most often highly effective, its use requires skill and practice, acceptance of the occasional failed block, and the knowledge and skill to implement alternative approaches when necessary.

Note: The current American Society of Anesthesiologists' Guidelines for Regional Anesthesia in Obstetrics are included in the Appendices of this book.

REFERENCES

1. Morrison D, Smedstad K. Continuous infusion epidurals for obstetric analgesia. *Can Anaesth Soc J* 1985;32:101–104.

2. Scott D, Walker L. Administration of continuous epidural analgesia. *Anaesthesia* 1963;18:82–83.

3. Spoerel W, Thomas A, Gerula G. Continuous epidural analgesia: Experience with mechanical injection devices. *Can Anaesth Soc J* 1970;17:37–51.

4. Zador G, Willdeck-Lund C, Nilsson B. Continuous drip lumbar epidural anesthesia with lidocaine for vaginal delivery. 1. Clinical efficacy and lidocaine concentrations in maternal, fetal and umbilical cord blood. *Acta Obstet Gynecol Scand* 1974;34(suppl):31–40.

5. Glover D. Continuous epidural analgesia in the obstetric patient: A feasibility study using a mechanical infusion pump. *Anaesthesia* 1977;32:499–503.

6. Evans K, Carrie L. Continuous epidural infusion of bupivacaine in labour: A simple method. *Anaesthesia* 1979;34:310–315.

7. Matouskova A, Hanson B, Elmen H. Continuous mini-infusion of bupivacaine into the epidural space during labor. III. A clinical study of 225 parturients. *Acta Obstet Gynecol Scand* 1979;83(suppl):43–52.

8. Davies A, Fettes I. A simple safe method for continuous infusion epidural analgesia in obstetrics. *Can Anaesth Soc J* 1981;28:484–487.

9. Taylor H. Clinical experience with continuous epidural infusion of bupivacaine at 6 ml per hour in obstetrics. *Can Anaesth Soc J* 1983;30:277–285.

10. Rosenblatt R, Wright R, Denson D, Raj P. Continuous epidural infusions for obstetric analgesia. *Reg Anesth* 1983;8:10–15.

11. Abboud T, Afrasiabi A, Sarkis F, et al. Continuous infusion epidural analgesia in parturients receiving bupivacaine, chloroprocaine, or lidocaine–maternal, fetal, and neonatal effects. *Anesth Analg* 1984;63:421–428.

12. Chestnut D, Bates J, Choi W. Continuous infusion epidural analgesia with lidocaine: Efficacy and influence during the second stage of labor. *Obstet Gynecol* 1987;69:323–327.

13. Chestnut D, Owen Bates J, Ostman L, Choi W, Geiger M. Continuous infusion epidural analgesia during labor: A randomized, double-blind comparison of 0.0625% bupivacaine/0.0002% fentanyl versus 0.125% bupivacaine. *Anesthesiology* 1988;68:754–759.

14. Phillips G. Continuous epidural analgesia in labor: The effect of adding sufentanil to 0.125% bupivacaine. *Anesth Analg* 1988;67:462–465.

15. Chestnut D, Vandewalker G, Owen C, Bates J, Choi W. The influence of continuous epidural bupivacaine analgesia on the second stage of labor and method of delivery in nulliparous women. *Anesthesiology* 1987;66:774–780.

16. Cohen SE, Yeh JY, Riley ET, Vogel TM. Walking with labor epidural analgesia: The impact of bupivacaine concentration and a lidocaine-epinephrine test dose. *Anesthesiology* 2000;92:387–392.

17. Greene B. A 26-gauge lumbar puncture needle: Its value in the prophylaxis of headache following spinal analgesia for vaginal delivery. *Anesthesiology* 1950;11:464–469.

18. Halpern S, Preston R. Postdural puncture headache and spinal needle design. *Anesthesiology* 1994;81:1376–1383.

19. Hood DD, Dewan DM. Anesthesia outcome in the morbidly obese parturient. *Anesthesiology* 1993;79:1210–1218.

20. Arkoosh VA, Palmer CM, Van Maren GA, et al. Continuous intrathecal labor analgesia—safety and efficacy [abstract]. *Anesthesiology* 1998;89:A1041.

21. Peterson D, Borup J, Chestnut D. Continuous spinal anesthesia: Case review and discussion. *Reg Anesth* 1983;8:109–113.

22. Kallos T, Smith T. Continuous spinal anesthesia with hypobaric tetracaine for hip surgery in lateral decubitus. *Anesth Analg* 1972;51:766–773.

23. Denny N, Masters R, Pearson D, et al. Postdural puncture headache after continuous spinal anesthesia. *Anesth Analg* 1987;66:791–794.

24. Rigler M, Drasner K. Distribution of catheter-injected local anesthetic in a model of the subarachnoid space. *Anesthesiology* 1991;75:684–692.

25. Rigler M, Drasner K, Krejcie T, et al. Cauda equina syndrome after continuous spinal anesthesia. *Anesth Analg* 1991;72:275–281.

26. Ross BK, Coda B, Heath CH. Local anesthetic distribution in a spinal model: A possible mechanism of neurologic injury after continuous spinal anesthesia. *Reg Anesth* 1992;17:69–77.

27. Lambert LA, Lambert DH, Strichartz GR. Irreversible conduction block in isolated nerve by high concentrations of local anesthetics. *Anesthesiology* 1994;80:1082–1093.

28. Schneider M, Ettlin T, Kaufmann M, et al. Transient neurologic toxicity after hyperbaric subarachnoid anesthesia with 5% lidocaine. *Anesth Analg* 1993;76:1154–1157.

29. Collis RE, Baxandall ML, Srikantharajah ID. Combined spinal epidural (CSE) analgesia: Technique, management and outcome of 300 mothers. *Int J Obstet Anesth* 1994;3:75–81.

30. Palmer CM, Cork RC, Hays R, et al. The dose-response relationship of intrathecal fentanyl for labor analgesia. *Anesthesiology* 1998;88:355–361.

31. Norris MC, Grieco WM, Borkowski M, et al. Complications of labor analgesia: Epidural versus combined spinal epidural techniques. *Anesth Analg* 1994;79:529–537.

32. Rawal N, VanZundert A, Holmström B, et al. Combined spinal-epidural technique. *Reg Anesth* 1997;22:406–423.

33. Bloom SL, McIntire DD, Kelly MA, et al. Lack of effect of walking on labor and delivery. *N Engl J Med* 1998;339:76–79.

34. Nageotte MP, Larson D, Rumney PJ, et al. Epidural analgesia as compared with combined spinal epidural analgesia during labor in nulliparous women. *N Engl J Med* 1997;337:1715–1719.

35. Parry MG, Fernando R, Bawa GPS, Poulton BB. Dorsal column function after epidural and spinal blockade: Implications for the safety of walking following low dose regional analgesia for labour. *Anaesthesia* 1998;53:383–403.

36. Pickering AE, Parry MG, Ousta B, Fernando R. Effect of combined epidural ambulatory labor analgesia on balance. *Anesthesiology* 1999;91:436–441.

37. McLeod A, Fernando R, Page F, Whitehouse A, England AJ. An assessment of maternal balance and gait using computerized posturography. Paper presented at: Annual Meeting of the Society for Obstetric Anesthesia and Perinatology; 1999; Denver, CO.

38. Douglas MJ. Walking epidural analgesia in labor. *Can J Anaesth* 1998;45:607–611.

39. Eisenach JC. Combined spinal-epidural analgesia in obstetrics. *Anesthesiology* 1999;91:299–302.

40. Campbell DC, Camann WC, Datta S. The addition of bupivacaine to intrathecal sufentanil for labor analgesia. *Anesth Analg* 1995;81:305–309.

41. Cohen SE, Cherry CM, Holbrook RH Jr, et al. Intrathecal sufentanil for labor analgesia: Sensory changes, side effects and fetal heart rate changes. *Anesth Analg* 1993;77:1155–1160.

42. Riley ET, Ratner EF, Cohen S. Intrathecal sufentanil for labor analgesia: Do sensory changes predict better analgesia and greater hypotension? *Anesth Analg* 1997;84:346–351.

43. Honet JE, Arkoosh VA, Norris MC, et al. Comparison among intrathecal fentanyl, meperidine and sufentanil for labor analgesia. *Anesth Analg* 1992;75:734–739.

44. Clarke VT, Smiley RM, Finster M. Uterine hyperactivity after intrathecal injection of fentanyl for analgesia during labor: A cause of fetal bradycardia [letter]? *Anesthesiology* 1994;81:1083.

45. Nielsen PE, Erickson JR, Abouleish EL, et al. Fetal heart rate changes after intrathecal sufentanil or epidural bupivacaine for labor analgesia: Incidence and clinical significance. *Anesth Analg* 1996;83:742–746.

46. Palmer CM, Maciulla JC, Cork RC, et al. The incidence of fetal heart rate changes after intrathecal fentanyl labor analgesia. *Anesth Analg* 1999;88:577–581.

47. Eberle RL, Norris MC, Eberle AM, et al. The effect of maternal position on fetal heart rate during epidural or intrathecal labor analgesia. *Am J Obstet Gynecol* 1998;149:150–155.

48. Kahn L, Hunter E. Combined spinal epidural (CSE) analgesia, fetal bradycardia and uterine hypertonus [letter]. *Reg Anesth* 1998;23:111–112.

49. Riley ET, Vogel TM, El-Sayed Y, et al. Patient selection bias contributes to an increased incidence of fetal bradycardia after combined spinal/epidural analgesia for labor [abstract]. *Anesthesiology* 1999;91:A1054.

50. Fogel ST, Daftary AR, Norris MC, et al. The incidence of clinically important fetal heart rate abnormalities: Combined spinal-epidural vs. epidural anesthesia for labor [abstract]. *Reg Anesth* 1999;24:A75.

51. Norris MC. Intrathecal opioids and fetal bradycardia: Is there a link? *Int J Obstet Anesth* 2000;9:264–269.

52. Albright GA, Forster RM. The safety and efficacy of combined spinal and epidural analgesia/anesthesia (6,002 blocks) in a community hospital. *Reg Anesth* 1999;24:117–125.

53. Sinclair JC, Fox HA, Lentz JF, Fuld GL, Murphy J. Intoxication of the fetus by a local anesthetic: A newly recognized complication of maternal caudal anesthesia. *N Engl J Med* 1965;273:1173–1177.

54. Paech MJ, Godkin R, Webster S. Complications of obstetric epidural analgesia and anaesthesia: A prospective analysis of 10,995 cases. *Int J Obstet Anesth* 1998;7:5–11.

55. Asling JH, Shnider SM, Margolis AJ, Wilkinson GL, Way EL. Paracervical block anesthesia in obstetrics. II. Etiology of fetal bradycardia following paracervical block anesthesia. *Am J Obstet Gynecol* 1970;107:626–634.

56. Manninen T, Aantaa R, Salonen M, Pirhonen J, Palo P. A comparison of the hemodynamic effects of paracervical block and epidural anesthesia for labor analgesia. *Acta Anaesthesiol Scand* 2000;44:441–445.

57. Ralston D, Shnider S. The fetal and neonatal effects of regional anesthesia in obstetrics. *Anesthesiology* 1978;48:34–64.

58. Ranta P, Jouppila P, Spalding M, Kangas-Saarela T. Paracervical block–a viable alternative for labor pain relief? *Acta Obstet Gynecol Scand* 1995;74:122–126.

59. Bonica J. *Principles and Practice of Obstetric Analgesia and Anesthesia.* Philadelphia: Davis; 1967:520–526.

60. Hunter CJ. Uterine motility studies during labor: Observations on bilateral sympathetic nerve block in the normal and abnormal first stage of labor. *Am J Obstet Gynecol* 1983;85:681–686.

61. James FI. Clinical obstetrical anesthesia: Labor and delivery. In: American Society of Anesthesiologists Annual Refresher Course Lectures. Chicago, IL; 1978:126A.

62. Leighton B, Halpern S, Wilson D. Lumbar sympathetic blocks speed early and second stage induced labor in nulliparous women. *Anesthesiology* 1999;90:1039–1046.

63. Eisenach JC. Obstetric anesthesia: What have you done for us lately? *Anesthesiology* 1999;91:907–908.

64. American Society of Anesthesiologists. Practice guidelines for obstetrical anesthesia: A report by the American Society of Anesthesiologists Task Force on Obstetrical Anesthesia. *Anesthesiology* 1999;90:600–611.

65. Douglas MJ. Platelets, the parturient and regional anesthesia. *Int J Obstet Anesth* 2001;10:113–120.

66. American Society of Regional Anesthesia. *Recommendations for Neuraxial Anesthesia and Anticoagulation.* Chicago: American Society of Regional Anesthesia; 1998.

67. Horlocker TT, Heit JA. Low molecular weight heparin: Biochemistry, pharmacology, perioperative prophylaxis regimens, and guidelines for regional anesthetic management. *Anesth Analg* 1997;85:874–885.

68. Carr MF, Hehre FW. Inadvertent lumbar puncture. *Anesth Analg* 1962;41:349–353.

69. Kenepp NB, Gutsche BB. Inadvertent intravascular injections during lumbar epidural anesthesia [letter]. *Anesthesiology* 1981;54:172–173.

70. Abraham RA, Harris AP, Maxwell LG, Kaplow S. The efficacy of 1.5% lidocaine with 7.5% dextrose and epinephrine as an epidural test dose for obstetrics. *Anesthesiology* 1986;64:116–119.

71. Leighton B, Norris M, DeSimone C, Rosko T, Gross J. The air test as a clinically useful indicator of intravenously placed epidural catheters. *Anesthesiology* 1990;73:610–613.

72. Michael S, Richmond MN, Birks RJS. A comparison between open-end (single hole) and closed-end (three lateral holes) epidural catheters. *Anaesthesia* 1989;44:578–580.

73. Reynolds F. Epidural catheter migration during labour [letter]. *Anaesthesia* 1988;43:69.

74. Mulroy MF, Norris MC, Liu SS. Safety steps in epidural injection of local anesthetics: Review of the literature and recommendations. *Anesth Analg* 1997;85:1346–1356.

75. Norris MC, Fogel ST, Dalman H, et al. Labor epidural analgesia without an intravascular "test dose." *Anesthesiology* 1998;88:1495–1501.

76. Norris MC, Ferrenbach D, Dalman H, et al. Does epinephrine improve the diagnostic accuracy of aspiration during labor epidural analgesia? *Anesth Analg* 1999;88:1073–1076.

77. Birnbach DJ, Chestnut DH. The epidural test dose in obstetric patients: Has it outlived its usefulness? *Anesth Analg* 1999;88:971–972.

78. Poblete B, Van Gessel EF, Gaggero G, Gamulin Z. Efficacy of three test doses to detect epidural catheter misplacement. *Can J Anesth* 1999;46:34–39.

79. Prince GD, Shetty GR, Miles M. Safety and efficacy of a low volume extradural test dose of bupivacaine in labour. *Br J Anaesth* 1989;62:503–508.

80. Stonham J, Moss P. The optimal test dose for epidural anesthesia. *Anesthesiology* 1983;58:389–390.

81. Fargas-Babjak A, McChesney J, Morison DH. The efficacy of bupivacaine 0.75 per cent as an epidural test dose. *Can Anaesth Soc J* 1980;27:500–501.

82. Okell RW, Sprigge JS. Unintentional dural puncture: A survey of recognition and management. *Anaesthesia* 1987;42:1110–1113.

83. Abouleish EI, Elias M, Nelson C. Ropivacaine-induced seizure following extradural anaesthesia: A case report. *Br J Anaesth* 1998;80:843–844.

84. Morton CP, Bloomfield S, Magnusson A, Jozwiak H, McClure JH. Ropivacaine 0.75% for extradural anaesthesia in elective Caesarean section: An open clinical and pharmacokinetic study in mother and neonate. *Br J Anaesth* 1997;79:3–8.

85. McClure JH, Morton CPJ. Ropivacaine test dose in extradural anaesthesia. *Br J Anaesth* 1997;79:813–817.

86. Dresner M, Adams M, Klien H. Ropivacine test dose in extradural anaesthesia. [letter]. *Br J Anaesth* 1997;79:813.

87. Moore D, Batra M. The components of an effective test dose prior to epidural block. *Anesthesiology* 1981;55:693–696.

88. Van Zundert A, Vaes L, De Wolf A. ECG monitoring of mother and fetus during epidural anesthesia. *Anesthesiology* 1987;66:584–585.

89. Colonna-Romano P, Lingaraju N, Godfrey SD, Braitman LE. Epidural test dose and intravascular injection in obstetrics: Sensitivity, specificity, and lowest effective dose. *Anesth Analg* 1992;75:372–376.

90. Colonna-Romano P, Salvage R, Lingaraju N, Seitman DT. Epinephrine-induced tachycardia is different from contraction-associated tachycardia in laboring patients. *Anesth Analg* 1996;82:294–296.

91. Cartwright P, McCarroll S, Antzaka C. Maternal heart rate changes with a plain epidural test dose. *Anesthesiology* 1986;65:226–228.

92. Leighton B, Norris M, Sosis M, et al. Limitations of epinephrine as a marker of intravascular injection in laboring women. *Anesthesiology* 1987;66:688–691.

93. Hood D, Dewan D, James F. Maternal and fetal effects of epinephrine in gravid ewes. *Anesthesiology* 1986;64:610–613.

94. DeSimone C, Leighton B, Norris M, Chayen B, Menduke H. The chronotropic effect of isoproterenol is reduced in term pregnant women. *Anesthesiology* 1988;69:626–628.

95. Schobel HP, Fischer T, Heuszer K, et al. Preeclampsia: A state of sympathetic overactivity. *N Engl J Med* 1996;335:1480–1485.

96. Leighton BL, Norris MC, De Simone CA, et al. Preeclamptic and healthy term pregnant patients have different chronotropic responses to isoproterenol. *Anesthesiology* 1990;72:392–393.

97. Gant NF, Daley GL, Chand S, et al. A study of angiotensin II pressor response throughout primigravid pregnancy. *J Clin Invest* 1973;52:2682–2689.

98. Roetman K, Eisenach J. Evaluation of lidocaine as an intravenous test dose for epidural anesthesia [abstract]. *Anesthesiology* 1988;69:A669.

99. Grice S, Eisenach J, Dewan D. Effect of 2-chloroprocaine test dosing on the subsequent duration of labor analgesia with epidural bupivacaine-fentanyl-epinephrine [abstract]. *Anesthesiology* 1988;69:A668.

100. Baker B, Longmire S, Jones M, et al. The epidural test dose in obstetrics reconsidered. In: Abstracts of Scientific Papers of the Annual Meeting of the Society for Obstetric Anesthesia and Perinatology; Halifax, Nova Scotia; 1987:69.

101. Cleaveland C, Rango R, Shand D. A standardized isoproterenol sensitivity test. *Arch Intern Med* 1972;130:47–52.

102. Leighton B, DeSimone C, Norris M, Chayen B. Isoproterenol is an effective marker of intravenous injection in laboring women. *Anesthesiology* 1989;71:206–209.

103. Gogarten W, Strümper D, Buerkle H, Van Aken H, Marcus MAE. Testing an epidural catheter in obstetrics: Epinephrine or isoproterenol? *Int J Obstet Anesth* 2001;10:40–45.

104. Leighton B, Gross J. Air: An effective indicator of intravenously located epidural catheters. *Anesthesiology* 1989;71:848–851.

105. Naulty J, Ostheimer G, Datta S, Knapp R, Weiss J. Incidence of venous air embolism during epidural catheter insertion. *Anesthesiology* 1982;57:410–412.

106. Leighton BL, Katsiris SE, Halpern SH, Wilson DB, Kronberg JE. Multiport epidural catheters: Can orifice location be tested? *Anesthesiology* 2000;92:1840–1842.

107. Shnider S. Experience with regional anesthesia for vaginal delivery. In: Shnider S, Moya F, eds. *The Anesthesiologist, Mother and Newborn.* Baltimore: Williams & Wilkins; 1974:38.

108. Bromage P. Physiology and pharmacology of epidural analgesia: A review. *Anesthesiology* 1967;28:592–622.

109. Marx G. Shock in the obstetric patient. *Anesthesiology* 1965;26:423–434.

110. Eckstein K, Marx G. Aortocaval compression and uterine displacement. *Anesthesiology* 1974;40:92–96.

111. Goodlin R. Aortocaval compression during cesarean section: A cause of newborn depression. *Obstet Gynecol* 1971;37:702–705.

112. Holmes F. The supine hypotensive syndrome: Its importance to the anaesthetist. *Anaesthesia* 1960;15:298–306.

113. Bieniarz J, Crottogini J, Curuchet E, et al. Aortocaval compression by the uterus in late human pregnancy. An arteriographic study. *Am J Obstet Gynecol* 1968;100:203–217.

114. Kerr M, Samuel E. Studies on the inferior vena cava in late pregnancy. *Br Med J* 1964;1:532–533.

115. DiFazio CA, Carron H, Grosslight KR, et al. Comparison of pH-adjusted lidocaine solutions for epidural anesthesia. *Anesth Analg* 1986;65:760–764.

116. Parnass S, Curran M, Becker G. Incidence of hypotension associated with epidural anesthesia using alkalinized and nonalkalinized lidocaine for cesarean section. *Anesth Analg* 1987;66:1148–1150.

117. Greiss FJ, Crandell D. Therapy for hypotension induced by spinal anesthesia during pregnancy. *JAMA* 1965;191:793–796.

118. Greiss FJ. Pressure flow relationship in the gravid uterine vascular bed. *Am J Obstet Gynecol* 1966;96:41–47.

119. Martin CJ, Gingerick B. Uteroplacental physiology. *J Obstet Gynecol Neonatal Nurs* 1976;5:16–25.

120. Adams F, Assali N, Cushman M, Westersten A. Interrelationships of maternal and fetal circulations. *Pediatrics* 1961;27:627–635.

121. Adamsons K, Myers R. Circulation in the intervillous space: Obstetrical considerations in fetal deprivation. In: Grunewald P, ed. *The Placenta*. Baltimore: University Park Press; 1975:158.

122. Lucas W, Kirschbaum T, Assali N. Spinal shock and fetal oxygenation. *Am J Obstet Gynecol* 1965;93:583–587.

123. Moya F, Thorndike V. Maternal hypotension and the newborn. *Proceedings of the Third World Congress of Anesthesiology, Sao Paulo, Brazil, 1964*.

124. Myers R. Two patterns of perinatal brain damage and their condition of occurrence. *Am J Obstet Gynecol* 1972;112:246–276.

125. Ebner H, Barcohana J, Bartoshuk A. Influence of postspinal hypotension on the fetal electrocardiogram. *Am J Obstet Gynecol* 1960;80:569–576.

126. Hon E, Reid B, Hehre F. The electronic evaluation of the fetal heart rate. II. Changes with maternal hypotension. *Am J Obstet Gynecol* 1960;79:209–215.

127. Bonica J, Hon E. Fetal distress. In: Bonica J, ed. *Principles and Practice of Obstetric Analgesia and Anesthesia*. Philadelphia: Davis; 1964:1252.

128. Zilianti M, Salazar J, Aller J, Aguero O. Fetal heart rate and pH of fetal capillary blood during epidural analgesia in labor. *Obstet Gynecol* 1970;36:881–886.

129. Moya F, Smith B. Spinal anesthesia for cesarean section: Clinical and biochemical studies of effects on maternal physiology. *JAMA* 1962;179:609–614.

130. Brizgyz R, Dailey P, Shnider S, Kotelko D, Levinson G. The incidence and neonatal effects of maternal hypotension during epidural anesthesia for cesarean section. *Anesthesiology* 1987;67:782–786.

131. Datta S, Alper M, Ostheimer G, Weiss J. Method of ephedrine administration and nausea and hypotension during spinal anesthesia for cesarean section. *Anesthesiology* 1982;56:68–70.

132. Abboud T, Blikian A, Noueihid R, et al. Neonatal effects of maternal hypotension during spinal anesthesia as evaluated by a new test [abstract]. *Anesthesiology* 1983;59:A421.

133. Leary E, Sabrine G, Sabrine A, Lyons G, Robinson. IV fluid and low dose epidural infusions–is IV fluid administration necessary [abstract]? *Br J Anaesth* 1999;82(suppl 1):A516.

134. Jackson R, Reid JA, Thorburn J. Volume preloading is not essential to prevent spinal-induced hypotension at Caesarean section. *Br J Anaesth* 1995;75:262–265.

135. Rout CC, Rocke DA, Levin J, Gouws E, Reddy D. A re-evaluation of the role of crystalloid preload in the prevention of hypotension associated with spinal anesthesia for elective cesarean section. *Anesthesiology* 1993;79:262–269.

136. Ueyama H, Yan-Ling H, Tanigami H, Mashimo T, Yoshiya I. Effects of crystalloid and colloid preload on blood volume in the parturient undergoing spinal anesthesia for elective cesarean section. *Anesthesiology* 1999;91:1571–1576.

137. Rout CC, Akoojee SS, Rocke DA, Gouws E. Rapid administration of crystalloid preload does not decrease the incidence of hypotension after spinal anaesthesia for elective Caesarean section. *Br J Anaesth* 1992;68:394–397.

138. Karinen J, Rasanen J, Alahuhta S, Jouppila R, Jouppila P. Effects of crystalloid and colloid preloading on uteroplacental and maternal haemodynamic state during spinal anaesthesia for caesarean section. *Br J Anaesth* 1995;75:531–535.

139. Cheek TG, Samuels P, Miller F, Tobin M, Gutsche BB. Normal saline i.v. fluid load decreases uterine activity in active labour. *Br J Anaesth* 1996;77:632–635.

140. Zamora JE, Rosaeg OP, Lindsay MP, Crossan ML. Haemodynamic consequences and uterine contractions following 0.5 or 1.0 litre crystalloid infusion before obstetric epidural analgesia. *Can J Anaesth* 1996;43:347–352.

141. Evans S, Crawford J, Stevens I, Durbin G, Daya H. Fluid therapy for induced labour under epidural analgesia: Biochemical consequences for mother and infant. *Br J Obstet Gynaecol* 1986;93:329–333.

142. Kenepp N, Shelley W, Gabbe S, et al. Fetal and neonatal hazards of maternal hydration with 5% dextrose before caesarean section. *Lancet* 1982;1:1150–1152.

143. Mendiola J, Grylack L, Scanlon J. Effects of intrapartum maternal glucose infusion on the normal fetus and newborn. *Anesth Analg* 1982;61:32–35.

144. Morton K, Jackson M, Gillmer M. A comparison of the effects of four intravenous solutions for the treatment of ketonuria during labour. *Br J Obstet Gynaecol* 1985;92:473–479.

145. Lanier W, Stangland K, Scheithauer B, Milde J, Michenfelder J. The effects of dextrose infusion and head position on neurologic outcome after complete cerebral ischemia in primates: Examination of a model. *Anesthesiology* 1987;66:39–47.

146. Wright R, Shnider S, Levinson G, Rolbin S, Parer J. The effect of maternal administration of ephedrine on fetal heart rate and variability. *Obstet Gynecol* 1981;57:734–738.

147. Huch A, Huch R. Transcutaneous noninvasive monitoring of PO2. *Hosp Pract* 1976;11:43–52.

148. Humphrey M, Chang A, Wood E, Morgan S, Hounslow D. A decrease in fetal pH during the second stage of labor when conducted in the dorsal position. *J Obstet Gynaecol Br Commonw* 1974;81:600–602.

149. Shnider S, deLorimier A, Holl J, Chapler F, Morishima H. Vasopressors in obstetrics. I. Correction of fetal acidosis with ephedrine during spinal hypotension. *Am J Obstet Gynecol* 1968;102:911–919.

150. Butterworth JI, Piccione WJ, Berrizbeitia L, et al. Augmentation of venous return by adrenergic agonists during spinal anesthesia. *Anesth Analg* 1986;65:612–616.

151. James FI, Greiss FJ, Kemp R. An evaluation of vasopressor therapy for maternal hypotension during spinal anesthesia. *Anesthesiology* 1970;33:25–34.

152. Shnider S, deLorimier A, Asling J, Morishima H. Vasopressors in obstetrics. II. Fetal hazards of methoxamine administration during obstetric spinal anesthesia. *Am J Obstet Gynecol* 1970;106:680–686.

153. Greiss FJ, Van Wilkes D. Effects of sympathomimetic drugs and angiotensin on the uterine vascular bed. *Obstet Gynecol* 1964;23:925–930.

154. Ramanathan S, Grant G. Vasopressor therapy for hypotension due to epidural anesthesia or cesarean section. *Acta Anaesthesiol Scand* 1988;32:559–565.

155. Moran D, Perillo M, Bader A, Datta S. Phenylephrine in treating maternal hypotension secondary to spinal anesthesia [abstract]. *Anesthesiology* 1989;71:A857.

156. Alahuhta S, Räsänen J, Jouppila P, Jouppila R, Hollmén AI. Ephedrine and phenylephrine for avoiding maternal hypotension due to spinal anaesthesia for caesarean section. *Int J Obstet Anesth* 1992;1:129–134.

157. Hall PA, Bennett A, Wilkes MP, Lewis M. Spinal anaesthesia for caesarean section: Comparison of infusions of phenylephrine and ephedrine. *Br J Anaesth* 1994;73:471–474.

158. Thomas DG, Robson SC, Redfern N, Hughes D, Boys RJ. Randomized trial of bolus phenylephrine or ephedrine for maintenance of arterial pressure during spinal anaesthesia for Caesarean section. *Br J Anaesth* 1996;76:61–65.

159. Ralston D, Shnider S, deLorimier A. Effects of equipotent ephedrine, metaraminol, mephentermine, and methoxamine on uterine blood flow in the pregnant ewe. *Anesthesiology* 1974;40:354–370.

160. Hughes S, Ward M, Levinson G, et al. Placental transfer of ephedrine does not affect neonatal outcome. *Anesthesiology* 1985;63:217–219.

161. Marx G, Cosmi R, Wollmen S. Biochemical status and clinical condition of mother and infant at cesarean section. *Anesth Analg* 1969;48:986–994.

162. Norris M. Hypotension during spinal anesthesia for cesarean section: Does it affect neonatal outcome? *Reg Anesth* 1987;12:191–193.

163. Moore D, Bridenbaugh L, Thompson G, Balfour R, Horton W. Factors determining dosages of amide-type local anesthetic drugs. *Anesthesiology* 1977;47:263–268.

164. Grimes D, Cates WJ. Deaths from paracervical anesthesia used for first-trimester abortion. *N Engl J Med* 1976;295:1397–1399.

165. Poppers P. Evaluation of local anesthetic agents for regional anaesthesia in obstetrics. *Br J Anaesth* 1975;47:322–327.

166. Adamson D. Continuous epidural anesthesia in the community hospital. *Can Anaesth Soc J* 1973;20:687–692.

167. Crawford J. The second thousand epidural blocks in an obstetric hospital practice. *Br J Anaesth* 1972;44:1277–1287.

168. Kandel P, Spoerel W, Kinch R. Continuous epidural analgesia for labour and delivery: Review of 1000 cases. *Can Med Assoc J* 1966;95:947–953.

169. Bush R. Caudal analgesia for vaginal delivery. II. Analysis of complications. *Anesthesiology* 1959;20:186–191.

170. Dogu T. Continuous caudal analgesia and anesthesia for labor and vaginal delivery. *Obstet Gynecol* 1969;33:92–97.

171. Epstein H, Sherline D. Single-injection caudal anesthesia in obstetrics. *Obstet Gynecol* 1969;33:496–500.

172. Gunther R, Bellville J. Obstetrical caudal anesthesia. II. A randomized study comparing 1 per cent mepivacaine with 1 per cent mepivacaine plus epinephrine. *Anesthesiology* 1972;37:288–298.

173. Youngstrom P, Boyd D, Rhoton F. Statistical process control (SPC) in obstetric anesthesia service: Six years experience [abstract]. *Anesthesiology* 1992;77:A1020.

174. Crawford JS. Some maternal complications of epidural analgesia for labour. *Anaesthesia* 1985;40:1219–1225.

175. Brown DL, Ransom DM, Hall JA, et al. Regional anesthesia and local anaesthetic-induced systemic toxicity: Seizure frequency and accompanying cardiovascular changes. *Anesth Analg* 1995;81:321–328.

176. Chadwick HS. An analysis of obstetric anesthesia cases from the American Society of Anesthesiologists Closed Claims Project database. *Int J Obstet Anesth* 1996;5:258–263.

177. Marx G. Cardiopulmonary resuscitation of late-pregnant women. *Anesthesiology* 1982;56:156.

178. American Heart Association. Advanced cardiac life support. *Special Resuscitation Situations.* 1997;11–8, 11–9.

179. American Heart Association and the International Liaison Committee on Resuscitation. Cardiac arrest associated with pregnancy. Guidelines 2000 for cardiopulmonary resuscitation and emergency cardiovascular care. *Circulation* 2000;102(suppl 1):247–249.

180. Morishima H, Adamsons K. Placental clearance of mepivacaine following administration to the guinea pig fetus. *Anesthesiology* 1967;28:343–348.

181. Philip J, Brown WJ. Total spinal anesthesia late in the course of obstetric bupivacaine epidural block. *Anesthesiology* 1976;44:340–341.

182. Reynolds F, Speedy HM. The subdural space: The third place to go astray. *Anaesthesia* 1990;45:120–123.

183. Ferguson S, Brighouse D, Valentine S. An unusual complication following combined spinal-epidural anaesthesia for caesarean section. *Int J Obstet Anesth* 1997;6:190–193.

184. Robbins PM, Fernando R, Lin GH. Accidental intrathecal insertion of an extradural catheter during combined spinal-extradural anesthesia for cesarean section. *Br J Anaesth* 1995;75:355–357.

185. Morgan B. Unexpectedly extensive conduction blocks in obstetric epidural analgesia. *Anaesthesia* 1990;45:148–152.

186. Collier C. Total spinal or massive subdural block? *Anaesth Intensive Care* 1982;10:92–93.

187. Labenow T, Keh-Wong E, Kristof K, et al. Inadvertent subdural injection: A complication of epidural block. *Anesth Analg* 1988;67:175–179.

188. Akamatsu T. Cardiovascular response to spinal anesthesia. In: Bonica J, ed. *Regional Anesthesia: Recent Advances and Current Status.* Philadelphia: FA Davis; 1969.

189. Wetstone D, Wong K. Sinus bradycardia and asystole during spinal anesthesia. *Anesthesiology* 1974;41:87–89.

190. Caplan R, Ward R, Posner K, Cheney F. Unexpected cardiac arrest during spinal anesthesia: A closed claims analysis of predisposing factors. *Anesthesiology* 1988;68:5–11.

191. Scull TJ, Carli F. Cardiac arrest after Caesarean section under subarachnoid block. *Br J Anaesth* 1996;77:274–276.

192. Hawthorne L, Lyons G. Cardiac arrest complicating spinal anaesthesia for caesarean section. *Int J Obstet Anesth* 1997;6:126–129.

193. Casady G, Moore C, Bridenbaugh L. Postpartum hypertension after use of vasoconstrictor and oxytocic drugs. *JAMA* 1960;172:1011–1015.

194. MacArthur C, Lewis M, Knox EG, Crawford JS. Epidural anaesthesia and long term backache after childbirth. *Br Med J* 1990;301:9–12.

195. MacArthur C, Lewis M, Knox EG. Investigation of long term problems after obstetric epidural anaesthesia. *Br Med J* 1992;304:1279–1282.

196. Svensson H, Andersson GBJ, Hagstad A, Jansson PO. The relationship of low back pain to pregnancy and gynecologic factors. *Spine* 1990;15:371–375.

197. Breen TW, Ransil BJ, Groves PA, Oriol NE. Factors associated with back pain after childbirth. *Anesthesiology* 1994;81:29–34.

198. Russell R, Dundas R, Reynolds F. Long-term backache after childbirth: Prospective search for causative factors. *Br Med J* 1996;312:1384–1388.

199. Macarthur AJ, Macarthur C, Weeks SK. Is epidural anesthesia in labor associated with chronic low back pain? A prospective cohort study. *Anesth Analg* 1997;85:1066–1070.

200. Patel AL, Fernando P, Gill P, et al. A prospective study of long-term backache after childbirth in primigravidae: The effect of ambulatory epidural analgesia during labor. *Int J Obstet Anesth* 1995;4:187.

201. Russell R. Assessment of motor blockade during epidural analgesia in labor. *Int J Obstet Anesth* 1992;1:230–234.

202. Cuerden C, Buley R, Downing JW. Delayed recovery from epidural block in labor: A report of four cases. *Anaesthesia* 1977;32:773–776.

203. Bromage PR. An evaluation of bupivacaine in epidural analgesia for obstetrics. *Can Anaesth Soc J* 1969;16:46–56.

204. Lund C, Hansen OB, Kehlet H, Mogensen T, Qvitzau S. Effects of etidocaine administered epidurally on changes in somatosensory evoked potentials after dermatomal stimulation. *Reg Anesth* 1991;16:38–42.

205. Bromage PR, Datta S, Dunford LA. Etidocaine: An evaluation in epidural analgesia for obstetrics. *Can Anaesth Soc J* 1974;21:535–545.

206. Loo CC, Dahlgren G, Irestedt L. Neurological complications in obstetric regional anaesthesia. *Int J Obstet Anesth* 2000;9:99–124.

207. Grove KH. Backache, headache and bladder dysfunction after delivery. *Br J Anaesth* 1973;45:1147–1149.

208. Olofsson CIJ, Ekblom AOA, Edman-Ordeberg GE, Irestedt LE. Post-partum urinary retention: A comparison between two methods of epidural analgesia. *Eur J Obstet Gynecol Reprod Biol* 1997;71:31–34.

209. Rawal N, Mollefors K, Axelsson K, Lingardh G, Widman B. An experimental study of urodynamic effects of epidural morphine and of naloxone reversal. *Anesth Analg* 1983;62:641–647.

210. Morrison LMM, Buchan AS. Comparison of complications with single-holed and multi-holed extradural catheters. *Br J Anaesth* 1990;64:183–185.

211. Narang UPS, Linter SPK. Failure of extradural blockade in obstetrics. *Br J Anaesth* 1988;60:402–404.

212. Beilin Y, Bernstein HH, Zucker-Pinchoff B. The optimal distance that a multiorifice epidural catheter should be threaded into the epidural space. *Anesth Analg* 1995;81:301–304.

213. D'Angelo R, Berkebile BL, Gerancher JC. Prospective examination of epidural catheter insertion. *Anesthesiology* 1996;84:88–93.

214. Hamilton CL, Riley ET, Cohen SE. Changes in the position of epidural catheters associated with the patient movement. *Anesthesiology* 1997;86:778–784.

215. Mets B, Broccoli E, Brown AR. Is spinal anesthesia after failed epidural anesthesia contraindicated for cesarean section? *Anesth Analg* 1993;77:629–631.

216. Goldstein MM, Dewan DM. Spinal anesthesia after failed epidural anesthesia [letter]. *Anesth Analg* 1994;79:1206–1207.

217. Gupta A, Sjöberg F, Bengtsson M. Spinal anaesthesia for caesarean section following epidural analgesia in labour: A relative contraindication. *Int J Obstet Anesth* 1994;3:153–156.

218. Kick O, Böhrer H. Unexpectedly high spinal anaesthesia following failed extradural anaesthesia for caesarean section. *Anaesthesia* 1993;48:271.

Shnider and Levinson's Anesthesia for Obstetrics,
edited by Samuel C. Hughes, et al.
Lippincott Williams & Wilkins,
Philadelphia, © 2001.

CHAPTER 9

INTRASPINAL ANALGESIA IN OBSTETRICS

PART I. OPIOIDS AND OTHER NON—LOCAL ANESTHETICS

JAMES C. EISENACH, M. D.

BASIC SCIENCE

Since their introduction in 1979 (1), the intraspinal (epidural and spinal) opioids rapidly have become an exciting addition to the field of obstetric anesthesia. This chapter reviews the physiologic and pharmacologic bases of intraspinal action of opioids and other nonlocal anesthetic analgesics; the benefits of using the intraspinal technique to treat labor, delivery, and postoperative pain; and the side effects produced by the use of this method. Although there are distinct advantages to the intraspinal technique, its use is not without a price. No other area in obstetric anesthesia has drawn as much attention in the last 20 years.

In order for pain to be perceived, the following chain of events must occur (Fig. 9.1): (1) stimulation of peripheral sensory nerve endings, leading to (2) generation of action potentials that are propagated centrally to the spinal cord; (3) synaptic transmission in the spinal cord, leading to activation of neurons projecting to the thalamus and other supraspinal centers; (4) synaptic transmission at these supraspinal sites, leading to activation of neurons projecting to several brain areas, resulting in the sensoriemotional experience of pain. Epidural injection of local anesthetics breaks this chain, primarily by causing conduction blockade at the level of the nerve roots and entry zone of fibers into the spinal cord dorsal horn. Unfortunately, conduction blockade with local anesthetics affects other fibers as well, leading to unwanted effects of numbness, sympathectomy, and motor block. Interest in the past 20 years has therefore focussed on defining mechanisms of synaptic transmission in the spinal cord and making clinical use of its modulation by opiates and other neurotransmitters. Implicit in this focus is the assumption that opioids and other agents will selectively dampen transmission of pain-related signals without affecting transmission of nonpainful sensory stimuli, and ideally do so with minimal side effects.

ENDOGENOUS OPIATES AND OPIATE RECEPTORS

The opiates have a long history of therapeutic relevance and still are among the most widely used drugs in medicine. Opioids have been used as anesthetics, analgesics, sedatives, antitussives, and antidiarrheals, typically administered as intravenous (IV), intramuscular, or oral agents. (Their systemic use in obstetrics is described in Chapter 7.) The discovery of opiate receptors combined with the discovery of endogenous opiate-like substances implied that exogenous opiates could be administered to specific sites (Table 9.1). The additional finding that opiate receptors were concentrated in discrete areas in the central nervous system (CNS) helped to explain the multiple actions of the opiates. When morphine was administered to superficial layers of the dorsal horn of the spinal cord, it was shown to produce a highly selective depressant action on nociceptive

pathways without affecting motor, sympathetic, or proprioceptive pathways (2). Opioids administered in minute doses to other receptor-laden areas in animals (e.g., the cortex) had no significant effect on nociceptive pathway action. Taken together, these outcomes indicated that opiate effects on a specific brain or other region dense with opiate receptors depended on the function routinely served by that region. We can therefore attempt to apply an opioid to a specific receptor site to obtain a specific and limited outcome, rather than administer systemic opioids that activate multiple receptors throughout the CNS and the periphery.

A wide variety of chemical compounds with opiate activity produce effects via recognition by a receptor. Opiates are thought to function in the spinal cord primarily by activating receptors presynaptically, thereby blocking the release of excitatory primary afferent neurotransmitters, including glutamate, substance P, and other tachykinins. It is clear that the use of intraspinal opiates engages an endogenous system composed of opiate receptors. Systemic opioids probably combine the effects of the supraspinal and direct spinal actions of the drugs administered.

Like many other neurotransmitter receptors, opiate receptors comprise a family of subtypes, with different anatomic locations and different physiologic effects (Tables 9.2 and 9.3). Several aspects of this division into distinct molecular entities have relevance to the use of intraspinal opiates in obstetrics and to drug development. First, clinically available agents are not specific to one subtype only. For example, morphine can act not only on both μ subtypes, but also at κ and δ subtypes at higher doses. Second, the role of κ-opioid receptors in spinal analgesia is somewhat controversial (3), and may change during pregnancy (4). Spinal injection of dynorphin, the naturally occurring κ-opioid agonist, does not result in analgesia, but rather long-lasting hyperalgesia (increased pain to a noxious stimulus) (5), and higher doses of this and other κ-agonists, such as butorphanol, produce overt spinal cord injury (6). On the other hand, pregnancy is associated with an increase in pain threshold, and this effect in rodents is due to activation of spinal κ-opioid receptors (4). Thus, although currently available κ-opioid agonists have not been shown to be useful for spinal analgesia in obstetrics, future, more selective κ-agonists could be.

Third, a problem with large doses of opioids in obstetrics, either epidurally or systemically, is alteration of fetal heart rate (FHR) pattern—either loss of variability with morphine and other μ-preferring agents, or a sinusoidal FHR pattern with butorphanol (7). Developmental studies indicate that the term fetus may have few, if any, δ-opioid receptors, and that these develop postnatally (8). Thus, δ-opioid specific agonists might have few or no effects on the fetal CNS, and hence the FHR pattern. A better understanding of opiate receptors and their subtypes may ultimately lead to specific drug development and unique clinical application in the future.

149

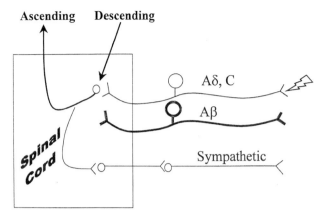

Figure 9.1. Pain transmission is accomplished by stimulation of peripheral afferents, specifically A-delta and C fibers, to conduct impulses to the spinal cord, where transmission occurs to neurons projecting to supraspinal sites. The spinal transmission of nociceptive information is under both descending and intrinsic modulation.

Table 9.1. ENDOGENOUS OPIATES AND OPIATE RECEPTORS: AN OUTLINE OF TERMS

Opiate receptor	Specific sites on cell membranes, primarily in the CNS, that interact with opiate drugs or endogenous opiate-like substances. There are five or more different types of opiate receptors and probably a subpopulation of those five types.
Endogenous opiates	Naturally occurring substances (opioid peptides) isolated in humans and having opiate-like properties. The term *endorphin* is often used generically to describe any endogenous opiate, but is perhaps best applied to those isolated from the pituitary gland.
Enkephalins	Two short-chain peptides isolated from the CNS that have opiate activity (methionine–and leucine–enkephalin). They interact with opiate receptors and function as neurotransmitters.
β-Lipotropin	A pituitary peptide containing 91 amino acids. It may break down to form active subunits.
β-Endorphin	A fragment of β-lipotropin (amino acids 61–91) having potent opiate activity. It has been synthesized and manufactured for intraspinal application on an experimental basis.

NON—OPIATE SPINAL ANALGESICS

In addition to opiates, a host of other neurotransmitters has been identified that inhibits synaptic transmission of nociceptive stimuli in the spinal cord and thus effects pain relief or analgesia

(Table 9.4, Fig. 9.2). Three of these—α_2-adrenergic, cholinergic, and adenosine agents—have been applied to the treatment of labor pain in humans. Following is a brief review of their pharmacology.

α_2-Adrenoceptors are located both on the afferent fiber terminals in the spinal cord (9), where they inhibit excitatory neurotransmitter release (10), and on the projecting spinal neurons, where they produce hyperpolarization and diminished response to excitatory neurotransmission (11). In both cases, these receptors are postsynaptic to the noradrenergic terminals, which reach the spinal cord from neurons with cell bodies in the pons and medulla (12). Intraspinal administration of α_2-adrenergic agonists produces analgesia in a variety of preclinical models of acute and chronic pain, without otherwise affecting sensation and without causing motor block (13). α_2-Adrenergic agonists do, however, decrease blood pressure, in part by sympathoinhibition at the level of the spinal cord, and in part by redistribution and actions in the brain (14). Large doses of α_2-adrenergic agonists decrease FHR (15), presumably due to fetal transfer and direct and indirect (via baroreflexes) actions on heart rate control. Finally, α_2-adrenergic agonists produce dose-dependent sedation by redistribution and effects on a brainstem nucleus, the locus ceruleus (16). Although α_2-adrenoceptor stimulation in the uterus could theoretically reduce uterine blood flow and enhance myometrial contractions, these effects have not been observed in preclinical models (15).

Cholinergic receptors, both muscarinic and nicotinic, are present in the spinal cord dorsal horn (17, 18), and their stimulation results in analgesia without other sensory blockade (19, 20). Spinal injection of the cholinesterase inhibitor neostigmine produces analgesia in several preclinical models of acute and chronic pain (21, 22). Interestingly, neostigmine is a more potent analgesic in female than male humans and animals (23), reflecting dual stimulation of both muscarinic and nicotinic receptors in females, but only muscarinic receptors in males. Neostigmine enhances analgesia from α_2-adrenergic agonists, since these agonists stimulate spinal acetylcholine release (Fig. 9.3). Spinal cholinergic receptor activation increases sympathetic nervous system activity, leading to an increase in blood pressure and heart rate (24). In animals, hypotension from spinally injected local anesthetics is attenuated or abolished by addition of neostigmine (25), presumably reflecting this sympathoinhibition. Unlike opioids, neostigmine and cholinergic agonists do not depress respiration, and unlike opiates and α_2-adrenergic agonists, they do not produce sedation, except at supratherapeutic doses (26).

Adenosine receptors, primarily of the A1 subtype, are also in the dorsal horn of the spinal cord, and their stimulation results in analgesia (27). Unlike the previously discussed receptors, however, adenosine receptors are more powerful inhibitors of spinal sensory synaptic transmission following induction of hypersensitivity, such as after nerve injury or peripheral inflammation, than in the normal state (28). Thus, whether adenosine itself or synthetic adenosine agonists would be effective for relief

Table 9.2. RECEPTORS, SUBPOPULATION, AND POSTULATED TYPES

		Activators	
Type	Physiologic Response	*Endogenous*	*Exogenous*
μ	Miosis, analgesia; bradycardia; respiratory depression	Met-Leu-enkephalin β-endorphin	Morphine
κ	Sedation; no respiratory depression	Dynorphin	Ethylketocyclazocine; bremazocine
σ	Excitatory symptoms; tachycardia; hypertonia; tachypnea	?	Phencyclidine; SKF10047
δ	Analgesia?	Met-Leu-enkephalin β-endorphin	DADL[a]; Dezocine? (μ and δ)
ϵ	?		

[a] α-leu$_5$-enkephalin.

Table 9.3. OPIATE RECEPTOR AND RESPONSE

Opiate Receptor Site	Physiologic and Pharmacologic Response
Medullary and pontine respiratory centers	Respiratory depression
Thalamus	
Lateral thalamus	Discrete, localized pain
Medial thalamus	Poorly localized, deep pain
(receptor density greater in medial thalamus)	
Substantia gelatinosa (dorsal horn of spinal cord)	First site in CNS for integration of sensory information (analgesia achieved)
Solitary nuclei	Depression of cough reflex; orthostatic hypotension
Area postrema (chemoreceptor trigger area)	Nausea and vomiting
Amygdala	Emotional behavior; euphoria
Gastrointestinal tract	Decreased motility (constipation)

Adapted from Snyder SH. Opiate receptors in the brain. *N Engl J Med* 1977; 296:266–271.

of labor pain is uncertain. Adenosine itself has been administered intrathecally to humans, the only side effect being transient lumbar pain (29). A trial of intrathecal adenosine in labor is underway in Sweden at the time of this writing (Sollevi, personal communication). Since adenosine has an extremely short half-life in blood, any systemically absorbed adenosine following intraspinal administration would likely have minimal or no effects in the mother or fetus. In addition to the inhibition of excitatory influences in the spinal cord by opioids, α_2-adrenergic agonists, and adenosine, there are numerous secondary meninges in the spinal cord (Fig. 9.2)

PRACTICAL CONSIDERATIONS

Aside from efficacy, two other preclinical observations are crucial to the clinical use of intraspinal agents in obstetrics. First is adequate testing for safety, related to both potential local neurotoxicity and effects on uterine perfusion, myometrial contractions, and direct effects on the fetus. It would clearly be unethical to proceed with clinical application without these assurances. Such studies have been performed for morphine, fentanyl, sufentanil, alfentanil, meperidine, clonidine, neostigmine, and adenosine (30–32). There is some concern over neurotoxicity from large doses of butorphanol in sheep (6), and this agent is associated with a sinusoidal FHR pattern (7).

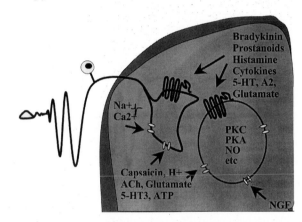

Figure 9.2. Excitatory influences in the spinal cord, which can be inhibited by opioids, α_2-adrenergic agonists, and adenosine. Peripheral nociceptors are excited by tissue injury or inflammation, resulting in release of excitatory neurotransmitters in the spinal cord (especially glutamate and substance P). This results in the generation of a variety of second messengers, including activation of protein kinases C (pK_c) and A (pK_a), generation of nitric oxide (*NO*), and release of prostaglandins, cytokines, and various nerve growth factors (*NGF*). Excitatory influences on this system include voltage gated Na and Ca channels, capsaicin and hydrogen ion sensitive channels, acetylcholine (ACH), especially nicotinic acetylcholine, receptors and serotonin (5-HT), bradykinin, and adenosine 2 (A2) receptors.

Table 9.4. SOME NEUROTRANSMITTER SYSTEMS PROVIDING ANALGESIA AFTER INTRATHECAL INJECTION IN ANIMALS AND CLINICALLY-USED DRUGS WHICH HAVE BEEN TESTED FOR EFFICACY (BUT NOT NECESSARILY SAFE) IN ANIMALS

Neurotransmitter	Receptor	Drugs
Acetylcholine	Cholinergic	Neostigmine
Adenosine	A1-purinergic	Adenosine
Enkephalin	μ-Opioid	Morphine, Fentanyl, Sufentanil
GABA	GABA	Midazolam
Glutamate	NMDA	Ketamine
Norepinephrine	α2-Adrenergic	Clonidine, Dexmedetomidine
Prostaglandins	Prostaglandins	Indomethacin, ketorolac, aspirin
Glycine	Glutamate	No clinically used drugs
Neuropeptide Y	NPY	No clinically used drugs
Nitric Oxide	Guanylate cyclase	No clinically used drugs
Protons	VR-1	No clinically used drugs
Serotonin	5HT-1,2,3	No clinically used drugs
Substance P	NK-1	No clinically used drugs

GABA	γ-amino-butyric acid	5-HT serotonin
NMDA	n-methyl-d-aspartate	NK-1 neurokinin-1
NPY	neuropeptide Y	
VR-1	vanilloid receptor 1	

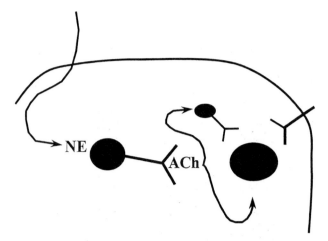

Figure 9.3. Interaction between α_2-adrenergic and cholinergic systems in the spinal cord. Descending noradrenergic pathways release norepinephrine (*NE*) in the spinal cord, which stimulates cholinergic interneurons to release acetylcholine (*ACh*). ACh acts in both direct and indirect ways to inhibit the response of projecting neurons in the spinal cord, which receive nociceptive information.

A second, important consideration is evidence that the compound to be injected would reach its site of action in the spinal cord in an efficient manner. In this regard, considerable information is available for morphine (33) and clonidine (34).

PHARMACOKINETICS AND PHARMACODYNAMICS

When injected epidurally, opiates must cross the dura, arachnoid, and pia membranes to reach their site of action in the spinal cord. It has been demonstrated that it is the arachnoid membrane that forms the primary barrier to drug transfer from epidural space to spinal cord (35). The dura, a coarsely woven structure of collagen fibers, is important to the integrity of the spinal space, but provides no real barrier to the movement of small molecules. In contrast, the arachnoid layer, comprised of cells connected by tight junctions, is analogous in many ways to the blood-brain barrier. For a drug to traverse the arachnoid, it must first partition into the lipid bilayer cell membrane, then traverse the cell itself, which is a hydrophilic space, then partition into another cell membrane before exiting into cerebrospinal fluid (CSF) (Fig. 9.4). In the absence of active transport mecha-

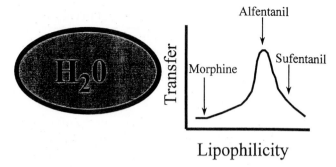

Figure 9.5. Effect of lipophilicity on rate of transfer of drug across the arachnoid membrane. As lipophilicity increases, rate of transfer does as well since drugs must cross the lipid-rich cell membrane to reach the cerebrospinal fluid (CSF). However, with further increases in lipophilicity, the drug is less able to cross the cell or to leave the membrane and enter CSF, and rate of transfer decreases. (Adapted from Bernards CM, Hill HF. Physical and chemical properties of drug molecules governing their diffusion through the spinal meninges. *Anesthesiology* 1992;77:750–756.)

nisms, this puts severe constraints on the physicochemical characteristics of a molecule to traverse this barrier. If it is too hydrophilic (morphine), transfer to CSF will be very inefficient, as it cannot cross the lipid bilayer. On the other hand, if it is too lipophilic (sufentanil), it cannot cross the water-filled barrier of the intracellular compartment, or will not exit the cell membrane. Indeed, it may never reach the arachnoid, partitioning instead into epidural fat. As such, the efficiency of drug transfer across meninges is biphasic with respect to lipid—solubility, with poor CSF bioavailability of highly lipid soluble drugs like fentanyl and sufentanil (Fig. 9.5). Thus, any analgesic effect of these drugs after epidural administration, particularly over prolonged periods of time, is mostly due to actions from systemic absorption and redistribution, not a spinal effect. On the other hand, with bolus (36) or brief infusions (37) of epidural fentanyl, as are commonly performed in obstetric anesthesia, there is evidence for a spinal effect. Thus, it is logical to use these agents for epidural analgesia in brief (< 6 hours) obstetric settings.

Once drug enters the CSF from transfer across the meninges, or from direct injection in the case of spinal administration, it is distributed in a variety of ways (Fig. 9.6). First, it can exit CSF

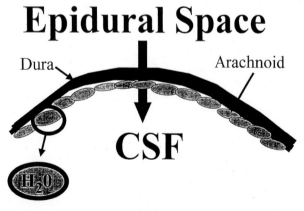

Figure 9.4. Transfer of drugs from epidural to spinal (intrathecal) space. Drug must cross the coarsely woven dura, which is not a barrier, diffuse into the cell membranes of the arachnoid cellular layer through the water-containing cell, through the cell membrane on the spinal side, and then into the water-filled cerebrospinal fluid space.

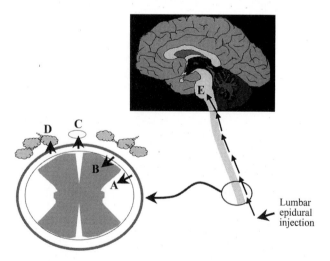

Figure 9.6. Movement of drug after lumbar epidural injection. Drug can cross the meninges and move cephalad (and caudad) in cerebrospinal fluid (CSF). As it crosses over the spinal cord, drug can enter the lipid-rich white mater (**A**), enter the gray mater, wherein lies the site of drug action for analgesia (**B**), or exit back into the epidural space to enter veins (**C**) or fat (**D**). Drug can pass further cephalad in CSF to the brainstem, and penetrate to areas of respiratory control (**E**).

Table 9.5. MOLECULAR WEIGHT, pKa, LIPID SOLUBILITY, AND RELATIVE POTENTIAL FOR CNS ENTRY FOR VARIOUS OPIOID AGENTS[a]

Opioid	Molecular Weight	pKa[b]	Octanol Water Partition Coefficient	Relative Potential for CNS Entry[c]	Onset of Analgesia	Duration of Analgesia
Morphine	285	7.9	1.4	1	Delayed	Prolonged
Meperidine	247	8.5	39	12	Rapid	Intermediate
Fentanyl	336	8.4	816	155	Rapid	Short
Sufentanil	386	8.0	1727	133	Rapid	Short
Alfentanil	417	6.5	89	10	Rapid	Short
Methadone	309	9.3	116	—	Rapid	Intermediate
Lidocaine	271	7.9	2.9[d]	—	—	—
Bupivacaine	324	8.1	27.5[d]	—	—	—

[a] Adapted from Hug Jr CC. Pharmacokinetics of new synthetic narcotic analgesics. In FG Estafanous, ed. Opioids in Anesthesia. Boston, Butterworth, 1984, p 52.
[b] At 37°C.
[c] Apparent partition coefficient at pH 7.4 multiplied by the free fraction of drug in plasma and divided by the value for morphine.
[d] n-Heptane/pH 7.4 buffer, partition coefficient.

to the epidural space in the opposite manner to that described earlier. Indeed, results from human tissues at autopsy and systematic studies in animals suggest that the vast majority of spinally administered sufentanil rapidly leaves the CSF compartment to enter epidural fat, from where it is slowly absorbed into the systemic circulation. Second, drug can diffuse within CSF, both cranially and caudad. Experience with local anesthetics suggests that such drug movement is rapid, since lumbar injection of isobaric bupivacaine can achieve within 10 minutes upper thoracic to low cervical drug effects. Preliminary studies in volunteers at Wake Forest University School of Medicine demonstrate that this is also true of opioids—morphine and fentanyl move rapidly and similarly in CSF. This has been demonstrated previously both in dogs (38) and in humans (39). Thus, although there is a concentration gradient decreasing from the site of injection, if drug remains in CSF it rapidly moves cephalad. Third, drug can penetrate the spinal cord to reach its site of action in the dorsal horn gray matter. Once again, the efficiency of this process depends on physicochemical characteristics of the drug, especially lipid solubility. It has been demonstrated that, for the extremely lipid-soluble opioid sufentanil, almost all the drug partitions into the axon-rich white mater on the surface and superficial layer of the spinal cord (33, 35, 40). Of clinically used opiates, morphine is the best at penetrating to gray matter without getting "sucked up" in the "sponge" of white mater.

The above considerations for opioids explain initial experience with their clinical use and provide guidance with regard to other drugs (Table 9.5). Epidural morphine would be expected to be more potent than IV administration, should have a slow onset of action (slow penetration of the cord), and should have extensive rostral spread (long residence time in CSF). In contrast, epidural sufentanil would be expected to be no more potent than IV administration, have a rapid onset of action, and have minimal dermatomal spread since the drug is acting by systemic absorption rather than at a spinal site. With spinal administration, morphine becomes yet more potent, dermatomally extensive, and long lasting, and, with large doses (5 to 10 μg), sufentanil can have some spinal effect. Interestingly, extensive dermatomal spread, although with brief duration, can be observed with spinal injection of fentanyl and sufentanil. This probably reflects the large dose of drug administered, allowing enough time in CSF for the normal, rapid spread, then rapid penetration of the cord. There is now significant clinical experience in obstetric anesthesia with intraspinal opioids and other nonlocal anesthetics.

REFERENCES

1. Wang JK, Nuss LA, Thomas JE. Pain relief by intrathecally applied morphine in man. *Anesthesiology* 1979;50:149–151.
2. Yaksh TL. Spinal opiate analgesia: Characteristics and principles of action. *Pain* 1981;11:293–346.
3. Leighton GE, Rodriguez RE, Hill RG, Hughes J. K-Opioid agonists produce antinociception after i.v. and i.c.v. but not intrathecal administration in the rat. *Br J Pharmacol* 1988;93:553–560.
4. Sander HW, Portoghese PS, Gintzler AR. Spinal kappa-opiate receptor involvement in the analgesia of pregnancy: Effects of intrathecal nor-binaltorphimine, a kappa-selective antagonist. *Brain Res* 1988;474:343–347.
5. Long JB, Martinez-Arizala A, Ecchevarria EE, Tidwell RE, Holaday JW. Hindlimb paralytic effects of prodynorphin-derived peptides following spinal subarachnoid injection in rats. *Eur J Pharmacol* 1988;153:45–54.
6. Rawal N, Nuutinen P, Prithvi Raj P, et al. Behavioral and histopathologic effects following intrathecal administration of butorphanol, sufentanil, and nalbuphine in sheep. *Anesthesiology* 1991;75:1025–1034.
7. Hatjis CG, Meis PJ. Sinusoidal fetal heart rate pattern associated with butorphanol administration. *Obstet Gynecol* 1986;67:377–380.
8. Zhu, YX, Hsu MS, Pintar JE. Developmental expression of the m, kappa, and delta opioid receptor mRNAs in mouse. *J Neurosci* 1998;18:2538–2549.
9. Stone LS, Broberger C, Vulchanova L, et al. Differential distribution of a2A and a2C adrenergic receptor immuno-reactivity in the rat spinal cord. *J Neurosci* 1998;18:5928–5937.
10. Kuraishi Y, Hirota N, Sato Y, Kaneko S, Satoh M, Takagi H. Noradrenergic inhibition of the release of substance P from the primary afferents in the rabbit spinal dorsal horn. *Brain Res* 1985;359:177–182.
11. North RA, Yoshimura M. The actions of noradrenaline on neurones of the rat substantia gelatinosa in vitro. *J Physiol* 1984;349:43–55.
12. Roy G, Philippe E, Gaulin F, Guay G. Peripheral projections of the chick primary sensory neurons expressing gamma-aminobutyric acid immunoreactivity. *Neuroscience* 1991;45:177–183.
13. Yaksh TL. Pharmacology of spinal adrenergic systems which modulate spinal nociceptive processing. *Pharmacol Biochem Behav* 1985;22:845–858.
14. Eisenach JC, Tong C. Site of hemodynamic effects of intrathecal a2-adrenergic agonists. *Anesthesiology* 1991;74:766–771.
15. Eisenach JC, Castro MI, Dewan M, Rose JC. Epidural clonidine analgesia in obstetrics: Sheep studies. *Anesthesiology* 1989;70:51–56.
16. Correa-Sales C, Rabin BC, Maze M. A hypnotic response to dexmedetomidine, an a2 agonist, is mediated in the locus coeruleus in rats. *Anesthesiology* 1992;76:948–952.
17. Khan IM, Yaksh TL, Taylor P. Epibatidine binding sites and activity in the spinal cord. *Brain Res* 1997;753:269–282.

18. Höglund AU, Baghdoyan HA. M2, M3 and M4, but not M1, muscarinic receptor subtypes are present in rat spinal cord *J Pharmacol Exp Ther* 1997;281:470–477.

19. Yaksh TL, Dirksen R, Harty GJ. Antinociceptive effects of intrathecally injected cholinomimetic drugs in the rat and cat. *Eur J Pharmacol* 1985;117:81–88.

20. Damaj MI, Fei-Yin M, Dukat M, Glassco W, Glennon RA, Martin BR. Antinociceptive responses to nicotinic acetylcholine receptor ligands after systemic and intrathecal administration in mice. *J Pharmacol Exp Ther* 1998;284:1058–1065.

21. Abram SE, Winne RP. Intrathecal acetyl cholinesterase inhibitors produce analgesia that is synergistic with morphine and clonidine in rats. *Anesth Analg* 1995;81:501–507.

22. Hwang JH, Hwang KS, Leem JK, Park PH, Han SM, Lee DM. The antiallodynic effects of intrathecal cholinesterase inhibitors in a rat model of neuropathic pain. *Anesthesiology* 1999;90:492–499.

23. Chiari A, Tobin JR, Pan HL, Hood D, Eisenach JC. Sex differences in cholinergic analgesia. I. A supplemental nicotinic mechanism in normal females. *Anesthesiology* 1999;91:1447–1454.

24. Sundaram K, Murugaian J, Krieger A, Sapru H. Microinjections of cholinergic agonists into the intermediolateral cell column of the spinal cord at T1–T3 increase heart rate and contractility. *Brain Res* 1989;503:22–31.

25. Carp H, Jayaram A, Morrow D. Intrathecal cholinergic agonists lessen bupivacaine spinal-block-induced hypotension in rats. *Anesth Analg* 1994;79:112–116.

26. Hood DD, Eisenach JC, Tuttle R. Phase I safety assessment of intrathecal neostigmine in humans. *Anesthesiology* 1995;82:331–343.

27. Sawynok J, Sweeney MI, White TD. Classification of adenosine receptors mediating antinociception in the rat spinal cord. *Br J Pharmacol* 1986;88:923–930.

28. Sollevi A. Adenosine for pain control. *Acta Anaesthesiol Scand* 1997;41:135–136.

29. Rane K, Segerdahl M, Goiny M, Sollevi A. Intrathecal adenosine administration—A phase 1 clinical safety study in healthy volunteers, with additional evaluation of its influence on sensory thresholds and experimental pain. *Anesthesiology* 1998;89:1108–1115.

30. Sabbe MB, Grafe MR, Mjanger E, Tiseo J, Hill HF, Yaksh TL. Spinal delivery of sufentanil, alfentanil, and morphine in dogs: Physiologic and toxicologic investigations. *Anesthesiology* 1994;81:899–920.

31. Yaksh TL, Rathbun M, Jag J, Mirzai T, Grafe M, Hiles RA. Pharmacology and toxicology of chronically infused epidural clonidine HCl in dogs. *Fundam Appl Toxicol* 1994;23:319–335.

32. Yaksh TL, Grafe MR, Malkmus S, Rathbun ML, Eisenach JC. Studies on the safety of chronically administered intrathecal neostigmine methylsulfate in rats and dogs. *Anesthesiology* 1995;82:412–427.

33. Bernards CM, Hill HF. Physical and chemical properties of drug molecules governing their diffusion through the spinal meninges. *Anesthesiology* 1992;77:750–756.

34. Eisenach J, Detweiler D, Hood D. Hemodynamic and analgesic actions of epidurally administered clonidine. *Anesthesiology* 1993;78:277–287.

35. Bernards CM, Hill HF. Morphine and alfentanil permeability through the spinal dura, arachnoid, and pia mater of dogs and monkeys. *Anesthesiology* 1990;73:1214–1219.

36. Liu SS, Gerancher JC, Bainton BG, Kopacz J, Carpenter RL. The effects of electrical stimulation at different frequencies on perception and pain in human volunteers: Epidural versus intravenous administration of fentanyl. *Anesth Analg* 1996;82:98–102.

37. D'Angelo R, Gerancher JC, Eisenach JC, Raphael BL. Epidural fentanyl produces labor analgesia by a spinal mechanism. *Anesthesiology* 1998;88:1519–1523.

38. Stevens RA, Petty RH, Hill HF, et al. Redistribution of sufentanil to cerebrospinal fluid and systemic circulation after epidural administration in dogs. *Anesth Analg* 1993;76:323–327.

39. Gourlay GK, Murphy TM, Plummer JL, Kowalski SR, Cherry A, Cousins MJ. Pharmacokinetics of fentanyl in lumbar and cervical CSF following lumbar epidural and intravenous administration. *Pain* 1989;38:253–259.

40. Ummenhofer WC, Arends RH, Shen DD, Bernards C. Comparative spinal distribution and clearance kinetics of intrathecally administered morphine, fentanyl, alfentanil and sufentanil. *Anesthesiology* 2000;92:739–753.

PART II CLINICAL APPLICATIONS

SAMUEL C. HUGHES, M. D.

The concept of intraspinal opioids is simple: long-lasting analgesia produced with minimal doses of opioids. This is potentially achieved by the almost direct, selective application of opioids (epidural or spinal) to the dorsal horn of the spinal column, resulting in analgesia without the systemic effects of opioids. The reality, however, includes specific side effects related to intraspinal opioids. The goal is to achieve a balance between administering enough opioid to allow the beneficial effects and avoiding higher doses that have increased side effects. It is only recently, for example, that the appropriate intrathecal dose of morphine for postoperative analgesia after cesarean section has been extensively evaluated (1, 2). Similarly, although the lipid—soluble opioids, fentanyl, and sufentanil have been increasingly used as intrathecal agents in labor with the combined spinal-epidural (CSE) technique, appropriate dose-response studies only have been recently performed (3, 4); however, the dose and combinations continue to be controversial (5). Use of the CSE technique has added a new clinical choice for obstetric analgesia and allowed significant investigation into pain mechanisms and possible drug combinations to achieve analgesia in labor (6–8). The remainder of this chapter examines the use of intraspinal opioid analgesia for labor, delivery, and intra- and postoperative cesarean section pain, and the side effects accompanying the use of this technique.

LABOR AND DELIVERY

When Wang et al. (9) demonstrated the successful and safe use of 0.5 to 1 mg intrathecal morphine for patients with chronic pain, the implications for obstetrics were clear. They had achieved 10 to 24 hours of analgesia with no sympathetic or motor blockade using very low doses of morphine. In general, the use of systemic opioids in obstetrics is limited by the possibility of maternal respiratory depression, orthostatic hypotension, nausea, vomiting, delayed gastric motility, decreased uterine activity when administered during early labor, and placental transfer of opioids resulting in neonatal respiratory depression. However, these problems are dose related, and some may be avoided or significantly ameliorated with the use of low-dose intraspinal opioids.

Intrathecal Opioids

Morphine

In an early investigation, the intrathecal application of as little as 0.5 mg morphine was successful in relieving the pain of the first stage of labor (Fig. 9.1) (10). In contrast, for nonobstetric patients, as much as 20 mg morphine has been used to relieve some forms of pain (11, 12). The ideal dose of morphine for analgesia during labor has not been determined and its use remains limited, but 0.025 to 0.1 mg morphine appears to be the appropriate range. High cerebrospinal fluid (CSF) levels of opioids can be achieved with as little as 0.25 mg intrathecal morphine, suggesting that the lower dose range may be useful (Fig. 9.2) (13). Significant side effects of nausea, vomiting, and pruritus have limited its use in obstetric analgesia, but it was the first drug investigated (14).

Early Clinical Experience

Scott et al. were the first to use intrathecal morphine (1.5 mg) to provide pain relief during labor (15). Although the study was small (n = 12), they made several important observations that are still relevant. First, patients obtained pain relief but "felt

contractions," demonstrating that opioid blockade of pain is not as complete as that achieved using local anesthetics. This effect potentially benefits patients who want pain relief but also fuller participation in the delivery experience. Second, they observed that 1.5 mg intrathecal morphine did not provide adequate pain relief for the second stage of labor. *Intraspinal opioids (except meperidine) achieve analgesia, not surgical anesthesia!* If surgical manipulation during labor and delivery is necessary (e.g., use of forceps or an episiotomy), local anesthetics would have to be administered via the epidural or spinal route (or other technique) to provide further analgesia or anesthesia. Compared with the flexibility offered by initially using a continuous epidural route, single-injection intrathecal administration has distinct disadvantages. One early investigator overcame this problem by following single-bolus injection of intrathecal morphine with placement of an epidural catheter to permit administration of local anesthetic if needed for delivery (16). The use of CSE has made this approach easier and will be discussed in detail. This allows for the easy intrathecal application of opioids and possibly other drugs, followed by the placement of an epidural catheter for later use as needed. However, CSE has only recently had more extensive applications, and our initial experience with intrathecal opioids was with the "single-shot" spinal. One limitation of the "single-shot" intrathecal technique is the slow onset of analgesia with morphine. Although early reports suggested a rapid onset, 30 to 45 minutes usually is required with morphine alone (Fig. 9.1). This is an unacceptable delay when the patient is in extreme pain. One possible approach to the problem is to combine a local anesthetic with morphine. Local anesthetics clearly have a potentiating effect on spinal morphine antinociception (17). Another approach might be to administer intrathecal opioids during early labor, perhaps when the cervix is 3 to 4 cm dilated with mild-to-moderate pain; this would allow for the onset of morphine's effects in early labor. While this may be effective in unique situations—for example, a patient with pulmonary hypertension—the slow onset and side effects have limited the use of morphine for labor analgesia.

The combination of 0.25 mg intrathecal morphine and 25 μg fentanyl administered through a long spinal needle placed through an epidural needle proved effective (18). The epidural catheter was then placed after the intrathecal injection to allow for the subsequent addition of a local anesthetic, which is generally needed in the second stage of labor (if not before) and also can be used if a surgical delivery is required. Bupivacaine 0.125% (or more dilute epidural solutions) has been demonstrated to be more effective if the patient had previously received intrathecal morphine (19). More recently, low-dose epidural infusions of fentanyl have been shown to produce analgesia by a primary spinal action (20). The combination of intrathecal morphine and fentanyl was first described by Leighton et al., but it is not analgesic *nirvana* (Fig. 9.3) (18). However, this study did demonstrate that lipid—soluble agents brought about rapid, profound—if short-lived—analgesia, and they are now used commonly with CSE techniques.

Limitations of Intrathecal Morphine

Intrathecal morphine has significant side effects, specifically the potential for delayed respiratory depression. While this appears extremely rare, it must be considered if this technique is to be used. Patients must be appropriately monitored for 12 to 24 hours for late onset of respiratory depression, and equipment for emergency resuscitation must be immediately available. Other side effects include nausea, vomiting, urinary

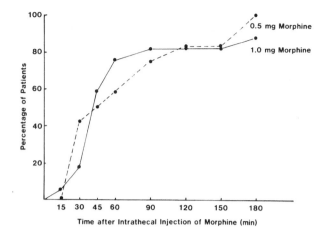

Figure 9.1. Onset of pain relief with intrathecal morphine. (Reprinted by permission from Abboud TK, Shnider SM, Dailey PA, et al. Intrathecal administration of hyperbaric morphine for the relief of pain in labor. *Br J Anaesth* 1984;56:1351–1360.)

retention, and pruritus (Table 9.1) (10). Pruritus is the most common of these side effects and may range from a mild facial itching to a generalized, highly irritating itch that requires immediate treatment. Aggressive treatment with naloxone (0.04 to 0.1 mg IV, repeated as necessary), including the possible use of a naloxone infusion (0.2 to 0.4 mg/h), diphenhydramine, nalbuphine, or small dose propofol bolus may decrease the pruritus and allow successful labor analgesia (14). Postdural puncture headaches (PDPH) were common (10, 21) with the initial use of

intrathecal morphine for labor. Thus, the early use of intrathecal opioids for labor analgesia, specifically morphine and fentanyl, was intriguing but generally considered to be impractical owing to the many side effects and the limitations of a single-shot spinal. However, these concerns have been resolved to a large extent (Table 9.2), and the use of intrathecal opioids has come full circle.

Intrathecal opioids and local anesthetics or other additives (via CSE, most commonly) are not routine in all centers at this time, but CSE may confer special benefits, for example, to parturients in whom the cardiovascular effects of routine regional anesthesia are undesirable. For certain cardiac patients, complications arise when there is a decrease in systemic vascular resistance during regional anesthesia (22). This can be avoided with the use of intraspinal opioids. Studies in animal models (23, 24) document that few, if any, cardiovascular effects accompany the use of epidural morphine (Fig. 9.4). Hypotension does occur in 10% to 15% of patients when fentanyl or sufentanil are combined with a local anesthetic and administered with CSE (25, 26). Several case reports of patients with complex cardiac problems demonstrate that intrathecal morphine can be used successfully (22, 27–30). The use of intrathecal opioids might benefit women with preeclampsia, although more investigation in these patients is necessary. In general, obstetric patients with aortic stenosis, tetralogy of Fallot, Eisenmenger's syndrome, coarctation of the aorta, or pulmonary hypertension might be considered candidates for the intraspinal technique, with or without an epidural catheter placed at the same time. The early clinical experience with intrathecal opioids and the development of finer spinal needles have led to the more routine use of CSE for labor analgesia.

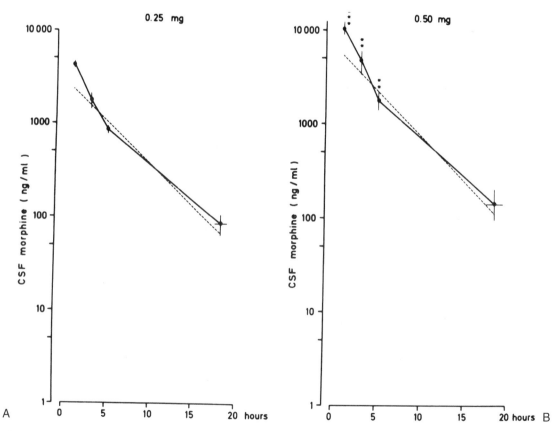

Figure 9.2. CSF morphine concentration contrasted with time plots following a single intrathecal dose of either (*A*) 0.25 mg or (*B*) 0.50 mg morphine in five and six patients, respectively. Values shown are mean ± SEM. The dotted line represents the regression line obtained by a monoexponential fit to the individual data points. Statistical evaluation by Student's t test. Statistical differences vs. the 0.25-mg group: **$P < .01$; ***$P < .001$. (Reprinted by permission from Nordberg G, Hedner T, Mellstrand T, Dahlström B. Pharmacokinetic aspects of intrathecal morphine analgesia. *Anesthesiology* 1984;60:448–454.)

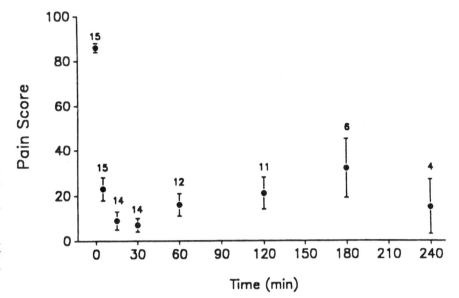

Figure 9.3. Mean ± SEM pain scores (0 = no pain, 100 = worst imaginable pain) after intrathecal injection of fentanyl (25 μg) and morphine (0.25 mg) for pain relief during labor. The number of patients still laboring under intrathecal opioid analgesia appears above each value. (Redrawn from Leighton BL, DeSimone CA, Norris MC, Ben-David B. Intrathecal narcotics for labor revisited: The combination of fentanyl and morphine intrathecally provides rapid onset of profound, prolonged analgesia. *Anesth Analg* 1989;69:122–125.)

Table 9.1. PERCENTAGES OF PATIENTS HAVING ADVERSE SIDE EFFECTS AFTER INTRATHECAL INJECTION OF 0.5 mg OR 1 mg MORPHINE*

Side Effects	Morphine		Combined Data (n = 30) (%)
	0.5 mg (n = 12) (%)	1 mg (n = 18) (%)	
Pruritus†	58	94	80
Nausea/vomiting	50	56	53
Urinary retention	42	44	43
Drowsiness/dizziness	33	50	43
Respiratory depression	0	6	3
Headache	0	5	3

* This table demonstrates the incidence of side effects demonstrated by one study, but is representative of what might be expected. Pruritus is the most common side effect. Incidence of urinary retention is very high and probably related to labor and delivery.
† $P = .02$ (0.5 mg vs. 1 mg).
Adapted from Abboud TK, Shnider SM, Dailey PA, et al. Intrathecal administration of hyperbaric morphine for the relief of pain in labor. *Br J Anaesth* 1984;56:1351–1360.

Table 9.2. INTRATHECAL OPIOIDS FOR LABOR AND DELIVERY: PROBLEMS ENCOUNTERED AND RESOLUTIONS

Problems Encountered With Initial Experience	Resolutions That Have Led to Increase in Spinal Techniques
1. Slow onset with intrathecal morphine (30–90 min)	Intrathecal fentanyl or sufentanil rapid onset (2–5 min); local anesthetic
2. Limitations of "single-shot" intrathecal injection	CSE technique
3. PDPH 15–30% historically with standard cutting spinal needles	Pencil-point, noncutting spinal needles with low incidence of PDPH
4. Side effects include pruritus, nausea, vomiting, respiratory depression	Lower dose of opioids, treatment (naloxone, nalbuphine, etc.), and use of routine monitoring

CSE = combined spinal-epidural technique; PDPH = postdural puncture headache.

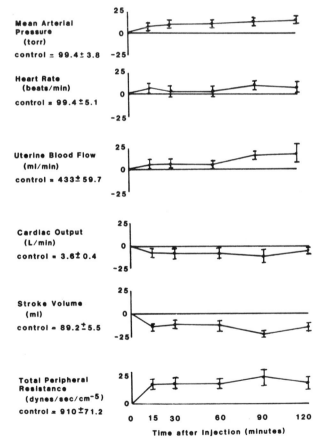

Figure 9.4. Following the injection of 20 mg epidural morphine in the pregnant ewe, there were no significant changes in maternal cardiovascular parameters or uterine blood flow. Not shown are fetal data that demonstrated no change in blood pressure, heart rate, or acid-base status. (Data from Rosen MA, Hughes SC, Curtis JD, Norton M, Levinson G, Shnider SM. Effects of epidural morphine on uterine blood flow and acid-base status in the pregnant ewe [abstract]. *Anesthesiology* 1982;57:A383.)

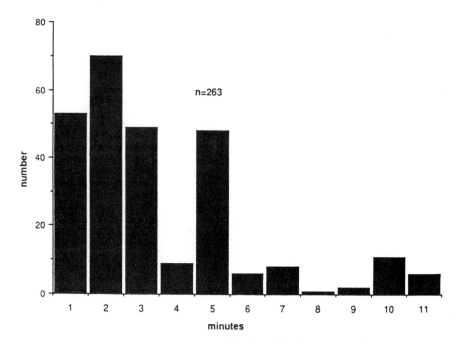

Figure 9.5. Time in minutes to first painless contraction following subarachnoid injection of 2.5 mg bupivacaine and 25 μg fentanyl. (Reprinted by permission from Collis RE, Baxandall ML, Srikantharajah ID, Edge G, Kadim MY, Morgan BM. Combined spinal epidural (CSE) analgesia: Technique, management, and outcome of 300 mothers. *Int J Obstet Anesth* 1994; 3:75–81.)

Combined Spinal-Epidural for Labor Analgesia

The use of CSE technique for labor analgesia has increased rapidly over the last few years. There has been extensive use of CSE for surgical procedures as well as labor analgesia (7). While CSE is not used commonly for cesarean section in the United States, there has been extensive experience in other parts of the world (Chapter 11: Table 11.8). This led to the introduction of this technique to the labor ward. An early large report of women who had received CSE for labor (n = 300) indicated that the technique could be very useful. The intrathecal application of bupivacaine (2.5 mg) and fentanyl (25 μg) provided rapid analgesia in 2 to 5 minutes in most women (Fig. 9.5) (6), although the spinal portion of the technique failed in 32 cases (10%). The epidural catheter provided successful analgesia for these patients. In the group with successful analgesia from the intrathecal injection (n = 268), an epidural top-up was required in most women (n = 245) within 90 minutes (mean) (Fig. 9.6) (6); however, the range was quite variable. There was no motor

blockade in 97% of the women, and approximately 50% chose to stand, walk, or sit in a rocking chair at some time during labor. Analgesia was maintained with 10 to 15 mL 0.1% bupivacaine and 0.0002% fentanyl. These results are very similar to the extensive investigation by Norris et al. (31) In an investigation undertaken by Campbell et al., the intrathecal preparation injected was sufentanil 10 μg and bupivacaine 2.5 mg (32). Bupivacaine alone provided analgesia for 70 ± 34 minutes and sufentanil for 114 ± 26 minutes, compared with 148 ± 27 minutes when administered together to nulliparous parturients requesting labor analgesia (Fig. 9.7). There was no evidence of motor blockade, excessive somnolence, fetal heart rate (FHR) abnormalities or PDPH in any of the patients. *However, pruritus was reported in 80% to 86% of the patients who received sufentanil.* The authors did a further study with the bupivacaine (2.5 mg) and sufentanil (10 μg) combination and compared it to a similar solution to which epinephrine (0.2 mg) had been added. The duration of intrathecal labor analgesia was significantly prolonged

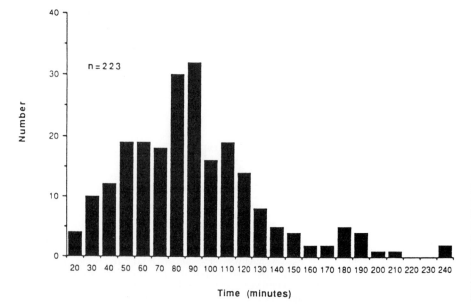

Figure 9.6. Time in minutes to first epidural top-up after subarachnoid block with 2.5 mg bupivacaine and 25 μg fentanyl (mean = 90 minutes; median = 86 minutes; mode = 95 minutes). (Reprinted by permission from Collis RE, Baxandall ML, Srikantharajah ID, Edge G, Kadim MY, Morgan BM. Combined spinal epidural (CSE) analgesia: Technique, management, and outcome of 300 mothers. *Int J Obstet Anesth* 1994;3:75–81.)

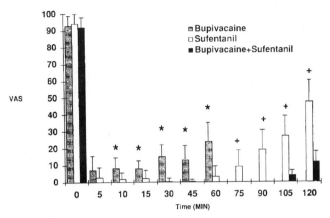

Figure 9.7. Visual analog scale (*VAS*) pain scores on the *y* axis, and time after the intrathecal injection of the study solution on the *x* axis. *Time 0* represents scores reported immediately prior to the intrathecal injection of the study solution. Data are mean ± SD; *$P < .02$ compared to either sufentanil or the combination of bupivacaine and sufentanil; +$P < .02$ compared to the combination of bupivacaine and sufentanil. (Reprinted by permission from Campbell DC, Camann WR, Datta S. The addition of bupivacaine to intrathecal sufentanil for labor analgesia. *Anesth Analg* 1995;81:305–309.)

by the addition of epinephrine (188 ± 25 minutes vs. 145 ± 23 minutes, $P < .0001$) (Fig. 9.8) (33). However, 100% of the women who received sufentanil plus bupivacaine could ambulate, while only 80% (NS) of those who received sufentanil, bupivacaine, and epinephrine were able to ambulate. Thus, the increased duration of action achieved with the addition of epinephrine must be weighed with the possibility of increased motor blockade, particularly if ambulation is a goal. Lower doses of epinephrine may not have this effect. There has now been extensive experience with this technique, and it is widely practiced (31, 34–44).

Few studies have tried to establish a dose-response curve with the several combinations suggested; however, the most common approach reported is a combination of fentanyl 25 μg or sufentanil 10 μg plus bupivacaine 2.5 mg followed by a dilute solution of bupivacaine (Table 9.3). The CSE technique has allowed investigators to establish a dose response for fentanyl (4, 45) and sufentanil (3, 5) when used as the sole intrathecal agent for

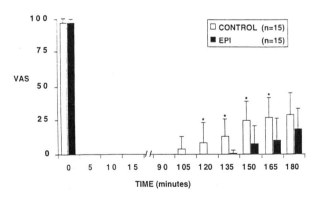

Figure 9.8. Visual analog scale (*VAS*) pain scores are on the *y* axis, and time (in minutes) after the intrathecal administration of the study solution on the *x* axis. *Time 0* represents VAS scores reported immediately before the intrathecal administration of the study solution. Data are expressed as mean ± SD; *$P < .05$. (Reprinted by permission from Campbell DC, Banner R, Crone LA, Hickman WG, Yip RW. Addition of epinephrine to intrathecal bupivacaine and sufentanil for ambulatory labor analgesia. *Anesthesiology* 1997;86:525–531.)

Table 9.3. COMBINED SPINAL-EPIDURAL FOR LABOR: POSSIBLE DRUG COMBINATIONS

Intrathecal

1) Fentanyl 10–25 μg
   or
   Sufentanil 2.5–10 μg
2) Bupivacaine 1–2.5 mg
3) Epinephrine 25–200 μg

Epidural

1) Bupivacaine 0.0625–0.125% at 10–15 mL/h
   or
2) Bupivacaine (as above) + fentanyl 1–2 μg/mL
   or
   Sufentanil 0.2–0.33 μg/mL

labor. In nulliparous women who received intrathecal sufentanil alone for labor analgesia, the median effective dose (ED$_{50}$) was 1.8 ± 0.6 μg and the calculated ED$_{95}$ was 15.3 ± 13.9 μg (3). When fentanyl was studied in a similar population, the median effective dose was 14 μg (confidence interval [CI], 13 to 15 μg), and the data indicated that there was no benefit to increasing the dose beyond 25 μg (Fig. 9.9) (4).

Side effects must be considered as well. With increasing doses of intrathecal opioids, the incidence of pruritus, sedation, nausea and vomiting increase, as well as other possible side effects (31). With refinement of CSE, lower doses of the drugs currently in use or the application of other drugs for neuromodulation may allow for adequate analgesia with fewer side effects.

Side Effects of CSE Technique

The side effects and complications that are encountered with the CSE technique are similar to those that result from either epidural or intrathecal opioids and are discussed later in this chapter. However, there are several unique concerns as well (31, 33).

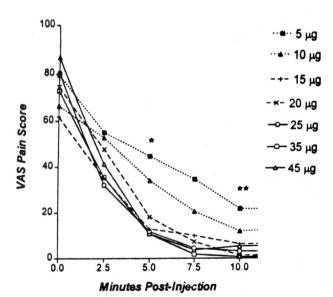

Figure 9.9. Pain scores after fentanyl injection. Mean visual analog pain scores recorded after intrathecal injection in all groups. *$P < .05$: 5-μg group vs. 15-μg through 45-μg groups, and 10-μg group vs. 25-μg through 45-μg groups. **$P < .05$, 5-μg group vs. 15-μg through 45-μg groups, 10-μg group vs. 20-μg and 35-μg groups. (Reprinted by permission from Palmer CM, Cork RC, Hays R, Van Maren G, Alves D. The dose-response relation of intrathecal fentanyl for labor analgesia. *Anesthesiology* 1998;88:355–361.)

Pruritus, as noted earlier, occurs in 80% of patients who receive intrathecal sufentanil (32). Although pruritus with lipid-soluble opioids is of shorter duration than that caused by morphine, it may be dose dependent (20, 45), and it is extremely common. **Hypotension** occurs in 5% to 10% of patients who receive intrathecal fentanyl or sufentanil (25, 26), and the incidence may increase with the addition of local anesthetics or other agents. The decrease in blood pressure probably results from pain relief and is likely related to a decrease in maternal catecholamines, particularly epinephrine (26, 46). **Fetal bradycardia** occasionally may occur with the onset of analgesia from intrathecally administered opioids (47–49), although this is controversial. The incidence of fetal bradycardia after routine epidural analgesia or analgesia achieved with intrathecal opioids (CSE) has been reported to be similar (48, 50, 51) or occur in greater frequency than with intrathecal opioids (49, 52, 53). Conversely, the large study by Collis et al. (6) noted that approximately one third of those patients with abnormal FHR tracings prior to CSE had improvement in their FHR patterns with CSE.

In a randomized investigation that compared analgesia with CSE vs. intravenous (IV) meperidine, an intent-to-treat analysis of 1223 women indicated that there was no increase in the rate of cesarean delivery for dystocia (CSE, 3.5% vs. IV meperidine, 4%; *P* not significant) or in the overall cesarean delivery rate (CSE, 6% vs. IV meperidine, 5.5%) (54). However, there was profound fetal bradycardia necessitating cesarean delivery in 8 of 400 parturients who received CSE vs. 0 of 352 who received IV meperidine (*P* < .01), but the method of fetal monitoring differed between the two groups. Despite this, the neonatal outcomes were similar. In a larger, retrospective study (n = 2560), there was no difference in the incidence of emergency cesarean delivery after CSE with intrathecal sufentanil (10 to 15 μg) vs. systemic medication or no medication (n = 1140) for labor analgesia (1.3% vs. 1.4%) (55). The authors noted that emergency cesarean delivery for fetal distress within 90 minutes of CSE occurred only in association with complicating obstetric factors.

While the concern for potential fetal bradycardia resulting from the CSE technique remains controversial, a possible mechanism was suggested in an early report (47). Clarke et al. suggested that uterine hyperactivity after intrathecal fentanyl (50 μg) was caused by a rapid decrease in maternal catecholamines. Thus, rapid onset in maternal analgesia may play a role. A decrease in maternal plasma epinephrine but not norepinephrine was demonstrated in a study comparing intrathecal fentanyl (25 μg) vs. epidural lidocaine (1.5%) for labor analgesia (56). While the decline in epinephrine was similar in both groups, there was a more rapid fall in epinephrine after intrathecal fentanyl (Fig. 9.10). In an animal model, it has been demonstrated that decreasing epinephrine but not norepinephrine will result in increased uterine activity (57a). Thus, the rapid onset of analgesia and a decline in maternal plasma epinephrine may cause an increase in uterine tone in some parturients and, potentially, fetal bradycardia. This will remain an area of controversy until further investigation is completed. However, the management of nonreassuring FHR changes includes maternal position change, and administration of oxygen and IV fluids.

In addition to the efficacy of β-agonist (terbutaline) administration, IV nitroglycerin (60 to 90 μg initially) has been shown to be effective in treating fetal bradycardia associated with uterine hyperactivity (58). A second dose of nitroglycerin was necessary in 38% of patients (total dose, 180 μg). Hypotension was minimal and brief. Fetal bradycardia was associated with an oxytocin infusion in 62% of the cases and spontaneous labor in 38%. Some clinicians would administer nitroglycerin 200 μg IV or 400 to 800 μg sublingual spray as the initial treatment, but this has not been prospectively evaluated. Nitroglycerin administration may prove useful if uterine hyperactivity is suspected after CSE.

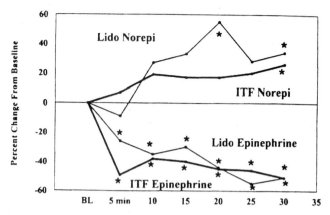

Figure 9.10. Percent change in maternal epinephrine and norepinephrine (*Norepi*) levels from baseline (*BL*) values. The intrathecal fentanyl group is indicated as *ITF* and the epidural lidocaine group as *Lido*. Data are mean ± SD. *Significantly different from baseline within the group. (Reprinted by permission from Cascio M, Pygon B, Bernett C, Ramanathan S. Labour analgesia with intrathecal fentanyl decreases maternal stress. *Can J Anaesth* 1997;44:605–609.)

Respiratory depression after intrathecal and epidural opioids is a rare but serious complication. Delayed respiratory depression has been reported in the early clinical experience with this technique (59). Respiratory depression has been noted after both intrathecal fentanyl (60) and sufentanil (61–65), although the latter is strikingly more frequently described. Maternal respiratory depression may occur more frequently if IV opioids have been given prior to intrathecal opioid administration. Respiratory depression also appears to be dose related (45, 66). Respiratory depression after intrathecal fentanyl (rare) or sufentanil comes on rapidly (5 to 30 minutes) and is easily treated with oxygen and naloxone (0.05 to 0.1 mg IV) as needed. Mild sedation or drowsiness is fairly common, but respiratory depression requiring IV naloxone and oxygen is highly unusual. Monitoring vital signs and mental alertness are necessary, and monitoring oxygen saturation with pulse oximetry can be useful.

High cervical sensory blocks have been reported with patients complaining of dysphagia or dyspnea (67, 68). This is very transient and can be treated with small doses of IV naloxone. **Meningitis** and **epidural abscess** have been reported with the use of CSE (69–71) but also after conventional spinal or epidural techniques (Chapter 23). The incidence of **PDPH** requiring an epidural blood patch has been reported to be the same when comparing epidural vs. the CSE technique (31). In one large series, there were no cases of PDPH after CSE (72). Surprisingly, with an epidural needle in place, passage of a spinal needle with the needle-through-needle technique does not always result in a successful dural puncture (6, 7). This may be explained in several ways (Fig. 9.11). The spinal needle should extend 10 to 15 mm beyond the tip of the epidural needle and the equipment used should be evaluated with this consideration in mind. In one recent large review, the spinal needle insertion had a failure rate of only 0.5% (55). If this occurs, proceeding with an epidural is usually successful.

When placing an epidural catheter with the CSE technique (after a dural puncture), there is concern that the catheter will penetrate the dura. While this has been reported, it is extremely rare (7). In one review of more than 11,500 patients with the CSE technique, there were no cases of *late* epidural migration. However, a handful of epidural catheters penetrating into the subarachnoid space were noted with *initial* epidural placement. While epiduroscopy studies have demonstrated that it is extremely difficult (if not impossible) to pass a 16- or 18-gauge epidural catheter through a hole made in the dura with a 25-gauge spinal needle (73), the possibility of subarachnoid,

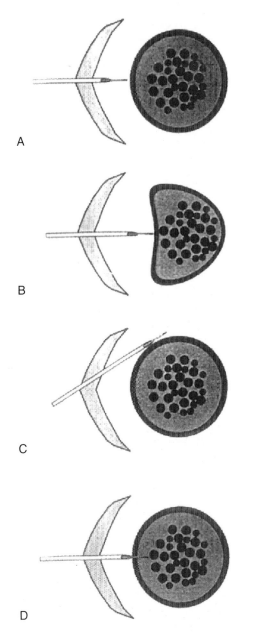

A

B

C

D

Figure 9.11. Figure showing various possibilities for combined spinal-epidural block failure due to incorrect technique (*A–C*) and correct position of epidural and spinal needle (*D*). *A*: Length of spinal needle protruding from tip of epidural needle is too short (or epidural needle is not introduced far enough into epidural space). *B*: Tip of spinal needle "tents" the dura but fails to pierce it (possibly a greater risk with "pencil-point" needles). *C*: Malposition of epidural needle. *D*: Correct position of epidural and spinal needles. (Reprinted by permission from Rawal N, Van Zundert A, Holmström B, Crowhurst JA. Combined spinal-epidural technique. *Reg Anesth* 1997;22:406–423.)

subdural, or IV placement of any "epidural" catheter exists. These dangers are not unique to the CSE technique, which has a remarkable safety record (7). Also, it should be noted that an epidural solution given immediately (within 5 minutes) after an intrathecal injection can increase the sensory level of the spinal agents previously administered (74, 75), but this is not clinically significant in most circumstances (76).

Walking Epidurals

Much of the focus on the CSE technique relates to the desire to decrease the broad motor effects of the traditional epidural,

which uses more concentrated local anesthetic solutions. One of the goals has been to allow the patient to ambulate, or at least achieve greater ease in patient care and greater patient satisfaction with increased patient mobility. There has also been an association made between conventional lumbar epidural analgesia and an increased rate of operative deliveries (see Chapter 3). This has resulted in the use of even more dilute local anesthetic solutions for lumbar epidural analgesia during labor, as well as encouraging the use of CSE techniques, and renewed investigation of the effects of walking during labor. Bloom et al., in a study of over 1000 parturients who did not receive regional analgesia for labor, failed to show any benefit on the progress in labor from "walking" compared with parturients who did not walk (77). There were no differences in labor progress, need for oxytocin augmentation, use of analgesics, or instrumental or surgical delivery rates. In an investigation by Nageotte et al. (78), 761 nulliparous women were evaluated at term gestation, comparing continuous lumbar epidural analgesia (bupivacaine 0.125% + fentanyl 2 μg $\cdot$ mL^{-1}, 10 mL./h) with CSE (sufentanil, 10 μg intrathecal + continuous infusion of bupivacaine 0.0625% + fentanyl 2 μg $\cdot$ mL^{-1}, 12 mL./h) for pain relief in labor. Among the group who received CSE analgesia, some were discouraged from walking while others were encouraged to walk. Patients with the standard epidural analgesia were not allowed to walk. There were no significant differences in the overall rate of cesarean section, incidence of dystocia, patients' or nursing staffs' assessment of the adequacy of analgesia, or the overall satisfaction between the groups. However, fewer women who received CSE required instrumental deliveries (CSE ambulation discouraged, 28% vs. CSE ambulation encouraged, 33%) compared with the standard epidural group (40%). Among the women who received CSE analgesia, there were no differences between the women who walked and those who did not, including the requirement for instrumental deliveries. Thus, the benefits of walking remain poorly documented and controversial.

Maternal Safety and Walking

The CSE technique is associated with mild hypotension and some degree of motor block in parturients. While these concerns may be minimal for most women, the patient must be carefully evaluated before ambulation is allowed (Table 9.4) (79). In the initial large study of this technique that created a great deal of interest in "walking," 131 of 275 parturients stood up out of bed and 76 sat in a rocking chair (6). Only 65 parturients actually walked, all in the company of a midwife. Of the initial group, 11 had severe motor block despite the low-dose CSE approach, and an additional 38 developed motor weakness at some time with the epidural infusion. The authors stressed the need to carefully evaluate the patients before ambulating.

Recent research has focused on more sophisticated evaluation of patients who have received epidural or CSE analgesia for labor, to include evaluating dorsal column sensory

---

Table 9.4. SUGGESTED CRITERIA FOR "WALKING EPIDURALS"

1. No obstetrical contraindications
2. No change in lying-to-sitting blood pressure (< 10%)
3. Ability to perform straight-leg raise
4. Ability to do one or more partial deep-knee bends at bedside
5. Someone is available to walk with the patient (partner, nurse, midwife)

Each hospital will need to consider its own criteria to allow patients to ambulate with regional anesthesia.
Adapted from Douglas MJ. Walking epidural analgesia in labour. *Can J Anaesth* 1998;45:607–611.

deficits (80) and computerized dynamic posturography (81). In the first instance, 90% or more of patients receiving low-dose bupivacaine/fentanyl analgesia (CSE or epidural) had normal lower limb motor power and dorsal column function (80). In the second study, women who received CSE (bupivacaine 2.5 mg/fentanyl 5 μg) were compared with pregnant women of similar gestation but not in labor using posturographic testing, which measures balance (80). The investigators concluded that balance function is preserved even in the presence of mild sensory deficits. If there was no clinical evidence of motor blockade, balance function was preserved. Investigation in this area is ongoing and intriguing (82). If the patient is allowed to ambulate, careful guidelines must still be considered (Table 9.4) (79).

At University of California San Francisco (UCSF), we allow ambulation after intrathecal opioid administration alone, but we do not allow ambulation with regional analgesic techniques that include the use of local anesthetics. Both patients and nursing staff have appreciated the use of more dilute epidural solutions and CSE techniques. However, this approach does not always provide satisfactory analgesia, and more concentrated epidural solutions should be used as indicated. While the CSE technique is appealing, it is not universally effective. Furthermore, epidural analgesic techniques with dilute solutions of local anesthetic agents and opioids may provide comparable results to those achieved with CSE techniques (39, 80, 81, 83).

PROGRESS IN LABOR

Intrathecal opioids could potentially effect the course of labor either directly or indirectly. Baraka et al. demonstrated that neither 1 nor 2 mg of intrathecal morphine affected the rate of cervical dilation (16). Two other studies reported a similar lack of effect of intrathecal morphine on progress in labor (10, 84). Epidural opioids have been reported to have no effect (85). However, Abouleish et al. noted a *prolonged* first but not second stage of labor after intrathecal morphine administration (0.2 mg) (19), while epidural fentanyl was reported to actually shorten labor (86). Various hypotheses were proposed, including (a) hypothalamic-pituitary level action of morphine, (b) a spinal cord site of action resulting in an effect similar to that of morphine upon micturition, and (c) direct uterine opioid receptor effects (18, 19, 87, 88).

As CSE techniques are used more frequently, some anecdotal reports suggest that a more rapid progression of labor occurs. When comparing CSE to epidural analgesia in laboring nulliparous women, investigators found no difference in the overall cesarean section rate or the incidence of dystocia (78). It was noted, however, that there was a slightly greater incidence of instrumental deliveries in those parturients who received epidural analgesia (40%) vs. those who received CSE (28% when walking was discouraged vs. 33% when walking was encouraged). Another randomized trial comparing CSE with epidural analgesia found no difference in mode of delivery (41). When comparing CSE labor analgesia with the parturient remaining in bed with the same analgesia and the parturient encouraged to walk for at least 20 minutes each hour, there was no significant difference in duration of labor or mode of delivery (89).

More recently, Tsen et al. noted that intrathecal sufentanil (10 μg) administered to nulliparous parturients in early labor resulted in more rapid cervical dilation compared with administration of standard labor epidural analgesia (Table 9.5) (90). The CSE group experienced a mean initial cervical dilation rate that was twice that of the epidural group, and this persisted for the first stage of labor. This shortened the time to full cervical dilation by 78 minutes in the CSE group. While this remains a controversial finding, the potential mechanism may be a rapid decrease in maternal circulating epinephrine, a known tocolytic, while norepinephrine remains elevated after CSE. It has been postulated that norepinephrine can increase uterine tone and can cause uterine hypertonia (47, 56, 57). However, as demon-

Table 9.5. PROGRESS OF LABOR

	Combined Spinal-Epidural*	Epidural
Onset of labor to analgesia (h)	10.0 ± 5.2	11.6 ± 8.9
Analgesia to full cervical dilation (h)	3.8 ± 2.6	5.1 ± 2.6[†]
Full cervical dilation to delivery (h)	1.8 ± 1.2	2.2 ± 1.5
Initial cervical dilation rate (cm/h)[‡]	2.1 ± 2.1	1.0 ± 1.0[†]
Mean cervical dilation rate[§]	2.3 ± 2.6	1.3 ± 0.7[†]
Mode of delivery (%)		
Spontaneous vaginal	68	66
Instrumental vaginal	16	16
Cesarean section	16	18

* Times and cervical dilation rates are shown as mean ± SD.
[†] $P < .05$ for difference between analgesic groups (see text for statistical details).
[‡] Initial cervical dilation rate = (first cervical examination after analgesia − last cervical examination before analgesia)/time between examinations.
[§] Mean cervical dilation rate = (10 − last cervical examination before analgesia)/time between examinations.
Reprinted by permission from Tsen LC, Thue B, Datta S, Segal S. Is combined spinal-epidural analgesia associated with more rapid cervical dilation in nulliparous patients when compared with conventional epidural analgesia? *Anesthesiology* 1999;91:920–925.

strated previously, the effects of regional analgesia and progress in labor are difficult to study carefully, and this will likely remain controversial.

Epidural Opioids

The use of continuous epidural infusions of local anesthetic solutions containing opioids has become standard for labor analgesia. When Behar et al. reported that good pain relief was achieved with epidural morphine (2 mg) in 1979, their finding stimulated consideration of its particular relevance for labor and delivery (91). The possibility of providing effective obstetric analgesia with such a small amount of opioid without resultant sympathectomy or motor blockade was very intriguing. The *continuous epidural* technique, if effective, would have a distinct advantage over single injection intrathecal administration because it would be readily adaptable to changing clinical situations, for example, a decision to perform a cesarean section.

Although one of the first reports following that of Behar et al. sounded optimistic (92), subsequent reports of epidural opioids were not encouraging. Most investigators have reported generally unsatisfactory results using low-dose epidural morphine or other opioids as sole agents for analgesia during labor. Husemeyer et al. (93) tried to repeat the work of Behar et al. (91) using 2 mg preservative-free epidural morphine for women in labor, and found that it provided no appreciable pain relief. Overall, investigators using 2 to 5 mg epidural morphine or equivalent doses of meperidine have demonstrated that these doses are inadequate (93–98). These findings contrast sharply with the effectiveness of 0.5 mg intrathecal morphine for labor analgesia reported initially (10) or 3 to 7.5 mg epidural morphine for postoperative analgesia. Studies performed by Hughes et al. at UCSF (99) suggested a dose response. At relatively similar doses, intrathecal injection introduces more morphine into the CSF than epidural administration (Table 9.6), indicating that epidural morphine doses must be much higher than intrathecal doses to achieve similarly effective analgesia.

Hughes et al. compared the effectiveness of preservative-free epidural morphine at doses of 2.0, 5.0, and 7.5 mg with that of

Table 9.6. INTRASPINAL MORPHINE AND CEREBROSPINAL FLUID CONCENTRATION

Site of Administration and Dose	Concentration (Time After Administration)	
	1 h	*18 h*
Epidural, 2–6 mg	200–1000 ng/mL	25–40 ng/mL
Spinal, 0.25–0.50 mg	4000–10,000 ng/mL	180–200 ng/mL

Adapted from Nordberger G, Hedner T, Mellstrand T, Dahlström B. Pharmacokinetic aspects of intrathecal morphine analgesia. *Anesthesiology* 1984;60:448–454.

bupivacaine 0.5%. Morphine 2 and 5 mg was ineffective, but at 7.5 mg it produced satisfactory analgesia in 7 of 11 patients (Fig. 9.12) (99). Analgesia produced by 0.5% bupivacaine (no longer commonly used for labor) was superior, although repeated doses were necessary and resulted in the expected significant motor and sympathetic blockade. Figure 9.12 also demonstrates the analgesia achieved with intrathecal administration of morphine from a subsequent study (10). As much as 10 mg epidural morphine was administered with only modest success (100, 101), with significant side effects that included nausea, vomiting, pruritus, and increased drowsiness. As epidural opioid doses increase, placental transfer of opioids also must be considered (Fig. 9.13). The slow-onset, high-dose requirement and significant side effects led most investigators to try other opioids as epidural agents.

Epidural meperidine (85), fentanyl (102), sufentanil (103), alfentanil (104), and lofentanil also have been used for analgesia for labor and delivery. These more lipophilic agents have a rapid onset but shorter duration of action than morphine. According to one study, 100 mg epidural meperidine provided satisfactory analgesia for obstetric patients for only 160 ± 90.3 minutes (85). Epidural fentanyl also was found to be somewhat effective but for a short duration. Analgesia of such short duration may be significantly related to systemic absorption. Epidural sufentanil was reported to provide significant dose-related

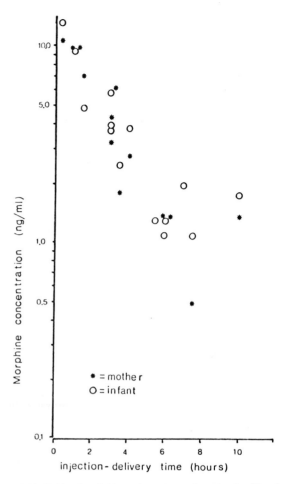

Figure 9.13. Epidural opioids and newborn drug levels. (Reprinted by permission from Nybell-Lindahl G, Carlsson C, Ingemarsson I, Westgren M, Paalzow L. Maternal and fetal concentrations of morphine after epidural administration during labor. *Am J Obstet Gynecol* 1981;139:20–21.)

analgesia for labor at doses as low as 5.0 μg (Fig. 9.14) with no neonatal complications. However, all patients had received an epidural lidocaine-epinephrine test dose, and the success of epidural sufentanil was most probably the product of the combination of local anesthetic, opioid, and the α₂-effects of epinephrine. Epidural alfentanil in large doses (30 μg · kg⁻¹) in contrast to smaller doses (105, 106) has led to neonatal hypotonia, and the high doses should be avoided (104). Thus, it is clear that epidural opioids alone have proven singularly unsuccessful as epidural agents. This was clearly demonstrated in a study in which women in active labor received sufentanil 10 μg, either intrathecally, epidurally diluted to 10 mL, or intravenously. The patients received no local anesthetics initially, and no epidural test dose. The epidural and IV sufentanil achieved minimal analgesia, while intrathecal sufentanil achieved excellent analgesia with a mean duration of 84 minutes (Fig. 9.15) (34). The excellent success of the application of intrathecal sufentanil encouraged the use of the CSE technique. However, the combination of an epidural local anesthetic and a lipid-soluble opioid became the focus of many investigators.

LOCAL ANESTHETICS AND LIPID-SOLUBLE OPIOIDS

Justins et al. suggested that 80 μg fentanyl added to 3 mL 0.5% bupivacaine provided a faster onset and longer duration of analgesia than a similar volume and concentration of bupivacaine

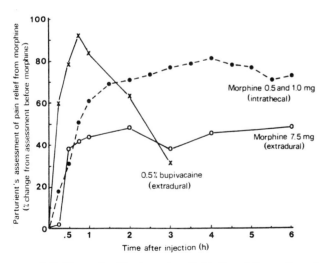

Figure 9.12. Maternal subjective pain relief before delivery after administration of contrasting 10 mL 0.5% epidural bupivacaine, 7.5 mg epidural morphine, or 0.5 and 1.0 mg intrathecal morphine. (Reprinted by permission from Hughes SC, Rosen MA, Shnider SM, Abboud TK, Stefani SJ, Norton M. Maternal and neonatal effects of epidural morphine for labor and delivery. *Anesth Analg* 1984;63:319–324; and Abboud TK, Shnider SM, Dailey PA, et al. Intrathecal administration of hyperbaric morphine for the relief of pain in labour. *Br J Anaesth* 1984;56:1351–1360.)

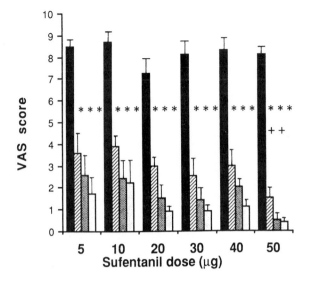

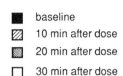

* p < 0.0001
+ p < 0.05

Figure 9.14. Effect of various dosages of epidural sufentanil alone for labor analgesia. All patients received a lidocaine with epinephrine test dose prior to injection of epidural sufentanil. There was a highly significant reduction in visual analog scale scores at 10, 20, and 30 minutes at all doses ($P < .0001$). (Modified from Steinberg R, Powell G, Hu X, Dunn S. Epidural sufentanil for analgesia for labor and delivery. *Reg Anesth* 1989;14:225–228.)

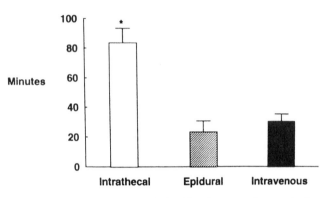

Figure 9.15. Duration of analgesia (median, interquartile range) after sufentanil administration. *$P < .001$; intrathecal vs. epidural and intravenous. (Reprinted by permission from Camann WR, Denney RA, Holby ED, Datta S. A comparison of intrathecal, epidural, and intravenous sufentanil for labor analgesia. *Anesthesiology* 1992;77:884–887.)

come variables are influenced by many other, more significant variables than dilute epidural opioids.

A large review of an obstetric service that modified its epidural labor analgesia practice from administration of local anesthetics alone to local anesthetics with opioids purported such benefits, but the service also "switched" from using 0.5% bupivacaine for labor to using more dilute local anesthetics (113). However, the ease of nursing care and patient satisfaction are sufficient to consider dilute infusions of a local anesthetic with a lipid-soluble opioid. While some patients may ultimately require more concentrated local anesthetic solutions (0.125% or 0.25% bupivacaine), initiation of the epidural with a more dilute solution has proved very popular.

Chestnut et al. reported that a continuous epidural infusion of 0.0625% bupivacaine with 0.0002% fentanyl (2 μg · mL^{-1}) at 12.5 mL/h produced analgesia that was similar to that achieved with an infusion of 0.125% bupivacaine alone (111). Further, D'Angelo et al. recently demonstrated that epidural, but not IV, fentanyl reduced epidural bupivacaine requirements

and saline (107). This landmark study and one that followed (Fig. 9.16) (108) have led to scores of recipes and variations on this basic theme of bupivacaine (variable concentrations and volumes) plus an opioid (most popularly fentanyl or sufentanil).

The use of a very low volume of bupivacaine (3 mL of 0.5%) (107) was an unusual approach that has been repeated by others (109, 110). It is not surprising that an opioid might "improve" such blocks. However, the claim of *rapid onset* of pain relief was not well documented, and a later report seemed to refute this suggestion (Fig. 9.17) (86). Comparing two techniques in which a block is established with bupivacaine 0.2% to 0.25% followed by a 12.5 mL/h infusion of either 0.125% or 0.0625% bupivacaine with 2 μg · mL^{-1} fentanyl, the addition of fentanyl did not improve the mean pain scores or the patients' assessment of the quality of analgesia during the first or second stage of labor; however, the more dilute bupivacaine solution with fentanyl led to less motor blockade (Fig. 9.18) (111). More dilute local anesthetic solutions with fentanyl have a particular appeal during the second stage of labor (112). One clear benefit is the finding of less motor blockade—that is, epidural fentanyl or sufentanil will allow use of a more dilute solution of bupivacaine (0.0625% vs. 0.125%) and spare motor block (111). While most patients seem to prefer these techniques because of the decreased motor block, it is not clear that there are significant benefits beyond this, such as a lower incidence of forceps delivery, length of second stage, or rate of cesarean section. It is likely that these out-

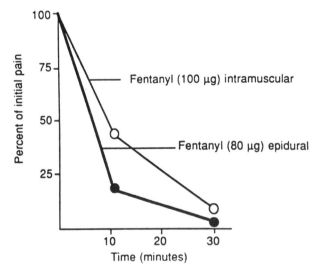

Figure 9.16. Changes in pain score after the first epidural injection of 0.5% bupivacaine in the intramuscular fentanyl group (-0-) and in the epidural fentanyl group (-•-). (Reprinted by permission from Justins DM, Knott C, Luthman J, Reynolds F. Epidural versus intramuscular fentanyl analgesia and pharmacokinetics in labour. *Anaesthesia* 1983;38:937–942.)

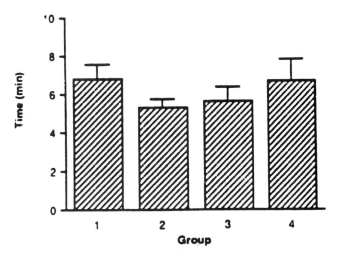

Figure 9.17. Epidural fentanyl/bupivacaine mixtures for obstetric analgesia. Whether patients received bupivacaine 9 mL 0.25% (group 1), bupivacaine 9 mL 0.25% plus fentanyl 50 μg (group 2) or 100 μg (group 3), or bupivacaine 0.068% plus fentanyl 100 μg (group 4), the onset time of analgesia was the same. Thus, even high-dose fentanyl (100 μg; group 3) with a concentrated local anesthetic (bupivacaine 0.25%) did not have a faster onset when compared to plain bupivacaine 0.25% (group 1). (Reprinted by permission from Cohen SE, Tan S, Albright GA, Halpern J. Epidural fentanyl/bupivacaine mixtures for obstetric analgesia. *Anesthesiology* 1987;67:403–407.)

in laboring women and concluded that the epidural was effective primarily through a spinal mechanism (20). It is also now clear that epidural fentanyl and sufentanil decrease epidural bupivacaine requirements in a dose-related manner (Fig. 9.19) (114–116).

In studies of sufentanil, Phillips (117) and other investigators (118–120) hoped that sufentanil's higher lipid solubility (1727 vs. 816) and proposed greater receptor affinity relative to that of fentanyl would confer an advantage. However, this does not seem to be the case when one examines the effects of comparable doses of these two agents. When given epidurally for labor, a bolus of sufentanil 30 μg plus bupivacaine 0.25% was required to achieve a significant difference in analgesia compared with bupivacaine 0.25% alone. The addition of 10 or 20 μg sufentanil to bupivacaine demonstrated no significant difference. Surely, routine doses as high as 30 μg sufentanil for labor analgesia are questionable. Many solutions of sufentanil and local anesthetics have now been evaluated for labor analgesia (116, 121–124). When more dilute solutions of bupivacaine are used (0.01% to 0.0625%) with sufentanil 0.25 to 1 $\mu g \cdot mL^{-1}$, effective analgesia can be achieved with a decreased motor block (83, 125–127). While it has been claimed that sufentanil provides better analgesia with fewer neonatal neurobehavioral effects, this is unlikely to be the case (128). It is likely that fentanyl 1 to 2 $\mu g \cdot mL^{-1}$ and sufentanil 0.25 to 0.33 $\mu g \cdot mL^{-1}$, as commonly used with dilute bupivacaine 0.0625% to 0.125% at 10 to 15 mL/h, are very similar, equally effective, and safe for the fetus and newborn, even with prolonged infusions (129–131). Repeated large

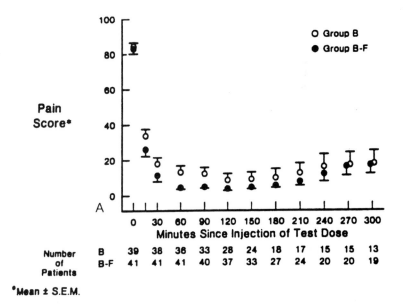

A

Number	B	39	38	36	33	28	24	18	17	15	15	13
of												
Patients	B-F	41	41	41	40	37	33	27	24	20	20	19

*Mean ± S.E.M.

Figure 9.18. Continuous infusion epidural analgesia during labor. *A*: Mean ± SEM pain scores over time during the first stage of labor. *B*: Patient assessment of analgesia quality during first stage of labor. Patients received either bupivacaine (0.125%, group B) or bupivacaine and fentanyl (0.0625% bupivacaine plus 2 mg · mL⁻¹ fentanyl, groups B through F). Both groups had similar onset and good quality analgesia, as judged by a visual analogue pain scale and the patients' verbal responses. While groups B through F had less motor loss (more dilute local anesthetic), this was achieved by giving 25 mg/h fentanyl. (Reprinted by permission from Chestnut DH, Owen CL, Bates JN, Ostman LG, Choi WW, Geiger MW. Continuous infusion epidural analgesia during labor: A randomized, double-blind comparison of 0.0625% bupivacaine/0.0002% fentanyl vs. 0.125% bupivacaine. *Anesthesiology* 1988;68:754–759.)

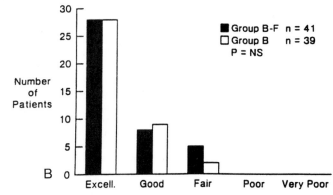

B

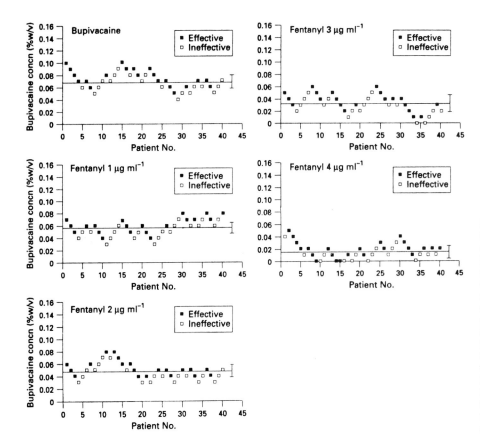

Figure 9.19. EC$_{50}$ of bupivacaine (effective concentration in 50% of subjects or minimum local anesthetic concentration [MLAC]), fentanyl 1, 2, 3, and 4 $\mu g \cdot mL^{-1}$, as determined by the technique of up-down sequential allocation. The MLACs of bupivacaine were 0.069%, 0.05%, 0.048%, 0.031%, and 0.015%, respectively. There was a reduction in MLAC of 18%, 31% ($P = .03\%$), 55% ($P < .0001$), and 72% ($P < .0001$) with fentanyl 1, 2, 3, and 4 $\mu g \cdot mL^{-1}$, respectively. Error bars represent 95% confidence interval. Testing interval was 0.01%. (Reprinted by permission from Lyons G, Columb M, Hawthorne L, Dresner M. Extradural pain relief in labour: Bupivacaine-sparing by extradural fentanyl is dose dependent. *Br J Anaesth* 1997;78:493–497.)

bolus doses of fentanyl (100 μg) or sufentanil (20 to 30 μg) are not recommended, however. If pain relief is not achieved with the solutions suggested, a more concentrated local anesthetic solution is likely needed, particularly for an instrumental delivery or surgical procedure. Other agents suggested include alfentanil, which does not appear to offer any benefit over other agents and is not recommended (104–106, 132, 133). Epidural butorphanol (134–136) at doses of 2 to 3 mg has resulted in maternal somnolence, potential dysphoria, and a sinusoidal FHR pattern in 100% of fetuses whose mothers received the 3 mg dose (135, 137). While butorphanol is a lipid-soluble agent with strong κ-receptor activity with potentially good effect upon visceral pain, it does not appear to offer advantages over fentanyl and sufentanil. Finally, epidural meperidine has been shown to be effective when used with or without a local anesthetic in labor (138–140). However, it has not been shown to be more effective than fentanyl or sufentanil. Meperidine has the unique property of acting like a local anesthetic; at the dose of approximately 1 mg · kg^{-1} administered intrathecally, it can provide both anesthesia for surgery and postoperative pain relief. As an epidural agent (25 mg), it will decrease or prevent the shivering that occurs during labor (140, 141). Of considerable importance, it must be remembered that a preservative-free solution must be used. Meperidine is not widely used for epidural analgesia during labor and delivery.

Morphine should not be forgotten as a potential additive to epidural local anesthesia. Administration of 2 mg epidural morphine in early labor (cervical dilation of 3 cm), followed by bupivacaine when contractions become more painful, significantly prolonged the duration of analgesia (142). However, this advantage may have limited utility with continuous infusions. Intrathecal morphine 0.2 mg has similar positive results (19) and deserves more consideration, but in a lower dose range (0.025 to 0.1 mg).

Current practice includes the widespread use of epidural fentanyl or sufentanil with dilute bupivacaine or ropivacaine solutions. A suggested approach is listed in Table 9.7. The solutions

used will vary depending on the parturient's needs, the obstetric plan, and whether the CSE technique is used. The trend in many obstetric centers is for more dilute epidural solutions.

A recent study suggested that initiating an epidural for labor (no CSE) with 15 mL bupivacaine 0.125% and sufentanil 10 μg in divided doses (3 mL as "test dose," followed by 12 mL as a slow bolus) *without* the often-used 1.5% lidocaine-epinephrine test dose was very effective and allowed ambulation (83). This was followed by an infusion of 0.0625% bupivacaine with 0.33 $\mu g \cdot mL^{-1}$ sufentanil at 13.5 to 15 mL/h, which allowed 86% of the parturients to walk at 30 minutes. If the lidocaine test-dose was administered, only 36% were able to walk. Also, if more

Table 9.7. CONTINUOUS EPIDURAL INFUSIONS FOR LABOR ANALGESIA: SUGGESTED SOLUTIONS

Drugs	Bupivacaine	Bupivacaine + Fentanyl	Bupivacaine + Sufentanil
Initiation of epidural (Divided doses)*			
Bupivacaine	0.0625–0.25%	0.0625–0.25%	0.0625–0.25%
Opioid	—	1–5 μg/mL	0.2–2 μg/mL
Volume	10–15 mL	10–15 mL	10–15 mL
Infusion			
Bupivacaine	0.125–0.25%	0.0625–0.25%	0.0625–0.25%
Opioid	—	1–2 μg/mL	0.2–0.33 μg/mL
Volume	10–15 mL/h	10–15 mL/h	10–15 mL/h

* A test dose with 1.5% lidocaine (3 mL) and epinephrine (15 μg) may be used prior to the epidural, or the initial solution chosen, given in divided doses, may serve as the test dose. If dilute solutions of bupivacaine with fentanyl or sufentanil are used to minimize motor blockade, the lidocaine test dose is often not used because it will increase the motor block achieved. Ropivacaine or levobupivacaine, in equipotent doses, may be substituted for bupivacaine.

Table 9.8. EPIDURAL OPIOIDS AND LOCAL ANESTHETICS FOR LABOR: A SUGGESTED TECHNIQUE AND REGIMEN*

1. Establish a solid block to T10 with bupivacaine 0.125–0.25% bupivacaine or lidocaine 1.5% (usually 10 mL in divided doses, with or without epinephrine). A bolus of fentanyl (50 μg?) or sufentanil (10–20 μg?) may be added to the local anesthetic.

2. Continuous infusion of bupivacaine 0.0625–0.125%[†] plus fentanyl 1–2 μg $\cdot$ mL^{-1} or sufentanil 0.2–0.33 μg $\cdot$ mL^{-1} at a rate of 10–15(15) mL/h. Adjust level by changing volume.

3. Top-up doses as needed for pain of 5 mL bupivacaine 0.125–0.25% plain, or 10 mL lidocaine 1.5% plain.

* An alternative regimen is described in Chapter 8, Table 8.3.
[†] More dilute solutions may be effective in some patients (e.g. , bupivacaine 0.03125% or 0.0625% with fentanyl 1–3 μg $\cdot$ mL^{-1}.

dilute bupivacaine solutions were used to initiate neural blockade, inadequate analgesia was achieved and more local anesthetic was required, precluding early ambulation. The authors concluded that ambulation during labor is not restricted to the CSE technique. There are numerous approaches to providing routine labor analgesia with epidural opioids (Table 9.8).

Patient-Controlled Epidural Analgesia

Epidural analgesia for labor is most often provided by a continuous infusion technique, supplemented with "top-up" bolus doses as needed for break-through pain. Patient-controlled epidural analgesia (PCEA) allows the patient to titrate the dose administered and theoretically avoids inadequate or excessive analgesia. PCEA may also decrease the number of interventions or additional time spent by the anesthesiologist to provide "top-ups" or administer additional local anesthetic. Routine continuous infusion techniques require at least one "top-up" for 25% (143) to 80% (144) of labor epidurals and more than one "top-up" in 25% (143) to 46% (145). This occurred even when bupivacaine 0.125% and fentanyl 1 μg $\cdot$ mL^{-1} was administered at 14 to 16 mL/h, with a need for intervention of 71%. In addition, it has been claimed that smaller, titrated doses of local anesthetic may with PCEA provide additional maternal safety, but this has not been documented.

Most studies have found that PCEA does not improve analgesia compared with continuous infusion (144–150) or intermittent top-up techniques (144, 146, 148, 151–153), and that these techniques were equally effective. While two studies (152, 154) have suggested increased maternal satisfaction with PCEA, most investigators have found no difference (145, 146, 148, 151, 155, 156). No investigator has demonstrated differences in maternal safety comparing PCEA with the more common techniques. Further, while two fairly large studies (144, 148) suggest PCEA reduces motor blockade, most investigators have found no difference (147, 149, 150, 152, 153, 155, 156, 156a). There are also conflicting results when attempting to evaluate the potential reduction in practitioner interventions with PCEA. While conserving the practitioner's time is an admirable goal, patient contact may lead to greater safety, potentially greater effectiveness of epidural analgesia, and patient satisfaction. Regardless of the acute need for intervention, the anesthesia practitioner must remain readily available to manage potential complications or the changing clinical requirements of the obstetric patient.

The most common clinical PCEA technique is administration of a basal infusion rate at 6 mL/h with 5-mL bolus doses with a 10-minute lockout period. This has been shown to decrease interventions by the anesthesiologist when compared to PCEA with no basal rate or PCEA with a 3-mL/h basal rate (147). The most appropriate bolus volume, lockout period, or maximum hourly dose has not been thoroughly investigated; however, the

technique outlined here is quite effective. Ropivacaine 0.125% has been found to be clinically indistinguishable from bupivacaine in a PCEA study (157). Clonidine 4.5 μg $\cdot$ mL^{-1} has been recently investigated as an adjuvant to bupivacaine 0.0625% and fentanyl 2 μg $\cdot$ mL^{-1} and found to improve analgesia and reduce the supplementation rate (158). However, this is an area that will need further investigation because clonidine remains an investigational drug for obstetric anesthesia. Clinical experience with PCEA suggests that any local anesthetic solution that provides good analgesia in labor when administered by continuous infusion can be equally effective when administered by PCEA.

Maternal and neonatal safety is similarly good with either PCEA or continuous epidural infusions when used for analgesia during labor. Although prolonged analgesia can be provided with either technique with minimal need for intervention by the anesthesiologist, regular evaluations to assess the appropriateness and effectiveness of the epidural blockade are recommended.

Continuous Spinal Analgesia

Continuous spinal analgesia can be provided using a standard epidural catheter and administering either local anesthetic, opioid, or a combination to provide labor analgesia. While this may have unique benefits when a routine epidural is extremely difficult to place (e.g., morbid obesity, previous spinal surgery), the chief disadvantage is the high incidence of PDPH. However, the introduction of spinal microcatheters (28 to 32 gauge) that would pass through a small-gauge spinal needle allowed significant investigation with this technique (158a, 159). Using 22-gauge spinal needles and 28-gauge polyurethane spinal catheters, the continuous spinal technique was used to evaluate intrathecal fentanyl, meperidine, and sufentanil for labor (159). While this technique has interesting investigational and potential clinical applications, several clinical reports of permanent neurologic sequelae were reported in association with spinal catheters, both small-bore and standard epidural catheters used intraspinally (see Chapter 5) (160–163). It has been suggested that the neurologic injuries are related to the nonuniform spread of local anesthetics (161, 163). Based on the available evidence, the Food and Drug Administration (FDA) decided to remove the small-bore catheters from clinical use (164). However, dilute local anesthetics and opioids used for labor analgesia appear to be safe and can be administered through a standard epidural catheter placed in the intrathecal space if this approach is chosen or necessary to achieve analgesia. There is ongoing FDA-approved research of small-bore catheter use for labor analgesia.

In a multicenter, FDA-approved study using a 22-gauge ramped Sprotte® spinal needle with a 28-gauge polyurethane catheter, preliminary results suggest a continuous intrathecal sufentanil solution of 5 μg $\cdot$ mL^{-1} administered at 1 mL/h can provide effective analgesia for patients in labor (165). These results are limited by the preliminary nature of the study. However, the dose of sufentanil appears to be greater than expected in this author's view. Finally, if a local anesthetic is required for further labor analgesia or anesthesia for operative delivery, caution is urged because of the potential for maldistribution of the local anesthetic (see Chapter 5). Thus, further investigation of this technique will be required before the use of spinal microcatheters in obstetric anesthesia becomes available.

The Lipid-Soluble Agents: Additives to Improve an Epidural

There may be unique indications for combining a lipid-soluble agent with a local anesthetic for analgesia during labor or delivery. Fentanyl 50 μg or sufentanil 5 to 10 μg added to a top-up dose for low-back pain unrelieved by plain bupivacaine

0.0625% to 0.125% may produce adequate analgesia. This is achieved without the further motor blockade that would result from increasing the concentration of the local anesthetic. This approach might have implications for the second stage of labor (112). Although the single dose of epidural fentanyl 50 to 100 μg or sufentanil 10 to 20 μg may be helpful as part of a top-up dose or at the start of labor, they would be inappropriate for repeated top-up doses. Ultimately, opioids must not be used to cover a poor epidural block, and clinicians must accept that some patients will need a more concentrated local anesthetic instead of larger doses of epidural opioids. During cesarean delivery with epidural anesthesia, the use of epidural fentanyl 1 μg · kg^{-1}, or approximately 100 μg, may be beneficial to alleviate the pain often experienced with exteriorization of the uterus or closing of the peritoneum (166). This application is extremely popular, but the benefits are probably subtle compared with those of a solid epidural or spinal anesthetic (167).

POSTOPERATIVE PAIN MANAGEMENT
Epidural Opioids

The use of epidural opioids to relieve the postoperative pain of cesarean delivery has been extremely successful. The approval of preservative-free morphine (Duramorph) by the FDA in 1984 led to its widespread use and ultimately changed postoperative pain management for our nonobstetric anesthesia colleagues and patients as well (168).

In 1979, Wolfe and Nicholas (169) reported that **fentanyl** 100 μg diluted with 8 mL 0.9% sodium chloride administered via an epidural catheter successfully relieved postoperative pain in 20 patients who had undergone elective cesarean section. Although time has shown epidural fentanyl alone to be less than ideal for postoperative analgesia (170, 171), this work led to substantial changes in pain management (168, 172, 173).

In another early study it was suggested that morphine 10.3 ± 2.5 mg was required following upper abdominal surgery and 7.5 ± 2.1 mg following lower abdominal surgery (174). Several investigators found 2 mg epidural morphine effective for chronic pain and some postoperative and traumatic pain, but inadequate for postcesarean pain (175–177). Rosen et al. found 2 mg epidural morphine inadequate for postcesarean pain, but 5 and 7.5 mg were equally effective (Fig. 9.20) (178).

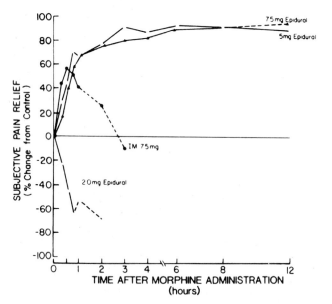

Figure 9.20. Epidural morphine relief of postoperative pain of cesarean delivery. (Reprinted by permission from Rosen MA, Hughes SC, Shnider SM, et al. Epidural morphine for relief of postoperative pain after cesarean delivery. *Anesth Analg* 1983;62:666–672.)

Although epidural **morphine** 4 to 5 mg has become the routine approach for postcesarean analgesia in many institutions, a wide variety of drugs have been examined. Epidural fentanyl remains a common approach to pain management in postcesarean section patients and has been widely investigated (79, 169–171, 179, 180). However, many believe that the systemic effects achieved by absorption from the epidural space (not unlike an intramuscular [IM] injection) explain much of fentanyl's effects (Fig. 9.21) (74). The analgesic effects of epidural lidocaine 2% with 1:200,000 epinephrine or epidural bupivacaine 0.5% alone generally outlast the effects of epidural fentanyl. Epidural fentanyl still has its adherents (179, 181), despite the work by Malinow et al. (182), who demonstrated that "analgesia…after a single epidural dose of fentanyl is of clinically insignificant duration after the use of lidocaine or bupivacaine anesthesia for cesarean section." Other investigators have found that a single dose of fentanyl added to 2% lidocaine and epinephrine (probably the most common epidural agent for cesarean section) has minimal or no effect on postoperative pain (183, 184). The use of patient-controlled analgesia (PCA) by Sevarino et al. (184) for postoperative pain management after epidural lidocaine and fentanyl (vs. lidocaine and saline) further demonstrated the minimal contribution of epidural fentanyl to postoperative pain relief. Several authors have suggested some contribution to improved intraoperative conditions when epidural fentanyl (1 μg · kg^{-1}) is added to 2% lidocaine for cesarean section (166). The potential intraoperative benefits of epidural fentanyl when added to bupivacaine were first noted in 1983 by Milon et al. (185) However, these investigators used approximately 1.7 μg · kg^{-1} epidural fentanyl and, as in many similar studies, one wonders if the same dose of fentanyl given intramuscularly would provide similar effects (179, 186). Indeed, an epidural dose of 1.7 μg · kg^{-1} fentanyl resulted in umbilical arterial plasma concentrations as high as 0.8 ng/mL (185). The effects on the newborn always must be considered, and some prefer to administer epidural opioids after the umbilical cord is clamped. (This is discussed later in the section on fetal effects of epidural opioids.) However, if the epidural block is not fully effective and IV opioids are considered necessary, epidural fentanyl is a good alternative. Administer 1 μg · kg^{-1} fentanyl through the epidural catheter, diluted to a volume of 10 to 15 mL with more local anesthetic or saline (187).

It has been demonstrated that the duration of analgesia in postcesarean section patients with 50 μg fentanyl is significantly improved by increasing the volume of injectate (187). Fentanyl is probably most effective when administered by a continuous infusion technique, for example, with dilute bupivacaine (0.1%) and epinephrine (0.5 μg/mL) (188). However, the use of a continuous infusion technique appears to be uncommon for postcesarean section analgesia and is rarely necessary in this author's view.

It has been suggested that lipid-soluble agents potentiate the effect of morphine, providing a more rapid onset, resulting in the use of lower doses of morphine, with fewer side effects, and a duration of analgesia equivalent to that obtained with larger doses of morphine alone (189). This alternative is appealing but remains to be documented in a large series of patients. The application of significant amounts of a lipid-soluble opioid should produce a rapid onset of analgesia. However, Sinatra et al. (190) could not demonstrate a potentiating effect of sufentanil 30 μg added to 3 mg morphine epidurally; the duration of analgesia was longer with 5 mg epidural morphine. The mean time before use of PCA in the morphine-only group was 13 hours compared with 2.8 hours in the sufentanil and morphine group (i.e., sufentanil did not potentiate the morphine). The use of PCA is a valuable tool when evaluating the effectiveness of agents used for pain control, because the patient determines when and how much drug to administer. The lack of potentiation demonstrated by Sinatra et al. has been confirmed by others, but the

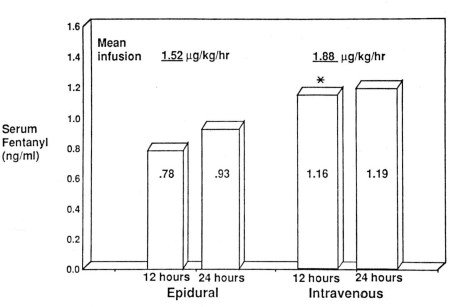

Figure 9.21. In a randomized double-blind comparison of epidural vs. intravenous (IV) fentanyl infusions for analgesia for cesarean section, no clinical advantage to the epidural infusion over IV infusion could be demonstrated. While the serum fentanyl levels were significantly higher in the IV group at 12 hours, there was no difference by 24 hours. The infusion rates were obviously quite similar. (Reprinted by permission from Ellis DJ, Millar WI, Reisner LS. A randomized double-blind comparison of epidural versus intravenous fentanyl infusion for analgesia after cesarean section. *Anesthesiology* 1990;72: 981–986.)

combination remains popular, with the consensus that fentanyl or other lipid-soluble agents improve intraoperative conditions (immediate effect) while morphine provides postoperative analgesia (long-term effect).

Epidural **sufentanil** also has been widely investigated in obstetrics, as well as in other postoperative pain management situations (118, 191, 192–194). The primary benefit of epidural sufentanil is its rapid onset and profound analgesia. Whether the analgesia is "better" than that achieved with fentanyl is unlikely, and sufentanil has the many limitations of fentanyl (as previously discussed), including a brief duration of action in the epidural space (2 to 5 hours) (118, 191). Rosen et al. at UCSF demonstrated at least 50% pain reduction in 15 minutes, but the duration of analgesia was brief compared with epidural morphine (Table 9.9) (191).

Sufentanil is approximately 5 to 10 times more potent than fentanyl when administered parentally. The ratio of analgesic potency of epidural sufentanil to fentanyl is approximately 5:1. When administered in equipotent doses epidurally, there is likely little difference. However, sufentanil is a reasonable agent to initiate a block for cesarean section or in an acute pain situation, to "top-up" a patchy epidural block, or perhaps to administer after delivery (after verifying epidural placement intraoperatively) to help blunt the pain of uterine exteriorization. Profound respiratory depression has occurred with epidural

sufentanil, and patients must be monitored carefully in the acute period after administration. No caregiver should administer this drug (or other opioids) unless he or she is capable of managing acute respiratory depression. Also concerning is the effect of higher doses of sufentanil (50 to 100 μg) on central temperature control. If the patient's central temperature drops, there is no shivering. The risk of asymptomatic hypothermia has been raised by several authors, but appears not to be a concern when reasonable epidural doses are used (25 to 30 μg) (195, 196). Smaller doses of epidural opioids may decrease the shivering that does occur with epidural anesthesia. The dose of epidural sufentanil for postoperative pain is probably 30 μg diluted to a volume of approximately 10 to 15 mL. Sufentanil can be given as a continuous infusion, but 15 μg/h may be needed (197), and continuous sufentanil alone without a local anesthetic is not commonly used.

Meperidine is another agent that is widely used epidurally (198–203). It is a unique opioid because it has local anesthetic properties. It is also very lipid soluble and has a rapid onset of action. A dose of 50 mg in 10 mL saline provides analgesia lasting approximately 3 to 4 hours, a duration similar to that with IM meperidine (200). Meperidine has been evaluated in doses ranging from 12.5 to 100 mg epidurally (202, 203), and it has been concluded that 25 mg in 5 mL saline was the optimal dose, while doses of 50 mg or greater offered no benefit. Epidural

Table 9.9. ONSET AND DURATION OF ANALGESIA WITH EPIDURAL MORPHINE AND SUFENTANIL

	Morphine Sulfate (5 mg)	Sufentanil (30 μg)	Sufentanil (40 μg)	Sufentanil (60 μg)
Onset of 50% pain relief (min)	52* (24–80)	15 (15–19)	15 (15–15)	15 (15–15)
Onset of 50% pain relief (min)	90* (60–202)	30 (15–38)	30 (15–45)	15 (15–19)
Duration of first dose (h)	26.4* (17.3–31.5)	3.9 (2.8–5.2)	4.5 (2.7–6.2)	5.6 (4.4–7.2)
Duration of second dose (h)	—	3.5 (2.5–5.9)	5.5 (3.9–7.0)	5.2 (4.1–6.6)

There are 10 patients in each group. Values are median with semiquartile range in parentheses.
*$P < .05$ compared to each sufentanil group.
Reprinted with permission from Rosen MA, Dailey PA, Hughes SC, et al. Epidural sufentanil for postoperative analgesia after cesarean section. *Anesthesiology* 1988;68:448–454.

meperidine provides a more rapid onset of analgesia than the IM route of administration, but its short duration of action is a limiting factor, especially compared with the success and longer duration of epidural morphine. The longer duration of epidural morphine allows for a single injection of the drug at the end of surgery and removal of the catheter in the operating room. Many other epidural opioids, including **diamorphine** (204–206), **phenoperidine** (206), **butorphanol** (207–209), **alfentanil** (210–212), **hydromorphone** (213–220), **buprenorphine** (221–226), **nalbuphine** (220, 227), **methadone** (204), and **lofentanil** (221), have been evaluated for postoperative analgesia, but none offer an advantage over morphine or fentanyl, the most commonly used epidural agents in the United States (206, 209–215).

Some of these agents have significant disadvantages, including a shorter duration of action compared to morphine, the requirement of administration by a continuous infusion technique, antagonism of opioid receptors, and in the case of lofentanil (never released commercially) and buprenorphine, resistance to naloxone that could lead to catastrophic respiratory depression. Butorphanol can lead to excessive sedation, most likely from activation of κ-receptors, and in sufficient doses may be neurotoxic when administered intrathecally (230, 231). Epidural ketamine and droperidol have been combined with morphine for postoperative pain management (232–236); however, neurotoxicity studies for many epidural agents are few and results are questionable.

In conclusion, while there are clinical uses for epidural fentanyl, sufentanil, or meperidine, the clear success with epidural morphine has made it the epidural agent of choice in the obstetric population for postoperative analgesia (180, 228, 229, 237–239).

Experience With Epidural Morphine

When Kotelko et al. (238) and Leicht et al. (239) reviewed the experience at UCSF with 5 mg epidural morphine for analgesia in healthy women undergoing cesarean delivery, they found that we achieved good to excellent analgesia lasting 24 to 36 hours for 84.6% of the patients (Table 9.10). Satisfactory postcesarean analgesia using a similar low-dose epidural technique has been reported at other centers as well (240, 241–243). Fuller et al. reported satisfactory analgesia and no serious complications with 5 mg epidural morphine in a large retrospective study (n = 4216), although they ultimately recommended using morphine 3.0 mg (180). Palmer et al. evaluated the optimal dose of epidural morphine for postoperative analgesia in cesarean section patients using PCA for additional analgesia. They administered epidural morphine in doses ranging from 1.25 to 5 mg and concluded that there was little benefit beyond 3.75 mg morphine (229). In my view, this supports the common use of 4 to 5 mg epidural morphine (single dose) in clinical practice. In our review of 1000 patients who received 5 mg epidural morphine, it should be noted that 5.9% reported pain relief as none to poor, despite the successful use of the epidural for cesarean section (Table 9.10). Thus, with lower doses of epidural morphine there is a greater

Table 9.10. EPIDURAL MORPHINE AFTER CESAREAN SECTION—1000 PATIENTS

Good to excellent pain relief (none or poor = 5.9%)	84.6%
Duration of analgesia	22.9 h
	SD 13.8
Patients requiring only oral analgesics	44%
Patients requiring NO subsequent analgesics	16%

Data from experience at University of California San Francisco; and from Leicht CH, Hughes SC, Dailey PA, Shnider SM, Rosen MA. Epidural morphine sulfate for analgesia after cesarean section: A prospective study of 1,000 patients [abstract]. *Anesthesiology* 1986;65:A366.

Table 9.11. EPIDURAL MORPHINE AFTER CESAREAN SECTION—1000 PATIENTS

Pruritus			
None	38.8%		
Mild	20.3%	*Treated*	28.6%
Moderate	35.5%		
Severe	3.9%		
Nausea	20.4%	*Treated*	10.5%
Vomiting	14.8%		
Respiratory depression	0.4%	*"Obviously real"*	0.1%

Data from experience at University of California San Francisco; and from Leicht CH, Hughes SC, Dailey PA, Shnider SM, Rosen MA. Epidural morphine sulfate for analgesia after cesarean section: A prospective study of 1,000 patients [abstract]. *Anesthesiology* 1986;65:A366.

need for additional analgesia and intervention. The administration of 4 to 5 mg epidural morphine is now standard practice for many anesthesiologists, and there is a long history of use to support the safety and effectiveness of this dose range.

Preservative-free morphine sulfate 4 to 5 mg is added through the epidural catheter once the neonate is delivered. This is administered in the operating room at the time of delivery to allow the analgesic to take effect before the local anesthetic has diminished; epidural onset may take as long as 60 minutes and is still improving at 90 minutes. The experience of 1000 consecutive patients at UCSF who received epidural morphine after cesarean section is shown in Table 9.10.

The most common side effect encountered is pruritus, which occurs in approximately 60% of patients. The most significant side effect is delayed respiratory depression (Table 9.11). To avoid this risk, the degree of somnolence and adequacy of ventilation are carefully assessed at frequent intervals (Table 9.12). Although some authors suggest that precise monitoring might include continuous measurement of end-tidal CO_2, the use of an impedance apnea monitor, pulse oximetry, or intensive care units, attentive nursing on the postpartum unit has proven satisfactory and adequate in this patient population. Experience over the last 20 years substantiates this approach.

The package insert for epidural morphine stresses that facilities using this drug must be equipped with resuscitative equipment, oxygen, naloxone, and appropriate resuscitative drugs. Moreover, patients must be carefully monitored for 12 to 24 hours following administration of the drug. Chronically ill or debilitated patients may be at particular risk for delayed respiratory depression. In addition, the depressant effects of morphine may be potentiated by the presence of other central nervous system depressants. Generalized sedation is a serious sign (rare), and such patients should be watched more closely. However, these comments apply as well to patients given opioids by IV, IM, or other routes.

A thoughtful approach combined with thorough knowledge of the subject is necessary when using any newer drug or technique. Clearly, good monitoring is the key to the safe use of epidural morphine or any opioid by any route of administration.

Intrathecal Opioids

The use of intraspinal opioids initially was limited to the epidural route of administration. This followed from (a) the initial success of epidural morphine in parturients, (b) the extensive investigation of various epidural dosing regimens and drugs, and (c) the initial reports of severe side effects with intrathecal opioids. The latter, no doubt, was related to the very high doses of intrathecal morphine given to patients (2 to 20 mg). Not surprisingly, the side effects were significant and clinicians shied away from the use of intrathecal opioids. Clearly, these problems were related to misunderstanding the dose requirements.

Table 9.12. EPIDURAL ANALGESIA ORDERS*

I. ANALGESIA:
  A. The patient has received the following epidural/intrathecal opiates. **Route**: Epidural or Intrathecal (circle)
      ●Preservative-free Morphine: _____ mg injected @ Date_____ Time_____
            ●Fentanyl: _____ mcg injected @ Date_____ Time_____

  B. Start continuous infusion via epidural catheter:

      ●Preservative-free **Morphine**: _____ mg/cc @ _____ mg/hr)
  OR   ●**Hydromorphine**: _____ mg/cc @ _____ mg/hr) **TOTAL CC/HR =**
  OR   ●**Fentanyl**: _____ mcg/cc @ _____ mcg/hr) _____cc/hr
  PLUS   ●**Bupivacaine**: _____ mg/cc @ _____ mg/hr)
  C. Morphine Sulfate 1-2 mg IV q 1 hour PRN pain. (*Hold IV Morphine if Sedation Scale > 3 or RR < 8.*)
  D. No other opiates, sedatives, hypnotics to be given except by order of Anesthesia service.

II. MONITORING: (applies to non-ventilated patients)
  A. For single epidural/intrathecal opiate injection, monitor and record RR q 1 hour ×24 hours.
  B. For continuous infusion, monitor and record RR q 1 hour ×24 hours at stable dose then per routine.
  C. For continuous infusion, monitor and record sedation scale q1h ×24 hours at stable continuous infusion then per routine (while awake).
      Sedation   **1** = Anxious/Agitated   **3** = Sedated, but responsive   **5** = Asleep, Sluggish response
      Scale: **2** = Cooperative   **4** = Asleep, but responsive   **6** = Asleep, Unresponsive
  D. For single injection or continuous, monitor analgesic effect q1h ×24 hours then per routine (while awake).
      Analgesia scale: 0-10   0 = no pain   10 = worst possible pain
  E. If bupivacaine is administered, monitor patient for presence of skin numbness and leg weakness q8h ×24 hours at stable dose then per routine.

III. MANAGEMENT OF SIDE EFFECTS:
  A. **Respiratory depression**:
      1) Administer naloxone 0.1 mg IV STAT if RR <8/min or sedation scale ≥4.
    Repeat dose q 1-2 minutes ×3 PRN.
  B. **Nausea, Vomiting, and/or Itching**:
      1) Diphenhydramine 25 mg IV or IM q2h prn itching.
      2) Naloxone 0.04 - 0.08 mg IV q 15 minutes ×3 prn severe itching.
        NOTE DOSE: Dilute Naloxone to a minimum volume 0.04 in 1 cc with Normal Saline.
      3) Droperidol 0.625 mg IV or IM q4h prn nausea.

IV. NOTIFY ANESTHESIA SERVICE (DESIGNATED BEEPER NO.) IF:
  A. Inadequate pain relief: Pain Score > 4/10 or > 3 doses of IV Morphine per shift.
  B. RR ≤ 8/min, shallow paradoxical or obstructed breathing.
  C. Sedation scale level 4 or greater.
  D. Systolic BP _____.
  E. Severe itching, nausea, vomiting, unrelieved by Naloxone.
  F. Sensory anesthesia and/or leg weakness.
  G. No urine output by 6 hours in patients without indwelling urinary catheters.

V. OTHER:
  A. Examine catheter site through transparent dressing q Shift. Notify Anesthesia Service for redness, fluid collection, tubing/catheter problems.
  B. Label dressing, tubing, bag and infusion device with "Epidural."
  C. Maintain IV access as ordered by primary service <u>OR</u> lock IV and flush q Shift with Normal Saline.
  D. Patient to be allowed out of bed only with assistance while infusion running.

V. PHYSICIAN TO BE NOTIFIED @ DESIGNATED Beeper # _____

VI. When epidural catheter is removed, discontinue all above orders.
  DESIGNATED PHYSICIAN: _____ am/pm_____ID#_____
                    Date/Time   Print Name   Signature
  RN_____ am/pm_____
                    Date/Time   Print Name   Signature
  LVN/UNIT CLERK_____ am/pm_____
                    Date/Time   Print Name   Signature

*These orders were developed for the Postoperative Pain Service and for use in labor and delivery when intraspinal opioids are used. (San Francisco General Hospital, San Francisco, CA)

Intrathecal morphine now has been investigated more thoroughly and has proven to be a very reasonable choice for postcesarean section analgesia (2, 244–250). Intrathecal fentanyl (251–253), sufentanil (254, 255), methadone (256), meperidine (257), and diamorphine (258), among other opioids, also have been studied, but intrathecal morphine clearly has become the preferred agent for postoperative analgesia.

Abouleish et al. evaluated 856 women undergoing cesarean section in a prospective study administering 0.2 mg intrathecal morphine for postoperative analgesia (245). The mean duration of analgesia was 14 hours, shorter than that achieved with 4 to 5 mg epidural morphine (22.9 hours) (239), but 58% of the women "did not require additional analgesics for 24 hours.

Uchiyama did a dose-response study administering intrathecal morphine 0.05, 0.1, and 0.2 mg for pain relief after cesarean section (248). They noted that 0.1 and 0.2 mg were equally effective (Fig. 9.22) and that the duration of analgesia was approximately 28 hours in each group, although there was a wide variation in individual response. The patients who received morphine 0.1 mg had fewer side effects, and that dose is commonly recommended (250). Palmer et al. performed a similar but more extensive dose-response study, administering morphine 0.025, 0.05, 0.075, 0.10, and 0.5 mg intrathecally for postcesarean analgesia (Fig. 9.23) (2). PCA morphine use provided access to additional analgesics. The authors concluded that even 0.075 mg intrathecal morphine provided significant analgesia and that there was "little

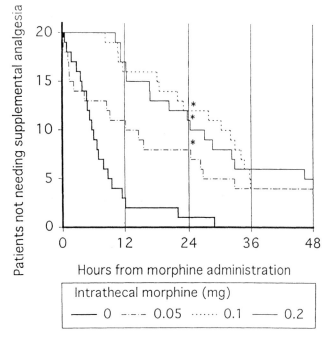

Figure 9.22. Time to first postoperative supplemental analgesic. The number of patients needing no analgesics during the first 24-hour period in groups 2, 3, and 4 were significantly higher compared with group 1. *P < .05 compared with group 1. (Reprinted by permission from Uchiyama A, Ueyama H, Nakano S, Nishimura M, Tashiro C. Low dose intrathecal morphine and pain relief following caesarean section. *Int J Obstet Anesth* 1994;3:87–91.)

justification for the use of more than 0.1 mg for postcesarean analgesia" (2). However, Gerancher et al. were unable to determine with meaningful precision a dose of intrathecal morphine for postcesarean section analgesia (259). Intrathecal morphine (0.1 to 0.5 mg) was administered using an up-down sequential allocation method. They were unable to arrive at an ED$_{50}$ and attributed this to patient variability.

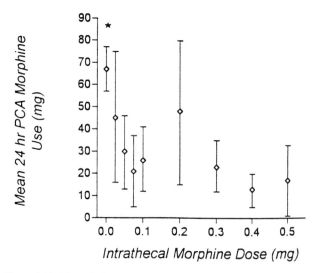

Figure 9.23. Mean 24-hour patient-controlled morphine use for each group (mean ± 95% confidence interval). *P < .05 vs. 0.075-, 0.1-, 0.3-, 0.4-, and 0.5-mg groups. (Reprinted by permission from Palmer CM, Emerson S, Volgoropolous D, Alves D. Dose-response relationship of intrathecal morphine for postcesarean analgesia. *Anesthesiology* 1999;90:437–444.)

When considering the extensive and increasing experience with intrathecal morphine, it is this author's view that the appropriate dose of intrathecal morphine for postcesarean section analgesia is 0.1 to 0.25 mg. There is wide variation between individual patients' analgesic requirements, patient population, and tolerance for the chief side effect, pruritus. Further, it is clear that while very low doses (0.075 mg or less) may be fairly effective, this will likely increase the frequency of interventions in the immediate postoperative period to achieve adequate, effective analgesia in many patients. Conversely, increasing the dose beyond 0.25 mg seems unnecessary and has now been shown to be of no benefit.

Intrathecal Fentanyl and Sufentanil: Postoperative Analgesia

Intrathecal fentanyl has been shown to provide analgesia, but of very brief duration. It was initially suggested that as little as 6.25 μg is an appropriate dose for postoperative pain management (251). However, clinical experience and investigation have demonstrated that minimal or only brief postoperative analgesia can be achieved with intrathecal fentanyl as a single agent (262). Belzarena et al. investigated women receiving intrathecal bupivacaine for elective cesarean section with fentanyl 0.25, 0.5, or 0.75 μg · kg^{-1} (252). The duration of analgesia (mean ± SD) ranged from 305 ± 89 minutes with 0.25 μg · kg^{-1} to 787 ± 161 minutes with 0.75 μg · kg^{-1} fentanyl. At the two higher doses, there were both decreased respiratory rate and increased pruritus and nausea. Dahlgren et al. (253) reported that fentanyl 10 μg added to intrathecal bupivacaine 12.5 mg for cesarean section increased the time of effective analgesia (visual analog scale [VAS] score ≤4) from 121 ± 29.1 minutes to 181 ± 38.4 minutes. However, when this is compared to intrathecal morphine, which can achieve 12 to 24 hours of analgesia, intrathecal fentanyl provides minimal postoperative analgesia alone. This is also true for sufentanil.

Intrathecal sufentanil 20 μg administered with bupivacaine for cesarean section achieved approximately 3 hours of postoperative analgesia (255). Dahlgren et al. noted that there was little difference between intrathecal sufentanil 2.5 μg and 5 μg when it was added to hyperbaric bupivacaine for cesarean section (253). The duration of action was approximately 3 hours, but there was a greater incidence of pruritus postoperatively (95%) with the larger dose. This study did demonstrate that either fentanyl (10 μg) or sufentanil (2.5 or 5.0 μg) added to bupivacaine decreased the incidence of intraoperative antiemetics administered vs. plain bupivacaine. Many clinicians add fentanyl 10 to 25 μg or sufentanil 2.5 to 10 μg to bupivacaine to improve the quality of intraoperative analgesia, although studies are conflicting (252, 260). Intrathecal fentanyl 15 μg has also been shown to improve the duration of lidocaine by 30 minutes in cesarean section patients compared to plain hyperbaric lidocaine (261). Conversely, Olöfsson et al. concluded that the addition of fentanyl 10 μg intrathecally or 100 μg epidurally failed to significantly improve anesthesia for cesarean section with either intrathecal bupivacaine (12.5 mg) or epidural bupivacaine (100 mg) (263). It is this author's practice to add intrathecal fentanyl 25 μg to morphine 0.1 to 0.25 mg and hyperbaric bupivacaine 12.5 to 15 mg for spinal anesthesia for cesarean section. It appears that the patients have less intraoperative pain, particularly with exteriorization of the uterus (practiced routinely by our surgeons), and a smoother transition to effective postoperative analgesia achieved with morphine. However, this has not been demonstrated in a large study. Intrathecal bupivacaine alone is a highly effective agent for spinal anesthesia (rapid onset, solid spinal block) and intrathecal morphine provides prolonged analgesia. Thus, the addition of lipophilic agents may be only a small, subtle improvement appreciated in only selected patients.

Table 9.13. OPIOIDS FOR POSTOPERATIVE ANALGESIA AFTER CESAREAN SECTION

Drug	Epidural Dose	Intrathecal Dose	Onset (min)	Duration (h)	Comment
Morphine	2–5 mg	0.1–0.25 mg	30–60	12–24	Slow onset but long duration
Fentanyl	50–100 μg	10–25 μg	5	2–3	Rapid onset, short duration; systemic action prominent with epidural administration
Sufentanil	30–50 μg	2.5–5 μg	5	2–3	Very similar to fentanyl (see above)
Meperidine	25–50 mg	10 mg (as additive to local); 1 mg $\cdot$ kg^{-1} (sole agent for surgery)	15–20	4–6	Rapid onset; intermediate duration; can decrease "shivering"

Intrathecal meperidine 10 mg has been shown to be effective for postoperative analgesia, but the duration of action is only 4 to 5 hours (257, 264). Meperidine is unique among the opioids, as stated previously, in that it has local anesthetic properties. It has been administered as the sole anesthetic agent for cesarean section (1 mg $\cdot$ kg^{-1}), but the duration of action is only approximately 40 minutes and it has little clinical application in this author's view (257, 264). If meperidine is to be used as an intrathecal or epidural agent, it must be preservative free. There is extensive laboratory and clinical experience with morphine, fentanyl, and sufentanil, which "can reasonably assure the safety of limited intrathecal doses of these drugs" (265).

In conclusion, intrathecal morphine, fentanyl, and sufentanil are now well-established choices for pain management (Table 9.13). Monitoring and treatment of side effects should be no different than those described for epidural morphine. Intrathecal opioids are effective and a safe choice for postoperative pain management in the obstetric patient.

Spinal Distribution and Clearance: Kinetics of Intrathecally Administered Opioids and Explanation of Clinical Results

In an animal study (pigs) of equal doses of morphine, alfentanil, fentanyl, and sufentanil, the extent of opioid distribution within the CSF, spinal cord, epidural space, and the systemic circulation after intrathecal injection were studied (172). The investigators demonstrated through model simulations that the integral exposure of the spinal cord to these opioids was highest for morphine. This was because of the low spinal cord distribution volume of morphine and slow clearance into plasma. The exposure of the spinal cord to fentanyl, sufentanil, or alfentanil was relatively low but for different reasons (Fig. 9.24). Fentanyl, for example, distributes rapidly from the intrathecal space into the epidural space and epidural fat, while sufentanil has a high spinal cord volume of distribution in the white mater. Since the spinal cord opioid receptors are in the gray mater, which is surrounded by white mater, it is hypothesized that much of the sufentanil is sequestered and relatively little reaches the opioid receptors. While this was an animal study, it helps explain the clinical differences when these drugs are applied in humans. The effective and prolonged action of intrathecal morphine for postoperative pain management is clarified by this study.

Does the Choice of Local Anesthetic Affect the Efficacy of Epidural Morphine?

A review of the use of epidural morphine by Kotelko et al. (266) revealed that the intraoperative use of 2-chloroprocaine for anesthesia adversely affected the successful use of epidural morphine for postoperative analgesia. They speculated that the 2-chloroprocaine solution (pH 2.7) lowers pH in the epidural space to such an extent that morphine remains highly ionized, which delays its onset and reduces its potency. However, their results contrast with those of Youngstrom et al. (240), who found that cesarean delivery patients anesthetized with 2-chloroprocaine and given 4 mg epidural morphine for postoperative pain experienced pain relief lasting 20 hours. Multiple studies have debated the possibility of 2-chloroprocaine antagonism of epidural morphine or fentanyl (182, 267–273). Of the numerous case studies and comments reporting adverse effects of the use of 2-chloroprocaine, the work by Eisenach et al. (269) is most intriguing. They demonstrated that a small test dose of 2-chloroprocaine vs. 2% lidocaine, followed by anesthesia with 0.5% bupivacaine, reduced the efficacy of postoperative analgesia with epidural morphine (5.0 mg). Thus, 2-chloroprocaine may, in fact, have a unique antagonistic effect upon intraspinal opioids. It has been suggested that the metabolite chloroaminobenzoic acid may act specifically at μ-receptors

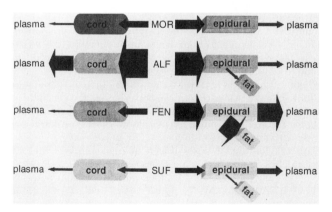

Figure 9.24. Schematic comparison of the median (morphine and sufentanil) or geometric mean (alfentanil and fentanyl) transfer and elimination rate constants. The thickness of the arrow is proportional to the rate constant estimate, i.e., the thicker the arrow, the higher the rate of transfer or elimination. The intensity of the shading of the compartments increases with increasing integral exposure of the spinal cord to the freely diffusable drug in the spinal cord extracellular fluid space. Thus, intrathecal morphine administration leads to the highest integral exposure of the spinal cord. (Reprinted by permission from Ummenhofer WC, Arends RH, Shen DD, Bernards CM. Comparative spinal distribution and clearance kinetics of intrathecally administered morphine, fentanyl, alfentanil, and sufentanil. *Anesthesiology* 2000;92:739–753.)

to antagonize the action of opioids, but this has never been proven. The mechanism of action is uncertain.

Epinephrine and Epidural Opioids

The addition of epinephrine to a local anesthetic solution offers the advantages of increasing the duration of action, lowering the peak serum local anesthetic level, and increasing the intensity of neural blockade, all of which might be beneficial for the patient given epidural opioids. As early as 1904, it was demonstrated that analgesia could be achieved with epinephrine alone, and by 1950, in parturients (274).

The latter study by Priddle and Andros involved several experiments, including administration of 1.0 mg epinephrine (1 mL of 1:1000) mixed with 1 mL 5% dextrose to parturients for labor analgesia. The result was complete pain relief. This approach is not recommended. The potential for neural damage from profound and prolonged vasoconstriction is very real. However, when combined with epidural and intrathecal agents, epinephrine clearly potentiates analgesia. We now know this potentiation to be mediated through α_2-adrenoreceptors and the inhibition of substance P and dorsal horn neurons (275–279).

It has been demonstrated in cats that spinally administered epinephrine suppresses noxiously evoked activity in the dorsal horn (280). These investigators suggested that adrenergic agonists "may act in a multiplicative fashion with spinally administered opioids to produce a profound suppression of noxiously evoked activity" (280). More recently, however, it has been demonstrated in a rat model that the neurotoxicity of intrathecally administered lidocaine is increased by the addition of epinephrine (280a). The authors suggested that, given the narrow therapeutic index of spinal lidocaine (Chapter 5), "the use of lidocaine with epinephrine should be reconsidered." While the use of intrathecal epinephrine has a long history of clinical safety and usefulness, further investigation is needed and ongoing at UCSF. The use of epinephrine, and now clonidine and its analogs, makes further use of our increasing knowledge of intraspinal mechanisms of pain transmission. Investigations by Eisenach (277, 279, 281–284) and others (285–291) may lead to the routine clinical use of clonidine or similar drugs in obstetric anesthesia. Intrathecal clonidine (150, 300, and 450 μg) has been shown to decrease pain in a dose-dependent fashion in women undergoing cesarean section (292). While analgesia lasting approximately 7 to 14 hours (range) was achieved, sedation was also dose dependent. When intrathecal clonidine (7.5 μg) was added to bupivacaine and fentanyl (12.5 μg) in cesarean section patients, there was a modest increase in the time to request for first analgesia (215 ± 79 minutes vs. 183 ± 80 minutes), but there was also a significant increase in sedation (293). The use of α-adrenergic agonists has been extensively reviewed, and it is suggested that clonidine, "added to local anesthetics for epidural, spinal, or peripheral blocks, prolongs and intensifies anesthesia for surgery" (279). In laboring patients, intrathecal clonidine in doses of 15 to 50 μg combined with local anesthetics or opioids, or both, has been studied (294). However, sedation and stability of blood pressure remain potential concerns. Adequate dose response studies in obstetric patients have not been done, and benefits remain unclear (291). More importantly, in the United States, both epidural and intrathecal clonidine remain largely prohibited by the FDA in obstetric patients with a **"Black Box" warning** in the clonidine package insert. The warning reads: *"Epidural clonidine is not recommended for obstetrical, postpartum, or perioperative pain management. The risks of hemodynamic instability, especially hypotension and bradycardia, from epidural clonidine may be unacceptable in these patients. However, in a rare obstetrical, postpartum, or perioperative patient, potential benefits may outweigh the possible risks"* (294). Thus, at least in the United States, it is suggested that the administration of epidural or intrathecal clonidine in laboring patients incurs additional medicolegal risks until further investigation demonstrates the

usefulness and safety of clonidine (294). In this author's view, there is little clear benefit to clonidine as either an epidural or an intrathecal agent for obstetric analgesia, and its use is not recommended at this time. Further FDA-approved research is ongoing and may ultimately demonstrate purposeful clinical applications for clonidine.

COMPLICATIONS OF INTRASPINAL OPIOIDS

The chief side effects of intraspinal opioids are pruritus, nausea, vomiting, somnolence, urinary retention, and respiratory depression. The reported incidence of side effects varies greatly, possibly because of the smaller number of patients and absence of controls in earlier studies. The most extensive early study of the side effects of epidural morphine was conducted by Reiz and Westberg (295). They clearly outlined the potential problems with the use of the technique, but reported a significantly lower incidence of side effects than encountered by others. In a study of 1200 patients, they found a 17% incidence of nausea and vomiting. Following use of a standard morphine solution, the incidence of pruritus was 15% but decreased to 1% with preservative-free morphine. However, a large review (n = 1000) of patients receiving epidural morphine for postcesarean analgesia at UCSF revealed a 60% incidence of pruritus, a finding consistent with most others (Table 9.11) (239).

Bromage et al. (296) reported a significantly higher incidence of side effects when 1:200,000 epinephrine was added to 10 mg epidural morphine than with administration of the same dose of morphine without epinephrine. While this finding represented only three volunteer patients without surgical pain, the results of this early work generally have been supported by others (31, 33, 297). Bromage et al. (296) also reported a decrease in peak plasma morphine levels from 44 ± 12.9 ng·mL^{-1} to 13.7 ± 6.7 ng·mL^{-1} with epidural morphine solutions containing epinephrine.

When evaluating intrathecal sufentanil 10 mg with bupivacaine 2.5 mg, Campbell et al. noted that the incidence of pruritus was 90% (33). When epinephrine 0.2 mg was added, the incidence of pruritus was 100%. Both intrathecal and epidural sufentanil and fentanyl can cause significant pruritus (2, 31). In a large review of clinical experience with CSE for labor analgesia (n = 1022) by Norris et al., the incidence of pruritus with intrathecal opioids (sufentanil 10 μg most often) was 41.4% (Fig. 9.25) (31).

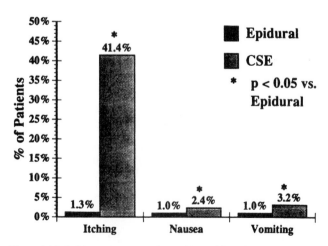

Figure 9.25. Itching, nausea, and vomiting within 60 minutes of induction of epidural or combined spinal-epidural labor analgesia. (Reprinted by permission from Norris MC, Grieco WM, Borkowski M, et al. Complications of labor analgesia: Epidural versus combined spinal epidural techniques. *Anesth Analg* 1994;79:529–537.)

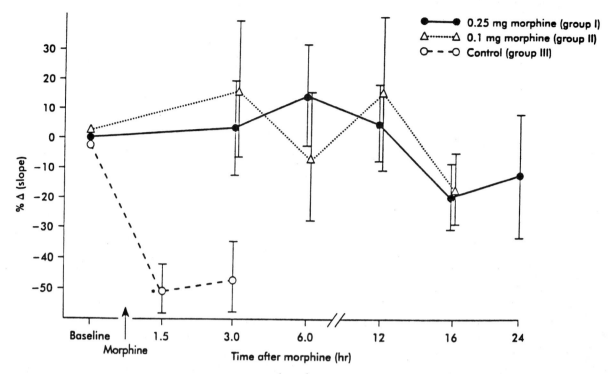

Figure 9.26. Percent change in CO_2 response slopes ($L \cdot min \cdot mm^{-1} Hg^{-1}$) from baseline values after patients received intrathecal or subcutaneous morphine (control). (Reprinted by permission from Abboud TK, Dror A, Mosaad P, et al. Minidose intrathecal morphine for the relief of postcesarean section pain: Safety, efficacy, and ventilatory responses to carbon dioxide. *Anesth Analg* 1988;67:137–141).

Vasoconstriction of veins by epinephrine leads to increased CSF and central levels of opioid, i.e., a slower systemic uptake of opioid. This may produce greater analgesia but also will increase side effects. Clearly, side effects from intraspinal opioids are dose related (114, 298). Use of the lowest effective dose that achieves adequately prolonged analgesia will decrease side effects and risks of adverse outcome (1, 2, 229).

RESPIRATORY DEPRESSION
Delayed Respiratory Depression

The most serious side effect, delayed respiratory depression (i.e., late onset of respiratory depression), has occurred with the use of both epidural and spinal opioids since the first use of this technique, and has occurred with both morphine and the lipid-soluble agents (59, 60, 63–65, 217, 299–312). All opioids, whether administered as IV, IM, intrathecal, or epidural agents, can cause and have caused respiratory depression. All patients who receive opioids should be monitored with this in mind (59, 313). Respiratory depression may occur when epidurally administered opioid reaches its peak plasma level (similar to absorption from IM injection) and cause relatively respiratory depression immediately or, more seriously, 6 or more hours after the initial administration of opioid. When intrathecal lipophilic opioids are administered, respiratory depression may occur within minutes and has been reported with both fentanyl and sufentanil (60, 63, 64).

Respiratory depression can and does occur in obstetric patients (59, 239). In a retrospective study of delayed respiratory depression in nonobstetric patients, the Swedish Society of Anesthesiologists estimated that, in 6000 to 9000 patients, the incidence of respiratory depression was 0.25% to 0.40% with epidural opioids and 4% to 7% with intrathecal opioids (314). Respiratory depression appeared to be related to the age of the patient (with increased incidence in those 70 years of age or older), the presence of pulmonary disease, the addition of systemic opioids, or the thoracic administration of epidural

morphine. The dose of opioid also has been shown to be important. In an early report, 1.0 mg intrathecal morphine was reported to cause respiratory depression (301). This dose now seems quite large, and morphine 0.1 to 0.25 mg is more likely to be used (postcesarean analgesia). Regardless of the dose administered, all patients given epidural or intrathecal morphine must be monitored for respiratory depression (Table 9.12) (59, 239).

Abboud et al. evaluated the CO_2 response in cesarean section patients receiving 0.1 or 0.25 mg intrathecal morphine or 8 mg subcutaneous morphine (246). Intrathecal morphine at these now commonly used doses did not affect the CO_2 response or minute ventilation, while both outcomes were depressed for 3 hours after subcutaneous morphine (Fig. 9.26).

Reports of respiratory depression are numerous and no longer unusual (Table 9.14) (60, 63, 64, 168, 217, 229, 239, 299–310, 312, 315, 316). The literature concerning the respiratory response to opioids administered by various routes demonstrates that with analgesia comes some degree of respiratory depression (45, 66, 246, 317–320). Respiratory depression is more common if prior IV opioids have been administered or excessive doses of intraspinal opioids are used (310, 311, 321, 322).

Profound respiratory depression with as little as 100 μg epidural fentanyl has been reported (307). Respiratory depression may occur at a rate of approximately 0.1% to 0.25% in cesarean section patients given epidural morphine. A nursing staff that is capable of and allowed to administer IM opioids has the necessary skills and general knowledge to monitor patients who have received epidural or intrathecal opioids. After staff education concerning the specific side effects of epidural or intrathecal opioids, monitoring these patients in the routine obstetric postpartum wards is appropriate.

Clinical experience suggests that the period when the patient is at greatest risk for delayed respiratory depression is 4 to 8 hours after the epidural or intrathecal administration of opioids. A biphasic ventilatory response to epidural morphine has been suggested, with initial respiratory depression caused by the serum level, and depression occurring at 8 hours due to

Table 9.14. RESPIRATORY DEPRESSION: HOW MUCH OF A PROBLEM?

	Patients (n)*	Respiratory Depression
Cesarean section—UCSF experience (prospective study) Leicht et al. (239)	1000	4 (0.4%)†
General surgery Stenseth et al. (316)	1085	10 (0.9%)
National survey—all patients Rawal et al. (315)	15,100	13 (0.9%)
General surgery Ready et al. (168)	623	4 (0.6%)
Cesarean section Fuller et al. (180)	4880	12 (0.25%)

UCSF = University of California San Francisco.
* In these papers, the patients with respiratory depression (both simple decreased respiratory rate and clear depression [see Fig. 9.27] all recovered with no sequelae. Many were simply observed, whereas some required naloxone and oxygen therapy.
† In the study at UCSF, only one of these four patients, or 0.1%, had true respiratory depression.

movement in the CSF (323). This was also suggested by Camporesi et al. (324), who demonstrated that CO_2 response curves in volunteers were maximally depressed at 0.5 hour following IV administration of morphine and at 6 to 10 hours following epidural administration. This is likely to be similar with the administration of intrathecal morphine as well. Although it is probably still prudent to monitor for 24 hours after epidural or intrathecal morphine, the risk period probably does not extend beyond 12 hours, assuming the patient is alert and free of other side effects at that time (Fig. 9.27). Patients who become unusually sedated and drowsy should be monitored more closely.

Providing pain relief always invites risk, and perhaps no medical intervention is without risk. However, the potential for respiratory depression must be a key caveat to the use of opioids whether the route is intraspinal, IM, or IV (59).

Pruritus

The most common side effect of intraspinal opioids is pruritus (Table 9.11), which is usually nonsegmental and highly variable in nature. Onset occurs shortly after analgesia develops.

Although many patients do not complain of this condition and thus appear asymptomatic, when asked they respond affirmatively. The cause of pruritus is unknown and does not appear to be related to histamine release (176). Treatment may include IV administration of naloxone (10 to 200 μg) or diphenhydramine (25 to 50 mg), although the latter regimen seems best suited to inducing sleep so the patient no longer "cares" about the itching. It also has been suggested that nalbuphine (10 mg subcutaneously) will decrease pruritus (325, 326). IV nalbuphine 2.5 to 5 mg also may be very helpful in decreasing pruritus (326–328). IV propofol 10 mg has been reported to relieve pruritus (329–331). In patients given 1 mg morphine for labor and delivery pain, Baraka et al. found a 100% incidence of pruritus (16). As noted earlier, even the small intrathecal doses of fentanyl or sufentanil used in CSE for labor analgesia can lead to a 90% to 100% incidence of pruritus. Since side effects are dose related and thus intensify with increasing levels of opioid in CSF, the onset of pruritus probably is related to the rostral spread of opioids in the CSF. The treatment of pruritus must be prompt and aggressive if the patient is to achieve satisfactory analgesia without complaint. The lower doses, particularly of intrathecal morphine used currently, have decreased side effects.

Herpes Simplex Virus

It has been suggested that there is a relationship between epidural morphine, facial pruritus, and herpes labialis (herpes simplex virus-1 [HSV-1] or cold sores) that may combine to reactivate oral HSV-1. This was first noted by Carden (332), after spinal morphine was administered to children for enuresis, and again in two interesting studies in patients undergoing cesarean section (333, 334). Several studies provide support for a central or "ganglion-trigger" mechanism (335–338). However, it must be remembered that exposure to UV light, immunosuppression, or trauma may reactivate HSV-1. It is not known if reactivation of HSV-1 occurs in labor following intraspinal opioids. It does not appear to be a major clinical problem. Some suggest that patients with a history of herpes labialis should be warned of a possible reactivation of their infection, although this is not universally followed. This author is unaware of any serious maternal or neonatal complications arising from reactivation of HSV-1.

Urinary Retention

Urinary retention is a minor but annoying side effect. Although not always apparent and difficult to judge in the obstetric

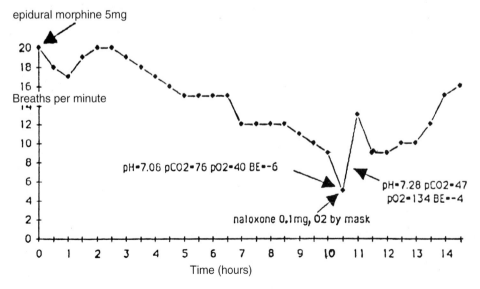

Figure 9.27. **Time sequence of respiratory depression in one patient.** This represents the respiratory rate (RR) of an obstetric patient who received 5 mg epidural morphine after a cesarean section. The patient became progressively sedate and had a decreasing RR. She was given naloxone and recovered uneventfully. (Reprinted by permission from Leicht CH, Hughes SC, Dailey PA, Shnider SM, Rosen MA. Epidural morphine sulfate for analgesia after cesarean section: A prospective report of 1000 patients [abstract]. *Anesthesiology* 1986;65:A366.)

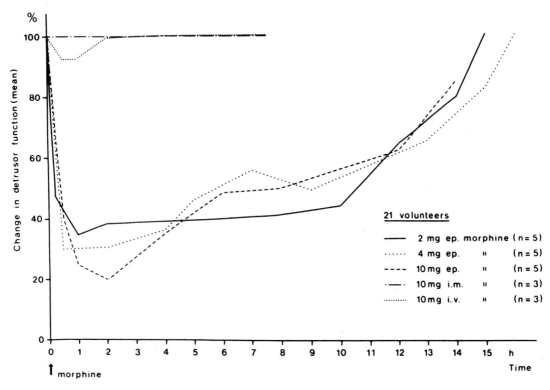

Figure 9.28. The urodynamic effects of epidural and intravenous morphine in male volunteers. Detrusor muscle function depression persisted for many hours following even 2 mg epidural morphine. This does not occur with systemic opioids, and a local spinal cause (i.e., opiate receptors) is probable. (Reprinted by permission from Rawal N, Möllefors K, Axelsson K, Lingardh G, Widman B. An experimental study of urodynamic effects of epidural morphine and of naloxone reversal. *Anesth Analg* 1983;62:641–647.)

population, the reported incidence among nonobstetric patients is 15% to 90% and may be higher in men (295, 339). There is evidence that the cause of urinary retention is the rapid onset of detrusor muscle relaxation produced by the local sacral spinal action of opioids (Fig. 9.28) (340), and there is a series of interesting studies investigating this mechanism (341–344). Onset occurs with analgesia and thus appears earlier than pruritus, nausea, and vomiting, which are centrally mediated. If necessary, urinary retention can be treated with naloxone, but patient ambulation or performing a single-straight urinary catheterization often relieves the problem. Since a Foley catheter commonly is placed in the cesarean section patient, and often in patients in labor, urinary retention is less of a problem in obstetric anesthesia.

Nausea and Vomiting

Nausea and vomiting are side effects whose causes are difficult to separate from surgical events or pregnancy itself. Nausea may result from allowing the patient to resume oral intake of food sooner, owing to the patient's general sense of well-being after achieving significant pain relief. Although the incidence of these effects is variable, the onset is predictable. Small doses of an antiemetic or naloxone can be used to treat them while maintaining analgesia. Metoclopramide (10 mg IV) is recommended by some, whereas others administer droperidol (0.625 mg IV). Several investigators have found moderate success with transdermal scopolamine patches (1.5 mg scopolamine) placed behind the patient's ear (345–347). Common side effects of this method include dry mouth (67%), drowsiness (18%), and occasionally blurred vision. The use of scopolamine patches may be a reasonable choice, but are uncommonly used.

Metoclopramide 10 mg IV is very effective in treating nausea and vomiting, and it has few side effects. It has been given to nursing women to improve lactation (348). It may also enhance analgesia by inhibiting acetylcholinesterase, but this is unproven (349). Thus, metoclopramide seems a safe and rea-

sonable choice. Ondansetron also is effective for intraspinal-induced nausea and vomiting, but its use may be limited because of its present cost (349a). Dolasetron 12.5 mg IV is a less-expensive alternative that might also be considered. Nalbuphine 2.5 to 5 mg IV may be useful, and propofol 10 to 20 mg IV has also been found to be helpful.

Side Effects and Use of Naloxone

Almost all side effects of intraspinal opioids can be decreased or relieved completely by administering naloxone intravenously. Analgesia can be maintained if the dosage of naloxone is titrated carefully (40 to 100 μg IV). Because central opiate receptors in the brain appear to be responsible for most of the side effects of intraspinal opioids (urinary retention excluded), high blood flow to the brain delivers enough naloxone to reverse side effects. The relatively low blood flow to the dorsal horn, which is dense with opiate-laden receptors, allows analgesia to continue. Dailey et al. found a significantly decreased incidence of pruritus in obstetric patients given a continuous infusion of 0.4 to 0.6 mg/h naloxone following 1 mg intrathecal morphine during labor (Table 9.15) (84). Analgesia was maintained despite the naloxone infusion (Fig. 9.29). Similar work with human volunteers and surgical patients demonstrated that a naloxone infusion of 5 to 10 μg · kg^{-1} increased minute ventilation and respiratory frequency to preepidural morphine levels and decreased end-tidal CO_2, which had increased in response to the epidural opioid (350). Lower doses of naloxone (1 μg · kg^{-1}) have been shown to be effective in the elderly, but may not be effective if significant respiratory depression or other side effects are in need of treatment (351). Intravenous naloxone should be titrated to effect to treat side effects; 0.1 to 0.6 mg/h is the more likely dose range. However, if the dose of naloxone reaches 10 μg · kg^{-1}, the duration of analgesia may be shortened by about 25% (352).

Table 9.15. INTRAVENOUS NALOXONE DECREASES SIDE EFFECTS AFTER INTRATHECAL MORPHINE (1 MG)

Side Effect	Saline Infusion (%) (n = 17)	Naloxone Infusion (%) (n = 23)	Statistical Significance
Pruritus	35	9	$P < .05$
Vomiting	53	26	NS
Drowsiness/ dizziness	65	35	NS

Adapted from Dailey PA, Brookshire GL, Shnider SM, et al. Naloxone decreases side effects after intrathecal morphine for labor. *Anesth Analg* 1985;64:658–666.

Although IV infusion of naloxone may help to reduce the side effects of intraspinal opioids, and may even prevent respiratory depression if given in higher doses, the routine use of this technique cannot be recommended for obstetrics, if only because of the inconvenience. Furthermore, although the effects on the newborn of clinical doses of naloxone appear to be benign, there is evidence in animal models that very high levels of naloxone may reduce the resistance of the fetus to hypoxic stress (353). There is no evidence of this vulnerability in humans: parenteral doses as high as 200 μg · kg^{-1} have been given to neonates without detectable adverse effects (354). However, naloxone does cross the placenta (355), and may increase the number and amplitude of FHR accelerations and affect fetal behavior (347).

Intravenous naloxone also may cause serious maternal problems and is to be used cautiously. In the nonobstetric literature, there are multiple case reports of pulmonary edema and cardiac arrest after naloxone administration (356–361). Although this problem seems unlikely in the obstetric setting and has not been reported, the use of opioid antagonists should not be undertaken without some consideration. Oral naltrexone (6 mg) has been suggested as a possible prophylactic drug to treat pruritus (362, 363), and an IV antagonist, nalmefene, may prove useful (364). The latter may be effective in reversing respiratory depression for 4 hours or more. Further investigation is needed in this area before these drugs can be recommended for routine use. Antagonism of side effects by the agonist-antagonist nalbuphine also might be considered; however, there are conflicting results and its use is not without risks (325, 365–368). A case report of naloxone-precipitated *acute opioid withdrawal* syndrome illustrates the potential risks with even small doses of naloxone (369). IV naloxone 0.14 mg was administered to a patient in divided doses to treat pruritus following epidural morphine 2.0 mg for postcesarean section analgesia. The patient became restless, agitated and tachypneic, and lacrimation and rhinorrhea were noted. The patient was opioid naïve, and this response was attributed to *acute* opioid withdrawal. While this appears to be extremely uncommon, naloxone or the longer-acting derivatives are not without potential risks.

NEONATAL EFFECTS OF INTRASPINAL OPIOIDS

The effects of opioids on the newborn are well known. Concern for the newborn, in part, stimulated the initial interest in the use of the intraspinal opioids: low-dose effective analgesia would pose less risk to the newborn, while providing adequate pain relief to the mother. The safe and effective use of intrathecal morphine has been demonstrated in the gravid rat and rabbit, and was supported by the early clinical reports (15, 16, 370). Newborns delivered of mothers given 2, 5, and 7.5 mg epidural morphine had high Apgar and Neurologic and Adaptive Capacity Scores, and normal values for umbilical arterial and venous blood-gas tensions (99). Nevertheless, the rapid placental transfer of epidural opioids is to be expected, and the clinician

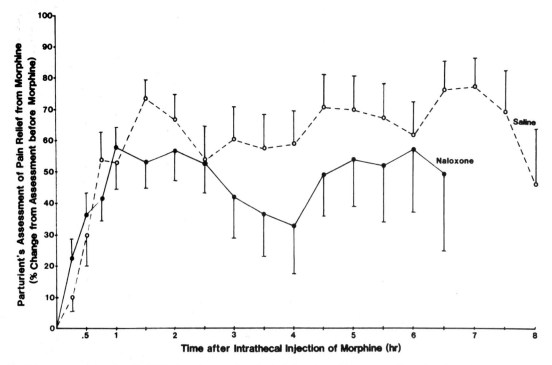

Figure 9.29. Predelivery maternal pain relief following the intrathecal administration of 1 mg morphine. One hour later, an intravenous bolus of naloxone 0.4 mg was given, followed by a naloxone infusion of 0.4 to 0.6 mg/h. (Reprinted by permission from Dailey PA, Brookshire GL, Shnider SM, et al. Naloxone decreases side effects after intrathecal morphine for labor. *Anesth Analg* 1985;64:658–666.)

should limit the dose given during labor to that which has been proven safe and effective (Fig. 9.13). Whether it is morphine, fentanyl, sufentanil, or another opioid, placental transfer occurs, and both maternal and fetal safety limit the amount of epidural opioid that should be given.

Early investigators documented the safe use of intrathecal morphine (10, 15, 16). Given the fairly low doses of intrathecal morphine (0.5 to 1 mg) initially used, neonatal safety is not a surprising finding (10). Dailey et al. also found that a continuous infusion of naloxone in the mother did not adversely affect the infant (84). During labor, there was no change in FHR or variability resulting from either intrathecal morphine injection or continuous naloxone infusion in the mother. At the time of delivery, the mean plasma concentration of naloxone was 1.92 ± 0.28 ng$\cdot$mL^{-1} in the umbilical venous blood. This is a relatively low concentration, especially when considering the typically high dose of naloxone used in pediatric resuscitation.

Dailey et al. also determined that the β-endorphin concentrations in the umbilical venous blood were not significantly different when saline rather than naloxone was infused (84). The β-endorphin levels were 78.7 ± 15.9 fmol/mL in newborns of mothers given saline, and 57.0 ± 8.2 fmol/mL in newborns of mothers given naloxone. These levels decreased as analgesia developed, but increased at delivery to preintrathecal morphine levels. The physiologic significance of plasma β-endorphin levels during labor and delivery is unknown; increased plasma β-endorphin levels resulting from stress are not associated with increased β-endorphin levels in the brain or CSF (371).

Epidural Fentanyl and Sufentanil

The increasing use of epidural fentanyl and sufentanil for labor analgesia has increased the concerns regarding fetal effects. If 10 to 20 μg/h sufentanil is to be used (as some authors have suggested) or 10 to 40 μg/h fentanyl plus potential bolus injections (50 to 100 μg) to treat incomplete pain relief (as some clinicians now practice), then the effects on the newborn must be considered. All opioids cross the placenta, including the lipid-soluble opioids. Neurobehavioral changes (short term) can be seen with all opioids. The investigation of IV alfentanil and meperidine in monkeys in labor found behavioral differences for up to 72 hours and possibly longer (372, 373). There is also concern that the umbilical plasma opioid levels measured and so often quoted as "low" may not be as important as brain tissue opioid levels. In dogs, the high lipid content of the brain and the significant lipid solubility of fentanyl result in higher opioid concentrations in the brain (ng/gm brain tissue) than in plasma (ng$\cdot$mL^{-1} serum) (372). Hypocarbia (hyperventilation with incomplete pain relief) also leads to higher brain fentanyl levels in dogs. Furthermore, there is accumulation of fentanyl in the sheep fetus when the ewe receives fentanyl (373). Despite these findings, in clinical practice the addition of fentanyl (1 to 3 μg$\cdot$mL^{-1}) or sufentanil (0.2 to 1 μg$\cdot$mL^{-1}) to local anesthetics for infusion during labor has proven to be safe and effective (129–131). While a safe upper limit of the total cumulative epidural fentanyl dose administered during labor has not been established, maximum doses of fentanyl 300 to 400 μg during labor have not proven to significantly affect the newborn (129, 131). While a mild reduction in the Neurologic and Adaptive Scores in babies whose mothers had received epidural fentanyl has been demonstrated (128), long clinical experience and clinical investigation (127, 129, 130, 374) have demonstrated the safety of epidural opioids. The current use of CSE in labor involves very small doses of intrathecal opioids, which would be expected to have no direct effect on the fetus or newborn. Fernando et al. (375) evaluated the neonatal outcome and placental transfer of fentanyl after CSE technique for labor analgesia. The patients received

intrathecal fentanyl 25 μg and bupivacaine 2.5 mg followed by an epidural infusion of bupivacaine 0.1% with 2 μg$\cdot$mL^{-1} fentanyl at 10 to 15 mL/h. Using this now fairly standard approach, the authors concluded that CSE appeared to have a negligible effect upon the neonatal condition.

Monitoring of Patients

Monitoring of patients who have received clinical doses of epidural or intrathecal opioids for labor as described in this chapter can be easily performed on the labor ward as part of the patient's usual obstetric care. After receiving lipid-soluble opioids, for example, fentanyl 2 μg$\cdot$mL^{-1} added to a local anesthetic solution for labor, monitoring for 4 hours after the solution is discontinued is adequate. Even shorter periods may be quite safe. However, after a larger bolus epidural injection of sufentanil (20 to 30 μg) or fentanyl (100 μg), respiratory depression can occur acutely or within the first 60 to 90 minutes, and monitoring must be appropriate. There are case reports involving administration of gross amounts of opioids (400 mg epidural morphine or 100 μg intrathecal sufentanil), and careful preparation and dilution of epidural and intrathecal drugs is vital. As we mix more drugs for obstetric regional anesthesia, such as opioids, epinephrine, sodium bicarbonate, possibly clonidine, and other drugs, we must be extremely cautious. Concerns regarding drug concentration and potential neurotoxicity of opioids or various combinations cannot be ignored (see below) (162, 265).

In summary, the use of epidural opioid-containing solutions has become routine for labor analgesia and is extremely effective and safe when used as suggested (Table 9.7). The use of intrathecal opioids has unique advantages and potential risks, but its use is also very routine in many centers. The fetus and newborn may benefit from these newer approaches to labor analgesia, because even more dilute solutions of several drugs have proven highly effective and may offer increased maternal and fetal safety by decreasing the amount of a local anesthetic or opioid that might have otherwise been administered.

Potential Neurotoxicity and Other Side Effects of Intraspinal Opioids

When using intraspinal opioids, the potential for opioid irritation of neural tissue must always be considered. There is ample evidence that morphine has no deleterious effect on neural tissue (265, 287, 376–380). However, as Hodgson et al. noted, limited animal safety data are available on several drugs used intrathecally or epidurally (Table 9.16) (265). Fentanyl, for example, has been investigated in laboratory studies and it appears benign, but there have been little data reported in the literature. However, it has had long clinical experience and appears safe. Clinicians are urged to be cautious when considering any new agent or combination of agents for intraspinal use. Many agents were suggested without adequate study of possible neurotoxicity (381). Even low doses of intrathecal butorphanol may cause neurotoxicity, and thus this does not seem to be an appropriate epidural agent in this author's view (Fig. 9.30) (230). Epidural droperidol, for example, was recently reported to decrease the side effects associated with the use of epidural morphine for analgesia after cesarean section (382). While the effects of droperidol in this situation have been controversial and extensively discussed in the literature (383–386), it appears that there has been little attention given to the potential of neurotoxicity. As noted earlier, it has been demonstrated in an animal model that intrathecal epinephrine increases the neurotoxicity of lidocaine (280a). This model may prove useful to more carefully study the intrathecal drugs commonly used in obstetric anesthesia.

Table 9.16. EVIDENCE OF NEUROTOXICITY OF SPINAL ANALGESICS

Drug	Animal Data			Human Data		
	Histologic	Physiologic	Behavioral	Histologic	Physiologic	Clinical
Opioids						
Hydrophilic						
Morphine	−*	−	−	−	−	−
Meperidine	NA	NA	NA	NA	NA	NA
Hydromorphone	NA	NA	NA	−†	NA	NA
Lipophilic						
Fentanyl	NA	NA	NA	NA	NA	−‡
Sufentanil	+/−	NA	−	NA	NA	−§
Alfentanil	−	NA	−	NA	NA	NA
Remifentanil	NA	NA	NA	NA	NA	NA
Partial agonists						
Butorphanol	+	NA	+	NA	NA	NA
Nalbuphine	+/−	NA	−	NA	NA	NA
α2-agonists						
Clonidine	−	−	−	−†	−	NA
AChE inhibitors						
Neostigmine‖	−	−	−	NA	NA	−
GABA agonists						
Midazolam	+/−	+	−	NA	NA	−
Baclofen	−	NA	−	NA	NA	−
NMDA antagonists						
Ketamine¶	+/−	+	+/−	NA	NA	NA
Amitriptyline	−	−	−#	NA	NA	NA
Somatostatin	+/−	+	+/−	+/−	NA	NA
NSAIDs						
Ketorolac**	NA	NA	NA	NA	NA	NA
Lysine acetylsalicylic acid	+/−	+	+/−	NA	NA	NA
Steroids						
Methylprednisolone††	−	NA	−	NA	NA	+/−
Triamcinolone††	−	NA	−	NA	NA	+/−

+ = studies support neurotoxicity; − = studies refute neurotoxicity; +/− = studies are inconsistent; AChE = acetylcholinesterase; GABA = γ-amino butyric acid; NA = no studies available; NMDA = N-methyl-D-aspartate; NSAIDs = nonsteroidal antiinflammatory drugs.
*Large-dose, high-concentration, long-term spinal morphine may be neurotoxic.
†Neurohistopathology performed on a single cancer patient.
‡Fentanyl safety based on clinical experience, not formal neurotoxicity testing.
§Sufentanil associated with transient muscle rigidity with epinephrine; safety based on clinical use only.
‖Neostigmine formulated with or without methly- and propylparabens.
¶Ketamine preserved with benzethonium chloride or chlorbutanol.
#Sedation and seizure followed by death in one animal receiving an intrathecal cervical superclinical dose.
**Ketorolac contains 10% alcohol solvent.
††These depot steroid preparations contain 3% polyethylene glycol and > 1% benzyl alcohol.
Hodgson PS, Weal JM, Pollock JE, et al. The neutoxicity of drugs given intrathecally (Spinal). *Anesth Analg* 1999;88:797–809.

Unusual complications have been associated with the use of intraspinal opioids. One case involved a cancer patient in whom chronic administration of very large doses of opioids was discontinued when good analgesia was provided with 1 mg intrathecal morphine; the patient then manifested opioid withdrawal (387). Although this is not likely to be a common problem in the obstetric population, it might well occur in chronic pain patients treated with long-term opioid therapy before the use of intraspinal opioids. Epidural butorphanol has caused withdrawal in an obstetric patient with a "silent" opioid abuse history. A unique syndrome of *acute withdrawal* in an obstetric patient after the single use of opioid was recently reported (369). An early report suggested the synergistic action of droperidol and epidural opioid (388), but this was not substantiated in a large review (239). When additional opioids, sedatives, or tranquilizers are given to a patient who has received intraspinal opioids, increased monitoring of the patient is required. Another rare but potential problem was suggested by a case report of an anaphylactic reaction to epidural fentanyl (389), but this ultimately was most likely a latex allergy. Although the analgesia achieved with intraspinal opioids is very real, so are the side effects. In most cases, these can be treated quite easily, but they must be acknowledged as part of the reason we use intraspinal opioids.

CONCLUSION

This technique is now well established in labor and delivery and for postoperative pain management. In labor, ever more dilute epidural solutions of local anesthetics and lipid-soluble opioids in larger volumes possibly provide excellent analgesia and decreased motor block, and may allow patients to ambulate (83). The use of the CSE technique offers unique advantages and is now widely used (6, 7). However, from the earliest use of CSE, it was clear that the side effects must be considered (31), and some caution is necessary until experience increases (294). The pain relief obtained with intraspinal opioids is superior to that provided by traditional methods, and intraspinal opioids have now been successfully used for over 20 years at UCSF and many other centers. Patients can potentially ambulate antepartum, and care for their newborn and interact with family members immediately postpartum. Intraspinal opioids have established a firm place in obstetric anesthesia last 20 years for both labor analgesia and postoperative pain management.

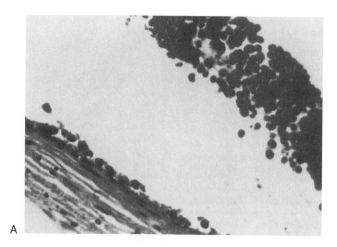

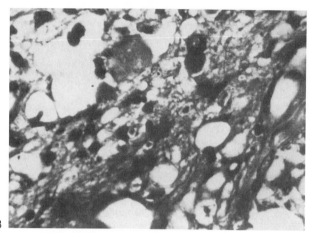

Figure 9.30. *A*: Section at level of catheter up. Inflammatory changes suggestive of suppurative meningitis due to irritating effect of small dose ($0.075 \ \text{mg} \cdot \text{kg}^{-1}$) of intrathecal butorphanol (electron microscopy × 400). *B*: Axonal and neuronal degeneration following small dose intrathecal butorphanol. Hemorrhages near catheter insertion: section at level of catheter insertion (electron microscopy × 400). (Reprinted by permission from Rawal N, Nuutinen L, Raj PP, et al. Behavioral and histopathologic effects following intrathecal administration of butorphanol, sufentanil, and nalbuphine in sheep. *Anesthesiology* 1991;75:1025–1034.)

REFERENCES

1. Dahl J, Jeppesen I, Jorgensen H, et al. Intraoperative and postoperative analgesic efficacy and adverse effects of intrathecal opioids in patients undergoing cesarean section with spinal anesthesia. *Anesthesiology* 1999;91:1919–1927.
2. Palmer CM, Emerson S, Volgoropolus D, et al. Dose-response relationship of intrathecal morphine for postcesarean analgesia. *Anesthesiology* 1999;90:437–444.
3. Arkoosh VA, Cooper M, Norris MC, et al. Intrathecal sufentanil dose response in nulliparous patients. *Anesthesiology* 1998;89:364–370.
4. Palmer CM, Cork RC, Hays R, et al. The dose-response relationship of intrathecal fentanyl for labor analgesia. *Anesthesiology* 1998;88:355–361.
5. Mardirosoff C, Dumont L. Two doses of intrathecal sufentanil (2.5 and 5 μg) combined with bupivacaine and epinephrine for labor analgesia. *Anesth Analg* 1999;89:1263–1266.
6. Collis RE, Baxandall ML, Srikantharajah ID. Combined spinal epidural (CSE) analgesia: Technique management and outcome of 300 mothers. *Int J Obstet Anesth* 1994;3:75–81.
7. Rawal N, VanZundert A, Holmström B, et al. Combined spinal-epidural technique. *Reg Anesth* 1997;22:406–423.
8. Nelson KE, D'Angelo R, Foss ML, et al. Intrathecal neostigmine and sufentanil for early labor analgesia. *Anesthesiology* 1999;91:1293–1298.
9. Wang JK, Nauss LA, Thomas JE. Pain relief by intrathecally applied morphine in man. *Anesthesiology* 1979;50:149–151.
10. Abboud TK, Shnider SM, Dailey PA, et al. Intrathecal administration of hyperbaric morphine for the relief of pain in labor. *Br J Anaesth* 1984;56:1351–1360.
11. Samii K, Chauvin M, Viars P. Postoperative spinal analgesia with morphine. *Br J Anaesth* 1981;53:817–820.
12. Cousins MJ, Mather LE, Glynn CJ, Wilson PR, Graham JR. Selective spinal analgesia [letter]. *Lancet* 1979;1:1141–1142.
13. Nordberg G, Hedner T, Mellstrand T, Dahlstrom B. Pharmacokinetic aspects of intrathecal morphine analgesia. *Anesthesiology* 1984;60:448–454.
14. Caldwell L, Rosen M, Shnider S. Subarachnoid morphine and fentanyl for labor analgesia: Efficacy and side effects. *Reg Anesth* 1994;12:2–8.
15. Scott PV, Bowen FE, Cartwright P, et al. Intrathecal morphine as sole analgesic during labour. *Br Med J* 1980;281:351–353.
16. Baraka A, Noueihid R, Hajj S. Intrathecal injection of morphine for obstetric analgesia. *Anesthesiology* 1981;54:136–140.
17. Akerman B, Arwestrom E, Post C. Local anesthetics potentiate spinal morphine antinociception. *Anesth Analg* 1988;67:943–949.
18. Leighton BL, DeSimone CA, Norris MC, Ben-David B. Intrathecal narcotics for labor revisited: The combination of fentanyl and morphine intrathecally provides rapid onset of profound, prolonged analgesia. *Anesth Analg* 1989;69:122–125.
19. Abouleish E, Rawal N, Shaw J, Lorenz T, Rashad N. Intrathecal morphine 0.2 mg versus epidural bupivacaine 0.125% or their combination: Effects on parturients. *Anesthesiology* 1991;74:711–716.
20. D'Angelo R, Gerancher JC, Eisenach JC, et al. Epidural fentanyl produces labor analgesia by a spinal mechanism. *Anesthesiology* 1998;88:1519–1523.
21. Bonnardot JP, Maillet M, Colau JC, Millot F, Deligne P. Maternal and fetal concentrations of morphine after intrathecal administration during labour. *Br J Anaesth* 1982;54:487–489.
22. Power KJ, Avery AF. Extradural analgesia in the intrapartum management of a patient with pulmonary hypertension. *Br J Anaesth* 1989;63:116–120.
23. Rosen MA, Hughes SC, Curtis JD, et al. Effects of epidural morphine on uterine blood flow and acid-base status in the pregnant ewe [abstract]. *Anesthesiology* 1982;57:A383.
24. Craft JB Jr, Bolan JC, Coaldrake LA, et al. The maternal and fetal cardiovascular effects of epidural morphine in the sheep model. *Am J Obstet Gynecol* 1982;142:835–839.
25. Cohen SE, Cherry CM, Holbrook RH Jr, et al. Intrathecal sufentanil for labor analgesia: Sensory changes, side effects and fetal heart rate changes. *Anesth Analg* 1993;77:1155–1160.
26. Riley ET, Ratner EF, Cohen S. Intrathecal sufentanil for labor analgesia: Do sensory changes predict better analgesia and greater hypotension? *Anesth Analg* 1997;84:346–351.
27. Ahmad S, Hawes D, Dooley S, Faure E, Brunner E. Intrathecal morphine in a parturient with a single ventricle. *Anesthesiology* 1981;54:515–517.
28. Abboud TK, Raya I, Noueihid R, Daniel J. Intrathecal morphine for relief of labor pain in a parturient with severe pulmonary hypertension. *Anesthesiology* 1983;59:477–479.
29. Robinson DE, Leicht CH. Epidural analgesia with low-dose bupivacaine and fentanyl for labor and delivery in a parturient with severe pulmonary hypertension. *Anesthesiology* 1988;68:285–288.
30. Copel JA, Harrison D, Whittemore R, Hobbins JC. Intrathecal morphine analgesia for vaginal delivery in a woman with a single ventricle: A case report. *J Reprod Med* 1986;31:274–276.
31. Norris MC, Grieco WM, Borkowski M, et al. Complications of labor analgesia: Epidural versus combined spinal epidural techniques. *Anesth Analg* 1994;79:529–537.
32. Campbell DC, Camann WC, Datta S. The addition of bupivacaine to intrathecal sufentanil for labor analgesia. *Anesth Analg* 1995;81:305–309.
33. Campbell DC, Banner R, Crone LA, Gore-Hickman W, Yip RW. Addition of epinephrine to intrathecal bupivacaine and sufentanil for ambulatory labor analgesia. *Anesthesiology* 1997;86:525–531.
34. Camann WR, Denney RA, Holby ED, Datta S. A comparison of intrathecal, epidural, and intravenous sufentanil for labor analgesia. *Anesth Analg* 1992;77:884–887.
35. Stacey RGW, Watt S, Kadim MY, Morgan BM. Single space combined spinal-extradural technique for analgesia in labour. 1993;71:499–502.

36. Camann WR, Minzter BH, Denney RA, Datta S. Intrathecal sufentanil for labor analgesia: Effects of added epinephrine. *Anesthesiology* 1993;78:870–874.

37. Grieco WM, Norris MC, Leighton BL, et al. Intrathecal sufentanil labor analgesia: The effects of adding morphine or epinephrine. *Anesth Analg* 1993;77:1149–1154.

38. Collis RE, Baxandall ML, Srikantharajah ID, Edge G, Kadim MY, Morgan BM. Combined spinal epidural analgesia with ability to walk throughout labour. *Lancet* 1993;341:767–768.

39. Buggy D, Hughes N, Gardiner J. Posterior column sensory impairment during ambulatory extradural analgesia in labour. *Br J Anaesth* 1994;73:540–542.

40. D'Angelo R, Anderson M, Philip J, Eisenach J. Intrathecal sufentanil compared to epidural bupivacaine for labor analgesia. *Anesthesiology* 1994;80:1209–1215.

41. Collis RE, Davies DWL, Aveling W. Randomised comparison of combined spinal-epidural and standard epidural analgesia in labour. *Lancet* 1995;345:1413–1416.

42. Fernando R, Prior C. Posterior column sensory impairment during ambulatory extradural analgesia in labour. *Br J Anaesth* 1995;74:349–350.

43. Plaat F, Alsaud S, Crowhurst JA, Singh R. Selective sensory blockade with low-dose combined spinal/epidural (CSE) allows safe ambulation in labour. A pilot study. *Int J Obstet Anesth* 1996;5: 220.

44. Parry M, Bawa G, Poulton B, Fernando R. Comparison of dorsal column functions in parturients receiving epidural and combined spinal epidural (CSE) for labour and elective caesarean section. *Int J Obstet Anesth* 1996;5:213.

45. Herman NL, Choi KC, Affleck PJ, et al. Analgesia, pruritus, and ventilation exhibit a dose-response relationship in parturients receiving intrathecal fentanyl during labor. *Anesth Analg* 1999;89:378–383.

46. Shnider SM, Abboud TK, Artal R, et al. Maternal catecholamines decrease during labor after lumber epidural anesthesia. *Am J Obstet Gynecol* 1983;147:13–15.

47. Clarke VT, Smiley RM, Finster M. Uterine hyperactivity after intrathecal injection of fentanyl for analgesia during labor: A cause of fetal bradycardia [letter]? *Anesthesiology* 1994;81:1083.

48. Nielsen PE, Erickson JR, Abouleish EL, et al. Fetal heart rate changes after intrathecal sufentanil or epidural bupivacaine for labor analgesia: Incidence and clinical significance. *Anesth Analg* 1996;83:742–746.

49. Palmer CM, Maciulla JC, Cork RC, et al. The incidence of fetal heart rate changes after intrathecal fentanyl labor analgesia. *Anesth Analg* 1999;88:577–581.

50. Eberle RL, Norris MC, Eberle AM, et al. The effect of maternal position on fetal heart rate during epidural or intrathecal labor analgesia. *Am J Obstet Gynecol* 1998;149:150–155.

51. Albright GA, Forster RM. Does combined spinal-epidural analgesia with subarachnoid sufentanil increase the incidence of emergency cesarean delivery? *Reg Anesth* 1997;22:400–405.

52. Kahn L, Hunter E. Combined spinal epidural (CSE) analgesia, fetal bradycardia and uterine hypertonus [letter]. *Reg Anesth Pain Med* 1998;23:111–112.

53. Riley ET, Vogel TM, El-Sayed Y, et al. Patient selection bias contributes to an increased incidence of fetal bradycardia after combined spinal/epidural analgesia for labor [abstract]. *Anesthesiology* 1999;91:A1054.

54. Gambling DR, Sharma SK, Ramin SM, et al. Study of combined spinal-epidural analgesia versus intravenous meperidine during labor. *Anesthesiology* 1998;90:1336–1344.

55. Albright GA, Forster RM. The safety and efficacy of combined spinal and epidural analgesia/anesthesia (6,002 blocks) in a community hospital. *Reg Anesth Pain Med* 1999;24:117–125.

56. Cascio M, Pygon B, Bernett C, Ramanathan S. Labour analgesia with intrathecal fentanyl decreases maternal stress. *Can J Anaesth* 1997;44:605–609.

57. Segal S, Csavoy AN, Datta S. The tocolytic effect of catecholamines in the gravid rat uterus. *Anesth Analg* 1998;87:864–869.

57a. Norris MC. Intrathecal opioids and fetal brady cardia: is there a link? *Int J Obstet Aneg* 2000;9:264–269.

58. Mercier FJ, Dounos M, Bouaziz H, et al. Intravenous nitroglycerine to relieve intrapartum fetal distress related to uterine hyperactivity: A prospective observational study. *Anesth Analg* 1997;84:1117–1128.

59. Hughes S. Respiratory depression following intraspinal narcotics: Expect it! *Int J Obstet Anesth* 1997;6:145–146.

60. Palmer CM. Early respiratory depression following intrathecal fentanyl-morphine combination. *Anesthesiology* 1991;74:1153–1155.

61. Hays RL, Palmer CM. Respiratory depression after intrathecal sufentanil during labor. *Anesthesiology* 1994;81:511–512.

62. Baker MN, Sarna MC. Respiratory arrest after a second dose of intrathecal sufentanil. *Anesthesiology* 1995;83:231–232.

63. Greenhalgh CA. Respiratory arrest in a parturient following intrathecal injection of sufentanil and bupivacaine. *Anaesthesia* 1996;51:173–175.

64. Jaffee JB, Drease GE, Kelly T, Newman LM. Severe respiratory depression in the obstetric patient after intrathecal meperidine or sufentanil. *Int J Obstet Anesth* 1997;6:182–184.

65. Ferouz F, Norris MC, Leighton BL. Respiratory arrest after intrathecal sufentanil. *Anesth Analg* 1997;85:1088–1090.

66. Norris MC, Fogel ST, Holtman B. Intrathecal sufentanil (5 vs. 10 μg) for labor analgesia: Efficacy and side effects. *Reg Anesth Pain Med* 1998;23:252–257.

67. Hamilton CL, Cohen SE. High sensory block after intrathecal sufentanil for labor analgesia. *Anesthesiology* 1995;83:1118–1121.

68. Currier DS, Levin DR, Campbell C. Dysphagia with intrathecal fentanyl. *Anesthesiology* 1997;87:1570–1571.

69. Harding SA, Collis RE, Morgan BM. Meningitis after combined spinal-extradural anaesthesia in obstetrics. *Br J Anaesth* 1994;73:544–547.

70. Cascio M, Heath G. Meningitis following a combined spinal-epidural technique in a laboring term parturient. *Can J Anaesth* 1996;43:399–402.

71. Schroter J, Wa Djamba D, Hoffmann V, Bach A, Motsch J. Epidural abscess after combined spinal epidural block. *Can J Anaesth* 1997;44:300–304.

72. Brownridge P. Spinal anaesthesia in obstetrics [letter]. *Br J Anaesth* 1991;67:663.

73. Holmström B, Rawal N, Axelsson K, Nydahl P-A. Risk of catheter migration during combined spinal epidural block-percutaneous epiduroscopy study. *Anesth Analg* 1995;80:747–753.

74. Bernard ST, Carrie LES. Epidural versus combined spinal epidural block for cesarean section. *Acta Anaesthesiol Scand* 1988;32:595–596.

75. Bernards CM, Kopacz DJ, Michel MZ. Effect of needle puncture on morphine and lidocaine flux through the spinal meninges of the monkey in vitro. Implications for combined spinal-epidural anesthesia. *Anesthesiology* 1994;80:853–858.

76. Leighton BL, Arkoosh VA, Huffnagle S, et al. The dermatomal spread of epidural bupivacaine with and without prior intrathecal sufentanil. *Anesth Analg* 1996;83:526–529.

77. Bloom SL, McIntire DD, Kelly MA, et al. Lack of effect of walking on labor and delivery. *N Engl J Med* 1998;339:76–79.

78. Nageotte MP, Larson D, Rumney PJ, et al. Epidural analgesia as compared with combined spinal epidural analgesia during labor in nulliparous women. *N Engl J Med* 1997;337:1715–1719.

79. Douglas MJ. Walking epidural analgesia in labor. *Can J Anaesth* 1998;45:607–611.

80. Parry MG, Fernando R, Bawa GPS, Poulton BB. Dorsal column function after epidural and spinal blockade: Implications for the safety of walking following low dose regional analgesia for labour. *Anaesthesia* 1998;53:382–387.

81. Pickering AE, Parry MG, Ousta B, Fernando R. Effect of combined epidural ambulatory labor analgesia on balance. *Anesthesiology* 1999;91:436–441.

82. Davies J, Fernando R, Verma S, et al. Postural stability following regional analgesia for labor. Annual meeting of the obstetric Anesthetists Association, May 2001: Edinburgh, Scotland.

83. Cohen SE, Yeh JY, Riley ET, Vogel TM. Walking with labor epidural analgesia: The impact of bupivacaine concentration and a lidocaine-epinephrine test dose. *Anesthesiology* 2000;92:387–392.

84. Dailey PA, Brookshire GL, Shnider SM, et al. Naloxone decreases side effects after intrathecal morphine for labor. *Anesth Analg* 1984;64:658–666.

85. Baraka A, Maktabi M, Noueihid R. Epidural meperidine-bupivacaine for obstetric anesthesia. *Anesth Analg* 1982;61:652–656.

86. Cohen SE, Tan S, Albright GA, Halpern J. Epidural fentanyl/bupivacaine mixtures for obstetric analgesia. *Anesthesiology* 1987;67:403–407.

87. Bicknell RJ, Leng G, Russell JA, Dyer RG , Mansfield S, Zhao BG. Hypothalamic opioid mechanisms controlling oxytocin neurones during parturition. *Brain Res Bull* 1988;20:743–749.

88. Sivalingam T, Pleuvry BJ. Actions of morphine pethidine and pentazocine on the oestrus and pregnant rat uterus in vitro. *Br J Anaesth* 1985;57:430–433.

89. Collis RE, Harding SA, Morgan BM. Effect of maternal ambulation on labour with low-dose combined spinal-epidural analgesia. *Anaesthesia* 1999;54:535–539.

90. Tsen LC, Thue B, Datta S, Segal S. Is combined spinal-epidural analgesia associated with more rapid cervical dilation in nulliparous patients when compared with conventional epidural analgesia? *Anesthesiology* 1999;91:920–925.

91. Behar M, Magora F, Olshwang D, Davidson JT. Epidural morphine in treatment of pain. *Lancet* 1979;1:527–528.

92. Booker PD, Wilkes RG, Bryson TH, Beddard J. Obstetric pain relief using epidural morphine. *Anaesthesia* 1980;35:377–379.

93. Husemeyer RP, O'Connor MC, Davenport HT. Failure of epidural morphine to relieve pain in labour. *Anaesthesia* 1980;35:161–163.

94. Writer WDR, James FM III, Wheeler AS. Double-blind comparison of morphine and bupivacaine for continuous epidural analgesia in labor. *Anesthesiology* 1981;54:215–219.

95. Magora F, Olshwang D, Eimerl D, et al. Observations on extradural morphine analgesia in various pain conditions. *Br J Anaesth* 1980;52:247–252.

96. Crawford JS. Forum: Experiences with epidural morphine in obstetrics. *Anaesthesia* 1981;36:207–209.

97. Perriss BW. Epidural opiates in labour. *Lancet* 1979;2:422.

98. Perriss BW. Epidural pethidine in labour. *Anaesthesia* 1980;35:380–382.

99. Hughes SC, Rosen MA, Shnider SM, et al. Maternal and neonatal effects of epidural morphine for labor and delivery. *Anesth Analg* 1984;63:319–324.

100. Von Hartung H-J, Wiest W, Klose R, Bauknect H, Hettenbach A. Epidurale morphin-injektion zur schmerzbekampfung in der geburtshilfe. *Fortschr Med* 1980;98:500.

101. Dick W, Traub E, Moller RM. Epidural morphine in obstetric anesthesia. *Obstet Anesth Digest* 1982;2:29–31.

102. Carrie LES, O'Sullivan GM, Seegobin R. Epidural fentanyl in labour. *Anaesthesia* 1981;36:965–969.

103. Steinberg RB, Powell G, Hu X, Dunn SM. Epidural sufentanil for analgesia for labor and delivery. *Reg Anesth* 1989;14:225–228.

104. Heytens L, Cammu H, Camu F. Extradural analgesia during labour using alfentanil. *Br J Anaesth* 1987;59:331–337.

105. Huckaby T, Gerard K, Scheidlinger J, Johnson MD, Datta S. Continuous epidural infusion of alfentanil-bupivacaine for labor and delivery [abstract]. *Anesthesiology* 1989;71:A846.

106. Ahn NN, Karambelkar D, Cannelli G, Rudy TE. Epidural alfentanil and bupivacaine analgesia during labor [abstract]. *Anesthesiology* 1989;71:A845.

107. Justins DM, Francis D, Houlton PG, Reynolds F. A controlled trial of extradural fentanyl in labor. *Br J Anaesth* 1982;54:409–414.

108. Justins DM, Knott C, Luthman J, Reynolds F. Epidural versus intramuscular fentanyl analgesia and pharmacokinetics in labour. *Anaesthesia* 1983;38:937–942.

109. Vella LM, Willats DG, Knott C, et al. Epidural fentanyl in labour. *Anaesthesia* 1985;40:741–747.

110. Deprats R, Mandry J, Grandjean H, et al. Analgesie peridurale au cours du travail. Étude comparative de l'association fentanyl-marcaïne et de la marcaïne seule. *J Gynecol Obstet Biol Reprod* (Paris) 1983;12:901–905.

111. Chestnut DH, Owen CL, Bates JN, et al. Continuous infusion epidural analgesia during labor: A randomized, double-blind comparison of 0.0625% bupivacaine/0.0002% fentanyl versus 0.125% bupivacaine. *Anesthesiology* 1988;68:754–759.

112. Chestnut DH, Laszewski LJ, Pollack KL, et al. Continuous epidural infusion of 0.0625% bupivacaine-0.0002% fentanyl during the second stage of labor. *Anesthesiology* 1990;72:613–618.

113. Naulty JS, Smith R, Ross R. Effect of changes in labor analgesia practice on labor outcome [abstract]. *Anesthesiology* 1989;69:A660.

114. Lyons G, Columb M, Hawthorne L, Dresner M. Extradural pain relief in labour: Bupivacaine sparing by extradural fentanyl is dose dependent. *Br J Anaesth* 1997;78:493–496.

115. Polteg LS, Columb MO, Wagner DS, Nauchton NN. Dose-dependent reaction in minimum local analgesic concentration of bupivacaine by sufentanil for epidural analgesia in labor. *Anesthesiology* 1998;89:626–632.

116. Vertommen JD, Vandermeulen E, Van Aken H, et al. The effects of the addition of sufentanil to 0.125% bupivacaine on the quality of analgesia during labor and on the incidence of instrumental deliveries. *Anesthesiology* 1991;74:809–814.

117. Phillips G. Epidural sufentanil/bupivacaine combinations for analgesia during labor: Effect of varying sufentanil doses. *Anesthesiology* 1987;67:835–838.

118. Donadoni R, Rolly G, Noorden H, Vanden Bussche G. Epidural sufentanil for postoperative pain relief. *Anaesthesia* 1985;40:634–638.

119. Niemegeers CJ, Schellenkens KHL, Van Bever WFM, Janssen PAJ. Sufentanil, a very potent and extremely safe intravenous morphine-like compound in mice, rats, and dogs. *Arzneimittelforschung* 1976;26:1551–1556.

120. Leysen JE, Gommeren W, Niemegeers CJE. (3H) sufentanil, a superior ligand for m-opiate receptors: Binding properties and regional distribution in rat brain and spinal cord. *Eur J Pharmacol* 1983;87:209–255.

121. Phillips G. Combined epidural sufentanil and bupivacaine for labor analgesia. *Reg Anesth* 1987;12:165–168.

122. Naulty JS, Ross R, Bergen W. Epidural sufentanil-bupivacaine for analgesia during labor and delivery [abstract]. *Anesthesiology* 1989;71:A842.

123. Phillips G. Continuous infusion epidural analgesia in labor: The effect of adding sufentanil to 0.125% bupivacaine. *Anesth Analg* 1988;67:462–465.

124. Van Steenberge A, Debroux HC, Noorduin H. Extradural bupivacaine with sufentanil for vaginal delivery. *Br J Anaesth* 1987;59:1518–1522.

125. Cohen S, Amar D, Pantuck CB, et al. Epidural analgesia for labour and delivery: Fentanyl or sufentanil. *Can J Anaesth* 1996;43:341–346.

126. Russell R, Reynolds F. Epidural infusions for nulliparous women in labour: A randomised double-blind comparison of fentanyl-bupivacaine and sufentanil/bupivacaine. *Anaesthesia* 1993;48:856–861.

127. Russell R, Reynolds F. Epidural infusion of low-dose bupivacaine and opioid in labour: Does reducing motor block increase the spontaneous delivery rate? *Anaesthesia* 1996;51:266–273.

128. Loftus JR, Hill H, Cohen SE. Placental transfer and neonatal effects of epidural sufentanil and fentanyl administered with bupivacaine during labor. *Anesthesiology* 1995;83:300–308.

129. Bader AM, Fragneto R, Terui K. Maternal and neonatal fentanyl and bupivacaine concentrations after epidural infusion during labor. *Anesth Analg* 1995;81:829–832.

130. Elliott RD. Continuous infusion epidural analgesia for obstetrics: Bupivacaine versus bupivacaine-fentanyl mixture. *Can J Anaesth* 1991;38:303–310.

131. Porter J, Bonello E, Reynolds F. Effects of epidural fentanyl on neonatal respiration. *Anesthesiology* 1998;89:79–85.

132. Fernando E, Shevde K, Eddi D. A comparative study of epidural alfentanil and fentanyl for labor pain relief [abstract]. *Anesthesiology* 1989;71:A846.

133. Carp H, Johnson MD, Datta S, Ostheimer GW. Continuous epidural infusion of alfentanil and bupivacaine for labor and delivery [abstract]. *Anesthesiology* 1988;69:A687.

134. Abboud TK, Reyes A, Steffens Z, et al. Bupivacaine/butorphanol/epinephrine for epidural anesthesia in obstetrics: Maternal and neonatal effects. *Reg Anesth* 1989;14:219–224.

135. Hunt CO, Naulty JS, Malinow AM, Datta S, Ostheimer GW. Epidural butorphanol-bupivacaine for analgesia during labor and delivery. *Anesth Analg* 1989;68:323–327.

136. Rodriguez J, Abboud TK, Reyes A, et al. Continuous infusion epidural analgesia during labor: A randomized, double-blind comparison of 0.0625 bupivacaine/0.002% butorphanol versus 0.125% bupivacaine [abstract]. *Anesthesiology* 1989;71:A840.

137. Hatjis CG, Meis PJ. Sinusoidal fetal heart rate pattern associated with butorphanol administration. *Obstet Gynecol* 1986;67:377–380.

138. Jaffe RA, Rowe MA. A comparison of the local anesthetic effects of meperidine, fentanyl, and sufentanil on dorsal root axons. *Anesth Analg* 1996;83:776–781.

139. Handley G, Perkins G. The addition of pethidine to epidural bupivacaine in labour: Effect of changing bupivacaine strength. *Anaesth Intensive Care* 1992;20:151–155.

140. Brownridge P, Plummer J, Mitchell J, Marshall P. An evaluation of epidural bupivacaine with and without meperidine in labor. *Reg Anesth* 1992;17:15–21.

141. Brownridge P. Shivering related to epidural blockade with bupivacaine in labour, and the influence of epidural pethidine. *Anaesth Intensive Care* 1986;14:412–417.

142. Niv D, Rudick V, Golan A, Chayen MS. Augmentation of bupivacaine analgesia in labor by epidural morphine. *Obstet Gynecol* 1986;67:206–209.

143. Sia AT, Chong JL. Epidural 0.2% ropivacaine for labour analgesia: Parturient-controlled or continuous infusion? *Anaesth Intensive Care* 1999;27:154–158.

144. Tan S, Reid J, Thorburn J. Extradural analgesia in labour: Complications of three techniques of administration. *Br J Anaesth* 1994;73:619–623.

145. Viscomi C, Eisenach JC. Patient-controlled epidural analgesia during labor. *Obstet Gynecol* 1991;77:348–351.

146. Purdie J, Reid J, Thorburn J, Ashbury AJ. Continuous extradural analgesia: Comparison of midwife top-ups, continuous infusions and patient controlled administration. *Br J Anaesth* 1992;68:580–584.

147. Ferrante FM, Rosinia FA, Gordon C, Datta S. The role of continuous background infusions in patient-controlled epidural analgesia for labor and delivery. *Anesth Analg* 1994;79:80–84.

148. Collis RE, Plaat FS, Morgan BM. Comparison of midwife top-ups, continuous infusion and patient-controlled epidural analgesia for maintaining mobility after a low-dose combined spinal-epidural. *Br J Anaesth* 1999;82:233–236.

149. Lysak SZ, Eisenach JC, Dobson II CE. Patient-controlled epidural analgesia during labor: A comparison of three solutions with a continuous infusion control. *Anesthesiology* 1990;72:44–49.

150. Ferrante FM, Lu L, Jamison SB, Datta S. Patient-controlled epidural analgesia: Demand dosing. *Anesth Analg* 1991;73:547–552.

151. Paech MJ, Pavy TJG, Sims C, et al. Clinical experience with patient-controlled and staff-administered intermittent bolus epidural analgesia in labour. *Anaesth Intensive Care* 1995;23:459–463.

152. Gambling DR, McMorland GH, Yu P, Laszlo C. Comparison of patient-controlled epidural analgesia and conventional intermittent "top-up" injections during labor. *Anesth Analg* 1990;70:256–261.

153. Vandermeulen EP, Van Aken H, Vertommen JD. Labor pain relief using bupivacaine and sufentanil: Patient controlled epidural analgesia versus intermittent injections. *Eur J Obstet Gynecol Reprod Biol* 1995;59(suppl):S47–S54.

154. Curry PD, Pacsoo C, Heap DG. Patient-controlled epidural analgesia in obstetric anaesthetic practice. *Pain* 1994;57:125–128.

155. Gambling DR, Huber CJ, Berkowitz J, et al. Patient-controlled epidural analgesia in labour: Varying bolus dose and lockout interval. *Can J Anaesth* 1993;40:211–217.

156. Paech MJ. Patient-controlled epidural analgesia in labour—is a continuous infusion of benefit? *Anaesth Intensive Care* 1992;20:15–20.

156a. Ferrante FM, Barber MJ, Segal M, Hughes NJ, Datta S. 0.0625% Bupivacaine with 0.0002% fentanyl via patient-controlled epidural analgesia for pain of labor and delivery. *Clin J Pain* 1995;11:121–126.

157. Owen MD, D'Angelo R, Gerancher JC, et al. 0.125% Ropivacaine is similar to 0.125% bupivacaine for labor analgesia using patient-controlled epidural infusion. *Anesth Analg* 1998;86:527–531.

158. Paech MJ, Pavy TJG, Orlikowski CEP, Evans SF. Patient-controlled epidural analgesia in labor: The addition of clonidine to bupivacaine-fentanyl. *Reg Anesth Pain Med* 2000;25:34–40.

158a. Huckaby T, Skerman JH, Hurley RJ, Lambert DH. Sensory analgesia for vaginal deliveries. A preliminary report of continuous spinal anesthesia with a 32-gauge catheter. *Reg Anesth* 1991;16:150–153.

159. Honet JE, Arkoosh VA, Norris MC, et al. Comparison among intrathecal fentanyl, meperidine, and sufentanil for labor analgesia. *Anesth Analg* 1992;75:734–736.

160. Drasner K, Rigler ML. Repeat injection after a "failed spinal": At times, a potentially unsafe practice [letter]. *Anesthesiology* 1991;75:713–714.

161. Drasner K, Rigler ML, Sessler DI, Stoller ML. Cauda equina syndrome following intended epidural anesthesia. *Anesthesiology* 1992;77:582–585.

162. Rigler ML, Drasner KD. Distribution of catheter injected local anesthetic in a model of the subarachnoid space. *Anesthesiology* 1991;75:684–692.

163. Ross BK, Coda B, Heath CH. Local anesthetic distribution in a spinal model: A possible mechanism of neurologic injury after continuous spinal anesthesia. *Reg Anesth* 1992;17:69–77.

164. Department of Health and Human Services. Food and Drug Administration Safety Alert: Cauda equina syndrome associated with use of small-bore catheters in continuous spinal anesthesia. May 29, 1992.

165. Arkoosh VA, Palmer CM, Van Maren GA, et al. Continuous intrathecal labor analgesia: Safety and efficacy [abstract]. *Anesthesiology* 1998;89:A1041.

166. Preston PG, Rosen MA, Hughes SC, et al. Epidural anesthesia with fentanyl and lidocaine for cesarean section: Maternal effects and neonatal outcome. *Anesthesiology* 1988;68:938–943.

167. Breen TW, Janzen JA. Epidural fentanyl and cesarean section: When should fentanyl be given? *Can J Anaesth* 1992;39:317–322.

168. Ready LB, Oden R, Chadwick HS, et al. Development of an anesthesiology-based postoperative pain management service. *Anesthesiology* 1988;68:100–106.

169. Wolfe MJ, Nicholas ADG. Selective epidural analgesia. *Lancet* 1979;1:150–151.

170. Ellis DJ, Millar WI, Reisner LS. A randomized double-blind comparison of epidural versus intravenous fentanyl infusion for analgesia after cesarean section. *Anesthesiology* 1990;72:981–986.

171. Loper KA, Ready LB, Downey M, et al. Epidural and intravenous fentanyl infusions are clinically equivalent after knee surgery. *Anesth Analg* 1990;70:72–75.

172. Ummenhofer WC, Arends RH, Shen DD, Bernards CM. Comparative spinal distribution and clearance kinetics of intrathecally administered morphine, fentanyl, alfentanil, and sufentanil. *Anesthesiology* 2000;92:739–753.

173. Shafer SL, Eisenach J. Location, location, location [editorial]. *Anesthesiology* 2000;92:641–643.

174. Bromage PR, Camporesi E, Chestnut D. Epidural narcotics for postoperative analgesia. *Anesth Analg* 1980;59:473–480.

175. Chayen MS, Rudick V, Borvine A. Pain control with epidural injection of morphine. *Anesthesiology* 1980;53:338–339.

176. Rawal N, Sjöstrand U, Dahlström B. Postoperative pain relief by epidural morphine. *Anesth Analg* 1981;60:726–731.

177. Yu CM, Youngstrom PC, Cowan RI, Set S. Post-cesarean epidural morphine: Double-blind study [abstract]. *Anesthesiology* 1980;53:A216.

178. Rosen MA, Hughes SC, Shnider SM, et al. Epidural morphine for pain relief of postoperative pain after cesarean delivery. *Anesth Analg* 1983;62:666–672.

179. Naulty JS, Datta S, Ostheimer GW, Johnson MD, Burger G. Epidural fentanyl for postcesarean delivery pain management. *Anesthesiology* 1985;63:694–698.

180. Fuller JG, McMorland GH, Douglas MJ, Palmer L. Epidural morphine for analgesia after cesarean section: A report of 4880 patients. *Can J Anaesth* 1990;37:636–640.

181. King MJ, Bowden MI, Cooper GM. Epidural fentanyl and 0.5% bupivacaine for elective cesarean section. *Anaesthesia* 1990;45:285–288.

182. Malinow AM, Mokriski BLK, Wakefield ML, et al. Choice of local anesthetic affects post-cesarean epidural fentanyl analgesia. *Reg Anesth* 1988;13:141–145.

183. Mahesh KT, Heavner JE. Post cesarean section analgesia requests are independent of when epidural fentanyl is given. *Anesth Analg* 1990;70:S255.

184. Sevarino FB, McFarlane C, Sinatra RS. Epidural fentanyl does not influence intravenous PCA requirements in the post-caesarean patient. *Can J Anaesth* 1991;38:450–453.

185. Milon D, Bentue-Ferrer D, Noury D, et al. Anésthesie péridurale pour césarienne par association bupivacaïne-fentanyl. *Ann Fr Anesth Reanim* 1983;2:273–279.

186. Gaffud MP, Bansal P, Lawton C, Velasquez N, Watson WA. Surgical analgesia for cesarean delivery with epidural bupivacaine and fentanyl. *Anesthesiology* 1986;65:331–334.

187. Birnbach DJ, Johnson MD, Arcario T, et al. Effect of diluent volume on analgesia produced by epidural fentanyl. *Anesth Analg* 1989;68:808–810.

188. Cohen S, Lowenwirt I, Pantuck C, et al. Bupivacaine 0.01% and/or epinephrine 0.5 μg/mL improves epidural fentanyl analgesia after cesarean section. *Anesthesiology* 1998;89:1354–1361.

189. Naulty JS, Parmet J, Pate A, et al. Epidural sufentanil and morphine for post-cesarean delivery analgesia [abstract]. *Anesthesiology* 1990;73:A965.

190. Sinatra RS, Savarino FB, Chung JH, et al. Comparison of epidurally administered sufentanil, morphine, and sufentanil-morphine combination for postoperative analgesia. *Anesth Analg* 1991;72:522–527.

191. Rosen MA, Dailey PA, Hughes SC, et al. Epidural sufentanil for postoperative analgesia after cesarean section. *Anesthesiology* 1988;68:448–454.

192. Cohen SE, Tan S, White PF. Sufentanil analgesia following cesarean section: Epidural vs. intravenous administration. *Anesthesiology* 1988;68:129–134.

193. Whiting WC, Sandler AN, Lau LC, et al. Analgesic and respiratory effects of epidural sufentanil in patients following thoracotomy. *Anesthesiology* 1988;69:36–43.

194. Vertommen JD, Van Aken H, Vandermeulen E, et al. Maternal and neonatal effects of adding epidural sufentanil to 0.5% bupivacaine for cesarean delivery. *J Clin Anesth* 1991;3:371–376.

195. Johnson MD, Sevarino FB, Lema MJ. Cessation of shivering and hypothermia associated with epidural sufentanil. *Anesth Analg* 1989;68:70–71.

196. Sevarino FB, Johnson MD, Lema MJ, Datta S, Ostheimer GW, Naulty JS. The effect of epidural sufentanil on shivering and body temperature in the parturient. *Anesth Analg* 1989;68:530–533.

197. Rosen MA, Hughes SC, Shnider SM, et al. Continuous epidural sufentanil for postoperative analgesia. *Anesth Analg* 1990;70:S331.

198. Glynn CJ, Mather LE, Cousins MJ, Graham JR, Wilson PR. Peridural meperidine in humans: Analgetic response, pharmacokinetics and transmission into CSF. *Anesthesiology* 1981;55:520–526.

199. Brownridge P, Frewin DB. A comparison study of techniques of postoperative analgesia caesarean section and lower abdominal surgery. *Anaesth Intensive Care* 1985;13:123–130.

200. Perriss BW, Latham BV, Wilson IH. Analgesia following extradural and IM pethidine in post-caesarean section patients. *Br J Anaesth* 1990;64:355–357.

201. Sjöström S, Hartvig P, Persson P, Tamsen A. Pharmacokinetics of epidural morphine and meperidine in humans. *Anesthesiology* 1987;67:877–888.

202. Ngan Kee WD, Lam KK, Chen PP, Gin T. Epidural meperidine after cesarean section: A dose-response study. *Anesthesiology* 1996;85:289–294.

203. Ngan Kee WD, Lam KK, Chen PP, Gin T. Epidural meperidine after cesarean section: The effect of diluent volume. *Anesth Analg* 1997;85:380–384.

204. Haynes SR, Davidson I, Allsop JR, Button DA. Comparison of epidural methadone with epidural diamorphine for analgesia following caesarean section. *Acta Anaesthesiol Scand* 1993;37:375–380.

205. Semple AJ, Macrae DJ, Munishankarappa S, Burrow LM, Milne MK, Grant IS. Effect of the addition of adrenaline to extradural diamorphine analgesia after caesarean section. *Br J Anaesth* 1988;60:632–638.

206. Macrae DJ, Munishankarappa S, Burrow LM, Milne MK, Grant IS. Double-blind comparison of the efficacy of extradural diamorphine, extradural phenoperidine and IM diamorphine following caesarean section. *Br J Anaesth* 1987;59:354–359.

207. Palacios QT, Jones MM, Hawkins JL, et al. Postcesarean section analgesia: A comparison of epidural butorphanol and morphine. *Can J Anaesth* 1991;38:24–30.

208. Camann WR, Loferski BL, Fanciullo GJ, et al. Does epidural butorphanol offer any clinical advantage over the intravenous route? *Anesthesiology* 1992;76:216–220.

209. Abboud TK, Moore M, Zhu J, et al. Epidural butorphanol or morphine for the relief of post-cesarean section pain: Ventilatory responses to carbon dioxide. *Anesth Analg* 1987;66:887–893.

210. Chrubasik J, Wüst H, Schulte-Mönting J, Thon K, Zindler M. Relative analgesic potency of epidural fentanyl, alfentanil, and morphine in treatment of postoperative pain. *Anesthesiology* 1988;68:929–933.

211. Penon C, Negre I, Ecoffey CF, et al. Analgesia and ventilatory response to carbon dioxide after intramuscular and epidural alfentanil. *Anesth Analg* 1988;67:313–317.

212. Dann WL, Hutchinson A, Cartwright DP. Maternal and neonatal responses to alfentanil administered before induction of general anaesthesia for caesarean section. *Br J Anaesth* 1987;59:1392–1396.

213. Chestnut DH, Choi WW, Isbell TJ. Epidural hydromorphone for postcesarean analgesia. *Obstet Gynecol* 1986;68:65–69.

214. Dougherty TB, Baysinger CL, Gooding DJ. Epidural hydromorphone for postoperative analgesia after delivery by cesarean section. *Reg Anesth* 1986;11:118–122.

215. Dougherty TB, Baysinger CL, Henenberger JC, Gooding DJ. Epidural hydromorphone with and without epinephrine for postoperative analgesia after cesarean delivery. *Anesth Analg* 1989;68:318–322.

216. Henderson SK, Matthew EB, Cohen H, Avram MJ. Epidural hydromorphone: A double-blind comparison with intramuscular hydromorphone for postcesarean section analgesia. *Anesthesiology* 1987;66:825–830.

217. Wüst HJ, Bromage PR. Delayed respiratory arrest after epidural hydromorphone. *Anaesthesia* 1987;42:404–406.

218. Halpern SH, Arellano R, Preston R, et al. Epidural morphine vs. hydromorphone in post-caesarean section patients. *Can J Anaesth* 1996;43:595–598.

219. Chaplan SR, Duncan SR, Brodsky JB, Brose WG. Morphine and hydromorphone epidural analgesia. A prospective, randomized comparison. *Anesthesiology* 1992;77:1090–1094.

220. Parker RK, Holtmann B, White PF. Patient-controlled epidural analgesia: Interactions between nalbuphine and hydromorphone. *Anesth Analg* 1997;84:757–763.

221. Bilsback P, Rolly G, Tampubolon O. Efficacy of the extradural administration of lofentanil, buprenorphine or saline in the management of postoperative pain: A double-blind study. *Br J Anaesth* 1985;57:943–948.

222. Lanz E, Simko G, Theiss D, Glocke MH. Epidural buprenorphine: A double blind study of postoperative analgesia and side effects. *Anesth Analg* 1984;63:593–598.

223. Jensen FM, Jensen NH, Holk IK, Ravnborg M. Prolonged and biphasic respiratory depression following epidural buprenorphine. *Anaesthesia* 1987;42:470–475.

224. Knape JT. Early respiratory depression resistant to naloxone following epidural buprenorphine. *Anesthesiology* 1986;64:382–384.

225. Simpson KH, Madej TH, Mcdowell JM. Comparison of extradural buprenorphine and extradural morphine after caesarean section. *Br J Anaesth* 1988;60:627–631.

226. Cohen S, Amar D, Pantuck CB. Continuous epidural-PCA postcesarean section: Buprenorphine-bupivacaine 0.03% [abstract]. *Anesthesiology* 1990;73:A975.

227. Camann WR, Hurley RH, Gilbertson LI, et al. Epidural nalbuphine for analgesia following caesarean delivery: Dose response and effect of local anaesthetic choice. *Can J Anaesth* 1991;38:728–732.

228. Hughes SC. Intraspinal narcotics for analgesia after cesarean section. *Curr Opin Anaesth* 1989;2:295–302.

229. Palmer CM, Nogami WM, Von Maren G, et al. Post cesarean epidural morphine: A dose response study. *Anesth Analg* 2000;90:887–891.

230. Rawal N, Nuutinen L, Raj PP, et al. Behavioral and histopathologic effects following intrathecal administration of butorphanol, sufentanil, and nalbuphine in sheep. *Anesthesiology* 1991;75:1025–1034.

231. Eisenach J. Opioid antagonist adjuncts to epidural morphine for postcesarean analgesia: Maternal outcomes [letter]. *Anesth Analg* 1994;79:611.

232. Ravat F, Dorne R, Baechle JP, et al. Epidural ketamine or morphine for postoperative analgesia. *Anesthesiology* 1987;66:819–822.

233. Naji P, Farschtschian M, Wilder-Smith O, Wilder-Smith C. Epidural droperidol and morphine for postoperative pain. *Anesth Analg* 1990;70:583–588.

234. Kawana Y. Epidural ketamine for postoperative pain relief after gynecologic operations: A double-blind study and comparison with epidural morphine. *Anesth Analg* 1988;67:798–802.

235. Van der Auwera D, Verborgh C, Camu F. Epidural ketamine for postoperative analgesia. *Anesth Analg* 1987;66:1340.

236. Brock-Utne JG, Rubin J, Nankowitz RJ. Epidural ketamine for control of postoperative pain [letter]. *Anesth Analg* 1986;65:990.

237. Loper KA, Ready LB, Nessly MN, Wild BS. Epidural morphine provides safe and effective analgesia on hospital wards. *Anesth Analg* 1990;70:S248.

238. Kotelko DM, Dailey PA, Shnider SM, et al. Epidural morphine analgesia after cesarean delivery. *Obstet Gynecol* 1984;63:409–413.

239. Leicht CH, Hughes SC, Dailey PA, Shnider SM, Rosen MA. Epidural morphine sulfate for analgesia after cesarean section: A prospective report of 1000 patients [abstract]. *Anesthesiology* 1986;65:A366.

240. Youngstrom PC, Cowan RI, Suthheimer C, Eastwood DW, Yu JCM. Pain relief and plasma concentrations from epidural and intramuscular morphine in post-cesarean patients. *Anesthesiology* 1982;57:404–409.

241. Coombs DW, Danielson DR, Pageau MG, Rippe E. Epidurally administered morphine for postcesarean analgesia. *Surg Gynecol Obstet* 1982;153:385–388.

242. Carmichael FJ, Rolbin SH, Hew EM. Epidural morphine for analgesia after cesarean section. *Can Anaesth Soc J* 1982;29:359–363.

243. Binsted RJ. Epidural morphine after cesarean section. *Anaesth Intensive Care* 1983;11:130–134.

244. Chadwick HS, Ready LB. Intrathecal and epidural morphine sulfate for postcesarean analgesia: A clinical comparison. *Anesthesiology* 1988;68:925–929.

245. Abouleish E, Rawal N, Fallon K, Hernandez D. Combined intrathecal morphine and bupivacaine for cesarean section. *Anesth Analg* 1988;67:370–374.

246. Abboud TK, Dror A, Mosaad P, et al. Minidose intrathecal morphine for the relief of post-cesarean section pain: Safety, efficacy, and ventilatory responses to carbon dioxide. *Anesth Analg* 1988;67:137–143.

247. Zakowski MI, Ramanathan S, Sharnick, Turndorf H. Uptake and distribution of bupivacaine and morphine after intrathecal administration in parturients: Effects of epinephrine. *Anesth Analg* 1992;74:664–669.

248. Uchiyama A, Ueyama H, Nakano S, et al. Low dose intrathecal morphine and pain relief following caesarean section. *Int J Obstet Anesth* 1994;3:87–91.

249. Sibilla C, Albertazzi R, Zatelli R, et al. Pain relief after caesarean section: Comparison of different techniques of morphine administration. *Int J Obstet Anesth* 1994;3:203–207.

250. Milner AR, Bogod DG, Harwood RJ. Intrathecal administration of morphine for elective Caesarean section. A comparison between 0.1 mg and 0.2 mg. *Anaesthesia* 1996;51:871–873.

251. Hunt CO, Naulty JS, Bader AM, et al. Perioperative analgesia with subarachnoid fentanyl-bupivacaine for cesarean delivery. *Anesthesiology* 1989;71:535–540.

252. Belzarena SD. Clinical effects of intrathecally administered fentanyl in patients undergoing cesarean section. *Anesth Analg* 1992;74:653–657.

253. Dahlgren G, Hulstrand C, Jakobsson J, et al. Intrathecal sufentanil, fentanyl, or placebo added to bupivacaine for cesarean section. *Anesth Analg* 1997;85:1288–1293.

254. Donadoni R, Vermeulen H, Noorduin H, Rolly G. Intrathecal sufentanil as a supplement to subarachnoid anaesthesia with lignocaine. *Br J Anaesth* 1987;59:1523–1527.

255. Courtney MA, Hauch M, Bader AM, et al. Perioperative analgesia with subarachnoid sufentanil administration. *Reg Anesth* 1992;17:274–278.

256. Jacobson L, Chabal D, Brody MC, Ward RJ, Ireton RC. I. Intrathecal methadone and morphine for postoperative analgesia: A comparison of the efficacy, duration and side effects. *Anesthesiology* 1989;70:742–746.

257. Thi TVN, Orliaguet G, Ngu TH, Bonnet P. Spinal anesthesia with meperidine as the sole agent for cesarean delivery. *Reg Anesth* 1994;19:386–389.

258. Graham D, Russell IF. A double-blind assessment of the analgesic sparing effect of intrathecal diamorphine (0.3 mg) with spinal anaesthesia for elective C/S. *Int J Obstet Anesth* 1997;6:224–230.

259. Gerancher JC, Floyd H, Eisenach J. Determination of an effective dose of intrathecal morphine for pain relief after C/S. *Anesthesiology* 1999;88:346–351.

260. Yee I, Carstoniu J, Halpern S, Pittini R. A comparison of two doses of epidural fentanyl during Caesarean section. *Can J Anaesth* 1993;40:722–725.

261. Palmer CM, Voulgaropoulos D, Aves D. Subarachnoid fentanyl augments lidocaine spinal anesthesia for cesarean delivery. *Reg Anesth* 1995;20:389–394.

262. Sibilla C, Albertazzi P, Zatelli R, Mertinello R. Perioperative analgesia for cesarean section: Comparison of intrathecal morphine and fentanyl alone or in combination. *Int J Obstet Anesth* 1997;6:43–48.

263. Olöfsson C, Ekblom A, Sköldefors E, Waglund B, Irestedt L. Anesthetic quality during cesarean section following subarachnoid or epidural administration of bupivacaine with or without fentanyl. *Acta Anaesthesiol Scand* 1997;41:332–338.

264. Kafle SK. Intrathecal meperidine for elective Caesarean section: A comparison with lidocaine. *Can J Anaesth* 1993;40:718–721.

265. Hodgson PS, Weal JM, Pollock JE, Liu SS. The neurotoxicity of drugs given intrathecally (spinal). *Anesth Analg* 1999;88:797–809.

266. Kotelko DM, Thigpen JW, Shnider SM, et al. Postoperative epidural morphine analgesia after various local anesthetics [abstract]. *Anesthesiology* 1983;59:A413.

267. Naulty JS, Hertwig L, Hunt CO, et al. Duration of analgesia of epidural fentanyl following cesarean delivery: Effects of local anesthesia drug selection [abstract]. *Anesthesiology* 1986;65:A180.

268. Hughes SC, Wright RG, Murphy D, et al. The effect of pH adjusting 3% 2-chloroprocaine on the quality of post-cesarean section analgesia with epidural morphine [abstract]. *Anesthesiology* 1988;69:A689.

269. Eisenach JC, Schlairet TJ, Dobson CE, et al. Effect of prior anesthetic solution on morphine analgesia. *Anesth Analg* 1991;73:119–123.

270. Phan CQ, Machernis EA, Lobo WD, Azar I, Lear E. The effect of alkalinization of 2-chloroprocaine on the onset and the quality of epidural morphine analgesia [abstract]. *Anesthesiology* 1989;71:A891.

271. Phan CQ, Machernis EA, Zung N, Azar I, Lear E. The quality of epidural morphine-fentanyl analgesia following epidural anesthesia with 2-chloroprocaine [abstract]. *Anesthesiology* 1989;71:A835.

272. Ackerman WE, Juneja MM. 2-chloroprocaine decreases the duration of analgesia of epidural fentanyl. *Anesth Analg* 1989;68:S2.

273. Durkan WJ, Baker LT, Leicht C. Postoperative epidural morphine analgesia after 3% 2-chloroprocaine (nesacaine-MPF) or lidocaine epidural anesthesia [abstract]. *Anesthesiology* 1989;71:A834.

274. Priddle HD, Andros GJ. Primary spinal anesthetic effects of epinephrine. *Anesth Analg (Curr Res)* 1950;29:156–162.

275. Kuraishi Y, Hirota N, Sato Y, et al. Noradrenergic inhibition of the release of substance P from the primary afferents in the rabbit spinal dorsal horn. *Brain Res* 1985;359:177–182.

276. Fleetwood-Walker SM, Mitchell R, Hope PH, Molony V, Iggo A. An alpha-2 receptor mediates the selective inhibition by noradrenaline of nociceptive responses of identified dorsal horn neurones. *Brain Res* 1985;334:243–254.

277. Eisenach JC, Lysak SZ, Vicsomi CM. Epidural clonidine analgesia following surgery: Phase I. *Anesthesiology* 1989;71:640–646.

278. Kitahata LM. Spinal analgesia with morphine and clonidine. *Anesth Analg* 1989;68:191–193.

279. Eisenach JC, Dekock M, Klinscha W. Alpha$_2$-adrenergic agonists for regional anesthesia: A clinical review of clonidine (1984–1995). *Anesthesiology* 1996;85:655–674.

280. Collins JG, Kitahata LM, Matsumoto M, Homma E, Suzukawa M. Spinally administered epinephrine suppresses noxiously evoked activity of WDR neurons in the dorsal horn of the spinal cord. *Anesthesiology* 1984;60:269–275.

280a. Hashimoto K, Hampl KF, Nakamura Y, Bollen AW, Feiner J, Drasner K. Epinephrine increases the neurotoxicity potential of intrathecally-administered lidocaine in the rat. *Anesthesiology* 2001;94:876–883.

281. Eisenach JC, Dewan DM, Rose JC, Angelo JM. Epidural clonidine produces antinociception, but not hypotension, in sheep. *Anesthesiology* 1987;66:496–501.

282. Eisenach JC, Castro MI, Dewan DM, Rose JC, Grice SC. Intravenous clonidine hydrochloride toxicity in pregnant ewes. *Am J Obstet Gynecol* 1988;160:471–476.

283. Eisenach JC, Castro MI, Dewan DM, Rose JC. Epidural clonidine analgesia in obstetrics. Sheep studies. *Anesthesiology* 1989;70:51–56.

284. Eisenach JC, Rauck RL, Buzzanell C, Lysak SZ. Epidural clonidine analgesia for intractable cancer pain: Phase I. *Anesthesiology* 1989;71:647–652.

285. Leimdorfer A, Metzner WRT. Analgesia and anesthesia induced by epinephrine. *Am J Physiol* 1949;157:116–121.

286. Reddy SVR, Maderdrut JL, Yaksh TL. Spinal cord pharmacology of adrenergic agonist-mediated antinociception. *J Pharmacol Exp Ther* 1980;213:525–533.

287. Yaksh TL, Reddy SVR. Studies in the primate on the analgesic effects associated with intrathecal actions of opiates, a-adrenergic agonists and baclofen. *Anesthesiology* 1981;54:451–467.

288. Post C, Gordh T, Minor B, Archer T, Freedman J. Antinociceptive effects and spinal cord tissue concentrations after intrathecal injection of guanfacine or clonidine into rats. *Anesth Analg* 1987;66:317–324.

289. Huntoon M, Eisenach JC, Boese P. Epidural clonidine after cesarean section: Appropriate dose and effect of prior local anesthetic. *Anesthesiology* 1992;76:187–193.

290. Chung C-J, Kim J-S, Park H-S, et al. The efficacy of intrathecal neostigmine, intrathecal morphine, and their combination for cesarean section analgesia. *Anesth Analg* 1998;87:341–346.

291. D'Angelo R, Evans E, Dean LA, Gaver R, Eisenach JC. Spinal clonidine prolongs labor analgesia from spinal sufentanil and bupivacaine. *Anesth Analg* 1999;88:573–576.

292. Filos K, Goudas LC, Patroni O, et al. Hemodynamic and analgesic profile after intrathecal clonidine: A dose response study. *Anesthesiology* 1994;81:591–601.

293. Benhammou D, Thorin D, Brichant J-F, et al. Intrathecal clonidine and fentanyl with hyperbaric bupivacaine improves analgesia during cesarean section. *Anesth Analg* 1998;87:609–613.

294. D'Angelo R. Should we administer epidural or spinal clonidine during labor [editorial]? *Reg Anesth Pain Med* 2000;25:3–4.

295. Reiz S, Westberg M. Side-effects of epidural morphine. *Lancet* 1980;2:203–204.

296. Bromage PR, Camporesi EM, Durant PA, Nielsen CH. Influence of epinephrine as an adjuvant to epidural morphine. *Anesthesiology* 1983;58:257–262.

297. Boas RA. Hazards of epidural morphine. *Anaesth Intensive Care* 1980;8:377–378.

298. Lu JK, Schafer PG, Gardner TL, et al. The dose-response pharmacology of intrathecal sufentanil in female volunteers. *Anesth Analg* 1997;85:372–379.

299. Christensen V. Respiratory depression after extradural morphine. *Br J Anaesth* 1980;52:841.

300. Davies GK, Tolhurst-Cleaver CL, James TL. CNS depression from intrathecal morphine. *Anesthesiology* 1980;52:280.

301. Glynn CJ, Mather LE, Cousins MJ, Wilson PR, Graham JR. Spinal narcotics and respiratory depression. *Lancet* 1979;2:356–357.

302. Jones RDM, Jones JG. Intrathecal morphine: Naloxone reversed respiratory depression but not analgesia. *Br Med J* 1980;281:645.

303. Liolios A, Anderson FH. Selective spinal analgesia. *Lancet* 1979;2:357.

304. Scott DB, McClure J. Selective epidural analgesia. *Lancet* 1979;1:1410–1411.

305. London SW. Respiratory depression after single epidural injection of local anesthetic and morphine. *Anesth Analg* 1987;66:797–799.

306. Streinstra R, Van Poorten F. Immediate respiratory arrest after caudal epidural sufentanil. *Anesthesiology* 1989;71:993–994.

307. Brockway MS, Noble DW, Sharwood-Smith GH, McClure JH. Profound respiratory depression after extradural fentanyl. *Br J Anaesth* 1990;64:243–245.

308. Krane BD, Kreutz JM, Johnson DL, Mathson JE. Alfentanil and delayed respiratory depression: Case studies and review. *Anesthesiology* 1990;70:557–561.

309. Katsiris S, Williams S, Leighton BL, Halpern S. Respiratory arrest following intrathecal injection of sufentanil and bupivacaine in a parturient. *Can J Anaesth* 1998;45:880–883.

310. Lu J, Manullang T, Staples M, et al. Maternal respiratory arrests, severe hypotension, and fetal distress after administration of intrathecal sufentanil and bupivacaine after intravenous fentanyl. *Anesthesiology* 1997;87:170–172.

311. Atkinson P, Huffnagle H, Arkoosh V, et al. How common is respiratory depression in laboring patients who receive intrathecal sufentanil alone or following IV opioids [abstract]? *Anesthesiology* 1997;87:A828.

312. Roseag OP, Suderman V, Yarnell RW. Early respiratory depression during caesarean section following epidural meperidine. *Can J Anaesth* 1992;39:71–74.

313. Brose WG, Cohen SE. Oxyhemoglobin saturation following cesarean section in patients receiving epidural morphine, PCA, or IM meperidine analgesia. *Anesthesiology* 1989;70:948–953.

314. Gustafsson LL, Schildt B, Jacobsen K. Adverse effects of extradural and intrathecal opiates: Report of a nationwide survey in Sweden. *Br J Anaesth* 1982;54:479–486.

315. Rawal N. Present state of extradural and intrathecal opioid analgesia in Sweden. *Br J Anaesth* 1987;59:791–799.

316. Stenseth R, Sellevold O, Breivik H. Epidural morphine for postoperative pain: Experience with 1085 patients. *Acta Anaesthesiol Scand* 1985;29:148–156.

317. Daley MD, Sandler AN, Turner KE, Vosu H, Slavchenko P. A comparison of epidural and intramuscular morphine in patients following cesarean section. *Anesthesiology* 1990;72:289–294.

318. Wheatly RG, Somerville ID, Sapsford DJ, Jones JG. Postoperative hypoxaemia: Comparison of extradural, IM and patient-controlled opioid analgesia. *Br J Anaesth* 1990;64:267–275.

319. Cohen SE, Labaille LT, Benhamou D, Levron JC. Respiratory effects of epidural sufentanil after cesarean section. *Anesth Analg* 1992;74:677–682.

320. Herman NL, Calicott R, Van Decar TK, et al. Determination of the dose-response relationship for intrathecal sufentanil in laboring patients. *Anesth Analg* 1997;84:1256–1261.

321. Ferouz F, Norris MC, Leighton BL. Risk of respiratory arrest after intrathecal sufentanil. *Anesth Analg* 1997;85:1088–1090.

322. Dahl JB, Jacobson JB. Accidental epidural narcotic overdose. *Anesth Analg* 1990;70:321–322.

323. Kafer ER, Brown JT, Scott D, et al. Biphasic depression of ventilatory responses to CO2 following epidural morphine. *Anesthesiology* 1983;58:418–427.

324. Camporesi EM, Nielsen CH, Bromage PR, Durant PAC. Ventilatory CO2 sensitivity after intravenous and epidural morphine in volunteers. *Anesth Analg* 1983;62:633–640.

325. Davies G, From R. A blinded study using nalbuphine for prevention of pruritus induced by epidural fentanyl. *Anesthesiology* 1988;69:763–765.

326. Morgan PJ, Mehta S, Kapala DM. Nalbuphine pretreatment in cesarean section patients receiving epidural morphine. *Reg Anesth* 1991;16:84–88.

327. Chalmers PC, Lang CM, Greenhouse BB. The use of nalbuphine in association with epidural narcotics. *Anesthesiol Rev* 1988;15:21–27.

328. Cohen SE, Ratner EF, Kreitzman TR, et al. Nalbuphine is better than naloxone for treatment of side effects after epidural morphine. *Anesth Analg* 1992;75:747–752.

329. Borgeat A, Wilder-Smith OH, Saiah M, Rifat K. Subhypnotic doses of propofol relieve pruritus induced by epidural and intrathecal morphine. *Anesthesiology* 1992;76:510–512.

330. Saiah M, Borgeat A, Wilder-Smith OH, Rifat K, Suter PM. Epidural-morphine- induced pruritus: Propofol versus naloxone. *Anesth Analg* 1994;78:1110–1113.

331. Beilin Y, Bernstein HH, Zucker-Pinchott B, et al. Subhypnotic doses of propofol do not relieve pruritus induced by intrathecal morphine after cesarean section. *Anesth Analg* 1998;86:310–313.

332. Cardan E. Herpes simplex after spinal morphine. *Anaesthesia* 1984;39:1031.

333. Gieraerts R, Navalgund A, Vaes L, et al. Increased incidence of itching and herpes simplex in patients given epidural morphine after cesarean section. *Anesth Analg* 1987;66:1321–1324.

334. Crone LA, Conly JM, Clark KM, et al. Recurrent herpes simplex virus labialis and the use of epidural morphine in obstetric patients. *Anesth Analg* 1988;67:318–323.

335. Crone LA, Conly JM, Storgard C, et al. Herpes labialis in parturients receiving epidural morphine following cesarean section. *Anesthesiology* 1990;73:208–213.

336. Ugolini G, Kuypers HG, Simmons A. Retrograde transneuronal transfer of herpes simplex virus type 1 (HSV 1) from motoneurones. *Brain Res* 1987;422:242–256.

337. Ugolini G, Kuypers HG, Strick PL. Transneuronal transfer of herpes virus from peripheral nerves to cortex and brainstem. *Science* 1989;243:89–91.

338. Scott PV, Fischer HBJ. Spinal opiate analgesia and facial pruritus: A neural theory. *Postgrad Med J* 1986;58:531–535.

339. Weddel SJ, Ritter RR. Epidural morphine: Serum levels and pain relief [abstract]. *Anesthesiology* 1980;53:A419.

340. Rawal N, Mollefors K, Axelsson K, Lingardh G, Widman B. An experimental study of urodynamic effects of epidural morphine and of naloxone reversal. *Anesth Analg* 1983;62:641–647.

341. Durant P, Yaksh T. Micturition in the unanesthetized rat: Effects of intrathecal capsaicin, N-vanillylnonanamide, 6-hydoxydopamine and 5,6-dihydroxytryptamine. *Brain Res* 1988;451:301–308.

342. Durant P, Lucas P, Yaksh T. Micturition in the unanesthetized rat: Spinal vs. peripheral pharmacology of the adrenergic system. *J Pharmacol Exp Ther* 1988;245:426–435.

343. Durant P, Yaksh T. Drug effects on urinary bladder tone during spinal morphine-induced inhibition of the micturition reflex in unanesthetized rats. *Anesthesiology* 1988;68:325–334.

344. Dray A. Epidural opiates and urinary retention: New models provide new insights. *Anesthesiology* 1988;68:323–324.

345. Loper KA, Ready LB, Dorman BH. Prophylactic transdermal scopolamine patches reduce nausea in postoperative patients receiving epidural morphine. *Anesth Analg* 1989;68:144–146.

346. Bailey PL, Streisand JB, Pace NL, et al. Transdermal scopolamine reduces nausea and vomiting after outpatient laparoscopy. *Anesthesiology* 1990;72:977–988.

347. Kotelko DM, Rottman RL, Wright WC, et al. Transdermal scopolamine decreases nausea and vomiting following cesarean section in patients receiving epidural morphine. *Anesthesiology* 1989;71:675–678.

348. Ehrenkranz RA, Ackerman BA. Metoclopramide effect on faltering milk production by mothers of premature infants. *Pediatrics* 1986;78:614–620.

349. Rosenblatt WHO, Cioffi AM, Sinatra RS, Silverman DG. Metoclopramide-enhanced analgesia for prostaglandin-induced termination of pregnancy. *Anesth Analg* 1992;75:760–763.

349a. Pan PH, Moore C, Fragneto R, Ross V, Justis G. Efficacy and cost-effectiveness of prophylactic ondansetron versus metoclopramide for cesarean section patients under epidural anesthesia. Abstract presented at: Annual Meeting of the Society for Obstetric Anesthesia and Perinatology; May 2000; Montreal, Canada.

350. Rawal N, Wattwil M. Respiratory depression after epidural morphine: An experimental and clinical study. *Anesth Analg* 1984;63:8–14.

351. Johnson A, Bengtsson M, Soderlind K, Löfstrom JB. Influence of intrathecal morphine and naloxone intervention on postoperative ventilatory regulation in elderly patients. *Acta Anaesthesiol Scand* 1992;36:435–444.

352. Rawal N, Schött U, Dahlström B, et al. Influence of naloxone infusion on analgesia and respiratory depression following epidural morphine. *Anesthesiology* 1986;64:194–201.

353. Young RSK, Hessert TR, Pritchard GA, Yagel SK. Naloxone exacerbates hypoxic-ischemic brain injury in the neonatal rat. *Am J Obstet Gynecol* 1984;50:52–56.

354. Wiener PC, Hogg MIJ, Rosen M. Effects of naloxone on pethidine-induced neonatal depression. *Br Med J* 1977;2:228–231.

355. Hibbard BM, Rosen M, Davies D. Placental transfer of naloxone. *Br J Anaesth* 1986;58:45–48.

356. Flacke JW, Flacke WE, Williams GD. Acute pulmonary edema following naloxone reversal of high-dose morphine anesthesia. *Anesthesiology* 1977;47:376–378.

357. Andree RA. Sudden death following naloxone administration. *Anesth Analg* 1980;59:782–784.

358. Taff RH. Pulmonary edema following naloxone administration. *Anesth Analg* 1983;59:576–577.

359. Prough DS, Raymond R, Baumgarner J, Shannon G. Acute pulmonary edema in healthy teenagers following conservative doses of intravenous naloxone. *Anesthesiology* 1984;60:485–486.

360. Partridge BL, Ward CF. Pulmonary edema following low-dose naloxone administration. *Anesthesiology* 1986;65:709–710.

361. Wride SRN, Smith RER, Courtney PG. A fatal case of pulmonary edema in a healthy young male following naloxone administration. *Anaesth Intensive Care* 1989;17:374–377.

362. Mok MS, Shuai SP, Lee C, Lee TY, Lippmann M. Naltrexone pretreatment attenuates side effects of epidural morphine [abstract]. *Anesthesiology* 1986;65:A200.

363. Abboud TK, Afrasiabi A, Davison J, et al. Prophylactic oral naltrexone with epidural morphine: Effect on adverse reactions and ventilatory responses to carbon dioxide. *Anesthesiology* 1990;72:233–237.

364. Knoieczko KM, Jones JG, Barrowcliffe MP, Jordan C, Altman DG. Antagonism of morphine-induced respiratory depression with nalmefene. *Br J Anaesth* 1988;61:318–323.

365. Morgan PJ, Mehta S. Prophylactic nalbuphine in cesarean section patients treated with epidural morphine. *Anesth Analg* 1989;68:S203.

366. Des Marteau JK, Cassot AL. Acute pulmonary edema resulting from nalbuphine reversal of fentanyl-induced respiratory depression. *Anesthesiology* 1986;65:237.

367. Blaise GA, McMichan JC, Nugent M, Hollier LH. Nalbuphine produces side-effects while reversing narcotic-induced respiratory depression. *Anesth Analg* 1986;65:S19.

368. Penning JP, Samson B, Baxter A. Nalbuphine reversal epidural morphine induced respiratory depression. *Anesth Analg* 1986;65:S119.

369. Sun HL. Naloxone-precipitated acute opioid withdrawal syndrome after epidural morphine. *Anesth Analg* 1998;86:544–545.

370. Yaksh TL, Wilson PR, Kaiko RF, Inturrisi CE. Analgesia produced by a spinal action of morphine and effects upon parturition in the rat. *Anesthesiology* 1982;51:386–392.

371. Steinbrook RA, Carr DB, Datta S, Naulty JS, Lee C, Fisher J. Dissociation of plasma and cerebrospinal fluid beta-endorphin-like immunoactivity levels during pregnancy and parturition. *Anesth Analg* 1982;61:893–897.

372. Golub MS, Eisele JH, Donald JM. Obstetric analgesia and infant outcome in monkeys: Infant development after intrapartum exposure to meperidine or alfentanil. *Am J Obstet Gynecol* 1988;159:1280–1286.

373. Golub MS, Eisele JH, Donald JM. Obstetric analgesia and infant outcome in monkeys: Neonatal measures after intrapartum exposure to meperidine or alfentanil. *Am J Obstet Gynecol* 1988;158:1219–1225.

374. Bailey CR, Ruggier R, Findley IL. Diamorphine-bupivacaine mixture compared with plain bupivacaine for analgesia. *Br J Anaesth* 1994;72:58–61.

375. Fernando R, Bonello E, Gill P, et al. Neonatal welfare and placental transfer of fentanyl and bupivacaine during ambulatory combined spinal epidural analgesia for labour. *Anaesthesia* 1997;52:517–524.

376. Abouleish E, Barmada MA, Nemoto EM, Tung A, Winter P. Acute and chronic effects of intrathecal morphine in monkeys. *Br J Anaesth* 1981;53:1027–1032.

377. Yaksh TL, Rudy TA. Chronic catheterization of the spinal subarachnoid space. *Physiol Behav* 1976;17:1031–1036.

378. Sabbe MB, Grafe MR, Mjanger E, et al. Spinal delivery of sufentanil, alfentanil, and morphine in dogs: Physiologic and toxicologic investigations. *Anesthesiology* 1994;81:899–920.

379. Yaksh TL, Noueihed RY, Durant PA. Studies of the pharmacology and pathology of intrathecally administered 4-anilinopiperidine analogues and morphine in the rat and cat. *Anesthesiology* 1986;64:54–68.

380. Wagemans MF, van der Valk P, Spoelder EM, Zuurmond WW, de Lange JJ. Neuro-histopathological findings after continuous intrathecal administration of morphine or a morphine/bupivacaine mixture in cancer pain patients. *Acta Anaesthesiol Scand* 1997;41:1033–1038.

381. Yaksh T, Collins JG. Studies in animals should precede human use of spinally administered drugs. *Anesthesiology* 1989;70:4–6.

382. Horta H, Ramos L, Concalves Z, et al. The inhibition of epidural morphine-induced pruritus by epidural droperidol. *Anesth Analg* 2000;90:638–641.

383. Carvelho JCA, Mathias RS, Senra WG, et al. Systemic droperidol and epidural morphine in the management of postoperative pain [letter]. *Anesth Analg* 1991;72:416.

384. Sanansilp V, Areewatana S, Tonsukchai N. Droperidol and the side effects of epidural morphine after cesarean section. *Anesth Analg* 1998;86:532–537.

385. Rainov NG, Gutjahr T, Burkert W. Intra-operative epidural morphine, fentanyl, and droperidol for control of pain after spinal surgery: A prospective, randomized, placebo-controlled, and double-blind trial. *Acta Neurochir* 1996;138:33–39.

386. Bach V, Carl P, Ravio O, et al. Potentiation of epidural opioids with epidural droperidol. *Anaesthesia* 1986;41:1116–1119.

387. Tung AS, Tenicela R, Winter PM. Opiate withdrawal syndrome following intrathecal administration of morphine. *Anesthesiology* 1980;53:340.

388. Cohen SE, Rothblatt AJ, Albright GA. Early respiratory depression with epidural narcotic and intravenous droperidol. *Anesthesiology* 1983;59:559–560.

389. Zucker-Pinchoff B, Ramanathan S. Anaphylactic reaction to epidural fentanyl. *Anesthesiology* 1989;71:599–601.

Shnider and Levinson's Anesthesia for Obstetrics,
edited by Samuel C. Hughes, et al.
Lippincott Williams & Wilkins,
Philadelphia, © 2001.

CHAPTER 10

INHALATION ANALGESIA AND ANESTHESIA FOR LABOR AND VAGINAL DELIVERY

STEVE M. YENTIS, M.B., B.Sci, M.D., F.R.C.A. AND SHEILA E.
COHEN, M.B., Ch.B., F.F.A.R.S.

James Simpson, Professor of Midwifery in Edinburgh, Scotland (Fig. 10.1a), is credited with the first use of inhalation analgesia in obstetrics in 1847, when he introduced ether for vaginal delivery (1). Although it met with considerable resistance from church leaders of the time, acceptance of the principle of abolishing pain during childbirth was assured when Queen Victoria was administered chloroform to good effect by Dr. John Snow (Fig. 10.1b) during the birth of her 8th and 9th children in 1853 and 1857. Since then, almost every new inhalation anesthetic agent has at some time been studied for obstetric analgesia for labor. However, few (except nitrous oxide) have been adopted to any great extent.

The first use of nitrous oxide dates from 1881, when Stanislav Klikovich (Fig. 10.1c), a Polish physician working in Russia, studied the effects of premixed 80% nitrous oxide in oxygen on laboring women. He concluded it was safe and effective, and that uterine contractions were unaffected (2). It is interesting that despite his work, administration of the more dangerous nitrous oxide/air mixtures was the technique adopted in the early 1900s. Indeed, although nitrous oxide/oxygen was reintroduced in the 1940s through 1950s, it was not until 1961 that Tunstall described the use of premixed nitrous oxide/oxygen for labor (3).

The current use of inhalation agents during childbirth is difficult to ascertain, since few data are available in the literature. However, those reports that do exist suggest wide variation between countries (Table 10.1); the reasons for this are unclear but are likely related to historical, economical, practical, and cultural differences, and variations in the availability of alternative methods of pain relief. In the United Kingdom, adoption of nitrous oxide/air apparatus by the Central Midwives Board in 1936 led to wide use of this agent, which persists today, although the gas has been presented in its premixed form with oxygen (Entonox®, BOC) since 1963. Nitrous oxide is presently the most widely used inhalation agent during labor and vaginal delivery.

It is important to define the terms inhalation analgesia and inhalation anesthesia. *Inhalation analgesia* refers to the inhalation of subanesthetic concentrations of anesthetic agents to provide pain relief for labor and/or delivery. The mother remains awake with protective laryngeal reflexes intact. It is administered by an anesthesiologist or other qualified persons or by the patient herself, and may be used alone or to supplement other methods of analgesia. *Inhalation anesthesia* refers to the administration of inhalation agents to produce general anesthesia.

INDICATIONS FOR INHALATION ANALGESIA AND ANESTHESIA

Some women choose not to have regional analgesia because of a fear of needles and complications, or they believe they will be unable to participate in the delivery. In such cases the choice of analgesic techniques for the first stage of labor includes psychoprophylactic techniques; use of inhalation agents, opioids, or other systemic drugs; or paracervical block. Although opioids and other systemic drugs are easily administered, they have the potential to cause neonatal respiratory and neurobehavioral depression. The relatively high incidence of fetal bradycardia after inhalational analgesia has led to the infrequent use of this technique. Inhalation techniques are often seen as an acceptable alternative (4, 12), and it is critical that those administering paracervical block are specifically educated in the technique and its potential hazards.

We do not recommend the use of *general anesthesia* for vaginal delivery. It is not recommended unless there is a specific indication. For example, if acute fetal distress occurs during the second stage of labor and operative vaginal delivery is indicated, general anesthesia may rarely be the most satisfactory technique because of the rapidity with which it can be instituted. If regional techniques are contraindicated (see Chapter 8) and inhalation analgesia or low-dose ketamine is inadequate to allow for a safe, controlled delivery, general anesthesia may be necessary (Table 10.2). Probably the most common indication for general anesthesia for vaginal delivery has been the necessity for rapid uterine relaxation (see Chapter 8), although with increased experience with nitroglycerin (glyceryl trinitrate) as an acute uterine relaxant, this indication may no longer hold (13, 14). General anesthesia may not be necessary.

INHALATION ANALGESIA
Principles

Inhalation analgesia is an attractive option since pregnancy causes a reduction in functional residual capacity and an increase in minute ventilation, resulting in more rapid equilibration between inspired and alveolar concentrations of inhaled agents. In addition, the pregnant woman has reduced requirements for anesthetics, making her more susceptible to their effects (15, 16). The features of any inhalation agent that might make it suitable for use during labor are related to the nature of labor pain and the agent's blood-gas solubility, potency, and side effects. Typically, individual contractions increase in intensity over 30 to 40 seconds before reaching their peak and then decrease over another 30 to 40 seconds. Pain is felt about 10 to 20 seconds after the onset of the contraction and lasts about 40 to 60 seconds. Thus, for intermittent administration and in order to be effective for individual contractions, the agent must have a very low blood-gas solubility such that inhalation at the onset of each contraction rapidly results in analgesic blood levels, with a rapid fall in blood levels at the end of each contraction when inhalation of the agent ceases (Figure 10.2a). An agent with high blood-gas solubility will require more time to achieve adequate blood levels (more than one contraction), while blood levels fall more slowly after cessation of inhalation, resulting in residual drug effects between contractions and cumulation

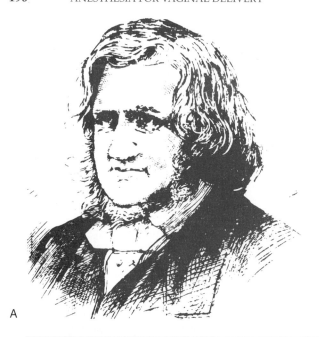

A

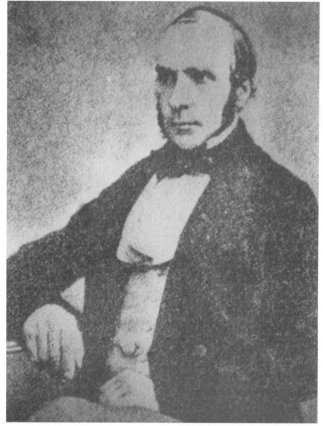

B

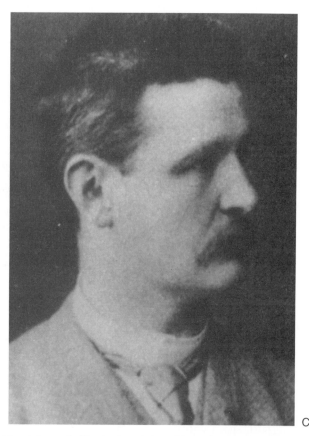

C

Figure 10.1. *A*: James Young Simpson; *B*: John Snow; *C*: Stanislav Klikovich. (*A* and *B*, supplied by the Association of Anaesthetists of Great Britain and Ireland; *C*, reproduced from Richards W, Parbrook GD, Wilson J. Stanislav Klikovich [1853–1910]. Pioneer of nitrous oxide and oxygen analgesia. *Anaesthesia* 1976;31:933–940, with permission [original picture published in Bogdanov AP. *Materials for the history of scientific and applied activities in Russia in the realms of zoology and allied branches of knowledge during the last 35 years, 1850–88.* Moscow: M. Volchaninova; 1892]).

(Figure 10.2b). An alternative approach is to administer the agent *continuously* during labor; once adequate blood levels are attained (depending again on the solubility) analgesia is provided for each contraction, although once again this results in residual effects between contractions.

Whatever its solubility, the agent's potency determines the inspired concentration required to be effective (with consequent important considerations relating to the equipment used to administer it). The agent's side effects also influence whether the agent will be a useful tool in clinical practice (i.e., whether higher concentrations may be safely administered and whether residual effects between contractions are acceptable). Ideally, the agent should have analgesic properties at concentrations well below those required to induce anesthesia, since an

Table 10.1. REPORTED USE OF NITROUS OXIDE

Investigator	Year	Country	Use of Inhalation Agents
Gibbs et al. (4)	1986	United States*	9%
Lind et al. (5)	1986	Norway	42%
Steer (6)	1993	United Kingdom	60%
Kangas-Saarela (7)	1994	Finland	56%
Schneider et al. (8)	1995	Switzerland	<10%
Capogna et al. (9)	1996	United Kingdom†	50%
		Belgium‡	1%
Beke et al. (10)	1997	Hungary	5%
Garcia et al. (11)	1998	United Kingdom	76%

* For delivery only: inhalation analgesia used in 6% of women and general anesthesia in 3%.

† Single hospital only.

‡ Two hospitals only.

Table 10.2. GENERAL ANESTHESIA FOR VAGINAL DELIVERY: A SUGGESTED TECHNIQUE*

1. Administer 30 mL 0.3 M sodium citrate.
2. Start an intravenous infusion.
3. Apply a pulse oximeter, blood pressure cuff, and electrocardiograph.
4. Preoxygenate for 3 min using at least 8 L/min oxygen, ensuring a tight seal with the facemask. If time is limited, taking 3 vital capacity breaths is an acceptable alternative.
5. When delivery is imminent and forceps are about to be applied, administer a "sleep" dose of thiopental and suxamethonium 1.5 mg/kg at the start of the next uterine contraction. A trained assistant should apply cricoid pressure until the trachea has been sealed by the cuff of the tracheal tube.
6. Verify the tracheal tube's position using capnography.
7. Administer 50% nitrous oxide in oxygen with 0.5% isoflurane (up to 3% isoflurane may be used if uterine relaxation is required. Caution and constant monitoring are required since cardiovascular depression may be severe. An alternative to high inspired concentrations of volatile agent is nitroglycerin (glyceryl trinitrate) 100 μg intravenously or 400 μg sublingually, repeated as necessary (13, 14). Sevoflurane 1%, desflurane 3%, or halothane 0.5% are suitable alternatives to isoflurane.
8. Use neuromuscular blockade as required. After delivery, the inspired concentration of agent should be reduced and an opioid given if perineal suturing is required. Administration of an oxytocin infusion may be necessary after delivery if high concentrations of volatile agent have been administered.
9. Extubate the trachea when the patient is fully awake.

* General anesthesia is not recommended except in special circumstances when rapid delivery is required and alternative methods of analgesia (including regional anesthesia) are inadequate or contraindicated. Examples include acute fetal distress during the second stage of labor, intrauterine manipulations requiring uterine relaxation, or an uncontrollable patient whose physical activity represents a danger to herself or the neonate.

accidental overdose may lead to respiratory depression, airway obstruction, or aspiration pneumonitis.

Finally, the effects of an inhalation agent on the fetus and neonate should be considered. First, the amount passing to the fetus is affected by its solubility and means of administration. For example, an insoluble agent breathed intermittently is rapidly expired by the mother with little cumulation into the fetus, whereas fetal transfer is greater whenever blood levels are maintained continuously, e.g., by continuous administration of a soluble agent. For each agent, greater placental transfer is likely with prolonged administration and with the use of higher inspired concentrations. Second, the side effects of the particular agent are important. These may be indirect (on maternal

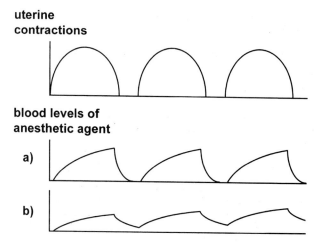

uterine contractions

blood levels of anesthetic agent

a)

b)

Figure 10.2. Schematic diagram of the effect of blood-gas solubility on uptake of an inhalational agent inhaled intermittently during labor. Contractions are shown at the top, blood levels of an insoluble agent are shown in *a*, and those of a soluble agent in *b*. In each case, inspiration begins when contractions become painful and continues until pain recedes. (Redrawn from Moir DD, Thorburn J. *Obstetric Anaesthesia and Analgesia.* 3rd ed. London: Bailliere Tindall; 1986.)

cardiac output and uteroplacental blood flow, maternal respiration, uterine activity, etc.) or direct (on the fetal cardiovascular system, neonatal neurobehavior, etc.). Fetal side effects may thus be apparent before delivery or manifest in the early postpartum period. An interesting early observation was that the parturient offered inhalation analgesia might hyperventilate in an attempt to maximize its benefit, with the potential risk of hypocapnia and placental vasoconstriction (17). However, this phenomenon may be no different than that seen with hyperventilation during painful labor. Third, the neonatal excretion of any drug that has transferred during labor is important; this also depends on the agent's solubility and the ability of the neonate to achieve adequate ventilation following delivery.

Equipment and Methods of Administration

Inhalation agents may be delivered using standard anesthetic equipment (Table 10.3) or using devices specifically designed for intermittent inhalation (Table 10.4). A standard anesthetic machine can be used to deliver nitrous oxide or volatile agents (or both). It produces continuous flow of gases and therefore results in continuous inhalation if the face mask is kept applied to the patient's face, and may result in environmental pollution if used for intermittent inhalation. The anesthesia machine provides continuous delivery and higher concentrations of inhalation agents, and results in higher blood concentrations of agents compared with intermittent inhalation. Anesthetic machines are therefore usually reserved for relatively short, intense periods, e.g., for delivery of the baby or forceps delivery. A suggested technique is outlined in Table 10.3.

Nitrous Oxide

Nitrous oxide is often used as a premixed 1:1 mixture with oxygen (in several countries including the United Kingdom, Canada, Australia, South Africa, and the United States), available commercially as Entonox®. In the United States, a 50% nitrous oxide in oxygen mixture is administered using a blending device (Nitronox®). Entonox® is manufactured utilizing the Poynting effect (named after the English physicist who described it), by which gaseous oxygen is bubbled through liquid nitrous oxide with vaporization of the liquid to form a gaseous mixture. Entonox® is supplied in cylinders that may be connected to a central manifold and then to a piped gas supply

Table 10.3. INHALATION ANALGESIA USING AN ANESTHETIC MACHINE: A SUGGESTED TECHNIQUE

1. Administer 30 mL 0.3M sodium citrate.
2. Apply a pulse oximeter and check the blood pressure.
3. Start an intravenous infusion.
4. Instruct the parturient in the technique. She needs to be aware that the gas may help, but that it may make her feel dizzy, nauseated, or sleepy.
5. Inhalation should begin 30 sec before the next contraction (if regular) or the moment a contraction is felt (if irregular), and cease when the contraction starts to recede.
6. Introduce the inhalational agent gradually, instructing the patient to take slow deep breaths and concentrate on her breathing. Maintain verbal contact with the patient and be reassuring.
7. Begin with 0.3% isoflurane or 30% nitrous oxide in oxygen, increasing the concentration gradually (allowing several contractions at each setting) until a satisfactory effect is achieved up to 0.5% isoflurane or 50% nitrous oxide in oxygen (up to 70% nitrous oxide is acceptable for a few breaths). Lower concentrations of isoflurane and nitrous oxide should be used if administered concurrently (e.g., 0.2% and 30%, respectively).
8. Stop administration immediately and change to 100% oxygen if unacceptable sedation or arterial desaturation occurs.
9. During the second stage of labor, 2–3 deep breaths should be taken before each push.
10. The obstetrician should consider pudendal block or infiltration of the perineum with local anesthetic for additional analgesia.

---

or supplied freestanding to the delivery suite. Three sizes of Entonox® cylinders are available, containing 500, 2000, or 5000 L of gas; they are colored blue with blue/white shoulders. At temperatures above −7°C (pseudocritical temperature), both nitrous oxide and oxygen remain in the gaseous phase, but at temperatures below this the nitrous oxide may liquify, resulting in liquid nitrous oxide at the cylinder's base with gaseous oxygen above. Use of a normal cylinder in this condition results in a high concentration of oxygen initially followed by almost pure nitrous oxide as the oxygen is exhausted. Cylinders may therefore contain an internal tube from the outlet, which draws gas from the lower part of the cylinder, so that in case of liquification, liquified nitrous oxide containing about 20% dissolved oxygen is delivered. Warming and repeated inversion of the cylinders can be used to reconstitute the gaseous mixture. In climates where temperatures commonly fall below the pseudocritical temperature,

Table 10.4. INTERMITTENT INHALATION ANALGESIA USING ENTONOX®: THE TECHNIQUE AS USED IN THE UNITED KINGDOM AND ELSEWHERE

1. Instruct the parturient in the technique. She needs to be aware that the gas may help, but that it may make her feel dizzy or nauseated.
2. In the United States, IV *infusion* is usually established, pulse oximetry is applied, and adequate scavenging of exhaled gases must be in place. (Administration of opioids must be done with caution and by knowledgeable personnel.)
3. Inhalation should begin 30 sec before the next contraction (if regular) or the moment a contraction is felt (if irregular), and cease when the contraction starts to recede.
4. The patient should take slow deep breaths, and concentrate on her breathing. Maintain verbal contact with the patient and be reassuring.
5. Remove the mask or mouthpiece between contractions and instruct the patient to breathe normally.
6. During the second stage of labor, 2–3 deep breaths should be taken before each push.
7. The obstetrician should consider pudendal block or infiltration of the perineum with local anesthetic for additional analgesia.

IV = intravenous.

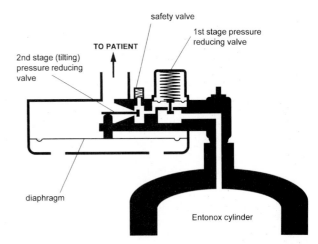

Figure 10.3. Diagram of an Entonox® two-stage pressure-reducing valve. The valve may be fitted to a piped gas outlet or (as shown here) a cylinder. (Redrawn from Ward CS. *Anaesthetic Equipment.* 2nd ed. London: Bailliere Tindall; 1985; and Davis PD, Parbrook GD, Kenny GNC. *Basic Physics and Measurement in Anaesthesia.* 4th ed. Oxford: Butterworth-Heinemann; 1995.)

special precautions should apply to the storage and handling of the cylinders.

Most use of Entonox® is with intermittent "on-demand" systems, reflecting the noncontinuous nature of labor pain, although continuous administration using simple face masks or nasal cannulae has also been used. The most common device consists of a two-stage pressure-reducing valve incorporated into a single housing (Figure 10.3). The first-stage pressure reduction delivers a lower pressure to the second-stage valve; when the parturient creates a negative pressure by breathing in, the large diaphragm moves upwards and tilts a rod, which constitutes the second-stage valve. Gas is thus delivered as long as the parturient makes inspiratory efforts. The valve is adjusted so that minimal negative pressure is required to activate gas flow. An expiratory valve is placed at the distal end of the delivery tubing so that the mouthpiece or face mask does not have to be removed from the face between breaths (Figure 10.4). Nasal cannulae have been used to provide a background level of gas in between contractions, supplemented by intermittent inhalation via a mouthpiece during contractions (18), although this is not routine practice.

For intermittent inhalation of nitrous oxide, given its low blood-gas solubility (0.47), it should be possible to achieve maximal blood levels of the gas within a short time of beginning inhalation. Interestingly, Klikovich reported in 1881 that the best results were obtained by inspiring the gas 30 to 60 seconds before each contraction, with an inspiratory pause before exhaling (2). Theoretical calculations by Waud and Waud suggest that a 50-second period of inhalation is required before each contraction, continuing until halfway between contractions (19). Given the unpredictable pattern of most women's contractions, a compromise is usually reached whereby inspiration of the gas begins the moment each contraction is initially felt, continuing until the peak has passed. Maximal analgesia may thus not be obtained. Slow deep breaths are more efficient than short shallow ones. This technique is something that many parturients find difficult to do, and it is therefore helpful if they have practiced the breathing technique beforehand, or at least during early labor when contractions are not so painful. Nitrous oxide concentration delivered is limited by the fixed performance of the delivery device, which is, however, an inherent safety feature of this technique. If administered by an anesthetist with an anesthesia machine, a faster onset of analgesia may be achieved by temporarily increasing the inspired concentration but with the risk of increased side effects.

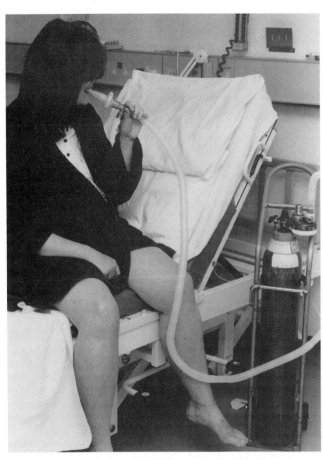

Figure 10.4. Patient using Entonox® equipment.

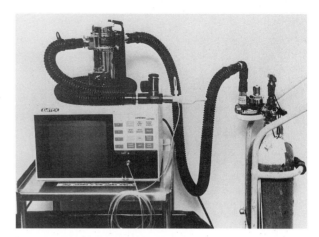

Figure 10.5. Equipment for using isoflurane with Entonox® equipment. (Reproduced with permission from Wee MYK, Hasan MA, Thomas TA. Isoflurane in labor. *Anaesthesia* 1993;48:369–372.)

Volatile Agents

Specific devices for intermittent inhalation of volatile agents during labor and vaginal delivery have been designed, although these are rarely used now. In the United Kingdom, the best known of these were the Emotril and Tecota trichloroethylene vaporizers and the Cardiff methoxyflurane inhaler. All three were temperature-compensated draw-over vaporizers suitable for self-administration by the mother and were popular for a time, although their respective agents were withdrawn for reasons unrelated specifically to obstetric practice. Other draw-over vaporizers have been used, including the hand-held Duke and Cyprane devices. To be suitable for draw-over inhalation analgesia, such a vaporizer should be unaffected by temperature and the parturient's minute volume and peak flow, both of which may vary widely during labor. Trichloroethylene and methoxyflurane were administered in air in concentrations of 0.2% to 0.5%. Since both agents had high blood-gas partition coefficients (9 and 13, respectively), analgesia was relatively slow in onset with cumulation even if inhaled intermittently. More recently, Entonox® has been inhaled from a standard on-demand Entonox® valve and passed through an isoflurane draw-over vaporizer to produce 0.2% to 0.25% isoflurane and 50% nitrous oxide in oxygen (Fig. 10.5) (20, 21). A similar concentration of isoflurane has been added to a nitrous oxide/oxygen mixture in a single cylinder and has been reported as being effective when inhaled through a standard Entonox® valve (22). Desflurane and sevoflurane have particularly low blood-gas solubilities (0.42 and 0.69, respectively), which might make them especially suited for intermittent inhalation. Desflurane requires a special vaporizer because of its low boiling point (23°C) and is thus unsuitable for draw-over use, although use

of desflurane delivered using an anesthetic machine has been described (23).

Maternal Effects

Analgesia

Nitrous Oxide. Surprisingly, it is difficult to find clear objective evidence of nitrous oxide's analgesic efficacy. Westling et al. found improved analgesia with intermittent 70% nitrous oxide compared with 40%, supporting a dose-related analgesic effect (24). However, a comparison of 50% and 70% nitrous oxide by intermittent inhalation performed 30 years ago found little difference in efficacy between the two concentrations (12). Approximately 70% of parturients rated their analgesia as good or better, while 90% reported the gas "helped." McAneny and Doughty found that self-administration of between 50% and 80% nitrous oxide produced complete pain relief in 8% to 14% of parturients, unrelated to inspired concentration (25). Using Entonox®, Rosen et al. obtained complete relief of pain in 11% of women, with 30% reporting little or no relief (26). A more recent report involving several thousand women using intermittent Entonox® found that 40% described the gas as helpful while 38% described it as unhelpful (27). Carstoniu et al. have recently challenged accepted wisdom by comparing premixed nitrous oxide/oxygen with compressed air in a double-blind, randomized, crossover study (28). There was no difference in visual analog pain scores over five successive contractions between the two gas mixtures, although most subjects were able to distinguish nitrous oxide and chose to continue with it. A study from Oulu, Finland, also found little benefit as demonstrated by visual analog pain scores from a variety of analgesic techniques, including intermittent inhalation of 50% nitrous oxide and meperidine (Figure 10.6), despite 72% and 83% of users, respectively, reporting good or moderate pain relief (29). This finding suggests that nitrous oxide, like opioids, may make parturients feel better without necessarily reducing objectively measured pain (30). Continuous administration may provide more consistent analgesia than intermittent inhalation (24). One possible reason for this might be the relatively low arterial concentrations of nitrous oxide achieved with intermittent inhalation. The mean concentration required for analgesia without loss of consciousness has been found to be 41.2% using continuous administration (31), whereas 50% nitrous oxide given intermittently only achieves an arterial concentration equivalent to breathing 26.4% (32). Intermittent inhalation of Entonox® achieves analgesic levels of nitrous oxide faster when 5 L/min is also administered continuously

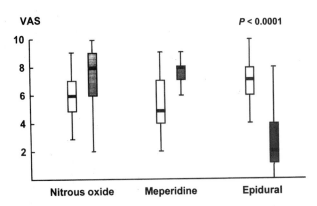

Figure 10.6. Visual analog pain scores (*VAS*) before (*clear*) and after (*shaded*) different analgesic interventions in labor. The graph shows median, interquartile range, and range. (Drawn from Ranta P, Jouppila P, Spalding M, Kangas-Saarela T, Hollmen A, Jouppila R. Parturients' assessment of water blocks, pethidine, nitrous oxide, paracervical and epidural blocks in labour. *Int J Obstet Anesth* 1994;4:193–198.)

via nasal cannulae, compared to intermittent inhalation alone or together with continuous administration of oxygen (18). (Environmental contamination remains a problem with this technique.)

Taken together, these studies suggest that about a third of parturients gain no benefit from self-administered inhalation of nitrous oxide, with the remainder deriving variable benefit. Few data exist on the use of higher concentrations administered by an anesthesiologist using an anesthetic machine. Despite its use for over 100 years, we do not appear to be any closer to quantifying nitrous oxide's analgesic effects in labor (33).

Volatile Agents.   Most volatile agents in common use have relatively poor analgesic qualities, limiting their usefulness. Other problems include their uterine relaxant effects at high inspired concentrations, and the risk of accidental overdosage and induction of general anesthesia, with its attendant hazards. If the agent is a poor analgesic, high concentrations must be administered to achieve an analgesic effect, increasing the risk of uterine relaxation and induction of anesthesia. Anesthetic requirements are reduced in pregnancy (15, 16), which makes mothers more susceptible to inhalation analgesia but also makes inadvertent induction of general anesthesia more likely. Two agents with powerful analgesic properties were trichloroethylene (Trilene®) and methoxyflurane (Penthrane®), which, despite being relatively soluble in blood, both enjoyed popularity as inhalation analgesics during the 1960s and 1970s but are no longer available, and are thus of historic interest only. Their high potency compensated, to a degree, for their other, less desirable properties.

The use of halothane in obstetric anesthesia has declined in recent years with the advent of newer agents. Halothane is considered too potent to be useful for inhalation analgesia without producing anesthesia. Although it has been useful for general anesthesia when rapid, profound uterine relaxation is needed, it is doubtful whether halothane is a better myometrial relaxant than the other inhalation agents. Furthermore, its slower elimination and potential for causing cardiac arrhythmias are also disadvantages. It has been safely used for cesarean section, although it is increasingly superseded by the newer inhalation agents.

Studies of enflurane have produced conflicting results, some suggesting a useful analgesic effect (34–36) and others finding unacceptable depression of consciousness with little analgesia (37). Neonatal condition appears unaffected by brief maternal inhalation of low concentrations of enflurane (34). Like halothane, enflurane causes dose-dependent uterine relaxation; thus, enflurane and halothane share many characteristics, and indications for their use in obstetric anesthesia are similar. An advantage of enflurane over halothane is that its effects are more rapidly reversible because of its lower blood solubility. On the other hand, a potential disadvantage of enflurane is its increased biotransformation and production of fluoride ions in morbidly obese subjects (38), although this has not been described in obstetrics (34).

Isoflurane has become popular in obstetrics because of its low blood-gas solubility (1.4), cardiovascular stability, and lack of hepatic and renal toxicity. At equipotent concentrations, its effect on uterine contractility is similar to that of halothane and enflurane (39). Isoflurane has been found to provide useful analgesia during labor comparable to that produced by nitrous oxide without producing adverse effects as long as concentrations under 0.7% are used (34, 40, 41). At higher concentrations, increased drowsiness occurs (41). During the second stage of labor, concentrations of 0.2% to 0.7% isoflurane result in analgesia similar to that produced by 30% to 60% nitrous oxide, with high rates of acceptance by patients, obstetricians, and anesthesiologists, low incidence of amnesia, similar amounts of blood loss, and similar neonatal outcomes (40). Wee et al. have described the use of Entonox® with isoflurane 0.2%, which resulted in lower pain scores than Entonox® alone although with greater drowsiness (20). Similar results have been obtained by Tunstall et al. (21, 22). Isoflurane is also widely used for general anesthesia performed for cesarean section (see Chapter 11) and would thus appear to be suitable for inhalation anesthesia for operative vaginal delivery if indicated.

Desflurane and sevoflurane have received surprisingly little attention in the literature despite their low blood-gas solubility and potential suitability for obstetrics. One study compared 1.0% to 4.5% desflurane and 30% to 60% nitrous oxide, both delivered continuously using an anesthetic machine during the second stage of labor (42). Concentrations of 2% desflurane produced comparable analgesia to 46% nitrous oxide, with no maternal or fetal adverse effects in either group other than a 23% incidence of amnesia in the desflurane group. This high incidence of amnesia may limit desflurane's usefulness in labor. Desflurane and sevoflurane have been used for cesarean section with maternal and fetal effects comparable to enflurane (42) and isoflurane (43), respectively. Preliminary work indicates that sevoflurane has less uterine relaxant action than isoflurane and halothane at equivalent minimum alveolar concentration (MAC) doses (44), although whether this has clinical significance is debatable. Preliminary results of studies in the pregnant sheep model suggest that sevoflurane preserves maternal hemodynamic stability, while causing greater increases in uterine blood flow than does isoflurane (45). Apart from these studies and individual case reports of sevoflurane for cesarean section (46, 47), there has been little other published work on sevoflurane in clinical obstetric practice despite its attractive properties of low blood-gas solubility, pleasant smell, and low irritability. Concerns about interaction between sevoflurane and soda-lime in circle systems at low-gas flows (48) are controversial and not reflected in the United Kingdom, where no restriction on use of low flows exists in the product license sheet, unlike in the United States.

Other Maternal Effects

Maternal Consciousness.   Even nitrous oxide's weak anesthetic properties may be enough to induce loss of consciousness in some parturients, especially at higher concentrations. Thus, 3% to 5% of women may become unconscious breathing intermittent 70% to 80% nitrous oxide compared with 1% or less at 50% gas (12, 25). In addition, "inadequate cooperation" has been reported in 9% of parturients at 50% nitrous oxide increasing to 17% of women at 80% gas (25). Despite this potential risk, use of Entonox® appears to be safe, as experience of its use over many years would testify (12, 25, 49–53). Depressed consciousness and induction of anesthesia is more of a concern with the volatile agents, which are much more potent as anesthetic agents than nitrous oxide. Thus, careful attention must be paid when administering these agents, firstly to ensure low concentrations are delivered and secondly to monitor the mother's level of consciousness.

Maternal Oxygenation. Studies into maternal oxygenation during intermittent nitrous oxide inhalation have produced conflicting results. While some have found no evidence of hypoxemia between contractions (28) or mild hypoxemia only (54), others have found frequent episodes of arterial desaturation, in some cases to less than 70% using pulse oximetry (55). It would appear that the respiratory depressant effect of opioids is additive (56); thus, studies not controlled for concurrent opioid administration are more likely to observe hypoxemia (54, 55, 57). It is interesting that only one of these studies that was randomized and double-blind found no hypoxemia and even a higher arterial saturation in the nitrous oxide/oxygen group than in the control group given compressed air (28). However, there is evidence that hypocapnia following hyperventilation, for example, resulting from painful contractions, may be followed by a period of hypoventilation, and that this may be exacerbated by nitrous oxide (58, 59). Despite this, in countries where use of nitrous oxide is common, routine monitoring using pulse oximetry is rare. In the United States, the use of pulse oximetry with nitrous oxide is recommended. One advantage of volatile agents over nitrous oxide is the ability to deliver them in effective concentrations together with high concentrations of oxygen, since they are much more potent. This may be especially useful in parturients with cardiorespiratory disease, or when maternal oxygen administration is indicated (e.g., the compromised fetus requiring urgent instrumental delivery).

Uterine Relaxation. Uterine relaxation resulting from use of inhalational agents may prolong labor and, more importantly, may result in increased blood loss following delivery. Nitrous oxide is devoid of uterine effects, as originally demonstrated by Klikovich, who inserted a tube into the uterus and measured intrauterine pressure (2). This is in contrast to the volatile agents. All of the volatile agents studied cause *in vitro* and *in vivo* dose-related uterine relaxation, more marked in pregnancy (39, 60, 61), with halothane, enflurane, and isoflurane equally depressant when used in equipotent concentrations (39). However, the general opinion is that little clinical effect results from use of low concentrations, at which oxytocics are able to overcome any relaxant effect (60, 61) (see Chapter 3). In a comparison of desflurane with nitrous oxide during the second stage of labor, no difference in peripartum blood loss was found between the two groups, although the number of patients studied was small (42). Whether further studies support the suggestion that sevoflurane has less uterine relaxant action than other agents (44), and whether this has any clinical significance when sevoflurane is used for labor or vaginal delivery, remains to be seen. The use of a volatile agent with a low blood-gas solubility and thus more rapidly reversible uterine effects would seem to be an additional attraction of using sevoflurane or desflurane.

Cardiovascular Effects. Although traditionally held to have no cardiovascular effects when used for labor and vaginal delivery, a recent study of intermittent 40% and 70% nitrous oxide and continuous 40% nitrous oxide in labor found a dose-related reduction in heart rate, cardiac output, and blood pressure that was greatest with continuous administration and that persisted between contractions (59). Since pain relief was also dose-dependent and greatest with continuous inhalation, it is possible that these cardiovascular effects were related to relief of pain rather than to a direct effect of the gas, although this could not be excluded. The volatile agents have well-known cardiovascular effects, but in the low concentrations used for labor and vaginal delivery these are unlikely.

Nitrous oxide may inhibit methionine synthetase after prolonged exposure (>24 hours) although inhibition may occur after shorter periods in cobalamin-deficient subjects (62). Such

patients cannot be reliably identified clinically, but although biochemical evidence of methionine synthetase inhibition has been reported after obstetric analgesia with nitrous oxide (63), intermittent inhalation in labor has not been associated with clinical manifestations of methionine synthetase inhibition (62).

Neonatal Effects

Placental transfer of all inhalation agents occurs rapidly, because they are highly lipid soluble, nonionized, and of fairly low molecular weight. Anesthetic levels increase rapidly in the fetal brain, and in general the degree of fetal and neonatal depression is directly proportional to the depth and duration of maternal anesthesia (64). Neonatal depression may result from direct drug effects or from physiologic changes induced in the mother, such as hypoventilation or hypotension.

Early studies suggested adverse effects of nitrous oxide on the fetus, although most involved cesarean section under general anesthesia, in which the deleterious effects probably arose from catecholamine production associated with light anesthesia in the absence of volatile agents rather than from the nitrous oxide itself (65, 66). Inhalation of nitrous oxide for analgesia during labor has not been associated with adverse effects including depression of neurobehavioral scores, despite rapid passage into the fetus and the theoretical risk of neonatal diffusion hypoxia, and limitation of the available space in the lung for oxygen (34, 67). Intermittent administration of 50% nitrous oxide results in negligible maternal (and presumably fetal) arterial levels by the start of the next contraction (32), unlike the situation in which nitrous oxide is inhaled continuously (Figure 10.7).

Animal and human studies have demonstrated that the fetus is more sensitive to volatile anesthetic agents (i.e., has lower MAC) than is the mother (68, 69). While in utero exposure to volatile agents for brief durations or at low concentrations (e.g., during labor) has minimal neonatal effects (34, 35, 40–42), prolonged or profound exposure not surprisingly leads to increasing fetal hypotension and acidosis (68, 70–72). Similar considerations apply to the stressed fetus, in whom maternal exposure before delivery should be limited in duration and amount if possible (73–75). Having said this, a benefit of inhalation analgesia with a volatile agent is the high inspired concentration of oxygen that is possible when using this technique. Thus, for example, Piggot et al. demonstrated higher umbilical venous partial pressures of oxygen and the decreased need for neonatal resuscitation

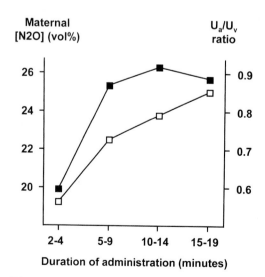

Figure 10.7. Mean maternal nitrous oxide concentration ([N_2O]; ■) and umbilical arterial-venous ratio of nitrous oxide (U_a/U_v ratio; □) following continuous maternal administration of nitrous oxide. (Drawn from data in Marx GF, Joshi CW, Orkin LR. Placental transmission of nitrous oxide. *Anesthesiology* 1970;32:429–432.)

following emergency cesarean section when 100% oxygen with 1.5 MAC isoflurane was administered, rather than 50% nitrous oxide (76).

Environmental Considerations

It has long been suspected that chronic exposure to inhaled anesthetic agents may increase the rates of miscarriage in health care workers, although the evidence for this is controversial (77, 78). Maximal permitted levels of nitrous oxide have been set at 25 parts per million (ppm) in the United States and 100 ppm in Sweden and the United Kingdom; levels exceeding 100 ppm have been found in delivery suites using nitrous oxide without scavenging, although levels may vary widely (79–81). This may be one factor affecting the low use of nitrous oxide in the United States, where an anesthetic machine with a scavenging device is usual for delivering nitrous oxide, rather than unscavenged Entonox® systems commonly used elsewhere in the world. Continuous administration of nitrous oxide by face mask or nasal cannulae clearly risks greater pollution since gas is delivered throughout the respiratory cycle instead of only during inspiration, and this may explain the low use of this method of delivery in comparison to on-demand administration. Concern has also been expressed about the contribution of inhalation agents, especially nitrous oxide, to global warming and depletion of atmospheric ozone (78).

SUMMARY

Inhalation analgesia with nitrous oxide continues to be a popular and simple method of providing pain relief during labor and vaginal delivery, although with considerable regional variation in its use. The use of volatile agents is less widespread, possibly related to the limitations of the current agents and their methods of administration. Because of its noninvasiveness and simplicity, inhalation analgesia is likely to continue to be a useful adjunct to other methods of analgesia or as the sole technique used, despite its relative lack of efficacy. An inhalation agent with low blood-gas solubility, profound analgesic effects, and lack of uterine relaxant actions would be an ideal agent for labor, providing rapid onset and offset. None of the currently available agents fulfill these criteria. Inhalation anesthesia is rarely used for vaginal delivery because of the risks associated with its use in the parturient and is unlikely to increase in use, given this fact and the increasing popularity of regional anesthesia. However, it remains an option in special circumstances, although the basic requirements for safe airway management should not be forgotten.

REFERENCES

1. Rae SM, Wildsmith JA. So just who was James "Young" Simpson? *Br J Anaesth* 1997;79:271–273.
2. Richards W, Parbrook GD, Wilson J. Stanislav Klikovich (1853–1910). Pioneer of nitrous oxide and oxygen analgesia. *Anaesthesia* 1976;31:933–940.
3. Tunstall ME. Use of a fixed nitrous oxide and oxygen mixture from one cylinder. *Lancet* 1961;2:964.
4. Gibbs CP, Krischer J, Peckham BM, Sharp H, Kirschbaum TH. Obstetric anesthesia: A national survey. *Anesthesiology* 1986;65:298–306.
5. Lind B, Hoel TM. Alleviation of labour pain in Norway. An interview investigation in 1969 and 1986. *Acta Obstet Gynecol Scand* 1989;68:125–129.
6. Steer P. The methods of pain relief used. In: Chamberlain G, Wraight A, Steer P, eds. *Pain and Its Relief in Childbirth.* Edinburgh: Churchill Livingstone; 1993:49.
7. Kangas-Saarela T, Kangas-Karki K. Pain and pain relief in labour: Parturients' experiences. *Int J Obstet Anesth* 1994;3:67–74.
8. Schneider M, Graber J, Thorin D, Castelanelli S. A survey of current obstetric anaesthesia practice in Switzerland. *Int J Obstet Anesth* 1995;4:207–213.
9. Capogna G, Alahuhta S, Celleno D, et al. Maternal expectations and experiences of labour pain and analgesia: A multicentre study of nulliparous women. *Int J Obstet Anesth* 1996;5:229–235.
10. Beke A, Takacs Gy, Sziller I, Fedak L, Papp Z. Obstetric anaesthesia in Hungary. *Int J Obstet Anesth* 1997;6:235–238.
11. Garcia J, Redshaw M, Fitzsimons B, Keene J. *First Class Delivery. A National Survey of Women's Views of Maternity Care.* London: Audit Commission; 1998:20.
12. Report to the Medical Research Council of the Committee on Nitrous Oxide and Oxygen Analgesia in Midwifery. Clinical trials of different concentrations of oxygen and nitrous oxide for obstetric analgesia. *Br Med J* 1970;1:709–713.
13. Vinatier D, Dufour P, Berard J. Utilization of intravenous nitroglycerin for obstetrical emergencies. *Int J Gynaecol Obstet* 1996;55:129–134.
14. Riley ET, Flanagan B, Cohen SE, Chitkara U. Intravenous nitroglycerin: A potent uterine relaxant for emergency obstetric procedures. *Int J Obstet Anesth* 1996;5:264–268.
15. Chan MTV, Mainland P, Gin T. Minimum alveolar concentration of halothane and enflurane are decreased in early pregnancy. *Anesthesiology* 1996;85:782–786.
16. Gin T, Chan MTV. Decreased minimum alveolar concentration of isoflurane in pregnant humans. *Anesthesiology* 1994;81:829–832.
17. Fadl ET, Utting JE. A study of maternal acid-base state during labour. *Br J Anaesth* 1969;41:327–337.
18. Arthurs GJ, Rosen M. Self-administered intermittent nitrous oxide analgesia for labour. Enhancement of effect with continuous nasal inhalation of 50% nitrous oxide (Entonox). *Anaesthesia* 1979;34:301–309.
19. Waud BE, Waud DR. Calculated kinetics of distribution of nitrous oxide and methoxyflurane during intermittent administration in obstetrics. *Anesthesiology* 1970;32:306–316.
20. Wee MYK, Hasan MA, Thomas TA. Isoflurane in labor. *Anaesthesia* 1993;48:369–372.
21. Arora S, Tunstall ME, Ross JA. Self-administered mixture of Entonox and isoflurane in labour. *Int J Obstet Anesth* 1992;1:188–202.
22. Tunstall ME, Ross JAS. Isoflurane, nitrous oxide and oxygen analgesic mixtures. *Anaesthesia* 1993;48:919.
23. Abboud TK, Swart F, Zhu J, Donovan MM, Dasilva EP, Yakal K. Desflurane analgesia for vaginal delivery. *Acta Anaesthesiol Scand* 1995;39:259–261.
24. Westling F, Milsom I, Zetterstrom H, Ekstrom-Jodal B. Effects of nitrous oxide oxygen inhalation on the maternal circulation during vaginal delivery. *Acta Anaesthesiol Scand* 1992;36:175–181.
25. McAneny TM, Doughty AG. Self-administration of nitrous oxide/oxygen in obstetrics. *Anaesthesia* 1963;18:488–497.
26. Rosen M, Mushin WW, Jones PL, Jones EV. Field trial of methoxyflurane, nitrous oxide, and trichloroethylene as obstetric analgesia. *Br Med J* 1969;3:263–267.
27. Wraight A. Coping with pain. In: Chamberlain G, Wraight A, Steer P, eds. *Pain and Its Relief in Childbirth.* Edinburgh: Churchill Livingstone; 1993:82.
28. Carstoniu J, Levytam S, Norman P, Daley D, Katz J, Sandler AN. Nitrous-oxide in early labor–safety and analgesic efficacy assessed by a double-blind, placebo-controlled study. *Anesthesiology* 1994;80:30–35.
29. Ranta P, Jouppila P, Spalding M, Kangas-Saarela T, Hollmen A, Jouppila R. Parturients' assessment of water blocks, pethidine, nitrous oxide, paracervical and epidural blocks in labour. *Int J Obstet Anesth* 1994;4:193–198.
30. Olofsson C, Ekblom A, Ekman-Ordeberg G, Hjelm A, Irestedt L. Lack of analgesic effect of systemically administered morphine or pethidine on labour pain. *Br J Obstet Gynaecol* 1996;103:968–972.
31. Jones PL, Rosen M, Mushin WW, Jones EV. Methoxyflurane and nitrous oxide as obstetric analgesics. I. A comparison by continuous administration. *Br Med J* 1969;3:255–259.
32. Latto IP, Molloy MJ, Rosen M. Arterial concentrations of nitrous oxide during intermittent patient-controlled inhalation of 50% nitrous oxide in oxygen (Entonox) during the first stage of labour. *Br J Anaesth* 1973;45:1029–1034.
33. Irestedt L. Current status of nitrous oxide for obstetric pain relief. *Acta Anaesthesiol Scand* 1994;38:771–772.
34. Stefani SJ, Hughes SC, Shnider SM, et al. Neonatal neurobehavioral effects of inhalation analgesia for vaginal delivery. *Anesthesiology* 1982;56:351–355.
35. Abboud TK, Shnider SM, Wright RG, et al. Enflurane analgesia in obstetrics. *Anesth Analg* 1981;60:133–137.

36. McGuinness C, Rosen M. Enflurane as an analgesic in labour. *Anaesthesia* 1984;39:24–26.

37. Westmoreland RT, Evans JA, Chastain GM. Obstetric use of enflurane (Ethrane). *South Med J* 1974;67:527–530.

38. Strube PJ, Hulands GH, Halsey MJ. Serum fluoride levels in morbidly obese patients: Enflurane compared with isoflurane anesthesia. *Anaesthesia* 1987;42:685–689.

39. Munson ES, Embro WJ. Enflurane, isoflurane and halothane and isolated human uterine muscle. *Anesthesiology* 1977;46:11–14.

40. Abboud TK, Gangolly J, Mosaad P, Crowell D. Isoflurane in obstetrics. *Anesth Analg* 1989;68:388–391.

41. McLeod DD, Ramayya GP, Tunstall ME. Self-administered isoflurane in labour. *Anaesthesia* 1985;40:424–426.

42. Abboud TK, Zhu J, Richardson M, Peres da Silva E, Donovan M. Desflurane: A new volatile anesthetic for cesarean section. Maternal and neonatal effects. *Acta Anaesthesiol Scand* 1995;39:723–726.

43. Gambling DR, Sharma SK, White PF, Van Beveren T, Bala AS, Gouldson R. Use of sevoflurane during elective cesarean birth: A comparison with isoflurane and spinal anesthesia. *Anesth Analg.* 1995;81:90–95.

44. Yamakage M, Mori T, Tsujiguchi N, Kawana S, Namiki A. Inhibitory effects of halothane, isoflurane, and sevoflurane on contractility and intracellular Ca^{2+} concentration of pregnancy myometrium in rats [abstract]. *Anesthesiology* 1998;89:A1050.

45. Stein D, Masaoka T, Wlody D, et al. The effects of sevoflurane on uterine blood flow and fetal well being in sheep. In: Abstracts of Scientific Papers of the Annual Meeting of the Society for Obstetric Anesthesia and Perinatology; Boston, MA; 1991.

46. Schaut DJ, Khona R, Gross JB. Sevoflurane inhalation induction for emergency cesarean section in a parturient with no intravenous access. *Anesthesiology* 1997;86:1392–1394.

47. Hara K, Saito Y, Morimoto N, Sakura S, Kosaka Y. Anaesthetic management of caesarean section in a patient with myelodysplastic syndrome. *Can J Anaesth* 1998;45:157–163.

48. Strum DP, Johnson BH, Eger EI II. Stability of sevoflurane in soda lime. *Anesthesiology* 1987;67:779–781.

49. Report on Confidential Enquiries into Maternal Deaths, 1982–84. London: Her Majesty's Stationery Office; 1989.

50. Report on Confidential Enquiries into Maternal Deaths, 1985–87. London: Her Majesty's Stationery Office; 1991.

51. Report on Confidential Enquiries into Maternal Deaths, 1988–90. London: Her Majesty's Stationery Office; 1994.

52. Report on Confidential Enquiries into Maternal Deaths, 1991–93. London: Her Majesty's Stationery Office; 1996.

53. Report on Confidential Enquiries into Maternal Deaths, 1994–96. London: Her Majesty's Stationery Office; 1998.

54. Davies JM, Hogg M, Rosen M. Maternal arterial oxygen tension during intermittent inhalation analgesia. *Br J Anaesth* 1975;47:370–378.

55. Reed PN, Colquhoun AD, Hanning CD. Maternal oxygenation during normal labour. *Br J Anaesth* 1989;62:316–318.

56. Zelcer J, Owers H, Paull JD. A controlled oximetric evaluation of inhalational, opioid and epidural analgesia in labour. *Anaesth Intensive Care* 1989;17:418–421.

57. Deckardt R, Fembacher PM, Schneider KT, Graeff H. Maternal arterial oxygen saturation during labor and delivery: Pain-dependent alterations and effects on the newborn. *Obstet Gynecol* 1987;70:21–25.

58. Northwood D, Sapsford DJ, Jones JG, Griffiths D. Nitrous oxide sedation causes post-hyperventilation apnoea. *Br J Anaesth* 1991;67:7–12.

59. Einarsson S, Senqvist O, Bengtsson A, Noren H, Bengson JP. Gas kinetics during nitrous oxide analgesia for labor. *Anaesthesia* 1996;51:449–452.

60. Marx GF, Kim YO, Lin CC, Halevy S, Schulman H. Postpartum uterine pressure under halothane or enflurane anesthesia. *Obstet Gynecol* 1978;51:695–698.

61. Abadir AR, Humayun SG, Calvello D, Gintautas J. Effects of isoflurane and oxytocin on gravid human uterus in vitro. *Anesth Analg* 1987;66:S1.

62. Guttormsen AB, Refsum H, Ueland PM. The interaction between nitrous oxide and cobalamin. *Acta Anaesthesiol Scand* 1994;38:753–756.

63. Landon MJ, Creagh-Barry P, McArthur S, Charlett A. Influence of vitamin B12 status on the inactivation of methionine synthase by nitrous oxide. *Br J Anaesth* 1992;69:81–86.

64. Moya F. Volatile inhalation agents and muscle relaxants in obstetrics. *Acta Anaesthesiol Scand* 1966;25(suppl):368–375.

65. Hay DM. Nitrous oxide transfer across the placenta and condition of the newborn at delivery. *Br J Obstet Gynaecol* 1978;85:299–302.

66. Stenger VG, Blechner JN, Prystowsky H. A study of prolongation of obstetric Anesthesia. *Am J Obstet Gynecol* 1969;103:901–907.

67. Marx GF, Joshi CW, Orkin LR. Placental transmission of nitrous oxide. *Anesthesiology* 1970;32:429–432.

68. Bachman CR, Biehl DR, Sitar D, Cumming M, Pucci W. Isoflurane potency and cardiovascular effects during short exposures in the foetal lamb. *Can Anaesth Soc J* 1986;33:41–47.

69. LeDez KM, Lerman J. The minimum alveolar concentration (MAC) of isoflurane in preterm neonates. *Anesthesiology* 1987;67:301–307.

70. Palahniuk RJ, Shnider SM. Maternal and fetal cardiovascular and acid-base changes during halothane and isoflurane anesthesia in the pregnant ewe. *Anesthesiology* 1974;41:462–472.

71. Biehl DR, Tweed WA, Cote J, Wade JG, Sitar D. Effect of halothane on cardiac output and regional flow in the fetal lamb in utero. *Anesth Analg* 1983;62:489–492.

72. Biehl DR, Yarnell R, Wade JG, Sitar D. The uptake of isoflurane by the foetal lamb in utero: Effect on regional blood flow. *Can Anaesth Soc J* 1983;30:581–586.

73. Cheek DBC, Hughes SC, Dailey PA, et al. Effect of halothane on regional cerebral blood flow and cerebral metabolic oxygen consumption in the fetal lamb in utero. *Anesthesiology* 1987;67:361–366.

74. Yarnell R, Biehl DR, Tweed WA, Gregory GA, Sitar D. The effect of halothane anaesthesia on the asphyxiated foetal lamb *in utero. Can Anaesth Soc J* 1983;30:474–479.

75. Baker BW, Hughes SC, Shnider SM, Field DR, Rosen MA. Maternal anesthesia and the stressed fetus: Effects of isoflurane on the asphyxiated fetal lamb. *Anesthesiology* 1990;72:65–70.

76. Piggott SE, Bogod G, Rosen M, Rees AD, Harmer M. Isoflurane with either 100% oxygen or 50% nitrous oxide in oxygen for caesarean section. *Br J Anaesth* 1990;65:325–329.

77. Buring JE, Hennekens CH, Mayrent SL, Rosner B, Greenberg ER, Colton T. Health experiences of operating room personnel. *Anesthesiology* 1985;62:325–330.

78. Dale O, Husum B. Nitrous oxide: At threat to personnel and global environment? *Acta Anaesthesiol Scand* 1994;38:777–779.

79. Munley AJ, Railton R, Gray WM, Carter KB. Exposure of midwives to nitrous oxide in four hospitals. *Br Med J* 1986;293:1063–1064.

80. Mills GH, Singh D, Longan M, O'Sullivan J, Caunt JA. Nitrous oxide exposure on the labour ward. *Int J Obstet Anesth* 1996;5:160–164.

81. Newton C, Fitz-Henry J, Bogod D. The occupational exposure of midwives to nitrous oxide–a comparison between two labour suites. *Int J Obstet Anesth* 1999;8:7–10.

THREE

OBSTETRIC COMPLICATIONS

Shnider and Levinson's Anesthesia for Obstetrics,
edited by Samuel C. Hughes, et al.
Lippincott Williams & Wilkins,
Philadelphia, © 2001.

CHAPTER 11

ANESTHESIA FOR CESAREAN SECTION

SAMUEL C. HUGHES, M.D. GERSHON LEVINSON, M.D.
AND MARK A. ROSEN, M.D.

Delivery of a baby by cesarean section has become increasingly common. In the 1950s and 1960s, 4% to 6% of deliveries were via the abdominal route. The most common indications were cephalopelvic disproportion, uterine dystocia, hemorrhage, and acute fetal distress. Currently, cesarean section rates between 20% and 25% are common; in high-risk centers with disproportionately increased incidences of pregnancy-induced hypertension, diabetes, Rh isoimmunization, prematurity, and other high-risk problems, the rates are even higher. There are wide differences in cesarean section rates between different countries (Fig. 11.1) (1); however, the annual rate of increase for all countries is significantly higher than in the past (2)

A number of factors account for the increased cesarean section rate. It has become commonly accepted that serious trauma to the baby can be eliminated by avoiding potentially difficult midforceps or vaginal breech deliveries and performing a cesarean section instead. The widespread use of electronic fetal monitoring prior to and during labor (see Chapters 36 and 37) has made it easier to identify a fetus in jeopardy and promptly deliver the baby by the abdominal route. The clinical impression that cesarean section is less traumatic for the tiny fetus and some cases of multiple gestations, and concerns over potential lawsuits in cases of poor neonatal outcome, have also encouraged obstetricians to perform cesarean sections with less positive indications than in the past (Fig. 11.2).

Although several reports indicate that maternal mortality is higher with cesarean birth vs. vaginal delivery, it is still a very rare occurrence. Reported rates are between 0 and 105 cases per 100,000 operations (3–6). In comparison, the mortality from automobile accidents in women of childbearing age is approximately 20 per 100,000 women. Despite the marked increase in cesarean births beginning in the 1970s, there was a decline in overall maternal and perinatal mortality (Fig 11.3, 11.4) (7, 8). Thus, when there is concern for potential for fetal morbidity, obstetricians often opt for cesarean delivery. Examples of some common indications for cesarean delivery are listed in Table 11.1.

CHOICE OF ANESTHESIA

The choice of anesthesia for cesarean section depends on the reason for the operation, the degree of urgency, the desires of the patient, and the judgment of the anesthesiologist. There is no one ideal method of anesthesia for cesarean section; the advantages and disadvantages of spinal, epidural, and general anesthesia are discussed in this chapter and suggested methods for these techniques are outlined. The anesthesiologist must choose the method that he or she believes (a) is safest and most comfortable for the mother, (b) is least depressant to the newborn, and (c) provides the optimal working conditions for the obstetrician.

Surveys indicate that conduction anesthesia is the most commonly used anesthetic for cesarean section (Fig 11.5) (9–13).

Spinal anesthesia appears to be the preferred technique nationwide (11). In one university hospital, general anesthesia is used in only 3% to 5% of cesarean sections, spinal in about 46% and epidural in about 50% (13a). The high use of epidural anesthesia for cesarean section in part reflects the fact that many of the patients already had functioning epidural anesthetics in place for labor. Data from the American College of Obstetricians and Gynecologists and the American Society of Anesthesiologists, as well as the experience of two University hospitals, has shown a very marked decrease in use of general anesthesia and an increase in the use of spinal and epidural anesthesia. (Fig. 11.6 and Table 11.2).

REGIONAL ANESTHESIA

Epidural or spinal anesthesia for cesarean section allows the mother to remain awake, minimizes or completely avoids the problems associated with airway management (such as failed tracheal intubation and maternal aspiration), and avoids possible neonatal drug depression from general anesthetics.

In the pregnant woman, the dose of local anesthetic required to achieve a given level with spinal anesthesia is approximately 50% to 70% of the dose required for nonpregnant women (14). With epidural anesthesia, some authors have reported that dose requirements are also reduced (Fig. 11.7) (15, 16). On the other hand, other studies suggest that with equal amounts of local anesthetic, there is no significant difference in sensory levels in pregnant and nonpregnant patients (Table 11.3) (17). Clinical observation suggests that it is difficult to establish a higher segmental level of anesthesia with additional incremental epidural doses of local anesthetic after administration of a large dose of local anesthetic. Animal data reveal neural susceptibility to blockade is enhanced during pregnancy (17a). This has been corroborated in a study of median nerve blocks comparing pregnant to nonpregnant women (17b).

Choice of Regional Technique

Spinal anesthesia has many advantages over epidural anesthesia for cesarean section. The technique is simpler to perform and the presence of cerebrospinal fluid (CSF) provides a more certain end point, and consequently spinal anesthesia has a higher degree of success than epidural anesthesia. With spinal anesthesia, the onset of anesthesia is more rapid, allowing the surgical incision to be made sooner and producing a shorter total operating room time (18). The rapid onset of anesthesia with subarachnoid anesthetics allows spinal anesthesia to be used for all but the most urgent emergency cesarean sections.

Spinal anesthesia produces a more profound block than epidural anesthesia, and the need for supplementary intravenous (IV) analgesics and anxiolytics is decreased (18). Because the dose of local anesthetic used with spinal anesthesia is small, there is little chance of maternal toxicity and very minimal

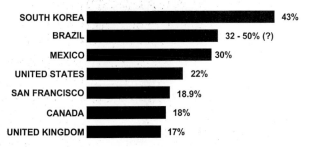

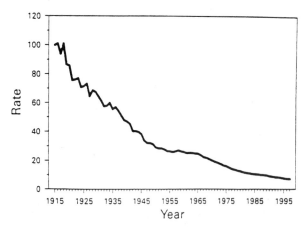

Figure 11.1. Cesarean section rates as reported by various health organizations and professional groups (1998 to 2000). The rate in Brazil is likely higher since in many public hospitals the cesarean section rate is 50%, rising to 85% or more in some units. Delivery by cesarean section is increasing in many countries around the world.

Figure 11.3. At the beginning of the 20th century, for every 1000 births, 6 to 9 women died in the United States of pregnancy-related complications. This has declined by almost 99% to <0.1 reported deaths per 1000 live births (7.7 deaths per 100,000 live births in 1997). Healthier mothers and babies. Centers for Disease Control and Prevention. *MMWR* 1999;48:849.

placental transfer of drug to the fetus. The current use of small-gauge spinal needles with noncutting pencil-point tips has reduced the incidence of postdural puncture headache (PDPH) to a very low level.

In a recent questionnaire study, 46 of 59 reporting anesthesia departments in Sweden used spinal anesthesia in more than 90% of all elective cesarean sections, and 29 of the 59 departments used spinal anesthesia in more than 80% of emergency cesarean sections (19). Some anesthesiologists prefer the continuous epidural technique because they believe hypotension occurs less precipitously with epidural anesthesia and, consequently, is easier to prevent or treat (20). However, with appropriate prehydration, uterine displacement, and the rapid administration of vasopressors, hypotension with spinal anesthesia is minimized or easily managed.

Although currently available local anesthetics reliably produce predictable levels of spinal anesthesia in most patients, the anesthetic level may be more controllable with continuous epidural anesthesia. If the initial dose does not produce a satisfactory sensory block, more drug can be injected through the epidural catheter. Continuous epidural techniques allow administration of additional local anesthetic to extend the duration

of anesthesia. With a continuous epidural technique, the anesthetic level can develop slowly, a potential advantage in patients with certain medical problems. Continuous spinal anesthesia, not commonly used, would provide the same advantage of extending the distribution or duration of the block and slowly titrating the level of anesthesia (21). A suggested technique for regional anesthesia for cesarean section is outlined in Tables 11.4, 11.5, and 11.6. The rationale for these recommendations is discussed below.

Preparation for Regional Block

During administration of spinal or epidural anesthesia, a total spinal or a toxic reaction from IV local anesthetic administration may occur. Total spinal results in hypotension, unconsciousness, and respiratory arrest, and IV local anesthetic toxicity can

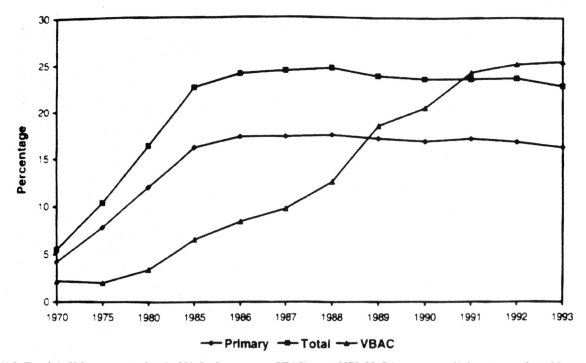

Figure 11.2. Trends in U.S. cesarean and vaginal birth after cesarean (VBAC) rates, 1970–93. *Primary cesarean birth rates* = number of first cesareans per 100 deliveries to women who had no previous cesarean delivery; *Total cesarean birth rate* = number of cesareans per 100 deliveries; *VBAC rate* = number of vaginal births per 100 deliveries to women with a previous cesarean delivery. (Reprinted by permission from Porreco RP, Thorpe JA. The cesarean birth epidemic: Trends, causes, and solutions. *Am J Obstet Gynecol* 1996;175:369–374.

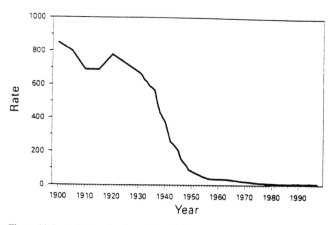

Figure 11.4. At the beginning of the 20th century, for every 1000 births, approximately 100 infants died before age 1 year. This has declined by 70% to 7.2 per 1000 live births from 1900–97. Healthier mothers and babies. Centers for Disease Control and Prevention. *MMWR* 1999;48:850.

cause convulsions, hypoxia, and cardiovascular collapse. Before starting a regional anesthetic for cesarean delivery, the anesthesiologist must be fully prepared to manage these potential complications. The anesthesia machine, laryngoscope, airways, endotracheal tubes, suction apparatus, monitoring equipment, and agents to induce general anesthesia and treat hypotension and other potential complications must be immediately available. Treatment of these complications is discussed in Chapters 5 and 8.

For some women, elective cesarean delivery is associated with anxiety and apprehension. More urgent, nonelective cesarean deliveries can exacerbate the concern a woman may have for the welfare of her baby and herself. In preparation for anesthesia and surgery, a compassionate, understanding, and professional demeanor by the anesthesiologist can significantly contribute to diminishing a woman's fear and worry. Although compassionate verbal reassurance is ordinarily sufficient before anesthetic administration, and sedative drugs are typically avoided until after delivery, some women may benefit from sedative medications.

Supplemental Medication for Anxiety

Treatment of maternal anxiety can facilitate performance of regional block and, with attainment of an adequate sensory level, provide the mother with a more pleasant delivery. Low doses of IV midazolam (0.5 to 4 mg), diazepam (2 to 8 mg), or an opioid (e.g., fentanyl 25 to 100 μg) can be used with minimal neonatal effects (22–24). However, amnesia, acceptable for a nonobstetric patient, may be undesirable for a woman undergoing cesarean delivery.

Table 11.1. COMMON INDICATIONS FOR CESAREAN SECTION

Previous section
Dystocia
Failure to progress
Malpresentation
Failure of induction
Fetal intolerance of labor
Fetal distress or nonreassuring fetal status
Prolapsed umbilical cord
Failed forceps or vacuum delivery
Hemorrhage
Placenta previa
Severe pregnancy-induced hypertension
Chorioamnionitis, herpes genitalis (active)
Breech presentation

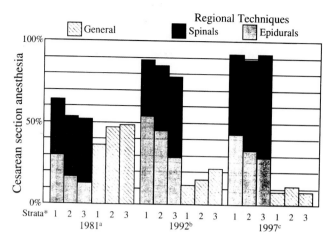

Figure 11.5. These data demonstrate the declining use of general anesthesia and the increasing use of regional anesthesia for cesarean section. Spinal anesthesia is increasingly used if an epidural has not been previously placed in labor. *a*: Gibbs CP, Krischer J, Peckham BM, Sharp H, Kirschbaum TH. Obstetric anesthesia: A national survey. *Anesthesiology* 1986;65:298–306. *b*: Hawkins JL, Gibbs CP, Orleans M, et al. Obstetric anesthesia work force study, 1981 versus 1992. *Anesthesiology* 1997;87:135–143. *c*: Hawkins JL, Beaty BR, Gibbs CP. Update on U.S. obstetric anesthesia practices [abstract]. *Anesthesiology* 1999;91:A1060. *Strata refer to size of delivery service. (Stratum I, >1500 births/year; Stratum II, 500–1499 births/year; Stratum III, <500 births/year.)

Antacid Administration

The hazards of aspiration pneumonitis and the use of oral antacids and other agents to minimize the likelihood and severity of aspiration are discussed fully in Chapter 22. Approximately 30% of women undergoing elective scheduled cesarean section will have significant amounts of acidic contents in their stomach unless they have received antacid within 1 hour before surgery (25). Because a small proportion of patients receiving a regional anesthetic will require a general anesthetic, we believe it is prudent to medicate **all** patients with a nonparticulate, oral antacid prior to cesarean section. The administration of an H$_2$-receptor antagonist or proton pump inhibitor can further reduce gastric

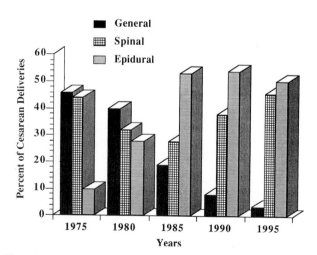

Figure 11.6. Type of anesthesia for cesarean delivery: The Brigham and Women's Hospital experience. Note the decreased use of general and increased used of epidural anesthesia. During 1975–95, cesarean sections under general anesthesia decreased from 46% to 3.6%. The popularity of spinal anesthesia gradually decreased, but recently its use has been increasing. (Modified from Ostheimer GW, ed. *Manual of Obstetric Anesthesia.* 2nd ed. London: Churchill Livingstone; 1992; and Tsen LC, Pitner WR, Camaan WR. General anesthesia for cesarean section at a tertiary care hospital 1990–1995: Indications and implications. *Int J Obstet Anesth* 1998;7:147–152.)

Table 11.2. TYPE OF ANESTHESIA USED FOR CESAREAN SECTION AT UNIVERSITY OF CALIFORNIA SAN FRANCISCO

| Year | Percentage of Total | | |
	Epidural (%)	Spinal (%)	General (%)
1985	83	1	16
1986	84	2	14
1987	84	1	15
1988	86	1	13
1989	82	4	14
1990	85	14	11
1991	67	19	14
1992	60	23	17
1993	59	25	16
1994	56	25	19
1995	55	28	17
1996	55	27	18
1997	49	31	20
1998	61	26	13
1999	59	28	13

During this 15-year period, the use of spinal anesthesia for cesarean section has significantly increased, but at this high-risk referral center, the need for general anesthesia has not declined.

acidity (26, 27), and the administration of metoclopramide perhaps accelerates gastric emptying, increases lower esophageal sphincter tone, and has an antiemetic effect (28).

Supplemental Oxygen

Parturients receiving a spinal or epidural anesthetic for cesarean delivery should be given supplemental oxygen. The use of nasal prongs or a clear plastic face mask is more acceptable to most parturients than an anesthesia face mask. The added maternal oxygen can increase fetal oxygenation. In healthy women undergoing elective cesarean section with a regional anesthetic, increasing inspired maternal oxygen concentrations from 21%

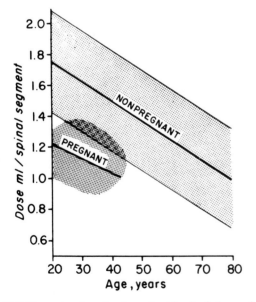

Figure 11.7. Regression lines for dose of epidural solution and age in nonpregnant women and in pregnant women at term. The gravida obviously requires much less drug. (Reprinted by permission from Bonica JJ, ed. *Principles and Practice of Obstetric Analgesia and Anesthesia.* Vol 1. Philadelphia: Davis; 1967:624; modification by Bonica JJ, from Bromage PR. Continuous lumbar epidural analgesia for obstetrics. *Can Med Assoc J* 1961;85:1136–1140.)

Table 11.3. COMPARISON OF SPREAD OF EPIDURAL ANESTHESIA IN PREGNANT AND NONPREGNANT WOMEN

	Volume of Bupivacaine 0.75% (mL)	Most Cephalad Thoracic Dermatome Anesthetized to Pinprick
Nonpregnant (n = 32)	15	5.7 ± 1.7
Pregnant (n = 60)	15	5.5 ± 1.2
Nonpregnant (n = 29)	20	4.7 ± 1.7
Pregnant (n = 29)	20	4.2 ± 1.5

Although bupivacaine 0.75% is no longer recommended for use in obstetrics, the findings in this study are still relevant.
Adapted from Grundy EM, Zamora AM, Winnie AP. Comparison of spread of epidural anesthesia in pregnant and nonpregnant women. *Anesth Analg* 1978;57:544–546.

to 100% resulted in an increase in umbilical venous Po_2 from 28 to 47 mm Hg and umbilical artery Po_2 from 15 to 25 mm Hg, respectively (Fig. 11.8) (29). The increased maternal oxygenation also provides additional maternal safety should complications of hypoventilation or hypotension occur. We routinely administer supplemental oxygen to increase maternal alveolar oxygen and maximize maternal oxygen saturation.

Prevention of Maternal Hypotension

Arterial hypotension is the most common immediate complication of spinal or epidural anesthesia for cesarean delivery. Pregnant women are particularly susceptible to hypotension following sympathetic blockade, an expected consequence of a regional block for cesarean section, either spinal or epidural. Most clinicians define hypotension as a decrease in systolic blood pressure greater than 25% from baseline values, or a systolic blood pressure less than 100 mm Hg.

Physiology of Hypotension. Hypotension results from sympathetic blockade, which decreases systemic vascular resistance and increases venous capacitance, resulting in peripheral venous pooling of blood and decreased cardiac preload (decreased central venous pressure and pulmonary artery occlusion pressure). The extent of preganglionic sympathetic fiber paralysis, which transmit motor impulses to smooth muscle of the arterial and venous vasculature, is related to the extent of the regional anesthetic. Consequently, the hemodynamic alterations following regional anesthesia vary with differing levels of regional blockade (Fig. 11.9) (30). The peripheral pooling of blood caused by sympathetic blockade to large veins and venules increases venous capacitance, decreases venous return to the heart and decreases cardiac output. However, cardiac output must increase to maintain blood pressure in compensation for the decrease in cardiac afterload.

Table 11.4. PREPARATION FOR REGIONAL ANESTHESIA FOR CESAREAN SECTION

1. Before starting the block, check resuscitation equipment and drugs:
   (a) oxygen delivery system and the anesthesia machine;
   (b) airways; (c) laryngoscope; (d) endotracheal tubes; (e) thiopental, propofol, or benzodiazepine for possible convulsion; (f) ephedrine for hypotension; and (g) suction apparatus.
2. Administer a nonparticulate oral antacid within 1 h of induction of anesthesia.
3. Transport the patient to the operating room with uterine displacement.
4. Measure baseline vital signs.
5. Administer intravenously 1000–2000 mL dextrose-free balanced salt solution rapidly.
6. Administer supplemental oxygen by facemask or nasal prongs.

Table 11.5. REGIONAL ANESTHESIA FOR CESAREAN SECTION: A SUGGESTED TECHNIQUE

Spinal anesthesia

Use small-gauge, pencil-point (noncutting) spinal needle.

Local anesthetic options:

1. Bupivacaine 12–15 mg (1.6–2 mL bupivacaine 0.75% in 8.25% dextrose)
2. Lidocaine 60–75 mg (1.2–1.5 mL lidocaine 5% in 7.5% glucose, diluted with equal volumes of CSF) (see Chapter 5) *or*
3. Tetracaine 8–10 mg hyperbaric tetracaine (0.8–1 mL 1% tetracaine with equal volumes of 10% dextrose in water)

Intrathecal opioid options—added to above local anesthetics

1. Fentanyl 10–25 μg (0.2–0.5 mL fentanyl 50 μg/mL solution)
2. Morphine 0.1–0.25 mg (0.2–0.5 mL preservative-free morphine, 5 mg/10 mL)
3. Both fentanyl and morphine in above doses

Epinephrine option—0.1–0.2 mg epinephrine may prolong and/or improve the quality of the block

Epidural anesthesia

Local anesthetic options:

1. 1.5–2.0% lidocaine
2. 0.5% bupivacaine
3. 3.0% 2-chloroprocaine

Epinephrine added to lidocaine at a concentration of 1:200,000.

Test Dose: Use a test dose that includes an adequate amount of local anesthetic to reliably detect intrathecal injection within 3–5 min administration, along with epinephrine 15 μg to detect intravascular injection. The authors prefer using lidocaine 45 mg with epinephrine 15 μg. Observe for heart rate increase within 60 sec or evidence of spinal blockade within 3–5 min. If test dose produces negative results, administer up to 20 mL local anesthetic in fractional increments of no more than 5 mL/30 sec. Inject additional drug as required through catheter to obtain sensory blockade up to fourth thoracic dermatome. Alternatively, if the local anesthetic is injected through the needle, an additional test dose should be administered through the catheter before its use.

pH adjustment options:

1. Add 1 mL (1 mEq) sodium bicarbonate (8.4%) to 10 mL lidocaine or chloroprocaine *or*
2. Add 0.1 mL (0.1 mEq) sodium bicarbonate to 20 mL bupivacaine

Epidural opioid options:

1. Fentany 50–100 μg or sufentanil 10–20 μg may be added to the local anesthetics to potentiate intraoperative analgesia.
2. Morphine 4–5 mg may be administered through the epidural catheter following delivery.

Position patient with left uterine displacement. Slight (10-degree) Trendelenburg tilt may improve venous return.

Monitor blood pressure every minute for first 20 min, then every 5 min for duration of surgery.

Monitor ECG and oxygen saturation.

CSF = cerebrospinal fluid; ECG = electrocardiogram.

Quantitative differences exist among the data of detailed circulatory mechanisms from various studies of spinal anesthesia (31). In general, reductions occur in arterial resistance, stroke volume, heart rate, cardiac output, and arterial blood pressure. Decreased vascular tone in the venous capacitance vessels is a primary factor for arterial hypotension induced by spinal anesthesia. Decreased resistance in pre- and postcapillary resistance vessels (arterial and postarteriolar circulation) appears to be a secondary factor for arterial hypotension in studies of human volunteers and patients (32).

There are differences in the vasodilation of the arterial circulation compared to the venous circulation induced by regional anesthetic sympathectomy. For areas affected, this is limited to no residual venous tone following sympathetic denervation.

Table 11.6. MANAGEMENT OF COMPLICATIONS OF REGIONAL ANESTHESIA FOR CESAREAN SECTION

1. If systolic blood pressure rapidly falls, or falls by 30% or below 100 mm Hg, ensure left uterine displacement and increase IV infusion rate. If blood pressure is not rapidly restored, administer 10–15 mg ephedrine IV; repeat if necessary.
2. Treat anxiety and incomplete or "spotty" anesthesia, if necessary, with one or more of the following agents prior to delivery of the infant: (a) 1–2 mg midazolam; (b) fentanyl up to 1 mg · kg^{-1} IV; (c) 40% nitrous oxide (by mask); (d) 0.25 mg · kg^{-1} ketamine IV; (e) 10–20 mL 0.5% lidocaine intraperitoneally.
3. If analgesia is inadequate, proceed to general anesthesia with endotracheal intubation.
4. If supplementation to spinal or epidural blockade is necessary after delivery, administer small doses of IV opioids, *or*
5. Metoclopramide (10 mg IV), droperidol (0.5 mg IV), ondansetron (4 mg IV), or dolasetron (12.5 mg IV) may be administered to reduce the likelihood of nausea and vomiting.

IV = intravenous.

However, arterial and arteriolar vasodilation, which follows sympathetic denervation, is rarely maximal in affected areas. These vessels maintain some intrinsic tone, probably due to the simultaneous paralysis of vasodilator sympathetic fibers. Of course, depending on the level of the regional anesthetic, compensatory reflex vasoconstriction takes place in those parts where the sympathetic nerves are unaffected, initiated by a decrease in blood pressure acting on receptors in the carotid sinus and aortic arch.

Prophylactic Treatment for Hypotension. The authors reviewed results of 583 consecutive cesarean sections performed under epidural anesthesia at the University of California San Francisco (UCSF) (33). The overall incidence of hypotension was 29%. Hypotension occurred more frequently in women not in labor (36%) than in those who were in labor (24%) (Fig 11.10) (33). With prehydration and uterine displacement, intramuscular (IM) prophylactic ephedrine administered 15 minutes

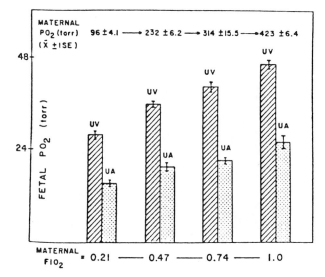

Figure 11.8. Histograms showing umbilical vein (*UV*) and umbilical artery (*UA*) Po_2 levels at different maternal levels of Fio_2. Maternal Pao_2 levels at four levels of Fio_2 are shown at top. Values are mean ± 1 SE (n = 10). (Reprinted by permission from Ramanathan S, Gandhi S, Arismendy J, Chalon J, Turndorf H. Oxygen transfer from mother to fetus during cesarean section under epidural anesthesia. *Anesth Analg* 1982;61:576–581.)

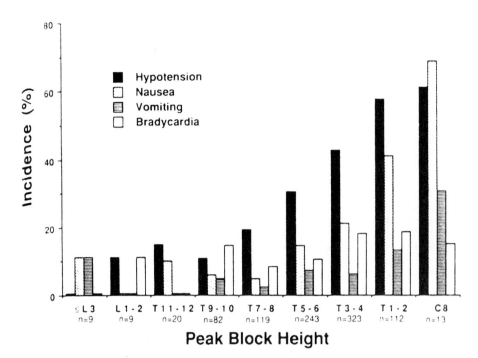

Figure 11.9. Incidence of hypotension, nausea, vomiting, and bradycardia in relation to the peak sensory block height during spinal anesthesia. Increasing sensory block height correlated with an increasing incidence of hypotension ($P = .0001$), nausea ($P = .0001$), vomiting ($P = .001$), and bradycardia ($P = .03$). (Reprinted by permission from Carpenter R, Caplan R, Brown D, et al. Incidence and risk factors for side effects of spinal anesthesia. *Anesthesiology* 1992;76:906–912.)

before the block did not appear to provide additional protection against hypotension. In all cases, maternal hypotension was promptly recognized and treated, and umbilical cord blood gas values and newborns were not affected by maternal hypotension.

While the use of prophylactic ephedrine to prevent hypotension has not been demonstrated to be useful in epidural anesthesia, it was thought that this would not be true for spinal anesthesia, where the onset of the sympathetic block is widely considered to be more rapid (34, 35).

Measures employed to reduce the incidence and severity of maternal hypotension associated with spinal or epidural anesthesia for cesarean delivery include (1) patient positioning to avoid aortocaval compression and promote cardiac preload; (2) prehydration to expand blood volume, increase cardiac preload, and thereby avoid the sudden decreases in cardiac preload; and (3) prophylactic or immediate use of appropriate vasopressors. Leg elevation and/or compressive leg wrapping (36) and the use of colloid or dextran rather than crystalloid

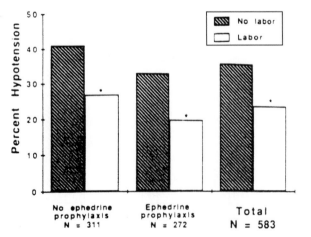

Figure 11.10. The incidence of hypotension divided according to the presence or absence of labor and the use of intramuscular prophylactic ephedrine. Single asterisk (*) indicates significant difference between nonlaboring and laboring mothers ($P < .05$). (Reprinted by permission from Brizgys RV, Dailey PA, Shnider SM, Kotelko DM, Levinson G. The incidence and neonatal effects of maternal hypotension during epidural anesthesia for cesarean section. *Anesthesiology* 1987;67:782–786.)

for prehydration (37–39) are additional measures currently not widely practiced.

PATIENT POSITIONING. When the parturient lies in the supine position after a regional anesthetic, her gravid uterus compresses the inferior vena cava and further decreases venous return to the heart. With sympathetic blockade she may not be able to compensate adequately for the venous obstruction. A decrease in blood pressure is associated with a comparable decrease in uterine blood flow and placental perfusion, and may lead to fetal hypoxia and acidosis. Therefore, the patient should not be permitted to lie in the supine position either in transit to the operating room or after the block is performed. After regional blockade, the patient should be positioned with left uterine displacement (LUD) to prevent aortocaval compression.

The Trendelenburg position may be useful in increasing venous return. It is speculated that head-down tilt can increase cardiac output by increasing venous return. However, studies have questioned the benefit of this simple maneuver. Investigators were unable to demonstrate a beneficial effect from 15-degree head-down tilt for 10 minutes immediately after spinal block with 3 mL hyperbaric 0.5% bupivacaine (with no effect on the lowest value of the systolic blood pressure) (40). In another study, head-down tilt of 10 degrees was useful only when systemic blood pressure had decreased by more than 30% from control values (41). Prophylactic head-down tilt resulted in a higher cephalad spread of analgesia but did not result in a reduced incidence of hypotension (41).

PREHYDRATION. Crystalloid administration by IV infusion shortly before inducing a regional anesthetic has been a mainstay of therapy to minimize the incidence and severity of hypotension, based on favorable previous studies (42). IV infusions for increasing cardiac preload should not contain dextrose, to prevent maternal and fetal hyperglycemia and subsequent neonatal hyperinsulinemia and hypoglycemia.

The value of crystalloid administration in increasing cardiac preload and reducing the incidence or severity of hypotension associated with spinal anesthesia has been questioned. In one study, patients undergoing elective cesarean section were randomized to receive no prehydration or 20 mL · kg^{-1} crystalloid over 15 to 20 minutes before spinal anesthesia. The incidence of hypotension was 55% among the women who received prehydration compared with 71% among the women who did not (43). Numerous studies using both crystalloid prehydration and uterine displacement have failed to completely eliminate hypotension as a consequence of spinal anesthesia for cesarean section.

Crystalloid preloading decreases but does not eliminate the incidence of hypotension. The increase in central venous pressure is probably transient due to a relatively short intravascular half-life of crystalloid, with rapid extravascular equilibration (44–46, 48). Crystalloid administration is probably benign for the majority of healthy pregnant women. However, it can be potentially unsafe for some, as the volumes advocated by some authorities have increased from 1000 to 1500 mL, to 30 mL · kg^{-1} and more, further decreasing colloid osmotic pressure, which decreases postpartum, and increases the risk of pulmonary edema.

It has been demonstrated that colloid may be superior for volume preloading (47, 48), by sustaining an increased blood volume, cardiac preload, and cardiac output, due to a longer intravascular half-life. However, despite volume expansion with colloid great enough to result in a significant increase in cardiac output, the incidence of hypotension associated with spinal anesthesia is not eliminated (48). Furthermore, colloid is expensive, may increase the risk of pulmonary edema after delivery with the autotransfusion of blood from the contracted uterus, and has a (small) risk of inducing an anaphylactoid reaction.

Perhaps volume replacement is not the most effective compensation for the preload reduction induced by spinal anesthesia. Leg wrapping after spinal anesthesia injection may be more successful. The beneficial effects of leg wrapping and simple leg elevation were differentiated in studies that determined a reduced incidence of hypotension (18% vs. 53%) that resulted only when the legs were wrapped, not simply elevated (39%) (36, 49). The efficacy of pneumatic compression devices on the lower extremities to prevent hypotension during spinal anesthesia for cesarean section revealed a reduced incidence of hypotension to 48% vs. 83% in the control group (50). However, use of leg wrapping or pneumatic compression techniques is labor intensive and not widely practiced.

VASOPRESSORS. Following institution of the block, the patient's blood pressure should be monitored every minute for the first 20 minutes and then every 5 minutes for the duration of surgery. Some anesthesiologists monitor blood pressure every minute until the baby is born. If hypotension occurs (either a systolic pressure of less than 100 mm Hg or a fall of 30% from preanesthetic levels), LUD should be increased and fluids rapidly infused. If hypotension is not corrected within 30 to 60 seconds, a dose of ephedrine (5 to 15 mg intravenously) should be administered.

Ephedrine is the vasopressor most commonly used for spinal or epidural anesthetic-induced maternal hypotension among patients undergoing cesarean section. This is based on ephedrine's combined α- and β-mimetic effects, which do not cause uterine vasoconstriction (see Fig. 2.18) (51, 52). Pure α-agonists have traditionally been avoided due to concern about their effects on uterine blood flow. In the experimental animal, ephedrine restores uterine blood flow toward normal when used to treat spinal hypotension. Prophylactic ephedrine has no adverse effect on uterine blood flow (see Fig. 2.19) (53, 54). Animal model studies have shown that methoxamine, phenylephrine, angiotensin, and levarterenol do not preserve uterine blood flow when used to treat hypotension following spinal anesthesia, and result in fetal hypoxemia (52). Ephedrine, mephentermine, and metaraminol improve uterine blood flow, but only ephedrine as a prophylactic infusion did not decrease uterine blood flow. Furthermore, ephedrine, but not phenylephrine, improves venous return in an animal model of spinal anesthesia (55).

In animal studies, pregnancy is associated with decreases in the efficacy of a variety of vasopressors on the uterine artery, but without consistent changes in the carotid artery (56). Differential sensitivity of the vasoconstricting action of adrenergic agents during pregnancy has been confirmed in laboratory studies of vascular endothelial rings (57). Pregnancy enhances vasocon-

strictor efficacy for both metaraminol and ephedrine in femoral vascular endothelial rings, and decreases constriction in uterine vascular endothelial arterial rings. However, the ratio of contraction produced at the femoral vs. the uterine endothelial rings during pregnancy was greater for ephedrine than metaraminol. Ephedrine appears to spare uterine perfusion during pregnancy due to more selective constriction of systemic vasculature compared with uterine vasculature, with more effectiveness than metaraminol (57).

Phenylephrine has been safely used for treatment of maternal hypotension due to epidural anesthesia for cesarean section (58). In a comparison of phenylephrine and ephedrine for prevention of maternal hypotension following spinal anesthesia for cesarean delivery, phenylephrine was found to be as effective as ephedrine and appeared to have no adverse neonatal effects (35).

Doppler velocimetry has been used to study the clinical effects of IV vasopressors on the maternal uterine and placental arcuate arteries, and the fetal umbilical, renal, and middle cerebral arteries during spinal anesthesia (59, 60). Fetal myocardial function was assessed by M-mode echocardiography. Comparisons were made of ephedrine to phenylephrine in a randomized study design, with both agents used as a prophylactic infusion supplemented with small boluses for systolic blood pressures that decreased by more than 10 mm Hg from baseline. Ephedrine infusions had no significant impact on Doppler velocimetry recordings. However, phenylephrine infusions significantly increased the uterine and placental arcuate arteries' blood flow velocity waveform indices and decreased vascular resistance in the fetal renal arteries. Despite these observations, no differences were found among the neonates between the two groups, suggesting tolerance among healthy fetuses (59). To date, studies have not evaluated the effects of ephedrine vs. phenylephrine among women whose fetuses are compromised by hypotension.

The authors recommend ephedrine administration for treatment of hypotension resulting from regional anesthesia for cesarean delivery. Various techniques of ephedrine administration have been used, studied, and reported, including prophylactic IM injection or IV bolus administration, prophylactic IV infusion, and immediate use at onset of hypotension. The efficacy and incidence of side effects (including reactive hypertension), the unpredictable absorption by the IM route, and the potential for adverse neonatal outcome have been studied (34, 61–65).

Recommendations. The authors recommend minimizing the incidence and/or severity of hypotension associated with regional anesthesia for cesarean section by (1) avoiding aortocaval compression by the gravid uterus; (2) providing adequate volume as a preload (when possible) to establish mild hypervolemia, but avoiding excessive fluid bolus volumes; (3) administering ephedrine by prophylactic IV bolus or promptly when systolic blood pressure begins to decrease; (4) using leg elevation and Trendelenburg positioning for moderate or severe hypotension; (5) ensuring immediate availability of phenylephrine for hypotension unresolved by appropriate doses of ephedrine; and (6) ensuring immediate availability of epinephrine for unresolving severe hypotension associated with bradycardia.

Prevention of Postdural Puncture Headache

One of the most annoying complications of spinal anesthesia or accidental dural puncture during attempted epidural anesthesia is PDPH. This subject is discussed in Chapter 23 and is briefly reviewed below.

Using the smallest needle possible can minimize the incidence of PDPH (66–87). Insertion of the needle with the bevel parallel to the longitudinal fibers of the dura appears to produce a smaller rent and a lower incidence of headache. The microscopic arrangement of dural fibers probably minimizes the size of the dural hole if the needle bevel is directed parallel to the

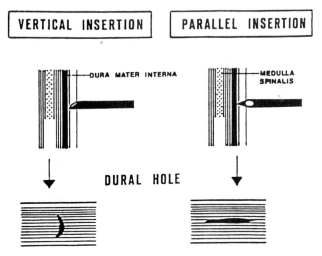

Figure 11.11. Types of needle insertion by lumbar punctures. In vertical vs. parallel insertion, the bevel of the spinal needle is inserted through the dura mater interna perpendicular to (vs. parallel to) the longitudinal dural fibers. The number of severed dural fibers is greater by vertical insertion. (Reprinted by permission from Mihic DN. Post-dural headache and relationship of needle bevel to longitudinal dural fibers. *Reg Anesth* 1985;10:76–81.)

longitudinal axis of the vertebral column (Fig. 11.11) (88). A study in which patients were assigned to either parallel or perpendicular insertion of the spinal needle bevel found a highly significant reduction in the incidence of headache if parallel insertion was employed (89). Similarly, with epidural needles, the incidence of headache after accidental dural puncture was significantly lower with parallel insertion of the needle (90).

"Pencil-point" needles (Fig. 11.12), which spread rather than cut dural fibers, are associated with a lower incidence of spinal headache (75, 79, 91–94). The Whitacre needle has a conical-

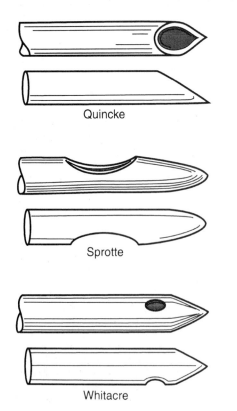

Figure 11.12. Comparison of Quincke point (*top*), Sprotte (*center*), and Whitacre (*bottom*) needles.

shaped solid tip with a lateral eye. The Sprotte needle has an oval-shaped solid tip and a lateral opening that is larger than the Whitacre. Both needles come in various sizes, ranging from 22 to 27 gauge. The 22-gauge needles are firmer and easier to insert than the smaller ones, which usually require an introducer. However, as with the cutting needle, larger sizes produce more headaches.

Based on an in vitro study, it has been postulated that, if the dura mater is punctured at an acute angle, the resulting holes in the dura and arachnoid would not be opposed, creating a flap valve that would reduce fluid leak (80). However, two randomized, prospective trials comparing the incidence of spinal headache between the midline and paramedian approach failed to validate this hypothesis (95, 96).

Subarachnoid Block: Anesthetic Solutions

The most popular drugs for spinal anesthesia for cesarean section are bupivacaine 0.75% in dextrose 8.25%, and lidocaine 5% in glucose 7.5%. Lidocaine rapidly produces a profound sensory and motor block usually lasting 45 to 75 minutes. For cesarean section with speedy surgeons, this agent is ideal. However more dilute solutions of lidocaine (1.5%) are increasingly used (Chapter 5, Table 5.6). For most cesarean, sections bupivacaine is appropriate. For unusually long cesarean sections, tetracaine 1% mixed with dextrose with epinephrine may be necessary. The effect of the addition of epinephrine to bupivacaine or lidocaine solutions is controversial, with some investigators claiming no clinically useful purpose (97), and others finding improved and prolonged sensory and motor block (98, 99). Clonidine has also been shown to improve intraoperative analgesia when added to bupivacaine and fentanyl, but may increase sedation (100, 101).

A number of reports have indicated that bupivacaine is superior to tetracaine in that it has a faster onset, has a lesser motor block (102), produces fewer failed blocks (99), and results in greater patient satisfaction (98). These findings, however, are debated by others (103, 104). Nonetheless, bupivacaine has become the spinal local anesthetic of choice.

Several studies have evaluated the subarachnoid spread of hyperbaric bupivacaine in the term parturient (105–107). Initially, Norris et al. chose a uniform dose of 12 mg to administer to 50 parturients (105), and in a subsequent study 15 mg was used (106). In these studies, it was apparent that it was *not* necessary to vary the dose of injected hyperbaric bupivacaine according to the patient's age, height, weight, body mass, or vertebral column length. For either dose, these variables did not affect the level of anesthesia. For very reliable blocks, many anesthesiologists are using the larger dose of 15 mg (108). This dose will produce a high level of sensory block (up to T2), with occasional patients showing analgesic levels of C2 (Fig. 11.13). The Trendelenburg position (10 degrees) may be important to ensure adequate venous return, but care must be taken that the drug does not spread cephalad to the medullary respiratory center. Lower doses of bupivacaine (9 mg) have been reported to be successful, but the combined spinal-epidural (CSE) technique was used (109).

Fentanyl, sufentanil, and morphine have been administered into the subarachnoid space immediately before, after, or combined with local anesthetic administration of hyperbaric bupivacaine 0.5% and 0.75%. Subarachnoid fentanyl in doses of 6.25 μg or greater significantly increases the duration and intensity of analgesia (110). In another report, intrathecal fentanyl (10 μg) added to bupivacaine (12.5 mg) did not significantly improve the quality of the spinal anesthetic (111). High doses (37.5 to 60 μg) do not clearly provide additional prolongation of analgesia, but do increase the incidence of side effects, notably pruritus (112). However, no respiratory depression was reported in patients for cesarean section, even with 60 μg. Improved intraoperative analgesia is achieved in the authors' view with a low

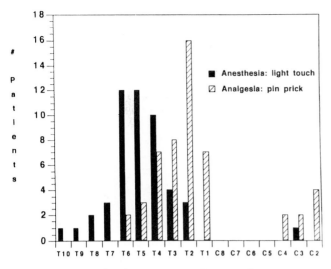

Figure 11.13. Maximum cephalad extent of analgesia to pin prick and anesthesia to light touch in 52 term parturients following subarachnoid injection of 15 mg hyperbaric bupivacaine and 0.15 mg morphine. (Adapted from Norris MC. Patient variables and the subarachnoid spread of hyperbaric bupivacaine in the term patient. *Anesthesiology* 1990;72:478–482.)

incidence of side effects with fentanyl 10 to 25 μg, although this remains controversial (112). Subarachnoid sufentanil 10 to 20 μg mixed with 10.5 mg hyperbaric bupivacaine 0.75% has also been demonstrated to improve intraoperative analgesia (113). In another study, the addition of intrathecal sufentanil (2.5 or 5 μg) to bupivacaine (12.5 mg) significantly increased the duration of the spinal blockade for cesarean section (114). However, only morphine produces a clinically relevant reduction in postoperative pain and analgesic consumption (112).

Subarachnoid morphine in doses of 0.1 to 0.25 mg combined with 0.75% hyperbaric bupivacaine improves intraoperative analgesia and prolongs postoperative pain relief (18 to 27 hours), with minor side effects such as pruritus and nausea and vomiting (115–118). A recent study failed to find the effective dose of intrathecal morphine for pain relief after cesarean delivery (119), while another study suggested that there is little justification for the use of more than 0.1 mg for postcesarean analgesia (120). However, doses of 0.1 to 0.25 mg intrathecal morphine are most commonly used. Even morphine (0.1 mg) administered into the subarachnoid space achieves significant CSF concentrations and good analgesia, but has the potential for rostral spread, resulting in late respiratory depression (121). Close monitoring to avoid respiratory depression and related side effects is necessary.

Epidural Anesthesia: Anesthetic Solutions

The use of epidural anesthesia for cesarean section has increased, most likely due to the increased use of epidurals for labor analgesia. In contrast to spinal blockade, local anesthetics primarily affect nerve roots rather than spinal cord, and the distribution of the regional block is volume dependent. Epidural anesthesia requires large doses of local anesthesia, which crosses the placenta and potentially affects the fetus and neonate. This subject is discussed extensively in Chapters 4 and 5.

The commonly used epidural local anesthetics for cesarean section include lidocaine (1.5% to 2%), bupivacaine (0.5%), ropivacaine (0.5% to 0.75%), and 2-chloroprocaine (3%). Each has advantages and potential disadvantages, and differs in speed of onset and duration of action. 2-Chloroprocaine has the most rapid onset and shortest duration. Bupivacaine has the slowest onset and the longest duration. Bupivacaine 0.5% is effective for

Table 11.7. CONTENTS (mg/mL) OF TWO SOLUTIONS OF 2-CHLOROPROCAINE

	Astra Nesacaine® 2%*	Astra Preservative-Free Nesacaine-MPF® 3%*
Chloroprocaine	20	30
Na-Metabisulfite or Bisulfite	—	—
Sodium chloride	4.7	3.3
Disodium EDTA	0.11	—
Methylparaben	1	—
pH	2.7–4.0	2.7–4.0

* Nesacaine® is prepared as 1% and 2% solutions, which are *not* used for lumbar or caudal blocks. They may be used to produce local anesthesia by infiltration and peripheral nerve block. Nesacaine-MPF® is preservative free and without EDTA and is indicated for epidural block. It is supplied in 2% and 3% solutions. Data from *Physicians Desk Reference.* Montvale, NJ: Medical Economics Co Inc; 1999.

cesarean section anesthesia, but in addition to the very slow onset, some authors find the block not dense enough. The 0.75% concentration has a faster onset and provides better surgical conditions, but because of the cardiac arrests associated with its accidental intravascular injection, this concentration is no longer recommended for use in obstetrics.

2-Chloroprocaine 3% rapidly produces profound anesthesia and is a good choice for cesarean section anesthesia. 2-Chloroprocaine is useful for cesarean section because of its rapid onset of surgical anesthesia. This characteristic, in addition to its short half-life in both maternal and fetal serum, makes this an attractive local anesthetic for situations of fetal distress and the need for urgent cesarean section. Earlier, more acidic preparations that contained high concentrations of the antioxidant sodium bisulfite were considered neurotoxic (122, 123). Preparations that contained disodium EDTA (Table 11.7) were reported to cause severe paralumbar muscle pain (124–126). This has been postulated to be muscle spasm resulting from acute lowering of tissue calcium due to active chelation by the sodium salts of EDTA. Current preparations of 2-chloroprocaine contain no antioxidant or preservative.

There are other potential problems with 2-chloroprocaine. The rapid onset of the block may be associated with a higher incidence of hypotension (127). 2-Chloroprocaine may interfere with the efficacy of subsequent epidural opioids or bupivacaine (128–132). This does not appear to be an effect of pH (128, 133), but may be due to a metabolite of 2-chloroprocaine.

The authors routinely use lidocaine 2%, and add epinephrine (1:200,000) just before administration. This will contain less antioxidant and has a higher pH than commercially prepared solutions.

Test Dose

Aspiration through the epidural needle or catheter is a fundamental aspect of a testing regimen. However, if aspiration fails to reveal CSF or blood, it does not preclude intravascular or subarachnoid location. Therefore, the anesthesiologist must test dose before administering the full therapeutic dose of local anesthetic, which would be harmful if accidentally administered to the blood or CSF. The test dose must contain an amount of local anesthetic sufficient to produce a perceptible, but safe spinal block if injected into the subarachnoid space. This dose is usually too small to allow recognition of an intravascular injection; thus, either a second test dose with a larger local anesthetic dose can be administered, or epinephrine (15 to 20 μg) can be added to the first test dose of local anesthetic. The larger dose of local anesthetic, if IV, will likely produce suggestive symptoms.

Epinephrine, if IV, likely will produce a rapid acceleration in heart rate of about 20 to 30 beats per minute within 30 seconds. When equivocal, repeat test dose after a negative aspiration can be very useful. Some clinicians object to the use of epinephrine as a test dose because of its unreliability among obstetric patients in labor, whose heart rate may not be stable, and possible adverse effects on uterine blood flow. Controversy regarding the preferred test dose has been discussed fully in Chapter 8.

When using a continuous catheter technique, the authors recommend test doses be given through the catheter prior to a therapeutic dose and before reinforcing doses because epidural catheters have been reported to migrate into the CSF, or into an epidural vein. Finally, since no test dose regimen is fully sensitive or specific, the full therapeutic dose of local anesthetic should be administered slowly in fractional, incremental doses rather than by rapid bolus injection, while carefully observing for adverse effects of intrathecal injection or systemic toxicity.

Epinephrine

Epinephrine is frequently added to local anesthetics to decrease systemic absorption and peak blood levels, intensify the motor block, prolong the duration of the anesthetic, and increase the intensity of sensory block (134–137). Some have avoided epinephrine in obstetrics, concerned that the α-adrenergic effects of epinephrine may decrease uterine blood flow, and that its β-mimetic effects may decrease maternal blood pressure, decrease uterine activity, and prolong labor (138–145). Absorbed epinephrine from the epidural space probably does not have significant effects on uterine blood flow (146–148). In pregnant ewes, epidural epinephrine (100 μg) did not decrease uterine blood flow (147). Epidural anesthesia with epinephrine 1:200,000 did not alter human intervillous blood flow (148).

The β-mimetic effects of systemically absorbed epinephrine have been shown to minimally decrease blood pressure, decrease uterine contractility, and prolong labor (140–144). For labor analgesia, the addition of epinephrine (except for the test dose) is unnecessary and can be avoided due to the small amounts of drug used, the lack of need for an intense motor block, or for prolonging a continuous infusion. For cesarean delivery, since larger doses of local anesthetic are used and more intense motor and sensory block is desired, the addition of epinephrine 1:200,000 can be advantageous.

Alkalinization of Local Anesthetics

Alkalinization of local anesthetic solutions has been advocated to speed the onset, prolong the duration, and intensify the quality of epidural local anesthetic blockade. As pH increases, the proportion of the nonionized lipid-soluble form of the local anesthetic increases; therefore, the drug should be more quickly available at the site of action. Clinical studies have shown that alkalinization of lidocaine is effective (149, 150), but studies of 2-chloroprocaine and bupivacaine have been contradictory (151–156). The onset of anesthesia (loss of sensation to tetanic stimulation at L2) in patients undergoing cesarean section or orthopedic procedures with pH-adjusted epidural lidocaine (1.5%) has been studied (149). Three pH values of lidocaine were studied: 4.55, 6.35, and 7.20. The onset of anesthesia was significantly more rapid in the higher pH groups (Fig. 11.14). A potential side effect of pH-adjusted local anesthetics is a higher incidence of hypotension subsequent to the more rapid onset of epidural anesthesia. A larger decrease in blood pressure was found in patients who received pH-adjusted 2% lidocaine for epidural anesthesia for cesarean section when compared with those who received the commercial preparation (Fig. 11.15) (157). Hypotension also developed more quickly in these patients. Possible adverse effects of hypotension on uteroplacental blood flow suggest that alkalinized lidocaine be used with caution in high-risk obstetric patients.

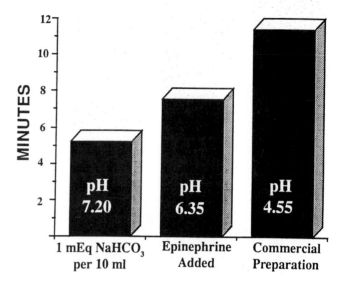

Figure 11.14. Times for onset of surgical anesthesia as measured with a nerve stimulator and the pH of the lidocaine epidural solution used. The patients received either a commercial preparation of lidocaine with epinephrine 1:200,000 (pH 4.55), plain lidocaine to which epinephrine was added to a final concentration of 1:200,000 (pH 6.35), or a commercially prepared solution of lidocaine with epinephrine 1:200,000 plus 1 mEq NaHCO₃ added per 10 mL solution (pH 7.20). (Modified with permission from DiFazio CA. Comparison of pH-adjusted lidocaine solutions for epidural anesthesia. *Anesth Analg* 1986;65:760–764.)

The usual recommended recipes are to add 2 mL 8.4% bicarbonate solution to 20 mL lidocaine or 2-chloroprocaine and 0.1 to 20 mL bupivacaine (158). If excess bicarbonate is added, precipitation may occur. This is especially true with bupivacaine, for which the margin of error is very small. Visible precipitation has been noted after only 0.2 mL 7.5% bicarbonate (0.18 mEq) was added to 30 mL 0.5% bupivacaine (159).

Epidural Opioids

Epidural fentanyl (50 to 100 μg) has been found to potentiate intraoperative analgesia (160–163), decrease nausea and vomiting

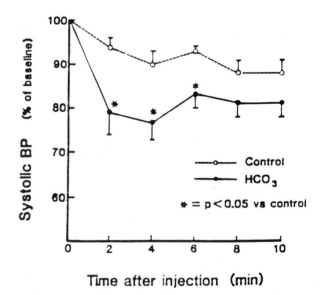

Figure 11.15. Time course of average systolic blood pressure (*BP*) readings (mean ± SEM) expressed as a percentage of the baseline value. (Reprinted by permission from Parnass SM, Curran MJA, Becker GL. Incidence of hypotension associated with epidural anesthesia using alkalinized and nonalkalinized lidocaine for cesarean section. *Anesth Analg* 1987;66:1148–1150.)

during uterine manipulation (161), and decrease requirements for supplemental opioid medication (162, 163) with no adverse maternal (160–163) or neonatal effects (163–165). Several studies have evaluated the neonatal respiratory rates and neurobehavioral status following epidural fentanyl (100 μg) used before the infant was delivered at cesarean section and have found no adverse effects (166–168). Larger doses have been given during epidural infusions for labor (53 to 400 μg or a mean of 184 μg) and had no adverse effect on neonatal ventilation or neurobehavioral scores (164–168).

The volume of diluent used with epidural fentanyl can affect its efficacy. Volumes greater than 10 mL appear to be necessary to provide complete analgesia (164). Other investigators who studied epidural meperidine (25 mg) found no difference in the effects of a 5 or 10 mL volume of diluent (169).

The addition of sufentanil (20 to 30 μg) to 0.5% bupivacaine with epinephrine 1:200,000 produced significantly better intraoperative anesthesia and longer postoperative analgesia compared with bupivacaine alone, with minimal maternal side effects and no adverse neonatal effects (170). The anesthetic potency of epidural sufentanil to epidural fentanyl is approximately 5:1, and when equianalgesic doses are administered there is no difference in onset, quality, or duration of analgesia (171, 172). The rapid onset of epidural sufentanil may be very helpful when acute pain relief is required (173). However, the systemic uptake of both fentanyl and sufentanil after epidural administration is significant, and its suitability as a neuraxial drug is questioned. Several studies suggest that the plasma concentrations achieved with epidural fentanyl are responsible for the postoperative analgesia achieved (see Chapter 9) (174, 175).

Epidural morphine is widely used to provide postoperative cesarean section analgesia. Five milligrams epidural morphine provides effective, safe, and prolonged (24-hour) analgesia after cesarean delivery with only mild and easily treatable side effects (176). In a prospective study of 1000 patients given 5 mg epidural morphine (177), it was found that 85% obtained good to excellent postoperative analgesia lasting 23 hours. Sixteen percent required no additional analgesia before discharge, and 44% required only oral analgesics. Side effects included moderate to severe pruritus (29%) and nausea or vomiting (20%), and one patient had severe respiratory depression (0.1%) that responded promptly to oxygen and IV naloxone. A later Canadian retrospective study of nearly 5000 patients confirmed these results (178). The patients received 2 to 5 mg epidural morphine with a mean duration of 23 hours. In another study, an attempt at determining an optimal dose suggested that no benefit was gained above 3.75 mg (179). The authors commonly use 4 to 5 mg epidural morphine. In our initial study of 1000 patients, all of whom had adequate epidurals for cesarean section, 5.9% had no or poor analgesia with 5.0 mg epidural morphine, requiring additional analgesics. If the dose of epidural morphine is decreased below 3 to 4 mg, the clinician can expect increasing demands for additional analgesia in the postoperative period (178). Studies of potential respiratory depression following the use of epidural morphine compared to IM morphine or patient-controlled analgesia (PCA) following cesarean section have been performed by a number of investigators (180–184). Although mild decreases in oxygen saturation have been seen, no maternal morbidity has been reported. In the review by Fuller et al. (178), there were 12 cases of respiratory depression (respiratory rate <10) noted by routine nursing observation with no adverse outcomes, which is similar to our experience at UCSF. It appears that all routes of opioid administration have depressant effects upon respiratory effort when given for postoperative pain (IV, IM, or intraspinal) (181). Thus, these reports (177, 178) and others (185, 186) confirm the efficacy of epidural morphine for analgesia after cesarean section and other surgeries, and suggest that its use is safe when basic monitoring criteria are rigidly followed and treatment is expeditiously instituted.

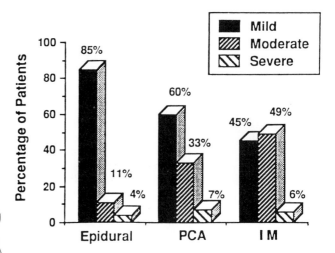

Figure 11.16. Postcesarean section pain relief. Amount of pain. (Modified with permission from Harrison DM, Sinatra R, Morgese L, Chung JH. Epidural narcotic and patient-controlled analgesia for post-cesarean section pain relief. *Anesthesiology* 1988;68:454–457.)

Epidural morphine (3 to 5 mg) is often combined with fentanyl (25 to 50 μg) or sufentanil (10 to 25 μg) to achieve a rapid onset and prolonged duration of analgesia. This may provide improved intraoperative analgesia as well (187). Epidural morphine has been compared to PCA for postoperative pain relief. Both provide excellent analgesia (87–89, 184, 188, 189), epidural morphine more so than PCA (Fig. 11.16) (184, 188). PCA produces more sedation (Fig. 11.17), and epidural morphine more pruritus (Fig. 11.18) (189). Patient-controlled epidural analgesia is used in some centers. Numerous drugs (with variable techniques or "recipes") have been used, to include morphine (190), meperidine (191), fentanyl (192), and sufentanil (193). While these techniques have proven effective, they are not used commonly for postoperative analgesia after cesarean section. Finally, the use of epidural morphine for postcesarean section pain relief appears to be safe for the neonate who breastfeeds (194). With either epidural or intrathecal morphine for postoperative pain relief, the newborn is exposed to a significantly smaller dose of opioids than with IM and IV opioids.

Dosage

In the pregnant woman, the dose of local anesthetic required to achieve a given level with spinal anesthesia is approximately 50% to 70% of the dose required for nonpregnant women (14, 16). With epidural anesthesia, some authors have reported

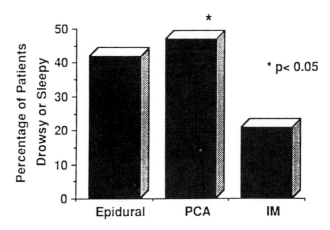

Figure 11.17. Postcesarean section pain relief. Incidence of sedation. (Modified with permission from Harrison DM, Sinatra R, Morgese L, Chung JH. Epidural narcotic and patient-controlled analgesia for post-cesarean section pain relief. *Anesthesiology* 1988;68:454–457.)

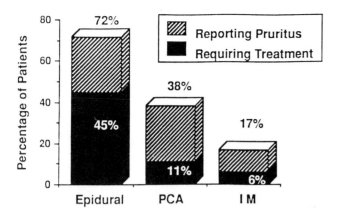

Figure 11.18. Postcesarean section pain relief. Incidence of pruritus. (Modified with permission from Harrison DM, Sinatra R, Morgese L, Chung JH. Epidural narcotic and patient-controlled analgesia for postcesarean section pain relief. *Anesthesiology* 1988;68:454–457.)

that dose requirements are also reduced (Fig. 11.7) (15, 16). On the other hand, other studies suggest that with equal amounts of local anesthetic, there is no significant difference in sensory levels in pregnant and nonpregnant patients (Table 11.3) (17). Clinical observation suggests that it is difficult to establish a higher segmental level of anesthesia with additional incremental epidural doses of local anesthetic after administration of a large dose of local anesthetic. Animal data reveal neural susceptibility to blockade is enhanced during pregnancy (195, 196). This has been corroborated in a study of median nerve blocks comparing pregnant to nonpregnant women (197).

Combined Spinal-Epidural Anesthesia

The earliest use of the CSE technique was by a surgeon in the United States in 1937 (198, 199). The technique consisted of the injection of procaine through a fine spinal needle into the epidural space and then subarachnoid. The first reported use for cesarean section anesthesia was in 1981 by Brownridge, who placed and tested an epidural catheter at the L1 to L2 interspace and then performed a spinal at the L3 to L4 interspace (double interspace technique) (200). The spinal anesthetic was adequate in 90% of the patients, but the catheter was available to reinforce or extend the spinal blockade as necessary and for postoperative analgesia. The current, more common, technique is the needle-through-needle approach (single interspace technique), which was described by Carrie in 1984 for cesarean section (201). The CSE technique is commonly used for labor analgesia and is described in more detail in Chapters 8 and 9. While CSE is not widely used for cesarean section in the United States, there is extensive literature documenting its safe use and potential benefits as well as risks (198–211).

Combined Spinal-Epidural Technique. While there are several special CSE kits and unique equipment provided by various manufacturers, the procedure can be easily performed using an 18-gauge Tuohy or Hustead epidural needle, for example, and a long (127 mm or greater) 24- or 26-gauge pencil-point spinal needle. The spinal needle can be added to a routine epidural tray or kit as needed, but must be long enough to extend at least 13 to 15 mm beyond the epidural needle. At San Francisco General Hospital, we commonly add a 24-gauge, 127-mm Gertie Marx® needle (International Medical Development, Park City, UT). Others commonly used are 26- or 29-gauge spinal needles (Table 11.8). While the smaller spinal needles may have a low incidence of PDPH with successful placement, ease of use must also be considered.

CSE for cesarean section can be performed easily by placing the epidural needle in the usual manner, followed by inserting the spinal needle through the epidural needle. A slight resistance will be felt as the spinal needle passes the tip of the

epidural needle, followed by a "pop" as the dura is penetrated. A recommended subarachnoid dose of 12 to 15 mg hyperbaric bupivacaine is then administered to achieve an adequate block for cesarean section and the spinal needle removed. An epidural catheter is then placed and secured. With this approach the epidural catheter is used to reinforce the spinal if needed (rarely), or to extend the length of the anesthetic if required. It can also be used for postoperative epidural analgesia. The purported advantage is the rapid onset and solid analgesia of a spinal technique with the flexibility offered by an epidural catheter. An alternative technique, the *sequential CSE* suggests administering a lower dose of bupivacaine (7.5 to 10 mg) initially, followed by additional epidural local anesthetic as needed to achieve a T4 level. In a further study using this approach, bupivacaine (7.5 mg) given intrathecally achieved a T7 (median) level with a range of T2 to L1 (205). All patients required additional epidural anesthetic (approximately 10 mL) to achieve a satisfactory surgical blockade. The authors suggest the CSE technique may be particularly advantageous in high-risk patients.

Davies et al (212). compared CSE to epidural anesthesia for cesarean section. The authors noted that the CSE technique was associated with earlier onset, more intense motor block, and lower-patient anxiety, as well as higher satisfaction before the start of surgery. There were no significant differences between the groups in the incidence and severity of hypotension, nausea, postpartum backache, pain, or headache, or overall satisfaction. While the occurrence of PDPH is a theoretical concern with this technique, it has not proven to be a problem in most reports (Table 11.8). Recently, Yun et al. (213) reported that the severity and duration of hypotension with CSE for cesarean section was greater if the spinal was placed with the patient in the sitting position vs. the lateral **decubitus** position. This may be related to the delay in the patient assuming the **recumbent** position because of epidural catheter placement. While hypotension appeared to be easily managed with CSE for cesarean section, the authors suggested the position used for induction be considered when there is greater maternal or fetal risk of hypotension.

While the use of the CSE technique may have unique advantages for labor analgesia (Chapters 8 and 9), the authors do not believe the CSE technique is necessary or indicated for routine use for cesarean section anesthesia. There is both increased risk and cost related to the CSE technique for only marginal benefits, although this remains controversial. Spinal anesthesia for cesarean section as described in this chapter has proven to be very satisfactory and efficient. In unique medical or surgical situations the *sequential CSE* may find purposeful application;

Table 11.8. INCIDENCE OF POSTDURAL PUNCTURE HEADACHE FOLLOWING CSE FOR CESAREAN SECTION

No.	Cesarean Section Patients Studied: Reference	PDPH (%)	Spinal Needle Gauge
130	202	0	29
100	452	0	26
>1000	453	0	26
400	209	0.5	—
150	211	1.3	26
100	210	1	26
300	203	0.7	26
80	208	0	26
22	213	None reported	24
59	212	6.8	26
21	205	0	26

CSE = combined spinal-epidural; PDPH = postdural puncture headache. Adapted with permission from Rawal N. Combined spinal-epidural technique. *Reg Anesth* 1997;22:406–423.

however, it is not a technique we prefer for routine cesarean section anesthesia.

Management of Complications

Despite the best efforts to minimize the incidence and severity of hypotension associated with regional anesthesia for cesarean delivery, profound hypotension with serious maternal and neonatal morbidity can occur. Continual frequent monitoring of blood pressure during the initiation of the block, prompt recognition of hypotension, and rapid intervention are necessary to avoid sequelae. The authors recommend administration of fluids and ephedrine by IV bolus promptly when systolic blood pressure begins to decrease. If this does not restore moderate or severely decreased blood pressure, elevate the legs or place the patient in Trendelenburg position. If hypotension is still not solved with appropriate doses of ephedrine (5 to 25 mg), phenylephrine (50 to 100 μg) is administered in low doses. When severe hypotension is associated with significant bradycardia, immediate administration of epinephrine may be indicated.

High or Total Spinal, Total Epidural

A very high or total spinal anesthetic can result from an accidental subarachnoid injection of local anesthetic intended for epidural administration or cephalad spread of a subarachnoid block. Signs include hypotension, complete sensory and motor block, bradycardia, apnea, loss of protective airway reflexes, and unconsciousness. The clinician should immediately establish an airway, ventilate with oxygen, and treat the compromised cardiovascular system. Endotracheal intubation, positive pressure ventilation, and prompt administration of vasopressors are usually indicated.

Total epidural can result from extensive spread of local anesthetic in the epidural space. Although the patient can become hypotensive and bradycardic, and respiratory embarrassment may result from motor blockade of the phrenic nerve, the patient may not completely lose consciousness unless profoundly hypotensive. Use of muscle relaxants and/or hypnotic agents to facilitate tracheal intubation is based on judgment. Otherwise, management is similar to that of a total spinal.

Local Anesthetic Toxicity

When large doses of local anesthetics are accidentally injected into an epidural vein, the patient will likely suffer central nervous system and possibly cardiovascular system toxicity. Manifestations include convulsions, unconsciousness, cardiac arrhythmias, and cardiovascular collapse. Immediate management of the airway and ventilation with oxygen are necessary to minimize sequelae. Some advocate the use of a small dose of a barbiturate, propofol, or benzodiazepine to facilitate termination of the convulsion. Arrhythmias and cardiovascular collapse can require significant cardiac stimulation (epinephrine) or closed-chest massage and defibrillation. Resuscitation after bupivacaine-induced cardiotoxicity, with a wide complex ventricular bradyarrhythmia may be very difficult; the recommended treatment is IV bretylium (214).

Failed Regional Block

If the sensory block is not satisfactory, supplementation of analgesia can be safely achieved by administration of low-dose opioid, inhaled nitrous oxide in oxygen, or incremental administration of low-dose IV ketamine (0.1 to 0.25 mg · kg^{-1}) (215), providing the mother remains awake and maintains her laryngeal reflexes. If the sensory level is inadequate, the regional block can be reinforced with additional local anesthetic when indicated, or general anesthesia should be induced with endotracheal intubation.

Repeating a spinal anesthetic after a previous failed spinal anesthetic or after a patchy epidural anesthetic is controversial.

The risk of high or total spinal, or persistent neurologic injury (e.g., cauda equina syndrome) is unpredictable and uncertain. Repetition of an epidural anesthetic must take into consideration the total dose of local anesthetic agents and careful monitoring for systemic toxicity.

Postdural Puncture Headache

This subject is discussed extensively in Chapter 23, but will be briefly outlined below. The occurrence of accidental dural puncture associated with epidural anesthesia will, of course, vary with the experience of the anesthesiologist. In training centers, the incidence reported is usually less than 2% but varies from 0.4% (216) to 6% (216, 217). If a dural puncture occurs after the use of an 18-gauge needle and the epidural technique is abandoned, almost 80% of patients develop a headache. However, if an epidural anesthetic is administered using another interspace (directing the catheter away from the dural hole), approximately 55% of patients develop a headache. The local anesthetic solution in the epidural space likely reduces the pressure gradient between the subarachnoid and epidural space, decreasing CSF leak and promoting dural healing. Local anesthetic injected into the epidural space following an accidental dural puncture may rarely result in a high spinal block (218, 219). Slow injection of fractionated doses and frequent monitoring of anesthetic dermatome levels and vital signs are recommended.

Prophylactic Saline or Blood. Some investigators have suggested that instillation of preservative-free salt solution through the epidural catheter after the epidural anesthetic has been allowed to wear off decreases the incidence of spinal headache (220–222). Administration of a prophylactic epidural blood patch via either the epidural catheter or spinal needle has been suggested (223, 224). Randomized, prospective trials of immediate blood patch, given through an epidural catheter, have found this to be of value (217, 225–228).

Bedrest and Hydration. Evidence suggests that prophylactic bed rest does not reduce the likelihood of developing PDPH. In a study of 100 neurology patients having diagnostic lumbar punctures with an 18-gauge needle, half were allowed to ambulate immediately after the puncture and half were kept in bed for 24 hours (229). The incidence and duration of the spinal headache was similar in both groups (Fig. 11.19). Likewise, increased hydration after dural puncture has little or no effect on the incidence of subsequent headache. Animal studies have shown that relatively large increases in fluid intake do not

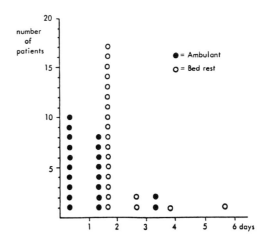

Figure 11.19. Time of onset of spinal headache in neurology patients following diagnostic lumbar puncture (18-gauge needle) who were either allowed to ambulate at will immediately following the block or were kept on bed rest for a 24-hour period. Duration of the headache was also similar in both groups. (Reprinted by permission from Carbaat PAT, van Crevel H. Lumbar puncture headache: Controlled study on the preventive effect of 24 hours' bed rest. *Lancet* 1981;2:1133–1135.)

Table 11.9. THERAPEUTIC BLOOD PATCH EPIDURAL FOR DURAL PUNCTURE HEADACHE

Investigator	No. of Patients	Success Rate (%)
Gormley (238)	7	100
DiGiovanni et al. (239, 454)	108	94
Glass and Kennedy (240)	50	94
Vondrell and Bernards (242)	60	96.5
Ostheimer et al. (245)	185	98.5
Abouleish et al. (246)	118	97.5
Loeser et al. (247)	31	96
Stride and Cooper (216)	135	64
		(Initial success was 90%, but headache returned in 30% of these patients.)
Williams et al. (249)	41	34
		(Blood patch was partially successful in an additional 54%.)

Personal communication cited in DiGiovanni AJ, Galbert MW, Wahle WM. Epidural injection of autologous blood for postlumbar-puncture headache. II. Additional clinical experiences and laboratory investigation. *Anesth Analg* 1972;51:226–232.

increase CSF production (230). The incidence of PDPH is independent of fluid intake (231).

Caffeine Therapy. IV or oral caffeine sodium benzoate has been reported to be effective therapy for PDPH (232). The mechanism is believed to be related to cerebral vasoconstriction. IV caffeine sodium benzoate (500 mg) relieves headaches in the majority of patients, but there is a very high recurrence rate. Camann et al. (233) demonstrated a beneficial effect of oral caffeine (300 mg) on headache, although there was a significant recurrence rate of 30%. Seizures were reported in a postpartum patient with elevated blood pressure after treatment of spinal headache with blood patch and caffeine sodium benzoate (234). Caffeine is a central nervous system stimulant and may have been an etiologic factor. Oral theophylline (300 mg) in a sustained release tablet has also been reported to ameliorate spinal headache (235, 236).

Epidural Blood Patch. A blood patch epidural using autologous blood can be performed in patients suffering from severe refractory PDPH (237). Using a rigidly aseptic technique, 15 to 20 mL blood is withdrawn via a venipuncture and immediately placed into the epidural space at the site of the dural rent. The reported success rate has been as high as 100% (Table 11.9) (238–248), but some studies suggest epidural blood patch may be less efficacious in the obstetric population. In one study of epidural blood patches performed in 48 patients who had had accidental dural punctures with a 16-gauge Touhy needle, the first patch produced complete and permanent relief in 33%, partial relief in 50%, and no relief in 12%. Twenty-nine percent of the patients required a second patch, of which 50% were completely successful, 36% were partially successful, and 14% gave no relief (249). Similarly, a review of 135 blood patches in 122 patients showed only 64% had complete and permanent relief of their PDPH after one patch (216). A long-term follow-up of 118 patients for 2 years has indicated that epidural blood patch is without serious complication. The occurrence of meningitis, adhesive arachnoiditis, or cauda equina syndrome is extremely rare (250), but nevertheless, strict aseptic technique and careful postprocedure monitoring are essential (251, 252). Backache is the most common complication. It is seldom severe or incapacitating and usually disappears within 48 hours, although it may occasionally last up to 3 months.

Successful epidural anesthesia following prior epidural blood patch has been reported (253). Although a high incidence of poor analgesia in patients with previous accidental dural punctures has been reported, it does not appear to be related to whether or not the patient was originally treated with a blood patch epidural (254). Experience with blood patch epidurals in human immunodeficiency virus (HIV)—positive patients demonstrates its safety (255–257).

The use of epidural dextran 40 in a volume of 20 to 30 mL has been suggested as an alternative to autologous blood. Complete relief has been reported to occur within 2 hours with no major complications (258). This may be useful in patients in whom autologous blood is contraindicated or unacceptable.

GENERAL ANESTHESIA

In contrast to regional anesthesia, general anesthesia has the advantages of a more rapid induction, less hypotension and cardiovascular instability, and better control of the airway and ventilation. Some patients are terrified of "needles in the back" or the prospect of being awake during major abdominal surgery. In addition, general anesthesia may be preferable for patients with preexisting neurologic or lumbar disc disease, coagulopathies, or infections. Although there are few contraindications to general anesthesia, due to the risk of airway management, most anesthesiologists prefer to avoid it.

Reduced Anesthetic Requirements

Anesthetic requirements are decreased during pregnancy. In the experimental animal, minimum alveolar concentration (MAC) for halothane, isoflurane, or methoxyflurane is 25% to 40% lower in pregnant animals than in nonpregnant animals (Table 11.10) (259). In women at an early gestational age, the MAC for isoflurane is about 72% that of nonpregnant women (260). Also, the reduced maternal functional residual capacity results in a faster rate of equilibration between inspired and alveolar (brain) gas tension. Therefore, the rate of induction of anesthesia is much more rapid in the pregnant patient, and overdose may easily occur.

Premedication

Although verbal reassurance is usually sufficient before anesthetic administration, treatment of maternal anxiety can be used with minimal neonatal effects. Low doses of IV midazolam (0.5 to 4 mg), diazepam (2 to 8 mg), or an opioid (e.g., fentanyl 25 to 100 μg) can be used with minimal neonatal effects (22–24).

Preparation and Equipment

If general anesthesia is used, important considerations include (a) prevention of aspiration pneumonitis; (b) having a plan of action for failed intubation; (c) prevention of supine

Table 11.10. MINIMAL ALVEOLAR CONCENTRATION (MAC) PRESENTED AS PERCENT END-TIDAL ANESTHETIC CONCENTRATION

	Nonpregnant* Ewes (n = 6)	Pregnant* Ewes (n = 6)	Change (%)
Halothane	0.97 ± 0.04	0.73[†] ± 0.07	−25
Isoflurane	1.58 ± 0.07	1.01[‡] ± 0.06	−40
Methoxyflurane	0.26 ± 0.02	0.18[§] ± 0.01	−32

* Mean ± SE
[†] $P < .001$
[‡] $P < .01$
[§] $P < .025$
Reprinted by permission from Palahniuk RJ, Shnider SM, Eger EI II. Pregnancy decreases the requirements for inhaled anesthetic agents. *Anesthesiology* 1974;41:82–83.

Table 11.11. GENERAL ANESTHESIA FOR CESAREAN SECTION: A SUGGESTED TECHNIQUE

1. Administer a nonparticulate oral antacid within 1 h of induction.
2. Maintain uterine displacement.
3. Start infusion with a large-bore IV catheter.
4. Preoxygenate for 3 minutes.
5. When the surgeon is ready to begin, an assistant should apply cricoid pressure (and maintain until position of endotracheal tube is verified and trachea is sealed by inflated cuff).
6. Administer thiopental 4–5 mg·kg^{-1} and succinylcholine 1–1.5 mg·kg^{-1}, wait 30–60 sec, then intubate trachea.
7. Administer N_2O (50%) + O_2 (50%) at high flow rates, with 0.5 MAC of halogentated agent. Use muscle relaxant as necessary.
8. Avoid maternal hyperventilation.
9. After delivery, anesthesia may be deepened by increasing the N_2O concentration, or administering opioids, barbiturates, or propofol. The halogenated hydrocarbon may be continued.
10. Extubate the trachea when the patient is fully awake.

IV = intravenous; MAC = minimal alveolar concentration.

hypotension; (d) maintenance of normal maternal ventilation and oxygenation; and (e) minimizing the duration of general anesthesia. Management of general anesthesia for cesarean section is outlined in Table 11.11.

Prevention of Aspiration

Aspiration of gastric contents during general anesthesia is a major cause of maternal morbidity and mortality and is discussed in Chapter 22. Routine administration of antacid prior to induction significantly raises gastric pH (261). However, use of antacids will not diminish the risk of aspiration of particulate matter.

The risk of regurgitation and aspiration is decreased by (a) rapid endotracheal intubation; (b) avoiding positive-pressure ventilation prior to intubation, which could inflate the stomach and make the patient more prone to regurgitate; (c) use of cricoid pressure (Sellick maneuver) to occlude the esophagus and prevent passive regurgitation during endotracheal intubation (262); and (d) extubating the patient only after she is fully awake and able to protect her airway.

We do not routinely administer a nondepolarizing muscle relaxant prior to succinylcholine to prevent fasciculations. A nondepolarizing muscle relaxant may make intubation more difficult since it prolongs the onset time of succinylcholine paralysis and reduces the duration and intensity of the block. It has been noted that pregnant women do not have intense fasciculations or post-succinylcholine muscle pain (263), possibly due to increased progesterone levels. Furthermore, pregnant women have less abdominal muscle tone and presumably will have less rise in intragastric pressure with fasciculations. Finally, and most significantly, it has been demonstrated in *nonpregnant* patients that, with fasciculations, the rise in the pressure in the lower esophageal junction is *greater* than the rise in intragastric pressure. Thus, the barrier pressure, which prevents passive regurgitation, actually increases with fasciculations (264). However, it is unclear whether this latter study can be applied to pregnant women.

Since morbidity and mortality are markedly increased when the volume of aspirate exceeds 0.4 mL·kg^{-1} and the pH is less than 2.5 (261), an effort is made to routinely increase maternal gastric pH and decrease gastric volume. Routine administration of an antacid prior to induction significantly raises gastric pH. Particulate or colloidal antacids are avoided since they themselves may cause severe physiologic insult and pulmonary damage if aspirated (265, 266). Sodium citrate (0.3 molar), a clear nonparticulate antacid, is effective and relatively benign if aspirated (267, 268). Commercial preparations of sodium citrate are readily available and appear to be safe and effective

(269, 270). Sodium citrate 15 to 30 mL is effective if administered in one dose 10 to 15 minutes before anesthesia, but the duration of action is quite short (40 minutes to 1 hour).

Preanesthetic administration of a histamine H$_2$-receptor antagonist such as cimetidine or ranitidine has been suggested to decrease gastric acidity and volume (271–273). Both of these drugs require an interval of at least 1 to 2 hours after oral administration and 45 to 60 minutes after IV or IM administration to be effective. Omeprazole, a proton pump inhibitor, also reduces gastric acidity but requires 40 minutes to be effective after IV administration (274). These drugs are probably not indicated routinely, with the possible exceptions of *elective* cesarean sections under general anesthesia or when the parturient has an unusual problem such as peptic ulcer disease or morbid obesity. Metoclopramide is an antiemetic that increases stomach emptying and raises gastroesophageal sphincter tone (28, 275–279). Because of its possible beneficial effects on gastroesophageal sphincter tone and gastric volume, its use might be considered in parturients with unusual problems predisposing to gastric regurgitation (280). Some clinicians routinely administer this drug because of its possible antiemetic effects.

Failed Intubation

Failed or difficult intubation is the leading cause of anesthetic-related maternal mortality (8, 281). The incidence of failed intubation in obstetrics is much greater than in the surgical patient (282–285). Postulated reasons are the presence of full dentition, increased incidence of laryngeal and pharyngeal edema, obstruction to laryngoscope placement by large pendulous breasts, and failure to allow adequate time for succinylcholine to be effective. Physical characteristics associated with difficulty in airway management and intubation are short muscular necks, receding lower jaws (micrognathia) with obtuse mandibular angles, protruding upper incisors, poor mobility of the mandible, long high-arched palate with a long narrow mouth, and increased alveolar mental distance (anterior depth of the mandible). Management of the difficult airway to include failed intubations is discussed in Chapter 21. However, a general approach to the patient is presented here.

Carefully performed preoperative evaluation of the patient will frequently alert the anesthesiologist to a potentially difficult intubation (286–288).

1. Viewing the patient from the lateral and anterolateral positions should identify patients with maxillary overgrowth (protruding upper incisors) or receding mandible (micrognathia).
2. Viewing and palpating the neck anteriorly allows the anesthesiologist to estimate the mandibular space. The space anterior to the larynx determines how easily the laryngeal axis will line up with the pharyngeal axis during laryngoscopy. Also, when there is a large mandibular space, the tongue does not have to be pulled maximally forward to reveal the larynx, and visualization is much easier. The mandibular space is most easily evaluated by measuring the thyromental distance with either a ruler or number of finger breadths (Fig. 11.20). The normal measurement is 6.5 cm or greater. If the distance is 6 to 6.5 cm without other anatomic problems, laryngoscopy and intubation are difficult, but usually possible. A distance of less than 6 cm suggests that laryngoscopy may be impossible (289). Other reports have confirmed the value of this measurement in predicting difficult intubation (290).
3. Flexing and extending the neck maximally will identify limitations that might prevent optimal alignment of the oral, pharyngeal, and laryngeal axes. The normal atlantooccipital joint allows 35 degrees of extension (291).
4. The relation of the size of the tongue to that of the oral cavity is estimated by visual examination of the oral pharynx. The patient sits upright with the head in the neutral

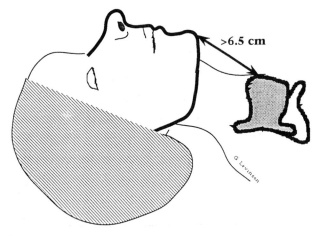

Figure 11.20. The distance from the thyroid notch to the tip of the chin is measured with the neck fully extended. If the distance is less than 6.5 cm, visualization of the vocal cords by direct laryngoscopy may be difficult or impossible.

position. She is asked to open her mouth as widely as possible (normal maximum mandibular opening is 5 to 6 cm) (292) and to protrude her tongue to a maximum. The observer sits opposite at eye level and inspects the pharyngeal structures. The airway is then classified according to the structures seen. If the soft palate, faucial pillars, and uvula are fully visualized, exposure of the glottis on direct laryngoscopy is usually easy. If the uvula is masked by the base of the tongue, some difficulty in exposing the glottis can be anticipated. If only the soft palate is visible or, indeed, if the soft palate is also masked by the base of the tongue, visualization of the glottis may not be possible using the conventional laryngoscope (Fig. 11.21) (285, 293, 294). If possible difficulty in intubating the parturient is suspected, an alternative to the usual rapid-sequence intubation should be used. This may include regional anesthesia, awake nasal intubation, or awake fiberoptic intubation. The "Practice Guidelines for Obstetric Anesthesia" suggest that "the availability of equipment for the management of airway emergencies is associated with reduced maternal complications" (295).

Despite careful preoperative evaluation, there still may be times when, following rapid-sequence induction, the anesthesiologist is unable to intubate the patient. A plan to manage a failed intubation is shown in Figure 11.22. Persistent attempts at intubation and repeated doses of succinylcholine should be avoided. Maternal hypoxia and chances of aspiration are more likely during prolonged attempts at intubation. A call for help should be initiated, cricoid pressure maintained, and the patient ventilated by mask with 100% oxygen. The surgical team should be apprised of the problem and emergency equipment, includ-

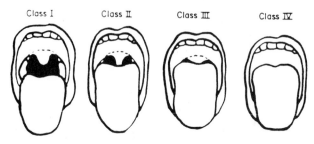

Figure 11.21. Pictorial classification of the pharyngeal structures as seen during examination of the oral pharynx. Class III and IV have been associated with difficulty in visualizing the larynx. (Modified with permission from Samsoon GLT, Young JRB. Difficult tracheal intubation: A retrospective study. *Anaesthesia* 1987;42:487–490.)

ing a laryngeal mask (LMA) prepared (296, 297). Preparations to establish an emergency airway would include a cricothyrotomy kit or surgical equipment and equipment for transtracheal jet ventilation (TTJV) (297).

If the indications for cesarean section are not immediately life-threatening to the mother or fetus, the mother should be allowed to awaken and anesthesia continued with either an awake intubation or a regional block. If there is an immediate life-threatening maternal or fetal problem, a judgment must be made concerning the relative risks of proceeding. If mask ventilation is relatively easy, general anesthesia without intubation may be an acceptable alternative. The preferred anesthetic agent for this approach, the method of ventilation, and decisions about subsequent attempts at intubation after delivery of the baby are controversial. Under any circumstance, adequate maternal oxygen and ventilation should be maintained, adequate depth of anesthesia provided, and cricoid pressure continuously applied.

If ventilation is difficult or impossible, the mother should be allowed to awaken or an LMA should be placed if possible (296, 298). An esophageal tracheal Combitube is another possibility. If placement of the LMA with cricoid pressure (CP) is not possible, CP may be released and the LMA tried again. If an airway is not established and ventilation is not possible, a cricothyrotomy or TTJV must be attempted (299). After adequate oxygenation is established, a cricothyroidotomy or tracheostomy may be performed, a cuffed tracheal tube may be inserted, and anesthesia and surgery should proceed. Under extreme circumstances, some anesthesiologists may choose to proceed with cesarean section under local anesthesia while maternal airway management is in progress. The laryngeal mask airway is shown in Chapter 21 (see Fig. 21.15) and the controversies discussed. The use of an LMA for general anesthesia for cesarean section is indicated only in the "cannot intubate, cannot ventilate" situation because of the risk of aspiration in LMA placement or use. The laryngeal mask is not designed for use in either apneic patients or patients with full stomachs (299–304). However, it may be lifesaving and is a vital part of emergency airway management.

Preoxygenation

Oxygen consumption at term is 20% higher than in the nonpregnant state (305). In addition, functional residual capacity is reduced 20% at term gestation due to upward displacement of the diaphragm (306). With reduced functional residual capacity, and increased oxygen consumption, the pregnant patient is more likely to become hypoxic during induction of anesthesia than is the nonpregnant patient. During a 1-minute period of apnea (due to paralysis after preoxygenation), a parturient will sustain a 150 mm Hg reduction in Pao_2, in contrast to a 50 mm Hg reduction in a nonpregnant woman) (307). Occasionally, difficult laryngoscopy and several attempts at intubation are encountered. Thus, maternal hypoxia is less likely with preoxygenation before induction. The usual method of preoxygenating before induction of general anesthesia is to have the patient breathe 100% oxygen for 3 to 5 minutes using a tight-fitting face mask. It has been demonstrated that having pregnant woman take four maximally deep inspirations of 100% oxygen within 30 seconds of induction of anesthesia is as effective in raising maternal Pao_2 as the standard 3-minute preoxygenation (Table 11.12) (308, 309). However, the duration of apnea in these patients was relatively brief ($Paco_2$ rose only 8 to 9 mm Hg). In a similar study of nonpregnant patients, oxygen saturation decreased more rapidly among the subjects preoxygenated with four breaths compared to those preoxygenated for 3 minutes (Table 11.13) (310). Eight maximal capacity breaths over a 60-second period may be as effective or more so than four deep breaths over the same time period or 3 minutes of tidal volume breathing (311, 312).

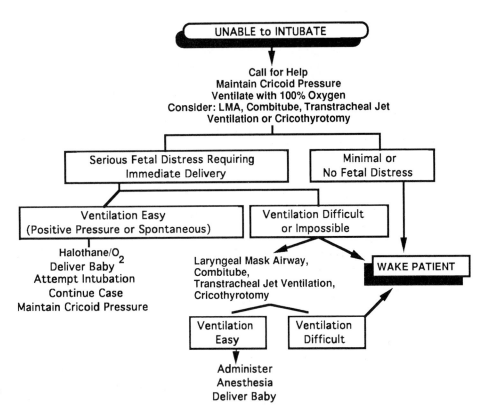

Figure 11.22. Algorithm for management of the difficult intubation.

Table 11.12. MATERNAL BLOOD GAS VALUES WITH PREOXYGENATION FOR CESAREAN SECTION

	Blood Gas	3 Min (n = 8)	4 Deep Breaths (n = 9)
		100% Oxygen	
Baseline	Pa_{O_2}	101	103
	Pa_{CO_2}	31	32
After preoxygenation	Pa_{O_2}	376	408
	Pa_{CO_2}	32	31
After intubation	Pa_{O_2}	264	313
	Pa_{CO_2}	40	40

Modified from Norris MC, Dewan DM. Preoxygenation for cesarean section: A comparison of two techniques. *Anesthesiology* 1985;62:827–829.

Reduced Anesthetic Requirements

Anesthetic requirements are decreased during pregnancy. In the experimental animal, MAC for halothane, isoflurane, or methoxyflurane is 25% to 40% less in pregnant animals than in nonpregnant animals (Table 11.10) (259). Among women, at an early gestational age, the MAC for isoflurane is about 68% that of the nonpregnant women (260). Also, the reduced maternal functional residual capacity results in a faster rate of equilibration between inspired and alveolar (brain) gas tension. Therefore, the rate of induction of anesthesia is much more rapid in the pregnant patient, and overdose may easily occur.

Maternal Ventilation

When anesthetized, excessive positive-pressure ventilation (maternal Pa_{CO_2} less than 20 mm Hg) may result in fetal hypoxemia and acidosis (313). The etiologic factors include reduced uterine and umbilical blood flow and increased affinity of maternal hemoglobin for oxygen (Bohr effect), resulting in less placental transfer of oxygen (Figs. 11.23, 11.24, and 11.25). The anesthe-

siologist should try to maintain a normal maternal Pa_{CO_2}, which at term gestation ranges between 30 and 33 mm Hg.

Maternal and Fetal Effects of Anesthetic Agents

Thiopental

Thiopental rapidly crosses the placenta, and it is not possible to deliver the baby before the drug is transferred to the fetus. After a single maternal IV dose, the drug can be detected in umbilical venous blood within 30 seconds (Fig. 5.13) (314). Thiopental reaches its peak concentration in umbilical venous blood in 1 minute and in umbilical arterial blood in 2 to 3 minutes. At delivery, the umbilical vein/maternal vein ratio is close to 1 (315). Why, then, is the neonate not affected? The fetal brain will not be exposed to high concentrations of barbiturate if the induction dose is less than $4 \text{ mg} \cdot \text{kg}^{-1}$. With this dose, umbilical arterial levels of thiopental are much lower than the umbilical venous levels (Fig. 11.26) (316).

Table 11.13. TIME TO ARTERIAL DESATURATION FOR SUBJECTS PREOXYGENATED WITH TWO DIFFERENT TECHNIQUES

Saturation (%)	3 Min (n = 6)	4 Breaths (n = 6)
97	7.9	5.6
95	8.4	6.0
93	8.6	6.3
90	8.9	6.8

Subjects were not pregnant. Pregnant patients would be expected to desaturate more quickly because of their decreased functional residual capacity (FRC) and increased oxygen consumption.
Modified from Gambee AM, Hertzka RE, Fisher DM. Preoxygenation techniques: Comparison of three minutes and four breaths. *Anesth Analg* 1987;66:468–470.

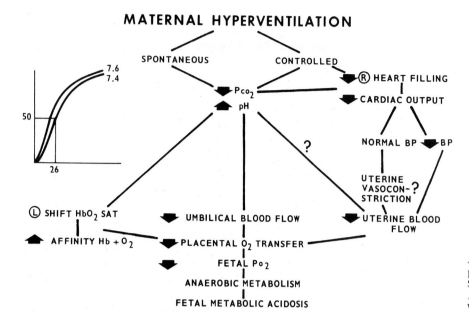

Figure 11.23. Pathophysiology of maternal hyperventilation. (Reprinted by permission from Shnider SM, Moya F, eds. *The Anesthesiologist, Mother and Newborn.* Baltimore, MD: Williams & Wilkins; 1973:98.)

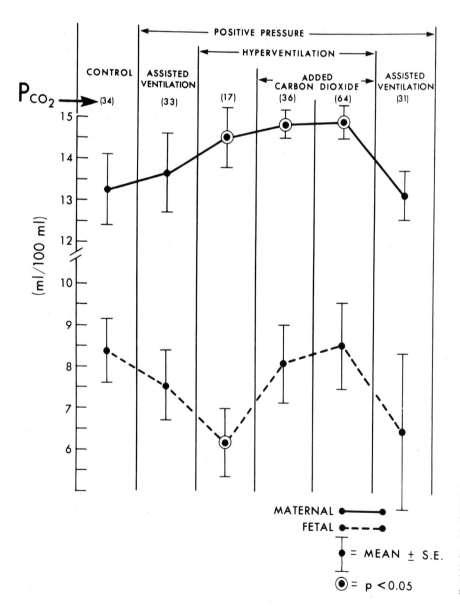

Figure 11.24. Changes from control values in mean maternal and fetal arterial oxygen content during five periods of positive pressure ventilation. Mean maternal $Paco_2$ during each period is indicated at the top of the figure. (Reprinted by permission from Levinson G, Shnider SM, deLorimier AA, Steffenson JL. Effects of maternal hyperventilation on uterine blood flow and fetal oxygenation and acid-base status. *Anesthesiology* 1974;40:340–347.)

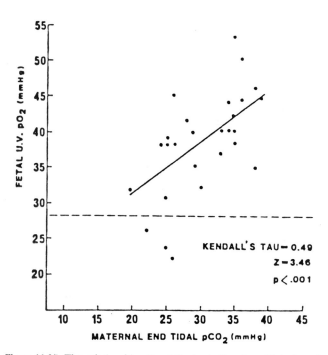

Figure 11.25. The relationship of umbilical vein Po$_2$ (mm Hg) plotted against maternal end-tidal Pco$_2$ (mm Hg). The *horizontal broken line* indicates the normal value of fetal umbilical vein Po$_2$ (28 mm Hg) in 27 healthy patients undergoing cesarean section under general anesthesia. (Reprinted by permission from Cook PT. The influence on foetal outcome of maternal carbon dioxide tension at caesarean section under general anaesthesia. *Anesth Intensive Care* 1984;12:296–302.)

Blood from the placenta either passes through the liver or traverses the ductus venosus into the inferior vena cava. Therefore, most of the thiopental is either cleared by the liver or diluted by blood from the lower extremities and viscera. Uptake of thiopental by fetal liver is probably not a significant factor in the observed resistance of the fetal brain to maternally administered barbiturate following a single IV injection. Other reasons for lack of neonatal depression after a sleep dose of thiopental are swift decline of the drug concentration in maternal blood due to redistribution, nonhomogeneity of blood in the intervillous space, and progressive dilution in the circulation due to shunting. There is no advantage to delaying delivery until the thiopental has redistributed in the mother or fetus. It should be stressed that, after large doses of thiobarbiturate (8 mg·kg^{-1}), babies are depressed (314).

Two studies compared induction of general anesthesia with thiopental 4 mg·kg^{-1} and ketamine 1 mg·kg^{-1}. In the first study, the authors evaluated postoperative analgesia requirements (317), and in another study, detection of maternal awareness by electroencephalogram (EEG) spectrum analysis was evaluated (318). Both of these studies confirmed the safety and effectiveness of thiopental for both the mother and newborn but suggested that use of ketamine resulted in lower postoperative morphine requirements (317) and lesser degree of awareness as judged by EEG spectrum analysis. However, none of the patients actually recalled any events during surgery (318). We recommend use of thiopental 4 to 5 mg·kg^{-1} for induction of general anesthesia for cesarean section.

Ketamine

Ketamine is sometimes used for induction of anesthesia in patients with possible hypovolemia or with acute asthma. The drug produces minimal respiratory depression and usually increases

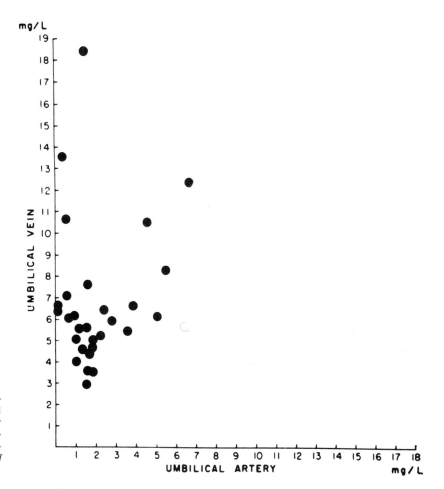

Figure 11.26. Relationship between the concentration of thiopental in umbilical artery and umbilical vein at birth. (Reprinted by permission from Finster M, Mark LC, Morishima HO, et al. Plasma thiopental concentrations in the newborn following delivery under thiopental-nitrous oxide anesthesia. *Am J Obstet Gynecol* 1966;95:621–629.)

arterial blood pressure 10% to 25%. Undesirable hypertension may occur, and the drug should not be given to patients with high blood pressure. In the bleeding hypotensive patient, cardiovascular stimulation is desirable, and ketamine may be the preferred induction agent for general anesthesia. Emergent delirium and hallucinations are common with high doses in unpremedicated patients (319). Premedication with, or co-administration of, diazepam or midazolam decreases the incidence of psychomimetic side effects (320, 321).

Because ketamine has vasopressor effects and many vasoactive compounds decrease uterine blood flow, several investigators have examined the effects of ketamine on uterine perfusion. In both pregnant ewes and monkeys, the increase in maternal blood pressure was not associated with a reduction in uterine blood flow (322–324). Ketamine produces a dose-related oxytocic effect on uterine tone when administered during the second trimester of pregnancy (see Fig. 3.19) (325, 326). However, when ketamine ($2 \mathrm{mg} \cdot \mathrm{kg}^{-1}$) is administered at term for cesarean section, no increase in intrauterine pressure is noted (see Fig. 3.20).

Ketamine crosses the placenta rapidly but does not produce neonatal depression unless used in doses above $1 \mathrm{mg} \cdot \mathrm{kg}^{-1}$ (see Fig. 7.24) (327, 328). At higher doses, low Apgar scores and neonatal muscular hypertonicity have been reported. In several instances, even with endotracheal intubation, ventilation of the infant has been difficult because of excessive muscle tone.

When ketamine is used in a single IV dose of $1 \mathrm{mg} \cdot \mathrm{kg}^{-1}$ for induction of general anesthesia for cesarean section, neonatal neurobehavioral test scores are slightly higher than after thiopental ($4 \mathrm{mg} \cdot \mathrm{kg}^{-1}$) (329). The Apgar scores and fetal acid-base status at birth are similar after ketamine or thiopental anesthesia (317, 318, 330, 331). However, it is unlikely that ketamine will replace thiopental as the routine induction agent of choice because of ketamine's psychotomimetic properties. On the other hand, ketamine has been considered to have an advantage over thiopental in the severely hypotensive, hypovolemic parturient or the patient with severe asthma (332, 333). The relationship between EEG (spectral edge frequency [SEF] 90) and the occurrence of awareness, defined as response to verbal command, was studied in 50 women undergoing general anesthesia for elective cesarean section. One arm of the patient was isolated with a tourniquet prior to induction of anesthesia. In those women receiving ketamine ($1 \mathrm{mg} \cdot \mathrm{kg}^{-1}$), there was a significant decrease in awareness (hand movement in response to verbal command) and a lower SEF 90 compared with the group who received thiopental ($4 \mathrm{mg} \cdot \mathrm{kg}^{-1}$). However, no mother had recall of surgical events with either agent (318). Ketamine in doses greater than $1 \mathrm{mg} \cdot \mathrm{kg}^{-1}$ may result in an unacceptably high incidence of neonatal depression.

Some authors have suggested that anesthesia be induced with ketamine (0.5 to $0.7 \mathrm{mg} \cdot \mathrm{kg}^{-1}$) combined with a smaller dose of thiopental ($2 \mathrm{mg} \cdot \mathrm{kg}^{-1}$). Reputed advantages of this approach are fewer hemodynamic effects, ability to use 100% oxygen, less maternal recall, and better neonatal neurobehavioral scores. However, a study comparing the induction of anesthesia with thiopental ($4 \mathrm{mg} \cdot \mathrm{kg}^{-1}$) or a combination of thiopental ($2 \mathrm{mg} \cdot \mathrm{kg}^{-1}$) and ketamine ($0.5 \mathrm{mg} \cdot \mathrm{kg}^{-1}$) did not demonstrate any advantage in regard to maternal recall, hemodynamic responses, or neonatal neurobehavioral scores (334).

Propofol

Propofol is an IV anesthetic agent that has become very popular. Desirable properties of the drug include rapid induction followed by rapid recovery with a low incidence of postoperative side effects. The drug has not yet been approved for obstetric anesthesia, and clinical experience in obstetric anesthesia is somewhat limited.

Studies in pregnant sheep indicate that anesthetic induction and maintenance with propofol has no direct adverse effects

on ovine uterine blood flow or fetal well-being (335). Uterine blood flow transiently decreased during induction and intubation with thiopental, but remained stable during induction with propofol. However, administration of succinylcholine resulted in transient but severe maternal bradycardia when propofol was used for induction of anesthesia. A number of clinical studies have compared propofol (1.5 to $2.8 \mathrm{mg} \cdot \mathrm{kg}^{-1}$) to thiopental (4 to $5 \mathrm{mg} \cdot \mathrm{kg}^{-1}$) for induction of cesarean section anesthesia (336–346). Propofol induction did not produce more hypotension than did thiopental. With both drugs, arterial blood pressure rose significantly with endotracheal intubation, but the increase was less with propofol. Increases in heart rate accompanying intubation were similar for both drugs, although in one small study, two of six patients developed severe bradycardia following administration of propofol and succinylcholine (347). This report is very similar to the work in our laboratory at UCSF in the sheep model noted earlier, in which propofol exaggerated the effects of succinylcholine on maternal heart rate, causing severe bradycardia during induction (335). This effect suggests that combining propofol with succinylcholine may have potential maternal risk, which could limit the usefulness of propofol. Placental transfer of propofol appears to be similar to thiopental (umbilical cord venous blood/maternal arterial blood 0.70) (337). The neonatal condition as appraised by Apgar scores, umbilical cord acid-base status, and Neurologic and Adaptive Capacity score (NACS) has been reported to be comparable to thiopental induction in most studies, but there have been some reports of lower Apgar scores, muscular hypotonus, and transient somnolence after propofol administration (336). Continuous infusions of propofol have been used ($100 \mu \mathrm{g} \cdot \mathrm{kg}^{-1} \cdot \mathrm{min}^{-1}$) and IV induction ($2.5 \mathrm{mg} \cdot \mathrm{kg}^{-1}$) with no newborn neurobehavioral effects (348, 349). However, higher infusion rates ($150 \mu \mathrm{g} \cdot \mathrm{kg}^{-1} \cdot \mathrm{min}^{-1}$) were associated with depressed neurobehavioral scores (344, 345, 348, 349). Until further investigation clarifies these contradictory findings, thiopental remains the induction agent of choice for cesarean section. Furthermore, the limited shelf-life of propofol, once drawn into a syringe is considerably shorter than that for thiopental (350).

Etomidate

Etomidate, a carboxylated imidazole, has minimal effects on cardiorespiratory function when used for the induction of anesthesia in a dose of $0.3 \mathrm{mg} \cdot \mathrm{kg}^{-1}$. It undergoes a rapid hydrolysis that leads to a quick recovery. It is not a popular induction agent for cesarean section despite a favorable report (351). This is probably due to the high incidence of pain on injection and the involuntary muscle movements in unpremedicated patients (352, 353). It also suppresses cortisol production in the neonate, although the clinical relevance is uncertain (354). Thus, etomidate is rarely used in obstetric anesthesia.

Muscle Relaxants

Muscle relaxants are commonly used prior to delivery to facilitate rapid endotracheal intubation and provide optimum operating conditions in a lightly anesthetized patient. Muscle relaxants have low lipid solubility and are highly ionized at physiologic pH. When conventional doses are administered clinically, insignificant placental transfer occurs (355–359).

Succinylcholine administered to the mother in high doses (2 to $3 \mathrm{mg} \cdot \mathrm{kg}^{-1}$) is detectable in fetal blood and may cause alterations in the electromyograph (360), but it has no depressant effects on neonatal ventilation. Only with maternal administration of massive doses ($10 \mathrm{mg} \cdot \mathrm{kg}^{-1}$) does enough placental transfer occur to cause neonatal depression (361). Despite reduced plasma pseudocholinesterase in parturients (362, 363), metabolism of moderate doses of succinylcholine is usually not

Table 11.14. TIME TO TWITCH RECOVERY AFTER SUCCINYLCHOLINE

	Succinylcholine (mg)	Twitch Recovery (min)		
		10%	50%	90%
Nonpregnant women (n = 15)	144	10.2	11.9	13.3
Cesarean sections (n = 10)	148	9.9	11.5	12.9

Adapted from Blitt CD, Petty WC, Alberternst EE, Wright BJ. Correlation of plasma cholinesterase activity and duration of action of succinylcholine during pregnancy. *Anesth Analg* 1977;56:78–81.

prolonged (Table 11.14) (364). In some patients, however, pseudocholinesterase levels are so low that they result in a prolonged block (362). Also, in patients with atypical cholinesterase, prolonged maternal and neonatal respiratory depression has been reported (365). After injection of an intubating dose of succinylcholine (1 to 1.5 mg·kg^{-1}), return of neuromuscular function should be ensured before additional relaxant is administered.

Nondepolarizing muscle relaxants may be administered in small doses to prevent fasciculations from succinylcholine and in larger doses to maintain muscle relaxation during surgery. Because these nondepolarizing relaxants are easily reversible, the authors prefer them to a continuous infusion of succinylcholine. Pancuronium and curare had been the more commonly used relaxants, but atracurium, vecuronium, rocuronium, and mivacurium have become the preferred agents because of their shorter duration of action (357–359, 366–371). As with curare (372) and pancuronium (373), placental transfer does occur (with similar umbilical/maternal venous ratios of approximately 0.1 to 0.2) (357–359, 369). With clinical doses (curare, 0.2 mg·kg^{-1}, pancuronium or vecuronium, 0.05 mg·kg^{-1}, atracurium, 0.5 mg·kg^{-1}, rocuronium, 0.6 mg·kg^{-1}, or mivacurium, 0.15 mg·kg^{-1}), there are no adverse neonatal effects of these drugs as measured by Apgar scores, umbilical cord acid-base status, or neonatal neurobehavioral scores.

Intubation can be achieved with either vecuronium (0.2 mg·kg^{-1}) or rocuronium (0.6 mg·kg^{-1}), for example, when succinylcholine is contraindicated. However, intubating conditions were achieved in approximately 175 seconds (370) and 79 seconds (369), respectively, times that are longer than that required with succinylcholine. If the dose of rocuronium is increased to 0.9 to 1.2 mg·kg^{-1}, an onset of action similar to succinylcholine can be achieved, but the duration of action is also prolonged (367). Rapacuronium has been evaluated for rapid-sequence induction for cesarean section (2.5 mg·kg^{-1}) and achieved intubating conditions as rapidly and effectively as succinylcholine (371). However, the duration of action is two to three times that of succinylcholine. Rapacuronium (1.5 mg·kg^{-1}) has been suggested as a suitable alternative to succinylcholine (374), but this dose has not been studied in the parturient. Rapacuronium has a longer duration of action than Asuccinylcholine and this would be a disadvantage should a failed intubation occur. However, because of its possible association with brochospasm, rapacuronium was voluntarily withdrawn from the market by the manufacturer, Organor, in March, 2001. The rapid onset of succinylcholine and short duration of action work very well to facilitate intubation in obstetric anesthesia when a rapid-sequence induction is required.

In the clinical doses commonly used, only very small amounts of muscle relaxants reach the fetus and there is no effect upon the fetal outcome. Maternal safety and surgical requirements should determine the neuromuscular agents used for cesarean section.

Nitrous Oxide

Nitrous oxide is the most popular inhalation agent in obstetric anesthesia. It produces no significant uterine relaxation. It is rapidly transferred across the placenta, but fetal tissue uptake during the first 20 minutes reduces the fetal arterial concentration and subsequent neonatal depression (see Fig. 10.7) (375, 376). In earlier studies, it was found that longer duration of anesthesia with nitrous oxide was associated with a more anesthetized newborn (377, 378). However, these studies were performed using 70% rather than the currently more common 50% nitrous oxide, and the effect of the time from induction to delivery was more exaggerated. With current techniques, using 50% nitrous oxide and 0.5 MAC halogenated agent, the time from induction to delivery may not be as critical. Nevertheless, most clinicians still believe the duration of anesthesia prior to delivery should be as brief as possible. This can be accomplished by delaying induction of anesthesia until the patient is prepped and draped and the obstetrician is ready to begin the operation. The use of nitrous oxide for surgery during pregnancy has been controversial, particularly in the first trimester. This is discussed in Chapter 13. However, it should be noted that clinical studies support the safety and lack of adverse effect of nitrous oxide on assisted reproductive techniques and for surgery during pregnancy, even in the first trimester (379–383). Therefore, the brief exposure for a cesarean section is unlikely to have adverse fetal effects even if induction to delivery times are prolonged (375, 384).

Halogenated Agents

The use of low-dose halogenated agents such as isoflurane (0.75%), halothane (0.5%), sevoflurane (1.0%), desflurane (2% to 4%), and enflurane (1.0%) as supplements to nitrous oxide anesthesia is very common. Associated with the use of low-dose halogenated agents has been the reduction of nitrous oxide concentration from 70% to 50% before delivery of the newborn. The halogenated agents (a) decrease the likelihood of maternal postoperative recall and awareness of intraoperative events; (b) permit higher maternal inspired oxygen tension; (c) may improve uterine blood flow; (d) do not result in increased uterine bleeding; and (e) do not depress the newborn. A clinical study confirmed a 28% decrease in MAC of isoflurane in pregnant women at 8 to 12 weeks of gestation compared with nonpregnant women (260). While the other halogenated agents have not been studied in humans, a similar reduction has been found in animal studies. There is no clear benefit to the use of sevoflurane (385) or desflurane (386) as volatile agents for cesarean section; thus, the authors routinely use isoflurane.

In an attempt to evaluate the potential effects of general anesthesia upon the compromised fetus, Cheek et al. used an adjustable uterine artery occluder to create hypoxia and acidosis in fetal lambs (387). General anesthesia in the ewe with 1% halothane did not abolish the fetal response to asphyxia. Regional cerebral blood flow, cerebral oxygen supply, and lower cerebral metabolic oxygen consumption were maintained. In a similar study of isoflurane in the ewe, while the increase in blood flow to the fetal brainstem and total brain was blunted, the balance between cerebral oxygen supply and demand remained favorable (388). While caution is necessary when extrapolating animal studies to clinical experience, these studies and others suggest that general anesthetic agents in common use have no unique adverse effects on the compromised fetus and can safely be used for cesarean section with general anesthesia (389–391).

Higher Maternal Oxygen. Maternal hyperoxia should improve fetal oxygenation and neonatal clinical condition at birth. In a study of 75 healthy women undergoing elective cesarean section under general anesthesia, oxygen tension, saturation, and oxygen content of fetal blood increased significantly with increases in maternal inspired oxygen concentration until maternal Pao$_2$ reached approximately 300 mm Hg (Table 11.15) (392). The

Table 11.15. IMPROVEMENT IN UMBILICAL VENOUS AND UMBILICAL ARTERIAL BLOOD OXYGEN TENSIONS AND NEONATAL CONDITION AT BIRTH WITH INCREASING MATERNAL OXYGEN TENSION

Maternal arterial P_{O_2} (mm Hg)	61–100	101–160	181–240	241–300	301–360	361–420	421–520
Number	13	12	3	10	19	11	7
Umbilical venous P_{O_2} (mm Hg)	29	31	29	35	38	41	41
Umbilical artery P_{O_2} (mm Hg)	16	20	21	23	25	26	25
Time necessary for infant to establish sustained respiration (sec)	62	54	33	27	11	13	14
Number of infants with Apgar score of 6 or less	4	2	1	0	0	0	0

There was no further change as maternal arterial P_{O_2} rose above 300 mm Hg.
Modified from Marx GF, Mateo CV. Effects of different oxygen concentrations during general anaesthesia for elective caesarean section. *Can Anaesth Soc J* 1971;18:587–593.

clinical condition of the newborn was also better in the higher oxygen groups. It was noted that there was no additional fetal or neonatal benefit if the maternal oxygen tension was above 300 mm Hg.

Other investigators (393, 394) compared anesthesia with either 50% oxygen (balance nitrous oxide and halogenated agent) to anesthesia with 100% oxygen and halogenated agent. The use of 100% oxygen significantly improved fetal oxygenation with particular benefit in emergent cases. Women receiving 100% oxygen received higher concentrations of isoflurane (1.8% initially, decreasing to 1.2%). There was no maternal awareness and no increased blood loss (394). Babies born to mothers who received 100% oxygen required less resuscitation than those whose mothers received 50% oxygen.

Improved Uterine Blood Flow. Anesthetic agents modify sympathetic activity. In pregnant sheep, noxious stimulation during nitrous oxide–oxygen anesthesia was associated with an increase in maternal blood pressure, a decrease in uterine blood flow, and an increase in plasma norepinephrine compared to the unstimulated awake animal (395). By contrast, noxious stimulation during nitrous oxide–oxygen anesthesia supplemented with either 0.5% halothane or 1% enflurane did not increase plasma catecholamines. Blood pressure remained unchanged in both

groups, and uterine blood flow increased with halothane but did not change with enflurane (Fig. 11.27).

Uterine Bleeding. The main concerns associated with the administration of halogenated agents are that they may decrease uterine muscle tone and that postpartum blood loss will increase. The halogenated agents produce a dose-related decrease in uterine contractility and tone (396–400). However, several studies have failed to demonstrate increased blood loss with low-dose halothane 0.1% to 0.8% (Tables 11.16 and 11.17) (401–406), enflurane 0.5% to 1.5% (407), or isoflurane 0.75% during cesarean section. At these low concentrations, the uterus in the immediate postpartum period is responsive to oxytocin stimulation (400). One study (408) demonstrated that the addition of halogenated agents was associated with a greater fall in postpartum hematocrit and an increased requirement for blood transfusion. However, it is apparent that, in this retrospective analysis, the group receiving halogenated agent was not comparable to the other groups. When higher concentrations of halogenated agents are used, (393, 394) blood loss is still not clinically significantly increased, and their regimens, as described in Table 11.18, may be useful when high-inspired maternal oxygen concentrations are indicated. There is no evidence to suggest that use of sevoflurane or desflurane as a maintenance agent for

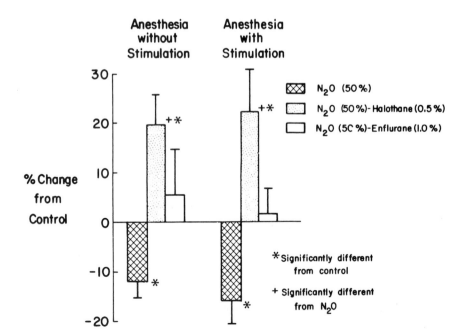

Figure 11.27. Uterine blood flow changes during anesthesia in the pregnant ewe with and without noxious stimulation. The three anesthetics administered for 1 hour each were nitrous oxide 50%, nitrous oxide 50% plus halothane 0.5%, and nitrous oxide 50% plus enflurane 1.0%. (Reprinted by permission from Shnider SM, Wright RG, Levinson G, et al. Plasma norepinephrine and uterine blood flow changes during endotracheal intubation and general anesthesia in the pregnant ewe. In: Abstracts of Scientific Papers of the Annual Meeting of the American Society of Anesthesiologists; Chicago, IL; 1978:115.)

Table 11.16. INFLUENCE OF ANESTHESIA ON BLOOD LOSS IN 145 CESAREAN SECTIONS

	Anesthetic			
	$N_2O:O_2$ (70:30) (50 Cases)	$N_2O:O_2$ (50:50) + 0.5% Halothane (50 Cases)	$N_2O:O_2$ (50:50) + 0.8% Halothane (25 Cases)	Epidural Analgesia (20 Cases)
Loss (mean ± SD) (mL)	792 ± 388	688 ± 206	702 ± 294	378 ± 146

Reprinted by permission from Moir DD. Anaesthesia for caesarean section: An evaluation of a method using low concentrations of halothane and 50 percent of oxygen. *Br J Anaesth* 1970;42:136–142.

cesarean section leads to increased blood loss, but these agents have not been studied extensively.

Neonatal Depression. A potential hazard of the use of these potent inhalational agents is neonatal depression. However, clinical experience supports the viewpoint that the slight increase in maternal anesthetic depth is not reflected in the clinical condition of the neonate at birth (393, 394, 401–405, 407, 409–412). The anesthetic plan should strive to avoid clinical situations that may cause fetal acidosis or hypoxemia. This includes use of LUD to prevent aortocaval compression and maternal hypotension, use of at least 50% oxygen prior to delivery, and avoiding excessive maternal hyperventilation. While the authors prefer regional anesthesia for cesarean section when possible, a well-conducted general anesthetic should have no long-term effects on the newborn. A recent survey in Germany found that general anesthesia is used for 61% of *elective cesarean sections,* 83% of urgent cases, and 98% of emergency cases, apparently with good success (413).

Maternal Awareness

Several surveys have reported a high incidence of maternal awareness of surgery and birth with subsequent unpleasant experiences such as nightmares following general anesthetics using only nitrous oxide–oxygen relaxant technique for vaginal delivery or cesarean section (Table 11.19) (346, 401–404, 407, 409, 410, 414–416). The incidence of awareness appears to vary inversely with the concentration of nitrous oxide. For example, in one study, approximately 9% of women who received 67% nitrous oxide in oxygen were aware of the delivery, whereas 26% were aware if 50% nitrous oxide was used (414). Maternal awareness has been reported to be essentially ablated if a low concentration (0.5 MAC) of a volatile agent is administered with 50% nitrous oxide in the interval between induction and delivery (e.g., halothane, 0.5%; isoflurane, 0.6%; sevoflurane, 1.0%; des-

flurane, 3.0%) (401–405, 407, 409–411). Other techniques to reduce awareness during the induction—to—delivery interval include repeat boluses of thiopental, ketamine, benzodiazepine, or propofol. In all circumstances, an adequate induction dose of thiopental or propofol must be administered to minimize the occurrence of awareness. We routinely use low concentrations of volatile agents with 50% nitrous oxide after tracheal intubation.

If a patient experiences awareness of intraoperative events, it is important to discuss the patient's experience and feelings in a candid fashion after the occurrence. The patient may benefit from an explanation, particularly the withdrawn or frightened patient. Referral for therapy may minimize the incidence of associated posttraumatic neurosis, nightmares, and anxiety.

REGIONAL VS. GENERAL ANESTHESIA: CONDITION OF THE NEWBORN

A neonate is conventionally evaluated by Apgar score, acid-base status, and neurobehavioral examination. Although it is widely believed that regional anesthesia is safer for the newborn, many studies indicate that either technique can result in vigorous, well-oxygenated babies.

Apgar Score

The anesthesiologist, Virginia Apgar, was the first to point out that babies were more vigorous following cesarean section under conduction (spinal) than general (cyclopropane) anesthesia (417). Since then, numerous studies have confirmed these findings. For example, the Collaborative Project (a research study involving 15 medical centers) demonstrated that among normal gravidas undergoing elective repeat cesarean section, more than five times as many neonates were depressed at 1 minute (Apgar 0 to 3) when delivery occurred under general anesthesia compared with regional anesthesia (418). Moreover,

Table 11.17. HEMATOCRIT VALUES BEFORE AND AFTER CESAREAN SECTION

Anesthetic Technique	Hematocrit (Preoperative)	Hematocrit Postoperative Day 1	Postoperative Postoperative Day 2
Halothane predelivery (n = 22)	37.7 ± 9.1	31.8 ± 4.3	31.4 ± 4.4
Halothane pre- and postdelivery (n = 20)	36.9 ± 3.9	30.8 ± 4.6	29.6 ± 4.3
Epidural (n = 23)	37.9 ± 9.1	33.1 ± 4.6	31.7 ± 4.1

Effect of low-dose halothane during cesarean section on intraoperative blood loss as estimated by postpartum hematocrit changes. Patients received (a) nitrous oxide and halothane 0.5% predelivery and nitrous oxide and opioid postdelivery; (b) nitrous oxide with halothane 0.5% throughout the operation; (c) epidural anesthesia.
Reprinted by permission from Thirion A-V, Wright RG, Messer CP, Rosen MA, Shnider SM. Maternal blood loss associated with low dose halothane administration for cesarean section [abstract]. *Anesthesiology* 1988;69:A693.

Table 11.18. EFFECT OF VARIOUS ANESTHETIC REGIMENS ON BLOOD LOSS AND CHANGE IN HEMOGLOBIN OVER 48 HOURS FOLLOWING CESAREAN SECTION*

	N$_2$O/O$_2$:50:50, Halothane 0.5%		100% O$_2$, Halothane 1.1% × 5 min, then Halothane 0.75%		100% O$_2$, Enflurane 2.5% × 5 min, then Enflurane 1.7%		100% O$_2$, Isofluran 1.8% × 5 min, then Isoflurane 1.2%	
	Elective	Emergent	Elective	Emergent	Elective	Emergent	Elective	Emergent
Mean blood loss	619	896	689	740	874*	610	613	641
SD	87	559	197	191	317	270	205	145
Mean maximum derease in Hb (%)	5.5	13.1	7.4	21.4	8.3	12.8	11.4*	15.6
SD	2.8	5.3	5.3	10.3	5.6	7.5	4.8	7.2

Hb = hemoglobin.
*$P < .05$ compared to N$_2$O:O$_2$–50:50, halothane 0.5% (elective).
Modified with permission from Bogod DG, Rosen M, Rees GAD. Maximum F$_{IO_2}$ during caesarean section. *Br J Anaesth* 1988;61:255–262.

in this study, three times as many newborns had depressed Apgar scores at 5 minutes after general anesthesia in contrast to regional anesthesia. The investigators believed this prolonged depression probably represented inadequate management of the newborn. In early work at UCSF, it was noted that after general anesthesia (thiopental induction followed by 70% nitrous oxide), neonates at 5 minutes of age were as vigorous as neonates whose mothers received regional anesthesia. However, there was a higher incidence of depressed newborns at 1 minute of age among those neonates exposed to general anesthesia, but they responded rapidly to stimulation and assisted ventilation. (Table 11.20). The initial lower Apgar scores among the babies exposed to general anesthesia was probably due to transient sedation rather than asphyxia. This transient sedation can be markedly reduced with current anesthetic techniques that include higher concentrations of inspired oxygen and reduced concentrations of nitrous oxide (50%), combined with low-dose halogenated agents (0.5 MAC), continuous lateral tilt, and reasonably expeditious delivery times (less than 10 to 15 minutes from induction to delivery [I-D interval], and less than 3 minutes from uterine incision to delivery [U-D interval]). While I-D intervals with general anesthesia are often very short in community practice (2 to 5 minutes), longer intervals can occur. In those cases, effective ventilation of the newborn with 100% oxygen will most often lead to high 5-minute Apgars and excellent newborn outcome.

Table 11.19. MATERNAL AWARENESS OF SURGERY AND BIRTH AFTER BARBITURATE-RELAXANT INDUCTION

Anesthetic	Incidence of Awareness (%)
Nitrous oxide: 50% (405, 411, 414, 415)	12–26
Nitrous oxide: 67–75% (401, 409, 414, 415)	4–10
Nitrous oxide: 33% + methoxyflurane (410)	3.5
Nitrous oxide: 25–40% + halothane 0.3–0.5% (402)	0
Nitrous oxide: 50% + halothane 0.1–0.65% (401, 403–405, 411)	0
Nitrous oxide: 50% + enflurane 0.5–1.5% (405, 407, 411)	0
Nitrous oxide: 50% + isoflurane 0.5–0.75% (411, 385)	0
Nitrous oxide: 50% + sevoflurane 1% (385)	0
Nitrous oxide: 50% + desflurane 3% (386)	0

In a review of 3940 cesarean deliveries between 1975 and 1983 (419), multivariate analysis revealed the risk of poor neonatal outcome was greater after general than regional anesthesia. The investigators found that general anesthesia, whether for elective or emergency cesarean section, was an independent risk factor for low Apgar scores after controlling for numerous other variables. Furthermore, analysis of the elective cesarean group found significantly higher Apgar scores at 1-minute after regional anesthesia. Although the infants born to mothers who received general anesthesia had lower 1-minute Apgar scores and required more active respiratory resuscitation, to include oxygen by mask after birth, there was marked improvement in the 5-minute Apgar scores. After multivariate analysis to control for numerous neonatal risks, the investigators concluded that infants delivered by cesarean section under general anesthesia were more likely to be depressed and more likely to require active resuscitation than those delivered by regional anesthesia. However, the ultimate neonatal outcomes were similar. When comparing general to regional anesthesia for cesarean delivery, others observed no difference in neonatal Apgar scores at 1 and 5 minutes (420, 421).

With any technique, babies delivered shortly after the induction of general anesthesia are as vigorous as those born with regional anesthesia (Tables 11.21 and 11.22). Early studies at UCSF found that neonatal depression after general anesthesia is related to the duration of anesthesia, which is in agreement with numerous other studies (376, 377, 422, 423). For example, Stenger et al. (376) reported a 15% incidence of depressed neonates when the mean duration of nitrous oxide anesthesia was 15 minutes and a 54% incidence when the duration was 36 minutes. Finster and Poppers (377) found that if the duration of anesthesia was less than 10 minutes, the mean Apgar score was 7.7, but it decreased to 6.8 in the group delivered between 11 and 20 minutes, and to 6.3 when the duration of anesthesia before delivery exceeded 21 minutes.

Thus, when general anesthesia is chosen, expeditious delivery of the newborn is preferred to minimize neonatal depression. If a prolonged operating time is anticipated, regional anesthesia may be preferable. In contrast to general anesthesia, the

Table 11.20. ELECTIVE CESAREAN SECTION: CLINICAL CONDITION OF NEWBORN

	Apgar Score: 7–10 (%)	
	1 Min	5 Min
Spinal (n = 151)	92	97
Epidural (n = 327)	91	99
General (n = 163)	69	97

Table 11.21. ELECTIVE CESAREAN SECTION: DURATION OF GENERAL ANESTHESIA (N$_2$O:O$_2$): ANTEPARTUM AND APGAR SCORES

	Apgar Score: 7–10	
Minutes of Anesthesia	No.	%
<5	16	88
6–10	47	74
11–20	36	69
21–30	20	50
31–60	11	36

Reprinted by permission from Rolbin SH, Levinson G, Shnider SM. Current status of anesthesia for cesarean section. *Weekly Anesthesiology Update.* Vol. 1. 1977: lesson 7.

authors have found that a prolonged duration of *epidural* anesthesia does not result in depressed neonates (Table 11.22). In addition, the hypotension so common with regional anesthesia, when properly and promptly treated, does not result in low Apgar scores (Table 11.23). This has been demonstrated for *spinal* anesthesia as well, which is increasingly the choice for cesarean section (18, 424, 425).

Acid-Base Status

Numerous investigators have compared fetal acid-base status in umbilical cord blood sampled from a doubly-clamped segment immediately after elective cesarean section delivery (42, 378, 409, 426–428). Differences between the techniques are minimal and not clinically significant. With any well-conducted anesthetic technique, a healthy fetus delivered by cesarean section with reasonably expeditious I-D times and U-D times less than 3 minutes should have neonatal acid-base values in the normal range. Even with prolonged general anesthesia and depressed Apgar scores (i.e., sleepy babies), fetal acid-base status is normal and effective ventilation and resuscitation should lead to a good outcome.

If fetal hypoxia and acidosis are found with elective cesarean section, a number of etiologic factors may exist. With general anesthesia, maternal hypoxia, excessive hyperventilation, aortocaval compression, or anesthetic overdose leading to hypotension can cause fetal asphyxia. With regional anesthesia, unrecognized, inadequate, or delayed treatment of hypotension may be the cause of fetal acidosis. *With either technique, a prolonged **U-D** time has been found to correlate directly with fetal hypoxia and acidosis.* Crawford and Davies (429) studied cesarean section with general anesthesia, and found that the condition of the infant, both clinical and biochemical (acid-base), was directly related to the time that elapsed from the initial uterine incision to completion

Table 11.22. ELECTIVE CESAREAN SECTION: DURATION OF EPIDURAL ANESTHESIA ANTEPARTUM AND APGAR SCORES

	Apgar Score: 7–10	
Minutes of Anesthesia	No.	%
< 20	20	85
21–30	44	93
31–60	214	92
61–120	40	90
> 20	5	100

Reprinted by permission from Rolbin SH, Levinson G, Shnider SM. Current status of anesthesia for cesarean section. *Weekly Anesthesiology Update.* Vol. 1. 1977: lesson 7.

Table 11.23. ELECTIVE CESAREAN SECTION: HYPOTENSION AND CONDITION OF INFANT

		No.	Apgar Score 7–10 (%)	
Spinal	Hypotension	104	91	
	No hypotension	47	100	NS
Epidural	Hypotension	102	88	
	No hypotension	227	93	NS

NS = no statistically significant difference between hypotension and no hypotension.

of delivery. This was confirmed by Datta et al. (430), who found both general and spinal anesthesia were associated with a significantly lower pH in the baby and a higher incidence of depressed Apgar scores if U-D intervals exceeded 3 minutes. Prolonged U-D intervals during regional anesthesia results in elevated fetal umbilical artery norepinephrine concentrations and associated fetal acidosis (431). Thus, the obstetrician should try to minimize the U-D interval whenever possible. Documentation on the anesthetic record of the I-D and U-D times is recommended.

Neurobehavioral Examination

Even when neonates are not depressed at birth as ascertained by low Apgar scores, more subtle neurobehavioral changes in the subsequent neonatal period may occur. This is discussed fully in Chapter 37. Using the early neonatal behavioral scale on infants delivered by cesarean section, Scanlon et al. (432) reported that infants born after general anesthesia with nitrous oxide were more depressed 6 to 8 hours later compared with those born after regional anesthesia. Palahnuik (409), Hodgkinson (433), and Abboud (420) et al. reported similar results. In all studies, the neurobehavioral effects were subtle and essentially disappeared by 24 hours of age. Hollmén et al. (434) found that neurobehavioral scores were lower in infants born after epidural rather than general anesthesia, but several of the mothers had hypotension that was not promptly treated. Abboud et al. found that hypotension from spinal anesthesia, when promptly treated, did not result in babies with depressed neurobehavioral scores (435). In a further study comparing epidural anesthesia and general anesthesia, the investigators found no difference in Apgar scores or neurobehavioral examinations of the newborn (420). In contrast, a study by Mahajan et al. of 90 healthy women undergoing elective cesarean section with either general, spinal, or epidural anesthesia found significantly higher NACS at 15 minutes and 2 hours when spinal anesthesia was used (436). However, the acid-base status and Apgar scores were similar in all groups, and the NACS was good in all neonates at the 24-hour examination. The reliability and validity of the NACS examination has been recently questioned (437), and the results reported by Mahajan seem to suggest no real clinical difference in newborn outcome regardless of anesthetic technique (438).

EMERGENCY CESAREAN SECTION

Sudden, unexpected complications occurring during late pregnancy or labor that adversely affect the mother or fetus may necessitate an immediate emergency cesarean section. Such complications include massive bleeding, prolapsed umbilical cord, or severe fetal distress. When the condition of the mother or fetus is in immediate jeopardy, general anesthesia is usually selected, but under some circumstances extension of an existing epidural or administration of a subarachnoid block may be appropriate. Choice of anesthesia for fetal distress remains controversial and will be discussed.

For some emergency cesarean sections in which neither the mother nor the fetus is in imminent danger, immediate delivery is not crucial. Examples include repeat cesarean section in early labor, failure of induction of labor, failure of labor to progress, failure of an instrumental vaginal delivery, chorioamnionitis, malpresentation of the fetus, and mild-to-moderate fetal distress. In these situations, either regional or general anesthesia may be administered, but currently regional anesthesia is most commonly selected.

Fetal distress is an imprecise and nonspecific term (439), but is commonly used to describe a clinical situation in which fetal well-being may be compromised by fetal hypoxia or asphyxia in the intrauterine environment. How reliably the fetal heart rate predicts adverse neonatal outcome and how dependably its interpretation dictates the speed at which the fetus should be delivered are controversial. However, fetal distress is a common indication for emergency cesarean section. Fetal hypoxia is a decrease in fetal oxygen tension (umbilical venous Po_2 <15 mm Hg), and fetal asphyxia is a decrease in fetal oxygen tension and an increase in carbon dioxide tension (umbilical venous Pco_2 >40 mm Hg). The fetal response to asphyxia includes redistribution of cardiac output to increase blood flow to vital organs–brain, heart, adrenal glands–thereby maintaining oxygen uptake by these organs. Blood flow to other organs is decreased, and the resulting anaerobic metabolism produces lactic acid and a metabolic acidosis. When asphyxia is prolonged or severe, the fetus may no longer be able to provide the increased blood flow to the vital organs, and cerebral and myocardial oxygen consumption will no longer be maintained.

Fetal distress is probably best defined as "progressive fetal asphyxia that, if not corrected or circumvented, will result in decompensation of the physiologic responses... and cause permanent central nervous system and other damage or death" (440). In a 1998 American College of Obstetricians and Gynecologists (ACOG) Committee Opinion (No. 197), it was stated that "the term *fetal distress* is imprecise and nonspecific" (439). The Committee went on to suggest that the term *fetal distress* be replaced with *nonreassuring fetal status*, followed by a further description of the findings (e.g., repetitive variable decelerations, fetal bradycardia, etc.). The Committee further noted that the term *fetal distress* may result in an unnecessarily urgent delivery under general anesthesia.

Anesthesia for cesarean delivery of the distressed fetus should rapidly provide suitable operating conditions for the obstetrician without (1) unduly jeopardizing maternal safety, (2) increasing fetal asphyxia, or (3) compromising fetal compensatory mechanisms. The rapidity required for delivery is usually determined by the obstetrician's assessment of the severity of the fetal asphyxia. With rare exceptions, there is usually sufficient time to provide anesthesia by either general anesthesia, extension of an existing labor epidural, or administration of a spinal anesthetic.

Traditionally, general anesthesia has been chosen because of (1) the belief that there is less likelihood of adverse maternal hemodynamic changes that could further compromise uteroplacental circulation, and (2) the belief that anesthesia can be more rapidly achieved with general than with spinal or epidural anesthesia. Several studies have shown that, in fact, regional anesthesia can be safely administered.

Regional vs. General Anesthesia

Marx et al. (441) studied the fetal biochemical and neonatal clinical data in 126 emergency cesarean sections performed for fetal distress. The etiology of the fetal distress (late or variable decelerations, persistent bradycardia or tachycardia, acidosis, thick meconium) was not significantly different between the anesthetic groups. The choice of anesthetic technique was determined by the wishes of the mother. General anesthesia was administered to 71, subarachnoid block to 33, and extension of an existing epidural to 22 parturients. The umbilical cord blood gas values were similar in all groups, while the 1-minute

Apgar scores were significantly higher in the regional anesthesia groups. The authors concluded that "regional analgesia provides maternal and fetal advantages even in the presence of fetal distress" (441). This has led many anesthesiologists to consider spinal anesthesia or extension of an epidural block for urgent cases where there are no obvious contraindications, such as maternal cardiovascular instability, extremely low platelet count, or patient refusal (441, 442).

Ramanathan et al. (443) studied 443 patients undergoing emergency cesarean section for fetal distress. Fetal distress consisted of (1) severe persistent bradycardia, (2) persistent late decelerations, (3) severe repetitive variable decelerations, or (4) loss of beat-to-beat variability. General anesthesia was administered to 322 patients, and existing labor epidurals were extended for 121 patients. There were no significant differences among Apgar scores, umbilical pH, or cord blood gases in any of the four fetal distress groups.

In a more recent review covering cesarean sections at the Brigham and Women's Hospital in Boston, only 3.6% of all cesarean sections were performed with general anesthesia, while 46% were performed with spinal anesthesia, and 50.4% with epidural anesthesia (444). Obviously, epidural blocks were extended or spinal anesthesia was used for many emergency cesarean sections, although this was not specifically detailed.

Despite the necessity for speed when administering anesthesia for fetal distress, careful technique is still necessary. Rapid preanesthetic assessment of the mother is essential. Potential problems with intubation or airway maintenance or technical difficulties with block placement will obviously affect the choice of anesthetic technique. Similarly, the presence of maternal hypovolemia, hemorrhage, or coagulopathy is an important consideration for choice of anesthetic technique.

Good communication between obstetric care providers and the obstetric anesthesia providers is vital for maternal and fetal safety, and necessary to consistently achieve the best possible outcome. ACOG has advised the obstetric care team to "be alert to the presence of risk factors that place the parturient at increased risk for complications from emergency general or regional anesthesia." This recommendation goes on to identify important risks to the parturient and recommends that the obstetrician inform and consult with the anesthesia provider regarding these factors ("ACOG Committee Opinion–Anesthesia for Emergency Deliveries" No. 104, first published in 1992, and reaffirmed in 1998). See Chapter 21, Appendix.

Morgan et al. (445) reviewed their experience with 360 consecutive emergency cesarean sections. In this prospective study, it was noted that 87% of these emergency cesarean sections could be anticipated. Assessment of the parturient by the obstetrician, midwife, and anesthesiologist early in labor allowed the timely placement of an epidural block to those who seemed likely to require a cesarean delivery. Cesarean section was performed with an epidural in 70% (251) of the patients. Spinal anesthesia for cesarean section was uncommon at this institution at the time of the study, and its use would have avoided still further general anesthetics. There were no significant differences in neonatal outcome between the general and epidural anesthesia groups.

Appropriate resuscitation drugs and equipment must be present. Adequate prehydration (as time permits) and aggressive use of ephedrine to correct and/or prevent maternal hypotension are necessary. Fetal monitoring should be continued, and if deterioration in the fetal condition occurs before the regional block is established, general anesthesia may still be necessary.

Extension of a Preexisting Labor Epidural: How Fast?

Several authors have investigated the speed of onset of an adequate epidural blockade for cesarean section with a preexisting,

Table 11.24. EXTENSION OF EPIDURAL BLOCKADE FOR EMERGENCY CESAREAN SECTION

Author	Ref	Agent for Labor	Agent Administered	Speed of Onset
Price et al. 1991 (n = 36)	(449)	0.25% bupivacaine by 10 mL bolus doses	2% lidocaine + 1:200,000 epinephrine 20 mL over 3–4 min	92% ready for surgery within 10 min 100% within 12.5 min
Gaiser et al. 1994 (n = 29)	(448)	Not noted	3% 2-chloroprocaine, 24 ± 6.0 mL	9 ± 5 min*
(n = 80)		Not noted	1.5% lidocaine with sodium bicarbonate and epinephrine 1:200,000, 24.6 ± 5.5 mL	12 ± 5 min
Gaiser et al. 1998 (n = 8)	(447)	0.125% bupivacaine 1:400,000	3% 2-chloroprocaine + sodium bicarbonate 25 mL	T_4 senory level 3.1 ± 0.3 min†
(n = 10)			1.5% lidocaine + sodium bicarbonate 1:200,000 epinephrine, 25 mL	4.4 ± 1.6 min
Lucas et al. 1999 (n = 30)	(446)	0.1% bupivacaine + fentanyl 2 μg·mL^{-1}	20 mL injected over 3 min bupivacaine 0.5%	T_4 sensory level (range) 14 min (11–19.3)‡
(n = 30)			Lidocaine 2% + 1:200,000 epinephrine	10 min (9–18.5)‡
(n = 30)			Bupivacaine 0.5% + lidocaine 2% 50:50 mixture + 1:200,000 epinephrine	12 min (8.8–17)‡

* $P < .05$
† $P < .005$
‡ No significant difference between groups

well-functioning labor epidural (Table 11.24) (446–449). The factors that determine the onset include the local anesthetic agent administered, the addition of bicarbonate, the speed of injection, and the density and dermatomal spread of the preexisting blockade.

For extension of a labor epidural block, adequate doses of rapidly acting local anesthetics should be administered. The authors most often select either 2-chloroprocaine 3%, or lidocaine 2% with NaHCO$_3$ (1 mEq/10 mL) and epinephrine 1:200,000 to produce rapid anesthesia. For subarachnoid block, either lidocaine 60 to 75 mg or bupivacaine 12 to 15 mg (with fentanyl 10 to 25 μg and morphine 0.1 to 0.25 mg) is satisfactory. Time may not allow the addition of intrathecal opioids in emergent situations.

While catheter migration or unrecognized misplacement of a catheter is rare, the rapid administration of local anesthetic without the usual careful regimen of testing requires that the clinician remain alert to the possible complications. Unexpected IV or intrathecal injection of a large dose of local anesthetic can occur, and the clinician must be prepared to proceed with emergency resuscitation. A recent report demonstrated that a subdural (but not subarachnoid) catheter used for labor analgesia provided good analgesia for labor with dilute bupivacaine 0.04%, epinephrine 1:600,000, and fentanyl 1.7 μg·mL^{-1}, but created a life-threatening emergency when the catheter was used later for cesarean section (450). When the epidural block was slowly extended with lidocaine 2%, epinephrine 1:200,000, and fentanyl 5 μg·mL^{-1} after a 3-mL test dose, a high block resulted within 10 minutes requiring urgent intubation. A total of 15 mL had been administered in an incremental fashion. Rapid extension without test dosing and incremental dosing of this subdural catheter (later proven by computed tomography) might have resulted in a catastrophic clinical situation. The increased use of the CSE technique in labor, as well as the use of very dilute local anesthetic solutions for a labor epidural, increase the likelihood that epidural catheters are not *well tested*. This increases the risk of a catastrophic outcome, or failed block, when rapid extension of a labor epidural is used for an urgent cesarean section. This is a significant risk if the subdural cannulation rate is as high as 0.82%, as has been suggested (451).

Rapid extension of an epidural block facilitates the use of regional anesthesia for emergency cesarean section and avoids administration of a general anesthetic, which has inherent risks. However, the clinician must understand that omitting an epidural test dose to hasten the onset of block for potential fetal benefit incurs additional risk to the mother. This should not be undertaken without careful consideration.

Maternal Benefits and Safety

The choice of anesthesia for cesarean section depends on the reason for the operation, the degree of urgency, and the desires of the patient. Many women prefer a regional anesthetic for cesarean section even in an urgent or stat situation. When regional anesthesia can be safely provided, it should be given consideration. However, the real benefit is the potential for decreased maternal morbidity and mortality. The report by Hawkins et al. (8) concerning anesthesia-related maternal mortality has clearly demonstrated the risks involved in general anesthesia. Maternal death from complications of general anesthesia for cesarean section increased from 20 deaths per million with general anesthesia (1979–84) to 32.3 deaths per million with general anesthesia (1985–90). In the same study period, deaths from regional anesthesia for cesarean section decreased from 8.6 to 1.9 per million regional anesthetics. In this review, 82% of the deaths occurred during cesarean section, while only 5% occurred during regional anesthesia for labor (13% listed as unknown). Unfortunately, this study was conducted without a review of the medical records, which were unavailable (281). The type of anesthesia was not identified in 20% of women who died, and the type of anesthesia was not identified in 40% of women whose cause of death was listed as cardiac arrest on the death certificate. The methods used to estimate the number of deaths and the number of cesarean sections have limitations of validity of the survey data. The authors may have underestimated the use of general anesthesia during the years 1985–90, which would result in an overstatement of the relative risk of general anesthesia. However, airway management remains a significant area of risk, along with obesity, *urgent* or *stat* surgery, and hypertensive diseases. While general anesthesia for *urgent* or *stat* cesarean deliveries remains an appropriate choice in numerous critical obstetric situations, the increasing use of regional anesthesia appears to have decreased maternal mortality related to anesthesia. No one method of anesthesia is ideal for cesarean section. The anesthesiologist must choose the method that provides the appropriate balance of maternal safety, fetal benefit, and suitable working conditions for the obstetrician. Maternal safety is achieved by using techniques that minimize risk, and ideally that provide optimal comfort. Fetal benefit includes minimizing further fetal depression and rapidly inducing anesthesia to facilitate delivery and newborn resuscitation. In a Committee opinion, ACOG has stated, "Performing a cesarean delivery for a nonreassuring fetal heart rate pattern does not necessarily preclude the use of regional anesthesia" (439).

Both the American Society of Anesthesiologists (ASA) and the American College of Obstetricians and Gynecologists (ACOG) have developed committee opinions or optimal goals that address the provision of care for emergency cesarean section. Both the "Optimal Goals for Anesthesia Care in Obstetrics," approved by the ASA House of Delegates in October 2000, and the "ACOG Committee Opinion–Anesthesia for Emergency Deliveries (No. 104)," first published in 1992 and reaffirmed in 1998, appear in the Appendix C of this book.

Both of these societies suggest that, when necessary, emergency cesarean deliveries should have the capability of beginning within 30 minutes. However, more recently, an ACOG Practice Bulletin, "Clinical Management Guidelines for Obstetrician-Gynecologists: Vaginal Birth After Cesarean Delivery" (VBAC) (No. 5, July 1999), recommends that physicians be "immediately" available to provide emergency care and institutions be equipped to respond to emergencies when VBAC is attempted because uterine rupture can be catastrophic. Anesthesia, obstetric and nurse personnel, and the necessary support services must be prepared to function within these guidelines. See Appendix C.

Anesthesia for cesarean section in the presence of some of the more common and significant obstetric and medical complications is discussed in the following chapters: preeclampsia-eclampsia, Chapter 16; placenta previa, abruptio placentae, and ruptured uterus, Chapter 20; parturients with cardiac disease, Chapter 26; the diabetic parturient, Chapter 28; parturient with HIV disease, Chapter 33 and the drug-addicted parturient, Chapter 34. Numerous medical conditions are discussed elsewhere in this book and may have unique considerations when planning anesthesia for a cesarean section.

REFERENCES

1. Notzon FC. International differences in the use of obstetric interventions. *JAMA* 1990;263:3286–3291.
2. Notzon FC, Placek PJ, Taffel SM. Comparisons of national cesarean-section rates. *N Engl J Med* 1987;316:386–389.
3. Evrard J, Gold EM. Cesarean section and maternal mortality in Rhode Island: Incidence and risk factors, 1965–1975. *Obstet Gynecol* 1977;50:594–597.
4. Rubin GL, Peterson HB, Rochat RW, McCarthy BJ, Terry JS. Maternal death after cesarean section in Georgia. *Am J Obstet Gynecol* 1981;139:681–685.
5. Petitti DB, Cefalo RC, Shapiro S, Whalley P. In-hospital maternal mortality in the United States: Time trends and relation to method of delivery. *Obstet Gynecol* 1982;59:6–12.
6. Frigoletto RJ, Ryan KJ, Phillippe M. Maternal mortality rate associated with cesarean section: An appraisal. *Am J Obstet Gynecol* 1980;136:969–970.
7. Bottoms SF, Rosen MG, Sokol RJ. Current concepts–the increase in the cesarean birth rate. *N Engl J Med* 1980;302:559–563.
8. Hawkins JL, Koonin LM, Palmer SK, Gibbs CP. Anesthesia-related deaths during obstetric delivery in the United States, 1979–1990. *Anesthesiology* 1997;86:277–284.
9. Gibbs CP, Krischer J, Peckham BM, Sharp H, Kirschbaum TH. Obstetric anesthesia: A national survey. *Anesthesiology* 1986;65:298–306.
10. Hicks JS, Levinson G, Shnider SM. Obstetric anesthesia training centers in the U.S.A.–1975. *Anesth Analg* 1976;55:839–845.
11. Hawkins JL, Gibbs CP, Orleans M, et al. Obstetric anesthesia work force survey: 1981 versus 1992. *Anesthesiology* 1997;87:135–143.
12. Hawkins JL, Beaty BR, Gibbs CP. Update on U.S. obstetric anesthesia practices [abstract]. *Anesthesiology* 1999;91:A1060.
13. Johnson RO, Lyons GR, Wilson RC, et al. Training in obstetric general anesthesia: A vanishing art? *Anaesthesia* 2000;55:163–183.
13a. Tsen LC, Pitner R, Camann WR. General anesthesia for cesarean section at a tertiary care hospital 1990–1995: Indications and implications. *Int J Obstet Anesth* 1998;7:147–152.
14. Assali NS, Prystowsky H. Studies on autonomic blockade. II. Observations on the nature of blood pressure fall with high selective spinal anesthesia in pregnant women. *J Clin Invest* 1950;29:1367–1375.
15. Bromage PR. Continuous lumbar epidural analgesia for obstetrics. *Can Med Assoc J* 1961;85:1136–1140.
16. Fagraeus L, Urban BJ, Bromage PR. Spread of epidural analgesia in early pregnancy. *Anesthesiology* 1983;58:184–187.
17. Grundy EM, Zamora AM, Winnie AP. Comparison of spread of epidural anesthesia in pregnant and nonpregnant women. *Anesth Analg* 1978;57:544–546.
17a. Flanagan HL, Datta S, Lambert DH, et al. Effect of pregnancy on bupivacaine-induced conduction blockade in the isolated rabbit vagus nerve. *Anesth Analg* 1987;66:123–126.
17b. Butterworth JF IV, Walker FO, Lysak SZ. Pregnancy increases median nerve susceptibility to lidocaine. *Anesthesiology* 1990;72:962–965.
18. Riley ET, Cohen SE, Macario A, et al. Spinal versus epidural anesthesia for cesarean section: A comparison of time efficiency costs, charges, and complications. *Anesth Analg* 1995;80:709–712.
19. Irestedt L. Spinal anesthesia for cesarean section. *Acta Anaesthesiol Scand* 1998;113(suppl):21–23.
20. Robson SC, Boys RJ, Rodeck C, Morgan B. Maternal and fetal hemodynamic effects of spinal and extradural anesthesia for elective caesarean section. *Br J Anaesth* 1992;68:54–59.
21. Arkoosh VA, Palmer CM, Van Marea GA, et al. Continuous intrathecal labor analgesia: Safety and efficacy [abstract]. *Anesthesiology* 1998;89:A1041.
22. Kanto J, Sjowall S, Erkkola R, et al. Placental transfer and maternal midazolam kinetics. *Clin Pharmacol Ther* 1983;33:786–791.
23. Eisele JH, Wright R, Rogge P. Newborn and maternal fentanyl levels at cesarean section. *Anesth Analg* 1982;61:179–180.
24. Kan RE, Hughes SC, Rosen MA, Kessin C, Preston PG, Lobo EP. Intravenous remifentanil: Placental transfer, maternal and neonatal effects. *Anesthesiology* 1998;88:1467–1474.
25. Roberts RB, Shirley MA. The obstetrician's role in reducing the risk of aspiration pneumonitis with particular reference to the use of oral antacids. *Am J Obstet Gynecol* 1976;124:611–617.
26. Rout CC, Rocke DA, Gouws E. Intravenous ranitidine reduces the risk of acid aspiration of gastric contents at emergency cesarean section. *Anesth Analg* 1993;76:156–161.
27. Lin CJ, Huang CL, Hsu HW, Chen TL. Prophylaxis against acid aspiration in regional anesthesia for elective cesarean section: A comparison between oral single-dose ranitidine, famotidine, and omeprazole assessed with fiberoptic gastric aspiration. *Acta Anaesthesiol Scand* 1996;34:179–184.
28. Chestnut DH, Vandewalker GE, Owen CL, Bates JN, Choi WW. Administration of metoclopramide for prevention of nausea and vomiting during epidural anesthesia for elective cesarean section. *Anesthesiology* 1987;66:563–566.
29. Ramanathan S, Gandhi S, Arismendy J, Chanon J, Turndorf H. Oxygen transfer from mother to fetus during cesarean section under epidural anesthesia. *Anesth Analg* 1982;61:576–581.
30. Carpenter RL, Caplan RA, Brown DL, et al. Incidence and risk factors for side effects of spinal anesthesia. *Anesthesiology* 1992;76:906–912.
31. Mark JB, Steele SME. Cardiovascular effects of spinal anesthesia. *Int Anesthesiol Clin* 1989;27:31.
32. Shimosato S, Etsten B. The role of the venous system in cardiocirculatory dynamics during spinal and epidural anesthesia in man. *Anesthesiology* 1969;30:619.
33. Brizgys RV, Dailey PA, Shnider SM, Kotelko DM, Levinson G. The incidence and neonatal effects of maternal hypotension

during epidural anesthesia for cesarean section. *Anesthesiology* 1987;67:782–786.

34. Gutsche BB. Prophylactic ephedrine preceding spinal analgesia for cesarean section. *Anesthesiology* 1976;45:462–465.

35. Moran D, Perillo M, LaPorta R, Bader A, Datta S. Phenylephrine in the prevention of hypotension following spinal anesthesia for cesarean delivery. *J Clin Anesth* 1991;3:301–305.

36. Bhagwanjee S, Rocke DA, Rout CC, Koovarjee RV, Brijball R. Prevention of hypotension following spinal anaesthesia for elective caesarean section by wrapping of the legs. *Br J Anaesth* 1990;65:819.

37. Mathru M, Rao TLK, Kartha RK, Shanmugham M, Jacobs HK. Intravenous albumin administration for prevention of spinal hypotension during cesarean section. *Anesth Analg* 1980;59:655.

38. Murray AM, Morgan M, Whitwam JG. Crystalloid versus colloid for circulatory preload for epidural caesarean section. *Anaesthesia* 1988;44:463.

39. Wennberg E, Frid I, Haljamae H, Noren H. Colloid (3% dextran 70) with or without ephedrine infusion for cardiovascular stability during extradural caesarean section. *Br J Anaesth* 1992;69:13.

40. Sinclair CJ, Scott DB, Edstrom HH. Effect of the Trendelenburg position on spinal anaesthesia with hyperbaric bupivacaine. *Br J Anaesth* 1982;54:497.

41. Miyabe M, Namiki A. The effect of head-down tilt on arterial blood pressure after spinal anesthesia. *Anesth Analg* 1993;76:549.

42. Marx GF, Cosmi EV, Wollman SB. Biochemical status and clinical condition of mother and infant at cesarean section. *Anesth Analg* 1969;48:986–993.

43. Rout CC, Rocke DA, Levin J, Gouws E, Reddy D. A re-evaluation of the role of crystalloid preload in the prevention of hypotension associated with spinal anesthesia for elective cesarean section. *Anesthesiology* 1993;79:262–269.

44. Rout CC, Akoojee SS, Rocke DA, Gouws E. Rapid administration of crystalloid preload does not decrease the incidence of hypotension after spinal anaesthesia for elective caesarean section. *Br J Anaesth* 1992;68:394–397.

45. Karinen J, Räsänen J, Alahuhta S, Jouppila R, Jouppila P. Effect of crystalloid and colloid preloading on uteroplacental and maternal haemodynamic state during spinal anaesthesia for Caesarean section. *Br J Anaesth* 1995;75:531–535.

46. Park GE, Hauch MA, Curlin F, Datta S, Bader AM. The effects of varying volumes of crystalloid administration before cesarean delivery on maternal hemodynamics and colloid osmotic pressure. *Anesth Analg* 1996;83:299–303.

47. Riley ET, Cohen SE, Rubenstein AJ, Flanagan B. Prevention of hypotension after spinal anesthesia for cesarean section: Six percent hetastarch versus lactated Ringer's solution. *Anesth Analg* 1995;81:838–842.

48. Ueyama H, He YL, Tanigami H, Mashimo T, Yoshiya I. Effects of crystalloid and colloid preload on blood volume in the parturient undergoing spinal anesthesia for elective cesarean section. *Anesthesiology* 1999;91:1571–1576.

49. Rout CC, Rocke DA, Gouws E. Leg elevation and wrapping in the prevention of hypotension following spinal anaesthesia for elective caesarean section. *Anaesthesia* 1993;48:304.

50. Goudie TA, Winter AW, Ferguson DJM. Lower limb compression using inflatable splints to prevent hypotension during spinal anaesthesia for caesarean section. *Acta Anaesthesiol Scand* 1988;32:541.

51. James FM, Greiss FC, Kemp RA. An evaluation of vasopressor therapy for maternal hypotension during spinal anesthesia. *Anesthesiology* 1970;33:25–34.

52. Shnider SM, deLorimier AA, Holl JW, Chapler FK, Morishima HO. Vasopressors in obstetrics. I. Correction of fetal acidosis with ephedrine during spinal anesthesia. *Am J Obstet Gynecol* 1968;102:911–919.

53. Ralston DH, Shnider SM, deLorimier AA. Effects of equipotent ephedrine, metaraminol, mephentermine, and methoxamine on uterine blood flow in the pregnant ewe. *Anesthesiology* 1974;40:354–370.

54. Hollmén AI, Jouppila R, Albright GA, Jouppila P, Vierola H, Koivula A. Intervillous blood flow during caesarean section with prophylactic ephedrine and epidural anaesthesia. *Acta Anaesthesiol Scand* 1984;28:396.

55. Butterworth JF, Piccione W, Berrizbeitia LD, et al. Augmentation of venous return by adrenergic agonists during spinal anesthesia. *Anesth Analg* 1986;65:612–616.

56. Weiner CP, Martinez E, Chestnut DH, Ghodsi A. Effect of pregnancy on uterine and carotid artery response to norepinephrine,

57. Tong C, Eisenach JC. The vascular mechanism of ephedrine's beneficial effect on uterine perfusion during pregnancy. *Anesthesiology* 1992;76:792.

58. Ramanathan S, Grant GJ. Vasopressor therapy for hypotension due to epidural anesthesia for cesarean section. *Acta Anaesthesiol Scand* 1988;32:559–565.

59. Alahuhta S, Rasanen J, Jouppila P, Jouppila R, Hollmen A. Ephedrine and phenylephrine for avoiding maternal hypotension due to spinal anaesthesia for caesarean section. *Int J Obstet Anesth* 1992;1:129.

60. Wright PMC, Iftikhar M, Fitzpatrick KT, Moore J, Thompson W. Vasopressor therapy for hypotension during epidural anesthesia for cesarean section: Effects on maternal and fetal flow velocity ratios. *Anesth Analg* 1992;75:56–63.

61. Datta S, Alper MH, Ostheimer G, Weiss JB. Method of ephedrine administration and nausea and hypotension during spinal anesthesia for cesarean section. *Anesthesiology* 1982;56:68.

62. Kang YG, Abouleish E, Caritis S. Prophylactic intravenous ephedrine infusion during spinal anesthesia for cesarean section. *Anesth Analg* 1982;61:839.

63. Gajraj NM, Victory FA, Pace NA, Van Elstraete AC, Wallace DH. Comparison of an ephedrine infusion with crystalloid administration for prevention of hypotension during spinal anesthesia. *Anesth Analg* 1993;76:1023.

64. King S, Rosen MA. Prophylactic ephedrine and hypotension associated with spinal anesthesia for cesarean delivery. *Int J Obstet Anesth* 1998;7:18–22.

65. Coppejans HC, Hoffman VH, Vercauteren MP, et al. Prevention of hypotension by a single 5-mg dose of ephedrine during spinal anesthesia in prehydrated cesarean delivery patients. *Anesth Analg* 2000;90:324–327.

66. Arner O. Complications following spinal anesthesia: Their significance and technique to reduce their incidence. *Acta Chir Scand* 1952;167(suppl):7.

67. Greene BA. A 26-gauge lumbar puncture needle: Its value in the prophylaxis of headache following spinal analgesia for vaginal delivery. *Anesthesiology* 1950;11:464–469.

68. Harris LM, Harmel MH. The comparative incidence of postlumbar puncture headache following spinal anesthesia administered through 20 and 24 gauge needles. *Anesthesiology* 1953;14:390–397.

69. Krueger JE. Etiology and treatment of postspinal headaches. *Anesth Analg* 1953;32:190–198.

70. Hart JR, Whitacre RJ. Pencil-point needle in prevention of postspinal headache. *JAMA* 1951;147:657–658.

71. Ebner H. An evaluation of spinal anesthesia in obstetrics. *Anesth Analg* 1959;38:378–387.

72. Phillips OC, Nelson AT, Lyons WB, Graff TD, Haris LC, Frazier, TM. Spinal anesthesia for vaginal delivery: A review of 2016 cases using Xylocaine. *Obstet Gynecol* 1959;13:437–441.

73. Myers L, Rosenberg M. The use of the 26-gauge spinal needle: A survey. *Anesth Analg* 1962;41:509–515.

74. Tarrow AB. Solution to spinal headaches. *Int Anesth Clin* 1963;1:877–887.

75. Cesarini M, Torrielli R, Lahaye F, Meme JM, Cabiro C. Sprotte needle for intrathecal anaesthesia for caesarean section: Incidence of post-dural puncture headache. *Anaesthesia* 1990;45:656–658.

76. Flatten H, Rodt SA, Vamnes J, Rosland J, Wisborg T, Koller ME. Postdural puncture headache—a comparison between 26 and 29 gauge needles in young patients. *Anaesthesia* 1989;44:147–149.

77. Lesser P, Bembridge M, Lyons G, MacDonald R. An evaluation of a 30-gauge needle for spinal anaesthesia for caesarean section. *Anaesthesia* 1990;45:767–768.

78. Barker P. Are obstetrical headaches avoidable? *Anaesth Intensive Care* 1990;18:553–554.

79. Snyder GE, Person DL, Flor CE, Wilden RT. Headache in obstetrical patients; comparison of Whitacre needle versus Quincke needle [abstract]. *Anesthesiology* 1989;71:A860.

80. Ready LB, Cuplin S, Haschke RH, Nessly M. Spinal needle determinants of rate of transdural fluid leak. *Anesth Analg* 1989;69:457–460.

81. Cruickshank RH, Hopkinson JM. Fluid leak through dural puncture sites. *Anaesthesia* 1989;44:415–418.

82. Lambert DH, Hurley RJ, Hertwig L, Datta S. Role of needle gauge and tip configuration in the production of lumbar puncture headache. *Reg Anesth* 1997;22:66–72.

83. Corbey MP, Bach AB, Lech K, Frørup AM. Grading of severity of postdural puncture headache after 27-gauge Quincke and Whitacre needles. *Acta Anaesthesiol Scand* 1997;41:779–784.

84. Douglas MJ, Ward ME, Campbell DC, Bright SB, Merrick PM. Factors involved in the incidence of post-dural puncture headache with the 25 gauge Whitacre needle for obstetric anesthesia. *Int J Obstet Anesth* 1997;6:220–223.

85. Buettner J, Wresch K-P, Klose R. Postdural puncture headache: Comparison of 25-gauge Whitacre and Quincke needles. *Reg Anesth* 1993;18:166–169.

86. Sitzman BT, Uncles DR. The effects of needle type, gauge, and tip bend on spinal needle deflection. *Anesth Analg* 1996;82:297–301.

87. Halpern S, Preston R. Postdural puncture headache and spinal needle design: Metaanalysis. *Anesthesiology* 1994;81:1376–1383.

88. Fink BR, Walker S. Orientation of fibers in human dorsal lumbar dura mater in relation to lumbar puncture. *Anesth Analg* 1989;69:768–772.

89. Mihic D. Postspinal headache and relationship of needle bevel to longitudinal dural fibers. *Reg Anesth* 1985;10:76–81.

90. Norris MC, Leighton BL, DeSimone CA. Needle bevel direction and headache after inadvertent dural puncture. *Anesthesiology* 1989;70:729–731.

91. Hart JR, Whitacre RJ. Pencil-point needle in prevention of spinal headache. *JAMA* 1981;147:657–658.

92. Cappe BE. Prevention of post spinal headache with a 22-gauge pencil-point needle and adequate hydration. *Anesth Analg* 1960;39:463–465.

93. Sprotte G, Schedel R, Pajunk H. An atraumatic needle for single shot regional anaesthesia. *Reg Anesth* 1987;10:104–108.

94. Kreuscher HP, Sandmann G. Prevention of postspinal headache by using Whitacre's pencil-point needle. *Reg Anesth* 1989;12:43–45.

95. Stasiuk R, Jenkins L. Post-spinal headache; a comparison of midline and laminar approaches. *Can J Anaesth* 1990;37:S58.

96. Jorgensen N. Post-dural puncture headache is more common with the paramedian approach. *Anesth Analg* 1991;72:S131.

97. Chambers WA, Littlewood DG, Scott DB. Spinal anesthesia with hyperbaric bupivacaine: Effect of added vasoconstrictors. *Anesth Analg* 1982;61:49–52.

98. Abouleish E. Epinephrine improves the quality of spinal hyperbaric bupivacaine for cesarean section. *Anesth Analg* 1987;66:395–400.

99. Moore DC. Spinal anesthesia: Bupivacaine compared with tetracaine. *Anesth Analg* 1980;59:743–750.

100. Benhamou D, Thorin D, Brichant J-F, Dailland P, Milon D, Schneider M. Intrathecal clonidine and fentanyl with hyperbaric bupivacaine improves analgesia during cesarean section. *Anesth Analg* 1998;87:609–613.

101. Eisenach JC, Dekock M, Klinscha W. a2-Adrenergic agonists for regional anesthesia: A clinical review of clonidine (1984–1995). *Anesthesiology* 1996;85:655–674.

102. Santos A, Pedersen H, Finster M, Edström H. Hyperbaric bupivacaine for spinal anesthesia in cesarean section. *Anesth Analg* 1984;63:1009–1013.

103. Logan MR, McClure JH, Wildsmith JAW. Plain bupivacaine: An unpredictable spinal anesthetic agent. *Br J Anaesth* 1986;58:292–296.

104. Russell IF. Spinal anesthesia for cesarean section. *Br J Anaesth* 1983;55:309–313.

105. Norris MC. Height, weight and the spread of hyperbaric bupivacaine in the term parturient. *Anesth Analg* 1988;67:555–558.

106. Norris MC. Patient variables and the subarachnoid spread of hyperbaric bupivacaine in the term parturient. *Anesthesiology* 1990;72:478–482.

107. Hartwell BL, Aglio LS, Hauch MA, Datta S. Vertebral column length and the spread of hyperbaric subarachnoid bupivacaine in the term parturient. *Reg Anesth* 1991;16:17–19.

108. De Simone CA, Leighton BL, Norris MC. Spinal anesthesia for cesarean delivery. A comparison of two doses of hyperbaric bupivacaine. *Reg Anesth* 1995;20:90–94.

109. Sarvela PJ, Halonen PM, Kortilla KT. Comparison of 9 mg of intrathecal plain and hyperbaric bupivacaine both with fentanyl for cesarean delivery. *Anesth Analg* 1999;89:1257–1262.

110. Hunt CO, Naulty JS, Bader AM, et al. Perioperative analgesia with subarachnoid fentanyl-bupivacaine for cesarean delivery. *Anesthesiology* 1989;71:535–540.

111. Olofsson C, Ekblom A, Skoldefors E, Waglund B, Irestedt L. Anesthetic quality during cesarean section following subarachnoid or epidural administration of bupivacaine with or without fentanyl. *Acta Anaesthesiol Scand* 1997;41:332–338.

112. Dahl JB, Jeppesen IS, Jorgensen H, Wetterslev, Moiniche S. Intraoperative and postoperative analgesic efficacy and adverse effects of intrathecal opioids in patients undergoing cesarean section with spinal anesthesia. *Anesthesiology* 1999;91:1919–1927.

113. Courtney MA, Bader AM, Hartwell B, Hauch M, Grennan MJ Datta S. Perioperative analgesia with subarachnoid sufentanil administration. *Reg Anesth* 1992;17:274–278.

114. Dalhgren G, Hultstrand C, Jakobsson J, et al. Intrathecal sufentanil, fentanyl, or placebo added to bupivacaine for cesarean section. *Anesth Analg* 1997;85:1288–1293.

115. Abboud TK, Dror A, Mosaad P, et al. Mini-dose intrathecal morphine for the relief of post-cesarean section pain: Safety, efficacy, and ventilatory responses to carbon dioxide. *Anesth Analg* 1988;67:137–143.

116. Abouleish E, Rawal N, Fallon K, Hernandez D. Combined intrathecal morphine and bupivacaine for cesarean section. *Anesth Analg* 1988;67:370–374.

117. Chadwick SH, Ready LB. Intrathecal and epidural morphine sulfate for post-cesarean analgesia: A clinical comparison. *Anesthesiology* 1988;68:925–929.

118. Stenkamp SJ, Easterling TR, Chadwick HS. Effect of epidural and intrathecal morphine on the length of hospital stay after cesarean section. *Anesth Analg* 1989;68:66–69.

119. Gerancher JC, Floyd H, Eisenach J. Determination of an effective dose of intrathecal morphine for pain relief after cesarean section. *Anesth Analg* 1999;88:346–351.

120. Palmer CM, Emerson S, Volgoropolous D, et al. Dose-response relationship of intrathecal morphine for postcesarean analgesia. *Anesthesiology* 1999;99:437–444.

121. Swart M, Sewell J, Thomas D. Intrathecal morphine for caesarean section; assessment of pain relief, satisfaction and side effects. *Anaesthesia* 1997;52:373–377.

122. Wang BC, Hillman DE, Spielholz NI, Turndorf H. Chronic neurological deficits and Nesacaine-CE: An effect of the anesthetic, 2-chloroprocaine, or the antioxidant, sodium bisulfite? *Anesth Analg* 1984;63:445–447.

123. Gissen AJ, Datta S, Lambert D. The chloroprocaine controversy: Is chloroprocaine neurotoxic? *Reg Anesth* 1984;9:135–145.

124. Fibuch EE, Opper SE. Back pain following epidurally administered Nesacaine-MPF. *Anesth Analg* 1989;69:113–115.

125. McLoughlin TM, DiFazio CA. More on back pain after Nesacaine-MPF. *Anesth Analg* 1990;71:562–563.

126. Stevens RA, Chester WL, Artuso JD, Bray JG, Nellestein JA. Back pain after epidural anesthesia with chloroprocaine in volunteers: Preliminary report. *Reg Anesth* 1991;16:199–203.

127. James FI. Chloroprocaine vs. bupivacaine for lumbar epidural analgesia for elective cesarean section. *Anesthesiology* 1980;52:488–491.

128. Chestnut DH. The influence of pH-adjusted 2-chloroprocaine on the quality and duration of subsequent epidural bupivacaine analgesia during labor: A randomized, double-blind study. *Anesthesiology* 1989;70:437–441.

129. Naulty JS, Hertwig L, Hunt CO. Duration of analgesia of epidural fentanyl following cesarean delivery: Effects of local anesthetic drug selection [abstract]. *Anesthesiology* 1986;65:A180.

130. Malinow AM, Mokriski BLK, Wakefield ML, et al. Anesthetic choice affects postcesarean epidural fentanyl analgesia. *Anesth Analg* 1988;67:S138.

131. Ackerman WE, Juneja MM. 2-chloroprocaine decreases the duration of analgesia of epidural fentanyl. *Anesth Analg* 1989;68:S2.

132. Camann WR, Gartigan PM, Gilbertson LI, et al. Chloroprocaine antagonism of epidural opioid analgesia: A receptor-specific phenomenon? *Anesthesiology* 1990;73:860–863.

133. Hughes SC, Wright RG, Murphy D, et al. The effect of pH adjusting 3% 2-chloroprocaine on the quality of post-cesarean section analgesia with epidural morphine [abstract]. *Anesthesiology* 1988;69:A689.

134. Ssakura S, Sumi M, Morimoto N, Saito Y. The addition of epinephrine increase intensity of sensory block during epidural anesthesia with lidocaine. *Reg Anesth Pain Med* 1999;24:541–546.

135. Bromage PR, Robson JG. Concentrations of lignocaine in the blood after intravenous, IM epidural and endotracheal administration. *Anaesthesia* 1961;16:461.

136. Mather LE, Tucker GT, Murphy TM, Stanton-Hicks DA, Bonica JJ. The effects of adding adrenaline to etidocaine and lignocaine in extradural anaesthesia. II. Pharmacokinetics. *Br J Anaesth* 1976;48:989–994.

137. Scott DB, Jebson PJR, Braid DP, Örtengren B, Frisch P. Factors affecting plasma levels of lignocaine and prilocaine. *Br J Anaesth* 1972;44:1040–1049.
138. Rosenfeld CR, Barton MD, Meschia G. Effects of epinephrine on distribution of blood flow in the pregnant ewe. *Am J Obstet Gynecol* 1976;124:156–163.
139. Wallis KL, Shnider SM, Hicks JS, Spivey HT. Epidural anesthesia in the normotensive pregnant ewe: Effects on uterine blood flow and fetal acid-base status. *Anesthesiology* 1976;44:481–487.
140. Rucker MP. The action of adrenaline on the pregnant uterus. *South Med J* 1925;18:412–418.
141. Gunther RE, Bauman J. Obstetrical caudal anesthesia. I. A randomized study comparing 1% mepivacaine with 1% lidocaine plus epinephrine. *Anesthesiology* 1969;31:5–19.
142. Gunther RE, Bellville JW. Obstetrical caudal anesthesia. II. A randomized study comparing 1 per cent mepivacaine with 1 per cent mepivacaine plus epinephrine. *Anesthesiology* 1972;37:288–298.
143. Matadial L, Cibils LA. The effect of epidural anesthesia on uterine activity and blood pressure. *Am J Obstet Gynecol* 1976;125:846–854.
144. Zador G, Englesson S, Nilsson BA. Continuous drip epidural anesthesia in labour. II. Influence on labour and foetal acid-base status. *Acta Obstet Gynecol* 1974;34(suppl):41–49.
145. Marx GF, Elstein ID, Schuss M, et al. Effects of epidural block with lignocaine and lignocaine-adrenaline on umbilical artery velocity wave ratios. *Br J Obstet Gynaecol* 1990;95:517–520.
146. Levinson G, Shnider SM, Krames E, Ring G. Epidural anesthesia for cesarean section: Effects of epinephrine in the local anesthetic solution. In: Abstracts of Scientific Papers of the Annual Meeting of the American Society of Anesthesiologists; Chicago, IL; 1975:285.
147. deRosayro AM, Hahrwold ML, Hill AB. Cardiovascular effects of epidural epinephrine in pregnant sheep. *Reg Anesth* 1981;6:4–7.
148. Albright GA, Jouppila R, Hollmén AI, Jouppila P, Vierola H, Kiovula A. Epinephrine does not alter human intervillous blood flow during epidural anesthesia. *Anesthesiology* 1981;54:131–135.
149. DiFazio CA, Carron H, Grosslight KR, Moseicki JC, Bolding WR, Johns RA. Comparison of pH-adjusted lidocaine solutions for epidural anesthesia. *Anesth Analg* 1986;65:760–764.
150. Galindo A. pH-adjusted local anesthetics: Clinical experience. *Reg Anesth* 1983;8:35–36.
151. Douglas MJ. The effect of pH adjustment of bupivacaine on epidural anesthesia for cesarean section [abstract]. *Anesthesiology* 1986;65:A380.
152. McMorland GH, Douglas MJ, Jeffrey WK, et al. Effect of pH-adjustment of bupivacaine on onset and duration of epidural analgesia in parturients. *Can Anaesth Soc J* 1986;33:537–541.
153. Tackley RM. Alkalinized bupivacaine and adrenaline for epidural caesarean section. *Anaesthesia* 1988;43:1019–1021.
154. Benhamou D, Labaille T, Bonhomme L, Perrachon N. Alkalinization of epidural 0.5% bupivacaine for cesarean section. *Reg Anesth* 1989;14:240–243.
155. Glosten B, Dailey PA, Preston PG, et al. pH-adjusted 2-chloroprocaine for epidural anesthesia in patients undergoing postpartum tubal ligation. *Anesthesiology* 1988;68:948–950.
156. Ross BK. Evaluation of epidural pH-adjusted 2% 2-chloroprocaine for labor analgesia [abstract]. *Anesthesiology* 1987;67:A629.
157. Parnass SM, Curran MJA, Becker GL. Incidence of hypotension associated with epidural anesthesia using alkalinized and nonalkalinized lidocaine for cesarean section. *Anesth Analg* 1987;66:1148–1150.
158. Peterfreund RA, Datta S, Ostheimer GW. pH adjustment of local anesthetic solutions with sodium bicarbonate: Laboratory evaluation of alkalinization and precipitation. *Reg Anesth* 1989;14:265–270.
159. Ikuta PT. pH adjustment schedule for the amide local anesthetics. *Reg Anesth* 1989;14:229–235.
160. Naulty JS, Datta S, Ostheimer GW, Johnson MD, Burger GA. Epidural fentanyl for postcesarean delivery pain management. *Anesthesiology* 1985;63:694–698.
161. Ackerman WE, Juneja MM, Colclough GW, Kaczorowski DM. Epidural fentanyl significantly decreases nausea and vomiting during uterine manipulation in awake patients undergoing cesarean section [abstract]. *Anesthesiology* 1988;69:A679.
162. Gaffud MP, Bansal P, Lawton C, Velasquez N, Watson WA. Surgical analgesia for cesarean delivery with epidural bupivacaine and fentanyl. *Anesthesiology* 1986;65:331–334.

163. Preston PG, Rosen MA, Hughes SC, et al. Epidural anesthesia with fentanyl and lidocaine for cesarean section: Maternal effects and neonatal outcome. *Anesthesiology* 1988;68:938–943.
164. Arcario T, Vartikar J, Johnson MD, et al. Effect of diluent volume on analgesia produced by epidural fentanyl [abstract]. *Anesthesiology* 1987;67:A441.
165. Porter J, Bonello E, Reynolds F. Effect of epidural fentanyl on neonatal respiration. *Anesthesiology* 1998;89:79–85.
166. Benlabed M, Midgal M, Dreizzen E, et al. Neonatal pattern of breathing after cesarean section with or without epidural fentanyl [abstract]. *Anesthesiology* 1989;69:A651.
167. Schlesinger TS, Miletich DJ. Epidural fentanyl and lidocaine during cesarean section: Maternal efficacy and neonatal safety using impedance monitoring [abstract]. *Anesthesiology* 1988;69:A649.
168. Capogna G, Celleno D, Tomassetti M, Castantino P, Feo GD, Nisini R. Epidural versus intravenous fentanyl for cesarean section delivery: Neonatal neurobehavioral effects. *Reg Anesth* 1988;13:S17.
169. Ngan Kee WD, Lam KK, Chen PP, Gin T. Epidural meperidine after cesarean section: The effect of diluent volume. *Anesth Analg* 1997;85:380–384.
170. Vertommen JD, Van Aken H, Vandermeulen E, et al. Maternal and neonatal effects of adding sufentanil to 0.5% bupivacaine for cesarean delivery. *J Clin Anesth* 1991;3:371–376.
171. Madej TH, Stunin L. Comparison of epidural fentanyl with sufentanil. *Anaesthesia* 1987;42:1156–1161.
172. Grass JA, Sakima NT, Schmidt R, et al. A randomized, double-blind, dose response comparison of epidural fentanyl versus sufentanil analgesia after cesarean section. *Anesth Analg* 1997;85:365–371.
173. Rosen MA, Dailey PA, Hughes SC, et al. Epidural sufentanil for postoperative analgesia after cesarean section. *Anesthesiology* 1988;68:448–452.
174. Loper KA, Ready LB, Sandler A. Epidural and intravenous fentanyl infusions are clinically equivalent following knee surgery. *Anesth Analg* 1990;70:72–75.
175. Ellis JD, Millar WL, Reisner LS. A randomized, double-blind comparison of epidural versus intravenous fentanyl infusion for analgesia after cesarean section. *Anesthesiology* 1990;72:981–986.
176. Rosen MA, Hughes SC, Shnider SM, et al. Epidural morphine for relief of postoperative pain after cesarean delivery. *Anesth Analg* 1983;62:666–672.
177. Leicht CH, Hughes SC, Dailey PA, Shnider SM, Rosen MA. Epidural morphine sulfate for analgesia after cesarean section: A prospective report of 1000 patients [abstract]. *Anesthesiology* 1986;65:A366.
178. Fuller JG, McMorland GH, Douglas J, Palmer L, Constantine LV. Epidural morphine for analgesia after caesarean section: A report of 4,880 patients. *Can J Anaesth* 1990;37:636–640.
179. Palmer CM, Petty JV, Nogami WN, et al. What is the optimal dose of epidural morphine for post cesarean section analgesia [abstract]? *Anesthesiology* 1996;85:A909.
180. Turner K, Sandler AN, Vosu H, Daley D, Slaveehenko P, Lau L. Respiratory pattern in post-cesarean section patients after epidural or intramuscular morphine. *Anesth Analg* 1989;68:S296.
181. Brose WG, Cohen SE. Oxyhemoglobin saturation following cesarean section in patients receiving epidural morphine, PCA or im meperidine analgesia. *Anesthesiology* 1989;70:948–953.
182. Choi HJ, Little MS, Fujita RA, Garber SZ, Tremper KK. Pulse oximetry for monitoring during ward analgesia: Epidural morphine versus parenteral narcotics [abstract]. *Anesthesiology* 1986;65:A371.
183. Östman LP, Owen CL, Bates JM, Scamman FL, Davis K. Oxygen saturation in patients the night prior to and the night after cesarean section during epidural morphine analgesia [abstract]. *Anesthesiology* 1988;69:A691.
184. Cohen SE, Subak LL, Brose WG, Halpern J. Analgesia after cesarean delivery: Patient evaluations and cost of five opioid techniques. *Reg Anesth* 1991;16:141–149.
185. Rawal N, Arner S, Gustofsson LL. Present state of extradural and intrathecal opioid analgesia in Sweden. *Br J Anaesth* 1987;59:791–799.
186. Ready LB, Loper KA, Nessly M, Wild L. Postoperative epidural morphine is safe on surgical wards. *Anesthesiology* 1991;75:452–456.
187. Dottens M, Rifat K, Morel DR. Comparison of extradural administration of sufentanil, morphine, and sufentanil-morphine combination after cesarean section. *Br J Anaesth* 1992;69:9–12.
188. Harrison DM, Sinatra R, Morgese L, Chung JH. Epidural narcotic and patient-controlled analgesia for post-cesarean section pain relief. *Anesthesiology* 1988;68:454–457.

189. Eisenach JC, Grice SC, Dewan DM. Patient-controlled analgesia following cesarean section: A comparison with epidural and intramuscular narcotics. *Anesthesiology* 1988;68:444–448.

190. Chrubasik J, Wust H, Schulte-Monting J, et al. Relative analgesic potency of epidural fentanyl, alfentanil, and morphine in treatment of postoperative pain. *Anesthesiology* 1988;68:929–933.

191. Ngee Kee WD, Lam KK, Chen PP, Gin T. Comparison of patient-controlled epidural analgesia with patient-controlled intravenous analgesia using pethidine or fentanyl. *Anaesth Intensive Care* 1997;25:126–132.

192. Cooper DW, Ryall DM, McHardy FE, et al. Patient-controlled extradural analgesia with bupivacaine, fentanyl, or a mixture of both, after caesarean section. *Br J Anaesth* 1996;76:611–615.

193. Sinatra RS, Severino FB, Paige D, et al. Patient controlled analgesia with sufentanil: A comparison of intravenous versus epidural administration. *J Clin Anesth* 1996;8:123.

194. Bernstein J, Patel N, Moszczynski Z, Parker F, Ramanathan S, Turndorf H. Colostrum morphine following epidural administration. *Anesth Analg* 1989;68:S23.

195. Flanagan HL, Datta S, Lambert DH, et al. Effect of pregnancy on bupivacaine-induced conduction blockade in the isolated rabbit vagus nerve. *Anesth Analg* 1987;66:123–126.

196. Datta S, Lambert DH, Gregus S, et al. Differential sensitivity of mammalian nerve fibers during pregnancy. *Anesth Analg* 1983;62:1070–1072.

197. Butterworth JI, Walker FV, Ly Sak ZK. Pregnancy increases median nerve susceptibility to lidocaine. *Anesthesiology* 1990;72:962–965.

198. Rawal N. Combined spinal-epidural technique. *Reg Anesth* 1997;22:406–423.

199. Soresi A. Episubdural anesthesia. *Anesth Analg* 1937;16:306–310.

200. Brownridge P. Epidural and subarachnoid analgesia for elective caesarean section. *Anaesthesia* 1981;36:70.

201. Carrie LES, O'Sullivan GM. Subarachnoid bupivacaine 0.5% for caesarean section. *Eur J Anaesth* 1984;1:275–283.

202. Carrie LES. Extradural spinal or combined spinal block for obstetric surgical anaesthesia. *Br J Anaesth* 1990;65:225–233.

203. Kumar CM. Combined subarachnoid and epidural block for caesarean section. *Can Anaesth Soc J* 1987;34:329–330.

204. Rawal N. Single segment combined subarachnoid and epidural block for caesarean section. *Acta Anaesthesiol Scand* 1988;32:61–66.

205. Thorán T, Holmström B, Rawal N, Schollia J, Lindeberg S, Skeppner G. Sequential combined spinal epidural block versus spinal block for cesarean section: Effects on maternal hypotension and neurobehavioral function of the newborn. *Anesth Analg* 1994;78:1087–1092.

206. Randalls B, Broadway JW, Browne DA, Morgan BM. Comparison of four subarachnoid solutions in a needle-through-needle technique for elective caesarean section. *Br J Anaesth* 1991;66:314–318.

207. Swami A, McHale S, Abbott P, Morgan B. Low dose spinal anesthesia for cesarean section using combined spinal-epidural (CSE) technique (abstract). *Anesth Analg* 1993;76:S423.

208. Fan S-Z, Susetio L, Wang Y-P, Liu C-C. Low dose of intrathecal hyperbaric bupivacaine combined with epidural lidocaine for cesarean section–a balance block technique. *Anesth Analg* 1994;78:474–477.

209. Dennison B. Combined subarachnoid and epidural block for caesarean section. *Can Anaesth Soc J* 1987;34:105–106.

210. Lyons G, Macdonald R, Mikl B. Combined epidural spinal anesthesia for caesarean section: Through the needle or in separate spaces? *Anaesthesia* 1992;47:199–201.

211. Westbrook JL, Donald F, Carrie LES. An evaluation of a combined spinal epidural needle set utilizing a 26-gauge, pencil point spinal needle for caesarean section. *Anaesthesia* 1992;47:990–992.

212. Davies JD, Paech MJ, Welch H, et al. Maternal experience during epidural or combined spinal-epidural anesthesia for cesarean section: A prospective, randomized trial. *Anesth Analg* 1997;85:607–613.

213. Yun EM, Marx GF, Santos AC. The effects of maternal position during induction of combined spinal-epidural anesthesia for cesarean delivery. *Anesth Analg* 1998;87:614–618.

214. Kasten GW, Martin ST. Bupivacaine cardiovascular toxicity: Comparison of treatment with bretylium and lidocaine. *Anesth Analg* 1985;64:911–916.

215. Akamatsu TJ, Bonica JJ, Rehmet R, Eng M, Ueland K. Experiences with the use of ketamine for parturition. I. Primary anesthetic for vaginal delivery. *Anesth Analg* 1974;53:284–287.

216. Stride PC, Cooper DM. Dural taps revisited: A 20-year survey from Birmingham Maternity Hospital. *Anaesthesia* 1993;48:247–255.

217. Berger C, Crosby E, Grodecki W. North American study of the management of dural puncture occurring during labour epidural analgesia. *Can J Anaesth* 1998;45:110–114.

218. Hodgkinson R. Total spinal block after epidural injection into an interspace adjacent to an inadvertent dural perforation. *Anesthesiology* 1981;55:593–594.

219. Leach A, Smith GB. Subarachnoid spread of epidural local anaesthetic following dural puncture. *Anaesthesia* 1988;43:671.

220. Crawford JS. The prevention of headache consequent upon dural puncture. *Br J Anaesth* 1972;44:598–599.

221. Craft JJ, Epstein BS, Coakley CC. Prophylaxis of dural-puncture headache with epidural saline. *Anesth Analg* 1973;52:228–231.

222. Smith BE. Prophylaxis of epidural wet tap headache. In: Abstracts of Scientific Papers of the Annual Meeting of the American Society of Anesthesiologists; San Francisco, CA; 1979:119.

223. Ozdil T, Powell WF. Postlumbar puncture headache: An effective method of prevention. *Anesth Analg* 1965;44:542–545.

224. Gutterman P, Bezier H. Prophylaxis of post myelogram headache. *J Neurol* 1978;49:869–871.

225. Quaynor H, Corbey M. Extradural blood patch–why delay? *Br J Anaesth* 1985;57:538–540.

226. Cheek TG, Banner R, Sauter J, Gutsche BB. Prophylactic extradural blood patch is effective. *Br J Anaesth* 1988;61:340–342.

227. Ackerman W, Juneja M, Kaczorowski D. The attenuation of a postdural puncture headache with a prophylactic blood patch in labor patients. *Anesth Analg* 1989;68:S1.

228. Colonna-Romano P, Shapiro BE. Unintentional dural puncture and prophylactic epidural blood patch in obstetrics. *Anesth Analg* 1989;69:522–523.

229. Carbaat PAT, van Crevel H. Lumbar puncture headache: Controlled study on the preventive effect of 24 hours' bed rest. *Lancet* 1981;2:1133–1135.

230. McLeskey CH, Hornbein TF, Pavlin EG. Hydration and postspinal headache. In: Abstracts of Scientific Papers of the Annual Meeting of the American Society of Anesthesiologists; San Francisco, CA; 1976:455–456.

231. Dieterich M, Brandt T. Incidence of post-lumbar puncture headache is independent of fluid intake. *Eur Arch Psychiatry Neurol Sci* 1988;237:194–196.

232. Sechzer P, Abel L. Post-spinal analgesia headache treated with caffeine: Evaluation with the demand method. *Curr Ther Res* 1978;24:307–312.

233. Camann W, Murray R, Mushlin PS, Lambert DH. Effects of oral caffeine on post-dural puncture headache: A double-blind placebo controlled trial. *Anesth Analg* 1990;70:181–184.

234. Bolton VE, Leicht CH, Scanlon TS. Postpartum seizure after epidural blood patch and intravenous caffeine sodium benzoate. *Anesthesiology* 1989;70:146–149.

235. Fuerstein T, Zeides A. Theophylline relieves headache following lumbar puncture. *Klin Wochenschr* 1986;64:216–218.

236. Schwalbe S, Schiffmiller M, Marx G. Theophylline for postdural puncture headache [abstract]. *Anesthesiology* 1991;75:A1082.

237. Duffy PT, Crosby ET. The epidural blood patch. Resolving the controversies. *Can J Anaesth* 1999;46:878–886.

238. Gormley JB. Treatment of postspinal headache. *Anesthesiology* 1960;21:565–566.

239. DiGiovanni AJ, Galbert MW, Wahle WM. Epidural injection of autologous blood for postlumbar-puncture headache. II. Additional clinical experiences and laboratory investigation. *Anesth Analg* 1972;51:226–232.

240. Glass PM, Kennedy WJ Jr. Headache following subarachnoid puncture: Treatment with epidural blood patch. *JAMA* 1972;219:203–204.

241. DuPont FS, Shire RD. Epidural blood patch: An unusual approach to the problem of post-spinal anesthetic headache. *Mich Med* 1972;71:105–107.

242. Vondrell JJ, Bernards WC. Epidural "blood patch" for the treatment of postspinal headaches. *Wis Med J* 1973;72:132–134.

243. Blok RJ. Headache following spinal anesthesia: Treatment by epidural blood patch. *J Am Osteopath Assoc* 1973;73:128–130.

244. Balagot RC, Lee T, Liu C, Kwan BK, Ecanow B. The prophylactic epidural blood patch [letter]. *JAMA* 1974;228:1369–1370.

245. Ostheimer GW, Palahniuk RJ, Shnider SM. Epidural blood patch for postlumbar-puncture headache [letter]. *Anesthesiology* 1974;41:307–308.

246. Abouleish E, de la Vega S, Blendinger J, Tiong-Oen T. Long-term follow-up of epidural blood patch. *Anesth Analg* 1975;54:459–463.

247. Loeser EA, Hill GE, Bennett GM, Sederberg JH. Time vs. success rate for epidural blood patch. *Anesthesiology* 1978;49:147–148.
248. Abouleish E. Epidural blood patch for the treatment of chronic postlumbar-puncture cephalgia. *Anesthesiology* 1978;49:291–292.
249. Williams EJ, Beaulieu P, Fawcett WJ, Jenkins JG. Efficacy of epidural blood patch in the obstetric population. *Int J Obstet Anesth* 1999;8:105–109.
250. Coates MB. Combined subarachnoid and epidural techniques. *Anaesthesia* 1982;37:89–90.
251. Berga S, Trierweiler MW. Bacterial meningitis following epidural anesthesia for vaginal delivery: A case report. *Obstet Gynecol* 1989;74:437–439.
252. Harding SA, Collis RE, Morgan BM. Meningitis after combined spinal-extradural anaesthesia in obstetrics. *Br J Anaesth* 1994;73:545–547.
253. Naulty JS, Herold R. Successful epidural anesthesia following epidural blood patch. *Anesth Analg* 1978;57:272–273.
254. Ong BY, Graham CR, Ringaert KR, Cohen MM, Palahniuk RJ. Impaired epidural analgesia after dural puncture with and without subsequent blood patch. *Anesth Analg* 1990;70:76–79.
255. Bevacqua B, Slucky A. Epidural blood patch in a patient with HIV infection [letter]. *Anesthesiology* 1991;74:952–953.
256. Frame W, Lichtmann M. Blood patch in the HIV-positive patient [letter]. *Anesthesiology* 1990;73:1297.
257. Tom DJ, Gulevich SJ, Shapiro HM, et al. Epidural blood patch in the HIV-positive population. *Anesthesiology* 1992;76:943–947.
258. Barrios-Alarcon J, Aldrete JA, Paragas-Tapia D. Relief of postlumbar puncture headache with epidural dextran 40: A preliminary report. *Reg Anesth* 1989;14:78–80.
259. Palahniuk RJ, Shnider SM, Eger EI II. Pregnancy decreases the requirements for inhaled anesthetic agents. *Anesthesiology* 1974;41:82–83.
260. Gin T, Chan MT. Decreased minimum alveolar concentration of isoflurane in pregnant humans. *Anesthesiology* 1994;81:829–832.
261. Roberts RB, Shirley MA. Reducing the risk of acid aspiration during cesarean section. *Anesth Analg* 1974;53:859–868.
262. Sellick BA. Cricoid pressure to control regurgitation of stomach contents during induction of anesthesia. *Lancet* 1961;2:404–406.
263. Thind GS, Bryson THL. Single dose suxamethonium and muscle pain in pregnancy. *Br J Anaesth* 1983;55:743–745.
264. Smith G, Dalling R, Williams TIR. Gastro-oesophageal pressure gradient changes produced by induction of anaesthesia and suxamethonium. *Br J Anaesth* 1978;50:1137–1143.
265. Gibbs CP, Hempling RE, Wynne JW, Hood CI. Antacid pulmonary aspiration [abstract]. *Anesthesiology* 1979;51:A290.
266. Eyler SW, Cullen BF, Murphy ME, Welch WD. Antacid aspiration in rabbits: A comparison of Mylanta and Bicitra. *Anesth Analg* 1982;61:288–292.
267. Gibbs CP, Spohr L, Schmidt D. The effectiveness of sodium citrate as an antacid. *Anesthesiology* 1982;57:44–46.
268. Abboud TK, Curtis JP, Shnider SM, Earl S, Henriksen EH. Comparison of the effects of sodium citrate and Gelusil on gastric acidity and volume. *Anesth Analg* 1982;61:167.
269. Gibbs CP, Banner TC. Effectiveness of Bicitra as a preoperative antacid. *Anesthesiology* 1984;61:97–99.
270. Chen CT, Toung TJR, Haupt HM, Hutchins GM, Cameron JL. Evaluation of Alka-Seltzer Effervescent in gastric acid neutralization. *Anesth Analg* 1984;63:325–329.
271. Pickering BG, Palahniuk RJ, Cumming M. Cimetidine premedication in elective cesarean section. *Can Anaesth Soc J* 1980;27:33–35.
272. Williams JG. H₂ receptor antagonists and anaesthesia. *Can Anaesth Soc J* 1983;30:264–269.
273. Manchikanti L, Kraus JW, Edds SP. Cimetidine and related drugs in anesthesia. *Anesth Analg* 1982;61:595–608.
274. Rocke DA, Rout CC, Gouws E. Intravenous administration of the proton pump inhibitor omeprazole reduces the risk of acid aspiration at emergency cesarean section. *Anesth Analg* 1994;78:1093–1098.
275. Brock-Utne JG, Rubin J, Downing JW, Dimopoulos CE, Moshal MG, Naicker M. The administration of metoclopramide with atropine: A drug interaction effect on the gastroesophageal sphincter in man. *Anaesthesia* 1976;31:1186–1190.
276. McNeill MJ, Ho ET, Kenny GNC. Effect of I.V. metoclopramide on gastric emptying after opioid premedication. *Br J Anaesth* 1990;64:450–452.
277. Brock-Utne JG, Dow TGB, Welman S, Dimopoulos GE, Moshal MG. The effect of metoclopramide on lower oesophageal sphincter tone. *Anaesth Intensive Care* 1978;6:26–29.
278. Murphy DF, Nally B, Gardiner J, Unwin A. Effect of metoclopramide on gastric emptying before elective and emergency caesarean section. *Br J Anaesth* 1984;56:1113–1116.
279. Wyner MB, Cohen SE. Gastric volume in early pregnancy. *Anesthesiology* 1982;57:209–212.
280. Orr DA, Bill KM, Gillan KRW, et al. Effects of omeprazole with and without metoclopramide in elective obstetric anesthesia. *Anaesthesia* 1993;48:114–119.
281. Chestnut DH. Anesthesia and maternal mortality. *Anesthesiology* 1997;86:273–284.
282. Lyons G. Failed intubation. *Anaesthesia* 1985;40:759–762.
283. Lyons G, MacDonald R. Difficult intubation in obstetrics. *Anaesthesia* 1985;40:1016.
284. Cormack RS, Lehane J. Difficult tracheal intubation in obstetrics. *Anaesthesia* 1984;39:1105–1111.
285. Samsoon GLT, Young JRB. Difficult tracheal intubation: A retrospective study. *Anaesthesia* 1987;42:487–490.
286. McIntyre JR. The difficult tracheal intubation. *Can J Anaesth* 1987;34:204–213.
287. Wilson ME, Spigekhalter D, Robertson JA, Lesser P. Predicting difficult intubation. *Br J Anaesth* 1988;61:211–216.
288. Rocke DA, Murray WB, Rout CC, Gouws E. Relative risk analysis of factors associated with difficult intubation in obstetric anesthesia. *Anesthesiology* 1992;77:67–73.
289. Patil VU, Stehling LC, Zauder HL. *Fiberoptic Endoscopy in Anesthesia.* Chicago, IL: Year Book Medical Publishers; 1983.
290. Mathew M, Hanna LS, Aldrete JA. Pre-operative indices to anticipate difficult tracheal intubation. *Anesth Analg* 1989;68:S187.
291. Brechner VL. Unusual problems in the management of airways. I. Flexion-extension mobility of the cervical spine. *Anesth Analg* 1968;47:362–373.
292. Finucane BT, Santora AH. Evaluation of the airway prior to intubation, *Principles of Airway Management.* Philadelphia: Davis; 1988:69–83.
293. Mallampati SR. Clinical signs to predict difficult tracheal intubation (hypothesis). *Can Anaesth Soc J* 1983;30:316–317.
294. Mallampati SR, Gatt SP, Gugino LD, et al. A clinical sign to predict difficult tracheal intubation: A prospective study. *Can Anaesth Soc J* 1985;32:429–434.
295. American Society of Anesthesiology. Practice Guidelines for Obstetric Anesthesia: A report by the American Society of Anesthesiologists Task Force on Obstetrical Anesthesia. *Anesthesiology* 1999;90:600–611.
296. Brain AIJ. Three cases of difficult intubation overcome by laryngeal mask airway. *Anaesthesia* 1985;40:353–355.
297. Benumof JL, Scheller MS. The importance of transtracheal jet ventilation in the management of the difficult airway. *Anesthesiology* 1989;71:769–778.
298. Benumof JL. Laryngeal mask airway and the ASA difficult airway algorithm. *Anesthesiology* 1996;84:686–698.
299. Brimacombe J, Berry A. The laryngeal mask airway for obstetric anaesthesia and neonatal resuscitation. *Int J Obstet Anesth* 1994;3:211–218.
300. Tunstall ME, Sheikh A. Failed intubation protocol: Oxygenation without aspiration. *Clin Anaesthesiol* 1986;4:171–187.
301. McClune S, Regan M, Moore J. Laryngeal mask airway for caesarean section. *Anaesthesia* 1990;45:227–228.
302. O'Sullivan G, Stoddart PA. Failed tracheal intubation. *Br J Anaesth* 1991;67:225.
303. King TA, Adams AP. Failed tracheal intubation. *Br J Anaesth* 1990;65:400–414.
304. Ansermino JM, Blogg CE, Carrie LES. Failed tracheal intubation at caesarean section and the laryngeal mask. *Br J Anaesth* 1992;68:54–59.
305. Widlund G. Cardio-pulmonary function during pregnancy: A clinical-experimental study with particular respect to ventilation and oxygen consumption among normal cases in rest and after work tests. *Acta Obstet Gynecol Scand* 1945;25(suppl):1–125.
306. Cugell DW, Frank NR, Gaensler ER, Badger TL. Pulmonary function in pregnancy. I. Serial observations in normal women. *Am Rev Tuberc* 1953;67:568–597.
307. Archer GJ Jr, Marx GF. Arterial oxygen tension during apnoea in parturient women. *Br J Anaesth* 1974;46:358–360.
308. Norris MC, Dewan DM. Preoxygenation for cesarean section: A comparison of two techniques. *Anesthesiology* 1985;62:827–829.
309. Norris MC, Kirkland MR, Torjman MC, et al. Denitrogenation in pregnancy. *Can J Anaesth* 1989;36:523–525.

310. Gambee AM, Hertzka RE, Fisher DM. Preoxygenation techniques: Comparison of three minutes and four breaths. *Anesth Analg* 1987;66:468–470.

311. Baraka AA, Taha SK, Aouad MT, El-Khatib MF, Kawabani NI. Preoxygenation, comparison of maximal breathing and tidal volume breathing techniques. *Anesthesiology* 1999;91:612–616.

312. Benumof JL. Preoxygenation: Best method for both efficacy and efficiency [editorial]. *Anesthesiology* 1999;91:603–605.

313. Levinson G, Shnider SM, deLorimier AA, Steffenson JL. Effects of maternal hyperventilation on uterine blood flow and fetal oxygenation and acid-base status. *Anesthesiology* 1974;40:340–347.

314. Kosaka Y, Takahashi T, Mark LC. Intravenous thiobarbiturate anesthesia for cesarean section. *Anesthesiology* 1969;31:489–506.

315. Bach V, Carl P, Ravlo O, et al. A randomized comparison between midazolam and thiopental for elective cesarean section anesthesia. III. Placental transfer and elimination in neonates. *Anesth Analg* 1989;68:238–247.

316. Finster M, Mark LC, Morishima HO, et al. Plasma thiopental concentrations in the newborn following delivery under thiopental-nitrous oxide anesthesia. *Am J Obstet Gynecol* 1966;95:621–629.

317. Ngan Kee WD, Khaw KS, Ma ML, Mailand PA, Gin T. Postoperative analgesic requirement after cesarean section: A comparison of anesthetic induction with ketamine or thiopental. *Anesth Analg* 1997;85:1294–1298.

318. Gaitini L, Vaida S, Collins G, Somri M, Sabo E. Awareness detection during caesarean section under general anaesthesia using EEG spectrum analysis. *Can J Anaesth* 1995;42:377–381.

319. Bovill JG, Dundee JW, Coppell DL, Moore J. Current status of ketamine anaesthesia. *Lancet* 1971;1:1285–1288.

320. Dich-Nielsen J, Holasek J. Ketamine as induction agent for caesarean section. *Acta Anaesthesiol Scand* 1982;26:139–142.

321. Reich DL, Silvay G. Ketamine: An update on the first twenty-five years of clinical experience. *Can J Anaesth* 1989;36:186–197.

322. Levinson G, Shnider SM, Gildea J, deLorimier AA. Maternal and foetal cardiovascular and acid base changes during ketamine anaesthesia. *Br J Anaesth* 1973;45:1111–1115.

323. Eng M, Berges PU, Bonica JJ. The effects of ketamine on uterine blood flow in the monkey. In: Abstracts of Scientific Papers of the Annual Meeting of the Society for Gynecological Investigation; Atlanta, GA; 1973:48.

324. Craft JB Jr, Coaldrake LA, Yonekura ML, et al. Ketamine, catecholamines, and uterine tone in pregnant ewes. *Am J Obstet Gynecol* 1983;146:429–434.

325. Galloon S. Ketamine for obstetric delivery. *Anesthesiology* 1976; 44:522–524.

326. Oats JN, Vasey DP, Waldron BA. Effects of ketamine on the pregnant uterus. *Br J Anaesth* 1979;51:1163–1166.

327. Little B, Chang T, Chucot L, et al. Study of ketamine as an obstetric agent. *Am J Obstet Gynecol* 1972;113:247–260.

328. Janeczko GF, El-Etr AA, Younes S. Low-dose ketamine anesthesia for obstetrical delivery. *Anesth Analg* 1974;53:828–831.

329. Hodgkinson R, Marx GF, Kim SS, Miclat NM. Neonatal neurobehavioral tests following vaginal delivery under ketamine, thiopental and extradural anesthesia. *Anesth Analg* 1977;56:548–553.

330. Pelz B, Sinclair DM. Induction agents for caesarean section: A comparison of thiopentone and ketamine. *Anaesthesia* 1973;28:37–42.

331. Downing JW, Mahomedy MC, Jeal DE, Allen PJ. Anaesthesia for caesarean section with ketamine. *Anaesthesia* 1976;31:883–892.

332. Corssen G, Gutierrez J, Reves JG, Huber FC. Ketamine in the anesthetic management of asthmatic patients. *Anesth Analg* 1972;51:588–596.

333. White PF, Way WH, Trevor AJ. Ketamine–its pharmacology and therapeutic uses. *Anesthesiology* 1982;56:119–136.

334. Schultetus RR, Hill CR, Dharamraj CM, Banner TE, Berman LS. Wakefulness during cesarean section after anesthetic induction with ketamine, thiopental, or ketamine and thiopental combined. *Anesth Analg* 1986;65:723–728.

335. Alon E, Ball RH, Gille MH, et al. Effects of propofol on maternal and fetal cardiovascular and acid-based variables in the pregnant ewe. *Anesthesiology* 1993;78:562–576.

336. Celleno D, Capogna G, Tomassetti M, et al. Neurobehavioral effects of propofol on the neonate following elective caesarean section. *Br J Anaesth* 1989;62:649–654.

337. Dailland P, Cockshott ID, Lirzin JD, et al. Intravenous propofol during cesarean section: Placental transfer, concentrations in breast milk, and neonatal effects–a preliminary study. *Anesthesiology* 1989;71:827–834.

338. Dailland P, Jaquinot P, Lirzin JD, et al. Neonatal effects of propofol administered maternally for anesthesia for cesarean section. *Cahiers d'Anesthesiologie* 1989;37:429–433.

339. Flynn RJ, Moore J, Sharpe TDE. A comparative study of propofol and thiopental as induction agents for cesarean section. *Anesth Analg* 1989;68:S321.

340. Valtonen M, Kanto J, Rosenberg P. Comparison of propofol and thiopentone for induction of anaesthesia for elective caesarean section. *Anaesthesia* 1989;44:758–762.

341. Moore J, Bill KM, Flynn RJ, McKeating KT, Howard PJ. A comparison between propofol and thiopentone as induction agents in obstetric anaesthesia. *Anaesthesia* 1989;44:753–757.

342. Gin T, Gregory MA, Oh TE. The hemodynamic effects of propofol and thiopentone for induction of caesarean section. *Anaesth Intensive Care* 1990;18:175–179.

343. Gin T, Gregory MA, Chan K, Oh TE. Maternal and fetal levels of propofol at caesarean section. *Anaesth Intensive Care* 1990;18:180–184.

344. Yau G, Gin T, Ewart MC, Kotur CF, Leung RK, Oh TE. Propofol for induction and maintenance of anaesthesia at caesarean section. A comparison with thiopentone/enflurane. *Anaesthesia* 1991;46:20–23.

345. Gin T, Yau G, Chan K, Gregory MA, Oh TE. Disposition of propofol infusions for caesarean section. *Can J Anaesth* 1991;38:31–36.

346. Abboud TK, Zhu J, Richardson M, Peres da Silva E, Donovan M. Intravenous propofol vs. thiamylal-isoflurane for caesarean section, comparative maternal and neonatal effects. *Acta Anaesthesiol Scand* 1995;39:205–209.

347. Baraka AS. Severe bradycardia following propofol-suxamethonium sequence. *Br J Anaesth* 1988;61:482–483.

348. Gin T, Gregory MA. Propofol during caesarean section. *Anesthesiology* 1990;73:789.

349. Gregory MA, Gin T, Yau G, Leung RK, Chan K, Oh TE. Propofol infusion anaesthesia for caesarean section. *Can J Anaesth* 1990;37:514–520.

350. American Society of Anesthesiology. *Recommendations for Infection Control for the Practice of Anesthesiology*. Park Ridge, IL: American Society of Anesthesiology; 1998:10–14.

351. Downing JW, Buley RJR, Brock-Utne JG, Houlton PC. Etomidate for induction of anaesthesia at caesarean section: Comparison with thiopentone. *Br J Anaesth* 1979;51:135–139.

352. Suresh MS, Solanki DR, Andrews JJ, Hedges P, Nguyen S. Comparison of etomidate with thiopental for induction of anesthesia at cesarean section [abstract]. *Anesthesiology* 1985;65:A400.

353. Laughlin TP, Newberg LA. Prolonged myoclonus after etomidate anesthesia. *Anesth Analg* 1985;64:80–82.

354. Reddy BK, Pizer B, Bull PT. Neonatal serum cortisol suppression by etomidate compared with thiopentone for elective caesarean section. *Eur J Anaesth* 1988;5:171–176.

355. Cohen EN, Paulson WJ, Wall J, Elert B. Thiopental, curare, and nitrous oxide anesthesia for cesarean section with studies on placental transmission. *Surg Gynecol Obstet* 1953;97:456–462.

356. Moya F, Kvisselgaard N. The placental transmission of succinylcholine. *Anesthesiology* 1961;22:1–6.

357. Dailey PA, Fisher DM, Shnider SM, et al. Pharmacokinetics, placental transfer, and neonatal effects of vecuronium and pancuronium administered during cesarean section. *Anesthesiology* 1984;60:569–574.

358. Demetriou M, Depoix JP, Diakite B, Fromentin M, Duvaldestin P. Placental transfer of Org NC45 in women undergoing cesarean section. *Br J Anaesth* 1982;54:643–645.

359. Flynn PJ, Frank M, Hughes R. Use of atracurium in caesarean section. *Br J Anaesth* 1984;56:599–605.

360. Drabkova J, Crul JF, Van Der Kleijn E. Placental transfer of 14C-labelled succinylcholine in near-term Macaca mulatta monkeys. *Br J Anaesth* 1973;45:1087–1095.

361. Kvisselgaard N, Mya F. Investigation of placental thresholds to succinylcholine. *Anesthesiology* 1961;22:7–10.

362. Shnider SM. Serum cholinesterase activity during pregnancy, labor and puerperium. *Anesthesiology* 1965;26:335–339.

363. Leighton BL, Cheek TG, Gross JB, et al. Succinylcholine pharmacodynamics in peripartum patients. *Anesthesiology* 1986;64:202–205.

364. Blitt CD, Petty WC, Alberternst EE, Wright BJ. Correlations of plasma cholinesterase activity and duration of action of succinylcholine during pregnancy. *Anesth Analg* 1977;56:78–81.

365. Baraka A, Haroun S, Bassili M, Abu-Haider G. Response of the newborn to succinylcholine injection in homozygote atypical mothers. *Anesthesiology* 1975;43:115–116.

366. Baraka A, Noueihid R, Sinno H, Wakid N, Agoston S. Succinylcholine vecuronium (Org NC45) sequence for cesarean section. *Anesth Analg* 1983;62:909–913.

367. Magorian T, Flannery FB, Miller RD. Comparison of rocuronium, succinylcholine, and vecuronium for rapid-sequence induction of anesthesia in adult patients. *Anesthesiology* 1993;79:913–918.

368. Hodgson RE, Rout CC, Rocke DA, Louw NJ. Mivacurium for caesarean section in hypertensive parturients receiving magnesium sulphate therapy. *Int J Obstet Anesth* 1998;7:12–17.

369. Abouleish E, Abboud T, Lechevalier T, Zhu J, Chalian A, Alford K. Rocuronium (Org 9426) for caesarean section. *Br J Anaesth* 1994;73:336–341.

370. Hawkins J, Johnson T, Kabicek M, et al. Vecuronium for rapid sequence intubation for cesarean section. *Anesth Analg* 1990;71:185–190.

371. Abboud TK, Bikhazi G, Mroz L, et al. Org 9487 vs. succinylcholine in rapid sequence induction for cesarean section patients: Maternal and neonatal effects [abstract]. *Anesthesiology* 1997;87:A906.

372. Kivalo I, Saarikoski S. Placental transmission and foetal uptake of 14C-dimethyltubocurarine. *Br J Anaesth* 1972;44:557–561.

373. Abouleish E, Wingard LJ Jr, de la Vega S, Uy N. Pancuronium in caesarean section and its placental transfer. *Br J Anaesth* 1980;52:531–536.

374. Miguel R, Witkowski T, Nagashima H, et al. Evaluation of neuromuscular and cardiovascular effects of two doses of rapacuronium (Org 9487) versus mivacurium and succinylcholine. *Anesthesiology* 1999;91:1648–1654.

375. Marx GF, Joshi CW, Orkin LR. Placental transmission of nitrous oxide. *Anesthesiology* 1970;32:429–432.

376. Stenger VG, Blechner JN, Prystowsky H. A study of prolongation of obstetric anesthesia. *Am J Obstet Gynecol* 1969;103:901–907.

377. Finster M, Poppers PJ. Safety of thiopental used for induction of general anesthesia in elective cesarean section. *Anesthesiology* 1968;29:190–191.

378. Shnider SM. Anesthesia for elective cesarean section. In: Shnider SM, ed. *Obstetrical Anesthesia: Current Concepts and Practice.* Baltimore: Williams & Wilkins; 1970:94.

379. Rosen MA, Roizen MF, Eger EI II, et al. The effect of nitrous oxide on in vitro fertilization success rate. *Anesthesiology* 1987;67:42–44.

380. Vincent RD, Syrop CS, Van Voorhis BJ, et al. An evaluation of the effects of anesthetic technique on reproductive success after laparoscopic pronuclear stage transfer (PROST): Propofol-nitrous oxide versus isoflurane-nitrous oxide. *Anesthesiology* 1995;82:352–358.

381. Beilin Y, Bodian CA, Mukherjee T, et al. The use of propofol, nitrous oxide, or isoflurane does not affect the reproductive success rate following gamete intrafallopian transfer (GIFT): A multicenter pilot trial/survey. *Anesthesiology* 1999;90:36–41.

382. Crawford JS, Lewis M. Nitrous oxide in early human pregnancy. *Anaesthesia* 1986;41:900–905.

383. Mazze RI, Kallen B. Reproductive outcome following anesthesia and operation during pregnancy: A registry of 5,405 cases. *Am J Obstet Gynecol* 1989;161:1178–1185.

384. Stefani SJ, Hughes SC, Shnider SM, et al. Neonatal neurobehavioral effects of inhalation analgesia for vaginal delivery. *Anesthesiology* 1982;56:351–355.

385. Gambling DR, Sharma SK, White PF, et al. Use of sevoflurane during elective caesarean birth: A comparison with isoflurane and spinal anesthesia. *Anesth Analg* 1995;81:90–95.

386. Abboud TK, Zhu M, Peres E. Desflurane: A new volatile anesthetic for cesarean section. Maternal and neonatal effects. *Acta Anaesthesiol Scand* 1995;39:723–726.

387. Cheek DB, Hughes SC, Dailey PA, et al. Effect of halothane on regional cerebral blood flow and cerebral metabolic oxygen consumption in the fetal lamb in utero. *Anesthesiology* 1987;67:361–366.

388. Baker BW, Hughes SC, Shnider SM, Field DR, Rosen MA. Maternal anesthesia and the stressed fetus: Effects of Isoflurane on the asphyxiated fetal lamb. *Anesthesiology* 1990;72:65–70.

389. Yarnell R, Biehl DR, Tweed WA, et al. The effect of halothane anaesthesia on the asphyxiated foetal lamb *in utero*. *Can Anaesth Soc J* 1983;30:474–479.

390. Swartz J, Cummings M, Pucci W, Biehl D. The effects of general anaesthesia on the asphyxiated foetal lamb in utero. *Can Anaesth Soc J* 1985;32:577–582.

391. Leicht CH, Baker BW, Rosen MA, et al. The effect of ketamine or sodium pentothal rapid sequence induction on the asphyxiated fetal lamb [abstract]. *Anesthesiology* 1986;65:A387.

392. Marx GF, Mateo CV. Effects of different oxygen concentrations during general anesthesia for elective caesarean section. *Can Anaesth Soc J* 1971;18:587–593.

393. Bogod DG, Rosen M, Rees GAD. Maximum FIO$_2$ during caesarean section. *Br J Anaesth* 1988;61:255–262.

394. Piggott SE, Bogod DG, Rosen M, Rees GAD, Harmer M. Isoflurane with either 100% oxygen or 50% nitrous oxide in oxygen for caesarean section. *Br J Anaesth* 1990;65:325–329.

395. Shnider SM, Wright RG, Levinson G, et al. Plasma norepinephrine and uterine blood flow changes during endotracheal intubation and general anesthesia in the pregnant ewe. In: Abstracts of Scientific Papers of the Annual Meeting of the American Society of Anesthesiologists; Chicago, IL; 1978:115.

396. Naftalin NJ, Phear WPC, Goldberg AH. Halothane and isometric contractions of isolated pregnant rat myometrium. *Anesthesiology* 1975;42:458–463.

397. Naftalin NJ, McKay DM, Phear WPC, Goldberg AH. The effects of halothane on pregnant and nonpregnant human myometrium. *Anesthesiology* 1977;40:15–19.

398. Munson ES, Maier WR, Caton D. Effects of halothane, cyclopropane and nitrous oxide on isolated human uterine muscle. *J Obstet Gynaecol Br Commonw* 1969;76:27–33.

399. Munson ES, Embro WJ. Enflurane, isoflurane, and halothane and isolated human uterine muscle. *Anesthesiology* 1977;46:11–14.

400. Marx GF, Kim YI, Lin CC, Halevy S, Schulman H. Postpartum uterine pressures under halothane or enflurane anesthesia. *Obstet Gynecol* 1978;51:695–698.

401. Moir DD. Anaesthesia for caesarean section: An evaluation of a method using low concentrations of halothane and 50 percent of oxygen. *Br J Anaesth* 1970;42:136–142.

402. Galbert MW, Gardner AE. Use of halothane in a balanced technique for cesarean section. *Anesth Analg* 1972;51:701–704.

403. Wilson J. Methoxyflurane in caesarean section. *Br J Anaesth* 1973;45:233.

404. Latto IP, Waldron BA. Anaesthesia for caesarean section. *Br J Anaesth* 1977;49:371–378.

405. Abboud TK, Kim SH, Henriksen EH, et al. Comparative maternal and neonatal effects of halothane and enflurane for cesarean section. *Acta Anaesthesiol Scand* 1985;29:663–668.

406. Thirion A-V, Wright RG, Messer CP, Rosen MA, Shnider SM. Maternal blood loss associated with low dose halothane administration for cesarean section [abstract]. *Anesthesiology* 1988;69:A693.

407. Coleman AJ, Downing JW. Enflurane anesthesia for cesarean section. *Anesthesiology* 1975;43:354–357.

408. Gilstrap LC, Hauth JC, Hankins C, Patterson AR. Effect of type of anesthesia on blood loss at cesarean section. *Obstet Gynecol* 1987;69:328–332.

409. Palahniuk RJ, Scatliff J, Biehl D, Wiebe H, Sankaran K. Maternal and neonatal effects of methoxyflurane, nitrous oxide and lumbar epidural anaesthesia for caesarean section. *Can Anaesth Soc J* 1977;24:586–596.

410. Crawford JS, Burton OM, Davies P. Anaesthesia for section: Further refinement of a technique. *Br J Anaesth* 1973;45:726–731.

411. Warren TM, Datta S, Ostheimer GW, et al. Comparison of the maternal and neonatal effects of halothane, enflurane and isoflurane for cesarean delivery. *Anesth Analg* 1983;62:516–520.

412. Shyken JM, Smeltzer JS, Baxi LV, et al. A comparison of the effect of epidural, general, and no anesthesia on acid-base volumes by stage of labor and type of delivery. *Am J Obstet Gynecol* 1990;163:802–807.

413. Stomer UM, Messerschmidt A, Wulf H. Anaesthesia for caesarean section—a German study. *Acta Anaesthesiol Scand* 1998;42:678–684.

414. Crawford JS. Awareness during operative obstetrics under general anesthesia. *Br J Anaesth* 1971;43:179–182.

415. Wilson J, Turner DJ. Awareness during caesarean section under general anaesthesia. *Br M J* 1969;1:280–283.

416. Abboud TK, D'Onofrio L, Reyes A, et al. Isoflurane or halothane for cesarean section: Comparative maternal and neonatal effects. *Acta Anaesthesiol Scand* 199 ;3:578–581.

417. Apgar V, Holaday DA, James LS, Prince CE, Weisbrot IM. Comparison of regional and general anesthesia in obstetrics. *JAMA* 1957;105:2155–2161.

418. Benson RC, Shubeck F, Clarke WM, et al. Fetal compromise during elective cesarean section. *Am J Obstet Gynecol* 1965;91:645–651.

419. Ong BY, Cohen MM, Palahniuk RJ. Anesthesia for cesarean section: Effects on neonates. *Anesth Analg* 1989;68:270–275.

420. Abboud TK, Nagapppala S, Murakawa K, et al. Comparison of the effects of general and regional anesthesia for cesarean section on neonatal neurologic and adaptive capacity scores. *Anesth Analg* 1985;64:996–1000.

421. Downing JW, Houlton PC, Barclay A. Extradural analgesia for cesarean section: A comparison with general anesthesia. *Br J Anaesth* 1979;51:367–373.

422. Kalappa R, Ueland K, Hansen JM, Eng M, Parer JT. Maternal acid-base status during cesarean section under thiopental, N$_2$O and succinylcholine anesthesia. *Am J Obstet Gynecol* 1971;109:411–420.

423. Hodges RJ, Tunstall ME. The choice of anaesthesia and its influence on perinatal mortality in caesarean section. *Br J Anaesth* 1961;33:572–588.

424. Caritic SN, Abouleish E, Edelston DI, et al. Fetal acid-based state following spinal or epidural anesthesia for cesarean section. *Obstet Gynecol* 1980;56:610–615.

425. Hodgson CA, Wauchob TD. A comparison of spinal and general anesthesia for elective caesarean section: Effect on neonatal condition at birth. *Int J Obstet Anesth* 1994;3:25–30.

426. Datta S, Brown WU Jr. Acid-base status in diabetic mothers and their infants following general or spinal anesthesia for cesarean section. *Anesthesiology* 1977;47:272–276.

427. Fox GS, Smith JB, Namba Y, Johnson RC. Anesthesia for cesarean section: Further studies. *Am J Obstet Gynecol* 1979;133:15–19.

428. James FM, Crawford JS, Hodgkinson R, Davies P, Naiem H. A comparison of general anesthesia and lumbar epidural analgesia for elective cesarean section. *Anesth Analg* 1977;56:228–235.

429. Crawford JS, Davies P. A return to trichloroethylene for obstetric anesthesia. *Br J Anaesth* 1975;47:482–489.

430. Datta S, Ostheimer GW, Weiss JB, Brown WU Jr, Alper MH. Neonatal effect of prolonged anesthetic induction for cesarean section. *Obstet Gynecol* 1981;58:331–335.

431. Bader AM, Datta S, Arthur GR, Benvenuti E, Courtney M, Hauch M. Maternal and fetal catecholamines and uterine incision-to-delivery interval during elective cesarean section. *Obstet Gynecol* 1990;75:600–603.

432. Scanlon JW, Shea E, Alper MH. Neurobehavioral responses of newborn infants following general or spinal anesthesia for cesarean section. In: Abstracts of Scientific Papers of the Annual Meeting of the American Society of Anesthesiologists; Chicago, IL; 1975:91.

433. Hodgkinson R, Bhatt M, Kim SS, Grewal G, Marx GF. Neonatal neurobehavioral tests following cesarean section under general and spinal anesthesia. *Am J Obstet Gynecol* 1978;132:670–674.

434. Hollmén AI, Jouppila R, Koivisto M, et al. Neurologic activity of infants following anesthesia for cesarean section. *Anesthesiology* 1978;48:350–356.

435. Abboud TK, Blikian A, Noueihid R, Nagappala S, Afrasiabi A, Henriksen EH. Neonatal effects of maternal hypotension during spinal anesthesia as evaluated by a new test [abstract]. *Anesthesiology* 1983;59:A421.

436. Mahajan J, Mahajan RP, Singh MM, et al. Anaesthetic technique for elective caesarean section and neurobehavioral states of newborns. *Int J Obstet Anesth* 1992;2:89–93.

437. Brockhurst NJ, Littleford JA, Halpern SH. The neurologic and adaptive capacity score: A systemic review of its use in obstetric anesthesia research. *Anesthesiology* 2000;92:237–246.

438. Camann WR. Use and abuse of neonatal neurobehavioral testing. *Anesthesiology* 2000;92:3–5.

439. American College of Obstetricians and Gynecologists. *Inappropriate Use of the Terms Fetal Distress and Birth Asphyxia*. Washington, DC: American College of Obstetricians and Gynecologists; 1998;197.

440. Parer JT, Livingston EG. What is fetal distress? *Am J Obstet Gynecol* 1990;162:1421–1427.

441. Marx GF, Luykx WM, Cohen SE. Fetal-neonatal status following caesarean section for fetal distress. *Br J Anaesth* 1984;56:1009–1013.

442. Mokriski BK, Naulty JS. General or regional anesthesia for emergent/urgent cesarean section for fetal distress. *Anesth Rev* 1993;20:69–74.

443. Ramanathan J, Ricca DM, Sibai BM, Angel JJ. Epidural vs general anesthesia in fetal distress with various abnormal fetal heart rate patterns. *Anesth Analg* 1988;67:S180.

444. Tsen LC, Pitner R, Camann WR. General anesthesia for cesarean section at a tertiary care hospital 1990–1995: Indications and implications. *Int J Obstet Anesth* 1998;7:147–152.

445. Morgan BM, Magni V, Goroszenuik T. Anaesthesia for emergency caesarean section. *Br J Obstet Gynaecol* 1990;97:420–424.

446. Lucas DN, Ciccone GK, Yentis SM. Extending low-dose epidural analgesia for emergency caesarean section. *Anaesthesia* 1999;54:1173–1177.

447. Gaiser RR, Cheek TG, Adams HK, Gutsche BB. Epidural lidocaine for cesarean delivery of the distressed fetus. *Int J Obstet Anesth* 1998;7:27–31.

448. Gaiser RR, Cheek TG, Gutsche BB. Epidural lidocaine versus 2-chloroprocaine for fetal distress requiring urgent cesarean section. *Int J Obstet Anesth* 1994;3:208–210.

449. Price ML, Reynolds F, Morgan BM. Extending epidural blockade for emergency caesarean section. *Int J Obstet Anesth* 1991;1:13–18.

450. Forrester DJ, Mukherju SK, Mayer DC, Spielman FJ. Dilute infusion for labor obscure subdural catheter and life-threatening block at cesarean delivery. *Anesth Analg* 1999;89:1267–1268.

451. Lubenow T, Keh-Wong E, Kristof K, Ivankovich O, Ivankovich AD. Inadvertent subdural injection: A complication of an epidural block. *Anesth Analg* 1988;67:175–179.

452. Rawal N, Schollin J, Wesstrom G. Epidural versus combined spinal epidural block for caesarean section. *Acta Anaesthesiol Scand* 1988;32:61–66.

453. Brownridge P. Spinal anaesthesia in obstetrics [letter]. *Br J Anaesth* 1991;67:663.

454. DiGiovanni AJ, Dunbar BS. Epidural injections of autologous blood for postlumbar puncture headache. *Anesth Analg* 1970;49:268–271.

Shnider and Levinson's Anesthesia for Obstetrics,
edited by Samuel C. Hughes, et al.
Lippincott Williams & Wilkins,
Philadelphia, © 2001.

CHAPTER 12

ANESTHESIA FOR POSTPARTUM STERILIZATION

STEPHEN H. ROLBIN, M.D., C.M., F.R.C.P. (C) AND
PAMELA J. MORGAN, M.D., F.R.C.P. (C)

I. POSTPARTUM TUBAL STERILIZATION

Surgical sterilization has become an increasingly common method of birth control. After rising from 16% to 42% between 1965 and 1988, the prevalence of surgical sterilization among women 15 to 44 years of age remained stable at 41% in 1995 (1). It is both a highly effective and safe technique. These factors, as well as societal and attitudinal changes, have made tubal sterilization a common and acceptable procedure. Estimates are that more than 1,000,000 sterilization operations are performed annually in the United States (2, 3).

Most tubal sterilizations are elective and are not performed at the time of childbirth (3). These procedures are referred to as "interval" sterilizations. Not only is the total number of procedures increasing, but also the incidence relative to the population and live births. This trend has developed from a broadening of the general indications for carrying out such procedures.

Tubal sterilization is associated with a mortality of 1.5 per 100,000 procedures, which is a lower rate than that associated with pregnancy (10 per 100,000). The widespread use of laparoscopic surgery has resulted in laparoscopic techniques being used in 38% of all female sterilization procedures and 60% of interval procedures (2).

The advantage of postpartum sterilization is that the fallopian tubes are more easily accessible because of the altered anatomy produced by the enlarged uterus, resulting in a simpler surgical procedure than when complete involution of the uterus has taken place. Currently, criteria for performing postpartum tubal ligation are based on the wishes and consent of the woman and her partner. Rates of serious complications such as bowel laceration or blood vessel injury are lower during a minilaparotomy than during elective laparoscopy (4). Puerperal sterilization usually does not lengthen the hospital stay and obviously eliminates the need for rehospitalization. This should reduce the patient's stress and total medical bills. However, postpartum sterilization is an elective procedure and should be done only when maternal conditions are safe (5). Often, patients with complications of pregnancy or medical conditions are advised to have sterilization performed when a complete involution of the uterus has taken place (i.e., 6 months after delivery). Even after such a delay, several patient factors increase the risk of complications 2-fold or more: diabetes mellitus, previous abdominal or pelvic surgery, lung disease, a history of pelvic inflammatory disease, and obesity (6).

In recent years, there has been a tendency to consider postpartum tubal ligation as a semiurgent operation (i.e., within hours of delivery). The hope is that infection would be reduced with immediate postpartum tubal ligation. It is believed that performing this procedure more than 48 hours after delivery is not prudent because bacteria, present in the uterus, may increase the risk of infection. A survey conducted among obstetric anesthesiologists expressed concern about aspiration of gastric contents should general anesthesia be given (7). Indeed, 4 out of 30 anesthesiologists had encountered aspiration of gastric contents in patients with general anesthesia administered in the postpartum period. The consensus from this survey was that immediate postpartum tubal ligation could be performed safely under a continuous epidural anesthetic that had been effective for labor and delivery, but that the risk of aspiration should limit the induction of general anesthesia in the immediate postpartum period.

This statement is not as straightforward as it seems. The successful use of an epidural catheter for tubal ligation is greater if the surgery is done immediately after delivery. One study found that 92% of women received satisfactory intraoperative anesthesia using in situ epidural catheters (8). The success rate was over 90% until 24 hours had passed, at which time it fell to 80%. Of greater concern is a second study that found that only 74% of women received satisfactory intraoperative analgesia using in situ catheters (9). If the catheter was used within 4 hours of delivery, successful anesthesia was obtained for 95% of patients vs. 67% in the group that had surgery more than 4 hours after delivery.

The rate of gastric emptying is delayed in women who have received systemic opioids during labor (10–12). Epidural or subarachnoid administration of opioids will also delay gastric emptying (13). Some have not found an effect of epidural opioids; however, this may be due to the use of low doses of fentanyl (13). The effects may be very different during a long labor, when the cumulative dose will be much greater (14). Ultrasound examination of the stomach contents of women in the postpartum period has shown that a significant number of women have delayed gastric emptying (15). The parturient must be treated as a patient with a full stomach and appropriate precautions taken.

II. TUBAL LIGATION VS. LAPAROSCOPIC STERILIZATION

Tubal ligation and laparoscopic coagulation are the two commonly used methods for postpartum sterilization. In contrast to interval procedures, postpartum sterilization is more commonly done by tubal ligation than by laparoscopic procedures (4). There are over 100 variations of these techniques. Of these, only a few are in common use today (16). Tubal ligation is easily accomplished in the immediate puerperal period, requires less experience than laparoscopic coagulation, and does not depend on expensive equipment (17). Results of a multicenter, multinational, randomized study of minilaparotomy with tubal ligation compared with laparoscopy have concluded that minilaparotomy is the preferred method of choice when done away from a major institution (4).

Postpartum laparoscopy has been found to be safe, practical, and acceptable by many authorities (18, 19). However, follow-up of these patients has shown a higher complication rate, and therefore it is no longer performed in the immediate puerperium, even though convalescence may be more rapid and comfortable (20, 21). There have been several reports of laparoscopic tubal ligation that stress the safety and simplicity of these procedures (22–26). They can be performed under local anesthesia with sedation and are quick, safe, inexpensive, and easy to perform (27). Although postpartum laparoscopic tubal coagulation has its advocates, most obstetricians favor the use of postpartum tubal ligation.

III. PHYSIOLOGIC CHANGES OF PREGNANCY AND THE PUERPERIUM

Pregnancy, labor, and delivery are associated with major physiologic changes, many of which extend into the postpartum period. Every maternal organ system undergoes major change during the course of pregnancy in order to accommodate the developing fetus. Details of these changes can be found elsewhere in the text. The cardiovascular and gastrointestinal alterations may have profound effects on the maternal response to surgery in the puerperium.

Cardiovascular Changes

In the first 2 to 3 days postpartum, there is a 15% to 30% increase in blood volume resulting from elimination of the placental circulation, an increase in venous return, and a shift of fluid from the interstitial compartment into the circulation (28). Cardiac output increases dramatically immediately postpartum, with values as high as 75% above predelivery levels (29). A decrease in both heart rate and stroke volume accounts for the reduction in cardiac output over the ensuing hours and days (30–32). The use of both Doppler and M-mode echocardiography has allowed researchers to examine the issue of when these cardiovascular parameters return to normal. Robson et al. performed serial hemodynamic studies at 2, 6, 12, and 24 weeks postpartum (32). Cardiac output declined by 33% at 24 weeks after delivery, with 28% of the decrease occurring by the second postpartum week. Reductions in both stroke volume and heart rate accompanied the decrease in cardiac output. No differences were noted between lactating and nonlactating women (32). Capeless et al. compared the changes in cardiovascular status in women before pregnancy and serially after conception until 12 weeks postpartum (33). These investigators reported that using M-mode echocardiography, left ventricular end-diastolic volume and stroke volume remain elevated over their values before conception when measured in the same patient population before and after a normal pregnancy (33).

Increases in cardiac output, blood volume, and hemodilution result in better perfusion of the alveoli. These changes result in a reduced arterial to end-tidal carbon dioxide tension difference during anesthesia for tubal ligation, which persists for 8 days following delivery (34).

In summary, women presenting for surgery in the immediate postpartum period continue to demonstrate alterations in cardiovascular parameters, which must be taken into consideration by the anesthesiologist.

Gastrointestinal Changes

Several factors predispose the pregnant patient to gastric retention and regurgitation. The large term uterus mechanically obstructs the duodenum and progesterone decreases intestinal motility and relaxes the gastroesophageal sphincter. Pain and analgesic drugs may delay gastric emptying.

The risk of aspiration in parturients has been well recognized since Mendelson first described a syndrome associated with aspiration of gastric acid (35). There is a notable difference in the risk for death in the obstetric population between general and regional anesthesia, a risk ratio that has increased from the period 1979–84 to 1985–90 (36). Of the 67 deaths associated with general anesthesia, 33 were specifically attributed to acid aspiration. Confidential Enquiries into Maternal Deaths in the United Kingdom has reported an increase in the number of deaths attributed to anesthesia, although the actual numbers are small (37). Another issue that is extremely important is that of maternal morbidity, which is poorly quantitated. Not all peripartum women who aspirate during the course of a general anesthetic will die. The assessment of international data regarding the admission of obstetric patients to an intensive care unit, as well as an evaluation of the reasons for the admission, may address the issues surrounding maternal morbidity during delivery and the puerperium.

In conclusion, serious consideration must be given to the risk-benefit ratio of postpartum sterilization, especially with the use of general anesthesia. The controversy surrounding this issue has led to a number of studies examining when the postpartum stomach becomes "safe."

Gastric Reflux

Gastroesophageal reflux, the incidence of which is increased during pregnancy, is a well- recognized risk factor for acid aspiration. In a study of 17 term parturients, Vanner, using a reflux provocation test with lower esophageal pH monitoring, demonstrated a significant number of reflux episodes in these patients (38). Gastroesophageal reflux decreased progressively by the second postpartum day, although no control population was used, so the results are difficult to interpret.

Gastric emptying plays a crucial role in the risk of aspiration in the pregnant population and can be assessed with a paracetamol absorption test. Macfie et al. did not demonstrate any difference in gastric emptying between nonpregnant and pregnant women during the first, second, or third trimester (39). The patients in the study were assessed in the sitting position. The same technique was used by Gin et al. to determine gastric emptying in the immediate postpartum period and 6 weeks later (40). Gastric emptying was found to be rapid, and there was no difference between the first and third postpartum day. At 6 weeks, gastric emptying was still rapid, but the metabolism of paracetamol appeared to be slower than immediately postpartum (40). Whitehead, using the paracetamol technique, did a controlled study of gastric emptying in nonpregnant women, women at various gestational ages, and postpartum women. As compared to nonpregnant controls, there were no differences in the gastric emptying times of women at different gestational ages but a significant delay in mothers within 2 hours after delivery (41). However, four of the patients in this group had received intramuscular meperidine during labor. There was no significant delay on the second postpartum day.

Applied potential tomography, which involves placing electrodes around the epigastrium as a measure of gastric emptying, was used in a serial manner on women at 37 to 40 weeks, 2 to 3 days postpartum, and at 6 weeks (42). No significant change over time was noted.

Ultrasound has also been used to examine stomach contents. Carp et al. demonstrated that high-resolution ultrasonography is capable of noninvasively identifying the stomach contents of parturients (43). A subsequent study by Jayaram et al. compared stomach contents and gastric emptying of women in the postpartum period with those of nonpregnant women (15). Initially, the presence or absence of solid food particles was compared between patients presenting for postpartum tubal ligation and gynecologic surgery. Gastric emptying of solid food was then compared between nonpregnant controls and women in the postpartum period. Eleven of 28 patients who were to undergo tubal ligation compared with none of the gynecology patients were found to have solid food in their stomachs. Nineteen of 20 women in the postpartum group had food in the stomach 4 hours after a meal compared to four of 21 in the nonpregnant group (Table 12.1). The authors concluded that the postpartum period carries the risk of a delay in gastric

Table 12.1. GASTRIC EMPTYING IN POSTPARTUM AND NONPREGNANT VOLUNTEERS

Variable	Nonpregnant[*] (n = 21)	Postpartum[*] (n = 20)	P
Age (yr)	34.1 ± 5.7	25.0 ± 5.0	.0001[†]
BMI	24.1 ± 4.8	26.5 ± 4.9	.11
Food particles in stomach at 4 h (n)	4	19	.0001[†]
Time from last opioid medication to ultrasound examination (h)	N/A	14.5 ± 6.9	
Time from delivery to ultrasound examination	N/A	9.0 ± 6.3	

BMI = body mass index.
* Values are mean ± SD.
† Difference is statistically significant.
Reprinted by permission from Jayaram A, Bowen MP, Deshpande S, Carp HM. Ultrasound examination of the stomach contents of women in the postpartum period. *Anesth Analg* 1997;84:525.

emptying. Additionally, Lam et al. have demonstrated that the ingestion of water 2 to 3 hours before postpartum sterilization did not alter gastric pH or volume as compared to fasted and nonpregnant controls (44).

Opioids and Gastric Emptying

Opioids have long been known to affect the smooth muscle of the gastrointestinal tract (10, 45). O'Sullivan et al. have demonstrated that women receiving intramuscular meperidine and promethazine during labor had slower gastric emptying rates than women who did not receive these drugs (10). Recently, studies have focused on the effects of epidural and intrathecal opioids on gastric emptying. The addition of a bolus dose of fentanyl 100 μg to 0.375% bupivacaine resulted in delayed gastric emptying in laboring women (46). Porter reported similar results with doses of fentanyl greater than 100 μg administered as an epidural infusion with 0.125% bupivacaine (14). Geddes administered 100 μg epidural fentanyl following cesarean section (47). Gastric emptying was slower in the first 45 minutes following surgery. In a study using an epidural infusion of 0.125% bupivacaine and 0.0002% fentanyl vs. bupivacaine alone, no difference was detected between the groups (48). Intrathecal fentanyl 25 μg slowed gastric emptying more than 50 μg epidural fentanyl or bupivacaine alone in a study by Kelly (13). Although some controversy exists, it would seem prudent to consider that gastric emptying may be affected by the administration of neuraxial fentanyl in a dose-related manner.

α_2 Agonists, clonidine, and dexmedetomidine, have also been investigated. Clonidine had no effect on gastric emptying when given as an intramuscular injection in gynecologic patients compared to morphine (49). When used in combination with morphine, dexmedetomidine did not significantly alter the effect on gastric emptying in rats (50).

Pharmacologic Therapy

The pH and volume of gastric contents affect the outcome in patients with aspiration pneumonitis. Drugs that can alter either or both of these parameters have been widely investigated. In high-risk patients, such as those presenting for cesarean section, nonparticulate antacids are routinely administered in many centers (51–53). Other drugs, including H_2 and dopamine antagonists and proton pump inhibitors, may be used for additional prophylaxis.

H_2 receptor antagonists, ranitidine or cimetidine, inhibit gastric acid secretion and reduce gastric volume. In a large study of 595 patients presenting for emergency cesarean section under general anesthesia, Rout documented gastric pH and volume in patients who were randomized to receive either 50 mg

intravenous (IV) ranitidine or placebo (54). All patients received 30 mL 0.3M sodium citrate upon entry to the operating room. The results demonstrated that the addition of 50 mg IV ranitidine to regimens including sodium citrate reduced the risk of aspiration if 30 minutes had passed between the time of drug administration and intubation (54). No patient in the study developed aspiration pneumonitis, although one patient aspirated gastric contents.

Metoclopramide, a dopamine antagonist, has been used as a prokinetic agent in an attempt to decrease gastric volume in high-risk patients. Centers with a vast experience with this drug do not routinely include it in their prophylactic regimen, suggesting that there is little benefit from the addition of this drug (52, 55, 56).

Omeprazole, a new antisecretory agent, decreases gastric secretion by inhibiting the activity of H+/K+ adenosine triphosphatase (ATPase) (57). Oral omeprazole 40 mg has been shown to be effective in reducing intragastric volume and acidity when given the night before and the morning of elective cesarean section (58). This regimen is not practical in many centers where women are not admitted the night before surgery, nor can it be adapted for the emergency situation. IV omeprazole 40 mg reduces the risk of acid aspiration provided that at least 30 minutes has elapsed from the time of administration to intubation (59). The fact that omeprazole is much more expensive than ranitidine must be considered.

Rout et al. in Natal, South Africa, have had a vast experience with the administration of general anesthesia for cesarean section. Their practice includes the routine administration of a nonparticulate antacid to women presenting for emergency cesarean section and the addition of 50 mg IV ranitidine only in high-risk situations (54).

Conclusion

How does the obstetric anesthesiologist proceed when a patient is scheduled for a postpartum sterilization procedure? The American Society of Anesthesiology Practice Guidelines for Obstetrical Anesthesia suggest that "The patient planning to have an elective postpartum tubal ligation (PPTL) within 8 hours of delivery should have no oral intake of solid foods during labor and postpartum until the time of surgery." Epidural, spinal, and general anesthesia can be effectively provided without affecting maternal complications. If the patient has a functioning epidural catheter in situ, the catheter can be reactivated for the surgical procedure. The anesthesiologist should be aware that an epidural catheter placed for labor may be more likely to fail with longer postdelivery time intervals. If no regional anesthetic technique was used for labor or delivery, we recommend the use of either spinal or epidural anesthesia. If general anesthesia is used, rapid sequence induction, cricoid pressure, and appropriate airway management are mandatory. Prophylactic sodium citrate, 30 mL 0.3 M solution, should be given to all patients. Some clinicians also administer 50 mg IV ranitidine.

The exact timing of postpartum tubal ligations must be flexible. Hospital costs, patients' length of stay, and other financial concerns dictate the practice of many physicians. It seems reasonable that surgery may proceed 8 to 12 hours postpartum provided that the patient is otherwise healthy and hemodynamically stable, opioid effects have worn off, nil per os status is acceptable, the condition of the neonate has been assessed and deemed to be normal, and surgery can be performed at a time when it does not compromise other aspects of patient care in the labor and delivery area.

IV. PHYSIOLOGIC CHANGES INDUCED BY LAPAROSCOPY

Carbon dioxide or nitrous oxide can be used for inducing pneumoperitoneum, but carbon dioxide remains a more popular choice. Its high solubility results in a rapid absorption of any remaining postoperative gas and may be safer if the gas is accidentally intravenously injected (60). Nitrous oxide is associated with less diaphragmatic and peritoneal irritation and diminishes shoulder pain in the postoperative period (61). This advantage has resulted in nitrous oxide being commonly used when the surgery is performed with local anesthesia or regional blockade.

Anesthesia for a patient undergoing laparoscopy with CO_2 insufflation involves several important considerations. Rising intraabdominal pressure by gas insufflation may result in altered ventilatory and cardiac parameters and may encourage reflux of gastric contents.

Minute ventilation decreases during pneumoperitoneum associated with laparoscopic procedures. This can lead to respiratory acidosis if appropriate ventilatory changes are not undertaken (62). Other respiratory effects of abdominal insufflation of gas include decreases in dynamic lung compliance and total respiratory compliance (62, 63). The fall in total respiratory compliance is position dependent, worsening with head-down tilt and recovering immediately upon deflation in patients positioned in a head-up tilt (63). A study by Tan et al. demonstrated that a 30% increase in minute ventilation, achieved by increasing tidal volume to more than $10 \text{ mL} \cdot \text{kg}^{-1}$ eliminated the increased CO_2 load during pelvic laparoscopy (64). Further work by Wahba et al. has indicated that $P_{ET}CO_2$ may not accurately reflect $PaCO_2$ during laparoscopic cholecystectomy. Their conclusions were that if $P_{ET}CO_2$ is <41 mm Hg, it can be used as an index of $PaCO_2$, provided that the anesthesiologist recognizes that an increased $(Pa-P_{ET})CO_2$, which reflects reduced cardiac output, may exist in some patients (65). Although not in widespread use, transcutaneous $PaCO_2$ monitoring may more accurately reflect arterial carbon dioxide tension than end-tidal monitoring (66). The respiratory changes in pregnancy will affect the anesthetic management of women undergoing laparoscopic sterilization. $PaCO_2$ should be maintained at a level of 32 to 34 mm Hg and the F_{IO_2} adequate to maintain oxygen saturations above 97%.

Significant hemodynamic effects can be demonstrated during pneumoperitoneum. In the healthy parturient presenting for tubal coagulation, these changes will likely be well tolerated. However, a woman with serious cardiac dysfunction may be seriously compromised, and a laparoscopy may not be an appropriate surgical approach. Reduced blood volume in the postpartum period also contributes to the occurrence of hypotension (19, 20, 61). Hemodynamic changes during pneumoperitoneum are position dependent. In the horizontal position, increases were noted in mean arterial pressure, central venous pressure, and pulmonary capillary wedge pressure (67). When a head-down tilt was adopted, a 40% further increase in filling pressures was noted. Cardiac output decreased, the effect being greatest with increasing time (68). In a head-up position, used during laparoscopic cholecystectomy, cardiac index was noted to decrease by 50% in healthy patients (69). It is important to note that in most situations, the insufflation pressure should be maintained at less than 20 mm Hg.

Serious complications from laparoscopic surgery can occur. Subcutaneous emphysema, pneumothorax, pneumomediastinum, and venous gas emboli have been reported (70–72). The gas may pass retroperitoneally through congenital foraminae, through defects in the diaphragm, or weak points of the aortic or esophageal hiatus. These infrequent but potentially fatal complications of laparoscopy must be ruled out whenever a patient becomes hypoxic, difficult to ventilate, or hypotensive.

V. ANESTHETIC MANAGEMENT
Local Anesthesia for Postpartum Sterilization

Local anesthesia for surgical procedures is reported to have the advantage of rapid onset, ease of administration, rapid recovery time, and less nausea, vomiting, and other postoperative side effects. A review of the literature concerning the Kenyan experi-

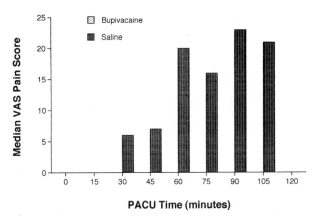

Figure 12.1. Data represent median pain scores on a visual analog scale (*VAS*) at 15-minute intervals in the postanesthesia care unit (PACU). The bupivacaine group had significantly lower pain scores than the saline group 30 to 90 minutes postoperatively, and maintained a median pain score of 0 throughout. (Reprinted by permission from Wittels B, Faure EAM, Chavez R, et al. Effective analgesia after bilateral tubal ligation. *Anesth Analg* 1998;87:621.)

ence with minilaparotomy under local anesthesia demonstrated the technique to be relatively safe, simple, effective, and well accepted (73). Bordahl et al. compared local anesthesia to general anesthesia for laparoscopic sterilization in a randomized, prospective study of 150 women. Local analgesia with IV sedation was highly acceptable to both patients and surgeons, and was associated with a substantial reduction in anesthesia costs, quicker postoperative recovery, and fewer side effects (74). The authors commented, however, on the necessity of anesthetic attendance during the procedure. Other authors agree with the findings of Bordahl and support the use of local anesthesia with IV sedation for laparoscopic sterilization (22, 24, 75). Although nitrous oxide rather than carbon dioxide has been suggested to decrease pain during laparoscopic tubal occlusion, a recent randomized, double-blind study refuted this statement (76). The investigators noted no difference in intraoperative or postoperative pain between nitrous oxide and carbon dioxide pneumoperitoneum.

The safety and cost-effectiveness of surgical contraception under local anesthesia makes this option appropriate, especially in developing countries (77).

The use of local anesthetic infiltration is especially useful in reducing postoperative pain after postpartum tubal ligation. Wittels et al. found that the infiltration of skin and uterine tubes with 0.5% bupivacaine resulted in better postoperative analgesia compared with placebo (Fig. 12.1) (78).

Regional Anesthesia for Postpartum Sterilization

The administration of uncomplicated regional anesthesia for postpartum surgery avoids the complications associated with general anesthesia. Either spinal or epidural anesthesia may be used.

For postpartum tubal ligation, a sensory level of T4 is needed to ensure that visceral pain is adequately blocked during exposure and manipulation of the fallopian tubes (79). This results in excellent surgical conditions and patient satisfaction. A block to T10 might be adequate, but some patients will be uncomfortable if more than the usual stimulation is necessary to locate the tubes.

Pregnancy is associated with certain physiologic changes that necessitate the modification of the doses of anesthetic drugs administered for spinal or epidural anesthesia. It is accepted that the dose of local anesthetic required to obtain any level of block is reduced by one third in the last trimester of pregnancy (80–82).

Table 12.2. BLOOD PRESSURE FALL IN NORMOTENSIVE PATIENTS FOLLOWING HIGH SPINAL ANESTHESIA (DERMATOME LEVELS T2–C3)

	Systolic	Diastolic
Nonpregnant (n = 5)	7%	4%
Term pregnant (n = 12)	43%	53%
36–48 h postpartum (n = 10)	12%	12%

Adapted from Assali NS, Prystowsky H. Studies on autonomic blockade: Comparison between the effects of tetraethylammonium chloride (TEAC) and high selective spinal anesthesia on blood pressure of normal and toxemic pregnancy. *J Clin Invest* 1950;29:1354–1366.

The Spread of Local Anesthetic Agents With Spinal or Epidural Anesthesia

Assali and Prystowsky used a continuous spinal technique with 0.2% procaine in 10 women both before and after delivery. They noted that 36 to 48 hours postpartum there was a 3- to 4-fold increase in the amount of anesthetic required to produce the same sensory level, and there also was a marked decrease in the cardiovascular effects (Table 12.2) (80). When equivalent doses of spinal anesthetic drugs (tetracaine 5 mg, dextrose 50 mg) were compared in full-term pregnant and healthy young gynecologic patients, there was a faster onset, higher level, and longer duration of blockade in the parturients (83). Marx studied spinal anesthesia in postpartum women undergoing tubal ligation and found a progressive decline in the duration of blockade over the first 3 days postpartum (83). More recently, Abouleish et al. found that postpartum tubal ligation patients required 30% or more (bupivacaine 0.75% in 8.25% dextrose) per segment than did elective repeat cesarean section patients (84). Similarly, Brooks and Mandel found that there was a progressive decrease in the dermatomal spread of epidural anesthesia beginning during the first 18 hours postpartum compared with antepartum cesarean section patients (Fig. 12.2) (85). Epidural dose requirements were not significantly different from those in nonpregnant patients after 36 hours postpartum.

The mechanism for the increased spread of epidural or spinal anesthesia in term pregnant women has not been proven. Increased blood flow to the highly vascular pia mater may result in increased penetration of nerve roots by local anesthetic agents, resulting in a more rapid onset of blockade. Distention of epidural veins has been implicated in the increased spread of anesthetic solution. Elevated intraabdominal pressure and inferior vena cava compression from the pregnant uterus have been suggested as likely causes during labor. However, the reduced dose requirement and reduced capacity of the intrathecal space do not appear to be directly related to uterine obstruction of the inferior vena cava. The reduced dose requirements persist even with adequate left uterine displacement and in the full-lateral position. In addition, the exaggerated lumbar lordosis of pregnancy may contribute to the increased cephalad spread of anesthetic solutions.

It would appear that uptake of epidural anesthetic agents occurs by similar mechanisms in both pregnant and nonpregnant patients. However, there is an increased spread of epidural anesthesia starting in the first trimester of pregnancy (86). This occurs at a time when mechanical factors are unlikely to play a significant role. A possible explanation is that these findings are attributable to hormonal changes (87). Datta et al., in examining the wider dermatomal spread of local anesthetics after epidural or spinal anesthesia, noted that the plasma as well as the cerebrospinal fluid (CSF) concentrations of progesterone were higher in term pregnancy and in the immediate (12 to 18 hours) postpartum period. An interesting finding is that, although elevated, the plasma and CSF progesterone concentrations were

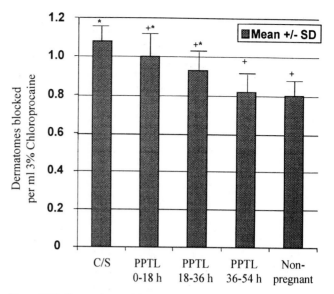

Figure 12.2. Comparison of the number of dermatomes blocked per mL 3% 2-chloroprocaine with epidural anesthesia in pregnant patients having cesarean deliveries (*C/S*), postpartum patients having postpartum tubal ligations (*PPTL*) at various intervals after delivery, and nonpregnant patients undergoing gynecologic procedures. +Significant at *P* < .02 from C/S group; *significant at *P* < .01 from nonpregnant group. (Reprinted by permission from Brooks GZ, Mandel ALZ. The early postpartum dermatomal spread of epidural 2-chloroprocaine. In: Abstracts of Scientific Papers of the Annual Meeting of the Society for Obstetric Anesthesia and Perinatology; San Antonio, TX; 1984:25.)

three and eight times lower in postpartum patients than in term parturients, while the segmental dose requirements for intrathecal lidocaine were the same in both groups. There was, however, an equal and lower segmental dose requirement for lidocaine in the term and immediate postpartum period compared with nonpregnant patients. These authors speculate that the increase in progesterone levels that may alter neuronal function is one of the factors responsible for these observations (87).

Fagraeus et al. have postulated that hyperventilation associated with pregnancy results in an alkalosis that is compensated for by lowered bicarbonate levels. This would result in decreased buffering capacity, allowing the local anesthetic agent to remain as a salt with a prolonged duration of action. This, in turn, would result in an increase in the time needed to reach complete analgesia; also, the drug would have time to spread further within the epidural space. The decreased buffering capacity during pregnancy might account for both the increased spread of local anesthetics and the increased time needed to achieve analgesia (86).

Dose Requirements for Spinal or Epidural Anesthesia in the Parturient

There is no clear recommendation about the dosage requirements for spinal or epidural anesthesia in the first 1 or 2 postpartum days. Age, height, weight, body mass index, and vertebral column length may affect the spread of subarachnoid local anesthetics. However, height has little effect on the spread of intrathecal lidocaine (88). The variation in the spread of the block was found to be large, and the use of patient height to adjust the dose would provide no clinically significant benefit.

In the past, Marx has used a subarachnoid dose of 6 mg hyperbaric tetracaine with satisfactory results (83). McKenzie recommended at least 75 mg 5% lidocaine, with a dosage range of 60 to 90 mg depending on the patient's height, to obtain anesthesia at the T10 level in the patient undergoing postpartum tubal ligation. Tetracaine 6 to 9 mg with 10% glucose achieves similar blockade heights (60).

The use of 5% lidocaine has become controversial because of concerns related to transient radicular irritation (TRI) (89).

Table 12.3. THE RATES OF POSTDURAL PUNCTURE HEADACHE AFTER SPINAL AND EPIDURAL ANESTHESIA IN OBSTETRIC PATIENTS

Group	Needle	Postpartum Headache	No. of Anasthetics	% PDPH
A*	26 guage Quincke	117	2256	5.2
B*	27 guage Quincke	21	852	2.5
C†	25 guage Whitacre	111	1000	1.1
D*	17 guage Epidural	278	21,578	1.3

PDPH = postdural puncture headache.
A vs. B, A vs. D, B vs. C, B vs. D
* P < .05.
C vs. D
† Not significant:
Reprinted by permission from Hurley RJ, Lambert D, Hertwig L, Datta S. Post dural puncture headache in the obstetric patient: Spinal vs. epidural anesthesia [abstract]. *Anesthesiology* 1992;77:A1018.

Table 12.4. NUMBERS, CASE FATALITY RATES, AND RISK RATIOS OF ANESTHESIA-RELATED DEATHS DURING CESAREAN SECTION DELIVERY BY TYPE OF ANESTHESIA: UNITED STATES, 1979–1984 AND 1985–1990

	Time Span	General	Regional
No. of Deaths	1979–1984	33	19
	1985–1990	32	9
Case Fatality Rate	1979–1984	20.0*	8.6†
	1985–1990	32.3*	1.9†
Risk Ratio	1979–1984	2.3	Referent
	1985–1990	16.7	Referent

* Per million general anesthetics for cesarean section.
† Per million regional anesthetics for cesarean section.
Modified by permission from Hawkins JL, Koonin LM, Palmer SK, Gibbs, CP. Anesthesia-related deaths during obstetric delivery in the United States, 1979–1990. *Anesthesiology* 1997;86:281.

This has been suggested by human as well as animal studies (90–93). The incidence of TRI is greater with lidocaine than with bupivacaine (94). Reducing the concentration of lidocaine to 2% does not prevent the occurrence of TRI (94, 95). In non-pregnant patients, spinal anesthesia can be achieved with lidocaine concentrations as low as 0.9% (96). Details of effective doses and the safety of lower concentrations of lidocaine for spinal anesthesia are currently being investigated, and no firm recommendations can be made at this point.

The authors recommend a block to about the T4 to T6 level to ensure patient comfort and ideal operating conditions. To obtain this, lidocaine has been suggested due to its short duration of action (61). Although lidocaine used for a single subarachnoid injection has never been associated with permanent neurologic deficit, we would prefer to use an alternative. Recent investigations in humans have suggested that other agents are suitable. Hyperbaric bupivacaine for spinal anesthesia may have a similar duration of block and time to discharge (94). Similar findings have been reported with 1.5% mepivacaine (97).

It is worth noting that the incidence of postspinal headaches is no different after spinal anesthesia with a 25-gauge Whitacre needle than after a planned epidural (Table 12.3) (98). The incidence is significantly lower than has been reported with the use of nonblunted spinal needles in the nonpregnant patient (99). There has been some interest related to the use of preservative-free intrathecal meperidine as an alternative to local anesthetic for postpartum tubal ligation. The dose that has been suggested is 1 mg/kg in 10% dextrose or saline, and the onset time is 3 to 5 minutes (100, 101). Although intrathecal preservative-free meperidine as the sole anesthetic agent has been reported to provide adequate anesthesia for postpartum tubal ligation, a shorter recovery room stay, and less postoperative pain, its use has not been widely adopted. Precise recommendations for the dose of epidural anesthetics are not known. Ghosh and Tipton reported on 48 patients who achieved satisfactory epidural anesthesia for tubal ligation surgery within 10 hours (mean 2 hours) of delivery (102). They used 10 to 15 mL 0.5% bupivacaine. The dose was arbitrarily chosen and sensory levels were not reported. Since dosage requirements are variable, some recommend using an epidural catheter and starting with doses similar to that used in pregnancy. If further anesthetic is needed, it can be easily added.

General Anesthesia for Postpartum Sterilization

Postpartum sterilization is an elective surgical procedure, and some clinicians are reluctant to provide general anesthesia. Complications of general anesthesia, more specifically airway management problems, account for 52% of anesthetic-related deaths during obstetric delivery in the United States. The case-fatality risk ratio for general anesthesia rose from 2.3 times that for regional anesthesia before 1985 to 16.7 times that after 1985 (Table 12.4) (36). Sterilization procedures, per se, are associated with a very low mortality. An international collaborative study reported that the mortality (adjusted for individuals lost to follow-up) is 13 per 100,000 sterilizations for interval procedures, 53.3 per 100,000 for postabortion procedures, and 43.4 per 100,000 after vaginal delivery (103).

If a patient is to undergo general anesthesia in the postpartum period, a number of considerations must be addressed. Altered physiologic and pharmacologic responses should be anticipated. Prophylactic antacids should be administered and the patient treated with "full-stomach" precautions. The routine use of a rapid sequence induction technique, with preoxygenation, cricoid pressure, and monitoring of both oxygen saturation and capnography, is essential. Finally, the anesthesiologist must prevent patient movement caused by light anesthesia or inadequate muscle relaxation during the moment of coagulation of the fallopian tubes.

Induction Agents

Thiopental has a long history of safety and efficacy as an induction agent in the obstetric patient. Although maternal bradycardia and lower neurologic and Adaptive Capacity scores have been reported when a prolonged infusion to delivery time occurred, (104–109) Gin et al. demonstrated that pharmacokinetic variables for propofol are similar in patients undergoing cesarean section and those in the immediate postpartum period (110). Some clinicians prefer propofol for its purported advantage of a faster recovery, particularly for briefer procedures such as postpartum tubal ligation.

Muscle Relaxants

Succinylcholine remains the muscle relaxant of choice to facilitate tracheal intubation during a rapid sequence induction unless a specific contraindication exists. Levels of plasma cholinesterase decrease during pregnancy, with a further fall in the postpartum period (111). This does not appear to have a significant effect on the length of action of succinylcholine (112). Metoclopramide may prolong the effects of succinylcholine in the postpartum period (113, 114). Monitoring of neuromuscular function with a nerve stimulator will assist the anesthesiologist in the determination of the state of neuromuscular blockade.

Prolonged neuromuscular blockade has been reported with the use of mivacurium, rocuronium, and vecuronium, but not atracurium, in the postpartum period (115–118). Changes in

Table 12.5. TIME COURSE OF ACTION AFTER ADMINISTRATION OF ROCURONIUM 600 μg/kg IN POSTPARTUM AND NONPREGNANT PATIENTS

	Onset[*]	Duration 25%[†] (min)	Induced recovery[‡] (min)
Postpartum	95 ± 30	31.1 ± 3.6	4.8 ± 0.9
Nonpregnant	91 ± 28	24.9 ± 4.0	3.2 ± 0.6
P	.624	< .001	.003

[*] Values are given as mean ± SD.
[†] Time from end of injection of rocuronium until recovery of twitch height to 25%.
[‡] Time required from 25% to 75% recovery of twitch height after reversal with neostigmine and atropine.
Reprinted by permission from Pühringer FK, Sparr HJ, Mitterschiffthaler G, Agoston S, Benzer A. Extended duration of action of rocuronium in postpartum patients. *Anesth Analg* 1997;84:353.

plasma cholinesterase are responsible for prolonging the action of mivacurium and altered liver blood flow, as well as hormonal effects that account for elimination changes of vecuronium and rocuronium. These changes are rarely clinically significant since the increase in length of action is usually only a few minutes (Table 12.5) (116, 117, 119). Neither metoclopramide nor H_2 agonists prolong the effect of nondepolarizing muscle relaxants, although mivacurium may be affected (118). Close monitoring of neuromuscular response with a nerve stimulator is important.

Inhalation Agents

It is a well-recognized fact that minimum alveolar concentration (MAC) decreases during pregnancy. A study of 24 patients undergoing tubal ligation in the postpartum period showed a decrease in the MAC of isoflurane in the first 12 hours postpartum. This decrease appeared to return to nonpregnant values 12 to 25 hours after delivery (120). A recent study by Song et al. compared fast-track eligibility after laparoscopic tubal ligation between the maintenance of anesthesia with propofol, desflurane, and sevoflurane (121). Desflurane and sevoflurane were noted to have a higher percentage of outpatients eligible for fast-tracking compared to those who received propofol for maintenance. These patients were not postpartum, but the newer inhalation agents may have advantages for surgery in the postpartum period.

VI. NEONATAL EFFECTS OF MATERNALLY ADMINISTERED DRUGS

Breast-feeding is considered the optimal method of infant feeding (122). More than 50% of babies being discharged from hospital in the United States are breastfed, and the number is increasing (123). The increasing frequency of breast-feeding and the awareness of health needs by the consumer have led to both patient and health care professionals questioning the safety and potential toxicity of drugs excreted in breast milk.

Most drugs administered to the mother are secreted in the breast milk (124). Factors involved in the transfer from plasma to milk include those of lipid solubility, ionization, concentration, degree of protein binding, and special transport mechanisms. In general, water- soluble drugs are excreted in higher concentration into colostrum, whereas lipid-soluble drugs are excreted in greater concentration into breast milk. The amount of drug that is absorbed by the newborn is usually small.

There is very little information and no evidence that any anesthetic agent given on a single-dose basis is secreted in clinically significant amounts. Most anesthetics are cleared rapidly from the mother, and it is permissible to allow breast-feeding as soon as is practical after surgery (125–127). However, repeated or long-term administration of drugs such as opioids and benzodiazepines may cause adverse effects in premature infants (127). Opioids, such as codeine, meperidine, and morphine in therapeutic doses given by any route result in insignificant levels in breast milk (124, 127, 128). However, the accumulation of normeperidine in breast milk is associated with depression of neurobehavioral scores (78). There are no effects from acetaminophen, codeine, and morphine in the recommended doses (129). Fentanyl has also been assessed. Total doses of 50 to 400 μg of epidural fentanyl were given to mothers in labor. There was a lack of fentanyl excretion in breast milk (124, 130–132). Its short half-life (185 minutes) and its rapid renal clearance explain this finding (124). All infants had normal Apgar scores at birth and normal neurobehavior assessment scores (130–132). IV fentanyl (2 μg/kg) has also been used for postpartum tubal ligation (133). Fentanyl concentrations in umbilical venous blood or colostrum were small, and therefore IV fentanyl is felt to be safe in breast-feeding women.

Early work found that bottle-fed infants had less weight gain than the breast-fed infants (134). While some epidural agents may affect neurobehavioral testing, such tests have neither been shown to have any effect on outcome measures in the neonate nor been shown to be a valid marker for breast-feeding success. A recent abstract assessed the neonate's sucking ability using a Whitney gauge (a simple calibrated chinstrap mercury strain gauge detecting and recording the newborn's jaw movements during sucking). Epidural 0.25% bupivacaine with or without fentanyl had no effect on the sucking characteristics of 116 neonates compared with neonates whose mothers had nonmedicated delivery (135). It has been observed that 3 days of continuous epidural infusion of 0.25% bupivacaine for postcesarean section pain relief improves the amount of breast-feeding and the weight gain of the newborn (136). In contrast, and of particular interest, was the observation that maternally administered IV fentanyl significantly depressed neonatal sucking. A recent report on the effects of epidural fentanyl revealed little effect on respiration (137).

Alfentanil has been assessed for use during postpartum tubal ligation and is excreted into the breast milk. Its short half-life (98 minutes) and high protein binding result in it being a safe drug for breast-feeding women (124). Sufentanil is probably safe because it has never been detected in breast milk. The clinical significance of drug milk levels of these opioids to the nursing infant is probably minimal (123, 124). It has been suggested that opioids found in breast milk can cause or contribute to unexplained episodes of apnea, bradycardia, and cyanosis occurring during the first week of life in full-term infants (138). However, much more investigation needs to be done to confirm this suggestion (139). Other investigators have reported that a relationship between maternal labor analgesia and delay in the initiation of breast-feeding in healthy neonates exists. They report that even small doses of alphaprodine, when administered 1 to 3 hours before delivery, may delay effective breast-feeding for hours or even days (139). For most drugs, however, the quantity excreted in the milk is insufficient to have any clinical effects (128, 129, 140).

In response to concerns raised in a review of pain medications during labor, a study of 189 women was done (141). In this study, neither parental opioids nor epidural labor analgesia using local anesthetics and opioids was associated with a reduced incidence of breast-feeding either in hospital or at 6 weeks postpartum (Table 12.6) (142).

Thiopental is found in breast milk but probably has insignificant effects on the newborn (124, 127, 128, 140). The concentration of propofol administered for induction of general anesthesia at cesarean section is very low in breast milk or colostrum. In addition, propofol is rapidly cleared from the neonatal circulation, so that exposure through breast milk is negligible and should have minimal effect on healthy newborns (143–147). Until further investigations clarify other contradictory

Table 12.6. LEVEL OF SIGNIFICANCE OF THE EFFECTS OF ANALGESIC DRUGS GIVEN INTRAPARTUM ON BREASTFEEDING AT 6 WEEKS POSTPARTUM

Factor	P
Neuraxial fentanyl	.53
Neuraxial sufentanil	.63
Duration of epidural analgesia	.41
Exposure to lidocaine for labor or cesarean section	.89
Exposure to bupivacaine	.95

Adapted by permission from Halpern S, Levine T, MacDonell J, Katsiris S, Leighton B. Effect of labor analgesia on breastfeeding success. *Birth* 1999;26:83–88.

findings, (109, 144–147) thiopental remains the agent of choice. Neonatal exposure to inhalational agents has minimal effects, if any, on breast-feeding. Theoretically, based on their pharmacokinetic profiles, the levels of enflurane, isoflurane, sevoflurane, and desflurane are all expected to be minimal (124, 127, 148). The risk to the newborn is very low.

All benzodiazepines appear in human milk. High or repeated clinical doses might be expected to exert a possible effect on the newborn (124, 127, 148, 149). Diazepam, in particular, should be avoided in the neonatal period (128). It has been reported that appreciable plasma levels of active substances are found in the neonate for up to 10 days after a single maternal dose of diazepam (149, 150). Most authorities strongly advise against its use (128, 149–153). Others disagree, and state that the excretion of diazepam into the breast milk is sufficiently small and that it does not warrant interruption of breast-feeding (126, 148). The risk of problems is probably greater if daily doses are being given. Similarly, there is probably an increased risk if the infant is premature or has a low birth-weight (127).

Midazolam and its active metabolite hydroxymidazolam are excreted in low concentration in breast milk and have a short plasma half-life of 2 to 5 hours in the neonate. No drug effect has been observed. Lorazepam has only a slight passage into the breast milk and has been demonstrated to be safe as an oral premedicant in nursing mothers (124, 127).

Atropine causes decreased lactation with large doses, even though it may not be appreciably excreted. In addition, evidence is lacking that a single dose of atropine could cause anticholinergic side effects in infants. Theoretically, glycopyrrolate would not be expected to cross into breast milk in any significant amount. Neostigmine and pyridostigmine are safe because the quantity in breast milk is low and gastrointestinal absorption is minimal. There is no information about the excretion of edrophonium in breast milk (124).

Many aspects of drug pharmacokinetics are impaired in the premature infant, including differences in absorption, metabolism, distribution, and elimination. Although evidence is lacking, it is commonly believed that the blood-brain barrier is more permeable in the premature infant. These factors may or may not be clinically relevant when a premature infant is given breast milk (148, 154).

VII. SUMMARY

The peripartum period is a time of change in both maternal physiology and pharmacology. Postpartum sterilization is an elective surgical procedure, and the necessity of performing this procedure immediately postpartum requires an assessment of the risk-benefit ratio. Patient preference, as well as institutional financial constraints, may influence the decision. Choice of an anesthetic technique should be individualized, based on anesthetic and/or obstetric considerations and patient preference. The authors most commonly prefer regional anesthetic techniques.

Patients who are healthy, are hemodynamically stable, and have had nothing by mouth for 8 hours are at low risk for complications related to surgical tubal ligation. The obstetric anesthesiologist should ensure that no recent opioids have been administered and that a full preoperative assessment has been performed. The use of perioperative antacids is warranted. Other prophylactic drugs such as ranitidine or proton pump inhibitors may also be administered. In all cases, despite the anesthetic technique chosen, equipment and drugs must be available should an emergency general anesthetic be required. Careful attention to monitoring of vital signs, including oxygen saturation, capnography, and neuromuscular blockade when muscle relaxants are used, is essential in postpartum tubal ligations as in all general anesthetics for surgical procedures.

Breast-feeding is considered the optimal method of feeding the newborn. There is very little information and no evidence that any anesthetic agent given as a single dose is secreted in clinically significant amounts in breast milk, and therefore breast-feeding should not be discontinued if the mother has received these drugs (1).

REFERENCES

1. Chandra A. Surgical Sterilization in the United States: Prevalence and Characteristics, 1965–95. National Center for Health Statistics. *Vital Health Stat* 1998.
2. Committee on Technical Bulletins of the American College of Obstetricians and Gynecologists. Sterilization. ACOG Technical Bulletin No. 113; 1988.
3. Talundi T. Tubal sterilization. *N Engl J Med* 1997;336:796–797.
4. World Health Organization. Minilaparotomy or laparoscopy for sterilization: A multicenter, multinational randomized study. *Am J Obstet Gynecol* 1982;143:645–652.
5. Committee on Technical Bulletins of the American College of Obstetricians and Gynecologists. Maternal and fetal medicine. ACOG Technical Bulletin No. 105; 1992.
6. Destefano F, Greenspan JR, Dicker RC, Peterson HB, Strauss LT, Rubin GL. Complications of internal laparoscopic tubal sterilization. *Obstet Gynecol* 1983;61:153–158.
7. Society for Obstetric Anesthesia and Perinatology. Bilateral tubal ligation–an emergency? *Society for Obstetric Anesthesia and Perinatology Newsletter* July 1, 1973.
8. Goodman EJ, Dumas SD. The rate of successful reactivation of epidural catheters for postpartum tubal ligation surgery. *Reg Anesth Pain Med* 1998;23:258–261.
9. Vincent RD, Reid RW. Epidural anesthesia for tubal ligation using epidural catheters placed during labour. *J Clin Anesth* 1993;5:289–291.
10. O'Sullivan GM, Sutton AJ, Thompson SA, Carrie LE, Bullingham RE. Noninvasive measurement of gastric emptying in obstetric patients. *Anesth Analg* 1987;66:505–511.
11. Nimmo WS, Wilson J, Prescott LF. Narcotic analgesics and delayed gastric emptying during labour. *Lancet* 1975;1:890–893.
12. Nimmo WS. Gastric emptying and analgesia. *Can J Anaesth* 1989;36:S45–S47.
13. Kelly MC, Carabine UA, Hill DA, Mirakhur RK. A comparison of the effect of intrathecal and extradural fentanyl on gastric emptying in laboring women. *Anesth Analg* 1997;85:834–838.
14. Porter JS, Bonello E, Reynolds F. The influence of epidural administration of fentanyl infusion on gastric emptying in labour. *Anaesthesia* 1997;52:1151–1156.
15. Jayaram A, Bowen MP, Deshpande S, Carp HM. Ultrasound examination of the stomach contents of women in the postpartum period. *Anesth Analg* 1997;84:522–526.
16. Cunningham FG, MacDonald PC, Gant NF, et al., eds. Surgical contraception. In: *Williams Obstetrics*. 20th ed. Stamford, CT: Appleton & Lange, 1997:1375–1381.
17. Chi IC, Petta CA, McPheeters M. A review of safety, efficacy, pros and cons, and issues of puerperal tubal sterilization—an update. *Adv Contracep* 1995;11:187–206.
18. Clark DH, Schneider GT, McManus S. Tubal sterilization: Comparison of outpatient laparoscopy and postpartum ligation. *J Reprod Med* 1974;13:69–70.
19. Keith L, Webster A, Lash A. A comparison between puerperal and nonpuerperal laparoscopic sterilization. *Int Surg* 1971;56:325–330.

20. Keith L, Webster A, Houser K, Procknicki L, Lash A, Barton J. Laparoscopy for puerperal sterilization. *Obstet Gynecol* 1972; 39:616–621.

21. Rennie AL, Richard JA, Milne MK, Dalrymple DG. Postpartum sterilization: An anaesthetic hazard? *Anaesthesia* 1979;34: 267–287.

22. Hatasaka HH, Sharp HT, Dowling DD, Teahon K, Peterson CM. Laparoscopic tubal ligation in a minimally invasive surgical unit under local anesthesia compared to a conventional operating room approach under general anesthesia. *J Laparoendosc Adv Surg Tech A* 1997;7:295–299.

23. Schnepper FW. Sterilization by open laparoscopy in a private office. *J Am Assoc Gynecol Laparosc* 1997;4:469–472.

24. DeQuattro N, Hibbert M, Buller J, et al. Microlaparoscopic tubal ligation under local anesthesia. *J Am Assoc Gynecol Laparosc* 1998;5: 55–58.

25. Hibbert ML, Buller JL, Seymour SD, Poore SE, Davis GD. A microlaparoscopic technique for Pomeroy tubal ligation. *Obstet Gynecol* 1997;90:249–251.

26. Reichert JA, Nagel LW, Solberg NS. Sterilization for family planning in a third world country. *Minn Med* 1997;80:27–30.

27. Taneepanichskul S, Intaraprasert S, Chaturachinda K. Modified minilaparotomy technique at interval female sterilization. *Contraception* 1997;55:351–353.

28. Frisoli G. Physiology and pathology of the puerperium. In: Iffy L, Kaminetzky H, eds. *Principles and Practice of Obstetrics and Perinatology.* New York: John Wiley & Sons, 1981:1657.

29. Cunningham FG, MacDonald PC, Gant NF. The puerperium. In: *Williams Obstetrics.* 18th ed. New York: Appleton & Lange; 1989: 245–256.

30. Ueland K, Hansen JM. Maternal cardiovascular dynamics. III. Labor and delivery under local and caudal analgesia. *Am J Obstet Gynecol* 1969;103:8–18.

31. Robson SC, Dunlop W, Hunter S. Haemodynamic changes during the early puerperium. *Br Med J* 1987;294:1065.

32. Robson SC, Hunter S, Moore M, Dunlop W. Haemodynamic changes during the puerperium: A Doppler and M-mode echocardiographic study. *Br J Obstet Gynaecol* 1987;94:1028–1039.

33. Capeless EL. When do cardiovascular parameters return to their preconception values? *Am J Obstet Gynecol* 1991;165:883–886.

34. Shankar KB, Moseley H, Kumar Y, Vemul V, Krishnan A. Arterial to end-tidal carbon dioxide tension difference during anaesthesia for tubal ligation. *Anaesthesia* 1987;42:482–486.

35. Mendelson CL. The aspiration of stomach contents into the lungs during obstetric anesthesia. *Am J Obstet Gynecol* 1946;52:191–205.

36. Hawkins JL, Koonin LM, Palmer SK, Gibbs CP. Anesthesia-related deaths during obstetric delivery in the United States, 1979–1990. *Anesthesiology* 1997;86:277–284.

37. Harmer M. Maternal mortality—is it still relevant? *Anaesthesia* 1997;52: 99–100.

38. Vanner RG, Goodman NW. Gastro-oesophageal reflux in pregnancy at term and after delivery. *Anaesthesia* 1989;44:808–811.

39. Macfie AG, Magides AD, Richmond MN, Reilly CS. Gastric emptying in pregnancy. *Br J Anaesth* 1991;67:54–57.

40. Gin T, Cho AMW, Lew JKL, et al. Gastric emptying in the postpartum period. *Anaesth Intensive Care* 1991;19:521–524.

41. Whitehead EM, Smith M, Dean Y, O'Sullivan G. An evaluation of gastric emptying times in pregnancy and the puerperium. *Anaesthesia* 1993;48:53–57.

42. Sandhar BK, Elliott RH, Windram I, Rowbotham DJ. Peripartum changes in gastric emptying. *Anaesthesia* 1992;47:196–198.

43. Carp H, Jayaram A, Stoll M. Ultrasound examination of the stomach contents of parturients. *Anesth Analg* 1992;74:683–687.

44. Lam KK, So HY, Gin T. Gastric pH and volume after oral fluids in the postpartum patient. *Can J Anaesth* 1993;40:218–221.

45. Jaffe JH, Martin WR. Opioid analgesics and antagonists. In: Gilman AG, Goodman LS, Gilman A, eds. *The Pharmacological Basis of Therapeutics.* 7th ed. New York: Macmillan; 1985:502–504.

46. Wright PMC, Allen RW, Moore J, Donnelly JP. Gastric emptying during lumbar extradural analgesia in labour; effect of fentanyl supplementation. *Br J Anaesth* 1992;68:248–251.

47. Geddes SM, Thorburn J, Logan RW. Gastric emptying following Caesarean section and the effect of epidural fentanyl. *Anaesthesia* 1991;46:1016–1018.

48. Zimmermann DL, Breen TW, Fick G. Adding fentanyl 0.0002% to epidural bupivacaine 0.125% does not delay gastric emptying in laboring parturients. *Anesth Analg* 1996;82:612–616.

49. Asai T, McBeth C, Stewart JIM, Williams J, Vaughan RS, Power I. Effect of clonidine on gastric emptying of liquids. *Br J Anaesth* 1997;78:28–33.

50. Asai T, Mapleson WW, Power I. Interactive effect of morphine and dexmedetomidine on gastric emptying and gastrointestinal transit in the rat. *Br J Anaesth* 1998;80:63–67.

51. Rowe TF. Acute gastric aspiration: Prevention and treatment. *Semin Perinatol* 1997;21:313–319.

52. Stuart JC, Kan AF, Rowbottom SJ, Yau G, Gin T. Acid aspiration prophylaxis for emergency Caesarean section. *Anaesthesia* 1996;51:415–421.

53. Tordoff SG, Sweeney BP. Acid aspiration prophylaxis in 288 obstetric anaesthetic departments in the United Kingdom. *Anaesthesia* 1990;45:776–780.

54. Rout C, Rocke DA, Gouws E. Intravenous ranitidine reduces the risk of acid aspiration of gastric contents at emergency cesarean section. *Anesth Analg* 1993;76:156–161.

55. Gin T. Intravenous omeprazole before emergency Cesarean section [correspondence]. *Anesth Analg* 1995;80:848–849.

56. Orr DA, Bill KM, Gillon KRW, Wilson CM, Fogarty DJ, Moore J. Effects of omeprazole, with and without metoclopramide in elective obstetric anaesthesia. *Anaesthesia* 1993;48:114–119.

57. Wallmark B, Jarestem B-M, Larsson H, Ryberg B, Brandstrom A, Fellenius E. Differentiation among inhibitory actions of omeprazole, cimetidine, and SCN on gastric acid secretion. *Am J Physiol* 1983;245(suppl 1):G64–G71.

58. Gin T, Ewart MC, Yau G, Oh TE. Effect of oral omeprazole on intragastric pH and volume in women undergoing elective Caesarean section. *Br J Anaesth* 1990;65:616–619.

59. Rocke DA, Rout CC, Gouws E. Intravenous administration of the proton pump inhibitor omeprazole reduces the risk of acid aspiration at emergency cesarean section. *Anesth Analg* 1994;78:1093–1098.

60. McKenzie R. Postpartum tubal ligation. In: Abouleish E, ed. *Pain Control in Obstetrics.* Philadelphia: Lippincott; 1977:411–425.

61. Fishburne JI, Keith L. Anesthesia. In: Phillips J, ed. *Laparoscopy.* Baltimore: Williams & Williams; 1977:69–85.

62. Iwasaka H, Miyakawa H, Yamamoto H, Kitano T, Taniguch K, Honda N. Respiratory mechanics and arterial blood gases during and after laparoscopic cholecystectomy. *Can J Anaesth* 1996;43:129–133.

63. Oikkonen M, Tallgren M. Changes in respiratory compliance at laparoscopy: measurements using side stream spirometry. *Can J Anaesth* 1995;42:495–497.

64. Tan PL, Less TL, Tweed WA. Carbon dioxide absorption and gas exchange during pelvic laparoscopy. *Can J Anaesth* 1992;39:677–681.

65. Wahba RWM, Mamazza J. Ventilatory requirements during laparoscopic choleysfectomy. *Can J Anaesth* 1993;40:206–210.

66. Bhavani-Shankar K, Steinbrook RA, Mushlin PS, Freiberger D. Transcutaneous PCO_2 monitoring during laparoscopic cholecystectomy in pregnancy. *Can J Anaesth* 1998;45:164–169.

67. Odeberg S, Ljungqvist O, Svenberg T, et al. Haemodynamic effects of pneumoperitoneum and the influence of posture during anesthesia for laparoscopic surgery. *Acta Anaesthesiol Scand* 1994;35:276–283.

68. Hirvonen EA, Nuutinen LS, Kauko M. Hemodynamic changes due to Trendelenburg positioning and pneumoperitoneum during laparoscopic hysterectomy. *Acta Anaesthesiol Scand* 1985;39:949–955.

69. Joris JL, Noirot DP, Legrand MJ, Jacquet NJ, Lamy ML. Hemodynamic changes during laparoscopic cholecystectomy. *Anesth Analg* 1993;76:1067–1071.

70. Hynes SS, Marshall RL. Venous gas embolism during gynaecological laparoscopy. *Can J Anaesth* 1992;39:748–749.

71. Klopfenstein CE, Gaggero G, Mamie C, Morel P, Forster A. Laparoscopic extraperitoneal inguinal hernia repair complicated by subcutaneous emphysema. *Can J Anaesth* 1995;42:523–525.

72. Wahba RW, Tessler MJ, Kleiman SJ. Acute ventilatory complications during laparoscopic upper abdominal surgery. *Can J Anaesth* 1996;43:77–83.

73. Ruminjo JK, Lynam PF. A fifteen-year review of female sterilization by minilaparotomy under local anesthesia in Kenya. *Contraception* 1997;55:249–260.

74. Bordahl PE, Raeder JC, Nordentoft J, Kirste U, Refsdal A. Laparoscopic sterilization under local or general anesthesia? A randomized study. *Obstet Gynecol* 1993;81:137–141.

75. Poindexter AN, Abdul-Malak M, Fast JE. Laparoscopic tubal sterilization under local anesthesia. *Obstet Gynecol* 1990;75:5–8.

76. Lipscomb GH, Summitt RL Jr, McCord ML, Ling FW. The effect of nitrous oxide and carbon dioxide pneumoperitoneum on operative and postoperative pain during laparoscopic sterilization under local anesthesia. *J Am Assoc Gynecol Laparosc* 1994;2:57–60.

77. Jack KE, Chao CR. Female voluntary surgical contraception via minilaparotomy under local anesthesia. *Int J Gynaecol Obstet* 1992;39:111–116.

78. Wittels B, Glosten B, Faure EAM, et al. Postcesarean analgesia with both epidural morphine and intravenous patient-controlled analgesia: Neurobehavioral outcomes. *Anesth Analg* 1997;85:600–606.

79. Moore DC. Method of administration of single-dose spinal (subarachnoid) anesthesia for some of the common surgical procedures. In: Moore DC, ed. *Regional Block*. 4th ed. Springfield, IL: Charles C Thomas; 1973:380–387.

80. Assali NS, Prystowsky H. Studies on autonomic blockade: Comparison between the effects of tetraethylammonium chloride (TEAC) and high selective spinal anesthesia on blood pressure of normal and toxemic pregnancy. *J Clin Invest* 1950;29:1354–1366.

81. Bromage PR. Spread of analgesia solutions in the epidural space and their site of action: A statistical study. *Br J Anaesth* 1962;34:161–178.

82. Sharrock NE, Greenidge J. Epidural dose responses in pregnant and nonpregnant patients [abstract]. *Anesthesiology* 1979;51:A298.

83. Marx GF. Regional analgesia in obstetrics. *Der Anaesth* 1972;21:84–91.

84. Abouleish EI. Postpartum tubal ligation requires more bupivacaine for spinal anesthesia than does cesarean section. *Anesth Analg* 1986;65:897–900.

85. Brooks GZ, Mandel ALZ. The early postpartum dermatomal spread of epidural 2-chlorprocaine [abstract]. Presented at: Annual Meeting of the Society for Obstetric Anesthesia and Perinatology; San Antonio, TX. 1984:25.

86. Fagraeus L, Urban BJ, Bromage PR. Spread of epidural analgesia in early pregnancy. *Anesthesiology* 1983;58:184–187.

87. Datta S, Hurley RJ, Naulty JS, Sern P, Lambert DH. Plasma and cerebrospinal fluid progesterone concentrations in pregnant and nonpregnant women. *Anesth Analg* 1986;65:950–954.

88. Huffnagle SL, Norris MC, Leighton BL, Arkoosh VA, Elgart RL, Huffnagle HJ. Do patient variables influence the subarachnoid spread of hyperbaric lidocaine in the postpartum patient? *Reg Anesth* 1994;19:330–334.

89. Douglas MJ. Neurotoxicity of lidocaine—does it exist [editorial]? *Can J Anaesth* 1995;42:181–185.

90. Hampl KF, Schneider MC, Thorin D, Ummenhofer W, Drewe J. Hyperosmolarity does not contribute to transient radicular irritation after spinal anesthesia with hyperbaric 5% lidocaine. *Reg Anesth* 1995;20:363–368.

91. Drasner K, Sakura S, Chan VW, Bollen AW, Ciriales R. Persistent sacral neurologic deficit induced by intrathecal local anesthetic infusion in the rat. *Anesthesiology* 1994;80:847–852.

92. Lambert LA, Lambert DH, Strichartz GR. Irreversible conduction block in isolated nerve by high concentrations of local anesthetics. *Anesthesiology* 1994;80:1082–1093.

93. Tarkkila P, Huhtula J, Tuominen M. Transient radicular irritation after spinal anaesthesia with hyperbaric 5% lidocaine. *Br J Anaesth* 1995;74:328–329.

94. Pollock JE, Neal JM, Stephenson CA, Wiley CE. Prospective study of the incidence of transient radicular irritation in patients undergoing spinal anesthesia. *Anesthesiology* 1996;84:1361–1367.

95. Hampl KF, Schneider MC, Pargger H, Gut J, Drewe J, Drasner K. A similar incidence of transient neurologic symptoms after spinal anesthesia with 2% and 5% lidocaine. *Anesth Analg* 1996;83:1051–1054.

96. Peng PW, Chan VW, Perlas A. Minimum effective anaesthetic concentration of hyperbaric lidocaine for spinal anaesthesia. *Can J Anaesth* 1998;45:122–129.

97. Liguori GA, Zayas VM, Chisholm MF. Transient neurologic symptoms after spinal anesthesia with mepivacaine. *Anesthesiology* 1998;88:619–623.

98. Hurley RJ, Lambert D, Hertwig L, Datta S. Post dural puncture headache in the obstetric patient: Spinal vs epidural anesthesia [abstract]. *Anesthesiology* 1992;77:A1018.

99. Vandam LD, Dripps RD. Long-term follow-up of patients who received 10,098 spinal anesthetics. *JAMA* 1956;161:586–591.

100. Curran C, Dickerson SE, Bailey SL. Efficacy of intrathecal meperidine as the sole anesthetic for postpartum tubal ligation [abstract]. *Anesthesiology* 1992;77:A1004.

101. Honet JE, Costello DT, Norris MC. Spinal anesthesia for postpartum tubal ligation: Meperidine vs lidocaine [abstract]. *Anesthesiology* 1991;75:A859.

102. Ghosh AK, Tipton RH. Early postpartum tubal ligation under epidural analgesia. *Br J Obstet Gynaecol* 1976;83:731–732.

103. Rochat RW, Bhiwandiwala PP, Feldblum PJ, Peterson HB. Mortality associated with sterilization: Preliminary results of an international collaborative study. *Int J Gynaecol Obstet* 1986;24:274–284.

104. Abboud TK, Zhu J, Richardson M, Peres da Silva E, Donovan M. Intravenous propofol vs thiamylal-isoflurane for caesarean section, comparative maternal and neonatal effects. *Acta Anaesthesiol Scand* 1995;39:205–209.

105. Alon E, Ball RH, Gillie MH, Parer JT, Rosen MA, Shnider SM. Effects of propofol and thiopental on maternal and fetal cardiovascular and acid-base variables in the pregnant ewe. *Anesthesiology* 1993;78:562–576.

106. Ganansia MF, Francois TP, Ormezzano X, Pinaud ML, Lepage JY. Atrioventricular Mobitz I block during propofol anesthesia for laparoscopic tubal ligation. *Anesth Analg* 1989;69:524–525.

107. Gin T, Gregory MA, Oh TE. The haemodynamic effects of propofol and thiopentone for induction of caesarean section. *Anaesth Intensive Care* 1990;18:175–179.

108. Gin T, O'Meara ME, Leung RK, Tan P, Yau G. Plasma catecholamines and neonatal condition after induction of anaesthesia with propofol or thiopentone at caesarean section. *Br J Anaesth* 1993;70:311–316.

109. Yau G, Gin T, Ewart MC. Propofol for induction at caesarean section. *Anaesthesia* 1991;46:20–23.

110. Gin T, Yau G, Jong W, Tan P, Leung RK, Chan K. Disposition of propofol at caesarean section and in the postpartum period. *Br J Anaesth* 1991;67:49–53.

111. Evans RT, Wroe JM. Plasma cholinesterase changes during pregnancy. Their interpretation as a cause of suxamethonium-induced apnoea. *Anaesthesia* 1980;35:651–654.

112. Leighton BL, Cheek TG, Gross JB. Succinylcholine pharmacodynamics in peripartum patients. *Anesthesiology* 1986;64:202–205.

113. Kao YJ, Turner DR. Prolongation of succinylcholine block by metoclopramide. *Anesthesiology* 1989;70:905–908.

114. Kao YJ, Tellez J, Turner DR. Dose-dependent effect of metoclopramide on cholinesterases and suxamethonium metabolism. *Br J Anaesth* 1990;65:220–224.

115. Guay J, Grenier Y, Varin F. Clinical pharmacokinetics of neuromuscular relaxants in pregnancy. *Clin Pharmacokinet* 1998;34:483.

116. Khuenl-Brady KS, Koller J, Mair P, Pühringer F, Mitterschiffthaler G. Comparison of vecuronium- and atracurium-induced neuromuscular blockade in postpartum and nonpregnant patients. *Anesth Analg* 1991;72:110–113.

117. Pühringer FK, Sparr HJ, Mitterschiffthaler G, Agoston S, Benzer A. Extended duration of action of rocuronium in postpartum patients. *Anesth Analg* 1997;84:352–354.

118. Ward SJ, Rocke DA. Neuromuscular blocking drugs in pregnancy and the puerperium. *Int J Obstet Anesth* 1998;7:251–260.

119. Gin T, Derrick JL, Chan MT, Chui PT, Mak TW. Postpartum patients have slightly prolonged neuromuscular block after mivacurium. *Anesth Analg* 1998;86:82–85.

120. Zhou HH, Norman P, DeLima LGR, Mehta M, Bass D. The minimum alveolar concentration of isoflurane in patients undergoing bilateral tubal ligation in the postpartum period. *Anesthesiology* 1995;82:20–24.

121. Song D, Joshi GP, White PF. Fast-track eligibility after ambulatory anesthesia: A comparison of desflurane, sevoflurane, and propofol. *Anesth Analg* 1998;86:267–273.

122. American Academy of Pediatrics. Work group on breastfeeding and the use of human milk. *Pediatrics* 1997;100:308–312.

123. Yaffe SJ. Introduction. In: Briggs GG, Freeman RK, Yaffe SJ. *Drugs in Pregnancy and Lactation*. 4th ed. Baltimore: Williams & Wilkins; 1994.

124. Lee JJ, Rubin P. Breast feeding and anaesthesia. *Anaesthesia* 1993;48:616–625.

125. Bond G, Holloway AM. Anaesthesia and breast-feeding–the effect on mother and infant. *Anaesth Intensive Care* 1992;20:426–430.

126. Borgatta L, Jenny RW, Gruss L, Ong C, Barad D. Clinical significance of methohexital, meperidine and diazepam in breast milk. *J Clin Pharmacol* 1997;37:186–192.

127. Spigset O. Anesthetic agents and excretion in breast milk. *Acta Anaesthesiol Scand* 1994;38:94–103.

128. Feilberg VL, Rosenborg D, Christensen CB, Morgensen JV. Excretion of morphine in human breast milk. *Acta Anaesthesiol Scand* 1989;33:426–428.

129. Findlay JWA, De Angelis RL, Kearney MF, Welch RM, Findlay JM. Analgesic drugs in breast milk and plasma. *Clin Pharmacol Ther* 1981;29:625–633.

130. Bader AM, Fragneto R, Terui KK, Arthur D, Loferski B, Datta S. Maternal and neonatal fentanyl and bupivacaine concentrations after epidural infusion during labor. *Anesth Analg* 1995;81:829–832.

131. Fernando R, Bonello E, Gill P, Urquhart J, Reynolds F, Morgan B. Neonatal welfare and placental transfer of fentanyl and bupivacaine during ambulatory combined spinal epidural analgesia for labour. *Anaesthesia* 1997;52:517–524.

132. Leuschen MP, Wolf LJ, Rayburn WF. Fentanyl excretion in breast milk. *Clin Pharm* 1990;9:336–337.

133. Steer PL, Biddle CJ, Marley WS, Lantz RK, Salik PI. Concentration of fentanyl in colostrum after an analgesic dose. *Can J Anaesth* 1992;39:231–235.

134. Abouleish EE, Donck AV, Meeuis H, Taylor F. Effect of anaesthesia for delivery on the weight on infants during the first 5 days of life. *Br J Anaesth* 1978;50:569–574.

135. Kotelko DM, Faulk DL, Rottman RL, et al. A controlled comparison of maternal analgesia: Effects on neonatal nutritional sucking behavior [abstract]. *Anesthesiology* 1995;83:A298.

136. Hirose M, Hara Y, Hosokawa T. The effect of postoperative analgesia with continuous epidural bupivacaine after cesarean section on the amount of breast feeding and infant weight gain. *Anesth Analg* 1996;82:1166–1169.

137. Porter J, Bonello E, Reynolds F. Effect of epidural fentanyl on neonatal respiration. *Anesthesiology* 1998;89:79–85.

138. Naumburg EG, Meny RG. Breast milk opioids and neonatal apnea. *Am J Dis Child* 1988;142:11–12.

139. Mathews MK. The relationship between maternal labour analgesia and delay in the initiation of breast-feeding in healthy neonates in the early neonatal period. *Midwifery* 1989;5:3–10.

140. Andersen LW, Qvist T, Hertz J, Mogensen F. Concentrations of thiopentone in mature breast milk and colostrum following an induction dose. *Acta Anaesthesiol Scand* 1987;31:30–32.

141. Walker M. Do labor medications affect breastfeeding? *J Human Lactation* 1997;13:131–137.

142. Halpern S, Levine T, Wilson D, MacDonell J, Katsiris SE, Leighton BL. Effect of labor analgesia on breastfeeding success. *Birth.* 1999;26:83–88.

143. Dailland P, Cockshott ID, Lirzin JD, et al. Intravenous propofol during cesarean section: Placental transfer, concentrations in breast milk and neonatal effects. A preliminary study. *Anesthesiology* 1989;71:827–834.

144. Gin T, Gregory MA. Propofol during caesarean section. *Anesthesiology* 1990;73:789.

145. Gregory MA, Gin T, Yau G, Leung RK, Chan K, Oh TE. Propofol infusion anesthesia for caesarean section. *Can J Anaesth* 1990;37:514–520.

146. Gin T, Yau G, Chan K, Gregory MA, Oh TE. Disposition of propofol infusions for caesarean section. *Can J Anaesth* 1991;38:31–36.

147. Celleno D, Capogna G, Tomassetti M, Constantino P, DeFeo G, Nisini R. Neurobehavioral effects of propofol on the neonate following elective caesarean section induction. *Br J Anaesth* 1989;62:649–654.

148. Kanto J. Risk-benefit assessment of anaesthetic agents in the puerperium. *Drug Saf* 1991;6:285–301.

149. Summerfield RJ, Nielsen MS. Excretion of lorazepam into breast milk. *Br J Anaesth* 1985;57:1042–1043.

150. Cole AP, Hailey DH. Diazepam and active metabolite in breast milk and their transfer to the neonate. *Arch Dis Child* 1975;50:741–742.

151. Kanto JH. Use of benzodiazepines during pregnancy, labour and lactation, with particular reference to pharmacokinetic considerations. *Drugs* 1982;23:354–380.

152. Erkkola R, Kanto J. Diazepam and breastfeeding. *Lancet* 1972;1:1235–1236.

153. Rathmell JP, Viscomi CM, Ashburn MA. Management of nonobstetric pain during pregnancy. *Anesth Analg* 1997;85:1074–1087.

154. Atkinson HC, Begg EJ, Darlow BA. Clinical pharmacokinetic considerations. *Clin Pharmacokinet* 1988;14:217–240.

Shnider and Levinson's Anesthesia for Obstetrics,
edited by Samuel C. Hughes, et al.
Lippincott Williams & Wilkins,
Philadelphia, © 2001.

CHAPTER 13

ANESTHESIA FOR SURGERY DURING PREGNANCY

GERSHON LEVINSON, M.D.

The incidence of surgery during pregnancy reportedly ranges from 0.3% to 2.2% (1–5). In addition, the incidence of unrecognized pregnancy in menstruating women presenting for ambulatory, nonobstetric surgery has been reported to be 0.3% (6). Based on these reports it has been estimated that each year in the United States up to 75,000 pregnant women may receive an anesthetic for surgery during pregnancy. These women require special attention in their anesthetic management if maternal morbidity and fetal wastage are to be avoided (Fig. 13.1). The basic objectives in the anesthetic management of pregnant women undergoing surgery are: **(a) maternal safety; (b) avoidance of teratogenic drugs; (c) avoidance of intrauterine fetal asphyxia; and (d) prevention of preterm labor.**

MATERNAL SAFETY

The physiologic changes that occur during pregnancy are discussed in Chapter 1. Many of these changes are due to hormonal factors, as well as to the mechanical effects of the enlarging uterus, and occur during the first and second trimesters. The changes of greatest relevance to the anesthesiologist are summarized below.

Alveolar ventilation is increased about 25% by the fourth month of pregnancy and rises progressively to 70% at term (Fig. 13.2) (7). End-tidal Pco_2 falls to 33 mm Hg by the third month of pregnancy (Fig. 13.3) (7). Functional residual capacity is decreased 10% at 6 months and 20% at term (Fig. 13.4) (8). Oxygen consumption increases significantly during midpregnancy (Fig. 13.5) due to the developing placenta, fetus, and uterine muscle.

In animal studies the anesthetic requirement for halogenated agents is decreased up to 40% by the second trimester (9, 10). In humans the MAC of isoflurane is reduced by 28% in pregnant women at 8 to 12 weeks of gestation compared to nonpregnant women (11). Similarly, the MAC of halothane and enflurane are decreased 27% and 30% respectively at 8 to 13 weeks of gestation.(Fig. 13.6) (12). The dose of thiopental for hypnosis is 17% less and that for anesthesia 18% less in pregnant women at 7 to 13 weeks of gestation compared with that in nonpregnant women (Fig. 13.7) (13). Furthermore in rats, and most likely other species, there is a progressive increase in the pain threshold throughout pregnancy (Fig. 13.8) (14), likely due to a progressive increase in endogenous endorphins in the substantia gelatinosa, which can be blocked by naltrexone administration (Fig. 13.9). **Induction of and emergence from anesthesia is more rapid because of the increased ventilation, decreased functional residual capacity and decreased anesthetic requirement.** The possibility of anesthetic overdose is therefore increased. The increased oxygen consumption and decreased functional residual capacity make the pregnant patient more likely to become hypoxic with respiratory obstruction or difficult endotracheal intubation. Even during rapid endotracheal intubation (30 seconds of apnea) arterial Po_2 can fall 50 to 60 mm Hg in mothers who are not preoxygenated.

Cardiac output and stroke volume are increased 35% to 40% (see Figure 26.2) (15–17) and blood volume is increased 20%

to 30% by 20 to 24 weeks of gestation (18, 19). Cardiac output increases 1000 mL/min by 8 weeks of gestation (Fig. 13.10) primarily because of stroke volume rather than heart rate (Fig. 13.11) (20). Inferior vena caval occlusion, although most pronounced in women near term, is also significant during the second trimester (Fig. 13.12) despite the apparently small size of the uterus. Lateral tilt to prevent supine hypotension and uterine hypoperfusion should be used for all surgical procedures if possible.

The increase in femoral venous pressure shown in Figure 13.12 is likely also reflected in the epidural veins and may be relevant in partially explaining the reduced dosage of local anesthetic necessary to achieve a given level of spinal or epidural anesthesia during pregnancy. Because of epidural venous engorgement the size of the subarachnoid and epidural spaces may be decreased, and less local anesthetic is required to produce a given level of anesthesia. However, this explanation for reduced local anesthetic requirement in pregnancy does not explain a number of other findings. Fagraeus et al. (21) showed that in women having epidural anesthesia during early pregnancy (8 to 12 weeks of gestation), a given dose of local anesthetic produced a significantly higher anesthetic level than in nonpregnant women (Fig. 13.13). In fact, the dose requirement was similar to that found in pregnant women at term. This early in pregnancy, because of the small uterine size, venous engorgement is not prominent. Similarly, the space-occupying effects of distended epidural veins at term are not likely to occur in rats because of their natural semiprone position. Nevertheless, in pregnant rats both somatic and visceral antinociceptive effects of epidural lidocaine were potentiated compared with those in nonpregnant rats (22).

Datta (23) and Flanagan (24) et al. compared the effects of local anesthetics on nerve conduction in the isolated vagus nerve from pregnant and nonpregnant rabbits. The onset of block was significantly faster in nerves from pregnant animals. Other investigators (25) demonstrated that the median nerve of pregnant women in the third trimester is more susceptible to conduction block induced by lidocaine than that of nonpregnant women.

There are most likely multiple factors explaining the increased effect of local anesthetics during pregnancy. These studies indicate that during pregnancy either nerve fibers have increased sensitivity to local anesthetics or there is enhanced diffusion of the local anesthetic to the membrane receptor site. **Therefore, when administering regional anesthesia the amount of local anesthetic should be reduced by 25% to 30% during any stage of pregnancy lest an excessively high level of anesthesia occur.**

It is unclear precisely at which point in gestation a pregnant woman becomes more susceptible to regurgitation and aspiration under anesthesia. Plasma gastrin levels, believed to be of placental origin, were found to be elevated in one unconfirmed study throughout gestation but were especially high in the second half (26). Using a paracetamol absorption technique, Macfie et al. (27) measured the rate of gastric emptying in pregnancy. They studied four groups of patients: nonpregnant controls, first trimester patients presenting for termination of

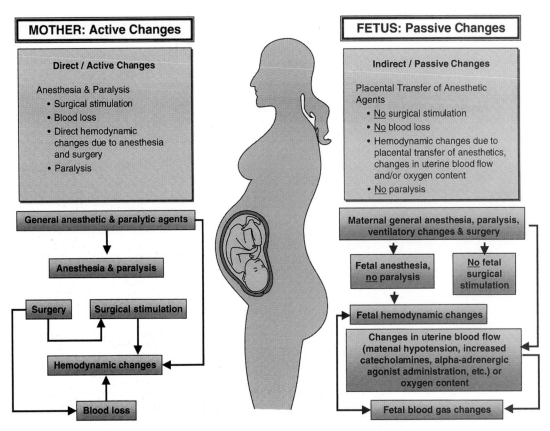

Figure 13.1. The effects of anesthetic and paralytic agents and surgery on the mother and fetus. (Reprinted by permission from Rosen MA. Management of anesthesia for the pregnant surgical patient. *Anesthesiology* 1999;91:1159–1163.)

pregnancy, second trimester patients presenting for prostaglandin termination of pregnancy, and patients presenting for elective Cesarean section. No significant delay in gastric emptying was demonstrated in any of the three trimesters of pregnancy compared with the control group. Wyner and Cohen (28) have shown that women under 20 weeks of gestation do not have increased gastric volumes or decreased pH compared to nonpregnant women. Nonetheless, in both groups more than a third of the women had a gastric volume greater than 25 mL with a pH less than 2.5. Other studies have indicated that during pregnancy lower esophageal sphincter tone is decreased, predisposing the pregnant woman to passive regurgitation. This reduced

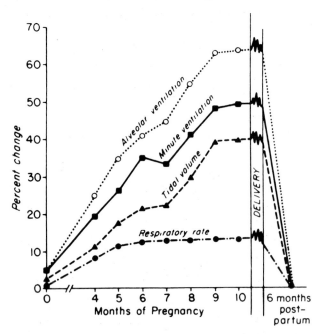

Figure 13.2. Changes in respiratory parameters during pregnancy. (Reprinted by permission from Bonica JJ, ed. *Principles and Practice of Obstetric Analgesia and Anesthesia*. Vol 1. Philadelphia: Davis; 1967:22.)

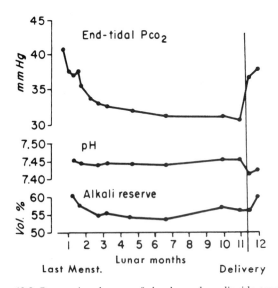

Figure 13.3. Progressive changes of alveolar carbon dioxide tensions, pH, and alkali reserve throughout pregnancy. (Reprinted by permission from Bonica JJ, ed. *Principles and Practice of Obstetric Analgesia and Anesthesia*. Vol 1. Philadelphia: Davis; 1967:28.)

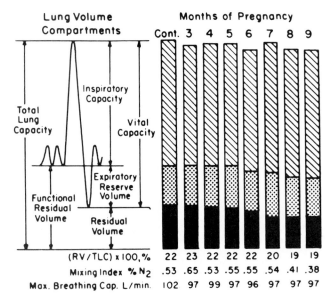

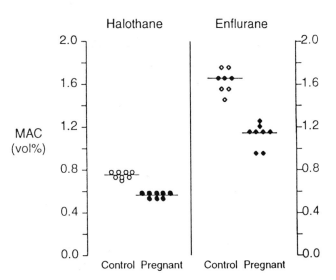

Figure 13.4. Serial measurements of lung compartments, pulmonary mixing index, and maximum breathing capacity during normal pregnancy. *RV* = residual volume; *TLC* = total lung capacity. (Reprinted by permission from Bonica JJ, ed. *Principles and Practice of Obstetric Analgesia and Anesthesia.* Vol 1. Philadelphia: Davis; 1967:25.)

Figure 13.6. Individual minimum alveolar concentrations (*MAC*) for halothane in pregnant women (*solid circles*) and nonpregnant women (*open circles*), and enflurane in pregnant women (*solid diamonds*) and nonpregnant women (*open diamonds*). (Reprinted by permission from Chan MTV, Mainland P, Gin T. Minimum alveolar concentration of halothane and enflurane are decreased in early pregnancy. *Anesthesiology* 1996;85:782–768.)

sphincter tone is especially apparent in women with symptoms of heartburn, and has been documented to be present as early as 15 weeks of gestation (28). Some suggest that all pregnant patients undergoing anesthesia should be premedicated with an oral antacid. Certainly, the author believes, any pregnant woman undergoing surgery during the third trimester or any time during pregnancy if she has symptoms of esophagitis should be intubated rapidly after induction of general anesthesia and pre-

treated with oral antacid. However, airway management during the second trimester remains controversial.

TERATOGENICITY OF ANESTHETICS

Teratogenicity, either morphologic, biochemical, or behavioral, may be induced at any stage of gestation by exogenous agents and detected at birth or later. To produce a defect, a teratogenic

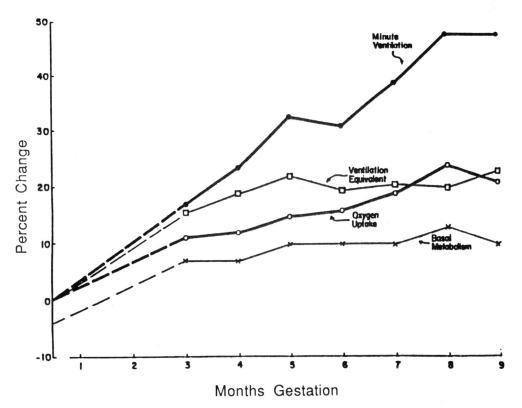

Figure 13.5. Percentage of changes in minute ventilation, oxygen uptake, basal metabolism, and the ventilation equivalent for oxygen at monthly intervals throughout pregnancy. (Reprinted by permission from Prowse CM, Gaensler EA. Respiratory and acid-base changes during pregnancy. *Anesthesiology* 1965;26:381–392.)

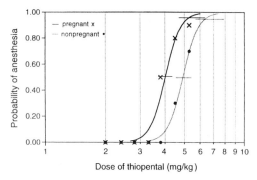

Figure 13.7. Calculated dose-response curves (log dose scale) for anesthesia in pregnant and nonpregnant women. The 95% confidence intervals for the median effective doses (ED$_{50}$s and ED$_{95}$s) also are displayed, slightly offset for clarity. Raw data are shown by X (*pregnant group*) and *filled circles* (*nonpregnant group*). (Reprinted by permission from Gin T, Mainland P, Chan MTV, et al. Decreased thiopental requirements in early pregnancy. *Anesthesiology* 1997;86:73–78.)

drug must be given in an appropriate dosage, during a particular developmental stage of the embryo, in a species or individual with a particular genetic susceptibility (Fig. 13.14).

The critical stages of organ development in humans are illustrated in Figure 13.15. Each organ and each system undergoes a critical stage of differentiation during which vulnerability to teratogens is greatest and specific malformations can be produced. For example, the period of sensitivity of the heart is 18 to 40 days and the limbs 24 to 34 days. Variations in genetic susceptibility may make interpretation of teratogenic studies difficult. Drugs may have a marked effect in one species and little teratogenic effect in another. Even in the same species different strains may respond differently. Thalidomide, which produces gross malformations in humans and rabbits, is safe in rats (29). Of the women who took thalidomide during the susceptible period, over 75% delivered normal babies (29).

Almost all commonly used anesthetics and premedicant drugs are teratogenic in some animal species. However, the applicability of these animal studies to humans has not been determined.

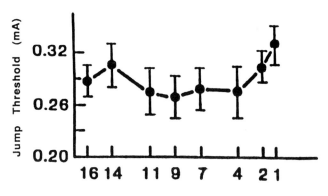

Days prior to parturition

Figure 13.9. Mean jump thresholds of pregnant rats implanted with two naltrexone pellets, presented as a function of days before parturition. Testing began 1 day after implantation. Each *point* represents the mean threshold of 7 rats ± SE. (Reprinted by permission from Gintzler A. Endorphin-mediated increases in pain threshold during pregnancy. *Science* 1980;210:193–195.)

Systemic Medications

Animal Studies

Numerous anomalies have been reported after pentobarbital or phenobarbital administration to mice, but not rats or rabbits (30–32). For example, a single dose of thiamylal caused teratogenic and growth-suppressing defects in the offspring of mice (31). Chlorpromazine, prochlorperazine, imipramine, and amphetamines given to pregnant rats and rabbits have been shown to be teratogenic and produce permanent changes in brain levels of norepinephrine, dopamine, 5-hydroxytryptamine, and their metabolites in the offspring (33–35).

Methadone is teratogenic in mice (36) but not in rats or rabbits (37). In hamsters the number of abnormal fetuses from females injected with a single dose of diacetylmorphine (heroin), phenazocine, pentazocine, propoxyphene, and methadone

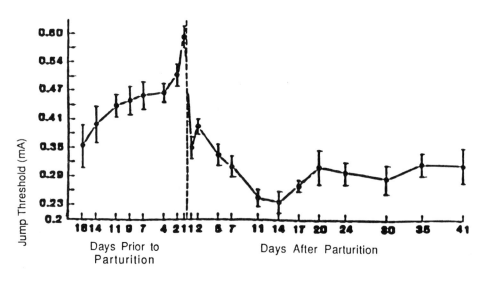

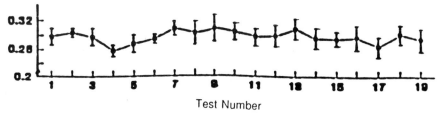

Figure 13.8. Mean jump threshold in pregnant rats as a function of days before and after parturition (*dashed line*). Each *point* represents the mean threshold of 8 rats ± SE. (Reprinted by permission from Gintzler A. Endorphin-mediated increases in pain threshold during pregnancy. *Science* 1980;210:193–195.)

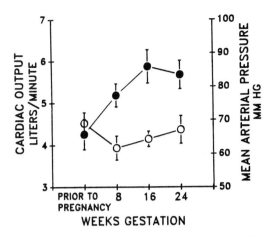

Figure 13.10. Cardiac output (*filled circles*) and mean arterial pressure (*open circles*) components of systemic vascular resistance are presented for 4 study periods. (Reprinted by permission from Capeless EL, Clapp JF. Cardiovascular changes in early phase of pregnancy. *Am J Obstet Gynecol* 1989;161:1449–1453.)

increased as the maternal dose increased (38). Morphine and meperidine produced an increase in the number of fetal anomalies only to a certain dose level. With multiple doses of diacetyl-morphine and methadone the incidence of anomalies increased further. Curiously, in this study, the opioid antagonists, nalorphine, naloxone, and levallorphan blocked the teratogenic effects. The authors postulated that hypoxia and hypercarbia induced by the unantagonized opioids may have actually been the teratogens rather than the opioids per se.

This is supported by studies of the new opioids: fentanyl, sufentanil, and alfentanil in rats in which respiratory depression did not develop (39, 40). Fentanyl in doses up to 500 μg/kg/day (from preconception to throughout pregnancy), sufentanil 100 μg/kg/day, or alfentanil 8000 μg/kg/day (each from day 5 through day 20 of pregnancy) were not teratogenic.

Human Studies

Three retrospective studies have suggested an association between ingestion of minor tranquilizers during pregnancy and an increased risk of congenital anomalies.

One study examined the prenatal records of over 19,000 live births to determine the incidence of severe anomalies in chil-

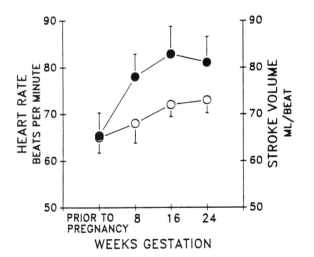

Figure 13.11. Stroke volume (*filled circles*) and heart rate (*open circles*) components of cardiac output are presented for four study periods. (Reprinted by permission from Capeless EL, Clapp JF. Cardiovascular changes in early phase of pregnancy. *Am J Obstet Gynecol* 1989;161:1449–1453.)

dren whose mothers had taken either meprobamate (Equinal, Miltown), chlordiazepoxide (Librium), "other drugs," or no drugs (41). The incidence of anomalies when meprobamate or chlordiazepoxide was prescribed during the first 6 weeks of gestation was significantly higher (12.1% and 11.4%, respectively) than when one of the other drugs (4.6%) or no drug (2.6%) was given. When the tranquilizers were administered later in pregnancy no differences were seen in the incidence of anomalies among the four groups. The study was not controlled for the presence of other risk factors for delivery of a child with congenital anomalies, and the findings for chlordiazepoxide were based on only four very different anomalies (duodenal atresia with Meckel's diverticulum, spastic diplegia with deafness, microcephaly, and mental deficiency) and did not reach the 5% level of statistical significance. However, the findings for meprobamate did reach a higher level of significance and, in addition, showed a preponderance of anomalies involving the heart (five of eight cases).

A second study from the Finnish Register of Congenital Malformations (1967–1971) reported an association of cleft palate with maternal ingestion of three groups of drugs: tranquilizers (diazepam and meprobamate), salicylates, and opioids (42). The study compared the use of these drugs during the first trimester in mothers of 590 children with oral clefts and found that intake of these drugs was significantly greater in these mothers than in controls: antianxiety agents, 6.2% in study mothers vs. 2.9% in control mothers; opioids, 6.7% vs. 2.2%; and salicylates, 14.9% vs. 5.6%.

A third study was based on interviews of 278 mothers of children with selected birth defects who had been exposed to a variety of drugs during the first trimester of pregnancy (43). Mothers of infants with cleft lips with or without cleft palate reported use of diazepam four times more frequently than mothers of infants with other defects.

In contrast to these three studies a fourth investigation failed to find an increased risk of congenital malformation associated with the use of minor tranquilizers during early pregnancy (44). A total of 50,282 pregnancies were reviewed and the incidence of malformations in 1870 children exposed in utero to meprobamate or chlordiazepoxide was compared to the incidence in 48,412 unexposed children. No differences in the groups were found.

Nonetheless, the Food and Drug Administration (FDA Drug Bulletin September-November 1975) has stated that, "while these data do not provide conclusive evidence that minor tranquilizers cause fetal abnormalities they do suggest an association. Since the use of these drugs during the first trimester of pregnancy is rarely a matter of urgency, benefit-risk considerations are such that their use during this period should almost always be avoided." This long-standing, relative contraindication and general concern about benzodiazepine use particularly in the first trimester has been recently dispelled (44a). The editors use preoperative medication for women to treat pain or anxiety when needed to include benzodiazepine and opioids (44b).

Anesthetics

Animal Studies

When **nitrous oxide** 80% was administered to chicken eggs for 6 hours on days 3, 4, or 5 of incubation, there was no increased rate of congenital anomalies (45). The combination of nitrous oxide and mild hypoxia (10% oxygen) for 6 hours produced more anomalies than mild hypoxia alone (45). When nitrous oxide 50% was administered to pregnant rats for 1 or 2 days a high incidence of intrauterine fetal death and a significant increase in skeletal malformations were found (46). When rats were exposed to 70 to 75% nitrous oxide, nitrogen, xenon (an anesthetic slightly more potent than nitrous oxide), or 0.6% halothane for 24 hours on day 9 of pregnancy, only nitrous oxide

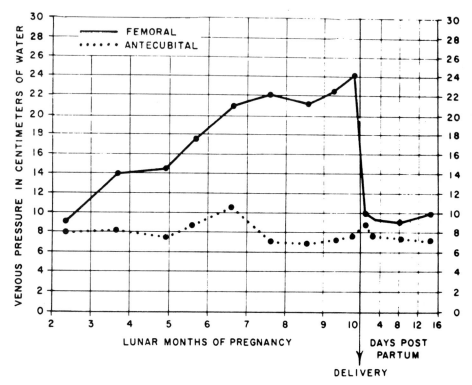

Figure 13.12. Venous pressure during pregnancy in the femoral and antecubital veins. (Reprinted by permission from Bonica JJ, ed. *Principles and Practice of Obstetric Analgesia and Anesthesia.* Vol 1. Philadelphia: Davis; 1967:17.)

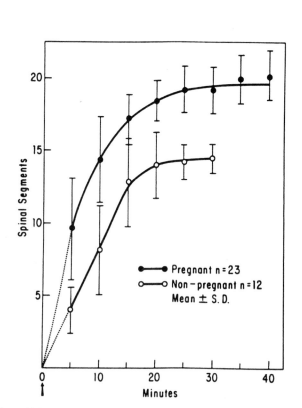

Figure 13.13. Rate of spread of epidural analgesia in nonpregnant and pregnant women in their first trimester. A line of best fit has been drawn. Injection time is denoted by the *arrow* at time zero. (Reprinted by permission from Fagraeus L, Urban BJ, Bromage PR. Spread of epidural analgesia in early pregnancy. *Anesthesiology* 1983;53:184–187.)

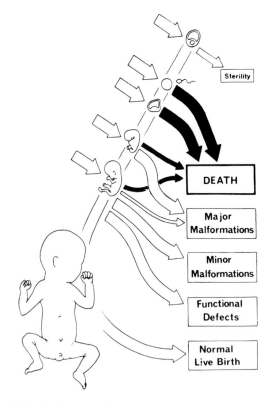

Figure 13.14. The influence of teratogenic factors on gametogenesis and various stages of embryonic and fetal development. During the preimplantation period, strong teratogenic agents kill the embryo. During embryogenesis, from day 13 to day 60, teratogenic agents are embryotoxic or produce major congenital malformations. During the following fetal period, minor morphologic and functional malformations can be produced. (Reprinted by permission from Tuchmann-Duplessis H. The effects of teratogenic drugs. In: Phillipp E, Barnes J, Newton M, eds. *Scientific Foundations of Obstetrics and Gynaecology.* Philadelphia: Davis; 1970.)

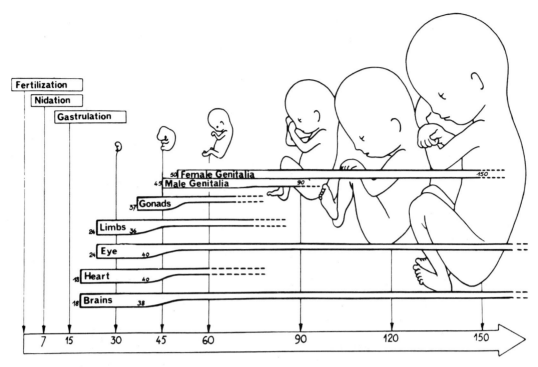

Figure 13.15. The timing of the morphogenesis of various organs, corresponding to the critical periods of teratogenic susceptibility. (Reprinted by permission from Tuchmann-Duplessis H. The effects of teratogenic drugs. In: Phillipp E, Barnes J, Newton M, eds. *Scientific Foundations of Obstetrics and Gynaecology.* Philadelphia: Davis; 1970.)

caused major anomalies (47, 48). On the other hand, continuous administration of 50 to 75% nitrous oxide for 24 hours on day 8 to 9 of gestation is teratogenic in rats (49). Mazze et al. (50) administered 50% nitrous oxide to mice for 4 hours each day on days 6 through 15 of pregnancy and did not show an increased incidence of anomalies. Similarly, Pope et al. (51) showed that, in rats, 50% nitrous oxide for 8 h/d throughout gestation was not teratogenic. These and other studies (52–55) indicate that, in chickens and rodents, exposure to nitrous oxide for up to 12 hours during each day of gestation is not teratogenic, but extreme conditions will produce teratogenic effects.

One of the major concerns regarding the use of nitrous oxide for surgery during pregnancy relates to the adverse effects of nitrous oxide on DNA synthesis. In fact, some believe that nitrous oxide is contraindicated during the first two trimesters of pregnancy (49). Nitrous oxide inactivates vitamin B_{12}, the essential cofactor for the enzyme methionine synthetase. The temporary inactivation of methionine synthetase interferes with folate metabolism, the conversion of uridine to thymidine, and thereby impairs DNA synthesis (Fig. 13.16). While the temporary inactivation of methionine synthetase does not appear to be clinically significant in the nonpregnant surgical patient, there is concern that the use of nitrous oxide may be potentially deleterious to the developing fetus. Indeed, Baden et al. (56, 57) showed that in rats maternal exposure to nitrous oxide produced a marked decrease in fetal methionine synthetase activity. The decreased methionine synthetase activity persisted for up to 72 hours.

It has been suggested that nitrous oxide toxicity can be prevented by pretreatment with folinic acid (formyltetrahydrofolate) (58–61). This suggestion has not been fully supported by animal studies. Indeed, the hypothesis that methionine synthetase inhibition is the mechanism of nitrous oxide teratogenicity has been questioned. One study showed that in rats, folinic acid administration reduced the incidence of skeletal abnormalities (but did not eliminate them) produced by exposure to 70% to 75% nitrous oxide on day 9 of pregnancy (61). Other studies have failed to substantiate this (62–64). In these studies the volatile anesthetics, isoflurane and halothane, administered

with N_2O prevented adverse reproductive effects in rats without preventing inhibition of methionine synthetase activity. Furthermore, treatment with folinic acid, which should have reversed the effects of N_2O on DNA production, did not prevent adverse reproductive effects (63, 64). In another study (65) using a whole-embryo rat culture system, it was demonstrated that supplemental methionine, but not folinic acid, almost completely prevented nitrous oxide-induced teratogenicity. These results suggest that decreased methionine rather than tetrahydrofolate plays the major role in nitrous oxide-induced teratogenicity other than situs inversus.

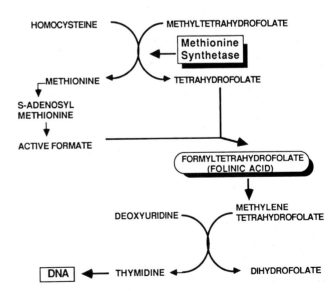

Figure 13.16. Nitrous oxide directly blocks the transmethylation reaction by which methionine is synthesized from homocystine and methyltetrahydrofolate. Nitrous oxide oxidizes vitamin B_{12}, the cofactor of the enzyme methionine synthetase. This action of nitrous oxide thus interferes with the production of DNA.

The sympathomimetic effects of nitrous oxide have also received attention as a possible cause of some malformations, especially situs inversus, the incidence of which is known to be markedly increased by α-adrenergic agonists. It has been postulated that the adverse reproductive effects of nitrous oxide are due to decreased uterine blood flow but phenoxybenzamine, an α-adrenergic antagonist did not prevent nitrous oxide teratogenicity (66). Fujinaga and Baden (65) demonstrated that nitrous oxide had an additive effect on phenylephrine-induced situs inversus that was blocked by prazosin (α-adrenergic antagonist). Results from the current and previous studies suggest that nitrous oxide stimulates α-adrenergic receptors in the embryo, but that the effects are weak and will only result in situs inversus in susceptible animals. Clearly, the etiology of nitrous oxide teratogenicity remains to be elucidated. **It should be emphasized that it is only teratogenic in animals under relatively extreme conditions not likely to be encountered clinically.**

Halothane in low concentrations for 12 to 48 hours produced numerous anomalies in rat fetuses (67). In mice, 3 hours of halothane 1.5% markedly increased the incidence of cleft palates and paw defects (68). In hamsters, 3 hours of halothane 0.6% in midgestation increased the number of abortions (55). The exposure of cell cultures to halothane produces marked inhibition in DNA synthesis, abnormal cell divisions, and bizarre multinucleated cells (69). Other investigators using rats, rabbits, and mice have not shown teratogenic effects of halothane (70–72).

Enflurane produces more cleft palates and other skeletal and visceral anomalies in fetuses of mice exposed to enflurane (1% volume) on days 6 and 15 of gestation (73).

Isoflurane (0.6%), in a similar study in mice, produced an incidence of cleft palate which was six times greater than that obtained with enflurane (12.2% vs. 1.9%) (74). Because mice have a tendency to develop cleft palates following a large variety of treatments and manipulations, it is likely that the findings in the two previous studies were species specific and of questionable significance for humans. The same investigators, therefore, studied pregnant rats given 0.75 MAC of halothane, enflurane, isoflurane, and 0.55 MAC nitrous oxide for 6-hour periods at three different stages of gestation (72). There were no major or minor teratologic effects produced by any of the anesthetics. Nitrous oxide exposure did result in an increase in fetal resorptions.

Methoxyflurane, diethyl ether, cyclopropane, and **fluroxene,** anesthetic agents no longer commonly used, have all been shown to be teratogenic in chick embryos (75, 76).

Muscle relaxants do not cross the placenta in significant amounts. Curare has been shown to cause musculoskeletal deformities when injected into the incubating chick embryo (77). Because of their respiratory effects, muscle relaxants are difficult to test in vivo. Using an in vitro rat whole embryo culture system d-tubocurarine, pancuronium, atracurium, and vecuronium were studied (78). Teratogenicity was only found at doses greater than 100 times the paralyzing dose in humans.

Local anesthetics act by stabilizing cell membranes and conceivably might affect cell mitosis and embryogenesis. In vivo studies have not shown teratogenic effects in rats (79, 80) and mice (81). In vitro studies in mice (82) and in chicks (83, 84) have shown lidocaine to cause neural tube closure defects. To reconcile these conflicting findings, Fujinaga studied the effects of lidocaine on rat embryos cultured in vitro (85). In the presence of 250 μM lidocaine, embryos showed an increased incidence of situs inversus compared with the control group but were otherwise normal. At 375 μM, embryos showed slight growth retardation but no significant morphologic abnormalities. At 500 μM, all viable embryos showed severe morphologic abnormalities. (In humans peak plasma lidocaine levels reach approximately 1 to 5 μg/mL with epidural anesthesia and approximately 1 μg/mL with spinal anesthesia. An in vitro concentration of approximately 1 μM is equivalent to about 0.24 μg/mL

plasma concentration.) In this study lidocaine caused teratogenic effects only at concentrations that vastly exceed those that are clinically relevant. Lidocaine did not cause neural tube closure defects at any concentrations evaluated.

Cocaine, however, has been shown to be teratogenic in mice (86) and rats (87). The teratogenicity of cocaine in humans is discussed fully in Chapter 34.

Human Studies

Human studies have consisted of large retrospective, epidemiologic surveys of adverse reproductive outcomes either in groups chronically exposed to low levels of anesthetic gases or in women who have undergone surgery during their pregnancy. Both these approaches have significant limitations. Studies on the adverse effects of exposure to waste anesthetic gases are frequently deficient due to lack of comparable control groups, lack of confirmation and verification of reported adverse outcomes, low response rates to questionnaires, lack of details on duration and amounts of actual exposure to waste gases, and lack of information on other factors associated with people exposed to waste anesthetic gases, such as exposure to hepatitis B virus, radiation, and methylmethacrylate, all of which are potentially teratogenic. Shortcomings of surveys of women that have undergone surgery during pregnancy include many of the above limitations as well as relatively small sample sizes, a multiplicity of drugs administered, and the unknown implications of the surgical condition that necessitated the original need for anesthesia.

Table 13.1 summarizes the major studies of the effects of waste anesthetic gases on reproductive outcome. The most consistent finding is the increased risk of spontaneous abortion in female personnel exposed to waste anesthetic gases. The incidence of miscarriage among the exposed women is approximately 25% to 30% greater than in nonexposed women (88–93).

Buring et al. (94) noted that this increase is relatively small and well within the range that might be due to uncontrolled confounding variables. As noted by Mazze and Lecky (95) epidemiologists usually consider increases in incidence of less than 200% to 300% as possibly due to other factors. Furthermore, a 30% increase is almost insignificant when one considers that the incidence of spontaneous abortions is increased at least 250% in women who consume more than three alcoholic drinks daily (96), and that cigarette smokers have an 80% increased risk of spontaneous abortions compared to nonsmokers (97).

The likelihood of exposure to waste anesthetic gases in operating rooms or dental offices producing major congenital anomalies is less certain. The studies with the most significant findings were the American Society of Anesthesiologists (ASA) Ad Hoc Committee on Occupational Diseases Among Operating Room Personnel (92) and the American Dental Association Survey (89). Both these studies showed borderline statistically significant increases in the incidence of congenital anomalies among some exposed personnel. These findings have been challenged, however (98). For example, the failure to find a dose-related effect of nitrous oxide in exposed dental assistants makes the alleged association between anesthetic gases and anomalies suspect. Furthermore, the incidence of anomalies in offspring of exposed assistants was no greater than that in the wives of unexposed (male) dentists. One might conclude, therefore, that other factors account for the results.

Several surveys of women who had received anesthesia for operations during pregnancy have failed to indict any anesthetic as a teratogen (1, 2, 4, 5, 99–102). Smith (2) retrospectively reviewed the neonatal outcomes of 67 women who had undergone surgery during pregnancy. Eleven of these women received an anesthetic during the first trimester. No congenital anomalies were found.

Shnider and Webster (1) reviewed the records of 147 women who received anesthesia for surgery during pregnancy: 47 during the first trimester, 58 during the second, and 42 during

Table 13.1. RESULTS OF MAJOR STUDIES ON EFFECTS OF WASTE ANESTHETIC GASES ON REPRODUCTIVE OUTCOME

Study	Subjects	No. of Pregnancies	Miscarriage Rate (%)	No. of Live Births	Congenital Abnormality (%)
Cohen et al. (89)	Operating room nurses	36	27.7	26	NG*
	General duty nurses	34	5.2	31	NG
	Female anesthesiologists	37	37.8	23	NG
	Other female MDs	58	10.3	52	NG
Cohen et al. (80)	Dental chairside assistants				
	No N_2O exposure	3197	8.1	2882	3.6
	N_2O exposure	701	16.0[†]	579	5.5[†]
	N_2O + halogenate exposure	93	24.6[†]	68	7.7
	No N_2O exposure	3184	8.1	2882	3.6
	N_2O—light exposure	407	14.2[†]	341	5.7[†]
	N_2O—heavy exposure	400	19.1[†]	316	5.2
	Wives of dentists				
	No N_2O exposure	5709	6.7	5277	4.9
	N_2O—light exposure	2104	7.7[†]	1890	4.6
	N_2O—heavy exposure	1328	10.2[†]	1177	4.8
Knill-Jones et al. (90)	Female anesthetists	737	18.2	599	6.5
	Other female MDs	2150	14.7[†]	1817	4.9
Rosenberg and Kirves (91)	Operating room nurses	257	19.5	NG	NG
	Other nurses	150	11.4[†]	NG	NG
ASA Ad Hoc Committee (92)	Anesthesiologists	468	17.1	384	5.9
	Other MDs	308	8.9[†]	276	3.0
	Nurse anesthetists	1826	17.0	1480	9.6
	Other nurses	1948	15.1	1629	7.6[†]
Axelsson and Rylander (93)	Operating room and anesthesia nurses	139	15.1	114	4.4
	Other nurses	573	11.0	434	2.1

* Not given.

[†] $P < .05$.

ASA = American Society of Anethesiologists; MD = medical doctor; NG = not given.

the third. These women were compared to 8926 women who delivered during this time period. The incidence of congenital anomalies was not significantly different in these groups. These investigators also reviewed the statistics from 61,000 patients who participated in the National Collaborative study. The incidence of birth defects in women who had not undergone surgery during pregnancy (60,000 women) was 5.02% compared to 6% in the 50 women undergoing appendectomy, a statistically insignificant difference.

Brodsky et al. (4) reported the incidence of anomalies in women having general anesthesia for surgery during pregnancy. Their survey was of 187 women having surgery and anesthesia during the first trimester and 100 women having surgery during the second trimester. These women were compared to a control group of 8654 women who had neither surgery during pregnancy nor occupational exposure to waste anesthetic gases. Brodsky et al. found no association between surgery during early pregnancy and congenital anomalies in live-born offspring. They did find an increase in the incidence of spontaneous abortions. In the first trimester the incidence of miscarriage was 8.0% in anesthetized women and 5.1% in control women. In the second trimester, the incidences were 6.5% for women having had anesthesia and surgery and 1.4% for women in the control group.

Duncan et al. (102) reviewed the incidence of congenital anomalies and spontaneous abortions in 2565 women who had undergone surgery during pregnancy. These women were matched to a similar number of control pregnancies by maternal age and area of residence.

There was no significant difference in the rate of congenital anomalies between study and control groups. There was a significant increase (two times) in spontaneous abortions in women

undergoing surgery in the first or second trimesters with general anesthesia and having gynecologic procedures. The risk was still increased (one and a half times) for procedures anatomically remote from the uterus. While it was concluded that general anesthesia was associated with a higher incidence of abortion, there were very few major procedures performed under regional anesthesia. It was not possible to determine from their data whether it was the magnitude or nature of the surgical procedure, rather than the anesthetic, which was responsible for the increased risk of abortion.

In the largest survey to date, Mazze and Källén (5) linked data from three Swedish health care registries, the Medical Birth Registry, the Registry of Congenital Malformations, and the Hospital Discharge Registry, for the years 1973–1981. Adverse outcomes examined were the incidences of (a) congenital anomalies, (b) stillborn infants, (c) infants dead at 168 hours, and (d) infants with very low and low birth weights. There were 5405 operations in the population of 720,000 pregnant women (operation rate, 0.75%). Of these, 2252 were performed in the first trimester, and 65% received general anesthetics, almost all of which included nitrous oxide. The results are summarized in Figure 13.17.

The incidence of congenital malformations and stillbirths were not increased in the offspring of women having an operation. However, the incidences of very low and low-birth-weight infants were increased; these were the result of both prematurity and intrauterine growth restriction. The incidence of infants born alive but dying within 168 hours was increased. No specific types of anesthesia or operation were associated with increased incidences of adverse reproductive outcomes. The cause of these outcomes was not determined. These adverse outcomes did not occur as a consequence of immediate delivery after operation because in most cases delivery was delayed by weeks to months.

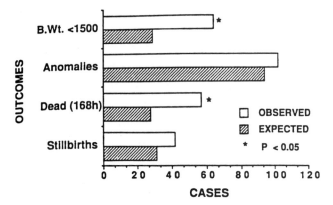

Figure 13.17. Total number of observed and expected adverse outcomes among women having nonobstetric operations during pregnancy. Incidence of infants with birth weights < 1500 g and of infants born alive and dying within 168 hours of birth were significantly increased (P < .05). (Reprinted by permission from Mazze RI, Källén B. Reproductive outcome after anesthesia and operation during pregnancy: A registry study of 5405 cases. *Am J Obstet Gynecol* 1989;161:1178–1185.)

However, the incidence of premature birth was increased by 46% (7.4% vs. 5.13%); intrauterine growth restriction was also a factor in reduced birth weight. Thus, it is clear that there is significant risk to the fetus when an operation is performed during pregnancy, but it is unclear whether the hazard is due to the surgery, the pathology for which the surgery was necessary, or the anesthetic. In a subsequent report (103), these investigators reviewed the outcome of the subset of 778 women whose surgical procedure was appendectomy. Significant findings included: a decrease in mean birth weight of 78 ± 24 g, an increased risk of delivery during the first week after appendectomy if the operation was performed after 23 weeks of gestation, no further increased risk of delivery after one week, no increase in the number of stillborn infants, and no increase in the number of congenitally malformed infants. Further indication of the safety of nitrous oxide, as used clinically, comes from studies of in vitro fertilization procedures, in which ova were retrieved under general (nitrous oxide) or local anesthesia and showed no differences in pregnancy rates (104–106). Two other reviews of exposure to nitrous oxide during cervical cerclage also showed no effects of the agent on fetal outcome (107, 108).

Two studies have shown an association between first trimester anesthesia exposure and central nervous system defects (109, 110). In the first study there was a small increase in the number of infants with neural tube defects born from mothers who had undergone surgery during the first trimester. It was unclear whether this increase was due to anesthetic technique, surgery, the maternal pathology or chance association. The second study failed to corroborate the increased incidence of neural tube defects but did find a very strong association between reported anesthesia exposure and the combination of hydrocephalus and eye defects (especially cataracts). Again the available data made chance association the most likely explanation for these findings. It is difficult to evaluate the biologic plausibility of both these studies as the types of outcomes reported in these studies have not been observed elsewhere, and the two studies do not support each other. This author does not believe these studies are clinically relevant.

Thus, studies to date indicate that surgery and anesthesia during pregnancy are in all likelihood not associated with an increased incidence of congenital anomalies but may produce a slightly increased risk of miscarriage. However, in all studies to date the number of women receiving an anesthetic during their pregnancy is in fact too small to state categorically that anesthetics are not teratogenic. Sullivan (111) has calculated the number of patients that must be exposed to a suspected teratogen to prove the drug's teratogenicity. For example, if an anesthetic doubled the incidence of an anomaly such as anencephaly, which has a spontaneous incidence of 1 per 1000, then 23,000 women would have to have been exposed to the anesthetic to have a statistically significant result. Of course, if an anesthetic had the teratogenicity of thalidomide, which increases the normal incidence of anomalies by 50,000 to 500,000 times, then a smaller number of anesthetic exposures would demonstrate teratogenicity. Clearly no anesthetic is such a potent teratogen.

Oxygen and Carbon Dioxide

Alterations in arterial blood gases frequently occur under anesthesia. In the experimental animal, hyperoxia, hypoxia, and hypercapnia may be teratogenic.

In mice (112), rabbits (113), rats (114), and chicks (115) congenital anomalies have been reported after exposure to hypoxia during organogenesis. The possible teratogenicity of hyperoxia is controversial. In hamsters, 100% oxygen at 2 atmospheres pressure for 3 hours, or 3 atmospheres pressure for 2 hours, resulted in a significant number of congenital anomalies (116). These defects included spina bifida, exencephaly, and limb defects. Hyperbaric oxygen administered to rabbits during late pregnancy resulted in retrolental fibroplasia, retinal detachment, microphthalmia, and stillbirth (117). Although it is clear from these studies that hyperbaric oxygen is teratogenic, high concentrations of oxygen at normal atmospheric pressure have not been found to be teratogenic in the experimental animal (118).

Prolonged periods of hypercarbia are associated with congenital anomalies in rats and rabbits. Carbon dioxide 6% and oxygen 20% administered to rats for 24 hours resulted in a high incidence of cardiac anomalies (119). In rabbits prolonged continuous inhalation of 10 to 13% carbon dioxide resulted in a high incidence of vertebral column malformations (118).

In humans, brief exposures of hypoxia, hyperoxia, hypercarbia, and hypocarbia have not been proven to be teratogenic, although isolated case reports alleging such an association have been published (120–122). Chronic hypoxemia, as occurs in people living at high altitude, is also not associated with an increased risk of anomalies.

Maternal Emotional Stress and Trauma

A number of factors that may be encountered in the pregnant patient having surgery have been suggested as being potentially teratogenic. Maternal anxiety and stress (123–129), maternal immobilization (130), and mechanical trauma such as falls, blows to the abdomen, automobile accidents, and bullet wounds (131–135) have all been implicated in case reports. The significance of these factors as teratogens is uncertain, because large epidemiologic studies have not been done.

Behavioral Teratology

The term "behavioral teratology" was first used by Werboff and Gottlieb (136) to describe the adverse action of a drug on "the behavior or functional adaptation of the offspring to its environment." Reserpine, chlorpromazine, and meprobamate administered to rats produced alterations of behavior in the offspring that persisted during adulthood (137–140). Other drugs, such as bromides (141), barbiturates (142), and salicylates (143) all impaired maze-learning ability in rat offspring.

Halogenated agents have also been shown to produce behavioral effects in rodents. Smith et al. (144) reported the behavioral effects of halothane in rat offspring. Pregnant female rats were anesthetized with halothane 2.5% for 5 minutes followed by 1.2% for 115 minutes during either the first, second, or third trimester. Their offspring were then tested at approximately 75 days postdelivery, which developmentally corresponds to young adulthood in humans. Learning deficits and changes in foot-shock sensitivity were found in the litters of mothers exposed during the first and second trimesters but not during the third.

Chalon et al. (145) have shown that mice twice exposed to halothane (1% or 2% for 30 minutes) or enflurane (2% or 4% for 30 minutes) in utero have significant learning defects. Second-generation offspring, born to dams exposed to 2% halothane in utero late in pregnancy and sired by normal unexposed males, also learned consistently slower than control mice (146).

The effect of lidocaine on postnatal development was studied in rats (147). Injections of lidocaine, 6 mg/kg of body weight, were given intramuscularly daily, on days 10 and 11 of gestation. No clinical dysfunction or behavioral changes could be related to maternal lidocaine administration. No cognitive dysfunction was evident in the offspring of lidocaine-treated animals.

It seems that in some rodents, subteratogenic doses of some psychoactive compounds produce behavioral deficits while not producing gross morphologic changes. This effect has not been demonstrated in humans. At present there is no evidence that anesthesia administered to a pregnant woman adversely affects later mental or neurologic development of her infant (148).

Transplacental Carcinogenesis

Concern regarding the potential for anesthetic agents administered to a pregnant woman to induce cancer in her baby is based on a number of observations. Oral administration of large doses of chloroform (149, 150) or trichloroethylene (151) produced cancer of the liver or kidney in mice. Halothane has been shown to interfere with the synthesis of DNA (152, 153) and may also produce abnormal products of cell division.

Using an in vitro microbial assay system employing two histidine-dependent mutants of *Salmonella typhimurium*, (154) Baden et al. (155, 156) showed that fluroxene was mutagenic but that halothane, enflurane, methoxyflurane, and isoflurane were not. In the experimental animal more than 30 different chemical compounds have been shown to be capable of inducing cancer in offspring when administered to the mother during gestation (157). It seems that the fetus is often more susceptible than the mother to carcinogenic compounds.

In a small pilot study (158), it was reported that isoflurane administered to mice during gestation produced hepatic neoplasms in the offspring. Because this study had methodologic flaws (test and control animals were treated differently), the studies were repeated and expanded to include enflurane, halothane, nitrous oxide, and methoxyflurane (159). All treatment and control groups had a similar number of neoplastic lesions. ***There was no indication that any anesthetic agent was carcinogenic.***

AVOIDANCE OF INTRAUTERINE FETAL ASPHYXIA

Intrauterine fetal asphyxia is avoided by maintaining normal maternal Pao_2, $Paco_2$, and uterine blood flow. Fetal oxygenation is directly dependent on maternal arterial oxygen tension, oxygen-carrying capacity (hemoglobin content), oxygen affinity, and uteroplacental perfusion. Maternal hypoxia will result in fetal hypoxia and, if uncorrected, fetal demise.

Maternal Oxygenation

Common causes of maternal hypoxia during anesthesia for operations during pregnancy, as well as during childbirth include laryngospasm, airway obstruction, improperly positioned endotracheal tube, inadequate ventilation, and low inspired oxygen in the anesthetic gas mixture. Common causes of hypoxia during regional anesthesia include severe toxic reactions or excessively

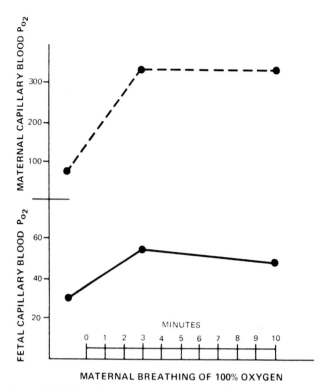

Figure 13.18. Effect of maternal inhalation of 100% oxygen in one case. At 3 and 10 minutes, fetal Po_2 was significantly above the baseline level. (Reprinted by permission from Wood C. Use of fetal blood sampling and fetal heart rate monitoring. In: Adamsons K, ed. *Diagnosis and Treatment of Fetal Disorders.* New York: Springer-Verlag; 1968:169.)

high spinal or epidural blocks with maternal hypoventilation. The usual careful anesthetic management should prevent the occurrence or continuation of significant maternal and fetal hypoxia.

Elevated maternal oxygen tensions commonly occur during anesthesia. In studies with isolated preparations of human placental and umbilical vessels, vasoconstriction occurs if high oxygen tensions are administered (160–162). Therefore, it had been feared that elevated oxygen tensions would decrease uteroplacental blood flow and fetal oxygenation. Studies of fetal scalp capillary Po_2, measured by sampling fetal blood (163) or using a transcutaneous oxygen electrode (164) have shown that increasing maternal Pao_2 will increase fetal Po_2 (Fig. 13.18). If the normal placental-fetal circulation has been significantly compromised by conditions such as umbilical cord compression or maternal hypotension, then increasing maternal oxygenation will not be reflected in the fetus. In no studies has maternal hyperoxia resulted in fetal hypoxia (163–166).

A rise in maternal Pao_2 even to 600 mm Hg seldom produces a fetal Pao_2 above 45 mm Hg and never above 60 mm Hg. The reasons for this large maternal-fetal oxygen tension gradient are high oxygen consumption of the placenta and uneven distribution of the maternal and fetal blood flow in the placenta. Thus, maternal hyperoxia cannot produce in utero retrolental fibroplasia or premature closure of the ductus arteriosus.

Maternal Carbon Dioxide

Fetal $Paco_2$ is also directly related to maternal $Paco_2$. There is evidence that low maternal $Paco_2$ or high maternal pH may be deleterious to the fetus for a number of reasons. Maternal hypocapnia produced by excessive positive pressure ventilation may increase mean intrathoracic pressure, decrease venous return to the heart, and lead to a fall in uterine blood flow (see Figure 2.22) (167). Maternal respiratory or metabolic alkalosis also decreases umbilical blood flow because of direct vasoconstriction (168). In addition, maternal alkalosis shifts the maternal oxyhemoglobin dissociation curve to the left, thereby increasing the affinity of maternal hemoglobin for oxygen, resulting in the release of less oxygen to the fetus at the placenta. Thus, fetal hypoxia and metabolic acidosis can occur as a result of maternal hyperventilation during anesthesia.

Maternal hypercapnia, as may occur with spontaneous ventilation and deep levels of anesthesia, will be associated with fetal respiratory acidosis. Moderate elevations of fetal Pa_{CO_2} are probably not detrimental, but severe fetal acidosis may produce myocardial depression.

Maternal Hypotension

Maternal hypotension from deep general anesthesia, sympathectomy, hypovolemia, or vena caval compression will cause a fall in uterine blood flow and may lead to fetal asphyxia. Hypotension and regional anesthesia are discussed in Chapter 8. With a general anesthetic–for example, halothane–a small fall in blood pressure that may occur with light anesthesia is not associated with significant reductions in uterine blood flow because of the concomitant decrease in uterine vascular resistance (169). Deep levels of halothane anesthesia resulting in significant hypotension (30% to 40% below control) will produce a fall in uterine blood flow and fetal asphyxia. In monkeys, deep halothane anesthesia producing prolonged maternal hypotension to a mean arterial pressure of 40 mm Hg or lower regularly produced fetal asphyxia, brain damage, or death (170). Fetal Pa_{O_2} fell from a normal control value of 30 to 15 mm Hg, fetal pH fell from 7.30 to 7.10 or lower, fetal bradycardia occurred, and with severe asphyxia (pH 7) lasting several hours, myocardial failure and fetal death occurred. With less severe asphyxia permanent brain damage occurred with lesions similar to those of human cerebral palsy.

Uterine Vasoconstriction and Hypertonus

Uterine vasoconstriction from endogenous or exogenous sympathomimetics increases uterine vascular resistance and decreases uterine blood flow. Sympathetic discharge and adrenal medullary activity may be encountered in the anxious unpremedicated patient or during light general anesthesia (174). Vasoactive drugs such as methoxamine, phenylephrine, or dopamine may reduce uterine blood flow (175–180). Uterine hypertonus is also associated with an increase in uterine vascular resistance and will decrease uterine blood flow. Drugs that increase uterine tone are ketamine in single intravenous doses above 1.1 mg·kg^{-1} (Figs. 13.19 and 13.20) (181), toxic doses of local anesthetics (182, 183), or α-adrenergic vasopressors.

PREVENTION OF PRETERM LABOR

Several anecdotal reports have suggested that anesthesia and operations during pregnancy may result in preterm labor during the postoperative period (184, 185). In these reports intra-abdominal procedures in which uterine manipulation or retraction was necessary most often resulted in preterm labor. Ovarian cystectomy, especially in the first trimester, has a high incidence of abortion. This is not inevitable; in many operations on the ovary, pregnancies have proceeded normally to term. Neurosurgical, orthopedic, thoracic, or plastic surgery procedures were not associated with preterm labor.

Whether anesthetics can stimulate or inhibit the onset of preterm labor is unknown. There is little information on the effects of anesthesia on oxytocin, prostaglandins, follicle-stimulating hormone, estrogen, or progesterone levels in the uterus or blood. Some commonly used anesthetic agents, such as halothane and enflurane, decrease uterine tone and inhibit uterine contractions. On this basis, some have suggested that

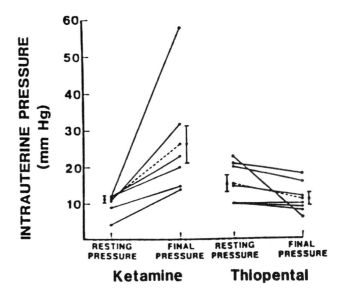

Figure 13.19. Changes in intrauterine pressure following administration of ketamine (2 mg·kg^{-1}) or thiopental (4 mg·kg^{-1}) to patients in the second trimester undergoing therapeutic abortions. *Solid lines* indicate individual patients; *dashed lines* are mean changes ± SEM. (Reprinted by permission from Oats JN, Vasey DP, Waldron BA. Effects of ketamine on the pregnant uterus. *Br J Anaesth* 1979;51:1163–1166.)

these agents be used during advanced pregnancy when uterine manipulation is anticipated. However, *in no study has any one anesthetic agent or technique been found to be associated with a higher or lower incidence of preterm delivery.*

As previously stated, some anesthetic agents—such as ketamine in doses greater than 1.1 mg·kg^{-1}—and some vasopressors do increase uterine tone and should probably be avoided when possible. Rapid intravenous injection of anticholinesterase agents, such as neostigmine or edrophonium, may directly stimulate acetylcholine release and theoretically could increase uterine tone and stimulate preterm labor. Neostigmine, when used to reverse the effects of muscle relaxants, should be administered slowly and be preceded by adequate doses of atropine.

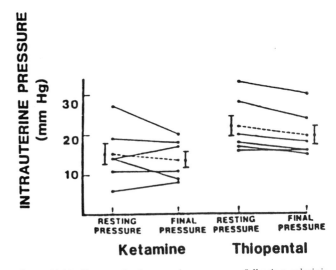

Figure 13.20. Changes in intrauterine pressure following administration of ketamine (2 mg·kg^{-1}) or thiopental (4 mg·kg^{-1}) to patients at term undergoing cesarean section. *Solid lines* indicate individual patients; *dashed lines* are mean changes ± SEM. (Reprinted by permission from Oats JN, Vasey DP, Waldron BA. Effects of ketamine on the pregnant uterus. *Br J Anaesth* 1979;51:1163–1166.)

Laparoscopic Surgery

Operative laparoscopy in general surgery and gynecology has become increasingly popular. The minimally-invasive surgery produces less post-operative pain and therefore less post-operative opioids and other analgesics are required, shorter hospitalizations and quicker return to normal activities. Recently, case reports have indicated that laparoscopic procedures can be performed safely during all trimesters of pregnancy (186, 187). The most common laparoscopic procedure performed during pregnancy is cholecystectomy. (Acute cholecystitis and appendicitis are the two most frequent nonobstetric emergencies occurring during pregnancy.) Other common laparoscopic procedures are appendectomy, ovarian torsion and management of adnexal masses.

In the largest review of laparoscopy during pregnancy, Reedy et al. (188) evaluated differences in five fetal outcome variables for patients undergoing laparoscopy versus laparotomy in singleton pregnancies between 4 and 20 weeks of gestation. A total of 2181 laparoscopies and 1552 laparotomies were reviewed. There were no significant differences between laparoscopy and laparotomy in infant birth weights, gestational duration, intrauterine growth restriction, infant death at one year, or fetal malformations.

When laparoscopic surgery is performed during pregnancy some additional precautions should be observed. To prevent accidental puncture of the uterus, especially as gestational age increases, most surgeons suggest using the open Hasson technique rather than the Verres needle to obtain access to the abdominal cavity (189). Adequate muscle relaxation should be provided and insufflation limited so that intra-abdominal pressure is kept low and does not exceed 15 mm Hg.

Maternal end tidal carbon dioxide should be monitored and ventilation adjusted to avoid respiratory acidosis. It has been suggested that prolonged respiratory acidosis during carbon dioxide insufflation is a cause of post-operative spontaneous abortion and preterm labor (184) and some have suggested the substitution of nitrous oxide gas for insufflation (44b) or the use of continuous transcutaneous P_{CO_2} monitoring during laparoscopy (190). Carbon dioxide is currently the gas of choice for pneumoperitoneum for a number of reasons including that it is noncombustible and, unlike nitrous oxide, it does not support combustion. Adjusting maternal ventilation to maintain end tidal carbon dioxide in the 30 to 35 mm Hg range should avoid excessive hypercarbia and fetal acidosis.

The lower extremity stasis commonly found in pregnancy combined with the pregnancy-induced increased levels of fibrinogen and Factors VII and XII, and the decreased venous return from the increased abdominal pressure produced by the pneumoperitoneum and the reverse Trendelenburg position frequently used during laparoscopic surgery all significantly increase the risk of deep venous thrombosis and thromboembolism. The use of anti-embolic devices such as intermittent pneumatic compression stockings is recommended.

Intraoperative transvaginal ultrasonography may be the most effective means of monitoring the fetus. Transabdominal ultrasound monitoring often fails during abdominal insufflation (191). If fetal distress develops, as indicated by fetal tachycardia, the pneumoperitoneum should be desufflated, the mother should be taken out of reverse Trendelenburg, lateral tilt assured and increased maternal oxygen provided.

RECOMMENDATIONS FOR ANESTHETIC MANAGEMENT (FIG. 13.21)

1. *Elective surgery* should be deferred until after delivery when the physiologic changes of pregnancy have returned toward normal. Women of childbearing age scheduled for elective surgery should be carefully queried regarding the possibility of pregnancy.
2. *Urgent surgery*—that is, operations that are essential but can be delayed without increasing the risk of permanent disability—should be deferred until the second or third trimester. *At present, no anesthetic drug—premedicant, intravenous induction agent, inhalation agent, or local anesthetic—has been PROVEN to be teratogenic in HUMANS.* However, despite the lack of proof, it is prudent to minimize or eliminate fetal exposure to drugs during the vulnerable first trimester.
3. *Emergency surgery*—that is, operations that cannot be delayed without increasing maternal morbidity or mortality—may be necessary during the first trimester. They are ideally performed under regional block if the contemplated surgery and maternal condition allow. Teratogenicity of local anesthetics in animals or humans has not been reported.
4. With *spinal anesthesia* fetal exposure to local anesthetic is much less than with other regional blocks.
5. *During the preoperative visit*, great effort should be made to allay maternal anxiety and apprehension. In describing

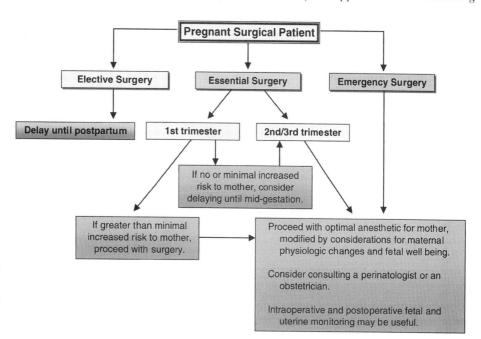

Figure 13.21. Summary recommendations for management of the pregnant surgical patient. (Reprinted by permission from Rosen MA. Management of anesthesia for the pregnant surgical patient. *Anesthesiology* 1999;91:1159–1163.)

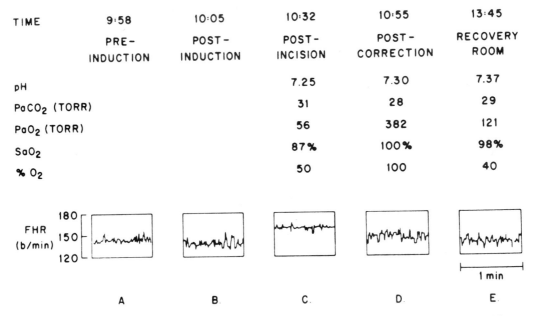

TIME	9:58 PRE-INDUCTION	10:05 POST-INDUCTION	10:32 POST-INCISION	10:55 POST-CORRECTION	13:45 RECOVERY ROOM
pH			7.25	7.30	7.37
$PaCO_2$ (TORR)			31	28	29
PaO_2 (TORR)			56	382	121
SaO_2			87%	100%	98%
% O_2			50	100	40

1 min

A   B   C   D   E.

Figure 13.22. Serial samples of fetal heart rate in a patient undergoing eye surgery. *A* and *B*: Baseline fetal heart rate of 140 beats per minute with normal beat-to-beat variability; *C*: Fetal tachycardia and stabilization of the beat-to-beat interval during inadvertent maternal hypoxemia (maternal $PaO_2 = 56$ mm Hg); *D*: After correction of maternal ventilation there is a return to baseline fetal heart rate and variability; *E*: Normal baseline postoperatively. (Reprinted by permission from Katz JD, Hook R, Barash PG. Fetal heart rate monitoring in pregnant patients undergoing surgery. *Am J Obstet Gynecol* 1976;125:267–269.)

risks and hazards to the parturients, the lack of documented teratogenicity can be presented. The likelihood of first trimester miscarriage increases from 5.1% without surgery to 8% with surgery (4), and the incidence of premature delivery increases from 5.13% without surgery to 7.47% with surgery (5).

6. *If general anesthesia* is necessary during the first trimester there is no proof that any well-conducted technique is superior to any other. Adequate oxygenation and avoidance of hyperventilation are mandatory.

7. *During pregnancy* patients may be at increased risk of aspiration, and the usual safeguards to prevent aspiration pneumonitis should be performed.

8. Aortocaval compression during the second and third trimesters should be prevented by avoiding the supine position. The left lateral tilt position should be used whenever possible.

9. *Ideally, continuous fetal heart rate monitoring* during surgery should be employed after the 16th week of gestation. This may provide an indication of abnormalities in maternal ventilation or uterine perfusion (Fig. 13.22).

10. *Continuous monitoring of uterine activity* during the postoperative period can detect the onset of preterm labor. Tocolytic therapy, instituted early, may prevent preterm delivery.

REFERENCES

1. Shnider SM, Webster GM. Maternal and fetal hazards of surgery during pregnancy. *Am J Obstet Gynecol* 1965;92:891–900.
2. Smith BE. Fetal prognosis after anesthesia during gestation. *Anesth Analg* 1963;42:521–526.
3. Smith BE. Teratogenic capabilities of surgical anesthesia. *Adv Teratol* 1968;3:127–179.
4. Brodsky JB, Cohen EN, Brown BW Jr, Wu ML, Whitcher C. Surgery during pregnancy and fetal outcome. *Am J Obstet Gynecol* 1980;138:1165–1167.
5. Mazze RI, Källém B. Reproductive outcome after anesthesia and operation during pregnancy: A registry study of 5405 cases. *Am J Obstet Gynecol* 1989;161:1178–1185.
6. Manley S, de Kelaita G, Joseph NJ, Salem MR, Heyman HJ. Preoperative pregnancy test in ambulatory surgery. Incidence and impact of positive results. *Anesthesiology* 1995;83:690–693.
7. Cugell DW, Frank NR, Gaensler EA, Badger TL. Pulmonary function in pregnancy. I. Serial observations in normal women. *Am Rev Tuberc* 1953;67:568–597.
8. Prowse CM, Gaensler EA. Respiratory and acid-base changes during pregnancy. *Anesthesiology* 1965;26:381–392.
9. Palahniuk RJ, Shnider SM, Eger EI II. Pregnancy decreases the requirement for inhaled anesthetic agents. *Anesthesiology* 1974;41:82–83.
10. Strout CD, Nahrwold ML. Halothane requirement during pregnancy and lactation in rats. *Anesthesiology* 1981;55:322–323.
11. Gin T, Chan MTV. Decreased minimum alveolar concentration of isoflurane in pregnant humans. *Anesthesiology* 1994;81:829–832.
12. Chan MT, Mainland P, Gin T. Minimum alveolar concentration of halothane and enflurane are decreased in early pregnancy. *Anesthesiology* 1996;85:782–786.
13. Gin T, Mainland P, Chan MT, Short TG. Decreased thiopental requirements in early pregnancy. *Anesthesiology* 1997;86:73–78.
14. Gintzler AR. Endorphin-mediated increases in pain threshold during pregnancy. *Science* 1980;210:193–195.
15. Lees MM, Taylor SH, Scott DB, Kerr MG. A study of cardiac output at rest throughout pregnancy. *J Obstet Gynaecol Br Commonw* 1967;74:319–328.
16. Lees MM, Scott DB, Kerr MG, Taylor SH. The circulatory effects of recumbent postural changes in late pregnancy. *Clin Sci* 1967;32:453–465.
17. Ueland K, Novy MJ, Peterson EN, Metcalfe J. Maternal cardiovascular dynamics. IV. The influence of gestational age on the maternal cardiovascular response to posture and exercise. *Am J Obstet Gynecol* 1969;104:856–864.
18. Pritchard JA. Changes in blood volume during pregnancy and delivery. *Anesthesiology* 1965;26:393–399.
19. Ueland K. Maternal cardiovascular dynamics. VII. Intrapartum blood volume changes. 1976;126:671–677.
20. Capeless EL, Clapp JF. Cardiovascular changes in the early phase of pregnancy. *Am J Obstet Gynecol* 1989;161:1449–1453.
21. Fagraeus L, Urban B, Bromage P. Spread of epidural analgesia in early pregnancy. *Anesthesiology* 1983;58:184–187.
22. Kaneko M, Saito Y, Kirihara Y, Kosaka Y. Pregnancy enhances the antinociceptive effects of extradural lignocaine in the rat. *Br J Anaesth* 1994;72:657–661.
23. Datta S, Lambert DH, Gregus J, Gissen AJ, Covino BG. Differential sensitivities of mammalian nerve fibers during pregnancy. *Anesth Analg* 1983;62:1070–1072.
24. Flanagan HL, Datta S, Lambert DH, Gissen AJ, Covino BG. Effects of pregnancy on bupivacaine-induced conduction blockage in the isolated rabbit vagus nerve. *Anesth Analg* 1987;66:123–126.

25. Butterworth JF, Walker FO, Lysak SZ. Pregnancy increases median nerve susceptibility to lidocaine. *Anesthesiology* 1990;72:962–965.

26. Attia RR, Eberd AM, Fischer JE. Gastrin. Placental, maternal and plasma cord levels: Its possible role in maternal residual gastric acidity. In: Abstracts of Scientific Papers of the Annual Meeting of the American Society of Anesthesiologists; San Francisco, CA; 1976:547.

27. Macfie AG, Magides AD, Richmond MN, Reily CS. Gastric emptying during pregnancy. *Br J Anaesth* 1991;67:54–57.

28. Wyner MB, Cohen S. Gastric volume in early pregnancy. *Anesthesiology* 1982;57:209–212.

29. Tuchmann-Duplessis H. Influence of certain drugs on the prenatal development. *Int J Gynaecol Obstet* 1970;8:777–797.

30. Setala K, Nyyssonen O. Hypnotic sodium pentobarbital as a teratogen for mice. *Naturwissenschaften* 1964;51:413.

31. Tanimura T. The effect of thiamylal sodium administration to pregnant mice upon the development of their offspring. *Acta Anat Nippon* 1965;40:323.

32. Goldman AS, Yakovac WC. Prevention of salicylate teratogenicity in immobilized rats by central nervous system depressants. *Proc Soc Exp Biol Med* 1964;115:693–696.

33. Roux C. Action teratogene de la prochlorperazine [Teratogenic action of prochlorperazine]. *Arch Franc Pediatr* 1959;16:968–971.

34. Robson JM, Sullivan FM. The production of foetal abnormalities in rabbits by imipramine. *Lancet* 1963;1:638–639.

35. Tonge SR. Permanent alterations in catecholamine concentration in discrete areas of brain in the offspring of rats treated with methylamphetamine and chlorpromazine. *Br J Pharmacol* 1973;47:425–427.

36. Jurand A. Teratogenic activity of methadone hydrochloride in mouse and chick embryos. *J Embryol Exp Morphol* 1973;30:449–458.

37. Markham JK, Emmerson JL, Owen NV. Teratogenicity studies of methadone HCl in rats and rabbits. *Nature* 1971;233:342–343.

38. Geber WF, Schramm LC. Congenital malformations of the central nervous system produced by narcotic analgesics in the hamster. *Am J Obstet Gynecol* 1975;123:705–713.

39. Fujinaga M, Stevenson JB, Mazze RI. Reproductive and teratogenic effects of fentanyl in Sprague-Dawley rats. *Teratology* 1986;34:51–57.

40. Fujinaga M, Mazze RI, Jackson EC, Baden JM. Reproductive and teratogenic effects of sufentanil and alfentanil in Sprague-Dawley rats. *Anesth Analg* 1988;67:166–169.

41. Milkovich L, van den Berg BJ. Effects of prenatal meprobamate and chlordiazepoxide hydrochloride on human embryonic and fetal development. *N Engl J Med* 1974;291:1268–1271.

42. Saxen I, Saxen L. Association between maternal intake of diazepam and oral clefts. *Lancet* 1975;2:498.

43. Safra MJ, Oakley GP. Association between cleft lip with or without cleft palate and prenatal exposure to diazepam. *Lancet* 1975;2:478–480.

44. Hartz SC, Heinomen OP, Shapiro S, Siskind V, Slone D. Antenatal exposure to meprobamate and chlordiazepoxide in relation to malformations, mental development, and childhood mortality. *N Engl J Med* 1975;292:726–728.

44a. Koren G, Pastuszak A, Ito S. Drugs in pregnancy [review]. *N Engl J Med* 1998;338:1128–1137.

44b. Rosen MA. Management of anesthesia for the pregnant surgical patient. *Anesthesiology* 1999;91:1159–1163.

45. Smith BE, Gaub MI, Moya F. Teratogenic effects of anesthetic agents: Nitrous oxide. *Anesth Analg* 1965;44:726–732.

46. Fink BR, Shepard TH, Blandau RJ. Teratogenic activity of nitrous oxide. *Nature* 1967;214:146–148.

47. Lane GA, Nahrwold ML, Tait AR, Taylor-Busch M, Cohen PJ. Anesthetics as teratogens: Nitrous oxide is fetotoxic, xenon is not. *Science* 1980;210:899–901.

48. Lane GA, DuBoulay PM, Tait AR, Taylor-Busch M, Cohen PJ. Nitrous oxide is teratogenic: Halothane is not [abstract]. *Anesthesiology* 1981;55:A252.

49. Mazze RI, Wilson AI, Rice SA, Baden JM. Reproduction and fetal development in rats exposed to nitrous oxide. *Teratology* 1984;30:259–265.

50. Mazze RI, Wilson AI, Rice SA, Baden JM. Reproduction and fetal development in mice chronically exposed to nitrous oxide. *Teratology* 1982;26:11–16.

51. Pope WDB, Halsey MJ, Lansdown ABG, Simmonds A, Bateman PE. Fetotoxicity in rats following chronic exposure to halothane, nitrous oxide or methoxyflurane. *Anesthesiology* 1978;48:11–16.

52. Coate WB, Kapp RW Jr, Lewis TR. Chronic exposure to low concentrations of halothane-nitrous oxide: Reproductive and cytogenetic effects in the rat. *Anesthesiology* 1979;50:310–318.

53. Doenicke A, Wittmann R, Heinrich H, Pausch J. L'effet abortif de l'halothane [The abortive effect of halothane]. *Anesth Analg Rean* 1975;32:41–46.

54. Doenicke A, Wittman R. Effet teratogene de l'halothane sur le foetus de rat [Teratogenic effect of halothane on the fetus of the rat]. *Anesth Analg Rean* 1975;32:47–51.

55. Bussard DA, Stoelting RK, Peterson C, Ishaq M. Fetal changes in hamsters anesthetized with nitrous oxide and halothane. *Anesthesiology* 1974;41:275–278.

56. Baden JM, Rice SA, Serra M, Kelley M, Mazze RI. Thymidine and methionine syntheses in pregnant rats exposed to nitrous oxide. *Anesth Analg* 1983;62:738–741.

57. Baden JM, Serra M, Mazze RI. Inhibition of fetal methionine synthetase by nitrous oxide. *Br J Anaesth* 1984;56:523–526.

58. Nunn JF, Chanarin I. Nitrous oxide inactivates methionine synthetase. In: Eger EI II, ed. *Nitrous Oxide/N_2O*. New York: Elsevier; 1985:211–233.

59. Deacon R, Chanarin I, Perry J, Lumb M. Impaired deoxyuridine utilization in the B_{12}-inactivated rat and its correction by folate analogues. *Biochem Biophys Res Commun* 1980;93:516–520.

60. O'Sullivan H, Jannings F, Ward K, McCann S, Scott JM, Weir DG. Human bone marrow biochemical function and megaloblastic hematopoiesis after nitrous oxide anesthesia. *Anesthesiology* 1981;55:645–649.

61. Keeling PA, Rocke DA, Nunn JF, Monk SJ, Lumb MJ, Halsey MJ. Folinic acid protection against N_2O teratogenicity in the rat. *Br J Anaesth* 1986;58:524–534.

62. Fujinaga M, Baden JM, Yhap EO, Mazze RI. Reproductive and teratogenic effects of nitrous oxide, isoflurane and their combination in Sprague-Dawley rats. *Anesthesiology* 1987;67:960–964.

63. Mazze RI, Fujinaga M, Baden JM. Halothane prevents nitrous oxide teratogenicity in rats, folinic acid does not. *Teratology* 1988;38:121–127.

64. Fujinaga M, Baden JM, Mazze RI. Halothane and isoflurane prevent the teratogenic effects of nitrous oxide, folinic acid does not [abstract]. *Anesthesiology* 1987;67:A456.

65. Fujinaga M, Baden JM. Methionine prevents nitrous oxide-induced teratogenicity in rat embryos grown in culture. *Anesthesiology* 1994;81:184–189.

66. Fujinaga M, Baden JM, Suto A, Myatt JK, Mazze RI. Preventive effects of phenoxybenzamine on N_2O-induced reproductive toxicity in Sprague-Dawley rats [abstract]. *Anesthesiology* 1990;73:A920.

67. Bashford AB, Fink BR. The teratogenicity of halothane in the rat. *Anesthesiology* 1968;29:1167–1173.

68. Smith BE, Usubiaga LE, Lehrer SB. Cleft palate induced by halothane anesthesia in C-57 black mice. *Teratology* 1971;4:242.

69. Sturrock JE, Nunn JF. Mitosis in mammalian cells during exposure to anesthetics. *Anesthesiology* 1975;43:21–23.

70. Kennedy GL, Smith SH, Keplinger ML, Calandra JC. Reproductive and teratologic studies with halothane. *Toxicol Appl Pharmacol* 1976;35:467–474.

71. Warton RS, Mazze RI, Baden JM, Hitt BA, Dooley JR. Fertility, reproduction and postnatal survival in mice chronically exposed to halothane. *Anesthesiology* 1978;48:167–174.

72. Mazze RI, Fujinaga M, Rice SA, Harris SB, Baden JM. Reproductive and teratogenic effects of nitrous oxide, halothane, isoflurane and enflurane in Sprague-Dawley rats. *Anesthesiology* 1986;64:339–344.

73. Wharton RS, Mazze RI, Wilson AI. Reproductive and fetal development in mice chronically exposed to enflurane. *Anesthesiology* 1981;54:505–510.

74. Mazze RI, Wilson AI, Rice SA, Baden JM. Fetal development in mice exposed to isoflurane. *Teratology* 1985;32:339–345.

75. Smith BE, Gaub MI, Moya F. Investigations into the teratogenic effects of anesthetic agents: The fluorinated agents. *Anesthesiology* 1965;26:260–261.

76. Anderson NB. The teratogenicity of cyclopropane in the chicken. *Anesthesiology* 1968;29:113–122.

77. Drachman DB, Coulombre AJ. Experimental clubfoot and arthrogryposis multiplex congenita. *Lancet* 1962;2:523–526.

78. Fujinaga M, Baden JM, Mazze RI. Developmental toxicity of nondepolarizing muscle relaxants in cultured rat embryos [abstract]. *Anesthesiology* 1991;75:A850.

79. Fujinaga M, Mazze RI. Reproductive and teratogenic effects of lidocaine in Sprague-Dawley rats. *Anesthesiology* 1986;65:626–632.

80. Ramazzotto LG, Curro FA, Paterson JA, Tanner P, Coleman M. Toxicological assessment of lidocaine in the pregnant rat. *J Dent Res* 1985;164:1214–1217.

81. Martin LVH, Jurand A. The absence of teratogenic effects of some analgesics used in anaesthesia. Additional evidence from a mouse model. *Anaesthesia* 1992;47:473–476.

82. O'Shea KS, Kaufman MH. Neural tube closure defects following in vitro exposure of mouse embryos to Xylocaine. *J Exp Zool* 1980;214:235–238.

83. Lee H, Nagele RG. Neural tube defects caused by local anesthetics in early chick embryos. *Teratology* 1985;31:119–127.

84. Lee H, Bush KT, Nagele RG. Time-lapse photographic study of neural tube closure defects caused by xylocaine in the chick. *Teratology* 1988;37:263–269.

85. Fujinaga M. Assessment of teratogenic effects of lidocaine in rat embryos cultured in vitro. *Anesthesiology* 1998;89:1553–1559.

86. Mahalik MP, Gautieri RF, Mann DE. Teratogenic potential of cocaine hydrochloride in CF-1 mice. *J Pharm Sci* 1980;69:703–706.

87. Fantel AG, MacPhail BJ. The teratogenicity of cocaine. *Teratology* 1982;26:17–19.

88. Cohen EN, Bellville JW, Brown BW Jr. Anesthesia, pregnancy, and miscarriage. *Anesthesiology* 1971;35:343–347.

89. Cohen EN, Brown BW Jr, Wu ML, et al. Occupational disease in dentistry and chronic exposure to trace anesthetic gases. *JADA* 1980;101:21–31.

90. Knill-Jones RP, Rodrigues LV, Moir DD, Spence AA. Anesthetic practice and pregnancy: Controlled survey of women anesthetists in the United Kingdom. *Lancet* 1972;1:1326–1328.

91. Rosenberg P, Kirves A. Miscarriages among operating theatre staff. *Acta Anaesthesiol Scand* 1973;53:S37–S42.

92. Ad Hoc Committee on the Effect of Trace Anesthetics on the Health of Operating Room Personnel (Cohen EN, chairman). American Society of Anesthesiologists. Occupational disease among operating room personnel. *Anesthesiology* 1974;41:321–340.

93. Axelsson G, Rylander R. Exposure to anesthetic gases and spontaneous abortion: Response bias in a postal questionnaire study. *Int J Epidemiol* 1982;11:250–256.

94. Buring JE, Hennekens CH, Mayrent SL, Rosner B, Greenberg ER, Colton T. Health experiences of operating room personnel. *Anesthesiology* 1985;62:325–330.

95. Mazze RI, Lecky JH. The health of operating room personnel [editorial]. *Anesthesiology* 1985;62:226–228.

96. Harlap S, Shiono PH. Alcohol, smoking and incidence of spontaneous abortions in the first and second trimester. *Lancet* 1980;2:173–176.

97. Kline J, Stein ZA, Susser M, Warburton D. Smoking: A risk factor for spontaneous abortion. *N Engl J Med* 1977;297:793–796.

98. Baden JM. Mutagenicity, carcinogenicity, and teratogenicity of nitrous oxide. In: Eger EI II, ed. *Nitrous Oxide/N₂O*. New York: Elsevier; 1985:235–247.

99. Lloyd TS. The safety of surgical operations during pregnancy. *South Med J* 1965;58:179–184.

100. Jacobs WM, Cooley D, Goen GP. Cardiac surgery with extracorporeal circulation during pregnancy: Report of 3 cases. *Obstet Gynecol* 1965;25:167–169.

101. Meffert WG, Stansel HC Jr. Open heart surgery during pregnancy. *Am J Obstet Gynecol* 1968;102:1116–1120.

102. Duncan PG, Pope WDB, Cohen MM, Greer N. The safety of anesthesia and surgery during pregnancy. *Anesthesiology* 1986;64:790–794.

103. Mazze RI, Källén B. Appendectomy during pregnancy: A Swedish registry study of 778 cases. *Obstet Gynecol* 1991;77:835–840.

104. Belasich-Allart JC, Hazout A, Guillet-Rosso F, Glissant M, Testart J, Frydman R. Various techniques for oocyte recovery in an in vitro fertilization and embryo transfer program. *J In Vitro Fertil Embryo Transfer* 1985;2:99–104.

105. Rosen MA, Roizen MF, Eger EI II, et al. The effect of nitrous oxide on in vitro fertilization success rate. *Anesthesiology* 1987;67:42–44.

106. Beilin Y, Bodian CA, Mukherjee T. The use of propofol, nitrous oxide, or isoflurane does not affect the reproductive success rate following gamete intrafallopian transfer (GIFT): A multicenter pilot trial/survey. *Anesthesiology* 1999;90:3641.

107. Crawford JS, Lewis M. Nitrous oxide in early human pregnancy. *Anaesthesia* 1986;41:900–905.

108. Aldridge LM, Tunstall ME. Nitrous oxide and the fetus: A review and the results of a retrospective study of 175 cases of anaesthesia for insertion of Sirodkhar suture. *Br J Anaesth* 1986;58:1348–1356.

109. Källén B, Mazze RI. Neural tube defects and first trimester operations. *Teratology* 1990;41:717–720.

110. Sylvester GC, Khourt MJ, Lu X, Erickson JD. First-trimester anesthesia exposure and the risk of central nervous system defects: A population-based case-control study. *Am J Public Health* 1994;84:1757–1760.

111. Sullivan FM. Animal tests to screen for human teratogens. *Pediatrics* 1974;53(suppl):822–823.

112. Ingalls TH, Curley FJ, Prindle RA. Anoxia as a cause of fetal death and congenital defect in the mouse. *Am J Dis Child* 1950;80:34–45.

113. Degenhardt KH. Durch O₂-mangel induzierte fehlbildungen der axialgradienten bei kaninchen. *Z Naturforsch* 1954;9:530.

114. Haring OM. The effects of prenatal hypoxia on the cardiovascular system in the rat. *Arch Pathol* 1965;80:351–356.

115. Grabowski CT. Teratogenic significance of ionic and fluid imbalance. *Science* 1963;142:1064–1065.

116. Ferm BH. Teratogenic effects of hyperbaric oxygen. *Proc Soc Exp Biol Med* 1964;116:975–976.

117. Fujikura T. Retrolental fibroplasia and prematurity in newborn rabbits induced by maternal hyperoxia. *Am J Obstet Gynecol* 1964;90:854–858.

118. Grote W. Storung der embryonalentwicklung bei erhohtem CO₂- und O₂-partialdruck und bei unterdruck. *Z Morphol Anthropol* 1965;56:165.

119. Haring OM. Cardiac malformations in rats induced by exposure of the mother to carbon dioxide during pregnancy. *Circ Res* 1960;8:1218–1227.

120. Ballabriga A, Samso Dies J, Bado JV. Estudios electroencefalogradicos sobre la anoxia fetal y neonatal en los animales de experimentacio [Electroencephalographic studies on fetal and neonatal hypoxia in experimental animals]. *Med Clin* 1957;3:164.

121. Pitt DB. A study of congenital malformations. II. *Aust N Z J Obstet Gynaecol* 1962;2:82–90.

122. Warkany J, Kalter H. Congenital malformations. *N Engl J Med* 1961;265:1046–1052.

123. Abramson JH, Ansuyah RS, Mbambo V. Antenatal stress and the baby's development. *Arch Dis Child* 1961;36:42–49.

124. Davis A, DeVault S, Talmadge M. Anxiety, pregnancy and childbirth abnormalities. *J Consult Psychol* 1961;25:74–77.

125. Davis A, DeVault S. Maternal anxiety during pregnancy and childbirth abnormalities. *Psychosom Med* 1962;24:464–470.

126. Crist T, Hulka JF. Influence of maternal epinephrine on behavior of offspring. *Am J Obstet Gynecol* 1970;106:687–691.

127. Ferreira AJ. Emotional factors in prenatal environment. *J Nerv Ment Dis* 1965;141:108–118.

128. Geber WF. Developmental effects of chronic maternal audiovisual stress on the rat fetus. *J Embryol Exp Morphol* 1966;16:1–16.

129. Geber WF, Anderson TA. Abnormal fetal growth in the albino rat and rabbit induced by maternal stress. *Biol Neonate* 1967;11:209–215.

130. Goldman AS, Yakovac WC. The enhancement of salicylate teratogenicity by maternal immobilization in the rat. *J Pharmacol Exp Ther* 1963;142:351–357.

131. Hinden E. External injury causing foetal deformity. *Arch Dis Child* 1965;40:80–81.

132. Ozan HA, Gonzalez AA. Post-traumatic fetal epilepsy. *Neurology* 1963;13:541–542.

133. Torpin R, Miller GT, Culpepper BW. Amniogenic fetal digital amputations associated with clubfoot. *Obstet Gynecol* 1964;24:379–384.

134. Turner EK. Teratogenic effects of the human foetus through maternal emotional stress: Report of a case. *Med J Aust* 1960;2:502–503.

135. Wiedemann HR. Schadigungen der frucht in der schwangerschaft. *Med Monatsschr* 1955;9:141–148.

136. Werboff J, Gottlieb JS. Drugs in pregnancy: Behavioral teratology. *Obstet Gynecol Surv* 1963;18:420–423.

137. Werboff J. Effects of prenatal administration of tranquilizers on maze learning ability. *Am Psychol* 1962;17:397.

138. Hoffield DR, McNew J, Webster RL. Effect of tranquilizing drugs during pregnancy on activity of offspring. *Nature* 1968;218:357–358.

139. Clarke CVH, Gorman D, Vernadakis A. Effects of prenatal administration of psychotropic drugs on behavior of developing rats. *Dev Psychobiol* 1970;3:225–235.

140. Young RD. Effects of differential early experiences and neonatal tranquilization on later behavior. *Psychol Rep* 1965;17:675–680.

141. Harned BK, Hamilton HC, Cole BB. The effect of administration of sodium bromide to pregnant rats on the learning ability of the offspring. II. Maze test. *J Pharmacol Exp Ther* 1974;82:215.

142. Armitage SG. The effects of barbiturate on the behavior of rat offspring as measured on learning and reasoning situations. *J Comp Physiol Psychol* 1952;45:146–152.

143. Butcher RE, Boorhees CV, Kimmel CA. Learning impairment from maternal salicylate treatment in rats. *Nature New Biol* 1972;236:211–212.

144. Smith RF, Bowman RE, Katz J. Behavioral effects of exposure to halothane during early development in the rat: Sensitive period during pregnancy. *Anesthesiology* 1978;49:319–323.

145. Chalon J, Tang C-K, Ramanathan S, Eisner M, Katz R, Turndorf H. Exposure to halothane and enflurane affects learning function of murine progeny. *Anesth Analg* 1981;60:794–797.

146. Chalon J, Hillman D, Gross S, Eisner M, Tang C-K, Turndorf H. Intrauterine exposure to halothane increases murine postnatal autotolerance to halothane and reduces brain weight. *Anesth Analg* 1963;62:565–567.

147. Teiling AKY, Mohammed AK, Minor BG, et al. Lack of effects of prenatal exposure to lidocaine on development of behavior in rats. *Anesth Analg* 1987;66:533–541.

148. Committee on Drugs of the American Academy of Pediatrics and the Committee on Obstetrics and Maternal and Fetal Medicine of the American College of Obstetricians and Gynecologists. Effect of medication during labor and delivery on infant outcome. *Pediatrics* 1978;62:402–403.

149. Eschenbrenner AB, Miller E. Induction of hepatomas in mice by repeated oral administration of chloroform with observations on sex differences. *J Natl Cancer Inst* 1945;5:251.

150. Report of Carcinogenesis Bioassay of Chloroform. Bethesda, MD: Carcinogenesis Program; Division of Cancer Cause and Prevention; National Cancer Institute; 1976.

151. National Cancer Institute. Carcinogenesis Bioassay of Trichloroethylene. CAS No. 79-01-6. National Cancer Institute Tech. Rep. Series No. 2. Washington, DC: U.S. Department of Health, Education and Welfare; Publ. No. (NIH) 76-802; February 1976.

152. Jackson SH. The metabolic effect of halothane on mammalian hepatoma cells in vitro. II. Inhibition of DNA synthesis. *Anesthesiology* 1973;39:405–409.

153. Sturrock J, Nunn JF. Effects of halothane on DNA synthesis and the presynthetic phase (G1) in dividing fibroblasts. *Anesthesiology* 1976;45:413–420.

154. Ames BN. The detection of chemical mutagens with enteric bacteria. In: Lollaender A, ed. *Chemical Mutagens: Principles and Methods for Their Detection.* New York: Plenum; 1971:267.

155. Baden JM, Brinkenhoff BS, Wharton RS, Hitt BA, Simmon VF, Mazze RI. Mutagenicity of volatile anesthetics: Halothane. *Anesthesiology* 1976;45:311–318.

156. Baden JM, Kelley M, Wharton RS, Hitt BA, Simmon VF, Mazze RI. Mutagenicity of halogenated ether anesthetics. *Anesthesiology* 1977;46:346–350.

157. Tomatis L. Transplacental carcinogenesis. In: Raven RW, ed. *Modern Trends in Oncology.* London: Butterworth; 1973:99.

158. Corbett TH. Cancer and congenital anomalies associated with anesthetics. *Ann NY Acad Sci* 1976;271:58–66.

159. Eger EI II, White AE, Brown CL, Biana CG, Corbett LH, Stevens WC. A test of carcinogenicity of enflurane, isoflurane, halothane, methoxyflurane, and nitrous oxide in mice. *Anesth Analg* 1978;57:678–694.

160. Nyberg R, Westin B. The influence of oxygen tension and some drugs on human placental vessels. *Acta Physiol Scand* 1957;39:216–227.

161. Panigel M. Placental perfusion experiments. *Am J Obstet Gynecol* 1962;84:1664–1683.

162. Tominaga T, Page EW. Accommodation of the human placenta to hypoxia. *Am J Obstet Gynecol* 1966;94:679–691.

163. Khazin AF, Hon EH, Hahre FW. Effects of material hyperoxia on the fetus. I. Oxygen tension. *Am J Obstet Gynecol* 1971;109:628–637.

164. Walker A, Madderin L, Day E, Renow P, Talbot J, Wood C. Fetal scalp tissue oxygen measurements in relation to maternal dermal oxygen tension and fetal heart rate. *J Obstet Gynaecol Br Commonw* 1971;78:1–12.

165. Neuman W, McKinnon L, Phillips L, Paterson P, Wood C. Oxygen transfer from mother to fetus during labor. *Am J Obstet Gynecol* 1967;99:61–70.

166. Gare DJ, Shime J, Paul WM, Hoskins M. Oxygen administration during labor. *Am J Obstet Gynecol* 1969;105:954–961.

167. Levinson G, Shnider SM, deLorimier AA, Steffenson JL. Effects of maternal hyperventilation on uterine blood flow and fetal oxygenation and acid-base status. *Anesthesiology* 1974;40:340–347.

168. Motoyama EK, Rivard G, Acheson F, Cook CD. The effect of changes in maternal pH and PCO_2 on the PO_2 of fetal lambs. *Anesthesiology* 1967;28:891–903.

169. Palahniuk RJ, Shnider SM. Maternal and fetal cardiovascular and acid-base changes during halothane and isoflurane anesthesia in the pregnant ewe. *Anesthesiology* 1974;41:462–472.

170. Brann AW, Myers RE. Central nervous system finding in the newborn monkey following severe in utero partial asphyxia. *Neurology* 1975;25:327–338.

171. Adamsons K, Mueller-Heubach E, Myers RE. Production of fetal asphyxia in the rhesus monkey by administration of catecholamines to the mother. *Am J Obstet Gynecol* 1971;109:248–262.

172. Rosenfeld CR, Baron MD, Meschia G. Effects of epinephrine on distribution of blood flow in the pregnant ewe. *Am J Obstet Gynecol* 1976;124:156–163.

173. Shnider SM, Wright RG, Levinson G, et al. Uterine blood flow and plasma norepinephrine changes during maternal stress in the pregnant ewe. *Anesthesiology* 1979;50:524–527.

174. Shnider SM, Wright RG, Levinson G, et al. Plasma norepinephrine and uterine blood flow changes during endotracheal intubation and general anesthesia in the pregnant ewe. In: Abstracts of Scientific Papers of the Annual Meeting of the American Society of Anesthesiologists; Chicago, IL; 1978:115.

175. James FM III, Greiss FC Jr, Kemp RA. An evaluation of vasopressor therapy for maternal hypotension during spinal anesthesia. *Anesthesiology* 1970;33:25–34.

176. Shnider SM, de Lorimier AA, Asling JH, Morishima HO. Vasopressors in obstetrics. II. Fetal hazards of methoxamine administration during obstetric spinal anesthesia. *Am J Obstet Gynecol* 1970;106:680–686.

177. Ralston DH, Shnider SM, de Lorimier AA. Effects of equipotent ephedrine, metaraminol, mephentermine and methoxamine on uterine blood flow in the pregnant ewe. *Anesthesiology* 1974;40:354–370.

178. Callender K, Levinson G, Shnider SM, Feduska NJ, Biehl DR, Ring G. Dopamine administration in the normotensive pregnant ewe. *Obstet Gynecol* 1978;51:586–589.

179. Eng M, Berges PU, Ueland K, Bonica JJ, Parer JT. The effects of methoxamine and ephedrine in normotensive pregnant primates. *Anesthesiology* 1971;35:354–360.

180. Greiss FC Jr, Gobble FL Jr. Effect of sympathetic nerve stimulation on the uterine vascular bed. *Am J Obstet Gynecol* 1967;97:962–967.

181. Oates JN, Vasey DP, Waldron BA. Effects of ketamine on the pregnant uterus. *Br J Anaesth* 1979;51:1163–1166.

182. Evans JA, Chastain GM, Philips JM. The use of local anesthetic agents in obstetrics. *South Med J* 1969;62:519–524.

183. Greiss FC Jr, Still JC, Anderson SC. Effects of local anesthetic agents on the uterine vasculatures and myometrium. *Am J Obstet Gynecol* 1976;124:889–899.

184. Amos JD, Schorr SJ, Norman PF. Laparoscopic surgery during pregnancy. *Am J Surg* 1996;171:435–437.

185. Reedy MB, Galan HL, Richards WE, Preece CK, Wetter PA, Kuehl TJ. Laparoscopy during pregnancy: A survey of laparoendoscopic surgeons. *J Reprod Med* 1997;42:33–38.

186. Steinbrook RA, Brooks DC, Datta S. Laparoscopic cholecystectomy during pregnancy: Review of anesthetic management, surgical considerations. *Surg Endosc* 1996;10:511–515.

187. Constantino GN, Vincent GJ, Mucalian GG, Kliefoth WL Jr. Laparoscopic cholecystectomy in pregnancy. *J Laparoendosc Surg* 1994;4:161–164.

188. Reedy MB, Källén B, Kuehl TJ. Laparoscopy during pregnancy: A study of five fetal outcome parameters with the use of the Swedish Health Registry. *Am J Obstet Gynecol* 1997;177:673–679.

189. Curet MJ, Allen D, Josloff RK, et al. Laparoscopy during pregnancy. *Arch Surg* 1996;131:546–551.

190. Bhavani-Shankar K, Steinbrook RA, Mushlin PS, Freiberger D. Transcutaneous PCO_2 monitoring during laparoscopic cholecystectomy in pregnancy. *Can J Anaesth* 1998;45:164–169.

191. Hart RO, Tamadon A, Fitzgibbons RJ, Fleming A. Open laparoscopic cholecystectomy in pregnancy. *Surg Laparosc Endosc* 1993;3:13–16.

Shnider and Levinson's Anesthesia for Obstetrics,
edited by Samuel C. Hughes, et al.
Lippincott Williams & Wilkins,
Philadelphia, © 2001.

CHAPTER 14

ANESTHESIA FOR FETAL PROCEDURES AND SURGERY

MARK A. ROSEN, M. D.

The Fetal Treatment Center at the University of California San Francisco (UCSF) performed the first surgery on a human fetus in 1981, on a fetus at 21 weeks of gestation with bilateral urinary obstruction due to a posterior urethral valve. We have performed extensive animal experimentation (numerous procedures on rabbits, approximately 2000 procedures on pregnant sheep, and over 500 fetal surgical procedures on pregnant monkeys) to establish the pathophysiology of a variety of fetal disease processes, and the feasibility of in utero intervention for improved outcome. In the past 2 decades, the multidisciplinary team at UCSF has pioneered substantial advances, improvements, and refinements in clinical criteria for surgical candidate selection, and techniques for surgical and anesthetic management (1). However, the goal has always focused on improving neonatal outcome without compromising maternal safety. The Center has undertaken surgical correction of a variety of congenital malformations that, if untreated, would lead to fetal or neonatal demise or significant postnatal morbidity. Between 1981 and 2000, we performed over 175 operations on fetuses for a variety of different abnormalities, the most common of which are listed in Table 14.1 (Fig. 14.1).

Fetal treatment originated with Liley's successful intraperitoneal blood transfusion to a fetus affected with erythroblastosis fetalis (2). Poorly documented, unsuccessful attempts were later made to effect complete exchange blood transfusions by directly accessing the fetal circulation with in utero fetal surgery (3). Treatment of fetal lung immaturity to avoid respiratory distress syndrome of prematurity was the next fetal disease treated; treatment consisted of administration of glucocorticoids to the fetus via the mother to increase fetal surfactant production. Subsequently, with improvements in the high resolution of ultrasonography, intravascular (umbilical cord vessels) blood transfusions to fetuses for erythroblastosis fetalis replaced the intraperitoneal technique. Diagnosis of many other fetal disorders by sonography, fetal echocardiography, fetoscopy, chorionic villous sampling, amniocentesis, and fetal blood sampling (cordocentesis) led to the use of other in utero therapeutic interventions such as placement of a percutaneous vesicoamniotic shunt for bilateral hydronephrosis. Additionally, a variety of techniques were performed for selective termination of an abnormal twin fetus, including hysterotomy (sectio parva) for monochorionic twins with reversed arterial perfusion sequence (e.g. acardiac/anencephalic twin). Further developments in fetal diagnosis, including single-shot rapid acquisition magnetic resonance imaging (MRI) (4) continue to improve our knowledge of the fetus, fetal and placental abnormalities, and the intrauterine environment.

Despite more than two decades of experience, fetal therapy, and particularly fetal surgery, remains a new field of medicine. The majority of fetal therapy procedures consist of relatively noninvasive fetal treatments such as administration of medications, hormones, or blood. The compelling rationale for prenatal correction of certain anatomic defects led to the development of the Fetal Treatment Center at UCSF. Success in these endeavors relies on a multidisciplinary team consisting of obstetricians, perinatologists, geneticists, sonologists, pediatric (fetal) surgeons, anesthesiologists, neonatologists, specialized nurses, social workers, and many other support personnel, who meet weekly to discuss fetal cases referred to the Center. Fetal surgery via hysterotomy (5) or endoscopy (6) requires special attention to the management of anesthesia for both mother and fetus, and intraoperative fetal monitoring for successful outcome.

With the continued improvements in technique and technical improvement in instrumentation, the future of fetal therapy includes the possibility of correcting an increasing variety of anatomic malformations and treating other prenatally diagnosed fetal diseases, including genetic disorders. Liley wrote, "For a variety of disorders, the physician and the parents are no longer helplessly dependent on what time, luck, and intrauterine life present with at birth. . . . Some day, for a wider range of fetal illness, we may be able to offer a brighter prospect than the present dismal alternatives of neonatal death, abnormality, or abortion" (7).

Advances in technology affecting fertilization, embryo transfer, and various types of fetal treatment continue to receive widespread attention within the scientific community, as well as the popular news media. At the core of this interest is a change in our perception of the fetus as secluded from medical treatment, to recognition of the fetus as a patient, an individual for whom medical treatment has become possible. Improvements in the diagnostic capabilities of high-resolution ultrasonography, MRI, computed tomography, fetoscopy, and cytogenetic and biochemical testing of amniotic fluid have increased our ability to recognize and delineate more precisely fetal anatomy and anomalies.

THERAPEUTIC ALTERNATIVES FOR FETAL MANAGEMENT

Only certain fetal anomalies are amenable to in utero intervention to achieve improved outcome. Most correctable malformations diagnosed in utero are best managed by appropriate medical and surgical therapy after delivery at term; some examples are listed in Table 14.2. Although a diagnosis of correctable malformation may not suggest a therapeutic alternative, it does provide time to coordinate appropriate prenatal and postnatal care, including transportation of the fetus to a medical center while in utero rather than as a newly delivered, fragile neonate. Prenatal diagnosis of serious malformations that are neither correctable nor compatible with normal postnatal life provides the choice of terminating the pregnancy (Table 14.3).

Examples of fetal malformations that may benefit from intervention in utero include deficiencies in pulmonary surfactant, anemia caused by erythroblastosis, hypothyroidism, other nutritional and metabolic deficiencies, and inherited defects potentially curable by stem cell transplantation (Table 14.4) (8–10). However, correction of an anatomic malformation in utero can be technically more difficult than providing a missing substrate, hormone, medication, or stem cell transplantation to the fetus.

Certain malformations may influence the timing of delivery, particularly when early correction of the malformation can help minimize progressive impairment (Table 14.5). In these cases, the abnormality becomes more severe with continued gestation.

Table 14.1. FETAL SURGICAL PROCEDURES AT UNIVERSITY OF CALIFORNIA SAN FRANCISCO

Congenital diaphramatic hernia
Congenital cystic adenomatoid malformation
Urinary tract obstruction
Sacrococcygeal teratoma
Twin-twin transfusion syndrome
Selective termination (acardiac/acephalic twin)
Fetal heart block (pacemaker insertion)
Myelomeningocele

Table 14.2. FETAL MALFORMATIONS DETECTABLE IN UTERO BUT BEST CORRECTED AFTER DELIVERY AT TERM

Esophageal, duodenal, jejunoileal, and anorectal atresias
Meconium ileus (cystic fibrosis)
Enteric cysts and duplications
Small intact omphalocele
Small intact meningocele, myelomeningocele, and spina bifida
Unilateral hydronephrosis
Craniofacial, extremity, and chest wall deformities
Cystic hygroma
Small sacrococcygeal teratoma
Benign cysts: e.g., ovarian, mesenteric

Modified from Harrison MR. The rationale for fetal treatment: Selection, feasibility, and risk. In Harrison MR, Evans MI, Adzick NS, Holzgreve W, eds. The Unborn Patient—The Art and Science of Fetal Therapy. 3rd ed. Philadelphia: WB Saunders, 2001:40.

Table 14.3. FETAL MALFORMATIONS OFTEN MANAGED BY SELECTIVE ABORTION

Anencephaly, porencephaly, encephalocele, and giant hydrocephalus
Severe anomalies associated with chromosomal abnormalities
    (e.g., trisomy 13, trisomy 18)
Renal agencies or bilateral polycystic kidney disease
Inherited, nontreatable chromosomal, metabolic, and hematologic
    abnormalities (e.g., Tay-Sachs disease)
Lethal bone dysplasias (e.g., recessive osteogenesis imperfecta)

Modified from Harrison MR. The rationale for fetal treatment: Selection, feasibility, and risk. In Harrison MR, Evans MI, Adzick NS, Holzgreve W, eds. The Unborn Patient—The Art and Science of Fetal Therapy. 3rd ed. Philadelphia: WB Saunders, 2001:40.

Table 14.4. FETAL DEFICIENCIES AND MALFUNCTIONS THAT MAY BENEFIT FROM MEDICAL TREATMENT IN UTERO

Deficient pulmonary surfactant
Anemia
Endocrine deficiency (hypothyroidism, goiter, adrenal hyperplasia)
Metabolic block (B_{12}-dependent methylmalonic acidemia,
    biotin-dependent multiple carboxylase deficiency)
Nutritional deficiency (intrauterine growth retardation)
Cardiac arrhythmias
Inherited defects potentially curable by stem cell transplantation

Modified from Harrison MR. The rationale for fetal treatment: Selection, feasibility, and risk. In Harrison MR, Evans MI, Adzick NS, Holzgreve W, eds. The Unborn Patient—The Art and Science of Fetal Therapy. 3rd ed. Philadelphia: WB Saunders, 2001:42.

Table 14.5. FETAL MALFORMATIONS THAT MAY BENEFIT FROM INDUCED PRETERM DELIVERY FOR EARLY NEONATAL CORRECTION

Obstructive hydrocephalus
Obstructive hydronephrosis
Amniotic band malformations
Gastroschisis or ruptured omphalocele
Intestinal volvulus and meconium ileus causing intestinal
    ischemia and/or necrosis
Hydrops fetalis
Intrauterine growth retardation
Arrhythmias causing cardiac failure

Modified from Harrison MR. The rationale for fetal treatment: Selection, feasibility, and risk. In Harrison MR, Evans MI, Adzick NS, Holzgreve W, eds. The Unborn Patient—The Art and Science of Fetal Therapy. 3rd ed. Philadelphia: WB Saunders, 2001:41.

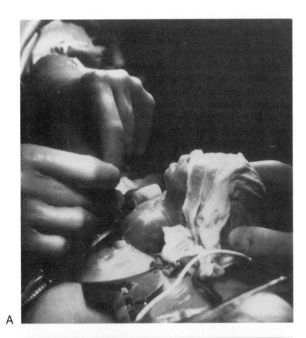

A

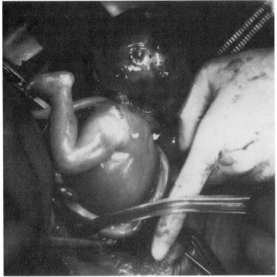

B

Figure 14.1. Surgical exposure of fetus. *A*: The fetal upper torso extrudes from the uterus. A temporary tracheal occlusion procedure is being performed on a fetus with severe congenital diaphragmatic hernia and liver herniation at 26 weeks of gestation. *B*: The lower fetal torso with a large sacrococcygeal teratoma is exposed by hysterotomy. The umbilical cord is not disturbed. This large teratoma is being excised from this 24-week fetus. The tumor is dark and mottled because the blood supply has been occluded by a tourniquet around its base before resection. (Modified with permission from Harrison MR. Fetal surgery. *Am J Obstet Gynecol* 1996;174:1255–1264.)

Table 14.6. FETAL MALFORMATIONS THAT MAY REQUIRE CESAREAN DELIVERY

Conjoined twins
Giant omphalocele or gastroschisis
Large hydrocephalus, sacrococcygeal teratoma, cystic
  hygroma, meningomyelocele
Malformations requiring preterm delivery when labor is
  inadequate or in the presence of fetal distress

Modified from Harrison MR. The rationale for fetal treatment:
Selection, feasibility, and risk. In Harrison MR, Evans MI, Adzick NS,
Holzgreve W, eds. The Unborn Patient—The Art and Science of Fetal
Therapy. 3rd ed. Philadelphia: WB Saunders, 2001:41.

However, the risks of prematurity with preterm delivery must be
evaluated against the risks of continued gestation. Elective cesarean delivery is appropriate for fetal malformations that cause
dystocia but are correctable after delivery (Table 14.6). It is also
appropriate when the fetal abnormality requires preterm delivery and adequate labor cannot be induced or cannot be tolerated by the fetus.

RATIONALE FOR INVASIVE INTRAUTERINE FETAL THERAPY

Intrauterine intervention has become a reasonable therapeutic alternative for certain correctable fetal abnormalities with
predictable, life-threatening developmental consequences. Fetal surgery is reasonable when it would provide a more successful outcome than therapy after birth, and the fetal or neonatal
outcome without therapy was significant enough to justify the
risk of surgery for the mother. Examples include congenital diaphragmatic hernia, congenital bilateral hydronephrosis, and
cystic pulmonary adenomatoid malformations associated with
hydrops, correction of which may prevent irreversible organ
damage or fetal demise. Prenatal correction of malformations
that cause high- or low-output cardiac failure, such as complete
heart block, large sacrococcygeal teratomas, or twin-twin transfusion syndromes, also may prevent fetal demise. Nonimmune hydrops fetalis due to fetal thoracic lesions (congenital cystic adenomatoid malformation, pulmonary sequestration, fetal pleural
effusion, and pericardial teratomas) and sacrococcygeal teratoma have a very poor prognosis, and often require rather immediate intervention to salvage the fetus (Table 14.7) (11, 12).

Table 14.7. ANATOMIC MALFORMATIONS THAT MAY BENEFIT FROM PRENATAL SURGICAL CORRECTION, CURRENTLY OR IN THE FUTURE

Bilateral obstructive hydronephrosis
Diaphragmatic hernia
Tracheal atresia-stenosis
Congenital cystic pulmonary adenomatoid malformation
Obstructive hydrocephalus
Cardiac abnormalities (particularly those that interfere with
  development, such as pulmonary-aortic obstuction)
Sacrococcygeal teratoma
Complete heart block
Neural tube defects
Skeletal abnormalities
Craniosynostosis
Cleft lip and palate
Twin-twin transfusion syndromes
Meningomyelocele

Modified from Harrison MR. The rationale for fetal treatment:
Selection, feasibility, and risk. In Harrison MR, Evans MI, Adzick NS,
Holzgreve W, eds. The Unborn Patient—The Art and Science of Fetal
Therapy. 3rd ed. Philadelphia: WB Saunders, 2001:43.

Before invasive therapy is considered, the natural history of
the malformations must be known, including the pathophysiology and prognosis. Furthermore, the lesion must be correctable
or palliative with a feasible technique that has a predictable outcome. The fetus must be evaluated thoroughly to ensure an accurate diagnosis has been made, to assess the severity of the lesion,
and to ensure the absence of associated congenital anomalies
that would contraindicate invasive management.

To appreciate some of the developments that have taken
place to date, it is illustrative to consider one malformation and
follow the approaches undertaken for its correction. **Congenital
diaphragmatic hernia** (CDH) occurs about 1 in 2400 births and
is characterized by herniation of abdominal contents into a
hemithorax, usually the left. When this occurs early in gestation,
it prevents normal lung development and leads to pulmonary
hypoplasia, pulmonary hypertension, and hypoxia at birth
with a poor prognosis. Data gathered by the Fetal Treatment
Center suggest that the mortality of CDH diagnosed before
25 weeks of gestation is about 60% even when those neonates
receive optimal postnatal support, including extracorporeal
membrane oxygenation (13).

Experimental work began with animal models. At first a fetal
lamb model was used to demonstrate technical feasibility and
physiologic soundness of the approach (14). However, the biology of gestation in sheep is quite different from humans and the
sheep uterus is very quiescent (i.e., not susceptible to preterm
labor or abortion following hysterotomy) and could not be used
to determine the safety and applicability of fetal intervention in
humans. Therefore, we investigated a primate model because
the primate uterus is very susceptible to both preterm labor and
late-gestation fetal loss after intervention (15).

The rhesus monkey has a similar spontaneous rate of preterm
labor and fetal loss as humans. In early experiments, it was noted
that halothane provided excellent uterine relaxation as well as
anesthesia for the pregnant monkey (16). This was confirmed
in subsequent primate experiments (17) and established the
primary anesthetic approach still used today, relying on volatile
agents to provide maternal and fetal anesthesia, as well as the
intense uterine relaxation required for in utero surgery.

The first step in addressing the problem of CDH was to
identify the pathophysiology of the disease. Fetal lambs had
balloons inflated in a hemithorax at various times during gestation. Fetal outcome resembled human CDH, with pulmonary
hypoplasia, pulmonary vascular changes similar to the changes
seen with persistent fetal circulation, and poor survival (14).
Deflation of the balloons prior to term led to improved survival
and histologic changes demonstrating catch-up growth and
development (18, 19).

The next step was to demonstrate the practicality of performing fetal surgery. Experimental creation of a diaphragmatic hernia in fetal lambs at midgestation consistently resulted
in pulmonary hypoplasia at term gestation. A second operation 20 days later to correct the lesion was performed. Lessons
were learned about intraabdominal and intrathoracic pressure
changes that affected fetal outcome. The increased fetal intraabdominal pressure compromised blood flow through the ductus
venosus, leading to fetal death. The technique was therefore
modified to include placement of an abdominal silo for the intestinal contents (similar to a gastroschisis repair); the evacuated
hemithorax was filled with fluid to prevent mediastinal shift after repair. After making these adjustments, survival improved,
demonstrating the feasibility of fetal surgery (20). These techniques were later applied to human operations (21–23).

CONGENITAL DIAPHRAGMATIC HERNIA: HUMAN RESULTS

The extensive animal work led to the development of a surgical approach that became a standard for our patients. This approach involved complete repair of the fetal defect through an

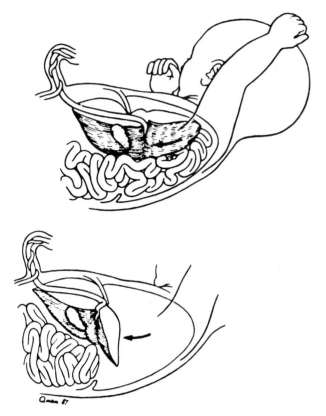

Figure 14.2. Attempts to reduce the herniated fetal liver (*arrows*) cause fetal deterioration and demise; autopsy and angiogram studies have documented kinking of the umbilical vein with compromise of venous return. (Reprinted by permission from Harrison MR, Langer JC, Adzick NS, et al. Correction of congenital diaphragmatic hernia in utero. V. Initial clinical experience. *J Pediatr Surg* 1990;25:47–57.)

open uterus, reducing the herniated abdominal contents out of the hemithorax, grafting a closure of the defective or absent diaphragm, and closing the abdominal wall with a silo to prevent increased intraabdominal pressure that could interfere with ductus venous blood flow. The initial experiences with human fetuses demonstrated no maternal mortality and no apparent effect on future maternal reproductive potential. However, there was a high incidence of preterm labor, and most significantly, if the fetal liver had herniated into the thorax early in gestation, the fetal surgical repair was nearly impossible. Manipulation of the liver, necessary for reduction of the liver into the abdomen, occluded the umbilical venous return to the fetus, leading to decreased cardiac output, bradycardia, and measurable fetal oxygen desaturation (Fig. 14.2) (21, 24, 25).

Having established that the diagnosis of CDH before 25 weeks was associated with a worse prognosis, and that liver herniation made the repair nearly impossible, the question of selection criteria became very important (26). There are certainly neonates with CDH who do well after birth and require minimal support, presumably reflecting late bowel herniation and relatively normal pulmonary development. On the other hand, it became apparent from the fetal surgery experience that if the fetal liver had herniated into the thorax early in gestation, the fetal surgical repair was nearly impossible.

We conducted a National Institutes of Health (NIH) trial for fetuses with CDH without herniated livers, and demonstrated the safety and technical feasibility of the treatment, but with no difference in neonatal outcome, making the additional risk to the mother and fetus inappropriate (27). A retrospective analysis noted a correlation of the ratio between the lung-to-head size, lung-to-head ratio (LHR), made sonographically, with postnatal

survival (28). The LHR was corroborated in a prospective trial, predicting survival among fetuses with left-sided congenital diaphragmatic hernias (29). It became apparent that open uterine correction of fetal CDH was not feasible for the fetuses in whom it could provide the most benefit (the most severe), and did not improve neonatal outcome among fetuses in whom the surgery was feasible (the less severe). In addition, a retrospective study revealed that fetuses with CDH and liver herniation into the hemithorax have a much worse prognosis than similarly afflicted fetuses without liver herniation (30).

TRACHEAL OCCLUSION

The fetal lung produces fluid that normally passes out the trachea into the amniotic fluid. Experimental animal work demonstrated that if the lung fluid was drained, pulmonary hypoplasia resulted, and if the trachea was occluded, the fluid accumulated, accelerating lung growth and pulmonary hyperplasia (31–36). Experimental work at the Fetal Treatment Center corroborated these findings, utilizing both intratracheal and external tracheal occlusion devices (37, 38). Experimental animal studies suggest that fetal lung growth after tracheal ligation is not solely a pressure phenomenon, but humoral factors present in lung fluid play a role in the exaggerated lung growth (39). Additionally, animal studies suggest blood flow velocity in the pulmonary artery, significantly reduced with pulmonary hypoplasia, is normalized by fetal tracheal occlusion and results in normal fetal physiologic response to changes in oxygen tension at term gestation (40).

This knowledge and experimentation offered the Fetal Treatment Center an alternative approach for intervention in the fetus with poor prognosis (liver herniation and low LHR) (Fig. 14.3). Initially, for human fetal surgery, an intratracheal plug was used. However, one fetus developed tracheomalacia, and another fetal trachea was incompletely occluded. Subsequent patients received external spring-loaded aneurysm clips placed on the trachea, but these were associated with problems as well, including damage to the trachea and, rarely, damage to the recurrent laryngeal nerves (6, 41). Currently, we use a detachable balloon, placed in the trachea for complete occlusion. We are currently conducting an NIH-sponsored, randomized trial of intratracheal balloon placement compared with postnatal therapy.

Concurrent with abandoning the open uterine approach for direct CDH repair, there was a desire to decrease the invasiveness of fetal surgery and reduce potential maternal morbidity, which led to the development of endoscopic techniques to avoid open hysterotomy (42). Less invasive techniques appear to be associated with less uterine irritability and less preterm labor. Most of our procedures are now performed endoscopically through the uterus, after a small maternal laparotomy incision is made. Minimal uterine invasiveness may also decrease the concentration of drugs needed for uterine relaxation intraoperatively, decreasing the likelihood of maternal hypotension and decreasing the potential for adverse fetal impact.

EXIT PROCEDURE

At birth, tracheal occlusion poses an obvious problem for the fetus. The occluding device must be removed before tracheoscopy and bronchoscopy are performed to inspect the trachea, and resuscitation can proceed. Endotracheal intubation is performed under controlled circumstances, and surfactant is often administered. To allow the time that these procedures require while uteroplacental gas exchange is preserved, a surgical and anesthetic modification of a general anesthetic approach to cesarean section was adopted, the ex utero intrapartum treatment (EXIT) procedure (43, 44).

Hysterotomy is made with a stapling devise developed at UCSF, to ensure uterine hemostasis during fetal manipulation

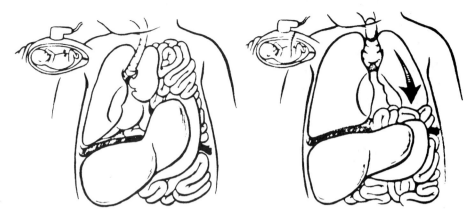

Figure 14.3. Anatomic depiction of the sonographic findings of fetuses whose lungs enlarge after tracheal obstruction. Before repair (*left*), the lobe of the liver, stomach, and intestines fill the left chest. Little change is seen in the first week after occlusion, but over the next several weeks (*right*), the lungs gradually enlarge, partially reducing the viscera out of the chest and shifting the mediastinum back toward its normal midline position. The trachea becomes dilated below the obstruction. (Modified with permission from Harrison MR, Adzick NS, Flake AW, et al. Correction of congenital diaphragmatic hernia in utero. VIII. Response of the hypoplastic lung to tracheal occlusion. *J Pediatr Surg* 1996;31:1339–1348.)

(U.S. Surgical Corporation, Norwalk, CT) (45). The deep inhaled halogenated anesthetic technique provides the necessary uterine relaxation, despite uterine incision, and partial or full delivery of the fetus. This is crucial to prevent placental disruption from the endometrium, maintaining placental perfusion and oxygenation of the fetus while the surgeon secures the fetal airway. Unlike the typical cesarean delivery, there is no attempt to limit induction of anesthesia to delivery time; rather, anesthesia is induced well in advance to ensure adequate concentrations of inhalational anesthetic for surgical tocolysis. Careful maintenance of maternal mean arterial pressure with fluids and ephedrine is necessary to avoid fetal compromise.

Nitroglycerin boluses (50 to 100 μg) are used if supplemental uterine relaxation is required. Nitric oxide donor agents have long been known to provide uterine relaxation (46). Obstetric anesthesiologists previously used inhaled amyl nitrate for acute relaxation. Nitric oxide donor agents similar to nitroglycerin provide potent tocolysis in nonhuman primates (47). In the past decade, obstetric anesthesiologists rediscovered nitric oxide donor agents. Nitroglycerin has been reported to provide uterine relaxation in clinical cases of delivery of an entrapped fetal head during vaginal breech delivery, at cesarean section, for breech extraction, for manual removal of a retained placenta, for reduction of a prolapsed (inverted) uterus, and for external version, among others (48–54). Despite the compelling clinical experience, the mechanism of action for uterine relaxation is unclear (increased uterine compliance vs. decrease in uterine contractile force), and the mechanism actually may be independent of nitric oxide (55). For other obstetric indications such as uterine hyperstimulation in labor (not fetal surgery), we use the sublingual spray as a readily available, convenient method of nitroglycerin administration.

We administer intramuscular (IM) pancuronium and fentanyl to the fetus, and monitor the fetus by placement of a pulse oximeter probe on the fetal hand. Subsequently, after the fetal airway is secured with an endotracheal tube, surfactant administered (when indicated), and ventilation through the tracheal tube results in an increasing oxygen saturation, the umbilical cord is clamped. After the cord is clamped, the maternal anesthetic is revised to a primarily opioid/nitrous oxide anesthetic, with oxytocin administration to facilitate the increased uterine tone and avoid postpartum hemorrhage. The average blood loss for EXIT procedures has not exceeded average blood loss for routine cesarean sections at UCSF. We have also managed the mother's anesthetic after the cord is clamped by activating a previously placed epidural catheter for surgical anesthesia, and used it to provide postoperative epidural analgesia.

The EXIT procedure has also been employed by our group and others for fetuses that have a predictably compromised airway, such as an obstructing mass (cystic hygroma, cervical teratoma, hemangioma, large thyroid goiter), that would benefit from careful inspection and tracheal intubation or tracheostomy at the time of birth (56–63). This technique has now been used for removal of tracheal clips by other groups (62). We have used the EXIT procedure to perform an intrapartum fetal thoracotomy and removal of a large chest mass (congenital cystic adenomatoid malformation). Using this technique, we have safely maintained fetal well-being and operating conditions for more than 2 hours. The fetal safety of this technique is apparent by monitoring the fetal oxygen saturation and heart rate, and by obtaining normal cord blood gases immediately after the cord is clamped. Another group reports improved outcome from "fetal stabilization" for antenatally diagnosed diaphragmatic hernia patients, with fetal "anesthetization" before airway management decreasing the incidence of persistent pulmonary hypertension and improving the survival rate of patients with severe CDH (64).

OTHER CORRECTABLE FETAL ABNORMALITIES

Malformations other than CDH are also treated, both clinically and experimentally (65). This includes congenital cystic adenomatoid malformations, sacrococcygeal teratomas, congenital bilateral hydronephrosis, twin-twin transfusion syndromes (66), and congenital heart diseases (67, 68). Correction of these anatomic malformations in utero may prevent irreversible organ damage. Malformations that cause high- or low-output cardiac failure such as complete heart block, twin-twin transfusion syndromes, large sacrococcygeal teratomas, and structural cardiac defects may benefit from prenatal correction. Intervention is useful for selective delivery (sectio parva) of an abnormal twin that jeopardizes the well-being of the normal twin, such as an acardiac, anencephalic fetus that places the normal twin at risk of a high-output cardiac failure (69). For the twin-twin transfusion syndrome, in which a shared placental circulation can be devastating to both twins, laser surgical photocoagulation of the communicating circulation may allow survival of one or both twins who are otherwise fated to succumb (70–71).

Congenital bilateral hydronephrosis caused by urethral obstruction (most often by posterior urethral valves in male fetuses) is another example of an anatomically simple lesion with potentially devastating consequences for the developing fetus if uncorrected before birth (Fig. 14.4) (73–80). Hydronephrosis can be detected relatively early because fluid-filled masses are particularly easy to detect with sonography and because the associated decreased fetal urine output results in oligohydramnios, a common obstetric indication for sonography.

Persistent urinary tract obstruction impairs fetal renal development, with the severity of parenchymal damage dependent on the degree and duration of obstruction. The resulting oligohydramnios caused by fetal urinary tract obstruction is associated with pulmonary hypoplasia, and skeletal, facial,

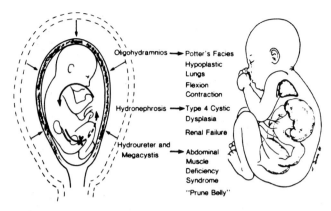

Figure 14.4. Developmental consequences of fetal urethral obstruction, with obstructed fetal urinary flow, hydronephrosis, hydroureter, megacystis, and oligohydramnios. (Reprinted with permission from Harrison MR, Filly RA, Parer JT, et al. Management of the fetus with a urinary tract malformation. *JAMA* 1981;246:635–639.)

and abdominal wall deformities. Severe hypoplasia may prevent neonatal survival.

Preterm delivery of the fetus allows for early urinary tract decompression ex utero; however, fetal pulmonary immaturity limits the efficacy of this approach. Physiologically, the ideal therapy is early decompression of the urinary tract with continued gestation in utero. Vesicoamniotic catheters allow urine to drain from the bladder into the amniotic fluid, thereby decompressing the urinary tract and allowing for continued fetal renal and pulmonary development. It may also restore normal amniotic fluid dynamics and prevent the occurrence of the severe sequelae of oligohydramnios. However, these catheters have frequent problems, including difficulty with percutaneous placement, occlusion, and in utero displacement.

Our clinical series in which fetal vesicostomy was performed via hysterotomy to decompress the fetal obstructive uropathy (bladder marsupialization or bilateral ureterostomies) confirms that development of fatal pulmonary hypoplasia can be prevented if amniotic fluid dynamics are restored, and that relief of the obstruction may obviate further renal damage, allowing nephrogenesis to proceed normally. However, detection before the occurrence of irreversible renal damage remains problematic (81, 82).

Fetal surgery has potentially unique advantages. The intrauterine environment supports rapid wound healing (without scarring before midgestation), and the umbilical circulation can provide the nutritional and respiratory fetal requirements. The immature fetal immune system may facilitate certain invasive procedures. Other potentially correctable defects include certain cardiac abnormalities, gastroschisis, cleft lip (83), cleft palate (84–86), craniofacial and craniosynostosis abnormalities (87, 88), as well as skeletal anomalies correctable by allogenic bone grafting (89, 90). Treatment of these anomalies is under investigation in animal models, including assessment of techniques for extracorporeal circulation in fetal lambs (91).

Until recently, only life-threatening malformations were considered for fetal treatment. With improvement in techniques and the introduction of less invasive techniques, application of fetal intervention for nonfatal fetal lesions is currently being undertaken, such as myelomeningocele, in which the goals are preventing or ameliorating the associated neurologic deficits and hydrocephalus. Early results of nonrandomized studies suggest that intrauterine repair decreases the incidence of hindbrain herniation and shunt-dependent hydrocephalus in infants with spina bifida, but increases the incidence of preterm delivery, and does not decrease the incidence of paraparesis or urinary incontinence (92–96). Some question whether myelomeningocele is ready to take its place as a legitimate indication for fetal surgery

until there is evidence of greater success in neonatal outcome, and fewer obstetric complications (Table 14.7) (97).

RISKS OF FETAL SURGERY

Fetal surgery has risks. These risks include those common to all surgical procedures, such as infection, blood loss, and the risk of blood transfusion. One unique consideration is the potential impact of procedures on future reproductive capabilities for the mother. Studies on nonhuman primates after fetal surgery indicate no decrease in fertility or increase in pregnancy loss in mothers who previously underwent fetal surgical procedures (15). For human fetal surgery, we have had no maternal deaths, but a few serious complications, and morbidity related to preterm labor and its management, including pulmonary edema (98).

Because fetal surgery takes place around midgestation, hysterotomy is not in the lower uterine segment, and delivery after fetal surgery and all future pregnancies must be by cesarean section. For endoscopic procedures, this may not be required. A few patients had uterine scar disruptions when labor progressed before the planned cesarean section was performed (in all circumstances, maternal and neonatal outcomes were excellent). Scar dehiscence is now rare, with improved techniques of opening and closing the uterus. However, amniotic fluid leaks, premature rupture of membranes, and chorioamniotic membrane separation (99) occur with a relatively high incidence. Fortunately, the ability to carry and deliver subsequent pregnancies does not appear to be jeopardized by fetal surgery (100).

Fetal surgery does not appear to place surviving neonates at a greater risk of poor outcome beyond those already identified related to prematurity and lung disease (101). The incidence and spectrum of neurologic injury to the fetus after open fetal surgery was 7 of 33 patients. The major abnormalities identified were periventricular hemorrhage, intraventricular hemorrhage, and periventricular leukomalacia. These injuries were most likely related to sudden changes in cerebral blood flow induced by the fetal surgical procedure itself (causing fetal bradycardia or hypotension), by maternal hemodynamic changes, changes in maternal oxygenation, administration of tocolytic drugs, or neonatal changes in hemodynamics or ventilation (102). Studies of the neurodevelopmental outcome of surviving newborns after open fetal surgeries revealed that many children have a favorable outcome. However, those fetuses with the most tenuous medical status had the most developmental delays; those that required intensive postnatal care, experienced intracranial hemorrhage, or required prolonged respiratory support had a worse neurologic and developmental prognosis.

ANESTHETIC CONSIDERATIONS

Many of the anesthetic considerations for fetal procedures and surgery are identical to those for nonobstetric surgery during pregnancy (Table 14.8). They include concern for maternal safety, avoidance of teratogenic drugs and fetal asphyxia, and

---

Table 14.8. ANESTHETIC CONSIDERATIONS FOR FETAL SURGERY

Basic objectives for pregnant women undergoing surgery
    Maternal safety
    Avoidance of teratogenic drugs
    Avoidance of intrauterine fetal asphyxia
    Prevention of preterm labor
Objectives unique to fetal surgery
    Fetal anesthesia and amnesia
    Increased requirement for fetal monitoring
    Increased likelihood of preterm labor
    Uterine relaxation for surgical exposure

prevention of preterm delivery. The anesthesiologist must be familiar with the alterations in physiology induced by pregnancy and their clinical anesthetic implications. These basic considerations are extremely important, and recently have been reviewed (54) and are discussed in Chapters 1 and 13.

Providing anesthesia for hysterotomy and fetal intervention poses unique challenges related to providing care for two patients, mother and fetus, and providing "surgical tocolysis." Fetal surgery is distinguished from other nonobstetric surgeries performed during pregnancy by an increased concern for fetal anesthesia and fetal monitoring, a significantly greater likelihood of intra- or postoperative preterm labor, and often the requirement for intense uterine relaxation ("surgical tocolysis") to safely accommodate surgical exposure through a hysterotomy.

For the minimally invasive fetoscopic procedures, particularly those that do not involve surgery on the fetus (including those that involve surgery on the placenta, e.g., twin-twin transfusion syndrome), the goals and anesthetic requirements are more basic. From nonhuman primate experiments, we know that preterm labor and subsequent delivery is minimal for those animals that underwent procedures with minimal uterine manipulation compared with those that underwent hysterotomy. Furthermore, halogenated anesthetic agents were very effective in halting the uterine electromyographic activity associated with increases in intraamniotic pressure seen on emergence from anesthesia, whereas ritodrine infusions or indomethacin were not effective (103).

Unlike maternal surgery, during fetal procedures, the fetus is not an innocent bystander for whom we attempt the least anesthetic interference. Instead, the fetus can be the primary patient and may benefit from anesthesia, with close monitoring of anesthetic effects to ensure well-being.

For many percutaneous procedures, such as fetal blood sampling or intrauterine blood transfusion, local anesthetic infiltration of the maternal abdominal wall or regional anesthesia can be sufficient. When intravenous (IV) sedation and anxiolysis are required, opioids and benzodiazepines can be safely administered. We routinely administer supplemental oxygen during procedures involving IV sedation and have "standby" readiness for rapid intervention for fetal distress (i.e., induction of general anesthesia for emergency cesarean section) if the fetus is at a viable gestational age. Mothers fast overnight, receive an oral antacid before the procedure, and are monitored in a fashion suitable for general anesthetic administration. We use incremental doses of IV midazolam (0.5 mg) and/or fentanyl (25 μg) and/or low-dose propofol infusions to achieve the desired level of conscious sedation.

More invasive fetal treatments that do not involve hysterotomy, such as minimally invasive fetoscopy, placement of vesicoamniotic or thoracoamniotic shunt catheters, or percutaneous endoscopic laser ablation of placental vessels, involve procedures similar to those for intrauterine blood transfusion (Fig. 14.5) (104, 105). Despite sonographic guidance, however, larger-sized needles or catheters and multiple placement attempts can be required. Adequate maternal anesthesia may be obtained with local anesthetic infiltration of the maternal abdomen, and the fetus may be sedated via placental transfer of drugs administered to the mother (including opioids and benzodiazepines). However, infiltration of the maternal abdomen with local anesthetic may be unsatisfactory for maternal comfort when needle placement requires multiple attempts. We have successfully used spinal, epidural, or general anesthetic technique as an alternative. In addition, it is important to consider the potential for fetal analgesic requirements and immobility.

Fetal sedation by placental transfer of maternally administered medication does not ensure an anesthetized or immobile fetus. Excessive fetal activity may render the procedure technically difficult, infeasible, or unsafe for the fetus. Fetal movement can be dangerous to the fetus because displacement of a needle or catheter may lead to bleeding, trauma, or compromise of the

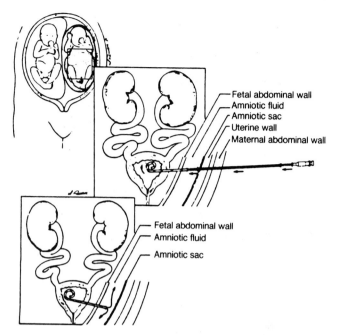

Figure 14.5. Shunt catheter placement for decompression of obstructed fetal urinary bladder. The catheter is pushed off the introducer needle so as to leave one end of the catheter in the fetal bladder and the other in the amniotic cavity. (Modified with permission from Harrison MR, Golbus MS, Filly RA, Nakayama DK, deLorimier AA. Fetal surgical treatment. *Pediatr Ann* 1982;11:896–903.)

umbilical circulation. When fetal movement and/or analgesia is not controlled by placental transfer of maternally administered IV medication, general anesthesia may be used that will anesthetize both mother and fetus. Additionally, fetal anesthesia and control of fetal movement can be safely achieved by direct IM or intravascular administration of opioids and/or neuromuscular blocking agents to the fetus. Pancuronium (0.05 to 0.1 mg · kg^{-1} IV or 0.3 mg · kg^{-1} IM) has been used for fetal paralysis during intravascular transfusions (106–112). We have used either IV or IM pancuronium (0.1 to 0.25 mg · kg^{-1}) for its longer duration and its vagolytic properties, which help maintain fetal heart rate (FHR), or vecuronium in comparable doses, to achieve paralysis of a shorter duration, about 1 to 2 hours (113). If regional anesthesia has been used for the mother, we also administer parenteral opioid (fentanyl) to the fetus in relatively large doses (25 μg · kg^{-1}) to provide analgesia and attenuate or abolish autonomic and stress responses for potentially painful procedures on the fetus.

The subjective phenomenon of pain, and the necessity or benefit of fetal "amnesia" for surgical intervention has not been adequately assessed in the human fetus. The question at what stage of gestation is it possible for the human fetus to be aware of its surroundings and, in particular, to be aware of pain remains unanswered. The answer involves knowledge of neural development and integration of the sensory system in the developing brain and its structures and functions necessary for awareness. There had been widespread belief that the human neonate and fetus were not capable of perceiving pain and that they possessed higher thresholds for nociceptive stimuli. Some theorized that this higher threshold would be adaptive for the pain associated with birth.

Evidence of memories of pain in human neonates is only anecdotal. However, detailed hormonal studies in preterm neonates undergoing surgery under minimal anesthesia revealed the marked release of catecholamines, growth hormone, glucagon, cortisol, aldosterone, and other corticosteroids, and the suppression of insulin secretion (114–116). Furthermore, these

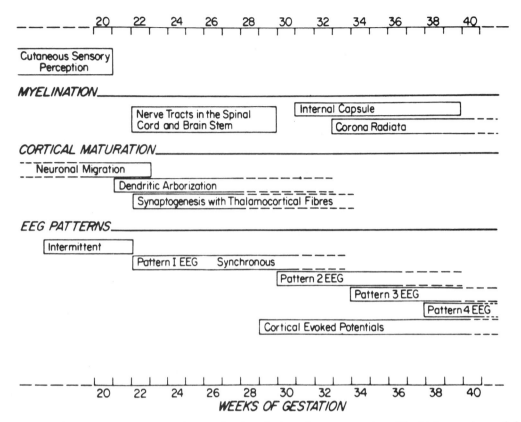

Figure 14.6. Development of cutaneous sensory perception, myelination of pain pathways, maturation of the fetal neocortex, and electroencephalogram patterns in the human fetus and neonate. (Reprinted by permission from Anand KJS, Hickey PR. Pain and its effects in the human neonate and fetus. *N Engl J Med* 1987;317:1321–1329.)

endocrine and metabolic responses to stress are abolished by administering anesthetics to preterm neonates (117). In addition, surgical manipulation of a nonanesthetized fetus results in varying degrees of autonomic nervous system stimulation, variations in heart rate, increased hormonal activity (118), and increased motor activity that can be ablated by anesthesia. Later in gestation, a fetus will respond to environmental stimuli such as noises, light, music, pressure, touch, and cold (119, 120). Information about the development of perceptual mechanisms of pain (Fig. 14.6) and the response of human preterm neonates to pain provides a physiologic rationale to support the philosophic rationale of providing fetal anesthesia (121). Pediatricians are well aware that preterm babies respond to heel sticks, perhaps with a level of response that is less than term gestation babies.

The fetal response to noxious stimuli may represent reflex rather than conscious response at earlier gestational ages. Before thalamic connections exist to the cortex (beginning at about 22 weeks), it seems doubtful that physiologic or pharmacologic responses to noxious stimuli by the fetus involve consciousness. Further, in terms of development, feedback mechanisms to dampen response to noxious stimuli do not fully develop until after 40 weeks of gestation, and some of the ways in which fetal nerve cells work and the spinal cord pathways used may be quite different than adults. However, even reflex response to noxious stimuli may affect sensory development. Perhaps the effect of trauma to the developing nervous system should be avoided. Consequently, along with the requirement for fetal immobility during some procedures, fetal "amnesia" may be an important goal of fetal anesthesia.

For procedures involving hysterotomy or endoscopy (e.g., repair of congenital cystic adenomatoid malformations; diaphragmatic hernia repair or tracheal balloon placement; selective termination of an anencephalic, acardiac, or monochorionic twin; or treatment of twin-twin transfusion syndromes), we use halogenated inhalation anesthetics to produce maternal and

fetal anesthesia and to provide the necessary uterine relaxation for surgery. Prior to inducing general anesthesia, we typically place a lumbar epidural catheter. Except for nonparticulate oral antacids, premedication or adjuvant anesthetic agents are routinely avoided for supplementation of the inhalation agent. This facilitates administration of maximal doses of the halogenated agent, which may be required for uterine relaxation. The dose of the halogenated agent is limited by the stability of the maternal cardiovascular system.

Avoidance of fetal asphyxia is best accomplished by assuring maternal oxygenation and organ perfusion. During fetal surgery, along with high concentrations of inspired halogenated agent, we administer a maximal FIO_2 and maintain adequate maternal blood pressure, sometimes using appropriate vasopressors, to ensure adequate uterine blood flow. Maintaining normal fetal temperature is also important. With fetal exposure, hypothermia can develop quickly. We expose as little of the fetus as possible, and use a system of continuous irrigation with warmed lactated Ringer's solution to prevent fetal hypothermia. For endoscopic techniques, a continuous infusion of a warmed lactated Ringer's solution not only provides thermal stability for the fetus, but it also improves visibility for the surgeons. High volume infusate must be composed of lactated Ringer's solution (not normal saline), because there can be maternal absorption of fluids and electrolytes. Furthermore, the volumes infused and withdrawn, and intraamniotic pressures must be carefully monitored to avoid uterine overdistention.

The hysterotomy is made with a stapling devise, to ensure uterine hemostasis and seal the membranes. The hysterotomy is closed using fibrin glue to create a watertight seal. Amniotic fluid is restored with warm lactated Ringer's solution, with volume assessed by ultrasonography.

During closure of the hysterotomy, magnesium sulfate therapy is administered, initially as a bolus-loading dose (4 to 6 g over 20 minutes), then sustained as a continuous infusion (2 g/h).

After the initial bolus dose of magnesium sulfate is administered, the halogenated agent is discontinued and the epidural catheter is tested and incrementally dosed with local anesthetics in concentrations and volumes appropriate for surgery, and parenteral opioids and nitrous oxide in oxygen are administered. This regimen facilitates tracheal extubation when the mother is fully awake, capable of protecting her airway, is comfortable, and precludes the coughing or straining with extubation that may jeopardize the integrity of the watertight uterine closure.

We provide postoperative analgesia with low concentrations of epidural local anesthetic infusions (with or without opioids) or use IV patient-controlled analgesia devices to administer opioids. This may offer an additional benefit by reducing maternal stress. In the nonhuman primate experiments, stress was a significant factor in amplification of the risk of uterine activity after hysterotomy and fetal surgery (103).

The danger of teratogenic effects from anesthetic drugs poses a potential risk. In genetically susceptible animal species, many of the commonly used anesthetic drugs induce teratogenic effects at specific stages of gestational development (see Chapter 13). In humans, however, no anesthetic agent appears to be safer or more teratogenic than another. However, the human studies have been too few to confirm that anesthetic agents are nonteratogenic, and it is unlikely that such studies could ever be conducted to provide statistically significant results.

Various procedures and techniques may affect fetal physiologic functions. The relationship between these procedures and altered fetal physiology is not precisely understood. For example, uterine incision, fetal manipulation, and anesthetic management each may affect fetal and placental circulation by several mechanisms, sometimes producing fetal compromise. Increased uterine activity, maternal hypotension, maternal hypocarbia, or hyperventilation may interfere with uterine and umbilical blood flow. Fetal manipulation may affect umbilical blood flow by direct compression or by inducing responses that affect fetal circulation.

FETAL CARDIOVASCULAR CIRCULATION

The fetal cardiovascular circulation is adapted for use of the placenta as the organ for oxygen uptake and carbon dioxide elimination. Therefore, it has a large placental blood flow and very small pulmonary blood flow. It is also adapted for existence in a low-oxygen environment and provides the cerebral circulation with blood that has greater oxygen content than that perfusing the lower body. Fetal cardiovascular circulation allows for mixing of blood between the right and left sides of the heart. Approximately one third of the relatively well-oxygenated inferior vena caval blood (which includes the blood returning from the placenta) is deflected by the christa dividens in the right atrium and shunted through the foramen ovale into the left atrium. Two thirds of the inferior vena caval blood passes from the right atrium to the right ventricle. Almost all poorly oxygenated superior vena caval blood also passes from the right atrium to the right ventricle. A conduit between the main pulmonary artery and the aorta, the ductus arteriosus, shunts approximately 90% of the right ventricular output ejected into the pulmonary artery. The left ventricular output, which includes the relatively well-oxygenated inferior vena caval blood (deflected through the foramen ovale) and the small amount of blood that perfuses the pulmonary circulation, is ejected into the aorta and perfuses the head and upper extremities. Figures 14.7 and 14.8 depict the circulation of the fetal lamb with normal blood pressures, oxygen saturations, and blood flows for the various vessels and cardiac chambers.

Cardiac output has two main determinants: heart rate and stroke volume. Fetal cardiac output, measured in terms of combined left and right ventricular output, is directly related to heart rate (122), which is probably the most important determinant

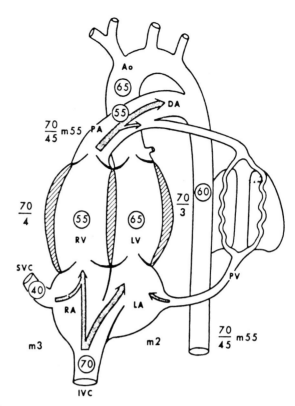

Figure 14.7. The fetal circulation. *Figures in circles* within the chambers and vessels represent percent oxygen saturation levels. *Figures alongside chambers and vessels* are pressures in mm Hg relative to an amniotic pressure level of zero. m = mean pressure; *Ao* = aorta; *DA* = ductus arteriosus; *PA* = pulmonary artery; *RV, LV* = right and left ventricle; *RA, LA* = right and left atrium; *IVC* = inferior vena cava. Data are obtained from late-gestation lambs. (Reprinted by permission from Rudolph AM, ed. *Congenital Diseases of the Heart.* Chicago, IL: Year Book Medical Publishers; 1974:3.)

of fetal cardiac output. Stroke volume is a function of preload, afterload, and myocardial contractility. Fetal myocardial contractility is probably maximally stimulated, with limited capacity to increase stroke volume. Fetal myocardial muscle strips are less compliant than those of adult hearts and have a greater resting tension, but a diminished response for increasing myocardial tension when stimulated (123). In fetal lambs, augmentation of preload has little effect on increasing cardiac output. Volume loading increases cardiac output by only 15% to 20% (124).

To function properly, the fetal circulation depends on a high venous return (125). Because the heart rate is predominant in regulating fetal cardiac output, baroreceptor and chemoreceptor responsiveness have important regulatory roles. Baroreflex activity exists by midgestation and increases in sensitivity as gestation advances (126). Chemoreflex activity from the aortic and carotid chemoreceptors in fetal lambs has been elicited and studied in utero (127–130). However, most of the information about the chemoreceptor role in the regulation of circulation has been obtained from anesthetized or short-term studies in fetal animals. A method for selectively denervating the aortic and carotid chemoreceptor and baroreceptor in fetal lambs in utero was developed which facilitates investigation of their roles in both normal fetal cardiovascular regulation and fetal response to stress (131).

Because the fetus has a limited capacity to increase cardiac output in response to stress, oxygen delivery to vital organs must be maintained by redistribution of blood flow. Cerebral blood flow in the fetal lamb is twice that in the adult, although both cerebral metabolic rates are similar (132, 133). These characteristics of fetal blood flow may represent a protective advantage for the fetus.

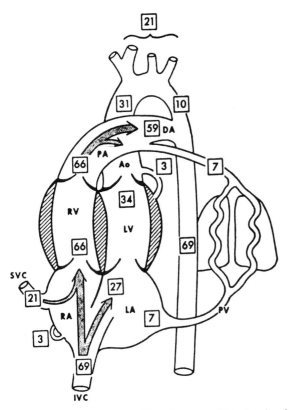

Figure 14.8. The fetal circulation. *Figure in squares* within the chambers and vessels represents percentages of the combined ventricular output that return to the fetal heart, percentages ejected by each ventricle, and percentages flowing through the main vascular channels. SVC = superior vena cava; *PV* = pulmonary vein; other abbreviations as in legend to Figure 14.7. Data are obtained from late gestation lambs. (Reprinted by permission from Rudolph AM, ed. *Congenital Diseases of the Heart.* Chicago, IL: Year Book Medical Publishers; 1974:8.)

Among the factors that may modulate cerebral blood flow are cerebral metabolic rate, arterial carbon dioxide tension ($Paco_2$), arterial oxygen content, blood pressure, and autoregulation (134–136). In fetal lambs, increases in cerebral metabolic rate or $Paco_2$ and decreases in arterial oxygen content are associated with increased cerebral blood flow. Cerebral blood flow autoregulation has been demonstrated to preserve cerebral blood flow in the normoxic fetal lamb when systemic blood pressures range 20% above or below normal values. However, autoregulation in response to hypotension may be incomplete, and the mechanism of autoregulation may depend on arterial oxygen concentration (137).

EFFECTS OF ANESTHESIA ON THE FETAL CARDIOVASCULAR CIRCULATION

The effects of inhalation anesthetic agents on the cardiovascular system of the fetus have been investigated, yet there is much to be learned. In fetal lambs, the concentration of halothane required to prevent movement in response to painful stimuli is much lower than that for adult sheep or newborn lambs (Table 14.9) (138). Although placental transfer of inhaled agents occurs rapidly, fetal levels of the halogenated agents remain lower than do maternal levels for a significant period after administration of these agents to the mother (Figs. 14.9 and 14.10). Reports conflict on the fetal effects when the mother has received halothane or isoflurane. In one study, maternal anesthesia with halothane 0.7% or isoflurane 1% (1 minimum alveolar concentration [MAC] for sheep) caused a mild decrease in fetal blood pressure with no change in fetal pulse rate, oxygen level, or acid-base status; however, anesthesia with halothane 1.5% or

Table 14.9. FETAL ANESTHETIC REQUIREMENT (MINIMUM ALVEOLAR CONCENTRATION) FOR HALOTHANE IN SHEEP (MEAN ± SE)

Blood Concentration at Minimum Alveolar Concentration* (mg/L)	
Theoretical (Calculated)	End-Tidal Concentration*(%)
Mothers 133 ± 5	0.69 ± 0.25
Fetuses 49 ± 28	0.33 ± 0.29

* Maternal and fetal values are significantly different (*P* < .001). Modified from Gregory GA, Wade JG, Biehl DR, Ong BY, Sitar D. Fetal anesthetic requirement (MAC) for halothane. *Anesth Analg* 1983;62:9–14.

isoflurane 2% (i.e., "deep anesthesia") caused decreases in fetal blood pressure, heart rate, oxygen saturation, and base excess, with progressive fetal acidosis (139). Other studies established that maternal anesthesia with halothane 1.5% caused a decrease in fetal arterial pressure after a few minutes (primarily because of a decrease in peripheral vascular resistance), with no change in pulse rate, cardiac output, oxygen, acid-base status, or blood flow to the fetal brain or other major fetal organs (Figs. 14.11, 14.12, and 14.13) (140, 141). Yet, another study demonstrated that maternal anesthesia with 2.0% isoflurane produced no significant decline in fetal blood pressure, but did produce a decrease in fetal cardiac index and the development of progressive fetal acidosis (142).

Deep inhalation anesthesia (2 MAC) may result in progressive fetal acidosis, whereas light anesthesia (1 MAC) or brief fetal exposure to deep anesthesia seems safe. Whether adverse responses result from direct impairment of fetal myocardial contractility, redistribution of fetal blood flow, or changes in uterine perfusion is uncertain. Also, the applicability of these studies is limited because the combined impact of fetal anesthesia, intrauterine manipulation, and fetal stress on maternal and fetal cardiovascular stability and regional blood flow remains unknown. The progressive fetal hypoxia may have resulted from failure to maintain uterine blood flow by increasing preload and providing appropriate vasopressors when halogenated agents were administered. In fact, uterine perfusion may increase with administration of halogenated agents if blood pressure is maintained, owing to uterine vessel vasodilation (139).

In nonanesthetized experimental animals, fetal asphyxia induced by occlusion of the umbilical circulation results in fetal

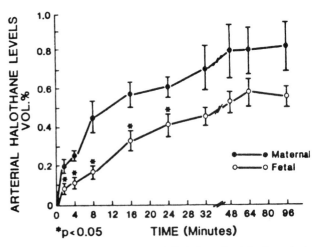

Figure 14.9. Maternal and fetal arterial halothane levels in sheep during maternal administration of 1.5% halothane (mean ± SE). (Reprinted by permission from Biehl DR, Cote J, Wade JG, et al. Uptake of halothane by the foetal lamb in utero. *Can Anaesth Soc J* 1983;30:24–27.)

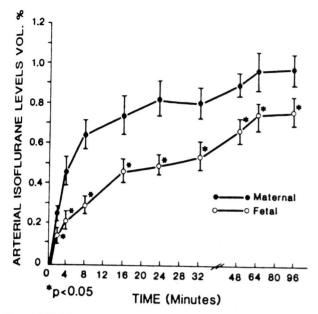

Figure 14.10. Maternal and fetal arterial isoflurane levels in sheep during maternal administration of 2.0% isoflurane (mean ± SE). (Reprinted by permission from Biehl DR, Yarnell R, Wade JG, Sitar D. The uptake of isoflurane by the foetal lamb in utero: Effect on regional blood flow. *Can Anaesth Soc J* 1983;30:581–586.)

bradycardia and hypertension, with decreased cardiac output and increased cerebral blood flow mediated partially by the fetal α- and β-adrenergic systems (68–72, 143–147). Reports on the effects of maternal halothane administration on the asphyxiated fetus are conflicting. In one study, maternal halothane administration did not further compromise fetal well-being. The blood pressure of the anesthetized fetus declined to values that were normal compared with those of the awake asphyxiated fetus; however, because the pulse rate increased, the cardiac output remained unchanged. Oxygenation did not deteriorate, and cerebral blood flow remained elevated (148). In another study, halothane administered to the mother of a severely acidotic fetus caused further aggravation of fetal acidosis and oxygen desaturation (149). Cerebral blood flow decreased as fetal blood pressure decreased.

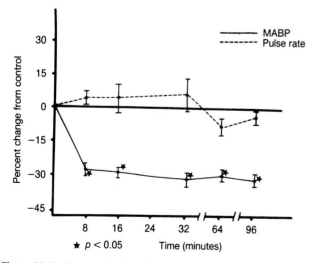

Figure 14.11. Changes in fetal sheep mean arterial blood pressure (*MABP*) and pulse rate during maternal administration of 1.5% halothane, expressed as percent change from control levels (mean ± SE). (Reprinted by permission from Biehl DR, Tweed WA, Cote J, et al. Effect of halothane on cardiac output and regional flow in the fetal lamb in utero. *Anesth Analg* 1983;62:489–492.)

FETAL MONITORING

Fetal asphyxia, hypoxia, or distress can be most effectively recognized, predicted, and avoided by fetal monitoring. Monitoring is also crucial to assess fetal response to corrective maneuvers. Methods for monitoring fetal well-being include fetal blood gases, pH, glucose, and electrolyte determinations, and measurements of FHR, blood pressure, and umbilical blood flow. Invasive methods and vascular access used in experimental fetal preparations require indwelling catheters that currently have limited application for clinical fetal surgery. However, capillary blood samples can be obtained for blood gas determinations, and vascular access can be achieved for fluid, blood, or drug administration during prolonged procedures involving a hysterotomy. On several occasions at UCSF, we have established vascular access in fetuses undergoing surgery and administered fluid or blood for resuscitation. Experimental techniques at accessing the fetal blood vessels on the surface of the placenta in the rhesus monkey for reliable, long-term vascular access have been successful (150, 151). In the future, more information may be used from detailed waveform analysis of the fetal electrocardiogram (ECG). New devices will become available for monitoring myometrial electrical activity and mechanical contractility and the fetal electroencephalogram. Additionally, devices will become available for continuous monitoring of fetal arterial oxygen saturation, such as the fetal pulse oximeter for labor (Nellcor N-400, Mallinckrodt Nellcor, Pleasanton, CA), Po_2 and Pco_2, and for monitoring fetal cerebral oxygenation, blood volume, and blood flow by near-infrared spectroscopy (152). We have experimented with the use of an implantable radiotelemeter for monitoring uterine activity and FHR (153).

The author has used FHR monitoring, pulse oximetry, and intermittent blood gas determinations as relatively noninvasive methods of assessing fetal well-being during fetal surgery. FHR can be monitored with a standard internal fetal electrode and a reference electrode on the maternal abdomen, both connected to a maternal ground plate and processed by an FHR cardiotachometer (16). However, the signal obtained is of low amplitude and is overwhelmed by movement artifact, rendering the conventional display of the beat-to-beat heart rate unreliable. The author has found that direct monitoring of the fetus by ECG is more reliable than the standard internal fetal electrode. Modified insulated atrial pacing wires are used as ECG leads. The bare wire at the distal end is sutured subcutaneously onto the fetal thorax for open uterus fetal surgery using the attached curved needles. The proximal end of the insulated wire is attached to a coaxial shielded cable, connecting the three leads to a cardiotachometer. The cardiotachometer was modified by increasing gain to allow for signal amplification and by the addition of a fixed low-pass frequency filter and variable high-pass frequency filter, which substantially reduce motion artifact. The ECG lead wires are stabilized to minimize capacitive coupling and changes in voltage offset between the fetal skin and the ECG lead wire. This allows for a more reliable display of the fetal ECG with visible P and QRS complexes (Fig. 14.14).

Plethysmography combined with spectrophotometric oximetry (pulse oximetry) also has proved very useful. A noninvasive sensor contains two low-voltage, low-intensity, light-emitting diodes as light sources, and a photodiode as a light receiver. Changes in the absorption of red light, relative to a change in the absorption of infrared light, indicate the arterial hemoglobin oxygen saturation (154). For open fetal surgical procedures and EXIT procedures, we use neonatal digital sensors wrapped around the fetal arm, leg, or (preferably) palmar arch. This is held in place with sterile, sticky plastic and covered with sterile aluminum foil to prevent artifact from the intense ambient surgical lighting. Alternatively, in the early 1980s, we developed a flat sensor for placement over any exposed fetal part so light could

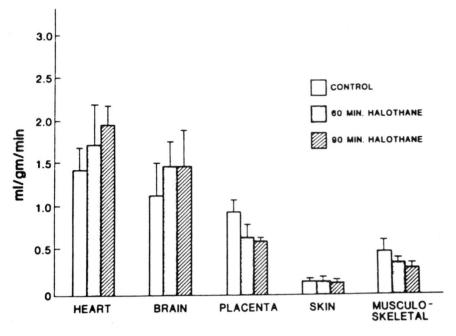

Figure 14.12. Fetal sheep regional blood flow during maternal administration of 1.5% halothane (mean ± SE). Values were obtained at control and after 60 and 90 minutes of halothane anesthesia using the labeled microsphere injection technique. (Reprinted by permission from Biehl DR, Tweed WA, Cote J, et al. Effect of halothane on cardiac output and regional flow in the fetal lamb in utero. *Anesth Analg* 1983;62:489–492.)

be measured predominantly by reflectance rather than transmission. This has become the foundation for fetal pulse oximetry in labor (155–157). We used a monitor that was modified by the addition of special circuits to reduce noise (low-noise amplifiers), also now used in the commercial fetal pulse oximeter, Nellcor N-400. We used a computer data collection system connected to the monitor to allow visualization of both red and infrared pulse signals and their respective percentages of modulation. Thus, qualitative and quantitative assessment of signal strength and reliability was possible (Figs. 14.15, 14.16, and 14.17). Intraoperative fetal pulse oximetry with the Nellcor N-400 monitor has been demonstrated as a very reliable monitoring parameter in the fetal lamb model (158).

Use of readily available, conventional pediatric sensors and conventional instruments calibrated for higher saturation can be useful for heart rate monitoring if the waveform is analyzed for reliability of the data. Although relative trends in oxygen-related quantities may be inferred from the data provided by conventional oximeters, they may not be precise (Fig. 14.18). The influence of fetal hemoglobin is insignificant, and the neonatal monitors used for pulse oximetry in the range of 75% to 100% saturation are reasonably reliable. However, oximeters calibrated for human adults underestimate the arterial oxygen saturation at the 25% level. At lower saturations, numeric modeling suggests that sensors with two different wavelengths than currently available provide better performance (159). These different wavelengths are incorporated into the Nellcor N-400 fetal oximeter.

Additionally, intraoperative sonography (Accuson, Mountain View, CA) using a sterile sleeve on the sonographic probe is important for monitoring the fetus, particularly for endoscopic procedures for which other monitors cannot be applied to the fetus. FHR, ventricular volume, and contractility can be determined by visualization of the heart, or heart rate can be ascertained by Doppler assessment of blood flow through the umbilical cord. However, in many circumstances, the sterile transducer cannot be positioned continuously because it interferes with the surgical field.

INTRAOPERATIVE UTERINE RELAXATION ("SURGICAL TOCOLYSIS") AND PREVENTION OF PRETERM LABOR

The human uterine wall has a thick, muscular layer that is sensitive to stimulation or manipulation. Because uterine stimulation increases the likelihood of inducing uterine contraction, the risk of preterm labor accompanies invasive fetal intervention. After incision, strong uterine contractions can occur; these have resulted in high incidences of postoperative abortion in experimental preparations using nonhuman primate fetuses. Strong uterine contractions may impede uterine blood flow or induce partial placental separation, which interferes with umbilical-placental blood flow; both of these compromise fetal well-being. A uterine contraction can displace a percutaneous intrauterine needle placed for intrauterine transfusion or shunt catheter placement. Prevention and treatment of preterm labor

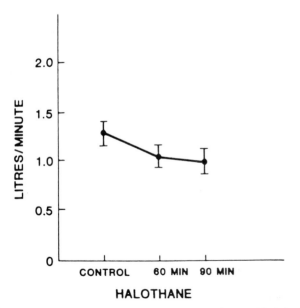

Figure 14.13. Fetal sheep cardiac output calculated using labeled microsphere injection technique during maternal administration of 1.5% halothane (mean ± SE). Values were obtained at control and after 60 and 90 minutes of halothane anesthesia. (Reprinted by permission from Biehl DR, Tweed WA, Cote J, et al. Effect of halothane on cardiac output and regional flow in the fetal lamb in utero. *Anesth Analg* 1983;62:489–492.)

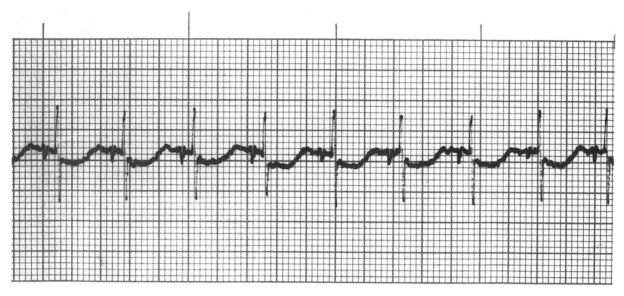

Figure 14.14. Electrocardiogram obtained using atrial pacing wires from a 25-week gestation fetus undergoing open repair of congenital diaphragmatic hernia (paper chart speed = 25 mm/min).

are critically important in the management of patients undergoing fetal intervention.

Tocolytic therapy includes a variety of drugs. The agents most commonly used for tocolysis are β-adrenergic agonists and magnesium sulfate, which prevent or inhibit preterm labor. Tocolysis is usually not necessary after simple percutaneous umbilical blood sampling or intrauterine transfusions. However, for more invasive percutaneous procedures (such as shunt catheter placement), magnesium or low-dose β-adrenergic agonist tocolytic agents can be administered intravenously for prophylactic control of uterine irritability.

For procedures involving hysterotomy and endoscopy, halogenated agents are used intraoperatively to inhibit uterine contractility and to provide the uterine relaxation necessary for surgery (5). We use a regimen of tocolysis that includes preoperative administration of indomethacin by suppository, intraoperative anesthetic by inhalation of halogenated agent (end-tidal concentrations of approximately 3 MAC), supplemented when necessary by bolus doses of nitroglycerin (50 to 100 μg) (48, 53, 160), and postoperative tocolysis by magnesium, supplemented by terbutaline (a β-adrenergic agonist) if necessary. After several days, tocolytic therapy is shifted to continuous subcutaneous infusion or oral administration of terbutaline, which the patient continues after hospital discharge. Depending on uterine activity, the postoperative regimen is supplemented by use of indomethacin or calcium-channel blocking agents.

At times, the halogenated agent alone does not provide the complete uterine relaxation required intraoperatively. Furthermore, concern had been raised that either the fetus was inadequately anesthetized to block the autonomic response to stress, or the halogenated agent adversely affected fetal myocardial contractility during prolonged procedures (24). For several years, we tried using an alternative anesthetic and tocolytic technique during repair of fetal diaphragmatic hernias. For maternal anesthesia, we administered nitrous oxide, fentanyl, and 0.25% inspired concentration of isoflurane. The patient was paralyzed, her lungs mechanically ventilated, and fluids administered to maintain a normal central venous pressure. We achieved intraoperative and postoperative uterine relaxation by administration of nitroglycerin at doses up to 20 μg $\cdot$ kg$^{-1}\cdot$min^{-1}, and we maintained mean arterial pressure above 60 mm Hg, using ephedrine when needed. Before uterine incision, the surgeon administered fentanyl 50 μg and pancuronium 0.3 mg intramuscularly to the fetus by ultrasound guidance. Although successful,

we weren't impressed that this technique offered any advantages (161). We no longer employ this technique.

Once closure of the uterus is begun, a bolus loading dose of magnesium sulfate (4 g) followed by a continuous infusion (2 g/h) is used for transition between intra- and postoperative

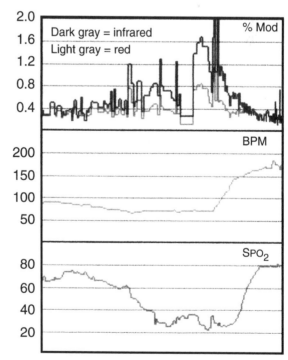

Figure 14.15. Two-minute tracing showing fetal heart rate (FHR) (beats per minute [BPM]; scale 0 to 250), oxygen saturation (SpO$_2$; scale 0% to 100%), and modulation of red and infrared light signals (light gray = red, dark gray = infrared; scale, 0% to 2%) in a 24-week gestation fetus undergoing open diaphragmatic hernia repair. Note that the decrease in FHR from about 90 BPM to 70 BPM precedes the decrease in oxygen saturation from about 70% to 22%, and recovery in FHR to about 160 BPM precedes the recovery in oxygen saturation. This may represent a transport delay in propagation of blood to the peripheral SpO$_2$ sensor. FHR may be a better monitor than SpO$_2$ for acute changes.

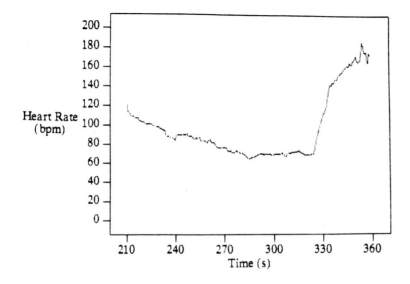

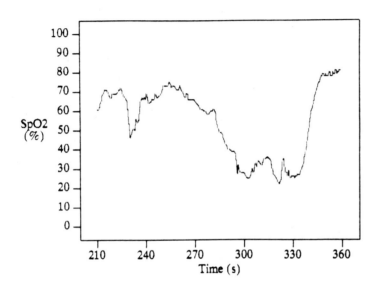

Figure 14.16. Graphic representation of the data in Figure 14.15 showing fetal heart rate (*bpm*) and oxygen saturation (SpO₂) more precisely detailed over the 120-second period.

tocolysis. The magnesium could be administered earlier. The continuous IV magnesium sulfate infusion is maintained for postoperative tocolysis, supplemented by β-adrenergic agonists if necessary. Intraoperatively, IV fluids are restricted to minimize the risk of postoperative pulmonary edema associated with administration of magnesium sulfate and β-adrenergic agonists.

The "surgical tocolysis" provided by deep inhalation anesthesia and sometimes supplemented by nitroglycerin could significantly increase the risk of maternal hemorrhage during uterine incision. To reduce the risk, surgical techniques have been developed that employ a stapling device for hemostasis and sealing of the membranes during hysterotomy. This same stapling device is used for EXIT procedures as well.

Magnesium sulfate infusions supplemented by terbutaline are the mainstay of our postoperative tocolytic management. Indomethacin (a prostaglandin synthetase inhibitor) is used pre- and postoperatively for the more invasive fetal surgical procedures. Although there have been case reports of prenatal closure of the ductus arteriosus and persistent fetal circulation associated with the use of prostaglandin synthetase inhibitors for tocolysis, these effects are rare when used to treat mothers before 34 weeks of gestation for limited durations. Fetal echocardiography is utilized postoperatively to detect early evidence of adverse cardiovascular changes due to indomethacin, at which time this agent is discontinued. Indomethacin use also has been associ-

ated with decreased fetal urine output caused by potentiation of the peripheral effects of antidiuretic hormone. In addition, neonatal bleeding and renal impairment could result from prolonged indomethacin therapy.

There is extensive experience with the use of calcium-channel blockers for tocolysis. They are rarely used for initial tocolytic management in fetal surgery unless contraindications exist to the use of other agents. All tocolytic agents have maternal, fetal, and neonatal side effects. A more complete discussion of tocolytic agents and anesthetic interactions can be found in Chapter 17.

THE FUTURE OF FETAL TREATMENT

The medical complexities associated with fetal surgery transcend the diagnosis and treatment of fetal disease. Fetal treatment presents technical options that have not yet been fully evaluated clinically. The options raise complex social, ethical, and legal issues that go beyond those customary for therapeutic intervention. Although the rationale for and intent of improving fetal health by in utero procedures are within the scope of traditional medicine, we must distinguish innovative therapy from experimentation.

The rationale for fetal surgery has become well established, yet many issues remain to be resolved. Issues of safety, efficacy,

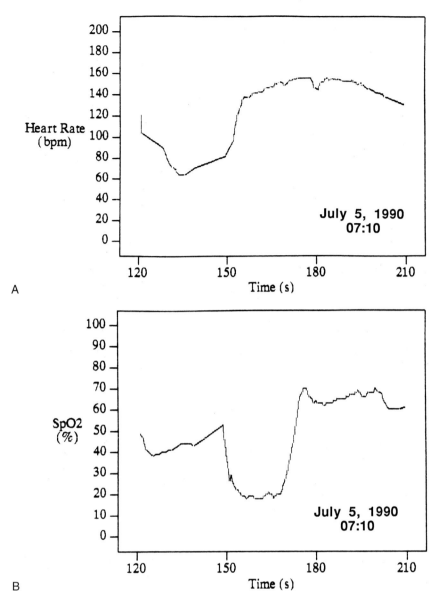

Figure 14.17. Data similar to Figure 14.16 from the same fetus a few minutes earlier, showing an acute decrease in fetal heart rate (FHR) (*A*) with associated decrease in fetal saturation (*B*). Note that the onset of the desaturation detected in the fetal hand is delayed relative to the onset of the bradycardia. Similarly, the recovery in FHR precedes the onset of rapid increase in saturation. This most likely represents a transport delay of blood from the heart to the fetal hand.

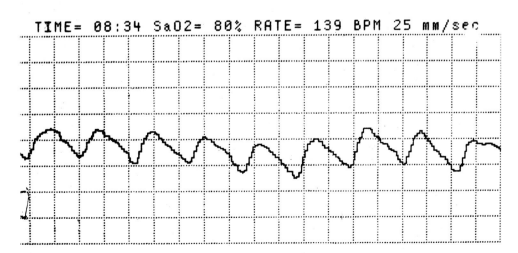

Figure 14.18. Pulse oximetry tracing from a 25-week gestation fetus undergoing open congenital diaphragmatic hernia repair.

cost-effectiveness, and resource allocation must be balanced with societal expectations, availability of therapy, and issues of potential long-range applications, implications, and consequences of intervention. The sensitivity, specificity, and appropriate use of prenatal diagnostic testing are crucially important.

Fetal treatment also raises unique and complicated ethical and legal questions about maternal rights and fetal needs. Treating a potentially viable fetus as a patient in its own right requires a consideration of the mother's medical interests, because it is her body that is the site of treatment. Who will act as medical advocate for each patient—mother and fetus—if preserving the health of one places the other at risk? Some of these questions must be resolved in the face of conflicting legal interpretations of the assumed responsibilities of parents, forced bodily intrusion, and legal termination of pregnancy. Could legal injunctions force fetal treatment in opposition to a mother's wishes, a situation analogous to overriding parental refusal of necessary treatment for a child? What are the liabilities (civil and criminal) once a therapy becomes established as safe and effective for intended purposes? These are complex issues, and parents must be provided with complete information about the nature of the procedure, its potential benefits for the fetus, and the risks inherent for both patients before an informed consent can be obtained. Parents should also be offered alternative therapies, if any, and informed of their expected consequences. The rights and safety of the mother must always be placed above those of the fetus.

Innovative treatment of the fetus must be tested in the rigorous nonhuman primate model, carefully evaluated in light of our uncertainties, and undertaken with caution. Before offering fetal procedures to patients, the UCSF Fetal Treatment Center established that intervention would not be considered until the natural history of the disease was defined (e.g., evaluating serial sonograms in untreated cases), and the pathophysiology, and feasibility and safety of intervention were established in nonhuman primate models. The UCSF Fetal Treatment Center founded the International Fetal Medicine and Surgery Society, which sets general and specific guidelines for fetal treatment and maintains a voluntary registry of fetal surgical procedures.

Fetal surgical and anesthetic techniques and tocolytic management must undergo continued improvement. The future of fetal surgery depends on advances in our ability to control preterm labor and technical innovation to allow the use of less invasive methods for repair of fetal defects. The risks and benefits of various anesthetic agents and techniques, and the effectiveness and safety of fetal monitoring must continue to be evaluated. We must learn, however, to distinguish fetuses that may benefit from invasive therapy from those that will not, intervening only when there is a reasonable probability of benefit.

REFERENCES

1. Albanese CT, Harrison MR. Surgical treatment for fetal disease. The state of the art. *Ann N Y Acad Sci* 1998;847:74–85.
2. Liley AW. Intrauterine transfusion of foetus in haemolytic disease. *Br Med J* 1963;2:1107–1109.
3. Adamsons K. Fetal surgery. *N Engl J Med* 1966;275:204–206.
4. Coakley FV, Hricak H, Filly RA, Barkovich AJ, Harrison M. Complex fetal disorders: Effect of MR imaging on management—preliminary clinical experience. *Radiology* 1999;213:691–696.
5. Harrison MR, Golbus MS, Filly RA, et al. Fetal surgery for congenital hydronephrosis. *N Engl J Med* 1982;306:591–593.
6. Vanderwall KJ, Skarsgard ED, Filly RA, Eckert J, Harrison MR. Fetendo-clip: A fetal endoscopic tracheal clip procedure in a human fetus. *J Pediatr Surg* 1997;32:970–972.
7. Liley AW. Foreword. In: Harrison MR, Golbus MS, Filly RA, eds. *The Unborn Patient: Prenatal Diagnosis and Treatment.* 2nd ed. Philadelphia: WB Saunders; 1991.
8. Harrison MR, Golbus MS, Filly RA, Nakayama DK, deLorimier AA. Fetal surgical treatment. *Pediatr Ann* 1982;11:896–903.
9. Harrison MR, Golbus MS, Filly RA. Management of the fetus: A correctable congenital defect. *JAMA* 1981;246:774–777.
10. Harrison MR. Fetal surgery. *Am J Obstet Gynecol* 1996;174:1255–1264.
11. Bullard KM, Harrison M. Before the horse is out of the barn: Fetal surgery for hydrops. *Semin Perinatol* 1995;19:462–473.
12. Bruch SW, Adzick NS, Reiss R, Harrison MR. Prenatal therapy for pericardial teratomas. *J Pediatr Surg* 1997;32:1113–1115.
13. Harrison MR, Adzick NS, Estes JM, Howell LM. A prospective study of the outcome for fetuses with diaphragmatic hernia. *JAMA* 1994;271:382–384.
14. Harrison MR, Jester JA, Ross NA. Correction of congenital diaphragmatic hernia in utero. I. The model: Intrathoracic balloon produces fatal pulmonary hypoplasia. *Surgery* 1980;88:174–182.
15. Adzick NS, Harrison MR, Glick PL, et al. Fetal surgery in the primate. III. Maternal outcome after fetal surgery. *J Pediatr Surg* 1986;21:477–480.
16. Harrison MR, Anderson J, Rosen MA, et al. Fetal surgery in the primate. I. Anesthetic, surgical, and tocolytic management to maximize fetal-neonatal survival. *J Pediatr Surg* 1982;17:115–122.
17. Nakayama DK, Harrison MR, Serono-Ferre M, Villa RL. Fetal surgery in the primate. II. Uterine electromyographic responses to operative procedures and pharmacologic agents. *J Pediatr Surg* 1984;19:333–339.
18. Harrison MR, Bressack MA, Churg AM, deLorimier AA. Correction of congenital diaphragmatic hernia in utero. II. Simulated correction permits fetal lung growth with survival at birth. *Surgery* 1980;88:260–268.
19. Adzick NS, Outwater KM, Harrison MR, et al. Correction of congenital diaphragmatic hernia in utero. IV. An early gestational fetal lamb model for pulmonary vascular morphometric analysis. *J Pediatr Surg* 1985;20:934–942.
20. Harrison MR, Ross NA, deLorimier AA. Correction of congenital diaphragmatic hernia in utero. III. Development of a successful surgical technique using abdominoplasty to avoid compromise of umbilical blood flow. *J Pediatr Surg* 1981;16:934–942.
21. Harrison MR, Langer JC, Adzick NS, et al. Correction of congenital diaphragmatic hernia in utero. V. Initial clinical experience. *J Pediatr Surg* 1990;25:47–57.
22. Harrison MR, Adzick NS, Longaker MT, et al. Successful repair in utero of a fetal diaphragmatic hernia after removal of herniated viscera from the left thorax. *N Engl J Med* 1990;322:1582–1584.
23. Harrison MR, Adzick NS, Flake AW, Jennings RW. The CDH two-step: A dance of necessity. *J Pediatr Surg* 1993;28:813–816.
24. Harrison MR, Adzick NS, Flake AW, et al. Correction of congenital diaphragmatic hernia in utero. VI. Hard-earned lessons. *J Pediatr Surg* 1993;28:1411–1418.
25. MacGillivray TE, Jennings RW, Rudolph AM, et al. Vascular changes with in utero correction of diaphragmatic hernia. *J Pediatr Surg* 1994;29:992–996.
26. Mychaliska GB, Bullard KM, Harrison MR. In utero management of congenital diaphragmatic hernia. *Clin Perinatol* 1996;23:823–841.
27. Harrison MR, Adzick NS, Rosen MA, et al. Correction of congenital diaphragmatic hernia in utero. VII. A prospective trial. *J Pediatr Surg* 1997;32:1637–1642.
28. Metkus AP, Filly RA, Stringer MD, et al. Sonographic predictors of survival in fetal diaphragmatic hernia. *J Pediatr Surg* 1996;31:148–152.
29. Lipshutz GS, Albanese CT, Feldstein VA, et al. Prospective analysis of lung-to-head ratio predicts survival for patients with prenatally diagnosed congenital diaphragmatic hernia. *J Pediatr Surg* 1997;32:1634–1636.
30. Albanese CT, Lopoo J, Goldstein RB, et al. Fetal liver position and perinatal outcome for congenital diaphragmatic hernia. *Prenat Diagn* 1998;18:1138–1142.
31. Alcorn D, Adamson TM, Lambert TF, et al. Morphological effects of chronic tracheal ligation and drainage in the fetal lamb lung. *J Anat* 1977;123:649–660.
32. Wilson JM, DiFiore JW, Peters CA. Experimental fetal tracheal ligation prevents the pulmonary hypoplasia associated with fetal nephrectomy: Possible application for congenital diaphragmatic hernia. *J Pediatr Surg* 1993;28:1433–1440.
33. Hedrick MH, Estes JM, Sullivan KM, et al. Plug the lung until it grows (PLUG): A new method to treat congenital diaphragmatic hernia in utero. *J Pediatr Surg* 1994;29:612–617.
34. DiFiore JW, Fauza DO, Slavin R, Peters CA, Fackler JC, Wilson JM. Experimental fetal tracheal ligation reverses the structural

and physiologic effects of pulmonary hypoplasia in congenital diaphragmatic hernia. *J Pediatr Surg* 1994;29:248–257.

35. Hashim E, Laberge JM, Chen MF, Quillen E. Reversible tracheal obstruction in the fetal sheep: Effects on tracheal fluid pressure and lung growth. *J Pediatr Surg* 1995;30:1172–1177.

36. Beierle EA, Langham MR, Cassin S. In utero lung growth in fetal sheep with diaphragmatic hernia and tracheal stenosis. *J Pediatr Surg* 1996;31:141–146.

37. Bealer JF, Skarsgard ED, Rosen M, et al. The "PLUG" odyssey: Adventures in experimental fetal tracheal occlusion. *J Pediatr Surg* 1995;30:361–364.

38. Vanderwall KJ, Sruch SW, Neuli M, et al. Fetal endoscopic ("Fetendo") tracheal clip. *J Pediatr Surg* 1996;31:1101–1104.

39. Papdakis K, Luks FI, De Paepe ME, Piasecki GJ, Wesselhoeft CW. Fetal lung growth after tracheal ligation is not solely a pressure phenomenon. *J Pediatr Surg* 1997;32:347– 351.

40. Sylvester KG, Rasanen J, Kitano Y, Flake AW, Crumblehome TM, Adzick NS. Tracheal occlusion reverses the high impendence to flow in the fetal pulmonary circulation and normalizes its physiological response to oxygen at full term. *J Pediatr Surg* 1998;33:1071–1075.

41. Harrison MR, Adzick NS, Flake AW, et al. Correction of congenital diaphragmatic hernia in utero. VIII. Response of the hypoplastic lung to tracheal occlusion. *J Pediatr Surg* 1996;31:1339–1348.

42. Harrison MR, Mychaliska GB, Albanese CT, et al. Correction of congenital diaphragmatic hernia in utero. IX. Fetuses with poor prognosis (liver herniation and low lung-to-head ratio) can be saved by fetoscopic temporary occlusion. *J Pediatr Surg* 1998;33:1017–1023.

43. Schulman SR, Jones BR, Slotnick N, Schwartz MZ. Fetal tracheal intubation with intact uteroplacental circulation. *Anesth Analg* 1993;76:197–199.

44. Mychaliska GB, Bealer JF, Rosen MA, et al. Operating on placental support: The ex utero intrapartum treatment procedure. *J Pediatr Surg* 1997;32:227–231.

45. Bond SJ, Harrison MR, Slotnick RN, Anderson J, Flake AW, Adzick NS. Cesarean delivery and hysterotomy using an absorbable stapling device. *Obstet Gynecol* 1989;74:25–28.

46. Kumar D, Zourlas PA, Barnes AC. In vivo effect of amyl nitrate on human pregnant uterine contractility. *Am J Obstet Gynecol* 1965;91:1061–1068.

47. Jennings RW, MacGillvray TE, Harrison MR. Nitric oxide inhibits preterm labor in the rhesus monkey. *J Matern-Fetal Med* 1993;2:170–175.

48. Peng ATC, Gorman RS, Shulman SM, et al. Intravenous nitroglycerin for uterine relaxation in the postpartum patient with retained placenta. *Anesthesiology* 1989;71:172–173.

49. DeSimone CA, Norris M. Intravenous nitroglycerin for uterine relaxation aids manual extraction of a retained placenta [letter]. *Anesthesiology* 1990;73:787.

50. Rolbin SH, Hew EM, Bernstein A. Uterine relaxation can be lifesaving [letter]. *Can J Anaesth* 1991;38:939–940.

51. Greenspoon JS, Kovacic A. Breech extraction facilitated by glyceryl trinitrate sublingual spray [letter]. *Lancet* 1991;338:124–125.

52. Mayer DC, Weeks SK. Antepartum uterine relaxation with nitroglycerin at Cesarean delivery. *Can J Anaesth* 1992;39:166–169.

53. Altabef KM, Spencer JT, Zinberg S. Intravenous nitroglycerin for uterine relaxation of an inverted uterus. *Am J Obstet Gynecol* 1992;166:1237–1238.

54. Rosen MA. Management of anesthesia for the pregnant surgical patient. *Anesthesiology* 1999;91:1159–1163.

55. Langevin PB, Katovich MJ, Wood CE, James CF, Langevin SO. The effect of nitroglycerin on the gravid uterus in sheep and rabbits. *Anesth Analg* 2000;90:337–343.

56. Catalano PJ, Urken ML, Alvarez M, Norton K, Wedgewood J, Holzman I. New approach to the management of airway obstruction in "high risk" neonates. *Arch Otolaryngol Head Neck Surg* 1992;118:306–309.

57. Langer JC, Tabb T, Thompson P, Paes BA, Caco CC. Management of prenatally diagnosed tracheal obstruction: Access to the airway in utero prior to delivery. *Fetal Diagn Ther* 1992;7:12–16.

58. Schwartz MZ, Silver H, Schulman S. Maintenance of the placental circulation to evaluate and treat an infant with massive head and neck hemangioma. *J Pediatr Surg* 1993;28:520–522.

59. Tanaka M, Sato S, Naito H, Nakayama H. Anesthetic management of a neonate with prenatally diagnosed cervical tumour and upper airway obstruction. *Can J Anaesth* 1994;41:236–240.

60. Skarsgard ED, Chitkara U, Krane EJ, Riley ET, Halamek LP, Dedo HH. The OOPS procedure (operation on placental support): In utero airway management of the fetus with prenatally diagnosed tracheal obstruction. *J Pediatr Surg* 1996;31:826–828.

61. Liechty KW, Crumbleholme TM, Flake AW, et al. Intrapartum airway management for giant fetal neck masses: The EXIT (ex utero intrapartum treatment) procedure. *Am J Obstet Gynecol* 1997;177:870–874.

62. Gaiser RR, Cheek TG, Kurth CD. Anesthetic management of cesarean delivery complicated by ex utero intrapartum treatment of the fetus. *Anesth Analg* 1997;84:1150–1153.

63. Waldman JD, Chilton L, Golmes G, Plowden J, Mathewson JW. Placenta-dependent systemic oxygenation; a case report of transposition with no septal defects. *Prenat Neonat Med* 1997;2:152–155.

64. Sachiyo S, Tomoaki T, Yamanouchi T, et al. Fetal stabilization for antenatally diagnosed diaphragmatic hernia. *J Pediatr Surg* 1999;34:1652–1657.

65. Albanese CT, Harrison MR. Surgical treatment for fetal disease: The state of the art. *Ann N Y Acad Sci* 1998;847:74–85.

66. Ville Y, Hyett J, Hecher D, et al. Preliminary experience with endoscopic laser surgery for severe twin-twin transfusion syndrome. *N Engl J Med* 1995;332:224–227.

67. Hanley FL. Fetal cardiac surgery. *Adv Card Surg* 1994;5:47–74.

68. Kohl T, Szabo Z, Suda K, et al. Fetoscopic and open transumbilical fetal cardiac catheterization in sheep: Potential approaches for human fetal cardiac intervention. *Circulation* 1997;95:1048–1053.

69. Robie GF, Payne GG Jr, Morgan MA. Selective delivery of an acardiac, acephalic twin. *N Engl J Med* 1989;320:512–513.

70. DeLia JE, Cruikshank DP, Keye WR. Fetoscopic neodymium:YAG laser occlusion of placental vessels in severe twin-twin transfusion syndrome. *Obstet Gynecol* 1990;75:1046–1053.

71. Ville Y, Hyett J, Hecher K, et al. Preliminary experience with endoscopic laser surgery for severe twin-twin transfusion syndrome. *N Engl J Med* 1995;332:224–227.

72. Milner R, Crombleholme TM. Troubles with twins: Fetoscopic therapy. *Semin Perinatol* 1999;23:474–483.

73. Harrison MR, Filly RA, Parer JT, et al. Management of the fetus with a urinary tract malformation. *JAMA* 1981;246:635–639.

74. Harrison MR, Ross NA, Noall RA, deLorimier AA. Correction of congenital hydronephrosis in utero. I. The model: Fetal urethral obstruction produces hydronephrosis and pulmonary hypoplasia in fetal lambs. *J Pediatr Surg* 1983;18:247–256.

75. Harrison MR, Nakayama DK, Noall RA, deLorimier AA. Correction of congenital hydronephrosis in utero. II. Decompression reverses the effects of obstruction on the fetal lung and urinary tract. *J Pediatr Surg* 1982;17:965–974.

76. Glick PL, Harrison MR, Noall RA, Villa RL. Correction of congenital hydronephrosis in utero. III. Early mid-trimester ureteral obstruction produces renal dysplasia. *J Pediatr Surg* 1983;18:681–687.

77. Glick PL, Harrison MR, Adzick NS, et al. Congenital hydronephrosis in utero. IV. In utero decompression prevents renal dysplasia. *J Pediatr Surg* 1984;19:649–657.

78. Nakayama DK, Glick PL, Villa RL, Noall R, Harrison MR. Experimental pulmonary hypoplasia due to oligohydramnios and its reversal by relieving thoracic compression. *J Pediatr Surg* 1983;18:347–353.

79. Sauer L, Harrison MR, Flake AW. Does an expanding fetal abdominal mass produce pulmonary hypoplasia. *J Pediatr Surg* 1987;22:508–512.

80. Golbus MS, Harrison MR, Filly RA, Callen RA, Katz M. In utero treatment of urinary tract obstruction. *Am J Obstet Gynecol* 1982;142:383–388.

81. Harrison MR, Golbus MS, Filly RA, et al. Fetal hydronephrosis: Selection and surgical repair. *J Pediatr Surg* 1987;22:556–558.

82. Crombleholme TM, Harrison MR, Langer JC, et al. Early experience with open fetal surgery for congenital hydronephrosis. *J Pediatr Surg* 1988;23:1114–1121.

83. Stelnicki EJ, Lee S, Hoffman W, et al. A long-term, controlled-outcome analysis of in utero versus neonatal cleft lip repair using an ovine model. *Plast Reconstr Surg* 1999;104:607–615.

84. Hallock GG. In utero cleft lip repair in A/J mice. *Plast Reconstr Surg* 1985;75:785–790.

85. Weinzweig J, Panter KE, Pantaloni M, et al. The fetal cleft palate. I. Characterization of a congenital model. *Plast Reconstr Surg* 1999;103:419–428.

86. Weinzweig J, Panter KE, Pantaloni M, et al. The fetal cleft palate. II. Scarless healing after in utero repair of a congenital model. *Plast Reconstr Surg* 1999;104:1356–1364.

87. Stelnicki EJ, Vanderwall K, Hoffman WY, Harrison MR, Glowacki J, Longaker MT. A new in utero sheep model for unilateral coronal craniosynostosis. *Plast Reconstr Surg* 1998;101:278–286.

88. Stelnicki EJ, Vanderwall K, Harrison MR, Longaker MT, Kaban LB, Hoffman WY. The in utero correction of unilateral coronal craniosynostosis. *Plast Reconstr Surg* 1998;101:287–296.

89. Hodgen GD. Antenatal diagnosis and treatment of fetal skeletal malformations: With emphasis on in utero surgery for neural tube defects and limb bud regeneration. *JAMA* 1981;246:1079–1083.

90. Michejda M, Hodgen GD. In utero diagnosis and treatment of non-human primate fetal skeletal anomalies. *JAMA* 1981;246:1093–1097.

91. Hawkins JA, Paape KL, Adkins TP, et al. Extracorporeal circulation in the fetal lamb: Effects of hypothermia and perfusion rate. *J Cardiovasc Surg* 1991;32:295–300.

92. Meuli-Simmen C, Meuli M, Adzick NS, et al. Latissimus dorsi flap procedures to cover myelomeningocele in utero: A feasibility study in human fetuses. *J Pediatr Surg* 1997;32:1154–1156.

93. Tulipan N, Bruner JP. Myelomeningocele repair in utero: A report of three cases. *Pediatr Neurosurg* 1998;28:177–180.

94. Bruner JP, Richards WO, Tulipan NB, et al. Endoscopic coverage of fetal myelomeningocele in utero. *Am J Obstet Gynecol* 1999;180:153–158.

95. Bruner JP, Tulipan N, Pachall RL, et al. Fetal surgery for myelomeningocele and the incidence of shunt-dependent hydrocephalus. *JAMA* 1999;282:1819–1825.

96. Sutton LN, Adzick NS, Bilaniuk LT, Johnson MP, Crombleholme TM, Flake AW. Improvement in hindbrain herniation demonstrated by serial fetal magnetic resonance imaging following fetal surgery for myelomeningocele. *JAMA* 1999;282:1826–1831.

97. Simpson J. Fetal surgery for myelomeningocele. *JAMA* 1999;282:1873–1874.

98. Longaker MT, Golbus MS, Filly RA, Rosen M, Chang SW, Harrison MR. Maternal outcome after open fetal surgery. *JAMA* 1991;265:737–741.

99. Graf JL, Bealer JF, Gibbs DL, Adzick NS, Harrison MR. Chorioamniotic membrane separation: A potentially lethal finding. *Fetal Diagn Ther* 1997;12:81–84.

100. Farrell JA, Albanese CT, Jennings RW, Kilpatrick SJ, Bratton BJ, Harrison MR. Maternal fertility is not affected by fetal surgery. *Fetal Diagn Ther* 1999;14:190–192.

101. Gibbs DL, Piecuch RE, Graf JL, Leonard CH, Farrell JA, Harrison MR. Neurodevelopmental outcome after open fetal surgery. *J Pediatr Surg* 1998;33:1254–1256.

102. Bealer JF, Raisanen J, Skarsgard ED, et al. The incidence and spectrum of neurological injury after open fetal surgery. *J Pediatr Surg* 1995;30:1150–1154.

103. Cauldwell CB, Rosen MA, Jennings RW. Anesthesia and monitoring for fetal intervention. In: Harrison MR, Evans M, Adzick NS, Holzgreve W, eds. *The Unborn Patient: The Art and Science of Fetal Therapy.* 3rd ed. Philadelphia: WB Saunders; 2000.

104. Manning F, Harrison MR, Rodeck C, and the International Fetal Medicine Surgery Society. Report of the International Fetal Surgery Registry: Catheter shunts for fetal hydronephrosis and hydrocephalus. *N Engl J Med* 1986;315:336–340.

105. Spielman FJ, Seeds JW, Corke BC. Anaesthesia for fetal surgery. *Anaesthesia* 1984;39:756–759.

106. Seeds JW, Corke BC, Spielman FJ. Prevention of fetal movement during invasive procedures with pancuronium bromide. *Am J Obstet Gynecol* 1986;155:818–819.

107. Moise KJ, Carpenter RJ, Deter RL, Kirshon B. The use of fetal neuromuscular blockade during intrauterine transfusions. *Am J Obstet Gynecol* 1987;157:874–879.

108. Copel JA, Grannum PA, Harrison D, Hobbins JC. The use of intravenous pancuronium bromide to produce fetal paralysis during intravascular transfusion. *Am J Obstet Gynecol* 1988;158:170–171.

109. Byers JW, Aubry RH, Feinstein SJ, et al. Intravascular neuromuscular blockade for fetal transfusion. *Am J Obstet Gynecol* 1988;158:677.

110. Pielet BW, Socol ML, MacGregor SN, Dooley SL, Minogue J. Fetal heart rate changes after fetal intravascular treatment with pancuronium bromide. *Am J Obstet Gynecol* 1988;159:640–643.

111. Moise KJ, Deter RL, Kirshon B, et al. Intravenous pancuronium bromide for fetal neuromuscular blockade during intrauterine transfusion for red-cell alloimmunization. *Obstet Gynecol* 1989;74:905–908.

112. Chestnut DH, Weiner CP, Thompson CS, McLaughlin GL. Intravenous administration of d-tubocurarine and pancuronium in fetal lambs. *Am J Obstet Gynecol* 1989;160:510–513.

113. Leveque C, Murat I, Toubas F, et al. Fetal neuromuscular blockade with vecuronium bromide: Studies during intravascular intrauterine transfusion in isoimmunized pregnancies. *Anesthesiology* 1992;76:642–644.

114. Anand KJS, Brown MJ, Bloom SR, Aynsley-Green A. Studies on the hormonal regulation of fuel metabolism in the human newborn infant undergoing anaesthesia and surgery. *Horm Res* 1985;22:115–128.

115. Anand KJS, Brown MJ, Causon RC, Christofides ND, Bloom SR, Aynsley-Green A. Can the human neonate mount an endocrine and metabolic response to surgery? *J Pediatr Surg* 1985;20:41–48.

116. Anand KJS. Hormonal and metabolic function of neonates and infants undergoing surgery. *Curr Opin Cardiol* 1986;1:681–689.

117. Anand KJS, Sippell WG, Aynsley-Green A. Randomized trial of fentanyl anaesthesia in preterm neonates undergoing surgery: Effects on the stress response. *Lancet* 1987;1:243–248.

118. Rose JC, Macdonald AA, Heymann MA, Rudolph AM. Developmental aspects of the pituitary-adrenal axis response to hemorrhagic stress in lamb fetuses in utero. *J Clin Invest* 1978;61:424–432.

119. Liley AW. The foetus as a personality. *Aust N Z J Psych* 1972;6:99–105.

120. Smyth CN. Exploratory methods for testing the integrity of the foetus and neonate. *J Obstet Gynaecol Br Commonw* 1965;72:920–935.

121. Anand KJS, Hickey PR. Pain and its effects in the human neonate and fetus. *N Engl J Med* 1987;317:1321–1329.

122. Rudolph AM, Heymann MA. Cardiac output in the fetal lamb: The effects of spontaneous and induced changes of heart rate on right and left ventricular output. *Am J Obstet Gynecol* 1976;124:183–192.

123. Friedman WF. The intrinsic physiologic properties of the developing heart. *Prog Cardiovasc Dis* 1972;15:87–111.

124. Gilbert RD. Control of fetal cardiac output during changes in blood volume. *Am J Physiol* 1980;238:H80–H86.

125. Gilbert RD. Determinants of venous return in the fetal lamb. *Gynecol Invest* 1977;8:233–245.

126. Shinebourne EA, Vapaavuori EK, Williams RL, Heymann MA, Rudolph AM. Development of baroreflex activity in unanesthetized fetal and neonatal lambs. *Circ Res* 1972;31:710–718.

127. Dawes GS, Duncan SLB, Lewis BV, Merlet CL, Owen-Thomas JB, Reeves JT. Hypoxaemia and aortic chemoreceptor function in foetal lambs. *J Physiol* 1969;201:105–116.

128. Dawes GS, Duncan SLB, Lewis BV, Merlet CL, Owen-Thomas JB, Reeves JT. Cyanide stimulation of the systemic arterial chemoreceptors in foetal lambs. *J Physiol* 1969;201:117–128.

129. Dawes GS, Lewis BV, Milligan JE, Roach MR, Talner NS. Vasomotor responses in the hind limbs of foetal and newborn lambs to asphyxia and aortic chemoreceptor stimulation. *J Physiol* 1968;195:55–81.

130. Goodwin JW, Milligan JE, Thomas B, Taylor JR. The effect of aortic chemoreceptor stimulation on cardiac output and umbilical bloodflow in the fetal lamb. *Am J Obstet Gynecol* 1973;116:48–56.

131. Itskovitz J, LaGamma EF, Rudolph AM. Baroreflex control of the circulation in chronically instrumented fetal lambs. *Circ Res* 1983;52:589–596.

132. Jones MD, Rosenberg AA, Simmons MA, Molteni RA, Koehler RC, Traystman RJ. Oxygen delivery to the brain before and after birth. *Science* 1982;216:324–325.

133. Makowski EL, Schneider JM, Tsoulos NG, Colwill JR, Battaglia FC, Meschia G. Cerebral blood flow, oxygen consumption and glucose utilization of fetal lambs in utero. *Am J Obstet* 1972;114:292–303.

134. Jones MD Jr, Sheldon RE, Peeters LL, Meschia G, Battaglia FC, Makowski EL. Fetal cerebral oxygen consumption at different levels of oxygenation. *J Appl Physiol* 1977;43:1080–1084.

135. Rosenberg AA, Jones MD, Traystman RJ, Simmons MA, Molteni RA. Response of cerebral blood flow to changes in PCO2 in fetal, newborn and adult sheep. *Am J Physiol* 1982;242:H862–H866.

136. Tweed WA, Cote J, Wade JG, Gregory G, Mills A. Preservation of fetal brain blood flow relative to other organs during hypovolemic hypotension. *Pediatr Res* 1982;16:137–140.

137. Tweed WA, Cote J, Pash M, Lou H. Arterial oxygenation determines autoregulation of cerebral blood flow in the fetal lamb. *Pediatr Res* 1983;17:246–249.

138. Gregory GA, Wade JG, Biehl DR, et al. Fetal anesthetic requirement (MAC) for halothane. *Anesth Analg* 1983;62:9–14.

139. Palahniuk RJ, Shnider SM. Maternal and fetal cardiovascular and acid-base changes during halothane and isoflurane anesthesia in the pregnant ewe. *Anesthesiology* 1974;41:462–472.

140. Biehl DR, Cote J, Wade JG, et al. Uptake of halothane by the foetal lamb in utero. *Can Anaesth Soc J* 1983;30:24–27.

141. Biehl DR, Tweed WA, Cote J, et al. Effect of halothane on cardiac output and regional flow in the fetal lamb in utero. *Anesth Analg* 1983;62:489–492.

142. Biehl DR, Yarnell R, Wade JG, Sitar D. The uptake of isoflurane by the foetal lamb in utero: Effect on regional blood flow. *Can Anaesth Soc J* 1983;30:581–586.

143. Cohn HE, Sacks EJ, Heymann MA, Rudolph AM. Cardiovascular responses to hypoxemia and acidemia in fetal lambs. *Am J Obstet Gynecol* 1974;120:817–824.

144. Peeters LL, Sheldon RE, Jones MD, Makowski EL, Meschia G. Blood flow to fetal organs as a function of arterial oxygen content. *Am J Obstet Gynecol* 1979;35:637–646.

145. Reuss ML, Parer JT, Harris JL, Krueger TR. Hemodynamic effects of alpha-adrenergic blockade during hypoxia in fetal sheep. *Am J Obstet Gynecol* 1982;142:410–415.

146. Court DJ, Parer JT, Block BSB, Llanos AJ. Effects of beta-adrenergic blockade on blood flow distribution during hypoxaemia in fetal sheep. *J Dev Physiol* 1984;6:349–358.

147. Johnson GN, Palahniuk RJ, Tweed WA, Jones MV, Wade JG. Regional cerebral blood flow changes during severe fetal asphyxia produced by slow partial umbilical cord compression. *Am J Obstet Gynecol* 1979;135:48–52.

148. Yarnell R, Biehl DR, Tweed WA, Gregory GA, Sitar D. The effect of halothane anaesthesia on the asphyxiated foetal lamb in utero. *Can Anaesth Soc J* 1983;30:474–479.

149. Palahniuk RJ, Doig GA, Johnson GN, Pash MP. Maternal halothane anesthesia reduces cerebral blood flow in the acidotic sheep fetus. *Anesth Analg* 1980;59:35–39.

150. Hedrick MH, Jennings RW, MacGillivray TE, et al. Endoscopic placental vessel catheterization for chronic fetal vascular access. *Surg Forum* 1992;43:504–505.

151. Hedrick MH, Jennings RW, MacGillivray TE, et al. Chronic fetal vascular access. *Lancet* 1993;342:1086–1087.

152. International Symposium on Intrapartum Surveillance. Nottingham, England; 1990.

153. Jennings RW, Adzick NS, Longaker MT, et al. Radiotelemetric fetal monitoring during and after open fetal operation. *Surg Gynecol Obstet* 1993;176:59–64.

154. Yelderman M, New W. Evaluation of pulse oximetry. *Anesthesiology* 1983;59:349–352.

155. Gardosi JO, Schram CM, Symonds EM. Adaptation of pulse oximetry for fetal monitoring during labour. *Lancet* 1991;1:1265–1267.

156. Johnson N, Johnson VA, Fisher J, Jobbings B, Bannister J, Lilford RJ. Fetal monitoring with pulse oximetry. *Br J Obstet Gynaecol* 1991;98:36–41.

157. Nijland R, Nierlich S, Jogsma HW, et al. Validation of reflectance pulse oximetry: An evaluation of a new sensor in piglets. *J Clin Monit* 1997;13:43–49.

158. Luks FI, Johnson BD, Papadakis K, et al. Predictive value of monitoring parameters in fetal surgery. *J Pediatr Surg* 1998;33:1297–1301.

159. Mannheimer PD, Casciani JR, Fein ME, Nierlich SL. Wavelength selection for low-saturation pulse oximetry. *Trans Biomed Eng* 1997;44:148–158.

160. Segal S, Csavoy AN, Datta S. Placental tissue enhances uterine relaxation by nitroglycerin. *Anesth Analg* 1998;86:304–309.

161. Cauldwell CB, Rosen MA, Harrison MR. The use of nitroglycerin for uterine relaxation during fetal surgery [abstract]. *Anesthesiology* 1995;82:A929.

Shnider and Levinson's Anesthesia for Obstetrics,
edited by Samuel C. Hughes, et al.
Lippincott Williams & Wilkins,
Philadelphia, © 2001.

CHAPTER 15

ANESTHESIA FOR ABNORMAL POSITIONS AND PRESENTATIONS, SHOULDER DYSTOCIA, AND MULTIPLE BIRTHS

SUSAN R. GORMAN MALONEY, M.D. AND GERSHON
LEVINSON, M.D.

Presentation refers to the portion of the fetus that is felt through the cervix on vaginal examination. A cephalic presentation can be vertex, brow, or face. **Position** describes the relation of a specific part of the fetus (occiput for vertex presentations, sacrum for breech, acromiom for shoulder) to the mother's pelvis (i.e., right occiput anterior). Fetuses with breech and vertex presentations are both described as having a longitudinal **lie**, meaning the fetal spine lies longitudinally against the maternal spine. At delivery, approximately 90% of single gestation fetuses present as a cephalic vertex presentation, either occiput transverse or anterior. All other presentations and positions (including a transverse lie) are considered abnormal. When compared with single gestation vertex deliveries, both multiple gestations and abnormally positioned single gestations are associated with a higher risk of maternal, fetal, and neonatal morbidity and mortality (1–5). Sometimes even single gestation vertex deliveries can present unexpected and serious anatomic challenges, as is the case with shoulder dystocia. Management of women with these complicated pregnancies and deliveries presents several unique problems for the obstetrician and anesthesiologist.

PERSISTENT OCCIPUT POSTERIOR

Early in labor, it is common for the occiput to be in the transverse or posterior position. Later in active labor, the fetus descends and the occiput usually undergoes normal internal rotation, that is, the face turns inward, to face the woman's sacrum and perineum. With this, the occiput comes to lie beneath the pubic symphysis. If this rotation does not occur, the persistent occiput posterior (OP) position often results in a more prolonged and painful labor than the occiput anterior position. The head in the OP position does not fit as well into the pelvis, resulting in prolonged or arrested descent and slowed cervical dilation. The occiput also exerts increased pressure on the posterior sacral nerves. The resulting severe back pain is often referred to as "back" labor in popular literature. Spontaneous delivery requires more uterine and abdominal work.

Etiology

Obstetricians do not know why some fetuses fail to rotate internally and thereby persist in their OP position. There is some debate as to whether epidural analgesia with higher concentrations of local anesthetic may contribute to the persistence of the OP position. There is insufficient evidence from controlled-randomized trials to make this determination. Any evidence of an association between the use of epidural analgesia and persistence of OP position from retrospective studies may simply reflect the greater need women with preexisting persistent OP positions have for the strong analgesia provided by an epidural.

Obstetric Management

While spontaneous delivery may occur, especially in a multipara with a large pelvis, the obstetrician will sometimes perform manual or forceps-assisted rotation and extraction. A recent survey of the American College of Obstetricians and Gynecologists fellows revealed that more than half of the respondents have abandoned mid-pelvic operative deliveries (6). Midforceps rotations have largely fallen out of favor due to their association with increased birth trauma, intracranial hemorrhage, and birth asphyxia (7). Many obstetricians will still use vacuum or forceps to assist vaginal delivery of an OP fetus that has descended to a +3 station (the fetal presenting part at 3 centimeters distal to the internal ischial spines).

Anesthetic Considerations

If the vertex is known to be in the OP position during the first stage of labor, some believe that regional techniques that profoundly relax the perineal muscles should be avoided until spontaneous internal rotation occurs. Still others believe that for some persistent OP fetuses, relaxing the pelvic muscles of an "overly tense" pelvic floor can allow the fetus to properly descend and rotate. This divergence of opinion is due to the paucity of clinical studies specifically examining the effect of epidural analgesia on the pelvic floor musculature and the further effect this has on the outcome of labor. There are some studies which suggest an increased need for forceps or vacuum assistance of delivery associated with epidural use (8–10) but whether persistent OP position accounted for part of this increased need was not examined.

Analgesia may be provided using a lumbar epidural infusion with as low a concentration of local anesthetic as is effective for pain relief. The anesthesiologist should titrate the concentration and volume of local anesthetic to the pain relief needs of each individual woman. Often 0.0625% to 0.125% bupivacaine with 1.5 to 2 $mg \cdot mL^{-1}$ of fentanyl at an infusion rate of 10 to 16 mL/hr is effective. If the woman remains uncomfortable, despite having an adequate T10-L1 distribution of sensory block, the anesthesiologist can increase the concentration of local anesthetic in the infusion. The anesthesiologist may also administer either fentanyl (50 to 100 μg) or sufentanil (10 to 20 μg) through the epidural catheter in a 10-mL volume of preservative-free saline or 0.125% to 0.25% bupivacaine as an additional bolus. Low concentrations of local anesthetics administered by infusion usually does not produce relaxation of the levator ani muscles, which may play an important role in producing internal rotation.

If the fetus does not spontaneously rotate from its OP position, and the obstetrician plans to assist delivery with forceps rotation, complete analgesia and perineal relaxation is important for maternal and fetal safety. Perineal relaxation allows for more precise placement of the forceps about the fetal head and

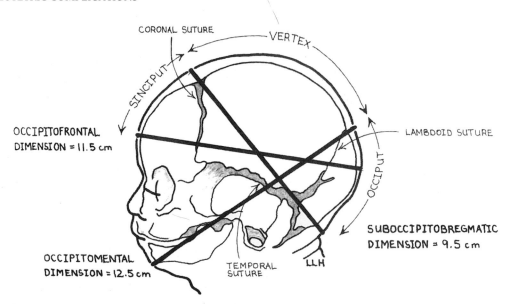

CORONAL SUTURE

VERTEX

SINCIPUT

OCCIPITOFRONTAL
DIMENSION = 11.5 cm

LAMBDOID SUTURE

OCCIPUT

SUBOCCIPITOBREGMATIC
DIMENSION = 9.5 cm

OCCIPITOMENTAL
DIMENSION = 12.5 cm

TEMPORAL
SUTURE

LLH

Figure 15.1. Diameters of the fetal head. (Redrawn by Halton LL, from Cunningham FG, MacDonald PC, Gant NF, et al. In: *Williams Obstetrics*, 18th ed. East Norwalk, CT: Appleton & Lange, 1989:93.)

reduces the risk of vaginal wall lacerations for the mother. Extending an existing lumbar epidural block to the perineum with 3% 2-chloroprocaine or 1.5% to 2.0% lidocaine should provide the optimal conditions for an atraumatic delivery thus lowering the risk of maternal and neonatal morbidity. Usually, a large-volume bolus of 10 to 15 mL is required to reach the sacral roots. For a woman without a preexisting epidural, establish a low spinal anesthetic with 40 to 60 mg of lidocaine or 7.5 mg of bupivacaine intrathecally. A forceps delivery without adequate anesthesia exposes mother and fetus to increased risks of lacerations and head trauma, respectively. Vacuum application and delivery can be carried out safely with minimal or no anesthesia. However, using a nitrous oxide/oxygen mixture by mask inhalation or additional local anesthetic through an existing epidural for perineal analgesia allows the procedure to be carried out with greater maternal comfort.

FACE OR BROW POSITIONS AND SHOULDER PRESENTATIONS

Most fetuses with cephalic presentation and a face or brow position are delivered by cesarean section because of cephalopelvic disproportion. Figure 15.1 demonstrates the increased presenting diameter of the fetal head along the occipitofrontal dimension (as for brow presentations) and occipitomental dimension (as for face presentations) as compared with the optimal (smallest) presenting diameter along the suboccipitobregmatic dimension (as for occiput anterior presentations.) Similarly, most fetuses in a transverse lie with a shoulder presentation are delivered by elective cesarean section. Rarely, the obstetrician will perform internal podalic version and extraction (Fig. 15.2) and deliver the baby vaginally as a breech presentation. Under these circumstances the obstetrician can often perform these intrauterine manipulations safely between contractions with epidural anesthesia providing pelvic and perineal muscle relaxation and nitroglycerin (NTG) providing additional uterine relaxation. Sometimes the uterine smooth muscle requires general anesthesia with a halogenated agent for adequate relaxation. The authors discuss situations such as this in the section on breech deliveries below.

Breech Presentation

In approximately 3.5% of pregnancies, the breech rather than the vertex presents first (11). There are three main types

of breech presentations: frank, complete, and incomplete (Fig. 15.3). A frank breech is one in which the lower extremities are flexed at the hips and extended at the knees so that the feet are against the face (the equivalent of the "pike" position in diving). A complete breech is one in which the fetal lower extremities are flexed at both the hips and knees so that the buttocks with the feet along side them present at the cervix (the equivalent of the "lotus" position in yoga). An incomplete breech presentation is one in which one or both fetal lower extremities are extended and one or both feet present in the vagina or introitus. This type is also referred to as a single or double footling breech presentation. Frank breech is present in about 60% of breech deliveries, incomplete breech in about 30%, and complete breech in approximately 10%.

Etiology

The causes of breech presentation are unknown, but several associated abnormalities are thought to predispose to this

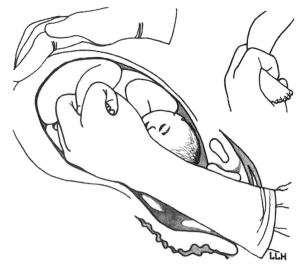

Figure 15.2. Internal podalic version. If at all possible, both feet are grasped because this technique makes the turning much easier. The insert shows a closer view of an obstetrican grasping the fetal ankles. (Redrawn by Halton LL, from Pritchard JA, MacDonald PC, Gant NF, et al. In: *Williams Obstetrics*, 17th ed. New York: Appleton-Century-Crofts, 1985:865.)

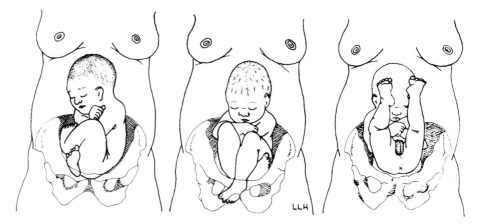

Figure 15.3. Types of breech presentation. left, complete breech; right, frank breech; middle, incomplete breech. (Redrawn by Halton LL., from Seeds JW. Malpresentations. In: *Obstetrics: normal and problem pregnancies*, 2nd ed. New York: Churchill Livingstone, 1991:551.)

presentation. During the first 35 weeks of pregnancy, the fetus often changes its presentation, as part of normal intrauterine fetal activity. It is believed that as the fetus approaches term it tends to accommodate to the shape of the uterine cavity, assuming a longitudinal lie with a vertex presentation. When the fetus is premature, its smaller size requires less accommodation. For this reason, breech presentation occurs more frequently in premature than full-term fetuses (11–13). A breech presentation may also result from interference with the normal process of accommodation between the fetal head, uterine cavity, and maternal pelvis. Placenta previa, uterine anomalies, pelvic tumors, fetal congenital anomalies—especially hydrocephalus and anencephaly—can all interfere with accommodation in this fashion. Additionally, uterine relaxation associated with great parity, multiple fetuses, and polyhydramnios can permit the fetus to maintain a nonvertex presentation by rendering such accommodation unnecessary (11).

Obstetric Management of Breech Presentations

The diagnosis of breech presentation is usually made by manual examination and confirmed by ultra-sound examination. There is a growing trend now to deliver all breeches by cesarean section. Consequently, the leading cause for primary elective cesarean section in many maternity units is breech presentation. However, many obstetricians believe it is safe to deliver selected breeches vaginally (11, 14–17). Guidelines for vaginal breech deliveries are listed in Table 15.1. In most centers, sometime between 36 weeks and the onset of active labor, external cephalic version (ECV) is attempted to convert a breech to a vertex presentation. ECV involves applying pressure to the mother's abdomen to turn the fetus either forward or backward in a somersault to achieve a vertex presentation (18).

Anesthetic Considerations for External Cephalic Version

Version is frequently performed with the aid of tocolytic agents (18). Studies show that use of tocolytics may improve the success rate of ECV in primiparous patients. Anesthesia has not been recommended for this procedure lest it mask injury and possible rupture of the uterus resulting from too much applied pressure. Indeed, one study of 68 second attempts at version under epidural anesthesia, after attempted ECV with beta-agonist had failed, resulted in successful version in 27/68 attempts, but also in complications in two of the 68 attempts (19). A quality assurance study of a series of ECV attempts with and without regional anesthesia showed that use of regional anesthesia was associated with a higher success rate of ECV and a decreased cesarean section rate. The study also showed that use of regional anesthesia for ECV was associated with an increased incidence of maternal hypotension and fetal bradycardia (20). Some randomized-control trials demonstrated an increase in ECV success and no increase in complications with use of epidural anesthesia (21, 22). Conversely, another randomized-clinical trial using spinal anesthesia showed no benefit or detriment (23).

When analyzing studies that show no complications, it is important to remember that a failure to demonstrate a significant increase in harm is not the same as proof of safety. The upper end of the 95% confidence interval for risk of a bad outcome may be estimated from a series that demonstrates few or no complications. The chance of complications may be as high as $(3 + n/N)$, where n is the number of complications in the series and N is the total number of subjects in the series (24). Therefore, although one randomized-controlled trial using ECV (21) revealed no complications, even from this very favorable study the absolute risk increase of complications attributable to epidural use in ECV must be estimated from 0% to as high as 8% to 9%.

For these reasons, the authors believe use of anesthesia to facilitate ECV is reasonable only under very specific circumstances. The version should be attempted between 37 and 38 weeks of gestation in the operating room under ultrasound guidance and fetal monitoring. There must also be a pre-established management plan for immediate cesarean section in the event of an unsuccessful attempt or any complication from such attempt.

Obstetric Management of Vaginal Breech Delivery

Breeches can be delivered vaginally in several different ways. During spontaneous breech delivery, the maternal efforts alone expel the infant. The obstetrician supports the infant, but

Table 15.1. CONSIDERATIONS FOR VAGINAL DELIVERY OF A BREECH PRESENTATION

Facilities:	Capability of emergency cesarean delivery
Obstetrician:	Experience in vaginal breech delivery
Anesthesia:	Anesthesiologist present for delivery, epidural catheter preferable
Type of breech:	Frank most favorable
Fetal size:	Optimal estimated weigth < 4 kg, but > 2.5 kg
Head position and size:	Exclusion of hyperextension and macrocephaly
Pelvis:	Adequate dimensions (various criteria) by computed tomography pelvimetry
Labor:	Normal progression in dilation, effacement, and descent

Adapted from Laros RK Jr, Flanagan TA, Kilpatrick SJ. Management of term breech presentation: a protocol of external cephalic version and selective trial of labor. *Am J Obstet Gynecol* 1995;172:1916–1923; and ACOG Technical Bulletin. *Management of the breech presentation.* 1986; No. 95:1.

performs no other traction or manipulation. Partial breech extraction, also called assisted breech delivery, refers to spontaneous delivery of the fetus as far as the umbilicus, with the obstetrician extracting the remainder of the body with or without forceps application to the after-coming head. When the entire body of the infant is extracted with intrauterine manipulation by the obstetrician, the delivery is termed a total breech extraction. This method of delivery is more commonly employed in delivery of the second or third of a multiple gestation, in which case the uterine cavity is still large and relaxed from its previous co-occupants.

Maternal, Fetal, and Neonatal Hazards

Breech deliveries are associated with increased maternal morbidity, regardless of delivery method. Compared to vertex presentations there is increased risk to the mother of cervical lacerations, perineal injury, shock due to intrapartum and postpartum hemorrhage, retained placenta, and infection for vaginal breech deliveries. The incidence of maternal complications is even greater with cesarean deliveries (3, 11, 25, 26).

There are several reasons for the increased perinatal morbidity and mortality associated with fetuses having a breech presentation. These fetuses are more likely to suffer intracranial hemorrhage from head trauma and asphyxia from cord compression. During spontaneous breech delivery, the uncontrolled expulsion of the fragile fetal head can result in tentorial tears and brain damage. Preterm infants with their soft craniums, fragile brain structures, decreased clotting ability and increased head versus body disproportion are at even greater risk. Indeed, preterm infants who undergo spontaneous breech delivery have a higher mortality than those delivered with the assistance of Piper forceps to protect their after-coming head (Fig. 15.4). However, intrauterine manipulation and improper placement of forceps can also result in fetal trauma and cord compression in delivery of breech infants.

Prolapse of the umbilical cord in breech presentations is a significant cause of increased fetal mortality. The gestational age of the baby has no effect on the incidence of cord prolapse, but the type of breech presentation does. The incidence of cord prolapse is 0.5% in vertex presentations, 0.5% with frank breech presentations, and 10% with incomplete or complete breech presentations (11). The frequency of umbilical cord prolapse is probably increased for complete and incomplete breeches because the presenting part fails to fill the lower uterine segment. While the cranium and buttocks both provide an adequate "plug" for the hole created by the dilating cervix, a combination of feet and legs do not.

Head entrapment is the most feared complication of an attempted vaginal breech delivery. Preterm infants are at greatest risk for this. Their buttocks and torsos are small and thus able to pass through a small cervical opening that may not be dilated enough to accommodate the disproportionately larger after-coming head. For this reason, many obstetricians will not attempt vaginal breech deliveries on infants with estimated fetal weights of less than 2,500 grams (Table 15.1).

The neonatal prognosis is significantly worse in breech deliveries, but it is unclear what portion of this increased morbidity is the result of the delivery itself. That is, some of the excess morbidity may be the result of the same unknown initial problem, such as a preexisting neuromuscular disorder, that caused the fetus to maintain a breech presentation in the first place. Also, some of the morbidity, such as congenital hip dislocations, may be the result of the intrauterine state of a sustained breech position. Cesarean delivery would not prevent such morbidity. Injury still occurs more frequently in breech than cephalic presentations, whether delivery is vaginal or cesarean (27). Perinatal mortality, even adjusted for prematurity and congenital anomalies, is still higher in breech presentations 1% to 2% versus 0.2% to 0.3% for all deliveries (27–30). The obstetric literature includes research studies that demonstrate a decrease in neonatal morbidity and mortality with elective cesarean delivery for breech births as well as studies that fail to indicate cesarean sections provide any benefit (3, 15, 16, 25, 29, 31, 32). A consistent finding is that nonelective, emergent cesarean deliveries have the highest rates of maternal and neonatal morbidity and mortality.

Anesthetic Considerations in Breech Delivery

If the breech is to be delivered by elective primary cesarean section, either regional or general anesthesia may be used. With both spinal and epidural anesthesia, extracting the infant through the uterine incision may be difficult. For this reason, NTG in sublingual spray form (400 μg per metered dose) or IV form (diluted to 50 to 100 μg · mL^{-1}) should be immediately available for breech deliveries. NTG can provide uterine relaxation within 30 to 60 seconds of administration. Doses of 50 to 200 μg IV or one to two sublingual doses of 400 μg each are often sufficient to facilitate delivery (33–36). If more relaxation is needed, the anesthesiologist should give more NTG and treat any resulting hypotension aggressively with ephedrine. If uterine contractions remain a problem, the anesthesiologist

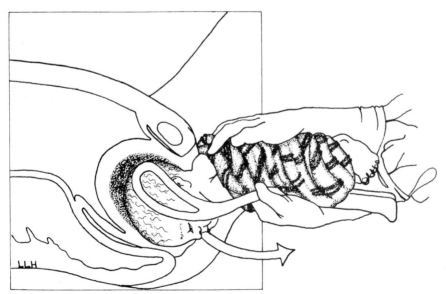

Figure 15.4. Vaginal breech delivery with piper forceps. (Redrawn by Halton LL, from Seeds JW. Malpresentations. In: *Obstetrics: Normal and Problem Pregnancies*, 2nd ed. New York: Churchill Livingstone, 1991:557.)

must be prepared to induce general anesthesia rapidly. After intubating the trachea, administration of isoflurane or another halogenated agent for uterine relaxation is indicated.

If an emergency cesarean section is required for fetal distress or prolapsed umbilical cord, general anesthesia is often necessary. A decision between regional and general techniques in these cases should result from the anesthesiologist's assessment of the time required to achieve adequate regional anesthesia and anticipated difficulty of intubation for general anesthesia, as well as the obstetrician's assessment of the fetal reserve. As with all decisions in obstetric anesthesia, communication between the obstetric and anesthetic care providers is essential.

If the breech is to be delivered vaginally, an anesthesiologist should be immediately available. They can assist by providing adequate analgesia for labor and delivery, but can also rapidly provide perineal and uterine relaxation or anesthesia for an emergency cesarean section. For vaginal breech delivery, most obstetricians use the partial breech extraction method. At the end of the second stage of labor the woman should be able to expel her baby until the umbilicus is seen, whereupon the obstetrician can extract the arms and deliver the after-coming head manually or with Piper forceps (Fig 15.4).

Labor is often managed, for example, with an epidural infusion of 0.0625% to 0.125% bupivacaine and 1.5 to 2 $\mu g \cdot mL^{-1}$ fentanyl. The delivery is then managed with a perineal dose of local anesthetic through the epidural catheter. Ten to 15 milliliters of 3% 2-chloroprocaine or 1.5% to 2% lidocaine with 1 mEq of bicarbonate added to each 10 milliliters of lidocaine for more rapid onset are both reasonable choices. Use of fast-acting agents is important because perineal relaxation is neither needed nor desirable until the very end of the second stage of labor, whereupon it is needed almost immediately to facilitate assisted delivery of the neonate's head.

In the past, some obstetricians avoided major regional anesthesia because of concern over prolonging the first or second stages of labor and decreasing the ability of the mother to push effectively. They feared an increased need for total breech extractions and thus, increased risk of traumatic delivery. More recently, many obstetricians have come to favor the use and even request the placement of epidural catheters in their patients attempting a vaginal breech delivery. They have found that epidural analgesia allows for an alert, cooperative mother who is able to avoid early pushing against an incompletely dilated cervix. This is important because women with a fetus in the breech presentation often experience rectal pressure earlier than those with a vertex presentation. Also with epidural analgesia these women can still push effectively during the second stage with proper anesthetic management and labor coaching. Epidural analgesia provides better pain relief compared with other methods of analgesia and has the flexibility to provide maximal perineal and pelvic floor relaxation for delivery of the after-coming head.

Several retrospective studies have provided reassurance by demonstrating that the incidence of complete breech extraction

was not increased with regional anesthesia, although some studies showed the second stage lengthened slightly (37–40). In one study (39), 94 vaginal breech deliveries managed with epidural anesthesia were compared to 277 vaginal breech deliveries managed without epidural anesthesia. Although the 1-minute Apgar scores were lower in the full-term breech infants born under epidural anesthesia, the 5-minute Apgar scores, perinatal morbidity, and maternal complications were similar in both groups. The other studies cited found no difference or decreased perinatal morbidity in the epidural groups across all categories measured.

Occasionally, epidural analgesia does not provide adequate anesthesia or perineal muscle relaxation for delivery of the after-coming head. The anesthesiologist may need to rapidly induce general anesthesia with thiopental, succinylcholine, and endotracheal intubation. In these situations halogenated agents are not always necessary because application of Piper forceps may not actually require uterine relaxation, but rather the perineal muscle relaxation provided by succinylcholine.

On the other hand, during breech deliveries, the lower uterine segment may contract and trap the after-coming head. In these cases, NTG or a halogenated agent like isoflurane will relax the uterine smooth muscle and facilitate delivery. When used with epidural analgesia for perineal relaxation, intravenous or sublingual NTG will generally provide adequate uterine relaxation to the lower uterine segment for delivery of the after-coming head without general anesthesia (33–36). Sometimes NTG will fail to provide adequate relaxation. For these rare circumstances, the anesthesiologist should induce general anesthesia, using a rapid sequence technique with cricoid pressure, and intubate the trachea, just as one would for an emergency cesarean delivery. After intubation, controlled ventilation with a halogenated agent will provide uterine relaxation with rapid onset and reversibility.

The intrauterine manipulations required for complete breech extraction can often be performed safely between contractions. For complete breech extractions, perineal anesthesia from an epidural and uterine relaxation with NTG or even general anesthesia with isoflurane may also be required.

Because of the increased risk of need for emergent cesarean section or induction of general anesthesia for vaginal delivery, all breech deliveries should be performed in a room appropriately equipped for either situation. Important information concerning breech deliveries is summarized in Table 15.2.

SHOULDER DYSTOCIA

While the preceding sections discussed the management of problems resulting from abnormal positions and presentations, occasionally normal occiput anterior presentations can develop problems after delivery of the baby's head. These problems may be mild, resulting in a slight delay (greater than 60 seconds) in head to body delivery time. Mild shoulder dystocias such as these may not require ancillary obstetric maneuvers.

Table 15.2. ANESTHETIC CONSIDERATIONS FOR BREECH PRESENTATION

Risk Factors	Anticipated Problems	Preparations
Too much room	Cord prolapse	Epidural for labor
Preterm		
Polyhydramnios	Perinatal fetal trauma with assisted vaginal delivery	2% 2-chloroprocaine, 2% lidocaine with bicarbonate for perineal dose
2nd twin after delivery of 1st		
	Head entrapment	Nitroglycerin for uterine relaxation
Not enough room	Difficult extraction at cesarean	Intubation and general anesthesia with isoflurane to relax uterus and/or for cesarean
Uterine anomalies		
Placenta previa		
Cannot tum, regardless		
Fetal abnormality		

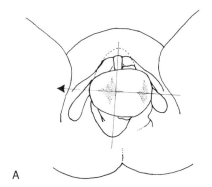
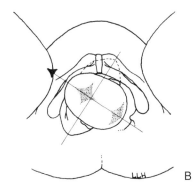

Figure 15.5. **A:** Initial anterior posterior position of the shoulder girdle. **B:** Normal oblique position of the shoulder girdle following delivery of the fetal head. Failure of the shoulder girdle to rotate from the anterior posterior to the oblique position can result in a shoulder dystocia. (Redrawn by Halton LL, from Naef RW, Martin JN. Intrapartum and postpartum emergencies: emergent management of shoulder dystocia. *Obstet Gynecol Clin North Am* 1995;22:248–251.)

Alternatively, these problems can be more severe with entrapment of the baby's anterior shoulder behind the maternal pubic symphysis. If there is an extended delay (beyond several minutes) in head to body delivery time, the baby's blood supply is compromised as the umbilical cord is compressed against its abdomen. Because of this risk of asphyxia, a severe shoulder dystocia, which is estimated to occur in slightly less than 1% of all births, (41) is an obstetric emergency.

Etiology and Epidemiology

When the fetus descends into the pelvis, its shoulders first enter in an anterior-posterior axis alignment (Fig. 15.5a). Later, the shoulders rotate into an oblique orientation (Fig. 15.5b). If the fetal trunk and shoulders do not rotate, the anterior shoulder does not easily pass out from under the pubic symphysis. A fetus' trunk can fail to rotate because of an increased resistance between the fetal skin and the maternal vaginal wall (maternal obesity), a large fetal chest (fetal macrosomia), or a precipitous labor that allows no time for proper trunk rotation (41).

Risk factors for dystocia can not always be identified before labor (42). While maternal diabetes and fetal macrosomia are the two risk factors most strongly associated with shoulder dystocia, even the combination of these two risk factors do not have a high positive predictive value. That is, the majority of diabetic mothers with babies greater than 4,250 grams do not experience shoulder dystocia with vaginal delivery (42). Furthermore, even though most of these women undergo elective cesarean section to prevent a possible dystocia, many cases of shoulder dystocia occur in nondiabetic women with babies less than 4,000 grams. Therefore, both the obstetrician and anesthesiologist should have well considered plans for the management of this emergency.

Obstetric Management

Obstetric management begins with recognizing the immediate warning signs such as a retraction of the head after initial delivery as the shoulder hangs up under the maternal pubis. This is often referred to as the "turtle sign." The obstetric care provider will then call for additional assistants to flex the maternal thighs against the abdomen in order to elevate the pubic symphysis and apply suprapubic pressure to displace the anterior fetal shoulder. This McRobert's maneuver is shown in Figure 15.6. Often the provider will cut an episiotomy to create more room for descent of the posterior shoulder. While it is important to deliver the fetus in a timely fashion (as delays can lead to asphyxia), strong traction on the fetal head and neck can result in damage to the brachial plexus or clavicle fracture. If numerous obstetric maneuvers with maximal pelvic relaxation (described below) fail, the obstetrician may attempt to replace the head into the vagina and deliver the baby by cesarean section (Zavanelli maneuver). Results of the Zavanelli maneuver have been reported in numerous case series. A 1999 critical review of several such reports showed the procedure to have a 92% success rate (43).

However, case series are far more likely to report successes than failures, and so this critical review may not reflect the true success rate of the procedure. Furthermore, because shoulder dystocias are usually responsive to more conservative maneuvers, few practitioners have any direct experience with the Zavanelli maneuver.

Anesthetic Considerations

Bony entrapment by the maternal pubic symphysis prevents delivery of the fetal anterior shoulder, however, there are several things the anesthesiologist can do to aid delivery. First, if the mother already has an epidural catheter in place, rapid injection of 15 milliliters of 3% 2-chloroprocaine or 2% lidocaine with sodium bicarbonate can rapidly provide significant perineal muscle relaxation. Because the risk of fetal asphyxia increases with time, the anesthesiologist should administer this perineal dose as soon as the possibility of a shoulder dystocia is

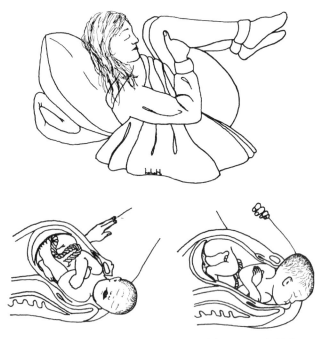

Figure 15.6. The McRoberts-maneuver. **Top:** The maternal thighs are flexed against the abdomen in order to elevate the pubic symphysis. **Bottom left:** With maternal thighs partially flexed, the anterior fetal shoulder remains trapped under the maternal pelvic bone. **Bottom right:** By sharply flexing the maternal thighs against the maternal abdomen, the fetal shoulder is able to pass under the elevated maternal pelvic bone. (Redrawn by Halton LL, from Naef RW, Martin JN. Intrapartum and postpartum emergencies: emergent management of shoulder dystocia. *Obstet Gynecol Clin North Am* 1995;22:248–252.)

Table 15.3. ANESTHETIC CONSIDERATIONS FOR SHOULDER DYSTOCIA

Risk Factors	Anticipated Problems	Preparations
Maternal diabetes Maternal obesity Fetal macrosomia Prolonged 2nd stage Precipitous labor Head retraction at perineum, "turtle sign"—immediate warning	Fetal asphyxia from umbilical cord compression against fetal abdomen	If epidural in place 3% 2-chloroprocaine or 2% lidocaine for perineal relaxation Succinylcholine for perineal relaxation—with induction drug, intubation, and ventilation equipment General anesthesia for emergency rescue cesarean

recognized. If the mother does not have an epidural in place, the anesthesiologist could induce general anesthesia with a hypnotic drug (sodium thiopental) and succinylcholine, followed by tracheal intubation for airway protection just as for any emergent cesarean delivery. This very rarely used approach entails risk for the mother and should not be attempted until all other more conservative maneuvers have been tried. Probably the real benefit of inducing general anesthesia is the pelvic muscle paralysis afforded by succinylcholine administration. Like the Zavanelli maneuver for obstetricians, induction of general anesthesia and paralysis of the mother is a method of last resort for the anesthesiologist. When the Zavanelli maneuver is attempted, the anesthesiologist can assist the obstetrician by administering NTG to relax the uterus. This may facilitate replacement of the fetal head back up into the vagina.

While maternal diabetes and fetal macrosomia are significant risk factors for shoulder dystocia, approximately 50% of all cases do not demonstrate these classic predisposing factors. For this reason, the anesthesia and obstetric care teams must be prepared to manage such emergencies. Important information concerning shoulder dystocia is summarized in Table 15.3.

MULTIPLE GESTATIONS

The incidence of twin and higher-order multiple gestations has increased significantly over the past 15 years with the rising use of fertility treatments such as ovulation-inducing drugs and in vitro fertilization with artificial implantation of multiple embryos. Therefore, the complications associated with multiple pregnancies have also become more common. The combined incidence of twins, triplets and higher-order multiple gestations is now more than 3% of all pregnancies (44). Many of the women with multiple pregnancies are older than 35 and, thus, are at even greater risk for obstetric complications.

The Mother

Preeclampsia-eclampsia, anemia, premature labor, prolonged labor, and antepartum and postpartum hemorrhage are more common in multiple gestations (45, 46). Despite the fact that maternal blood volume increases earlier in pregnancy and reaches levels approximately 40% greater than in single gestations, anemia still occurs more frequently and is more severe in multiple gestations (47). The larger uterus predisposes the parturient to more severe supine hypotension. The increase in uterine distension due to multiple gestation also leads to a more frequent occurrence of nausea and vomiting, dyspnea, leg edema, and varicosities. Blood loss during twin delivery is twice that of a single gestation. Manual extraction of the placenta is required twice as often (45). Intrauterine death of one fetus in a multiple gestation can cause maternal disseminated intravascular coagulopathy (1). Maternal mortality is two to three times higher in multiple gestations.

The Fetus

Fetuses in both mono and dizygotic twinning are at increased risk for intrauterine growth restriction from placental insufficiency and other causes (1). There are two circumstances in monozygotic twinning which pose special hazards to the fetuses. An anastomosis may be present between the two vascular systems, resulting in transfusion of blood from one fetus to the other. In such cases one twin may receive most of the blood and become polycythemic with cardiomegaly and heart failure, while the other twin may not receive enough blood to survive (twin–twin transfusion syndrome). Monoamniotic, monozygotic twins pose another hazard. This occurs in up to 4% of identical twins and is associated with a dramatically increased risk of fetal mortality (50% chance of intrauterine death) due to intertwining and occlusion of the umbilical vessels (48).

The Neonate

Preterm labor and preterm premature rupture of membranes are both more common in women with multiple pregnancies (1). Approximately 30% to 40% of all twins are premature (49). This increased incidence of premature delivery may be due to overdistension and thus, hyperirritability of the uterus and also the increased incidence of maternal complications such as preeclampsia-eclampsia. Fetal growth is independent of the number of fetuses in the uterus until 28 weeks of gestation. At this point a progressive weight lag develops when compared with single gestations. The neonatal death rate is higher in infants of multiple gestations, due mostly to prematurity. However, mature twins also have a higher mortality than mature single births (1). This is most likely due to a higher incidence of other factors that complicate multiple gestations, such as congenital anomalies, prolapsed umbilical cord, abnormal presentations and neonatal intracranial and visceral hemorrhage. The second twin is likely to be more depressed, asphyxiated, and requiring of resuscitation than the first (1, 50). The most significant risk factor for morbidity in the second twin is the period of potential hypoxemia caused either by contraction of the uterus or by premature separation of the placenta after the first infant has been delivered.

Obstetric Management

Any combination of presentations of the fetuses can occur but the most common are vertex-vertex or vertex-breech. Rarely, interlocking of body parts (Fig. 15.7) and resulting interference with engagement or delivery of one fetus by his/her twin can occur. The duration of labor is often shorter in multiple gestations because of the smaller fetal size and frequent effacement of the cervix before the onset of contractions. On the other hand, dysfunctional uterine contractions associated with an over-distended uterus may prolong labor in some cases.

For vertex-vertex twins, the American College of Obstetricians and Gynecologists recommends that cesarean delivery be

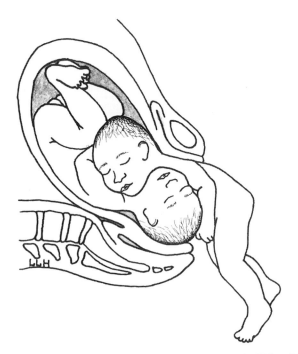

Figure 15.7. Interlocking twins: chin-to-chin. (Redrawn by Halton LL, from MacDonald JS. Other obstetric procedures. In: *Principles and Practice of Obstetric Analgesia and Anesthesia,* 1st ed. Philadelphia: FA Davis Co., 1969:1372.)

performed only for the same indications applied to singleton gestations. In a series of 362 twins, more than 80% of the vertex-vertex and 70% of the vertex-nonvertex twins were delivered vaginally (51). For vaginal delivery, continuous fetal heart rate monitoring of both infants is recommended. If this is not feasible, after delivery of the first infant, the second infant should then have continuous monitoring for immediate recognition of acute fetal asphyxia. In general, when the first twin is in a nonvertex position, cesarean delivery is the method of choice. Regardless of chosen delivery mode, personnel and equipment to resuscitate both infants should be available.

Anesthetic Considerations

The major considerations in regard to choice of anesthesia for multiple gestations are the frequent association with prematurity and breech presentation. The anesthesiologist may need to provide anesthesia for version, extraction and breech vaginal delivery, midforceps delivery, or cesarean delivery very rapidly. Therefore early intrapartum evaluation and preparation is essential. Just as for a singleton breech delivery, the anesthesiologist should insert a large intravenous cannula, ensure that blood is available, and be prepared to provide general anesthesia on an emergent basis.

For vaginal delivery, epidural analgesia is the method of choice for women with multiple gestation. Adequate perineal anesthesia prevents involuntary bearing down by the mother and possible uncontrolled delivery of a small first twin through an incompletely dilated cervix. Forceps deliveries, which are more frequent with multiple gestations, are easier to accomplish with the complete perineal relaxation provided by epidural anesthesia. Epidural anesthesia can also facilitate delivery of the second twin (4). As mentioned above in the section on breeches, after the first twin is delivered, the uterine cavity often remains enlarged and relaxed for a brief period of time. Because of this, the position of the second twin may change. The obstetrician may need to perform an internal podalic version and extraction (Fig. 15.2). In essence, the obstetrician reaches into the uterus, grasps the fetal ankles and pulls the baby out by its feet. Many experts also prefer epidural anesthesia for this version and ex-

Table 15.4. ANESTHETIC CONSIDERATIONS FOR MULTIPLE GESTATION

Anticipated Problems	Preparations
Maternal	Large-bore IV access
Advanced age	Epidural for labor
Supine hypotension	Blood available
Respiratory compromise	Uterine constriction agents in
Preeclampsia-eclampsia	room: oxytocin, methergine,
Dysfunctional labor	prostaglandin $F_{2\alpha}$
Postpartum hemorrhage	Nitroglycerin for uterine
Neonatal	relaxation
Prematurity	General anesthesia and
Twin-twin transfusion syndrome	resuscitation equipment
Congenital anomalies	Resuscitation equipment and
Breech presentation	personnel for each infant
2nd twin asphyxia at delivery	

traction. When internal podalic version and complete extraction are performed under epidural anesthesia, manipulations are made between contractions. Uterine relaxation makes internal podalic version easier. In one study of 22 cases (with success in 20) of internal podalic version of the second twin in transverse lie with unruptured membranes, IV NTG induced transient and prompt uterine relaxation (52). The techniques of using intravenous or sublingual NTG as well as general anesthesia with halogenated agents for uterine relaxation are discussed in the section on breech deliveries.

Just as in breech deliveries, lumbar epidural anesthesia using dilute local anesthetic combined with fentanyl or sufentanil provides complete pain relief but still preserves adequate strength in the abdominal muscles for the mother to push and thereby assist with delivery.

The woman with a multiple gestation is at greater risk for developing hypotension. The larger gravid uterus produces more aortocaval compression and increases the incidence and severity of maternal hypotension when combined with the sympathetic block of epidural anesthesia. Also, patients with sympathetic blockade will not vasoconstrict to maintain blood pressure in response to the increased blood loss seen at twin deliveries. Left uterine displacement during labor and delivery and adequate fluid and blood replacement are particularly important when caring for women with multiple pregnancies.

When a cesarean section is indicated, either regional or general anesthesia may be used. The available evidence does not favor one method over the other. The choice of anesthesia for cesarean delivery of a multiple gestation depends on the preference and experience of the anesthesiologist, the obstetrician, and the patient. After cesarean delivery, the previously distended uterus may require extra constriction agents in addition to the usual oxytocin, such as methergine or prostaglandin $F_{2\alpha}$ in order to prevent excessive postpartum blood loss.

Important information concerning multiple gestations is summarized in Table 15.4.

The obstetric anesthesiologist plays an important role in the care of women with pregnancies complicated by breech and other abnormal presentations, shoulder dystocia, and multiple gestation. Open and frequent communication between the anesthesiologist and obstetric team is essential for providing optimal clinical care in these difficult situations.

REFERENCES

1. American College of Obstetricians and Gynecologists. Special problems of multiple gestation. *Int J Gynaecol Obstet* 1999;64:323–333.
2. Stone J, Eddleman K, Patel S. Controversies in the intrapartum management of twin gestations. *Obstet Gynecol Clin North Am* 1999;26:327–343.

3. Roman J, Bakos O, Cnattingius S. Pregnancy outcomes by mode of delivery among term breech births: Swedish experience 1987–1993. *Obstet Gynecol* 1998;92:945–950.

4. De Veciana M, Major C, Morgan MA. Labor and delivery management of the multiple gestation. *Obstet Gynecol Clin North Am* 1995;22:235–246.

5. American College of Obstetricians and Gynecologists. Operative vaginal delivery. *Int J Gynaecol Obstet* 1994;47:179–185.

6. Bofill JA, Rust OA, Perry KG, et al. Operative vaginal delivery: a survey of fellows of ACOG. *Obstet Gynecol* 1996;88:1007–1010.

7. Cunningham FG, MacDonald PC, Gant NF. Dystocia due to abnormalities in presentation, position or development of the fetus. In: *Williams Obstetrics*, 18th ed. Norwalk, CT: Appleton & Lange, 1989;362–364.

8. Yancey MK, Pierce B, Schweitzer D, et al. Observations on labor epidural analgesia and operative delivery rates. *Am J Obstet Gynecol* 1999;180:353–359.

9. Nageotte MP, Larson D, Rumney PJ, et al. Epidural analgesia compared with combined spinal-epidural analgesia during labor in nulliparous women. *N Engl J Med* 1997;337:1715–1719.

10. Lyon DS, Knuckles G, Whitaker E, et al. The effect of instituting an elective labor epidural program on the operative delivery rate. *Obstet Gynecol* 1997;90:135–141.

11. Cunningham FG, MacDonald PC, Gant NF. Techniques for breech delivery. In: *Williams Obstetrics*, 18th ed. Norwalk, CT: Appleton & Lange, 1989:393–403.

12. Hill LM. Prevalence of breech presentation by gestational age. *Am J Perinatol* 1990;7:92–93.

13. Hickok DE, Gordon DC, Milberg JA, et al. The frequency of breech presentation by gestational age at birth: a large population-based study. *Am J Obstet Gynecol* 1992;166:851–852.

14. Daniel Y, Fait G, Lessing JB, et al. Outcome of 496 term singleton breech deliveries in a tertiary center. *Am J Perinatol* 1998;15:97–101.

15. Irion O, Hirsbrunner Almagbaly P, Morabia A. Planned vaginal delivery versus elective caesarean section: a study of 705 singleton term breech presentations. *Br J Obstet Gynaecol* 1998;105:710–717.

16. Albrechtsen S, Rasmussen S, Reigstad H, et al. Evaluation of a protocol for selecting fetuses in breech presentation for vaginal delivery or cesarean section. *Am J Obstet Gynecol* 1997;177:586–592.

17. Laros RK Jr, Flanagan TA, Kilpatrick SJ. Management of term breech presentation: a protocol of external cephalic version and selective trial of labor. *Am J Obstet Gynecol* 1995;172:1916–1923.

18. American College of Obstetricians and Gynecologists. External cephalic version. *Int J Gynaecol Obstet* 1997;59:73–80.

19. Rozenberg P, Goffinet F, de Spirlet M, et al. External cephalic version with epidural anaesthesia after failure of a first trial with betamimetics. *Br J Obstet Gynaecol* 2000;107:406–410.

20. Patel R, Ramanathan S. Regional anesthesia and external cephalic version: a quality assurance study. Presented at the Society for Obstetric Anesthesia and Perinatology 28th Annual Meeting, Tucson, 1996.

21. Schorr SJ, Speights SE, Ross EL, et al. A randomized trial of epidural anesthesia to improve external cephalic version success. *Am J Obstet Gynecol* 1997;177:1133–1137.

22. Neiger R, Hennessy MD, Patel M. Reattempting failed external cephalic version under epidural anesthesia. *Am J Obstet Gynecol* 1998;179:1136–1139.

23. Dugoff L, Stamm CA, Jones OW III, et al. The effect of spinal anesthesia on the success rate of external cephalic version: a randomized trial. *Obstet Gynecol* 1999;93:345–349.

24. Newman TB. If almost nothing goes wrong, is almost everything all right? Interpreting small numerators [Letter]. *JAMA* 1995;274:1013.

25. Diro M, Puangsricharern A, Royer L, et al. Singleton term breech deliveries in nulliparous and multiparous women: a 5-year experience at the University of Miami/Jackson Memorial Hospital. *Am J Obstet Gynecol* 1999;181:247–252.

26. Erkaya S, Tuncer RA, Kutlar I, et al. Outcome of 1040 consecutive breech deliveries: clinical experience of a maternity hospital in Turkey. *Int J Gynaecol Obstet* 1997;59:115–118.

27. Scorza WE. Intrapartum management of breech presentation. *Clin Perinatol* 1996;23:31–49.

28. Guyer B, MacDorman MF, Martin JA, et al. Annual summary of vital statistics—1997. *Pediatrics* 1998;102:1333–1349.

29. Gifford DS, Morton SC, Fiske M, et al. A meta-analysis of infant outcomes after breech delivery. *Obstet Gynecol* 1995;85:1047–1054.

30. Peters KD, Kochanek KD, Murphy SL. Deaths: final data for 1996. *Natl Vital Stat Rep* 1998;47:1–100.

31. Ismail MA, Nagib N, Ismail T, et al. Comparison of vaginal and cesarean section delivery for fetuses in breech presentation. *J Perinat Med* 1999;27:339–351.

32. Koo MR, Dekker GA, van Geijn HP. Perinatal outcome of singleton term breech deliveries. *Eur J Obstet Gynecol Reprod Biol* 1998;78:19–24.

33. Craig S, Dalton R, Tuck M, et al. Sublingual glyceryl trinitrate for uterine relaxation at Caeserean section—a prospective trial. *Aust N Z J Obstet Gynaecol* 1998;38:34–39.

34. DeSimone CA, Norris MC, Leighton BL. Intravenous nitroglycerin aids manual extraction of a retained placenta [Letter]. *Anesthesiology* 1990;73:787.

35. Peng AT, Gorman RS, Shulman SM, et al. Intravenous nitroglycerin for uterine relaxation in the postpartum patient with retained placenta [Letter]. *Anesthesiology* 1989;71:172–173.

36. Wessén A, Elowsson P, Axemo P, et al. The use of intravenous nitroglycerin for emergency cervico-uterine relaxation. *Acta Anaesthesiol Scand* 1995;39:847–849.

37. Bowen-Simpkins P, Fergusson IL. Lumbar epidural block and the breech presentation. *Br J Anaesth* 1974;46:420–424.

38. Crawford JS. An appraisal of lumbar epidural blockade in patients with a singleton fetus presenting by the breech. *J Obstet Gynaecol Br Commonw* 1974;81:867–872.

39. Confino E, Ismajovich B, Rudick V, et al. Extradural analgesia in the management of singleton breech delivery. *Br J Anaesth* 1985;57:892–895.

40. Breeson AJ, Kovacs GT, Pickles BG, et al. Extradural analgesia–the preferred method of analgesia for vaginal breech delivery. *Br J Anaesth* 1978;50:1227–1230.

41. Wagner RK, Nielsen PE, Gonik B. Shoulder dystocia. *Obstet Gynecol Clin North Am* 1999;26:371–383.

42. American College of Obstetricians and Gynecologists. Shoulder dystocia. *Int J Gynaecol Obstet* 1998;60:306–313.

43. Sandberg EC. The Zavanelli maneuver: 12 years of recorded experience. *Obstet Gynecol* 1999;93:312–317.

44. Ventura SJ, Martin JA, Curtin SC, et al. Births: final data for 1997. *Natl Vital Stat Rep* 1999;47:1–96.

45. Cunningham FG, MacDonald PC, Gant NF. In: *Williams Obstetrics*, 18th ed. Norwalk, CT: Appleton & Lange, 1989:629–652.

46. Doyle P. The outcome of multiple pregnancy. *Hum Reprod* 1996;11(Suppl 4):110–120.

47. Abrams B. Maternal nutrition. In: Creasy RK, Resnick R, eds. *Maternal-Fetal Medicine, Principles and Practice*, 3rd ed. Philadelphia: WB Saunders, 1994:162–170.

48. Adams DM, Chervenak FA. Intrapartum management of twin gestation. *Clin Obstet Gynecol* 1990;33:52–60.

49. Mokriski BK. Abnormal presentation and multiple gestation. In: Chestnut DH, ed. *Obstetric Anesthesia; Prinicples and Practice*, 2nd ed. St. Louis: Mosby, 1999:694–710.

50. Young BK, Suidan J, Antoine C, et al. Differences in twins: the importance of birth order. *Am J Obstet Gynecol* 1985;151:915–921.

51. Chervenak FA, Johnson RE, Youcha S, et al. Intrapartum management of twin gestation. *Obstet Gynecol* 1985;65:119–124.

52. Dufour P, Vinatier D, Vanderstichele S, et al. Intravenous nitroglycerin for internal podalic version of the second twin in transverse lie. *Obstet Gynecol* 1998;92:416–419.

53. American College of Obstetricians and Gynecologists. Management of the breech presentation. *ACOG Technical Bulletin* 1986;95.

Shnider and Levinson's Anesthesia for Obstetrics,
edited by Samuel C. Hughes, et al.
Lippincott Williams & Wilkins,
Philadelphia, © 2001.

CHAPTER 16

ANESTHETIC CONSIDERATIONS FOR THE HYPERTENSIVE DISORDERS OF PREGNANCY

ROBERT R. GAISER, M.D., BRETT B. GUTSCHE, M.D.
AND THEODORE G. CHEEK, M.D.

Hypertensive disease remains one of the most studied and complex dilemmas of pregnancy. Each year approximately 6% to 8% of pregnancies in the United States become complicated by hypertensive disease (1). Hypertension during pregnancy is associated with significant maternal, fetal, and neonatal morbidity and mortality. The terminology to describe hypertension in pregnancy is nonuniform and confusing, and "several overlapping terms are commonly applied to varying clinical manifestations of the same disease" (1–3). While a variety of classifications have been applied to this disorder in the past, two distinct entities are apparent: pregnancy-induced hypertension (PIH) and chronic hypertension (Table 16.1) (1, 4). PIH is a multiorgan disease process with elevated blood pressure. It is divided into clinical subsets depending on the end-organ effects, including preeclampsia, eclampsia, and HELLP (or **h**emolysis, **e**levated **l**iver enzymes, and **l**ow **p**latelets).

When PIH includes renal involvement and leads to proteinuria, it is traditionally referred to as preeclampsia (1). Preeclampsia is a disorder that occurs typically after the 20th week of gestation, except when associated with a hydatidiform mole, but rarely occurs before the 24th week. Preeclampsia is characterized by a triad of symptoms: hypertension, generalized edema, and proteinuria. While not part of the triad, hyperreflexia is usually present. The American College of Obstetricans and Gynecologists (ACOG) clinical definition of preeclampsia includes a sustained systolic blood pressure of at least 140 mm Hg or a sustained diastolic blood pressure of 90 mm Hg (1). Although increased systolic blood pressure of 30 mm Hg or diastolic of 15 mm Hg from second-trimester values was once thought to be of diagnostic value, this concept is no longer considered to be valid (1, 4). Some obstetricians have stated that edema is an unreliable sign of preeclampsia. Women with hypertension and proteinuria, without edema, can develop eclamptic convulsions (5–7). Furthermore, not all patients who develop eclampsia have antecedent hypertension. Preeclampsia usually abates within 48 hours of termination of pregnancy and delivery of the entire placenta. In fact, postpartum curettage has been studied and advocated as a means to hasten the resolution of this disease process (8). Eclampsia is another subset of PIH with central nervous system involvement leading to seizures or grand mal convulsions not related to other cerebral conditions. Although PIH has been called "preeclampsia-eclampsia" or "toxemia of pregnancy," these terms are no longer used to describe the condition.

Chronic hypertension is the presence of persistent maternal hypertension, regardless of cause, before the 20th week of gestation or beyond 6 weeks after delivery. This chapter is primarily concerned with PIH but will use the terms for the several recognized subsets (preeclampsia, eclampsia, and HELLP as well).

INCIDENCE AND ETIOLOGY OF PREGNANCY-INDUCED HYPERTENSION

In the United States, the incidence of PIH complicating pregnancy is often stated to be 6% to 8% (1), although a large study from 1979 to 1986 reported the incidence to be only 26 per 1,000 births (7). The incidence of eclampsia has been reported as 0.2 to 0.67 per 1,000 births, with maternal mortality of 0.4% to 11.9% and perinatal mortality of 20% to 30% (7–12).

PIH most often occurs in young primigravidas, with those under 20 years of age having five times the incidence of those over 20 years of age (9). There is no significant difference between its occurrence in blacks and whites, although there is a higher rate in unmarried vs. married women and in Medicaid vs. privately insured patients (9). These data may reflect differences in access to medical care or other issues (such as nutritional status) based on socioeconomic factors. There also may be variation in rates of PIH according to geographic location (9, 10). Although PIH occurs most frequently in young primigravidas, it is by no means limited to this group. From a study of 2,947 healthy women (11), randomized to receive aspirin (60 mg/day) or a placebo at 13 to 27 weeks, 156 women (5.3%) developed preeclampsia. In order of importance of a positive prediction were (a) systolic blood pressure at entry, (b) obesity before pregnancy, (c) number of previous abortions or miscarriages and, surprisingly, (d) an absence of smoking history. In an analysis of the women entering the above study with chronic hypertension, the predictive factors for development of preeclampsia were (a) preeclampsia in a previous pregnancy, (b) hypertension of at least 4 years' duration, and (c) a diastolic blood pressure of at least 100 mm Hg in early pregnancy. Factors found not to be associated with a higher incidence of preeclampsia were race (without superimposed chronic hypertension) (11, 12), advanced maternal age (>35 years) (10), and climactic factors (13). Aspirin did not significantly lower the incidence of preeclampsia (11, 12). Several studies of eclamptic patients have indicated that maternal morbidity and mortality increase with both age and parity (14, 15). From a series of 298 eclamptic patients, the onset of eclampsia occurred before delivery in 44%, during delivery in 37%, and after delivery in 19% (14). Among the hospitalized patients, eclampsia was manifested before delivery in 17%, during delivery in 52%, and after delivery in 34%. Of those developing eclampsia postpartum, 43% did so within 4 hours of delivery, and 86% within 24 hours. Risk factors, as currently understood, are listed in Table 16.2.

The incidence of PIH is markedly higher in conditions associated with rapid uterine enlargement, such as hydatidiform mole, multiple gestations, polyhydramnios, and diabetic mothers with a macrosomic fetus. A Canadian study found the incidence of preeclampsia to be 9.9% in 334 diabetic pregnancies compared

Table 16.1. CLASSIFICATION OF HYPERTENSIVE DISORDERS COMPLICATING PREGNANCY

Pregnancy-induced hypertension (PIH): Hypertension that develops as a consequence of pregnancy and regresses postpartum. Several clinical subsets are recognized, depending on end-organ effects:

1. Hypertension without proteinuria, pathological edema, or other obvious end-organ disease. The term PIH denotes this limited form, i.e., hypertension without end-organ disease, but is also used as a comprehensive term for the spectrum of disease.
2. Preeclampsia
   - Hypertension with renal involvement
   - Often subdivided into *mild* (diastolic blood pressure <100 mm Hg) or *severe* (diastolic blood pressure >110 mm Hg) but cannot rigidly separate. This is, however, useful as a clinical description.
3. Eclampsia
   - Hypertension with renal and CNS involvement (grand mal seizures)
4. HELLP
   - Hypertension with the clinical picture animated by hematologic and hepatic manifestations

Chronic hypertension: Chronic (coincidental) underlying hypertension that antecedes pregnancy and continues postpartum

Pregnancy-aggravated hypertension: Underlying hypertension worsened by pregnancy
   - Superimposed preeclampsia
   - Superimposed eclampsia

Transient hypertension: Hypertension that develops after the midtrimester of pregnancy is characterized by mild elevations of blood pressure and regresses after pregnancy. This term is still used by some and may be useful clinically. Some classification systems ignore the term and would refer to PIH without end-organ involvement.

There is little consensus on the definition of hypertensive disorders in pregnancy, and, thus, there are several parallel classifications. Adapted from Cunningham FG, MacDonald PC, Gant NF, eds. *Williams Obstetrics*, 20th ed. Norwalk, CT: Appleton & Lange, 1997:694.

to 4.3% in 16,534 nondiabetic controls (16). Perinatal mortality was 60 per 1,000 births compared to 3.3 per 1,000 births in nondiabetic preeclamptic mothers. The more severe the diabetes the higher the occurrence of preeclampsia. Poor control of hyperthyroidism increased the risks of both severe preeclampsia and low-birthweight infants (17). Social factors including job-related stress among pregnant workers (18, 19) and changes

Table 16.2. RISK FACTORS FOR THE DEVELOPMENT OF PREGNANCY-INDUCED HYPERTENSION[a]

Factor	Risk Ratio
Nulliparity	3:1
Age >40 years	3:1
African-American race	1.5:1
Family history of pregnancy-induced hypertension (PIH)	5:1
Chronic hypertension	10:1
Chronic renal disease	20:1
Antiphospholipid syndrome	10:1
Diabetes mellitus	2:1
Twin gestation	4:1
Angiotensinogen gene T235	
Homozygous	20:1
Heterozygous	4:1

[a] Low socioeconomic status and young maternal age are traditional risk factors. The actual independent contribution of these factors to the risk of PIH is questionable.
From ACOG Technical Bulletin. *Hypertension in pregnancy*. No. 219. 1996, with permission.

in paternity in later pregnancies among multiparas (20) also increased the incidence.

Etiology

The cause of PIH, a disorder known to occur only in humans, is yet to be elucidated. Whether the initiating factor of this disorder is immunologic, genetic, or simply a decrease in uterine blood flow is unknown. In normal pregnancy the spiral arteries of the myometrium lose their muscular wall and become distended. In preeclampsia some of these arteries do not lose their muscular wall and remain constricted (21). This results in increased uterine vascular resistance and causes as much as a 30% to 40% decrease in uterine blood flow, compared with normal pregnancies (22, 23). Maternal circulating serum nitrite levels, a metabolic product of the potent vasodilator nitric oxide, were decreased in patients with preeclampsia suggesting this contributes to the pathophysiologic changes (24). However, in the fetoplacental circulation total nitrites were increased, suggesting a compensatory response by the fetus to improve fetoplacental circulation (25).

Several investigators from UCSF and elsewhere have presented compelling evidence that damage to the vascular endothelial cells releases a peptide substance (fibronectin or endothelia) (26–41). The cause of endothelial cell damage resulting in the release of fibronectin has been postulated to be release of factors or mitogens from the poorly perfused placenta (27, 32). It has been suggested that the measurement of fibrinectin levels may not only indicate the severity of preeclampsia but may also predict its onset before the clinical signs and symptoms develop (33, 34). Endothelial cell injury, which may involve not only the maternal vascular endothelium but also the maternal myocardial endothelium (35) and the placental vascular endothelium (36), is associated with reduced synthesis of vasorelaxing substances, increased production of vasoconstrictors, and impaired synthesis of endogenous anticoagulants which favors platelet aggregation and activation of coagulation (28). Fibronectin or endothelia, the peptide released by damaged endothelial cells, causes vasoconstriction and loss of capillary endothelial integrity with leakage of fluid and protein and platelet aggregation (Fig. 16.1). Levels of fibrinogen elevated in PIH become markedly decreased by 48 hours after delivery, which

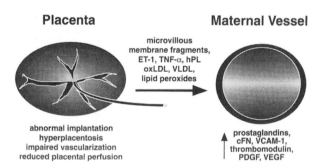

Figure 16.1. Proposed model of preeclampsia pathogenesis. Compromised implantation, hyperplacentosis, and/or impaired placental bed vascularization results in the functional reduction of placental perfusion. In response to this ischemic and/or hypoxic state, these plantae secrete or elaborate into the maternal circulation factors that directly or indirectly cause systemic vasular endothelial cell dysfunction. Possible candidates for such translational factors include placental microvillous membrane fragments, endothelin-1 (ET- 1), tumor necrosis factor-α (TNF-α), human placental lactogen (hPL), oxidized LDL (oxLDL), VLDL, and lipid peroxides. Activation of the systemic maternal vascular endothelium appears to result in increased secretion of vasopressors, procoagulants, cell adhesion molecules, and growth and permeability factors (e.g., prostaglandins [PGs], fibronectin [cFN], VCAM-1, thrombomodulin PDGF, and VEGF). From Lindeimer MD, Roberts JM, Cunningham FG, eds. Chelsey's Hypertensive Disorders in Pregnancy, 2nd ed. Stamford, CT, Appleton & Lange. 1999:419, with permission.

markedly could explain the rapid clinical improvement seen following delivery. In addition to fibronectin maternal serum levels of triglycerides, free fatty acids and malondialdehyde, which are elevated in preeclampsia, decrease with resolution of the disorder in the 48 hours following delivery (37). Decreased colloid oncotic pressures and proteinuria are highly correlated to elevated fibronectin levels, which suggests that endothelial injury, not proteinuria, is the primary mechanism of hypoproteinuria and reduced colloid oncotic pressure in preeclampsia (38). Yet maternal serum from severe preeclamptics was not cytotoxic to umbilical venous cell cultures exposed to it (39).

Preeclampsia is associated with an imbalance in the maternal production and circulating serum levels of two prostaglandins, prostacyclin and thromboxane (40). Thromboxane present in excess is associated with vasoconstriction, platelet aggregation, decreased uterine blood flow and increased uterine activity where prostacyclin present in decreased amounts has the opposite effects (40). This imbalance between thromboxane and prostacyclin may be related to endothelial cell injury (41) and to placental trophoblastic production of thromboxane (28, 41, 42). Low-dose aspirin (60 mg/day), which decreases the production of thromboxane without effecting that of prostacyclin was thought to protect against the development and severity of preeclampsia if started on a daily regimen in the early second trimester (42–48). Furthermore, its use was associated with neither adverse effects on the fetus (49) nor problems with epidural anesthesia or maternal-neonatal bleeding complications (50). Unfortunately, large multicenter studies have questioned the efficacy of low-dose aspirin as an effective means of preventing the development of preeclampsia, even in pregnancies at high risk (51–53). In preeclamptic mothers, an increase in placental production or progesterone was associated with decreased placental prostacyclin production (54).

As previously stated, **hypertension, proteinuria, and generalized edema** characterize preeclampsia, a recognized subset of PIH. Hypertension is defined as a sustained systolic blood pressure of at least 140 mm Hg or a sustained diastolic blood pressure of at least 90 mm Hg. Blood pressure may depend greatly on position, and measurements should be taken in a uniform manner with the proper cuff size. Although an increase in systolic blood pressure of 30 mm Hg or diastolic of 15 mm Hg from second trimester values had been thought to be of diagnostic value, this is no longer considered valid (1). Proteinuria is defined as the excretion of more than 0.3 g of protein per liter of urine in a 24-hour urine collection or the excretion of more than 1 g of protein per liter (+1 or +2 on "dipstick" test) in two catheterized or clean-catch midstream samples taken more than 6 hours apart (4). However, the results of random "dipstick" assessment of proteinuria may not correlate with those of a 24-hour urine collection (55). Edema must be generalized and not limited to just the ankles or legs, often present in normal gravidae in late pregnancy. The presence of two of the three signs usually allows for the diagnosis of preeclampsia, provided the pregnancy has progressed beyond the 20th week or if the signs and symptoms develop earlier in a molar pregnancy.

"Severe preeclampsia" is defined when any of the following conditions exist: (a) systolic blood pressure greater than 160 to 180 mm Hg, diastolic blood pressure greater than 110 mm Hg; (b) proteinuria in excess of 5 g/24 h (+3 or +4 by "dipstick" test); (c) oliguria of less than 500 mL in 24 h; (d) grand mal seizures (eclampsia); (e) headache or cerebral disturbances; (f) visual disturbances; (g) epigastric pain; (h) pulmonary edema or cyanosis, or (i) impared liver function of unclear etiology and thrombocytopenia (Table 16.3) (1). The development of preeclampsia in the early second trimester often indicates that it will rapidly progress to the severe category with significant perinatal mortality. If one or more grand mal convulsions not related to other conditions occurs in preeclampsia, eclampsia is diagnosed and the prognosis for both mother and fetus worsens significantly.

Table 16.3. CLINICAL MANIFESTATIONS OF SEVERE DISEASE IN PATIENTS WITH PREGNANCY-INDUCED HYPERTENSION

Blood pressure > 160–180 mm Hg systolic or > 100 mm Hg diastolic
Proteinuria > 5 g/24 h (normal < 300 mg/24 h)
Elevated serum creatinine
Grand mal seizures (eclampsia)
Pulmonary edema
Oliguria < 500 mL/24 h
Microangiopathic hemolysis
Thrombocytopenia
Hepatocellular dysfunction (elevated alanine aminotransferase, aspartase aminotransferase)
Intrauterine growth retardation of oligohydramnios
Symptoms suggesting significant end-organ involvement: headache, visual disturbances, or epigastric or right-upper quadrant pain

From ACOG Technical Bulletin. *Hypertension in pregnancy.* No. 219, 1996, with permission.

PATHOPHYSIOLOGY

The pathophysiology of PIH involves nearly every organ system. In the past, the primary pathophysiology was believed to be vasoconstriction and its consequences (56). Although vasoconstriction does play a role, viewing the disorder as the result of vasoconstriction is overly simplistic. Contrary to former beliefs, it appears that PIH is associated with a hyperdynamic cardiovascular state (Table 16.4) (57). The cardiovascular findings can vary considerably between preeclampsia and hypertensive parturients. In severe preeclamptic patients near term, pulmonary artery catheterization has shown normal or high cardiac indexes (58). Systemic vascular resistance itself was slightly elevated, if at all, in two studies (59, 60), as compared with normal pregnant women at 36 to 38 weeks' gestation (Table 16.4). These data suggest that increased blood pressure observed among preeclamptic women may result from an increased cardiac output rather than an increased systemic vascular resistance, as previously thought. In both studies, parturients had normal or hyperdynamic left ventricular function. Cardiac output is considerably elevated in preeclampsia, and this elevation may precede the hypertension and other findings associated with the disorder (Figs. 16.2 and 16.3) (57, 58). Interestingly, there is no correlation between the severity of the preeclampsia and the increase in cardiac output (61). Mild and severe preeclamptic parturients have similar increases in cardiac output. After delivery, left ventricular function may decrease temporarily to within the normal range, then increase again (62). Although it was previously believed that the central venous pressure (CVP) was low and tended to decrease with an increased severity of the disorder, more recent studies (59, 60) have demonstrated that CVP is essentially normal or very slightly elevated in patients with severe preeclampsia. The CVP may not correlate well with the pulmonary capillary occlusion pressure (PCOP), which tends to be normal (59). A low PCOP may more reliably reflect decreased vascular volume than a low CVP, although the CVP and PCOP may show some correlation (Figs. 16.4 and 16.5) (59). CVP is not reliable and has led some clinicians to discourage CVP monitoring in favor of PCOP monitoring (63–66). However, others think that CVP monitoring is a useful diagnostic and therapeutic tool, particularly when used to aid in vascular volume expansion (67–69). In most studies, a CVP of 6 mm Hg or less has not been associated with serious elevations of PCOP.

Plasma volume is markedly reduced among preeclamptic parturients compared with normal parturients (Table 16.5). Using red blood cells labeled with a nonradioactive isotope of chromium, the plasma volume, as well as the red cell volume, were determined in normal, preeclamptic, and nonproteinuria gestational hypertensive parturients. In parturients with

Table 16.4. COMPARISON OF CARDIOVASCULAR PARAMETER OF NORMAL NONPREGNANT, NORMAL PREGNANT, AND SEVERE PREECLAMPTIC WOMEN

	Normal Nonpregnant[a] (11–13 wks postpartum) ($n = 10$)	Normal Pregnancy[a] (36–38 wks gestation) ($n = 10$)	Severe Pregnancy-Induced Hypertension Before Delivery[b] ($n = 45$)	Severe Preeclampsia Before Delivery[c] ($n = 41$)	Severe Preeclampsia with Pulmonary Edema[d] ($n = 8$)
Mean arterial pressure (mm Hg)	86.4 ± 7.5	90.3 ± 5.8	138 ± 3	130 ± 2	136 ± 3
Central venous pressure (mm Hg)	3.7 ± 2.6	3.6 ± 2.5	4 ± 1	4.8 ± 0.4	11 ± 1
Pulmonary capillary wedge pressure (mm Hg)	6.3 ± 2.1	7.5 ± 1.8	10 ± 1	8.3 ± 0.3	18 ± 1
Cardiac output (liter/min)	4.3 ± 0.9	6.2 ± 1	7.5 ± 0.23	8.4 ± 0.2	10.5 ± 0.6
Systemic vascular resistance ($dyne \cdot cm \cdot sec^{-3}$)	$1,530 \pm 520$	$1,210 \pm 266$	$1,496 \pm 64$	$1,226 \pm 37$	964 ± 50
Systemic vascular resistance index ($dyne \cdot cm \cdot sec^{-3} \cdot M^2$)	—	—	$2,726 \pm 120$	$2,293 \pm 65$	—
Pulmonary vascular resistance ($dyne \cdot cm \cdot sec^{-3}$)	119 ± 47	78 ± 22	70 ± 5	65 ± 3	71 ± 9
Left ventricular stroke work index ($g \cdot m \cdot m^{-2}$)	41 ± 8	48 ± 6	81 ± 2	84 ± 2	87 ± 10

[a] Data are from 10 normal pregnancies at 36 to 38 weeks gestation and 11 to 13 weeks postpartum. (Adapted from Clark SL, et al. Central hemodynamic assessment of normal term pregnancy. *Am J Obstet Gynecol* 1989;161:1439–1442.)

[b] Data are taken from 45 patients with severe pregnancy-induced hypertension (PIH) near time of delivery. (Adapted from Cotton DB, Lee W, Huhta JC, et al. Hemodynamic profile of severe pregnancy-induced hypertension. *Am J Obstet Gynecol* 1988;158:523–529.)

[c] Data are from 41 patients with severe preeclampsia but no pulmonary edema shortly before delivery. (Adapted from Mabie WC, Ratts TE, Sibai BM. The central hemodynamics of preeclampsia. *Am J Obstet Gynecol* 1989;161:1443–1448.)

[d] Data are from eight patients with pulmonary edema superimposed on severe preeclampsia shortly before delivery. (Adapted from Mabie WC, Ratts TE, Sibai BM. The central hemodynamics of preeclampsia. *Am J Obstet Gynecol* 1989;161:1443–1448.)

preeclampsia, not gestational hypertension, all three components were decreased (70). The failure of the plasma volume to expand in midpregnancy (20 to 24 weeks) may foretell the future development of preeclampsia (71).

Colloid oncotic pressure may be decreased in preeclampsia and correlates with the decreased plasma protein levels (72). An animal model, somewhat resembling the severe preeclamptic human, has been produced in the near-term gravid ewe by repeated plasmapheresis resulting in a lowering of the plasma oncotic pressure (73). The decreased plasma oncotic pressure, coupled with capillary endothelial damage and marked vasoconstriction, may well account for the development of pulmonary edema that occurs in 2.9% of preeclamptic patients (74). Usually associated with pulmonary edema are other complicating factors including disseminated intravascular coagulopathy, sepsis, abruptio placentae, preexisting chronic hypertension, and excessive intravenous infusion of crystalloid, colloid, or both. Pulmonary edema usually occurs in the first few postpartum days and is seen more commonly in older multiparous patients with preexisting chronic hypertension. Increases in both the PCOP and CVP are associated with pulmonary edema (75, 76). The correlation between the two measurements is not constant and reliable in severe preeclampsia (77–79). However, those patients with pulmonary edema inevitably show a CVP of 6 mm Hg or greater. Not only are there increased circulating levels of renin, angiotensin, catecholamines, and atrial natriuretic factor in preeclampsia (80, 81), but there is evidence that the response to vasoactive drugs may be heightened, as compared with the normal gravida (82). Although the intravascular volume may be decreased, salt and water are retained in tissues, causing edema. There is evidence of cerebral edema in eclamptic patients (83). Blood viscosity is elevated, thereby aggravating the problem of decreased uteroplacental perfusion (84). The cardiovascular pathophysiology associated with preeclampsia in the peripartum period have been well summarized by the studies of both Cotton (59) and Mabie (60).

Severe preeclampsia and eclampsia may have associated coagulation abnormalities that involve primarily decreases in platelet number and function (85, 86). Although some investigators have found a low incidence of thrombocytopenia (87), others found thrombocytopenia (defined as a platelet count of less then $150,000/mm^3$) in as many as 50% of preeclamptic parturients in the third trimester (88). The etiology of the thrombocytopenia is believed to be related to platelet adherence to exposed collagen at sites of endothelial damage (89). There is increased platelet turnover secondary to aggregation stimulated by endothelial damage. While many anesthesiologists are uncomfortable providing epidural analgesia or anesthesia in patients with platelet counts of $<100,000/mm^3$ and the majority would not place an epidural with a platelet count of 50,000 to $80,000/mm^3$ (90), data are lacking for such a rigid stance (91, 92). Others have suggested coagulation be investigated with a bleeding time; however, its lack of efficacy and value have been demonstrated (93, 94). A reduced platelet count may be associated with intrauterine fetal growth retardation (95). Other less pronounced changes in coagulation include slightly prolonged partial thromboplastin time (statistically but not clinically significant) and an increased serum level of fibrin split products (Tables 16.6 and 16.7) (87, 88, 96).

The *"HELLP" syndrome*, which is associated with high maternal and fetal mortality and maternal morbidity, has been described in PIH (97). It usually occurs before 36 weeks' gestation. Patients complain of malaise (90%), epigastric pain (90%), and nausea and vomiting (50%) with some having a nonspecific viral flulike syndrome (98). Initially, hypertension and proteinuria may be very mild. The disorder is rapidly progressive, with development of disseminated intravascular coagulation (DIC) as well as liver and renal failure. Its diagnosis calls for immediate delivery, regardless of gestation, to prevent maternal and fetal death (99). Patients developing thrombocytopenia below $50,000/mm^3$ require as many as 11 postpartum days to achieve a platelet count in excess of $100,000/mm^3$. These severely affected patients require a longer period of diuresis to occur postpartum and may need plasma exchange. Patients having platelet counts of more than $50,000/mm^3$ experience a faster recovery and usually do not require plasma exchange (100). Commonly, platelet counts

NORMAL PREGNANCY

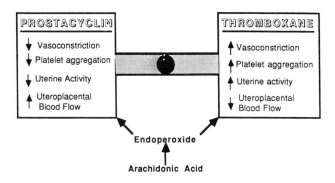

PREECLAMPSIA

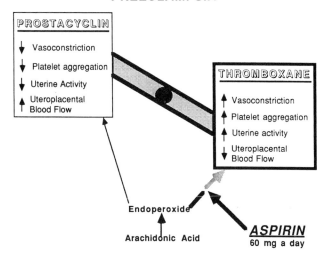

Figure 16.2. Comparison of the balance in the biological actions of prostacyclin and thromboxane in normal pregnancy with the imbalance of increased thromboxane and decreased prostacyclin in the preeclamptic patient. It was thought that if a patient was at risk for development of preeclampsia and given aspirin, 60 mg a day from the end of the first trimester throughout gestation, production of thromboxane would decrease without affecting prostacyclin production, thus attenuating the severity or even development of preeclampsia. Unfortunately, large studies have not confirmed this hypothesis except in patients with essential hypertension, who are at high risk for developing preeclampsia. (Modified from Walsh SW: Preeclampsia: An imbalance in placental prostacyclin and thromboxane production. *Am J Obstet Gynecol* 1985;152: 335–340).

reach their lowest level by 24 to 48 hours after delivery (101). When delivery does not result in recovery, some clinicians advocate plasmaphoresis of the mother (102). Platelet counts frequently decrease to levels below 50,000/mm^3 following delivery; such levels have been associated with epidural hematomas arising from previously administered epidural blocks for delivery (103).

The **upper airway edema** and laryngeal edema of normal pregnancy can be aggravated to the point of airway obstruction (104, 105). The lung volumes, capacities, and function are not significantly altered by preeclampsia (106). Respiratory depression from administration of magnesium, opioids, or sedatives may lead to hypoxia and hypercarbia. The oxygen-hemoglobin dissociation curve is shifted to the left, which may decrease oxygen availability to the fetus (107). This shift has been attributed to increased levels of carboxyhemoglobin resulting from an increased catabolism of circulating red blood cells (108). Plasma pseudo-cholinesterase activity is decreased compared with normal gravid women (109). This decrease is not due to the effect of magnesium used to treat the disorder (110).

Renal function is adversely affected by PIH and preeclampsia in PIH with significant renal involvement leading to proteinuria. Glomerular filtration rate and creatinine clearance decrease. Blood uric acid levels increase and may correlate with the severity of the disease (111). Renal blood flow is compromised. Large amounts of all serum proteins may be lost through the urine. Renal lesions are common and are characterized by swelling of capillary endothelial cells (a hallmark of the renal pathology in preeclampsia rarely seen in other conditions) (112). This endothelial lesion results in a disturbance of the glomerular basement membrane permeability, leading to the characteristic glomerular alteration of preeclamptic nephropathy (113). Acute renal failure with oliguria may occur in PIH, especially in patients having other complicating factors such as abruptio placentae with disseminated intravascular coagulopathy and hemorrhage, the "HELLP" syndrome, and superimposed essential hypertension (114). Some clinicians believe that patients with preeclampsia will experience a complete reversal of these renal pathologic changes, whereas others believe preeclampsia may be associated with the permanent lesions of focal glomerular sclerosis (115). Women with renal failure developing from preeclampsia superimposed on essential hypertension often suffer permanent renal damage, often requiring dialysis. When renal failure occurs in the antepartum period, delivery is usually associated with a rapid resolution. Oliguria and renal failure may occur in the absence of hypovolemia and marked continued hydration can result in pulmonary edema (116). These patients may suffer either from selective renal artery vasospasm or from frank volume overload with cardiac dysfunction (117). Thus, preeclamptic parturients with oliguria who do not respond to a modest fluid load may require pulmonary artery catheterization for correct diagnosis and proper treatment.

Hepatic involvement in preeclampsia is usually mild. However, in severe PIH or when preeclampsia is complicated by the "HELLP" syndrome, periportal hemorrhages, ischemic lesions, generalized swelling, and even subcapsular hematomas sometimes occur in the liver. The hepatic swelling produces epigastric pain. An elevation in liver enzyme levels is one of the hallmarks of the "HELLP" syndrome.

Hyperreflexia occurs, and **central nervous system** irritability often increases. Coma may develop even without eclampsia. An encephalopathy has been shown to accompany severe preeclampsia. It is characterized by headache, visual disturbances, altered mental status, and focal neurologic signs. Blood flow in the middle, anterior, and posterior cerebral arteries is decreased as measured by Doppler ultrasound (118). Many eclamptic patients have an increased intracranial pressure that can be exacerbated by hypercarbia, metabolic acidosis, and hypoxia (83). Of patients becoming eclamptic, 50% do so before labor, 33% in labor, and 17% postpartum.

Uterine activity is increased and the uterus can become hyperactive and markedly sensitive to oxytocin. Rapid labor with painful contractions are common. Preterm labor frequently occurs. Uterine and placental blood flow (intervillous blood flow) are markedly diminished by 50 to 70% (119) because of both increased vascular resistance and increased maternal blood viscosity secondary to the increased hematocrit (84). The placenta, which is often small, may show signs of premature aging and frequently exhibits infarcts, fibrin deposition, calcification, and abruption. The incidence of abruptio placentae is significantly increased in PIH and in mothers with pregnancies complicated by hypertension from other causes. The leading cause of *maternal death* in PIH is intracranial hemorrhage (120). Other causes of morbidity and mortality include congestive heart failure with pulmonary edema, pulmonary aspiration of gastric contents, postpartum hemorrhage, DIC, acute renal failure, ruptured liver, and septic shock (121).

In PIH, the *fetus* is at increased risk owing to the marginal placental function, which may become inadequate, particularly

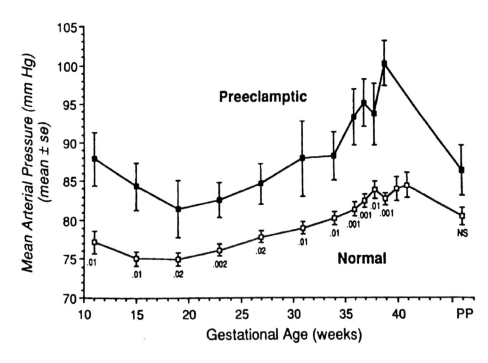

Figure 16.3. Cardiac output in the group with preeclampsia is elevated throughout pregnancy as compared with the group with normal blood pressure. PP, postpartum. (Adapted from Easterling TR, Benedetti TJ, Schmucker BC. Maternal hemodynamics in normal and preeclamptic pregnancies: a longitudinal study. *Obstet Gynecol* 1990;76:1061–1069.)

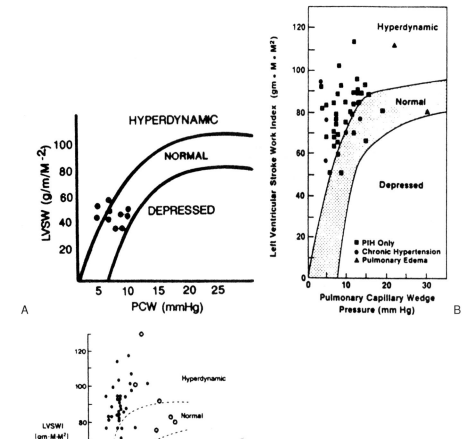

Figure 16.4. Left ventricular function expressed as pulmonary capillary wedge pressure (mm Hg) vs. left ventricular stroke work index (g mm^2). Note the vast majority of the patients afflicted with PIH or preeclampsia show a marked hyperdynamic left ventricular function. **A:** In normal gravid patients not in labor at 36 to 38 weeks' gestation. (From Clark SL, Cotton DB, Lee W, et al. Central hemodynamic assessment of normal term pregnancy. *Am J Obstet Gynecol* 1982;161:1439–1442, with permission.) **B:** In patients with severe pregnancy-induced hypertension shortly before delivery. (From Cotton DB, Lee W, Huhta JC, et al. Hemodynamic profile of severe pregnancy-induced hypertension (PIH). *Am J Obstet Gynecol* 1988;158:523–529, with permission.) **C:** In patients with severe preeclampsia shortly before delivery. (From Mabie WC, Ratts TE, Sibai BM. The central hemodynamics of severe preeclampsia. *Am J Obstet Gynecol* 1989;161:1443–1448, with permission.)

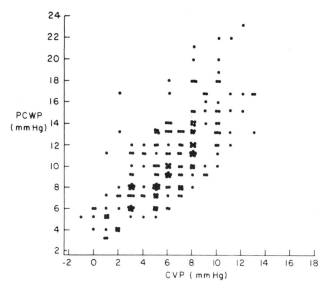

Figure 16.5. The relationship between the central venous pressure (CVP) and the pulmonary capilary wedge pressure (PCWP) in women with severe pregnancy-induced hypertension. Patients with the same data are represented by a single point. (From Cotton DB, Lee W, Huhta JC, et al. Hemodynamic profile of severe pregnancy-induced hypertension. *Am J Obstet Gynecol* 1988;158:523–529, with permission.)

in the presence of increased uterine activity. Aortocaval compression, induced hypotension from therapy or anesthesia, and the use of depressant drugs greatly increase the danger to the fetus. Both preterm and small-for-gestational age neonates born through thick meconium are common. The presence of small-for-gestational age and preeclampsia increase the risk of fetal acidosis and are strong predictors of the need for neonatal resuscitation (122). The leading causes of intrauterine mortality are placental infarction, followed by retardation of placental growth, abruptio placentae, and acute infection of amniotic fluid (123). Contrary to previous belief, the presence of PIH does not accelerate fetal lung or neurologic development (124). Severe maternal hypertension may be associated with an increased incidence of mental retardation and development of global and motor dysfunction (125). Perinatal morbidity and mortality are often related to preterm birth accompanied by respiratory distress, intracranial hemorrhage, small-for-gestational age neonate, and aspiration of meconium.

THERAPY

The definitive therapy for PIH is delivery of the fetus and the placenta. Until this can be accomplished, the obstetric objective is to control the disease process. The pregnancy is allowed to continue as long as the intrauterine environment is adequate to support growth and maturation of the fetus without endangering the mother. In more severe preeclamptic parturients, but in those who can be relatively well controlled, pregnancy may be continued until the fetus is of sufficient maturity and size to ensure survival following birth or until other factors indicate the need for delivery (126). In very severe preeclampsia, eclampsia, and the "HELLP" syndrome, the mother is quickly stabilized and the fetus delivered expeditiously, regardless of size and maturity. Indications for rapid delivery include any of the following conditions: (a) severe hypertension unresponsive to antihypertensives, (b) renal dysfunction with developing oliguria, (c) liver dysfunction, (d) development of coagulopathy or thrombocytopenia, (e) the onset of eclampsia, or (f) evidence of severe fetal compromise that could result in fetal demise. Prolonging gestation in these pregnancies is often disastrous, with a high fetal mortality and many maternal complications (127). As long as the fetus tolerates uterine contractions, induction and vaginal delivery is often possible and is not contraindicated in preeclampsia. However, cesarean section is indicated if the fetus is markedly premature but viable; if there are signs of a significantly compromised or rapidly worsening intrauterine environment, a worsening biophysical profile, or fetal distress; or if the mother's condition is rapidly deteriorating.

The general aims of therapy are to minimize vasospasm; to improve circulation, particularly to the uterus, placenta, and

Table 16.6. COAGULATION DETERMINATIONS IN ECLAMPSIA vs. NORMAL PREGNANCY[a]

	Eclamptic Women (n = 62)	Normal Women (n = 24)	P value
Platelets (10^3/mL)	266 ± 89^a	269 ± 54^a	NS
−2 SD < 161 × 10^3	10/62	1/24	
< 100 × 10^5	1/62	1/24	
Fibrinogen (mg/dL)	405 ± 98^a	437 ± 77^a	NS
−2 SD < 283 mg/dL	5/62	1/24	
Fibrin degradation products			
< 10 μg/mL	44/62	22/24	< 0.05
10–40 μg/mL	17/66	2/24	
> 40 μg/mL	1/62	0/24	
Partial thromboplastin time (sec)	29.8 ± 6.6^a	26.4 ± 1.8^a	< 0.001
Prothrombin time (sec)	11.2 ± 0.8^a	11.2 ± 0.6^a	NS

[a] Mean ± SD.
NS, not significant.
Adapted from Sibai BM, Anderson GD, McCubbin JH. Eclampsia II: clinical significance of laboratory findings. *Obstet Gynecol* 1982;59:153–157.

Table 16.5. TOTAL BLOOD VOLUME AND HEMATOCRITS IN NONPREGNANCY, NORMAL PREGNANCY, AND PREECLAMPSIA

	Nonpregnancy (n = 5)	Normal Pregnancy (n = 5)	Eclampsia (n = 5)
Total blood volume (mL)	3,035	4,425	3,530
Change from nonpregnant state	—	+47	+16
Hematocrit (%)	38.2	34.7	40.5

Blood volumes measured with chromium-51 in five eclamtic women, after recovery in the nonpregnant state, then again in a subsequent normal pregnancy. Note the minimal elevation of the total blood volume, but the increased hematocrit concentration in the eclamptic patients.
Adapted from Prichard JA, Cunningham GA, Prichard SA. The Parkland Memorial Hospital protocol for the treatment of eclampsia: evaluation of 245 cases. *Am J Obstet Gynecol* 1984;148:948–954.

Table 16.7. COAGULATION DETERMINATIONS IN NORMAL LATE THIRD TRIMESTER PREGNANCIES vs. NULLIPAROUS PREECLAMPSIA IN THIRD TRIMESTER WITH AND WITHOUT THROMBOCYTOPENIA ($<150,000$)[a]

	Normal Pregnant Controls ($n = 24$)	Nulliparous Preeclampsia with No thrombocytopenia ($n = 22$)	Nulliparous Preeclampsia with thrombocytopenia ($n = 22$)
Platelet count ($\times 10^3$ mL)	251 ± 60.6	199 ± 34	79.4 ± 40.6
Platelet associated IgG (fg IgG per platelet)	2.6 ± 1.1	3.9 ± 2.0	10.6 ± 12.2
Bleeding time (min)	4.4 ± 1.2	7.6 ± 4.6	13.0 ± 8.3
Thromboxane B_2 (ng/mL)	254 ± 135	120 ± 103	122 ± 94.3
Prothrombin time (sec)	12 ± 2	10.9 ± 0.6	10.5 ± 0.6
Activated partial thromboplastic time (sec)	33.5 ± 4.7	30.4 ± 4.4	33.5 ± 4.3
Fibrinogen (mg/dL)	449 ± 116	553 ± 199	452 ± 123

[a] Data expressed as mean $\pm$ SD.
Adapted from Burrows RF, Hunter DJS, Andrew M, et al. A prospective study investigating the mechanism of thrombocytopenia in preeclampsia. *Obstet Gynecol* 1987;70:334–338.

kidneys; to improve intravascular volume; to correct acid-base and electrolyte imbalances; and to decrease both CNS and reflex hyperactivity. Frequently, with early detection and proper therapy, the pathophysiologic changes of preeclampsia can be minimized and the pregnancy carried to near term. Therapy, as a rule, is symptomatic.

Hospitalization and bed rest in the lateral decubitus position (to prevent aortocaval compression and improve uterine blood flow) are often most effective. This therapy with adequate dietary intake frequently promotes diuresis and decreases blood pressure. The upright and supine positions, which favor aortocaval compression, seem to aggravate the condition. Preeclampsia is associated with water and salt retention and a few clinicians still favor fluid and salt restriction on the basis that hydration and salt may be associated with pulmonary and cerebral edema (128). However, the predominant opinion is that adequate hydration and intravascular volume expansion with a balanced salt solution is beneficial from the standpoint of lowering maternal blood pressure and improving placental and fetal blood flow (129–133). In the past, severe sodium restriction was recommended, a practice that frequently led to sodium depletion and possibly increased production of renin, angiotensin, and aldosterone (134). Evidence now favors an adequate sodium intake with minimal, if any, sodium restriction (135). Intravenous fluids should contain sodium, particularly if oxytocin is used, to prevent water intoxication and convulsions. The diet should be adequate and balanced with no attempt made at weight reduction. Diuretics, particularly the thiazide type, are not used to treat edema. The use of diuretics, usually furosemide, is reserved for acute therapy of pulmonary edema caused by congestive heart failure or other factors.

Early hospitalization involving bed rest, oral antihypertensives, and frequent fetal testing of severe preeclamptics was found to prolong gestation a mean of 15.4 days and reduce neonatal complications as compared to delivery within 48 hours of admission (136).

Magnesium Therapy

In North America and in many developing countries, parenterally administered magnesium is the first-line therapeutic drug in controlling PIH. In this decade our obstetric colleagues from the United Kingdom in greater number have begun to use magnesium for its anticonvulsant properties as a result of several clinical trials (137–141). It is an effective anticonvulsant, tocolytic and a mild generalized vasodilator. The mechanism of its antiseizure activity has been attributed to its depression of the central nervous system (142–147); however, the definitive mechanism remains unknown. Although many other anticonvulsants have been used, including barbiturates, diazepam, chlormethi-

azole, and particularly phenytoin sodium, none have proved superior to magnesium in either efficacy or lack of side effects (148–151).

Magnesium's tocolytic action makes it useful in preeclampsia when the uterus is often hyperactive and accompanied by a compromised intrauterine environment. However, despite this tocolytic action, magnesium therapy in preeclampsia does not appear to be associated with prolongation of either induced or spontaneous labor (138, 152, 153). Magnesium depresses both smooth muscle contractions and central nervous system catecholamine release (154–156). These properties may explain its mild and often significant beneficial effect on lowering maternal blood pressure and improving uterine blood flow (157–159). Magnesium is associated with cerebral arterial vasodilation which may relieve maternal cerebral ischemia associated with the disorder (160–162). Magnesium has also been found to lower levels of plasma endothelin-1 in preeclamptics, a substance present in elevated amounts which damages vascular endothelial cells (163). The beneficial and detrimental effects of magnesium sulfate are summarized in Table 16.8. Therapeutic maternal plasma levels of magnesium are in the range of 4 to 6 mEq $\cdot$ L^{-1} (2 mEq $\cdot$ L^{-1} = 2.4 mg $\cdot$ dL^{-1} = 1 mmol $\cdot$ L^{-1}) with toxicity occurring when plasma levels exceed 10 mEq $\cdot$ L^{-1} (Table 16.8).

Magnesium therapy is associated with both maternal and neonatal side effects. Serious toxicity may be the result of either absolute overdose or (more frequently) elevation of blood levels

Table 16.8. EFFECTS OF INCREASING PLASMA MAGNESIUM LEVELS

Plasma Levels (mg $\cdot$ dL^{-1})	Plasma Levels (mg $\cdot$ dL^{-1})	Effects
1.5–2.0	1.8–2.4	Normal plasma level
4.0–8.0	4.8–9.6	Therapeutic range
5.0–10	6.0–12.0	Electrocardiographic changes (P-Q interval prolonged, QRS complex widens)
10	12	Loss of deep tendon reflexes
15	18	Sinoatrial and atrioventricular block
15	18	Respiratory paralysis
25	30	Cardiac arrest

Four different systems of units for the reporting of magnesium concentrations are in use: 1.0 mEq $\cdot$ L^{-1} = 1.22 mg $\cdot$ dL^{-1} = 0.5 mmol $\cdot$ L^{-1} = 12.2 mg $\cdot$ L^{-1}.

following repeated doses or continuous infusion in the presence of decreased renal function. Overdose can lead to maternal weakness, respiratory insufficiency, and even cardiac failure. Fortunately, these complications do not usually arise until after the deep tendon reflexes are depressed, hence magnesium should be decreased or discontinued when such deep tendon reflex depression occurs. Magnesium overdose (e.g., apnea, obtundation) can be antagonized by intravenous administration of 1 g (10 mL) 10% calcium gluconate over 2 minutes. While this might lead to a seizure, it usually doesn't and airway management and cardiovascular status are obviously the first concern.

Magnesium and Muscle Relaxants

Magnesium in therapeutic dosages is associated with abnormal neuromuscular transmission, which correlates with increased serum magnesium levels and decreased serum calcium levels (164). Partial neuromuscular blockade has been associated with magnesium plasma levels in excess of 11 to 12 mEq · L^{-1} as magnesium attenuates the release of acetylcholine at the myoneural junction, decreases the sensitivity of the junction to acetylcholine, and lessens the excitability of the muscle membrane. An often quoted earlier in vitro study suggested that magnesium increased the degree of neuromuscular block of both succinylcholine and curare (Fig. 16.6) (165). However, other studies have questioned this. Levels of pseudocholinesterase are lower in preeclamptic parturients than normal parturients (166), but the administration of magnesium does not further lower pseudocholinesterase levels (164, 167). The onset and duration of a single intubating dose of succinylcholine was not significantly altered by magnesium 60 mg · kg^{-1} in normal individuals (168) nor in eclamptic patients receiving magnesium therapy (169). Thus, the initial dose of succinylcholine for intubation should not be decreased in the preeclamptic patient given magnesium and requiring general anesthesia. Repeated doses or continued infusion of magnesium may result in a prolonged neuromuscular blockade due to development of a phase II block.

Ghoneim and Long (165) first demonstrated in vitro that a bathing concentration of magnesium sulfate, 0.1 mg · mL^{-1}, decreased the dose response curve of curare by a factor greater than fourfold. In humans magnesium has been shown to increase markedly the potency and duration and to decrease the latency of the nondepolarizing muscle relaxants, specifically curare, vecuronium, rocuronium and mivacuronium (170–

173). Because of the marked interaction of the nondepolarizing muscle relaxants and magnesium, we avoid these relaxants or use them in very small incremental doses in patients receiving magnesium.

Magnesium: Other Side Effects

An earlier study demonstrated that magnesium in healthy parturients had little effect on the bleeding time, a test of dubious clinical value (174). More recent studies in gravid parturients receiving magnesium therapy, initiated for tocolysis (175) or for preeclampsia (176) found bleeding times modestly increased. Ravn et al. (177) demonstrated that magnesium administered to healthy volunteers also increased bleeding times and decreased platelet activity. However, despite the dubious clinical value of bleeding-time assessment, none of the above studies found changes that were likely to increase the hazard of neuroaxial blockade or be clinically sufficient to contraindicate epidural or subarachnoid block. An in vivo study on healthy volunteers using thromboelastography has recently shown that magnesium sulfate had no clinically significant effect (178).

Magnesium therapy in 294 preeclamptics or parturients in preterm labor was not associated with decreases in colloid osmotic pressure until it was continuously infused for nearly 48 hours (179). Pulmonary edema developed in only four preeclamptics, all four of whom had low colloid osmotic pressure before the infusion.

Magnesium rapidly crosses the placenta with both ionized and nonionized cord blood levels paralleling those in maternal blood (180). Atkinson et al. (181) found a statistically significant decrease in short-term fetal heart rate (FHR) variability with neither decrease in long-term variability nor in the number of FHR accelerations in the fetuses of preeclamptic mothers receiving magnesium. A subsequent study (182) found magnesium levels exceeding 4.6 mg · dL^{-1} in preeclamptics were associated with significant decreases in short-term FHR variability, long-term FHR variability and FHR accelerations. Therapeutic levels of magnesium in the mother are not associated with significant detrimental effects on the neonate (183–186). Hence, the cause of neonatal depression in mothers receiving magnesium is rarely due to the magnesium itself. With high maternal levels of magnesium, the newborn may exhibit decreased muscle tone, respiratory depression, and apnea. Intravenously administered calcium may partially overcome the neuromuscular blocking properties of magnesium in both mother and newborn.

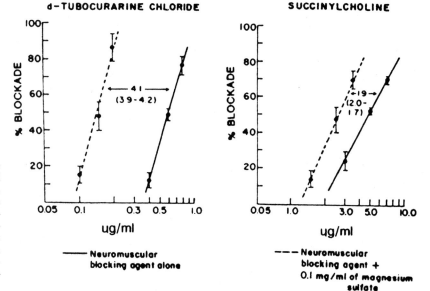

Figure 16.6. Dose-response curves of d-tubocurarine chloride and succinylcholine with and without added magnesium using a rat phrenic nerve preparation. Each point represents the mean of five observations with the standard error represented. Magnesium sulfate (0.1 mg · mL^{-1}) is a subminimal dose. The magnitude of the potentiation by magnesium is shown between the curves with their fiducial limits. (From Ghoneim MM, Long JP. Interaction between magnesium and other neuromuscular blocking agents. *Anesthesiology* 1970;32:23–27, with permission.)

However, the initial management of magnesium toxicity in the newborn is support of ventilation. Although the slow administration of calcium is safe in the newborn, its administration is more controversial in the mother because calcium may antagonize the anticonvulsant effects of magnesium. In cases of gross maternal magnesium overdose with respiratory or cardiac depression, it is important to support the mother's depressed ventilation and administer calcium. Because magnesium is excreted by the kidneys, it must be given with care and in reduced doses when urinary output is decreased or renal function impaired. Decreased renal excretion resulting from impaired renal function is a major cause of magnesium toxicity in preeclampsia.

Magnesium therapy is usually initiated by intravenous administration of 4 g over 20 minutes, followed by continuous infusion $(2 \text{ to } 3 \text{ g} \cdot \text{h}^{-1})$ administered by a controlled-infusion device. Two to four grams given more rapidly during eclamptic convulsions frequently terminate the convulsion. However, more commonly a small dose of thiopental or a benzodiazepine is used for immediate management of eclamptic seizures.

A summary of the benefits and side effects of magnesium is given in Table 16.8. Despite these side effects, its long record of safety and demonstrated efficacy have established magnesium as the initial drug of choice in the therapy of PIH (142, 143, 148, 185–187).

ANTIHYPERTENSIVE AGENTS

If maternal blood pressure exceeds either 180 mm Hg systolic or 110 mm Hg diastolic despite the administration of magnesium or other anticonvulsants and bed rest, antihypertensives are indicated. Generally, lower blood pressures are not treated in PIH. Antihypertensive therapy, although beneficial for the mother, does not appear to significantly improve fetal status or neonatal outcome in the term neonate (188–190). However, aggressive management of blood pressure with antihypertensive therapy at 28 to 32 weeks' gestation can prolong gestation, thereby improving the gestational age of the neonate at delivery, and decrease neonatal morbidity, decreasing admission of neonates to the intensive care unit, and decreasing the number of days spent in the unit by neonates admitted (136).

Hydralazine

Until recently, the most widely used antihypertensive drug for preeclampsia was hydralazine. It provides effective control of blood pressure with its primary action of decreasing precapillary arteriolar resistance (191). It is associated with an increased maternal cardiac output and tachycardia, which may interfere with its antihypertensive effect. Hydralazine is also associated with increased renal blood flow. Following intravenous administration, maximal effect is achieved in 20 to 30 minutes, with a duration of only 2 to 3 hours. Hydralazine was thought to increase placental blood flow (192). However, studies have shown that, for a significant number of parturients, it may decrease uterine blood flow (not necessarily related to placental blood flow) by as much as 25% (193, 194), and it may be associated with neonatal thrombocytopenia (195, 196). Although still widely used in PIH, hydralazine is being replaced by other antihypertensives. **Methyldopa** has been a popular antihypertensive for treatment of PIH, particularly in Europe. It may be useful in the chronically hypertensive parturient after initial control of hypertension has been accomplished with hydralazine or for prolonged control of hypertension in the postpartum period. Its lack of ill effects on the fetus and newborn is well established (197). **Clonidine** and *prazosin*, two additional alpha blockers, have been used with good results in preeclampsia (198).

Beta-Blockers

The use of β-blocking drugs in preeclampsia and hypertensive gravid parturients is becoming more common. Initially it was feared that **propanolol**, a nonselective beta-blocker, was associated with increased uterine activity, decreased uterine and placental blood flow, decreased fetal heart rate, decreased fetal tolerance to hypoxia, and adverse neonatal outcomes. Although well-controlled studies of beta-blockers versus placebo are lacking, considerable clinical testing appears to demonstrate the safety of these drugs for the gravid parturient and her fetus. Chronic use of cardioselective beta$_1$-adrenergic blockers, such as atenolol (199–201) and **metoprolol** (202), during pregnancy appears to be effective maternal antihypertensives without causing ill effects on the fetus. *Esmolol*, a rapid ultrashort-acting cardioselective beta$_1$-adrenergic blocker, is effective in treating tachycardia and hypertension in nongravid patients (203) and has been used in isolated gravid parturients with success. However, studies in the gravid ewe found it produced fetal beta-adrenergic blockade and hypoxemia in the fetus (204). Hence, additional studies are required before its routine use can be recommended in the preeclamptic parturient.

Labetalol is an effective antihypertensive that produces a nonselective beta-blockade and a selective postsynaptic alpha-blocker with a beta/alpha ratio of 3:1 to 7:1 following oral or intravenous administration, respectively (205). In addition, it may also produce vasodilation by beta$_2$-receptor stimulation (206). Its onset is rapid after intravenous injection and, it has an elimination half-life of 1.7 hours following oral ingestion in gravid parturients (207). Its administration in both gravid hypertensive animals (208, 209) and hypertensive mothers (194, 210–212) has not been associated with decreased uterine or placental perfusion, fetal bradycardia, fetal deterioration, or neonatal problems. A single case report describes a fetal death following labetalol administration. Upon closer examination, the dose administered was excessive (50 mg in a single intravenous dose), resulting in profound maternal hypotension (213). We agree with the authors who recommend titration of labetalol i.v. with 5 to 10 mg doses. It has a more rapid onset of action and lacks the side effects of tachycardia, nausea, headache, excessive hypotension, and decreased uterine blood flow associated with hydralazine (214, 215). Labetalol is becoming widely used for both the control of hypertension and for attenuation of acute hypertension associated with a rapid sequence induction of general anesthesia in the severely preeclamptic or eclamptic parturient. Caution must be used in the administration of beta-blockers to patients with bronchoconstrictive disorders and with compromised myocardial function because these drugs may cause bronchoconstriction and decreased ventricular function.

Calcium-Channel Blockers

The calcium-channel blockers, particularly **nifedipine**, are gaining importance as safe and effective antihypertensives in pregnancy, particularly in PIH. In addition to being relaxants of a vascular smooth muscle (thus decreasing systemic vascular resistance), they also are potent uterine relaxants and increase renal blood flow. Because of its lack of associated tachycardia, nifedipine is usually preferred over verapamil. It is usually administered by oral or sublingual routes. Its use in severe preeclampsia was shown to be more effective than that of hydralazine in lowering maternal blood pressure, prolonging pregnancy, and causing considerably less fetal distress (216, 217). Contrary to earlier reports, it is not associated with decreased uterine perfusion, fetal deterioration, or decreased fetal-placental blood flow (218). Nifedipine has also been found to effectively increase urinary output in antepartum and postpartum severe preeclamptic parturients (219). Nifedipine is a potent uterine muscle relaxant and is gaining popularity as a tocolytic; hence, postpartum hemorrhage may be more likely to occur if nifedipine is administered close to the time of delivery. When administered in the presence of magnesium, it is associated with a potentiated hypotensive response, which is possibly explained by the supposition that magnesium, like nifedipine, acts as a calcium-channel blocker (220, 221). Following oral ingestion in gravid parturients with PIH, peak blood levels were reached in 40 minutes, complete elimination occurred in 360 minutes, and a half-life of 54 minutes was found (222). Other calcium-channel blockers being investigated include nimodipine and nicardipine. *Nimodipine* is rapidly absorbed after oral administration and has significant maternal and fetal cerebral vasodilator activity (223). *Nicardipine* may be administered intravenously as a continuous infusion (224).

Rapid-Acting Antihypertensives

Other potent rapid-acting antihypertensives have been used primarily in acute hypertensive crises or to attenuate or treat the marked hypertensive response associated with laryngoscopy and intubation during induction of general anesthesia. Diazoxide, a thiazide derivative with no diuretic effect, has the disadvantage of often causing sudden uncontrolled hypotension associated with decreased uterine blood flow and fetal distress (225). In addition, diazoxide interferes with glucose metabolism and uric acid excretion and is a potent uterine relaxant; thus it may be associated with significant postpartum hemorrhage. It is rarely used in obstetrics today. Three other very potent and rapid-acting antihypertensives of short duration are *trimethaphan*, sodium *nitroprusside* (SNP), and *trinitroglycerin* (TNG). These are usually given as intravenous infusions for acute control of blood pressure during induction to and emergence from general anesthesia. Their use for this purpose is discussed later. When antihypertensives are given to the gravid parturient with severe preeclampsia or eclampsia, the fetal heart rate should be closely monitored. Sudden decreases in maternal blood pressure can rapidly produce fetal distress as the uteroplacental circulation becomes further compromised. One usually aims to produce only a partial return of maternal blood pressure to normal levels and/or diastolic pressure to below 110 mm Hg until after delivery. Another interesting possibility for antihypertensive control of PIH may be the use of *fenoldapam*. It is a dopamine D₁-like receptor agonist and a rapid-acting vasodilator. Although not yet studied for this purpose, this agent has a very favorable hemodynamic profile.

CONTROL OF CONVULSIONS

In eclampsia, the first priority is to control grand mal convulsions. Until this is accomplished, no attempt is made to deliver the fetus. Maternal mortality increases with the number of convulsions, the elevation of maternal blood pressure, and the age and parity of the parturient (14, 15, 226). Initially, intravenous administration of a rapid-acting anticonvulsant, such as a thiobarbiturate (thiopental, 50 to 100 mg), a benzodiazepine (diazepam, 2.5 to 5 mg, or midazolam, 1 to 2 mg), or magnesium (2 to 4 g) is used to terminate a convulsion. Further convulsions are prevented by continued intravenous administration of magnesium (2 to 4 g·h⁻¹) or another anticonvulsant, such as a benzodiazepine or chloromethiazole. Continued convulsions despite adequate magnesium therapy are often indicative of additional CNS pathology, such as venous thrombosis, intracerebral hemorrhage, or edema, and indicate the need for further evaluation. Oxygen should be administered during a seizure to protect the patient against hypoxia caused by diminished ventilation and increased maternal metabolism. If convulsions do not terminate rapidly, administer succinylcholine and intubate the trachea to prevent pulmonary aspiration and to ensure adequate ventilation. Postictal depression may require the support of ventilation to ensure adequate oxygenation and to prevent hypercapnia and respiratory acidosis. Because convulsions are often associated with metabolic acidosis, bicarbonate may be indicated after determination of arterial blood gases and pH. In severe preeclampsia or eclampsia, frank congestive cardiac failure and pulmonary edema may occur, for which a rapidly-acting, intravenously administered diuretic drug, such as furosemide, is given. If cerebral edema is suspected, an osmotic diuretic drug, such as mannitol, may be administered, but only in the presence of adequate urinary output. *Dexamethasone* (10 to 16 mg) may also be of use in this condition. Mechanical hyperventilation during the postpartum period may be initiated. Before birth, excessive maternal hyperventilation may result in fetal hypoxia and acidosis. Further therapy consists of controlling blood pressure. In severe preeclampsia or eclampsia, disseminated intravascular coagulation may develop, but usually resolves promptly following delivery.

Pritchard and co-workers treated 245 eclamptic parturients between 1955 and 1984 with only a single maternal death caused by an initial intravenous overdose of magnesium (227). All newborns in excess of 1,500 g survived. Essentially, only magnesium sulfate for convulsion control and the antihypertensive hydralazine were used. Fluids were restricted; diuretics were avoided; invasive maternal monitoring was rarely used; and once convulsions were controlled, rapid delivery was accomplished (usually by induction of labor and vaginal delivery).

More recently, a multicenter study (*n* = 327) of women with severe hypertensive disease compared those who did and did not receive epidural analgesia (227a). Epidural anesthesia use did not increase the frequencies of cesarean delivery, cesarean delivery for fetal distress or failure to progress, pulmonary edema, or renal failure among this group of parturients with severe hypertensive disease. This study and other work described in this chapter indicate that women with severe hypertensive disease during pregnancy can be safely managed with epidural analgesia and anesthesia.

MONITORING THE SEVERE PREECLAMPTIC OR ECLAMPTIC PATIENT

Before anesthesia for delivery is initiated, convulsions and severe hypertension should be treated. Although patients with mild preeclampsia may not require special monitoring, those severely afflicted with the disorder will require special considerations. Blood pressure should be monitored frequently. This usually is adequately accomplished with an automatic noninvasive blood pressure device. Such equipment possess good accuracy, and when necessary, can give readings every minute, although prolongation of such frequent readings is associated with patient discomfort and occasionally radial nerve palsies. Invasive direct arterial blood pressure monitoring is rarely required. We reserve it for patients with pulmonary edema, those on ventilators, and others who may require frequent arterial specimens for pH and blood gas analyses. In addition, direct arterial monitoring may be indicated in very unstable patients receiving continuous infusions of potent vasoactive drugs such as sodium nitroprusside.

CENTRAL VENOUS MONITORING

Central venous monitoring is often indicated in severe preeclamptic or eclamptic patients, particularly in those with marked hypertension or oliguria. As previously discussed, some obstetricians and anesthesiologists recommend the replacement of the CVP with the pulmonary artery catheter (65, 66, 77–79). They argue that, in the presence of left ventricular failure or another cardiac disease, the CVP may not accurately reflect intravascular volume (preload) or left ventricular function. They also correctly state that, with only the CVP, one can not reliably diagnose the effects and the various components of the cardiovascular system as they contribute to the clinical picture found in a particular patient. For example, is the severe hypertension observed caused by marked arterial vasoconstriction that is best treated with a vasodilator such as hydralazine or is it the result of a hyperdynamic left ventricle with an increased cardiac output that is treated best with a beta-blocker?

Although not directly related to obstetrics, two studies deserve special consideration in the decision regarding the pulmonary artery catheter. In the first study, a 31-question multiple-choice examination regarding knowledge and use of the pulmonary artery catheter was sent to 496 physicians. There was a direct correlation between the frequency of use of the pulmonary artery catheter and mean score (228). Differences in experience, training, and hospital affiliation accounted for 42% of the variability in test scores, with frequency of use having the strongest influence. While this study does not argue against the use of the pulmonary artery catheter, it does provide a warning to those physicians who use it less frequently. When a pulmonary artery catheter is indicated, one option is to seek assistance from more experienced colleagues. The other study (229) examined the association between the use of pulmonary artery catheters and outcome for patients in their first 24 hours in the intensive care unit. Through case matching, patients with pulmonary artery catheters had an increased mortality, longer stay in the intensive care unit, and higher hospital costs (10). It appeared that the pulmonary artery catheter was the only difference between patients and may have been associated with the increased mortality and increased utilization of resources. The decision regarding the need for placement of a pulmonary artery catheter must be carefully considered.

The management of parturients with pulmonary artery catheters on the labor suite is multidisciplinary, with the anesthesiologist or critical care physician assisting the obstetrician in the medical decisions. As the vast majority of PIH parturients have adequate left ventricular function and normal pulmonary artery pressures, one must weigh the risk of pulmonary artery catheterization against the usefulness of any additional information gained beyond that obtained from central venous catheterization. For PIH parturients, the authors restrict the use of pulmonary artery catheterization to those with refractory oliguria, cardiac lesions, or signs of congestive heart failure. Table 16.9 summarizes indications for pulmonary artery catheterization (65).

CONSIDERATIONS FOR DELIVERY

Delivery of a preterm neonate may be necessitated by deterioration of either the intrauterine environment or the condition of

---

Table 16.9. INDICATIONS FOR PULMONARY ARTERY CATHETER PLACEMENT IN THE SEVERE PREECLAMPTIC OR ECLAMPTIC PATIENT: FINDINGS AND THEIR THERAPY

1. Unresponsive or refractory hypertension
   a. Increased systemic vascular resistance (Rx: vasodilators)
   b. Increased cardiac output (Rx: decrease preload with nitroglycerin or decrease cardiac output with a betablocker)
2. Pulmonary edema
   a. Cardiogenic or left ventricular failure (Rx: afterload reduction or ionotrops)
   b. Increased systemic vascular resistance (Rx: afterload reduction)
   c. Noncardiogenic volume overload (Rx: diuretics, fluid restriction)
      Decreased colloid oncotic pressure (Rx: 25% albumin, fluid restriction)
3. Persistent arterial desaturation; unable to distinguish between cardiac or noncardiac origin
4. Oliguria unresponsive to modest fluid loading
   a. Low preload (Rx: crystalloid infusion)
   b. Severe increased systemic vascular resistance with low cardiac output (Rx: afterload reduction)
   c. Selective renal artery vasoconstriction

Adapted from Clark SB, Cotton DB. Clinical indications for pulmonary artery catheterization in the patient with severe preeclampsia. *Am J Obstet Gynecol* 1988;158:453–458.

---

the mother. When severe preeclampsia develops in the second trimester before 24 weeks' gestation despite aggressive obstetric management, the outcome of the fetus is dismal (less than 7% survival) and maternal complications are frequent (40%) (57). The expectant management of parturients with severe preeclampsia at 28 to 32 weeks' gestation was compared with those who delivered 48 hours following glucocorticoid administration (136). Expectant management consisted of bed rest, oral antihypertensives, and intensive antenatal fetal testing. With expectant management, the duration of gestation was prolonged by two weeks without increasing the incidence of eclampsia or abruptio placentae. Furthermore, expectant management decreased both the admission rate and the duration of stay of these neonates to the neonatal intensive care unit. If the fetus is in an unfavorable lie, delivery by cesarean section is usually chosen. If the fetus is dead or nonviable or if, conversely, it is of reasonable size (greater than 2,500 g) and tolerates labor, vaginal delivery with induction is usually indicated. Because the uterus of the preeclamptic parturient is markedly sensitive to oxytocin, induction and vaginal delivery are often possible though the cervix is not "ripe."

ANESTHESIA AND ANALGESIA
General Considerations

The parturient with PIH requires a reliable means of intravenous drug administration, such as that provided by at least an 18-gauge indwelling intravenous catheter. Intravenously administered fluids should not consist of dextrose in water alone, especially if oxytocin is used, because of the danger of water intoxication. Rather, isotonic- balanced salt solutions should be used. Rapid infusion of dextrose-containing solutions should be avoided or limited to a maximum of 125 mL·h^{-1} of 5% dextrose because neonatal hypoglycemia and hyperbilirubinemia are associated with the resultant maternal hyperglycemia (230). Urinary output should be monitored to help guide fluid replacement.

In the severely preeclamptic parturient, a CVP catheter may be of value for determining fluid and blood replacement, particularly if the parturient has refractory oliguria. To replenish intravascular volume before administration of an epidural block, balanced salt solutions or plasma expanders such as 5% or 25% albumin are given while the CVP is being monitored (231). The choice of the hydrating solution is open to debate. Rapid infusion of 2 liters of balanced salt solution, as is often given in a healthy parturient, may significantly lower the colloid oncotic pressure for 24 hours compared to the infusion of a colloid solution (232). Although this is tolerated by the normal parturient, the preeclamptic parturient with her often already lowered serum colloid pressure and damaged capillary endothelium may not tolerate such rapid crystalloid infusions, and may precipitate acute pulmonary edema (233, 234). Infusion of 500 or 1,000 mL of 5% albumin in severe preeclamptics has been found to increase cardiac output and decrease systemic vascular resistance with no effect or minimal lowering of mean arterial blood pressure (235). Hence, use of albumin infusions might be preferable in the severe preeclamptic parturient. Certainly, rapid intravenous hydration, particularly with crystalloid solutions, should be done with care and with constant monitoring of the CVP and urinary output, while observing for early signs and symptoms of pulmonary edema.

Maternal urinary output and protein excretion are important indicators of disease severity in the severe preeclamptic parturient and require accurate monitoring throughout the peripartum period. This requires an indwelling bladder catheter, especially during labor and for as long as several days following delivery. Continuous infusion of oxytocin has a marked antidiuretic effect, similar to an antidiuretic hormone. When infused at rates greater than 10 μu/min, it may markedly decrease urinary output, cause retention of free water, and result in hyponatremia and water intoxication. When oxytocin is infused, all intravenous solutions should be isotonic in regard to electrolyte content.

The parturient should be encouraged to remain on her left side to avoid aortocaval compressions. Supplemental oxygen during labor and delivery may be indicated because of the left-shifted maternal oxygen hemoglobin dissociation curve of the preeclamptic parturient (107, 108).

The choice of analgesia depends on the obstetric situation. Although opioids provide analgesia, they have no anticonvulsant and little antihypertensive effect. Tranquilizers, often used with opioids, should be given in small doses. Patient-controlled analgesia (PCA) with fentanyl or meperidine may provide satisfactory analgesia during the active phase of labor. For PCA, the initial intravenous loading dose of meperidine is 25 to 50 mg and/or fentanyl 1 $\mu g \cdot kg^{-1}$. Additionally, 10 to 15 mg of self-administered meperidine, or 25 to 50 μg of fentanyl every 20 minutes may be given. The doses and lock-out periods for PCA in obstetric anesthesia are not well defined. Paracervical block is not recommended in circumstances where uteroplacental blood flow may be compromised or in the presence of fetal bradycardia, acidosis or distress, and its use in the preeclamptic parturient delivering a viable newborn is not recommended. However, it provides first-stage maternal analgesia for a nonviable fetus, a postpartum dilation and evacuation, or repair of a cervical laceration.

At delivery, augmentation of nitrous oxide analgesia with a pudendal block or local infiltration of the perineum can provide satisfactory analgesia for most forceps deliveries. In the unlikely event that general anesthesia is required for vaginal delivery, care must be taken to avoid sudden severe maternal hypertension with tracheal intubation during a rapid-sequence intravenous induction. Such an event predisposes the mother to intracerebral hemorrhage and pulmonary hypertension with pulmonary edema.

Lumbar Epidural Analgesia: Benefits

The use of major conduction analgesia, particularly continuous lumbar epidural analgesia, in parturients with PIH has been often debated in the past. Today, the use of continuous lumbar epidural analgesia in the severe preeclamptic or eclamptic patient whose convulsions are under control is widely accepted and even recommended by both anesthesiologists and obstetricians (236–242). When not contraindicated by gross coagulation abnormalities, maternal septicemia, or marked untreated hypovolemia, continuous lumbar epidural analgesia offers the parturient with PIH many advantages. It can provide complete pain relief for labor and delivery without the need for depressant drugs. It provides ideal obstetric conditions for vaginal delivery, particularly for the preterm neonate. It is also suitable for operative vaginal delivery (vacuum extraction, forceps delivery) and can be extended rapidly for cesarean section.

During labor and delivery, continuous lumbar epidural analgesia decreases maternal oxygen requirements and prevents maternal hyperventilation associated with painful contractions (243, 244). This hyperventilation may further decrease uterine blood flow and cause maternal metabolic acidosis. Maternal circulating levels of catecholamines may be elevated in preeclampsia and may decrease uteroplacental perfusion; epidural analgesia significantly decreases the circulating level of epinephrine (245). In fact, epidural analgesia may entirely blunt the hemodynamic and neuroendocrine response to the pain of labor and delivery (246). It improves intervillous blood flow in severe preeclamptic parturients (Table 16.10) (241), and it appears to protect against eclamptic convulsions (237, 239). Because epidural analgesia stabilizes blood pressure at modestly lower levels, sudden hypertensive events associated with rapid-sequence induction of general anesthesia and intubation are avoided (Fig.16.7) (247–250). Such sudden hypertensive events are associated with pulmonary edema, cerebral edema, and

Table 16.10. BLOOD PRESSURE AND INTERVILLOUS BLOOD FLOW BEFORE AND AFTER EPIDURAL BLOCK IN NINE PATIENTS WITH SEVERE PREECLAMPSIA IN LABOR[a,b]

	Before Epidural	After Epidural	p Value
Systolic blood pressure (torr)	155 ± 15	155 ± 20	NS
Diastolic blood pressure (torr)	100 ± 16	100 ± 19	NS
Intervillous blood flow (mL/min/dL)	196 ± 120	320 ± 183	<0.01

[a] Mean ± SD.
[b] All Apgar scores at 1 and 5 min ≥ 8. Eight of nine patients had increases in intervillous blood flow following epidural block. One patient who gave birth to a 2,200-g newborn at 39 weeks' gestation had a decrease in intervillous blood flow from 72 to 68 mL/min/dL after epidural block and no fetal distress. All patients were prehydrated with 500 mL of Ringer's solution, were kept in 15-degree left lateral tilt, and had an epidural block initiated with 10 mL of 0.25% bupivacaine.
From Jouppila P, Jouppila R, Hollmen A, et al. Lumbar epidural analgesia to improve intervillous blood flow during labor in severe preeclampsia. *Obstet Gynecol* 1982;59;158–161, with permission.

intracranial hemorrhage (251, 252). Finally, the risk of pulmonary aspiration of gastric contents is minimized because the patient remains awake.

Concerns with epidural analgesia include the potential of sudden maternal hypotension that rapidly lead to fetal deterioration (253) and may further decrease an already compromised intervillous blood flow. Additionally, there is the concern about the use of regional anesthesia in the parturient at risk of developing a coagulopathy with the subsequent risk of epidural hematoma.

With proper technique, significant maternal hypotension and fetal distress can usually be avoided after lumbar epidural block (240). The percentage decrease in blood pressure is no greater in preeclamptic parturients than it is for normal parturients (Fig. 16.8) (236, 239, 247, 254). Graham and Goldstein demonstrated that cardiac output was not decreased by epidural block in severe preeclamptic patients (255). Newsome and co-workers found that, in severe preeclamptic patients, although epidural block for either vaginal delivery or cesarean section lowered the mean arterial pressure from 121 mm Hg to 98 mm Hg, there was no decrease in cardiac index, pulmonary vascular resistance, central venous pressure, or pulmonary capillary wedge pressure (79). Prevention of hypotension in severe preeclamptics does not require large amounts of intravenous hydration (256), but it does require the meticulous avoidance of aortocaval compression. Should hypotension occur, in addition to further uterine displacement and hydration, small intravenous doses of ephedrine (2.5 to 5 mg) are given as required to restore and maintain blood pressure. Hypotension associated with epidural block, if treated rapidly by the above means, was not associated with fetal or neonatal deterioration, even when the epidural block was used in cases of fetal distress for urgent cesarean section (257).

Animal and human studies have shown no evidence of diminished uterine or intervillous blood flow during epidural analgesia unaccompanied by hypotension (258–263). Studies in preeclamptic parturients having essential hypertension showed that intervillous blood flow was maintained or improved with the use of epidural analgesia (Table 16.11) (241). In contrast, induction of general anesthesia was associated with decreased uterine and intervillous blood flow in pregnant normotensive animals and humans (264, 265). When local anesthetics are properly used, they are not associated with convulsions and are not contraindicated in seizure disorders. Indeed, local anesthetics have been used successfully to terminate clinical status epilepticus

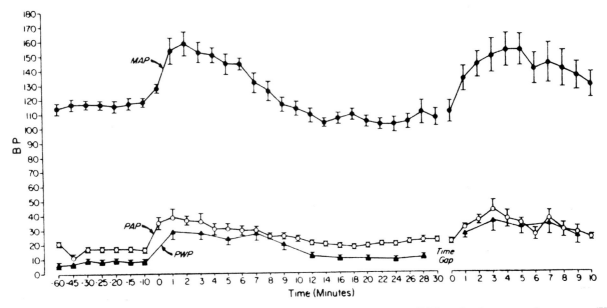

Figure 16.7. Mean and SEM of mean arterial pressure (MAP), mean pulmonary artery pressure (PAP), and pulmonary wedge pressure (PWP = PCWP) in eight patients with severe preeclampsia receiving general anesthesia for cesarean section. Anesthesia consisted of thiopental (3 mg·kg⁻¹), succinylcholine (100 mg), nitrous oxide (40%), 0.5% halothane, and a 0.2% succinylcholine infusion. (From Hodgkinson R, Husain FJ, Hayashi RH. Systemic and pulmonary blood pressure during cesarean section in parturients with gestational hypertension. *Can Anaesth Soc J* 1980;27:389–394, with permission.)

(266–268). A comparison of epidurals for cesarean section using lidocaine showed similar neonatal outcomes in normal compared with preeclamptic parturients as assessed by umbilical arterial and venous blood gases, Apgar scores, and early neurobehavioral scores at 4 and 24 hours, despite a modestly prolonged total body clearance of lidocaine in the neonates of preeclamptic mothers (18.5 + 4.7 vs. 14.1 + 1.3 μg·h·mL⁻¹) (269).

For most mothers with severe preeclampsia or controlled eclampsia, clinical experience and recent investigational work support the use of continuous lumbar epidural analgesia as the preferred method of analgesia for labor and vaginal delivery.

Similarly for cesarean section, spinal or epidural anesthesia may be preferable to general anesthesia in most circumstances.

Patient Preparation

Before instituting a continuous lumbar epidural block in a *severely preeclamptic* parturient, it is important that the patient's overall medical management, including state of hydration and management of hypertension, are well controlled. The absence of a severe coagulopathy must be confirmed. The use of a pulse oximeter during labor is helpful and gives an early indication of developing pulmonary edema or inadequate circulation.

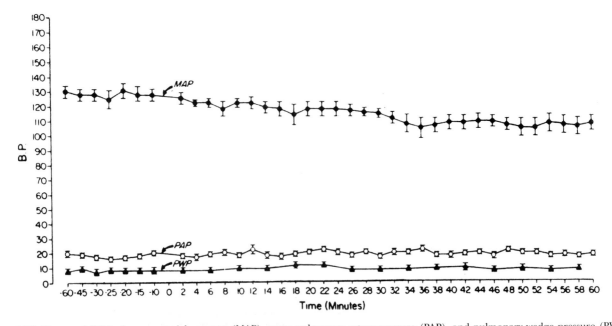

Figure 16.8. Mean and SEM of mean arterial pressure (MAP), mean pulmonary artery pressure (PAP), and pulmonary wedge pressure (PWP = PCWP) in 12 patients with severe preeclampsia receiving epidural analgesia for cesarean section. Bupivacaine, 0.75% (no longer recommended for use in obstetrics since 1983) was injected at time 0. (From Hodgkinson R, Husain FJ, Hagash RH. Systemic and pulmonary blood pressure during cesarean section. *Can Anaesth Soc J* 1980;27:389–394, with permission.)

Continuously recorded electronic monitoring of fetal heart rate and uterine contractions is mandatory because the parturient's ability to judge the frequency, strength, and duration of contractions may be decreased. Although a decrease in systolic blood pressure of 25% is usually without consequence in normal pregnancy (provided the systolic blood pressure does not fall below 100 mm Hg), such a decrease may not be tolerated if placental function is already compromised, as it is in preeclampsia. The fetal heart rate tracing will provide rapid and reliable signs if the decrease in maternal blood pressure is too great for the fetus to withstand. Before the block is initiated, limited prehydration (not exceeding a CVP of 6 cm of water if a CVP monitor is utilized) should be considered. Rapid volume administration may cause excessive hydration and pulmonary edema. A pulmonary artery catheter should be considered in parturients having (a) refractory hypertension, (b) oliguria not responding to a modest fluid load, (c) suspected left ventricular failure that is likely to progress to congestive heart failure, (d) signs of developing pulmonary edema, or (e) superimposed cardiac disease (Table 16.10).

Prehydration before an epidural or subarachnoid block in the severely preeclamptic parturient must be performed with great caution. The decreased colloid oncotic pressure and damaged capillary endothelial integrity predispose her to rapid development of pulmonary edema. Before an epidural block for labor, where only a T10 sensory level is sought, 500 mL of a balanced salt solution or 0.9% saline solution without dextrose is usually adequate to prevent hypotension, provided the parturient is not dehydrated. When an epidural block for cesarean section is sought (which requires a minimum upper sensory level of T4), larger amounts of prehydration are indicated. In the mild preeclamptic parturient, 1 to 2 liters of balanced salt solution is usually adequate. However, in more *severe preeclamptic* parturients with diastolic blood pressures in excess of 100 mm Hg, such rapid prehydration with crystalloid alone may not be adequate to prevent hypotension and may subject the parturient to pulmonary edema.

In these patients prior to the regional anesthetic, prehydration with 1,000 mL of a crystalloid solution followed by the use of additional fluids and vasopressors are necessary with the onset of a sympathectomy. It is usually possible to manage those patients without a CVP catheter.

Some clinicians prefer to monitor the CVP in these patients and administer colloid in addition to the crystalloid. Under these circumstances, if the CVP remains 0 or less following the administration of 1,000 mL of crystalloid, the authors usually administer either 5% or 25% albumin to elevate the CVP to a positive pressure before initiating the block and then extend the block slowly in steps with further hydration or ephedrine as required to prevent hypotension. A decreasing blood pressure following an epidural block is initially treated with a small intravenous injection of ephedrine (2.5 to 5.0 mg), then a bolus of 50 to 100 mL of 25% albumin. When such an epidural block is allowed to dissipate, the parturient must be observed for signs indicating the development of pulmonary edema. A rapidly rising central venous pressure, a falling oxygen saturation, or both are indicative of impending pulmonary edema.

Epidural Block for Vaginal Delivery

Because labor tends to be rapid and painful in the preeclamptic parturient, early placement of the epidural catheter and establishment of an adequate sensory block is indicated. This practice eliminates the need for opioid analgesia, which may have a depressant effect on the fetus. Following an appropriate test dose to detect unrecognized intravascular or subarachnoid injection, the block is initiated with a small volume (6 to 10 mL) of a dilute local anesthetic. If blood pressure remains stable, additional doses of local anesthetic may be repeated to provide complete

pain relief throughout the first stage of labor or more commonly, a continuous infusion of dilute local anesthetic with opioids is utilized (i.e. bupivacaine 0.0625% with fentanyl 1-2 $\mu g \cdot mL^{-1}$). We also add 1:400,000 epinephrine to the local anesthetic to improve the quality of the block. There is one case report of severe hypertension following the epidural administration of a local anesthetic with epinephrine (270), with several others documenting no ill effects of its use (271, 272). Some clinicians prefer a denser block and would use a more concentrated local anesthetic (i.e., bupivacaine 0.25%). This has the advantage of blocking all pain perception and allows for a more rapid initiation of a surgical block if needed.

With the onset of the second stage of labor, sufficient additional local anesthetic is injected to ensure complete perineal analgesia. Complete perineal analgesia may be desirable in parturients with severe preeclampsia because it allows for operative vaginal delivery. It prevents uncontrollable bearing-down by the parturient, an occurrence that is associated with sudden changes in the cardiovascular and the CNS, and it minimizes the likelihood of a precipitous delivery of a preterm or small neonate, an event that is associated with neonatal intracerebral hemorrhage.

Subarachnoid Block for Vaginal Delivery

If vaginal delivery is imminent, spinal anesthetia to a T10 sensory level or an injection of an opioid and a local anesthetic can safely provide rapid and complete analgesia for vaginal delivery. The use of a combined spinal-epidural technique would allow for extension of the block if necessary. The problem of sudden maternal hypotension is usually not great if the sensory level does not exceed T10, if left uterine displacement is ensured, and if the block is preceded with hydration. The disadvantages of a single subarachnoid injection can be solved by performing a combined spinal-epidural technique. If the need for cesarean section arises, the epidural catheter can be bolused with a local anesthetic. To produce the required T10 sensory level, hyperbaric lidocaine, bupivacaine, or tetracaine are all satisfactory. The addition of 25 μg fentanyl to the above solution will improve the quality and prolong the duration of the block.

CESAREAN SECTION
Regional Anesthesia

Cesarean section is often indicated in the parturient with PIH because of the deterioration of the intrauterine environment or the worsening of the mother's condition. If time allows and no contraindications (such as coagulation disorders) exist, the authors use continuous lumbar epidural anesthesia although the use of spinal anesthesia has gained wide acceptance (273). The authors do not consider eclampsia to be a contraindication to the use of epidural anesthesia for either vaginal delivery or cesarean section, if convulsions are controlled and the parturient is responsive. Medical therapy is continued, the parturient is monitored and prehydrated, and left uterine displacement is ensured. Following placement of the epidural catheter and injection of a suitable test dose, a T10 sensory level is obtained by injection of 8 to 10 mL of 1.5 to 2% lidocaine with epinephrine 1:200,000, 0.5% bupivacaine, or 0.5% ropivacaine. After the initial block is obtained and the maternal arterial and central venous pressures (if indicated) are stabilized, the sensory level is raised to a minimum T4 level in one or two stages by administering additional doses of local anesthetics. In the severely preeclamptic or eclamptic patient, an epidural block produced as described may require 30 minutes or longer to achieve, but is rarely associated with severe maternal hypotension or fetal deterioration. The addition of 50 to 100 μg fentanyl to the local anesthetic will (a) speed the onset of the block; (b) improve the quality of the block; (c) decrease visceral discomfort associated with uterine exteriorization, uterine interiorization, and peritoneal retraction; and

(d) prolong the duration of the block without demonstrable ill effects on the fetus. At the conclusion of surgery, epidural injection of preservative-free morphine, 4 mg will provide up to 24 hours of excellent postoperative analgesia. After delivery and during closure, small amounts of intravenous opioids and/or midazolam or diazepam are given if required for maternal sedation and comfort. In addition to the advantages discussed earlier, epidural anesthesia for cesarean section in the parturient with PIH eliminates the sudden maternal hypertension associated with induction to and emergence from general anesthesia, provides cardiovascular and CNS stability (Fig. 16.8), and provides effective postoperative analgesia without producing significant maternal depression by infusions of low concentrations of local anesthetics or epidural opioids.

Some anesthesiologists avoid subarachnoid block for cesarean section, fearing its use may be associated with sudden and profound hypotension. They also argue that the fluids administered to treat the hypotension leads to pulmonary edema. Wallace, et al. examined the use of regional anesthesia for parturients with severe preeclampsia (274). Eighty parturients with the diagnosis were randomized to receive either general, epidural, or spinal anesthesia for cesarean section. The authors noted no excessive hypotension nor excessive intravenous fluid administration in the spinal group. There were no serious maternal complications such as pulmonary edema. Furthermore, there was no difference in umbilical cord pH or Apgar scores among the groups, suggesting adequate placental perfusion. Other studies have also shown the safety of high spinal block for cesarean section in preeclamptic parturients. Twelve preeclamptics, six who were severe, received a subarachnoid block with 12.5 mg hyperbaric bupivacaine after only a liter of crystalloid prehydration. Hypotension was treated with further fluids and ephedrine. The incidence of hypotension to a decrease of 80% or less of control systolic pressure occurred in only two of the 12 patients, one of whom developed a C5 sensory block. Mean pulsatile uterine artery index rose insignificantly and all babies had Apgar scores of 7 or above at 5 minutes, and in seven newborns, when obtained, umbilical artery pH was 7.14 to 7.42 (275). A retrospective study of severe preeclamptics ($n = 103$) undergoing elective cesarean section with either spinal or epidural block revealed no difference in hemodynamic effects between the two groups (Fig. 16.9) (273). There were also no differences in Apgar scores, incidence of maternal intensive care unit admission, or postoperative pulmonary edema. The parturients who had spinal anes-

thesia did receive more i.v. crystalloid ($1,780 \pm 838$ mL) then those who had epidural anesthesia ($1,359 \pm 674$ mL). With great attention to detail, continuous monitoring of maternal blood pressure, and the use of small, repeated doses of intravenous ephedrine following adequate prehydration, one can safely use spinal anesthesia. Hyperbaric 0.75% bupivacaine (12 to 15 mg) reliably produces a T4 sensory level. The addition of fentanyl 15 to 25 μg or 0.2 mg of preservative-free morphine to the local anesthetic solution will improve the quality of the block, diminish visceral discomfort, and provide prolonged continuous pain relief in the postoperative period.

A truly emergent cesarean section in preeclampsia is often required for a nonreassuring fetal heart rate tracing. If the parturient's blood pressure is stable, not severely hypovolemic, has a functioning lumbar epidural catheter in place, the block can be quickly increased by injecting a rapid-acting local anesthetic (i.e., 3% 2-chloroprocaine or 2% lidocaine) as she is being prepared, without delaying surgery. In the true emergency, we do not hesitate to use subarachnoid block for the parturient with severe preeclampsia, if not contraindicated by other factors.

General Anesthesia

On rare occasions, general anesthesia is required for cesarean section in the parturient with severe preeclampsia. For a true, emergency cesarean section, there may not be enough time for a regional anesthetic, or a regional block may be contraindicated (e.g., bleeding disorder, patient refusal). The technique of general anesthesia must be modified in the severe preeclamptic parturient to allow for (a) increased upper airway edema, (b) interactions of anesthetic drugs with drugs used by the obstetrician, particularly magnesium, and (c) marked hypertensive responses to intubation, surgical stimulation, and later, extubation under light general anesthesia.

The increased upper airway edema associated with normal pregnancy is usually exacerbated in preeclampsia, at times to an extent that may seriously compromise the patient's airway (276, 277). Cases have been reported in which awake intubation or tracheotomy were required to maintain an open airway (278). Severe uvular edema obstructing vision of the posterior pharynx has also been observed. Before induction of general anesthesia, the airway must be thoroughly evaluated. If dysphonia, dysphoria, dyspnea, or respiratory distress are present, inspection of the larynx and vocal cords is mandatory with possible awake, fiberoptic intubation or tracheotomy required (see Chapter 21).

Because of the interaction of magnesium and muscle relaxants, the latter must be used with caution in preeclampsia. Defasciculation with a nondepolarizing muscle relaxant is unnecessary (279). For endotracheal intubation, succinylcholine ($1.5 \text{ mg} \cdot \text{kg}^{-1}$) ensures rapid and complete relaxation. Additional relaxants should not be given unless the surgical field and response to a nerve stimulator indicate the need. Any of the newer, shorter-acting muscle relaxants may be used if the dose effect is titrated with a nerve stimulator in place. The sensitivity to nondepolarizing muscle relaxants is markedly increased in parturients receiving magnesium (280–283), and reversal at the conclusion of surgery may be prolonged, so cautious dosing is appropriate. When nondepolarizing muscle relaxants are used, only very small doses are given while monitoring the relaxation achieved with a nerve stimulator. If, following delivery, one continues to administer two-thirds of the minimum alveolar concentration (MAC) of a potent inhalational agent combined with 50% to 70% nitrous oxide, supplemented as required with small doses of an opioid, additional doses of muscle relaxants are usually not required.

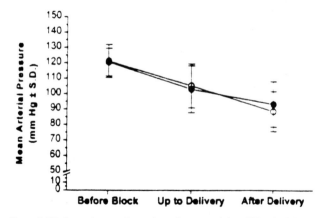

Figure 16.9. Severely preeclamptic patients receiving 103 spinal (open circles) or 35 epidural (closed circles) anesthetic procedures for cesarean section. Data are mean ± SD. Lowest mean blood pressures recorded do not differ between groups. **"Before Block,"** 20 min before regional anesthesia induction; **"Up to Delivery,"** period from regional anesthesia induction to delivery; **"After Delivery,"** period from delivery to the end of surgery. (From Hood DD, Curry R. Spinal versus epidural anesthesia for cesarean section in severely preeclamptic patients. *Anesthesiology* 1999;90:1276–1282, with permission.)

Endotracheal Intubation

Endotracheal intubation, surgical stimulation, and emergence from light-balanced general anesthesia in normal parturients

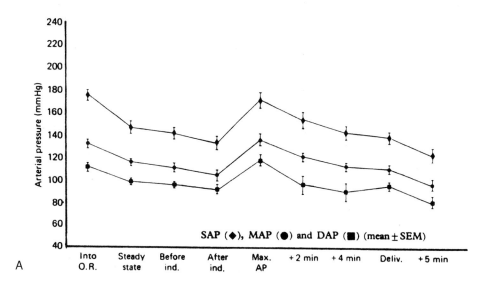

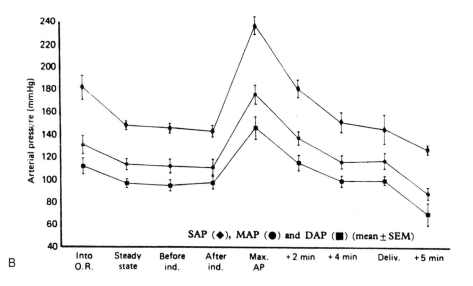

Figure 16.10. Responses of systolic arterial pressure (SAP), mean arterial pressure (MAP, and diastolic arterial pressure (DAP) in women undergoing cesarean section with general anesthesia, as follows: induction with lidocaine ($1\ mg \cdot kg^{-1}$), etomidate ($0.2\ mg \cdot kg^{-1}$), and succinylcholine (100 mg); intubation and maintenance with 50% nitrous oxide and 0.5% halothane. **A:** In 13 young (mean age 20 years), law-parity women. **B:** In seven older (mean age 30 years), multiparous women. Note the greater degree of hypertension in the group of older parturients. (From Connell H, Dalgleish JG, Downing JW. General anesthesia in mothers with severe preeclampsia-eclampsia. *Br J Anaesth* 1987;59:1375–1380, with permission.)

are accompanied by significant increases in blood pressure, maternal heart rate, and circulating catecholamines (284). These increases can be extreme in the parturient who has severe PIH (Fig. 16.7). In one study, elevation of the systolic pressure in hypertensive parturients averaged more than 56 mm Hg. Multiparous parturients older than 25 years of age appear to be at greatest risk for this severe blood pressure elevation (Fig. 16.10) (248). Means used to attenuate this response have included pretreatment with opioids, magnesium, lidocaine, or (more frequently) antihypertensives. One study found that pretreatment with $1.5\ mg \cdot kg^{-1}$ intravenous lidocaine before intubation was not effective in decreasing the hypertensive response in the preeclamptic parturient, even with the prior injection of magnesium (285). Lawes and co-workers (249) found intravenous fentanyl 200 μg and droperidol 5 mg effective in the attenuation of the hypertensive response to intubation in 19 of 25 hypertensive parturients, without ill effects on the neonate. Allen and co-workers observed that the administration of alfentanil ($10\ \mu g \cdot kg^{-1}$) 60 seconds before intubation prevented significant hypertension in 24 preeclamptics; however, 17 of the neonates required naloxone and four neonates had low 1-minute Apgar scores (285). We await studies examining the effect of remifentanil which may prove very useful (286).

Various antihypertensive drugs such as hydralazine, labetalol, nitroglycerin, and nitroprusside have been used to prevent and treat acute hypertension during general anesthesia in the parturient, particularly during induction and endotracheal intubation. A recent study in parturients with severe preeclampsia demonstrated a significant increase in middle cerebral artery flow velocity (V_m) and systemic hypertension with induction of general anesthesia for cesarean section (Fig. 16.11) (287). In patients with severe preeclampsia, any additional insult resulting from acute variations in cerebral blood flow may be deleterious. The advantages and disadvantages associated with each drug are outlined in Table 16.11. The anesthesiologist must be prepared to prevent and immediately treat any severe hypertension or (on occasion) hypotension that occurs during general anesthesia.

Cesarean section with the parturient receiving nitrous oxide and a muscle relaxant alone is often associated with maternal hypertension and recall of surgery. This practice also does not allow for administration of high concentration of inspired oxygen ($FIo_2 > 0.5$), which is shown to be beneficial for both normal and asphyxiated fetuses during general anesthesia (288, 289). Adding up to two-thirds MAC of a potent inhalational drug (e.g., 0.5% halothane, 0.7% isoflurane, or 3.0% desflurane) overcomes these problems and ensures maternal analgesia and amnesia. Indeed, in cases of severe fetal distress using

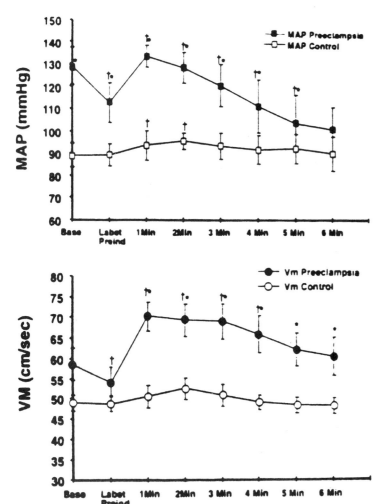

Figure 16.11. **A:** Mean arterial pressure (MAP) in the study (preeclampsia) and control groups at baseline (Base); after the administration of labetalol and before induction in the study group (Labet); before induction in the control group (Preind); and 1-6 min after tracheal intubation. *Significantly different between groups ($P < 0.05$). †Significantly different from baseline values ($P < 0.05$). **B:** Mean middle cerebral artery flow velocity (V_m) in the study (preeclampsia) and control groups at baseline (Base); after the administration of labetalol and before induction in the study group (Labet); before induction in the control group (Preind); and 1 to 6 min after tracheal intubation. *Significantly different between groups ($P < 0.05$). †Significantly different from baseline values ($P < 0.05$). (From Ramanathan J, Angel JJ, Bush AJ, et al. Changes in maternal middle cerebral artery blood flow velocity associated with general anesthesia in severe preeclampsia. *Anesth Analg* 1999;88:357–361, with permission.)

the potential inhalation anesthetics, initially at 1.5 MAC for the first minute, then a two-thirds MAC in oxygen alone until delivery, ensures adequate maternal amnesia and analgesia and maintains maternal oxygen saturation near 100%, desirable because of the left shift of the maternal oxygen hemoglobin dissociation curve in the preeclamptic parturient (107). Intravenous fentanyl and lidocaine may be useful to acutely lower maternal blood pressure and decrease the likelihood of CNS injury. The use of such low concentrations of potent inhalational drugs is not associated with decreased uterine activity, increased uterine bleeding, or neonatal depression (290–292). Ketamine, which is recommended for induction of general anesthesia in bleeding or asthmatic patients, is best avoided in preeclampsia because of its tendency to produce hypertension when full anesthetic doses (0.75 to 1 mg · kg^{-1}) are used for induction. Throughout general or regional anesthesia those parturients receiving magnesium should continue to receive it. Antihypertensive drugs should be given as required.

POSTPARTUM CARE OF MOTHER AND NEONATE

The neonate born of a PIH mother is at higher risk for prematurity, small-for-gestational-age size, asphyxiation, drug depression, and meconium aspiration. Levy et al. (122) identified predictors of neonatal resuscitation of the newborn. Preeclampsia significantly increased the possibility of the neonate having an umbilical arterial pH less than 7.15. However, there is a widely held belief that preeclampsia accelerates fetal maturation. Chari et al. (293) performed a matched cohort study

examining whether the presence of preeclampsia in the parturient advances the maturity in preterm infants. The Ballard score determines neonatal maturity by assessing neurologic and physical characteristics. Based upon this criteria, PIH was not associated with accelerated fetal neurologic and physical development. Immediate complications in the neonate include respiratory distress, instability of body temperature, poor feeding, hypoglycemia, and hypocalcemia. In the first days of life, intensive therapy is often required to ensure adequate monitoring and support. If available, it is prudent to admit the newborn of a severely preeclamptic or eclamptic mother directly to a neonatal intensive care unit rather than to the well-baby nursery.

The severely PIH parturient is prone to convulse or develop pulmonary edema within 24 hours of delivery. These events may occur as an epidural block dissipates. If magnesium has been given, it should be continued, usually for 48 hours postpartum, or other longer-acting oral anticonvulsants may be substituted. Likewise, antihypertensive therapy is continued (as necessary) with longer-acting preparations replacing intravenous infusions. The first 48 hours are as critical for such a patient as any other period of her prenatal course. Thus, in the severely PIH parturient, continued careful monitoring, therapy, and pain relief are required if convulsions and other problems are to be avoided. Kalur, et al. presented three cases with postpartum preeclampsia-induced shock and death (294). Common to these three cases, as well as the other cases reported, was profound hypotension in parturients with minimal blood loss at delivery and hyponatremia. The etiology of the syndrome is not know. The infusion of hypertonic saline may be of benefit in this unique subset of patients.

Table 16.11. ANTIHYPERTENSIVE DRUGS USED TO PREVENT OR TREAT EPISODES OF HYPERTENSION DURING GENERAL ANESTHESIA

	Administration and Dose	Onset and Duration of Action	Effect on Uterine and Placental Blood Flow	Special Properties Advantages	Disadvantages
Hydralazine Arterial vasodilator MW:160	IV bolus: 5–10 mg IV infusion: 20 mg·500 mL^{-1} (0.04 mg·mL^{-1})	Maximum effect requires 20–30 min after IV administration; duration ~2 h	Originally thought to improve; this is now questioned	1. Easy to administer; no special equipment or monitoring required 2. Maintains maternal cardiac output 3. Long history of safe use in obstetrics	1. Slow unreliable onset 2. Maternal tachycardia 3. ↓ placental blood flow; fetal distress 4. Neonatal thrombocytopenia 5. Maternal nausea, vomiting, headache
Labetalol β_1 and α blocker; ?-β_2 agonist MW: 365	IV boluses: 10–20 mg up to total of 1–3 mg·kg^{-1}	IV onset, 1–2 min; duration 2–3 h	Improves uterine and placental blood flow	1. Easy to administer; no special equipment or monitoring required 2. Little risk of overshoot 3. Improved placental blood flow 4. Few maternal side effects 5. Rapid onset	1. Large variation in effective dose 2. Alone, may not effectively ↓ BP 3. Use with caution in patients with asthma, chronic pulmonary obstructure disease, or compromised ventricular function
Nitroprusside Direct-acting arterial vasodilator MW: 298	Constant IV infusion: 0.05–10 µg·kg^{-1}·h^{-1} Infusion: 50 mg·500 mL^{-1} 5% dextrose in water (50 µg·mL^{-1})	Onset <1 min; duration only a few minutes	Dilates uterine artery in vitro; no ill effects unless severe hypotension present	1. Rapid onset and dissipation 2. Potent reliable antihypertensive 3. No ill effects on fetus	1. Unstable solution; must protect from light 2. Easy to overshoot; need A-line 3. ↑ intracranial pressure 4. Cyanide toxicity; not in short-term use and <3 µg·kg^{-1}·h^{-1} 5. Tachyphylaxis
Nitroglycerin Venodilator MW: 227 (used less commonly)	Constant IV infusion: 5–50 mg·min^{-1} Infusion: 25–50 mg·500 mL^{-1} (50–100 µg·mL^{-1})	Onset <2 min; duration only a few minutes	Questionable, depends on state of maternal hydration; has been associated with fetal deterioration	1. Rapid onset and dissipation	1. Need IV pump to administer 2. May need arterial line 3. Great variation in response, if well-hydrated not very effective (>60% failure rate) 4. ↑ intracranial pressure 5. ↓ cardiac index and O$_2$ delivery
Trimethaphan Ganglionic blocker MW: 597 (not in common use)	IV infusion: 1 mg·mL^{-1} IV boluses: 1–4 mg	IV onset <1 min: duration <5 min	Minimal, if no severe maternal hypotension	1. Reliable, rapid acting 2. Large molecular weight limits fetal transfer 3. Rapid dissipation	1. May require arterial line for BP monitoring 2. Interferes with action of pseudocholinesterase, resulting in prolonged duration of succinylcholine 3. Histamine release (?) 4. May cause mydriasis

MW, molecular weight; BP, blood pressure.

REFERENCES

1. American College of Obstetricians and Gynecologists. *Hypertension in pregnancy. ACOG Technical Bulletin no. 219.* Washington DC: ACOG, 1996.
2. Steer PJ. The definition of pre-eclampsia. *Br J Obstet Gynaecol* 1999;106:753–755.
3. North RA, Taylor RS, Schellenberg JC. Evaluation of definition of pre-eclampsia. *Br J Obstet Gynaecol* 1999;106:767–773.
4. Consensus Report. High blood pressure in pregnancy. *Am J Obstet Gynecol* 1990;163:1689–1712.
5. Chesley LC. Diagnosis of preeclampsia [Editorial]. *Obstet Gynecol* 1985;65:423–425.
6. Davey DA, MacGillivray I. The classification and definition of the hypertensive disorders of pregnancy. *Am J Obstet Gynecol* 1988;158:892–898.
7. Sibai BM. Pitfalls in the diagnosis and management of preeclampsia [Editorial]. *Am J Obstet Gynecol* 1988;159:1–5.
8. Magann EF, Martin JN Jr, Isaacs JD, et al. Immediate postpartum curettage: accelerated recovery from severe preeclampsia. *Obstet Gynecol* 1993;81:502–506.
9. Saftlas AF, Olson DR, Franks AL, et al. Epidemiology of preeclampsia and eclampsia in the United States, 1979–1986. *Am J Obstet Gynecol* 1990;163:460–465.
10. World Health Organization (WHO). International collaborative study of hypertensive disorders of pregnancy: geographic variation in the incidence of hypertension in pregnancy. *Am J Obstet Gynecol* 1988;158:80–83.
11. Sibai BM, Gordon T, Thom E, et al. Risk factors for preeclampsia in healthy nulliparous women: a prospective multicentered study. *Am J Obstet Gynecol* 1995;172:642–648.
12. Sibai BM, Lindheimer M, Hauth J, et al. Risk factors for preeclampsia, abruptio placentae, and adverse neonatal outcomes among women with chronic hypertension. *N Engl J Med* 1998;339:667–671.

13. Magann EF, Perry KG Jr, Morrison JC, et al. Climatic factors and preeclampsia-related hypertensive disorders of pregnancy. *Am J Obstet Gynecol* 1995;172:204–205.

14. Porapakkham S. An epidemiologic study of eclampsia. *Obstet Gynecol* 1979;54:26–30.

15. Moodley J, Naicker RS, Mankowitz E. Eclampsia—a method of management. *S Afr. Med J* 1983;63:530–535.

16. Garner PR, D'Alton ME, Dudley DK, et al. Preeclampsia in diabetic pregnancies. *Am J Obstet Gynecol* 1990;163:505–508.

17. Millar LK, Wing DA, Leung AS, et al. Low birthweight and preeclampsia in pregnancies complicated by hyperthyroidism. *Obstet Gynecol* 1994;84:946–949.

18. Klonoff-Cohen HS, Cross JL, Pieper CF. Job stress and preeclampsia. *Epidemiology* 1996;7:245–249.

19. Landsbergis PA, Hatch MC. Psychosocial work stress and pregnancy-induced hypertension. *Epidemiology* 1996;7:346–351.

20. Turpin LS, Simon LP, Eskenazi B. Changes in paternity: a risk factor for preeclampsia in multiparas. *Epidemiology* 1996;7:240–242.

21. Khong TY, DeWolfe F, Robertson WB, et al. Inadequate maternal vascular response to placentation in pregnancies complicated by preeclampsia and by small-for-gestational-age infants. *Br J Obstet Gynecol* 1986;93:1049–1059.

22. Ducey J, Schulman H, Farmakides G. A classification of pregnancy based on Doppler velocimetry. *Am J Obstet Gynecol* 1987;157:860–864.

23. Kaar K, Jouppila P, Kuikka J, et al. Intervillous blood flow in normal and complicated late pregnancy measured by means of an intravenous ^{133}Xe method. *Acta Obstet Gynecol Scand* 1980;59:7–10.

24. Seligman SP, Bugow JP, Claney RM, et al. The role of nitric oxide in the pathogenesis of preeclampsia. *Am J Obstet Gynecol* 1994;171:944–948.

25. Lyall F, Young A, Greer IA. Nitric oxide concentrations are increased in the fetoplacental circulation in preeclampsia. *Am J Obstet Gynecol* 1995;173:714–718.

26. Saleh AA, Bottoms SF, Welch RA, et al. Preeclampsia, delivery and the hemostatic system. *Am J Obstet Gynecol* 1987;157:331–336.

27. Rogers GM, Taylor RN, Roberts JM. Preeclampsia is associated with a serum factor cytotoxic to human endothelial cells. *Am J Obstet Gynecol* 1988;159:908–914.

28. Roberts JM, Taylor RN, Musci TJ, et al. Preeclampsia: an endothelial cell disorder. *Am J Obstet Gynecol* 1989;161:1200–1204.

29. Taylor RN, Varma M, Teng NH, et al. Women with preeclampsia have higher plasma endothelin levels than women with normal pregnancies. *J Clin Endocrinol Metab* 1990;71:1675–1677.

30. Liston WA, Kilpatrick DC. Preeclampsia—an endothelial cell disorder plus "something else" [Letter]. *Am J Obstet Gynecol* 1990;163:1365–1366.

31. Schrier RW, Briner VA. Peripheral arterial vasodilation and water retention in pregnancy: Implications for pathogenesis of preeclampsia-eclampsia. *Obstet Gynecol* 1991;77:632–639.

32. Musci TJ, Roberts JM, Rodgers GM, et al. Mitogenic activity is increased in the sera of preeclamptic women before delivery. *Am J Obstet Gynecol* 1988;159:1446–1451.

33. Halligan A, Bonnar J, Sheppard B, et al. Haemostatic, fibrinolytic and endothelial variables in normal pregnancies and preeclampsia. *Br J Obstet Gynaecol* 1994;101:488–492.

34. Jones I, Cowley D, Andersen M, et al. Fibronectin as a predictor of preeclampsia: a pilot study. *Aust N Z J Obstet Gynaecol* 1996;36:1–3.

35. Barton JR, Heitt AK, O'Connor WN, et al. Endomyocardial ultrastructural findings in preeclampsia. *Am J Obstet Gynecol* 1991;165:389–391.

36. Shanklin DR, Sibai BM. Ultrastructural aspects of preeclampsia. I. Placental bed and uterine boundary vessels. *Am J Obstet Gynecol* 1989;161:735–741.

37. Hubel CA, McLaughlin MK, Evans RW, et al. Fasting serum triglycerides, free fatty acids and malondialdehyde are increased in preeclampsia, are positively correlated and decrease within 48 hours post partum. *Am J Obstet Gynecol* 1996;174:975–982.

38. Bhatia RK, Bottoms SF, Saleh AA, et al. Mechanisms for reduced colloid osmotic pressure in preeclampsia. *Am J Obstet Gynecol* 1987;157:106–108.

39. Kupferminc MJ, Mullen TA, Russell TL, et al. Serum from patients with severe preeclampsia is not cytotoxic to endothelial cells. *J Soc Gynecol Invest* 1996;3:89–92.

40. Walsh SW. Preeclampsia: An imbalance in placental prostacyclin and thromboxane production. *Am J Obstet Gynecol* 1985;152:335–340.

41. Goodman RP, Killam AP, Brash AR, et al. Prostacyclin production during pregnancy: Comparison of production during normal pregnancy and pregnancy complicated by hypertension. *Am J Obstet Gynecol* 1982;142:817–822.

42. Nelson DM, Walsh SW. Aspirin differentially affects thromboxane and prostacyclin production by trophoblast and villous core compartments of human placental villi. *Am J Obstet Gynecol* 1989;161:1593–1598.

43. Wallenburg HCS, Dekker CA, Makovitz JW, et al. Low-dose aspirin prevents pregnancy-induced hypertension and preeclampsia in angiotensin-sensitive primigravidas. *Lancet* 1986;1:1–3.

44. Benigni A, Gregorini G, Frusca T, et al. Effect of low dose aspirin on fetal and maternal generation of thromboxane by platelets in women at high risk of pregnancy-induced hypertension. *N Engl J Med* 1989;321:357–362.

45. Lubbe WF. Prevention of preeclampsia by low-dose aspirin. *N Z Med J* 1990;103:237–238.

46. Peaceman AM, Rehnberg KA. The effect of aspirin and indomethacin on prostacyclin and thromboxane production by placental tissue incubated with immunoglobulin G fractions from patients with lupus anticoagulant. *Am J Obstet Gynecol* 1995;173:1391–1396.

47. Sibai BM, Caritis SN, Thom E, et al. Prevention of preeclampsia in healthy nulliparous pregnant women. *N Engl J Med* 1993;329:1213–1218.

48. Hauth JC, Goldberg RL, Parker CR Jr, et al. Low dose aspirin to prevent preeclampsia. *Am J Obstet Gynecol* 1998;168:1083–1093.

49. Anonymous. Low dose aspirin in pregnancy and early childhood development: follow up of the collaborative low dose aspirin study in pregnancy. CLASP collaborative group. *Br J Obstet Gynaecol* 1995;102:861–868.

50. Sibai BM, Caritis SN, Thom E, et al. Low dose aspirin in nulliparous women: safety of continuous epidural block and correlation between bleeding time and maternal-neonatal bleeding complications. *Am J Obstet Gynecol* 1995;172:1553–1557.

51. Gallery EDM, Ross MR, Hawkins M, et al. Low-dose aspirin in high-risk pregnancy? *Hypertens Preg* 1997;16:229–238.

52. Viinikki L, Hartikainen-Sorri AL, Lumme R, et al. Low dose aspirin in hypertensive pregnant women: effect on pregnancy outcome and prostacyclin-thromboxane imbalance in mother and newborn. *Br J Obstet Gynaecol* 1993;100:809–815.

53. Comments: low dose aspirin in prevention and treatment of intrauterine growth retardation and pregnancy-induced hypertension. *Lancet* 1993;341:396–400.

54. Walsh SW, Coulter S. Increased placental progesterone may cause decreased placental prostacyclin production in preeclampsia. *Am J Obstet Gynecol* 1989;161:1586–1592.

55. Meyer NL, Mercer BM, Friedman SA, et al. Urinary dipstick protein: a poor prediction of absent or severe proteinuria. *Am J Obstet Gynecol* 1994;170:137–141.

56. Speroff L. Toxemia of pregnancy: mechanism and therapeutic management. *Am J Cardiol* 1973;32:582–591.

57. Easterling TR, Benedetti TJ. Preeclampsia: a hyperdynamic disease model. *Am J Obstet Gynecol* 1989;160:1447–1453.

58. Easterling TR, Benedetti TJ, Schmucker BL. Maternal cardiac output in preeclamptic pregnancies: a longitudinal study. *Obstet Gynecol* 1990;76:1061–1069.

59. Cotton DB, Lee W, Huhta JC, et al. Hemodynamic profile of severe pregnancy-induced hypertension. *Am J Obstet Gynecol* 1988;158:523–529.

60. Mabie WC, Ratts TE, Sibai BM. The central hemodynamics of severe preeclampsia. *Am J Obstet Gynecol* 1989;161:1443–1448.

61. Scardo J, Kiser R, Dillon A, et al. Hemodynamic comparison of mild and severe preeclampsia: Concept of stroke systemic vascular resistance index. *J Matern Fetal Med* 1996;5:268–272.

62. Phelan JP, Yurth DA. Severe preeclampsia. I. Peripartum hemodynamic observations. *Am J Obstet Gynecol* 1982;144:17–22.

63. Tellez R, Curiel R. Relationship between central venous pressure and pulmonary capillary wedge pressure in severely toxemic patients. *Am J Obstet Gynecol* 1991;165:487.

64. Cotton DB, Longmire S, Jones MM, et al. Cardiovascular alterations in severe pregnancy-induced hypertension: effects of intravenous nitroglycerin coupled with blood volume expansion. *Am J Obstet Gynecol* 1986;154:1053–1059.

65. Clark SL, Cotton DB. Clinical indications for pulmonary artery catheterization in the patient with severe preeclampsia. *Am J Obstet Gynecol* 1988;158:453–458.

66. Clark SL. Reliance on central venous pressure with regard to fluid management in preeclampsia deemed dangerous. *Am J Obstet Gynecol* 1990;162:598.

67. Fliegner JR. Correction of hypovolemic and central venous pressure monitoring in the management of severe preeclampsia and eclampsia. *Am J Obstet Gynecol* 1987;156:1041–1042.

68. Woodward DG, Romanoff ME. Is central venous pressure monitoring "contraindicated" in patients with severe preeclampsia? *Am J Obstet Gynecol* 1989;161:837–839.

69. Goodlin RC. Pulmonary artery catheterization in severe preeclampsia. *Am J Obstet Gynecol* 1990;162:601–603.

70. Sliver HM, Seebeck M, Carlson R. Comparison of total blood volume in normal, preeclamptic, and nonproteinuric gestational hypertensive pregnancy by simultaneous measurement of red blood cell and plasma volumes. *Am J Obstet Gynecol* 1998;179:87–93.

71. Sibai BM, Abdella TN, Anderson GD, et al. Plasma findings in pregnant women with mild hypertension: therapeutic considerations. *Am J Obstet Gynecol* 1983;145:539–544.

72. Benedetti TJ, Carlson RW. Studies of colloid osmotic pressure in pregnancy-induced hypertension. *Am J Obstet Gynecol* 1979;135:308–311.

73. Joyce TH III, Longmire S, Tessem JH, et al. Creation of pregnancy induced hypertension model in the pregnant ewe. *Anesthesiology* 1987;67:A455.

74. Sibai BM, Mabie BC, Harvey CJ, et al. Pulmonary edema in severe preeclampsia-eclampsia: Analysis of 37 consecutive cases. *Am J Obstet Gynecol* 1987;156:1174–1179.

75. Strauss RG, Keefer JR, Burke T, et al. Hemodynamic monitoring of cardiogenic pulmonary edema complicating toxemia of pregnancy. *Obstet Gynecol* 1980;55:170–174.

76. Keefer JR, Strauss RJ, Civetta JM, et al. Non-cardiogenic pulmonary edema and invasive cardiac monitoring. *Obstet Gynecol* 1981;58:46–51.

77. Benedetti TJ, Cotton DB, Read JC, et al. Hemodynamic observations in severe preeclampsia with a flow-directed pulmonary artery catheter. *Am J Obstet Gynecol* 1980;136:465–470.

78. Cotton DB, Gonik B, Dorman K, et al. Cardiovascular alterations in severe pregnancy-induced hypertension. Relationship of central venous pressure to pulmonary capillary wedge pressure. *Am J Obstet Gynecol* 1985;151:762–764.

79. Newsome LR, Bramwell RS, Curling P. Severe preeclampsia: hemodynamic effects of lumbar epidural analgesia. *Anesth Analg* 1986;65:31–36.

80. Abboud T, Artal R, Sarkis R, et al. Sympathoadrenal activity, maternal, fetal and neonatal responses after epidural anesthesia in the preeclamptic patient. *Am J Obstet Gynecol* 1982;144:915–918.

81. August P, Lenz T, Ales KL, et al. Longitudinal study of the renin-angiotensin aldosterone system in hypertensive pregnant women: deviations related to the development of superimposed preeclampsia. *Am J Obstet Gynecol* 1980;163:1612–1621.

82. Leighton BL, Norris MC, DeSimone CA, et al. Preeclamptic and healthy term pregnant patients have different chronotropic responses to isoproterenol. *Anesthesiology* 1990;72:392–393.

83. Richards N, Noodley J, Graham DJ, et al. Active management of the unconscious eclamptic patient. *Br J Obstet Gynaecol* 1986;93:554–562.

84. Buchan PC. Preeclampsia: a hyperviscosity syndrome. *Am J Obstet Gynecol* 1982;142:111–112.

85. Kelton JG, Hunter DJS, Neame P. A platelet function defect in preeclampsia. *Obstet Gynecol* 1985;65:107–109.

86. deBoer K, Leconder I, Cate JW, et al. Placenta-type plasminogen activator inhibitor in preeclampsia. *Am J Obstet Gynecol* 1988;158:518–522.

87. Sibai BM, Anderson CD, McCubbin JH. Eclampsia II. Clinical significance of laboratory findings. *Obstet Gynecol* 1982;59:153–157.

88. Burrows RF, Hunter DJF, Andrew M, et al. A prospective study investigating the mechanism of thrombocytopenia in preeclampsia. *Obstet Gynecol* 1987;70:334–338.

89. Socol M, Wiener C, Louis G, et al. Platelet activation in preeclampsia. *Am J Obstet Gynecol* 1985;151:494–497.

90. Beilin Y, Bodian CA, Haddad EM, et al. Practice patterns of anesthesiologists regarding situations in obstetric anesthesia where clinical management is controversial. *Anesth Analg* 1996;83:735–741.

91. Rasmus KT, Rottman RL, Kotelko DM, et al. Unrecognized thrombocytopenia and regional anesthesia in parturients: a retrospective review. *Obstet Gynecol* 1989;73:943–946.

92. Beilin Y, Zahn J, Comerford M. Safe epidural analgesia in thirty parturients with platelet counts between 69,000 and 98,000 per milliliter. *Anesth Analg* 1997;85:385–388.

93. Channing-Rogers RP, Levin J. A critical review of the bleeding time. *Semin Thromb Hemostasis* 1990;16:1–120.

94. The bleeding time [Editorial]. *Lancet* 1991;337:1447–1448.

95. Trudinger BJ. Platelets and intrauterine growth retardation in preeclampsia. *Br J Obstet Gynaecol* 1976;83:284–286.

96. Prichard JA, Cunningham FG, Mason RG. Coagulation changes in eclampsia, their frequency and pathogenesis. *Am J Obstet Gynecol* 1976;124:855–864.

97. Weinstein L. Syndrome of hemolysis, elevated liver enzymes and low platelet count: A severe consequence of hypertension in pregnancy. *Am J Obstet Gynecol* 1982;142:159–167.

98. Sibai BM. The HELLP syndrome (hemolysis, elevated liver enzymes and low platelets): much ado about nothing. *Am J Obstet Gynecol* 1990;162:311–316.

99. VanDam PA, Renier M, Baekelandt TM, et al. Disseminated intravascular coagulation and the syndrome of hemolysis, elevated liver enzymes and low platelets in severe preeclampsia. *Obstet Gynecol* 1989;73:97–102.

100. Martin JN Jr, Blake PE, Lowry SI, et al. Pregnancy complicated by preeclampsia-eclampsia with the syndrome of hemolysis, elevated liver enzymes, and low platelet count: how rapid is postpartum recovery? *Obstet Gynecol* 1990;76:737–741.

101. Martin JN Jr, Blake PG, Perry KG Jr, et al. The natural history of HELLP syndrome: patterns of disease progression and regression. *Am J Obstet Gynecol* 1990;162:126–137.

102. Martin JN Jr, Files JC, Blake PG, et al. Plasma exchange for preeclampsia. I. Postpartum use for presently severe preeclampsia-eclampsia with HELLP syndrome. *Am J Obstet Gynecol* 1990;162:126–137.

103. Ramanathan J, Kahlil M, Sibai BM, et al. Anesthetic management of the syndrome of hemolysis, elevated liver enzymes, and low platelet count (HELLP) in preeclampsia, a retrospective study. *Reg Anesth* 1988;13:20–24.

104. Seager SJ, MacDonald R. Laryngeal edema and preeclampsia, a case report. *Anaesthesia* 1980;35:360–362.

105. Heller PJ, Scheider EP, Marx GF. Pharyngolaryngeal edema as a presenting symptom in preeclampsia. *Obstet Gynecol* 1983;62:523–524.

106. Rees GB, Pipkin FB, Symonds EM, et al. A longitudinal study of respiratory changes in normal human pregnancy with cross-sectional data on subjects with pregnancy-induced hypertension. *Am J Obstet Gynecol* 1990;162:826–830.

107. Kambam JR, Handte RE, Brown WV, et al. Effect of normal and preeclamptic pregnancies on oxyhemoglobin dissociation. *Anesthesiology* 1986;65:426–427.

108. Kambam JR, Entman S, Mouton S, et al. Effect of preeclampsia on carboxyhemoglobin levels: a mechanism for a decrease in P50. *Anesthesiology* 1988;68:433–434.

109. Kambam JR, Mouton S, Entman S, et al. Effect of preeclampsia on plasma cholinesterase activity. *Can J Anaesth* 1987;34:509–511.

110. Kambam JR, Perry SM, Entman S, et al. Effect of magnesium on plasma cholinesterase activity. *Am J Obstet Gynecol* 1988;159:309–311.

111. Fay RA, Bromham DR, Brooks JA, et al. Platelets and uric acid in the prediction of preeclampsia. *Am J Obstet Gynecol* 1985;152:1038–1039.

112. Gaber LW, Spargo BH, Lindheimer MD. Renal pathology in preeclampsia. *Clin Obstet Gynecol* 1987;1:971–995.

113. Gartner HV, Sammoun A, Wehrmann M, et al. Preeclamptic nephropathy—an endothelial lesion. A morphological study with a review of the literature. *Eur J Obstet Gynecol Reprod Biol* 1998;77:11–27.

114. Sibai BM, Villar MA, Mabie BC. Acute renal failure in hypertensive disorders of pregnancy: pregnancy outcome and remote prognosis in thirty-one consecutive cases. *Am J Obstet Gynecol* 1990;162:777–783.

115. Nochy D, Hinglais N, Jacquot C, et al. *De novo* focal glomerular sclerosis in preeclampsia. *Clin Nephrol* 1986; 24:221–227.

116. Lee W, Gonik B, Cotton DB. Urinary diagnosis indices in preeclampsia-associated oliguria: correlation with invasive hemodynamic monitoring. *Am J Obstet Gynecol* 1987;156:100–103.

117. Clark SL, Greenspoon JS, Aldahl D, et al. Severe preeclampsia with persistent oliguria: management of hemodynamic subsets. *Am J Obstet Gynecol* 1986;154:490–494.

118. Zunker P, Ley-Pozo J, Louwen F, et al. Cerebral hemodynamics in preeclampsia/eclampsia syndrome. *Ultrasound Obstet Gynecol* 1995;6:411–415.

119. Sibai BM, Spinnato JA, Anderson GD. Eclampsia V. The incidence of nonpreventable eclampsia. *Am J Obstet Gynecol* 1986;154:581–590.

120. Simolke GA, Cox SM, Cunningham FG. Cerebrovascular accidents complicating pregnancy and the puerperium. *Obstet Gynecol* 1991;78:37–42.

121. Lopez-Liera M. Complicated eclampsia: fifteen years' experience in a referral medical center. *Am J Obstet Gynecol* 1982;142:28–35.

122. Levy BT, Sawson JD, Toth PP, et al. Predictors of neonatal resuscitation, low Apgar scores, and umbilical artery pH among growth restricted neonates. *Obstet Gynecol* 1998;91:909–916.

123. Saftlas AF, Ofson DR, Franks AL. Epidemiology of preeclampsia and eclampsia in the United States, 1976–1986. *Am J Obstet Gynecol* 1990;163:460–465.

124. Chari RS, Friedman SA, Schiff E, et al. Is fetal neurologic and physical development accelerated in preeclampsia. *Am J Obstet Gynecol* 1996;174:829–832.

125. Taylor DJ, Howie PW, Davidson J, et al. Do pregnancy complications contribute to neurodevelopmental disability? *Lancet* 1985;1:713–716.

126. Odendaal HJ, Pattinson RC, Bam R, et al. Aggressive or expectant management for patients with severe preeclampsia between 28–34 weeks' gestation: a randomized controlled trial. *Obstet Gynecol* 1990;76:1070–1075.

127. Sibai BM, Taslimi M, Abdella TN, et al. Maternal and perinatal outcome of conservative management of severe preeclampsia in midtrimester. *Am J Obstet Gynecol* 1985;152:32–37.

128. Lindheimer MD, Katz AI. Preeclampsia: pathophysiology, diagnosis and management. *Am Rev Med* 1989; 40:233–250.

129. Sehgal NN, Hitt JR. Plasma volume expansion in the treatment of preeclampsia. *Am J Obstet Gynecol* 1980;138:165–168.

130. Gallery ED, Mitchell MD, Redman CW. Fall in blood pressure in response to volume expansion in pregnancy associated hypertension (pre-eclampsia): why does it occur? *Hypertension* 1984;2:177–182.

131. Siekmann U, Heilmann L, Klosa W, et al. Simultaneous investigations of maternal cardiac output and fetal blood flow during hypervolemic hemodilution in preeclampsia: preliminary observations. *J Perinatol Med* 1986;14:59–69.

132. Kirskon B, Moise KJ, Cotton DB, et al. Role of volume expansion in severe preeclampsia. *Surg Gynecol Obstet* 1988;167:367–371.

133. Belfort M, Akovic K, Anthony J, et al. The effect of acute volume expansion and vasodilatation with verapamil on uterine and umbilical Doppler indices in severe preeclampsia. *J Clin Ultrasound* 1994;22:317–325.

134. Page EW. On the pathogenesis of preeclampsia and eclampsia. *J Obstet Gynaecol Br Commonw* 1972;79:833–894.

135. Sims EAH. Pre-eclampsia and related complications of pregnancy. *Am J Obstet Gynecol* 1970;107:154–181.

136. Sibai BM, Mercer BM, Schiff E, et al. Aggressive versus expectant management of severe preeclampsia at 28-32 weeks' gestation: a randomized controlled trial. *Am J Obstet Gynecol* 1994;171:818–822.

137. Robson SC. Magnesium sulphate: the time of reckoning [Editorial]. *Br J Obstet Gynaecol* 1996;103:99–102.

138. Eclampsia Trial Collaborative Group. Which anticonvulsant for women with eclampsia? Evidence from the collaborative eclampsia trial. *Lancet* 1995;345:1455–1463.

139. Gulmezoglu AM, Duby L. Use of anticonvulsants in eclampsia and preeclampsia: survey of obstetricians in the United Kingdom and Republic of Ireland. *Br Med J (Clin Res Ed)* 1998;316:975–976.

140. Chien PF, Khan KS, Arnott N. Magnesium sulphate in the treatment of eclampsia and pre-eclampsia: an overview of the evidence from randomized trials. *Br J Obstet Gynaecol* 1996;103:1085–1091.

141. Bennett P, Edwards D. Use of magnesium sulphate in obstetrics [Editorial]. *Lancet* 1997;350:1491.

142. Moodley J. Magnesium sulphate in clinical practice: an obstetrician's viewpoint. *Int J Obstet Anesth* 1998;7:73–75.

143. James MFM. Magnesium in obstetric anesthesia. *Int J Obstet Anesth* 1998;7:115–123.

144. Shelly WC, Gutsche BB. Magnesium and seizure control [Letter]. *Am J Obstet Gynecol* 1980;136:146–147.

145. Thurnau GR, Kemp DB, Jarvis A. Cerebrospinal fluid levels of magnesium in patients with preeclampsia after treatment with magnesium sulfate: a preliminary report. *Am J Obstet Gynecol* 1987;157:1435–1438.

146. Mokriski BLK, Malinow AM, Martz DG, et al. $MgSO_4$ and EEG effects in preeclampsia. *Anesthesiology* 1988;69:A696.

147. Cotton DB, Hallak M, Janusz C, et al. Central anticonvulsant effects of magnesium sulfate on N-methyl-D-aspartate-induced convulsions. *Am J Obstet Gynecol* 1993;168:974–978.

148. Sibai BM. Magnesium sulfate is the ideal anticonvulsant in preeclampsia-eclampsia. *Am J Obstet Gynecol* 1990;162:1141–1145.

149. Friedman SA, Lim KH, Baker CA, et al. Phenytoin versus magnesium sulfate in preeclampsia: a pilot study. *Am J Perinatol* 1993;10:233–238.

150. Lucas MJ, Leveno KJ, Cunningham FG. A comparison of magnesium sulfate with phenytoin for the prevention of eclampsia. *N Engl J Med* 1995;333:201–205.

151. The Eclampsia Trial Trial Collaborative Group. Which anticonvulsant for women with eclampsia? Evidence from the Colloborative Eclampsia Trial. *Lancet* 1995;345:1455–1463.

152. Atkinson MW, Guinn D, Owen J, et al. Does magnesium sulfate affect the length of labor induction in women with pregnancy associated hypertension? *Am J Obstet Gynecol* 1995;173:1219–1222.

153. Witlin AG, Friedman SA, Sibai BM. The effect of magnesium therapy on the duration of labor in women with mild preeclampsia at term: a randomized, double-blind placebo-controlled trial. *Am J Obstet Gynecol* 1997;176:623–627.

154. Lipman J, James MFM, Erskine J, et al. Autonomic dysfunction in severe tetanus: magnesium sulfate as an adjunct to deep sedation. *Crit Care Med* 1987;15:987–988.

155. James MEM, Beer RE, Esser JD. Intravenous magnesium sulfate inhibits catecholamine release associated with tracheal intubations. *Anesth Analg* 1989;68:772–776.

156. Sipes SL, Weiner CP, Gellhaus TM, et al. The plasma renin-angiotensin system in preeclampsia: Effects of magnesium sulfate. *Obstet Gynecol* 1989;73:934–937.

157. Belfort MA, Saade GR, Moise KJ. The effect of magnesium sulfate on maternal and fetal blood flow in pregnancy induced hypertension. *Acta Obstet Gynaecol Scand* 1993;72:526–530.

158. Cotton DB, Gonik B, Dorman KF. Cardiovascular alterations in severe pregnancy-induced hypertension: acute effects of intravenous magnesium sulfate. *Am J Obstet Gynecol* 1984;148:162–165.

159. Scardo JA, Hogg BB, Newman RB. Favorable hemodynamic effects of magnesium sulfate in preeclampsia. *Am J Obstet Gynecol* 1995;173:1249–1253.

160. Sadeh M. Action of magnesium sulfate in the treatment of preeclampsia-eclampsia. *Stroke* 1989;20:1273–1275.

161. Belfort MA, Moise KJ Jr. Effect of magnesium sulfate on maternal brain blood flow in preeclampsia: a randomized, placebo-controlled study. *Am J Obstet Gynecol* 1992;167:661–666.

162. Belfort MA, Saade GR, Moise KJ Jr. The effect of magnesium sulfate on maternal retinal blood flow in preeclampsia: a randomized placebo-controlled study. *Am J Obstet Gynecol* 1992;167:1548–1553.

163. Mastrogiannis DS, Kalter CS, O'Brien WF, et al. Effect of magnesium sulfate on plasma endothelin-1 levels in normal and preeclamptic patients. *Am J Obstet Gynecol* 1992;167:1554–1559.

164. Ramanathan J, Sibai BM, Pillai R, et al. Neuromuscular transmission studies in preeclamptic women receiving magnesium sulfate. *Am J Obstet Gynecol* 1988;158:40–46.

165. Ghoneim MM, Long JP. Interaction between magnesium and other neuromuscular blocking agents. *Anesthesiology* 1970;32:23–27.

166. Kambam JR, Mouton S, Entman S, et al. Effect of preeclampsia on plasma cholinesterase activity. *Can J Anaesth* 1987;34:509–511.

167. Kambam JR, Perry SM, Entman S, et al. Effect of magnesium on plasma cholinesterase activity. *Am J Obstet Gynecol* 1988;159:309–311.

168. James MFM, Cork RC, Dennett JE. Succinylcholine pretreatment with magnesium sulfate. *Anesth Analg* 1986;65:373–376.

169. Baraka A, Yazigi A. Neuromuscular interaction of magnesium with succinylcholine-vecuronium sequence in the eclamptic parturient. *Anesthesiology* 1987;67:806–808.

170. Giesecke G, Morris RE, Dalton MD, et al. On magnesium, muscle relaxants, toxemic parturients and cats. *Anesth Analg* 1980;47:689–695.

171. Sinatra RS, Philip BK, Naulty JS, et al. Prolonged neuromuscular blockade with vecuronium in a patient treated with magnesium sulfate. *Anesth Analg* 1985;64:1220–1222.

172. Kussman B, Shorten G, Uppington J, et al. Administration of magnesium sulfate before rocuronium: effects on speed of onset and duration of neuromuscular block. *Br J Anaesth* 1997;79:122–124.

173. Hodgson RE, Rout CC, Rocke DA, et al. Mivacurium for caesarean section in hypertensive patients receiving magnesium sulfate therapy. *Int J Obstet Anesth* 1998;7:12–17.

174. Kelleher JF, Millar WL, Reisner LS. The effect of intravenous magnesium sulfate on the bleeding time in healthy volunteers. *Anesthesiology* 1989;71:A887.

175. Fuentes A, Rojas A, Porter KB, et al. The effect of magnesium sulfate on bleeding time in pregnancy. *Am J Obstet Gynecol* 1995;173:1246–1249.

176. Kyneczl-Leisure M, Cibilis LA. Increased bleeding time after magnesium sulfate infusion. *Am J Obstet Gynecol* 1996;175:1293–1294.

177. Ravn HB, Vissinger H, Kristensen SD, et al. Magnesium inhibits platelet activity—an infusion study in healthy volunteers. *Thromb Hemost* 1996;75:939–944.

178. Ames WA, McDonnell N, Potter D. The effect of ionised magnesium on coagulation using thromboelastography. *Anaesthesia* 1999;54:999–1006.

179. Yeast JD, Halberstadt C, Meger BA, et al. The risk of pulmonary edema and colloid osmotic pressure changes during magnesium sulfate infusion. *Am J Obstet Gynecol* 1993;169:1566–1571.

180. Mason BA, Standley CA, Whitly JE, et al. Fetal ionized magnesium levels parallel maternal levels during magnesium sulfate therapy for preeclampsia. *Am J Obstet Gynecol* 1996;175:213–217.

181. Atkinson MW, Belfort MA, Saade GR, et al. The relation between magnesium sulfate therapy and fetal heart rate variability. *Obstet Gynecol* 1994;83:967–970.

182. Hiett AK, Devoe LD, Brown HL, et al. Effect of magnesium on fetal heart rate variability using computer analysis. *Am J Perinatol* 1995;12:259–261.

183. Green KW, Key TC, Coen R, et al. The effects of maternally administered magnesium sulfate on the neonate. *Am J Obstet Gynecol* 1983;146:29–33.

184. Pruett KM, Kirshon B, Cotton DB, et al. The effects of magnesium sulfate therapy on Apgar scores. *Am J Obstet Gynecol* 1988;159:1047–1048.

185. Lewis R, Sibai B. Recent advances in the management of preeclampsia. *J Matern-Fetal Med* 1997;6:6–15.

186. Witlin AG, Sibai BM. Magnesium sulfate therapy in preeclampsia and eclampsia. *Obstet Gynecol* 1998;92:883–889.

187. Fawcett WJ, Haxby EJ, Male DA. Magnesium: physiology and pharmacology. *Br J Anaesth* 1993;83:302–320.

188. Pritchard JA, Cunningham FG, Prichard SA. The Parkland Memorial Hospital protocol for the treatment of eclampsia: evaluation of 245 cases. *Am J Obstet Gynecol* 1984;148:951–963.

189. Sibai BM, Mabie WC, Shamson R, et al. A comparison of no medication versus methyldopa or labetalol in chronic hypertension during pregnancy. *Am J Obstet Gynecol* 1990;162:960–967.

190. Sibai BM, Gonzalez AR, Mabie WC, et al. A comparison of labetalol plus hospitalization versus hospitalization alone in the management of preeclampsia remote from term. *Obstet Gynecol* 1987;70:323–327.

191. Paterson-Brown S, Robson SC, Redfern N, et al. Hydralazine boluses for the treatment of severe hypertension in preeclampsia. *Br J Obstet Gynaecol* 1994;101:409–413.

192. Jouppila P, Kirkinen P, Loivula A, et al. Effects of dihydralazine infusion on the fetoplacental blood flow and maternal prostanoids. *Obstet Gynecol* 1985;65:115–118.

193. Lunell NO, Lewander R, Nylund L, et al. Acute effect of dihydralazine on uteroplacental blood flow in hypertension during pregnancy. *Gynecol Obstet Invest* 1983;16:274–282.

194. Lipshitz J, Ahokas RA, Reynolds SL. The effect of hydralazine on placental perfusion in the spontaneously hypertensive rat. *Am J Obstet Gynecol* 1987;156:356–359.

195. Vink GJ, Moodley J. The effect of low-dose hydralazine on the fetus in the emergency treatment of hypertension in pregnancy. *S Afr Med J* 1982;62:475–477.

196. Lindheimer MD, Katz AI. Hypertension in pregnancy (current concepts). *N Engl J Med* 1985;313:675–680.

197. Cockburn J, Moar VA, Olmstead M, et al. Final report of study on hypertension during pregnancy: the effect of specific treatment on the growth and development of the children. *Lancet* 1982;1:647–649.

198. Horvath JS, Phippard A, Korda A, et al. Clonidine hydrochloride: a safe and effective antihypertensive in pregnancy. *Obstet Gynecol* 1985;66:634–638.

199. Rubin PC, Butters L, Clark DM, et al. Placebo-controlled trial of atenolol in treatment of pregnancy induced hypertension. *Lancet* 1983;1:431–434.

200. Rubin PC. Beta blockers in pregnancy. *Br J Obstet Gynaecol* 1987;94:292–293.

201. Mouton S, Liedholm H, Lingman G, et al. Fetal and uteroplacental haemodynamics during short term atenolol treatment of hypertension in pregnancy. *Br J Obstet Gynaecol* 1987;94:312–317.

202. Liedholm H, Melander A. Drug selection in treatment of pregnancy hypertension. *Acta Obstet Gynecol Scand* 1984;118:49–55.

203. Gold MI, Sacks DJ, Grosnoff DB, et al. Use of esmolol during anesthesia to treat tachycardia and hypertension. *Anesth Analg* 1989;68:101–104.

204. Eisenach JB, Castro MI. Maternally administered esmolol produced fetal β-adrenergic blockade and hypoxemia in sheep. *Anesthesiology* 1989;71:718–722.

205. MacCarthy PE, Bloomfield SS. Labetalol: a review of its pharmacology, pharmacokinetics, clinical uses and adverse effects. *Pharmacotherapy* 1983;3:193–219.

206. Baum T, Sybertz EJ. Pharmacology of labetalol in experimental animals. *Am J Med* 1983;75:15–23.

207. Rogers RC, Sherif AKL, Sibai BM. Nifedipine pharmacokinetics in pregnancy-induced hypertension. *Abstracts of Scientific Papers, Society for Obstetric Anesthesia and Perinatalogy, Houston.* 1990:63.

208. Akokas RA, Mabie WC, Sibai BM, et al. Labetalol does not decrease placental perfusion in the hypertensive term-pregnant rat. *Am J Obstet Gynecol* 1989;160:480–484.

209. Eisenach JC, Mandell G, Dewan DM. Maternal and fetal effects of labetalol in pregnant ewes. *Anesthesiology* 1991;74:292–297.

210. Jouppila P, Kirkinew PS, Loivula A, et al. Labetalol does not alter the placental and fetal blood flow or maternal prostanoids in preeclampsia. *Br J Obstet Gynaecol* 1986;93:543–547.

211. Ramanathan J, Sibai BM, Mabie WC, et al. The use of labetalol for attenuation of the hypertensive response to endotracheal intubation in preeclampsia. *Am J Obstet Gynecol* 1988;159:650–654.

212. Pickles CJ, Symonds EM, Piplin FB. The fetal outcome in a randomized double-blind controlled trial of labetalol versus placebo in pregnancy induced hypertension. *Br J Obstet Gynaecol* 1989;96:38–43.

213. Olsen KS, Beier-Helgersen R. Fetal death following labetalol administration in preeclampsia. *Acta Obstet Gynecol Scand* 1992;71:145–147.

214. Davey DA, Dommisse J, Garden A. Intravenous labetalol and intravenous dihydralazine in severe hypertension in pregnancy. In: Riley A, Symonds EM, eds. *The Investigation of Labetalol in the Management of Hypertension in Pregnancy.* Amsterdam: Exerpta Medica, 1982:51–61.

215. Mabie WC, Gonzalez AR, Sibai BM, et al. A comparative trial of labetalol and hydralazine in the acute management of severe hypertension complicating pregnancy. *Obstet Gynecol* 1987;70:328–333.

216. Walters BNJ, Redman CWG. Treatment of severe pregnancy associated hypertension with the calcium antagonist nifedipine. *Br J Obstet Gynaecol* 1984;91:330–336.

217. Fenakel K, Fenakel G, Appelman Z, et al. Nifedipine in the treatment of severe preeclampsia. *Obstet Gynecol* 1991;77:331–337.

218. Moretti MM, Fairlie FM, Akls S, et al. The effect of nifedipine therapy on fetal and placental Doppler waveforms in preeclampsia remote from term. *Am J Obstet Gynecol* 1990;163:184–188.

219. Barton JR, Hiett AK, Conover WB. The use of nifedipine during the postpartum period in patients with severe preeclampsia. *Am J Obstet Gynecol* 1990;162:788–792.

220. Waisman GD, Magorga LM, Camera MI, et al. Magnesium plus nifedipine: potentiation of hypotensive effect in preeclampsia. *Am J Obstet Gynecol* 1988;159:308–309.

221. Lindeman KS, Hirshman CA, Freed AN. Magnesium sulfate resembles a calcium channel blocker in airway smooth muscle. *Anesthesiology* 1988;69:A699.

222. Rogers RC, Sibai BM, Whybrew WD. Labetalol pharmacokinetics in pregnancy induced hypertension. *Am J Obstet Gynecol* 1990;162:362–366.

223. Belfort MA, Saade GR, Moise KJ Jr, et al. Nimodipine in the management of preeclampsia: maternal and fetal effects. *Am J Obstet Gynecol* 1993;172:1652–1654.

224. Carbonne B, Jannet D, Touboul C, et al. Nicardipine treatment of hypertension during pregnancy. *Obstet Gynecol* 1993;81:908–914.

225. Neuman J, Weiss B, Rabello Y, et al. Diazide for the acute control of severe hypertension complicating pregnancy: a pilot study. *Obstet Gynecol* 1979;53:50–53.

226. Lopez-Liera M. Complicated eclampsia: Fifteen years' experience in a referral medical center. *Am J Obstet Gynecol* 1982;142:28–35.

227. Prichard JA, Cunningham FG, Mason RG. Coagulation changes in eclampsia, their frequency and pathogenesis. *Am J Obstet Gynecol* 1976;124:855–864.

227a. Hogg B, Hauth JC, Caritis SN, et al. Safety of labor epidural anesthesia for women with severe hypertensive disease. *Am J Obstet Gynecol* 1999;181:1096–1101.

228. Iberti TJ, Fischer EP, Leibowitz AB, et al. A multicenter study of physicians' knowledge of the pulmonary artery catheter. *JAMA* 1990;264:2928–2932.

229. Connors AF Jr, Speroff T, Dawson NV, et al. The effectiveness of right heart catheterization in the initial care of critically ill patients. SUPPORT investigators. *JAMA* 1996;276:889–897.

230. Knepp NE, Kumar S, Shelley WC, et al. Fetal and neonatal hazards of maternal hydration with 5% dextrose before cesarean section. *Lancet* 1982;1:1150–1152.

231. Joyce TH III, Loon M. Preeclampsia: effect of albumin 25% infusion. *Anesthesiology* 1981;55:A313.

232. Jones MM, Longmire S, Cotton DB, et al. Influence of crystalloid versus colloid infusion on peripartum colloid osmotic pressure changes. *Obstet Gynecol* 1986;66:659–666.

233. Benedetti TJ, Kates R, Williams V. Hemodynamic observations in severe preeclampsia complicated by pulmonary edema. *Am J Obstet Gynecol* 1985;152:330–334.

234. Cotton DB, Jones M, Longmire SS, et al. Role of intravenous nitroglycerin in the treatment of severe pregnancy-induced hypertension complicated by pulmonary edema. *Am J Obstet Gynecol* 1986;154:91–93.

235. Wasserstrum N, Kirshon B, Willis RS, et al. Quantitative hemodynamic effects of acute volume expansion in severe preeclampsia. *Obstet Gynecol* 1989;73:545–550.

236. Moir DD, Victor-Rodriques L, Willocks J. Extradural analgesia during labour in patients with preeclampsia. *J Obstet Gynaecol Br Commonw* 1972;79:465–469.

237. Bigler von R, Stamm O. Die periduralanasthesis zur Verhinderung des eklamptischen Anfalls und als Therapie des eklamptischen Comas. *Gynaecologia* 1964;158:228–233.

238. Benedetti TJ, Benedetti JK, Steuchever MA. Severe preeclampsia: maternal and fetal outcome. Part B. Hypertension in pregnancy. *Clin Exp Hypertens* 1982;2/3:401–416.

239. Merrell DA, Kock MAT. Epidural anaesthesia as an anticonvulsant in the management of hypertensive and eclamptic patients in labour. *S Afr Med J* 1980;58:875–877.

240. Hodgkinson R, Husain FJ, Hayashi RH. Systemic and pulmonary blood pressure during caesarean section in parturients with gestational hypertension. *Can Anaesth Soc J* 1980;27:389–394.

241. Jouppila P, Jouppila R, Hollmen A, et al. Lumbar epidural analgesia to improve intervillous blood flow during labor in severe preeclampsia. *Obstet Gynecol* 1982;59:158–161.

242. Gutsche BB. The role of epidural anesthesia in preeclampsia (the experts opine) *Surv Anesth* 1986;30:304–311.

243. Sangoul F, Fox GS, Houle GL. Effect of regional anesthesia on maternal oxygen consumption during the first stage of labor. *Am J Obstet Gynecol* 1975;121:1080–1083.

244. Hagerdal M, Morgan CW, Sumner AE, et al. Minute ventilation and oxygen consumption during labor with epidural analgesia. *Anesthesiology* 1983;59:425–427.

245. Abboud T, Artal R, Sarkis F, et al. Sympathoadrenal activity, maternal, fetal and neonatal responses after epidural anesthesia in the preeclamptic patient. *Am J Obstet Gynecol* 1982;144:915–918.

246. Ramanathan J, Coleman P, Sibai B. Anesthetic modification of hemodynamic and neuroendocrine stress responses to cesarean delivery in women with severe preeclampsia. *Anesth Analg* 1991;73:772–779.

247. Moore TR, Key TC, Reisner LS, et al. Evaluation of the use of continuous lumbar epidural anesthesia for hypertensive pregnant women in labor. *Am J Obstet Gynecol* 1985;152:404–412.

248. Connell H. Dalgleish JG, Downing JG. General anaesthesia in mothers with severe preeclampsia/eclampsia. *Br J Anaesth* 1987;59:1375–1380.

249. Lawes EG, Downing JW, Duncan PW, et al. Fentanyl droperidol supplementation of rapid sequence induction in the presence of severe pregnancy-induced and pregnancy-aggravated hypertension. *Br J Anaesth* 1987;59:1381–1391.

250. Lavies NG, Meiklejohn BH, May AE, et al. Hypertensive and catecholamine response to tracheal intubation in patients with pregnancy-induced hypertension. *Br J Anaesth* 1989;63:429–434.

251. Fox EJ, Sklar GS, Hill CH, et al. Complications related to the pressor response to endotracheal intubation. *Anesthesiology* 1977;47:524–525.

252. Lopez-Llera M, Rubio Linares G, Hernandez-Horla JL. Maternal mortality rates in eclampsia. *Am J Obstet Gynecol* 1976;124:149–155.

253. Hon EH, Reid BL, Hehre FW. The electronic evaluation of fetal heart rate. II. Changes with maternal hypotension. *Am J Obstet Gynecol* 1960;79:209–215.

254. Greenwood PA, Lilford RJ. Effect of epidural analgesia on maximum and minimum blood pressures during first stage of labour in primagravidae with mild/moderate gestational hypertension. *Br J Obstet Gynaecol* 1986;93:260–263.

255. Graham C, Goldstein A. Epidural analgesia and cardiac output in severe preeclampsia. *Anaesthesia* 1980;35:709–712.

256. Wright JP. Anesthetic considerations in preeclampsia-eclampsia. *Anesth Analg* 1982;62:590–601.

257. Brizgys RV, Dailey PA, Shnider SM, et al. The incidence and neonatal effects of maternal hypotension during epidural anesthesia for cesarean section. *Anesthesiology* 1987;67:782–786.

258. Wallis KH, Shnider SM, Hicks JS, et al. Epidural anesthesia in the normotensive pregnant ewe: Effects on uterine blood flow and fetal acid base status. *Anesthesiology* 1976;44:481–487.

259. Jouppila R, Jouppila P, Kuikka J, et al. Placental blood flow during cesarean section under lumbar extradural analgesia. *Br J Anaesth* 1978;50:275–278.

260. Jouppila R, Jouppila P. Hollmen A. Effect of segmental extradural analgesia on placental blood flow during normal labour. *Br J Anaesth* 1978;50:563–567.

261. Husemeyer RP, Crawley JCW. Placental intervillous blood flow measured by inhaled 133Xe clearance in relation to induction of epidural analgesia. *Br J Obstet Gynaecol* 1979;86:426–431.

262. Houvinen K, Lehtovirta P, Forss M, et al. Changes in placental intervillous blood flow measured by the 133 xenon method during lumbar epidural block for elective cesarean section. *Acta Anaesthesiol Scand* 1979;23:529–533.

263. Jouppila R, Jouppila P, Hollmen A, et al. Epidural analgesia and placental blood flow during labour in pregnancies complicated by hypertension. *Br J Obstet Gynaecol* 1979;86:969–972.

264. Jouppila R, Jouppila P. Effects of induction of general anesthesia for cesarean section on intervillous blood flow. *Acta Obstet Gynecol Scand* 1979;58:249–253.

265. Palahniuk RJ, Cumming M. Foetal deterioration following thiopentone-nitrous oxide anaesthesia in the pregnant ewe. *Can Anaesth Soc J* 1977;24:361-3–70.

266. deJong RH. *Physiology and Pharmacology of Local Anesthesia.* Springfield, IL: Charles C. Thomas, 1970:211.

267. Bernhard CG, Bohm E.*Local Anesthetics as Anticonvulsants.* Stockholm: Almquist & Wiksel, 1966.

268. Richie JM, Greene NM. Local anesthetics. In: Gilman AG, Goodman LS, Gilman A, eds. *The Pharmacological Basis of Therapeutics*, 6th ed. New York: Macmillan, 1980:307.

269. Ramanathan J, Bottorff M, Jeter JN, et al. The pharmacokinetics and maternal and neonatal effects of epidural lidocaine in preeclampsia. *Anesth Analg* 1986;65:120–126.

270. Hadzik A, Vloka J, Patel N, et al. Hypertensive crisis after a successful placement of an epidural anesthetic in a hypertensive parturient (case report). *Reg Anesth* 1995;20:156–158.

271. Dror A, Abboud TK, Moore J. Maternal hemodynamic responses to epinephrine containing local anesthetics in mild preeclampsia. *Reg Anesth* 1988;13:107–111.

272. Heller PJ, Goodman C. Use of local anesthetics with epinephrine for epidural anesthesia in preeclampsia. *Anesthesiology* 1986;65:224–226.

273. Hood DD, Curry R. Spinal versus epidural anesthesia for cesarean section in severely preeclamptic patients: a retrospective survey. *Anesthesiology* 1999;90:1276–1292.

274. Wallace DH, Leveno KJ, Cunningham FG. Randomized comparison of general and regional anesthesia for cesarean delivery in pregnancy complicated by severe preeclampsia. *Obstet Gynecol* 1995;86:193–199.

275. Karineu J, Rasaneu J, Alahuhta S, et al. Maternal and utero-placental haemodynamic state in preeclamptic patients during

spinal anaesthesia for caesarean section. *Br J Anaesth* 1996;76:616–620.

276. Brock-Utne JC, Downing JW, Seedat F. Laryngeal oedema associated with preeclamptic toxemia. *Anaesthesia* 1977;32:556–560.

277. Jouppila R, Jouppila P, Hollmen A. Laryngeal oedema as an obstetric anaesthesia complication. *Acta Anaesthesiol Scand* 1980;24:97–98.

278. Kerri-Szanto M. Laryngeal oedema complicating obstetric anaesthesia. *Anaesthesia* 1978;33:272.

279. De Vore JS, Asrani R. Magnesium sulfate prevents succinylcholine-induced fasciculations in toxemia parturients. *Anesthesiology* 1980;52:76–77.

280. Lee C, Nguyen NB, Tran BK, et al. Quantification of magnesium-pancuronium interaction in the diaphragm and tibialis anterior. *Anesthesiology* 1982;57:A392.

281. Tran B, Nguyen B, Chung H, et al. Interaction between magnesium and vecuronium in rabbits. *Anesthesiology* 1984;61:A403.

282. Baraka A, Yazigi A. Neuromuscular interaction of magnesium with succinylcholine-vecuronium sequence in the eclamptic parturient. *Anesthesiology* 1987;67:806–808.

283. Gaiser RR, Seem EH. Use of rocuronium in a pregnant patient with an open eye injury, receiving magnesium medication for preterm labour. *Br J Anaesth* 1996;77:669–671.

284. Loughran PG, Moore J, Dundee JW. Maternal stress response associated with caesarean delivery under general and epidural anaesthesia. *Br J Obstet Gynaecol* 1986;93:943–949.

285. Allen RW, James MFM, Uys PF. Attenuation of the pressor response to tracheal intubation in the hypertensive proteinuric pregnant patient by lignocaine, alfentanil and magnesium sulfate. *Br J Anaesth* 1991;66:216–223.

286. Kan R, Hughes S, Rosen M, et al. Intravenous remifentanil: placental transfer, maternal and neonatal effects. *Anesthesiology* 1998;88:1467–1474.

287. Ramanathan J, Angel JJ, Bush AJ, et al. Changes in maternal middle cerebral artery blood flow velocity associated with general anesthesia in severe preeclampsia. *Anesth Analg* 1999;88:357–361.

288. Marx GF, Mateo CV. Effects of different oxygen concentrations during general anaesthesia or elective caesarean section. *Can Anaesth Soc J* 1971;18:587–593.

289. Morishima HO, Daniels SS, Richards RT, et al. The effect of increased maternal Pao_2 upon the fetus during labor. *Am J Obstet Gynecol* 1975;123:257–264.

290. Moir DD. Anaesthesia for caesarean section. An evaluation of a method using low concentrations of halothane and 50 percent of oxygen. *Br J Anaesth* 1970;42:136–142.

291. Marx GF, Kim YI, Lin CC, et al. Postpartum uterine pressures under halothane or enflurane anesthesia. *Obstet Gynecol* 1978;51:695–698.

292. Warren TM, Datta S, Ostheimer GW, et al. Comparison of maternal and neonatal effects of halothane, enflurane, and isoflurane for cesarean section delivery. *Anesth Analg* 1983;62:516–520.

293. Chari RS, Friedman SA, Schiff E, et al. Is fetal neurologic and physical development accelerated in preeclampsia? *Am J Obstet Gynecol* 1996;174:829–832.

294. Kalur JS, Martin JMN, Kirchner KA, et al. Postpartum preeclampsia induced shock and deaths. A report of three cases. *Am J Obstet Gynecol* 1991;165:1362–1368.

Shnider and Levinson's Anesthesia for Obstetrics,
edited by Samuel C. Hughes, et al.
Lippincott Williams & Wilkins,
Philadelphia, © 2001.

CHAPTER 17

ANESTHESIA FOR PRETERM LABOR AND DELIVERY

ANDREW M. MALINOW, M.D. AND PATRICIA A. DAILEY, M.D.

INTRODUCTION

Seven to eight percent of all deliveries in the United States occur preterm. Preterm deliveries are responsible for over 60% of perinatal morbidity and mortality (1–3). It is preterm delivery that is largely responsible for the relatively high perinatal mortality in the United States, as compared with other Western countries.

As gestational age or birth weight increases, the survival rate increases (1, 4). Survival at 6 months of age without major neurologic injury is 13% for an infant born at 23 weeks gestational age, 40% at 24 weeks gestational age and 70% at 26 to 27 weeks gestational age (5). An infant born at 32 week's gestational age and weighing 1,000 to 1,250 g has a predicted survival rate of near 100% (Fig. 17.1) (4). Thus, the prevention of preterm labor or the recognition and successful treatment of preterm labor has a significant impact on perinatal survival.

Preterm labor occurs in as many as 14% of all pregnancies that result in a live birth (6). Investigators currently are attempting to better define the causes of preterm labor. Concurrently, clinicians are giving emphasis to providing intensive antenatal care as well as education for patients at high risk for preterm labor prevention. Preterm labor prevention programs typically include weekly visits to the obstetric caregiver and nurse educator for a review of early symptoms and for examination of the cervix. The primary goal is the prevention of preterm labor; the secondary goal is the early recognition and treatment of preterm labor (Fig. 17.2) (7).

DEFINITIONS

The currently accepted definition of **preterm labor** is as follows: (*a*) pregnancy between 20 and 37 completed weeks from the last menstrual period; (*b*) regular uterine contractions of at least 30-second duration occurring at least once every 10 minutes; and (*c*) cervical effacement and/or dilation. The term premature infant has been replaced by **preterm infant**. A preterm infant has been defined as an infant delivered between 20 and 37 weeks after the first day of the last menstrual period (i.e., at least 3 weeks before the expected date of term delivery). In the past any infant weighing less than 2,500 g at delivery was considered to be preterm. But it is now recognized that some of these neonates are *small for gestational age (SGA)* and are not preterm. An infant who weighs less than 2,500 g at birth is now labeled as a *low-birth-weight infant*, regardless of gestational age. A *very low-birth-weight infant* is an infant that weighs less than 1,500 g at delivery.

A history of a previous preterm delivery, multiple gestation, or both represent two of the most significant risk factors for preterm labor and delivery (3). Many other obstetric and social factors are associated with preterm labor (Fig. 17.3). These associations do not necessarily represent cause-and-effect relationships. Subclinical chorioamnionitis may represent the cause of preterm labor in up to 40% of preterm births (3, 8). Microbes initiate an inflammatory response marked by increased prostaglandin production which may initiate preterm labor. In addition, microbes produce proteolytic enzymes (e.g., mucidases, sialidases) which may weaken the otherwise intact membranes leading to a preterm premature rupture of membranes. Infection with group B β-hemolytic streptococcus, gonorrhea, chlamydia and bacteroides have all been associated with preterm complications (8). There is clinical benefit to screen all patients, in an effort to detect subclinical colonization with some, if not all, of these microbes. If such colonization is detected, then appropriate antibiotic therapy is used to cure or suppress infection during pregnancy.

Recently, there has been interest in other modalities to screen for preterm labor. The association of fetal fibronectin in vaginal fluid with preterm labor has been investigated. The results of follow-up studies have not corroborated the initial enthusiasm for fibronectin as a predictive screening tool (poor specificity). However, the absence of fibronectin has a very high negative predictive value (greater than 95%) (8). Repeated vaginal exams have traditionally been a way to screen at-risk women for preterm labor. The use of vaginal ultrasound to measure crevical length (less than 3 cm at 24 to 28 weeks is predictive) or detect cervical funneling (dilation of the internal but not external cervical os) has also been investigated as a screening tool (8). Unfortunately, in most cases the cause of preterm labor is unclear; approximately 50% of preterm deliveries occur in women with no risk factors (3). Furthermore, not all preterm births result from preterm labor. As many as 20% to 25% of all preterm deliveries are performed for maternal (severe preeclampsia) or fetal indications (hemolytic anemia secondary to Rh sensitization). Advances in fetal therapy will hopefully decrease the frequency of fetal indications for preterm delivery.

INDICATIONS FOR TOCOLYTIC THERAPY

Once preterm labor has been diagnosed, a decision of whether to attempt inhibition of preterm labor must be made (Table 17.1). There are some situations in which the inhibition of preterm labor is relatively contraindicated. For example, most obstetricians have routinely avoided tocolytic therapy in women with ruptured membranes because of uncertainty regarding efficacy, as well as concern that such therapy might increase the risk of maternal and/or fetal infection (9, 10). In two different studies tocolytic therapy did not increase maternal or neonatal infectious complications. However, tocolytic therapy also did not result in improved neonatal outcome when compared with expectant management. One study (10) did suggest that a subgroup of patients with ruptured membranes at less than 28 weeks' gestation might benefit from tocolytic therapy.

The benefits of attempting to delay delivery of the preterm infant must be weighed against the maternal and fetal risks of therapy. Although the prognosis has improved during recent years, infants are still at high risk for intrapartum death, neonatal respiratory failure, and intraventricular hemorrhage. If inhibition of preterm labor is attempted, it may be for the *short-term*, to allow glucocorticoids administered to the mother to accelerate fetal lung maturity or to allow for arrangement of the

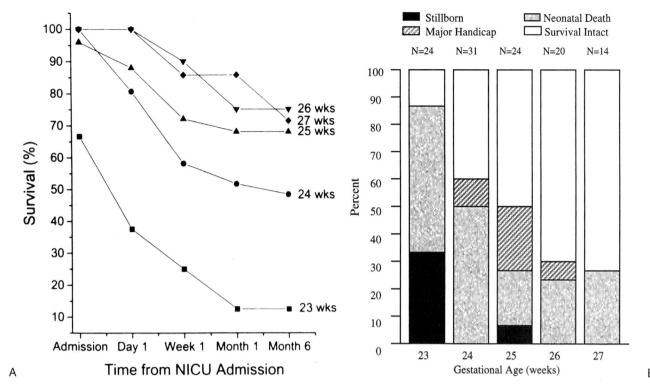

A

Time from NICU Admission

B

Gestational Age (weeks)

Figure 17.1. **A:** Infant survival curves by gestational age at delivery of 114 very premature infants delivered by Baylor College of Medicine Perinatal Service. **B:** Six-month outcome data. Major handicap denotes severe abnormalities on cranial ultrasound. Intact survival denotes absence of severe abnormalities on cranial ultrasound of 114 very premature infants delivered by Baylor College of Medicine Perinatal Service. (From Kramer WB, Saade GR, Goodrum L, et al. Neonatal outcome after active perinatal management of the very premature infant between 23 and 27 weeks' gestation. *J Perinatol* 1997;17:439–443, with permission.)

proper delivery setting (e.g., patient transport and assembly of neonatal specialists). Long-term inhibition of preterm labor will obviously allow further maturation of the fetus for weeks to months.

Tocolytic agents are occasionally used to manage intrapartum fetal distress while preparations are made for immediate delivery. Uterine contractions, by reducing placental blood flow, may exceed the reserve of an already compromised fetoplacental unit. Tocolytic agents may improve uteroplacental blood flow and fetal oxygenation by decreasing myometrial activity. Terbutaline (11), ritodrine (12), and magnesium sulfate (13) have all been used to manage intrapartum fetal distress; they appear most useful when there is evidence of uterine tachysystole. Recently, nitroglycerin, a nitric oxide (NO) donor, has been reported to be efficacious in instances where uterine quiescence is acutely needed, such as internal podalic version (14). L-Arginine-NO biochemistry will be a field surely exploited by investigators in the near future.

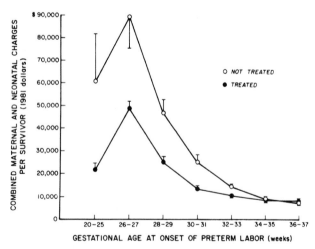

Figure 17.2. The combined maternal and neonatal charges per surviving infant (±SEM) relative to gestational age at onset of preterm labor. Charges were based on hospital charges and physicians' fees. Patients in the *treated group* received intravenous terbutaline or isoxsuprine. Patients in the *not treated group* received no β-adrenergic therapy and were allowed to deliver without gestational delay. (From Korenbrot CC, Aalto LH, Laros RK. The cost effectiveness of stopping preterm labor with β-adrenergic treatment. *N Engl J Med* 1984;310:691–696, with permission.)

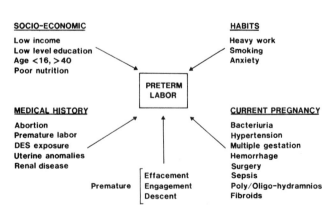

Figure 17.3. Obstetric and social factors associated with preterm labor. (From Creasy RK. Preterm labor and delivery. In: Creasy RK, Resnik R, eds. *Maternal-Fetal Medicine, Principles and Practice.* Philadelphia: WB Saunders, 1984:419, with permission.)

Table 17.1. CRITERIA FOR INHIBITION
OF PRETERM LABOR

Table 17.1. **CRITERIA FOR INHIBITION
OF PRETERM LABOR**

Long-term treatment
 1. Intact membranes
 2. Fetus < 2,500 g; 20–30 weeks
 3. Documented contractions
 4. Cervical change and > 80% effacement, or
   cervical dilation > 2 cm but less than 4 cm

Short-term treatment
 1. Postoperative
 2. Patient transfer
 3. Corticosteroid treatment
 4. Fetal distress: preparation for immediate delivery

Relative contraindications to treatment
 1. Ruptured amniotic membranes (long term)
 2. Fever of unknown origin/amnionitis
 3. Severe hemorrhage
 4. Fetal anomalies incompatible with life
 5. Maternal cardiac disease

Physiology of Uterine Contractions

The physiology of uterine contractions is reviewed in detail elsewhere (15, 16). Briefly, contraction of smooth muscle depends on the interaction of filaments of actin and myosin. The energy for this interaction comes from the hydrolysis of adenosine triphosphate (ATP), and the interaction depends on the phosphorylation of myosin by the enzyme myosin light-chain kinase. This enzyme requires activation by calmodulin, which in turn depends on a relatively high level of intracellular calcium ions for activation.

There are a number of steps in this cascade at which smooth muscle contraction can be inhibited (Fig. 17.4). β-Adrenergic agonists, prostaglandin synthetase inhibitors, and ethanol produce increased levels of cyclic AMP. Magnesium sulfate and calcium entry-blocking drugs probably prevent the increase in intracellular Ca^{2+} levels needed for the activation of calmodulin, which is necessary for activation of myosin light-chain kinase.

Inhibition of smooth muscle contraction is discussed in more detail in the sections on the mechanisms of action of specific tocolytic agents.

PREVENTION AND TREATMENT OF PRETERM LABOR
Efficacy of Pharmacologic Therapy

The use of pharmacologic therapy to inhibit or prevent preterm labor has become a standard obstetric practice. However, there are few prospective, randomized studies in which tocolytic agents are compared to placebo. Thus it is difficult to evaluate the efficacy and overall safety of tocolytic therapy. A review (17) of studies published between 1971 and 1979 noted that the mean effectiveness of drug therapy was 70% (with a range of 29% to 87%), whereas the mean effectiveness of placebo was

Maternal, fetal and neonatal side effects of drugs currently used for treating preterm labor are listed in Table 17.2. It is obvious that these drugs have important implications for the anesthesiologist because of their varying effects on fluid and electrolyte balance, as well as on the cardiovascular and respiratory systems. Despite aggressive tocolysis, preterm labor may still occur. Indeed it is not unusual for an attempted inhibition of labor to be unsuccessful and for labor to progress rapidly. The anesthesiologist may be asked to provide analgesia for labor or for an operative delivery by forceps or cesarean section. Thus an understanding of the effects of tocolytic drugs on anesthetic management is important.

Table 17.2. **SIDE EFFECTS OF DRUGS USED TO STOP LABOR**

Drug	Maternal Effects	Fetal and Neonatal Effects
β-Adrehergic agents	Hypotension Tachycardia Chest pain/tightness Pulmonary edema Congestive heart failure Arrhythmias (atrial and ventricular) Anxiety, nervousness Nausea and vomiting Headache Hyperglycemia Metabolic (lactic) acidosis	Tachycardia Hyperglycemia Increased free fatty acids Fetal asphyxia with large doses due to maternal hypotension or increased uterine vascular resistance resulting in decreased uterine blood flow Decreased incidence of respiratory distress syndrome (?)
Magnesium sulfate	Pulmonary edema Chest pain/tightness Nausea and vomiting Flushing Drowsiness Blurred vision Increased sensitivity to muscle relaxants	Hypotonia Drowsiness Decreased gastric motility Hypocalcemia
Prostaglandin synthetase inhibitors	Gastrointestinal irritation Inhibition of platelet function Reduced factor XII Depressed immune system	Premature closure of the ductus arteriosus Pulmonary hypertension
Calcium entry-blocking agents	Hypotension Reduced cardiac contractility Reduced cardiac conduction Inhibition of platelet aggregation Nitric oxide donors Headache Tachyphylaxis	Methemoglobinemia (?)

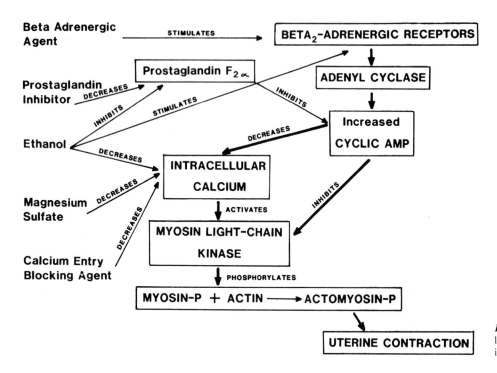

Figure 17.4. Principal site of pharmacologic action of drugs used to inhibit uterine contractility and stop preterm labor.

49% (27% to 71% range). In addition, the various clinical series have varying criteria for inclusion in the study and varying definitions of success of therapy. The high rate of success with placebo underscores the fact that not all preterm women with uterine contractions need pharmacologic tocolytic therapy. Some patients will experience cessation of contractions with bed rest and hydration alone. The use of real-time ultrasonography may help the obstetrician determine which patients need tocolytic therapy. Castle and Turnbull (18) reported their experience with real-time ultrasonography to establish the presence or absence of fetal breathing movement in patients with a diagnosis of preterm labor. Delivery occurred within 48 hours in 19 of 20 patients with no detectable fetal breathing, whereas pregnancy continued for at least 1 week in 25 of 34 patients with fetal breathing movements. Subsequently, others have confirmed the predictive value of fetal breathing movements in the diagnosis and assessment of preterm labor (19, 20).

Tocolytic agents used in modern obstetric practice include: (*a*) β-adrenergic agents; (*b*) magnesium sulfate; (*c*) prostaglandin synthetase inhibitors; and (*d*) calcium-entry blocking agents. The use of ethanol to treat preterm labor has been abandoned by most obstetricians in the United States and is not discussed in this chapter. Interested readers may refer to Chapter 18 on this subject published in the third edition of this text (21).

β-Adrenergic Agents

β-Adrenergic agents are the most commonly used drugs for the treatment (especially short term) of preterm labor. These agents may be administered intravenously, subcutaneously, or orally. All β-agonists have combined β_1 and β_2 effects (Table 17.3). The desired uterine tocolytic activity is a result of stimulation of β_2-receptors in uterine smooth muscle. Unfortunately, stimulation of β_1-receptors may result in marked increases in maternal heart rate and cardiac output. Hyperglycemia and hypotension are the major undesirable β_2-receptor effects (Fig. 17.5).

Ritodrine and terbutaline are two of the more β-receptor specific agents (22). At the present time, although only ritodrine is specifically approved for treatment of preterm labor, terbutaline is also used as a β-adrenergic tocolytic by many clinicians.

Table 17.3. SELECTIVE β-ADRENERGIC RECEPTOR STIMULATION[a]

	β_1	β_2
Uterine muscle	No effect	Relaxation
Cardiovascular		
Blood vessels	No effect	Vasodilation
Heart rate	Increase	No effect
Heart muscle (strength of contraction)	Stimulation	No effect
Cardiac output	Increase	No effect
Respiratory		
Bronchial muscle	No effect	Relaxation
Secretions	No effect	Slight increase
Central nervous system	?	Stimulation
Gastrointestinal	?	Relaxation
Metabolic		
Pancreas β cells	No effect	Insulin secretion
Liver	No effect	Glycogenolysis
Fat cells	Lipolysis	Gluconeogenesis

[a] All β-agonists when given systemically have combined β_1 and β_2 effects.

Mechanism of Action

Through the action of cyclic AMP and the calcium pump, the β-adrenergic agents inhibit the cellular regulatory mechanisms of myosin light-chain phosphorylation, resulting in relaxation of the smooth muscle of the uterus (Fig. 17.5) (23, 24). β-Agonists interact with β-adrenergic receptors located on the outer surface of the target cell. This complex then activates adrenyl cyclase, an enzyme located on the internal surface of the plasma membrane of the target cell. This stimulates the conversion of ATP to cyclic AMP (cAMP). Increased cAMP concentration diminishes myosin light-chain kinase activity through reduced intracellular calcium levels. When myosin phosphorylation is reduced, the actin-myosin interaction diminishes and the myometrium relaxes. cAMP also affects ion transport across cellular and mitochondrial membranes by acting on the Na^+-K^+ pump, resulting in hypokalemia caused by increased pumping of Na^+ out of the cell and K^+ into the cell.

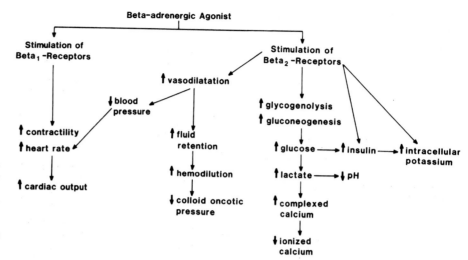

Figure 17.5. The cardiovascular and metabolic effects of β-adrenergic receptor stimulation. (From Cotton DB, Strassner HT, Lipson LG, et al. The effects of terbutaline on acid base, serum electrolytes, and glucose homeostasis during the management of preterm labor. *Am J Obstet Gynecol* 1981;141:617–624, with permission.)

Treatment Regimen

β-Adrenergic therapy should be initiated only after (*a*) obtaining baseline maternal weight, blood pressure, heart rate, and respiratory rate measurements; (*b*) performing a physical examination with emphasis on the heart and lungs; and (*c*) collecting urine for microscopic examination and culture. It is prudent to obtain a blood sample for analysis of white blood cell count, hemocrit and serum electrolytes. Some clinicians routinely obtain a baseline electrocardiogram. This allows for detection of an undiagnosed arrhythmia, which may be worsened by β-adrenergic therapy. It also provides a baseline electrocardiogram for comparison should the patient experience a cardiovascular complication of β-adrenergic therapy. However, in practice, the baseline electrocardiogram rarely affects the management of patients with no history of cardiovascular disease and no cardiovascular abnormality on physical examination.

The usual initial intravenous infusion rates are 0.05 to 0.1 mg · min^{-1} for ritodrine, and 0.01 mg · min^{-1} for terbutaline. Usual maximal infusion rates are .035 mg · min^{-1} for ritodrine and 0.08 mg · min^{-1} for terbutaline. Maternal blood pressure and heart rate are monitored closely.

Side Effects of β-Adrenergic Agents

Widespread use of β-adrenergic agents has resulted in cases of pulmonary edema, hypotension, myocardial ischemia, cardiac arrhythmia, cerebral vasospasm, and rarely maternal death (23). Isoxsuprine is more likely to cause maternal hypotension than ritodrine or terbutaline. Fortunately, isoxsuprine has been abandoned by most obstetricians in the United States.

Pulmonary Edema

Pulmonary edema is the most frequent serious complication of β-adrenergic tocolytic therapy. This complication occurs in approximately 1% of those patients who receive parenteral β-adrenergic therapy. Prolonged exposure to β-adrenergic therapy appears to be a risk factor for the development of pulmonary edema. The majority of published case reports have noted the development of pulmonary edema only after 24 hours, and in many cases after 48 hours, of therapy (24–28). Earlier case reports suggested that concurrent corticosteroid (e.g., dexamethasone, β methasone) administration predisposed patients to pulmonary edema (24, 29). However, these glucocorticoids have little mineralocorticoid activity, and at least one prospective study has not confirmed that glucocorticoid therapy is a risk factor for development of pulmonary edema (30).

Pulmonary edema may develop on a noncardiogenic basis as the result of "capillary leak" due to oncotic-hydrostatic pressure forces in the pulmonary circulation or on cardiogenic basis as the result of fluid overload and myocardial failure (23, 24, 31, 32).

Patients receiving β-adrenergic therapy are at significant risk for noncardiogenic pulmonary edema. Hydration (before and during tocolytic therapy), as well as sodium and water retention secondary to β-adrenergic receptor stimulation, all contribute to increase the risk of noncardiogenic pulmonary edema. β-Adrenergic activation stimulates antidiuretic hormone release (33) and exerts a direct action on renal tubular handling of sodium, resulting in enhanced tubular reabsorption of sodium (34). Because of the antinatriuretic effects of β-adrenergic stimulation, the amount of fluid retained during β-adrenergic therapy is greater when isotonic saline is administered than when dextrose is administered (23, 29). In a study comparing glucose and saline solutions as vehicles for ritodrine, (23) patients who received isotonic saline retained at least 1 liter of fluid more than did the glucose-treated patients. Seven of twelve patients in the saline group, but none in the glucose group, developed pulmonary congestion requiring treatment. Pregnant baboons, (35, 36) who were given ritodrine and lactated Ringer's solution retained 61% of administered fluid, as compared with 23% retained by animals who received lactated Ringer's solution alone. Ritodrine-treated animals also retained more sodium than did animals not treated with ritodrine. Ritodrine-treated animals had a significant increase in cardiac index, pulmonary capillary wedge pressure, and heart rate and a significant decrease in systemic vascular resistance. Colloid oncotic pressure decreased in both groups during a period of increased volume infusion. In ritodrine-treated animals, the lowest colloid oncotic pressures were seen concurrently with maximal wedge pressures, resulting in a colloid oncotic pressure-to-pulmonary capillary wedge pressure gradient favoring a net flux of water from pulmonary vasculature to pulmonary interstitium.

The circulatory effects of β-adrenergic receptor stimulation have been studied in unanesthetized chronically instrumented pregnant sheep (37). Ritodrine produces a significant increase in maternal heart rate and cardiac output and a decrease in systemic vascular resistance. Pulmonary arterial and pulmonary capillary wedge pressures tend to increase, despite a slight fall in the pulmonary vascular resistance (Fig. 17.5) (38). Theoretically, the shortened systolic ejection and diastolic filling times associated with the β-adrenergic-induced tachycardia may result in myocardial ischemia, a decrease in left ventricular compliance and an increase in pulmonary capillary wedge pressure, or both (39).

Benedetti (40) noted that there are few data that confirm that β-adrenergic tocolytic therapy actually results in myocardial failure. He also noted that pulmonary edema during tocolytic therapy is not unique to β-adrenergic therapy. He reviewed 12 patients who had pulmonary edema during tocolytic therapy between 1978 and 1985. Nine patients received either β-adrenergic therapy alone or in combination with magnesium sulfate. But three patients received magnesium sulfate alone. He hypothesized that "in patients who are at high risk for the development of pulmonary edema, there is an underlying infection associated with if not causing the preterm labor" (40). Such infections might include unrecognized amniotic fluid or urinary tract infection and may be associated with the release of endotoxin. Endotoxin has been shown to increase lung capillary permeability and to affect lung balance (41). Noncardiogenic pulmonary edema may occur secondary to increased lung capillary permeability. After *Escherichia coli* endotoxin administration, lung extravascular fluid volume increases at lower (pulmonary capillary minus plasma oncotic) pressure, as compared with control sheep or sheep receiving ritodrine infusion only. β-Adrenergic agents do not increase permeability. An increase in pulmonary capillary wedge pressure caused by β-adrenergic therapy, combined with the increased pulmonary capillary permeability caused by endotoxin, would predispose patients receiving β-adrenergic agents to pulmonary edema. A recent retrospective study (42) confirmed that tocolytic therapy for preterm labor was associated with an increased incidence of pulmonary edema in the presence of maternal infection. It is recommended that clinicians rule out underlying infection in patients receiving tocolytic therapy, even in those without clinical symptoms.

Hypoxia during pulmonary edema may be exacerbated by the inhibition of hypoxic pulmonary vasoconstriction by β-adrenergic agents. A study in dogs has demonstrated that ritodrine significantly inhibits hypoxic pulmonary vasoconstriction, the normal mechanism for diverting blood flow away from areas of hypoventilation (43). Thus the patient who develops pulmonary edema with gas exchange defects during ritodrine therapy may develop hypoxia out of proportion to the degree of radiologically apparent pulmonary edema as a result of the failure of the lung to autoregulate and effectively redistribute pulmonary perfusion.

To decrease the possibility of pulmonary edema during β-adrenergic therapy, total fluid intake (intravenous and oral) should be limited to 1.5 to 2.5 L/24 h. One approach is to administer the β-adrenergic agonist in a solution of 0.45 sodium chloride. Dextrose is not included in the intravenous fluids because of the hyperglycemia induced by the β-adrenergic agents. Daily weights, strict intake and output measurements, and hematocrit (i.e., hemodilution) are measured. The frequency of cardiovascular complications may be decreased by carefully limiting the dose of the β-adrenergic agent. Specifically, there is little tocolytic efficacy to be gained by giving more β-agonist than that necessary to increase the maternal heart rate by 20% to 30%. The authors also recommend the use of the pulse oximeter in patients receiving parenteral β-adrenergic tocolytic therapy. The pulse oximeter may facilitate early diagnosis of pulmonary edema by allowing the physician to detect early decreases in hemoglobin oxygen saturation.

If pulmonary edema develops, the drug infusion should be discontinued and supplemental oxygen administered. An arterial blood gas should be obtained to determine the degree of hypoxemia. Frequently, these measures are sufficient and no further intervention is necessary (24, 32). In a recent review of 58 cases of pulmonary edema associated with tocolytic therapy, the clinical response to conservative therapy was prompt (32). Only four of the 58 patients required intubation and mechanical ventilation.

With the discontinuation of β-adrenergic therapy, heart rate and blood pressure usually return toward pretherapy values over a 30- to 90-minute time period (Fig. 17.6) (37, 38, 44). If hypoxemia persists, further intervention including diuretics, chest radiographic examination, positive pressure ventilation, and central venous and pulmonary artery pressure monitoring may be necessary. The possibility of an unrecognized site of infection should be investigated, particularly if pulmonary arterial and pulmonary capillary wedge pressures are normal. Serum potassium values should be closely monitored if diuretics are administered.

Myocardial Effects

β-Adrenergic agents, including the β₂-selective agents, have potent inotropic and chronotropic effects on the maternal heart. Ritodrine therapy increases heart rate, stroke volume, left ventricular ejection fraction, and cardiac output, resulting

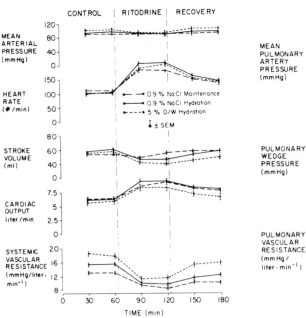
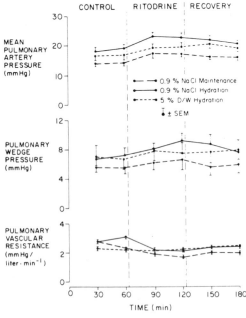

Figure 17.6. The effects of β-adrenergic receptor stimulation on systemic and pulmonary hemodynamics in unanesthetized, chronically instrumented pregnant sheep. Values represent mean ± 1 SE and are for the three different types of hydration. (From Kleinmen G, Nuwayhid B, Rudelstorfer R, et al. Circulatory and renal effects of β-adrenergic-receptor stimulation in pregnant sheep. *Am J Obstet Gynecol* 1984;149:865–874, with permission.)

in a greatly increased myocardial oxygen demand (37, 45). Premature ventricular contractions, premature nodal contractions, and atrial fibrillation have occurred in patients receiving β-adrenergic therapy (23). There have been some reports of myocardial ischemia, which appears to be subendocardial in location, usually manifesting as chest pain or tightness and ST-segment and T-wave changes on electrocardiogram, and resolving shortly after discontinuation of β-adrenergic therapy (28, 45–49). However, not all ST-segment and T-wave changes represent myocardial ischemia. Two recent studies noted frequent electrocardiographic changes during ritodrine therapy in asymptomatic patients (50, 51). Both studies concluded that these changes may represent "a physiologic expression of ritodrine-induced tachycardia or hypokalemia" (50).

Metabolic Effects

β-Adrenergic therapy produces a number of metabolic changes related to glucose, insulin, and potassium (Fig. 17.7) (23, 52–57). By stimulating adenyl cyclase on the membranes of liver cells, ritodrine activates hepatic phosphorylase, which mediates the production of glucose from stored glycogen. Hyperglycemia occurs rapidly, even in nondiabetic patients. Patients who are receiving dextrose-containing solutions or concurrent corticosteroid therapy or who are known to be diabetic are at increased risk for significant hyperglycemia and may require insulin. Insulin-dependent diabetic patients usually require a concomitant insulin infusion to prevent the development of diabetic ketoacidosis (23).

Both direct stimulation of pancreatic β cells by the β-adrenergic agent and increased levels of glucose result in increased serum insulin levels. *Hypokalemia* occurs as the result of the insulin-mediated movement of potassium, together with glucose, from the extracellular to the intracellular space and to direct stimulation of β_2-receptors in skeletal muscle leading to activation of Na$^+$-K$^+$ ATPase (54). Urinary excretion of potassium during β-adrenergic therapy is not increased. **Total body potassium levels appear to be maintained.** The influence of intravenous solution content on ritodrine-mediated metabolic changes in 25 patients who received ritodrine for treatment of preterm labor was evaluated (58). The use of the following was compared: (*a*) 5% dextrose in water; (*b*) 5% dextrose in 0.9 sodium chloride; (*c*) 5% dextrose in Ringer's lactate; (*d*) 0.9 sodium chloride; and (*e*) Ringer's lactate. Dextrose enhanced

the ritodrine-mediated decrease in the serum concentration of potassium. The researchers concluded that, of the five solutions evaluated in their study, Ringer's lactate appeared to be the best solution, whereas 5% dextrose in water was the least desirable.

The administration of supplemental potassium is controversial. Although it is postulated that hypokalemia results in hyperpolarization of nerve and conducting systems as the result of the alteration of the intracellular to extracellular potassium concentration ratio, no adverse effects caused by the hypokalemia have been reported. Restoration of serum potassium to normal levels is not recommended (23, 56, 57, 59). Rapid intravenous infusion of potassium can cause significant complications. Serum potassium concentrations usually return to normal within 3 hours of discontinuing β-adrenergic therapy (49, 57).

There have been four reported cases of terbutaline-associated hepatitis in pregnancy (60). In each case, discontinuation of terbutaline led to amelioration of enzymatic markers of liver damage.

Anesthetic Considerations

Patients who have recently received β-adrenergic agents to treat preterm labor or to acutely treat fetal distress before delivery may require anesthesia. Unfortunately, the half-lives of ritodrine and terbutaline in pregnant women are prolonged. For example, Kuhnert et al. (61) noted that the distribution phase and equilibrium phase half-lives for ritodrine in pregnant women are 32 ± 21 minutes and 17 ± 10 hours, respectively. As noted earlier, the cardiovascular effects of ritodrine and terbutaline persist for 30 to 90 min after their discontinuation (37, 38, 44). When anesthesia is required after administration of a β-adrenergic tocolytic agent, a delay to allow the tachycardia to subside is ideal. However, women with failed tocolysis frequently require urgent induction of anesthesia. A long delay may compromise the fetus.

There are no prospective clinical studies of anesthetic management after administration of a β-adrenergic tocolytic agent. The literature is limited to case reports (62–66), retrospective studies published in letter (67) and abstract form (68), and review articles and textbook chapters. Ravindran et al. (65) presented one case each of intraoperative pulmonary edema, sinus tachycardia, and ventricular arrhythmia after perioperative administration of terbutaline. They recommended that induction of general anesthesia be delayed at least 10 minutes after discontinuation of β-adrenergic infusion.

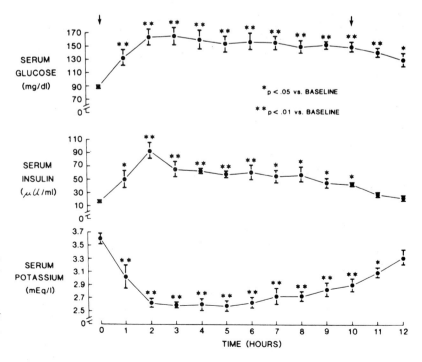

Figure 17.7. The levels of mean serum glucose, insulin, and potassium at baseline (left arrow), during 10 hours of infusion of terbutaline, and 2 hours after the infusion (right arrow) in six patients in preterm labor. (From Cotton DB, Strassner HT, Lipson LG, et al. The effects of terbutaline on acid base, serum electrolytes, and glucose homeostasis during the management of preterm labor. *Am J Obstet Gynecol* 1981;141:617–624, with permission.)

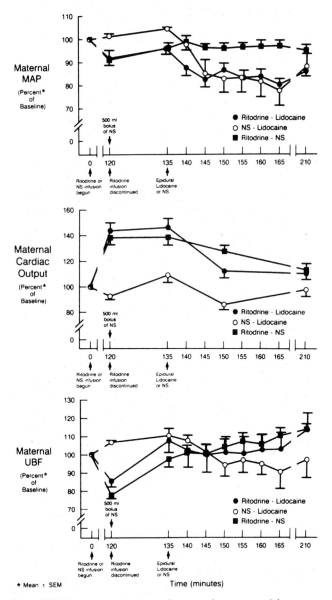

Figure 17.8. Response over time of maternal mean arterial pressure (MAP), cardiac output, and uterine blood flow after intravenous infusion of ritodrine or normal saline (NS) control for 2 hours, followed by epidural administration of lidocaine or NS control in gravid ewes. (From Chestnut DH, Pollack KL, Thompson CS, et al. Does ritodrine worsen maternal hypotension during epidural anesthesia in gravid ewes? *Anesthesiology* 1990;72:315–321, with permission.)

Shin and Kim (68) retrospectively noted that maternal hypotension occurred in two of three women who received *epidural anesthesia* within 30 minutes of discontinuation of ritodrine versus one of eight women in whom there was a delay of greater than 30 minutes ($P = 0.15$). They recommended that epidural anesthesia should "be deferred at least 30 minutes following discontinuation of ritodrine provided that such a delay does not jeopardize the fetus." (68) However, Chestnut et al. (69) observed that prior administration of ritodrine did not worsen maternal hypotension during epidural lidocaine anesthesia in gravid ewes (epinephrine was not included in the lidocaine solution) (Fig. 17.8). The inotropic and chronotropic activity of ritodrine seemed to protect cardiac output and uterine blood flow during epidural lidocaine anesthesia in that study. In practice, a delay of 15 minutes oftenwill result in sufficient slowing of the maternal heart rate to allow the physician to proceed with induction of regional anesthesia. Epidural anesthesia, with

its slower onset and greater flexibility, is theoretically preferred over spinal anesthesia, except when delivery is imminent. One should avoid aggressive hydration before induction of regional anesthesia in patients who have received long-term β-adrenergic tocolytic therapy. Frequently, these patients have a positive fluid balance and are at risk for the development of pulmonary edema if presented with a large fluid bolus. Instead, a modest fluid bolus (e.g., 250 to 500 milliliters of Ringer's lactate) should be given, followed by the induction of regional anesthesia. The volume of crystalloid should be titrated to maintain normal blood pressure.

If hypotension occurs, what vasopressor should be given? Ephedrine, a mixed α and β-agonist, is the preferred vasopressor in most cases of hypotension in obstetric anesthesia practice. The conventional wisdom is that ephedrine's β-agonist activity helps to maintain maternal cardiac output and uterine perfusion. Chestnut et al. (70, 71) hypothesized that, in a patient already receiving a β-agonist, any vasopressor effect from ephedrine should result from α-receptor stimulation. The accompanying uterine vasoconstriction would then result in decreased uterine blood flow. However, they noted that ephedrine aided restoration of uterine blood flow velocity in gravid guinea pigs rendered hypotensive by acute hemorrhage during terbutaline infusion (Fig. 17.9) (70). Ephedrine seemed to restore cardiac output despite the presence of preexisting β-receptor stimulation. Subsequently, they evaluated the prophylactic administration of various vasopressors to normotensive gravid guinea pigs after ritodrine infusion (71). Epinephrine and phenylephrine each significantly worsened uterine blood flow velocity (Fig. 17.10). Ephedrine clearly preserved uterine blood flow velocity, and mephentermine resulted in an intermediate response. McGrath et al. compared the maternal and fetal effects of maternally-administered ephedrine to phenylephrine in gravid ewes subjected to epidural anesthesia-induced hypotension during ritodrine infusion (72). Although ephedrine and phenylephrine were both adequate maternal arterial pressors, ephedrine was associated with increased uteroplacental blood flow without change in uterine vascular resistance. Phenylephrine administration did not increase (nor did it decrease) uteroplacental blood flow but did increase uterine vascular resistance (Fig. 17.11) (72). Collectively these studies suggest that ephedrine produces greater venoconstriction than arterial constriction (73).

One should use caution before extrapolating laboratory data to clinical practice. Nonetheless, these results suggest that ephedrine remains a satisfactory choice of vasopressor in patients who have recently received a β-adrenergic tocolytic agent. Some clinicians have expressed concern that ephedrine may worsen tachycardia or precipitate arrhythmia, administration of small doses of phenylephrine may represent a safe alternative (74, 75). Of course, prophylaxis of hypotension is preferable to treatment of hypotension. Shin and Kim (66) reported one case in which ventricular tachycardia and fibrillation developed after administration of ephedrine for treatment of hypotension (during epidural anesthesia for cesarean section) 30 minutes after discontinuation of ritodrine infusion.

If general anesthesia is required after discontinuation of the β-adrenergic agent, one should remember that tachycardia as a result of β-adrenergic therapy makes it difficult to estimate the depth of anesthesia and fluid status. The tachycardia may be interpreted as a sign of inadequate analgesia, which may result in an overdosage of anesthetics. Tachycardia may be interpreted as a sign of hypovolemia, which may result in excess fluid replacement. One should avoid using agents that exacerbate the tachycardia (e.g., atropine, glycopyrrolate, pancuronium) (76). Severe tachycardia and systolic hypertension have been reported in patients given ritodrine followed shortly thereafter with atropine premedication. Patients receiving β-adrenergic agonists have an increased incidence of arrhythmias. An intravenous bolus of lidocaine ($1 \text{ mg} \cdot \text{kg}^{-1}$) administered at the time of rapid

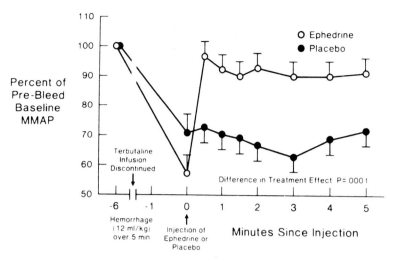

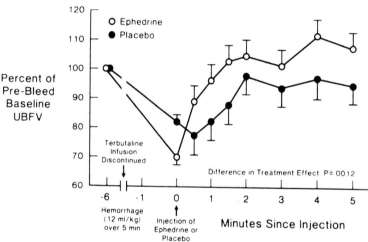

Figure 17.9. Response over time of maternal mean arterial pressure (MMAP) and uterine artery blood flow velocity (UBFV) after hemorrhage and intravenous administration of ephedrine, 1 mg/kg, or placebo (saline, 0.2 mL) in gravid guinea pigs. All values are expressed as mean (±SEM) percentage of the prebleed baseline. (From Chestnut DH, Weiner CP, Wang JP, et al. The effect of ephedrine upon uterine artery blood flow velocity in the gravid guinea pig subjected to terbutaline infusion and acute hemorrhage. *Anesthesiology* 1987;66:508–512, with permission.)

intravenous induction of anesthesia with thiopental and succinylcholine may theoretically reduce the incidence of ventricular ectopy. Hyperventilation should be avoided because this will increase the movement of potassium intracellularly and potentiate the hyperpolarization of the cell membrane (54). Isoflurane does not sensitize the myocardium to catecholamine-induced ventricular arrhythmias.

Magnesium Sulfate

Magnesium sulfate has emerged as the tocolytic agent of choice in most obstetric centers. The tocolytic effects of magnesium sulfate, were reported by Hall et al. (77) in 1959. They demonstrated that strips of myometrium excised from gravid human uteri exhibited reduced contractility in the presence of magnesium ion. They also reported that patients with pregnancy-induced hypertension who were treated with magnesium sulfate had a greater incidence of labor prolonged beyond 24 hours than did controls. Since the initial report of prolonged labor associated with magnesium sulfate, there have been a number of other reports of intravenous magnesium sulfate slowing uterine contractions, both when it is used for seizure prophylaxis in preeclampsia (78) and when it is used in the treatment of preterm labor (79–88). Although chest pain and pulmonary edema may occur, these complications occur less often with magnesium sulfate therapy than with β-adrenergic therapy. In light of certain reports questioning the efficacy of ritodrine tocolysis [especially in preterm pregnancies greater than 28 weeks gestational age (89)] and with the increased familiarity of its use for seizure prophylaxis in preeclamptic

pregnancies, intravenous magnesium sulfate is a commonly used tocolytic in North America.

Mechanism of Action

Magnesium probably works at a cellular level and a nerve transmission level to decrease uterine activity. The mechanism for the inhibitory effect of magnesium sulfate on smooth muscle activity remains uncertain. Like calcium, magnesium is intimately involved in the regulation of muscle contraction (interaction of actin and myosin) and neuromuscular transmission (release of acetylcholine at the neuromuscular junction). Extracellular magnesium effects uptake, binding, and distribution of cellular calcium in vascular smooth muscle (90). Iseri and French (91) described magnesium as "nature's physiologic calcium blocker." By competing with calcium for surface-binding sites on smooth muscle membranes, magnesium probably prevents the increase in the free intracellular calcium concentration that is necessary for myosin light-chain kinase activity. In addition, there is evidence that an increased magnesium ion concentration activates adenyl cyclase and synthesis of cAMP (90).

Magnesium also acts at the neuromuscular junction by decreasing the release of acetylcholine (by competing with calcium for binding sites on the acetylcholine vesicle) and by decreasing the sensitivity of the endplate to acetylcholine. In unanesthetized preeclamptic women receiving magnesium sulfate neuromuscular transmission is abnormal (92). The intensity of the abnormality correlates with increased serum concentrations of magnesium.

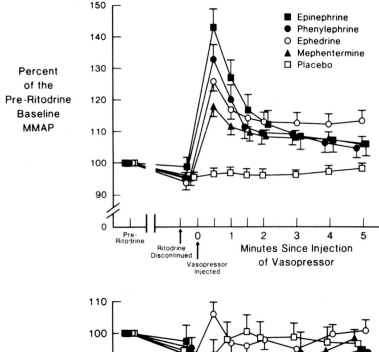

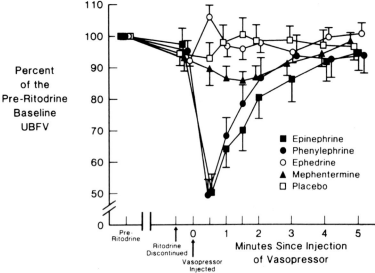

Figure 17.10. Response over time of maternal mean arterial pressure (MMAP) and uterine artery blood flow velocity (UBFV) after intravenous infusion of ritodrine and subsequent injection of epinephrine (0.001 mg · kg^{-1}), phenylephrine (0.01 mg · kg^{-1}), mephentermine (1 mg · kg^{-1}), ephedrine (1.0 mg · kg^{-1}), or placebo (saline, 0.2 mL) in gravid guinea pigs. Each value is expressed as the mean (±SEM) percentage of the pre-ritodrine baseline for that vasopressor. (From Chestnut DH, Ostman LG, Weiner CP, et al. The effect of vasopressor agents upon uterine artery blood flow velocity in the gravid guinea pig subjected to ritodrine infusion. *Anesthesiology* 1988;68:363–366, with permission.)

Treatment Regimen

Several clinical protocols have been described for the tocolytic use of magnesium sulfate (79–82). Serum magnesium concentrations between 5 and 7 mg/dL (4–6 mEq/L: 2 Equivalents = 24 grams) are usually sufficient to inhibit the contractions of patients in preterm labor. Higher (3 to 5 g/h) infusion rates of magnesium sulfate, resulting in correspondingly higher serum magnesium levels, are tolerated by some patients in an effort to effectively tocolyze triplet and higher-order multiple gestation (93). Table 17.4 lists serum magnesium concentrations obtained after intravenous administration of magnesium sulfate at various dosages.

Side Effects

Magnesium sulfate tocolysis has also been associated with some of the same side effects associated with β-adrenergic tocolysis, including pulmonary edema, chest pain, chest tightness, and nausea (82–94). Simultaneous administration of magnesium sulfate with a β-adrenergic agent may increase the likelihood of these side effects. Ferguson et al. (83) compared ritodrine alone with ritodrine and magnesium sulfate for tocolysis. Serious side effects (chest pain with or without electrocardiogram changes, chest pressure, adult respiratory distress syndrome) occurred more often in the magnesium sulfate-ritodrine group (46% of patients) than in the ritodrine-alone group (6% of patients). Of note was the fact that, in most of these patients, ritodrine was discontinued and magnesium sulfate alone was continued for tocolysis without sequelae.

Increasing serum magnesium concentrations greater than 7 mg/dL may result in profound muscle weakness, respiratory paralysis, impaired myocardial conduction and function, and even death. In the presence of impaired renal function, serum magnesium concentrations may rapidly reach toxic levels. Loss of deep tendon reflexes (corresponding to a serum level of 10 mg/dL) precedes respiratory embarrassment. Deep tendon reflexes should be clinically demonstrable at bedside exam and recorded on a regular basis during magnesium tocolysis. Intravenous calcium gluconate (1 g) or calcium chloride (300 mg) is an effective antidote for magnesium-induced respiratory weakness but does not provide protection of the airway in a compromised patient.

The conventional wisdom is that administration of magnesium sulfate incurs little risk of cardiovascular side effects. Indeed, bolus administration of magnesium sulfate typically results in only transient decreases in systemic vascular resistance and mean arterial pressure in preeclamptic women (95). These changes typically are not maintained by continuous magnesium sulfate infusion. Thus many clinicians consider magnesium

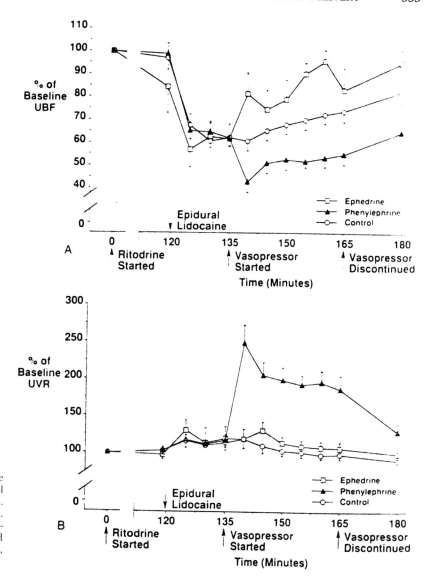

Figure 17.11. Uterine blood flow (UBF) over time for the ephedrine, phenylephrine, and NS control groups. All values are expressed as mean (±SEM). (From McGrath JM, Chestnut DH, Vincent RD, et al. Ephedrine remains the vasopressor of choice for treatment of hypotension during ritodrine infusion and epidural anesthesia. *Anesthesiology* 1994;80:1073–1081, with permission.)

Table 17.4. SERUM MAGNESIUM LEVELS OBTAINED AFTER INTRAVENOUS BOLUS FOLLOWED BY CONSTANT INFUSION[a]

MgSO$_4$ Therapy	No. of Samples	Magnesium in Serum (mg/dL)	
		Mean ± SD	*Range*
Baseline	17	1.8 ± 0.4	1.3–2.9
After 4-g bolus	35	3.5 ± 0.7	1.6–4.8
1 g/h	74	4.0 ± 0.8	2.3–5.7
2 g/h	536	5.1 ± 0.8	2.9–7.5
3 g/h	28	6.4 ± 1.4	4.1–12.0

[a] MgSO$_4$ intravenous bolus of 4 g followed by infusion started at 2 g/h with the rate changed on the basis of the patient's clinical response. From Elliott JP. Magnesium sulfate as a tocolytic agent. *Am J Obstet Gynecol* 1983;147:277–284, with permission.

sulfate to be the tocolytic agent of choice in patients at risk for hemorrhage (e.g., placenta previa). Benedetti (23) reported one case of prolonged hypotension after terbutaline therapy in a bleeding parturient. He concluded that use of β-adrenergic agents should be avoided in bleeding patients. Subsequently, he stated that "In most instances of suspected clinical abruption

and documented placenta previa, magnesium sulfate is an effective and safe alternative to βmimetic therapy. This agent has no significant vasodilatory properties and will not work against the body's own compensatory mechanisms in handling volume loss" (40).

Chestnut et al. (96) evaluated whether the intravenous infusion of ritodrine or magnesium sulfate altered the hemodynamic response to maternal hemorrhage, in gravid ewes. They noted that magnesium sulfate, but not ritodrine, worsened the maternal hypotensive response to hemorrhage (Fig. 17.12). They speculated that Mg^{2+} attenuated the compensatory cardiovascular response to hemorrhage. They also speculated that ritodrine's inotropic and chronotropic activity helped maintain maternal cardiac output and mean arterial pressure during hemorrhage.

Anesthetic Considerations

Should there be a delay between the discontinuation of magnesium sulfate and the administration of regional anesthesia? Suresh and Lawson (97) opined that magnesium sulfate "should be discontinued prior to initiation of lumbar epidural analgesia because magnesium can increase the likelihood of hypotension through its generalized vasodilating properties." However, many anesthesiologists safely give epidural anesthesia to preeclamptic women who *continue* to receive magnesium sulfate during

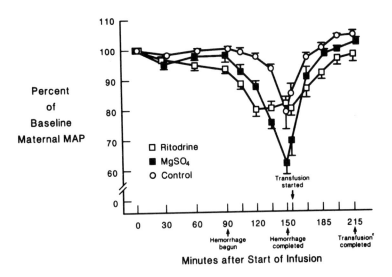

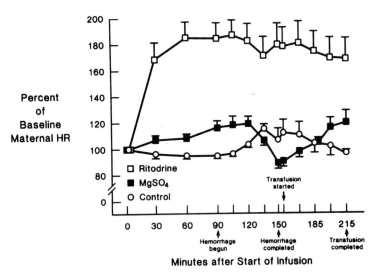

Figure 17.12. Response over time of maternal heart rate (HR) and mean arterial pressure (MAP) during intravenous administration of ritodrine (0.004 mg to $1/kg^{-1}/min^{-1}$), magnesium sulfate (4 g/h), or saline control, and maternal hemorrhage in gravid ewes. All values are expressed as mean (±SE) percentage of baseline. (From Chestnut DH, Thompson CS, McLaughlin GL, et al. Does the intravenous infusion of ritodrine or magnesium sulfate alter the hemodynamic response to hemorrhage in gravid ewes? *Am J Obstet Gynecol* 1988;159:1467–1473, with permission.)

anesthesia and surgery. Magnesium sulfate decreased maternal blood pressure but not uterine blood flow or fetal oxygenation during epidural lidocaine anesthesia in gravid ewes (Fig. 17.13) (98). Incremental doses of intravenous ephedrine should be injected as needed to support maternal arterial pressure (99). If applicable to humans, this study suggests that hypermagnesemia may interfere with maintenance of maternal blood pressure and increase the risk of modest hypotension during regional anesthesia in normotensive parturients. In the authors' judgement, it is not necessary for the anesthesiologist to withhold epidural anesthesia from women who have recently received magnesium sulfate for tocolysis. Although the slower onset of epidural anesthesia seems preferable to the faster onset of spinal anesthesia, spinal anesthesia has been safely given to women for urgent cesarean section of a preterm infant in many cases.

Patients who are receiving magnesium sulfate therapy are more sensitive to both the depolarizing and nondepolarizing muscle relaxants (100). These patients should not be "pretreated" with a nondepolarizing agent before receiving succinylcholine. However, because of individual patient variation, the dose of succinylcholine used for tracheal intubation should not be decreased below $1 \text{ mg} \cdot \text{kg}^{-1}$. If additional muscle relaxation is required, muscle relaxants should be administered in small increments and neuromuscular blockade monitored (101).

There is some evidence from nonpregnant patients that coincidental magnesium infusion decreases intra- and post-operative analgesic needs (102, 103). Although parenteral analgesics should not be withheld from a patient with painful preterm contractions, care should be given to titrate the dose of opioid to effect and not to administer an empiric dose because it "works well" in other patients.

Prostaglandin Synthetase Inhibitors

Prostaglandin synthetase inhibitors (PGSIs) have been suggested as an alternative to β-adrenergic agents for inhibition of preterm labor, particularly in patients with cardiac disease or hyperthyroidism (104). PGSIs alone have been shown to be effective in postponing preterm delivery (104–107) and PGSIs have been used to potentiate the tocolytic effects of β-adrenergic drugs (105, 106). However, some obstetricians avoid these agents because of concern regarding potential adverse effects on the fetus (Table 17.2).

Mechanism of Action

Prostaglandins $F_2\alpha$ and $E_2\alpha$ have a potent stimulatory action on the uterus. They not only activate myometrial contraction but also cause softening of the cervix (108). Prostaglandins are present in blood and amniotic fluid in low concentrations during pregnancy. However, during labor and spontaneous abortion, blood and amniotic fluid prostaglandin concentrations increase (109).

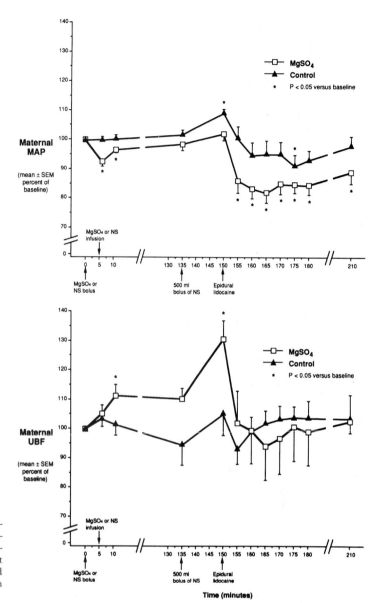

Figure 17.13. Response over time of maternal mean arterial pressure (MAP) and uterine blood flow after intravenous administration of magnesium sulfate (MgSO₄), followed by epidural administration of lidocaine in gravid ewes. (From Vincent RD, Chestnut DH, Sipes SL, et al. Magnesium sulfate decreases maternal blood pressure but not uterine blood flow during epidural anesthesia in gravid ewes. *Anesthesiology* 1991;74:77–82, with permission.)

Nonsteroidal anti-inflammatory analgesics such as aspirin, *indomethacin*, naproxen, ketorolac, *sulindac* and others inhibit the synthesis of prostaglandins by preventing the metabolic conversion of arachidonic acid (110). Of these drugs, indomethacin has received the most extensive evaluation as a tocolytic agent. Indomethacin may be administered either orally or rectally.

Effects

Prostaglandins are involved in maintaining prenatal patency of the ductus arteriosus. There is concern that the administration of PGSIs to the mother in preterm labor will produce premature closure of the ductus arteriosus in utero and result in neonatal pulmonary hypertension. This appears to be related to the gestational age of the fetus. Most adverse effects have been associated with use of PGSIs after 34 weeks' gestation. Studies (111, 112) have shown that the administration of PGSIs to pregnant rats in late gestation produces contraction of the fetal ductus arteriosus in utero; however, there was less decrease in ductal diameter as gestational age decreased. Administration of acetylsalicylic acid to fetal lambs in late gestation caused increased fetal pulmonary artery pressure as well as increased resistance to flow across the ductus arteriosus. These changes did not occur in early gestation (113, 114). Indomethacin is now frequently used to cause closure of patent ductus arteriosus in preterm

infants; however, it appears to be less effective in infants under 1,000 g. These observations collectively suggest that PGSIs might be safer to use earlier (24 to 28 weeks) than later in gestation. Niebyl and Witter (115) concluded that adverse neonatal effects are unlikely if indomethacin is used in short courses, is restricted to patients at less than 34 weeks' gestation, and is stopped at an appropriate interval before delivery. Other studies (116, 117) have also suggested that short-term administration of indomethacin before 34 weeks' gestation is safe for the fetus. Moise et al. (118) performed serial fetal echocardiography in 13 pregnant women who received indomethacin for treatment of preterm labor between 26 and 31 weeks' gestation. Evidence of ductal constriction in seven of fourteen fetuses led the authors to discontinue indomethacin. The authors concluded that indomethacin causes transient constriction of the ductus arteriosus in some fetuses, even after short-term maternal use. **Sulindac** causes only mild and transient ductal constriction perhaps due to its more limited placental transfer than indomethacin (119–121). In any case, right ventricular pressures can be followed by fetal Doppler studies, and therapy discontinued if early signs of fetal compromise are observed.

PGSIs also affect renal function. Indomethacin has been shown to decrease the glomerular filtration rate and to lower plasma renin activity. Long-term indomethacin administration to pregnant monkeys resulted in decreased fetal kidney size and increased fetal liver size (122). Oligohydramnios was common, probably resulting from renal vasoconstriction and antidiuretic effect associated with decreased renal prostaglandin $E_2\alpha$ synthesis. Kirshon et al. (123) observed that maternal administration of indomethacin results in decreased fetal urine output. Indeed, some obstetricians give indomethacin specifically to treat polyhydramnios. However, Wurtzel (124) observed that maternal administration of indomethacin does not significantly alter neonatal renal function.

PGSIs inhibit cyclooxygenase, the first enzyme in prostaglandin synthesis. The major product of prostaglandin synthesis in platelets is thromboxane A_2, a potent stimulator of platelet aggregation and a vasoconstrictor. Aspirin permanently inactivates the enzyme; the effect of aspirin remains for the lifetime of exposed platelets, and aggregation is abnormal up to 7–10 days following ingestion of aspirin. In contrast, indomethacin and most other PGSIs reversibly inhibit cyclooxygenase and only transiently interfere with platelet function (125).

Anesthetic Considerations

Aspirin may result in prolongation of the bleeding time (126, 127). Some anesthesiologists perform a bleeding time test before initiating regional anesthesia in patients who have recently received a PGSI to treat preterm labor. Williams et al. (128) reported one case of cervical epidural hematoma after steroid injection into the cervical epidural space of a patient who had been receiving indomethacin. This complication occurred after the seventh epidural steroid injection over a 2-year period. However, epidural hematoma is a very rare complication in obstetric patients, and the authors are unaware of any case of epidural hematoma after administration of epidural anesthesia to a parturient who was taking a PGSI. The anesthesiologist should assess all risks and benefits of regional anesthesia versus alternatives. In the absence of other risk factors for abnormal bleeding and coagulation, the authors perform regional anesthesia without first obtaining a bleeding time measurement in selected patients who have received a PGSI. Finally, PGSIs should be considered a potential factor in postoperative or postpartum bleeding resulting from inhibition of myometrial contraction (129).

Calcium Entry-Blocking Drugs

Calcium entry-blocking drugs are primarily used in the treatment of ischemic heart disease, hypertension, and paroxysmal supraventricular tachycardia, but they are potentially useful as tocolytic agents. Among the calcium-entry blocking drugs, nifedipine has received the most extensive evaluation for use as a tocolytic agent. *Nifedipine* has fewer effects on cardiac conduction and has more specific effects on myometrial contractility than some of the other calcium-entry blocking drugs. Ulmsten et al. (130) administered nifedipine to 10 patients in preterm labor with a gestational age of 33 weeks or less. The primary aim of treatment was to postpone delivery for 3 days to allow glucocorticoid treatment to accelerate fetal lung maturation. Delivery was postponed in all patients for at least 3 days. Nifedipine regularly caused transient facial flush and a moderate increase in heart rate; headache and dizziness sometimes occurred. However, no other serious side effects were observed in the mother, fetus, or neonate. Others (131–133) have reported that nifedipine seems both efficacious and safe when given for tocolysis in pregnant women. These studies have consistently noted that nifedipine is associated with less frequent and less severe cardiovascular side effects than occur with ritodrine. Using Doppler ultrasound, Mari et al. (134) observed that short-term oral administration of nifedipine did not affect either the fetal or uteroplacental circulation in pregnant women. Pirhonen et al. (135) noted that a single oral dose of nifedipine decreased uterine vascular resistance and did not affect fetal vascular resistance in pregnant

women. These studies conflict with other studies, (136, 137) which noted that administration of nifedipine or nicardipine (especially when given in high doses) decreased uterine blood flow and resulted in fetal hypoxemia and acidosis in laboratory animals. Further studies are needed before there is widespread clinical use of these agents for tocolysis in pregnant women. Given that the calcium entry blockers are a diverse group of drugs with different mechanisms of action, it is possible that some but not all of these agents are safe and appropriate for tocolysis.

Mechanism of Action

The contractility of smooth muscle (including myometrium) is directly related to the concentration of free calcium within the cytoplasm; a decrease in cytoplasmic free calcium decreases contractility. Calcium entry blockers act by altering net calcium uptake through cellular membranes by blockade of the aqueous voltage-dependent membrane channels selective for calcium or by affecting intracellular uptake and release mechanisms. The calcium entry blockers form a chemically diverse group, with unrelated chemical structure and differing pharmacologic and electrophysiologic profiles; thus it is unlikely that there is a single site of action (138, 139).

Side Effects

Ingestion of oral nifedipine during or just after discontinuation of magnesium infusion (perhaps in an attempt to switch the patient to an oral tocolytic) has been associated with respiratory muscle weakness (140), even at serum magnesium levels below what is associated with respiratory embarrassment (141). Support of the maternal airway as well as injection with intravenous calcium is appropriate therapy for such an episode.

Hypotension has also been reported in a preeclamptic patient ingesting nifedipine while on a magnesium sulfate infusion (142). Although, the baseline circulatory volume inherent in preeclampsia must have certainly contributed to this episode, an animal model using perfused, isolated rat-hearts has shown that the combination of nifedipine and magnesium sulfate potentiates the depressed cardiac performance associated with either therapy (143, 144).

Anesthetic Considerations

Experience with the calcium entry-blocking drugs suggests that the drugs may be continued until surgery (145). However, the effects of these drugs in combination with inhalation anesthetic agents (e.g., isoflurane) may exacerbate myocardial depression, conduction defects, and vasodilation (146). In addition, postpartum uterine atony may occur and may be unresponsive to oxytocin and prostaglandin 15 methyl $F_2\alpha$, leading to postpartum hemorrhage. The administration of the calcium entry-blocking drug nicardipine to rats has been shown to arrest labor; however, oxytocin and prostaglandin $F_2\alpha$ were ineffective in restoring uterine activity (147).

Nitroglycerin

Nitric oxide relaxes smooth muscle as well as uterine muscle. Nitroglycerin is a nitric oxide donor. If given in appropriate doses and delivered by an appropriate route, nitroglycerin should be an effective tocolytic agent. Lees et al. performed an open study of transdermal nitroglycerin including 13 women admitted in preterm labor (148). There has been no randomized-controlled trial of nitroglycerin as a long-term tocolytic. However, case reports and series are accumulating describing the intravenous and intraoral administration of nitroglycerin for intrapartum and postpartum relaxation to effect internal podalic and external version, replacement of an inverted uterus and removal of a placenta trapped by a contracted lower uterine segment (149).

Intravenous infusion of nitroglycerin has been used as an intra- and postoperative tocolytic in women undergoing surgery on an exteriorized fetus. Please refer to Chapter 14 for details.

THE PRETERM INFANT

The preterm fetus, especially the fetus of less than 30 weeks' gestation and weighing less than 1,500 g, is physiologically less well adapted than the fully mature full-term fetus to tolerate the stress of labor and delivery (150). The preterm fetus is more vulnerable to asphyxia during labor and delivery than is the term fetus, because of a lower hemoglobin concentration and thus a lower oxygen-carrying capacity. The preterm fetus is more susceptible to intracranial hemorrhage resulting from a soft, poorly calcified cranium and fragile dura mater, germinal matrix, and subependymal veins; the cerebral distortion resulting from molding of the fetal head may result in stretching and tearing of intracranial structures and hemorrhage. Preterm fetuses also have a relative deficiency of clotting factors that may accentuate their susceptibility to intraventricular hemorrhage; coagulation abnormalities are further exacerbated by hypoxia.

Cesarean Section or Vaginal Delivery

The safest method of delivery of the preterm infant, particularly one of less than 30 weeks' gestation and less than 1,500 g, is controversial. In the past only a minority of obstetricians performed a cesarean section before 30 weeks' gestation because of the poor prognosis for survival in the face of increased risk of maternal morbidity and mortality. Current obstetric management of the preterm infant includes intrapartum electronic fetal heart rate monitoring and aggressive attempts at minimizing delivery-related trauma. Obstetricians now perform cesarean delivery of very low-birth-weight infants for a variety of indications (e.g., fetal distress, breech presentation, intrauterine growth restriction, failure of labor to progress, and maternal conditions such as severe preeclampsia and antepartum hemorrhage). In some cases, obstetricians face the dilemma of deciding whether or not to perform an often classical cesarean section for fetal distress in patients with uncertain gestational age or in patients whose fetuses are on the borderline of extrauterine viability (living less than 25 weeks). In that case is it appropriate to subject the mother to the increased risk of cesarean section, recognizing the borderline viability of the fetus? In some cases of uncertain gestational age, the obstetrician may use ultrasound to obtain an estimated fetal weight.

Some, but not all, studies suggest that liberal or even routine performance of cesarean section may increase the survival of preterm infants (151–159), presumably because cerebral trauma and the intermittent hypoxia of labor are avoided. But most studies on the method of delivery of very low-birth-weight infants are retrospective and not well controlled. In a retrospective study of 109 singleton neonates with birth weights of 1,000 g or less, there was no difference in the frequency of neonatal morbidity or mortality between infants delivered vaginally and those delivered by cesarean section among those with birth weights from 751 to 1,000 g (151). Among the newborns with birth weights between 501 and 750 g, the vaginally delivered infants had an increased frequency of intraventricular hemorrhage, as compared with those born by cesarean section, but this was not statistically significant. Anderson et al. (158) performed a prospective study, evaluating the effects of the active phase of labor and the method of delivery on the frequency of germinal layer/intraventricular hemorrhage in 89 neonates with ultrasound-estimated fetal weights less than or equal to 1,750 g. They noted an increased incidence of germinal layer/intraventricular hemorrhage within 1 hour after delivery in the infants of women who experienced the active phase of labor, regardless of the method of delivery. The incidence of germinal layer/intraventricular hemorrhage beyond 1 hour

after delivery and the overall incidence of these complications were both similar in the vaginal delivery and the cesarean delivery groups. Thus they concluded that "The infant of the woman delivered by cesarean section before the active phase of labor is not protected from developing germinal layer/intraventricular hemorrhage; only the time at which the infant will develop hemorrhage is shifted to later in neonatal life." They also noted that there was an increased incidence of progression to more severe grades of hemorrhage (i.e., grades III and IV), regardless of the method of delivery, in those infants whose mothers experienced the active phase of labor. Thus they speculated that "abdominal delivery before the active phase of labor may prevent the most serious form of germinal layer/intraventricular hemorrhage rather than the overall frequency of hemorrhage" (158).

A meta-analysis of controlled trials examining the question of elective cesarean with selective (i.e., for obstetric reasons other than preterm) cesarean delivery showed the odds ratio "tended for all neonatal outcomes" to favor elective cesarean delivery (160). However, further examination of the confidence intervals revealed them to be wide, yielding no clear statistical significance. In addition, the odds ratio for maternal mortality with cesarean delivery was almost three times higher than with vaginal delivery.

It is clear that obstetricians now deliver a large percentage of preterm infants by cesarean section. Malloy et al. (159) examined birth and death certificate data from Missouri for the years 1980 to 1984. The cesarean section rate for infants weighing 2,500 to 7,000 g increased from 14 to 18% between 1980 and 1984. Meanwhile, the cesarean section rate for 1,500 to 2,499 g infants increased from 21% to 26%, and the cesarean section rate for very low-birth-weight infants (i.e., 500 to 1,499 g) increased from 24% to 44%. The first-day death rate was higher in those infants delivered vaginally; however, this difference was nullified by an excess of deaths in the next 6 days of life in the cesarean section group. Overall, there was no significant difference between the vaginal and cesarean section groups in survival beyond the first week. The authors concluded that "There is little evidence that the use of cesarean section for the delivery of very low-birth-weight infants, independent of maternal or fetal compromise, improves overall survival" (159). That is, this study suggests that there is no benefit to performing cesarean section just because the patient is preterm.

However, there is an increased risk of fetal distress during preterm labor. Also, patients with a preterm breech presentation are at risk for prolapse of the umbilical cord, entrapment of the fetal head behind an incompletely dilated cervix, or both. Entrapment of the head appears to be more common in infants weighing less than 1,500 g because the head is relatively larger than the buttocks or trunk. Many authors have recommended the routine use of cesarean section for delivery of breech infants weighing less than 1,500 g (152, 155–157, 161–163) resulting in an increase in the use of cesarean section for preterm breech delivery. In a retrospective study of infants born between 1974 and 1978, the risk of neonatal death was significantly higher for breech infants delivered vaginally than for those delivered by cesarean section. For the 1,000- to 1500-g birth-weight group the neonatal mortality for vaginal and cesarean breech deliveries was 433 and 170 neonatal deaths per 1,000 live births, respectively. However, there is no prospective, controlled study demonstrating that abdominal delivery of a fetus in breech presentation is safer than vaginal delivery in the perterm population. The apparent improvement in survival with cesarean section may be related to the change in the mode of delivery or may be due to other factors and perinatal maneuvers (164–170).

The controversy persists regarding the importance of continuous *electronic fetal heart rate (FHR) monitoring* of the preterm fetus. Luthy et al. (171) compared continuous electronic FHR monitoring and fetal blood gas sampling with periodic auscultation of the FHR in a multicenter randomized study of preterm singleton pregnancies with fetal weights between 700 and 1,750 g.

They noted no significant difference between the two groups in the incidence of perinatal or infant death, in the prevalence of low 5-minute Apgar scores, intrapartum acidosis, or intracranial hemorrhage, or in the frequency of cesarean section. In a follow-up study of the surviving children, Shy et al. (172) observed that the incidence of cerebral palsy was higher in the electronic FHR monitored group than in the group that was monitored by auscultation (20% versus 8%, $P < 0.03$). The authors concluded that "as compared with a structured program of periodic auscultation, electronic fetal monitoring does not result in improved neurologic development in children born prematurely" (172).

Maternal Anesthesia

There are no well controlled, prospective clinical studies on the use of analgesia and anesthesia during labor and delivery of the preterm fetus. In a Canadian study of 10 university teaching hospitals, the perinatal death rate for premature infants was 440 per 1,000 when no anesthesia was administered, as compared with 140 per 1,000 when conduction anesthesia was administered (173). These differences may reflect a large number of precipitous or poorly controlled deliveries with subsequent injury of the fetal head.

Wright et al. (174) retrospectively reviewed the neonatal outcome for 339 consecutive parturients who underwent preterm vaginal delivery over a 10-year period at their hospital. The study was limited to women who delivered singleton fetuses in a vertex presentation, with no congenital anomalies, between 25 and 36 weeks' gestation. The authors divided these 339 patients into those who received epidural or spinal anesthesia and those who received pudendal block, local perineal infiltration, or no anesthesia (i.e., the control group). They also divided the infants into three groups according to gestational age: 25 to 28 weeks, 29 to 32 weeks, and 33 to 36 weeks. Within these groups the authors noted no statistically significant differences between the regional and the control group in umbilical cord venous and arterial blood gas and pH values, Apgar scores,

or time to sustained respiration. There was a tendency toward more vigorous neonates in the 25 to 28 weeks' gestation group when regional anesthesia was used, but this difference was not statistically significant.

In selecting an analgesic technique it must be remembered that the preterm fetus and newborn are particularly susceptible to the depressant effects of transplacentally acquired systemic medications and local and general anesthetic agents as a result of: (a) less protein available for drug binding (175) and decreased drug affinity by the protein that is present; (176, 177) (b) increased levels of bilirubin, (178–180) which may compete with the drug for protein binding; (c) increased likelihood that the drug may attain high concentrations in the central nervous system because of a poorly developed blood-brain barrier; (183); (d) a higher incidence of asphyxia during labor and delivery (175, 182, 183); and (e) a decreased ability to metabolize and excrete drugs.

However, the capability of the fetus to metabolize drugs is greater than originally thought. In contrast to fetuses of other species, liver microsomes of human fetuses have significant amounts of cytochrome P-450, detectable as early as the 14th week of gestation, (184–186) to catalyze the oxidation of various drugs (187, 188). For example, even the preterm human fetus has the capability of metabolizing both ester- and amide-type local anesthetics (189–193). In fact, two studies noted that preterm fetal lambs are more resistant to toxic reactions than are term fetuses. Teramo et al. (194, 195) administered lidocaine to preterm fetal lambs either by continuous intravenous infusion or by bolus injection and found that, as long as the fetal arterial concentration of lidocaine remained below $7 \mu g \cdot mL^{-1}$, there were no fetal cardiovascular changes. On the other hand, concentrations of lidocaine of $11.6 \mu g \cdot mL^{-1}$ produced transient episodes of epileptiform high-voltage activity recorded in the electroencephalogram, followed immediately by hypertension associated initially with tachycardia (Fig. 17.14). Only with the bolus injection of 30 to 50 milligram of lidocaine did they observe an initial fetal bradycardia and hypotension (Fig. 17.15) (194). The amounts of lidocaine necessary to produce convulsive episodes

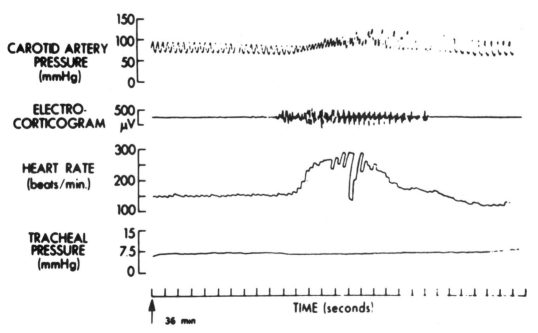

Figure 17.14. Fetal arterial pressure, electrocorticogram, heart rate, and tracheal pressure during one epileptiform burst following fetal infusion of 1.98 to $1.0 \text{ mg} \cdot \text{min}^{-1} \cdot \text{kg}^{-1}$ of lidocaine. The epileptiform activity precedes increases in blood pressure and heart rate by approximately 2 sec. The fetus had been paralyzed with succinylcholine. Thirty-six minutes indicates the time from the beginning of the infusion. (From Teramo K, Benowitz N, Heymann MA, et al. Effects of lidocaine on heart rate blood pressure, and electrocorticogram in fetal sheep. *Am J Obstet Gynecol* 1974;118:935–949, with permission.)

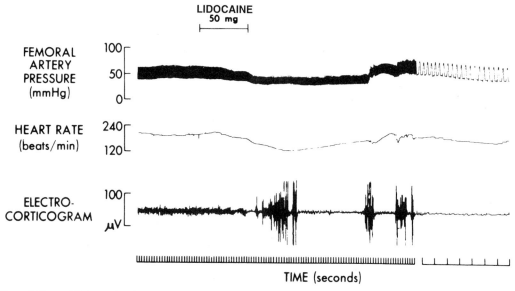

Figure 17.15. Effect of 50 mg (22.2 mg · kg⁻¹) of lidocaine injected as a bolus into the femoral vein of the fetal lamb in utero. (From Teramo K, Benowitz N, Heymann MA, et al. Effects of lidocaine on heart rate, blood pressure, and electrocorticogram in fetal sheep. *Am J Obstet Gynecol* 1974;118:935–949, with permission.)

depended on fetal gestational age: younger fetuses required far more lidocaine than did older fetuses (Fig. 17.16). Gestational age also influenced the fetal cardiovascular response: increases in blood pressure and heart rate in response to lidocaine were greater with advancing gestational age. Teramo et al. (195) suggested that the greater toxicity of local anesthetics in the older fetuses could be related to an increased propensity of the drug to enter the neural tissues or to the increased number and sensitivity of individual neurons.

Pedersen et al. (196) performed a study to evaluate whether gestational age affects the pharmacokinetics and pharmacodynamics of lidocaine in gravid ewes and fetal lambs. They gave lidocaine intravenously to gravid ewes for 180 minutes, to reach a steady-state maternal plasma lidocaine concentration of approximately 2 μg · mL⁻¹. There were no significant differences in steady-state plasma lidocaine concentrations between preterm (119 ± 1 days gestation or 0.8 of term pregnancy) and term (138 ± 1.2 days) fetuses. Tissue uptake of lidocaine tended to be higher in the preterm mothers than in the term mothers,

but these differences were significant only in the brain and the adrenal glands. Tissue uptake of lidocaine was similar in both groups of fetal lambs, except that it was higher in the lungs and liver in the term fetuses. Transplacental passage of lidocaine did not adversely affect fetal cardiac output, organ blood flow, or blood gas and acid-base values. The authors concluded that the pharmacokinetics and pharmacodynamics of lidocaine in the maternal and fetal sheep did not differ between the two gestational age studies.

However, as mentioned previously, preterm fetuses may still be at great risk for developing toxic reactions to local anesthetics and for experiencing increased depression after maternally administered opioid, sedative, and general anesthetic drugs because of low protein-binding capacities, (176, 177, 197–199) a poorly developed blood-brain barrier, 3 and a higher incidence of asphyxia during labor and delivery (175, 182, 183). In fact, asphyxia: (*a*) reduces the protein-binding capacity (199–201); (*b*) increases the normal maternal-fetal hydrogen ion difference, thereby causing "trapping" (i.e., weak bases, such as amide local anesthetics, and opioids administered to the mother, concentrate on the fetal side of the placental circulation when the fetal pH drops) (177, 201–205); (*c*) increases the blood-brain barrier permeability (206–208); and (*d*) enhances the myocardial depressant effects of local anesthetics (209–213). Recently Morishima et al. (214) subjected preterm fetal lambs (i.e., 119 ± 2 days gestation, or 0.8 of term pregnancy) to modest asphyxia by producing partial umbilical cord occlusion. They then gave either lidocaine or saline-control intravenously to the mothers for 180 minutes. At steady state, maternal and fetal plasma lidocaine concentrations were 2.32 ± 0.12 and 1.23 ± 0.17 μg · mL⁻¹, respectively, similar to those obtained during epidural anesthesia in humans. Asphyxia resulted in the typical fetal compensatory response (i.e., decreased fetal heart rate and increased blood flow to the fetal brain, heart, and adrenal glands). Asphyxia and saline did not result in additional deterioration of the fetal lamb, but asphyxia and lidocaine resulted in a significant increase in Paco₂ and significant decreases in fetal pH, mean arterial pressure, and blood flows to the brain, heart, and adrenal glands. These responses differed from the responses to lidocaine in the asphyxiated mature fetal lamb, as observed in an earlier study by the same group of investigators (215). The authors concluded that the preterm, immature fetal lamb "loses its cardiovascular adaptation to asphyxia

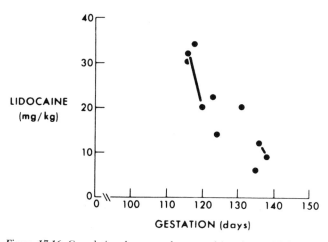

Figure 17.16. Correlation between the convulsive dose of lidocaine (mg/fetal weight) and gestational age in the lamb fetus. Points connected with a line represent data from the same fetus. (From Teramo K, Benowitz N, Heymann MA, et al. Gestational differences in lidocaine toxicity in the fetal lamb. *Anesthesiology* 1976;44:133–138, with permission.)

when exposed to clinically acceptable plasma concentrations of lidocaine obtained transplacentally from the mother." Of course, one should keep in mind that the authors did not compare the fetal response to lidocaine with the fetal response to other anesthetic, analgesic, or sedative drugs. Also the authors evaluated the effects of lidocaine-alone on the fetal response to asphyxia. That is, they did not consider the other potential benefits of epidural anesthesia, such as the decreased maternal stress response and the ability of epidural anesthesia to facilitate a smooth, controlled, atraumatic delivery of the preterm fetal head.

During labor, systemic analgesics should be given with caution. Bilirubin is competitively displaced by water-soluble organic anions that also bind to albumin, such as salicylates, sulfonamides, and benzoates (216). Preterm infants are already predisposed to the development of hyperbilirubinemia as a result of a decreased albumin-binding capacity for bilirubin (217).

During the latent phase of labor, emotional support and reassurance are often sufficient. If analgesia is necessary during the active phase, continuous lumbar epidural anesthesia is the anesthetic of choice. Minimal doses of local anesthetic can be used to provide segmental analgesia during the first stage, then extended to provide perineal relaxation and anesthesia during the second stage. 2-Chloroprocaine is rapidly metabolized and bupivacaine is highly protein bound, so fetal toxicity is minimal with either agent. Kuhnert et al. (218) observed no difference in the elimination of 2-chloroaminobenzoic acid (a major metabolite of 2-chloroprocaine) between preterm and term neonates.

The anesthesiologist should remember that patients in preterm labor may have a rapid active phase of the first stage of labor; these patients often deliver precipitously. Specific anesthetic requirements or vaginal delivery of the preterm infant include: (*a*) inhibition of inappropriate maternal expulsive efforts before complete cervical dilation, especially with a breech presentation; (*b*) avoidance of precipitous delivery, which results in rapid decompression of the fetal head and increased risk of intracranial bleeding; and (*c*) provision of a relaxed pelvic floor and perineum, which will facilitate a smooth, controlled delivery of the infant's head. This last factor is especially important in cases of breech presentation. Unfortunately, appropriate timing of regional anesthesia is more difficult with preterm labor than with term labor. The preterm parturient may have a latent phase of labor that is prolonged for hours or days by administration of a tocolytic agent. When tocolytic therapy fails, the patient typically is in advanced labor. For example, after a few strong contractions, she may have a cervical dilation of 5 or 6 centimeters, and delivery may be imminent. The anesthesiologist should remember that full cervical dilation represents the dilation sufficient to allow for retraction of the cervix over the fetal head. In the preterm parturient, 7 centimeters may constitute full cervical dilation, rather than 10 centimeters as at term. Thus the anesthesiologist may be asked to provide immediate epidural or spinal-epidural anesthesia.

When patients are admitted in preterm labor, if analgesia is not yet required but rapid progress of labor is anticipated, an epidural catheter can be placed early in labor and local anesthetic can be injected when needed. On occasion, when it appears that tocolysis has failed or delivery is imminent, one may begin epidural anesthesia in a preterm patient and labor may cease (219). If the original goal was to stop the labor, this is not a source of concern. One should not view epidural anesthesia as primary tocolytic therapy. Indeed, it is not clear that there is a cause and effect relationship between epidural anesthesia and cessation of labor, even in preterm parturients. But the authors consider it preferable to start epidural anesthesia early in preterm patients, recognizing that one may discontinue the epidural anesthesia (and in some cases even remove the catheter) when labor stops in some of those patients. If you wait until it is clear that preterm delivery is imminent, you will wait too long in some patients.

In cases where vaginal delivery is imminent, low spinal anesthesia (single-shot or as part of a combined spinal-epidural anesthetic) rapidly provides maximal perineal relaxation and analgesia. While pudendal block or even simple local infiltration of the perineum provides some analgesia for delivery, neither produces profound relaxation of the pelvic floor. Relaxation of the levator ani and bulbocavernous muscles helps reduce soft tissue resistance of the lower birth canal.

Most obstetricians agree that episiotomy is indicated in the vaginal delivery of a preterm infant and that the episiotomy should be performed before the fetal vertex begins to distend the perineum (220). Delivery of the head should be controlled to avoid rapid decompression of the head and intracranial bleeding. There is controversy regarding the role of forceps in the delivery of the preterm infant. Excessive compression with forceps or malplacement of forceps may fracture the fetal skull or tear the falx or tentorium. Many obstetricians use forceps only if there is a need to shorten the second stage of labor.

For cesarean section either lumbar epidural or spinal anesthesia is preferred to avoid the potential neonatal central system depression associated with general anesthesia.

After delivery the preterm neonate often requires extensive resuscitation as outlined in Chapter 39. These infants have a high incidence of birth asphyxia, respiratory distress, hypovolemia, hypoglycemia, anemia, and temperature instability.

REFERENCES

1. Brans YW, Escobedo MB, Hayashi RH, et al. Perinatal mortality in a large perinatal center: Five-year review of 31,000 births. *Am J Obstet Gynecol* 1984;148:284–289.
2. Gonik B, Creasy RK. Preterm labor: its diagnosis and management. *Am J Obstet Gynecol* 1986;154:3–8.
3. American College of Obstetricians and Gynecologists. *Preterm labor. ACOG Technical Bulletin no. 133.* 1989
4. Goldenberg RL, Nelson KG, Hale CD, et al. Survival of infants with low birth weight and early gestational age, 1979 to 1981. *Am J Obstet Gynecol* 1984;149:508–511.
5. Kramer WB, Saade GR, Goodrum L, et al. Neonatal outcome after active perinatal management of the very premature infant between 23 and 27 weeks gestation. *J Perinatol* 1997;17:439–443.
6. Bakketeig LS, Hoffman HJ. Epidemiology of preterm birth: results from a longitudinal study of births in Norway. In: MG Edler, Hendricks CH, eds. *Obstetrics and Gynecology. I. Preterm labor.* London: Butterworth,1981:17–46.
7. Iams JD. Current status of prematurity prevention. *JAMA* 1989;262:265–266.
8. Kurki T. A survey of etiological mechanisms and therapy of preterm labor. *Acta Obstet Gynecol Scand* 1998;77:137–141.
9. Garite TJ, Keegan KA, Freeman RK, et al. A randomized trial of ritodrine tocolysis versus expectant management in patients with premature rupture of membranes at 25 to 30 weeks of gestation. *Am J Obstet Gynecol* 1987;157:388–393.
10. Weiner CP, Renk K, Klugman M. The therapeutic efficacy and cost-effectiveness of aggressive tocolysis for premature labor associated with premature rupture of the membranes. *Am J Obstet Gynecol* 1988;159:216–222.
11. Arias F. Intrauterine resuscitation with terbutaline: a method for the management of acute intrapartum fetal distress. *Am J Obstet Gynecol* 1978;131:39–43.
12. Sheybany S, Murphy JF, Evans D, et al. Ritodrine in the management of fetal distress. *Br J Obstet Gynaecol* 1982;89:723–726.
13. Reece EA, Chervenak FA, Romero R, et al. Magnesium sulfate in the management of acute intrapartum fetal distress. *Am J Obstet Gynecol* 1984;148:104–106.
14. Smith GN, Brien JF. Use of nitroglycerin for uterine relaxation. *Obstet Gynecol Surv* 1998;53:559–565.
15. Huszar G. Biology and biochemistry of myometrial contractility and cervical maturation. *Semin Perinatol* 1981;5:216–235.
16. Huddleston JF. Preterm labor. *Clin Obstet Gynecol* 1982;25:123–136.
17. Hendricks CH. The case for nonintervention in preterm labor. In: Elder MG, Hendricks CH, eds. *Obstetrics and Gynecology. I. Preterm labor.* London: Butterworth, 1981:98.

18. Castle BM, Turnbull AC. The presence or absence of fetal breathing movements predicts the outcome of preterm labour. *Lancet* 1983;2:472–473.

19. Agustsson P, Patel NB. The predictive value of fetal breathing movements in the diagnosis of preterm labour. *Br J Obstet Gynaecol* 1987;94:860–863.

20. Schreyer P, Caspi E, Natan NB, et al. The predictive value of fetal breathing movement and Bishop score in the diagnosis of "true" preterm labor. *Am J Obstet Gynecol* 1989;161:886–889.

21. Chestnut DH, Dailey PA. Anesthesia for preterm labor. In: Shnider SM, Levinson G, eds. *Anesthesia for Obstetrics*, 3rd ed. Baltimore: Williams & Wilkins, 1993:337–364.

22. Lipshitz J, Baillie P, Davey DA. A comparison of the uterine β_2-adrenoreceptor selectivity of fenoterol, hexoprenaline, ritodrine, and salbutamol. *S Afr Med J* 1976;50:1969–1972.

23. Benedetti TJ. Maternal complications of parenteral β-sympathomimetic therapy for premature labor. *Am J Obstet Gynecol* 1983; 145:1–6.

24. Benedetti TJ, Hargrove JC, Rosene KA. Maternal pulmonary edema during premature labor inhibition. *Obstet Gynecol* 1982;59:33S–37S.

25. Elliott HR, Abdulla U, Hayes PJ. Pulmonary oedema associated with ritodrine infusion and β-methasone administration in premature labour. *Br Med J* 1978;2:799–800.

26. Stubblefield PG. Pulmonary edema occurring after therapy with dexamethasone and terbutaline for premature labor: a case report. *Am J Obstet Gynecol* 1978;132:341–342.

27. Jacobs MM, Knight AB, Arias F. Maternal pulmonary edema resulting from βmimetic and glucocorticoid therapy. *Obstet Gynecol* 1980;56:56–59.

28. Katz M, Robertson PA, Creasy RK. Cardiovascular complications associated with terbutaline treatment for preterm labor. *Am J Obstet Gynecol* 1981;139:605–608.

29. Tinga DJ, Aarnoudse JG. Post-partum pulmonary edema associated with preventive therapy for premature labor. *Lancet* 1979;1:1026.

30. Philipsen T, Eriksen PS, Lynggard F. Pulmonary edema following ritodrine-saline infusion in premature labor. *Obstet Gynecol* 1981;58:304–308.

31. Wheeler AS, Patel KF, Spain J. Pulmonary edema during β_2-tocolytic therapy. *Anesth Analg* 1981;60:695–696.

32. Pisani RJ, Rosenow EC. Pulmonary edema associated with tocolytic therapy. *Ann Intern Med* 1989;110:714–718.

33. Schrier RW, Lieberman R, Ufferman RC. Mechanism of antidiuretic effect of β-adrenergic stimulation. *J Clin Invest* 1972;51:97–111.

34. Bello-Reuss E. Effect of catecholamines on fluid reabsorption by the isolated proximal convoluted tubule. *Am J Physiol* 1980;238:F347–F352.

35. Hauth JC, Hankins GD, Kuehl TJ, et al. Ritodrine hydrochloride infusion in pregnant baboons. I. Biophysical effects. *Am J Obstet Gynecol* 1983;146:916–924.

36. Hankins GD, Hauth JC, Kuehl TJ, et al. Ritodrine hydrochloride infusion in pregnant baboons. II. Sodium and water compartment alterations. *Am J Obstet Gynecol* 1983;147:254–259.

37. Nuwayhid BS, Cabalum MT, Lieb SM, et al. Hemodynamic effects of isoxsuprine and terbutaline in pregnant and nonpregnant sheep. *Am J Obstet Gynecol* 1980;137:25–29.

38. Kleinman G, Nuwayhid B, Rudelstorfer R, et al. Circulatory and renal effects of β-adrenergic-receptor stimulation in pregnant sheep. *Am J Obstet Gynecol* 1984;149:865–874.

39. Hadi HA, Albazzaz SJ. Measurement of pulmonary capillary pressure during ritodrine tocolysis in term pregnancies: a new noninvasive technique. *Am J Perinatol* 1993;10:351–353.

40. Benedetti TJ. Life-threatening complications of β-mimetic therapy for preterm labor inhibition. *Clin Perinatol* 1986;13:843–852.

41. Gabel JC, Drake RE. Effect of endotoxin on lung fluid balance in unanesthetized sheep. *J Appl Physiol* 1984;56:489–494.

42. Hatjis CG, Swain M. Systemic tocolysis for premature labor is associated with an increased incidence of pulmonary edema in the presence of maternal infection. *Am J Obstet Gynecol* 1988;159:723–728.

43. Conover WB, Benumof JL, Key TC. Ritodrine inhibition of hypoxic pulmonary vasoconstriction. *Am J Obstet Gynecol* 1983;146:652–656.

44. Barden TP. Effect of ritodrine on human uterine motility and cardiovascular responses in term labor and the early postpartum state. *Am J Obstet Gynecol* 1972;112:645–652.

45. Hosenpud JD, Morton MJ, O'Grady JP. Cardiac stimulation during ritodrine hydrochloride tocolytic therapy. *Obstet Gynecol* 1983;62:52–58.

46. Michalak D, Klein V, Marquette GP. Myocardial ischemia: a complication of ritodrine tocolysis. *Am J Obstet Gynecol* 1983;146:861–862.

47. Ron-El R, Caspi E, Herman A, et al. Unexpected cardiac pathology in pregnant women treated with β-adrenergic agents (ritodrine). *Obstet Gynecol* 1983;61:10S–12S.

48. Tye K-H, Desser KB, Benchimol A. Angina pectoris associated with use of terbutaline for premature labor. *JAMA* 1980;244:692–693.

49. Ying Y-K, Tejani NA. Angina pectoris as a complication of ritodrine hydrochloride therapy in premature labor. *Obstet Gynecol* 1982;60:385–388.

50. Hendricks SK, Keroes J, Katz M. Electrocardiographic changes associated with ritodrine-induced maternal tachycardia and hypokalemia. *Am J Obstet Gynecol* 1986;154:921–923.

51. Faidley CK, Dix PM, Morgan MA, et al. Electrocardiographic abnormalities during ritodrine administration. *South Med J* 1990;83:503–506.

52. Cotton DB, Strassner HT, Lipson LG, et al. The effects of terbutaline on acid base, serum electrolytes, and glucose homeostasis during the management of preterm labor. *Am J Obstet Gynecol* 1981;141:617–624.

53. Spellacy WN, Cruz AC, Buhi WC, et al. The acute effects of ritodrine infusion on maternal metabolism: Measurements of levels of glucose, insulin, glucagon, triglycerides, cholesterol, placental lactogen, and chorionic gonadotropin. *Am J Obstet Gynecol* 1978; 131:637–642.

54. Brown MJ, Brown DC, Murphy MB. Hypokalemia from β_2-receptor stimulation by circulating epinephrine. *N Engl J Med* 1983;309:1414–1419.

55. Kauppila A, Tuimala R, Ylikorkala O, et al. Effects of ritodrine and isoxsuprine with and without dexamethasone during late pregnancy. *Obstet Gynecol* 1978;51:288–292.

56. Moravec MA, Hurlbert BJ. Hypokalemia associated with terbutaline administration in obstetrical patients. *Anesth Analg* 1980;59:917–920.

57. Hurlbert BJ, Edelman JD, David K. Serum potassium levels during and after terbutaline. *Anesth Analg* 1981;60:723–725.

58. Perkins RP, Varela-Gittings F, Dunn TS, et al. The influence of intravenous solution content on ritodrine-induced metabolic changes. *Obstet Gynecol* 1987;70:892–895.

59. Chestnut DH. Anesthesia for preterm delivery. In: Hood DD, ed. *Anesthesia in Obstetrics and Gynecology: Problems in Anesthesia*. Philadelphia: JB Lippincott, 1989:663.

60. Quinn PG, Sherman BW, Tavill AS, et al. Terbutaline hepatitis in pregancy; report of two cases and literature review. *Am J Gastroenterol* 1994;89:781–784.

61. Kuhnert BR, Gross TL, Kuhnert PM, et al. Ritodrine pharmacokinetics. *Clin Pharmacol Ther* 1986;40:656–664.

62. Knight RJ. Labour retarded with β-agonist drugs: a therapeutic problem in emergency anesthesia. *Anaesthesia* 1977;32:639–641.

63. Schoenfeld A, Joel-Cohen SJ, Duparc H, et al. Emergency obstetric anaesthesia and the use of β_2-sympathomimetic drugs. *Br J Anaesth* 1978;50:969–971.

64. Crowhurst JA. Salbutamol, obstetrics and anaesthesia: a review and case discussion. *Anaesth Intensive Care* 1980;8:39–43.

65. Ravindran R, Viegas OJ, Padilla LM, et al. Anesthetic considerations in pregnant patients receiving terbutaline therapy. *Anesth Analg* 1980;59:391–392.

66. Shin YK, Kim YD. Ventricular tachyarrhythmias during cesarean section after ritodrine therapy: interaction with anesthetics. *South Med J* 1988;81:528–530.

67. Suppan P. Tocolysis and anaesthesia for caesarean section [Letter]. *Br J Anaesth* 1982;54:1007.

68. Shin YK, Kim YD. Anesthetic considerations in patients receiving ritodrine therapy for preterm labor. *Anesth Analg* 1986;65:S140.

69. Chestnut DH, Pollack KL, Thompson CS, et al. Does ritodrine worsen maternal hypotension during epidural anesthesia in gravid ewes? *Anesthesiology* 1990;72:315–321.

70. Chestnut DH, Weiner CP, Wang JP, et al. The effect of ephedrine upon uterine artery blood flow velocity in the gravid guinea pig subjected to terbutaline infusion and acute hemorrhage. *Anesthesiology* 1987;66:508–512.

71. Chestnut DH, Ostman LG, Weiner CP, et al. The effect of vasopressor agents upon uterine artery blood flow velocity in the gravid guinea pig subjected to ritodrine infusion. *Anesthesiology* 1988;68:363–366.

72. McGrath JM, Chestnut DH, Vincent RD, et al. Ephedrine remains the vasopressor of choice for treatment of hypotension

during ritodrine infusion and epidural anesthesia. *Anesthesiology* 1994;80:1073–1081.

73. Lawson NW, Wallfisch HK. Cardiovascular pharmacology: a new look at the "pressors." In: Stoelting RK, Barash PG, Gallagher TJ, eds. *Advances in Anesthesia*. Chicago: Year Book Medical Publishers, 1986:195–270.

74. Ramanathan S, Grant GJ. Vasopressor therapy for hypotension due to epidural anesthesia for cesarean section. *Acta Anaesthesiol Scand* 1988;32:559–565.

75. Moran DH, Perillo M, Bader AM, et al. Phenylephrine in treating maternal hypotension secondary to spinal anesthesia. *Anesthesiology* 1989;71:A857.

76. Sheybany S. Ritodrine in the management of fetal distress. *Br J Obstet Gynaecol* 1982;89:723–726.

77. Hall DG, McGaughey HS Jr, Corey EL, et al. The effects of magnesium therapy on the duration of labor. *Am J Obstet Gynecol* 1959;78:27–32.

78. Hutchinson HT, Nichols MM, Kuhn CR, et al. Effects of magnesium sulfate on uterine contractility, intrauterine fetus, and infant. *Am J Obstet Gynecol* 1964;88:747–758.

79. Steer CM, Petrie RH. A comparison of magnesium sulfate and alcohol for the prevention of premature labor. *Am J Obstet Gynecol* 1977;129:1–4.

80. Spisso KR, Harbert GM Jr, Thiagarajah S. The use of magnesium sulfate as the primary tocolytic agent to prevent premature delivery. *Am J Obstet Gynecol* 1982;142:840–845.

81. Valenzuela G, Cline S. Use of magnesium sulfate in premature labor that fails to respond to β-mimetic drugs. *Am J Obstet Gynecol* 1982;143:718–719.

82. Elliott JP. Magnesium sulfate as a tocolytic agent. *Am J Obstet Gynecol* 1983;147:277–284.

83. Ferguson JE, Hensleigh PA, Kredenster D. Adjunctive use of magnesium sulfate with ritodrine for preterm labor tocolysis. *Am J Obstet Gynecol* 1984;148:166–171.

84. Petrie RH. Tocolysis using magnesium sulfate. *Semin Perinatol* 1981;5:266–274.

85. Harbert GM, Spisso KR. The management of preterm labor: use of magnesium sulfate. In: Zuspan FP, Christian CD, eds. *Reid's Controversy in Obstetrics and Gynecology*, 3rd ed. Philadelphia: WB Saunders, 1983:73–79.

86. Beall MH, Edgar BW, Paul RH, et al. A comparison of ritodrine, terbutaline, and magnesium sulfate for the suppression of preterm labor. *Am J Obstet Gynecol* 1985;153:854–859.

87. Hollander DI, Nagey DA, Pupkin MJ. Magnesium sulfate and ritodrine hydrochloride: A randomized comparison. *Am J Obstet Gynecol* 1987;156:631–637.

88. Wilkins IA, Lynch L, Mehalek KE, et al. Efficacy and side effects of magnesium sulfate and ritodrine as tocolytic agents. *Am J Obstet Gynecol* 1988;159:685–689.

89. The Canadian Preterm Labor Investigators Group. Treatment of preterm labor with the β adrenergic agonist ritodrine. *N Engl J Med* 1992;327:308–312.

90. Altura BM, Altura BT. Magnesium ions and contraction of vascular smooth muscles: relationship to some vascular diseases. *Fed Proc* 1981;40:2672–2679.

91. Iseri LT, French JH. Magnesium: nature's physiologic calcium blocker. *Am Heart J* 1984;108:188–193.

92. Ramanathan J, Sibai BM, Pillai R, et al. Neuromuscular transmission studies in preeclamptic women receiving magnesium sulfate. *Am J Obstet Gynecol* 1988;158:40–46.

93. Elliott JP, Radin TG. Serum magnesium levels during magnesium sulfate tocolysis in high-order multiple gestations. *J Reprod Med* 1995;40:450–452.

94. Elliot JP, O'Keefe DF, Greenberg P, et al. Pulmonary edema associated with magnesium sulfate and β-methasone administration. *Am J Obstet Gynecol* 1979;134:717–719.

95. Cotton DB, Gonik B, Dorman KF. Cardiovascular alterations in severe pregnancy-induced hypertension: acute effects of intravenous magnesium sulfate. *Am J Obstet Gynecol* 1984;148:162–165.

96. Chestnut DH, Thompson CS, McLaughlin GL, et al. Does the intravenous infusion of ritodrine or magnesium sulfate alter the hemodynamic response to hemorrhage in gravid ewes? *Am J Obstet Gynecol* 1988;159:1467–1473.

97. Suresh MS, Lawson NW. Anesthesia for parturients with toxemia of pregnancy. In: Datta SJ, Ostheimer GW, eds. *Common Problems in Obstetric Anesthesia*. Chicago: Year Book Medical Publishers, 1987:332–347.

98. Vincent RD, Chestnut DH, Sipes SL, et al. Magnesium sulfate decreases maternal blood pressure but not uterine blood flow during epidural anesthesia in gravid ewes. *Anesthesiology* 1991;74:77–82.

99. Sipes SL, Chestnut DH, Vincent RD, et al. Which vasopressor should be used to treat hypotension during magnesium sulfate infusion and epidural anesthesia. *Anesthesiology* 1992;77:101–108.

100. DeVore JS, Asrani R. Magnesium sulfate prevents succinylcholine induced fasciculations in toxemic parturients. *Anesthesiology* 1980;52:76–77.

101. Skaredoff MN, Roak ER, Datta SJ. Hypermagnesaemia and anaesthetic management. *Can Anaesth Soc J* 1982;29:35–41.

102. Koinig H, Wallner T, Marhofer P, et al. Magnesium sulfate reduces intra- and postoperative analgesic requirements. *Anesth Analg* 1998;87:206–210.

103. Tramer MR, Schneider J, Marti R-A, et al. Role of magnesium sulfate in postoperative analgesia. *Anesthesiology* 1996;84:340–347.

104. Neibyl JR. Prostaglandin synthetase inhibitors. *Semin Perinatol* 1981;5:274–287

105. Gamissans O, Cararach V, Serra J. The role of prostaglandin inhibitors, β-adrenergic drugs and glucocorticoids in the management of threatened pre-term labor. In: Jung H, Lamberti G, eds. *β-mimetic Drugs in Obstetrics and Perinatology: Third Symposium on β-mimetic Drugs*. New York: Thieme-Stratton, 1982:71–84.

106. Gamissans O, Canas E, Escofet J, et al. Prostaglandin synthetase inhibitors in the management of premature labor. In: *Proceedings of the Ninth World Congress of Gynecology and Obstetrics, Tokyo, 1979*. Amsterdam: Excerpta Medica, 1979:914–918.

107. Zuckerman H, Reiss U, Rubinstein I. Inhibition of human premature labor by indomethacin. *Obstet Gynecol* 1974;44:787–792.

108. Grieves S, Liggins GC. Phospholipase A activity in human and ovine uterine tissue. *Prostaglandins* 1976;12:229–241.

109. Karim SMM. Appearance of prostaglandin $F_2\alpha$ in human blood during labor. *Br Med J* 1968;4:618–621.

110. Vane JR. Inhibition of prostaglandin synthesis as a mechanism of action for aspirin-like drugs. *Nat New Biol* 1971;231:232–235.

111. Sharpe GL. Indomethacin and closure of the ductus arteriosus. *Lancet* 1975;1:693.

112. Sharpe GL, Larsson KS, Thalme B. Studies on closure of the ductus arteriosus. XII. In utero effect of indomethacin in rats and rabbits. *Prostaglandins* 1975;9:585–596.

113. Rudolph AM, Heymann MA. Hemodynamic changes induced by blockers of prostaglandin synthesis in the fetal lamb in utero. *Adv Prostaglandin Thromboxane Leukot Res* 1978;4:231–237.

114. Heymann MA, Rudolph AM. Effects of acetylsalicylic acid on the ductus arteriosus and circulation in fetal lambs in utero. *Circ Res* 1976;38:418–422.

115. Niebyl JR, Witter FR. Neonatal outcome after indomethacin treatment for preterm labor. *Am J Obstet Gynecol* 1986;155:747–749.

116. Dudley DKL, Hardie MJ. Fetal and neonatal effects of indomethacin used as a tocolytic agent. *Am J Obstet Gynecol* 1985; 151:181–184.

117. Morales WJ, Smith SG, Angel JL, et al. Efficacy and safety of indomethacin versus ritodrine in the management of preterm labor: a randomized study. *Obstet Gynecol* 1989;74:567–572.

118. Moise KJ, Huhta JC, Sharif DS, et al. Indomethacin in the treatment of premature labor. Effects on the fetal ductus arteriosus. *N Engl J Med* 1988;319:327–331.

119. Carlen SJ, O'Brien WF, O'Leary TD, et al. Randomized comparison of indomethacin and sulindac for the treatment of refractory preterm labor. *Obstet Gynecol* 1992;79:220–228.

120. Rasanen J, Jouppila P. Fetal cardiac function and ductus arteriosus during indomethacin and sulindac therapy for treatment of threatened preterm labor: a randomized study. *Am J Obstet Gynecol* 1995;173:20–25.

121. Kramer WB, Saade GA, Belfort M, et al. A randomized double-blind study comparing the fetal effects of sulindac to terbutaline during the management of preterm labor. *Am J Obstet Gynecol* 1999;180:396–401.

122. Novy MJ. Effects of indomethacin on labor, fetal oxygenation, and fetal development in Rhesus monkeys. *Adv Prostaglandin Thromboxane Leukot Res* 1978;4:285–300.

123. Kirshon B, Moise KJ Jr, Wasserstrum N, et al. Influence of short-term indomethacin therapy on fetal urine output. *Obstet Gynecol* 1988;72:51–53.

124. Wurtzel D. Prenatal administration of indomethacin as a tocolytic agent: effect on neonatal renal function. *Obstet Gynecol* 1990;76:689–692.

125. Kocsis JJ, Hernandovich J, Silver MJ, et al. Duration of inhibition of platelet prostaglandin formation and aggregation by ingested aspirin or indomethacin. *Prostaglandins* 1973;3:141–144.

126. Bick RL, Adams T, Schmalhorst WR. Bleeding times, platelet adhesion, and aspirin. *Am J Clin Pathol* 1976;65:69–72.

127. Benigni A, Gregorini G, Frusca T, et al. Effect of low-dose aspirin on fetal and maternal generation of thromboxane by platelets in women at risk for pregnancy-induced hypertension. *N Engl J Med* 1989;321:357–362.

128. Williams KN, Jackowski A, Evans PJD. Epidural haematoma requiring surgical decompression following repeated cervical epidural steroid injections for chronic pain. *Pain* 1990;42:197–199.

129. Lewis RB, Schulman JD. Influence of acetylsalicylic acid, an inhibitor of prostaglandin synthesis, on the duration of human gestation and labour. *Lancet* 1973;2:1159–1161.

130. Ulmsten U, Andersson K-E, Wingerup L. Treatment of premature labor with the calcium antagonist nifedipine. *Arch Gynecol* 1980;229:1–5.

131. Read MD, Wellby DE. The use of a calcium antagonist (nifedipine) to suppress preterm labour. *Br J Obstet Gynaecol* 1986;93:933–937.

132. Ferguson JE, Dyson DC, Holbrook RH, et al. Cardiovascular and metabolic effects associated with nifedipine and ritodrine tocolysis. *Am J Obstet Gynecol* 1989;161:788–795.

133. Ferguson JE, Dyson DC, Schutz T, et al. A comparison of tocolysis with nifedipine or ritodrine: analysis of efficacy and maternal, fetal, and neonatal outcome. *Am J Obstet Gynecol* 1990;163:105–111.

134. Mari G, Kirshon B, Moise KJ, et al. Doppler assessment of the fetal and uteroplacental circulation during nifedipine therapy for preterm labor. *Am J Obstet Gynecol* 1989;161:1514–1518.

135. Pirhonen JP, Erkkola RU, Ekblad UU, et al. Single dose of nifedipine in normotensive pregnancy: nifedipine concentrations, hemodynamic responses, and uterine and fetal flow velocity waveforms. *Obstet Gynecol* 1990;76:807–811.

136. Ducsay CA, Thompson JS, Wu AT, et al. Effects of calcium entry blocker (nicardipine) tocolysis in rhesus macaques: fetal plasma concentrations and cardiorespiratory changes. *Am J Obstet Gynecol* 1987;157:1482–1486.

137. Harake B, Gilbert RD, Ashwal S, et al. Nifedipine: effects on fetal and maternal hemodynamics in pregnant sheep. *Am J Obstet Gynecol* 1987;157:1003–1008.

138. Forman A, Andersson KE, Ulmsten U. Inhibition of myometrial activity by calcium antagonists. *Semin Perinatol* 1981;5:288–294.

139. Struyker-Boudier HAJ, Smits JFM, DeMey JGR. The pharmacology of calcium antagonists: a review. *J Cardiovasc Pharmacol* 1990;15:S1–S10.

140. Snyder SW, Cardwell MS. Neuromuscular blockade with magnesium sulfate and nifedipine. *Am J Obstet Gynecol* 1989;161:35–36.

141. BenAmi M, Giladi Y, Shalev E. The combination of magnesium sulphate and nifedipine; a cause of neuromuscular blockade. *Br J Obstet Gynecol* 1994;101:262–263.

142. Waisman GD, Mayorga LM, Camera MI, et al. Magnesium plus nefedipine; potentiation of hypotensive effect in preeclampsia? *Am J Obstet Gynecol* 1988;159:308–309.

143. Thorp JM, Spielman FJ, Valea FA, et al. Nifedipine enhances the cardiac toxicity of magnesium sulfate in the isolated perfused Sprague-Dawley rat heart. *Am J Obstet Gynecol* 1990;163:655–656.

144. Kurtzman JL, Thorp JM, Spielman FJ, et al. Do nifedipine and verapamil potentaite the cardiac toxicity of magnesium sulfate? *Am J Perinatol* 1993;10:450–452.

145. Reves JG, Kissin I, Lell WA, et al. Calcium entry blockers: uses and implications for anesthesiologists. *Anesthesiology* 1982;57:504–518.

146. Tosone SR, Reves JG, Kissin I. Hemodynamic response to nifedipine in dogs anesthetized with halothane. *Anesth Analg* 1983;62:903–908.

147. Csapo AI, Puri CP, Tarro S, et al. Deactivation of the uterus during normal and premature labor by the calcium antagonist nicardipine. *Am J Obstet Gynecol* 1982;142:483–491.

148. Lees C, Campbell S, Jauniaux E, et al. Arrest of preterm labor and prolongation of gestation with glyceril trintrate, a nitric oxide donor. *Lancet* 1994;343:1325–1326.

149. Smith GN, Brien JF. Use of nitroglycerin for uterine relaxation. *Obstet Gynecol Surv* 1998;53:559–565.

150. Bowes WA Jr. Delivery of the very low birth-weight infant. *Clin Perinatol* 1981;8:183–195.

151. Barrett JM, Boehm FH, Vaughn WK. The effect of type of delivery on neonatal outcome in singleton infants of birth weight of 1,000 g or less. *JAMA* 1983;250:625–629.

152. Smith ML, Spencer SA, Hull D. Mode of delivery and survival in babies weighing less than 2000 g at birth. *Br Med J* 1980;281:1118–1119.

153. Stewart AL, Reynolds EOR. Improved prognosis for infants of very low birthweight. *Pediatrics* 1974;54:724–735.

154. Stewart AL, Turcan DM, Rawlings G, et al. Prognosis for infants weighing 1,000 grams or less at birth. *Arch Dis Child* 1977;52:97–104.

155. Goldenberg RL, Nelson KG. The premature breech. *Am J Obstet Gynecol* 1977;127:240–244.

156. Ingemarsson I, Westgren M, Svenningsen NW. Long-term follow-up of preterm infants in breech presentation delivered by caesarean section. *Lancet* 1978;2:172–175.

157. Sachs BP, McCarthy BJ, Rubin G, et al. Cesarean section: risk and benefits for mother and fetus. *JAMA* 1983;250:2157–2159.

158. Anderson GD, Bada HS, Sibai BM, et al. The relationship between labor and route of delivery in the preterm infant. *Am J Obstet Gynecol* 1988;158:1382–1390.

159. Malloy MH, Rhoads GG, Schramm W, et al. Increasing cesarean section rates in very low-birth-weight infants: effect on outcome. *JAMA* 1989;262:1475–1478.

160. Grant A, Penn ZJ, Steer PJ. Elective or selective cesarean delivery of the small baby? a systematic review of the controlled trials. *Br J Obstet Gynaecol* 1996;103:1197–1200.

161. Lewis BV, Seneviratne HR. Vaginal breech delivery or cesarean section. *Am J Obstet Gynecol* 1979;134:615–618.

162. Duenhoelter JH, Wells CE, Reisch JS, et al. A paired controlled study of vaginal and abdominal delivery of the low birth weight breech fetus. *Obstet Gynecol* 1979;54:310–313.

163. Main DM, Main EK, Maurer MM. Cesarean section versus vaginal delivery for the breech fetus weighing less than 1500 grams. *Am J Obstet Gynecol* 1983;146:580–584.

164. Karp LE, Doney JR, McCarthy T, et al. The premature breech: trial of labor or cesarean section? *Obstet Gynecol* 1979;53:88–92.

165. Fairweather DUI, Stewart AL. How to deliver the under 1500-gram infant. In: Zuspan FP, Christian CD, eds. *Reid's Controversy in Obstetrics and Gynecology*, 3rd ed. Philadelphia: WB Saunders, 1983:154–164.

166. Woods JR Jr. Effects of low-birth-weight breech delivery on neonatal mortality. *Obstet Gynecol* 1979;53:735–740.

167. Mann LI, Gallant JM. Modern management of the breech delivery. *Am J Obstet Gynecol* 1979;134:611–614.

168. Bowes WA Jr, Taylor ES, O'Brien M, et al. Breech delivery: evaluation of the method of delivery on perinatal results and maternal morbidity. *Am J Obstet Gynecol* 1979;135:965–973.

169. Effer SB, Saigal S, Hunter DJS, et al. Effect of delivery method on outcomes in the very low-birth weight breech infant: is the improved survival related to cesarean section or other perinatal maneuvers? *Am J Obstet Gynecol* 1983;145:123–128.

170. Rosen MG, Chik L. The effect of delivery route on outcome in breech presentation. *Am J Obstet Gynecol* 1984;148:909–914.

171. Luthy DA, Shy KK, van Belle G, et al. A randomized trial of electronic fetal monitoring in preterm labor. *Obstet Gynecol* 1987;69:687–695.

172. Shy KK, Luthy DA, Bennett FC, et al. Effects of electronic fetal-heart-rate monitoring, as compared with periodic auscultation, on the neurologic development of premature infants. *N Engl J Med* 1990.322:588–593.

173. Ontario Perinatal Mortality Study Committee. *Second Report of the Perinatal Mortality Study in Ten University Teaching Hospitals, Three Reports, Sec. 1, 1961, suppl. to 2nd report.* Toronto: Department of Health, 1967: Tables 108–124.

174. Wright RG, Shnider SM, Thirion A-V, et al. Regional anesthesia for preterm labor and vaginal delivery: effects on the fetus and neonate. *Anesthesiology* 1988;69:A654.

175. Cook LN. Intrauterine and extrauterine recognition and management of deviant fetal growth. *Pediatr Clin North Am* 1977;24:431–454.

176. Mather LE, Long GJ, Thomas J. The binding of bupivacaine to maternal and foetal plasma proteins. *J Pharm Pharmacol* 1971;23:359–365.

177. Thomas J, Long G, Moore G, et al. Plasma protein binding and placental transfer of bupivacaine. *Clin Pharmacol Ther* 1976;19:426–434.

178. Boggs TR, Hardy JB, Frazier FM. Correlation of neonatal serum total bilirubin concentration and developmental status at age eight months. *J Pediatr* 1967;71:553–560.

179. Chez RA, Fleischman AR. Fetal therapeutics: challenges and responsibilities. *Clin Pharmacol Ther* 1973;14:754–761.

180. Cashore WJ, Stern L. Neonatal hyperbilirubinemia. *Pediatr Clin North Am* 1977;24:509–527.

181. Himwich WA. Physiology of the neonatal central nervous system. In: Stave U, ed. *Physiology of Perinatal Period*. New York: Appleton-Century-Crofts, 1970:725–728.

182. Jones MD Jr, Battaglia FC. Intrauterine growth retardation. *Am J Obstet Gynecol* 1977;127:540–549.

183. Low JA, Wood SL, Killen HL, et al. Intrapartum asphyxia in the preterm fetus <2000 gm. *Am J Obstet Gynecol* 1990;162:378–382.

184. Rane A, Sjoqvist F, Orrenius S. Cytochrome P-450 in human fetal liver microsomes. *Chem Biol Interact* 1971;3:305.

185. Yaffe SJ, Juchau MR. Perinatal pharmacology. *Ann Rev Pharmacol* 1974;14:219–238.

186. Alvares AP, Schilling G, Levin W, et al. Cytochromes P-450 and b5 in human liver microsomes. *Clin Pharmacol Ther* 1969;10:655–659.

187. Pelkonen O, Vorne M, Arvela P, et al. Drug metabolizing enzymes in human fetal liver and placenta in early pregnancy. *Scand J Clin Lab Invest* 1971;27(suppl):S116–S117.

188. Rane A, Sjoqvist F, Orrenius S. Drugs and fetal metabolism. *Clin Pharmacol Ther* 1973;14:666–672.

189. Vallner JJ. Binding of drugs by albumin and plasma protein. *J Pharm Sci* 1977;66:447–465.

190. Magno R, Berlin A, Karlsson K, et al. Anesthesia for cesarean section. IV. Placental transfer and neonatal elimination of bupivacaine following epidural analgesia for elective cesarean section. *Acta Anaesth Scand* 1976;20:141–155.

191. Shnider SM, Way EL. The kinetics of transfer of lidocaine (Xylocaine) across the human placenta. *Anesthesiology* 1968;29:944–950.

192. Meffin P, Long GL, Thomas J. Clearance and metabolism of mepivacaine in the human neonate. *Clin Pharmacol Ther* 1973;14:218–225.

193. Brown WU Jr, Bell GB, Lurie AO, et al. Newborn blood levels of lidocaine and mepivacaine in the first postnatal day following maternal epidural anesthesia. *Anesthesiology* 1975;42:698–707.

194. Teramo K, Benowitz N, Heymann MA, et al. Effects of lidocaine on heart rate, blood pressure, and electrocorticogram in fetal sheep. *Am J Obstet Gynecol* 1974;118:935–949.

195. Teramo K, Benowitz N, Heymann MA, et al. Gestational differences in lidocaine toxicity in the fetal lamb. *Anesthesiology* 1976;44:133–138.

196. Pedersen H, Santos AC, Morishima HO, et al. Does gestational age affect the pharmacokinetics and pharmacodynamics of lidocaine in mother and fetus? *Anesthesiology* 1988;68:367–372.

197. Burt RAP. The foetal and maternal pharmacology of some of the drugs used for the relief of pain in labour. *Br J Anaesth* 1971;43:824–836.

198. Scott DB. Analgesia in labour. *Br J Anaesth* 1977;49:11–17.

199. Tucker GT, Mather LE. Pharmacokinetics of local anaesthetic agents. *Br J Anaesth* 1975;47:213–224.

200. Tucker GT. Plasma binding and disposition of local anesthetics. *Int Anesthesiol Clin* 1975;13:33–59.

201. Shnider SM, Way EL. Plasma levels of lidocaine (Xylocaine) in mother and newborn following obstetrical conduction anesthesia: clinical applications. *Anesthesiology* 1968;29:951–958.

202. Ralston DH, Shnider SM. The fetal and neonatal effects of regional anesthesia in obstetrics. *Anesthesiology* 1978;48:34–64.

203. Brown WU Jr, Bell GC, Alper MH. Acidosis, local anesthetics, and the newborn. *Obstet Gynecol* 1976;48:27–30.

204. Dodson WE. Neonatal drug intoxication: local anesthetics. *Pediatr Clin North Am* 1976;23:399–411.

205. Biehl D, Shnider SM, Levinson G, et al. Placental transfer of lidocaine: effects of fetal acidosis. *Anesthesiology* 1978;48:409–412.

206. Lending M, Slobody LB, Mestern J. Effect of hyperoxia, hypercapnia and hypoxia on blood-cerebrospinal fluid barrier. *Am J Physiol* 1961;200:959–962.

207. Evans CAN, Reynolds JM, Reynolds ML, et al. The effect of hypercapnia and hypoxia on a blood-brain barrier mechanism in fetal and newborn sheep. *J Physiol* 1976;255:701–714.

208. Ritter DA, Kenny JD, Norton HJ, et al. A prospective study of free bilirubin and other risk factors in the development of kernicterus in premature infants. *Pediatrics* 1982;69:260–266.

209. Asling JH, Shnider SM, Margolis AJ, et al. Paracervical block anesthesia in obstetrics. II. Etiology of fetal bradycardia following paracervical block anesthesia. *Am J Obstet Gynecol* 1970;107:626–634.

210. Rosefsky JB, Petersiel ME. Perinatal deaths associated with mepivacaine paracervial block anesthesia in labor. *N Engl J Med* 1968;278:530–533.

211. Anderson KE, Gennser G, Nilsson E. Influence of mepivacaine on isolated human foetal hearts at normal or low pH. *Acta Physiol Scand* 1970;353(suppl):34–47.

212. Morishima HO, Heymann MA, Rudolph AM, et al. Transfer of lidocaine across the sheep placenta to the fetus: hemodynamic and acid-base responses of the fetal lamb. *Am J Obstet Gynecol* 1975;122:581–588.

213. Rosen MA, Thigpen JW, Shnider SM, et al. Bupivacaine cardiotoxicity in hypoxic-acidotic sheep. *Anesth Analg* 1985;64:1089–1096.

214. Morishima HO, Pedersen H, Santos AC, et al. Adverse effects of maternally administered lidocaine on the asphyxiated preterm fetal lamb. *Anesthesiology* 1989;71:110–115.

215. Morishima HO, Santos AC, Pedersen H, et al. Effect of lidocaine on the asphyxial responses in the mature fetal lamb. *Anesthesiology* 1987;66:502–507.

216. Seligman JW. Recent and changing concepts of hyperbilirubinemia and its management in the newborn. *Pediatr Clin North Am* 1977;24:509–527.

217. Kapitulnik J, Valaes T, Kaufman NA, et al. Clinical evaluation of Sephadex gel filtration in estimation of bilirubin binding in serum in neonatal jaundice. *Arch Dis Child* 1974;49:886–894.

218. Kuhnert BR, Kuhnert PM, Reese ALP, et al. Maternal and neonatal elimination of CABA after epidural anesthesia with 2-chloroprocaine during parturition. *Anesth Analg* 1983;62:1089–1094.

219. Melsen NC, Noreng MF. Epidural blockade in the treatment of preterm labour. *Anaesthesia* 1988;43:126–127.

220. Bishop EH, Israel SL, Briscoe CL. Obstetric influences on the infant's first year of life. *Obstet Gynecol* 1965;26:628–634.

Shnider and Levinson's Anesthesia for Obstetrics,
edited by Samuel C. Hughes, et al.
Lippincott Williams & Wilkins,
Philadelphia, © 2001.

CHAPTER 18

COAGULATION DISORDERS AND HEMOGLOBINOPATHIES IN THE OBSTETRIC AND SURGICAL PATIENT

RUSSELL K. LAROS, JR., M.D.

On occasion the obstetrician-gynecologist and anesthesiologist are confronted by the need to anesthetize and deliver or operate on a patient with a coagulation disorder or hemoglobinopathy. Most all patients with a hemoglobinopathy will have had the diagnosis made during the antepartum period. However, when the history suggests an undiagnosed abnormality of coagulation, a preoperative laboratory screen (platelet count, prothrombin time, partial thromboplastin time, fibrin degradation products (FDPs), and thrombin time) will usually indicate either normalcy or the need for further studies to specifically identify the abnormality. Although most bleeding disorders can be anticipated and diagnosed preoperatively by history and laboratory evaluation, on occasion they may present themselves for the first time dramatically during surgery. In either instance, a clear understanding of the coagulation mechanism, the laboratory evaluation of coagulation, and therapy of the common disorders of hemostasis is essential.

THE COAGULATION MECHANISM

The initial coagulation mechanism for thrombus formation in vivo is adhesion of platelets to the injured vessel walls (1). Exposed subendothelium in the injured tissue initiate adhesion, which is promptly followed by a change in shape of the platelet:

$$\text{Injury} + \text{platelets} \xrightarrow[\text{aggregation}]{\text{adhesion}} \text{platelet factors} + \text{ADP}$$

Both the platelet membrane and release of the contents of δ-, α-, and γ-granules are involved in platelet adhesion and aggregation as well as the initiation of the plasma phase of coagulation. The ADP released from platelets attracts more platelets to the area, resulting in platelet aggregation. The aggregation phenomenon tends to perpetuate itself, because newly attracted platelets in turn release ADP and attract additional platelets. Increasingly large amounts of platelet factors become available for initiation of the plasma phase of coagulation.

Table 18.1 details some of the properties of the coagulation factors (2). With the exception of fibrinogen, prothrombin, and calcium, the coagulation factors are trace proteins. Factor III is not listed in the table and is, in fact, the tissue factor thromboplastin. The preferred descriptive name and several common synonyms for the coagulation factors are as follows: V, proaccelerin or labile factor; VII, proconvertin or serum prothrombin conversion accelerator; VIII, antihemophilic factor or antihemophilic globulin; IX, plasma thromboplastin component or Christmas factor; X, Stuart factor or Prower factor; XI, plasma thromboplastin antecedent; XII, Hageman factor or glass or contact factor; and XIII, fibrin stabilizing factor.

The third column in the table indicates the site of biosynthesis for each factor. It is noteworthy that prothrombin, factor VII, factor IX, and factor X are dependent on vitamin K for their synthesis and, thus, are the factors depleted when a patient is receiving a vitamin K antagonist such as sodium warfarin. The biologic half-life is also listed for each factor and can be used to estimate roughly the frequency of replacement therapy needed during an acute bleeding problem.

The remainder of the coagulation process can be broadly divided into three phases: the extrinsic pathway, intrinsic pathway, and common pathway. The pathway of function for each of the plasma factors is also noted in Table 18.1.

The total coagulation scheme can be summarized by the following schematized seven equations:

1. $\text{Injury} + \text{platelets} \xrightarrow[\text{aggregation}]{\text{adhesion}} \text{platelet factors} + \text{ADP}$

2. $\text{Tissue thromboplastin} + \text{VII} \xrightarrow{\text{Ca}^{++}} \text{extrinsic activator}$

3. $\text{XII} + \text{XI} + \text{IX} + \text{PF3} + \text{VIII} \xrightarrow{\text{Ca}^{++}} \text{intrinsic activator}$

4. $\text{X} + \text{V} + \text{PF3} + \text{Ca}^{++} \xrightarrow[\substack{\text{intrinsic} \\ \text{activator}}]{\substack{\text{extrinsic} \\ \text{activator}}} \text{common activator}$

5. $\text{Prothrombin} \xrightarrow[\text{Ca}^{++}]{\text{common activator}} \text{thrombin}$

6. $\text{Fibrinogen} \xrightarrow{\text{thrombin}} \text{fibrin polymer}$

7. $\text{Fibrin polymer} + \text{VIII} \xrightarrow{\text{Ca}^{++}} \text{stabilized fibrin}$

The basic feature of coagulation is the conversion of circulating fibrinogen into a stabilized fibrin clot; it occurs in two steps. First, fibrinogen is enzymatically converted to fibrin monomer by the action of thrombin, and the fibrin monomeric units polymerize (equation 6). Next, the resulting fibrin clot is strengthened and further rendered insoluble by the action of Factor XIII (equation 7).

In order for fibrinogen to be converted to fibrin, thrombin must be generated from its precursor prothrombin. This reaction is catalyzed by a complex, common activator which consists of the activated form of factor X, factor V, calcium, and platelet factors (equation 5). The production of the common activator can occur as a result of two different pathways, the intrinsic and extrinsic. The intrinsic is so named because all its components are present in the circulating plasma (equation 3). This pathway is probably triggered by both endothelial damage and platelet factors. The extrinsic pathway is so named because it is triggered by tissue thromboplastin (equation 2).

Finally, the fibrinolytic system must be briefly considered. Fibrinolysis is the major physiologic means by which fibrin is disposed of after its hemostatic function has been fulfilled. The mechanism of fibrinolysis is schematically summarized by

Table 18.1. SOME PROPERTIES OF COAGULANT FACTORS

Factor	Biochemistry	Biosynthesis	Biologic Half-life (h)	Function
Fibrinogen (I)	Glycoprotein; MW 340,000; 3 globular subunits	Liver	72–120	Common pathway; fibrin precursor
Prothrombin (II)	Monomeric glycoprotein; MW 69,000	Liver; vitamin K[a]	67–106	Common pathway; proenzyme precursor of thrombin
Calcium (IV)	Ionic calcium	—		Extrinsic, intrinsic and common pathways
Factor V	Multimeric; MW 200,000–400,000	Liver	12–36	Common pathway
Factor VII	Monomeric glycoprotein; MW 63,000	Liver; vitamin K	4–6	Extrinisic pathway; proenzyme
Factor VIII	Multimeric glycoprotein; MW 330,000; circulates bound to multimeric von Willebrand factor	Probably by liver	10–14	Intrinsic pathway
Factor IX	Monomeric glycoprotein; MW 62,000	Liver; vitamin K	24	Instrinsic pathway; coenzyme
Factor X	Two-chain glycoprotein; MW 59,000	Liver; vitamin K	24–60	Common pathway; proenzyme
Facor XI pathway	Two-chain glycoprotein; MW 200,000	Liver	48–84	Intrinsic proenzyme
Factor XII	Monomeric glycoprotein; MW 80,000	Unknown	52–60	Intrinsic pathway; proenzyme
Factor XIII	Multimeric glycoprotein; MW 320,000; 4 subunits	Liver; megakaryocytes	72–168	Common pathway; proenzyme; transglutaminase
von Willebrand	Series of macromolecules; MW $1–15 \times 10^6$	Endothelial cells and megakaryocytes	12–36	Intrinsic pathway; Forms a stable complex with factor VIII

[a] Vitamin K required for synthesis.
MW, molecular weight.

equations 8 and 9:

8. $\text{Plasminogen} \xrightarrow{\text{activators}} \text{plasmin}$

9. $\begin{matrix}\text{Fibrin}\\\text{Fibrinogen}\\\text{Complement}\\\text{Factor VIII}\end{matrix} \xrightarrow{\text{plasmin}} \text{degradation products}$

Plasminogen is a β-globulin with a molecular mass of 81,000 daltons. It circulates in the plasma in concentrations of 10 to 20 mg/dL. It is activated by a heterogeneous group of substances termed "plasminogen activators" (equation 8). Activators reside within the lysozyme of most cells, and urokinase and streptokinase are examples of specifically identified activators. The activated form of plasminogen, plasmin, is a proteolytic enzyme with a wide spectrum of activity. It cleaves arginyl-lysine bonds in a large variety of substrates, including fibrinogen, fibrin, factor VIII, and various components of complement (equation 9). It has a very short life in plasma, owing to its inactivation by humoral antiplasmins.

There are also a number of plasma proteases that function as inhibitors of coagulation and fibrinolysis. They serve to control both the speed and extent of coagulation and fibrinolysis. The major inhibitor of the extrinsic phase is C1 inhibitor which inactivated factor VII$_a$ and kallikrein. The major inhibitor of the intrinsic phase is antithrombin III (ATIII) which inhibits factor IX$_a$, factor X$_a$, and thrombin. Other inhibitors are α_1-antitripsin, α_2-macroglobulin, and α_2-antiplasmin. Protein C is also a potent inhibitor of coagulation. Activated protein C (with its cofactor, protein S) reacts with factors V and VIII to destroy their coagulation property. The antithrombin scheme is summarized by the following four equations (2–5):

10. $\text{Thrombin} \xrightarrow{\text{ATIII}} \text{inactivated thrombin}$

11. $\begin{matrix}\text{IXa}\\\text{Xa}\\\text{XIa}\\\text{XIIa}\\\text{Kallikrein}\end{matrix} \xrightarrow{\text{ATIII}} \text{inactivated serine proteases}$

12. $\text{Protean C} \xrightarrow{\text{Thrombin}} \text{activated protein C}$

13. $\text{Activated Protein C} \xrightarrow{\text{Protein S}} \text{inactivated V and VIII: C complex}$

Factor V Leiden is the most recent genetic risk factor to be identified. In this disorder factor V has a molecular defect which substitutes glutamine for arginine at the activated protein C cleavage site. This factor V Leiden no longer degradable by active protein C but retains its procoagulant activity. ATIII, protein C, protein S deficiencies, and factor V Leiden are all inherited as autosomal dominant disorders. A significant number of venous thromboembolic events are associated by one of the above disorders. While there is currently no consensus about long-term anticoagulation, many pregnant women with hereditary thrombophilia will be anticoagulated throughout pregnancy and the puerperium, especially if they have had a prior venous thromboembolism.

Finally, the antiphospholipid-anticardiolipin antibody syndrome is associated with thrombosis, fetal wastage and early onset preeclampsia (3–8). Many patients with this syndrome will be treated with low-dose aspirin and adjusted-dose heparin during their pregnancy. If there is a history of thrombosis, anticoagulation should be continued postpartum.

LABORATORY METHODS FOR STUDY OF BLOOD COAGULATION

There is no single test suitable as an overall laboratory screening study of hemostasis and blood coagulation. Commonly, the combination of platelet count, activated partial thromboplastin time (aPTT), prothrombin time (PT), and thrombin time are used as a screening battery. Table 18.2 indicates which factors are measured by each study and indicates the normal value for the study in question. Bleeding times are not included on this list because they have limited clinical value (9). There are a large number of additional studies that define specific abnormalities of platelet function or allow measurements of a specific plasma clotting factor. The Rumpel-Leede test, platelet adhesiveness, platelet aggregation, whole blood prothrombin activation rate,

Table 18.2. SCREENING COAGULATION TESTS

Study	Measures	Normal Values
Platelet count	Number of platelets	$140–440 \times 10^9/\text{L}$
Partial thromboplastin time	II, V, VIII, IX, X, XI	24–36 sec
Prothrombin time	II, V, VII, X	11–12 sec
Thrombin time	I, II, circulating split products, heparin	16–20 sec
Fibrinogen	Fibrinogen	150–450 mg/dL
Fibrin degradation products	D-dimer and other degradation products	<20 ng/L

and clot retraction are all examples of studies that further define abnormalities of platelet function.

Precise levels of each circulating plasma factor can be defined by either the thromboplastin generation test or cross-correction studies with normal plasma and plasma known to be deficient in the factor being assayed. A specific assay for factor XIII is also available. Several accurate methods are now available for the quantitative assay of plasma fibrinogen. Normal values range from 160 to 415 mg · 100 mL^{-1} and are abnormal in acquired hypofibrinogenemia secondary to disseminated intravascular coagulation and in the hereditary afibrinogenemias and dysfibrinogenemias.

Studies used in the evaluation of fibrinolysis include the euglobulin clot lysis time and the demonstration of fibrin-fibrinogen degradation products by a variety of techniques. When thrombophilia is suspected, studies should not at the time of an acute thrombotic event. An exception is factor V Leiden which is tested for using a molecular diagnostic technique (4).

It is important to remember that the screening coagulation studies do not provide a specific etiologic diagnosis. Such a diagnosis is important because only then is it possible to optimally treat excessive bleeding should it occur during surgery. Furthermore, the presence of an adequate coagulation screen in a patient suspected of having a coagulation abnormality does not diminish the necessity of pursuing a specific diagnosis and making available specific therapy should it be needed.

In the past the bleeding time has proposed to be out as useful in predicting severe bleeding during surgical procedures and delivery. Several extensive reviews indicate that the utility of the bleeding time has not been enhanced by standardization of the method, that there is no clinically useful correlation between the bleeding time and platelet count in thrombocytopenic individuals, and that there is no evidence that the bleeding time is a predictor of the risk of either spontaneous or surgically induced hemorrhage (9, 10).

TREATMENT OF COAGULATION ABNORMALITIES

The author will not attempt to discuss all possible congenital and acquired coagulation disorders but only considers those most commonly seen by the obstetrician-gynecologist and anesthesiologist dealing with obstetric patients. Acquired disorders are far more common than congenital, and those seen most frequently include idiopathic thrombocytopenic purpura, disseminated intravascular coagulation, liver disease, and anticoagulant therapy. The congenital disorders seen most frequently are von Willebrand's disease and factor XI deficiency.

Table 18.3 suggests values of various coagulation factors which treatment with appropriate procoagulants should be carried out prior to surgery. None of these values should be considered to be absolute "trigger points" for treatment. A variety of clinical factors such as magnitude of planned surgery, medication history and blood pressure lability should also be considered in planning treatment (11, 12).

Table 18.3. ABNORMAL COAGULATION STUDIES AND SURGERY

Coagulation Study	Inadequate for Surgery
Platelets ($\times 10^9/\text{L}$)	<50
Prothrombin time (sec)	>18
Partial thromboplastin time (sec)	>60
Fibrinogen (mg/dL)	>100

Platelet Disorders

Thrombocytopenia is the most common platelet disorder and is due to either diminished production or increased destruction of platelets (see Chapter 23, Fig. 23.7). The severity of bleeding in thrombocytopenia is roughly proportional to the degree to which the platelet count has been lowered.

A specific diagnosis is obviously essential for the proper total management of a patient with thrombocytopenia. However, when hemorrhage is due to thrombocytopenia, platelet transfusions are frequently of value (13). The success of platelet transfusion therapy is dependent on the functional integrity of the transfused platelets, the underlying cause of the platelet defect in the recipient, and the presence and level of antiplatelet antibodies. Platelet transfusions are available both as platelet-rich plasma and platelet concentrates. When platelet concentrates are used, a relatively large number of platelets remain in the bag and can be harvested by adding a small amount of normal saline solution after evacuation of each bag to resuspend platelets remaining in the bag. One can expect an increase in platelet count of 5 to $10 \times 10^9/\text{L}$/unit of platelets transfused. The exact incremental rise and the length of platelet survival are dependent both on the underlying disease process and the freshness of the platelets.

The complications of platelet transfusion are less common and less serious than those accompanying transfusion of whole blood. They include bacterial contamination, infectious hepatitis, febrile transfusion reaction and post-transfusion purpura.

Management of **idiopathic thrombocytopenic purpura** (ITP) during pregnancy requires concern for both mother and fetus. (4–6, 14–16) ITP is an autoimmune disorder in which antiplatelet immunoglobulin (Ig)G is produced. The reticuloendothelial system is responsible for platelet destruction with the spleen being the primary site for both antibody production and platelet destruction. The diagnosis of ITP is made according to established criteria that include a normal blood count, except for thrombocytopenia, a normal bone marrow, with adequate or increased megakaryocytes, a blood smear showing an increased percentage of large platelets, normal coagulation studies, increased levels of platelet-associated IgG and no other obvious cause of thrombocytopenia.

The goal of treatment for patients with ITP is remission, not cure. Thus, therapy is stepwise: corticosteroids, then splenectomy, and, following that, consideration of immunosuppressive therapy or plasmapheresis. Each step is determined by the severity of the clinical situation. The management of ITP in pregnancy requires special consideration because the human placenta is known to have receptors for the F_c portion of the IgG molecule. Active transfers of IgG and antibodies from the mother to the fetus occur and causes neonatal thrombocytopenia in from 50% to 70% of neonates.

Most obstetricians and hematologists would agree that the overall management of pregnant women with this disorder should be similar to that of a nonpregnant individual. Initially one should employ corticosteroids such as prednisone in a dose of 0.5 to 1 mg · kg^{-1}. If a response to corticosteroids has not been achieved, splenectomy is indicated and should be carried out if at all possible during the middle trimester. Corticosteroids have been used for the last 30 years and owe their efficacy to both an immunosuppressive effect and a slowing of the rate of platelet destruction by the reticuloendothelial systems. By themselves, corticosteroids produce a transient remission in 75% of cases in adults, but a sustained remission in only 14% to 33% of cases. More recently immunosuppression with high dose serum immune globulin has been found to be useful and now is often used during pregnancy before resorting to splenectomy. Other agents include danazol, cyclophosphamide, azathioprine, vincristine and vinblastin. Danazol is relatively contraindicated if the patient is carrying a male fetus, and the various chemotherapeutic agents are only used as a last resort.

The major controversial issue in the management of ITP has been the mode of delivery. Because of the theoretic risks of intracranial hemorrhage to thrombocytopenic fetuses, many investigators have advocated cesarean section for all women with ITP. A review summarizes data on 165 cases (17). Of the 134 infants delivered vaginally, 50 (37%) either had or developed platelet counts below 100×10^9/L and 28 (21%) had counts below 30×10^9/L. Only 1 infant was described as having intracerebral bleeding and this was nonfatal. By contrast, of the 31 infants delivered by cesarean section, 17 (55%) had platelet counts below 10×10^9/L and 9 (29%) below 30×10^9/L. There were three serious hemorrhages, one of which was intracranial hemorrhage at 3 days of age. These data do not support the premise that delivery by cesarean section is beneficial for thrombocytopenic infants of women with ITP. A more recent report describing 31 pregnancies from 25 women with immune thrombocytopenic purpura managed at a single institution also concluded that the route of delivery may not affect the incidence of intracranial hemorrhage in infants with thrombocytopenia (15). A series of 55 pregnancies complicated by autoimmune thrombocytopenia also found that severe neonatal thrombocytopenia is an infrequent complication and that intracranial hemorrhage is a very rare event and is not related to the mode of delivery (18).

In an attempt to define those fetuses really at risk, Scott and associates (19) have suggested the use of fetal platelet counts obtained by fetal scalp blood sampling in early labor. They have documented the reliability of the technique and suggest cesarean section only for those infants with platelet counts proven to be below 30×10^9/L. An alternative technique is percutaneous umbilical cord blood sampling performed at 38 weeks' gestation (20, 21). Similarly, Samuels and associates (22) and Kelton and associates (23) have studied the value of platelet-associated IgG in predicting the significantly thrombocytopenic infant. Unfortunately, the antibody studies do not allow the prospective detection of those infants with marked thrombocytopenia.

Because there is no evidence substantiating that cesarean section offers benefits to a thrombocytopenic infant, the author believes that the decision on route of delivery should be based on obstetric indications alone. It is important to remember that neonatal alloimmune thrombocytopenia (NAIT) is a totally different disorder wherein there is an incompatibility between the mother and fetus with respect to platelet antigens. NAIT is analogous to Rh isoimmunization except that the sensitization is to platelet antigens and the maternal antibody crosses the placenta and interacts with the fetus' platelets rather than red blood cells. Fetal thrombocytopenia occurs earlier in pregnancy, is severe and is associated with intracranial hemorrhage in 10 to 20% of affected fetuses. The mother is not thrombocytopenic. Fetal risk is especially high when an older sibling has had an intracranial hemorrhage (24). Fetal blood sampling is used to make the diagnosis and treatment usually consists of administration of intravenous IgG weekly. Delivery is usually by cesarean section.

Five reports concern the use of epidural catheters in patients with platelet counts of less than 100×10^9/L without any neurologic sequelae (see Chapter 23) (25–30). Hew-Wing and associates conclude that "the current belief, that epidural anesthesia is contraindicated in patients whose platelet counts are below 100×10^9/L, has no supporting data" (28). The experience of Beilin and associates in 30 patients with platelet counts between 69 and 98×10^9/L supports this statement (29). A platelet count obtained several weeks before delivery is not reliable in predicting thrombocytopenia during labor in women with mild thrombocytopenia (30).

Acquired and Congenital Plasma Factor Disorders

Von Willebrand's disease (vWD) is inherited as an autosomal dominant trait and is characterized by abnormal bleeding of varying severity. The pathophysiologic basis for the disease is a marked decrease or absence of both clottable and antigenic factor VIII. Criteria for laboratory diagnosis are as yet not completely satisfactory but include slight to moderate reduction in the aPTT, a clottable factor VIII level 15% to 30% of normal, a prolonged bleeding time, abnormal platelet adhesiveness, a lack of ristocetin-induced platelet aggregation, and a factor VIII coagulant activity-to factor VIII antigen ratio of 1 (31–34). The factor VIII level should be checked periodically during the antenatal course and pretreatment reserved for patients with levels of less than 25% of normal. DDAVP (l-deamino-8-D-arginine-vasopressine) should be used instead of cryoprecipitate for cases known to be responsive (type I and some IIa). Treatment is begun when the patient presents in labor. A dose of 0.3 μg · kg^{-1} of DDAVP given over 30 minutes with the total dose not greater than 25 μg. Treatment is repeated every 12 hours with infusions being progressively less effective.

The specific treatment for serious hemorrhagic manifestations in patients with vWD who are not responsive to DDAVP is Pasteurized, fractionated fresh frozen plasma (Humate-P®, Alphanate®), cryoprecipitate or fresh frozen plasma. Serious bleeding (and thus treatment) is rare if the factor VIII level is greater than 25% of normal and/or the bleeding time is less than 15 minutes. If cesarean section is required for obstetrical reasons, treatment is indicated if the level is less than 40%. Cryoprecipitate, given in a dose 24 to 36 U/kg (0.24 to 0.39 bags/kg) is followed by half the dose every 12 hours for 3 to 8 days. If possible, treatment should begin 24 hours preoperatively to allow new factor VIII synthesis in addition to the elevation obtained from the therapeutic material. When unanticipated acute bleeding is encountered or immediate cesarean section planned, the initial therapeutic dose should be increased by approximately 50% and a second dose should be given approximately 12 hours later (35). Levels should be checked daily after vaginal delivery or cesarean section and therapy given if the level falls below 25% or bleeding occurs (36–39). The various glycine-precipitated antihemophiliac factors available for treatment of classical hemophilia should not be used in vWD. While they are effective at raising factor VIII levels, they do not correct the bleeding time or ristocetin platelet aggregation defect nor, in fact, clinical bleeding.

In **liver disease** virtually every hemostatic function may be impaired. Deficiencies of prothrombin and of factors VII, IX, and X generally result from decreased synthesis by the damaged liver (40). Factor V and fibrinogen are also synthesized by the liver; however, their levels are usually not so severely depressed. The diversity of the coagulation abnormality will be reflected in the laboratory studies by abnormalities in the aPTT, PT, and fibrinogen levels and by abnormal fibrinolysis.

Treatment consists of both vitamin K administration and procoagulant replacement therapy. Vitamin K can be administered as vitamin K_1 in a dose of 50 mg intramuscularly; it will produce improvement in approximately 30% of patients with liver disease. Replacement therapy is accomplished with fresh frozen plasma in a dose of 10 to 20 $mL \cdot kg^{-1}$ (40).

Factor XI deficiency (plasma thromboplastin antecedent deficiency) is a hereditary disorder transmitted as an incompletely recessive autosomal trait manifested either as a major defect in homozygous individuals with factor XI levels below 20% or as a minor defect in heterozygous individuals with levels ranging from 30% to 65% of normal (41). However, severity of bleeding does not always correlate with the level of factor XI (42–44). The aPTT is usually prolonged in individuals with factor XI deficiency, and the specific diagnosis is confirmed by demonstrating a factor XI level that is below 65% of normal.

Despite the fact that factor XI normally decreases during pregnancy (45), most gravidas do not encounter bleeding problems. In three series, 37 women went through 18 pregnancies without a major hemorrhage (33, 46). Therapy is based on maintaining the factor XI level above 40% for minor procedures (including delivery) and above 50% for major procedures. Treatment consists of a loading dose of fresh frozen plasma of 10 $mL \cdot kg^{-1}$ followed by a maintenance dose of 5 $mL \cdot kg^{-1}$/day. Several authors have reported successful management of factor XI women whose pregnancy was further complicated by the development of factor XI inhibitor (47, 48). **Disseminated intravascular coagulation** is really a syndrome produced as part of an underlying disease that in some way leads to initiation of the clotting mechanisms (49). In the area of obstetrics and gynecology, disseminated intravascular coagulation is seen in association with placental abruption (9), the dead fetus syndrome (50), amniotic fluid embolism (51), gram-negative sepsis (52), saline abortions (53), and severe preeclampsia-eclampsia (54–56).

Laboratory diagnosis is based on demonstrating consumption of procoagulants (57); *(a)* a decrease in fibrinogen, a decrease in platelet count, and variable prolongation of the PT and aPTT, *(b)* demonstration of circulating fibrin-fibrinogen degradation products [prolongation of the total clotting time (TCT) and a positive study for fibrin degradation products]; and *(c)* indirect evidence of obstruction of the microcirculation, such as abnormal red cell morphology (increased red cell fragmentation).

Treatment consists of: *(a)* treatment of the underlying disease, that is, removal of the source of thromboplastin whenever possible; *(b)* administration of procoagulants to replace factors that have been consumed; and (c) anticoagulant therapy with heparin to stop consumption and generation of split products. Heparin is administered in a dose of 500 to 1,000 units/h intravenously after a loading dose of 5,000 units. Laboratory control of heparin therapy may be difficult. However, unless the fibrinogen level is very low, an adequate end point can usually be obtained consisting of an increased TCT or activated clotting time to approximately 1.5 times the control value. Procoagulants can be administered in the form of fresh, platelet-rich plasma following the guidelines above for platelet transfusions. Platelet transfusions are particularly indicated if heparin is to be administered in the face of significant thrombocytopenia ($<30 \times 10^9$/L).

Finally, surgery or delivery in the **anticoagulated patient** must be considered. Patients receiving coumarin anticoagulants will generally withstand minor surgery if the PT is less than 35 seconds and major surgery if the PT is less than 18 seconds (INR less than 1.7). Correction of a bleeding disorder secondary to coumarin therapy is accomplished by withholding the drug and administering vitamin K_1 in a dose of 5 to 50 milligrams

intravenously. Although the larger doses of vitamin K_1 will speed the rate of return to normal, this is accomplished at the cost of making reanticoagulation with coumarin difficult for a week or more. When prompt correction is required, it can also be accomplished by administering fresh frozen plasma, 5 to 8 $mL \cdot kg^{-1}$.

In a number of situations it is desirable to have a patient fully anticoagulated with heparin during delivery or a surgical procedure. If adequate hemostasis becomes a problem, heparin can be discontinued and instantly counteracted by the administration of protamine sulfate in a dose of 50 milligrams intravenously. If bleeding continues following this dose and the thrombin time or activated clotting time is still prolonged, a second dose of 50 milligrams should be given and this regimen repeated as needed until correction is obtained.

HEMOGLOBINOPATHIES

Our understanding of the molecular genetics of the hemoglobinopathies and the ability to make specific diagnoses has unfolded rapidly over the past three decades (58–61). The hemoglobinopathies can be broadly divided into two general types. In the thalassemia syndromes, normal hemoglobin is synthesized at an abnormally slow rate. In contrast, the structural hemoglobinopathies occur because of a specific change in the amino acid content of hemoglobin. These structural changes may have either no effect or profound effects on the function of hemoglobin, including instability of the molecule, reduced solubility, methemoglobinemia, and increased or decreased oxygen affinity.

THALASSEMIA SYNDROMES

The thalassemia syndromes are named and classified by the type of chain that is inadequately produced. The two most common are α- and β-thalassemia, both of which affect the synthesis of hemoglobin A. Reduced synthesis of γ or δ chains and combinations in which two or more globin chains are affected are relatively rare. In each instance, the thalassemia is a quantitative disorder of globin synthesis (62).

α-Thalassemia

In α-thalassemia, one or more structural genes are physically absent from the genome. In the homozygous stage all four genes are deleted and no chains are produced. Thus the fetus is unable to synthesize normal hemoglobin F or any adult hemoglobins. This deficiency results in high output cardiac failure, hydrops fetalis, and stillbirth (63). Because hydrops is frequently associated with severe preeclampsia hydrops fetalis caused by α-thalassemia is a growing health care problem (64).

The most severe form of α-thalassemia compatible with extrauterine life is hemoglobin H disease, which results from deletion of three α genes. In these patients abnormally high quantities of both hemoglobin H (β_4) and hemoglobin Barts (γ_4) accumulate. Because hemoglobin H precipitates within the red cell, the cell is removed by the reticulo-endothelial system, leading to a moderately severe hemolytic anemia.

In α-thalassemia minor (α-thalassemia 1) two genes are deleted, leading to a mild, hypochromic, microcytic anemia that must be differentiated from iron deficiency. A single gene deletion (α-thalassemia 2) is clinically undetectable and is called the "silent carrier" state.

Thus, the α-thalassemias present in the adult as mild, hypochromic, microcytic anemias. Diagnosis is presumptive by exclusion of iron deficiency and β-thalassemia. A specific diagnosis of α-thalassemia trait can be made with restriction endonuclease techniques. However, these studies would only be applicable under special circumstances. Although α-thalassemia does not present a hazard to the adult, it does have serious genetic

Table 18.4. HEMATOLOGIC AND CLINICAL ASPECTS OF THE THALASSEMIA SYNDROMES

	Hemoglobin (Hb) Pattern[a]				
Condition	Hb Level	HbA$_2$	HbF	Other Hb	Clinical Severity
Homozygotes					
α-thalassemia	↓↓↓↓	0	0	80% Hb Barts, remainder Hb H and Hb Portland	Hydrops fetalis
β^+-thalassemia	↓↓↓	Variable	↑↑	Some Hb A	Moderately severe features of Cooley's anemia
β°-thalassemia	↓↓↓↓	Variable	↑↑↑	No Hb A	Severe Cooley's anemia
$\delta\beta^\circ$-thalassemia	↓↓	0	100%	No Hb A	Thalassemia intermedia
Heterozygotes					
α-thalassemia silent carrier	N	N	N	1–2% Hb Barts in cord blood at birth	N
α-thalassemia trait	↓	N	N	5% Hb Barts in cord blood at birth	Very mild
Hb H disease	↓↓	N	N	4–30% Hb H in adults; 25% Hb Barts in cord blood	Thalassemia intermedia
β^+-thalassemia	↓ to ↓↓	↑	↑	None	Mild
β°-thalassemia	↓ to ↓↓	↓	↑↑↑	None	Mild

[a] ↑, increase; ↓, decrease. Number of arrows indicates relative intensity. N, normal.

implications when a mating of two individuals with α-thalassemia trait occurs. Under these circumstances a specific diagnosis must be made using restriction endonuclease techniques or a DNA probe before undertaking antenatal diagnosis (65, 66). One fetus has been treated successfully with intrauterine intravascular exchange transfusions followed by neonatal bone marrow transplantation (67).

β-Thalassemia

In β-thalassemia, no gene deletions have been demonstrated. The best evidence to date suggests that underproduction of β globulin chains is caused by a quantitative reduction in messenger RNA leading to a decreased rate of transcription. In the homozygous β-thalassemia condition, a chain production is unimpeded and these highly unstable chains accumulate and eventually participate. Markedly ineffective erythropoiesis and severe hemolysis result in a condition known as thalassemia major or Cooley's anemia. The fetus is protected from severe disease by γ chain production. However, this protection disappears rapidly after birth, with the affected infant becoming anemic by 3 to 6 months of age. The infant has splenomegaly and requires blood transfusions every 3 to 4 weeks. Death generally occurs by the third decade of life and is usually secondary to myocardial hemochromatosis. Those female infants surviving until puberty are usually amenorrheic with severely impaired fertility (68, 69). However, there are a growing number of successful pregnancies reported in women with β-thalassemia major (70, 71).

β-Thalassemia minor results in a variable degree of illness depending on the rate of β-chain production. The characteristic findings include a relatively high red blood cell (RBC) count, moderate to marked microcytosis, and a peripheral smear resembling iron deficiency. Hemoglobin electrophoresis characteristically shows an elevation of hemoglobin A$_2$. β-Thalassemia trait does not impair fertility, and the incidences of prematurity,

low birth weight infants, and infants of abnormal size for gestational age are identical to those in normal women (72, 73).

Again, the mating of two individuals both heterozygous for β-thalassemia is an indication for antenatal diagnosis. A detailed program of prenatal identification and antenatal diagnosis has been described by Alger and associates (72). The clinical characteristics and hematologic findings of the various thalassemias are summarized in Table 18.4.

STRUCTURAL HEMOGLOBINOPATHIES

To date several hundred variants of α, β, γ, and δ chains have been identified. Most differ from normal chains by only one amino acid. The nomenclature and frequency of the commonest hemoglobinopathies in African-Americans are depicted in Table 18.5 (74). Diagnosis of a specific hemoglobinopathy requires identification of the abnormal hemoglobin utilizing hemoglobin electrophoresis.

Table 18.5. NOMENCLATURE AND FREQUENCY OF THE COMMONEST HEMOGLOBINOPATHIES IN ADULT AFRICAN-AMERICANS

Hemoglobinopathy	Abbreviated Name	Frequency
Sickle cell trait	Hb SA	1:122
Sickle cell anemia	Hb SS	1:708
Sickle cell-hemoglobin C disease	Hb SC	1:757
Hemoglobin C disease	Hb CC	1:4,790
Hemoglobin C trait	Hb CA	1:41
Hemoglobin S-β-thalassemia	Hb Sβ-thal	1:1,672
Hemoglobin S-high F	Hb S-HPFH	1:3,412

Sickle-Cell Trait

Women with sickle-cell trait do well during pregnancy and labor but caution must be observed when using anesthesia to assure good oxygenation. Because there is a two-fold increase in the rate of urinary tract infection, prenatal patients should be screened for asymptomatic bacteriuria (75–77). These patients may become iron deficient, and supplementation during pregnancy is indicated.

Sickle-Cell Anemia

Patients with sickle-cell anemia (SCA) suffer from lifelong complications in part caused by the markedly shortened life span of their red blood cells. Most observers feel that the prepregnancy course of an individual is a good index of how she will do during pregnancy. Although series reported before 1979 indicated a high perinatal mortality and incidence of infants weighing less than 2,500 grams (78, 79), recent series showed generally good fetal outcomes (80, 81). Virtually all of the signs and symptoms of SCA are secondary to either hemolysis, vasoocclusive disease, or an increased susceptibility to infection. Clinical manifestations may affect growth and development, with growth retardation and skeletal changes secondary to expansion of the marrow cavity. Painful crises may occur in the long bones, abdomen, chest, or back (82). The cardiovascular manifestations are those of a hyperdynamic circulation, and pulmonary signs may be secondary either to infection or vasoocclusion. In addition to painful vasoocclusive episodes, patients may exhibit hepatomegaly, signs and symptoms of hepatitis, cholecystitis, and painful splenic infarcts. Genitourinary signs include hyposthenuria, hematuria, and pyelonephritis.

Treatment for patients with sickle-cell anemia has been largely symptomatic, with the major objective being ending a painful crisis and combating infection. Urinary tract and pulmonary infections should be promptly diagnosed and vigorously treated with appropriate antibiotics. During the third trimester, fetal surveillance with either nonstress or stress tests should be carried out regularly.

In addition to red blood cell transfusion, three approaches to treatment have been carefully evaluated in the laboratory and clinically (82). Inhibition of hemoglobin S polymerization by a chemical agent would be an ideal approach. Unfortunately, no anti-sickling agent tested to date has a sufficient benefit as compared to its toxicity to warrant clinical use. Treatment with agents that lower the mean corpuscular hemoglobin concentration by causing an osmotic swelling of the cells is also useful. Clortrimazole is such an agent and has been used successfully in nonpregnant individuals. The third approach is the use of agents that increase hemoglobin F production within the red cells. Both the antineoplastic agents, 5-azacytidine and hydroxyurea, have been tested and found to significantly reduce the frequency and severity of painful crises. Unfortunately, none of these approaches have been used during pregnancy; however, clortrimazole should be safe and the risk-benefit ratio is probably favorable for hydroxyurea. Finally, bone marrow transplantation is a permanent cure for sickle-cell disease.

Transfusion therapy has been used widely for years in the treatment of symptomatic patients with SCA. More recently, partial exchange transfusions and/or prophylactic transfusions have been advocated (76, 83). The transfusion protocol utilized at the author's institution is outlined in Table 18.6. The objective of the partial exchange transfusion is to achieve a hematocrit of greater than 35% and a hemoglobin A level of greater than 40%. Exchange transfusion is repeated when the hematocrit falls to less than 25%, the hemoglobin A level to less than 20%, or crisis or labor occur.

A prospective, randomized study of 72 patients with SCA showed no significant difference in perinatal outcome between women treated with prophylactic transfusion and those

Table 18.6. PROTOCOL FOR PARTIAL EXCHANGE TRANSFUSION

I. Begin at 24–28 weeks of gestation
II. Baseline laboratory studies
  A. Hb, Hct, WBC, reticulocyte count
  B. Hb electrophoresis
III. Type and crossmatch blood: 4 units of fresh, buffy coat-poor, Hb S-free, washed, packed RBCs
IV. Exchange
  A. In morning
    1. Infuse 500 mL of crystalloid over 1–2 h
    2. Remove 500 mL by phlebotomy over same time period
    3. Infuse 2 units of packed RBCs over 1–2 h
  B. In afternoon: Repeat morning procedure
V. Repeat laboratory evaluation following morning
  A. Hb, Hct
  B. Hb electrophoresis
VI. Additional exchange (2–4 units) if
  A. Hct < 35%
  or
  B. Hb A level < 40%

Hb, hemoglobin; Hct, hematocrit; WBC, white blood cell; RBC, red blood cell.

transfused only if their hemoglobin fell below 6 g/dL or hematocrit below 18%.84 Sixty-six patients with sickle cell-hemoglobin C disease and 23 with sickle cell-β-thalassemia were only transfused for hematologic reasons and experienced similar perinatal outcomes. Prophylactic transfusion significantly reduced the incidence of painful crises and other sickle cell disease-related complications. However, the benefits attained must be balanced against a 25% incidence of alloimmunization and 20% delayed transfusion reaction.

By contrast, a retrospective study from the United Kingdom of 81 pregnancies concluded that prophylactic transfusion for women with SCA and a poor obstetric or hematologic history benefited from transfusion and experienced a lower incidence of maternal complications (85).

During labor and delivery, care must be taken to be sure that the patient is well oxygenated and well hydrated. Anesthesia-related hypovolemia and/or hypoxia is contraindicated. In an untransfused patient regional anesthesia should be administered with great caution (86). Careful fetal monitoring should be carried out throughout labor. However, if an exchange transfusion protocol has been utilized and the hemoglobin A level is greater than 40%, painful crises are distinctly unusual (84). Two reports from the Preoperative Transfusion in Sickle Cell Disease Study Group (87, 88) conclude that a conservative transfusion regimen was as effective in preventing perioperative complications. Unfortunately, only five of the 707 patients were pregnant.

Sickle-Cell Hemoglobin SC Disease

Women who are doubly heterozygous for both the hemoglobin S and the hemoglobin C genes are referred to as having hemoglobin SC disease (Hb SCD). Hemoglobin electrophoresis reveals approximately 60% hemoglobin C and 40% hemoglobin S. Patients with Hb SCD generally have a normal habitus, a healthy childhood, and a normal life span. If a systematic screening program has not been utilized, many women are first diagnosed during the latter part of pregnancy when a complication occurs. At the beginning of pregnancy, most women are mildly anemic and splenomegaly is present. Examination of a peripheral blood smear will show numerous target cells. Hemoglobin electrophoresis will ensure the correct diagnosis (89).

During pregnancy, 40% to 60% of patients with Hb SCD will behave as if they had sickle cell anemia. In contrast to patients with SCA, they frequently experience rapid and severe anemic crises due to splenic sequestration. Also, they have a greater

Table 18.7. VARIOUS GENOTYPES OF HEMOGLOBIN E AND THEIR PHENOTYPIC EXPRESSION

Hemoglobin Genotype	Degree of Anemia[a]	MCV[b]	Electrophoresis (%)				Phenotypic Expression
			$A + A_2$	E	F	S	
A/E	0	↓	68	30	<2	0	None
E/E	0 to +	↓↓	<4	94	<2	0	None
E/α-thal	+ to ++	↓	50	15	35	0	None
S/E	++	↓	0	40	0	60	None
E/β+-thal	++	↓↓	10	60	30	0	Splenomegaly
E/β°-thal	+++	↓↓	0	60	40	0	Splenomegaly

[a] Number of + symbols indicates relative severity.

[b] MCV, mean corpuscular volume; number of arrows indicates relative amount of decrease.

tendency to experience bone marrow necrosis with the release of fat-forming marrow emboli. The clinical manifestations of Hb SCD are otherwise similar to SCA but milder. The general management of symptomatic patients with Hb SCD is identical to that for patients with SCA. While several authors have reported good results with vigorous transfusion protocols for all patients with Hb SCD, the author has reserved exchange transfusion for those patients who are either symptomatic or whose hematocrit is less than 25%. Considerations for the management of labor are the same as with SCA.

The Transfusion in Sickle Cell Disease Study Group reported on surgery in 92 patients with Hb SCD and other sickle-variants (90). Four of the patients were pregnant. They concluded that preoperative transfusion should be used selectively. It is noteworthy that one of the two deaths occurred in a 35-year-old woman with Hb SCD who underwent a cesarean section for fetal distress. Her hemoglobin was 10 g/dL preoperatively and she was not transfused. A 50% placental abruption was discovered at surgery and she developed respiratory failure on the first postoperative day.

Hemoglobin S-β-Thalassemia

In this condition the patient is heterozygous for the sickle cell and the β-thalassemia gene. In addition to decreased β chain production, there is a variably increased production of hemoglobin F and hemoglobin A₂. Because of this variable production rate, hemoglobin electrophoresis reveals a spectrum of hemoglobin concentrations. Hemoglobin S may account for 70% to 95% of the hemoglobin present, with hemoglobin F rarely exceeding 20% (91). Because of the thalassemia influence, hemoglobin S concentration exceeds hemoglobin A concentration. This is in sharp contrast to patients with sickle-cell trait, in whom hemoglobin A levels exceed the concentration of hemoglobin S.

The diagnosis is made in an anemic patient by demonstrating increased hemoglobin A₂ and hemoglobin F levels in association with level of hemoglobin S exceeding that of hemoglobin A. The peripheral smear reveals hypochromia and microcytosis with anisocytosis, poikilocytosis, basophilic stippling, and target cells. The clinical manifestations of this disorder parallel SCA but are generally milder. Painful crises may occur; however, these patients have a normal body habitus and frequently enjoy an uncompromised life span. The author believes that the role of exchange transfusion should be similar to that in patients with Hb SCD. That is, exchange transfusion is reserved for the woman who experiences painful crises or whose anemia leads to a hematocrit of less than 25%.

Hemoglobin C Trait and Disease

Hemoglobin C trait is an asymptomatic trait without reproductive consequences. Target cells are found in the peripheral

smear but anemia is not present. Hemoglobin C disease is the homozygous state and is a mild disorder usually discovered during a medical evaluation. Mild hemolytic anemia with a hematocrit in the range of 25% to 35% is characteristic. The red blood cells show microspherocytes and characteristic targeting. There is no increased morbidity or mortality associated with pregnancy and no specific therapy is indicated.

Hemoglobin E Disease

The recent resettlement of individuals of Southeast Asian extraction has resulted in an increase in the number of persons with hemoglobin E trait and disease. The clinical and laboratory manifestations of the various hemoglobin E syndromes are outlined in Table 18.7 (92, 93). Most individuals have a mild, microcytic anemia that is of no clinical significance and requires no treatment. Those individuals homozygous for hemoglobin E have a greater degree of microcytosis and are frequently anemic. Target cells are prominent. Like hemoglobin C trait and disease, no specific therapy is required and reproductive outcome is normal.

REFERENCES

1. Shattil SJ, Bennett JS. Platelets and their membranes in hemostasis: physiology and pathophysiology. *Ann Intern Med* 1981;94:108–118.
2. Colman RW, Hirsh J, Marder VJ, et al. *Hemostasis and Thrombosis.* Philadelphia: J. B. Lippincott, 1987.
3. Bick RL, Kaplan H. Syndromes of thrombosis and hypercoagulability. *Med Clin North Am* 1998;82:409–458.
4. Florell SR, Rodgers GM. Inherited thrombotic disorders: an update. *Am J Hematol* 1997;54:53–60.
5. Rosendahl GR. Risk factors for venous thrombosis: prevalence, risk and interaction. *Semin Hematol* 1997;34:171–187.
6. American College of Obstetricians and Gynecologists. *Antiphospholipid syndrome. ACOG Educational Bulletin* 1988; no. 244.
7. Lockshin MD. Antiphospholipid antibody. Babies, blood clots, biology. *JAMA* 1997;277:1549–1551.
8. Khamashta MA, Cuadrado MJ, Mujuc F, et al. The management of thrombosis in the antiphospholipid-antibody syndrome. *N Engl J Med* 1995;332:993–997.
9. Rodgers RPC, Levin J. A critical reappraisal of the bleeding time. *Semin Thromb Hemost* 1990;16:1–20.
10. Lind SE. The bleeding time does not predict surgical bleeding. *Blood* 1991;77:2547–2552.
11. American Society of Anesthesiologists. *Transfusion Practices,* 3rd ed. Park Ridge, IL: Committee on Transfusion Medicine, 1998.
12. Development Task Force of the College of American Pathologists. Fresh-Frozen Plasma, Cryoprecipitate, and Platelets Administration Practice Guidelines: Practice parameter for the use of fresh-frozen plasma, cryoprecipitate, and platelets. *JAMA* 1994;271:777–781.
13. Cash JD. Platelet transfusion therapy. *Clin Hematol* 1972;1:395–411.
14. Laros RK Jr, Kagan R. Route of delivery for patients with immune thrombocytopenia purpura. *Am J Obstet Gynecol* 1984;148:901–908.

15. Cook RL, Miller RC, Katz VL, et al. Immune thrombocytopenic purpura in pregnancy: a reappraisal of management. *Obstet Gynecol* 1981;78:578–583.

16. Tarantino MD, Goldsmith G. Treatment of acute thrombocytopenic purpura. *Semin Hematol* 1998;35(suppl 1):28–35.

17. Kagan R, Laros RK Jr. Immune thrombocytopenia. *Clin Obstet Gynecol* 1983;26:537–546.

18. Payne SD, Resnik R, Moore TR, et al. Maternal characteristics and risk of severe neonatal thrombocytopenia and intracranial hemorrhage in pregnancies complicated by autoimmune thrombocytopenia. *Am J Obstet Gynecol* 1997;177:149–155.

19. Scott JR, Gruikshank DP, Kochenour NK, et al. Fetal platelet counts in the obstetric management of immunologic thrombocytopenic purpura. *Am J Obstet Gynecol* 1980;136:495–499.

20. Moise KL Jr, Carpenter RJ Jr, Cotton DB, et al. Percutaneous umbilical cord blood sampling in the evaluation of fetal platelet counts in pregnant patients with autoimmune thrombocytopenia purpura. *Obstet Gynecol* 1988;72:346–350.

21. Scioscia AL, Grannum PAT, Copel JA, et al. The use of percutaneous umbilical blood sampling in immune thrombocytopenic purpura. *Am J Obstet Gynecol* 1988;159:1066–1068.

22. Samuels P, Bussel JB, Braitman LE, et al. Estimation of the risk of thrombocytopenia in the offspring of pregnant women with presumed immune thrombocytopenic purpura. *N Engl J Med* 1990;323:229–235.

23. Kelton JG, Inwood MJ, Barr RM, et al. The prenatal prediction of thrombocytopenia in infants of mothers with clinically diagnosed immune thrombocytopenia. *Am J Obstet Gynecol* 1982;144:449–454.

24. Bussel JB, Zabusky MR, Berkowitz RL, et al. Fetal alloimmune thrombocytopenia. *N Engl J Med* 1997;337:22–26.

25. Waldman SD, Feldstein GS, Waldman HJ, et al. Caudal administration of morphine sulfate in anticoagulated and thrombocytopenic patients. *Anesth Analg* 1987;66:267–271.

26. Rolbin SH, Abbott D, Musclow E, et al. Epidural anesthesia in pregnant patients with low platelet counts. *Obstet Gynecol* 1988;71:918–920.

27. Rasmus KT, Rottman RL, Kotelko DM, et al. Unrecognized thrombocytopenia in parturients: A retrospective review. *Obstet Gynecol* 1989;71:943–946.

28. Hew-Wing R, Rolbin SH, Hew E, et al. Epidural anesthesia and thrombocytopenia. *Anaesthesia* 1989;44:775–782.

29. Beilin Y, Zahn J, Comerford M. Safe epidural analgesia in thirty parturients with platelet counts between 69,000 and 98,000 mm³. *Anesth Analg* 1997;85:385–388.

30. Simon L, Santi TM, Sacquin P, et al. Pre-anesthetic assessment of coagulation abnormalities in obstetric patients: usefulness, timing and clinical implications. *Br J Anaesth* 1997;78:678–683.

31. Veltkamp JJ, van Tilburg NH. Autosomal hemophilia. *Br J Haematol* 1984;26:141–152.

32. Weiss HJ, Hoyer LW, Rickles FR, et al. Quantitative assay of a plasma factor deficient in von Willebrand's disease that is necessary for platelet aggregation. *J Clin Invest* 1973;52:2708–2716.

33. Kadir RA, Lee CA, Sabin CA, et al. Pregnancy in women with von Willebrand's disease or factor XI deficiency. *Br J Obstet Gynaecol* 1998;105:314–321.

34. Sadler JE, Gralnick HR. Commentary: a new classification for von Willebrand disease. *Blood* 1994;84:676–679.

35. Shulman NR. The physiologic basis for therapy of classic hemophilia and related disorders. *Ann Intern Med* 1967;67:856–882.

36. Noller KL, Bowie EJW, Kempers RD, et al. Von Willebrand's disease in pregnancy. *Obstet Gynecol* 1973;41:865–872.

37. Krishanamurth M, Miotti AB. Von Willebrand's disease and pregnancy. *Obstet Gynecol* 1977;49:244–247.

38. Lipton RA, Ayromlooi J, Coller BS. Severe von Willebrand's disease during labor and delivery. *JAMA* 1982;248:1355–1357.

39. Cohen S, Goldiner PL. Epidural analgesia for labor and delivery in a patient with von Willebrand disease. *Reg Anesth* 1989;14:95–97.

40. Spector I, Corn M. Laboratory tests of hemostasis: the relation to hemorrhage in liver disease. *Arch Intern Med* 1967;119:577–582.

41. Leiba H, Ramot B, Many A. Heredity and coagulation studies in ten families with Factor XI deficiency. *Br J Haematol* 1965;11:654–665.

42. Rimon A, Schiffman S, Feinstein D, et al. Factor XI activity and Factor XI antigen in homozygous and heterozygous Factor XI deficiency. *Blood* 1976;48:165–174.

43. Purcell G, Nossel HL. Factor XI (PTA) deficiency. *Obstet Gynecol* 1970;35:69–74

44. Litz CE, Swaim WR, Dalmasso AP. Factor XI deficiency: genetic and clinical studies of a single kindred. *Am J Hematol* 1988;28:8–12.

45. Phillips LL, Rosano L, Skrodelis V. Changes in Factor XI levels during pregnancy. *Am J Obstet Gynecol* 1973;116:1114–1116.

46. Rapaport SI, Proctor RR, Patch MJ, et al. The mode of inheritance of PTA disease. *Blood* 1961;18:149–174.

47. Connelly NR, Brull SJ. Anesthetic management of a patient with factor XI deficiency and factor XI inhibitor undergoing a cesarean section. *Anesth Analg* 1993;76:1365–1366.

48. Ginsberg SS, Clyne LP, McPhedran P, et al. Successful childbirth by a patient with congenital factor XI deficiency and an acquired inhibitor. *Br J Haematol* 1993;84:172–174.

49. Laros RK Jr, ed. *Blood Disorders in Pregnancy*. Philadelphia, Lea & Febiger, 1986.

50. Sutton DMC, Hauser R, Kulaping S, et al. Intravascular coagulation in abruptio placentae. *Am J Obstet Gynecol* 1971;109:604–614.

51. Phillips LL, Skrodelis V, Kers TA. Hypofibrinogenemia and intrauterine fetal death. *Am J Obstet Gynecol* 1964;89:903–914.

52. Phillips LL, Davidson EC. Procoagulant properties of amniotic fluid. *Am J Obstet Gynecol* 1972;113:911–919.

53. Phillips LL, Skrodelis V, Quigley HJ. Intravascular coagulation in septic abortion. *Obstet Gynecol* 1967;30:350.

54. Laros RK Jr, Penner JA. Pathophysiology of disseminated intravascular coagulation in saline-induced abortion. *Obstet Gynecol* 1976;48:353–356.

55. Davidson EC, Phillips LL. Coagulation studies in the hypertensive toxemias of pregnancy. *Am J Obstet Gynecol* 1972;113:905–910.

56. Pritchard JA, Cunningham FG, Mason RA. Coagulation changes in eclampsia. *Am J Obstet Gynecol* 1976;124:855–864.

57. Carey MJ, Rodgers GM. Disseminated intravascular coagulation: clinical and laboratory aspects. *Am J Hematol* 1998;59:65–73.

58. Bunn HF, Forget BJ. *Human Hemoglobins*. Philadelphia: Saunders, 1986.

59. Weatherall DJ, Clegg JB. *The Thalassemia Syndromes*, 2nd ed. Oxford, U.K.: Blackwell Scientific, 1981.

60. Steinberg MH, Adams JG. Thalassemia: recent insights into molecular mechanisms. *Am J Hematol* 1982;12:81–92.

61. Beris P, Darbellay R, Extermann P. Prevention of β-thalassemia major and Hb Bart's hydrops fetalis syndrome. *Semin Hematol* 1995;32:244–261.

62. Kilpatrick SJ, Laros RK. Thalassemia in pregnancy. *Clin Obstet Gynecol* 1995;38:485–496.

63. Higgs DR, Vickers MA, Wilkie AOM, et al. A review of the molecular genetics of the human α-globin gene cluster. *Blood* 1989;73:1081–1104.

64. Chui DHK, Waye JS. Hydrops fetalis caused by α-thalassemia: an emerging health care problem. *Blood* 1998;7:2213–2222.

65. Miller JM. Alpha thalassemia minor in pregnancy. *J Reprod Med* 1982;27:207–209.

66. Kan YW, Golbus MS, Dozy AM. Prenatal diagnosis of alpha-thalassemia. *N Engl J Med* 1976;295:1165–1167.

67. Carr S, Rubin L, Dixon D, et al. Intrauterine therapy for homozygous α-thalassemia. *Obstet Gynecol* 1995;85:876–879.

68. Kazazian HH, Boehm CD. Molecular basis and prenatal diagnosis of β-thalassemia. *Blood* 1988; 72:1107–1116.

69. Fosburg MT, Nathan DG. Treatment of Cooley's anemia. *Blood* 1991;76:435–444.

70. Jensen CE, Tuck SM, Wonke B. Fertility in β-thalassemia major: a report of 16 pregnancies, preconceptual evaluation and a review of the literature. *Br J Obstet Gynaecol* 1995;102:625–629.

71. Kumar RM, Rizk DEE, Khuranna A. β-Thalassemia major and successful pregnancy. *J Reprod Med* 1997;42:294–298.

72. Alger LS, Golbus MS, Laros RK Jr. Thalassemia and pregnancy. *Am J Obstet Gynecol* 1979;134:662–673.

73. Fleming AF, Lynch W. Beta-thalassemia minor during pregnancy with particular reference to iron status. *J Obstet Gynaecol Br Common* 1967;76:451–457.

74. Motulsky AG. Frequency of sickling disorders in U.S. Blacks. *N Engl J Med* 1973;288:31–33.

75. Whalley PJ, Pritchard JA, Richards JR. Sickle cell trait and pregnancy. *JAMA* 1963;186:1132–1135.

76. Blattner P, Dar H, Nitowski HM. Pregnancy outcome in women with sickle cell trait. *JAMA* 1977;238:1392–1394.

77. Whalley PJ, Martin FG, Pritchard JA. Sickle cell trait and urinary tract infections during pregnancy. *JAMA* 1964;189:903–906.

78. Horger E. Sickle cell and sickle cell-hb C disease during pregnancy. *Obstet Gynecol* 1972;39:873–876.

79. Pritchard JA, Scott DE, Whalley PJ, et al. The effects of maternal sickle cell hemoglobinopathies and sickle cell trait on reproductive performance. *Am J Obstet Gynecol* 1973;117:662–670.

80. Morrison JC, Wiser WL. The use of prophylactic partial exchange transfusion in pregnancies associated with sickle cell hemoglobinopathies. *Obstet Gynecol* 1976;48:516–520.

81. Cunningham FG, Pritchard JA, Mason RA. Pregnancy and sickle cell hemoglobinopathies. *Obstet Gynecol* 1983;62:419–424.

82. Bunn HF. Pathogenesis and treatment of sickle cell disease. *N Engl J Med* 1997;11:762–769.

83. Francis RB, Johnson CS. Vascular occlusion in sickle cell disease: current concepts and unanswered questions. *Blood* 1991;77:1405–1414.

84. Koshy M, Burd L, Wallace D, et al. Prophylactic red-cell transfusion in pregnant patients with sickle cell disease. *N Engl J Med* 1988;319:1447–1452.

85. Howard RJ, Tuck SM, Pearson TC. Pregnancy in sickle cell disease in the U.K.: results of a multicentre survey of the effect of prophylactic blood transfusion on maternal and fetal outcome. *Br J Obstet Gynaecol* 1995;102:947–951.

86. Cunningham FG, Pritchard JA, Mason RA, et al. Prophylactic transfusion of normal red blood cells during pregnancy complicated by sickle cell hemoglobinopathies. *Am J Obstet Gynecol* 1979;135:994–1003.

87. Koshy M, Weiner SJ, Miller ST, et al. Surgery and anesthesia in sickle cell disease. *Blood* 1995;86:3676–3684.

88. Vichinsky EP, Haberkern CM, Neumayr L, et al. A comparison of conservative and aggressive transfusion regimens in the perioperative management of sickle cell disease. *N Engl J Med* 1995;333:206–213.

89. Maduska AL, Guinee WS, Heaton AJ, et al. Sickling dynamics of red blood cells and other physiologic studies during anesthesia. *Anesth Analg* 1975;54:361–364.

90. Neumayr L, Koshy M, Haberkern C, et al. Surgery in patients with hemoglobin SC disease. *Am J Hematol* 1998;57:101–108.

91. Finer P, Blair J, Rowe P. Epidural analgesia in the management of labor pain and sickle cell crisis—a case report. *Anesthesiology* 1988;68:799–800.

92. Wong SC, Ali MAM. Hemoglobin E disease. *Am J Hematol* 1982;13:15–21.

93. Ferguson JE, O'Reilly RA. Hemoglobin E and pregnancy. *Obstet Gynecol* 1985;66:136.

Shnider and Levinson's Anesthesia for Obstetrics,
edited by Samuel C. Hughes, et al.
Lippincott Williams & Wilkins,
Philadelphia, © 2001.

CHAPTER 19

AMNIOTIC FLUID EMBOLISM

VALERIE A. ARKOOSH, M.D.

Amniotic fluid embolism (AFE) is a rare but catastrophic complication of pregnancy. Meyer published the first report of this syndrome in 1926 (1). AFE, however, did not become widely recognized until the 1941 publication of a detailed report of eight parturients dying of sudden shock during labor and delivery (2). Since these original descriptions, numerous case reports have attributed sudden maternal death to AFE. Confounding all of these reports is the fact that AFE syndrome remains a diagnosis of exclusion. Review of recent literature suggests that the historical concept of an actual embolism of amniotic fluid producing the clinical syndrome is not accurate. More likely, AFE is an anaphylactoid type of reaction that occurs in susceptible patients. Despite numerous attempts at understanding AFE syndrome, the exact pathophysiology, pathogenesis, and a reliable means of diagnosis remain elusive.

INCIDENCE AND MORTALITY

Several surveys have attempted to quantify the incidence of and mortality due to this syndrome. The original article by Steiner and Lushbaugh estimated that AFE occurred in approximately one in 8,000 obstetric cases (2). More recent data suggests that the incidence is much lower. Amniotic Fluid Embolism (AFE) was the attributed cause of 7.8% ($n = 10$) of the maternal deaths in the United Kingdom between 1991 and 1993, equating to 4.3 deaths from AFE per million pregnancies (3). During the 2-year period between January 1, 1994 and December 31, 1995, signs and symptoms consistent with AFE occurred with a frequency of one per 20,646 deliveries in California (4). Even this incidence may in fact be lower than actually occurs as it is likely that minor episodes that spontaneously resolve are either not recognized or not reported.

Significant maternal mortality is associated with the occurrence of AFE. Early reviews describe a nearly 100% mortality (5–7). Recent advances in critical care medicine and an improved understanding of the syndrome appear to be having a positive impact on overall maternal survival. Maternal mortality was 61% in Clark's 1983 to 1995 national registry survey of 46 patients who met strict criteria for the diagnosis of AFE (Table 19.1) (8). However, only seven (15%) of the 46 patients survived neurologically intact. Of the fetuses in utero at the time of the event, 79% survived but only 39% were neurologically intact (8). In the more recent 1994 to 1995 California survey, maternal mortality was 26.4% (4). Maternal outcome was also improved with 87% of survivors discharged home without obvious sequelae.

CLINICAL PRESENTATION AND DIAGNOSIS

AFE has been reported to occur during first trimester curettage abortion (9–11), second trimester abortion with saline (12), prostaglandin or urea (10), amniocentesis (13), spontaneously during the third trimester, during labor, during cesarean delivery, postpartum (14), and with abdominal trauma (15, 16). Advanced maternal age, multiparity, a large fetus, meconium-stained fluid, oxytocin use, hyperstimulated labor, placental abruption, uterine rupture and intrauterine fetal death have historically been considered predisposing conditions for AFE (6).

However, in two recent reviews, none of these conditions correlated with AFE (8, 15), making prediction of patients at risk virtually impossible.

Supporting an immunologic basis for this syndrome, in Clark's national registry of 46 patients there was a significant relationship between AFE and male fetal sex. Additionally, 41% of women gave a history of allergy or atopy (8). Other findings of note include the lack of a relationship between oxytocin use or antecedent uterine hyperstimulation and AFE. Uterine hypertonus, however, frequently accompanied the symptoms of AFE. Given that uterine hypoxia may induce myometrial hypertonus, (17), Clark theorizes that hypertonus, associated with AFE is a result of the initial maternal hemodynamic response to a profound cardiovascular insult rather than the cause of AFE (8).

The classic triad of AFE includes acute hypoxia, hemodynamic collapse and coagulopathy without an obvious precipitating cause. Patients, however, can present with a broad range of signs and symptoms (Table 19.2). The time course of the appearance of symptoms is also highly variable. Patients may present with what initially appears to be an isolated coagulopathy (18) or isolated hypoxemia (19, 20). Related signs and symptoms may not manifest for several hours. The differential diagnosis of AFE includes pulmonary thromboembolism, venous air embolism, septic or hypovolemic shock, myocardial infarction, peripartum cardiomyopathy, uterine rupture, eclampsia, local anesthetic toxicity, placental abruption, cerebral vascular accident, aspiration pneumonia and anaphylaxis (Table 19.3).

Initial diagnosis of AFE must be based on a high index of suspicion and the clinical signs and symptoms of hypoxia, hypotension and coagulopathy. A chest radiograph may be normal or show diffuse pulmonary edema (21). Unfortunately, there is no definitive test to diagnose AFE in a clinically useful time period. In the late 1970s and early 1980s, the finding of fetal squamous cells in a blood sample aspirated from the distal port of a "wedged" pulmonary artery catheter was considered pathognomonic of AFE (22–25). Shortly thereafter, several case series described the presence of amniotic fluid material and squamous cells in the pulmonary aspirate of normal parturients (26–28). Squamous cells were also found, and considered a contaminant, in nonpregnant patients with central monitoring (29, 30). **Current consensus concludes that the presence of amniotic fluid material in the maternal pulmonary circulation is not pathognomonic for AFE.**

Japanese investigators have developed a monoclonal antibody directed against a glycoprotein found in meconium and amniotic fluid. This immunostaining is more sensitive than hematoxylin-eosin or Alcian blue staining in detecting amniotic fluid derived mucin in lung sections and can also be used to detect this mucin in maternal serum (31, 32). A noninvasive test detects the presence of zinc coproporphyrin, a component of meconium, in maternal plasma. A level above 35 nmol/L is diagnostic for AFE. These tests are currently not available in the United States.

If a postmortem diagnosis of AFE is sought, special tissue staining and analysis is often necessary. Staining with antiserum to human keratin, immunoperoxidase, rhodamine B fluorescence, and immunohistochemical analysis have all been described as sensitive methods of demonstrating squamous cells (33–36).

Table 19.1. AMNIOTIC FLUID EMBOLISM REGISTRY ENTRY CRITERIA

Acute hypotension or cardiac arrest

Acute hypoxia, defined as dyspnea, cyanosis, or respiratory arrest

Coagulopathy, defined as laboratory evidence of intravascular consumption or severe clinical hemorrhage in the absence of other explanations[a]

Onset of the above during labor, cesarean section, or dilation and evacuation or within 30 min postpartum

Absence of any other significant confounding condition or potential explanation for the signs and symptoms observed

Occurrence within 5 years of registry opening

---

[a] Patients meeting all other criteria, including abrupt cardiorespiratory arrest, who died before coagulopathy could be assessed were included in the primary analysis.
From Clark SL, Hankins GDV, Dudley DA, et al. Amniotic fluid embolism: analysis of the national registry. *Am J Obstet Gynecol* 1995;172:1158–1169, with permission.

PATHOPHYSIOLOGY

There are no animal models of AFE syndrome that mimic exactly the clinical symptoms seen in parturients suspected of having an AFE. Most animal models of AFE find pulmonary vasospasm and pulmonary hypertension accompanied by right heart failure to be the principal hemodynamic alteration in AFE syndrome (37–39). Although occasional case reports suggest that AFE in humans can be associated with noncardiogenic pulmonary edema (40, 41), the majority of human reports find mild to moderate increases in pulmonary artery pressure, variable increases in central venous pressure, increased pulmonary capillary wedge pressures and left ventricular dysfunction or failure to be the predominate hemodynamic abnormalities (42–47). However, unlike animal models in which pulmonary artery catheters are in place at the time of the event, central hemodynamic data

Table 19.2. SIGNS AND SYMPTOMS OF AMNIOTIC FLUID EMBOLISM

Sign/Symptom	No. of Patients	Percentage of Patients
Hypotension	46	100
Fetal distress (n = 30 fetuses in utero at time of event)	30	100
Pulmonary edema or adult respiratory distress syndrome	28	93
Cardiopulmonary arrest	40	87
Cyanosis	38	83
Coagulopathy (n = 38 patients surviving long enough to confirm diagnosis)	38	83
Dyspnea (n = 45. One patient already intubated at time of event)	22	49
Seizure	22	48
Uterine atony	11	23
Bronchospasm	7	15
Transient hypertension	5	11
Cough	3	7
Headache	3	7
Chest pain	1	2
Dysrhythmias		
Electromechanical dissociation	11	24
Bradycardia	10	22
Ventricular tachycardia of fibrillation	8	17
Asystole	6	13
Not described	3	7
None	8	17

Data from Clark SL, Hankins GDV, Dudley DA, et al. Amniotic fluid embolism: analysis of the national registry. *Am J Obstet Gynecol* 1995;172:1158–1169.

Table 19.3. DIFFERENTIAL DIAGNOSIS OF AMNIOTIC FLUID EMBOLISM

Pulmonary thromboembolism

Venous air embolism

Septic or hypovolemic shock

Myocardial infarction

Peripartum cardiomyopathy

Uterine rupture

Eclampsia

Local anesthetic toxicity

Placental abruption

Cerebral vascular accident

Aspiration pneumonia

Anaphylaxis

---

in humans is typically obtained more than one hour after the event and from the subset of women who have survived the initial insult. In the most carefully-conducted study to date, pregnant goats receiving autologous amniotic fluid ± meconium experienced maximal central hemodynamic effects within 10 minutes of amniotic fluid injection. These changes had generally resolved by 30 minutes (48). Changes included marked increase in pulmonary vascular resistance, systemic vascular resistance, systolic, diastolic and mean arterial blood pressure, systolic and diastolic pulmonary artery pressure. In the goats receiving amniotic fluid that contained meconium, there was also a marked increase in the pulmonary capillary wedge pressure and a fall in cardiac output to 40% of baseline at 10 minutes. Oxygenation was severely adversely effected by amniotic fluid containing meconium. Unlike the hemodynamic changes, which essentially resolved by 30 minutes, changes in oxygenation showed no signs of resolution at three hours after injection. One can hypothesize that similar immediate hemodynamic changes occur in parturients but go undetected due to the lack of central monitoring at the time of the event.

In an attempt to reconcile the animal and human data, Clark has suggested a biphasic clinical presentation in humans (49). Consistent with the animal models, parturients may experience pulmonary vasospasm with associated severe hypoxemia and right heart failure as the initial perturbation following exposure to amniotic fluid. This severe hypoxemia may explain why few women who survive an AFE do so neurologically intact (8). In those who do survive, these initial changes have resolved by the time that central hemodynamic monitoring is instituted. A secondary phase characterized by left ventricular failure, adult respiratory distress syndrome and disseminated intravascular coagulation then ensues (Table 19.4). Left ventricular

Table 19.4. HEMODYNAMIC INDICES IN PATIENTS WITH AMNIOTIC FLUID EMBOLISM

Case	MPAP (mm Hg)	PCWP (mm Hg)	PVR (dynes/s/cm^{-5})	LVWSI (g/m/M^2)
1	20	14	83	Clinical LVF
2	31	26	206	Clinical LVF
3	27	21	86	33
4	23	14	277	Nuclear scan: LVF
5	27	18		Clinical LVF
6	29	19	138	19
7	18	16	133	3
8	42	31	215	12
9	21	16	137	31

MPAP, mean pulmonary artery pressure; PCWP, pulmonary capillary wedge pressure; PVR, pulmonary vascular resistance; LVSWI, left ventricular stroke work index; LVF, left ventricular failure.
From Clark SL. Amniotic fluid embolism. In: Clark SL, Phelan JP, Cotton DB, eds. *Critical Care Obstetrics* Oradell, NJ: Medical Economics Books, 1987:320, with permission.

Table 19.5. BLOOD COAGULATION AND LABORATORY TESTS IN DISSEMINATED INTRAVASCULAR COAGULATION

	Normal Values during Pregnancy	Disseminated Intravascular Coagulation
Plasma fibrinogen	400–650 mg/dL	<150 mg/dL
Platelet count	150,000–300,000/mm^3	<50,000/mm^3
Thrombin time	15–20 sec	>100 sec
Prothrombin time	10–12 sec	>100 sec
Partial thromboplastin time	35–50 sec	>100 sec
Fibrin degradation products	<16 μg/mL	>200 μg/mL
Fibrin degradation product dillution	1:4	> 1:128
Red blood cell fragmentation	No	Yes

depression may be due to a decrease in coronary artery blood flow in the presence of AFE (50) or to a direct myocardial depressant effect of amniotic fluid.

Although coagulopathy (DIC) (Table 19.5) will develop in 40% to 50% of patients who survive the initial event, it does not occur in the majority of animal studies. Bleeding diathesis alone is the presenting symptom in 10% to 15% of AFE cases (49). Some patients will have only a subclinical coagulopathy manifested by a transient rise in fibrin split products or fall in platelet count. Coagulopathy is often compounded by uterine atony.

In sum, the typical clinical presentation is biphasic. The initial phase consists of severe hemodynamic instability or collapse with hypoxemia followed by (in those surviving) left ventricular failure, a variable elevation of pulmonary artery pressure and coagulopathy.

PATHOGENESIS

Given that fetal squamous cells and other amniotic fluid material is found in the maternal circulation of most parturients, the question of what triggers the clinical syndrome of AFE persists. Compounding the difficulty in answering this question has been the inability to produce a reliable animal model of human AFE. Several whole animal studies performed in the 1950s and 1960s documented hypoxia, pulmonary vasoconstriction and right heart failure following the intravascular injection of amniotic fluid. Most of these studies, however, gave human amniotic fluid stored for some period of time to a nonhuman species and some recipient animals were male or nonpregnant females. Looking at the studies that gave autologous amniotic fluid to pregnant animals, the results vary by species. In two studies of term-pregnant sheep, given their own amniotic fluid in 150 mL aliquots, there was an immediate and severe decrease in systemic vascular resistance accompanied by a significant increase in pulmonary vascular resistance (38, 39). Neither study found evidence of a direct depressant effect on myocardial contractility. Conversely, in two primate studies and one study in rabbits, all given autologous amniotic fluid, the infusion of amniotic fluid with or without meconium was completely innocuous (51–53), suggesting that it may not be amniotic fluid per se that causes the syndrome but, some abnormality within it. Using the pregnant goat model, left ventricular dysfunction and dysoxia were observed only with embolism of amniotic fluid containing meconium (48). In sum, the animal studies do little to clarify the etiology of the clinical syndrome seen in humans other than to suggest that there is an as yet unidentified humoral factor present in amniotic fluid that triggers the syndrome in some patients.

Results from in vitro studies are also inconsistent and vary with species. In humans, Verdernikov failed to detect any con-

tractile or relaxant effect of amniotic fluid supernatant on an isolated omental artery taken from term parturients at cesarean delivery (54). In gravid ewes, filtered ewe amniotic fluid did not produce any direct depressant effect on cardiac contractility in the isolated ewe heart (37). However, in the same animals, when the systemic and pulmonary circulations were isolated and perfused separately, amniotic fluid produced changes only on the circulation into which it was injected. Pulmonary vascular resistance increased 72% following injection into the pulmonary circulation with no change in the systemic circulation. Systemic vascular resistance decreased 32% following perfusion of the systemic circulation with no change in pulmonary vascular resistance. These authors also concluded that it is a humoral factor found in amniotic fluid that produces the reported changes in pulmonary and systemic vascular resistance.

Several mediators including endothelin and the *leukotrienes* have been suggested as the humoral factors causing the clinical syndrome. Endothelin is a highly-potent vasoconstrictor peptide present in amniotic fluid. It reaches maximum concentration in the amniotic fluid during labor. In both pregnant and nonpregnant rabbits intravenous injection of meconium-stained human amniotic fluid, whole raw amniotic fluid and the supernatant of amniotic fluid produces significant increases in circulating endothelin levels (55). Rabbits injected with the precipitate of amniotic fluid remaining after centrifugation experienced no change in endothelin levels. Endothelin produces sustained contraction of porcine coronary arteries and increases left atrial pressure and decreases cardiac output in a canine model (56, 57). Thus, these authors conclude that endothelin may mediate the early pathological changes in human AFE.

Given the similarities between the hemodynamic symptoms of AFE and those seen with anaphylaxis, leukotriene (slow-reacting substance) must also be considered a potential mediator. Human amniotic fluid injected into nonpregnant rabbits caused dyspnea, convulsions, urinary incontinence, shock and death (58). Extracts from the lungs of these animals all contained leukotriene. A second group of rabbits were given a selective 5-lipoxygenase inhibitor, which inhibits leukotriene production, prior to being injected with amniotic fluid. Some of these rabbits showed the same symptoms as the control group but none died. Leukotriene activity was not present in the lung extract from these animals. Interestingly, unlike the above study which found no change in endothelin levels following injection of amniotic fluid precipitate, the rabbits in this study that received amniotic fluid precipitate had the same symptoms as the amniotic fluid group. All died within 4 minutes and exhibited leukotriene-like activity in the lung extracts. Additional support for leukotriene as a mediator comes from an in vitro study showing that amniotic fluid surfactant enhances leukotriene production by both white blood cells and the lung (59).

The etiology of coagulopathy in AFE is also unclear and the studies somewhat confusing. In vitro studies of amniotic fluid have shown a shortened whole blood clotting time, a thromboplastin-like effect, induction of platelet aggregation, a release of platelet factor III, a direct factor X-activating factor, presence of tissue factor and activation of the complement cascade (49, 60, 61). Supernatant samples of human amniotic fluid from both midtrimester and third trimester pregnancies added to whole blood from nonpregnant volunteers resulted in accelerated clot initiation and propagation as measured by the thromboelastogram (62). Yet, one study concluded that although amniotic fluid has factor X-activating properties, the amount of procoagulant in clear amniotic fluid is insufficient to cause significant clinical intravascular coagulation (63).

In sum, the pathogenesis of amniotic fluid embolism remains unclear. No single unifying hypothesis can be drawn from the animal data, as many of the studies are contradictory. Interpretation is further complicated by the studies that use heterologous amniotic fluid and nongravid animals in the model. The applicability of these studies to the human AFE syndrome may be

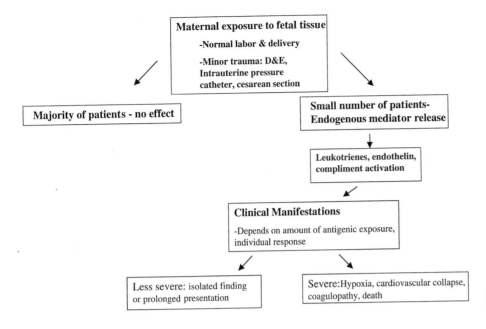

Figure 19.1. Proposed maternal immunologic response to amniotic fluid exposure.

limited. After extensive review of the 46 patients submitted to the national registry, Clark felt the data suggested that the AFE syndrome is, from a clinical standpoint, similar to anaphylaxis and septic shock and that there may be a common underlying mechanism (8). He proposes that AFE be described as **anaphylactoid syndrome of pregnancy**. The logic for this is as follows (Fig. 19.1): the hemodynamic and hematologic changes seen with AFE are clinically, very similar to those seen with anaphylaxis or septic shock; the syndrome occurs after maternal intravascular exposure to fetal tissue; the severity of symptoms varies, perhaps related to the degree of exposure and susceptibility of maternal fetal pairs.

TREATMENT

Treatment should be focused on reversing the triad of AFE syndrome: hypoxia, hemodynamic instability with left ventricular

Table 19.6. SUGGESTED TREATMENT APPROACH FOR AMNIOTIC FLUID EMBOLISM

1. Intubate and ventilate with 100% FIO_2.
2. Initiate CPR if indicated.
3. If undelivered, monitor fetus and deliver.
4. Provide aggressive volume and pressor support. Insert second intravenous and central venous line if possible. Pressor support might include:
   Dopamine 2–5 $\mu g \cdot kg^{-1} \cdot min^{-1}$
   Dobutamine 15–30 $\mu g \cdot kg^{-1} \cdot min^{-1}$
   Isoproterenol 0.05–0.10 $\mu g \cdot kg^{-1} \cdot min^{-1}$
   Norepinephrine 0.1–0.4 $\mu g \cdot kg^{-1} \cdot min^{-1}$—Epinephrine 0.15–0.30 $\mu g \cdot kg^{-1} \cdot min^{-1}$
5. Guide hemodynamic management with pulmonary artery catheter measurements as soon as possible.
6. Anticipate need for and treat coagulopathy (disseminated intravascular coagulation) with cryoprecipitate, fresh frozen plasma and blood.
7. Anticipate and treat left ventricular failure and adult respiratory distress syndrome

Data from Burrows A, Khoo SK. The amniotic fluid embolism syndrome: 10 years' experience at a major teaching hospital. *Aust N Z J Obstet Gynaecol* 1995;35:245–250; and Clark SL. Amniotic fluid embolism. *Clin Perinatol* 1986;13:801–811.

dysfunction and coagulopathy. There is no human data to support treatment regimens aimed at reversing pulmonary artery vasospasm or right heart failure. Management must be aggressive and is initially supportive (Table 19.6) (8, 15, 64). For parturients who are undelivered at the time of the event, keep in mind that delivery of the fetus is necessary to successfully perform CPR in the third trimester of pregnancy (65). Coagulopathy should be anticipated in those patients surviving the initial episode. Cryoprecipitate, fresh frozen plasma, platelets and blood are likely to be required. Cryoprecipitate, in particular, not only replaces fibrinogen but fibronectin, as well. Fibronectin is necessary for proper functioning of the reticuloendothelial system and is typically depleted following surgery, trauma, burns or sepsis. The reticuloendothelial system must remove any endogenous cellular debris from the lungs and other tissue areas, the lymphatic circulation and vascular compartment. Several case reports describe significant improvement in patient oxygenation following administration of cryoprecipitate (66–68).

Although there is no human data reporting the use of antihistamines in the treatment of AFE, an animal study suggests that this approach may be useful. In a 1970 study of rabbits injected with a standardized bolus of human amniotic fluid, rabbits treated with phenergan had decreased symptoms and improved survival compared with the control animals (69). Isolated case reports describe the successful use of innovative treatment approaches. One patient underwent cardiopulmonary bypass and pulmonary artery thromboembolectomy after a pulmonary perfusion scan demonstrated a massive embolism to the left lung (70). Microscopic examination of the thrombus revealed a high concentration of fetal squamous cells. In a case of AFE complicated by acute renal failure, continuous arteriovenous hemofiltration was used successfully to increase the cardiac index and improve arterial oxygenation (71). Although some authors in the 1970s and 1980s recommend the use of early heparinization in AFE (72–74), recent work does not recommend its use (15, 64).

SUMMARY

AFE syndrome is an infrequent, unpreventable and catastrophic complication of pregnancy. It is virtually impossible to predict which patients are at risk for AFE. There is growing data to support the hypothesis that the clinical syndrome represents an anaphylactoid response in susceptible patients to the entry of amniotic fluid into maternal circulation. It is unlikely that AFE is a true embolic event. Diagnosis must be based on a spectrum of clinical signs and symptoms. Even with immediate recognition and aggressive treatment, a high percentage of patients will succumb to the event or survive with permanent neurologic deficits. Nonetheless, intact survival is possible and a high index of suspicion should be maintained for this complication so that aggressive treatment can begin immediately.

REFERENCES

1. Meyer JR. Embolia pulmonar amnio caseosa. *Brasil Med* 1926;2: 301–303.
2. Steiner PE, Lushbaugh BS. Maternal pulmonary embolism by amniotic fluid. *JAMA* 1941;117:1245–1254.
3. Hibbard BM, Anderson MM, Drife JO, et al. *Report on confidential enquiries into maternal deaths in the United Kingdom, 1991–1993*. London: HMSO, 1996.
4. Gilbert WM, Danielsen B. Amniotic fluid embolism: decreased mortality in a population-based study. *Obstet Gynecol* 1999;93: 973–977.
5. Liban E, Raz S. A clinicopathologic study of fourteen cases of amniotic fluid embolism. *Am J Clin Pathol* 1969;51:477–486.
6. Peterson EP, Taylor HB. Amniotic fluid embolism. An analysis of 40 cases. *Obstet Gynecol* 1970;35:787–793.
7. Morgan M. Amniotic fluid embolism. *Anaesthesia* 1979;34:20–32.
8. Clark SL, Hankins GDV, Dudley DA, et al. Amniotic fluid embolism: analysis of the national registry. *Am J Obstet Gynecol* 1995;172:1158–1167.
9. Cates W, Boyd C, Halvorson-Boyd G, et al. Death from amniotic fluid embolism and disseminated intravascular coagulation after a curettage abortion. *Am J Obstet Gynecol* 1981;141:346–348.
10. Guidotti RJ, Grimes DA, Cates W. Fatal amniotic fluid embolism during legally induced abortion, United States, 1972 to 1978. *Am J Obstet Gynecol* 1981;141:257–261.
11. Lawson HW, Atrash HK, Franks AL. Fatal pulmonary embolism during legal induced abortion in the United State from 1972 to 1985. *Am J Obstet Gynecol* 1990;162:986–990.
12. Mirchandani HG, Mirchandani IH, Parikh SR. Hypernatremia due to amniotic fluid embolism during a saline-induced abortion. *Am J Forensic Med Pathol* 1988;9:48–50.
13. Hasaart THM, Essed GGM. Amniotic fluid embolism after transabdominal amniocentesis. *Eur J Obstet Gynecol Reprod Biol* 1983;16: 25–30.
14. Margarson MP. Delayed amniotic fluid embolism following cesarean section under spinal anaesthesia. *Anaesthesia* 1995;50:804–806.
15. Burrows A, Khoo SK. The amniotic fluid embolism syndrome: 10 years' experience at a major teaching hospital. *Aust N Z J Obstet Gynaecol* 1995;35:245–250.
16. Clark SL. Amniotic fluid embolism. *Crit Care Clin* 1991;7:877–882.
17. Paul RH, Koh BS, Bernstein SG. Changes in fetal heart rate: uterine contraction patterns associated with eclampsia. *Am J Obstet Gynecol* 1978;130:165–169.
18. Bastien JL, Graves JR, Bailey S. Atypical presentation of amniotic fluid embolism. *Anesth Analg* 1998;87:124–126.
19. Quance D. Amniotic fluid embolism: detection by pulse oximetry. *Anesthesiology* 1988;68:951–952.
20. Quinn A, Barrett R. Delayed onset of coagulopathy following amniotic fluid embolism: two case reports. *Int J Obstet Anesth* 1993;2:177–180.
21. Murphy KJ, Kazerooni EA, Braun MA, et al. Radiographic appearance of intrathoracic complications of pregnancy. *Can Assoc Radiol J* 1996;47:453–459.
22. Masson RG, Ruggieri J, Siddiqui MM. Amniotic fluid embolism: definitive diagnosis in a survivor. *Am Rev Respir Dis* 1979;120:187–192.
23. Masson RG, Ruggieri J. Pulmonary microvascular cytology: a new diagnostic application of the pulmonary artery catheter. *Chest* 1985;88:908–914.
24. Agia G, Wyatt L, Re E. Pulmonary microvascular cytology: a new diagnostic appliation of the pulmonary artery catheter [Letter]. *Chest* 1986;90:627–628.
25. Ricou B, Reper P, Suter PM. Rapid diagnosis of amniotic fluid embolism causing severe pulmonary failure. *Intensive Care Med* 1989;15:129–131.
26. Kuhlman K, Hidvegi D, Tamura RK, et al. Is amniotic fluid material in the central circulation or peripartum patients pathologic? *Am J Perinatol* 1985;2:295–299.
27. Lee W, Ginsburg KA, Cotton DB, et al. Squamous and trophoblastic cells in the maternal pulmonary circulation identified by invasive hemodynamic monitoring during the peripartum period. *Am J Obstet Gynecol* 1986;155:999–1001.
28. Clark SL, Pavlova Z, Greenspoon J, et al. Squamous cells in the maternal pulmonary circulation. *Am J Obstet Gynecol* 1986;154:104–106.
29. Lee KR, Catalano PM, Oritz-Giroux S. Cytologic diagnosis of amniotic fluid embolism. *Acta Cytol* 1986;30:177–182.
30. Giampaolo C, Schneider V, Kowalski BH, et al. The cytologic diagnosis of amniotic fluid embolism: A critical reappraisal. *Diagn Cytopathol* 1987;3:126–128.
31. Kobayashi H, Ohi H, Terao T, et al. Histological diagnosis of amniotic fluid embolism by monoclonal antibody TKH-2 that recognizes NeuAc alpha 2-6Ga1NAc epitope. *Hum Pathol* 1997;28:428–433.
32. Kobayashi H, Hidekazu O, Toshi T. A simple, noninvasive, sensitive method for diagnosis of amniotic fluid embolism by monoclonal antibody TKH-2 that recognizes NeuAc alpha 2-6Ga1NAc. *Am J Obstet Gynecol* 1993;168:848–853.
33. Garland IWC, Thompson WD. Diagnosis of amniotic fluid embolism using an antiserum to human keratin. *J Clin Pathol* 1983;36:625–627.
34. Ishiyama I, Mukaida M, Komuro E, et al. Analysis of a case of generalized amniotic fluid embolism by demonstrating the fetal isoantigen (A blood type) in maternal tissues of B blood type, using immunoperoxidase staining. *J Clin Pathol* 1986;85:239–241.
35. Shapiro SH, Wessely Z. Rhodamine B fluorescence as a stain for amniotic fluid squames in maternal pulmonary embolism and fetal lungs. *Ann Clin Lab Sci* 1988;18:451–454.
36. Lunetta P, Penttila A. Immunohistochemical identification of syncytiotrophoblastic cells and megakaryocytes in pulmonary vessels in a fatal case of amniotic fluid embolism. *Int J Legal Med* 1996;108: 210–214.
37. Rodgers BM, Staroscik RN, Reis RL. Effects of amniotic fluid on cardiac contractility and vascular resistance. *Am J Physiol* 1971;220: 1979–1982.
38. Reis RL, Pierce WS, Behrendt DM. Hemodynamic effects of amniotic fluid embolism. *Surg Gynecol Obstet* 1969;129:45–48.
39. Rodgers BM, Staroscik RN, Reis RL. Amniotic fluid embolism: effects on myocardial contractility and systemic and pulmonary vascular resistance. *Surg Forum* 1969;20:203–205.
40. Noble WH, St-Amand J. Amniotic fluid embolus. *Can J Anaesth* 1993;40:971–980.
41. Koegler A, Sauder P, Marolf A, et al. Amniotic fluid embolism: a case with non-cardiogenic pulmonary edema. *Intensive Care Med* 1994;20:45–46.
42. Clark SL, Montz FJ, Phelan JP. Hemodynamic alterations associated with amniotic fluid embolism: A reappraisal. *Am J Obstet Gynecol* 1985;151:617–621.
43. Clark SL, Cotton DB, Gonik B, et al. Central hemodynamic alterations in amniotic fluid embolism. *Am J Obstet Gynecol* 1988;158: 1124–1126.
44. Dib N, Tanvir B. Amniotic fluid embolism causing severe left ventricular dysfunction and death: Case report and review of the literature. *Cathet Cardiovasc Diagn* 1996;39:177–180.
45. Vanmaele L, Noppen M, Vincken W, et al. Transient left heart failure in amniotic fluid embolism. *Intensive Care Med* 1990;16:269–271.
46. Girard P, Mal H, Laine J, et al. Left heart failure in amniotic fluid embolism. *Anesthsiology* 1986;64:262–265.
47. van Haeften TW, Strack van Schijndel RJM, Thijs LG. Severe lung damage after amniotic fluid embolism; a case with hemodynamic measurements. *Neth J Med* 1989;35:317–320.
48. Hankins GDV, Synder RR, Clark SL, et al. Acute hemodynamic and respiratory effects of amniotic fluid embolism in the pregnant goat model. *Am J Obstet Gynecol* 1993;168:1113–1130.
49. Clark SL. New concepts in amniotic fluid embolism: a review. *Obstet Gynecol Surv* 1990;45:360–368.
50. Richards DS, Carter LS, Corke B, et al. The effect of human amniotic fluid on the isolated perfused rat heart. *Am J Obstet Gynecol* 1988;158:210–214.
51. Stolte L, van Kessel H, Seelen J, et al. Failure to produce the syndrome of amniotic fluid embolism by infusion of amniotic fluid and meconium into monkeys. *Am J Obstet Gynecol* 1967;98:694–697.
52. Adamsons K, Mueller-Heubach E, Myers RE. The innocuousness of amniotic fluid infusion in the pregnant rhesus monkey. *Am J Obstet Gynecol* 1971;109:977–984.

53. Spence MR, Mason KG. Experimental amniotic fluid embolism in rabbits. *Am J Obstet Gynecol* 1974;119:1073–1078.

54. Vedernikov YP, Saade GR, Zlatnik M, et al. The effect of amniotic fluid on the human omental artery in vitro. *Am J Obstet Gynecol* 1999;180:454–456.

55. El Maradny E, Kanayama N, Halim A, et al. Endothelin has a role in early pathogenesis of amniotic fluid embolism. *Gynecol Obstet Invest* 1995;40:14–18.

56. Yanagisawa M, Kurihara H, Kimmura S, et al. A novel potent vaso-constrictor peptide produced by vascular endothelial cells. *Nature* 1988;332:411–415.

57. Goetz KL, Wang BC, Madwed JB, et al. Cardiovascular, renal and endocrine responses to intravenous endothelin in conscious dogs. *Am J Physiol* 1988;255:1064–1068.

58. Azegami M, Mori N. Amniotic fluid embolism and leukotrienes. *Am J Obstet Gynecol* 1986;155:1119–1124.

59. Lee HC, Yamaguchi M, Ikenoue T, et al. Amniotic fluid embolism and leukotrienes—the role of amniotic fluid surfactant in leukotriene production. *Prostaglandins Leukot Essent Fatty Acids* 1992;47:117–121.

60. Lockwood CJ, Bach R, Guha A, et al. Amniotic fluid contains tissue factor, a potent initiator of coagulation. *Am J Obstet Gynecol* 1991;165:1335–1341.

61. Hammerschmidt DE, Ogburn PL, Williams JE. Amniotic fluid activates complement. *J Lab Clin Med* 1984;104:901–907.

62. Liu EHC, Shailaja S, Koh SCL, et al. An assessment of the effects on coagulation of midtrimester and final-trimester amniotic fluid on whole blood by thrombelastograph analysis. *Anesth Analg* 2000;90:333–336.

63. Phillips LL, Davidson EC. Procoagulant properties of amniotic fluid. *Am J Obstet Gynecol* 1972;113:911–919.

64. Clark SL. Amniotic fluid embolism. *Clin Perinatol* 1986;13:801–811

65. Oates S, Williams GL, Rees GAD. Cardiopulmonary resuscitation in late pregnancy. *Br Med J* 1988;297:404–405.

66. Rodgers GP, Heymach GJ. Cryoprecipitate therapy in amniotic fluid embolization. *Am J Med* 1984;76:916–920.

67. Kumar B, Christmas D. Plasma fibronectin levels in amniotic fluid embolism [Letter]. *Intensive Care Med* 1985;11:273–274.

68. Rodgers GP. Amniotic fluid embolism [Letter]. *JAMA* 1986;256:1893–1894.

69. Dutta D, Bhargava KC, Chakravarti RN, et al. Therapeutic studies in experimental amniotic fluid embolism in rabbits. *Am J Obstet Gynecol* 1970;106:1201–1208.

70. Esposito RA, Grossi EA, Coppa G, et al. Successful treatment of postpartum shock caused by amniotic fluid embolism with cardiopulmonary bypass and pulmonary artery thromboembolectomy. *Am J Obstet Gynecol* 1990;163:572–574.

71. Weksler N, Ovadia L, Stav A, et al. Continuous arteriovenous hemofiltration in the treatment of amniotic fluid embolism. *Int J Obstet Anesth* 1994;3:92–96.

72. Chung AF, Merkatz IR. Survival following amniotic fluid embolism with early heparinization. *Obstet Gynecol* 1973;42:809–814.

73. Strickland MA, Bates GW, Whitworth NS, et al. Amniotic fluid embolism: prophylaxis with heparin and aspirin. *South Med J* 1985;78:377–379.

74. Uszynski M. Heaprin therapy in the primary phase of amniotic fluid embolism. *Thromb Haemost* 1984;52:362.

Shnider and Levinson's Anesthesia for Obstetrics,
edited by Samuel C. Hughes, et al.
Lippincott Williams & Wilkins,
Philadelphia, © 2001.

CHAPTER 20

ANTEPARTUM AND POSTPARTUM HEMORRHAGE

WILLIAM R. CAMANN, M.D. AND DIANE R. BIEHL, M.D.

Hemorrhage in the obstetric patient remains a leading cause of maternal mortality (1–5). When maternal deaths from ectopic pregnancies and maternal hemorrhage are combined, bleeding is the leading cause of pregnancy-related maternal mortality (Fig. 20.1) (1, 3, 6). Better prenatal care, more accurate diagnostic methods, and the availability of intensive care during parturition has improved maternal outcome, but the precipitating factors for obstetric hemorrhage have not been eliminated. Thus, an understanding of the causes and management of obstetric hemorrhage is important for all anesthesiologists.

ANTEPARTUM HEMORRHAGE

A patient may bleed at any time during her pregnancy, but the most severe bleeding usually occurs in the third trimester. Two of the major causes are placenta previa and abruptio placentae.

Placenta Previa

The incidence of placenta previa varies between 1:345 and 1:53 deliveries (7, 8) and is higher in multiparous patients and in patients undergoing repeat cesarean sections (9). The recurrence risk is approximately 5%.

Placenta previa varies in degree and may be complete (37%), partial (27%), or low-lying (46%) (Fig. 20.2). The main sign is painless vaginal bleeding. The patient may bleed, then bleeding may stop spontaneously (the usual situation); however, sudden severe hemorrhage may recur at any time. Although placenta previa is the cause of vaginal bleeding in only about one-third of antepartum hemorrhages (10), all patients who present with vaginal bleeding in the third trimester should be considered to have placenta previa until disproved. If the diagnosis of placenta previa is suspected, the placenta can be located by means of B-scan ultrasonography (Figs. 20.3 and 20.4). Gray imaging has provided for even more accurate localization of placental position in low-lying or marginal implantation. The accuracy of this technique in the third trimester is about 95%. If the ultrasound examination is inconclusive, definitive diagnosis is made by direct examination of the cervical os. This procedure is usually done in the delivery room only after all preparations have been made to perform a cesarean section (i.e., "the double set-up") (Table 20.1). A vaginal examination is carried out to determine whether the placenta is covering or encroaching on the lower segment of the uterus and the cervical os.

Before term gestation, the patient is usually managed conservatively with bed rest hoping that bleeding will cease spontaneously. Once the patient is near-term gestation, fetal maturity is assessed by amniocentesis or other techniques (see Chapter 35, and the mother is delivered by cesarean section. If during pregnancy, the patient begins to bleed and does not stop spontaneously, emergency cesarean section must be carried out despite the gestational age of the fetus. The fetus becomes compromised quickly if maternal hypotension occurs (Fig. 20.5) (11). It is also possible for the placental bleeding to cause fetal exsanguination. The combination of maternal hypotension,

fetal exsanguination, and preterm delivery can be catastrophic to the newborn.

ANESTHETIC MANAGEMENT
"Double Set-Up"

The "double set-up" refers to a vaginal examination in an operating room prepared with all the personnel and equipment necessary to do an immediate cesarean section if profuse bleeding should occur. With advances in high-resolution ultra-sonography the double set-up is no longer commonly performed. However, on occasion it still may be utilized for definitive diagnosis. Before the vaginal examination, if the patient has already bled profusely, as manifested by postural or obvious hypotension, blood volume should be restored. A central venous pressure line can be useful in evaluating and treating hypovolemia.

During the vaginal examination for the diagnosis of placenta previa, sudden and severe maternal hemorrhage may occur, necessitating immediate emergency cesarean section. Therefore before the examination, with the patient in the lithotomy position, the abdomen is prepared and draped and all preparations for cesarean section are completed. At least one large bore intravenous line should be established and at least 2 units of red blood cells should be immediately available before examination of the patient.

Preparation for general anesthesia should include administration of a nonparticulate oral antacid within 15 to 30 minutes of the examination. A trained assistant should be present to provide cricoid pressure. The examination of the cervical os is then performed, and the diagnosis is made (Table 20.1).

Placenta Previa—Actively Bleeding

If the diagnosis of placenta previa is confirmed and the patient is actively bleeding, an emergency cesarean section under general anesthesia is performed immediately.

When the mother is bleeding copiously and may be in hemorrhagic shock, resuscitation of the mother may be extremely difficult. It may not be possible to correct completely the blood loss before surgery because the hemorrhaging will continue until the placenta is removed. Packed red blood cells and crystalloid or colloid should, nevertheless, be infused as rapidly as possible.

Induction of anesthesia is accomplished with either an appropriate dose of thiopental, propofol or ketamine (0.5 to 1 mg/kg) plus succinylcholine (1.5 mg $\cdot$ kg^{-1}) and endotracheal intubation. Ketamine stimulates the sympathetic nervous system centrally to increase heart rate and blood pressure. In the severely hypovolemic patient in whom peripheral vasoconstriction is already maximal, ketamine will not cause any increase in blood pressure. In fact, in these patients the direct cardiac depressant effect of ketamine may actually produce a decrease in blood pressure. In some severe situations with profound hypotension, endotracheal intubation should be facilitated with succinylcholine alone. The possibility of maternal recall should be secondary to maternal safety.

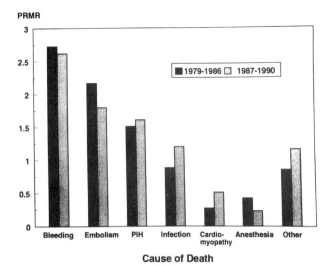

PRMR

Cause of Death

Figure 20.1. Cause-specific pregnancy-related mortality ratios (PRMR) for 1979–1986 and 1987–1990, United States. PRMR, pregnancy-related deaths per 100,000 live births; PIH, pregnancy-induced hypertension. Bleeding includes: ruptured ectopic, uterine rupture, abruptio placentae, retained placenta, uterine bleeding, and disseminated intravascular coagulation. (From Berg CJ, Atrash HK, Koonin LM, et al. Pregnancy-related mortality in the United States, 1987–1990. *Obstet Gynecol* 1996;88:161–167, with permission.)

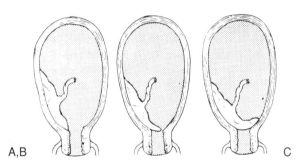

Figure 20.2. Types of placenta previa. **A:** Low implantation of placenta. **B:** Partial placenta previa. **C:** Total placenta previa. (From Bonica JJ, Johnson WL. Placenta praevia, abruptio placentae or rupture of the uterus. In: Bonica JJ, ed. *Principles and Practice of Obstetric Analgesia and Anesthesia.* Philadelphia: Davis, 1969:164, with permission.)

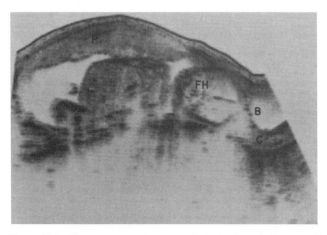

Figure 20.3. Ultrasonogram of an anteriorly implanted placenta. P, placenta; FH, fetal head; B, maternal bladder; C, cervix. (Courtesy of Dr. R. Filly, University of California San Francisco.)

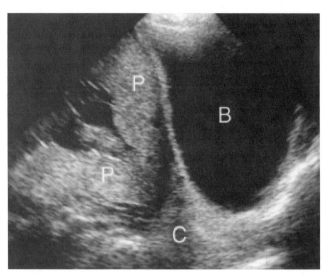

Figure 20.4. Longitudinal sonogram of a patient at 26 weeks' gestation showing complete placenta previa. P, placenta; B, bladder; C, cervix. (Courtesy of Dr. R. Filly, University of California San Francisco.)

Maintenance of anesthesia before delivery depends on the clinical condition of the mother. Initially, 100% oxygen is administered, or nitrous oxide up to 50% may be added as tolerated by the patient. A halogenated agent in a low dose may be used to supplement nitrous oxide to decrease the incidence of maternal recall if the cardiovascular system is stable. Muscle relaxants may be required to provide optimum operating conditions.

If the placenta is easily removed intact, the threat to the mother is much less. Blood volume, as assessed by blood pressure, central venous pressure, and urine output, is restored to normal, and anesthesia is maintained with either the inhalational agent or opioids and muscle relaxants.

The neonate may require intensive resuscitation at birth. These infants may be asphyxiated, acidotic, and hypovolemic. Immediate intubation and ventilation with 100% oxygen should be instituted, and an umbilical venous catheter should be placed for administration of fluids. An umbilical arterial catheter is also useful for monitoring blood pressure and blood gases (Chapter 38). Ideally, a neonatologist should be available to attend to the neonate. Transfer to an intensive care nursery for further close observation and treatment should be accomplished as soon as possible.

Placenta Previa—Not Bleeding

If the diagnosis of placenta previa is established by ultrasound or determined by vaginal examination with a double set-up and the patient is not currently bleeding, cesarean section is still

---

Table 20.1. ANTEPARTUM HEMORRHAGE: "THE DOUBLE SET-UP"

Preparation
    Two 16- or 18-gauge plastic catheters
    Blood pump IV set
    Blood for transfusion
    Oral antacid (nonparticulate)
    Oxygen
    Skilled assistant
Bleeding and cesarean section
    Treat hypovolemia
    Induce ketamine (1 mg · kg^{-1}) plus succinylcholine (1.5 mg · kg^{-1})
    Intubate: provide cricoid pressure
    O$_2$ or 50% N$_2$O and O$_2$ until baby delivered
    Awake extubation

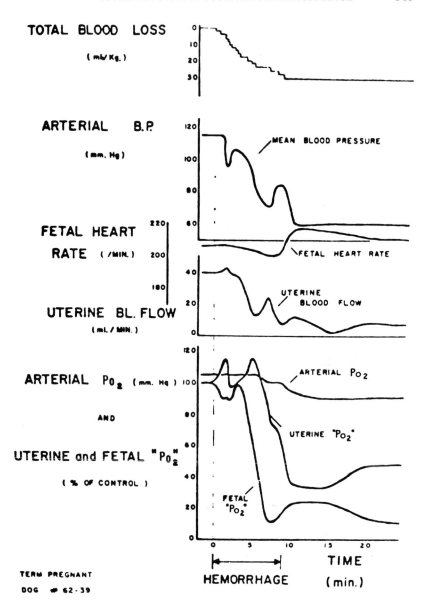

TOTAL BLOOD LOSS

(ml/Kg.)

ARTERIAL   B.P.

(mm. Hg)

MEAN BLOOD PRESSURE

FETAL HEART

RATE   (/MIN.)

FETAL HEART RATE

UTERINE BL. FLOW

(ml. / MIN.)

UTERINE
BLOOD FLOW

ARTERIAL PO_2 (mm. Hg)

AND

UTERINE and FETAL " PO_2 "

(% OF CONTROL)

ARTERIAL PO_2

UTERINE "PO_2"

FETAL
"PO_2"

TIME
(min.)

HEMORRHAGE

TERM PREGNANT

DOG # 62-39

Figure 20.5. Effects of acute hemorrhage in pregnant dogs. Rapid bleeding produced a prompt fall in mean material arterial blood pressure, a comparable fall in uterine blood flow, decreased fetal tissue PO$_2$, and fetal bradycardia. (Adapted from Romney SL, Gabel PV, Takeda Y. Experimental hemorrhage in late pregnancy. *Am J Obstet Gynecol* 1963;87:636.)

required. Despite the preparation of the patient for a general anesthetic as part of the double set-up, some believe that spinal or epidural anesthesia may be used if the patient requests it and if no evidence of hypovolemia is present. This is true regardless of whether the diagnosis is made by ultrasound or vaginal examination. Others believe that general anesthesia is usually preferable in patients with placenta previa because of the possible increased blood loss in these patients. If the placenta is anterior in the lower uterine segment the uterine incision will cut through the placenta. Tears in the lower uterine segment may also occur, which increases maternal blood loss.

Placenta Previa and Placenta Accreta

Placental implantation directly onto or into the myometrium gives rise to one of three conditions: *placenta accreta* is *onto* the myometrium; *placenta increta* is *into* the myometrium; and placenta percreta is penetration through the full thickness of the myometrium (Fig. 20.6) (9, 12). With placenta percreta implantations may occur onto bowel, bladder or other pelvic organs and vessels. Any of these placental implantations can produce a markedly adherent placenta, which cannot be removed without tearing the myometrium.

These abnormal placental implantations occur more frequently in patients with placenta previa. Placenta increta and

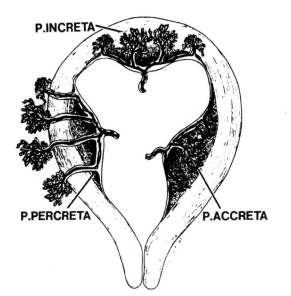

P.INCRETA

P.PERCRETA

P.ACCRETA

Figure 20.6. Classification of placenta accreta based on degree of penetration of myometrium. (From Kamani AAS, Gambling DR, Christilaw J, et al. Anaesthetic management of patients with placenta accreta. *Can J Anaesth* 1987;34:613–617.)

Table 20.2. PLACENTA PREVIA WITH PRIOR UTERINE INCISIONS—EFFECT ON INCIDENCE OF PLACENTA ACCRETA

Prior Cesarean Sections (n)	Patients with Placenta Previa (n = 286)	Placenta Previa Accreta (n = 29)	Percent
0	238	12	5
1	25	6	24
2	15	7	47
3	5	2	40
4	3	2	67

From Clark SL, Koonings PP, Phelan JP. Placenta previa/accreta and prior cesarean section. *Obstet Gynecol* 1985;66:89–92, with permission.

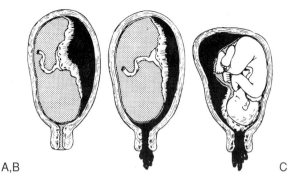

Figure 20.7. Abruptio placentae. **A:** Internal or concealed hemorrhage. **B:** External hemorrhage. **C:** Prolapse of the placenta. (From Bonica JJ, Johnson WL. Placenta praevia, abruptio placentae or rupture of the uterus. In: Bonica JJ, ed. *Principles and Practice of Obstetric Analgesia and Anesthesia.* Philadelphia: Davis, 1969:1166.)

percreta are rare but can be diagnosed antenatally by ultrasound. In the general obstetric population the incidence of placenta accreta is approximately 1:2,500 (12) and cannot be reliably diagnosed by ultrasonography. In patients with *placenta previa* and no prior cesarean sections, the incidence is 5% to 7% (9, 13, 14). However, the risk of placenta accreta in patients with placenta previa who have had a prior cesarean delivery is much greater (Table 20.2). With one prior uterine incision, the incidence of placenta accreta has been reported to be between 24% and 31%, and with two or more prior uterine incisions, the incidence rises to about 50%.

In patients with placenta previa and accreta, massive intraoperative blood loss is common. Reported average blood loss has ranged from 2,000 to 5,000 milliliters with some patients requiring more than 30 units of blood. Approximately 20% of these patients develop coagulopathies (15). Between 30% and 72% have required cesarean hysterectomy (9, 13–15).

Placenta accreta is not reliably diagnosed until the uterus is open. The anesthesiologist must keep in mind this possibility and be prepared to treat sudden massive blood loss. Despite the serious risks, the type of anesthesia chosen for patients with placenta previa and repeat cesarean section is still open to debate. Reviews suggest that regional anesthesia does not contribute to increased maternal morbidity (13, 16) and may be appropriate in many cases of placenta accreta.

For patients with placental increta the likelihood of massive intraoperative blood loss and cesarean hysterectomy are markedly higher than for placenta accreta. With placenta percreta maternal hemorrhage and death can occur despite adequate preparation and expert management. Cardiovascular collapse secondary to an amniotic-fluid like syndrome has been reported (17). If the diagnosis of placenta percreta is made antenatally uterine incision remote from the placenta can be made, umbilical cord clamped, baby delivered, the placenta allowed to remain in situ, and the uterus closed. A controlled hysterectomy can than be performed or the abdomen closed and the patients followed carefully with or without the administration of methotrexate to facilitate placental involution (18).

Abruptio Placentae

The term *abruptio placentae* refers to the separation of a normally implanted placenta after 20 weeks' gestation and before the birth of the fetus. The term marginal separation of the placenta refers to a mild form of abruptio placentae. The incidence of abruptio placentae varies from 0.2% to 2.4% (10). Maternal mortality is significant, probably 1.8% to 2.8% (9, 18). Perinatal mortality may be as high as 50% (19).

The etiology of abruptio placentae is not well defined but is associated with hypertensive disorders of pregnancy, high parity, uterine abnormalities (e.g., tumors), previous placental abruption (10, 20), and cocaine use (21). The clinical manifestations

of this disease depend primarily on the site and degree of placental separation and the amount of blood loss (Fig. 20.7). Bleeding from the abruption may appear through the vagina (external or revealed hemorrhage) or remain concealed in the uteroplacental unit (internal or concealed hemorrhage). The degree of revealed vaginal bleeding is often misleading, and concealed hemorrhage (retroplacental clot) provides one of the main problems for the anesthesiologist in caring for these patients on an emergency basis. The amount of blood loss is commonly underestimated, and as much as 4,000 milliliters of blood may be sequestered in the uterus. Abruptio placentae is classified as mild, moderate, or severe. In mild or moderate abruption there is usually no maternal hypotension or coagulopathies and no fetal distress. Severe abruption is characterized by maternal hypotension, uterine irritability, hypertonicity and pain, fetal distress or death, and clotting abnormalities. Of all abruptions, the mild to moderate types account for 85% to 90% and severe types account for 10% to 15%.

CLOTTING ABNORMALITIES ASSOCIATED WITH ABRUPTIO PLACENTAE

Besides the problem of hemorrhage in the mother, severe abruptio placentae may result in blood coagulation defects (22, 23). Two theories have evolved to explain the observed clotting defects:

1. Placental abruption causes circulating plasminogen to be activated, which enzymatically destroys circulating fibrinogen (fibrinolysis).
2. Thromboplastin from placenta and decidua triggers the activation of the extrinsic clotting pathway, causing thrombin to convert fibrinogen to fibrin (disseminated intravascular coagulation).

It is unlikely that either mechanism operates exclusively. In the clinical situation, the end result is hypofibrinogenemia, platelet deficiency, and decreased factors V and VIII. Once the clotting mechanism has been activated, degeneration products of the fibrin-fibrinogen system also appear in the circulation. The patient then manifests widespread bleeding from the intravenous sites, gastrointestinal tract, and subcutaneous tissues, as well as the uterus.

In all patients suspected of having abruptio placentae, clotting parameters should be determined. With sophisticated laboratory equipment, actual amounts of the clotting factors present in the blood and degradation products can be measured. However, the clinical situation is often acute, and treatment must be instituted before test results are known. For this reason, a simple clot observation test that can be performed in the delivery suite is often preferred. In this test, 5 milliliters of maternal venous blood are drawn into a clean glass test tube, shaken gently, and allowed to stand. If a clot does not form within 6 minutes or the clot is lysed within 1 hour, a clotting defect is probably present. If the clot fails to form within 30 minutes, the fibrinogen level is probably less than 100 mg/dL.

When the blood sample is drawn for the clot observation test, a sample also should be sent to the laboratory for complete analysis, including hemoglobin, hematocrit, platelet count, prothrombin time, partial thromboplastin time, fibrinogen level, and fibrin degradation product analyses. The complete results will be useful for the management of these patients both intrapartum and postpartum. Analyses should be repeated frequently to monitor treatment, because the clotting parameters may take several days to return to normal. The use of thromboelastography may prove useful in some cases of obstetric hemorrhage (24).

MANAGEMENT OF ABRUPTIO PLACENTAE

The definitive management of abruptio placentae is to empty the uterus. The method by which this is accomplished depends on (a) the degree of abruption; (b) the time in gestation at which abruption occurs; (c) the stability of the maternal cardiovascular and hematologic systems; and (d) the status of the fetus.

The diagnosis of mild or moderate abruption is usually made by excluding placenta previa with ultrasound examination. After the diagnosis, if the fetus is mature, an amniotomy is performed, labor is induced or augmented with oxytocin if necessary, the fetus is monitored continuously by electronic means and baseline clotting studies are obtained. If there are no signs of maternal hypovolemia or uteroplacental insufficiency and if clotting studies are normal, continuous lumbar epidural, caudal, or subarachnoid block may be used for labor and vaginal delivery.

For severe abruption and emergency cesarean section general anesthesia is usually selected. Regional anesthesia is contraindicated in patients with hypovolemic shock, severe coagulation abnormalities, or both. The induction and maintenance of general anesthesia are similar to the procedures used for actively-bleeding placenta previa, as outlined earlier.

At delivery intensive resuscitation of the newborn is usually required. These infants are usually severely asphyxiated and severely hypovolemic. In addition, they may also be premature.

After delivery of the infant and removal of the placenta, subsequent management of the mother may continue to be difficult. If blood has extravasated into the myometrium, the uterus may not contract and bleeding may continue. Oxytocin by infusion (e.g., 20 to 40 units per liter) should be started as soon as the infant is delivered. If this is not effective, intravenous ergot preparations (e.g., 0.2 mg methylergonovine) or prostaglandin (e.g., 15-methylprostaglandin F-2-alpha 250 μg i.v. or i.m.) may be administered. Hypogastric or internal iliac artery ligation, embolization, or hysterectomy may be required as a life-saving procedure for the mother (25–27).

Massive and rapid blood transfusion restores the depleted blood volume, maintains tissue perfusion, and prevents renal damage. If blood is not immediately available, crystalloid, albumin, hetastarch or plasmanate should be used to maintain the circulating blood volume. When necessary, fresh frozen plasma will restore factors V and VIII components, and in severe situations, platelet concentrate may also be required (6 to 12 units). Cryoprecipitate contains 23% of the fibrinogen in a unit of plasma and thus provides a concentrated fibrinogen and factor VIII in a small volume. Infusion of fibrinogen is no longer recommended because it may only aggravate the disseminated intravascular coagulation and it carries a high risk of transmitting serious viral illnesses.

During an apparently normal vaginal delivery, abruptio placentae may occur just before the birth of the infant. In this situation, the problems are maternal hemorrhage and fetal asphyxia. Clotting deficits do not usually become manifest. The anesthesiologist should resuscitate the mother by establishing intravenous access and supporting her circulation with crystalloid solution and blood when available. Intravenous infusion of oxytocin should begin as soon as the infant and placenta are delivered. General anesthesia may be required if operative vaginal or abdominal delivery of the infant is necessary.

These patients, regardless of the mode of delivery, are extremely susceptible to postpartum hemorrhage resulting from uterine atony. Frequent monitoring of maternal vital signs, urine output, and fundal firmness is necessary.

Other Causes of Antepartum Hemorrhage

Placenta previa and abruptio placentae account for one-half to two-thirds of all cases of antepartum hemorrhage. The remainder are due to cervical polyps, carcinoma, vaginal and vulvar varicosities, circumvallate placenta, and vasoprevia. The latter two causes do not present as much of a threat to the mother as to the fetus because the bleeding is primarily from fetal vessels. Other obstetric problems may give rise to hemorrhage as a result of derangement of the clotting mechanisms (see Chapter 18). Severe preeclampsia, maternal infection, amniotic fluid embolism, and intrauterine death may all result in disseminated intravascular coagulation and hemorrhage if the diagnosis is not established quickly and treatment instituted.

UTERINE RUPTURE

Uterine rupture is a potentially catastrophic obstetric complication that may occur antepartum, intrapartum or postpartum. The incidence of uterine rupture had declined during the 1980s, and in the United States, maternal mortality was calculated to be 0.1% when rupture occured (28). This decreased incidence was attributed to improved diagnostic and treatment facilities and the decline in grand multiparity. Causes include (a) separation of the uterine scar; (b) rupture of the myomectomy scar; (c) previous difficult deliveries; (d) rapid, spontaneous, tumultuous labor; (e) prolonged labor in association with excessive oxytocin stimulation or cephalopelvic disproportion; (f) weak or stretched uterine muscles, such as might be found in the grand multipara, in multiple gestation, or in polyhydramnios; and (g) traumatic rupture (iatrogenic) occurring from intrauterine manipulations, difficult forceps applications, and excessive suprafundal pressure.

Although the uterine rupture is usually found at the site of a previous operation or injury, reviews had indicated that maternal mortality was low in these circumstances because rupture is recognized and promptly treated (28–30). Traumatic rupture or spontaneous uterine rupture (with no uterine scar) carries a substantial incidence of maternal mortality due to obstetric hemorrhage, which may exceed 50%. Maternal death from rupture apparently occurs because the possibility is not considered, and blood transfusions are inadequate and laparotomy is delayed or not done. In the last 10 to 15 years, the incidence of uterine rupture has significantly increased, tripling in the state of Massachusetts between 1985 and 1995 (31). Other states have reported an approximate 25% increase in the incidence of uterine rupture over a 2 to 3 year period in the mid-1990s. The more recent increased incidence of uterine rupture may be due to the increased demand to reduce the cesarean section rate in the United States and other countries, particularly by vaginal birth after previous cesarean section (VBAC) (32). The occurrence of uterine rupture after a previous cesarean section is dependent on the type and location of the previous surgery. Table 20.3 demonstrates the estimated occurrence (33). An increased rate of uterine rupture among parturients with previous uterine scars has been reported in association with *induction* of labor using oxytocin, in comparison to the uterine rupture rate in spontaneously laboring women (2.3% vs. 0.7%: $P = 0.001$) (34). In this study, no significant increase was demonstrated in

Table 20.3. OCCURRENCE OF UTERINE RUPTURE DURING LABOR AFTER A PREVIOUS CESAREAN SECTION

Previous Section	Percentage
Classical uterine scar	4–9%
T-shaped incision	4–9%
Low-vertical incision	1–7%
Low-transverse incision	0.2–1.5%

From ACOG Practice Bulletin. Vaginal birth after previous cesarean delivery. Clinical Management Guidelines for Obstetricians and Gynecologists. No. 5. 1999, with permission.

the rate of uterine rupture among women with previous uterine scars in association with oxytocin *augmentation* of labor. In a recent review of over 500,000 deliveries in California during 1995, there were 392 uterine ruptures (0.07%) (35). However, in those patients with a prior cesarean section delivery, the incidence of uterine rupture was 0.43%. Trials of labor after previous cesarean section may be inappropriate in an environment without personnel and facilities to quickly respond and perform an emergency cesarean section when indicated. The American College of Obstetricians and Gynecologists (ACOG) has recently recommended based primarily on consensus and expert opinion that: "Because uterine rupture may be catastrophic, VBAC should be attempted in institutions equipped to respond to emergencies with physicians immediately available to provide emergency care" (see Appendix C) (33). Some have advocated that trials of labor not be mandated for women who have had a previous cesarean section and that efforts should be focused on reducing the primary cesarean section rate (31, 36). When a uterus ruptures during labor after previous cesarean section, if definitive management is delayed, maternal and fetal morbidity and mortality substantially increase.

Signs and symptoms depend on the extent of the rupture and include vaginal bleeding, severe uterine or lower abdominal pain, shoulder pain from subdiaphragmatic irritation by blood, disappearance of fetal heart tones, and severe maternal hypotension and shock. Anesthetic management for laparotomy, uterine repair, hysterectomy, or hypogastric ligation is similar to that outlined above for the actively bleeding, acutely hypovolemic patient.

TRIAL OF LABOR FOLLOWING CESAREAN SECTION

In the United States, 98% of all women who had cesarean sections were once delivered by cesarean in subsequent pregnancies, but a marked change occurred. In 1982, ACOG published specific guidelines on a trial of labor following cesarean section (37). This abrupt change in attitude has, in part, been due to the tremendous increase in cesarean sections in the 1980s and early 1990s. The guidelines specifically exclude patients who have had classic cesarean sections, but recommended that many patients who have lower segment transverse scars be considered candidates for a trial of labor in subsequent pregnancies.

Dehiscence of the lower segment transverse scar has been shown to be less catastrophic than rupture of the classical scar or spontaneous rupture of the uterus. Maternal hemorrhage, hypotension, and fetal demise are associated with rupture through the uterine muscle. In contrast, the lower uterine segment consists predominantly of connective tissue after 36 weeks' gestation. This part of the uterus does not contain placental tissue under normal circumstances. Fetal compromise with any scar dehiscence is less frequent than with classic uterine rupture.

The safety of both mother and fetus during a trial of labor can only be ensured, however, if the patient is carefully monitored in

a hospital that is equipped to perform an emergency cesarean section (33). Appropriate selection of patients for a trial of labor is necessary for a reasonable chance of successful vaginal delivery. Patients with a singleton fetus and vertex presentation are candidates, if no other maternal risk factors such as a placenta previa, marginal separation of the placenta, hypertension, or diabetes are present. A previous diagnosis of dystocia or failure to progress is not considered an absolute contraindication: 50% to 70% of patients with these diagnoses in previous pregnancies deliver vaginally after a trial of labor (33). With such nonrecurrent indications for cesarean section such as placenta previa, breech presentation, or preeclampsia, the success rate for vaginal delivery is 60% to 80% (31–33).

The advantages of vaginal delivery over cesarean section include decreased maternal blood loss, decreased febrile morbidity, and more rapid ambulation after delivery, as well as less well- defined psychologic benefits in terms of maternal-infant bonding and maternal sense of success and well-being. However, the alleged advantages of VBAC over elective cesarean have been questioned. A recent review found that complications (need for hysterectomy, uterine rupture, and operative injury) which occurred after trial of labor were more likely than after elective repeat cesarean section (38). ACOG has now issued a new practice bulletin on this topic, which discusses the risks and benefits of VBAC (see Uterine Rupture) (33). The risks of lowering the cesarean delivery rate in the United States include uterine rupture and fetal trauma and this topic is currently getting renewed consideration and is controversial (31, 36).

Anesthetic Management

Initially, when the recommendations for the management of a trial of labor were being developed, regional anesthetic techniques were considered to be contraindicated because it was believed that regional anesthesia might mask the hallmark sign of uterine rupture pain. Subsequent experience showed that dehiscence of the lower segment scar frequently did not cause pain. The most reliable method of detecting dehiscence was by the change in uterine tone and contraction pattern. Several reports have demonstrated that epidural anesthesia can be used safely in patients undergoing a trial of labor (31, 36, 38–43). Adequate pain relief may encourage more women to choose a trial of labor (33). It is prudent in this patient group to use the lowest effective concentrations and volumes of local anesthetic with continuous electronic monitoring of uterine contractions and fetal heart rate, as higher concentrations of local anesthetic may indeed mask the pain of uterine rupture (43). However, the most common sign of uterine rupture is a nonreassuring fetal heart rate (FHR) pattern with variable deceleration that may evolve into late deceleration, bradycardia and loss of FHR.

If a trial of labor is unsuccessful and cesarean section is required, the epidural block may be used for the cesarean section if both mother and fetus are stable. In the true emergency situation with suspected uterine scar rupture, fetal distress, or other maternal complications, such as cardiovascular instability, a general anesthetic to effect a rapid delivery is indicated. The anesthesiologist must also anticipate that cesarean hysterectomy may be required if a complicated rupture has occurred. The incidence of hysterectomy for uncontrollable hemorrhage in this group of patients is 0.001% (28).

POSTPARTUM HEMORRHAGE

The postpartum period is typically defined as the 6-week period after delivery of the infant. Postpartum hemorrhage occurs in 3% to 5% of all deliveries, and can occur within minutes after delivery. The main causes of postpartum hemorrhage include: retained products of conception, uterine atony, cervical, vaginal, uterine lacerations, and bleeding from the episiotomy site. Twenty percent of all patients who have antepartum hemorrhage will also bleed postpartum. Severe postpartum hemorrhage can occur with little or no warning. For this reason, immediately after delivery the anesthesiologist should observe the patient closely and be prepared to institute resuscitation of the mother and to give an anesthetic at a few seconds' notice.

Retained Placenta

The incidence of retained placenta is approximately 1% of all vaginal deliveries, and retained products of conception usually require manual exploration of the uterus. This can sometimes be accomplished without an analgesic and anesthetic, but the mother can be severely distressed and the obstetrician can encounter difficulty in exploring a uterus that is partially contracted. For these reasons, analgesia is often necessary. If the mother has an epidural or spinal block encompassing T10 to S4, manual removal of the placenta can be accomplished without pain.

If the parturient has not received a regional block before delivery, other analgesic maneuvers can be tried before administering general anesthesia. Intravenous sedation with benzodiazepines or ketamine ($0.1\ \mathrm{mg \cdot kg^{-1}}$), inhalation analgesia, or judicious use of opioids such as alfentanil or fentanyl can also be tried, but careful observation of the mother is essential to prevent oversedation and potential aspiration both during and after removal of the placenta.

In addition to providing analgesia or anesthesia, uterine relaxation can facilitate removal of the placenta. Administration of 50 to 100 μg nitroglycerin intravenously has been reported to result in uterine relaxation sufficient to remove the placenta (44). Because of the side effects of hypotension and headache, careful monitoring of maternal vital signs is required both during and after administration of nitroglycerin. Nitroglycerin is preferable to inhalation of amyl nitrite, however, since the administration is more controlled. An excellent review (44) summarizes the advantages of nitroglycerin for use in this setting. Avoidance of general anesthesia removes the risks and consequences of failed intubation and pulmonary aspiration of gastric contents. The onset of uterine relaxation is immediate and can be performed without an anesthesia machine or operating room. Maternal recovery is more rapid and sedation or unconsciousness is avoided. Although hypotension is a possibility, most reports indicate this is either rare, or of short duration and easily treated. The most common route of administration is intravenous, but nitroglycerin can also be given intranasally, sublingual or transdermal (45).

The mechanism of nitroglycerin (NTG) involves the effects of nitric oxide (NO) on uterine smooth muscle. However, in vitro preparations largely have failed to show a relaxant effect of NTG on isolated uterine muscle strips. A recent investigation indicates that a (as yet unidentified) factor from the placenta acts to enhance the effect of NTG, which may explain the variance between the clinical observations and in vitro studies (46).

Another difficulty rarely encountered is uterine inversion when the removal is attempted by traction on the umbilical cord without careful pressure applied to the uterus through the abdomen (47, 48). The uterus and placenta appear at the introitus, and severe hypotension and bradycardia may occur in the mother. This initial response is thought to be a vasovagal reflex, but hemorrhage from the placental site and endometrium also occurs. The treatment is to replace the uterus as quickly as possible with steady pressure before the cervix constricts and prevents replacement. The use of nitroglycerin can facilitate obstetric management of an inverted uterus. Previously, general anesthesia was recommended for this situation, but several recent reports describe the successful use of NTG (49, 50). Hypotension is certainly of concern, but NTG is rapid and prompt replacement of a relaxed uterus may, in many cases, avoid the need to institute general anesthesia. In rare cases, laparotomy

may be required to replace the inverted uterus. Once the uterus is replaced, an infusion of oxytocin is administered to maintain the increased uterine tone (contraction) and to prevent a recurrence of the inversion.

Uterine Atony

Uterine atony, in varying degrees, occurs in approximately 2% to 5% of all vaginal deliveries (51). Uterine atony is increased with multiparity, multiple births, polyhydramnios, large infants, retained placenta, operative intervention such as internal version and extraction and in the presence of chorioamnionitis. It may occur immediately or several hours after delivery of the infant.

Resuscitation of the mother necessitates: (a) replacement of blood loss initially with crystalloid and colloid solution, then with packed red blood cells as soon as possible; (b) intravenous infusion of oxytocin to cause contraction of the uterus; (c) general supportive measures (i.e., oxygen by face mask) with the patient in the Trendelenburg position; and (d) close monitoring of vital signs. Central venous pressure monitoring can be helpful when hemorrhage is profound.

When an oxytocin infusion and obstetric maneuvers (such as uterine massage) fail to result in appropriate uterine contractions, other pharmacologic therapies are available. When these drugs are used, their side effects must be considered (Table 20.4).

Ergot alkaloids: Methylergonovine (Methergine) or ergonovine (Ergotrate or Ergometrine) can be administered in a dose of 0.2 mg. The onset of action is rapid and the dose can be repeated if necessary. The ergot alkaloids can be administered intravenously or intramuscularly, but many clinicians suggest that, for safety concerns, the intramuscular route is preferable. However, extreme hypertension has been noted with both routes of administration. In the critical situation, diluting 0.2 mg of methylergonovine in 10 milliliters of saline and administering it in 1 to 2 milliliters boluses can be very effective. The effect is very rapid and the duration of action is 30 minutes to 2 hours. Use of methylergonovine is associated with a high incidence of nausea and vomiting, and this side effect should be expected in the awake patient receiving regional anesthesia. Other side effects include pulmonary (small) and coronary artery vasoconstriction and systemic hypertension. Myocardial infarction has been reported in postpartum women after ergonovine administration. Thus, careful monitoring of the ECG and blood pressure is mandatory. The drugs should be used with caution in patients with preexisting hypertension, preeclampsia, asthma, or coronary artery disease. Concomitant use of methylergonovine and other vasopressors (such as ephedrine or phenylephrine) can result in exaggerated hypertensive responses.

Prostaglandins: Prostaglandins of the E- and F-series result in uterine contraction. Prostaglandin E_2 is not marketed for this use in North America, but significant cardiovasculer side effects have been reported when used for induction of labor (49). Initially, prostaglandin $F_{2\alpha}$ was used, although now the most common agent is 15-methyl prostaglandin $F_{2\alpha}$ (Hemabate). The effects of the drugs are similar but 15-methyl prostaglandin $F_{2\alpha}$ is 10 times more potent than the parent compound and remains in the peripheral circulation much longer. This drug, in a dose of 250 μg, may be given intravenously, intramuscularly, or directly into uterine muscle and onset of action is rapid (53–56). Prostaglandin $F_{2\alpha}$ administration may lead to an increase in cardiac output and pulmonary pressure. The latter is a consistent finding and may be catastrophic in the patient with preexisting cardiac disease. Hankins et al. (57) reported development of arterial oxygen desaturation as measured by pulse oximetry after use of prostaglandin $F_{2\alpha}$ for treatment of uterine atony.

Table 20.4. SIDE EFFECTS OF DRUGS USED TO TREAT UTERINE ATONY

	Dose	Primary Route (Alternate)	Frequency of Dose	Cardiovascular	Renal	Respiratory	Gastrointestinal
Oxytoxin	10–40 U in 1,000 mL normal saline or lactated Ringer's solution	IV (IM, IMM)	Continuous IV infusion	IV bolus can cause ↓ SVR, ↓ MAP, ↑ HR, ↓PVR, [severe ↓ BP reported]. Dilution recommended to avoid problems [20–40 units/1 L i.v. fluid]	Antidiuretic effect; water intoxication possible with larger doses	—	Rare nausea and vomiting
Ergot alkaloids (ergonovine and methylergonovine)	0.2 mg	IM (IMM)	q 2–4 h	Hypertension; vasoconstriction; severe hypertension causing stroke or seizure; coronary artery vasospasm [myocardial infarction reported]	—	Rare bronchospasm; avoid in asthmatics, if possible	Nausea and vomiting
Protaglandin; 15 methyl prostaglandin F₂alpha	0.25 mg	IM (IMM)	q 15–90 min, not to exceed 8 doses	↑ CO, ↑ PVR (potentially severe and life-threatening with existing cardiac disease); no change SVR; severe hypo and hypertension reported (rare)	—	Bronchospasm; ↓ O₂ saturation	Nausea, vomiting, and diarrhea
Dinoprostone (PGE₂)	20 mg	PR	q 2 h	↓ SVR, ↓ MAP, ↑ CO, no change in PVR	—	Bronchodilation	Nausea, vomiting, and diarrhea

SVR, systemic vascular resistance; MAP, mean arterial pressure; HR, heart rate; PVR, pulmonary vascular resistance; CO, cardiac output; PR, per rectum; IM, intramuscular; IV, intravenous; IMM, intramyometrial.

Cardiovascular collapse, (58) transient severe hypertension, (59) and fatalities (60) have been reported after the use of prostaglandin F$_2\alpha$. Thus, close monitoring of the cardiovascular and pulmonary consequences of the drug is required. Despite their concerns, prostaglandin F$_2\alpha$ has proved highly effective in treating uterine atony. The dose may be repeated if needed based on clinical circumstances, however, severe bronchospasm and hypotension have been reported with a second dose (54). The recommended maximum dose is 2.0 mg with repeated doses given every 15 to 30 minutes.

If the above measures are not successful, internal iliac artery ligation or emergency hysterectomy may be required. The anesthetic considerations are very similar to those for placenta previa or abruptio placenta, without an infant to influence management. The patient in an unstable condition before surgery can be expected to lose anywhere from 2 to 18 liters of blood before completion of the hysterectomy (16).

Cervical and Vaginal Lacerations

Both of these conditions may result in hemorrhagic shock. One of the main problems with lacerations is that they can be undiagnosed because of other complications. Blood loss can be undetected if it occurs after the patient has been transferred to the recovery room. Resuscitation should be started and the patient should be transferred back to the delivery room. A careful search for the source of the bleeding may require a general anesthetic to allow the obstetrician to explore the uterus and examine the cervix and vaginal vault. If the bleeding source is not found, in rare cases laparotomy may be required.

Blood Loss and Cesarean Section

In most high-risk obstetric units, the incidence of cesarean sections is now 15% to 25%. Regardless of the indication for cesarean section, the anesthesiologist must remember that sudden hemorrhage can occur with any manipulation of the highly vascular full-term uterus. Blood loss during an "elective" cesarean section is estimated to be between 800 and 1,200 milliliters. However, it is rare that patients undergoing elective, uncomplicated cesarean delivery require transfusion. Despite this, obstetric patients receive 4% of the blood components used annually in the United States (61). No evidence supports the assertion that general anesthesia will result in increased blood loss at cesarean delivery (62, 63). During *repeat* cesarean sections, adhesions, varicosities in the uterus, or rupture of the previous scar, sudden and severe hemorrhage may occur. The anesthesiologist must be prepared to resuscitate a parturient in hemorrhagic shock.

Other Strategies

Blood salvage during cesarean delivery: Intraoperative blood salvage and reinfusion has become common in many surgical procedures when large blood loss is expected, such as certain cardiac, vascular and orthopedic operations. However, the use of this technology has never become popular in obstetrics owing to the fear of reinfusion of amniotic fluid and consequent development of the sequelae of amniotic fluid embolism (AFE). Blood salvage techniques incorporate extensive washing and filtration of blood, but it is not known if this removes the particular factors in amniotic fluid that are responsible for the AFE. In 1995, the National Heart, Lung, and Blood Institute of the National Institute of Health expressed concerns about the safety of blood salvaged at cesarean section (64). One report describes three patients who received 9 units of shed, salvaged, and washed blood without complications (65). Two recent series describe 15 and 139 patients, respectively, who received shed and washed blood at cesarean delivery without apparent adverse sequelae

(66, 67). It appears that the fears of use of cell-salvage in obstetrics may not be as valid as previously thought (68). However, the safety of this technique has still not been fully accepted for use during cesarean delivery, and more work is needed (61, 69). A recent case report noted a probably death resulting from salvaged blood cells reinfused at cesarean section. The patient died with the clinical diagnosis of amniotic fluid embolism (70). Moreover, as most obstetric hemorrhage is sudden and often unpredictable, it is not at all clear that intraoperative cell salvage would make an appreciable impact upon either homologous blood exposure or maternal mortality. The requirements for blood-salvage equipment, set-up, and personnel are not always readily available in many centers at all times, and emergent use is frequently unobtainable, even in the most well-equipped hospitals.

Acute hemodilution: Collection of blood immediately prior to surgery with maintenance of blood volume using infused crystalloid or colloid is known as acute normovolemic hemodilation (ANH). This blood is reinfused following surgery, allowing for blood loss during surgery to occur at a lower hematocrit, thus reducing loss of red cell mass. ANH has been successfully used in a variety of nonpregnant patients to reduce homologous transfusion requirements. The higher the initial hematocrit, the more red cell volume can be extracted preoperatively. The natural hemodilution and blood volume expansion of normal pregnancy may limit the effectiveness of ANH by lowering mean initial hematocrit. Nonetheless, one report does describe this technique in patients with placenta previa presenting for elective cesarean delivery (71). A volume of 750 to 1,000 milliliters of blood was removed preoperatively, with a decrease in mean hematocrit from 34% to 25%. The blood was later reinfused in all patients, and the procedure was well tolerated. Only one out of 38 patients required homologous transfusion.

Autologous donation: Patients who are undergoing repeat cesareans or who are at risk for bleeding complications during delivery may elect autologous blood donation during pregnancy (72). With the risk of transmission of serious viral illnesses in homologous blood transfusions, some patients donate their own blood before surgery. Several studies of pregnant patients who made autologous donations suggest that this is a low-risk procedure and merits consideration for use in obstetrics (73–75).

Management of Hemorrhage: Thromboelastography

Thromboelastography (TEG) is used frequently in liver transplantation and cardiac surgery to monitor coagulopathy and anticoagulent therapy (76). Some obstetric units have adopted this ward-based monitor and its use in obstetrics has been extensively reviewed (77). TEG measures the viscoelastic properties of blood. It can detect the increasing stickiness as fluid blood forms clot. The thromboelastogram is a real-time graphic display with either pen and ink or computer graphic. The graph formed demonstrates the entire process of coagulopathy to include rate and strength of clot formation and the ultimate decay.

Thromboelastography has been used to a limited extent to manage hemorrhage in obstetrics to include a case of disseminated intravascular coagulation (DIC) with placental abruption (24) and a coagulopathy after a forceps delivery (78). The obstetric experience is extremely small compared to liver transplantation where TEG has been used extensively to guide therapy for massive transfusion (79). While TEG has been used to evaluate or manage idiopathic thrombocytopenia purpura (ITP), (80) hemolysis of liver enzymes and low platelets (HELLP), (81) preeclampsia (82) and effects of low-dose aspirin (83) in parturients, there remains no firmly established place in clinical obstetric anesthesia. While TEG has clear potential use in the management of obstetric hemorrhage, it remains largely a research tool with further work needed to validate its use in parturients.

CONCLUSION

Hemorrhage remains a major factor contributing to maternal death in obstetrics and contributes significantly to perinatal mortality. The pregnant patient often bleeds unexpectedly and may exsanguinate in a matter of minutes; every anesthesiologist should be prepared to rapidly diagnose and treat hemorrhagic shock in the obstetric patient.

REFERENCES

1. Chichakli L, Atrash H, MacKay A, et al. Pregnancy-related mortality in the United States due to hemorrhage: 1979–1992. *Obstet Gynecol* 1999;94:721–725.
2. Department of Health and others. *Report on Confidential Enquiries into Maternal Deaths in the United Kingdom, 1994–1996*. London: HMSO, 1998.
3. Berg CJ, Atrash HK, Koonin LM, et al. Pregnancy-related mortality in the United States, 1987–1990. *Obstet Gynecol* 1996;88:161–167.
4. Drife J. Management of primary postpartum hemmorhage. *Br J Obstet Gynaecol* 1998;243:1–7.
5. American College of Obstetricians and Gynecologists. *Postpartum hemorrhage. ACOG Educational Bulletin no. 243.* 1998:1–7.
6. Center for Disease Control. Special focus: surveillance for reproductive health. *MMWR* 1997;46:SS-4.
7. Hibbard LT. Placenta previa. *Am J Obstet Gynecol* 1969;104:172–184.
8. Green-Thompson RW. The use of acute hemodilution in parturients undergoing cesarean section. *Clin Obstet Gynecol* 1982;9:479–515.
9. Clark SL, Koonings PP, Phelan JP. Placenta previa/accreta and prior cesarean section. *Obstet Gynecol* 1985;66:89–92.
10. Wilson RJ. Bleeding during late pregnancy. In: Wilson RJ, Carrington EC, Ledger WJ, eds. *Obstetrics and Gynecology*, 7th ed. St. Louis: CV Mosby, 1983:356–371.
11. Romney SL, Gabel PV, Takeda Y. Experimental hemorrhage in late pregnancy: effects on maternal and fetal hemodynamics. *Am J Obstet Gynecol* 1963;87:636–649.
12. Breen JL, Neubecker RT, Gregori CA, et al. Placenta accreta, increta and percreta: a survey of 40 cases. *Obstet Gynecol* 1977;49:43–47.
13. Stanco LM, Schrimmer DB, Paul RH, et al. Emergency peripartum hysterectomy and associated risk factors. *Am J Obstet Gynecol* 1993;168:879–883.
14. Singh PN, Rodrigues C, Gupta AN. Placenta previa and previous cesarean section. *Acta Obstet Gynecol Scand* 1981;60:367–368.
15. Read JA, Cotton DB, Miller FC. Placenta accreta: changing clinical aspects and outcomes. *Obstet Gynecol* 1980;56:31–34.
16. Chestnut DH, Dewan DM, Redick LF, et al. Anesthetic management for obstetric hysterectomy: a multi-institution study. *Anesthesiology* 1989;70:607–610.
17. Rashid A, Moir C, Butt J. Sudden death following cesarean section for placenta previa and accreta. *Am J Forensic Med Pathol* 1994;15:32.
18. Mathews N, McCowan L, Patten P. Placenta previa accreta with delayed hysterectomy, 1996. *Aust N Z J Obstet Gynaecol* 1996;36:476.
19. Hibbard BM, Jeffcoate TNA. Abruptio placenta. *Obstet Gynecol* 1966;27:155–167.
20. Abdella TN, Sibal BM, Hays Jr JM, et al. Relationship of hypertensive disease to abruptio placentae. *Obstet Gynecol* 1984;64:365–370.
21. Acker D, Sachs BP, Tracey KJ. Abruptio placenta associated with cocaine use. *Am J Obstet Gynecol* 1993;146:220–224.
22. Gilabert J, Estelles A, Aznar J, et al. Abruptio placentae and disseminated intravascular coagulation. *Acta Obstet Gynecol Scand* 1985;64:35–39.
23. Pritchard JA. Hematological problems associated with delivery, placental abruption, retained dead fetus and amniotic fluid embolism. *Clin Haematol* 1973;2:563–586.
24. Steer PL, Finley BE, Blumenthal LA. Abruptio placentae and disseminated intravascular coagulation: Use of thrombo elastography and sonoclot analysis. *Int J Obstet Anesth* 1994;3:229–233.
25. Evans S, McShane P. The efficacy of internal iliac artery ligation in obstetrical hemorrhage. *Surg Obstet Gynecol* 1985;160:250.
26. O'Leary JA. Uterine artery ligation in the control of post cesarean hemorrhage. *J Reprod Med* 1995;40:189–193.
27. Collins CD, Jackson JE. Pelvic arterial embolization following hysterectomy and bilateral internal iliac artery ligation for intractable primary postpartum hemorrhage. *Clin Radiol* 1995;50:710–714.
28. Megafu U. Factors influencing maternal survival in ruptured uterus. *Int J Obstet Gynecol* 1985;23:475–480.
29. Schrinsky DC, Benson RC. Rupture of the pregnant uterus: a review. *Obstet Gynecol Surv* 1978;33:217–232.
30. Ware HH. Rupture of the uterus. *Clin Obstet Gynecol* 1960;3:637–645.
31. Sachs B, Kobelin C, Castro M, et al. The risks of lowering the cesarean-delivery rate. *N Engl J Med* 1999;340:54–57.
32. Rageth JC, Juzi C, Grossenbacher H. Delivery after previous cesarean: a risk evaluation. *Obstet Gynecol* 1999;93:332–337.
33. ACOG. Vaginal birth after previous cesarean delivery. *ACOG Practice Bulletin. Clinical management guidelines for obstetricians and gynecologists.* 1999:5.
34. Zelop CM, Shipp TD, Repke JT, et al. Uterine rupture in induced or augmented labor in gravid women with one prior cesarean delivery. *Am J Obstet Gynecol* 1999;181:882–886.
35. Gregory K, Korst L, Cane P, et al. Vaginal birth after cesarean section and uterine rupture rates in California. *Obstet Gynecol* 1999;94:985–989.
36. FDA Public Health Advisory. *Need for caution when using vacuum assisted delivery devices.* Rockville, MD: FDA, May 21, 1998.
37. ACOG Committee on Obstetrics and Maternal/Fetal Medicine. American College of Obstetricians and Gynecologists' Guidelines for vaginal delivery after cesarean childbirth. *ACOG Newsltr* 1982;26:1.
38. McMahon MJ, Luther ER, Bowes WA, et al. Comparison of trial of labor with an elective second cesarean section. *N Engl J Med* 1996;335:689–695.
39. Lavin JP Jr. Vaginal delivery after cesarean birth: frequently asked questions. *Clin Perinatol* 1983;10:439–453.
40. Uppington J. Epidural analgesia and previous cesarean section. *Anaesthesia* 1983;38:336–341.
41. Rudnick V, Niv D, Hetman-Peri M, et al. Epidural analgesia for planned vaginal delivery following previous cesarean section. *Obstet Gynecol* 1984;64:621–623.
42. Kelly MC, Hill DC, Wilson DB. Low-dose epidural bupivacaine/fentanyl infusion does not mask uterine rupture. *Int J Obstet Anesth* 1997;6:52–54.
43. Rowbotham SJ, Critchley LA, Gin T. Uterine rupture and epidural analgesia during a trial of labor. *Anaesthesia* 1997;52:483–488.
44. Riley ET, Flanagan B, Cohen SE, et al. Intravenous nitroglycerin: a potent uterine relaxant for emergency obstetric procedures. Review of literature and report of three cases. *Int J Obstet Anesth* 1996;5:264–268.
45. Redick LF, Livingston E. A new preparation of nitroglycerin for uterine relaxation. *Int J Obstet Anesth* 1995;4:14–16.
46. Segal S, Csavoy AN, Datta S. Placental tissue enhances uterine relaxation by nitroglycerin. *Anesth Analg* 1998;86:304–309.
47. Platt LD, Druzing ML. Acute puerperal inversion of the uterus. *Am J Obstet Gynecol* 1981;141:187–190.
48. Watson P, Besch N, Bowes Jr. WA. Management of acute and subacute puerperal inversion of the uterus. *Obstet Gynecol* 1980;55:12–16.
49. Dawson NJ, Gabbott DA. Use of sublingual glyceryl trinitrate as a supplement to volatile inhalation anesthesia in a case of uterine inversion. *Int J Obstet Anesth* 1997;6:135–137.
50. Altabef KM, Spencer JT, Zinberg S. Intravenous nitroglycerin for uterine relaxation of an inverted uterus. *Am J Obstet Gynecol* 1992;166:1237–1238.
51. Herbert WNP, Afalo RC. Management of postpartum hemorrhage. *Clin Obstet Gynecol* 1984;27:139–148.
52. Hughes W, Hughes S. Hemodynamic effects of prostaglandin E_2. *Anesthesiology* 1989;70:713–716.
53. Buttino L Jr, Garite TJ. The use of 15 methyl F_2 alphaprostaglandin (Prostin 15 M) for the control of postpartum hemorrhage. *Am J Perinatol* 1986;3:241–243.
54. O'Leary AM. Severe bronchospasm and hypotension after 15-methyl prostaglandin F_2 alpha in atonic postpartum hemorrhage. *Int J Obstet Anesth* 1994;3:42–44.
55. Bigrigg A, Chui D, Chissell S, et al. Use of intramyometrial 15-methyl prostaglandin F_2 alpha to control atonic postpartum hemorrhage following vaginal delivery and failure of conventional therapy. *Br J Obstet Gynaecol* 1991;98:734–736.

56. Merrikay AO, Mariano JP. Controlling refractory atonic postpartum hemorrhage with hemabate sterile solution. *Am J Obstet Gynecol* 1990;162:205–208.

57. Hankins G, Berryman G, Scott R, et al. Maternal arterial desaturation with 15-methyl prostaglandin F_2 alpha for uterine atony. *Obstet Gynecol* 1988;72:367–370.

58. Douglas MJ, Farquharson DR, Ross PL, et al. Cardiovascular collapse following an overdose of prostaglandin F_2 alpha: a case report. *Can J Anaesth* 1989;36:466–469.

59. Mayhew J. Hypertension responsive to Dinoprost under anaesthesia. *Anesth Analg* 1986;65:1248.

60. Cates W, Grimes D, Haber R, et al. Abortion deaths associated with the use of prostaglandin F_2 alpha. *Am J Obstet Gynecol* 1977;127:219–222.

61. Fong J, Gurewitsch ED, Lump L, et al. Clearance of fetal products and subsequent immunoreactivity of blood salvaged at cesarean delivery. *Obstet Gynecol* 1999;93:968–972.

62. Camann WR, Datta S. Red cell use during cesarean delivery. *Transfusion* 1991;31:12–15.

63. Ekeroma AJ, Ansar A, Stirrat GM. Blood transfusion in obstetrics and gynaecology. *Br J Obstet Gynecol* 1997;104:278-2–84.

64. National Heart, Lung and Blood Institute. Expert Panel on the Use of Autologous Blood. Transfusion alert: use of autologous blood. *Transfusion* 1995;35:703–711.

65. Jackson SH, Lanser RE. Safety and effectiveness of intracesarean blood salvage. *Transfusion* 1993;33:181.

66. Rainaldi MP, Tazzari PL, Scagliarini G, et al. Blood salvage during cesarean section. *Br J Anaesth* 1998;80:195–198.

67. Rebarber A, Lanser SER, Jackson S, et al. The safety of intraoperative autologous blood collection and autotransfusion during cesarean section. *Am J Obstet Gynecol* 1998;179:712–720.

68. Catling SJ, Williams S, Fielding AM. Cell salvage in obstetrics: an evaluation of the ability of cell salvage combined with leucocyte depletion filtration to remove amniotic fluid from operative blood loss at caesarean section. *Int J Obstet Anesth* 1999;8:79–84.

69. Camann WR. Cell salvage during cesarean delivery: is it safe and valuable? Maybe, maybe not! *Int J Obstet Anesth* 1999;8:75–76.

70. Oei SG, Wingen CBM, Kerkkamp HEM. Cell salvage: how safe in obstetrics? *Int J Obstet Anesth* 2000;9:143.

71. Grange CS, Douglas MJ, Adams TJ, et al. The use of acute hemodilution in parturients undergoing cesarean section. *Am J Obstet Gynecol* 1998;178:156–160.

72. Palmer RH, Kane JG, Churchill WH, et al. Cost and quality in the use of blood bank service for normal deliveries, cesarean sections and hysterectomies. *JAMA* 1986;256:219–223.

73. Kruskall MS, Leonard S, Klapholz H. Autologous blood donation during pregnancy: analysis of safety and blood use. *Obstet Gynecol* 1987;70:938–941.

74. O'Dwyer G, Mylotte M, Sweeney M, et al. Experience of autologous blood transfusion in an obstetrics and gynecology department. *Br J Obstet Gynaecol* 1993;100:571–574.

75. Droste S, Sorenson T, Price T, et al. Maternal and fetal hemodynamic effects of autologous blood donation during pregnancy. *Am J Obstet Gynecol* 1992;167:89–93.

76. Mallett SV, Cox D. Thromboelastography. *Br J Anaesth* 1992;69:307–313.

77. Gorton H, Lyons G. Is it time to invest in a thromboelastograph? *Int J Obstet Anesth* 1999;8:171–178.

78. Sharma SK, Vera RL, Stegall WC, et al. Management of a postpartum coagulopathy using thromboelastography. *J Clin Anesth* 1997;9:243–247.

79. Gillies BSA. Thromboelastography and liver transplantation. *Semin Thromb Hemost* 1995;21:45–49.

80. Steer PL. Anaesthetic management of a parturient with thromboelastopenia using thromboelastography and sonoclot analysis. *Can J Anaesth* 1993;40:84–85.

81. Chadwick HS, Wall MH, Chandler W, et al. Thromboelastography in mild and severe preeclampsia. *Anesthesiology* 1993;79:A992.

82. Orlikowski CEP, Rocke DA, Murray WB, et al. Thromboelastographic changes in preeclampsia and eclampsia. *Br J Anaesth* 1996;77:157–161.

83. Payne AJ, Orlikowski CEP, Moodley J, et al. Thromboelastography as a measure of coagulation in high risk patients receiving low dose aspirin. *Obstet Gynecol* 1993;13:222–226.

FOUR

ANESTHETIC COMPLICATIONS

Shnider and Levinson's Anesthesia for Obstetrics,
edited by Samuel C. Hughes, et al.
Lippincott Williams & Wilkins,
Philadelphia, © 2001.

CHAPTER 21

DIFFICULT AIRWAY MANAGEMENT

ROBIN A. STACKHOUSE, M.D. AND CEDRIC R. BAINTON, M.D.

INTRODUCTION

The airway continues to be a significant management problem in the practice of obstetrical anesthesia. Difficult intubation, aspiration (often related to airway management) and a high incidence of substandard care are consistent findings in deaths directly attributable to anesthesia (1–5).

It is encouraging that the overall anesthesia-related maternal death rate is small and has decreased significantly in the United States in recent decades. Much of this decrease has been attributed to the greater use of regional anesthesia, which has a 16.7-fold lower death rate than that for general anesthesia (6, 7). In fact, 50% of anesthesia-related maternal mortality involves general anesthesia despite the fact that general anesthesia accounts for only 16% of anesthetics for cesarean delivery. Death rates for general anesthesia may actually be increasing (6). However, this may be due to a trend to reserve the use of general anesthesia for the most emergent cesarean sections. The risk of failed intubation in obstetrics has been estimated to have increased 8-fold compared to the general operating room, 1:250 in obstetrics compared to 1:2,000 in the surgical suite (8–11). As there is an attempt to lower cesarean section rates and a higher percentage are performed using regional techniques individual practitioners have less experience with general anesthesia in obstetrics (12, 13). Therefore, it is critically important to be aware of the problems (difficult airway management, aspiration), minimize the incidence of encountering problems, and be capable of instituting alternative management plans should difficulty be encountered. As Tunstall stated, the goal is "oxygenation without aspiration" (14).

Clearly, the suggestions of the American Society of Anesthesiologists' Task Force on Airway Management (15) need to be rigorously applied to the obstetric patient if mortality statistics are to improve. These suggestions include: careful history, thorough airway examination, thoughtful selection of an airway management approach, adequately skilled practitioners to perform the selected techniques, careful consideration of extubation techniques, and finally, appropriate education of the patient as to problems that can be expected to recur in future anesthetics.

This chapter discusses these airway principles as they apply to the practice of obstetrical anesthesia.

PHYSIOLOGIC CHANGES OF PREGNANCY

A thorough review of the physiologic changes of pregnancy can be found in Chapter 1. Changes that specifically impact airway management are elaborated here.

Airway/Respiratory Changes

Capillary engorgement and edema of the respiratory tract involves the nose, pharynx and larynx. This results in decreased space (partial obstruction) and increased risk of bleeding with standard airway management techniques (16–18).

Pulmonary changes include a decrease in residual volume (RV), expiratory reserve volume (ERV), and functional residual capacity (FRC) secondary to the cephalic displacement of the diaphragm by the expanding uterus. In up to one third of parturients, closing volume (CV) may be greater than FRC at term in the supine position (18). In addition, oxygen consumption ($MVRO_2$) increases by 20% (16). As a result of these physiologic changes, parturients are at greater risk for hypoxia during periods of apnea. After pre oxygenation, the partial pressure of oxygen (PO_2) decreases more rapidly in the parturient than in the nonpregnant patient (19). Consequently, the anesthesiologist has less time to manage a parturient's airway before desaturation occurs, and procedures outlined in the difficult airway algorithm must be instituted as will be discussed later in this chapter.

Gastrointestinal Changes

During pregnancy, the gastroesophageal barrier pressure (gastroesophageal junction pressure minus gastric pressure) decreases, the gastric acidity increases, and the intragastric pressure increases (especially with obesity, multiple gestations and polyhydramnios). Ultrasonography data suggests that gastric-emptying time is normal prior to the onset of labor, but solid foods may still be present in the stomach for as long as 8 to 24 hours after ingestion once labor begins (20). Parturients, particularly those in active labor, are at increased risk of reflux of gastric contents, and consequently at increased risk of aspiration when airway protective reflexes have been lost. The mortality risk from aspiration in an obstetrical patient is 10% to 25% (21).

AIRWAY ASSESSMENT
History

Has there been a problem in the past? What knowledge does the patient have of the problem? Are there records to review and personal physicians who can be consulted? It is essential to identify the problem and relate it to your examination (15, 22, 23).

Anatomic Examination
Oropharyngeal/Mandibular Space

Does the mouth open adequately? Are there malformations, swelling, edema, tumors, large tongue, temporomandibular joint disease, or other pathology? Is the patient obese? Are there signs of decreased oropharyngeal space such as assessory muscle use or drooling?

Mallampati (24, 25) hypothesized that the degree to which oropharyngeal structures could be visualized upon examination should correlate with the structures that could be seen on laryngoscopy and developed a scoring system. Samsoon and Young later modified this scoring to the Mallampati classification now in use (9). The observer should stand at eye level, using a light source and assess the patient's airway with the patient sitting, head in a neutral position, mouth open and tongue protruding maximally without phonating.

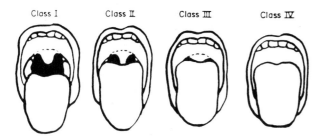

Figure 21.1. Mallampati classification. Pictorial classification of the pharyngeal structure s as seen when conducting the examination. (Adapted from Samsoon GLT, Young JRB. Difficult tracheal intubation: a retrospective study. *Anaesthesia* 1987;42:487–490.)

The airway is classified according to the structures seen:

Class I: soft palate, fauces, uvula, tonsillar pillars

Class II: soft palate, fauces, uvula

Class III: soft palate, base of uvula

Class IV: soft palate not visible (Fig. 21.1)

The Mallampati score has been correlated with the view of the laryngeal structures visible on laryngoscopy (26). Cormack and Lehane have classified the view achieved:

Grade 1: Most of the glottis is visible

Grade 2: Only the posterior extremity of the glottis is visible

Grade 3: No part of the glottis, only the epiglottis can be seen

Grade 4: Not even the epiglottis can be seen (Fig. 21.2)

Grades 3 and 4 views on laryngoscopy are associated with difficulty in intubation. Patients with a class IV airway should be considered at risk for difficult endotracheal intubation (6.6%). Those with a Class III airway are at intermediate risk (4.3%). Patients with Class I and II airways are seldom at risk for intubation difficulties (1.3%) (27).

Data suggests that Mallampati scores change during gestation with an increase in Class IV airways among patients between 12 and 38 weeks' gestation (28). This may be exacerbated by a prolonged second stage of labor (29). The trend toward a worsening Mallampati score is hypothesized to be due to increased pharyngeal edema and fatty infiltration of pharyngeal tissue (30). It is important to remember that the Mallampati score is based upon what can be seen with a direct line of sight. Thus, it is useful in defining the oral and upper portion of the pharyngeal space. However, where structures are hidden in the deep pharynx (laryngeal tonsils, laryngeal cysts, deep pharyngeal edema) the Mallampati score is misleading.

In cases where a difficult intubation is suspected, a more thorough examination may be needed. The evaluation of the oropharyngeal space may be made after topicalization of the airway in nonemergent situations.

The degree to which a patient can open their mouth (interincisor distance or gap), size and position of upper teeth, and the size of the mandible are components of the Mandibular space available to attain a line of vision (LOV) when performing laryngoscopy (Fig. 21.3). If the perpendicular distance between the LOV and the lower incisors is less than 2.5 centimeters or the interincisor gap is less than 5 centimeters, intubation may be difficult (30).

Atlanto-occipital Extension/Neck Mobility

Atlanto-occipital (A-O) extension is important in aligning the oral and pharyngeal axes during laryngoscopy. It may be affected by ankylosis, short/stocky neck, dwarfism, etc. The pharyngeal and laryngeal axes are brought into alignment by flexion of the neck. The three axes are optimally aligned when the patient is placed in the sniffing position (Fig. 21.4) (31). Atlanto-occipital extension can be measured by the angle that is traversed by the occlusal surface of the maxillary teeth when the head is extended maximally from the neutral position. Normal A-O extension is 35 degrees. A decrease of more than one-third correlates with difficult endotracheal intubation (32).

Sternomental/Thyromental Distance

The distance between the bony point of the mentum and either the thyroid (less than 6.5 to 7 cm) or the upper border of the manubrium (less than 12.5 to 13.5 cm) have been shown to correlate with difficult laryngoscopy (33–36). The sensitivity and specificity of these tests depend on what length is chosen as a cut-off point in determining risk of difficulty. If the larger length is chosen, the sensitivity (proportion of difficult intubations correctly predicted to be difficult) is increased, at the expense of specificity (proportion of easy intubations correctly predicted to be easy) (36).

Submandibular Compliance

Despite normal evaluations using the other airway criteria, difficulty may still be encountered if the compliance of the tissue in the submandibular space is compromised. This is the space into which the soft tissues must be displaced during laryngoscopy. Consequently, those processes that alter the compliance of this tissue (Ludwig's angina, tumor infiltration, scarring from radiation, burns, surgery) may affect visualization of the larynx regardless of normal physiognomy (22).

Body Habitus

Large breasts can project upwards to fill the space in which the laryngoscope handle must be placed. Thus, standard laryngoscopy will not be possible unless measures are taken to displace the breasts or special equipment is used such as a short-handled blade or a polio blade.

Cricothyroid Membrane

If the cricothyroid membrane can not be identified, the ability to perform successful cricothyrotomy will be unlikely and this emergency solution to airway control will be unavailable.

The studies of airway variables that correlate with difficult airway management have been quantified as to their sensitivity, specificity and positive-predictive values (proportion of predicted difficult intubations that actually prove to be difficult). Reported sensitivity and specificity of the tests varies between different studies. This may be a result of genetic variables in the different patient populations, variations in performing the assessments and variations in definition of difficult laryngoscopy. This leaves the clinician with a series of tests with a positive-predictive value of less than 30% (37).

Attempts have been made to improve the ability of predicting difficult laryngoscopy by combining those elements of the airway assessment, which are independent variables in predicting

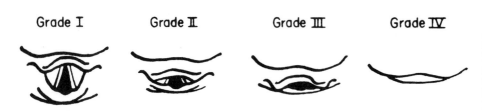

Figure 21.2. Laryngoscopic view classification. Laryngoscopic views obtained by modifying the drawings of Cormack and Lehane. (Adapted from Samsoon GLT, Young JRB. Difficult tracheal intubation: a retrospective study. *Anaesthesia* 1987;42:487–490.)

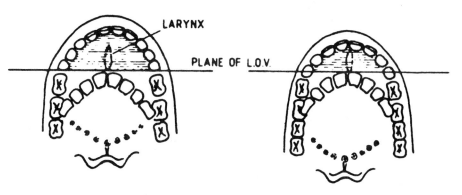

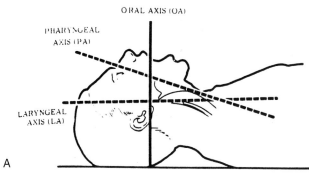

Figure 21.3. Laryngoscopic line of view. Schematic view of the mandible, plane of LOV, mandibular space (shaded area), and the position of the larynx. **A:** Large mandibular space. **B:** Small mandibular space. (Adapted from Bellhouse CP, Doré C. Criteria for estimating likelihood of difficulty of endotracheal intubation with the Macintosh laryngoscope. *Anaesth Intensive Care* 1988;16:329–337.)

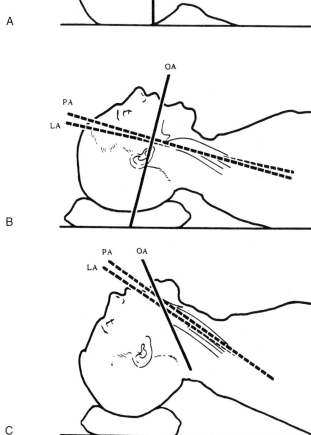

Figure 21.4. Alignment of oral, pharyngeal, and laryngeal axes. Schematic diagram demonstrating head position for endotracheal intubation. **A:** Neutral position. **B:** Elevation of the head approximately 10 cm aligns the laryngeal and pharyngeal axes. **C:** Subsequent extension of the head on the atlanto-occipital joint aligns the oral axis with the pharyngeal and laryngeal axes. (Adapted from Stone DJ, Gal TJ. Airway Management. In: Miller RD, ed. *Anesthesia*, 3rd ed. New York: Churchill Livingston, 1990:1265–1292.)

difficulty (Fig. 21.5) (27, 38). These scoring systems significantly increase the accuracy of predicting airway problems, but unfortunately become too complex to use clinically and only give a probability of difficulty and not a prediction in any given patient. Despite the limitations of a physical exam in predicting difficulty, current examinations and information about previous anesthetics are the best way of predicting and avoiding airway management problems. The airway exam should include: interincisor distance, oropharyngeal classification, mandibular space (length and compliance), range of motion of the head and neck, neck (length, thickness, muscularity, ease of identification of the cricothyroid membrane), teeth (size, degree of protuberance), configuration of the palate, breasts (degree to which they will affect laryngoscope placement), and any pathologic states (bleeding, edema, infection, masses) (39). An estimate of the ease of mask ventilation may be made based on factors such as whether the patient is edentulous, obese, or shows signs of airway obstruction (22).

GENERAL ANESTHESIA

The approach to airway management is determined by whether the patient's airway is known or predicted to be difficult and the urgency with which the patient requires anesthesia. In fact, the American College of Obstetricians and Gynecologists (ACOG) has published a committee opinion (see Appendix) which details the circumstances under which a parturient should receive antepartum consultations with a physician who is credentialed to provide general and regional anesthesia, a joint management plan formulated and consideration given to referral of the patient for delivery at a hospital that can manage such anesthesia on a 24-hour basis (40).

When antepartum assessment predicts a parturient to be at risk of difficult airway management, the delivery plan may involve early intervention with regional anesthesia or planned awake airway management followed by the induction of general anesthesia and elective cesarean section. Early placement of an epidural catheter with careful verification of its location and dosing can minimize the necessity for general anesthesia should an operative delivery become necessary. It is a calculated risk, however, because should complications of regional anesthesia or maternal/fetal complications occur, airway management under emergency circumstances may become necessary which puts the parturient at inordinate risk of aspiration and/or hypoxemia. Securing the airway under elective circumstances in an awake patient who is maintaining her own oxygenation and ventilation and is at minimal risk of aspiration (as she would be NPO for adequate duration) avoids the major risks of general anesthesia and should be assessed vis-à-vis the risk to the parturient of an operative delivery.

Aspiration Prophylaxis

The factors that determine the risk of aspiration include:

1. pH, volume, and composition (liquid vs. particulate) of gastric contents (21, 41–43)

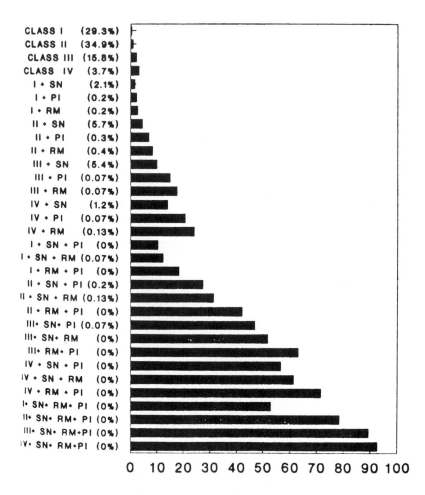

CLASS I (29.3%)
CLASS II (34.9%)
CLASS III (15.8%)
CLASS IV (3.7%)
I + SN (2.1%)
I + PI (0.2%)
I + RM (0.2%)
II + SN (5.7%)
II + PI (0.3%)
II + RM (0.4%)
III + SN (5.4%)
III + PI (0.07%)
III + RM (0.07%)
IV + SN (1.2%)
IV + PI (0.07%)
IV + RM (0.13%)
I + SN + PI (0%)
I + SN + RM (0.07%)
I + RM + PI (0%)
II + SN + PI (0.2%)
II + SN + RM (0.13%)
II + RM + PI (0%)
III+ SN+ PI (0.07%)
III+ SN+ RM (0%)
III+ RM+ PI (0%)
IV + SN + PI (0%)
IV + SN + RM (0%)
IV + RM + PI (0%)
I+ SN+ RM+ PI (0%)
II+ SN+ RM+ PI (0%)
III+ SN+ RM+PI (0%)
IV+ SN+ RM+PI (0%)

0 10 20 30 40 50 60 70 80 90 100

Figure 21.5. Probability of experiencing a difficult intubation. The probability of experiencing a difficult intubation (grades 3 and 4) for varying combinations of risk factors and the observed incidence of these combinations in the study population (percentage). SN, short neck; PI, protruding maxillary incisors; RM, receding mandible. (Adapted from Rocke DA, Murray, WB, Rout CC, et al. Relative risk analysis of factors associated with difficult intubation in obstetric anesthesia. *Anesthesiology* 1992;77:67–73.)

2. Gastric pressure
3. Forces inhibiting reflux of gastric contents into the pharynx (lower esophageal sphincter (LES) tone, upper esophageal sphincter (UES) tone and cricoid pressure (CP)

To minimize these risks, multiple prophylactic steps can be taken (see Chapter 22). Gastric contents with a pH of less than 2.5 and a volume of greater than 0.4 mL · kg^{-1} especially if particulate, pose the highest risk. It is now recommended that a nonparticulate antacid such as 0.3 M sodium citrate, 30 milliliters, be administered pre operatively. This is capable of neutralizing 255 mL of HCL with a pH of 1.0 and has a duration of action of 40 minutes to 1 hour. Histamine receptors (H2) blocking agents administered IV, are useful adjuncts, but require an average of 40 minutes to be effective. This may result in a negligible change in aspiration risk at the time of induction of anesthesia for an emergency case, but will decrease the risk of aspiration on emergence (44, 45). The proton pump inhibitor and antisecretory agent, omeprazole, also reduces gastric acidity, and requires 40 minutes to be effective (45–47). Metaclopramide, a prokinetic agent, decreases gastric volume within 30 to 60 minutes. It crosses the placenta but has not been shown to have any lasting adverse neurobehavioral effects on the newborn (46).

Barrier pressure to gastroesophageal reflux is normally 18 ± 2 mm Hg (48) (normal LESP = 24 ± 3; normal gastric pressure = 5 ± 2). In pregnancy, gastric pressure can rise to 35 mm Hg (49). Although LESP also rises to 35 to 44 cm H$_2$O (26 to 32 mm Hg) (16), the barrier pressure is reduced. Should reflux into the lower esophagus occur, the UES with a resting pressure of 38 mm Hg lends some protection against aspiration. When general anesthesia is induced, however, these pressure relationships change. UESP decreases to 8 mm Hg after sodium thiopental administration (50). Succinycholine

increases gastric pressure, but causes a greater increase in the gastroesophageal junction pressure and therefore does not worsen barrier pressure (51). As a result of the changing pressure relationship, pregnant women are at increased risk of aspiration on the induction of general anesthesia.

Cricoid pressure (CP), first described by Sellick, supplies the necessary barrier to regurgitation of gastric contents during the induction of anesthesia and prevents inflation of the stomach during positive-pressure ventilation (52). The cricoid cartilage is the only tracheal cartilage with a ring structure. When a pressure of 40 Newton's (N) is applied to the cricoid, fluids under a pressure of 100 cm H$_2$O (approximately 74 mm Hg) may be opposed (53). Although CP has been shown to reduce LESP by 50% (48), parturients are at risk of regurgitation whether the barrier pressure is further reduced or not. CP provides the required barrier. Despite Sellick's initial recommendation to remove nasogastric tubes (NG) prior to the induction of anesthesia to ensure efficacy of CP, it has been shown to be unnecessary (53).

The cricoid cartilage is identified by first palpating the neck for the more prominent thyroid cartilage. The cricoid cartilage is the next cartilaginous structure felt when palpating in a caudal direction. In women the thyroid cartilage may not be prominent, in this case, palpation of the tracheal cartilages starting at the sternal notch may help to identify the cricoid cartilage. As the fingers move cephalad on the neck, they will encounter a cartilage that is wider than those below. This is the cricoid cartilage (Fig. 21.6).

CP was originally described as anterior pressure with the thumb and index finger (52). A double-handed modification has been described (53) where the assistant's other hand is used for counter pressure behind the patient's neck to limit the change in head position that would occur with anterior pressure alone.

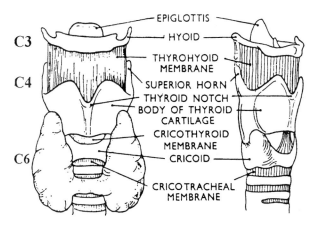

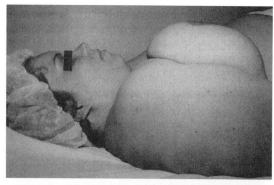

Figure 21.6. Anatomy of the airway. External frontal (left) and antero-lateral (right) views of the larynx. (Adapted from Ellis H, Feldman S. *Anatomy for Anesthesiologists*, 6th ed. Oxford, U.K.: Blackwell Scientific, 1993.)

Induction of General Anesthesia

When general anesthesia is to be used in obstetrics, the method of airway management will depend on the urgency of the procedure and the anticipated ease or difficulty of intubation and ventilation. For stat situations with no anticipated airway difficulties, the standard technique for initiation of general anesthesia as described in Chapter 11 is used.

As previously discussed, the parturient is at increased risk of difficult airway management (both intubation and ventilation), more rapid desaturation and aspiration. This mandates that conditions (positioning and pre oxygenation) be optimized such that the first attempt at airway management be the best attempt. All equipment for routine and emergency airway management should be immediately available (Table 21.1).

The patient should be positioned supine, with 15 degrees of left uterine displacement. The head and neck should be in the Magill or "sniff" position. In obese patients, or those with engorged breasts, standard positioning of the head on a small pillow may not optimize the head and neck position. The airway can be improved by creating a wedge-shaped support out of sheets or blankets that is placed under the shoulders and head (Fig. 21.7).

Preoxygenation should be performed with high-flow oxygen and a tight mask seal for 3 minutes, if time permits. This allows for maximal oxygenation and denitrogenation and therefore the greatest time to desaturation during apnea (54). When urgency of delivery dictates, four maximal capacity breaths affords a reasonable compromise (55, 56). However, eight maximal ca-

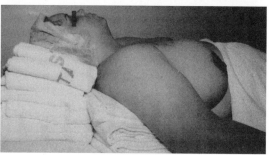

Figure 21.7. Positioning of the obese parturient. **A:** Obese pregnant woman in the supine position. **B:** The same patient positioned with the shoulders and occiput elevated so that the head assumes the 'sniffing' position.

pacity breaths over a 60-second period may be as effective, or more so, than 3 minutes of tidal volume breathing (57). Induction agents and muscle relaxants should have a rapid onset and short duration to allow for the return of spontaneous ventilation and consciousness should difficult airway management ensue. In the case of complete inability to ventilate, even a short-acting muscle relaxant, such as succinylcholine, may not wear off before serious hypoxia develops (Fig. 21.8) (58). However, succinylcholine is the muscle relaxant of choice, unless there is a contraindication to its use.

Laryngoscopy and intubation should be performed once muscle relaxation is achieved. Poor visualization of the larynx despite optimal laryngoscope placement may be improved with external laryngeal pressure. Pressing on the thyroid cartilage in a backward, upward and rightward direction is known as the BURP maneuver (59). Once the laryngoscopist determines the necessary pressure using their right hand, they instruct the assistant to duplicate the maneuver. Tracheal intubation is confirmed by auscultation over the apices of the lung and by the presence of end-tidal carbon dioxide (CO_2).

If tracheal intubation is unsuccessful on the first attempt, steps outlined in the difficult airway algorithm (modified for obstetrics) should commence (Fig. 21.9). At whatever time intubation is successful, the cesarean section may proceed. When the initial attempt at intubation fails, the clinician must make a judgment whether to attempt a second laryngoscopy directly, or attempt mask ventilation. An immediate second (best attempt) laryngoscopy is acceptable if oxygen desaturation has not occurred. Best attempt at laryngoscopy is defined as being performed by an experienced endoscopist, with the patient in optimal position with no significant muscle tone, using optimal external laryngeal manipulation, and perhaps a single change in laryngoscope blade type and/or size (60). If unsuccessful, ventilation should be attempted by face mask (FM), a call for assistance should be made. Once oxygen saturation has been restored, further attempts at laryngoscopy may be made. Numerous, repeated attempts at larynoscopies should be avoided because pharyngeal trauma will make ventilation progressively more difficult if not impossible (39). If ventilation by face mask

Table 21.1. EQUIPMENT FOR AIRWAY MANAGEMENT IN OBSTETRICS

Routine
    Laryngoscope (standard, polio), multiple blades
      (Mac 3, 4, Miller 2, 3)
    Endotracheal tubes (5.0–7.0)
    Oral airways (80, 90, 100 mm)
    Nasal airways (7, 8, 9)
    Laryngeal masks (size 3, 4)
    Esophageal tracheal combitube
    Stylets, bougie
Emergency
    Tube exchanger
    Cricothyrotomy kit
    Transtracheal Jet Ventilation equipment
    Lightwand, retrograde intubation equipment
Anticipated difficult: nonemergent airway
    Fiberoptic laryngoscope and accessory equipment/medications
    Fixed fiberoptic blades (Bullard, Wu Scope, Upsher)

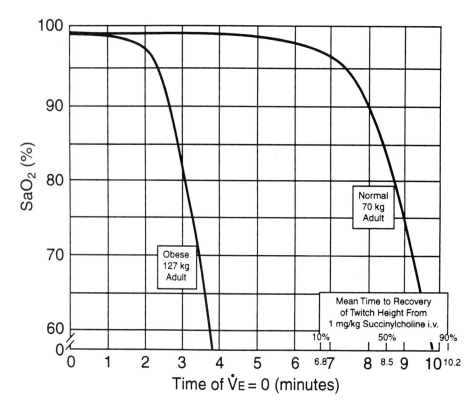

Figure 21.8. **Time to hemoglobin desaturation with initial $Fa_{O_2} = 0.87$.** Sa_{O_2} versus time of apnea in normal 70 kg adults versus obese adults. (Adapted from Benumof JL, Dagg R, Benumof R. Critical hemoglobin desaturation will occur before return to an unparalyzed state following 1 mg/kg intravenous succinylcholine. *Anesthesiology* 1997;87:979–982.)

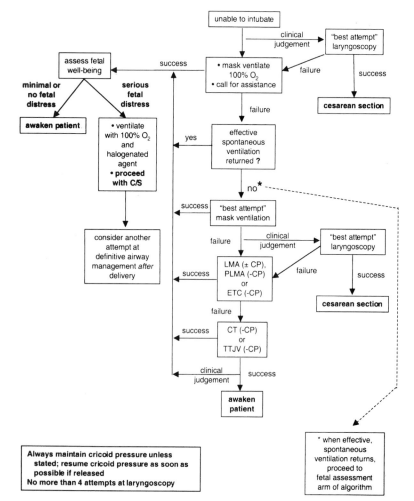

Figure 21.9. **Difficult airway management at cesarean section.** Failed intubation algorithm in obstetrics. CP, cricoid pressure; C/S, cesarean section; LMA, laryngeal mask airway; PLMA, ProSeal laryngeal mask airway (Laryngeal Mask Company, Henley-on-Thames, U.K.); ETC, esophageal tracheal combitube; CT, cricothyrotomy; TTJV, transtracheal jet ventilation.

is possible, and further attempts at intubation are futile or ill—advised, a decision must be made as to the risk/benefit ratio to the mother and fetus of continuing with cesarean section or awakening the mother. If ventilation with face mask alone is not possible, clinical judgement must be used to determine whether to quickly proceed to "optimal/best attempt" at laryngoscopy (if oxygen saturation is adequate) or a "best attempt" at mask ventilation. "Best attempt" mask ventilation is defined as two person additive/synergistic effort, optimal jaw thrust and mask seal, oropharyngeal airway and bilateral nasopharyngeal airways (39). In obstetrical patients, nasal airways must be placed with caution, secondary to the risk of epistaxis. If laryngoscopy was attempted but failed, "best attempt" ventilation should be made immediately. Upon institution of adequate mask ventilation and oxygenation, a decision is made as to whether further attempts at laryngoscopy have a reasonable chance of success or whether to allow spontaneous ventilation to return and either proceed with the cesarean section or awaken the patient. If attempts at ventilation have been unsuccessful, nonsurgical airway management techniques (laryngeal mask airway [LMA], ProSeal LMA [PLMA; Laryngeal Mask Company, Henley-on-Thames, U.K.], or esophageal-tracheal combitube [ETC]) should be tried. If airway management is successful, the decision is again at the point of proceeding with the surgical procedure or awakening the patient. If failure occurs, then a surgical airway (cricothyrotomy, transtracheal jet ventilation [TTJV], or tracheostomy) should be obtained. Cricothyrotomy and tracheostomy result in a definitive airway (an airway of adequate size [greater than 4.0 mm ID] with a cuff which would protect from aspiration and allow ventilation irrespective of pulmonary compliance) that can be used for surgical procedures. TTJV, with the risk of pneumothorax and aspiration, is not a definitive airway, and it would generally be advisable to awaken the patient.

If the decision to awaken the patient was made during the difficult airway management, it may still be necessary to proceed with a cesarean section. The options for anesthetic management would include awake intubation techniques or regional anesthesia.

When determining whether to proceed with a cesarean section in a parturient with an unprotected airway or to awaken the parturient, a number of questions should be considered. Does her life depend upon completion of surgery? Is fetal distress severe and showing no signs of recovering (e.g. placental abruptio, prolapsed cord)? Is fetal distress long-standing but not severe? Is the procedure elective? When maternal survival is the issue, there is no option but to proceed with surgery. Similarly, if the fetus is not in imminent jeopardy, then awakening the mother is the appropriate course. If the fetus is in imminent danger and the maternal airway has not been secured, those involved must use their clinical judgment and weigh the risks of fetal versus maternal morbidity and mortality (10, 30, 61).

Airway Management Techniques

Fiberoptic Intubation

Awake intubation techniques (flexible fiberoptic laryngoscopy, fiberoptic blades, and blind nasal intubation) require time to perform since topicalization and/or nerve blocks of the airway need to be performed in order for the patient to tolerate the procedure. They may be used when airway difficulty is anticipated or as a secondary plan after awakening a patient when there was a failure in airway management.

Fiberoptic nasal intubation is generally easier to perform than fiberoptic oral intubation because the angle of curvature of the ETT more closely matches that of the airway when approached through the nose. The nasal route also has the advantage of being more easily tolerated by patients because there isn't as

great a stimulus of the gag reflex. In pregnancy, however, there are disadvantages to the nasal approach. There is capillary engorgement and edema of the nasal mucosa. These result in an increased risk of nasal bleeding and a smaller diameter space through which the endotracheal tube must pass. Individual experience with fiberoptic laryngoscopy in obstetrics is limited, and the information on the subject consists predominantly of case reports and extrapolation from the literature on fiberoptic intubation in other clinical settings (62–67).

Factors which will impact the success and ease of fiberoptic laryngoscopy are: experience, presence of secretion and blood, adequacy of topical anesthesia and blocks, blurred view (fog, focus, secretions), pharyngeal space, time and presence of a fiberoptic channel that aims the scope toward the airway (22).

An antisialagogic (glycopyrrolate) should be administered to inhibit further secretion formation. If required, sedation is administered (midazolam, fentanyl) in minimum doses necessary to avoid neonatal depression. Topical anesthesia and blocks are then performed.

Neuroanatomy of the Airway

The trigeminal nerve, cranial nerve V (CN V), provides innervation to the nasal mucosa via the ophthalmic (V1) and maxillary (V2) divisions. V1 innervates through the anterior ethmoidal nerve. V2 becomes the infraorbital nerve, the nasopalatine nerve and the sphenopalatine ganglion (Fig. 21.10). Sensation to the posterior one third of the tongue, the soft palate, and oropharynx is supplied by the glossopharyngeal nerve (CN IX) (Fig. 21.11). Branches of the vagus nerve (CN X) provide sensation to the pharynx, larynx, and trachea via the superior

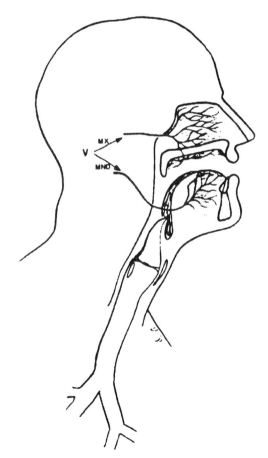

Figure 21.10. Trigeminal nerve. Sensory distribution of the maxillary (MX) and mandibular (MND) branches of the trigeminal nerve (V). (Adapted from Patil VU, Stehling LC, Zander HL. *Fiberoptic Endoscopy in Anesthesia.* St. Louis, Mosby, 1983.)

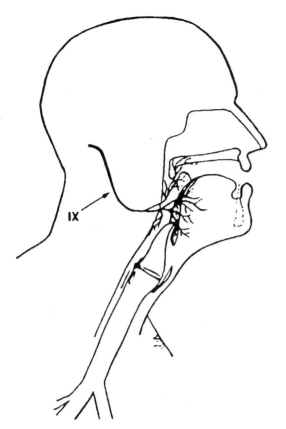

Figure 21.11. Glossopharyngeal nerve. Sensory distribution of the glossopharyngeal nerve (IX). (Adapted from Patil VU, Stehling LC, Zander HL. *Fiberoptic Endoscopy in Anesthesia.* St. Louis: Mosby, 1983.)

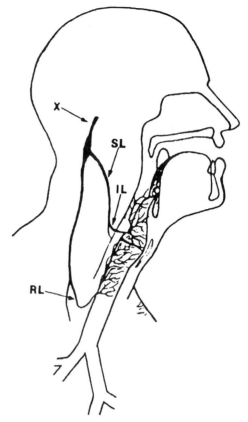

Figure 21.12. Vagus nerve. Sensory distribution of the vagus nerve. (Adapted from Patil VU, Stehling LC, Zander HL. *Fiberoptic Endoscopy in Anesthesia.* St. Louis, Mosby, 1983.)

laryngeal nerve (SLN) and the recurrent laryngeal nerve (RLN). The SLN provides sensory innervation to the lower pharynx and the true vocal cords. The external branch of the SLN, which separates from the internal branch posterior to where the internal branch passes through the thyrohyoid ligament, supplies motor fibers to the cricothyroid muscle. The remainder of the intrinsic muscles of the larynx are innervated by the RLN, which also provides sensation to the larynx below the vocal cords (Fig. 21.12) (22, 68, 69).

Topical Anesthesia/Nerve Blocks of the Airway

NOSE AND NASOPHARYNX. The mucosa of the nose needs to be both topicalized, for patient comfort, and vasoconstricted, to inhibit bleeding. The agents most commonly used for this purpose are 4% cocaine or 3% to 4% lidocaine with 0.25% neosynephrine. Both cocaine and neosynephrine pose the potential risk of decreasing uterine blood flow. It has been shown that intravenous doses of cocaine decrease uterine blood flow in a dose-dependent manner in gravid ewes. Doses of 0.7 mg·kg^{-1} result in a 15% decrease in uterine blood flow. Maximum decrement in uterine blood flow (40%) occurred with doses of greater than or equal to 1.4 mg·kg^{-1} (70). This has been corroborated by other studies (71, 72). Cocaine is absorbed from the nasal mucosa in 8 to 11 minutes and has a bioavailability of 60% to 80% (73, 74). When cocaine (160 mg) is applied on cotton pledgets, an average of 36% was absorbed in 12 patients undergoing elective nasal surgery (75). Assuming the absorption is equivalent in parturients, although it may be higher secondary to vascular engorgement, this would result in 0.7 mg·kg^{-1} being absorbed in a 70-kg patient. As shown by Foutz et al. (70), this could compromise fetal perfusion.

Data concerning the systemic absorption of neosynephrine is scarce. After administration of aqueous phenylephrine hydrochloride 2.5% solution in the eye, peak plasma levels occur

in less than 20 minutes and have hemodynamic consequences (76). The concentration used is 10 times that used for vasoconstriction in the nose. However, the volumes used were much less than those used for nasal vasoconstriction and the concentration of the drug that reaches the nose for absorption after ophthalmic application would be lower than what was administered. It is the author's experience that neosynephrine 0.25% administered intranasally can cause systemic hypertension. It may therefore adversely effect uteroplacental blood flow.

The use of 1% ephedrine dripped into the nostril for vasoconstriction has been reported for fiberoptic nasal intubation of a parturient at 38 weeks' gestation with a submandibular abscess (65). The baby wasn't delivered for another week, and no information about fetal tolerance of the procedure was given. There are no data on systemic absorption of ephedrine after nasal administration.

Whichever vasoconstrictor is chosen, care should be taken to use the minimum effective dose and to monitor maternal hemodynamic response and fetal heart rate response to the medication.

MOUTH/OROPHARYNX. Topicalization may be achieved by aerosolization of 2% to 4% lidocaine or by a block of the glossopharyngeal nerve at the base of the anterior tonsillar pillars. The tongue is retracted laterally to expose the palatoglossal arch (anterior tonsillar pillar). A small (25 to 27 gauge, 1/2 inch) needle is inserted to the depth of 0.5 cm at the base of the anterior pillar. Two milliliters of 2% lidocaine is injected after negative aspiration. This is repeated on the contralateral side (71). If a spray technique is used, awareness of absolute dose and potential for local anesthetic toxicity is required. Peak systemic levels occur between 20 and 40 minutes depending on the agent and how it is administered. Toxicity is rare, except in patients with impaired liver function, but may be increased in parturients who are already receiving local anesthetics through an epidural or who have a decreased seizure threshold (eclampsia).

LARYNX/TRACHEA.   There are numerous methods for topicalization of the larynx and trachea. An aerosol spray of 2% to 4% lidocaine is effective for both the larynx and trachea if the patient is prompted to take deep breaths to entrain the spray below the vocal cords. The particle size of the spray determines the spread of the local anesthetic. An atomizer connected to an oxygen source with 8 to 10 liters flow provides the optimal particle size for limiting the spread of local anesthesia (LA) distal to the trachea. Nebulizers generate particle sizes of 30 to 60 microns, (77) which results in the local anesthetic being entrained deeper into the tracheobronchial tree and in greater systemic absorption.

Lidocaine is the LA of choice secondary to its large margin of safety. Tetracaine toxicity from topical administration has been reported in doses as low as 40 milligrams (69, 78). Benzocaine can cause methemoglobinemia in clinical doses. Cetacaine is a mixture of tetracaine and benzocaine.

An alternative to the spray technique is a combination of bilateral superior laryngeal nerve (SLN) block and transtracheal block. The landmarks for the SLN are either the cornu of the hyoid or the thyroid (Fig. 21.13). The landmark is palpated with the nondominant hand. A small needle is advanced until it contacts either the cornu of the thyroid or hyoid. The needle is then "walked off" the cartilage/bone into the thyrohyoid membrane and 1.5 to 2.0 milliliters of 2% lidocaine is injected and the needle withdrawn. Block of the contralateral nerve is then performed.

A transtracheal block is performed by first identifying the cricothyroid membrane (as when applying CP). A 20-gauge angiocatheter attached to a syringe filled with 4 milliliters of 2% lidocaine is advanced through the cricothyroid membrane until air is aspirated. The needle is then withdrawn, air aspiration from the catheter is verified, the LA is injected, and the catheter withdrawn. Using an angiocatheter rather than a needle limits the risk of airway damage if the patient coughs during injection of the LA.

Trickle-down anesthesia has also been described in which 8 milliliters of 4% lidocaine in a 10-milliliter syringe is attached to a 14-gauge catheter. The patient's tongue is pulled forward using gauze. The LA is drizzled on the posterior surface of the tongue over 8 to 10 minutes (79). It is imperative that the patient not be allowed to retract their tongue during swallowing or the LA will not reach the larynx and topicalization will be inadequate.

Aspiration may be a concern if the airway is fully topicalized/blocked. However, if performed adequately, there should be no gag reflex and the upper esophageal sphincter will still be intact. This should minimize the risk of aspiration. The alternative is to topicalize/block in all distributions except that of the recurrent laryngeal nerve and to spray LA through the channel of the fiberoptic scope just before passing it through the vocal cords. This limits the period of aspiration risk, but will likely make the patient cough, and possibly reflux, or cause the endoscopist to lose their view of the airway.

Fiberoptic Laryngoscopy.   The endotracheal tube (ETT) is lubricated and passed either through the nose at a 90-degree angle to the plane of the face, or an appropriate size intubating oral airway (Berman, Ovassapian, Williams) until it is in the pharynx. The lubricated, focused and defogged fiberoptic scope is then passed through the ETT and into the airway. Adjustments of the ETT position may be required to help aim the scope toward the airway. Successful fiberoptic intubation requires that: space be maintained around the scope to give the widest field of view, secretions and blood be minimized, the target must always be kept in the center of the field of view, and the channel (ETT or oral airway) always aimed toward the airway. After passing the scope into the trachea, the ETT should be advanced over the fiberscope. If the ETT will not advance, the fiber has either exited the Murphy eye or the ETT is abutting the larynx. Rotate the ETT as you gently advance it and the bevel will become free of the obstruction. If the fiberscope was advanced out the Murphy eye, you will likely need to withdraw the ETT and the scope as a unit and begin again.

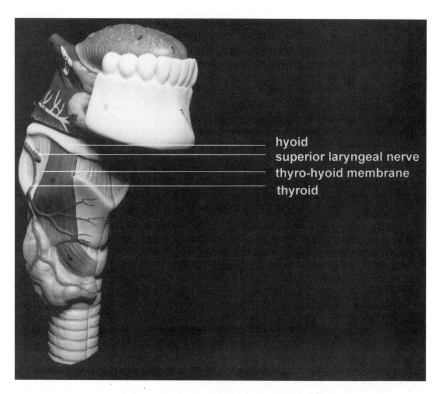

Figure 21.13. Anatomy for superior laryngeal nerve block.

hyoid
superior laryngeal nerve
thyro-hyoid membrane
thyroid

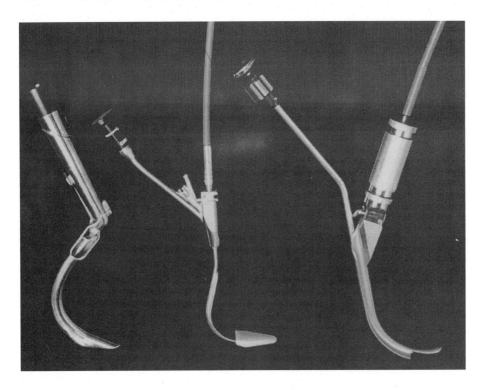

Figure 21.14. Rigid fiberoptic blades. **A:** Wu Scope. **B:** Bullard. **C:** Upsher.

Rigid fiberoptic devices such as the Bullard blade, the Upsher blade and the Wu scope system are alternatives to the flexible fiberoptic scope. The Wu scope has a tubular blade and can therefore maintain space in the pharynx if edema is present (Fig. 21.14).

Laryngeal Mask Airway

The LMA consists of a 12-millimeter ID shaft and a cuffed silicone rubber mask that seals in the hypopharynx. The proximal end of the cuff should rest at the base of the tongue. The distal end contacts the upper esophageal sphincter and the sides rest in the pyriform fossae (80, 81). A size 3 LM is appropriate for most women.

There are a growing number of case reports that document successful use of the LMA in obstetrics (82–88). Recent reports of the LMA being used for elective cesarean section using positive-pressure ventilation without adverse outcomes have appeared in abstract form, (89, 90) but not in a peer-reviewed journal and seems ill-advised to the authors. Positive-pressure ventilation with the laryngeal mask has been shown to generate a pressure-dependent leak, which results in gastric insufflation. Peak pressures of 15, 20, 25, and 30 cm H_2O generated leaks of 2.1%, 8.3%, 20.8%, and 35.4% respectively (91). The use of positive pressure ventilation can only be recommended until spontaneous ventilation returns. The major issues are how cricoid pressure effects placement of the LM; how the LM effects the efficacy of CP; and whether there is a safer alternative.

Effect of Cricoid Pressure on the Laryngeal Mask. The LMA can be successfully inserted and provide an unobstructed airway on the first attempt in 90% of patients. The success rate rises to as much as 98% if a second attempt is made (92). Providing an unobstructed airway, however, does not guarantee that the mask is seated as in Figure 21.15a. Radiologic (80, 81) and fiberoptic studies (93, 94) have shown that less than optimal placement of the LM may occur without any clinical evidence of airway obstruction. In 20% to 64% of patients the epiglottis will be within the cuff. In fact, the reason the mask was designed with fenestrations was to avoid airway obstruction from impaction of the epiglottis within the lumen. The cuff may be back-folded against the posterior pharyngeal wall resulting in a clear communication between the airway and the esophagus (Fig. 21.15b). The LM may also become impacted on the arytenoids without being detected clinically (Fig. 21.15c) (81).

The distal end of the LMA may be located as high as C4 or as low as T1 (80, 81). Because of this wide variation, it is easy to see how cricoid pressure (at the C6 level) could adversely effect LM placement. Studies designed to assess the extent of this effect have had widely disparate results (Table 21.2).

It is difficult to assess the significance of the results by Ansermino and Blogg (95). Their determinance of successful placement was not made on the basis of whether the LM provided an unobstructed airway, but on such criteria as outward movement of the LMA with cuff inflation, condensation in the tube and satisfactory compliance during manual ventilation. Therefore, their success rate may be artificially low. Brimacombe (92, 93) achieved 85% to 90% successful intubations when cricoid pressure was used, (96) whereas Asai et al. had only 50% success (94). The significant difference between these studies is the use of single-handed vs. double-handed cricoid pressure. The data indicates that double-handed pressure has a greater adverse effect on the ability to place the LM.

Cricoid pressure applied after LMA insertion, has been shown to dramatically decrease the ability to blindly intubate through the LM from 90% to 56% (97). When cricoid pressure was released, another 30% could be intubated blindly. As there is no statistical difference between 86% and 90%, these results would tend to indicate that the problem with intubation was the anatomic changes produced by cricoid pressure rather than malposition of the LM secondary to the cricoid pressure. It is preferable to use a technique that allows visualization. However, it appears that despite the ability to visualize the airway with a fiberoptic scope, intubation may not be possible in the presence of cricoid pressure. This is believed to be due to the anterior tilting of the larynx of 10 to 40 degrees that results from cricoid pressure and possibly from the closer apposition of the vocal cords (98). If intubation through the laryngeal mask is performed, it is advisable to use a long 6 mm I.D. endotracheal tube (ETT). Because of the length of the LMA shaft, only 8 cm can project beyond the fenestration. In the average woman, 8.1 cm is required to keep the ETT cuff from overlying the vocal cords (98). An Endotrol or a microlaryngeal ETT provide the required length.

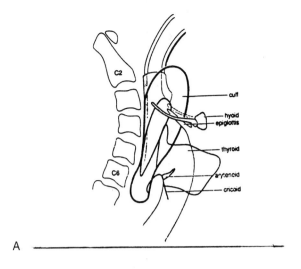

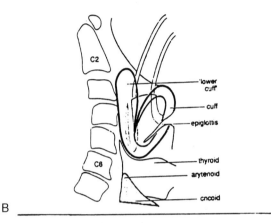

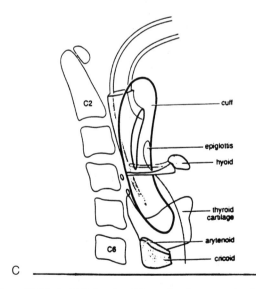

Figure 21.15. **A:** LMA in situ. Schematic of a properly placed LMA. **B:** Back-folding LMA with down-folded epiglottis. **C:** LMA anterior to the arytenoids and within the laryngeal inlet. All three placements resulted in functional LMA's. (Adapted from Nandi PR, Nunn JF, Charlesworth CH, et al. Radiologic study of the laryngeal mask. *Eur J Anaesthesiol* 1991;4(S):33–39.)

Effect of the Laryngeal Mask Airway on Cricoid Pressure.
Whether cricoid pressure is an effective barrier to regurgitated stomach contents with a LMA in situ was assessed in one cadaver study (99). After verifying correct placement of the LMA, cricoid pressure with a force of 43 Newton's was applied and found ef-

Table 21.2. THE NUMBER OF OCCASIONS ON WHICH LARYNGEAL MASK AIRWAY INSERTION IS SUCCESSFUL IN THE PRESENCE AND ABSENCE OF CRICOID PRESSURE

Authors	Cricoid Pressure		Sham Cricoid Pressure	
Heath and Allagain	50/50	(SH)		
Brimacombe	34/40	(SH)	37/40	
Ansermino and Blogg	3/20	(DH)	19/22	
Brimacombe et al.	45/50	(SH)	49/50	
Asai et al.	10/20	(DH)	19/20	
Total	142/180	79%	124/132	94%

SH, single-handed; DH, double-handed.
Adapted from Brimacombe J, Berry A. The laryngeal mask airway for obstetric anaesthesia and neonatal resuscitation *Int J Obstet Anesth* 1994;3: 211–218.

fective against a pressure of 7.84 kPa (60 mm Hg, 80 cm H_2O) of barium infused into the trachea. This is approximately twice the intra-gastric pressure that is reached even with twin gestations. As there is no way to ethically test for risk of aspiration in patients, this data is reassuring.

Laryngeal Mask and Aspiration. Aspiration is the second leading cause anesthetic-related of maternal mortality (100). Preoperative administration of medications such as nonparticulate antacids, H2-receptor blockers, and promotility agents help to decrease the morbidity and mortality, but the techniques that we utilize can also help to minimize this risk. Dye studies using ingested methylene blue capsules have been performed to assess the relative risk of esophageal reflux when either a LMA or a facemask (FM) and oral airway were used (101, 102). Both studies used subjects undergoing elective surgery who had no history that would put them at risk for reflux. Barker et al. (101) found a 0% incidence of pharyngeal staining with methylene blue in the FM group, but a 25% incidence of pharyngeal staining in the LMA groups El Mikatti, et al., however, used the same study design and found no staining in either the FM or LMA groups (102). Other data to help clarify the risk comes from reflux studies using esophageal pH probes (103, 104). In these studies, there was a 57% incidence of pH change consistent with reflux in the LMA group as compared with a 22% incidence in the FM group. This high incidence can be partially explained by data that estimate silent regurgitation to occur in 8% to 15% of people (105). In addition, lower esophageal sphincter (LES) tone has been measured when either a FM or a LMA was utilized (106). In this study, care was taken to allow adequate time for reflex changes in esophageal motility and LES tone to resolve prior to measurements being performed. The LES pressure decreased by 3.6 cm H_2O when a LMA was in place but increased by 2.2 cm H_2O when using a FM and oral airway. These studies indicate that the risk of reflux, and consequently, aspiration are higher if a LMA rather than a FM with oral airway is used.

Laryngeal Mask Airway Conclusions. Emergency airway management of difficult airways occurs frequently enough in obstetrics that every anesthesiologist must be prepared when the situation arises. If intubation and mask ventilation of the patient prove impossible, the use of the LMA may be life-saving. Because of the problems of placing the LM when cricoid pressure is maintained, and the increased risk of aspiration as compared with a FM, it can only be recommended in the emergency "cannot intubate, cannot ventilate" (CI/CV) situation. If a CI/CV situation occurs, the clinician must make the decision as to whether to release CP transiently on the first attempt at LMA placement. Releasing CP increases the probability of successful placement on the first attempt and may be considered if desaturation has already begun. CP should be re applied immediately after LM placement.

ProSeal Laryngeal Mask Airway

The ProSeal laryngeal mask airway (PLMA) is a new device, which was designed to overcome a major weakness of the standard LMA, that it does not isolate the airway from the esophogus. This has limited the use of the LMA when positive pressure ventilation is required or in patients at risk of aspiration (107). The PLMA has a number of modifications to the mask, which have resulted in an improved mucosal seal. The oropharyngeal leak pressure averages 10 cm H_2O higher with the PLMA than the standard LMA (108). This increased leak preassure is accomplished despite lower recorded mucosal pressures. This lessens the risk of ischemia to the mucosa and adjacent structures (109). The major design change of the PLMA is the addition of a second tube lateral to the airway tube that ends at the tip of the mask. This isolates the esophagus from the airway and has been shown in initial studies to eliminate reflux of esophageal fluids into the bowl of the mask if there is at least 10 milliliters of air in the cuff (108). Another study has shown the PLMA to be inserted successfully in 52 of 60 patients in an average of 20 seconds without using the introducer device. When the introducer device is used, the first attempt success rate rises to 59 of 60 attempts in an average of 15 seconds (110).

Isolation of the esophagus from the airway with the PLMA depends on proper placement. This raises the issue of whether the device will seat properly when cricoid pressure is being used. To date, there are no studies to answer this question. Extrapolating from data on the LMA, it is likely that cricoid pressure would adversely effect the positioning of the PLMA and therefore negate the possible advantage of this device over the LMA. Pending available data, the recommendation would be to release cricoid pressure while placing the PLMA. When optimally seated, there should be no evidence of an air leak through the esophageal vent tube.

Esophageal Tracheal Combitube

The esophageal tracheal combitube (ETC) is a double-lumen tube with an "esophageal" lumen, a "tracheal" lumen and a distal and proximal cuff. Two sizes are available. The smaller size should be used in patients between 4 and 5 feet tall.

The ETC is designed to be placed blindly by lifting the tongue and mandible while inserting the tube in a curved downward motion until the printed rings on the tube are between the patient's teeth. The proximal balloon is inflated with 100 milliliters of air, and the distal with 10 to 15 milliliters. Over 80% of the time, the tube will be in the esophagus (111). Ventilation should first be given through the longer blue lumen. If breath sounds are heard, and CO_2 is present, the tube is in the esophagus and ventilation should continue through that lumen. Otherwise, ventilation should be changed to the "tracheal" lumen. If ventilation is successful, the tube has passed into the trachea. If breath sounds still can't be heard, the tube is in the esophagus and the proximal cuff is occluding the airway. The tube should be withdrawn 3 centimeters and then ventilation attempted through the esophageal lumen (112).

The ETC has proven successful in emergency medical management, difficult airway management, and cardiopulmonary resuscitation (CPR) (111–115). It has been reported to generate higher oxygen tension than an ETT, possibly due to expiratory resistance (PEEP) through the perforations in the esophageal lumen (116). It also protects against aspiration because it isolates the esophagus from the esophageal lumen by the distal cuff when placed in the esophagus. Any reflux of gastric contents can be suctioned through the "tracheal" lumen when it is in the esophagus.

Disadvantages of the ETC include failure to ventilate if there is poor pulmonary compliance (degree not stated) and risk of esophageal rupture since esophageal cuff pressure can reach 10 kPa or 102 cm H_2O with recommended inflation volumes (117). It is a supraglottic device and therefore unable to alle-viate glottic problems such as massive edema or laryngospasm. It is contraindicated when there is an intact gag reflex or esophageal pathology.

Comparative data between the LMA and ETC are needed to better define which device has greater efficacy in various clinical scenarios. At the current time, the majority of clinicians have more familiarity and expertise with the LMA than the ETC, particularly in obstetric anesthesia.

Cricothyrotomy

Cricothyrotomy is a relatively fast and easy, although invasive, method of achieving definitive airway control. It can be accomplished more rapidly than a tracheotomy and as rapidly as transtracheal jet ventilation (TTJV). The anatomy for cricothyrotomy is much more familiar to anesthesia practitioners than that for a tracheotomy while the complication rate is lower under emergency circumstances (118). There are two main advantages to performing a cricothyrotomy over TTJV. First, it establishes a definitive airway that can be used for up to 72 hours, after which time the risk of subglottic stenosis and vocal cord dysfunction increases. Second, the diameter of the tube used for a cricothyrotomy allows for exhalation through the tube. With TTJV, the native airway must be maintained patent (no laryngospasm or other obstruction) or baurotrauma will occur rapidly and may be fatal when oxygen is delivered at 50 psi.

There are numerous commercial kits available for performing cricothyrotomy. It is our opinion that the Seldinger technique has the greatest chance for success with the least morbidity to produce a definitive airway, i.e., an adequate sized (greater than 4.0 mm ID) cuffed tube in situ which would protect from aspiration and allow for ventilation irrespective of pulmonary compliance. A Seldinger kit should include a needle, syringe, flexible wire and dilators, no. 10 scalpel blade, and a cuffed tracheostomy tube. The Seldinger technique is familiar to anesthesia providers who use it on a regular basis to achieve vascular access. The signs that are indicators of success for vascular access are simply transferred to the airway, for example:

1. The free flow of blood through the needle puncturing the blood vessel becomes a free flow of air through the needle puncturing the cricoid membrane.
2. The easy insertion of a flexible wire through the puncture needle into the blood vessel, without hesitation or hanging up, becomes the same, easy insertion of the flexible wire through the needle into the trachea. Easy advancement of this wire guarantees correct placement in the trachea, ensuring that the final device will be appropriately placed.
3. The free flow of blood through the catheter inserted into the blood vessel inserted into the flexible wire now becomes the free exchange of air both inhalation and exhalation, through the cuffed endotracheal tube inserted into the trachea over the flexible wire and dilator.

Proper identification of the cricothyroid membrane is critically important. This is done, as previously discussed for cricoid pressure. The thumb and middle finger of one hand immobilize the larynx while a needle (preferably 14 gauge or larger to minimize risk of piercing cartilage), attached to a syringe, is directed perpendicular to the membrane. The puncture is made in the lower one third of the membrane to avoid vascular structures. When the needle punctures the cricothyroid membrane, a change of resistance will be felt and air can be aspirated. If the needle is directed perpendicularly, it can not pass through the posterior wall of the trachea, as it would contact the signet-shaped posterior aspect of the cricoid ring first. Once the airway has been identified, the needle tip is angled caudally, the syringe is removed, and a wire (0.038 inch with flexible tip) passed through the needle. An incision is then made through the skin and cricothyroid membrane into the trachea. The scalpel is plunged downward with constant contact to the needle, the needle acting as a guide for the scalpel, into the trachea. A no. 10 scalpel blade makes the ideal incision size since the width of the blade that penetrates the cricothyroid membrane is approximately that of the tube being placed in the airway. This minimizes the force necessary for inserting the dilator/tube assembly. The needle is withdrawn and the dilator, with the tube, is advanced over the wire. The wire and dilator are withdrawn, leaving the cricothyrotomy tube in place.

Currently, no commercial kit combines all the desirable features of the "ideal" cricothyrotomy kit. Some commercial systems leave only a few millimeters of the device in the airway before the next insertion step is made, making it more likely that the final device will not be placed in the trachea. Also, most lack a cuffed-flexible tracheostomy tube. However, this can be easily fashioned from a standard ETT, trimmed to the proper length while preserving the pilot balloon. Such a kit must be assembled, sterilized and available at the anesthetizing location at all times. Practicing on models can perfect the technique. Nasco International (Fort Atkins, WI) makes a cricothyrotomy simulator that has a replaceable latex larynx. After only a few attempts, the technique can be easily performed in less than 30 seconds. It is the author's experience that the skills learned on the model ideally prepare the practitioner for performing the technique on patients.

Transtracheal Insufflation and/or Jet Ventilation

Transtracheal Jet Ventilation (TTJV) is a technique whereby oxygen under pressure can be injected directly into the trachea through a percutaneous catheter. Transtracheal catheters are placed by performing cricothyroid puncture and threading a catheter (12 to 16 gauge) into the airway. The catheter is connected to a pre-assembled, noncompliant system with tight (luer lock or equivalent) connections and a 50 psi oxygen source (119). A toggle valve or flow regulator is interposed between the O_2 source and catheter. The patient can be ventilated by insufflation with continuous O_2 flow (1 to 2 L/min) or by jet ventilation with intermittant bursts of oxygen released by the toggle valve with 0.5 to 1 second inflation time and a 1:3 inspiratory-to-expiratory ratio. Short catheters (angiocaths) have a higher risk of becoming dislodged submucosally thereby creating massive subcutaneous emphysema upon jet ventilation. Longer catheters (intracaths, 8 inches), with the tip placed near the carina, are preferred since they are less likely to be dislodged and O_2 delivery near the carina results in better oxygenation and CO_2 exchange with oxygen insufflation (120). All catheters can become kinked.

Absolute contraindications to TTJV include total expiratory obstruction of the native airway, airway disruption, and improperly placed catheters in any space other than the trachea. With airway obstruction, intrathoracic pressure rapidly increases with resultant baurotrauma and airway disruption. Oxygen injected through the ruptured airway or into subcutaneous areas can lead to pneumothorax, pneumomediastinum, subcutaneous emphysema, and airway and circulatory compromise (119). TTJV is a hazardous procedure which should be reserved to temporize a difficult problem where the operator can take time to be sure that the catheter is intratracheal. Cautious injection of O_2 assures that there is no subcutaneous leak.

Extubation

Prior to extubation, any issues that may result in the need for further airway management must be resolved.

1. Is there airway edema? This may be assessed by direct laryngoscopy, fiberoptic laryoscopy and by whether the patient can breathe around the endotracheal tube with the cuff deflated and the lumen occluded.

2. Is there hemodynamic instability?
3. Did the patient aspirate? Are there oxygenation problems?
4. Are there residual drug effects that may compromise the airway?
5. Are there any other co-existing medical problems which will result in a failed extubation?

When the answer to all these question are no, the patient must be assessed for level of consciousness. Localization to a noxious stimulus (reaching for the endotracheal tube) is not adequate. The patient must show purposeful responses. When there is on-going concern over the need for re intubation, extubation may be performed over an exchange catheter (some of which can be used for ventilation), or with a transtracheal catheter in place.

The chart should reflect the precise nature of the airway problem. Was the difficulty a result of problems with the oral opening, the pharyngeal space, A-O extension, neck compliance, blades used (document which were used), patient position, or level of experience of the intubator?

The American Society of Anesthesologists (ASA) recommends follow-up care for patients having airway management problems (15). The issues should be discussed with the patient and any responsible family member. As of 1992, a National Difficult Airway/Intubation Registry was established through the Medic Alert Foundation which is a nonprofit organization. There is a 24-hour emergency response center which can provide data on any registered individual.

CONCLUSION

By heeding the advice of the ASA Task Force on Difficult Airway Management, it should be possible to minimize, but not eliminate, the risks of airway management in obstetric practice. Be alert to historical and physical signs and symptoms of difficult airways (past and present), have proper equipment and trained personnel available, and be prepared to initiate alternative airway management techniques. There is still no universal method to predict the problem, nor the technology to overcome it. This can only be addressed by heightening the awareness of potential airway difficulties and increasing knowledge regarding management to reduce adverse outcomes.

REFERENCES

1. Department of Health and others. *Report on Confidential Enquiries into Maternal Deaths in the United Kingdom, 1988–90.* London: HMSO, 1994.
2. Department of Health and others. *Report on Confidential Enquiries into Maternal Deaths in the United Kingdom, 1991–93.* London: HMSO, 1996.
3. Department of Health and others. *Report on Confidential Enquiries into Maternal Deaths in the United Kingdom, 1994–96.* London: HMSO, 1998.
4. Willatts SM. Confidential enquiries into maternal deaths in the United Kingdom, 1991–1993. *Int J Obstet Anesth* 1997;6:73–75.
5. Willatts S. Anaesthetic lessons to be learned from confidential enquiries into maternal deaths. *Acta Anaesthesiol Scand* 1997;110: 25–26.
6. Hawkins JL, Koonin LM, Palmer SK, et al. Anesthesia-related deaths during obstetric delivery in the United States, 1979–1990. *Anesthesiology* 1997;86:277–284.
7. Chestnut DH. Anesthesia and maternal mortality. *Anesthesiology* 1997;86:273–276.
8. Lyons G. Failed intubation: six years' experience in a teaching hospital unit. *Anaesthesia* 1985;40:759–762.
9. Samsoon GLT, Young JRB. Difficult tracheal intubation: a retrospective study. *Anaesthesia* 1987;42:487–490.
10. Hawthorne L, Wilson R, Lyons G, et al. Failed intubation revisited: 17-yr experience in a teaching maternity unit. *Br J Anaesth* 1996;76:680–684.
11. Benumof JL. Laryngeal mask airway and the ASA difficult airway algorithm. *Anesthesiology* 1996;84:686–699.

12. Tsen L, Pitner R, Camann W. General anesthesia for cesarean section at a tertiary care hospital 1990–1995: indications and implications. *Int J Obstet Anesth* 1998;7:147–152.

13. Hawkins J, Giggs C. General anesthesia for cesarean section: are we really prepared? [Editorial]. *Int J Obstet Anesth* 1998;7:145–146.

14. Tunstall M. Failed intubation in the parturient [Editorial]. *Can J Anaesth* 1989;36:611–613.

15. American Society of Anesthesiologists. Practice guidelines for management of the difficult airway. A report by the American Society of Anesthesiologists' Task Force on Management of the Difficult Airway. *Anesthesiology* 1993;78:597–602.

16. Shnider S, Levinson G. Anesthesia for cesarean section. In: Shnider S, Levinson G, eds. *Anesthesia for Obstetrics,* 3rd ed. Baltimore: Williams & Wilkins, 1993:211–245.

17. Glassenberg R. General anesthesia and maternal mortality. *Semin Perinatol* 1991;15:386–396.

18. Lawlor M, Johnson C, Weiner M. Airway management in obstetric anesthesia. *Int J Obstet Anesth* 1993;3:225–232.

19. Archer GW, Marx GF. Arterial oxygen tension during apnoea in parturient women. *Br J Anaesth* 1974;46:358–360.

20. Carp H, Jayaram A, Stoll M. Ultrasound examination of the stomach contents of parturients. *Anesth Analg* 1992;74:683–687.

21. Rowe TF. Acute gastric aspiration: prevention and treatment. *Semin Perinatol* 1997;21:313–319.

22. Bainton CR. Airway management: a perspective. In: Bainton CR, ed. *New Concepts in Airway Management.* Boston: Little, Brown, 1994:1–30.

23. Bainton CR. Difficult intubations: what's the best test? *Can J Anaesth* 1996;43:541–543.

24. Mallampati SR. Clinical sign to predict difficult tracheal intubation (hypothosis). *Can J Anaesth* 1983;30:316.

25. Mallampati SR, Gatt SP, Gugino LD, et al. A clinical sign to predict difficulty intubation: a prospective study. *Can Anaesth Soc J* 1985;32:429–434.

26. Cormack RS, Lehane J. Difficult tracheal intubation in obstetrics. *Anaesthesia* 1984;39:1105–1111.

27. Rocke DA, Murray WB, Rout CC, et al. Relative risk analysis of factors associated with difficult intubation in obstetric anesthesia. *Anesthesiology* 1992;77:67–73.

28. Pilkington S, Carli F, Dakin MJ, et al. Increase in Mallampati score during pregnancy. *Br J Anaesth* 1995;74:638–642.

29. Farcon EL, Kim MH, Marx GF. Changing Mallampati score during labour. *Can J Anaesth* 1994;41:50–51.

30. Harmer M. Difficult and failed intubation in obstetrics. *Int J Obstet Anesth* 1997;6:25–31.

31. Stone DJ, Gal TJ. Airway management. In: Miller RD, ed. *Anesthesia,* 3rd ed. New York: Churchill Livingston, 1990:1265–1292.

32. Bellhouse CP, Dore C. Criteria for estimating likelihood of difficulty of endotracheal intubation with the Macintosh laryngoscope. *Anaesth Intensive Care* 1988;16:329–337.

33. Lewis M, Keramati S, Benumof JL, et al. What Is the best way to determine oropharyngeal classification and mandibular space length to predict difficult laryngoscopy? *Anesthesiology* 1994;81:69–75.

34. Frerk CM. Intubation through the laryngeal mask. *Anaesthesia* 1991;46:985–986.

35. Savva D. Prediction of difficult tracheal intubation. *Br J Anaesth* 1994;73:149–153.

36. Al Ramadhani, Mohamed LA, Rocke DA, et al. Sternomental distance as the sole predictor of difficult laryngoscopy in obstetric anaesthesia. *Br J Anaesth* 1996;77:312–316.

37. Butler PJ, Dhara SS. Prediction of difficult laryngoscopy: An assessment of the thyromental distance and Mallampati tests. *Anaesth Intensive Care* 1992;20:139–142.

38. Wilson ME, Spiegelhalter D, Robertson JA, et al. Predicting difficult intubation. *Br J Anaesth* 1988;61:211–216.

39. Benumof JL. ASA. Difficult airway algorithm: new thoughts and considerations. Presented at the Annual Meeting of the Society for Airway Management, Newport Beach, CA, 1997.

40. ACOG Committee Opinion on Obstetric: Maternal and Fetal Medicine. Anesthesia for emergency deliveries. *Int J Gynaecol Obstet* 1992;39:148.

41. Cheek TG, Gutsche BB. Pulmonary aspiration of gastric contents. In: Shnider S, Levinson G, eds. *Anesthesia for Obstetrics,* 3rd ed. Baltimore: Williams & Wilkins, 1993:407–429.

42. Mendelson CL. The aspiration of stomach contents into the lungs during obstetric anesthesia. *Am J Obstet Gynecol* 1946;52:191–205.

43. Roberts RB, Shirley MA. Reducing the risk of acid aspiration. *Anesth Analg* 1974;53:859–868.

44. Rout CC, Rocke DA, Gouws E. Intravenous ranitidine reduces the risk of acid aspiration of gastric contents at emergency caesarean section. *Anesth Analg* 1993;76:156–161.

45. Yau G, Kan AF, Gin TT, et al. A comparison of omeprazole and ranitidine for prophylaxis against aspiration in emergency caesarean section. *Anaesthesia* 1992;47:101–104.

46. Orr DA, Bill KM, Gillon KRW, et al. Effects of omeprazole, with and without metoclopramide, in elective obstetric anaesthesia. *Anaesthesia* 1993;48:114–119.

47. Rocke DA, Rout CC, Gouws E. Intravenous administration of the proton pump inhibitor omeprazole reduces the risk of acid aspiration at emergency cesarean section. *Anesth Analg* 1994;78:1093–1098.

48. Tournadre J-P, Chassard D, Berrada KR, et al. Cricoid cartilage pressure decreases lower esophageal sphincter tone. *Anesthesiology* 1997;86:7–9.

49. Vanner RG. Laryngeal mask airway in the failed intubation drill. *Int J Obstet Anesth* 1995;4:191–192.

50. Vanner RG, Pryle BJ, O'Dwyer JP, et al. Upper oesophageal sphincter pressure during inhalation anaesthesia. *Anaesthesia* 1992;47:950–954.

51. Gibbs CP, Modell JH. Management of aspiration pneumonitis. In: Miller RD, ed. *Anesthesia,* 3rd ed. New York: Churchill Livingston, 1990:1293–1319.

52. Sellick BA. Cricoid pressure to control regurgitation of stomach contents during induction of anaesthesia. *Lancet* 1961;2:404–406.

53. Salem MR. Rapid sequence induction facts and fiction. Presented at the Annual Meeting of the Society for Airway Management, Newport Beach, CA, 1997.

54. Gambee AM, Hertzka RE, Fisher DM. Preoxygenation techniques: comparison of three minutes and four breaths. *Anesth Analg* 1987;66:468–470.

55. Norris MC, Dewan DM. Preoxygenation for cesarean section: a comparison of two techniques. *Anesthesiology* 1985;62:827–829.

56. Norris MC, Kirkland MR, Torjman MC, et al. Denitrogeration in pregnancy. *Can J Anaesth* 1989;36:523–525.

57. Baraka A, Taha S, Aouad M, et al. Preoxygenation, comparison of maximal breathing and tidal volume breathing techniques. *Anesthesiology* 1999;91:612–616.

58. Benumof J, Dagg R, Benumof R. Critical hemoglobin desaturation will occur before return to an unparalyzed state following 1 mg/kg intravenous succinylcholine. *Anesthesiology* 1997;87:979–982.

59. Knill RL. Difficult laryngoscopy made easy with a "BURP." *Can J Anaesth* 1993;40:279–282.

60. Benumof JL. Difficult laryngoscopy: maintaining the best view. *Can J Anaesth* 1994;41:361–365.

61. Norman B. Failed tracheal intubation. *Br J Anaesth* 1996;77:559.

62. Burns AM, Dorje P, Lawes EG, et al. Anaesthetic management of caesarean section for a mother with pre-eclampsia, the Klippel-Feil syndrome and congenital hydrocephalus. *Br J Anaesth* 1988;61:350–354.

63. Broomhead CJ, Davies W, Higgins D. Awake oral fibreoptic intubation for caesarean section. *Int J Obstet Anesth* 1995;4:172–174.

64. D'Alessio JG, Ramanathan J. Fiberoptic intubation using intraoral glossopharyngeal nerve block in a patient with severe preeclampsia and HELLP syndrome. *Int J Obstet Anesth* 1995;4:168–171.

65. Fayek SS, Isaac PA, Shah J. Awake fiber optic intubation in a 38-week pregnant patient with submandibular abscess. *Int J Obstet Anesth* 1994;3:103–105.

66. Edwards RM. Fiberoptic intubation: a solution to failed intubation in a paturient? *Anaesth Intensive Care* 1994;22:718–719.

67. Ovassapian A, Krejcie TC, Yelich SJ, et al. Awake fiberoptic intubation in the patient at high risk of aspiration. *Br J Anaesth* 1989;62:13–16.

68. Boerner TF, Ramanathan S. Functional anatomy of the airway. In: Benumof JL, ed. *Airway Management: Principles and Practice.* St. Louis: Mosby–Year Book, 1996:3–21.

69. Ovassapian A. Anatomy of the airway, fiberoptic airway endoscopy. In: Ovassapian A, ed. *Anesthesia and Critical Care.* New York: Raven Press, 1990:15–24.

70. Foutz SE, Kotelko DM, Shnider SM, et al. Placental transfer and effects of cocaine on uterine blood flow and the fetus. *Anesthesiology* 1983;59:A422.

71. Woods JR, Plessinger MA, Clark KE. Effect of cocaine on uterine blood flow and fetal oxygenation. *JAMA* 1987;257:957–961.

72. Covert RF, Schreiber MD, Tebbett IR, et al. Hemodynamic and cerebral blood flow effects of cocaine, cocaethylene and benzoylecgonine in conscious and anesthetized fetal lambs. *J Pharmacol Exp Ther* 1994;270:118–126.

73. Barnett G, Hawks R, Resnick R. Cocaine pharmacokinetics in humans. *J Ethnopharmacol* 1981;3:353–366.

74. Jeffcoat A, Perex-Reyes M, Hill J, et al. Cocaine disposition in humans after intravenous injection, nasal insufflation (snoring), or smoking. *Drug Metab Dispos* 1989;17:153–159.

75. Greinwald JJ, Holtel M. Absorption of topical cocaine in rhinologic procedures. *Laryngoscope* 1996;106:1223–1225.

76. Kumar V, Schoenwald R, Barcellos W, et al. Aqueous vs. viscus phenylephrine. I. Systemic absorption and cardiovascular effects. *Arch Opthalmol* 1986;104:1189–1191.

77. Sanchez A, Trivech NS, Morrison DE. Preparation of the patient for awake intubation. In: Benumof JL, ed. *Airway Management: Principles and Practice.* St. Louis: Mosby–Year Book, 1996:159–182.

78. Ho R, Nanevicz T, Yee R, et al. Benzocaine-induced methemoglobinemia—two case reports related to transesophageal echocardiography premedicated. *Cardiovasc Drug Ther* 1998;12:311–312.

79. Ross BK. Fiberoptics in parturients: the technique. In: Sol Shnider MD, ed. *Obstetrical Anesthesia: 1995.* San Francisco: 1995:135–145.

80. Goudsouzian NG, Denman W, Cleveland R, et al. Radiologic localization of the laryngeal mask airway in children. *Anesthesiology* 1992;77:1085–1089.

81. Nandi PR, Nunn JF, Charlesworth CH, et al. Radiologic study of the laryngeal mask. *Eur J Anaesthesiol* 1991;4(S):33–39.

82. Chadwick IS, Vohra A. Anaesthesia for emergency caesarean section using the brain laryngeal airway. *Anaesthesia* 1989;44:261–262.

83. McClune S, Regan M, Moore J. Laryngeal mask airway for caesarean section. *Anaesthesia* 1990;45:227–228.

84. Storey J. The laryngeal mask for failed intubation at caesarean section. *Anaesth Intensive Care* 1992;20:118–119.

85. Priscu V, Priscu L, Soroker D. Laryngeal mask for failed intubation in emergency caesarean section. *Can J Anaesth* 1992;39:893.

86. McFarlane C. Failed intubation in an obese obstetric patient and the laryngeal mask. *Int J Obstet Anesth* 1993;2:183–184.

87. Hasham FM, Andrews PJD, Juneja MM, et al. The laryngeal mask airway facilitates intubation at cesarean section. A case report of difficult intubation. *Int J Obstet Anesth* 1993;2:181–182.

88. Lim W, Wareham C. The laryngeal mask in failed intubation. *Anaesthesia* 1990;41:689.

89. Liew E, Chan-Liao M. Experience of using laryngeal mask anesthesia for cesarean section. Presented at the 11th World Congress of Anesthesiology, Sydney, Australia, 1996:439.

90. Yang H, Suh B. Laryngeal mask airway in cesarean section. Presented at the 11th World Congress of Anesthesiology, Sydney, Australia, 1996:439.

91. Devitt JH, Wenstone R, Noel AG, et al. The laryngeal mask airway and positive-pressure ventilation. *Anesthesiology* 1994;80:550–555.

92. Brimacombe J. Cricoid pressure and the laryngeal mask airway. *Anaesthesia* 1991;46:986–987.

93. Brimacombe J, White A, Berry A. The effect of cricoid pressure on ease of insertion of the laryngeal mask airway. *Br J Anaesth* 1993;71:800–802.

94. Asai T, Barclay K, Power I, et al. Cricoid pressure impedes placement of the laryngeal mask airway and subsequent tracheal intubation through the mask. *Br J Anaesth* 1994;72:47–51.

95. Ansermino JM, Blogg CE. Cricoid pressure may prevent insertion of the laryngeal mask airway. *Br J Anaesth* 1992;69:465–467.

96. Brimacombe J, Berry A. The laryngeal mask airway for obstetric anaesthesia and neonatal resuscitation. *Int J Obstet Anesth* 1994;3:211–218.

97. Heath ML, Allagain J. Intubation through the laryngeal mask: a technique for unexpected difficult intubation. *Anaesthesia* 1991;46:545–548.

98. Asai T, Latto IP, Vaughan RS. The distance between the grille of the laryngeal mask airway and the vocal cords. *Anaesthesia* 1993;48:667–669.

99. Strang TI. Does the laryngeal mask airway compromise cricoid pressure? *Anaesthesia* 1992;47:829–831.

100. Department of Health and others. *Report on Confidential Enquiries into Maternal Deaths in the United Kingdom, 1985–87.* London: HMSO, 1991.

101. Barker P, Langton JA, Murphy PJ, et al. Regurgitation of gastric contents during general anaesthesia using the laryngeal mask airway. *Br J Anaesth* 1992;69:314–315.

102. El Mikatti N, Luthra AD, Healy TE, et al. Gastric regurgitation during general anaesthesia in the supine position with the laryngeal and face mask airways. *Br J Anaesth* 1992;68:529–530(P).

103. Owens T, Robertson P, Twomey K, et al. Incidence of gastroesophageal reflux with the laryngeal mask. *Anesthesiology* 1993;79:A1053.

104. Owens TM, Robertson P, Twomey C, et al. The incidence of gastroesophageal reflux with the laryngeal mask: A comparison with the face mask using esophageal lumen pH electrodes. *Anesth Analg* 1995;80:980–984.

105. Leach AB, Alexander CA. The laryngeal mask—an overview. *Eur J Anaesthesiol* 1991;4(S):19–31.

106. Rabey PG, Murphy PJ, Langton JA, et al. Effect of the laryngeal mask airway on lower oesophageal sphincter pressure in patients during general anaesthesia. *Br J Anaesth* 1992;69:346–348.

107. Brain AIJ, Verghese C, Strube PJ. The LMA 'ProSeal'—a laryngeal mask with an osopharyngeal vent. *Br J Anaesth* 2000;84:650–654.

108. Keller C, Brimacombe J, Kleinsasser A, et al. Does the ProSeal laryngeal mask airway prevent aspiration of regurgitated fluid? *Anesth Analg* 2000;91:1017–1020.

109. Keller C, Brimacombe J. Mucosal pressure and oropharyngeal pressure with the ProSeal versus laryngeal mask airway in anaesthetized paralysed patients. *Br J Anaesth* 2000;85:262–266.

110. Brimacombe J, Keller C. The ProSeal laryngeal mask airway—a randomized crossover study with the standard laryngeal mask airway in paralysed, anesthetized patients. *Anesthesiology* 2000;93:104–109.

111. Atherton GL, Johnson JC. Ability of paramedics to use the combitube in prehospital cardiac arrest. *Ann Emerg Med* 1993;22:1263–1268.

112. Frass M. Combitube: The role of combitube in emergency airway management. Society for Airway Management (SAM). Newport Beach, CA, 1997.

113. Frass M, Frenzer R, Rauscha F, et al. Evaluation of esophageal tracheal Combitube in cardiopulmonary resuscitation. *Crit Care Med* 1987;15:609–611.

114. Frass M, Frenzer R, Rauscha F, et al. Ventilation with the esophageal tracheal Combitube in cardiopulmonary resuscitation: promptness and effectiveness. *Chest* 1988;93:781–784.

115. Staudinger T, Tesinsky P, Klappacher G, et al. Emergency intubation with the Combitube in two cases of difficult airway management. *Eur J Anaesth* 1995;12:189–193.

116. Frass M, Johnson JC, Atherton GL, et al. Esophageal tracheal Combitube (ETC) for emergency intubation: Anatomical evaluation of ETC placement by radiography. *Resuscitation* 1989;18:95–102.

117. Mallick A, Quinn AC, Bodenham AR, et al. Use of the Combitube for airway maintenance during percutaneous dilatational tracheostomy. *Anaesthesia* 1998;53:249–255.

118. Melker R, Florete Jr. O. Percutaneous dilational cricothyrotomy and tracheostomy. In: Benumof JL, ed. *Airway management: principles and practice.* St. Louis: Mosby–Year Book, 1996.

119. Benumof JL, Scheller MS. The importance of transtracheal jet ventilation in the management of the difficult airway. *Anesthesiology* 1989;71:769–778.

120. Slutsky AS, Watson J, Leith D, et al. Tracheal insufflation of oxygen (trio) at low flow rates sustains life for several hours. *Anesthesiology* 1985;63:278–286.

Shnider and Levinson's Anesthesia for Obstetrics,
edited by Samuel C. Hughes, et al.
Lippincott Williams & Wilkins,
Philadelphia, © 2001.

APPENDIX

ANESTHESIA FOR EMERGENCY DELIVERIES

ACOG COMMITTEE OPINION: COMMITTEE ON OBSTETRICS:
MATERNAL AND FETAL MEDICINE*

NUMBER 104, MARCH 1992

Failed intubation and pulmonary aspiration of gastric contents continue to be leading causes of maternal morbidity and mortality from anesthesia. The risk of these complications can be reduced by careful antepartum assessment to identify patients at risk, greater use of regional anesthesia when possible, and appropriate selection and preparation of patients who require general anesthesia for delivery.

Antepartum Risk Assessment

The obstetric care team should be alert to the presence of risk factors that place the parturient at increased risk for complications from emergency general or regional anesthesia. These factors include, but are not limited to, marked obesity, severe facial and neck edema, extremely short stature, a short neck, difficulty opening the mouth, a small mandible, protuberant teeth, arthritis of the neck, anatomic abnormalities of the face or mouth, a large thyroid, asthma, serious medical or obstetric complications, and a history of problems with anesthetics.

When such risk factors are identified, a physician who is credentialed to provide general and regional anesthesia should be consulted in the antepartum period to allow for joint development of a plan of management including optimal location for delivery. Strategies thereby can be developed to minimize the need for emergency induction of general anesthesia in women for whom this would be especially hazardous. For those patients at risk, consideration should be given to the planned placement in early labor of an intravenous line and an epidural or spinal catheter, with confirmation that the catheter is functional. If the patient at unusual risk is identified (e.g., prior failed intubation), strong consideration should be given to antepartum referral of the patient to allow for delivery at a hospital which can manage such anesthesia on a 24-hour basis.

Emergency Anesthesia

The need for expeditious abdominal delivery cannot always be anticipated. When preparing for the rapid initiation of anesthesia, the maternal as well as the fetal status must be considered. Oral nonparticulate antacids should be administered immediately prior to the induction of general or major regional anesthesia to decrease the mother's risk of developing aspiration pneumonitis.

Although there are some situations in which general anesthesia is preferable to regional anesthesia, the risk of general anesthesia must be weighed against the benefit for those patients who have a greater potential for complications. Examples of circumstances in which a rapid induction of general anesthesia may be indicated include prolapsed umbilical cord with severe fetal bradycardia and active hemorrhage in a hemodynamically unstable mother.

In some cases, a nonreassuring fetal heart rate pattern is diagnosed as "fetal distress," and delivery is performed immediately. The term "fetal distress" is imprecise, nonspecific, and has little positive predictive value. The severity of the fetal heart rate abnormality should be considered when the urgency of the delivery and the type of anesthesia to be administered are determined. Cesarean deliveries that are performed for a nonreassuring fetal heart rate pattern do not necessarily preclude the use of regional anesthesia.

This document reflects emerging clinical and scientific advances as of the date issued and is subject to change. The information should not be construed as dictating an exclusive course of treatment or procedure to be followed. This document was published in *Int J Gynecol Obstet* 1992;39:148.

Shnider and Levinson's Anesthesia for Obstetrics,
edited by Samuel C. Hughes, et al.
Lippincott Williams & Wilkins,
Philadelphia, © 2001.

CHAPTER 22

PULMONARY ASPIRATION OF GASTRIC CONTENTS

THEODORE G. CHEEK, M.D. AND BRETT B. GUTSCHE, M.D.

Avoiding gastric content pulmonary aspiration among pregnant patients remains a fundamental goal for anesthesiologists. Although maternal anesthetic deaths are rare and the incidence of death is decreasing, preventable deaths such as those caused by aspiration should be viewed with continuing concern and sustained efforts made towards prevention.

This chapter provides an assessment of current data on aspiration risk, and reviews the conditions during pregnancy and labor that increase the risk of aspiration. It will also include a description of the recognition and treatment of aspiration pneumonitis and provide suggestions to decrease or avoid the occurrence of this life-threatening catastrophe.

EPIDEMIOLOGY OF ASPIRATION OF GASTRIC CONTENTS IN PREGNANCY

Data from the United States reveal that aspiration of gastric contents is still a leading cause of maternal anesthetic death, accounting for 33% of fatalities (Table 22.1) (1). Ongoing surveys from the United Kingdom show that over the last 40 years, the two leading causes of maternal anesthetic death, although decreasing, continue to be loss of airway control with anoxia and aspiration of gastric contents (Table 22.2) (2–4). Triennial mortality reports for 1988–93 in the United Kingdom (2, 3) show four maternal anesthetic deaths from anoxia and four from aspiration. The absence of death from aspiration in the 1994–96 period may either represent statistical periodicity or may provide evidence that increased awareness of maternal risk and improved attention to safety precautions and aspiration prophylaxis at induction of anesthesia have resulted in fewer deaths (4). One recent series estimated the overall incidence of aspiration during cesarean section anesthesia to be 1 in 1600 (5). In another report from Norway, the risk of intraoperative aspiration was 2/25,330 among gynecologic surgeries and 4/3680 among cesarean sections (6). Another study found pulmonary aspiration of gastric contents in 25 of 85,594 cases. The incidence was 4.1 times greater among emergency procedures than among elective procedures. In contrast, there were no aspirations among 30,199 patients receiving regional anesthesia (Table 22.3) (5–9). Estimates of the incidence of aspiration as a cause of maternal death vary widely and range from an earlier 100 annually in the United States (10) to less than 1 in 1 million deliveries in a more recent survey (4). Mortality following aspiration is estimated to be in the 4% to 5% range (11). Morbidity requiring mechanical ventilation or prolonged hospital stay ranges from 15% to 20% (11). The data arising from the United Kingdom over the past 3 decades suggest that reduction in anesthesia as a cause of mortality (from 12% to 0.8%), to include a significant decline in aspiration as a cause of maternal mortality (Fig. 22.1), has been achieved by attention to detail and refusal to compromise standards. Some would suggest that the risk of maternal aspiration is not as great as once believed (12–15), and others argue for relaxation of safety standards (16, 17). We believe that aspiration is a major threat to maternal well-being and that efforts to avoid aspiration have resulted in improved maternal outcome and should be steadfastly continued (18–20).

FACTORS THAT INCREASE THE RISK OF ASPIRATION

Gastrointestinal changes during pregnancy that increase the risk of maternal aspiration include slowed gastrointestinal transit, increased gastric volume, increased gastric acidity, and decreased gastroesophageal sphincter tone. Other factors that increase the aspiration risk during pregnancy include labor-related nausea, pain, fear, ketosis, numerous drugs and disease states, obesity, recent food ingestion, and loss of airway reflexes due to any cause. A more detailed review of the physiologic changes during pregnancy that alter the gastrointestinal system can be found in Chapter 1.

Gastric Emptying

An extensive summary of the studies concerning gastric emptying and their sometimes-conflicting results can be found in Table 22.4 (21–37). In general, techniques using radiographic examination, paracetamol absorption, or stomach ultrasound have often shown that gastric emptying may not be delayed during pregnancy. In contrast, it is clear that during labor, gastric emptying is slow to nonexistent. As elective cesarean sections continue to decrease, delayed gastric transit applies to the vast majority of women who receive anesthesia in the obstetric suite. However, controversy remains, and delayed gastric emptying has been reported as early as 8 to 14 weeks of gestation (29, 35). After delivery, gastric emptying also has been shown to be slow, especially in the immediate postpartum period (33, 37). The physiologic basis for these changes is found in the combined effects of increased plasma levels of progesterone and gastrin (38), decreased plasma levels of the hormone motilin (39), and mechanical displacement of the pylorus by the gravid uterus later in pregnancy. Pregnant women suffering from heartburn, which can indicate gastroesophageal junction dysfunction, may have even longer delays in gastric emptying. The stress response activated by fear, pain, starvation, and ketosis seen in labor has been shown to delay gastric emptying (28, 40). Contrasting opinions regarding gastric emptying during pregnancy (41) suggest that pregnancy is not associated with a consistent pattern of gastric emptying. Anesthetic management of pregnant patients, especially those in labor, must be approached as if the stomach is not empty, and thus pulmonary aspiration of gastric contents remains a risk.

Drugs and Gastric Emptying

The use of drugs, particularly opioids and sedatives, retards stomach emptying. Meperidine prolongs gastric emptying time by 5 hours or more in 70% of patients in labor (26, 42). This is antagonized by naloxone. Parenteral meperidine prolongs the antacid effect of sodium citrate because of decreased gastric emptying (27) but decreases the effectiveness of metoclopramide (26, 42, 43). Epidural analgesia during labor has little effect on gastric emptying (43). The addition of fentanyl 0.0002% to epidural infusions of local anesthetics does not

391

Table 22.1. CAUSES OF ANESTHESIA-RELATED DEATH DURING OBSTETRIC DELIVERY: UNITED STATES, 1979–90

	Type of Anesthesia	
Cause of Death	General (n = 67)	Regional (n = 33)
Airway Problems		
Aspiration	22 (33%)	0
Intubation problems	15 (22%)	0
Inadequate ventilation	10 (15%)	0
Respiratory failure	2 (3%)	0
Cardiac arrest during anesthesia	15 (22%)	2 (6%)
Local anesthetic toxicity		17 (52%)
High spinal/epidural		11 (33%)
Unknown	3 (4%)	2 (6%)

Adapted from Hawkins JL, Koonin LM, Palmer SK, Gibbs CP. Anesthesia-related deaths during obstetric delivery in the United States, 1979–1990. *Anesthesiology* 1997;86:273–276.

appear to delay gastric emptying during labor (44, 45), but a 100-μg epidural bolus does slow gastric transit (46–48). It has been reported that subarachnoid fentanyl but not epidural fentanyl decreased gastric emptying in labor, but this has not been substantiated (49).

Ritodrine and other mixed β-agonists employed as tocolytics for preterm labor may inhibit gastrointestinal motility (50). Intravaginal prostaglandin E$_2$ does not appear to affect gastric emptying (27). Magnesium may also decrease gastric transit.

Gastroesophageal Tone and Reflux, and Gastric Pressure

Heartburn during pregnancy occurs in 45% to 70% of women (51, 52), with a reported incidence of hiatal hernias of 27% (53). The heartburn is caused by gastric reflux as a result of a decreased competence of the lower esophageal sphincter (LES) (54, 55). Gastroesophageal reflux decreases markedly by the second postpartum day. The presence of heartburn indicates an increased risk of regurgitation, particularly when the supine position is assumed.

During pregnancy, the upward force of the uterus increases gastric pressure from 7.3 cm H$_2$O (normal) to 17.2 cm H$_2$O. Lithotomy and Trendelenburg positions can cause a further in-

crease in gastric pressure of 5.6 to 8.8 cm H$_2$O. The presence of twins, hydramnios, or gross obesity may be associated with intragastric pressures greater than 40 cm H$_2$O (56). Both fundal pressure (Fig. 22.2) and succinylcholine fasciculations can raise intragastric pressure significantly. During pregnancy, the LES tone usually rises from 35 to 44 cm H$_2$O, providing some protection from rising intragastric pressures. However, Lind et al. (57) found that parturients with heartburn experienced an average decrease in LES tone to 24 cm H$_2$O and required only a small rise in gastric pressure of 7.3 cm H$_2$O to cause LES opening and regurgitation. All pregnant women studied by Brock-Utne et al. (58) had decreased LES tone.

Medications that reduce LES tone include opioids, diazepam, and anticholinergics such as atropine and glycopyrrolate (59–64). However metoclopramide, 10 mg IV, increases LES tone in nonpregnant patients who receive either opioids or atropine (65, 66).

Gastric Acidity

Increased gastric acid secretion occurs during pregnancy (67, 68), caused by the markedly elevated plasma levels of the hormone gastrin (69). The elevated plasma levels of gastrin, together with very high placental tissue concentrations of gastrin, suggest placental production and/or storage of the hormone. Dehydration and starvation ketosis during labor may also increase gastric acid secretions. Oral alcohol, sometimes abused, markedly increases gastric secretions and acidity.

Combined Risk of Volume and pH

Mendelson (8) was one of the first to suggest that both volume and pH play a role in the severity of aspiration sequelae. Teabeaut suggested a gastric pH below 2.5 was associated with an increased incidence of acute symptoms of aspiration pneumonitis (70). Roberts and Shirley described a human "threshold volume" of 0.4 mL $\cdot$ kg^{-1} gastric fluid ($\approx$25 mL) and a pH lower than 2.5 that caused aspiration pneumonitis (71, 72). Using these criteria, Roberts and Shirley found that, regardless of the time of last meal or the time between the last meal and the onset of labor, 25% of parturients were at risk. They also found that 70% of women who were fasted before elective cesarean section were still at high risk for the complication of aspiration.

More recently, Raidoo et al. suggested that the volume of liquid at pH 2.5 required to cause pneumonia in primates is two times higher ($\approx$0.8 mL $\cdot$ kg^{-1}) than once thought (73). It is clear that the incidence and intensity of aspiration pneumonitis increase as pH decreases and aspirate volume increases

Table 22.2. ANESTHESIA AS A CAUSE OF MATERNAL DEATH, 1973–96

	Years					Totals
Causes	1973–78	1979–84	1985–90	1991–93	1994–96	1973–96
Pulmonary aspiration	24	15	4	1	0	44
Anoxia (failed intubation)	23	16	5	4	0	48
Drug misuse	8	4	0	0	0	12
Apparatus	4	2	0	0	0	6
Epidural/spinal	6	2	2	1	1	12
Miscellaneous	15	10	1	2	0	28
Total	80	49	12	8	1	150

Adapted from *Confidential Enquiries into Maternal Deaths in England and Wales (1994–1996)*. Reprinted by permission from Hibbard BM, Anderson MM, Drife JO, et al. *Report on Confidential Enquiries into Maternal Deaths in the United Kingdom, 1988–1990*. London: HMSO; 1994; Hibbard BM, Anderson MM, Drife JO, et al. *Report on Confidential Enquiries into Maternal Deaths in the United Kingdom, 1991–1993*. London: HMSO; 1996; and Drife J, Lewis G, Neilson J, et al. *Report on Confidential Enquiries into Maternal Deaths in the United Kingdom, 1994–1996*. London: HMSO; 1998.

Table 22.3. INCIDENCE OF PULMONARY ASPIRATION DURING ANESTHESIA

Type of Surgery	Study	No. of Cases	Aspirations	Incidence
Gynecologic	Soreide et al., 1996 (6)	25,330	2	1/12,665
General (all)	Mellin-Olsen et al., 1996 (7)	85,594	25	1/3424
General elective	Warner et al., 1993 (9)	202,061	67	1/3886
Emergency (all)	Warner et al., 1993 (9)	13,427	15	1/895
Regional (all)	Mellin-Olsen et al., 1996 (7)	30,199	0	0
Obstetric	Mendelson, 1946 (8)	44,016	66	1/667
All cesareans	Schneck et al., 1999 (11)	115,000/y	~72	1/1600
Cesarean (emergent)	Soreide et al., 1996 (6)	~3680	4	~1/920

The literature suggests that aspiration is more frequent with emergency surgery and cesarean section.

(Figs. 22.3–22.5) (8, 70, 74, 75). Elevated pH gastric fluid with or without particulate matter can also predispose patients to severe pneumonia (74). A number of authors provide data that the combined risk of pH <2.5 and gastric volume >25 mL is similar between pregnant term patients and nonpregnant patients. Whether or not this is ultimately proven, many of the other risk factors mentioned, particularly increased difficulty in airway management and decreased LES tone, place the parturient at much greater risk for aspiration than the general population. The goal of decreasing gastric volume and neutralizing pH prior to general anesthesia in the parturient remains an important part of anesthetic management.

PATHOPHYSIOLOGY AND TREATMENT OF PULMONARY ASPIRATION

The morbidity and mortality following aspiration depend on both the amount and the nature of aspirated matter. Three types of gastric material can be aspirated, each of which will cause a different clinical picture: (a) material with pH less than 2.5, causing a chemical pneumonitis or acid aspiration syndrome; (b) solid or particulate matter; and (c) fecal or other bacterially contaminated material, usually as a result of intestinal obstruction, perforation, or bowel infarct. In the parturient, the most common forms of pulmonary aspiration are those of acid and particulate aspiration; fecal aspiration in the obstetric population is rare.

Diagnostic and Therapeutic Considerations

The acute signs and symptoms of gastric fluid aspiration are often immediate and are described in Table 22.5. Signs and symptoms usually occur within the first 2 hours of aspiration in most patients (11, 76), although latency periods of 6 to 8 hours have been reported, especially during general anesthesia (77).

If aspiration is witnessed or suspected, particularly in an obtunded patient, the patient should be turned to the side and placed in the head-down position; the mouth and posterior pharynx should be suctioned; and the trachea should be intubated with a cuffed endotracheal tube. The trachea should be suctioned several times immediately after intubation. Ventilation with 100% oxygen between suctioning is recommended to prevent hypoxia.

There is abundant evidence from animal studies that positive-pressure ventilation markedly decreases mortality from acid aspiration (75, 77, 78). Cameron et al. (79) demonstrated in dogs that the immediate initiation of positive pressure ventilation after aspiration of 2 mL/kg 0.1 N HCl placed in the right main stem bronchus resulted in a 100% survival rate. When ventilation was delayed 24 hours, only 40% survived, suggesting the efficacy of early ventilation, even in the absence of severe symptoms.

Except in the aspiration of particulate matter, saline or bicarbonate tracheal lavage should not be performed because it may spread the material and extend the lung damage (77). When particulate matter has been aspirated, bronchoscopy for removal of solid material and reexpansion of atelectatic segments of lung should be performed as soon as initial resuscitation is accomplished. Some clinicians obtain a specimen of gastric contents to examine for the presence of particulate matter, analyze for pH, and possibly culture for the presence of bacteria and antibiotic sensitivities, although current recommendations suggest that these data are not useful for patient management. However, arterial blood gas determinations will indicate the need for increased inspired oxygen concentrations, ventilation, and the use of positive end-expiratory pressure. Chest radiographs taken as soon as possible after the incident and at regular intervals as

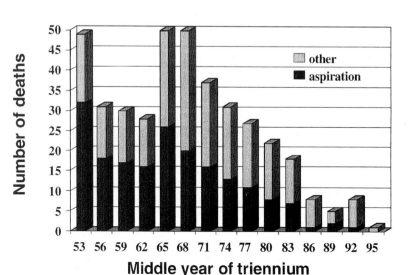

Figure 22.1. The Confidential Enquiries into Maternal Deaths (CEMD) has been compiled continuously since 1952. This figure represents maternal deaths due to anesthesia and aspiration (1952–1966). The midpoint of each triennial report is used as a reference point. Maternal mortality has declined significantly in the United Kingdom to include deaths directly associated with anesthesia and aspiration of gastric contents. (Data from CEMD summarized by Dr. G. O'Sullivan, St. Thomas' Hospital, London, England.)

Table 22.4. SUMMARY: STUDIES ON GASTRIC EMPTYING—PREGNANCY AND POSTPARTUM

Study	Method of Assessment	Gestation Period	Gastric Emptying
Hirscheimer et al., 1938 (21)	X-ray	Labor (10 subjects)	Delayed in 2 subjects
La Salvia and Steffen, 1950 (22)	X-ray	3rd trimester Labor Labor + opioids	No delay Slight delay Marked delay
Crawford, 1956 (23)	X-ray	Labor (12 subjects)	Delayed in 2 subjects
Hunt and Murray, 1958 (24)	Large volume test meal	3rd trimester Postpartum	No change No change
Davison et al., 1970 (25)	Double sampling test meal	3rd trimester Labor	?Delayed Delayed
Nimmo et al., 1975 (26)	Paracetamol absorption	Labor Labor + opioids	Slight delay Marked delay
O'Sullivan et al., 1987 (27)	Epigastric impedance	3rd trimester 1st h postpartum	No delay Delay if opioids used
Lewis and Crawford, 1987 (28)	Light breakfast (< 4 h) or NPO prior to CS	Term for cesarean Not in labor	73 mL vol, lower pH 33 mL vol
Simpson et al., 1988 (29)	Paracetamol	12–14 wk gestation	71 min peak pregnant 45 min peak nonpregnant
Macfie et al., 1991 (30)	Paracetamol	1st, 2nd, 3rd trimester	No change
Gin et al., 1991 (31)	Paracetamol	Postpartum day 1; 3 and 6 wk	No change
Sandhar et al., 1992 (32)	Applied potential tomography	37–40 wk 2–3 d postartum 6 wk postartum	No change No change No change
Whitehead et al., 1992 (33)	Paracetamol	1st, 2nd, 3rd trimester 1st 2 h postpartum 18–36 h postpartum	No delay Delayed No delay
Carp et al., 1992 (34)	Ultrasound examination stomach contents	Nonpregnant control 34 pregnant volunteers Laboring patients	Lack solids after 4 h Lack solids after 4 h 16/39 with solids despite NPO 8–24 h
Levy et al., 1994 (35)	Paracetamol	8–12 wk gestation Nonpregnant control	Delayed emptying No delay
Jayaram et al., 1997 (37)	Ultrasound examination stomach contents	Postpartum BTL Gynecologic surgery	11/28 had gastric food No food in stomach
Scrutton et al., 1999 (36)	Ultrasound examination stomach contents	Labor: water only Labor: light food	104 mL vomitus 309 mL vomitus

BTL = bilateral tubal ligation; CS = cesarean section; NPO = nothing by mouth.

appropriate will aid in determining the extent and progress of the pathologic process. A record of urinary output and continuous central venous pressure measurement will aid in fluid management. Any patient suspected of aspirating gastric material, particularly if symptoms of aspiration are present, should be placed in an intensive care environment for close monitoring and respiratory care until resolution of the process. Rapid early therapy is essential to minimize morbidity and mortality. One report of aggressive ventilation and rapid crystalloid volume restoration in 38 nonpregnant severe aspiration victims resulted in the survival of 30 (79%), with 5 deaths from cerebral hemorrhage and only 3 from respiratory complications (80).

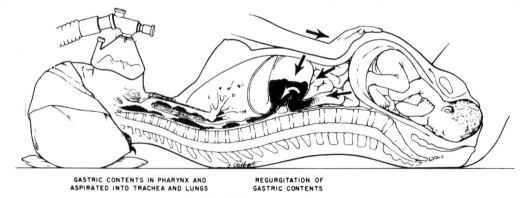

GASTRIC CONTENTS IN PHARYNX AND
ASPIRATED INTO TRACHEA AND LUNGS

REGURGITATION OF
GASTRIC CONTENTS

Figure 22.2. Regurgitation of gastric contents caused by marked increase in intraabdominal and intragastric pressure from an attempt to place pressure on the uterus during delivery. (Reprinted by permission from Bonica JJ, ed. In: *Principles and Practice of Obstetric Analgesia and Anesthesia.* Vol 1. Philadelphia: Davis; 1967:676.)

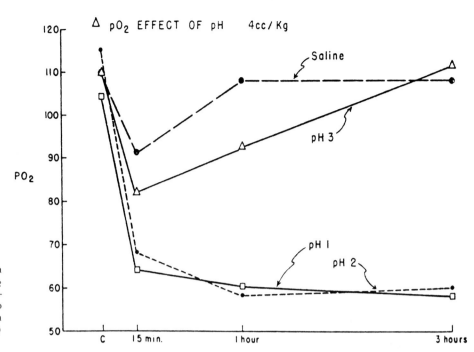

Δ pO$_2$ EFFECT OF pH   4cc/Kg

Figure 22.3. Effect of decreasing pH in a fixed volume of aspirated fluid on Po$_2$ in four animals. (Reprinted by permission from Awe WC, Fletcher WS, Jacob SW. The pathophysiology of aspiration pneumonitis. *Surgery* 1966;60:232–239.)

Acid Gastric Material

The most common form of pulmonary aspiration in the parturient is that of acid material resulting in a chemical pneumonitis characterized by bronchospasm, the development of a high alveolar-arterial oxygen gradient, and a pulmonary exudate resembling pulmonary edema fluid. This syndrome was described by Mendelson in 1946 (8) and now bears his name. Teabeaut (70) showed in rabbits that when the pH of aspirated material fell below 2.5, the typical clinical syndrome developed. Both Mendelson (8) and Bosomworth and Hamelberg (81) demonstrated that the pH of the aspirate, not gastric or enteric enzymes, was responsible for development of the syndrome.

Blood gases frequently show a marked hypoxemia with a Pao$_2$ of less than 50 mm Hg on room air. With the administration of high-inspired oxygen concentrations, a marked alveolar-arterial gradient (PA-ao$_2$) is found (Fig. 22.6). This is thought to represent impaired diffusion, pulmonary shunting, and pulmonary arteriolar vasoconstriction (82, 83). Initially, the Paco$_2$ may be normal or slightly below normal, but with the progression of the process, it may become slightly elevated. A metabolic acidosis is often seen as the condition worsens.

Abnormal chest radiographic examinations will appear in 85% to 90% of those who aspirate, usually between 12 and 24 hours after the insult. The chest radiograph shows soft mottled densities widely distributed over the peripheral areas but especially pronounced in the dependent lung areas, particularly of the right side. The initial picture resembles that of a "snow storm" over the lung fields (Fig. 22.7), usually assuming an alveolar pattern and occasionally a reticular pattern (76). Mediastinal shift is rare. As the process continues, a chest radiograph typical of pulmonary edema may develop. Atelectasis and pleural effusion also may be present.

The pathologic picture is best described as a severe chemical burn of the lung. Initially, there is decreased pulmonary compliance. Acid aspiration is followed by proteinaceous edema of the lung; transudation of a plasma-like substance, neutrophils, and fibrin; and disruption of the alveolar-capillary membrane with a decrease in pulmonary gas exchange efficiency. This is in part due to impaired surfactant production. There is acute bronchitis and bronchiolitis, sloughing of mucosa, and intra-alveolar hemorrhage. Types I and II alveolar cells undergo necrosis, and free laminated inclusion bodies are seen in the pulmonary transudate. Lung weight may be two or three times normal. An increase

in lung water and a decrease in lung volume and compliance follow. Initially no signs of infection are present, but with progression there may be an increase in polymorphonuclear leukocytes. Kennedy et al. (84) observed a biphasic pattern to acid pulmonary injury at 1 and 4 hours in a rat model. This suggested an initial direct physiochemical interaction or capsaicin-sensitive afferent nerve-mediated response. A second phase of acute inflammatory response and protein leak 4 to 6 hours later is mediated by neutrophils. This second phase appears to be enhanced by high levels of serine protease in alveolar fluid (85). Tumor necrosis factor (TNF) is emerging as an important mediator of acid-induced lung injury (86). Davidson et al. have shown that both acidic and nonacidic particulate aspirates produce a markedly increased response in TNF compared to tracheally instilled saline or pure HCl (87). In 24 to 36 hours after the initial insult, alveolar consolidation and airway damage are observed and may result in mucosal sloughing (88). Organization of a hyaline membrane may be seen (89).

Resolution of the lesion begins by about 72 hours, and by 2 to 3 weeks lung weight has returned to near normal. Permanent damage is usually minimal (90). When infection occurs, it may be gram-positive, gram-negative, or a mixture of bacteria. The pathophysiologic picture of pulmonary acid aspiration has been well reviewed by a number of authors (11, 76, 84, 91).

Particulate and Antacid Aspiration

Gastric contents are often a combination of fluid and particulate foodstuffs. The pulmonary response to aspiration of gastric particulate matter differs from aspiration of acid alone. The response to small food particles is a combination of hemorrhage and edema occurring soon after aspiration, followed more slowly by a granulomatous reaction with bronchiolar and alveolar damage (91, 92).

Aspiration of large particles or a large amount of particulate material can lead to immediate and complete obstruction of the airway with suffocation, unless the material can be removed by rapid intubation, suction, and possibly bronchoscopy. Instillation of small amounts (3 to 5 mL) of physiologic saline solution before suction may help dislodge particles. Clinically, this may be accompanied by coughing, tachypnea, cyanosis, and tachycardia. Breath sounds may be decreased over the involved areas. Chest radiograph initially shows atelectasis with homogeneous

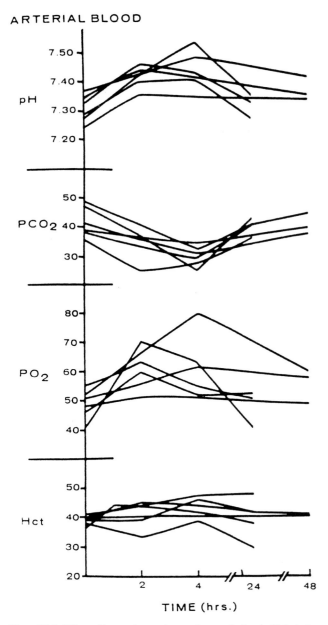

ARTERIAL BLOOD

Figure 22.4. Effect of increasing aspirate volume of a fixed pH. Intratracheal instillation of 1 mg · kg^{-1} 0.1 normal HCl on arterial pH, Po$_2$, and hematocrit. No spontaneous deaths occurred. Decrease in CO$_2$ caused by increase in spontaneous hyperventilation due to acid instillation. (Reprinted by permission from Greenfield LJ, Singleton RP, McCaffree DR, Coalson JJ. Pulmonary effects of experimental graded aspiration of hydrochloric acid. *Ann Surg* 1969;170:74–86.)

densities in affected areas. If involvement is sufficiently great, there will be a mediastinal shift. If the condition is untreated, pulmonary abscess may develop. Initial treatment includes immediate and repeated tracheobronchial suction, oxygenation, ventilation, and tracheal instillation of small amounts of saline to help dislodge material.

Encouragement of coughing may help dislodge the material. Except in cases in which only minimal amounts of material are aspirated, bronchoscopy should be performed as soon as possible after the incident for diagnosis and removal of foreign material. Initially, the fiberoptic bronchoscope may be used through the endotracheal tube to diagnose the presence of foreign material and to remove very small particulate matter under direct vision. The presence of large particulate matter or the development of atelectasis requires immediate bronchoscopy to remove

this material and allow reinflation of the atelectatic segments. Tracheal aspirates should be obtained at regular intervals, especially with the development of fever, for Gram's stain, culture, and sensitivity to allow rational antibiotic therapy.

The concept that severe lung lesions occur below a threshold of pH 2.5 has led many to conclude that the nonacidic aspirates are relatively benign. Although the effects are transient and less severe, aspiration of clear liquids such as saline and water can produce signs of pulmonary edema, epithelial damage, and a widening alveolar-arterial oxygen gradient. Aspiration of gastric fluids containing particulate antacids has been shown in humans to result in a clinical picture similar to that of acid aspiration (93) with pulmonary edema, impaired oxygenation, and pulmonary shunting, even when the pH of the aspirate was 6.5 (94, 95). Gibbs (95) and Eyler et al. (96) have shown that aspiration of insoluble particulate antacids in animals results in pulmonary lesions that are more severe and of longer duration than those produced by aspiration of similar volumes of hydrochloric acid (pH 1.6). Numerous reports of maternal death (97–99) following aspiration of insoluble antacid preparations indicate that such prophylaxis is an ineffective, as well as potentially dangerous, medical practice.

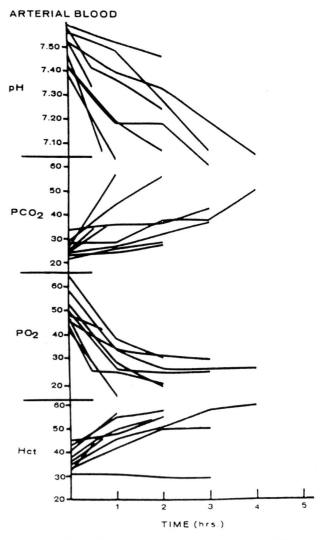

ARTERIAL BLOOD

Figure 22.5. Effect of increasing aspirate volume of a fixed pH. Intratracheal instillation of 3 mL · kg^{-1} 0.1 normal HCl on arterial pH, Po$_2$, and hematocrit. The rapid decline in arterial pH, Po$_2$, and CO$_2$ retention was usually associated with early death. (Reprinted by permission from Greenfield LJ, Singleton RP, McCaffree DR, Coalson JJ. Pulmonary effects of experimental graded aspiration of hydrochloric acid. *Ann Surg* 1969;170:74–86.)

Table 22.5. CLINICAL SIGNS AFTER ASPIRATION OF GASTRIC CONTENTS IN 50 PATIENTS

Latent Period	No.	%
0–1 h	48	96
2 h	2	4
Fever, total	47	94
99–102°F	24	48
>102°F	23	46
Tachypnea	39	78
Rales	36	72
Cough	18	36
Cyanosis	16	32
Wheezing	16	32
Apnea	15	30
Shock	12	24

Reprinted by permission from Bynum LJ, Pierce AK. Pulmonary aspiration of gastric contents. *Am Rev Respir Dis* 1976;114:1129–1136.

Steroid Therapy

Most authorities now discourage steroid administration following gastric aspiration, reporting that it has no benefit for treatment or reduction in mortality (100, 101).

Antibiotic Therapy

Because the incidence of infection is fairly low after aspiration, and infection may occur despite prophylaxis (82), most clinicians today oppose initiation of prophylactic antibiotic therapy at the time of acid aspiration (76, 88, 102). Regular cultures should be taken of the tracheal aspirate for Gram's stain, culture, and sensitivity. Appropriate antibiotics can then be rationally started on the basis of this information.

Experimental Treatment of Aspiration Pneumonitis

Attempts to counteract TNF and interleukin (IL)-mediated pneumonitis with anti-TNF and IL antibodies have not met with

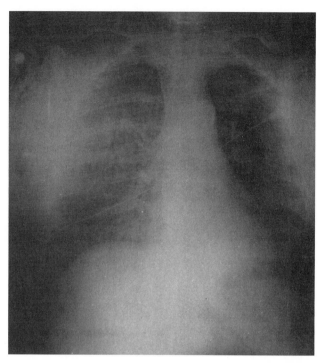

Figure 22.7. Acid aspiration (Mendelson's syndrome) with marked involvement of the right lung. Note the generalized soft, mottled densities and the absence of mediastinal shift.

persuasive success (87). This suggests both multiple mediators of the inflammatory response and separate pulmonary reactions to both acid and particulate matter.

Efforts to treat acid aspiration with inhaled nitric oxide (80 ppm for 5 hours) have been shown to increase lung injury in the rat, as do high-inspired oxygen concentrations (103).

Other approaches to limiting pulmonary damage due to aspiration with prostacyclin, prostaglandin $F_{2\alpha}$, nonsteroidal drugs, and surfactant have not been successful.

PREVENTION OF PULMONARY ASPIRATION IN THE OBSTETRIC PATIENT

"That which cannot be easily treated had better be prevented." These words by J. Alfred Lee summarize well the circumstances that surround pulmonary aspiration in the parturient. The first and most important step in the prevention of pulmonary aspiration is the recognition that every parturient is at risk for this catastrophe. Since pulmonary aspiration is usually associated with the use of general anesthesia, many claim general anesthesia is best avoided in the obstetric patient. Such a rigid policy not only denies the use of general anesthesia when it is indicated, but in addition gives no guarantee that aspiration will not occur. Nevertheless, the routine use of general anesthesia in obstetrics is best replaced by other forms of analgesia that preserve maternal consciousness. Clearly, these forms of analgesia are not without risk of aspiration. Deep maternal sedation with systemic opioids, tranquilizers, and sedatives may obtund the airway reflexes. Opioids are associated with nausea and vomiting. Regional anesthesia can lead to (a) local anesthetic toxicity with convulsions, followed by central nervous system (CNS) depression; (b) hypotension from sympathetic block compounded by aortocaval compression, also causing CNS depression; and (c) abdominal and intercostal muscle weakness, depressing the ability of the patient to cough and clear the airway. Inhalation analgesia, although it avoids neonatal depression and maintains upper airway reflexes, may accidentally advance to the stage of airway obstruction and airway reflex obtundation. The anesthetist must be aware that the patient may vomit, and if the mask

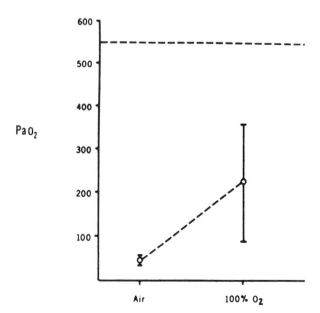

Figure 22.6. Response of mean PaO₂ to breathing 100% oxygen for 15 minutes in 12 patients. In all cases, the rise fell short of the generally accepted normal value of 500 mm Hg, indicating a right-to-left shunt-like effect. (Reprinted by permission from Lewis RT, Burgess JH, Hampson LG. Cardiorespiratory studies in critical illness: Changes in aspiration pneumonitis. *Arch Surg* 1971;103:335–340.)

Table 22.6. EVENTS SURROUNDING 4 CASES OF OBSTETRIC ASPIRATION (IN ~3680 CESAREAN SECTIONS)

Surgery	Anesthesia	Risk Factors	Mechanism
Semi-urgent	General with endotracheal intubation	Labor, recent food intake	Regurgitation at induction prior to laryngoscopy
Semi-urgent	General with endotracheal intubation	Labor, opioids, difficult intubation	Regurgitation at laryngoscopy and mask ventilation
Semi-urgent	General with endotracheal intubation	Labor, opioids	Regurgitation in early recovery phase
Semi-urgent	General with endotracheal intubation	Labor, opioids, recent food, difficult intubation	Vomiting during repeated intubation attempts

Adapted from Soreide E, Bjornestad E, Steen PA. An audit of perioperative aspiration pneumonitis in gynaecological and obstetric patients. *Acta Anaesthesiol Scand* 1996;40:14–19.

is not removed and the mouth suctioned, the vomitus can be inhaled. In reality all parturients in labor, especially those who receive any form of pharmacologic analgesia, require continuous monitoring and observation by qualified medical personnel if the catastrophe of aspiration is to be avoided. Typical events associated with obstetric aspiration are shown in Table 22.6.

General Anesthesia

When general anesthesia is required for the obstetric patient, her airway must be protected with a cuffed endotracheal tube placed either immediately after loss of consciousness or, less commonly, before induction. Although an intravenous (IV) rapid-sequence induction is usually employed, inhalation induction is not absolutely contraindicated.

It is rare that general anesthesia is required for vaginal delivery. Even difficult forceps deliveries can usually be accomplished with regional or a pudendal block supplemented by inhalation analgesia. General anesthesia for the parturient without intubation, except under the most unusual circumstances, is not acceptable practice. A rapid IV induction of anesthesia with thiopental and succinylcholine followed by immediate intubation of the trachea is recommended, as described in Chapters 11 and 21.

For a safe induction, the anesthetist requires a trained assistant to apply cricoid pressure, and to assist should difficulties arise. In any patient in whom difficult laryngoscopy and intubation are anticipated, intubation by direct visualization after topical anesthesia, fiberoptic bronchoscopy, or the blind nasal route is recommended. This might include patients with morbid obesity, hypoplastic mandible, limited range of neck motion, and limited temporomandibular joint mobility.

Position During Induction

Some authors recommend the head-up position for induction. However, we discourage this because it renders laryngoscopy and intubation more difficult, it increases the danger of hypotension, and pulmonary aspiration is more likely should vomiting occur. The patient is placed in the supine position on the delivery table and the right hip is elevated 10 to 15 degrees with folded sheets, a foam wedge, or inflatable bag, or the table is tipped 15 degrees to the left to minimize aortocaval compression. The head should be supported on a small pillow in the "sniffing" position. The sniffing position will give better visualization during laryngoscopy and will facilitate intubation.

Prevention of Muscle Fasciculations

The depolarizing muscle relaxant succinylcholine causes generalized muscle fasciculations and an immediate rise in intra-

gastric pressure (104–106). Pretreatment with a small dose of a nondepolarizing muscle relaxant such as curare (3 mg) will prevent the fasciculations and associated rise in intragastric pressure. Precurarization also avoids fasciculation-induced increases in maternal oxygen consumption prior to intubation, a potential benefit in the parturient with a decreased oxygen reserve (107). However, succinylcholine-induced muscle fasciculations are minimal among pregnant women and typically involve only the facial muscles. Furthermore, the use of a nondepolarizing relaxant to prevent fasciculations results in a longer latency period and requires a larger dose of succinylcholine to ensure adequate relaxation for laryngoscopy and intubation. The effect of muscle fasciculations on lower esophageal sphincter tone may be greater than that on intragastric pressure and may actually prevent passive regurgitation.

Cricoid Pressure (Sellick's Maneuver)

Pressing the cricoid cartilage dorsally and cephalad against the body of the sixth cervical vertebra will occlude the esophagus and prevent passive regurgitation of gastric contents during intubation (Fig. 22.8) (108). Cricoid pressure has been shown to be effective in preventing reflux of gastric contents into the posterior pharynx with gastric pressures as high as 50 to 94 cm H_2O (mean 74) (109). Potential hazards of the maneuver are excessive pressures with possible trauma to the larynx and lateral displacement of the larynx, making intubation or ventilation

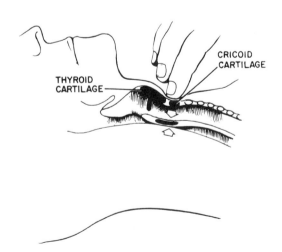

Figure 22.8. The technique of posterior pressure on the cricoid cartilage to occlude the esophagus can be effective in blocking regurgitation but not active vomiting. (Modified from Hamelberg W, Bosomworth PB, eds. *Aspiration Pneumonitis.* Springfield, IL: Charles C. Thomas; 1968.)

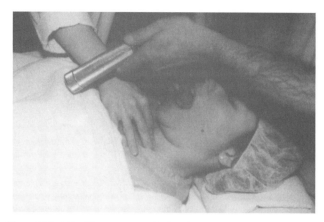

Figure 22.9. Cricoid pressure applied without neck support causes flexion of chin and hinders insertion of laryngoscope and visualization of retropharynx.

(when necessary) more difficult (110). When cricoid pressure is applied, support of the neck (usually with the operator's other hand) is essential to prevent flexion of the head and neck, which may render laryngoscopy and laryngeal visualization impossible (Figs. 22.9 and 22.10). This approach has been disputed by Cook (111), although it is not clear from his study whether other neck support was used or how much cricoid force was applied. Training is essential to properly execute cricoid pressure. An assistant can be easily trained by applying cricoid pressure to himself or herself while he or she attempts to swallow a mouthful of water. Adequate cricoid pressure is applied when the trainee finds swallowing impossible (Dr. Michael Rosen, personal communication). Herman et al. (112) have suggested teaching adequate cricoid pressure (20 to 40 N) with a life-size laryngotracheal model placed on an infant scale. Recent reports of cricoid pressure resulting in decreased lower esophageal sphincter tone reinforce the need to apply adequate pressure (113).

Relationship Between the Difficult Airway and Aspiration

A growing body of evidence points to failed intubation and inability to control the airway during emergency induction of general anesthesia as highly associated with gastric content aspiration (114–116). Most obstetric emergencies requiring rapid initiation of anesthesia can be managed by elevating and intensifying an already-functioning epidural catheter or expeditious placement of subarachnoid block. However, when an obstetric

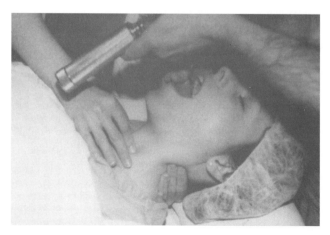

Figure 22.10. Cricoid pressure applied with posterior neck support allows extension of neck and promotes easier insertion of laryngoscope and visualization of retropharynx.

Table 22.7. DIFFICULT AIRWAY IN OBSTETRICS (ESTIMATES)

Study	Incidence of Failed Intubation
Obstetric	
Hawthorne et al., 1996 (117)	1/250 (teaching hospital)
Rocke et al., 1992 (119)	1/750 (teaching hospital)
Lyons and MacDonald, 1985 (118)	1/2130 (private practice)
General Surgical	
Samsoon and Young, 1987 (120)	1/2230 (total of 6/13,380)

emergency is of such urgency as to prohibit any delay required for regional block, or if conduction analgesia itself is strongly contraindicated, a rapid-sequence induction of general oral tracheal anesthesia is indicated, unless there are conditions that would make intubation difficult. Awake intubation must be increasingly considered as an important alternative to "crash" induction or a failed regional block. Several studies have suggested that the relative risk of failed intubation in obstetrics is between 1/250 and 1/750 (Table 22.7) (117–120).

PREVENTION OF DIFFICULT AIRWAY COMPLICATIONS

The combination of a difficult airway during emergency induction of general anesthesia in obstetrics and the predisposition of the pregnant patient to pulmonary aspiration of gastric contents remains an important consideration for anesthesiologists. Difficult airway recognition, prevention, and management are discussed in detail in Chapter 21. Early recognition of a potential difficult airway by either the obstetrician or anesthesiologist and a coordinated plan of management is important for optimal patient management. It has recently been reported that training obstetricians to evaluate the patient's airway can increase the early identification of the difficult airway. This can increase the obstetrician's request for anesthesia consultation and early use of regional analgesia (121). Although techniques for using LMA[TM]* or obturator airway when intubation is impossible (Figs. 22.11, 22.12) may allow for life-saving ventilation when

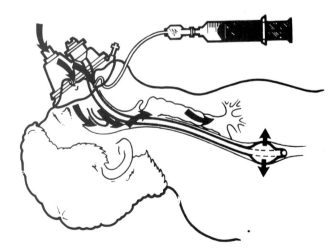

Figure 22.11. Esophageal gastric tube airway in place. (Reprinted by permission from Tunstall ME, Geddes C. Failed intubation in obstetric anaesthesia: An indication for the use of the "esophageal gastric tube airway." *Br J Anaesth* 1984;56:659–661.)

---

* *LMA* is a trademark of The Laryngeal Mask Company and all references herein to *LMA* are to this trademark.

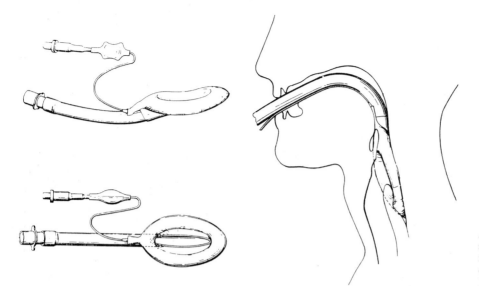

Figure 22.12. View of laryngeal airway and airway in place. (Reprinted by permission from Brain AIJ. The laryngeal mask: A new concept in airway management. *Br J Anaesth* 1983;55:801–805.)

mask ventilation is impossible (122, 123), these instruments may not prevent aspiration (124–131) and should not be used routinely in obstetric anesthesia. Management of the difficult airway encountered during induction of general anesthesia ranges from approaches such as the Tunstall failed intubation drill (132–135) and reference to the American Society of Anesthesiologists (ASA) guidelines on difficult airway management (136) to more updated approaches outlined in Chapters 11 and 21.

Awake Extubation

After the patient emerges from anesthesia, the endotracheal tube must be left in place until the patient is awake, is completely responsive to commands, and has no signs of muscle weakness. The patient may be placed in the lateral head-down (Trendelenburg) position. The mouth and posterior pharynx are suctioned. Extubation should take place with the patient breathing 100% oxygen. The lungs are inflated, and during inflation the tracheal tube cuff is deflated and the tube immediately removed. Deflation of the cuff and removal of the tube during positive pressure inflation of the lungs will tend to blow material that may have collected above the cuff up and out of the trachea. Reviews of prevention of aspiration during parturition continue to be published (122).

PROPHYLAXIS FOR ASPIRATION PNEUMONITIS

A number of approaches have been suggested to prevent pulmonary aspiration and pneumonitis. However, no approach is completely effective or should be solely relied upon to prevent aspiration or pneumonitis.

Fasting Orders During Labor and Gastric Volume

Few topics inspire such controversy as what should be permitted for oral intake during labor. The desire to foster maternal emotional comfort as well as nutritional requirements conflicts with the possibility that immediate anesthesia for delivery could be required at any time, with the remote but devastating risk of aspiration. It is easy for "maternal advocates" to call for an end to what may seem to be punitive nothing-by-mouth (NPO) orders, and advocate liberalized intake of liquid and solid nourishment during labor. They could argue that the occurrence of maternal aspiration is extremely rare and there are no large prospective studies associating restricted oral intake with improved maternal safety (16). These arguments were appropriately compared

by Chestnut and Cohen (18) to "a suggestion that the airlines relax safety standards, given the remarkable record of air safety during the last decade."

Due to the unproven efficacy of aspiration prophylaxis and conflicting data from clinical studies, clinical practice varies widely. In some hospitals, pregnant women are offered full meals during labor, whereas in other hospitals, even with prolonged labor women are fasted without IV infusions of glucose because it has been associated with maternal ketosis and possible hypotension (137, 138). A study by O'Sullivan et al. suggests that gastric emptying may not be as slow as once believed in pregnancy (27). An array of investigators suggest small volumes of oral liquid are not associated with increased gastric volume or lower pH prior to surgery in pregnant and nonpregnant patients (139–142). In contrast, Lewis and Crawford (28) compared patients who were given a light breakfast less than 4 hours before elective cesarean section to those who fasted. They found the gastric volume was increased among the patients who had eaten (73.4 mL vs. 33 mL) and there was a lower pH in the fed versus the fasted parturients.

Scrutton et al. compared women fed a standardized light diet during labor to women allowed only water (36). Ultrasound examination of the stomach 45 minutes after delivery showed significantly higher residual gastric volumes in those allowed to eat. Among those patients who vomited, the quantity of vomitus was significantly greater in those eating a light diet than those who consumed only water (309 ± 173 mL vs. 104 ± 83 mL). Although women allowed to eat had reduced ketones and nonesterified fatty acids, the investigators believed that the larger gastric volumes suggest eating policies in labor should be approached with caution. In addition, case reports continue to appear in the literature in which feeding a patient during labor can be associated with Mendelson's syndrome (143).

We believe that it is well advised to continue the practice of *presurgical* fasting of pregnant patients for 6 hours. In contrast, the parturient in labor with a functioning epidural does not need as rigid a fasting regime. For example, in our practice, most women in labor with a functioning epidural block are allowed ice chips and limited sips of clear oral liquid intake of 100 to 200 mL per hour. Our rationale is that the probability of general anesthesia among these parturients is very low. In our experience of more than 20 years and more than 10,000 cesarean sections, we have not had a maternal aspiration. However, the number of rapid sequence inductions for cesarean section during that time period was about 500, in part since every effort was made to use regional block or awake intubation in those considered at risk for difficult intubation.

The ASA has published a set of practice guidelines for obstetric anesthesia that include recommendations for oral intake

Table 22.8. FASTING GUIDELINES IN THE OBSTETRIC PATIENT

	Published Evidence	Task Force Opinion	Recommendation
Clear liquids	Insufficient evidence regarding fasting time and risk for emesis/reflux or aspiration during labor	Agree oral intake of clear liquid improves comfort/satisfaction	Uncomplicated labor: modest amounts of oral liquid, including water, fruit juice (no pulp), carbonated beverages, clear tea, and black coffee
		Equivocal regarding whether oral clear liquids during labor increase maternal risk for pulmonary aspiration	Patients with additional risk: obesity, difficult airway or higher cesarean section risk, nonreassuring fetal heartrate pattern; further oral restrictions—case by case
Solids	Insufficient data to address any particular fasting period for solids in parturients	Elective cesarean: NPO 6–8 h	Solid foods are to be avoided in laboring patient
		In labor, timing of delivery is uncertain. Fasting compliance is not always possible	Elective cesarean: fast consistent with usual hospital policy
			Both amount and time of food must be considered when timing surgery

NPO = nothing by mouth; OB = parturient.
Adapted from the American Society of Anesthesiologists Task Force on Obstetrical Anesthesia. Practice guidelines for obstetrical anesthesia. *Anesthesiology* 1999;90:600–611.

during labor and prior to cesarean section. These may be useful in crafting departmental/hospital parameters and assisting in clinical decision-making (Table 22.8, see Appendix B) (144, 145). Similarly, the American College of Obstetricians and Gynecologists has also recommended that only ice chips and small sips of clear liquids be consumed during labor (146).

Oral Antacid Therapy

After Taylor and Pryse-Davies (68) first showed the efficacy of oral magnesium trisilicate BPC to increase the gastric pH above 2.5, it became a widespread practice to administer suspensions of insoluble oral antacids every 3 to 4 hours in 15- to 30-mL doses to laboring women. Fortunately, this practice has been abandoned. Aspiration of insoluble antacids may result in severe and persistent lung pathologic conditions, as described earlier in this chapter. An alternative oral antacid, 0.3 M sodium citrate, was first recommended by Lahiri et al. (147), who found that 15 mL resulted in a very rapid neutralization of stomach contents. Gibbs et al. (95) showed that aspiration of sodium citrate in dogs produced a pulmonary histologic lesion that was much less severe compared to those lesions produced by aspiration of equal volumes of particulate antacids or acidic liquid. Arterial blood gas impairment and shunting, although present after aspiration of sodium citrate, are less severe than with acid aspiration (96). A dose of 30 mL 0.3 M sodium citrate is capable of neutralizing up to 255 mL hydrochloric acid with a pH of 1 (148). Neutralization of gastric acid by sodium citrate has been reported to last 40 minutes to 1 hour (148–150). The time required for an increase in pH is usually less than 5 minutes, compared with 30 minutes for the insoluble antacids (151).

The limitations of sodium citrate include systemic absorption and metabolic alkalosis after multiple doses, a laxative effect, and a disagreeable taste, requiring the addition of flavoring, which may decrease its effectiveness. Gillett et al. (152) found that 17% of both elective and emergency cesarean section patients still had a gastric pH <3 after receiving 30 mL oral 0.3 M sodium citrate. These findings may be explained by the excessive gastric volume or inadequate gastric mixing that is more prone to occur in the pregnant patient (153).

The properties of rapid mixing, effective neutralization of gastric acid, and lack of pulmonary damage if aspirated make sodium citrate 0.3 M (30 mL) the preferred antacid to administer before induction of general anesthesia in the obstetric pa-

tient. Its absorption from the gastrointestinal tract and its unpleasant taste make its routine use throughout labor ill advised. In our practice, we generally give sodium citrate (15 minutes prior to induction) only to those obstetric patients who are to undergo general anesthesia in elective cases and immediately upon learning general anesthesia will be required in emergency cases. Others, including the editors, administer oral antacid to all patients having a cesarean section.

Sodium bicarbonate 8.4%, 20 mL has been recommended as an effective antacid (154). However, it is not completely effective (155) and releases about 0.4 L intragastric gas.

Although helpful, oral antacid prophylaxis is not a panacea and will not protect all obstetric patients. It will not prevent the aspiration of solid or bacterially contaminated material. It may produce a false sense of security. In addition, it may not effectively neutralize gastric material when large volumes are present.

H$_2$-Receptor Antagonists and Proton Pump Inhibitors

Pharmacologic suppression of gastric acid production by histamine-receptor inhibition on the oxyntic cell as a form of aspiration prophylaxis in obstetrics was first studied by Pickering et al. (156). Both cimetidine (300 mg) and ranitidine (50 mg), when given orally the night before surgery and again 1 to 2 hours before anesthesia induction, are effective in reliably elevating gastric pH above 2.5 in most but not all parturients (157, 158). When these drugs are combined with metoclopramide, gastric volume is consistently less than 25 mL (159, 160).

When given just before emergency general anesthesia, the H$_2$ blockers are not effective in rapidly elevating gastric pH unless at least 30 minutes has elapsed (161). However, giving the H$_2$ blocker intramuscularly or intravenously along with 30 mL oral 0.3 M sodium citrate has been shown to reliably maintain the gastric pH above 2.5 for much longer than citrate alone. The acute use of the H$_2$ blockers does not appear to have any ill effects on the newborn (157). Likewise, the occasional CNS side effects seen in patients receiving chronic cimetidine are not seen in mothers after short-term administration. Rarely, the rapid IV use of both cimetidine and ranitidine may be associated with cardiovascular depression or arrhythmia (162, 163) that is not seen when these drugs are given orally or by intramuscular injection. The administration of both cimetidine and ranitidine has been reported to alter hepatic metabolic activity and to prolong the metabolism and elevate the blood levels of a number of drugs by inhibiting cytochrome P450 oxidation and redistribution. These drugs include amide local anesthetics, anticoagulants, propranolol, benzodiazepines, and theophylline (164–166). Subsequently, other investigators have questioned these earlier reports as they have found preoperative H$_2$ blockers have little or no effect on drug disposition in pregnancy (167–170).

Famotidine, an amidine derivative H$_2$-receptor antagonist, given prior to surgery as 20 mg (2 h orally [PO], or 1 h intramuscularly) or nizatidine (150 to 300 mg PO) will maintain pH between 5.7 and 7.2 and gastric volume below 10 mL in nonpregnant patients (171–173). Both drugs are reported to have negligible effects on hepatic blood flow, drug enzyme induction, and cholinesterase activity (174, 175), and minimal adverse hemodynamic effects (176, 177).

Particulate oral antacids have been shown to inhibit the bioavailability of both cimetidine and ranitidine (178). Earlier reports that H$_2$ blockers inhibited anticholinesterase activity are not clinically relevant. H$_2$ inhibitors do not affect the duration of neuromuscular block after depolarizing or nondepolarizing drugs (179–182).

Omeprazole (20 to 40 mg PO) and lansoprazole (15 to 30 mg PO) block the hydrogen ion pump of gastric oxyntic cells. Omeprazole has been studied more in obstetrics and appears to have a long duration of effect and minimal adverse reactions (183). Rout (161) and Rocke (184) et al. have conducted a large series on the antacid and volume reduction efficacy of ranitidine and omeprazole. They concluded ranitidine was slightly more effective than omeprazole if given 30 minutes or more before induction of anesthesia and was less expensive (161, 185). Omeprazole does not affect lidocaine kinetics (186). Comparison of new generation H$_2$ and proton pump inhibitors has been made in parturients without revealing important individual drug advantages (187–189).

Routine antacid prophylaxis (sodium citrate, H$_2$ or proton pump inhibitors) of all laboring women is not warranted for a number of reasons: (a) the vast majority of parturients will not require general anesthesia and hence are not at great risk of aspiration of gastric contents; (b) those requiring emergency general anesthesia can be adequately treated with 30 mL 0.3 M sodium citrate and an IV H$_2$ blocker plus metoclopramide shortly before induction; (c) the cost of routine prophylaxis administration would be significant; and (d) there is evidence that the elevated pH associated with presurgical prophylactic H$_2$ antagonists causes increased intragastric bacterial growth (190). If such material is aspirated, we may be "exchanging the aspiration of acid for the aspiration of colonized gastric contents" (191). In selected patients, such as those with acid reflux, obesity, diabetes, or preeclampsia, and those with a recognized difficult airway, it may be prudent to employ antacid prophylaxis in labor.

In our practice, H$_2$ inhibitor therapy is generally limited to elective cesarean section under general anesthesia or to those at higher risk for aspiration. Because of their latency, H$_2$ blockers administered shortly before induction of anesthesia will do little to protect the patient from acid aspiration during induction. In an obstetric emergency requiring general anesthesia, a combination of an H$_2$ inhibitor, metoclopramide, and sodium citrate prior to induction may be a sensible choice. Short-term protection is provided by sodium citrate, and longer-term protection is afforded by cimetidine in the event of aspiration during emergence from general anesthesia.

Emptying the Stomach Pharmacologically

The dopamine antagonists, characterized by metoclopramide, have come into clinical use. These increase gastroesophageal sphincter pressure and are effective antiemetics (192). Although these drugs do not block gastric acid secretion, they inhibit dopaminergic receptors, thus promoting gastric emptying and decreasing gastric volume in normal patients and in patients undergoing cesarean section (193). It appears these drugs act

on postganglionic nerves intrinsic to the wall of the intestinal tract, thereby releasing acetylcholine, which promotes peristalsis and increases lower esophageal sphincter tone. Centrally, metoclopramide blocks dopamine receptors and induces secretion of prolactin. Metoclopramide (10 mg IV), a derivative of procaine, increases stomach emptying over a 40- to 60-minute period. Unfortunately, the effectiveness of metoclopramide in increasing gastroesophageal sphincter tone is decreased by anticholinergics such as glycopyrrolate. Despite opioid antagonism to the gastric emptying effects of metoclopramide, studies have shown that the drug still has considerable efficacy in decreasing the gastric volume in laboring patients who have received opioids (65). Metoclopramide crosses the blood-brain barrier and the placenta (194). As a dopamine antagonist, metoclopramide is unlikely to produce sedation. However, in high doses it can produce extrapyramidal effects (which respond readily to diphenhydramine) and perhaps stress-induced tachycardia (195). Combined with an H$_2$ blocker, the dopamine antagonists reliably elevate gastric pH above 2.5 and lower gastric volume below 25 mL in normal nonpregnant patients undergoing elective surgery (160, 161). The usual dose of metoclopramide is 10 mg PO or IM about 1 hour prior to the induction of anesthesia, or 10 mg IV, which will have an effect within 1 to 3 minutes. Acute administration of dopamine antagonists prior to cesarean section has not produced adverse effects in either mother or newborn.

The use of emetics (i.e., apomorphine) or nasogastric tubes will not guarantee an empty stomach (196). The duration of apomorphine's emetic effect is unpredictable; it may continue into the induction period. If the stomach is distended, which is rare in the parturient, it may be decompressed by an orogastric tube intraoperatively before extubation.

Combination Antacid Prophylaxis

In recent years, most anesthetists have adopted a variation of H$_2$-receptor antagonist, proton pump inhibitor, dopamine-receptor inhibitor, and clear oral liquid antacid, such as that recommended long ago by Moir (197). Although there is disagreement regarding the most effective combination (198–200), a majority of surveyed anesthetists use some combination of the above (Table 22.9) (11, 201–206).

Anticholinergic Therapy

It has been suggested that the use of anticholinergics (atropine, scopolamine, and glycopyrrolate) protect against acid aspiration by decreasing the volume of gastric secretions and decreasing the amount of gastric acid secreted. Human studies have failed to demonstrate the effectiveness of anticholinergics in decreasing either the acidity or volume of gastric contents (207). An undesirable anticholinergic side effect is the decrease in lower esophageal sphincter resting tone, which could increase the incidence of gastric reflux in an already high-risk population. Anticholinergic therapy is not recommended for routine preoperative use during pregnancy and should be reserved for specific medical or anesthetic indications.

Postpartum Tubal Ligation

Demand for postpartum tubal sterilization (PPTL) continues because it is convenient for the patient and surgeon and technically simple (see Chapter 12). Recent ASA guidelines remain vague regarding risks, timing, and recommended anesthetic technique (144). Many patients can safely undergo this procedure provided an anesthesiologist is available to evaluate the patient and conduct the anesthetic in an appropriate environment. If surgery is performed in the first few hours or days after delivery, it is prudent to remember that the physiologic changes of pregnancy resolve at different rates. Epidural and spinal requirements may increase slightly within hours of delivery,

Table 22.9. INTERNATIONAL ASPIRATION PROPHYLAXIS PATTERNS

Study	Country	In Labor Routine Prophylaxis	Cesarean Elective Prophylaxis	Cesarean Emergency Prophylaxis
Burgess and Crowhurst, 1989 (203)	Australia	22%	85%	89%
Tordoff and Sweeney, 1990 (201)	UK	75%	99%	100%
Plumer and Rottman, 1993 (204)	US	62%	89%	87%
Benhamou, 1993 (205)	France	63%	51%	88%
Helbo-Hansen and Bang, 1993 (206)	Denmark	2%	29%	36%
Greiff et al., 1994 (202)	UK	57%	100%	100%
Schneck et al., 1997 (11)	Germany	7%	52%	68%

UK = United Kingdom; US = United States.
The vast majority of authors used an H_2 blocker and sodium citrate. Many used metoclopramide.

while general anesthesia requirements remain unchanged. Respiratory function may return to normal more rapidly than airway anatomy (208), cardiovascular changes, or gastric emptying. The anesthetic risk has not been determined for postpartum sterilization, although one study suggested a mortality rate of 3.6/100,000 (209). Compared to patients who undergo interval sterilization, a greater number of postpartum patients have solid food in their stomachs at least 6 hours after delivery (37). A delay in gastric emptying has also been associated with parenteral (26, 27) and neuraxial opioid administration during labor (33, 48).

Administration of general anesthesia within the first 8 to10 hours and probably within the first 1 to 2 weeks postpartum is still associated with many risks associated with the physiologic changes of pregnancy. Failed intubation due to airway anatomy changes will be higher than in nonpregnant patients (117–119). Recent food ingestion or opioid administration and the presence of obesity or diabetes also must be considered as increasing the risk of general anesthesia in the immediate postpartum period. Aspiration prophylaxis is recommended for patients undergoing PPTL.

Epidural or spinal block for PPTL, although suggested to decrease the risk of maternal mortality (1), are not always reliable and carry their own important risks. In hospitals with busy labor epidural services, reactivation of the indwelling labor catheter for PPTL is popular. Recent reports of high failure rates of reactivated catheters (210) contrast with reports of high success rates (211). Our own experience suggests that if the catheter is initially placed at an adequate depth (4 to 5 cm) and the catheter dressing is reflected and the catheter is checked for appropriate positioning prior to the PPTL, the incidence of success is greater than 90% and thus worth utilizing.

Spinal block for PPTL is a satisfactory alternative to epidural block. Dose requirements may increase by 8 to 24 hours postpartum (212). In our practice, the first choice of anesthesia for PPTL is to perform it either by using the indwelling epidural catheter immediately after delivery or by reactivation at least 8 hours later. Our second choice is spinal anesthesia. General anesthesia is uncommon but used when patients decline regional block and is performed after the patient has been NPO for 8 hours after delivery. A useful review of this subject was recently published by Bucklin and Smith (213).

CONCLUSION

Pulmonary aspiration of stomach contents, although rare, remains a leading cause of maternal morbidity and mortality. Most cases of aspiration among parturients are preventable by careful observation and expert anesthesia care during labor and delivery (Table 22.10). All parturients must be assumed to have full stomachs. Avoidance of general anesthesia, over-sedation, and hypotension will do much to eliminate pulmonary aspiration. When general anesthesia is required, a skilled anesthetist and a trained assistant are required, as are cricoid pressure and a

rapid securing of the airway. Preoperative antacid prophylaxis is recommended. Should pulmonary aspiration occur, prompt and proper therapy with continuous monitoring is required and is best accomplished in an intensive care setting if high mortality is to be avoided. There remain a number of areas worthy of study to improve prevention of maternal mortality. Many authorities have suggested that the trend away from general anesthesia for cesarean section has been instrumental in reducing maternal death and that this trend should continue (214–217). An increase in the availability and utilization of intensive care services for women experiencing anesthetic misadventure in obstetrics may contribute to improved outcome (216). Identification and assessment of near-miss critical incidents are not widely attempted and may prove effective in further improving our understanding and prevention of the causes of maternal anesthetic catastrophes (216). Others have suggested that anesthesiologists follow the example of airline pilot training and require regular hands-on practice with simulators of rare but devastating anesthetic occurrences (218).

In the end, the many points in this chapter are of less consequence than the root condition surrounding most aspiration and airway accidents. That is, the rush to anesthetize an unprepared parturient often not fully evaluated by an anesthesiologist creates a situation fraught with danger. Both anesthesiologists and obstetricians must consider the potential risk of this type of practice. Rescuing fetuses is important, but not at the expense of the mother's life. Informed, educated obstetricians will be much

Table 22.10. SUGGESTED MEANS OF PREVENTING PULMONARY ASPIRATION OR DECREASING ITS INCIDENCE

I. Avoid situations that could result in loss of maternal consciousness with an unprotected airway
  a. General anesthesia, when alternatives are appropriate
  b. Over-sedation
  c. Significant hypotension
  d. Local anesthetic toxicity
II. Use appropriate techniques for general anesthesia
  a. Intubation of all obstetric patients in 2nd half of pregnancy receiving general anesthesia
  b. Trained assistant for induction of anesthesia
  c. Defasciculation with nondepolarizer (suggested by some)
  d. Cricoid pressure before loss of consciousness until successful intubation
  e. Rapid production of relaxation with succinylcholine 1.5 mg/kg IV
  f. Extubation only when patient is fully awake, and capable of airway protection (awake extubation)
III. Careful observation of all obstetric patients receiving analgesia/anesthesia and appropriate management postpartum
IV. Assume all women in 2nd half of pregnancy from midgestation are at risk for gastric content aspiration

IV = intravenous.

more likely to consult the anesthetist in a timely fashion regarding parturients at high anesthetic risk. It is the responsibility of the anesthesiologist, when consulted, to evaluate the high-risk patient in a timely manner. Placement of an epidural block for labor may seem an ideal solution; however, this is not always possible or desired by the parturient. At a minimum, a plan can be established in consultation with the obstetrician to avoid a last-minute emergency cesarean section requiring general anesthesia. Also, the mother can receive IV and oral prophylaxis in anticipation of possible general anesthesia.

In a recent article on medical mistakes, a Harvard surgery resident wrote that it is the process as much as the individual physician that leads to medical error and misadventure (219). He singled out the specialty of anesthesia as one success story obtaining extraordinary results in correcting medical error.

If one considers the 3-fold increase of cesarean sections and the millions of legal abortions performed in the last 20 years, there has been an enormous reduction in anesthetic-related maternal mortality, for which obstetric anesthetists can take credit. Unfortunately, conditions that increase medical error still persist, and include poor communication among team members, haste, and inattention to detail. Efforts must continue to enhance early communication regarding high-risk and potential emergency obstetric parturients. Obstetric practice patterns that lead to excessive haste and inadequate time to assess critical patient details must be reduced to a minimum.

REFERENCES

1. Hawkins JL, Koonin LM, Palmer SK, Gibbs CP. Anesthesia-related deaths during obstetric delivery in the United States, 1979–1990. *Anesthesiology* 1997;86:273–276.
2. Hibbard BM, Anderson MM, Drife JO, et al. Report on Confidential Enquiries into Maternal Deaths in the United Kingdom, 1988–1990. London, England: HMSO;1994.
3. Hibbard BM, Anderson MM, Drife JO, et al. Report on Confidential Enquiries into Maternal Deaths in the United Kingdom, 1991–1993. London, England: HMSO;1996.
4. Drife J, Lewis G, Neilson J, et al. Report on Confidential Enquiries into Maternal Deaths in the United Kingdom, 1994–1996. London, England: HMSO;1998.
5. Schneck H, Wagner R, Scheller M, von Hundelshausen B, Kochs E. Anesthesia for cesarean section and acid aspiration prophylaxis. *Anesth Analg* 1999;88:63–66.
6. Soreide E, Bjornestad E, Steen PA. An audit of perioperative aspiration pneumonitis in gynaecological and obstetric patients. *Acta Anaesthesiol Scand* 1996;40:14–19.
7. Mellin-Olsen J, Fasting S, Gisvold SE. Routine preoperative gastric emptying is seldom indicated. A study of 85,594 anaesthetics with special focus on aspiration pneumonia. *Acta Anaesthesiol Scand* 1996;40:1184–1188.
8. Mendelson CL. Aspiration of stomach contents into lungs during obstetric anesthesia. *Am J Obstet Gynecol* 1946;52:191–205.
9. Warner MA, Warner ME, Weber JG. Clinical significance of pulmonary aspiration during the perioperative period. *Anesthesiology* 1993;78:56–62.
10. Merrill RB, Hingson RA. Studies of the incidence of maternal mortality from the aspiration of vomitus during anesthesia occurring in major obstetric hospitals in the United States. *Anesth Analg* 1951;30:121–135.
11. Schneck H, von Hundelshausen B, Wagner R, Scheller M, Kochs E. Prophylaxis against obstetric acid aspiration syndrome in the German Federal Republic in 1997. A review based on results of a federal survey. *Anasthesiologie, Intensivmedizin, Notfallmedizin, Schmerztherapie* 1999;34:204–213.
12. Stoelting RK. NPO and aspiration pneumonitis: Changing perspectives. In: American Society of Anesthesiologists Annual Refresher Course Lectures. Philadelphia, PA 1993:41–49.
13. Conklin K. Maternal physiological adaptations during gestation, labor and the puerperium. *Semin Anesth* 1991;10:221–234.
14. Gorback MS. Cut-off values and aspiration risk [letter]. *Anesth Analg* 1989;69:417.
15. Gorback MS. What we still don't know about the risk of aspiration. *Curr Rev Clin Anesth* 1991;11:215–219.
16. Elkington KW. At the water's edge: Where obstetrics and anesthesia meet [clinical commentary]. *Obstet Gynecol* 1991;77:304–308.
17. McKay S, Mahan C. How can aspiration of vomitus in obstetrics best be prevented? *Birth* 1988;15:222–235.
18. Chestnut DH, Cohen SE. At the waters edge: Where obstetrics and anesthesia meet [reply]. *Obstet Gynecol* 1991;77:965–966.
19. Gutsche BB, Domurat MF, Marx G, et al. Should parturients in labor receive prophylaxis to elevate gastric pH and decrease gastric volume [the expert's opinion]? *Surv Anesth* 1986;29:196–198.
20. Soreide E. Prevention of aspiration pneumonitis in the obstetric patient. *Acta Anaesthesiol Scand* 1997;110(suppl):23–24.
21. Hirscheimer A, January DA, Daversa JJ. An X-ray study of gastric function during labour. *Am J Obstet Gynecol* 1938;36:671–673.
22. La Salvia LA, Steffen EA. Delayed gastric emptying time in labor. *Am J Obstet Gynecol* 1950;50:1075–1081.
23. Crawford JS. Some aspects of obstetric anaesthesia. *Br J Anaesth* 1956;28:201–208.
24. Hunt JW, Murray SA. Gastric function in pregnancy. *J Obstet Gynaecol Br Commonw* 1958;65:78–83.
25. Davison JS, Davison MC, Hay DM. Gastric emptying time in pregnancy and labour. *Br J Obstet Gynaecol* 1970;77:37–41.
26. Nimmo WS, Wilson J, Prescott LF. Narcotic analgesics and delayed gastric emptying during labour. *Lancet* 1975;1:890–893.
27. O'Sullivan G, Sutton AJ, Thompson SA, Carrie LE, Bullingham RES. Non-invasive measurement of gastric emptying in obstetric patients. *Anesth Analg* 1987;66:505–511.
28. Lewis M, Crawford JS. Can one risk fasting the obstetric patient for less than 4 hours? *Br J Anaesth* 1987;59:312–314.
29. Simpson KH, Stakes AF, Miller M. Pregnancy delays paracetamol absorption and gastric emptying in patients undergoing surgery. *Br J Anaesth* 1988;60:24–27.
30. Macfie AG, Magides AD, Richmond MN, Reilly CS. Gastric emptying in pregnancy. *Br J Anaesth* 1991;67:54–57.
31. Gin T, Cho AMW, Lew JKL, et al. Gastric emptying in the postpartum period. *Anaesth Intensive Care* 1991;19:521–524.
32. Sandhar BK, Elliott RH, Windram I, Rowbotham DJ. Peripartum changes in gastric emptying. *Anaesthesia* 1992;47:196–198.
33. Whitehead EM, Smith M, Dean Y, O'Sullivan G. An evaluation of gastric emptying times in pregnancy and the puerperium. *Anaesthesia* 1993;48:53–57.
34. Carp H, Jayaram A, Stoll M. Ultrasound examination of the stomach contents of parturients. *Anesth Analg* 1992;74:683–687.
35. Levy DM, Williams OA, Magides AD, Reilly CS. Gastric emptying is delayed at 8–12 weeks' gestation. *Br J Anaesth* 1994;73:237–238.
36. Scrutton MJL, Metcalfe GA, Lowy C, Seed PT, O'Sullivan G. Eating in labour: A randomized controlled trial assessing the risks and benefits. *Anaesthesia* 1999;54:329–334.
37. Jayaram A, Bowen MP, Deshpande S, Carp HM. Ultrasound examination of the stomach contents of women in the postpartum period. *Anesth Analg* 1997;84:522–526.
38. Csapo A. Progesterone block. *Am J Anat* 1956;98:273–291.
39. Christofides ND, Ghatei MA, Bloom SR, Barbog C, Gillmer MDG. Decreased plasma motilin concentrations in pregnancy. *Br Med J* 1982;285:1453–1454.
40. Simpson KH, Stakes AF. Effect of anxiety on gastric emptying in preoperative patients. *Br J Anaesth* 1987;59:540–544.
41. O'Sullivan G. Gastric emptying during pregnancy and the puerperium. *Int J Obstet Anesth* 1993;2:216–224.
42. Holdsworth JD. Relationship between stomach contents and analgesia in labour. *Br J Anaesth* 1978;50:1145–1148.
43. Wilson J. Gastric emptying in labour: Some recent findings and their clinical significance. *J Int Med Res* 1978;6(suppl):54–62.
44. Zimmermann DL, Breen TW, Fick G. Adding fentanyl 0.0002% to epidural bupivacaine 0.125% does not delay gastric emptying in laboring parturients. *Anesth Analg* 1996;82:612–616.
45. Porter JS, Bonello E, Reynolds F. The influence of epidural administration of fentanyl infusion on gastric emptying in labour. *Anaesthesia* 1997;52:1151–1156.
46. Wright PMC, Allen RW, Moore J, Donnelly JP. Gastric emptying during lumbar extradural analgesia in labour: Effect of fentanyl supplementation. *Br J Anaesth* 1992;68:248–251.
47. Geddes SM, Thorburn J, Logan RW. Gastric emptying following cesarean section and the effect of epidural fentanyl. *Anaesthesia* 1991;46:1016–1018.
48. Ewah B, Yau K, Reynolds F, Carson RJ, Morgan B. Effect of opioids on gastric emptying. *Int J Obstet Anesth* 1993;2:125–128.

49. Kelly MC, Carabine UA, Hill DA, Mirakhur RK. A comparison of the effect of intrathecal and extradural fentanyl on gastric emptying in laboring women. *Anesth Analg* 1997;85:834–838.

50. Creasy RK. Preterm parturition. *Semin Perinatol* 1981;3:191–302.

51. Hart DM. Heartburn in pregnancy. *J Int Med Res* 1978;6(suppl):1–5.

52. Marrero JM, Goggin PM, de Caestecker JS, Pearce JM, Maxwell JD. Determinants of pregnancy heartburn. *Br J Obstet Gynaecol* 1992;99:731–734.

53. Mixson WJ, Woloshin HJ. Hiatus hernia in pregnancy. *Obstet Gynecol* 1956;8:249–260.

54. Castro L de P. Reflux esophagitis as the cause of heartburn in pregnancy. *Am J Obstet Gynecol* 1967;98:1–10.

55. Vanner RG, Goodman NW. Gastro-oesophageal reflux in pregnancy at term and after delivery. *Anaesthesia* 1989;44:808–811.

56. Spence AA, Moir DD, Finlay WEI. Observations on intragastric pressure. *Anaesthesia* 1967;22:249–256.

57. Lind JF, Smith A, McIver DR, Coopland AT, Crispin JS. Heartburn in pregnancy: A manometric study. *Can Med Assoc J* 1968;98:571–574.

58. Brock-Utne JG, Downing JW, Dimopoulos GE, Rubin J, Moshal MG. Effect of domperidone on lower esophageal sphincter tone in late pregnancy. *Anesthesiology* 1980;52:321–323.

59. Brock-Utne JG, Rubin J, Downing JW, et al. The administration of metoclopramide with atropine. *Anaesthesia* 1976;31:1186–1190.

60. Brock-Utne JG, Rubin J, Welman S, et al. The action of commonly used antiemetics on the lower oesophageal sphincter. *Br J Anaesth* 1978;50:295–298.

61. Brock-Utne JG, Rubin J, Welman S, et al. The effect of glycopyrrolate (Robinul) on the lower oesophageal sphincter. *Can Anaesth Soc J* 1978;25:144–146.

62. Hall AW, Moossa AR, Clark J, Cooley GR, Skinner DB. The effects of premedication drugs on the lower oesophageal high pressure zone and reflux status of rhesus monkeys and man. *Gut* 1975;16:347–352.

63. Hey UMF, Ostick DG, Mazumder JK, Lord WD. Pethidine, metoclopramide and the gastro-esophageal sphincter: A study in healthy volunteers. *Anaesthesia* 1981;36:173–176.

64. Cotton BR, Smith G. Comparison of the effects of atropine and glycopyrrolate on the lower oesophageal sphincter pressure. *Br J Anaesth* 1981;53:875–879.

65. McNeill MJ, Ho ET, Kenny GNC. Effect of IV metoclopramide on gastric emptying after opioid premedication. *Br J Anaesth* 1990;64:450–452.

66. Brock-Utne JG, Dow TGB, Welman S, Dimopoulos GE, Moshal MG. The effect of metoclopramide on lower oesophageal sphincter tone. *Anaesth Intensive Care* 1978;6:26–29.

67. Murray FA, Erskine JP, Fielding J. Gastric secretion in pregnancy. *J Obstet Gynaecol Br Commonw* 1957;64:373.

68. Taylor G, Pryse-Davies J. The prophylactic use of antacids in the prevention of the acid-pulmonary aspiration syndrome (Mendelson's syndrome). *Lancet* 1966;1:288–291.

69. Attia RR, Ebeid AM, Fischer JE, Goudsouzian NG. Maternal, fetal and placental gastrin concentrations. *Anaesthesia* 1982;37:18–21.

70. Teabeaut JR. Aspiration of gastric contents: An experimental study. *Am J Pathol* 1952;28:51–67.

71. Roberts RB, Shirley MA. Reducing the risk of acid aspiration during cesarean section. *Anesth Analg* 1974;53:859–868.

72. Roberts RB, Shirley MA. The obstetrician's role in reducing the risk of aspiration pneumonia with particular reference to the use of oral antacids. *Am J Obstet Gynecol* 1976;124:611–617.

73. Raidoo DM, Rocke DA, Brock-Utne JG, Marszalek A, Engelbrecht HE. Critical volume for pulmonary acid aspiration: Reappraisal in a primate model. *Br J Anaesth* 1990;65:248–250.

74. James CF, Modell JH, Gibbs CP, Kuck EJ, Ruiz BC. Pulmonary aspiration: Effects of volume and pH in the rat. *Anesth Analg* 1984;63:665–668.

75. Awe WC, Fletcher WS, Jacob SW. The pathophysiology of aspiration pneumonitis. *Surgery* 1966;60:232–239.

76. Bynum LJ, Pierce AK. Pulmonary aspiration of gastric contents. *Am Rev Respir Dis* 1976;114:1129–1136.

77. Hamelberg W, Bosomworth PP. Aspiration pneumonitis: Experimental studies and clinical observations. *Anesth Analg* 1964;43:669–677.

78. Booth DJ, Zuidema GD, Cameron JL. Aspiration pneumonia: Pulmonary arteriography after experimental aspiration. *J Surg Res* 1972;12:48–52.

79. Cameron JL, Sebor J, Anderson RP, Zuidema GD. Aspiration pneumonia: Results of treatment by positive-pressure ventilation in dogs. *J Surg Res* 1968;8:447–457.

80. Hickling KG, Howard R. A retrospective survey of treatment and mortality in aspiration pneumonia. *Intensive Care Med* 1988;14:617–622.

81. Bosomworth PP, Hamelberg W. Etiologic and therapeutic aspects of aspiration pneumonitis: Experimental study. *Surg Forum* 1962;13:158–159.

82. Lewis RT, Burgess JH, Hampson LG. Cardiorespiratory studies in critical illness: Changes in aspiration pneumonitis. *Arch Surg* 1971;103:335–340.

83. Morgan JG. Pathophysiology of gastric aspiration. *Int Anesthesiol Clin* 1977;15:1–11.

84. Kennedy TP, Johnson KJ, Kunkel RG, et al. Acute acid aspiration lung injury in the rat: Biphasic pathogenesis. *Anesth Analg* 1989;69:87–92.

85. Knight PR, Druskovich G, Tait AR, Johnson KJ. The role of neutrophils, oxidants and proteases in the pathogenesis of acid pulmonary injury. *Anesthesiology* 1992;77:772–778.

86. Goldman G, Wellborn R, Kobizek L, et al. Tumor necrosis factor-alpha mediates acid-aspiration induced systemic organ injury. *Ann Surg* 1990;212:513–519.

87. Davidson BA, Knight PR, Helinski JD, et al. The role of tumor necrosis factor-alpha in the pathogenesis of aspiration pneumonitis in rats. *Anethesiology* 1999;91:486–490.

88. Modell JH. Aspiration pneumonia. In: American Society of Anesthesiologists Annual Refresher Course Lectures. Philadelphia: Lippincott; 1983:163–170.

89. Greenfield LJ, Singleton RP, McCaffree DR, Coalson JJ. Pulmonary effects of experimental graded aspiration of hydrochloric acid. *Ann Surg* 1969;170:74–86.

90. Moran TJ. Experimental aspiration pneumonia. IV. Inflammatory and reparative changes produced by intratracheal injection of autologous gastric juice and hydrochloric acid. *Arch Pathol* 1955;60:122–129.

91. Churg A. Aspiration of gastric contents. *Anesthesiology* 1979;51:2–3.

92. Wynn JW, Reynolds JC, Hood DI, Auerbach D, Ondrasick J. Steroid therapy for pneumonitis induced in rabbits by aspiration of food stuff. *Anesthesiology* 1979;51:11–19.

93. Taylor G. Acid pulmonary aspiration syndrome after antacids: A case report. *Br J Anaesth* 1975;47:615–617.

94. Bond VR, Stoelting RK, Gupta CD. Pulmonary aspiration syndrome after inhalation of gastric contents containing antacids. *Anesthesiology* 1979;51:452–453.

95. Gibbs CP, Schwartz DJ, Wynne JW, Hood CI, Ruck EJ. Antacid pulmonary aspiration in the dog. *Anesthesiology* 1979;51:380–385.

96. Eyler SW, Cullen BF, Welch WD, Murphy M. Antacid aspiration in rabbits. *Anesth Analg* 1982;61:183–184.

97. Tompkinson J, Turnbull A, Robson G, et al. Report on Confidential Enquiries into Maternal Deaths in England and Wales, 1973–1975. London, England: HMSO; 1979.

98. Heaney GAH, Jones HD. Aspiration syndromes in pregnancy. *Br J Anaesth* 1979;51:266–267.

99. Whittington RM, Robinson JS, Thompson JM. Fatal aspiration (Mendelson's syndrome) despite antacids and cricoid pressure. *Lancet* 1979;2:228–230.

100. Bernard GR, Luce JM, Sprung CL, et al. High dose corticosteroids in patients with the adult respiratory distress syndrome. *N Engl J Med* 1987;317:1565–1570.

101. The Veterans Administration Systemic Sepsis Cooperative Study Group. Effect of high dose glucocorticoid therapy on mortality in patients with clinical signs of sepsis. *N Engl J Med* 1987;317:659–665.

102. Murray HW. Antimicrobial therapy in pulmonary aspiration. *Am J Med* 1979;66:188–190.

103. Nader N, Knight PR, Bobela I, et al. High dose nitric oxide inhalation increases lung injury after gastric aspiration. *Anesthesiology* 1999;91:741–749.

104. Andersen N. Changes in intragastric pressure following administration of suxamethonium: Preliminary report. *Br J Anaesth* 1962;34:363–367.

105. Miller RD, Way WL. Inhibition of succinylcholine-induced increased intragastric pressure by nondepolarizing muscle relaxants and lidocaine. *Anesthesiology* 1971;34:185–188.

106. Muravchick S, Burkett L, Gold MI. Succinylcholine-induced fasciculations and intragastric pressure during induction of anesthesia. *Anesthesiology* 1981;55:180–183.

107. Marx GF, Bassell GM. In defense of the use of d-tubocurarine prior to succinylcholine in obstetrics. *Anesthesiology* 1983;59:157.

108. Sellick BA. Cricoid pressure to control regurgitation of stomach contents during induction of anaesthesia. *Lancet* 1961;2:404–406.

109. Fanning GL. The efficacy of cricoid pressure in regurgitation of gastric contents. *Anesthesiology* 1970;32:553–555.

110. Allman KG. The effect of cricoid pressure application on airway patency. *J Clin Anesth* 1995;7:197–199.

111. Cook TM. Cricoid pressure: Are two hands better than one? *Anaesthesia* 1996;51:365–368.

112. Herman NL, Carter B, Van Decar TK. Cricoid pressure: Teaching the recommended level. *Anesth Analg* 1996;83:859–863.

113. Chassard D, Tournadre JP, Berrada KR, Bouletreau P. Cricoid pressure decreases lower oesophageal sphincter tone in anaesthetized pigs. *Can J Anaesth* 1996;43:414–417.

114. Gibbs CP, Rolbin SH, Norman P. Cause and prevention of maternal aspiration. *Anesthesiology* 1984;61:111–112.

115. Rubin GL, Peterson HB, Rochat RW, McCarthy BJ, Terry JS. Maternal death after cesarean section in Georgia. *Am J Obstet Gynecol* 1981;139:681–685.

116. Scott DB. Mendelson's syndrome. *Br J Anaesth* 1978;50:977–978.

117. Hawthorne L, Wilson R, Lyons G, Dresner M. Failed intubation revisited: 17-yr experience in a teaching maternity unit [see comments]. *Br J Anaesth* 1996;76:680–684.

118. Lyons G, MacDonald R. Difficult intubation in obstetrics. *Anaesthesia* 1985;40:1016.

119. Rocke DA, Murray WB, Rout CC, Gouws E. Relative risk analysis of factors associated with difficult intubation in obstetric anesthesia. *Anesthesiology* 1992;77:67–73.

120. Samsoon GLT, Young JRB. Difficult intubation: A retrospective study. *Anaesthesia* 1987;42:487–490.

121. Gaiser RR, McGonigal ET, Litts P, Cheek TG, Gutsche BB. Obstetricians ability to assess the airway. *Obstet Gynecol* 1999;93:648–652.

122. Rowe TF. Acute gastric aspiration: Prevention and treatment. *Semin Perinatol* 1997;21:313–319.

123. Gataure PS, Hughes JA. The laryngeal mask airway in obstetrical anesthesia. *Can J Anaesth* 1995;42:30–33.

124. Brimacombe J, Berry A. LMA for failed intubation [correspondence]. *Can J Anaesth* 1993;40:802–803.

125. Brimacombe J. Cricoid pressure and the laryngeal mask airway. *Anaesthesia* 1991;46:986–987.

126. Ansermino JM, Blogg CE. Failed trachea intubation at caesarean section and the laryngeal mask. *Br J Anaesth* 1992;69:465–467.

127. Cyana AM, Macleod DM. The laryngeal mask: Cautionary tales [letter]. *Anaesthesia* 1990;45:167.

128. Campbell JR. The laryngeal mask: Cautionary tales [letter]. *Anaesthesia* 1990;45:167.

129. Criswell J, John R. The laryngeal mask: Cautionary tales [letter]. *Anaesthesia* 1990;45:167.

130. Griffen RM, Hatcher IS. Aspiration pneumonia and the laryngeal mask airway. *Anaesthesia* 1990;45:1039–1040.

131. Koehi N. Aspiration and the laryngeal mask airway. *Anaesthesia* 1991;46:419.

132. Tunstall ME, Sheick A. Failed intubation protocol: Oxygenation without aspiration. *Clin Anesthesiol* 1986;4:171–188.

133. Tunstall ME. Failed intubation drill. *Anaesthesia* 1976;31:850.

134. Norman B. Failed tracheal intubation [letter]. *Br J Anaesth* 1996;77:559.

135. Rosen M. Difficult and failed intubation in obstetrics. In: Latto IP, Rosen M, eds. *Difficulties in Tracheal Intubation*. London, England: Bailliere Tindall; 1985.

136. American Society of Anesthesiologists. Task Force on Management of the Difficult Airway: Practice guidelines for management of the difficult airway. *Anesthesiology* 1993;78:597–602.

137. Marx GF, Domurat MF, Costin M. Potential hazards of hypoglycaemia in the parturient. *Can J Anaesth* 1987;34:400–402.

138. Marx GF, Desai PK, Habib NS. Detection and differentiation of metabolic acidosis in parturients. *Anesth Analg* 1980;59:929–931.

139. Miller M, Wishart HY, Nimmo WS. Gastric acid at induction of anaesthesia: Is a 4-hour fast necessary? *Br J Anaesth* 1983;55:1185–1187.

140. Hutchinson A, Maltby JR, Reid CRG. Gastric fluid volume and pH in elective inpatients: Coffee or orange juice versus overnight fast. *Can J Anaesth* 1988;35:12–15.

141. McGrady EM, MacDonald AG. Effect of the preoperative administration of water on gastric volume and pH. *Br J Anaesth* 1988;60:803–805.

142. Sutherland AD, Maltby JR, Sale JP, Reid CRG. The effect of preoperative oral fluid and ranitidine on gastric fluid volume and pH. *Can J Anaesth* 1987;34:117–121.

143. Boyle RK. Mendelson syndrome in the labour ward. *Aust N Z J Obstet Gynaecol* 1997;37:76–79.

144. American Society of Anesthesiologists. Task Force on Obstetrical Anesthesia: Practice guidelines for obstetrical anesthesia. *Anesthesiology* 1999;90:600–611.

145. American Society of Anesthesiologists. Task Force on Preoperative Fasting: Practice guidelines for preoperative fasting and the use of pharmacologic agents to reduce the risks of pulmonary aspiration. Application to healthy patients undergoing elective procedures. *Anesthesiology* 1999;90:896–905.

146. American Academy of Pediatrics/American College of Obstetricians and Gynecologists. *Guidelines for Perinatal Care.* 4th ed. Washington, DC: American College of Obstetricians and Gynecologists; 1997.

147. Lahiri SK, Thomas TA, Hodgson RMH. Single-dose antacid therapy for the prevention of Mendelson's syndrome. *Br J Anaesth* 1973;45:1143–1146.

148. Gibbs CP, Spohr L, Schmidt D. The effectiveness of sodium citrate as an antacid. *Anesthesiology* 1982;57:44–46.

149. Dewan DM, Floyd HM, Thistlewood JM, Bogard TD, Spielman FJ. Sodium citrate pretreatment in elective cesarean section patients. *Anesth Analg* 1985;64:34–37.

150. O'Sullivan GM, Bullingham RE. Does twice the volume of antacid have twice the effect in pregnant women at term? *Anesth Analg* 1984;63:752–756.

151. Gibbs CP, Banner TC. Effectiveness of Bicitra as a preoperative antacid. *Anesthesiology* 1984;61:97–99.

152. Gillett GB, Watson JD, Langford RM. Prophylaxis against acid aspiration syndrome in obstetric practice. *Anesthesiology* 1984;60:525.

153. Holdsworth JD, Johnson K, Mascall G, Gwynne Roulston R, Tomlinson PA. Mixing of antacids with stomach contents. *Anaesthesia* 1980;35:641–650.

154. Faure EAM, Lim HS, Block BS, Tan PL, Roizen MF. Sodium bicarbonate buffers gastric acid during surgery in obstetric and gynecologic patients. *Anesthesiology* 1987;67:274–277.

155. Mathews HM, Moore J. Sodium bicarbonate as a single dose antacid in obstetric anaesthesia. *Anaesthesia* 1989;44:590–591.

156. Pickering BG, Palahniuk RJ, Cumming M. Cimetidine premedication in elective cesarean section. *Can Anaesth Soc J* 1980;27:33–35.

157. Hodgkinson R, Glassenberg R, Joyce TH III, et al. Comparison of cimetidine (Tagamet) with acidity before elective cesarean section. *Anesthesiology* 1983;59:86–90.

158. McAuley DM, Moore J, Dundee JW, McCaughey W. Oral ranitidine in labor. *Anaesthesia* 1984;39:433–438.

159. Manchikanti L, Marrero TC, Roush JR. Preanesthetic cimetidine and metoclopramide for acid aspiration prophylaxis in elective surgery. *Anesthesiology* 1984;61:48–54.

160. Manchikanti L, Colliver JA, Marrero TC, Roush JR. Ranitidine and metoclopramide for prophylaxis of aspiration pneumonitis in elective surgery. *Anesth Analg* 1984;63:903–910.

161. Rout CC, Rocke DA, Gouws E. Intravenous ranitidine reduces the risk of acid aspiration of gastric contents at emergency cesarean section. *Anesth Analg* 1993;76:156–161.

162. Camarri E, Chirone E, Fanteria G, Zocchi M. Ranitidine induced bradycardia. *Lancet* 1982;2:160.

163. Mangiameli A, Condorelli G, Dato A. Cardiovascular response to the acute intravenous administration of the H2 receptor antagonists ranitidine and cimetidine. *Curr Ther Res* 1984;36:13–17.

164. Feely J, Wilkinson GR, Wood AJJ. Reduction of liver blood flow and propranolol metabolism by cimetidine. *N Engl J Med* 1981;304:692–695.

165. Feely J, Guy E. Ranitidine also reduces liver blood flow. *Lancet* 1982;1:169.

166. Feely J, Wilkinson GR, McAllister CB, Wood AJ. Increased toxicity and reduced clearance of lidocaine by cimetidine. *Ann Intern Med* 1982;96:592–594.

167. Flynn RJ, Moore J, Collier PS, Howard PJ. Effect of intravenous cimetidine on lignocaine disposition during extradural caesarean section. *Anaesthesia* 1989;44:739–741.

168. Flynn RJ, Moore J, Collier PS, Howard PJ. Single dose oral H2-antagonists do not affect plasma lidocaine levels in the parturient. *Acta Anaesthesiol Scand* 1989;33:593–596.

169. O'Sullivan GM, Smith M, Morgan B, Brighouse D, Reynolds F. H2 antagonists and bupivacaine clearance. *Anaesthesia* 1988;43:93–95.

170. Dailey PA, Hughes SC, Rosen MA, et al. Effect of cimetidine and ranitidine on lidocaine concentrations during epidural anesthesia for cesarean section. *Anesthesiology* 1988;69:1013–1017.

171. Abe K, Shibata M, Demizu A, et al. Effect of oral famotidine on pH and volume of gastric contents. *Anesth Analg* 1989;68:541–544.

172. Pattichis K, Louca LL. Histamine, histamine H_2 receptor antagonists, gastric acid secretion and ulcers: An overview. *Drug Metab Drug Interact* 1995;12:1–36.

173. Howden CW, Tytgat GN. The tolerability and safety profile of famotidine. *Clin Ther* 1996;18:36–54.

174. Ohnishi K, Saitoh N, Nomura F, et al. Effect of famotidine on hepatic hemodynamics and peptic ulcer. *Am J Gastroenterol* 1987;82:415–418.

175. Chermos AN. Pharmacodynamics of famotidine in humans. *Am J Med* 1986;81(suppl):3–7.

176. Omote K, Namiki A, Sumita S, et al. Comparative studies on hemodynamic effects of intravenous cimetidine, ranitidine and famotidine in intensive care unit patients. *Jpn J Anesthesiol* 1987;36:940–947.

177. Miyata K, Fujiwara A. Effect of famotidine on cardiovascular system and bronchoresistance in anesthetized dogs. *Clin Reports* 1987;21:221–230.

178. Mihaly GW, Marino AT, Webster LK, et al. High dose antacid (Mylanta II) reduces the bioavailability of ranitidine. *Br Med J* 1982;285:998–999.

179. Turner DR, Kao YJ, Bivona C. Neuromuscular block by suxamethonium following treatment with histamine type 2 antagonists or metoclopramide. *Br J Anaesth* 1989;63:348–350.

180. Kambam JR, Franks JJ. Cimetidine does not affect plasma cholinesterase activity. *Anesth Analg* 1988;67:69–70.

181. Hawkins JL, Adenwala J, Camp C, Joyce TH III. The effect of H2-receptor antagonist premedication on the duration of vecuronium-induced neuromuscular blockade in postpartum patients. *Anesthesiology* 1989;71:175–177.

182. McCarthy G, Mirakhur RK, Elliott P, Wright J. Effect of H2-receptor antagonist pretreatment on vecuronium and atracurium induced neuromuscular block. *Br J Anaesth* 1991;66:713–715.

183. Blum RA, Shi H, Karol MD, Greski-Rose PA, Hunt RH. The comparative effects of lansoprazole, omeprazole, and ranitidine in suppressing gastric acid secretion. *Clin Ther* 1997;19:1013–1023.

184. Rocke DA, Rout CC, Gouws E. Intravenous administration of the proton pump inhibitor omeprazole reduces the risk of acid aspiration at emergency cesarean section. *Anesth Analg* 1994;78:1093–1098.

185. Rocke DA, Rout DA. Response to letter. *Anesth Analg* 1995;80:848–849.

186. Noble DW, Bannister J, Lamont M, Andersson T, Scott DB. The effect of oral omeprazole on the disposition of lignocaine. *Anaesthesia* 1994;49:497–500.

187. McAllister JD, Moote CA, Sharpe MD, Manninen PH. Random double-blind comparison of nizatidine, famotidine, ranitidine and placebo. *Can J Anaesth* 1990;37(suppl):S22.

188. Atanasoff PG, Brull SJ, Weiss BM, et al. The time course of gastric pH changes induced by omeprazole and ranitidine: A 24-hour dose response study. *Anesth Analg* 1995;80:975–979.

189. Hett DA, Scott RC, Risdall JE. Lansoprazole in the prophylaxis of acid aspiration during elective surgery. *Br J Anaesth* 1995;74:614–615.

190. Laws HL, Palmer MD, Donald JM Jr, et al. Effects of preoperative medications on gastric pH, volume and flora. *Ann Surg* 1986;203:614–619.

191. Gorback MS. Preoperative H2-receptor antagonists. *Anesth Analg* 1990;71:205–206.

192. Chestnut DH, Vandewalker GE, Owen CL, Bates JN, Choi WW. Administration of metoclopramide for prevention of nausea and vomiting during epidural anesthesia for elective cesarean section. *Anesthesiology* 1987;66:563–566.

193. Murphy DF, Nally B, Gardiner J, Unwin A. Effect of metoclopramide on gastric emptying before elective and emergency caesarean section. *Br J Anaesth* 1984;56:1113–1116.

194. Bylsma-Howell M, McMorland GH, Rurak DW, et al. Placental transport of metoclopramide: Assessment of maternal and neonatal side effects. *Can Anaesth Soc J* 1983;30:487–492.

195. Eisenach JC, Dewan DM. Metoclopramide exaggerates stress-induced tachycardia in pregnant sheep. *Anesth Analg* 1996;82:607–611.

196. Brock-Utne JG, Rout C, Moodley J, Mayat N. Influence of preoperative gastric aspiration on the volume and pH of gastric contents in obstetric patients undergoing cesarean section. *Br J Anaesth* 1989;62:397–401.

197. Moir D. Cimetidine, antacids and pulmonary aspiration. *Anesthesiology* 1983;59:81–83.

198. Stuart JC, Kan AF, Rowbottom SJ, Yau G, Gin T. Acid aspiration prophylaxis for emergency cesarean section. *Anaesthesia* 1996;51:415–421.

199. Maltby JR, Elliott RH, Warnell I, et al. Gastric fluid volume and pH in elective surgical patients: Triple prophylaxis is not superior to ranitidine alone. *Can J Anaesth* 1990;37:650–655.

200. Mathews HML, Wilson CM, Thompson EM, Moore J. Combination treatment with ranitidine and sodium bicarbonate prior to obstetric anesthesia. *Anaesthesia* 1986;41:1202–1206.

201. Tordoff SG, Sweeney BP. Acid aspiration prophylaxis in 288 obstetric anaesthetic departments in the United Kingdom. *Anaesthesia* 1990;45:776–780.

202. Greiff JMC, Tordoff SG, Griffiths R, May AE. Acid aspiration prophylaxis in 202 obstetric anaesthetic units in the UK. *Int J Obstet Anesth* 1994;3:137–142.

203. Burgess RW, Crowhurst JA. Acid aspiration prophylaxis in Australian obstetric hospitals: A survey. *Anaesth Intensive Care* 1989;17:492–495.

204. Plumer MH, Rottman R. How anesthesiologists practice obstetric anesthesia [Responses of practicing obstetric anesthesiologists at the 1993 meeting of the Society for Obstetric Anesthesia and Perinatology]. *Reg Anesth* 1996;21:49–60.

205. Benhamou D. French obstetric anaesthetists and acid aspiration prophylaxis. *Eur J Anaesthesiol* 1993;10:27–32.

206. Helbo-Hansen HS, Bang U. Current Danish practice for aspiration prophylaxis in obstetric anesthesia: A survey. *Int J Obstet Anesth* 1993;2:233–235.

207. Christensen V, Skovsted P. Effects of general anaesthetics on pH of gastric contents of man during surgery: A survey of halothane, fluroxene and cyclopropane anesthesia. *Acta Anaesthesiol Scand* 1975;19:49–74.

208. Mackenzie AI. Laryngeal oedema complicating obstetric anaesthesia [letter]. *Anaesthesia* 1978;33:271–277.

209. Peterson HB, Destefano F, Greenspan JR, Ory HW. Mortality risk associated with tubal sterilization in United States hospitals. *Am J Obstet Gynecol* 1982;143:125–129.

210. Viscomi CM, Rathmell JP. Labor epidural catheter reactivation or spinal anesthesia for delayed postpartum tubal ligation: A cost comparison. *J Clin Anesth* 1995;7:380–383.

211. Goodman EJ, Dumas SD. The rate of successful reactivation of labor epidural catheters for postpartum tubal ligation surgery. *Reg Anesth* 1998;23:258–261.

212. Abouleish EI. Postpartum tubal ligation requires more bupivacaine for spinal anesthesia than does cesarean section. *Anesth Analg* 1986;65:897–900.

213. Bucklin B, Smith CV. Postpartum tubal ligation: Safety, timing, and other implications for anesthesia. *Anesth Analg* 1999;89:1269–1274.

214. Thomas TA. Maternal mortality. *Int J Obstet Anaesth* 1994;3:125–126.

215. Robinson APC, Lyons G. Morbidity and mortality from obstetric anesthesia in the 1990s. *Curr Opin Anaesthesiol* 1999;12:277–281.

216. Willatts S. Anaesthetic lessons to be learnt from confidential inquiries into maternal death. *Acta Anaesthesiol Scand* 1997;110:25–26.

217. Tsen LC, Pitner R, Camann WR. General anesthesia for cesarean section at a tertiary care hospital 1990–1995: Indications and implications. *Int J Obstet Anesth* 1998;7:147–152.

218. Gaba DM. Improving anesthesiologists' performance by simulating reality [editorial]. *Anesthesiology* 1992;76:491–494.

219. Gawande A. When doctors make mistakes. *New Yorker.* 1999:40–55.

Shnider and Levinson's Anesthesia for Obstetrics,
edited by Samuel C. Hughes, et al.
Lippincott Williams & Wilkins,
Philadelphia, © 2001.

CHAPTER 23

NEUROLOGIC COMPLICATIONS OF REGIONAL ANESTHESIA FOR OBSTETRICS

PHILIP R. BROMAGE, M.B., B.S., F.R.C.A., F.R.C.P.C.

> Maintaining a certain controlled level of anxiety—or at least concern—is helpful for optimal performance whenever a person is working in what is called a "safety-sensitive job."
> Moore-Ede, "The Twenty-Four Hour Society"

For the past 160 years, maternal neurologic injury has been recognized as a rare hazard of childbirth. Initial accounts described lower motor neuron injuries related to cephalopelvic disproportion and pressure on nerves and nerve trunks crossing the pelvic brim (1). A century later, it became evident that disproportion and difficult labor could cause ischemic injury to the spinal cord itself, through pressure of the fetal head on spinal branches of the internal iliac artery ascending from the pelvis to supply the lower part of the spinal cord, as shown in Figure 23.1 (2–4).

Developments in magnetic resonance imaging (MRI) have brought about an extraordinary revolution in our understanding of central nervous system pathology in relation to daily anesthesia practice. The ability to view the entire nervous system and its integuments in three dimensions and several discriminatory modes, and to be able to distinguish pus from blood, or fresh blood from old blood, has opened new opportunities for rapid, precise diagnosis and timely treatment of neurologic emergencies. Previously arcane and apparently uncommon conditions such as syringomyelia and Arnold-Chiari malformations have become more frequently noticed and recognized as possible reasons to avoid epidural or subarachnoid anesthesia, or as causes of postpartum neurologic complications that may be amendable to appropriate surgical correction (5–9).

In the meantime, invasive anesthetic techniques of epidural and subarachnoid block, and combinations of the two, have become commonplace for obstetric pain relief, with each technique carrying remote but potentially catastrophic risks of trauma, ischemia of the spinal cord, and infection of the epidural and subarachnoid spaces surrounding it. Recently, a third, unrelated force has emerged to disturb the balance of anesthetic risk and safe practice. Rising hospital costs and financial expediency have driven hospital managers and medical staffs to policies of accelerated hospital discharge—within 24 to 48 hours of vaginal delivery and 48 to 72 hours after cesarean section—before sites of needle trauma in the spinal canal have healed, and within the incubation period for infectious complications such as meningitis or epidural abscess. Postanesthetic visits, formerly done at the bedside a day or two after delivery, have now become a remote formality, sometimes conducted by telephone, often several days after discharge from hospital, and by a nurse who may have had little neurologic training and no personal contact with the patient. This shift in anesthetic practice patterns away from personal, hands-on postanesthetic contact comes at a price: sooner or later, delayed diagnosis and treatment of rare instances of evolving spinal sepsis or other postanesthetic neurologic complications will slip unnoticed through the fragile safety net of remote, third-party communication to end in tragic

outcome, thus potentially undermining a century of very successful medical effort to combine humane childbirth with maximum safety to mother and child.

While the profession as a whole may be slow to confront this danger, the individual anesthesiologist must adapt appropriately and improve performance in two ways. First, one can improve performance technically by reexamining personal markers of neurologic outcome (such as an inappropriately high incidence of accidental dural puncture during epidural needle placement) and modifying one's technique accordingly (10, 11). Second, one can improve performance by heightening neurologic consciousness during performance of neuraxial blockade and by always envisioning in one's mind's eye the anatomic path taken by invading needles, catheters, and injected solutions within the spinal canal. This exercise is aided if one familiarizes oneself with MRI appearances of needle trauma to the spinal cord in axial and sagittal views, and with the characteristics of nonanesthetic pathology, such as viral myelitis, and intrinsic lesions, such as Arnold-Chiari malformations and associated or independent syringomyelia. These mental processes and broadened etiologic visions are helpful in developing a safe attitude of creative pessimism, sound medical judgment, and appropriate technical performance in one's daily work. Further, it is beneficial to develop a close working relationship with colleagues in the departments of radiology and neurology, where help must be sought urgently in the event of an anesthetic-related complication (12).

Provision of safe, painless childbirth by subarachnoid or epidural blockade is an exercise in controlled neurologic suppression. Therefore, it is appropriate that the obstetric anesthesiologist cultivate the role of an applied neurologist in the daily routine selection and administration of neuraxial blockade and in postanesthetic follow-up. The legal consequences of neglecting those follow-up skills and obligations will be discussed in Chapter 25.

Neurologic complications of regional anesthesia for childbirth are most conveniently considered in three etiologic categories: (a) complications due primarily to intrinsic maternal factors associated with childbirth, or some coincidental pathology unrelated to childbirth or the anesthetic; (b) complications due entirely to extrinsic anesthetic factors; and (c) combinations of intrinsic nonanesthetic maternal factors and extrinsic anesthetic causes. Constant awareness of their potential existence performs three defensive safety functions in obstetric anesthesia practice:

1. As a stimulus to efficient neurologic insight in preanesthetic evaluation of all obstetric patients and in their postpartum follow-up.
2. As an aid to avoid ill-advised embroilment in any preexisting neurologic pathology when alternative means of analgesia or anesthesia may be more appropriate than neuraxial blockade.

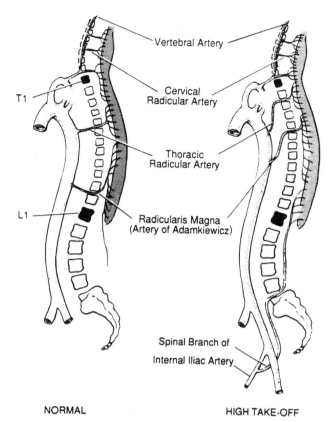

Figure 23.1. Diagram showing blood supply of the spinal cord. In about 85% of cases, the radicularis magna originates between T9 and L2, and provides the major blood supply to the thoracolumbar region. In about 15% of cases, the radicularis magna originates at about T5 (high takeoff), and the lower thoracolumbar region is supplied by a branch of the internal iliac artery entering by way of the intervertebral foramen between L5 and the sacrum. (Modified from Bromage PR, ed. Anatomy. In: *Epidural Analgesia.* Philadelphia: WB Saunders; 1978:52; Lazorthes G, Poulhes J, Bastide G, Chancolle AR, Zadel O. La vascularisation de la moelle épinière [étude anatomique et physiologique]. *Rev Neurol* 1962;106:535; and Lazorthes G, Gouaze A, Bastide G, Soutoul J-H, Zadeh O, Santini J-J. La vascularisation artérielle du renflement lombaire. Etude des variations et des suppléances. *Rev Neurol* 1966;114:109.)

3. As a stimulus to practice rigorous infection control and gentle, atraumatic, technical precision when administering regional anesthesia to obstetric patients.

The true incidence of postpartum maternal palsy is difficult to estimate, and it is even more difficult to separate intrinsic maternal causes of neurologic injury from nonmaternal, anesthetic-related factors. Large sample retrospective surveys of maternal obstetric injury gathered from multiple centers are subject to gross underestimation due to widely differing recording practices (13). Single-center studies are likely to be rewarding. At one university center, an 8-year sample of 23,827 deliveries between 1975 and 1983 uncovered almost identical incidences of neurologic defects after epidural (1:276) and general (1:289) anesthesia. In all of these cases, normal neurologic function returned within 72 hours, suggesting that the temporary injuries in both groups were caused by obstetric factors unrelated to anesthesia (14). Several large surveys of neurologic complications in obstetric epidural anesthesia are summarized in Table 23.1.

More recently, a prospective, multidisciplinary, in-hospital and postdischarge community audit of 48,066 deliveries in a single administrative district of Britain during 1991–92 revealed a total of 19 prolonged neurologic complications associated with pregnancy and delivery (a ratio of 1:2530 births). However, only one neurologic sequela attributable to anesthesia (a prolonged nerve root paresthesia) occurred in a subgroup of 13,007 mothers who received epidural anesthesia, and no sequelae arose in a smaller subgroup of 629 mothers who received subarachnoid anesthesia (a combined ratio of 1:13,636) (15). These remarkably reassuring data from Europe should not be taken as a signal to relax any aspect of preventive neurologic caution in current North American obstetric practice, where comparable methods of audit have not been applied and where a mix of published and unpublished case reports suggests areas of opportunity to improve current standards of outcome data collection and related anesthetic and administrative practices (12).

Cases that fall into the category of preexisting maternal pathology are uncommon, but awareness of their potential existence is important in order to avoid injudicious choice of regional anesthetic techniques that may mask the onset of an intrinsic neurologic complication and involve the anesthesiologist in subsequent litigation. Some conditions relevant to regional anesthesia have been well recognized for many years, while others have become apparent only within the past decade, since the remarkable diagnostic acuity of MRI technology has become widely available. Most of these preexisting conditions are uncommon. However, mild presenting symptoms or signs may exist prenatally to warn of potential trouble; the anesthesiologist should be alert to look for occult evidence that may be uncovered by a brief but efficient preanesthetic history and physical examination of the back and lower limbs. Preanesthetic screening formalities carried out by trained nursing assistants may augment, but cannot replace, the rapid hands-on physical examination by the responsible anesthesiologist of record.

INTRINSIC MATERNAL OBSTETRIC PALSY

Intrinsic causes of postpartum neurologic complications fall into the following categories that may exist singly or, very rarely, in combination. These must be a background against which the risks of neuraxial blockade should be weighed before one embarks on spinal or epidural anesthesia for vaginal or cesarean delivery:

1. Mechanical pressure of the fetal head on lumbosacral nerves descending across the pelvic brim (Fig. 23.2). The diagram illustrated in Figure 23.3 distinguishes central from peripheral nerve injury.
2. Pressure on nutrient arteries to the lower spinal cord ascending from iliac vessels within the pelvis.
3. Preexisting anomalies of the spinal canal and its vasculature.
4. Preexisting infections, or neoplasia affecting the central nervous system.

Pressure of Fetal Head on Nerve Structures or Spinal Nutrient Arteries in the Pelvis

Neural Structures

Although not commonly or routinely performed, some anesthesiologists suggest that during the routine preanesthetic visit a rapid check be done to exclude signs of preexisting neural compression injury. This suggested examination would include bilateral knee, ankle, and Babinski reflexes; ability to dorsiflex the ankle; and a check for hypalgesia over the anterior and posterior thigh and lateral calf. While this examination can be done in less than 3 to 4 minutes, it is not currently a routine practice.

Spinal Nutrient Arteries

In the early 1960s, the etiologic spectrum of maternal birth palsy was suddenly widened by the studies of Lazorthes et al. on the arterial supply to the spinal cord (2, 3). They demonstrated a dual supply to the conus medullaris, with the primary source coming

Table 23.1. SURVEY REPORTS OF NEUROLOGIC COMPLICATIONS IN OBSTETRIC EPIDURAL ANESTHESIA

Study	No. of Blocks	Neurologic Sequelae	Incidence
Kandel, 1966	1000	0	0
Crawford, 1972 (80)	1035	0	0
Holdcroft, 1976	1000	1 reversible neuropathy	10:10,000
Bleyaert, 1979	3000	0	0
Abouleish, 1981	1417	3 reversible neuropathies	21.2:10,000
Crawford, 1985 (171)	27000	2 neuropathies: 1 reversible, 1? recovery 1 epidural abscess: recovered 1 epidural hematoma: recovered 1 ? cauda equina syndrome: numbness and weakness of legs, bladder dysfunction; recovery 1 reversible VI cranial nerve palsy	2.2:10,000
Ong et al., 1987 (14)	9403	34 reversible neuropathies	36.2:10,000
Scott and Hibbard, 1990 (13)	505,000	38 neuropathies: only 1 permanent 1 permanent anterior spinal artery syndrome 1 epidural abscess: ? recovery 1 epidural hematoma: ? recovery 5 reversible cranial nerve palsy: III or VI 1 bilateral subdural cranial hematoma: recovered	0.9:10,000
Scott, 1995	108,133	38 reversible neuropathies	3.5:10,000
Holdcroft et al., 1995 (15)	13,007	1 reversible neuropathy	0.8:10,000
Paech, 1998	10,995	1 neuropathy: ? recovery	0.9:10,000

Reprinted by permission from Loo C, Dahlgren G, Irestedt L. Neurological complications in obstetric regional anaesthesia. *Int J Obstet Anesth* 2000;9:99–124.

from the long descending branch of the artery of Adamkiewicz (radicularis magna or arteria magna) and a secondary supply from the internal iliac arteries ascending via the iliolumbar and laterosacral arteries (Fig. 23.1). Lazorthes also showed that a reciprocal contribution is made by these two sources, depending on the vertebral level at which the artery of Adamkiewicz originates from the aorta. In approximately 85% of the population, this artery arises between T9 and L3 and supplies the bulk

of the conus medullaris, whereas the ascending contributions from the internal iliac arteries are relatively tenuous and probably expendable without causing permanent ischemic damage to the conus. In the remaining 15% of the population, the artery of Adamkiewicz has a high takeoff in the middle-to-upper thoracic region (average level: T5), and then the respective contributory roles of the two arterial supplies are reversed: a relatively slender supply descends from above, and a larger and relatively more

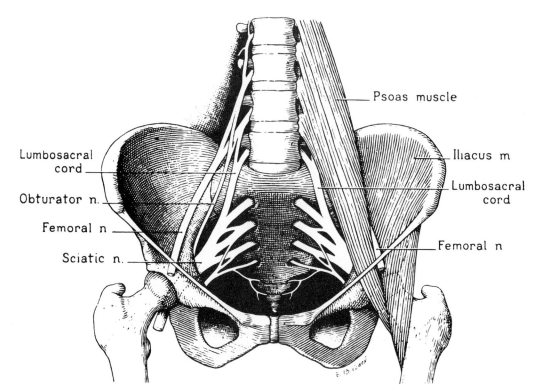

Figure 23.2. The relationship of the lumbosacral cord to the pelvis and the psoas major muscle. (Reprinted by permission from Cole JT. Maternal obstetric paralysis. *Am J Obstet Gynecol* 1946;52:374.)

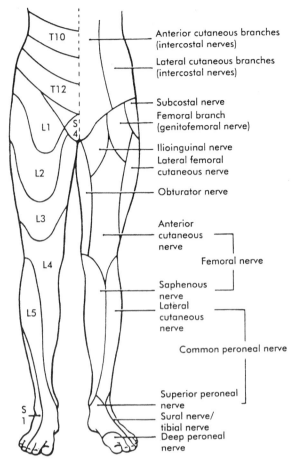

Figure 23.3. Anterior diagram of segmental (*left side*) and peripheral (*right side*) sensory nerve distributions useful in distinguishing central from peripheral nerve injury. (Reprinted by permission from Redick LF. Maternal perinatal nerve palsies. *Postgrad Obstet Gynecol* 1992;12:1–6.)

important component ascends from branches of the internal iliac artery that lie along the posterior wall of the pelvis and cross in front of the ala of the sacrum. It is in this 15% minority that the conus may be in danger of ischemic necrosis from prolonged compression by the fetal head, especially if any degree of disproportion exists and if labor is protracted and complicated by a difficult instrumental delivery.

More than a decade after these studies were published, in 1980 an interesting survey of maternal obstetric palsy from Nigeria corroborated the clinical implications of Lazorthes work to a remarkably precise degree. Bademosi et al. reviewed 34 cases of maternal palsy arising out of their obstetric population at the University of Ibadan in the 10-year period of 1966–76 (4). Of these 34 mothers, 29 recovered within 1 to 2 years. The remaining five mothers (i.e., 15%) did not recover and remained permanently paraplegic. Subsequent personal correspondence with the senior author revealed that none of the 34 patients had received subarachnoid or epidural anesthesia, thus eliminating the possibility that regional anesthesia might have contributed to the catastrophic outcome of the five permanently paralyzed patients.

The importance of these low takeoff spinal arteries as a rare mechanical cause of paralysis associated with epidural or subarachnoid anesthesia will be discussed later in the section "Direct Complications of Regional Anesthesia."

Maternal Congenital Anomalies of the Spine

Uncommon congenital abnormalities of the maternal spinal column must be kept in mind for two practical reasons. First, most of the anomalies occur in the lumbar region, where they increase the technical difficulties of subarachnoid or epidural puncture and where an associated low-lying spinal cord is at risk of accidental needle trauma. Second, associated anomalies of the underlying lumbar epidural vasculature, such as arteriovenous malformation (AVM), may include a collection of large, distended epidural veins that will bleed freely and give rise to an expanding epidural hematoma if lacerated by a spinal needle.

Spinal Dysraphism (Spina Bifida Occulta)

Incomplete closure of the distal neural crest is a common familial condition, ranging from a 17% incidence of spina bifida occulta without any other abnormality to rare cases of meningomyelocele in less that 0.1% of births (16). Between these extremes are infrequent cases of spina bifida occulta associated with a low-lying or tethered spinal cord extending below the normal termination at T12 to L1 vertebral level to as far as the L4 or L5 vertebra. Detectable cutaneous or subcutaneous stigmata such as local skin discoloration or a skin dimple, fat pad, or tuft of hair are usually present in such cases and should be sought as part of a routine preanesthetic examination of the back (17). The underlying lumbar epidural space is likely to be obliterated, and so a lumbar epidural block should not be attempted in these cases. Patients with a known history of spina bifida or signs of lumbar stigmata that may suggest a low-lying or tethered cord will also be at risk of lumbar subarachnoid puncture if the advancing needle cannot be halted instantly when cerebrospinal fluid (CSF) is encountered (18). In such cases, attempts to induce a subarachnoid block are ill advised. The "suck-and-see" technique (i.e., the loss-of-resistance to negative pressure test as described later in this chapter) may be used very cautiously and with firm manual control of the spinal needle to halt it as soon as the subarachnoid space is entered, just as if one were attempting to perform a cisternal puncture via the atlantooccipital approach (19).

Arteriovenous Malformations

Prior to 1980, AVMs of the spine were considered to be very rare and demonstrable only by the complicated and invasive technique of selective arteriography of the spinal cord. Now, in common with other congenital malformations of the central nervous system, they have become more frequently recognized and more reliably identified by their distinctive MRI signal on T2-weighting (20). Approximately 20% of spinal AVMs are accompanied by a cutaneous angioma in the same metameric distribution as a visible warning of their underlying presence (21). These intraspinal anomalies tend to become symptomatic in the latter part of pregnancy due to local vasodilation caused by a combination of hormonal changes, increased blood volume, and raised epidural venous pressure from partial occlusion of the inferior vena cava by the enlarged uterus (22, 23).

The neurologic risks of spinal AVMs in late pregnancy are determined largely by their simple relationships of tissue capillary flow to arterial pressure (P1), azygos venous pressure (P2), and local tissue pressure (P3), summarized in the equation:

$$\text{Tissue blood flow: } \alpha = \frac{\Delta P1 - P2}{P3}$$

All three of these pressures are critically important to spinal cord survival in the presence of a spinal AVM. Arterial pressure (P1) should be maintained near normal levels, while venous outflow pressure in the azygos system (P2) must be kept low by lateral posture to avoid inferior vena cava compression, and intraspinal pressure (P3) should not be raised by large-volume infusions of epidural medications (24).

For vaginal delivery, this author prefers to avoid regional anesthesia if the level of the AVM is such that a lumbar epidural or subarachnoid needle may traverse the lesion. Under these circumstances, a cesarean section under general anesthesia may be preferable. If the AVM is distant from the lumbar area, then careful induction of regional anesthesia with epidural block is acceptable and may allow a controlled vaginal delivery.

Similar determinants of tissue perfusion operate intracranially in late pregnancy and during delivery, when the risk of subarachnoid hemorrhage from intracranial vascular malformations is reported to increase 8-fold by the third trimester (25).

Because of these hemodynamic dangers, obstetric and anesthesia management must aim at preventing any bouts of sharply raised venous pressure from the expulsion efforts of natural labor. The choice of anesthesia in such cases is difficult and subject to much debate (see Chapter 29) (26).

Arnold-Chiari Syndrome

In normal subjects, the choice of subarachnoid or epidural anesthesia for cesarean section appears to be immaterial provided the procedures are performed skillfully and gently with appropriately sized needles chosen for each technique (9, 27). However, in patients with unrecognized Arnold-Chiari malformations, leakage of CSF through a spinal dural puncture wound as small as that produced by a 25-gauge needle may cause descent of the hindbrain into the foramen magnum, with resulting traction on the temporal meninges and severe, recurrent headaches (6a). In some cases, this form of "acquired" Chiari malformation may resolve spontaneously without serious harm, although a small, unilateral hygroma over one parietal region has been reported (28). In rare and more extreme cases, traction on the cranial meninges may lead to acute unilateral or bilateral subdural hematomas requiring urgent surgical decompression (27–33).

Until the advent of MRI, the concepts of postspinal puncture headache, the Arnold-Chiari syndrome, syringomyelia, and intracranial subdural hematoma seemed independent, unrelated entities in the context of complications arising from subarachnoid or epidural anesthesia. Now, those descriptive boundaries have become progressively blurred as technical advances in MRI have increasingly clarified the dynamic interrelationships between the base of the skull and its hindbrain contents. The practical anesthetic corollaries to this new, integrated knowledge have emerged as more technically demanding than commonly appreciated and may be summarized briefly:

1. The termination of spinal cord and its investing integuments may vary widely in vertebral level from T12 to L3 to 4. The textbook level of "T12 to L1" is only an approximation of the average. Therefore, firm manual control and rigid precision of needle advancement are mandatory safety measures that should conform to this range of anatomic uncertainty.
2. Varying degrees of lumbar dysraphism are common, and the underlying epidural space may be narrow and, in rare instances, even obliterated.
3. MRI evidence further indicates that subclinical degrees of Arnold-Chiari malformations at the base of the skull are more frequent than were thought, and should be considered (along with the rare secondary complication of intracranial subdural hematoma) in the differential diagnosis of all cases of postdural puncture headache (PDPH) and postspinal cranial nerve palsy.

DIRECT COMPLICATIONS OF REGIONAL ANESTHESIA

Walking Epidurals: Neuromuscular Coordination and Trauma

The benefit of pain-free, early ambulation after major surgical operations is well recognized. In thoracic and upper abdominal surgery, this is technically achievable by selective segmental blockade of the thoracic segments while the nerve supply to the legs is left unaffected (34). The beneficial effects of walking on uterine dynamics during the first stage of labor are controversial but less easily achieved, since the legs and the painful area of the lower abdomen and perineum share the same spinal segments. Consequently, the question arises: How can one maintain normal proprioception and neuromuscular control while providing effective segmental pain relief throughout active labor? The answer must lie in pharmacologic rather than anatomic separation of nociception and proprioception, which can be achieved to some degree through differential blockade within the dorsal horn of the spinal cord using appropriate epidural mixtures of very dilute local anesthetic agents, opioids, and α_2-adrenergic agonists. A number of obstetric epidural studies have examined these options with varying degrees of success (see Chapter 8 and 9) (35–41).

At present, attempts to achieve a reliable differential block tread a fine line. The balance between effective pain relief and stable, safe ambulation is not predictable. The risk of stumbling from lower limb incoordination with bodily injury demands very thorough neurologic assessment, patient's informed consent, and close attendance if ambulation after regional block techniques is to be permitted (40).

In this author's opinion it is prudent practice to insist that a separate and specific consent form be signed for ambulation after walking epidurals, and patients undertaking that exercise should be constantly observed to avoid an accidental injury.

Pressure Sores

Bedsores may seem an unlikely neurologic complication for young, healthy parturients, but decubitus ulcers can develop very rapidly in patients rendered insensitive and immobile by overenthusiastic postoperative epidural blockade, and are more prone to occur in diabetics with some degree of existing microangiopathy. A combination of sustained immobility, mild arterial hypotension, and intense sensory blockade has resulted in buttock or heel sores within 18 to 20 hours in healthy women of childbearing age (42, 43, 43a).

Uncomplicated cesarean sections usually do not cause sufficient postoperative pain to require very intense or prolonged postoperative epidural analgesia. Instead, subarachnoid morphine in a dose of 150 to 300 μg added to the spinal local anesthetic along with a modest dose of a short-acting opioid (e.g., sufentanil 5 to 10 μg or fentanyl 10–25 μg) is sufficient to provide excellent intraoperative analgesia and 18 to 24 hours of adequate postoperative analgesia (see Chapter 9). This is a simpler, less expensive, and more appropriate choice than adding continuous epidural management to a situation that does not usually call for greater analgesia.

Postpartum Backache

A survey of postpartum backache in a population of 11,701 deliveries from one hospital in Britain found that backache lasting for more than 6 weeks occurred in 10.5% of women delivered by natural childbirth. A similar incidence of backache occurred after delivery by elective cesarean section, regardless of whether general or epidural anesthesia was used (44). However, in those women who received epidural analgesia for labor and delivery or for cesarean section following a failed trial of labor, the incidence of prolonged backache rose to 18.9%. This highly significant difference was attributed to the combination of active labor and epidural anesthesia, and to the possibility of ligamentous damage arising from tolerance of potentially damaging postures and straining movements in the presence of segmental analgesia.

To appreciate the surprisingly powerful influence of epidural analgesia on the incidence of prolonged backache, it is important to understand the historic and pharmacologic implications of these data, which were gathered during an 8-year period commencing in 1978. At that time, many British anesthetists were still employing more concentrated solutions of local anesthetics for labor than were colleagues elsewhere. It was common for 0.375% or even 0.5% bupivacaine to be used throughout labor, although the 0.25% solution was more favored in North America and the 0.125% dilution was encouraged in Belgium (45).

Surgical concentrations of local anesthetics for epidural analgesia in labor cause an inappropriate degree of motor blockade in the affected parts, resulting in loss of tone in muscles of the pelvic floor once analgesia has spread downward to involve the sacral segments. Intense analgesia permits the mother to adopt and maintain postures that may place excessive strain on vertebral and sacroiliac joints, and that are likely to result in prolonged postpartum backache and disability. The current practice of multifaceted neuraxial analgesia with mixtures of dilute local anesthetics, opioids, and selective α_2-adrenergic agonists, such as clonidine, has avoided this specific problem by retaining effective motor power and coordination while providing adequate pain relief.

Two Canadian surveys of backache comparing nonepidural deliveries with epidural analgesia for labor and delivery in a population of 329 women found a slightly greater incidence of backache in the epidural group on the first postpartum day, but no significant difference 1 week later and 1 year later (10% in the epidural group vs. 14% in the nonepidural group) (46, 47).

Similarly, Breen et al. (48) surveyed 1042 women 1 to 2 months postpartum and found that the incidence of back pain was 44% in those who received epidural analgesia and 45% in those who did not. Through stepwise multiple logistic regression, postpartum back pain was found to be associated with a history of back pain, younger age, and greater weight. No statistically significant association was found between postpartum back pain and epidural anesthesia.

Chloroprocaine Backache

Temporary, severe backache lasting approximately 12 hours after epidural chloroprocaine led to a number of studies in patients and volunteers, which indicated that the backache was due to the added antioxidants, methylparaben, and EDTA and not to the chloroprocaine itself (49–53). The present formulation of chloroprocaine for epidural use contains neither methylparaben nor EDTA and appears to be free from the risk of drug-induced backache (see Chapter 5) (54).

Postdural Puncture Headache (PDPH)

In obstetric patients, the prevalence and intensity of PDPH are determined by four simple physical factors governing the volume of CSF lost through a puncture hole in the spinal meninges. The first factor is the size of the hole, determined by the caliber and design of the epidural or subarachnoid needle; 16- or 18-gauge epidural needles make the largest holes and cause the greatest CSF loss, while in vitro studies indicate that the pencil-point 27-gauge Whitacre needle or the 25-gauge Atraucan needle have the best combinations of technical reliability and low-volume CSF leak. Finer-caliber needles (29 gauge) are too unstable to be technically reliable in clinical practice (19, 55, 56). The second factor is the obliquity of the spinal needle track through the dura; an extreme 30-degree angle of insertion results in a partial overlap of the severed dural edges and creates a self-sealing track that tends to hold the dural puncture wound closed—a technique that can be demonstrated in vitro but is not easily accomplished in vivo (57). The third factor involves active labor and delivery, during which intense maternal expulsive efforts cause sharp increases of pressure in the epidural veins surrounding the dural sac, compressing the dura and forcing CSF through the dural puncture hole so that subarachnoid pressure falls (58). The fourth factor is the loss

Table 23.2. DIFFERENTIAL DIAGNOSIS OF POSTDURAL PUNCTURE HEADACHE

- Nonspecific
- Migraine
- Hypertension related
- Caffeine withdrawal
- Pneumocephalus
- Infection
- Cortical vein thrombosis
- Intracranial subarachnoid hemorrhage
- Increased intracranial pressure (e.g., mass lesions, pseudotumor cerebri)

of CSF, which allows the brain to sag downward within the skull, causing traction on the cranial meninges and symptoms of PDPH. Among the available regimens to treat PDPH, epidural blood patch has become established as the simplest and most reliable (59).

DIFFERENTIAL DIAGNOSIS OF POSTDURAL PUNCTURE HEADACHE

As in any therapeutic situation, diagnosis **must** precede treatment to avoid inappropriate, expensive, and potentially harmful mistakes. The postpartum patient may develop a nonspecific headache (e.g., tension headache), a migraine headache, or a headache related to hypertension or caffeine withdrawal. Evaluation of the postpartum patient with a headache should include an inquiry about headaches prior to delivery. In a study by Benhamou et al. (60), headaches were reported by 12% of postpartum patients who received epidural analgesia without dural puncture (n = 1058) and by 15% of 140 patients who delivered without epidural analgesia. Known dural puncture with loss-of-resistance techniques using air-filled syringes may cause a headache related to pneumocephalus with varying severity, but typically with an onset that is more temporally related to the dural puncture, which most often resolves after a few hours. However, the cardinal sign of PDPH due to low CSF pressure is unremitting, continuous cephalgia in the sitting or standing posture that is promptly relieved by recumbency. Absence of relief on lying down should signal the need to search for other, potentially more serious causes (see Table 23.2).

Infection

a. Meningitis: This headache often is accompanied by fever, leucocytosis, systemic signs of illness, and nuchal rigidity, and may cause lethargy and altered mental status. As contrary as it may seem for evaluation of a possible PDPH, performing a diagnostic lumbar puncture for definitive diagnosis is essential if meningitis is suspected.
b. Paranasal sinusitis: This usually follows an upper respiratory infection, with tenderness to pressure over the frontal, ethmoidal, or maxillary sinuses, possibly accompanied by a low fever and purulent nasal discharge.
c. Systemic viral infections: Tick fever or Epstein-Barr virus (infectious mononucleosis) may present as a severe headache before fever manifests, and may merit MRI investigation of the brain and spinal cord (61).

Cortical Vein Thrombosis

The estimated incidence of this rare condition ranges from 1:3000 to 1:6000 deliveries. Headache is throbbing and unrelieved by bed rest, with sweating, nausea, and occasionally focal seizures (62–65).

The incidence in the postpartum patient appears to be higher than in the general population. Diagnosis is made with one of several techniques to include computed tomography (CT),

MRI, or angiography. There is no clear treatment beyond symptomatic measures.

Intracranial Subarachnoid Hemorrhage

Subarachnoid hemorrhage from rupture of a cerebral aneurysm or AVM may occur at any time during the peripartum period. The severe headache, typically occipital, is usually associated with signs of meningeal irritation, alterations in level of consciousness, and focal neurologic signs. Prompt neurologic consultation and appropriate imaging studies are essential (see Chapter 29).

Intracranial Subdural Hematoma

The interrelationships between the Arnold-Chiari syndrome, syringomyelia, and intracranial subdural hematoma have been discussed earlier. They are mentioned again to emphasize the interrelationships that exist between CSF volume and normal hindbrain stability within the cranium in marginal, subclinical degrees of the Arnold-Chiari malformation. In such cases, active expulsive efforts during labor, unrestricted ambulation, and physical activity in the presence of a lumbar dural puncture wound may lead to downward sagging of the brainstem, and ultimately to the acute emergency of unilateral or bilateral subdural hematoma described earlier (28–33).

The clinical picture of "benign" PDPH and a potentially life-threatening subdural hematoma may be very similar, with occipital and upper cervical pain, nausea and vomiting, photophobia, and no localizing signs. The single clinical difference is the response to posture; in subdural hematoma, the headache is constant whether the patient is standing or lying down, while headache due to loss of CSF becomes less intense on recumbency. Unfortunately, this distinguishing sign is not absolute (65). A recent review noted eight cases of intracranial subdural hematoma after epidural anesthesia for parturients (65a). Rare cases of Chiari-I malformation, secondary to spontaneous spinal CSF leaks, will show precisely the same clinical features of symptomatic relief on recumbency, but patients will have a history of postural headache that existed **prior** to spinal puncture, and they may show thickening and edema of the cranial dura mater on T1-weighted MRI enhanced with intravenous gadolinium (66).

Acute subdural hematoma is associated with signs that may include headache, vomiting, somnolence, and mental status changes related to increased intracranial pressure (ICP). This can be a life-threatening emergency, calling for urgent confirmation by MRI of the skull followed by surgical decompression (trephination).

Increased Intracranial Pressure

Rare causes of headache in the postpartum period include mass lesions and pseudotumor cerebri, both of which may have significant symptomology related to increased ICP, including focal neurologic deficits, visual disturbances, seizures, and vomiting (see Chapter 29).

Risks of Developing Postdural Puncture Headache

During the informed consent process and discussion of the choice between subarachnoid and epidural block (or both), the patient may inquire about respective risks of PDPH with each technique. Two important variables are involved in formulating an answer to that question: first, the skill of the anesthesiologist performing the epidural puncture, and second, the caliber and design of the needle that creates the puncture wound, which will determine the rate of CSF loss from the spinal subarachnoid space.

Accidental dural puncture wounds with epidural needles of 16 to 18 gauge make the largest holes, with a 75% to 80% chance of PDPH that is sufficiently intense to require a blood patch (67). Published data from surveys of teaching institutions indicate that the frequency of accidental dural puncture during attempted epidural induction varies 15-fold, from 0.4% (68) to 6% (55), depending on technique and technical proficiency. Dural puncture wounds from these large-gauge epidural needles carry a 90% risk of PDPH, and 75% to 80% of those headaches are likely to be severe enough to require a therapeutic epidural blood patch (69). Therefore, anesthesia departments that experience a 6% accidental dural puncture rate must expect an associated blood patch rate of 4% to 5%, together with the expenses incurred in the process.

A much lower incidence and severity of PDPH is incurred by narrow-bore needles designed for subarachnoid anesthesia. Published rates of PDPH after spinal anesthesia vary from 5% to 6% with 26-gauge Quincke-tipped needles, to 1% to 2% with 25-gauge pencil-point Whitacre needles, and only 13% of these puncture wounds cause headaches severe enough to require a blood patch (67). Subarachnoid punctures with the 27-gauge Whitacre needle result in a much lower incidence (0.5%), severity, and duration of headache, which rarely requires a blood patch (70). There are several commercially produced pencil-point spinal needles with a similarly low incidence of PDPH.

These data suggest that in skilled hands and using the most appropriate needles, subarachnoid and epidural analgesia carry a degree of risk of PDPH and that both are approaching the same asymptote, with an irreducible incidence of PDPH of approximately 0.5% (Chapter 11, Table 11.8). However, in less-skilled hands, the choice of epidural analgesia with the larger 16- to 18-gauge needles may result in a 5% to 6% chance of accidental dural puncture (55). Under such circumstances, properly conducted subarachnoid anesthesia with a 27-gauge Whitacre needle or another pencil-point needle can produce equally good intraoperative and postoperative conditions and may be the better choice for cesarean section.

Treatment of Low-Pressure Postdural Puncture Headache

Because PDPH is brought on by standing or sitting and is relieved by recumbency, 24-hour bed rest once was enforced as a logical prophylactic measure after spinal anesthesia or accidental dural puncture. Enforced recumbency as an effective prophylactic measure was challenged as long ago as 1947. Cullen and Griffith studied the incidence of headache in 200 women after spinal anesthesia with a 22-gauge needle for delivery (71). The incidence (20%) and intensity of headache were precisely the same whether the mothers were allowed to adopt their position of choice or recumbency was strictly enforced. This observation went unnoticed until rediscovered in 1974, when the subject was again addressed in the same journal 27 years later (72). Since 1974, increasing evidence has accumulated that posture is not a factor influencing the incidence of headache, regardless of other variables such as needle size, age, and pregnancy (Fig. 23.4) (72–74).

One study using 25- and 26-gauge needles for subarachnoid anesthesia for vaginal delivery showed a 36% incidence of headache in patients kept at rest for 24 hours and a 22% incidence in those allowed out of bed after 6 hours (75). Contemporary obstetric practice favors adoption of the patient's position of choice, followed by early ambulation and a return to bed rest if headache arises, then active treatment with epidural blood patch if the headache persists.

Similarly, increased hydration has not been shown to increase the normal $0.35\ mL\cdot min^{-1}$ production of CSF, or prevent the development of PDPH or ameliorate its course once it develops. Therefore, the arcane dictum of bed rest and increased

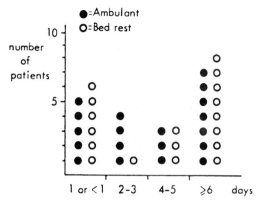

Figure 23.4. Spinal headache developed in 19 of 50 neurology patients following diagnostic lumbar puncture (18-gauge needle) who were allowed to ambulate at will immediately following the block. In a similar group of patients kept at bed rest for 24 hours, spinal headache developed in 18 of 50. Duration of the headache was also similar in both groups. (Reprinted by permission from Carbaat PAT, Van Crevel H. Lumbar puncture headache: Controlled study on the preventive effect of 24 hours' bed rest. *Lancet* 1981;2:1133–1135.)

hydration after known dural puncture is no longer routinely practiced. Therapies other than epidural blood patch have been tried, with variable success.

Methylxanthines

The theoretic support for using systemic caffeine is based on primate studies showing that acutely lowered CSF pressure causes venodilation (76). Caffeine redresses the balance by inducing cerebral vasoconstriction and reduction of cerebral blood flow in postdural puncture patients (77).

Oral caffeine, or theophylline 300 mg, is a simple, inexpensive palliative treatment reported to give symptomatic relief of PDPH, but insufficient relief to reduce the incidence of blood patch requirements (78, 79).

Epidural Saline Infusions

Epidural saline infusions to bolster the sagging spinal sack due to low CSF pressure have had a long but relatively unsuccessful history over the past 40 years. Following accidental dural puncture, an epidural catheter is left in place and 1 to 1.5 L isotonic Ringer's lactate or Hartmann's solution are infused over 24 hours. Relief is usually satisfactory for the first day, but continued infusion may give rise to severe interscapular pain, and headache often returns by the third or fourth day (80). Epidural saline infusions are seldom employed, except when epidural blood patch is contraindicated.

Epidural Dextran

A report of epidural dextran-40 in volumes of 20 to 30 mL claimed it relieved PDPH in 56 patients after other methods had failed. Relief occurred rather slowly—within 5 to 30 minutes in most patients, but up to 2 hours for others (81). Prophylactic epidural dextran injection has been reported to be highly efficacious (82). However, epidural dextran as an alternative to epidural blood patch has not found widespread acceptance or success.

Sumatriptan Succinate (Imitrex)

Sumatriptan, a serotonin-receptor agonist, is a potent vasoconstrictor that is effective in the treatment of migraine, and was reported to give relief in a series of six patients after deliberate spinal puncture with 20- or 22-gauge needles and accidental

puncture with large-bore epidural needles (83). Sumatriptan 6 mg was injected subcutaneously in all six patients. The drug is excreted in human breast milk and has been reported to cause coronary artery spasm in rare cases with preexisting coronary artery disease (84). Larger prospective studies are necessary before routine use of the drug can be recommended.

Adrenocorticotropic Hormone

Adrenocorticotropic hormone of 1.5 $U \cdot kg^{-1}$ by intravenous infusion is reported to produce relief of PDPH within 2 to 6 hours (85, 86). The mode of action is speculative but possibly due to retention of sodium and increased intravascular volume (87). Further investigation of this treatment is warranted, but routine use is not advocated at this time.

Epidural Blood Patch

Since its introduction by Gormley in 1960, autologous epidural blood patch has become recognized as the definitive treatment for PDPH (88). Three requirements are necessary for success. First, there should be a normal clotting profile. Second, the blood should be introduced close to or at the site of the puncture. Introduction of the blood one space below the dural rent ensures that the normal negative intrapleural pressure transmitted to the epidural space will draw the blood cephalad and spread it effectively over the hole. This has been demonstrated by MRI after epidural blood patch procedures (89, 90). Third, a sufficient volume of blood must be injected to accomplish two aims: to seal the hole, and to exert enough pressure around the dura to restore CSF pressure and relieve the headache immediately. The instant-relief characteristic of a successful blood patch seems to depend on the administration of rather generous volumes of autologous blood—in the range of 15 to 20 mL (91, 92). A recent review discusses several of the controversies related to this technique (92a).

Controversy still exists over the choice between delayed and prophylactic blood patch when a functioning epidural catheter is in place but a large dural hole is known to exist from an earlier accidental dural puncture. In obstetrics, the wait-and-see school of thought may anticipate a 35% to 85% chance of headache that will require active blood patch treatment sooner or later. The preventive school prefers to lessen the odds by injecting autologous blood through the catheter an hour or so after the epidural block has worn off and fluid has had an opportunity to resorb from the epidural space (93).

Evidence is accumulating that prophylactic epidural blood patching may have merit, with an incidence of post–blood-patch headache in the range of 10% to 21% (94–96). The technique is gaining in use, and according to a recent survey, it is performed in 25% of North American academic centers (55). The few patients who still suffer from headache after a prophylactic blood patch usually respond satisfactorily to a second blood patch.

However, like so many other interventions, prophylactic blood patch at the end of satisfactory epidural anesthesia is not without its own inherent complications. One case of immediate total spinal anesthesia has been reported following a 15-mL prophylactic epidural blood patch given at the conclusion of an operation in which the upper segmental level of analgesia did not rise above T4. Presumably, the compressive effects of the epidural blood on the outside of the dura forced local anesthetic-laden CSF up to medullary and midbrain levels (97).

Neurologic Safety of Epidural Blood Patch

Published accounts are reassuring. Despite a remarkable safety record, a blood patch is, in fact, an iatrogenic epidural hematoma, and, theoretically, excessive volumes of injected blood confined within the vertebral canal could impair spinal cord blood flow. However, in women of childbearing age, the intervertebral foramina are freely patent and elevated CSF pressures decline rapidly within 15 minutes of injection of a 15-mL blood patch (98). MRI monitoring of 18- to 20-mL blood patches confirms that blood passes outward through the intervertebral foramina, backward along the needle track into subcutaneous tissues, and inward through the dural puncture hole to form a thin layer within the dura (91, 99). This pattern of distribution carries the sinister possibility that a breach of aseptic technique during performance of an epidural blood patch may spread infection through the injected culture medium to create a combination of epidural and paraspinous abscess, as well as meningitis, a catastrophe that could end in paraplegia unless treated promptly and aggressively. To date, there are no published reports of such a serious complication, but the danger is always present, and aseptic precautions while performing an epidural blood patch should be correspondingly immaculate.

Epidural patch with fibrin glue has been suggested as an alternative to epidural blood patch. Fibrin glue is widely used in neurosurgery to obtain a watertight dural seal. At the present time, there are no reports of its use for the treatment of PDPH (100, 101).

Shivering

Shivering is an interesting and relatively harmless neurophysiologic accompaniment of labor in approximately 10% of normal deliveries. The incidence of this uncomfortable nuisance rises sharply to 20% to 70% in women receiving neuraxial blockade for labor or cesarean section, and is more common with subarachnoid than with epidural anesthesia because the shivering threshold is depressed and body core temperature falls faster and further by the rapid onset and greater intensity of subarachnoid blockade (102, 103). Some peripartum shivering-like tremor is nonthermoregulatory, and the etiology has been hypothesized to be multifactorial (104).

Bouts of shivering are suppressed and maternal comfort restored by epidural or subarachnoid administration of lipid-soluble opioids. Meperidine is the most effective in terms of relative dosage, and 25 mg epidural preservative-free meperidine is usually sufficient to abolish shivering within 15 minutes (105, 106), whereas larger doses of fentanyl (100 μg) (107) or sufentanil (50 μg) (108) are needed. It is postulated that this peculiar efficacy of meperidine may reside in its properties as both a μ- and a κ-receptor agonist within the spinal cord (106).

ENHANCED LOCAL ANESTHETIC ACTION IN PREGNANCY

Rostral Spread of Blockade

During pregnancy, rising levels of progesterone cause the entire nervous system, central and peripheral, to become more susceptible to general and local anesthetics (109, 110). Consequently, excessive rostral spread of subarachnoid and epidural blocks, accompanied by the appearance of *Horner's syndrome*, may be encountered even when the local anesthetic dosage has been reduced in proportion to the increased neural susceptibility of late pregnancy. The space-occupying effect of dilated epidural veins was formerly considered to be a major physical factor in this phenomenon of enhanced cephalad spread of spinal local anesthetics in late pregnancy. However, this factor is probably of minor importance compared with the hormonal effects of pregnancy that increase neural susceptibility to local anesthetics throughout the neuraxis.

Delayed rostral spread of segmental analgesia may be further exaggerated when a lipid- soluble opioid such as fentanyl or sufentanil is added to subarachnoid local anesthetics for cesarean section. Then, conservative doses of lidocaine (60 to 80 mg) or bupivacaine (10 to 11.25 mg) may show delayed

rostral spread as far as the second cervical dermatome (unpublished observations). The differential spinal block produced by such delayed rostral spread has some interesting features and accompanying dilemmas in clinical management. When hypalgesia to cold (ice cubes) reaches the chin, i.e., the second cervical dermatome, patients may complain of two symptoms that are likely to trigger hasty "crash" endotracheal intubation by trainees who are unfamiliar with the neuroanatomy and physiology of high segmental deafferentation. First, the patient may complain of a sensation of dyspnea: "I can't breathe, doctor." At this point, gentle application of a face mask and pneumotachometer will usually indicate that diaphragmatic motor power is intact and deep breaths of 600 to 1000 mL can be achieved, and that ventilatory support is not needed but verbal encouragement is required. Next, the patient may whisper, "I can't swallow." This indicates that segmental deafferentation has reached the upper cervical region, the neck strap muscles stabilizing the hyoid bone and innervated by the ansa hypoglossi (C1 to C3) are becoming deafferented, and the hyoid cannot be fixed securely enough to accomplish the first act of deglutition (elevation and fixation of the hyoid bone by contraction of the geniohyoid, mylohyoid, digastric, and stylohyoid muscles, accompanied by backward thrust of the tongue to direct a bolus of secretions into the posterior pharynx) (111).

At this point, and provided tidal volume is not impaired, the head should be turned to one side, again with appropriate verbal support, and mouth suction applied under a face mask delivering 100% oxygen, while the patient is reassured that all is well, that the situation is transient and under control, just as if she were having a tooth filled in a dental chair. With such routine and close monitoring by pulse oximetry and tidal volume, together with mouth suction as required, it is very rare indeed for this transient neuropharmacologic complication to require induction of general anesthesia and emergency endotracheal intubation.

Prolonged Neural Blockade

Unduly prolonged anesthetic blockade is a second corollary of the enhanced neural susceptibility of pregnancy. During the 2 decades from 1960 to1980, reports appeared of prolonged neural blockade lasting 10 to 48 hours after continuous epidural anesthesia for labor, all of which were followed by complete recovery (112–114). In each case, 0.5% concentrations of tetracaine or bupivacaine had been used, and those reports serve as a reminder of two important clinical considerations. First, the neuraxis of pregnant women is very susceptible to the action of local anesthetics, opioids, and other neuroactive agents, and dosage must always be modified accordingly. Second, prolonged, intense blockade is undesirable since it carries an inherent risk of masking any coincidental pathologic process, such as a simple nursing problem as a developing bedsore or an epidural hematoma, thereby delaying potentially urgent treatment to the point that recovery is jeopardized (115).

The Spinal Subdural Space

The subdural space is a potential space lying between the dura mater and the pia-arachnoid, extending from the skull to the caudal termination of the dural sac and outward within the dural root sleeves as they exit through the intervertebral foramina. Spinaloscopy in cadavers demonstrated that the subdural space is easily expansible by injected fluids (116). This potential space presents a navigational hazard en route to the epidural space lying outside the dura mater, or to the subarachnoid space lying inside the pia-arachnoid. Accidental injection into the subdural space creates a "sink" within which small volumes of hyperbaric spinal anesthetic agents may remain sequestered as osmotic irritants, or in which larger volumes of misplaced epidural solutions are able to spread rostrally, as a thin layer for many segments beyond their expected limit in the more capacious epidural space (117–120), and which may subsequently rupture into the subarachnoid space to create an extensive and potentially dangerous subarachnoid block (121).

Accidental entry into the subdural space is relatively uncommon during attempted epidural puncture, with an incidence of less that 0.8% (117), and is usually due to intermittent instead of continuous advance of the needle (122), or to ill-advised rotation of the epidural needle, when the arching needle point may scribe a cut in the dura, permitting direct access to the subdural space beyond (123–126). Accidental invasion of the subdural space occurs more often during attempted subarachnoid puncture, and past evidence from the radiologic literature serves to illustrate the nature and extent of accidental subdural distribution. When myelography was performed commonly, 4% to 13% of attempted myelograms were spoiled by accidental injection and sequestration of radiopaque dye in the spinal subdural space (127, 128). Dye could be seen outlining the subdural space of the cauda equina, and neurologic complications sometimes resulted from prolonged and close contact between the loculated dye and the neural elements of the cauda equina (129, 130).

Contemporary studies of subarachnoid anesthesia with hyperbaric spinal anesthetics also report a similar proportion of unsatisfactory block in which the extent of anesthesia fell significantly short of the intended segmental level (131), suggesting that the sequestration of small volumes of concentrated injectate in the subdural "sink" may be the common denominator of unsatisfactory results in both myelography and hyperbaric spinal anesthesia. Clinical data indicate that this may be so, since the complication of inadequate segmental spread is very unlikely to occur when the method of spinal needle insertion is modified to avoid the subdural space by routine use of the loss-of-resistance-to-negative-pressure test, or "suck-and-see" technique (19). The "suck-and-see" technique transmits a powerful vacuum of approximately minus 600 mm Hg to the advancing needle point, which clamps the arachnoid membrane onto the dura, thus collapsing the potential subdural space and ensuring instant appearance of CSF the moment the needle aperture enters the subarachnoid space. This powerful, unequivocal signal calls for immediate halt of the advancing needle, with confidence that the entire subarachnoid dose will reach its intended destination without any accidental losses en route. Moreover, immediate arrest of the needle's advance provides greater safety from trauma to the underlying cauda equina, or to the spinal cord when punctures are performed at vertebral levels above the termination of the cord.

Massive Subarachnoid Injection

In vitro studies show that uninjured human dura mater is tough and very resistant to penetration by epidural catheters (132). Catheter migration through the dura is extremely unlikely to occur in the absence of iatrogenic injury, usually by ill-advised rotation of the epidural needle, as described above (122–126). However, accidental transdural catheterization of the subarachnoid space and high segmental block has been reported following atraumatic epidural puncture without any apparent needle rotation (121).

Table 23.2 shows the distribution of diagnostic signs of dural puncture in one series of 3500 epidural blocks for labor, with a 0.6% incidence of unintentional dural taps, one third of which were not detected at the time of epidural induction (133). This possibility of occult subarachnoid catheterization emphasizes the need for close supervision, and for routine measurement and documentation of upper and lower segmental levels of analgesia during continuous epidural infusions to ensure that accidental subarachnoid spread of analgesia and accompanying arterial hypotension do not go unrecognized and untreated.

Toxic Intravenous Injection

Accidental intravascular injection of local anesthetic may occur from epidural injection sites commonly employed in obstetrics. During caudal block, needles passed into the sacral canal may pierce the thin cortical layer of a sacral vertebra and enter cancellous bone. From that point, in the marrow cavity, subsequent injections of a local anesthetic enter the circulation almost as rapidly as an accidental intravenous injection. Toxic reactions result very rapidly, and speed of onset is enhanced by the nature of the venous anatomy of the region (134). Spinal veins located mainly in the lateral parts of the vertebral canal drain into the vertebral venous plexus. This system serves as an essential bypass when the inferior vena cava is partially obstructed by the gravid uterus, and venous flow discharges via the azygos vein directly into the superior vena cava and the right atrium of the heart. Flow in the azygos system rises in direct proportion to the degree of caval obstruction, and this is greatest when the parturient is lying on her back with the gravid uterus compressing the inferior vena cava (2, 3). Under these circumstances, convulsions and cardiovascular depression may occur very rapidly from relatively small quantities of intravenous local anesthetic. Prevention of local anesthetic systemic reactions is discussed in Chapter 5 and includes careful aspiration of the epidural catheter prior to injection, the use of appropriate test doses, and injection of large doses in small increments (135–137).

Treatment of toxic convulsions from accidental intravenous injection of local anesthetic is along standard lines, i.e., turning the patient into the lateral posture to relieve caval obstruction and prevent inhalation of vomitus should be the first and most urgent maneuver, followed by oxygen hyperventilation and vasopressor therapy as indicated by clinical signs.

Recent anatomic studies have suggested another and potentially more catastrophic mechanism for massive accidental entry of injected epidural anesthetic into the general circulation. Cryomicrotome sections of the human lumbar vertebral canal reveal an important anatomic detail of the lacunae in the posterior surface of the lumbar vertebral bodies where the basivertebral vein exits to join the epidural venous plexus. The edges of these lacunae are sharp and roofed by a thin membrane contiguous with the posterior longitudinal ligament (138). It has been postulated that pressure from epidural injectates may invaginate this membrane over the sharp edges of the lacunae. Subsequent rupture at that point could allow local anesthetic to pour from the epidural space into the general circulation, causing an immediate toxic reaction (139). In the absence of some unrecognized pathology, such an outcome would be extremely unlikely in normal subjects, where an epidural bolus of 15 mL injected in 10 seconds will generate a brief peak pressure of only 15 to 20 cm H_2O, which dissipates rapidly within the next 10 seconds (140), an order of magnitude less than normal epidural pressures of 170 to 200 cm H_2O generated by strong coughing or bearing-down efforts (141). Injection of large volumes of local anesthetics should always be administered in divided doses; this will also decrease the likelihood of the problem.

CHRONIC NEUROLOGIC COMPLICATIONS
Iatrogenic Trauma

Due to a combination of anatomic variables, the spinal cord and its meningeal coverings are more vulnerable to needle trauma than is commonly reflected in the clinical performance of lumbar epidural or subarachnoid block. The surface anatomy of the spine and its bony landmarks are subject to normal variation in three respects. First, the notion that the cord ends at the level of the first lumbar interspace (L1 to L2) is merely an approximation to the mean of a range that extends from the upper border of T12 vertebral body to the L3 to L4 interspace. Second, the intercristal line (Tuffier's line), used as a landmark

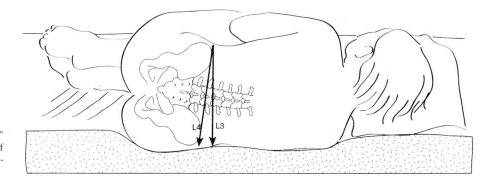

Figure 23.5. Cephalad shift of "apparent" intercristal line from lateral flexion of spine and lateral tilting of the broad female pelvic brim with lateral posture.

for the L4 to L5 interspace, may cross the midline half a segment higher at the spine of L4 (142). Third, the intercristal line may appear to be shifted even higher in patients lying in the lateral position due to lateral tilting of a broad female pelvis (see Fig. 23.5). Consequently, cephalad errors in the vertebral level of needle insertion are very common. Radiographic and postmortem studies indicate a 50% cephalad error of one interspace and a 5% error of two spaces (143), and very occasionally three spaces (144a), placing the site of puncture well cephalad to the termination of the cord (see Fig. 23.6).

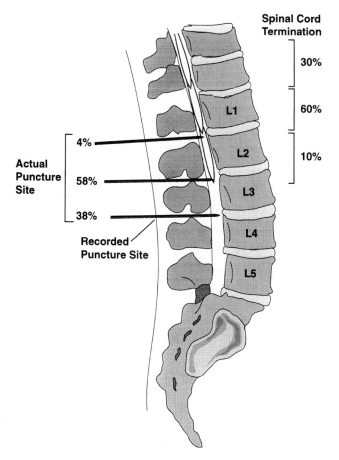

Figure 23.6. Lumbar puncture hazards to conus medullaris. The variations of the level of termination of the spinal cord are shown. The numbers (*right*) indicate the approximate percentage of each level that was found among 129 specimens. (Reprinted by permission from Bonica JJ, ed. *Principles and Practice of Obstetric Anesthesia.* Philadelphia: FA Davis; 1969;1:552.) The actual puncture sites of spinal needles are shown on *left* (radiologically recorded) compared to the recorded or assumed puncture site. (Reprinted by permission from Van Gessel EF, Forster A, Gamulin Z. Continuous spinal anesthesia: Where do spinal catheters go? *Anesth Analg* 1993;76:1004–1007.)

Such errors of needle placement are not inherently dangerous, provided that all other aspects of needle control are faultless and that the operator's grip on the advancing needle is sufficiently firm and controlled to halt the advance of the needle within a millimeter or so of receiving the appropriate signal to stop. In epidural puncture, this will be at the moment of loss-of-resistance. In subarachnoid puncture and using the "suck-and-see" technique, the signal comes abruptly at the instant when CSF suddenly spurts into the vacuum syringe (19). Failing the essential ability to halt the needle instantly, uncontrolled forward motion of the needle may pierce an underlying spinal cord, causing intense lancinating pain and some degree of objective neurologic deficit (144), or if the patient is under general anesthesia with warning reflexes obtunded, actual injection into the cord may result in a cavitational lesion and permanent paraplegia (145).

Catheter Trauma

Contemporary epidural catheters are available with soft, flexible tips that are extremely unlikely to cause vascular or neural trauma within the spinal canal. Very rarely, a wayward epidural catheter may cause indirect vascular injury to the spinal cord in the following manner: Approximately 2% to 4% of epidural catheters lodge in an intervertebral foramen and exit partially or completely into the paravertebral space beyond (146–148). If the existing catheter should happen to share the same foramen that contains the incoming anterior spinal artery, mechanical compression by a stiff catheter or reactive spasm of the artery may cause ischemia of the anterior two thirds of the lower spinal cord ("anterior spinal artery syndrome"). This is characterized by motor paralysis of one or both legs, with or without loss of pain and temperature sensation, but sparing of posterior column function subserving sensation of light touch and joint posture and vibration sense (149). This rare technical accident is reported to be completely reversible, provided it is recognized promptly and the catheter is withdrawn before permanent ischemic damage has occurred (150, 151). The introduction of reinforced, pliable catheters of soft polyurethane material has reduced the likelihood of such an unusual but extremely serious neurologic complication (152).

Complications of Vascular Origin

Epidural or subarachnoid needles and catheters commonly cause slight bleeding in the spinal canal, but this is clinically insignificant provided hemostasis is functioning normally. Neurologic complications from an expanding intraspinal hematoma are extremely rare in the absence of one or more of the following risk factors:

1. Intrinsic or extrinsic blood coagulation abnormalities (see Chapter 18).
2. Vascular anomalies of the spinal canal. As mentioned earlier in this chapter, cutaneous angiomas of the trunk often

communicate with an intraspinal component at the same segmental level and with epidural veins that have become distended over several segments in their role as an alternative pathway for venous return in late pregnancy (21–23).

3. Ankylosing spondylitis, complicated by spinal stenosis, and a tendency for difficult, traumatic spinal punctures (153). In addition, such patients may have received nonsteroidal antiinflammatory drugs that may interfere with platelet function and coagulation. Coagulopathies are discussed fully in Chapter 18. Readers are referred to that section for a full discussion of the difficult decisions regarding analgesic and anesthetic management for cesarean section that arise in toxemic patients with a falling platelet count (see Chapters 11 and 16).

Iatrogenic-Pneumatic Trauma: Loss-of-Resistance Test With Air

Identification of the epidural space by loss-of-resistance test (LORT) is technically more precise when performed with noncompressible fluid such as saline than with air in the "seeking" syringe (154). Prior to the introduction of disposable glass syringes and talc-free surgical gloves, the incidence of accidental dural puncture due to talc-jammed plungers became high enough to recommend air and a "bouncing-plunger" technique instead of saline as the more reliable of the two methods (155).

Unfortunately, the air-filled epidural technique carries its own set of pneumatic complications of the LORT if abused by injecting large volumes of air in excess of 10 to 15 mL into the epidural space, or if the dura is accidentally punctured and smaller volumes of air are injected into the subarachnoid space.

In young adults, epidural air is rapidly decompressed as it passes freely through patent intervertebral foramina, without causing harm other than one or more unblocked segments (156, 157) or paravertebral emphysema that will be clinically undetectable but evident on CT or MRI. However, large volumes of extradural air of 20 mL or more may travel rostrally to appear above the clavicles as subcutaneous emphysema of the neck (158). With even larger volumes of extradural air, 30 to 40 mL, and in patients with narrowed intervertebral foramina, the pneumatic pressure generated inside the vertebral canal may be severe enough to compress neural tissue or its venous outflow, leading to temporary paraplegia (159). In cases where the dura has been accidentally punctured at the outset, further attempts at localization with large boluses of air may lead to pneumocephalus with onset of severe headache (160–162) or transient cranial nerve palsy (163). However, the 3 to 5 mL air commonly used by many practitioners for the LORT should not lead to serious problems.

Complications of Vascular Origin: Hematoma

Preeclamptic patients are at risk of coagulation deficiencies that may cause uncontrolled intraspinal bleeding and spinal cord compression from vascular trauma by epidural or subarachnoid needles and catheters. Coagulation deficiencies and their clinical management are discussed fully in Chapter 18. Here it is necessary to stress only two practical aspects relating to clinical management.

First, currently available bedside and laboratory coagulation tests must be seen as only approximate rather than absolute guides to safe anesthetic practice. Formerly, carefully performed bleeding times have been shown to correlate reasonably well with the platelet count but not necessarily with platelet function, and a platelet count of 100,000 mm³ or more and a bleeding time of 10 minutes or less have been regarded as critical levels beyond which it is imprudent to place epidural catheters (164). Today, the bleeding time has been discarded by many authorities as an unreliable index (165, 166), and epidural catheters have been

placed harmlessly in some preeclamptic patients with platelet counts as low as 69,000 to 100,000 mm³ (167–169a). However, in a recent case report, an epidural hematoma was diagnosed in a patient with preeclampsia and a platelet count of 71,000 mm³ prior to surgery (170). There was no neurologic damage in the patient, but this is one of several cases of spinal hematomas reported in association with epidural anesthesia for obstetrics (Table 23.3) (170–179). A recent review of nerve injury with anesthesia noted the link between spinal cord damage and epidural hematomas (179a). However, when considering a platelet count prior to regional anesthesia, it should be remembered that maternal thrombocytopenia (platelet count $<150 \times 10^9/L$) may occur in an otherwise healthy parturient. In a study of 6770 women in late pregnancy, it was demonstrated that a platelet count $>115 \times 10^9/L$ in an otherwise healthy woman (i.e., no pregnancy-induced hypertension, idiopathic thrombocytopenic purpura, etc.) probably does not require further investigation (see Fig. 23.7). Some anesthesiologists consider a platelet count $>100 \times 10^9/L$ in an otherwise-healthy term pregnant woman as acceptable and not requiring further investigation.

Second, and most important, these existing data are too sparse to give any statistical assurance that the danger of intraspinal bleeding is sufficiently remote to safely dispense with anything but the most stringent postanesthetic surveillance in such cases (180). Therefore, clinical management and safety precautions should follow similar lines to those recommended for nonobstetric patients placed at comparable risk of intraspinal bleeding from thromboprophylaxis with low-molecular-weight heparin. That is to say, neurologic nursing care must be impeccable, with regular 4-hour checks of lower limb function from the time of epidural catheter insertion until at least 4 hours after catheter removal (181–183). Finally, it is prudent to consider the possibility that removal of the epidural catheter may disturb a tenuous clot around a damaged vein and restart intraspinal bleeding if the clotting processes are still subnormal at that time. Therefore, as a precaution, blood should be drawn and coagulation status evaluated prior to catheter removal in such cases (184).

Chemical Contaminants of the Subarachnoid and Epidural Spaces

As long as an epidural catheter is in place, the opportunity exists for accidental injection of a wrong and potentially harmful substance. Fortunately, the intact meninges present an effective but limited defense against chemical insults that would prove disastrous in the subarachnoid space. For example, epidural injections of 6% aqueous phenol have been used (under X-ray control) to relieve terminal cancer pain without any detectable, untoward results (185), whereas the same phenol solution would have disastrous results in the subarachnoid space.

Accidental epidural injections of a bizarre variety of incorrect solutions have been reported, including ephedrine, magnesium sulfate (186), thiopental on a number of occasions, potassium chloride, and phenol (187), with results that range from excellent analgesia with no detectable sequelae to permanent paraplegia in one patient after an epidural dose of 15 mL 11.25% potassium chloride (188). Two cases of accidental epidural parenteral nutrition enjoyed excellent postoperative analgesia, one lasting 24 hours after receiving an epidural infusion of 300 mL intralipid with an osmolality of 350 mOsm/kg over a 5-hour period (189). The other patient received 160 mL hypertonic amino acid mixture with an osmolality of 2000 mOsm/kg over a period of 2 hours and remained pain free for 27 hours (190). Neither patient appeared to suffer any neurologic sequelae. At the other extreme, one particularly scandalous case arose in Britain when a young photographic model was given an epidural top-up of paraldehyde during her first labor. Permanent and painful quadriplegia followed this extraordinary act of negligence (191).

Table 23.3. CASE REPORTS OF SPINAL HEMATOMA IN OBSTETRIC EPIDURAL ANESTHESIA

Study	Site of Hematoma/ Indication	Risk Factor for Hematoma	Presentation	Investigation	Treatment	Outcome
Ballin, 1981 (175)	?Epidural/ labor	Nil	24 h after operation: bilateral leg weakness and numbness, no bladder dysfunction	Plain X-ray	Conservative	Recovered
Newman, 1983 (176)	?Epidural/ labor	Nil	2 h after delivery: shooting pain, involuntary twitching and weakness of both legs, no urinary dysfunction	Plain X-ray	Conservative	Minimal weakness and paresthesia
Roscoe, 1984 (177)	Subdural/ labor	Ependymoma	3 d postpartum: backache numbness and weakness of legs, urinary retention, perianal numbness, decreased anal tone	Myelogram	Surgery 1 d after onset	Residual weakness of legs
Crawford, 1985 (171)	?Epidural/ labor	?	Several wk history of low backache and some motor and sensory loss in lower part of leg. Neurologist: resolving hematoma	?	Conservative	Recovered
Sibai, 1986 (170a)	?Lumbar/ labor	Preeclampsia	"Bleeding" with epidural catheter placement	None	Conservative	Recovered
Scott, 1990 (172)	Epidural	?	?	?	Surgery	Still improving
Lao, 1993 (178)	Subdural/ cesarean	Abnormal aPTT, preeclampsia	1 d postpartum: difficulty in walking, urinary retention, absent anal tone	MRI	Surgery 86 h postpartum	Full neurologic recovery
Yarnell, 1996 (179)	Epidural/ labor	Cholestasis of pregnancy, coagulopathy	12 h after epidural: backache, weakness and numbness of legs, numbness of perineum, absent anal tone	MRI	Surgery 16 h after onset	Mild weakness of right quadriceps
Yuen, 1999 (170)	Epidural/ cesarean section	Preeclampsia, 71×10^9 L platelets (?)	Seizure 1 h postpartum that spared lower limbs, motor sensory loss below L_1 noted; small lumbar hematoma and pneumoencephalus diagnosed (prolonged block or hematoma?—case unclear)	CT	Immediate surgery	No deficits

aPTT = activated partial thromboplastin time; CT = computed tomography; MRI = magnetic resonance imaging.
Modified from Loo CC, Dahlgren G, Irestedt L. Neurologic complications in obstetric regional anaesthesia. *Int J Obstet Anesth* 2000;9:99–124.

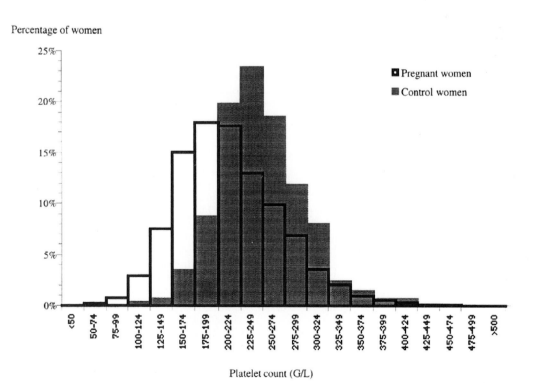

Figure 23.7. Histogram of platelet count of pregnant women (n = 6770) compared with nonpregnant women (n = 287). The histogram of platelet counts indicates a left shift during pregnancy. Among the pregnant women, 786 had a platelet count <150 × 10^9/L, but 738 women (94%) were diagnosed with gestational thrombocytopenia and had no other pathology. (Reprinted by permission from Boehlen F, Hohlfeld P, Extermann P, Perneger TV, De Moerloose P. Platelet count at term pregnancy: A reappraisal of the threshold. *Obstet Gynecol* 2000;95:29–33.)

Table 23.4. DIAGNOSTIC SIGNS IN 21 CASES OF UNINTENTIONAL DURAL PUNCTURE AMONG 3500 EPIDURAL BLOCKS FOR LABOR (0.6%)

CSF drip from needle	9/21
CSF aspirated from needle	3/21
Hypotension after test dose	2/21
No discernible sign of dural puncture at time of catheter insertion (retrospective diagnosis: postpuncture headache)	7/21

CSF = cerebrospinal fluid.
Reprinted by permission from Okell RW, Sprigge JS. Unintentional dural puncture: A survey of recognition and management. *Anaesthesia* 1987; 42:1110–1113.

All of these accidents occurred in the presence of an intact dura mater, shielding the delicate subarachnoid space. The pia-covered cord and spinal roots in the subarachnoid space are far more vulnerable to the direct effects of chemical contaminants than are the dural-covered elements in the epidural space. A hole in the dura from accidental dural puncture with a 16- or 18-gauge epidural needle allows epidural solutions to leak into the subarachnoid space, particularly if epidural pressure is raised by excessively rapid injection. Then, contaminants that might have been innocuous when excluded by an intact dura become potentially harmful. For example, accidental dural puncture occurred with a 16-gauge needle during attempted epidural analgesia for labor (192). After successful delivery and prior to removal of the epidural catheter, 40 mL 0.9% saline was injected into the epidural space as prophylaxis against a low CSF pressure headache. Unfortunately, the saline contained 1.5% benzyl alcohol as a preservative. Paraparesis of the lower limbs followed and gradually receded over a period of about 16 months. In this instance, the concentration of benzyl alcohol was not high enough to cause damage in the epidural space, and it must be concluded that the saline and preservative leaked into the subarachnoid space through the 16-gauge needle hole in the dura.

These examples of published wrongful injections represent only a fraction of unpublished cases, and they serve as reminders of the constant danger from this type of error, where the outcome depends on the nature, quantity, and speed of administration of the erroneous drug. The diagnostic signs of an unintentional dural block are summarized in Table 23.4. These accidents can be eliminated by appropriate managerial practices and ongoing, in-house education.

SPINAL INFECTIONS
Risk

The following four recent trends in obstetric anesthetic practice have contributed to increased opportunities for spinal infection to arise in the postpartum period. These risks must be met by heightened awareness of the need for rational aseptic precautions on the part of every anesthesiologist, followed by appropriate postpartum surveillance to identify and treat, in a timely fashion, any emerging symptoms and signs of developing meningitis or epidural abscess.

Asepsis

Fifty years ago, and prior to the introduction of broad-spectrum antibiotics, aseptic precautions during epidural or subarachnoid induction were as strict as for an elective surgical procedure. Nursing attendants wore surgical masks, and anesthesiologists wore cap and mask, scrubbed, and donned sterile gown and gloves (193, 194). Today, hand-washing has become cursory, the sterile gown has been discarded by most anesthesiologists, the cap by many, and even the surgical mask by significant numbers (195, 196). One recent survey of obstetric anesthesiologists in Britain revealed that 273 out of 539 respondents did not wear a

mask while performing either epidural or subarachnoid blocks (197), in spite of evidence that a fresh surgical mask does provide significant protection against droplet contamination (198, 199). Such a departure from established surgical asepsis appears imprudent, both as an inappropriate rejection of a simple, readily available precaution, and as a weakening of defense in the event of any subsequent alleged negligence arising from intraspinal infection. Case reports of spinal infection attributable to iatrogenic droplets are infrequent but well documented (200, 201).

In many obstetric facilities, the risk of droplet infection is further intensified by liberal visiting privileges during induction of epidural block, when the attending nurse and as many as three or four unmasked family members may be in close proximity to the "sterile field" in the labor room. It has been this author's practice to insist that clean surgical masks be worn by all medical and nursing attendants, and that visitors leave the labor room prior to preparation and performance of the block, unless suitably capped and masked.

Skin Disinfectants

The halide disinfectants chlorhexidine 0.5% in 80% alcohol and 10% aqueous povidone iodine have proved to be the most reliable agents for disinfection of the skin (202). However, even with these agents, skin disinfection is never perfect since colonies of gram-positive cocci residing in hair follicles and sweat glands may survive adequate contact with the disinfectant (203). Worse still, the actual disinfectant containers themselves may become colonized by bacteria after previous opening, and so single-use packets of disinfectant are now recommended for routine use (204).

Continuous Spinal-Epidural Technique

Preservation of the vulnerable subarachnoid space from iatrogenic infection has been a central rationale for the successful promotion of epidural analgesia as a safer and more versatile alternative to subarachnoid block in obstetric practice. Accordingly, accidental dural puncture has been regarded as an unfortunate and largely preventable lapse that is almost entirely avoidable by appropriate training and that need not occur more often than once in 200 cases (i.e., 0.5% incidence) in properly trained hands (205). Contemporary acceptance of increasingly high accidental dural puncture rates of 4% (10) and even higher (55) has opened the door to unquestioning acceptance of combining epidural catheterization with deliberate puncture of the dura to induce supplementary subarachnoid block as a powerful "two-pronged" maneuver to gain technical benefits of both epidural and subarachnoid medication of the spinal cord at one stroke. The profit aspect of this adventure in terms of rapid, profound anesthesia is unchallenged, and the incidental sacrifice of a safety barrier to the subarachnoid space has been accepted as an inconsequential loss.

The continuous spinal-epidural (CSE) technique is now widely practiced and acclaimed for obstetric and surgical procedures (see Chapter 9). The fact remains that the potential danger from septic invasion of the CSF has been increased by juxtaposition of an aditus, or walkway, for infection leading directly from the potentially infected skin surface to the immediate vicinity of the dural puncture wound, breaching the meningeal defenses surrounding the subarachnoid space.

This has an important bearing on diagnosis and appropriate clinical management if infection should arise. In the presence of an intact dura, the clinical signs and symptoms of an epidural abscess are quite different from meningitis, as summarized in Table 23.5. However, if infection starts inside the meninges, as meningitis, the incubation period is likely to be short, usually within 1 to 2 days, and sometimes as early as 12 hours after dural puncture (206, 207), and accompanied by early fever, cerebral symptoms, and cervical irritation manifest by nuchal

Table 23.5. DIAGNOSTIC FEATURES OF POSTPARTUM MENINGITIS AND EPIDURAL ABSCESS

	Meningitis	Epidural Abscess
Incubation period	28 h (average), 12–100 h (range)	6 d (average), 3–10 d (range)
Symptoms	Diffuse: headache, backache, malaise, photobia	Localized: severe lumbar pain at region of puncture site **Late sign:** radiating root pain
Signs		
Body temperature*	101.9°F (average), 99.5–103°F (range)	100.5°F (average), 98.9–102°F (range)
Mental	Confusion irritable, mania (rare), convulsions (rare)	
Physical†	Nuchal stiffness or rigidity, positive Kernig or Brudzinski signs	Tenderness over injection site; restricted straight leg raising (unilateral or bilateral) **Late paralytic signs:** urinary retention, absent rectal tone and reflex or lower limb reflexes
Investigations	Emergency lumbar puncture if: headache or neck stiffness **or** positive Kernig's sign + fever **or** mental state changes (i.e., 2 out of 4 cardinal signs)	**URGENT MRI OF SPINE**
Cerebrospinal fluid	Turbid, increased protein, decreased glucose polymorphonuclear leukocytosis	

MRI = magnetic resonance imaging.
*Nonsteroidal antiinflammatory drugs (NSAID's) may obtund fever and nuchal rigidity.
†Dural puncture wounds, whether accidental or intentional, as in combined spinal-epidural, permit sequential infection of both epidural and subarachnoid spaces, resulting in a confusing mixture of clinical symptoms and signs.
Meningitis references: 201, 204–218, 237.
Epidural Abscess references: 221–233, 237.

rigidity that must be distinguished from a low pressure, postlumbar puncture headache due to loss of CSF (208–219). All four of the cardinal signs of meningitis—headache, fever, mental confusion, and varying degrees of meningism, ranging from slight neck stiffness to a positive Kernig's sign—are seldom evident initially, but the presence of two or more of these signs are sufficient indication for urgent diagnostic lumbar puncture and CSF analysis (220). A raised CSF protein and a lowered glucose content with or without a polymorphonuclear pleocytosis are clear confirmatory signs of septic meningitis and indications for urgent chemotherapy (218–220). A lymphocytic pleocytosis in the CSF is more likely to indicate a rare coincidental viral infection unrelated to the dural puncture, such as Epstein-Barr viral encephalomyelitis that will not respond to chemotherapy and must run its course (61).

When infection originates outside the intact dura in the form of an epidural abscess, the incubation period is markedly extended to 4 days or longer, and fever and mental confusion are less prominent, or absent (see Table 23.5). In this situation, time becomes critical as the abscess develops and compresses adjacent neural tissues, with the probability of permanent paraplegia if surgical decompression by emergency laminectomy is not carried out within 8 to 12 hours (221–231).

These clinical distinctions of spinal sepsis become blurred in the presence of both an epidural catheter and a deliberate or accidental meningeal puncture wound. Then, rapid spread of infection from the epidural space to the subarachnoid space may result in a mixed constellation of fever, headache, and delirium from meningitis, along with backache and segmental radiating pain from the epidural abscess (216, 232–237). Each of these four warning signs of impending meningitis (headache, fever, stiff neck, and mental changes) is tenuous and easily suppressed by drugs—fever and neck rigidity by nonsteroidal antiinflammatory drugs (NSAIDs), headache and mental changes by opioids. Therefore, each sign must be given due weight in deciding whether to perform an emergency spinal puncture and CSF

analysis. While NSAIDs such as diclonefac are useful and appropriate analgesic drugs after cesarean section under general anesthesia (235), they are likely to suppress one or more of the cardinal signs of spinal sepsis after subarachnoid, epidural, or CSE blocks, and to introduce dangerous delays in appropriate treatment by "masking the mischief" (218, 236).

Contemporary reporting practices of postanesthetic adverse neurologic outcomes in North America allow only a partial estimate of their true prevalence. The task of tracing these cases through closed-claim files of liability insurance companies is protracted, incomplete, and immensely laborious (179a). Available European data suggest that their prevalence may be greater than is commonly acknowledged. For example, one Danish university hospital reported seven cases of meningitis or epidural abscess out of 100 epidural catheter insertions in a 17-month period, an incidence of 7% (238). However, this has not been the case in the United Kingdom and elsewhere, where the CSE technique is widely practiced (239).

The gravity of these potentially catastrophic neurologic dangers must be seen in perspective against recent developments in contemporary anesthetic practice. The power and versatility of the CSE technique have proven most attractive; however, the potential hazard of deliberately breaching the meningeal defenses must be considered.

Influence of Current Trends in Obstetric Practice and Hospital Administration

The last and increasingly serious risk of postanesthetic complication lies in rare neurologic sequelae that may arise after the mother has returned home, when any delays in readmission are likely to jeopardize prompt diagnosis and urgent treatment.

Performance of epidural or subarachnoid anesthesia for obstetric delivery carries the implicit responsibility for effective postanesthetic follow-up and containment of any anesthesia-related adverse sequelae. Efficient performance of that obligation has been hampered as the postpartum hospital stay has become progressively shortened to discharge at 24 to 36 hours after vaginal delivery and 36 to 72 hours after cesarean section—both discharge times being well within the range of incubation periods for either meningitis or epidural abscess, as shown in Table 23.5. Thus, the general adoption of such ultra-early discharge practices has bypassed customary postanesthetic precautions recommended for surveillance of neuraxial blockade in major surgical cases.

Here, the obstetric issue lies not in the magnitude of the surgery, but rather in the remote risks inseparable from major, invasive anesthetic techniques adopted for childbirth, coupled with contemporary hospital management practices of ultra-early postpartum discharge that hinder appropriate hands-on postanesthetic surveillance (240, 241). Since those risks remain operative for several days after the mother has returned home, the situation calls for creation of secure administrative procedures that will allow rapid readmission to the hospital with immediate investigation and timely treatment in the event of any postanesthetic neurologic complication that may arise.

Finally, it is necessary to return to the beginning of this chapter and reemphasize the possibility of "associated but unrelated" spinal pathology, when the cause of the postanesthetic neurologic catastrophe is unrelated to the anesthetic. In some instances where no regional anesthetic has been administered, the true, nonanesthetic cause may be quite obvious and no blame can possibly be attributed to the anesthetic (242), but in others the true cause may be more difficult to determine (243), and as observed in one such case:

"Had our patient received regional as opposed to general anesthesia, because of the close temporal relationship to the transverse myelitis, it would almost certainly have been implicated as a major etiologic factor and might well have been the subject of legal proceedings" (244).

REFERENCES

1. Beatty TE. Second Report of the New Lying-in Hospital, Dublin. *Dublin J Med Sci* 1838;12:273–313.
2. Lazorthes G, Poulhes J, Bastide G, Chancolle AR, Zadeh O. La vascularisation de la moelle épinière (étude anatomique et physiologique). *Rev Neurol* 1962;106:535–557.
3. Lazorthes G, Gouaze A, Bastide G, Soutoul J, Zadeh O, Santini J-J. La vascularization arterielle du renflement lombaire. Etudes des variations et des suppleances. *Rev Neurol* 1966;114:109–122.
4. Bademosi O, Osuntokum BO, Van der Werd HJ, Bademosi AK, Ojo OA. Obstetric neuropraxia in the Nigerian African. *Int J Gynaecol Obstet* 1980;17:611–614.
5. Lufkin RB, ed. Magnetic resonance contrast imaging. In: *The MRI Manual*. 2nd ed. Baltimore: Mosby; 1998:21–40.
6. Hullander RM, Bogard TD, Lievers D, Moran D, Dewan DM. Chiari I malformation presenting as recurrent spinal headache. *Anesth Analg* 1992;75:1025–1026.
6a. Penney DJ, Smallman JMB. Arnold-Chiari malformation and pregnancy. *Int J Obstet Anes* 2001;10:139–141.
7. Milhorat TH, Johnson WD, Miller JI, Bergland RM, Hollander-Sher J. Surgical treatment of syringomyelia based on magnetic resonance imaging criteria. *Neurosurgery* 1992;31:231–244.
8. Davies PRF, Loach AB. Spinal anaesthesia and spina-bifida occulta. *Anaesthesia* 1996;51:1158–1160.
9. Nel MR, Robson V, Robinson PN. Extradural anaesthesia for caesarean section in a patient with syringomyelia and Chiari type I anomaly. *Br J Anaesth* 1998;80:512–515.
10. Huffnagle SL, Morris MC, Arkoosh VA, et al. The influence of epidural needle bevel orientation on spread of sensory blockade in the laboring parturient. *Anesth Analg* 1998;89:326–330.
11. Bromage PR. The influence of epidural needle bevel on spread of sensory blockade in the laboring patient. *Anesth Analg* 1999;88:962.
12. Leape LL, Woods DD, Hatlie MJ, Kizer KW, Schroeder SA, Lundberg GD. Promoting patient safety and preventing error [editorial]. *JAMA* 1998;280:1444–1447.
13. Scott DB, Hibbard BM. Serious non-fatal complications associated with extradural blocks in obstetric practice. *Br J Anaesth* 1990;64:537–541.
14. Ong BY, Cohen MM, Esmail A, Cumming M, Kozody R, Palahniuk RJ. Paresthesia and motor dysfunction after labor and delivery. *Anesth Analg* 1987;66:18–22.
15. Holdcroft A, Gibberd FB, Hargrove RL, Hawkins DF, Dellaportas CI. Neurological complications associated with pregnancy. *Br J Anaesth* 1995;75:522–526.
16. Neville BGR. Neural tube defects: Spinal bifida. In: Walton J, ed. *Brain's Diseases of the Nervous System*. 10th ed. Oxford: University Press; 1993:462–463.
17. Morgenlander JC, Redick LF. Spina dysraphism and epidural anesthesia. *Anesthesiology* 1994;81:783–785.
18. Wood GG, Jacka MJ. Spinal hematoma following spinal anesthesia in a patient with spina bifida occulta. *Anesthesiology* 1997;87:983–984.
19. Bromage PR, Van Steenberge A, Fagraeus L, Van Zundert A, Corke BC. A loss-of- resistance-to-negative-pressure test for subarachnoid puncture with narrow-gauge needles. *Reg Anesth* 1993;18:155–161.
20. Gilbertson JR, Miller GM, Goldman MS, Marsh WR. Spinal dural arteriovenous fistulas: MR and myelographic findings. *Am J Neuroradiol* 1995;16:2049–2057.
21. Eastwood DW. Hematoma after epidural anesthesia: Relationship to skin and spinal angiomas. *Anesth Analg* 1991;73:352–354.
22. Symon L, Kuyama H, Kendall B. Dural arteriovenous malformations of the spine: Clinical features and surgical results in 55 cases. *J Neurosurg* 1984;60:238–247.
23. Redekop GJ, Del Maestro RF. Vertebral hemangioma causing spinal cord compression during pregnancy. *Surg Neurol* 1992;38:210–215.
24. Martin JT. Compartment syndromes: Concepts and perspectives for the anesthesiologist. *Anesth Analg* 1992;75:275–283.
25. Robinson JL, Hall CS, Sedzimir CB. Arteriovenous malformations, aneurysms and pregnancy. *J Neurosurg* 1974;41:63–70.
26. Ong BY, Littleford J, Segstro R, Paetkau D, Sutton I. Spinal anaesthesia for caesarean section in a patient with a cervical arteriovenous malformation. *Can J Anaesth* 1996;43:1052–1058.
27. Semple DA, McClure JH, Wallace EM. Arnold-Chiari malformation in pregnancy. *Anaesthesia* 1996;51:580–582.
28. Hart IK, Bone I, Hadley DM. Development of neurologic problems after lumbar puncture. *Br Med J* 1988;296:51–52.
29. Sathi S, Stieg PE. Acquired Chiari I malformation after multiple lumbar punctures: Case report. *Neurosurgery* 1993;32:306–309.
30. Diemunsch P, Balabaud VP, Petian C, et al. Hematome sous dural bilateral apres analgesia peridurale. *Can J Anaesth* 1998;45:328–331.
31. Benzon HT. Intracerebral hemorrhage after dural puncture and epidural blood patch: Nonpostural and noncontinuous headache. *Anesthesiology* 1984;60:258–259.
32. Brinquin L, Bonsignour JP, Hor F, Diraison Y, Tougouri M, Buffat JJ. Hematome sous-dural intracranien dans les suites d'une rachianesthesie. *La Presse Medicale* 1988;17:874–875.
33. Wyble SW, Bayhi D, Webre D, Viswanathan S. Bilateral subdural hematomas after dural puncture: Delayed diagnosis after false negative computed tomography scan without contrast. *Reg Anesth* 1992;17:52–53.
34. Bromage PR, ed. Postoperative analgesia: Early and ultra-early ambulation. In: *Epidural Analgesia*. Philadelphia: WB Saunders; 1978:456–457.
35. Breen TW, Shapiro T, Glass B, Foster-Payne D, Oriol NE. Epidural analgesia for labor in an ambulatory patient. *Anesth Analg* 1993;77:919–924.
36. O'Meary ME, Gin T. Comparison of 0.125% bupivacaine with 0.125% bupivacaine and clonidine as extradural analgesia in the first stage of labour. *Br J Anaesth* 1993;71:651–656.
37. Le Poulain B, De Kock M, Scholtes JL, Van Lierde M. Clonidine combined with sufentanil and bupivacaine with adrenaline for obstetric analgesia. *Br J Anaesth* 1993;71:657–660.
38. Buggy D, Hughes N, Gardiner J. Posterior column sensory impairment during ambulatory extradural analgesia in labour. *Br J Anaesth* 1994;73:540–542.
39. Chassard D, Mathon L, Dailler F, Golfier F, Tournadre JP, Bouletreau P. Extradural clonidine combined with sufentanil and 0.0625% bupivacaine for analgesia in labour. *Br J Anaesth* 1996;77:458–462.

40. Parry MG, Fernando R, Bawa GPS, Poulton BB. Dorsal column function after epidural and spinal blockade: Implications for the safety of walking following low-dose regional analgesia for labour. *Anaesthesia* 1998;53:382–403.

41. Claes B, Soetens M, Van Zundert A, Datta S. Clonidine added to bupivacaine- epinephrine-sufentanil improves epidural analgesia during childbirth. *Reg Anesth Pain Med* 1998;23:540–547.

42. Punt CD, Van Neer PAFA, de Lange S. Pressure sores as a possible complication of epidural analgesia. *Anesth Analg* 1991;73:657–659.

43. Smet IGG, Vercauteren MP, De Jongh RF, Vundelinckx GFM, Heylen RJ. Pressure sores as a complication of patient-controlled epidural analgesia after cesarean delivery: Case report. *Reg Anesth* 1996;21:338–341.

43a. Short J, Ryall EA. Pressure sores following epidural analgesia in labor. *Int J Obstet Anes* 2001;10:146–147.

44. Macarthur A, Macarthur C, Weeks SK. Epidural anaesthesia and low back pain after delivery: A prospective cohort study. *Br Med J* 1995;311:1336–1339.

45. Vanderick G, Geerinckx K, Van Steenberge AL, DeMuylder E. Bupivacaine 0.125% in epidural block analgesia during childbirth: Clinical evaluation. *Br Med J* 1974;46:838–844.

46. MacArthur C, Lewis M, Knox EG, Crawford JS. Epidural anaesthesia and long-term backache after childbirth. *Br Med J* 1990;301:9–12.

47. Macarthur AJ, Macarthur C, Weeks SK. Is epidural anesthesia in labor associated with chronic low back pain? A prospective cohort study. *Anesth Analg* 1997;85:1066–1070.

48. Breen TW, Ransil BJ, Groves PA, Oriol NE. Factors associated with back pain after childbirth. *Anesthesiology* 1994;81:29–34.

49. Fibuch EF, Opper SE. Back pain following epidurally administered Nesacaine-MPF. *Anesth Analg* 1989;69:113–115.

50. Hynson JM, Sessler DI, Glosten B. Back pain in volunteers after epidural anesthesia with chloroprocaine. *Anesth Analg* 1991;72:253–256.

51. Stevens RA, Chester WL, Artusio JD, et al. Back pain after epidural anesthesia with 2-chloroprocaine in volunteers. *Reg Anesth* 1991;16:199–203.

52. Stevens RA, Urmey WF, Urquhart BL, Kao T-C. Back pain after epidural anesthesia with chloroprocaine. *Anesthesiology* 1993;78:492–497.

53. Stevens RA. Back pain following epidural anesthesia with 2-chloroprocaine [editorial]. *Reg Anesth* 1997;22:299–302.

54. Nesacaine MPF (chloroprocaine HCl) injection USP [package insert]. In: *Physicians' Desk Reference.* 52nd ed. Montvale, NJ: Medical Economics; 1998:566.

55. Berger C, Crosby E, Grodecki W. North American survey of the management of dural puncture occurring during labour epidural analgesia. *Can J Anaesth* 1998;45:110–114.

56. Holst D, Mollman M, Ebel C, Hausmann R, Wendt M. In vitro investigation of cerebrospinal fluid leakage after dural puncture with various spinal needles. *Anesth Analg* 1998;87:1331–1335.

57. Hatalvi BI. The dynamics of postspinal headache. *Headache* 1977;17:64–67.

58. Ravindran RS, Viegas OJ, Tasch MD, Cline PJ, Deaton RL, Brown TR. Bearing down at the time of delivery and the incidence of spinal headache in parturients. *Anesth Analg* 1981;60:524–526.

59. Gielen M. Post dural puncture headache (PDPH): A review. *Reg Anesth* 1989;14:101–106.

60. Benhamou D, Hamza J, Ducot B. Postpartum headache after epidural analgesia without dural puncture. *Int J Obstet Anesth* 1995;4:17–20.

61. Donovan WD, Zimmerman RD. MRI findings of severe Epstein-Barr virus encephalomyelitis: Case report. *J Comput Assist Tomogr* 1996;20:1027–1029.

62. Younker D, Jones MM, Adenwala J, Citrin A, Joyce TH III. Maternal cortical vein thrombosis and the obstetric anesthesiologist. *Anesth Analg* 1986;68:1007–1012.

63. Gerwitz EC, Costin M, Marx GF. Cortical vein thrombosis may mimic postdural puncture headache. *Reg Anesth* 1987;12:188–190.

64. Ravindran RS, Zandstra GC, Viegas OJ. Postpartum headache following regional analgesia: A symptom of cerebral venous thrombosis. *Can J Anaesth* 1989;36:705–707.

65. Macon ME, Armstrong L, Brown EM. Subdural hematoma following spinal anesthesia. *Anesthesiology* 1990;72:380–381.

65a. Loo CC, Dahlgreen G, Irestedt L. Neurological complications in obstetric regional anesthesia. *Int J Obstet Anesth* 2000;9:99–124.

66. Atkinson JLD, Weinshenker BG, Miller GM, et al. Acquired Chiari I malformation secondary to spontaneous spinal cerebrospinal fluid leakage and chronic intracranial hypotension in seven cases. *J Neurosurg* 1998;88:237–242.

67. Lambert DH, Hurley RJ, Hertwig L, Datta S. Role of needle gauge and tip configuration in the production of lumbar puncture headache. *Reg Anesth* 1997;22:66–72.

68. Stride PC, Cooper GM. Dural taps revisited: A 20-year survey from Birmingham Maternity Hospital. *Anaesthesia* 1993;48:247–255.

69. Williams E, Beaulieu P, Jenkins G, Fawcett W. Efficiency of epidural blood patches in obstetrics. *Can J Anaesth* 1998;45:1031.

70. Lynch J, Kasper S-M, Strick K, et al. The use of Quincke and Whitacre 27-gauge needles in orthopedic patients: Incidence of failed spinal anesthesia and postdural puncture headache. *Anesth Analg* 1994;79:124–128.

71. Cullen WA, Griffith HR. Postpartum results of spinal anesthesia in obstetrics. *Anesth Analg* 1947;26:114–121.

72. Jones RJ. The role of recumbency in the prevention and treatment of postspinal headache. *Anesth Analg* 1974;53:788–796.

73. Carbaat PAT, van Grevel H. Lumbar puncture headache: Controlled study on the preventive effect of 24 hours' bed rest. *Lancet* 1981;1:1133–1135.

74. Cook PT, Davies MJ, Beavis RE. Bed rest and post lumbar puncture headache: The effectiveness of 24-hour recumbency in reducing the incidence of postlumbar puncture headache. *Anaesthesia* 1989;44:389–391.

75. Thornberry EA, Thomas TA. Posture and postspinal headache: A controlled trial in 80 patients. *Br J Anaesth* 1988;60:195–197.

76. Miyakawa Y, Meyer JS, Ishihara N, et al. Effect of cerebrospinal fluid removal on cerebral blood flow and metabolism in the baboon: Influence of tyrosine infusion and cerebral embolism on cerebrospinal fluid pressure autoregulation. *Stroke* 1977;8:346–351.

77. Dodd JE, Efird RC, Rauck RL. Cerebral blood flow changes with caffeine therapy for postdural headaches [abstract]. *Anesthesiology* 1989;71:A679.

78. Camann WR, Murray RS, Mushlin PS, Lambert DH. Effects of oral caffeine on postdural puncture headache. A double-blind, placebo controlled trial. *Anesth Analg* 1990;70:181–184.

79. Schwalbe SS, Schiffmiller MW, Marx GF. Theophylline for post-dural puncture headache [abstract]. *Anesthesiology* 1991;75:A1082.

80. Crawford JS. The prevention of headache consequent upon dural puncture. *Br J Anaesth* 1972;44:598–600.

81. Barrios-Alarcon J, Aldrete JA, Parajas-Topia D. Relief of postlumbar puncture headache with epidural dextran-40: A preliminary report. *Reg Anesth* 1989;14:78–80.

82. Salvador L, Carrero E, Castillo J, et al. Prevention of post dural puncture headache with epidural-administered Dextran 40 [letter]. *Reg Anesth* 1992;17:357–358.

83. Carp H, Singh PJ, Vadhera R, Jayaram A. Effects of the serotonin-receptor agonist sumatriptan on postdural puncture headache: Report of six cases. *Anesth Analg* 1994;79:180–182.

84. Sumatriptan Succinate (Imitrex). *Physicians' Desk Reference.* 52nd ed. Montvale, NJ: Medical Economics; 1998:1037.

85. Collier BB. Treatment for post dural puncture headache. *Br J Anaesth* 1994;72:366–367.

86. Foster P. ACTH treatment for post-lumbar puncture headache. *Br J Anaesth* 1994;73:429.

87. Kshatri KM, Foster PA. Adrenocorticotropic hormone infusion as a novel treatment for post dural puncture headache. *Reg Anesth* 1997;22:432–434.

88. Gormley JB. Treatment of postspinal headache. *Anesthesiology* 1960;21:565–566.

89. Beards SC, Jackson A, Griffiths AG, Horsman EL. Magnetic resonance imaging of extradural blood patches: Appearances from 30 minutes to 18 hours. *Br J Anaesth* 1993;71:182–188.

90. Vakharia SB, Thomas PS, Rosenbaum AE, et al. Magnetic resonance imaging of cerebrospinal fluid leak and tamponade effect of blood patch in postdural puncture headache. *Anesth Analg* 1997;84:585–590.

91. Szeinfeld M, Ihmeidan TH, Moser MM, Machado R, Klose KJ, Serafini AN. Epidural blood patch: An evaluation of the volume and spread of blood injected into the epidural space. *Anesthesiology* 1986;64:820–822.

92. Carrie LES. Epidural blood patch: Why the rapid response? *Anesth Analg* 1991;72:129–130.

92a. Duffy PJ, Crosby ET. The epidural patch. Resolving the controversies. *Can J Anaesth* 1999;46:878–886.

93. Ackerman WE, Colclough GW. Prophylactic epidural blood patch: The controversy continues. *Anesth Analg* 1987;66:913.

94. Cheek TG, Banner R, Sauter J, Gutsche BB. Prophylactic extradural blood patch is effective. *Br J Anaesth* 1988;61;340–342.

95. Trevedi NS, Eddi D, Shevde K. Prevention of headache following inadvertent dural puncture. *Reg Anesth* 1989;14(suppl):51S.

96. Colonna-Romano P, Shapiro BE. Unintentional dural puncture and prophylactic epidural blood patch in obstetrics. *Anesth Analg* 1989;69:522–523.

97. Lievers D. Total spinal anesthesia following prophylactic epidural blood patch. *Anesthesiology* 1990;73:1287–1289.

98. Coombs DW, Hooper D. Subarachnoid pressure with epidural blood "patch." *Reg Anesth* 1979;4:3–6.

99. Griffiths AG, Beards SC, Jackson A, Horsman EL. Visualization of extradural blood patch for post lumbar puncture headache by magnetic resonance imaging. *Br J Anaesth* 1993;70:223–225.

100. Gerritse BM, van Dongen RTM, Crul BJP. Epidural fibrin glue injection stops persistent cerebrospinal fluid leak during long-term intrathecal catheterization. *Anesth Analg* 1997;84:1140–1141.

101. Gil F, Garcia-Aguado R, Barcia JA, et al. The effect of fibrin glue patch in an in vitro model of postdural puncture leakage. *Anesth Analg* 1998;87:1125–1128.

102. Leslie K, Sessler DI. Reduction of shivering threshold is proportional to spinal block height. *Anesthesiology* 1996;84:1327–1331.

103. Saito T, Sessler DI, Fujita K, Ooi Y, Jeffrey R. Thermoregulatory effects of spinal and epidural anesthesia during Cesarean delivery. *Reg Anesth Pain Med* 1998;23:418–423.

104. Panzer O, Ghazanfari N, Sessler DI, et al. Shivering and shivering-like tremor during labor with and without epidural analgesia. *Anesthesiology* 1999;90:1609–1616.

105. Matthews NC, Corser G. Epidural fentanyl for shaking in obstetrics. *Anaesthesia* 1988;43:783–785.

106. Kurz A, Ikeda T, Sessler DI, et al. Meperidine decreases the shivering threshold twice as much as the vasoconstriction threshold. *Anesthesiology* 1997;86:1046–1054.

107. Wheelahan JM, Leslie K, Silbert BS. Epidural fentanyl reduces the shivering threshold during epidural lidocaine anesthesia. *Anesth Analg* 1998;87:587–590.

108. Sevarino FB, Johnson MD, Lema MJ, Datta S, Ostheimer GW, Naulty JS. The effect of epidural sufentanil on shivering and body temperature in the parturient. *Anesth Analg* 1989;68:530–533.

109. Flanagan HL, Datta S, Lambert DH, Gissen AJ, Covino BG. Effect of pregnancy on bupivacaine induced conduction blockade in the isolated rabbit vagus. *Anesth Analg* 1987;66:123–126.

110. Butterworth JF, Walker FO, Lysak SZ. Pregnancy increases median nerve susceptibility to lidocaine. *Anesthesiology* 1990;72:962–965.

111. Bannister LH, Berry MM, Collins P, Dyson M, Dussek JE, Ferguson MWJ, eds. Mechanism of deglutition. In: *Gray's Anatomy.* 38th ed. New York: Churchill Livingstone; 1995:1732–1733.

112. Bromage PR. An evaluation of bupivacaine in epidural analgesia for obstetrics. *Can Anaesth Soc J* 1969;16:46–56.

113. Pathy GV, Rosen M. Prolonged block with recovery after extradural analgesia for labour. *Br J Anaesth* 1975;47:520–522.

114. Cuerden C, Buley R, Downing JW. Delayed recovery after epidural block in labour: A report of four cases. *Anaesthesia* 1977;32:773–776.

115. Bromage PR. Masked mischief [editorial]. *Reg Anesth* 1993;18:143–144.

116. Blomberg RG. The lumbar subdural extra arachnoid space of humans: An anatomical study using spinaloscopy in autopsy cases. *Anesth Analg* 1987;66:177–180.

117. Lubenow T, Keh-Wong E, Kristof K, Ivankovich O, Ivankovich AD. Inadvertent subdural injection: A complication of an epidural block. *Anesth Analg* 1988;67:175–179.

118. Reynolds F, Speedy HM. The subdural space: The third place to go astray. *Anaesthesia* 1990;45:120–123.

119. McMenemin IM, Sissons CRJ, Brownridge P. Accidental subdural catheterization: Radiological evidence of a possible mechanism for spinal cord damage. *Br J Anaesth* 1992;69:417–419.

120. Hogan QH, Haddox JD. Headache from intracranial air after lumbar epidural injection: Subarachnoid or subdural? *Reg Anesth* 1992;17:303–305.

121. Elliott DW, Voyvodic F, Brownridge P. Sudden onset of subarachnoid block after subdural catheterization: A case of subarachnoid rupture? *Br J Anaesth* 1996;76:322–324.

122. Bromage PR. On rotating the epidural needle: In response [letter]. *Anesth Analg* 1996;82:430.

123. Woerth SD, Bullard JR, Alpert CC. Total spinal anesthesia. A late complication of epidural anesthesia. *Anesthesiology* 1977;47:380–381.

124. Meiklejohn BH. The effect of rotation of an epidural needle: An in vitro study. *Anaesthesia* 1987;42:1180–1182.

125. Asato F, Nakatani K, Matayoshi Y, Katekawa Y, Chinen K. Development of a subdural motor blockade. *Anaesthesia* 1993;48:46–49.

126. Duffy BL. "Don't turn the needle!" *Anaesth Intensive Care* 1993;21:328–330.

127. Hamby WB. Misplaced lipiodol: An analysis of 104 lipiodol spinograms. *Radiology* 1941;37:343–346.

128. Schultz EH, Brogdon BG. The problem of subdural placement in myelography. *Radiology* 1962;79:91–96.

129. Tainter EG, Grayson CE. Large volume myelography. *Ann NY Acad Sci* 1959;78:956–965.

130. Jones MD, Newton TH. Inadvertent extra-arachnoid injections in myelography. *Radiology* 1963;80:818–822.

131. Norris MC. Patient variables and the subarachnoid spread of hyperbaric bupivacaine in the term parturient. *Anesthesiology* 1990;72:478–482.

132. Hardy PAJ. Can epidural catheters penetrate dura mater? An anatomical study. *Anaesthesia* 1986;41:1146–1147.

133. Okell RW, Sprigge JS. Unintentional dural puncture: A survey of recognition and management. *Anaesthesia* 1987;42:1110–1113.

134. McGown RG. Accidental marrow sampling during caudal anaesthesia. *Br J Anaesth* 1972;44:613–615.

135. Leighton BL, Gross JB. Air: An effective indicator of intravenously located epidural catheters. *Anesthesiology* 1989;71:848–851.

136. Leighton BL, Norris MC, De Simone CA, Rosko T, Gross JB. The air test as a clinically useful indicator of intravenously placed epidural catheters. *Anesthesiology* 1990;73:610–613.

137. Handler JS, Bromage PR. Venous air embolism during cesarean delivery. *Reg Anesth* 1990;15:170–173.

138. Hogan QH. Lumbar epidural anatomy: A new look by cryomicrotome section. *Anesthesiology* 1991;75:767–775.

139. Hogan QH. Migration of an epidural catheter? *Anesth Analg* 1993;76:910–911.

140. Usubiaga JE, Wikinski JA, Usubiaga LE. Epidural pressure and its relation to spread of anesthetic solutions in the epidural space. *Anesth Analg* 1967;46:440–446.

141. Bromage PR, ed. Epidural pressures. In: *Epidural Analgesia.* Philadelphia: WB Saunders; 1978:160–175.

142. Hogan QH. Tuffier's line: The normal distribution of anatomic parameters. *Anesth Analg* 1994;78:194–195.

143. Van Gessel EF, Forster A, Gamulin Z. Continuous spinal anesthesia: Where do spinal catheters go? *Anesth Analg* 1993;76:1004–1007.

144. Greaves JD. Serious spinal cord injury due to haematomyelia caused by spinal anaesthesia in a patient treated with low-dose heparin. *Anaesthesia* 1997;52:150–154.

144a. Broadbent CR, Maxwell WB, Ferrie R, et al. Ability of anaesthetists to identify a marked lumber interspace. *Anaesthesia* 2000;55:1122–1126.

145. Bromage PR, Benumof JL. Paraplegia following intracord injection during attempted epidural anesthesia under general anesthesia. *Reg Anesth Pain Med* 1998;23:104–107.

146. Bridenbaugh DL, Moore DC, Bagdi P, Bridenbaugh PO. The position of plastic tubing in continuous block techniques: An X-ray study of 552 patients. *Anesthesiology* 1968;29:1047–1049.

147. Bromage PR, ed. Technical complications of epidural catheters. In: *Epidural Analgesia.* Philadelphia: WB Saunders; 1978:226–228.

148. Yoshii WY, Rottman RL, Rosenblatt RM, et al. Epidural catheter-induced traumatic radiculopathy in obstetrics: One center's experience. *Reg Anesth* 1994;19:132–135.

149. McLellan DL. Infarction and ischaemia of the spinal cord and cauda equina. In: Walton JN, ed. *Brain's Diseases of the Nervous System.* 10th ed. Oxford: University Press; 1993:511–512.

150. Richardson J, Bedder M. Transient anterior spinal cord syndrome with continuous postoperative epidural analgesia. *Anesthesiology* 1990;72:764–766.

151. Ben-David D, Vaida S, Collins G, et al. Transient paraplegia secondary to an epidural catheter. *Anesth Analg* 1994;79:598–600.

152. Banwell BR, Morley-Foster P, Krause R. Decreased incidents of complications in parturients with the Arrow (FlexTip Plus) epidural catheter. *Can J Anaesth* 1998;45:370–372.

153. Wulf H. Epidural anaesthesia and spinal haematoma. *Can J Anaesth* 1996;43:1260–1271.

154. Bromage PR, ed. Identification of the epidural space. In: *Spinal Epidural Analgesia.* Edinburgh: E&S Livingstone; 1954:48–52.

155. Bromage PR, ed. Identification of the epidural space. In: *Epidural Analgesia.* Philadelphia: WB Saunders; 1978:192–195.

156. Dalens B, Bazin JE, Haberer JP. Epidural air bubbles as a cause of incomplete analgesia during epidural anesthesia. *Anesth Analg* 1987;66:679–683.

157. Valentine SJ, Jarvis AP, Shutt LE. Comparative study of the effects of air or saline to identify the extradural space. *Br J Anaesth* 1991;66:224–227.

158. Thomas JE, Schachner S, Reynolds A. Subcutaneous emphysema as a result of loss- of-resistance identification of epidural space. *Reg Anesth* 1982;7:44–45.

159. Nay PG, Milasziewicz R, Jothilingham S. Extradural air as a cause of paraplegia following lumbar analgesia. *Anaesthesia* 1993;48:402–404.

160. Katz Y, Markovits R, Rosenberg B. Pneumocephalus after inadvertent intrathecal air injection during epidural block. *Anesthesiology* 1990;73:1277–1279.

161. Gonzalez-Carrasco FJ, Aguilar JL, Llubia C, Nogues S, Vidal-Lopez F. Pneumocephalus after accidental dural puncture during epidural anesthesia. *Reg Anesth* 1993;18:193–195.

162. Aida S, Taga K, Yamakura T, Enoh H, Shimoji K. Headache after attempted epidural block: The role of intrathecal air. *Anesthesiology* 1998;88:76–81.

163. Laviola S, Kirvela M, Spoto M-R, Tschuor S, Alon E. Pneumocephalus with intense headache and unilateral pupillary dilatation after accidental dural puncture during epidural anesthesia for cesarean section. *Anesth Analg* 1999;88:582–583.

164. Ramanathan J, Sibai BM, Vu T, Chauhan D. Correlation between bleeding times and platelet counts in women with pre-eclampsia undergoing Cesarean section. *Anesthesiology* 1989;71:188–191.

165. Rodgers CRP, Levin P. A critical reappraisal of the bleeding time. *Semin Thromb Hemost* 1990;16:1–20.

166. O'Kelly SW, Lawes EG, Luntley JB. Bleeding time: Is it a useful clinical tool? *Br J Anaesth* 1992;68:313–315.

167. Orlikowski CEP, Rocke DA, Murray WB, et al. Thromboelastography changes in pre-eclampsia and eclampsia. *Br J Anaesth* 1996;77:157–161.

168. Beilin Y, Zahn J, Comerford M. Safe epidural analgesia in thirty parturients with platelet counts between 69,000 and 98,000 mm³. *Anesth Analg* 1997;85:385–388.

169. Sharma SK, Philip J, Whitten CW, Padakandla UB, Landers DF. Assessment of changes in coagulation in parturients with preeclampsia using thromboelastography. *Anesthesiology* 1999;90:385–390.

169a. Boehlen F, Hohfeld P, Extermann P, Perneger T, De Moerloose P. Platelet count at term pregnancy: A reappraisal of the threshold. *Obstet Gynecol* 2000;95:29–33.

170. Yeun TST, Jua JSW, Tan TS. Spinal haematoma following epidural anaesthesia in a patient with eclampsia. *Anaesthesia* 1999;54:350–371.

170a. Sibai BM, Taslimi MM, El-Nazer A, et al. Maternal perinatal outcome associated with the syndrome of hemolysis, elevated liver enzymes, and low platelets in severe preeclampsia. *Am J Obstet Gynecol* 1986;155:501–509.

171. Crawford JS. Some maternal complications of epidural analgesia for labour. *Anaesthesia* 1985;40:1219–1225.

172. Scott DB, Hibbard BM. Serious non-fatal complications associated with extradural block in obstetric practice. *Br J Anaesth* 1990;64:537–541.

173. Ready LB, Plumer MH, Haschke RH, Austin E, Sumi SM. Neurotoxicity of intrathecal local anesthetics in rabbits. *Anesthesiology* 1985;63:364–370.

174. Renck H. Neurological complications of central nerve blocks. *Acta Anaesthesiol Scand* 1995;39:859–868.

175. Ballin NC. Paraplegia following epidural analgesia. *Anaesthesia* 1981;36:952–953.

176. Newman B. Postnatal paraparesis following epidural analgesia and forceps delivery. *Anaesthesia* 1983;38:350–351.

177. Roscoe MWA, Barrinton TW. Acute spinal subdural hematoma: A case report and review of literature. *Spine* 1984;9:672–675.

178. Lao TT, Halpern SH, MacDonald D, Huh C. Spinal subdural haematoma in a parturient after attempted epidural anaesthesia. *Can J Anaesth* 1993;40:340–345.

179. Yarnell RW, D'Alton ME. Epidural hematoma complicating cholestasis of pregnancy. *Curr Opin Obstet Gynecol* 1996;8:239–242.

179a. Cheney FW, Domino KB, Caplan RA, Posner KL. Nerve injury associated with anesthesia: A closed claims analysis. *Anesthesiology* 1999;90:1062–1069.

180. Hanley JA, Lippman-Hand A. If nothing goes wrong, is everything all right? *JAMA* 1983;249:1743–1745.

181. Sprung J, Cheng EY, Patel S. When to remove an epidural catheter in a parturient with disseminated intravascular coagulation. *Reg Anesth* 1992;17:351–354.

182. Vandermeulen EP, van Aken H, Vermylen J. Anticoagulants and spinal-epidural anesthesia. *Anesth Analg* 1994;79:1165–1177.

183. Horlocker TT. Regional anesthesia and analgesia in the patient receiving thromboprophylaxis. *Reg Anesth* 1996;21:503–507.

184. Liu SS, Mulroy MF. Neuraxial anesthesia and analgesia in the presence of standard heparin. *Reg Anesth* 1998;23(suppl 2):157–163.

185. Bromage PR, ed. Epidural chemical neurolysis: Technique. In: *Epidural Analgesia.* Philadelphia: WB Saunders; 1978:629–634.

186. Dror A, Henriksen E. Accidental epidural magnesium sulphate injection. *Anesth Analg* 1987;66:1020–1021.

187. Guiness JP, Cantees KK. Epidural injection of a phenol-containing ranitidine preparation. *Anesthesiology* 1990;73:553–555.

188. Shankar KB, Patel NV, Nishkala R. Paraplegia following epidural potassium chloride. *Anaesthesia* 1985;40:45–47.

189. Bickler P, Spear R, McKay W. Intralipid solution mistakenly infused into the epidural space. *Anesth Analg* 1990;71:712–713.

190. Patel PC, Sharif AMY, Fernando PUE. Accidental infusion of total parenteral nutrition solution through an epidural catheter. *Anesthesiology* 1984;39:383–384.

191. Brahams D. Record award for personal injuries sustained as a result of negligent administration of epidural anaesthetic. *Lancet* 1982;1:159.

192. Craig DB, Habib GG. Flaccid paraparesis following obstetrical anesthesia: Possible role of benzyl alcohol. *Anesth Analg* 1977;56:219–221.

193. Bromage PR, ed. Technique: Preliminary preparations. In: *Spinal Epidural Analgesia.* Edinburgh: E&S Livingstone; 1954:46–47.

194. Macintosh R, Lee JA. Sterilization: The operator. Technique of lumbar puncture. In: *Lumbar Puncture and Spinal Analgesia.* 3rd ed. Edinburgh: Churchill Livingstone; 1973:94–100.

195. Lee JJ, Parry H. Bacterial meningitis following spinal anaesthesia for Caesarean Section. *Br J Anaesth* 1991;66:383–386.

196. Yentis SM. Wearing of face masks for spinal anaesthesia. *Br J Anaesth* 1992;68:224.

197. Panikkar KK, Yentis SM. Wearing of masks for obstetrical regional anaesthesia. A postal survey. *Anaesthesia* 1996;51:398–400.

198. Philips BJ, Fergusson S, Armstrong P, Anderson FM, Wildsmith JAW. Surgical face masks are effective in reducing bacterial contamination caused by dispersal from upper airway. *Br J Anaesth* 1992;69:407–408.

199. McLure HA, Talboys CA, Yentis SM, Azadian BS. Surgical masks and downward dispersal of bacteria. *Anaesthesia* 1998;53:624–626.

200. North JB, Brophy BP. Epidural abscess: A hazard of spinal epidural anaesthesia. *Aust N Z J Surg* 1979;49:484–485.

201. Veringa E, van Belkum A, Schellekens H. Iatrogenic meningitis by *Streptococcus salivarius* following lumbar puncture. *J Hosp Infect* 1995;29:316–317.

202. Sakuragi T, Yanagisawa K, Dan K. Bacterial activity of skin disinfectants on methicillin resistant *Staphylococcus aureus. Anesth Analg* 1995;81:555–558.

203. Sato S, Sakuragi T, Dan K. Human skin flora as a potential source of epidural abscess. *Anesthesiology* 1996;85:1276–1282.

204. Birnbach DJ, Stein DJ, Murray O, Thys DM, Sordillo EM. Povidone iodine and skin disinfectants before initiation of epidural anesthesia. *Anesthesiology* 1998;88:668–672.

205. Bromage PR, ed. *Epidural Analgesia.* Philadelphia: WB Saunders; 1978:206–212, 716–722.

206. Aldebert S, Sleth JC. Bacterial meningitis after combined spinal and epidural anesthesia in obstetrics. *Ann Fr Anesth Reanim* 1996;15:687–688.

207. Newton JA, Lesnik TK, Kennedy CA. *Streptococcus salivarius* following spinal anaesthesia. *Clin Infect Dis* 1997;18:840–841.

208. Ready LB, Helfer D. Bacterial meningitis in parturients after epidural anesthesia. *Anesthesiology* 1989;71:988–990.

209. Berga S, Trierweiler MW. Bacterial meningitis following epidural anesthesia for vaginal delivery: A case report. *Obstet Gynecol* 1989;74:437–439.

210. Stallard N, Barry P. Another complication of the combined extradural-subarachnoid technique. *Br J Anaesth* 1995;75:370–371.

211. Roberts SP, Petts HV. Meningitis after obstetric anaesthesia. *Anaesthesia* 1990;45:376–377.

212. Harding SA, Collis RE, Morgan BM. Meningitis after combined spinal-extradural anaesthesia in obstetrics. *Br J Anaesth* 1994;73:545–547.

213. Liu SS, Pope A. Spinal meningitis masquerading as postdural puncture headache. *Anesthesiology* 1996;85:1493–1494.

214. Cascio M, Heath G. Meningitis following a combined spinal-epidural in a labouring term parturient. *Can J Anaesth* 1996;43:399–402.

215. Blackmore TK, Morley HR, Gordon DL. Streptococcus mitis-induced bacteremia and meningitis after spinal anesthesia. *Anesthesiology* 1993;78:592–594.

216. Bouhemad B, Dounas M, Mercier FJ, Benhamou D. Bacterial meningitis following combined spinal-epidural analgesia for labour. *Anaesthesia* 1998;53:292–295.

217. Davies L, Hargreaves C, Robinson PN. Postpartum meningitis. *Anaesthesia* 1993;48:788–789.

218. Laurila JJ, Kostamovaara PA, Alahuta S. *Streptococcus salivarius* meningitis after spinal anesthesia. *Anesthesiology* 1998;89:1579–1580.

219. Adams RD. Pyogenic infections of the central nervous system. In: Petersdorf RG, Adams RD, Braunwald E, Isselbacher KJ, Martin JB, Wilson JD, eds. *Harrison's Principles of Internal Medicine.* 10th ed. New York: McGraw-Hill; 1983:2084–2091.

220. Metersky ML, Williams A, Rafanan AL. Retrospective analysis: Are fever and altered mental status indications for lumbar puncture in a hospitalized patient who has not undergone neurosurgery? *Clin Infect Dis* 1997;25:285–288.

221. Ngan Kee WD, Jones MR, Thomas P, Worth RJ. Extradural abscess complicating extradural anaesthesia for caesarean section. *Br J Anaesth* 1992;69:647–652.

222. Tabo E, Ohkuma Y, Kimura S, et al. Successful percutaneous drainage of epidural abscess with epidural needle and catheter. *Anesthesiology* 1994;80:1393–1394.

223. Borum SE, McLeskey CH, Williamson JB, et al. Epidural abscess after obstetric epidural analgesia. *Anesthesiology* 1995;82:1523–1526.

224. Bromage PR. Spinal extradural abscess: Pursuit of vigilance. *Br J Anaesth* 1993;70:471–473.

225. Yuste M, Canet J, Garcia M, et al. An epidural abscess due to resistant *Staphylococcus aureus* following epidural catheterization. *Anaesthesia* 1997;52:163–165.

226. Kindler C, Seeberger M, Siegemund M, Schneider M. Extradural abscess complicating lumbar extradural anaesthesia and anal-

gesia in an obstetric patient. *Acta Anaesthesiol Scand* 1996;40:858–861.

227. Schroter J, Wa Djamba D, Hoffman V, et al. Epidural abscess after combined spinal- epidural block. *Can J Anaesth* 1997;44:300–304.

228. Knight JW, Cordingley JJ, Palazzo MGA. Epidural abscess following epidural steroid and local anaesthetic injection. *Anaesthesia* 1997;52:576–578.

229. Dysart RH, Balakrishnan V. Conservative management of extradural abscess complicating spinal-extradural anaesthesia for caesarean section. *Br J Anaesth* 1997;78:591–593.

230. Dhillon AR, Russell IF. Epidural abscess in association with obstetric epidural analgesia. *Int J Obstet Anesth* 1997;6:118–121.

231. Kindler CH, Seeberger MD, Staender SE. Epidural abscess complicating epidural anesthesia and analgesia [review]. *Acta Anaesthesiol Scand* 1998;42:614–620.

232. Tham EJ, Stoodley MA, Macintyre PE, Jones NR. Back pain following postoperative epidural analgesia: An indicator of possible spinal infection. *Anaesth Intensive Care* 1997;25:297–301.

233. Bollensen E, Menck S, Buzanoski J, Prange HW. Iatrogenic epidural spinal abscess. *Clin Invest* 1993;71:780–786.

234. McCartney C, MacLennan F. Do the risks of combined spinal-epidural analgesia in labour outweigh the benefits? *Anaesthesia* 1998;53:717–718

235. Bush DJ, Lyons G, Macdonald R. Diclofenac for analgesia after caesarean section. *Anaesthesia* 1992;47:1075–1077.

236. Bromage PR. Masked mischief. *Reg Anesth* 1996;21:62–63.

237. Sarubbi F, Vasquez J. Spinal epidural abscess associated with the use of temporary epidural catheters: Report of two cases and review. *Clin Infect Dis* 1997;25:1155–1158.

238. Holt HM, Andersen SS, Andersen O, Gahrn-Hansen B, Siboni K. Infections following epidural catheterization. *J Hosp Infect* 1995;30:253–260.

239. Rawal N, Van Zundert A, Holmström B, Crowhurst JA. Combined spinal- epidural technique. *Reg Anesth* 1997;22:406.

240. Bromage PR. Neurological complications of subarachnoid and epidural anaesthesia [editorial]. *Acta Anaesthesiol Scand* 1997;41:439–444.

241. Breivik H. Neurological complications in association with spinal and epidural analgesia–again. *Acta Anaesthesiol Scand* 1998;42:609–613.

242. Schreiner EJ, Lipson SF, Bromage PR, Camporesi EM. Neurological complications following general anaesthesia. *Anaesthesia* 1983;38:226–229.

243. Kitching A, Taylor S. A postoperative neurological problem. *Anaesthesia* 1989;44:695–696.

244. Gutowski NJ, Davies AO. Transverse myelitis following general anaesthesia. *Anaesthesia* 1993;48:44–45.

Shnider and Levinson's Anesthesia for Obstetrics,
edited by Samuel C. Hughes, et al.
Lippincott Williams & Wilkins,
Philadelphia, © 2001.

CHAPTER 24

ANESTHESIA-RELATED MATERNAL MORTALITY

JOY L. HAWKINS, M.D., GERARD M. BASSELL, M.B., B.S.,
AND GERTIE F. MARX, M.D.

THE SCOPE OF THE PROBLEM

"Reproductive" mortality is usually divided into pregnancy-related deaths (e.g., from abortion, ectopic pregnancy, and all other gestation-related causes) and contraception-related deaths (e.g., from oral drugs, intrauterine devices, and sterilization) (1). However, the postpartum duration included in this category varies widely. Although most reviews of pregnancy-related mortality have limited themselves to 6 weeks after delivery (2, 3), the Centers for Disease Control and Prevention (CDC) and others extend the period to 1 year (4). Because approximately 15% of pregnancy-related fatalities occur more than 6 weeks after parturition (for example, deaths due to peripartum cardiomyopathy) (5), extension of the tabulation period past that point should be the aim.

Pregnancy-related deaths have been classified as direct (i.e., due to true obstetric causes such as uterine hemorrhage); indirect (i.e., due to nonobstetric causes such as preexisting or incidental medical disease); or unrelated, such as an unplanned accident ("unplanned" because both suicide and homicide may be consequent to the pregnancy, i.e., indirect). In general, deaths from anesthesia have been classified as indirect (6). The International Classification of Diseases, 9th Division, Clinical Modification (ICD-9-CM) lists anesthesia as a separate cause of maternal mortality (Table 24.1).

The Maternal Mortality Rate is traditionally defined as the number of maternal deaths divided by the number of live births during the same reporting period. It provides a ratio, not a true rate, because the denominator does not include the entire population at risk for the outcome described by the numerator (i.e., not all deaths are associated with a "live birth"). In the United States the collection of maternal mortality statistics began in 1915, when mandatory registration of live births was instituted (see Figure 11.3). In the United Kingdom, triennial "Reports on Confidential Enquiries into Maternal Deaths in England and Wales" (CEMD) have been available since 1952. For international comparisons, England and Wales were chosen as a "standard" population for the following reasons: (a) there was dependable registration; (b) a large population with practically no annual fluctuations in the age-specific rate could be studied; (c) age distribution was nonextreme; and (d) mortality was of the same order as that in the Netherlands and Scandinavia (7). These CEMD reports cover between 1.9 and 2.7 million births per triennium. To date, 15 triennial reports have been published (14–28), the first for the years 1952–54, and the most recent for the period 1994–96. The maternal mortality data for the years 1985–87 were combined for the first time in a single report for the four countries comprising the United Kingdom (England, Wales, Scotland, and Northern Ireland) (25). This was made possible, even necessary, by the progressive decline in the number of maternal deaths in Scotland and Northern Ireland, which made maintenance of confidentiality in those countries difficult.

The U.S. maternal mortality was stable, at approximately 60 per 10,000, until the 1930s (6), when a progressive decline began that intensified following World War II. Since then, as in other developed nations, substantial reductions in mortality have been registered in the areas of infection, preeclampsia, and in-hospital hemorrhage so that the current U.S. rate has fallen to 7.5 per 100,000 (8, 9). Fatalities related to the administration of anesthesia have paralleled the overall reduction in pregnancy-related mortality (10–13). To exemplify these trends, maternal deaths over the 20-year period of 1946–65 were reviewed (11). The total obstetric mortality per 10,000 live births declined from 18.3 during 1946–50 to 13.7 during 1951–55, 9.6 during 1956–60, and 7.4 during 1961–65. The corresponding rates for anesthesia-related maternal mortality were reduced from 0.54 per 10,000 live births to 0.41, 0.28, and 0.19, respectively. Thus, the overall reduction in mortality over the 20-year term of the review was between 35% and 40% for both obstetric and anesthetic causes.

Similarly, during the first 45 years of the CEMD reports, pregnancy-related mortality decreased from 68 per 100,000 total births in 1952 to 9.9 in 1994–96 (14–28). The rate of decline has been maintained at approximately 20% per triennium. Recently, an encouraging trend has been apparent in the statistics from England and Wales. During the period 1970–96, the anesthesia-associated death rate (per million pregnancies) has fallen from 12.8 in the 1970–72 triennium to 10.5, 12.1, 8.7, 7.2, 1.9, 1.7, 3.5, and 0.5 during the subsequent triennia through 1996 (28). The contribution of anesthesia to the overall number of direct maternal deaths has declined as well from a high of 13% to a low of 0.8% in 1994–96. Although statistically accurate comparisons between the triennia cannot be made, the decreases in the anesthesia-associated death rate have occurred during a period when the number of anesthetics administered to gravidas has increased tremendously. Thus, the improvement is probably greater than that suggested by the falling death rate alone. In the most recent review of maternal mortality trends in Israel, overall maternal mortality decreased 25% between 1975 and 1995 (29). Anesthesia-related deaths fell from 11% in 1975–83 to 0% in 1990–95; i.e., there were no maternal deaths due to anesthesia in the most recent period studied.

Anesthesia-related maternal mortality rates are improving in the United States as well, but anesthesia remains a prominent cause of pregnancy-related mortality. In 1987, the CDC established an ongoing National Pregnancy Mortality Surveillance System, which monitors maternal deaths at the national level and conducts epidemiologic studies of the deaths of pregnant women (30). Retrospective data were collected on deaths for the period 1979–86; data collection has been prospective for deaths since 1987. Health departments in all 50 states, the District of Columbia, and New York City have provided the CDC with copies of death certificates (with patient and provider information removed) and, when available, the linked pregnancy

---

Table 24.1. THE INTERNATIONAL CLASSIFICATION OF DISEASES, 9TH REVISION, CLINICAL MODIFICATION (ICD-9-CM)

---

668   Complications of the administration of anesthetic or other sedation in labor and delivery
             Include: Complications arising from the administration of a general or local anesthetic,
                      analgesic, or other sedation in labor and delivery
             Exclude: Reaction to spinal block or lumbar puncture (349.0)
668.0   Pulmonary complications
             Inhalations or aspiration of stomach contents or secretions following anesthesia or
                sedation in labor and delivery
             Mendelson's syndrome
             Pressure collapse of lung
668.1   Cardiac complications
             Cardiac arrest or failure following anesthesia or other sedation in labor and delivery
668.2   Central nervous system complications
             Cerebral anoxia
668.8   Other complications of anesthesia or other sedation in labor and delivery
668.9   Unspecified complications of anesthesia and other sedation
349   Other and unspecified disorders of the nervous system
349.0   Reaction to spinal or lumbar puncture

---

outcome records (birth certificates and fetal death records) for all identified pregnancy-related deaths from 1979 to 1996. In addition, state maternal mortality review committees, the media, and individuals have reported cases not otherwise identified. The collection system is far from perfect, and it has been estimated that as many as 37% (31) of maternal deaths may be missed or misclassified because the relationship to pregnancy is not noted.

Deaths are considered pregnancy-related if they occur during pregnancy or within 1 year of pregnancy termination and result from (a) complications of the pregnancy itself, (b) a chain of events initiated by the pregnancy, or (c) the aggravation of an unrelated condition by the physiologic or pharmacologic effects of pregnancy (8). Clinical epidemiologists review each pregnancy-related death certificate and, when available (89% of anesthesia cases), the matched pregnancy outcome record. According to the system developed by the American College of

Obstetricians and Gynecologists (ACOG)/CDC Maternal Mortality Study Group, information on all deaths is reviewed by clinically experienced epidemiologists as to cause of death, associated obstetric conditions, and the outcome of pregnancy. Data are coded after review of all available information (including cause of death codes, notes and other information written on the certificate, linked birth and fetal death certificates, and any other information available).

In the United States, anesthesia is the sixth leading cause of maternal death behind hemorrhage, embolism, pregnancy-induced hypertension complications, infection, and cardiomyopathy (Fig. 24.1). From 1987 to 1990, anesthesia complications accounted for 2.5% of maternal deaths overall (8): 1.8% of "undelivered" deaths, 1.9% of ectopic deaths, 2.8% of live births, and 8.6% of abortion deaths (Table 24.2). When anesthesia deaths during 1979–90 were analyzed, the maternal mortality rates showed a similar decline to those in Great Britain, from

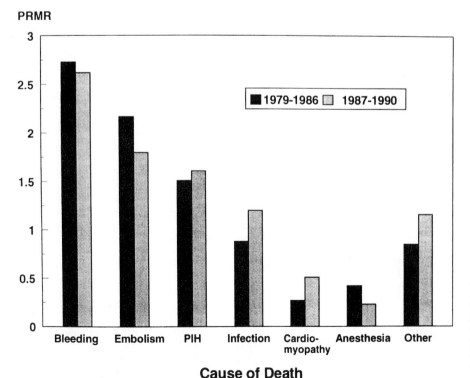

Figure 24.1. Cause-specific pregnancy-related mortality ratios (PRMR) for 1979–86 and 1987–90, United States. *PIH,* pregnancy-induced hypertension; *PRMR,* pregnancy-related deaths per 100,000 live births. (Reprinted by permission from Berg CJ, Atrash HK, Koonin LM, Tucker M. Pregnancy-related mortality in the United States, 1987–1990. *Obstet Gynecol* 1996; 88:161–167.)

Table 24.2. CAUSES OF PREGNANCY-RELATED DEATH BY OUTCOME OF PREGNANCY, UNITED STATES, 1987–90

	% Live Births	% Undelivered	% Ectopic	% Abortions	% Total
Hemorrhage	21	15	95	19	29
Embolism	23	34	1	11	20
PIH	24	5	0	1	18
Infection	12	13	1	49	13
Cardiomyopathy	6	3	0	0	6
Anesthesia	3	2	2	9	3

PIH = pregnancy-induced hypertension.
Reprinted by permission from Berg JC, Atrash HK, Koonin LM, Tucker M. Pregnancy-related mortality in the U.S., 1987–1990. *Obstet Gynecol* 1996;88:161–167.

Table 24.3. ANESTHESIA-RELATED MATERNAL MORTALITY RATES FOR THE UNITED STATES AND ENGLAND AND WALES BY TRIENNIUM, 1979–90

Triennium	United States*	England and Wales[†]
1979–81	4.3	8.7
1982–84	3.3	7.2
1985–87	2.3	1.9
1988–90	1.7	1.7

*Per million live births.
[†]Estimated rate per million maternities.
Reprinted by permission from Hawkins JL, Koonin LM, Palmer SK, Gibbs CP. Anesthesia-related deaths during obstetric delivery in the United States, 1979–1990. *Anesthesiology* 1997;86:277–284.

4.3 per million live births in the years 1979–81 to 1.7 per million live births in the years 1988–90 (Table 24.3) (32). A more striking finding was the difference in deaths associated with general vs. regional anesthesia. Although the number of maternal deaths due to general anesthesia remained constant over the period studied, the number of deaths associated with regional anesthesia declined markedly (Fig. 24.2). This occurred despite a large increase in the use of regional anesthesia for cesarean section

in virtually every hospital in the United States (33). The calculated risk ratio between deaths due to general and regional anesthesia was 2.3:1 in the earlier time period (1979–84) vs. 16.7:1 in the later time period (1985–90) (Table 24.4). Similarly, in the CEMD reports from 1967 to 1984, problems during general anesthesia accounted for 96% of anesthetic-related maternal mortality.

The decline in deaths associated with regional anesthesia occurred in the mid1980s, coincident with the withdrawal of 0.75% bupivacaine, and was probably due to increasing awareness of local anesthetic toxicity and use of test dosing. A review of almost 11,000 epidurals for obstetric cases (with data collected prospectively from 1989 to 1994) contained no maternal mortalities (34). The incidence of potentially life-threatening morbidity was 0.02%: eight unexpectedly high blocks and 3 patients with mild respiratory depression after postoperative epidural opioid. There was no major local anesthetic toxicity.

The calculated risk ratios show that general anesthesia is more likely to be associated with maternal mortality than is regional anesthesia in the obstetric patient. There are several reasons why that might be. First, during general anesthesia the airway must always be managed, and airway management is more difficult in the obstetric patient. Airway problems were by far the most common cause of anesthesia-related deaths. General anesthesia

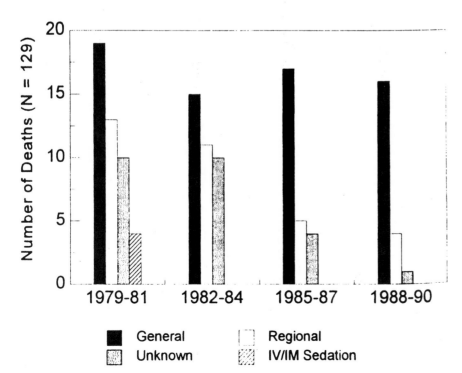

Figure 24.2. Anesthesia-related maternal deaths by types of anesthesia, United States, 1979–90 (Reprinted by permission from Hawkins JL, Koonin LM, Palmer SK, Gibbs CP. Anesthesia-related deaths during obstetric delivery in the United States, 1979–1990. *Anesthesiology* 1997;86:277–284.)

Table 24.4. NUMBERS, CASE FATALITY RATES, AND RISK RATIOS OF ANESTHESIA-RELATED DEATHS DURING CESAREAN SECTION DELIVERY BY TYPE OF ANESTHESIA, UNITED STATES, 1979–84 AND 1985–90

	No. of Deaths		Case Fatality Rate		Risk Ratio	
	1979–84	1985–90	1979–84	1985–90	1979–84	1985–90
General	33	32	20.0* (95% CI, 17.7–22.7)	32.3* (95% CI, 25.9–49.3)	2.3 (95% CI, 1.9–2.9)	16.7 (95% CI, 12.9–21.8)
Regional	19	9	8.6† (95% CI, 1.8–9.4)	1.9† (95% CI, 1.8–2.0)	Referent	Referent

CI = confidence interval.
*Per million general anesthetics for cesarean section.
†Per million regional anesthetics for cesarean section.
Reprinted by permission from Hawkins JL, Koonin LM, Palmer SK, Gibbs C. Anesthesia-related deaths during obstetric delivery in the United States, 1979–1990. *Anesthesiology* 1997,86:277–284.

is often chosen in emergencies, when preparation and examination of the patient are not optimal. General anesthesia is used in patients who have failed regional anesthesia (due to obesity) or have contraindications to its use (preeclampsia or HELLP syndrome [hemolysis, elevated liver enzymes, and low platelet count occurring in association with preeclampsia]), and these patients may have increased risk factors for a difficult airway as well. And finally, general anesthesia is not used as often in residency training programs on their obstetric rotations because regional anesthesia is preferred by anesthesiologists, patients, and obstetricians.

In England and Wales, during the years 1970–78, nearly 10 times as many deaths were related to general vs. regional anesthesia: 40 mortalities were caused by inhalation of gastric contents, of which 28 were due to intubation problems and only seven were due to complications of regional block (Table 24.5) (20–22). In the 1991–93 report (27), of the eight deaths directly attributable to anesthesia, seven occurred during or immediately after general anesthesia, and one occurred when epidural anesthesia was performed without an intravenous line and hypotension led to cardiac arrest. In the 1994–96 report, there was only one death related (indirectly) to anesthesia, a remarkable achievement (Table 24.6) (28).

Table 24.6. DEATH RATES PER MILLION BY CAUSE OF DEATH, MATERNITIES IN THE UNITED KINGDOM 1985–96

	Rate			
Cause	1985–87	1988–90	1991–93	1994–96
Thromboembolism	14.6	14.0	15.1	21.8
Pregnancy-induced hypertension	11.9	11.4	8.6	9.1
Hemorrhage	4.4	9.3	6.5	5.5
Amniotic fluid embolism	4.0	4.7	4.3	7.7
Early pregnancy	10.6	10.2	7.8	6.8
Sepsis	2.6	3.0	3.9	6.4
Anesthetic	2.6	1.7	3.5	0.5
Cardiac, indirect	10.1	8.9	16.0	17.7
Psychiatric, indirect				4.1
Total direct and indirect	99.6	100.9	98.9	121.9

Data represent a summary of recent triennial reports into maternal deaths in the United Kingdom. Table modified (with additions) from May A. Confidential Enquiries Into Maternal Deaths 1994–1996. *Int J Obstet Anesth* 1999;8:77–78.

Table 24.5. MATERNAL DEATHS DIRECTLY ATTRIBUTABLE TO ANESTHESIA

Cause	1973–75	1976–78	1985–87	1988–90	1991–93	1994–96
Inhalation of stomach contents during induction of anesthesia	9	4	1	1	0	0
Inhalation of stomach contents during difficult intubation	4	7	0	1	0	0
Hypoxia due to esophageal/ failed intubation	3	9	6	1	0	0
Misuse of drugs	4	3	0	0	0	0
Accidents with apparatus	2	2	0	0	0	0
Subarachnoid injection of anesthetic during attempted epidural block	2	1	0	0	0	0
Miscellaneous causes*	7	4	1	2	8	1
Total	31	30	8	5	8	1

*Miscellaneous causes included allergic reaction, inadequate reversal of muscle relaxant, intravenous overload, postoperative asphyxial episode, and mismanagement of epidural block in a patient with cardiac disease. The one death in the most recent report appears in the "miscellaneous" category since it exhibited features of excessive drug dosage, inappropriate management of regional block, misuse of drugs, and "unconventional" resuscitation.
Data from Confidential Enquiries Into Maternal Deaths in England and Wales reports 1973–1975, 1976–1978, 1985–1987, 1988–1990, 1991–1993, and 1994–1996 (21, 22, 25–28).

CAUSES OF ANESTHESIA-RELATED MATERNAL MORTALITY
Deaths Resulting From General Anesthesia
Pulmonary Aspiration of Gastric Contents

A review of maternal deaths in the United States found aspiration (usually accompanied by a difficult intubation) to be the leading cause of anesthesia-related maternal mortality (31). The anatomic and physiologic changes occurring in the gastrointestinal tract during pregnancy make regurgitation of gastric contents during anesthesia more likely in gravid women than in nonpregnant patients, and should pulmonary aspiration occur, its effects can be more severe. A number of phenomena of both mechanical and hormonal origin account for this. First, the rate of gastric emptying and transit time of bowel contents may be increased during pregnancy. These changes are heightened during labor by the effects of pain and anxiety, the recumbent position, and opioid medications used for the systemic relief of pain (35). Second, the likelihood of regurgitation is enhanced by the progressive pressure of the uterus and abdominal contents on the stomach, changing its axis from the vertical to the horizontal. At the same time, tonus at the gastroesophageal junction is decreased and pressure within the stomach is increased, particularly in the lithotomy position (36). Third, the hormonally induced reduction in gastric tone and motility make nausea, vomiting, and reflux more likely (37). Finally, although acid and pepsin secretions by the stomach are diminished during the major portion of pregnancy, toward term they tend to increase to above-normal levels (38). Thus, should pulmonary aspiration occur intrapartum, the severity of lung injury could well be greater than it would have been earlier in pregnancy. Therefore, parturients must always be considered to have a full stomach, and the gastric contents must be expected to be particularly hazardous.

Pulmonary aspiration of gastric contents can occur following either regurgitation, a passive process, or vomiting, an active one. The quality and volume of aspirate are the major determinants of the type and severity of sequelae. Thus, the inhalation of solid foodstuffs has the propensity for producing airway obstruction, varying degrees of pulmonary collapse, mediastinal shift, and reflex bronchospasm. Bronchoscopic removal of aspirated material allows for reinflation of collapsed pulmonary segments and is the appropriate therapeutic maneuver in this situation. Inhalation of liquid gastric juice, particularly with a pH of 2.5 or less, produces the pulmonary acid aspiration (Mendelson's) syndrome (39). Here, acid injury of the bronchial mucosa is the primary insult and causes bronchiolar spasm, peribronchiolar exudates, focal hemorrhages, and areas of parenchymal necrosis. Therapeutic intervention is aimed at ventilatory support; antibiotics and steroids are not indicated. Complete large airway obstruction or aspiration of a volume of acidic gastric juice sufficient to flood both lungs can result in hypoxic cardiac arrest.

Since the increased risk of pulmonary aspiration during the peripartum period was first recognized, significant advances have been made in its prevention. The hazards of aspirating gastric contents should be explained during "preparation for childbirth" classes, and women should be warned to avoid ingestion of all but small amounts of clear liquids once labor is imminent. The ACOG's *Guidelines for Perinatal Care*, 4th ed. (GPC) notes, "By early in the third trimester, patient education should include information about the following points: . . . The consequences of ingesting solid food after the onset of labor, given that a general anesthetic could be required for the delivery" (40). The incidence of vomiting caused by dehydration and ketosis has been reduced by the widespread use of intravenous hydration with dextrose-containing balanced salt solutions, and vomiting caused by emotional stress or opioid analgesics has been ameliorated by the employment of small doses of tranquilizers with antiemetic properties when indicated. GPC also states, "Patients in active labor should avoid oral ingestion of anything except sips

of clear liquids, occasional ice chips, or preparations for moistening the mouth and lips. When significant amounts of hydration and energy substrate are needed because of a long labor, they should be given by intravenous infusion" (39). The possibility of regurgitation can also be decreased by attending to those factors that make it more likely to occur. Thus, avoidance of further increases of intragastric pressure, relative to esophageal pressure, is of paramount importance unless the parturient's protective airway reflexes are known to be intact. The use of suprafundal pressure should be restricted to conscious parturients or those whose airway has been protected by a cuffed endotracheal tube.

Prevention of vomiting or regurgitation is only one of the series of maneuvers that can be expected to reduce the incidence of aspiration pneumonitis in pregnancy. Occlusion of the cervical esophagus with the cricoid cartilage (Sellick's maneuver) deters the passage of regurgitated contents into the nasopharynx and from there into the lower airway. This technique should be a component of all general anesthetics administered to gravidas from the mid–second trimester until 2 to 3 days postpartum. Pressure on the cricoid cartilage should be applied by a skilled assistant from the time of injection of the drug used for anesthetic induction, and should be maintained until the anesthesiologist has inflated the cuff of the endotracheal tube and demonstrated its proper placement with capnography. A modification of Sellick's maneuver offers two advantages. By placing the palm of the assistant's hand flat against the patient's anterior chest wall under the surgical drapes and using the palmar aspects of the index and middle fingers for the compression (Fig. 24.3), interference with the laryngoscope handle is avoided and large breasts are spread apart by the assistant's forearm (41). If appropriately skilled personnel adhere to these guidelines, "it is certain that gastric aspiration into the lungs during anaesthesia is preventable" (42).

Forestalling the passage of gastric contents into the airway is obviously the most important factor in avoiding the pulmonary aspiration syndrome. In recent years, however, much work has centered on methods of decreasing the volume and acidity of gastric contents in an attempt to lessen the severity of lung injury should they be inhaled. Oral administration of antacids during labor has been shown to decrease gastric juice acidity, and nonparticulate antacids may be less harmful to the pulmonary parenchyma than particulate ones if aspirated (43–45). GPC states, "Aspiration is a significant leading cause of anesthetic-related maternal mortality and morbidity, and the aspiration of acidic gastric contents with a pH of less than 2.5 is more harmful than the aspiration of less acidic gastric contents. Therefore, prophylactic administration of an antacid before induction of a major regional or general anesthetic is appropriate. Particulate

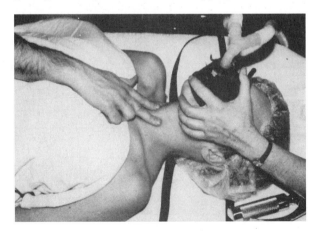

Figure 24.3. Modification of Sellick's maneuver. The assistant places the palmar surface of the hand to the anterior aspect of the patient's chest wall. The palmar aspects of the index and middle fingers, each slightly to either side of the middle of the arch of the cricoid cartilage, are used to press the cricoid posteriorly onto the esophagus.

antacids may be harmful if aspirated; a clear antacid, such as a solution of 0.3 mol/L sodium citrate or a similar preparation, may be a safer choice" (40). Maneuvers such as turning the gravida from side to side to ensure thorough mixing of the antacid with contents of both antral and fundal gastric pouches can further improve acid neutralization (46). Yet deaths caused by maternal aspiration pneumonitis still occur, even after the routine administration of oral antacids during labor (47).

Pharmacologic methods of aiding stomach emptying or reducing the volume and acidity of gastric contents have received much recent attention. Metoclopramide, a propulsive agent also used for diabetics with gastroparesis, can be helpful in decreasing gastric volume in pregnancy (48). Cimetidine, a H2 receptor antagonist, although efficient in reducing gastric volume and acidity (49), may impair hepatic metabolism of hypnotic or opioid drugs. Although cimetidine crosses the placenta this effect to the newborn, is probably not of clinical significance in single doses. Ranitidine and other histamine-2 receptor antagonists with a structure different from that of cimetidine do not adversely affect oxidative or conjugative metabolism (50). Despite their popularity, the value of histamine-2 receptor antagonists in reducing gastric volume and acidity during labor and their routine use to prevent acid-aspiration pneumonitis remain controversial.

Despite the dissemination of information concerning the pathophysiology of the acid-aspiration syndrome in pregnancy, fatalities continue to occur. More frequent use of regional analgesia during labor, vaginal delivery, and cesarean section can be expected to reduce the incidence of the syndrome. In those clinical situations in which conduction block cannot be used and general anesthesia is required, endotracheal intubation is mandatory with the precautions against regurgitation and aspiration outlined earlier to be used by skilled, knowledgeable operators.

Inability to Intubate the Trachea

Passage of an endotracheal tube has become an accepted part of the technique of general anesthesia in obstetrics, but "failure to achieve successful endotracheal intubation is now an important contributor to maternal death" (51). A recent analysis of anesthetic maternal mortalities found "airway problems" to be the most common category of causes (32). Anatomic abnormalities of the face, neck, or upper airway are the most common causes of difficulty in intubating the trachea. GPC provides a list of items that should alert the obstetric care provider to "increased risk from anesthesia and should be communicated to the anesthesia care provider in advance of delivery to permit formulation of a management plan" (40). Particular care must be taken in assessing the gravida's airway anatomy before induction of general anesthesia. If anatomic abnormalities are present, awake endotracheal intubation provides a safer alternative to the usual method (Table 24.7) (52).

Table 24.7. RELATIVE RISK FACTORS ASSOCIATED WITH DIFFICULTY AT TRACHEAL INTUBATION COMPARED WITH UNCOMPLICATED MALLAMPATI CLASS I = 1

Risk Factor	Relative Risk
Mallampati Class	
II	3.23
III	7.58
IV	11.30
Short neck	5.01
Receding mandible	9.71
Protruding maxillary incisors	8.00

Reprinted by permission from Rocke DA, Murray WB, Rout CC, Gouws E. Relative risk analysis of factors associated with difficult intubation in obstetric anesthesia. *Anesthesiology* 1992;77:67–73.

Pregnancy can pose additional problems in achieving safe isolation of the airway. The combination of large breasts and an increased anteroposterior thoracic diameter can severely reduce the room available for manipulation of the laryngoscope handle. These impediments can be ameliorated somewhat by holding or taping large breasts laterally and caudally. Also, a short laryngoscope handle (53) may allow an increased range of movement during difficult airway manipulation. Edema of the laryngeal mucosa occurs in all term-pregnant gravidas to some degree, but it is usually of greater amount and is more often the cause of problems in the preeclamptic woman and, occasionally, in healthy gravidas following prolonged, strenuous bearing-down efforts or during upper respiratory infections (54). If the preeclampsia is severe, swelling of the epiglottis may make visualization of the larynx more difficult than expected, but the more usual problem is a reduction in the caliber of the airway, resulting in an inability to pass an endotracheal tube of anticipated size. Routine endotracheal intubation in late pregnancy should be accomplished with a tube 0.5 to 1 mm smaller than that used for a similarly sized nonpregnant woman, and preeclamptic gravidas can be expected to require an even smaller tube if the airway is to be secured easily and atraumatically.

Despite the above precautions, difficulties with endotracheal intubation have been encountered after anesthesia has been induced. The incidence of failed intubation during obstetric anesthesia has been reported to be approximately eight times that encountered in surgical patients (55). Endobronchial intubation is more hazardous in the parturient because of the pregnancy-induced decrease in functional residual capacity (reducing oxygen storage) and increase in metabolic rate (increasing oxygen use) (56). It is of paramount importance to delay skin incision until successful endotracheal intubation has been confirmed by appropriate auscultation of the upper chest bilaterally, aided by proof of CO_2 exhalation by capnography (57). This allows for discontinuation of the anesthetic and a change in technique should intubation prove impossible. Under such circumstances, the parturient should be allowed to regain consciousness so that awake placement of the endotracheal tube can be tried or a regional technique chosen. If surgery has begun before the larynx has been intubated, or if the surgical indication is a maternal life-threatening one (e.g., severe hemorrhage, uterine rupture), the anesthetic can be continued by mask with maintenance of cricoid pressure or laryngeal mask airway (58) and assisted ventilation (but without further muscle relaxant). Safety of the airway must be guaranteed as soon as possible, however, either by passage of an endotracheal tube over a fiberoptic bronchoscope or through the laryngeal mask airway. Cricothyrotomy may be necessary in a "can't intubate–can't ventilate" situation. Every labor suite should have the instruments required for emergency tracheostomy, and each delivery room should be equipped with a means of providing temporary transtracheal ventilation (58). The American Society of Anesthesiologists' (ASA) difficult airway algorithm can be adapted for use in the obstetric patient (see Chapter 21) (57).

A review of general anesthesia use during cesarean section from a tertiary care hospital provides a telling case report of a failed intubation–failed ventilation scenario: "... a 39-year-old multiparous woman presented for elective cesarean section for a term fetus in a breech presentation during normal day shift hours (7 a.m.–3 p.m.). Multiple failed attempts at placing a spinal anesthetic in this 152 cm (5′), 68.5 kg (151 lb) woman with a class II airway resulted in the decision to proceed with general anesthesia. After preoxygenation, a rapid sequence induction, a total of five attempts at intubation with different laryngoscope blades, an unsuccessful mask airway, a failed Combitube placement, and an unsuccessful cricothyroidotomy, the parturient went into cardiopulmonary arrest. A surgical tracheostomy was completed and cardiac resuscitation accomplished, but the patient remained in a coma until death occurred 7 days later" (59).

Deaths Resulting From Regional Analgesia

Cardiovascular Collapse

There are several reasons for the precipitous decline in regional anesthetic deaths (Fig. 24.2). For example, the realization that gravidas require smaller amounts of local anesthetic than do nonpregnant women to produce a similar dermatome level has led to a decrease in the incidence of excessively high levels of spinal block. The occurrence of significant hypotension as a complication of sympathetic blockade has been reduced by the more widespread use of adequate intravenous fluid preloading and prevention of aortocaval compression by uterine displacement.

Decreased Drug Requirement. During pregnancy, a smaller dose of spinally or epidurally administered local anesthetic is required to achieve the desired level of neural blockade. Drug requirement falls to about two thirds of the usual dose by the third trimester. This phenomenon was first noted clinically but has since been confirmed by three separate studies. When continuous, selective spinal blockade with 0.2% procaine was compared in 10 women prepartum and again postpartum, at least twice the amount of local anesthetic was required to produce sensory analgesia to the fourth cervical dermatome when the measurements were taken approximately 48 hours after delivery (60). Also, when the spread of lumbar epidural analgesia was ascertained in a large number of surgical patients and gravid women after injection of various local anesthetics through wide-bore needles, pregnancy-related discrepancies in the extent of sensory levels were noted (61). For example, a nonpregnant woman of specific age and height in whom blockade to the tenth thoracic dermatome was achieved with 20 mL 2% lidocaine needed only 14 mL to produce the same extent of denervation when pregnant at term. Finally, in a comparison of the effects of equal doses of spinal anesthetic (hyperbaric tetracaine, 5 mg) administered under identical conditions to obstetric and young gynecologic patients, a significantly more rapid onset, higher level, and longer duration of blockade were produced in the parturients (62).

This altered response appears to be a direct consequence of the physiologic changes induced by gestation. Reduced buffer capacity caused by hyperventilation-induced compensated alkalemia may allow a local anesthetic to remain a salt for a longer time and, therefore, to persist in the compartment of injection for a prolonged period (63). The increased progesterone concentrations of pregnancy can affect smooth muscle behavior and the structure and function of neurons (64). Over the course of gestation, plasma progesterone undergoes a more than 30-fold increase from a nonpregnant level of less than $3 \, ng \cdot mL^{-1}$ to more than $100 \, ng \cdot mL^{-1}$. At the same time, cerebrospinal fluid concentrations rise from 0.4 to $3.0 \, ng \cdot mL^{-1}$ (65). Epidural venous distention can reduce the capacity of both the epidural and subarachnoid spaces, thus enhancing the spread of local anesthetic solutions, and retarded meningeal capillary circulation may delay drug absorption, thereby prolonging the duration of analgesia (66). The increased degree of lumbar lordosis that occurs during pregnancy may promote an exaggerated cephalad spread of the anesthetic. Inferior vena caval compression plays only an indirect role in that the resultant redistribution of a portion of the venous return to the paravertebral system of veins may produce a further diminution in epidural and subarachnoid space capacities (67). However, reduced drug requirement is unrelated to maternal position and persists despite immediate displacement of the uterus once the anesthetic has been injected. In fact, the decrease in drug requirement for regional block can be demonstrated as early as the latter part of the first trimester before the onset of aortocaval compression and is maintained into the early postpartum period. Thus, 23 women receiving epidural analgesia at 8 to 12 weeks of pregnancy had a drug requirement of $21.3 \pm 2.1 \, mg$ lidocaine per spinal segment, whereas in 12 nonpregnant con-

trols the corresponding amount was $27.1 \pm 2.4 \, mg$ ($P < .001$) (63). In women undergoing postpartum tubal ligation, analysis of the extent and duration of epidural or spinal blockade revealed a progressive decline in both variables over the first 3 postpartum days (67). It may be significant that the mother's venous distensibility undergoes an almost parallel decrease (68).

Intravenous Fluid Preloading. Sympathetic blockade produces postarteriolar pooling of blood, thereby decreasing effective circulating blood volume. When a large area of the vascular bed is denervated in this manner, venous return to the heart can be reduced. In addition, vascular tone depends more on sympathetic control during pregnancy than it does in the nongravid state. These factors, combined with the effects of the caval component of aortocaval compression, make the pregnant woman more susceptible to the arterial pressure–lowering effects of sympathetic blockade. Thus, hypotension is liable to develop at sensory levels of analgesia that would not cause hypotension in nonpregnant women.

Following the demonstration that intravenous fluid administration was effective in reversing the blood pressure fall occurring after spinal anesthesia in pregnant ewes (69), human studies in term-pregnant gravidas were undertaken. In women undergoing elective cesarean section under spinal anesthesia, 1 L lactated Ringer's solution, as an intravenous preload before injection of the anesthetic, reduced the incidence of significant hypotension (70). Other studies demonstrated that ephedrine was not predictably effective in treating block-induced hypotension unless acute intravenous hydration accompanied its use. This unreliability occurred even when large doses of the drug were administered. However, when concomitant fluid administration was employed, ephedrine proved to be effective both prophylactically and therapeutically (71).

Several investigations have indeed confirmed the efficacy of intravenous prehydration in reducing both the incidence of postblock hypotension and its deleterious effect on the uteroplacental circulation. In one study, maternal blood pressure and fetal heart rate were recorded in 104 parturients who received epidural analgesia during labor. Although all the women were lying on their left sides throughout, only 51 received an intravenous preload of 1 L balanced salt solution just before the local anesthetic was injected. Their incidence of maternal hypotension was significantly lower when compared with that in the nonhydrated gravidas (72). Another investigation employed the intravenous radioactive-xenon method to assess the effect of epidural block on placental intervillous blood flow (73). Thirty-eight healthy women scheduled for elective cesarean section were studied. Of these, 24 gravidas selected epidural block and were divided into two groups. The first 11 women received $10 \, ml \cdot kg^{-1}$ intravenously of a plasma expander within 10 minutes of institution of the block; the other 13 received no fluid preload. The remaining 14 parturients chose general anesthesia and functioned as controls; in them, anesthesia was induced at the conclusion of the blood flow measurements. When the epidural block was administered without a preceding intravenous fluid bolus, maternal mean arterial pressure and intervillous blood flow underwent significant decreases. In contrast, measurements of intervillous blood flow in the preloaded group were comparable to those in the control patients, and arterial pressures declined only to a slight degree. In yet another study, 60 women scheduled for elective cesarean section received 2 L balanced salt solution immediately before institution of an epidural block (74). Systolic blood pressure declined less than 10% from control levels in 78% of the women, and despite infusion of a relatively large volume of crystalloid solution, central venous pressure, measured in 20 of the gravidas, rose from an initial mean level of 4.05 ± 0.5 to a mean of $5.72 \pm 0.5 \, cm \, H_2O$ after the establishment of the epidural block. This confirms the safety of intravenous fluid preloading in healthy parturients.

However, more recent studies have not been able to show that fluid preload reliably prevents hypotension (75, 76). Rout et al. randomized patients to receive either no preload or 20 ml · kg^{-1} crystalloid administered over 15 to 20 minutes before spinal anesthesia for elective cesarean section (75). Hypotension occurred in 55% of preloaded patients and 71% of unpreloaded patients, a statistically significant difference of 16%. However, there was no difference in severity, timing, or duration of hypotension; amount of ephedrine given; or condition of the neonate. They concluded that hypotension cannot be eliminated by preloading and questioned whether administration of a fixed volume before spinal anesthesia for urgent cases should be considered mandatory. Ueyama et al. randomly allocated parturients to receive either 1.5 L crystalloid, 0.5 L colloid, or 1.0 L colloid prior to spinal anesthesia for elective cesarean section (76). Blood volume and cardiac output were measured noninvasively. Hypotension was prevented only in those patients exhibiting a significant increase in blood volume and cardiac output. The incidence of hypotension was 75% in the crystalloid group, 58% in the 0.5 L colloid group, and 17% in the 1.0 L colloid group. In short, there is no method guaranteed to prevent spinal hypotension. Maternal blood pressure must be followed closely following placement of the regional block and hypotension treated aggressively with ephedrine, or if needed, phenylephrine.

Adequate displacement of the uterus from the great vessels is a prerequisite both for the avoidance of block-induced hypotension and for the initiation of therapy if a fall in blood pressure occurs. It should be obvious that the aggressive administration of intravenous fluids and ephedrine will be to no avail unless there is unimpeded return of blood from the lower extremities to the right side of the heart. In the vast majority of gravidas, uterine displacement should be to the left (away from the vena cava). This can be achieved most efficiently by elevating the right hip with a wedge and tilting the delivery table to the left. During an episode of severe hypotension, it may also be useful to elevate the parturient's legs to facilitate venous return.

LOCAL ANESTHETIC TOXICITY

Since the introduction into clinical practice of the highly lipid-soluble and protein-bound amide local anesthetics, a number of cases of fatal cardiac arrest have occurred in pregnant women exposed to bupivacaine. Typically, cardiovascular collapse, often following a brief grand mal seizure, has followed unintended intravascular injection or rapid absorption of this potent, long-lasting drug from the epidural space during attempted lumbar or caudal epidural block (77). Electrocardiographic patterns have included asystole, ventricular tachycardia, ventricular fibrillation, and complete atrioventricular dissociation, sometimes with only P waves present. Difficult resuscitation has been the norm, with prolonged external cardiac compression and frequent countershock often required (78). All three commercially available concentrations of bupivacaine have been involved, albeit to different extents. The majority of cases have occurred with the 0.75% concentration.

A representative case was described as follows. A healthy gravida chose epidural anesthesia for her elective cesarean section at term. Sixty seconds after a test-dose of 4 mL 0.75% bupivacaine, the therapeutic dose of 16 mL was injected. Thirty seconds later, one severe convulsion developed and was followed instantaneously by cardiac asystole. Immediate endotracheal intubation, ventilation with 100% oxygen, and closed cardiac compression were undertaken while the baby was being delivered by cesarean section. Normal cardiac rhythm returned after approximately 20 minutes of external massage, two countershocks, intracardiac epinephrine, and intravenous bicarbonate (79).

In managing a catastrophe such as this, two important considerations must be borne in mind. First, external cardiac compression is most effective when performed with the patient in the supine position on an unyielding surface. During late pregnancy, however, this position produces aortocaval compression with a consequent decrease in venous return. This impediment to cardiac filling is detrimental to effective restoration of the circulation; thus, delivery of the infant must be considered an important part of the resuscitation attempt. In cases of cardiac arrest, the American Heart Association has stated the following: "Several authors now recommend that the decision to perform a perimortem cesarean section should be made rapidly, with delivery effected within 4 to 5 minutes of the arrest" (80). Should immediate delivery be deemed unsafe or impractical, the uterus should be manually displaced at the same time as external cardiac compression is initiated (81). Alternatively, a wooden frame (the Cardiff resuscitation wedge) or similar device that prevents aortocaval compression in pregnant women during cardiopulmonary resuscitation can be used (82).

Second, seizures induced by bupivacaine are accompanied by severe acidemia, hypoxemia, and hypercarbia (83). This makes hyperventilation with 100% oxygen and intravenous administration of sodium bicarbonate necessary components of the early management if resuscitation is to have a chance of success. Advanced cardiac life support (ACLS) protocols should be followed, including electric defibrillation when necessary. The ASA Guidelines for Obstetrical Anesthesia state, "Basic and advanced life-support equipment should be immediately available in the operative area of labor and delivery units. If cardiac arrest occurs during labor and delivery, standard resuscitative measures and procedures, including left uterine displacement, should be taken" (84).

Bupivacaine-induced seizures and cardiac arrest should be preventable. Carefully identify the epidural space. Aspirate the needle or catheter to identify blood or cerebrospinal fluid. Administer a test dose of sufficient magnitude to produce symptoms and signs of toxicity (e.g., tinnitus, agitation, metallic taste, facial paresthesias, sudden drowsiness). Dose the needle or catheter with incremental injections of the therapeutic dose, allowing sufficient time between aliquots to permit manifestations of either subarachnoid or intravascular placement. These are all means by which the technique of epidural block in obstetrics can be made safer.

The choice of a "marker" in the anesthetic solution is controversial in obstetric patients. When added to the test dose, epinephrine can produce an increase in heart rate if injected into an epidural vein. This tachycardia can be so short lived (20 seconds), however, that its recognition may be difficult and, in this regard, use of an electrocardiograph or pulse oximeter during injection of the local anesthetic is suggested. Even with such accurate measurement of the maternal heart rate, however, it is not possible to differentiate between the tachycardia caused by the intravenous injection of a small amount of epinephrine and that associated with uterine contractions (85). Another concern regarding the use of epinephrine as a marker is the possibility of its producing a decrease in uteroplacental blood flow in situations in which there is already some degree of (recognized or unrecognized) placental insufficiency. As evidence for this risk, epinephrine has been shown to decrease intervillous blood flow in gravid ewes in a dose-related manner (86). In addition, when human parturients received epinephrine (40 μg) as part of an epidural injection, fetal umbilical artery blood velocity systolic/diastolic ratios, a measure of vascular resistance, underwent marked change. Those fetuses with normal umbilical arterial resistance before the epidural injection were relatively unaffected. In contrast, when baseline resistance was high, epinephrine-containing epidural injections worsened the situation to the point of producing transient decelerations in the fetal heart rate in two of the six fetuses in this group (87).

At the request of the U. S. Food and Drug Administration, in August 1983 the three manufacturers of bupivacaine in North America recommended against the use of the 0.75% concentration in obstetric practice. Consequently, the highest concentration available for use in parturients is 0.5%. Unfortunately, the response of some anesthesiologists has been to increase the volume of the lower concentration to that which will produce an equivalent dose of drug (e.g., 30 mL 0.5% = 150 mg = 20 mL 0.75%). Thus, the risk to a patient under these circumstances has not been reduced (77).

UNRECOGNIZED EVENTS DURING REGIONAL BLOCKADE

Maternal deaths attributable to a lack of awareness of the expected symptoms or signs of high spinal or epidural block during cesarean section have occurred. The scenario has tended to follow a predictable pattern: After institution of regional blockade, symptoms of a higher-than-expected level have either been ignored or have engendered an inappropriate response. As might be expected, these incidents have not been reported in the medical literature, but have been represented in the type of closed claims analyses that are occasionally published (14–28, 88).

In a case with which one of the authors (Bassell) is familiar, the parturient complained of nausea within the first 5 minutes following the injection of a tetracaine (15 mg) spinal anesthetic for cesarean section. The anesthesia provider injected droperidol intravenously without measuring a brachial blood pressure or defining the level of sensory blockade. After repeated and progressively weaker patient complaints of dyspnea, diazepam (10 mg) was injected intravenously. Within a few minutes, respiratory arrest had occurred. Late resuscitation complicated by unrecognized esophageal intubation resulted in brain death. Unfortunately, the lack of clinical awareness underlying this event is not unique. Continuing the widespread deployment of sophisticated monitoring devices such as pulse oximeters and capnographs and requiring their use even when regional anesthesia is employed will prevent maternal deaths. Needless to say, their use during general anesthesia is mandatory (57).

CONCLUSION

Elimination of anesthetic-related maternal mortality requires the careful administration of the appropriate anesthetic by well-trained specialists. The inverse relationship between the experience and training of personnel who provide obstetric anesthesia and maternal mortality cannot be overemphasized (28, 89–91). As hospital services are consolidated, round-the-clock obstetric anesthesia provided by anesthesiologists in well-equipped, fully staffed labor suites should lead to improvements in maternal and fetal safety. The last 40 years have seen the birth of obstetric anesthesia as a recognized subspecialty with its own specialty groups, such as the Society for Obstetric Anesthesia and Perinatology (SOAP) and the Obstetric Anaesthetists Association (OAA). Anesthesiologists-in-training are receiving the type of instruction in obstetric anesthesia principles that allows them to face their responsibilities to parturients with knowledge, experience, and confidence. What has made anesthesia safer for the pregnant patient? As Lee and Singh have noted, we can speculate that the improved safety of anesthesia in obstetrics might be attributable to "(1) more providers with increased skills and interest; (2) the increased use of regional anesthesia and, as a consequence, a decreased use of general anesthesia; (3) improved aids for difficult intubation; [and] (4) more precise monitoring of respiratory and cardiovascular parameters during an anesthetic in a parturient" (92).

REFERENCES

1. Beral V. Reproductive mortality. *Br Med J* 1979;2:622–631.
2. Sachs BP, Oriol NE, Ostheimer GW, et al. Anesthetic-related maternal mortality, 1954 to 1985. *J Clin Anesth* 1989;1:333–338.
3. Endler GC, Mariona FG, Sokkol RJ, Stevenson LB. Anesthesia-related maternal mortality in Michigan, 1972 to 1984. *Am J Obstet Gynecol* 1988;159:187–193.
4. Koonin LM, Atrash HK, Lawson HW, Smith JC. Maternal mortality surveillance, United States, 1979–1986. *MMWR* 1991;40:1–13.
5. Rubin G, McCarthy B, Shelton J, Rochar RW, Terry J. The risk of childbearing re-evaluated. *Am J Public Health* 1981;71:712–716.
6. Green JR. Changing patterns of maternal mortality. Paper presented at: Anesthesia for the High-Risk Mother, Fetus and Newborn; 1983; San Francisco, CA.
7. Bonte JTP, Verbrugge HP. Maternal mortality: An epidemiological approach. *Acta Obstet Gynecol Scand* 1967;46:445–474.
8. Berg JC, Atrash HK, Koonin LM, Tucker M. Pregnancy-related mortality in the U. S., 1987–1990. *Obstet Gynecol* 1996;88:161–167.
9. Centers for Disease Control and Prevention. Maternal mortality—United States, 1982–1996. *JAMA* 1998;280:1042–1043.
10. Klein MD, Clahr J. Factors in the decline of maternal mortality. *JAMA* 1958;168:237–242.
11. Greiss FC Jr, Anderson SG. Elimination of maternal deaths from anesthesia. *Obstet Gynecol* 1967;29:677–681.
12. Crawford JS. The anaesthetist's contribution to maternal mortality. *Br J Anaesth* 1970;42:70–73.
13. Hodgkinson R. Maternal mortality. In: Marx GF, Bassell GM, eds. *Obstetric Analgesia and Anesthesia*. Amsterdam: Elsevier Scientific; 1980:375–395.
14. *Report on Confidential Enquiries Into Maternal Deaths in England and Wales, 1952–1954*. London, England: HMSO; 1957. No. 97.
15. *Report on Confidential Enquiries Into Maternal Deaths in England and Wales, 1955–1957*. London, England: HMSO; 1960. No. 103.
16. *Report on Confidential Enquiries Into Maternal Deaths in England and Wales, 1958–1960*. London, England: HMSO; 1963. No. 108.
17. *Report on Confidential Enquiries Into Maternal Deaths in England and Wales, 1961–1963*. London, England: HMSO; 1966. No. 115.
18. Arthure H, Tomkinson J, Organe G, Kuck M, Adelstein AM, Weatherall JAC. *Report on Confidential Enquiries Into Maternal Deaths in England and Wales, 1964–1966*. London, England: HMSO; 1970. No. 119.
19. Arthure H, Tomkinson J, Organe G, Bates M, Adelstein AM, Weatherall JAC. *Report on Confidential Enquiries Into Maternal Deaths in England and Wales, 1967–1969*. London, England: HMSO; 1972. No. 1.
20. *Report on Confidential Enquiries Into Maternal Deaths in England and Wales, 1970–1972*. London, England: HMSO; 1975. No. 11.
21. Tomkinson J, Turnbull A, Robson G, Cloake E, Adelstein AM, Weatherall JAC. *Report on Confidential Enquiries Into Maternal Deaths in England and Wales, 1973–1975*. London, England: HMSO; 1979. No. 14.
22. Tompkinson J, Turnbull A, Robson G, et al. *Report on Confidential Enquiries Into Maternal Deaths in England and Wales, 1976–1978*. London, England: HMSO; 1982. No. 26.
23. Turnbull AC, Tindall VR, Robson G, Dawson IMP, Cloake EP, Ashley JSA. *Report on Confidential Enquiries Into Maternal Deaths in England and Wales, 1979– 1981*. London, England: HMSO; 1986. No. 29.
24. Turnbull A, Tindall VR, Beard RW, et al. *Report on Confidential Enquiries Into Maternal Deaths in England and Wales, 1982–1984*. London, England: HMSO; 1989. No. 34.
25. Tindall VR, Beard RW, Sykes MK, et al. *Report on Confidential Enquiries Into Maternal Deaths in the United Kingdom, 1985–1987*. London, England: HMSO; 1991.
26. Hibbard BM, Anderson MM, Drife JO, et al. *Report on Confidential Enquiries Into Maternal Deaths in the United Kingdom, 1988–1990*. London, England: HMSO; 1994.
27. Hibbard BM, Anderson MM, Drife JO, et al. *Report on Confidential Enquiries Into Maternal Deaths in the United Kingdom, 1991–1993*. London, England: HMSO; 1996.
28. Lewis G, Drife J, Botting B, et al. *Report on Confidential Enquiries Into Maternal Deaths in the United Kingdom, 1994–1996*. London, England: HMSO; 1998.
29. Yoles I, Maschiach S, Berlovitz Y, Modan B. Maternal mortality in Israel in the years 1975–1995; causes and trends [abstract]. *Am J Obstet Gynecol* 1998;178(suppl):S210.
30. Ellerbrock TV, Atrash HK, Hogue CJR, Smith JC. Pregnancy mortality surveillance: A new initiative. *Contemp Obstet Gynecol* 1988;31:23–24.
31. Rochat RW, Koonin LM, Atrash HK, Jewett JF. Maternal mortality in the United States: Report from the Maternal Mortality Collaborative. *Obstet Gynecol* 1988;72:91– 97.
32. Hawkins JL, Koonin LM, Palmer SK, Gibbs CP. Anesthesia-related deaths during obstetric delivery in the United States, 1979–1990. *Anesthesiology* 1997;86:277–284.

33. Hawkins JL, Gibbs CP, Orleans M, Martin-Salvaj G, Beaty B. Obstetric anesthesia work force survey, 1981 versus 1992. *Anesthesiology* 1997;87:135–143.

34. Paech MJ, Godkin R, Webster S. Complications of obstetric epidural analgesia and anaesthesia: A prospective analysis of 10,995 cases. *Int J Obstet Anesth* 1998;7:5–11.

35. Nimmo WS, Wilson J, Prescott LF. Narcotic analgesics and delayed gastric emptying during labour. *Lancet* 1975;1:890–893.

36. Brock-Utne JG, Dow TGB, Welman S. The effect of metoclopramide on the lower oesophageal sphincter in late pregnancy. *Anaesth Intensive Care* 1978;6:26–29.

37. Vanner RG, Goodman NW. Gastro-oesophageal reflux in pregnancy at term and after delivery. *Anaesthesia* 1989;44:808–811.

38. Attia RR, Ebeid AM, Fischer JE. Maternal, fetal and placental gastrin concentrations *Anaesthesia* 1982;37:18.

39. Mendelson CL. The aspiration of stomach contents into the lungs during obstetric anesthesia. *Am J Obstet Gynecol* 1946;52:191–204.

40. American Academy of Pediatrics/American College of Obstetricians and Gynecologists. *Guidelines for Perinatal Care.* 4th ed. Washington, DC: American College of Obstetricians and Gynecologists; 1997.

41. Cowling J. Cricoid pressure: A more comfortable technique. *Anaesth Intensive Care* 1982;10:93–94.

42. Rosen M. Deaths associated with anaesthesia for obstetrics [editorial]. *Anaesthesia* 1981;36:145–146.

43. Roberts RB, Shirley MA. Reducing the risk of acid aspiration during cesarean section. *Anesth Analg* 1974;53:858–868.

44. Gibbs CP, Spohr L, Schmidt D. The effectiveness of sodium citrate as an antacid. *Anesthesiology* 1982;57:44–46.

45. Gibbs CP, Schwartz DJ, Wynne JW, Hood CI, Kuck EJ. Antacid pulmonary aspiration in the dog. *Anesthesiology* 1979;51:380–385.

46. Holdsworth JD, Johnson K, Mascall G, Roulston RG, Tomlinson PA. Mixing of antacids with stomach contents: Another approach to the prevention of the acid aspiration (Mendelson's) syndrome. *Anaesthesia* 1980;35:641–650.

47. Gillett GB, Watson JD, Langford RM. Prophylaxis against acid aspiration syndrome in obstetric practice [letter]. *Anesthesiology* 1984;60:525.

48. Cohen SE, Jasson J, Talafre ML. Does metoclopramide decrease the volume of gastric contents in patients undergoing cesarean section? *Anesthesiology* 1984;61:604–607.

49. Hodgkinson R, Glassenberg R, Joyce TH III, Coombs DW, Ostheimer GW, Gibbs CP. Comparison of cimetidine with antacid for safety and effectiveness in reducing gastric acidity before elective cesarean section. *Anesthesiology* 1983;59:86–90.

50. Abernethy DR, Greenblatt DJ, Eshelman FN, Shader RI. Ranitidine does not impair oxidative or conjugative metabolism: Noninteraction with antipyrine, diazepam and lorazepam. *Clin Pharmacol Ther* 1984;35:188–192.

51. Crawford JS. Difficulty in endotracheal intubation associated with obstetric anesthesia. *Anesthesiology* 1979;51:475.

52. Rocke DA, Murray WB, Rout CC, Gouws E. Relative risk analysis of factors associated with difficult intubation in obstetric anesthesia. *Anesthesiology* 1992;77:67–73.

53. Datta S, Briwa J. Modified laryngoscope for endotracheal intubation of obese patients. *Anesth Analg* 1981;60:120–121.

54. Jouppila R, Jouppila P, Hollmen A. Laryngeal oedema as an obstetric anaesthesia complication: Case reports. *Acta Anaesthesiol Scand* 1980;24:97–98.

55. Samsoon GLT, Young JRB. Difficult intubation: A retrospective study. *Anaesthesia* 1987;42:487–490.

56. American Society of Anesthesiologists. Standards for basic anesthetic monitoring: ASA Standards, Guidelines and Statements. Park Ridge, IL: American Society of Anesthesiologists; 2000:477.

57. American Society of Anesthesiologists. Practice Guidelines for Management of the Difficult Airway: A report by the American Society of Anesthesiologists' Task Force. *Anesthesiology* 1993;78:597–602.

58. Benumof JL, Scheller MS. The importance of transtracheal jet ventilation in the management of difficult airway. *Anesthesiology* 1989;71:769–778.

59. Tsen LC, Pitner R, Camann WR. General anesthesia for cesarean section at a tertiary care hospital 1990–1995: Indications and implications. *Int J Obstet Anesth* 1998;7:147–152.

60. Assali NS, Prystowsky H. Studies on autonomic blockade. I. Comparison between the effects of tetraethylammonium chloride (TEAC) and high selective spinal anesthesia on the blood pressure of normal and toxemic pregnancy. *J Clin Invest* 1950;29:1354–1360.

61. Bromage PR. Spread of analgesic solutions in the epidural space and their site of action: A statistical study. *Br J Anaesth* 1962;34:161–178.

62. Marx GF, Orkin LR, eds. *Physiology of Obstetric Anesthesia.* Springfield, IL: Charles C. Thomas; 1969:97–99.

63. Fagraeus L, Urban BJ, Bromage PR. Spread of epidural analgesia in early pregnancy. *Anesthesiology* 1983;58:184–187.

64. Flanagan HL, Datta S, Lambert DH. Effect of pregnancy on bupivacaine-induced conduction blockade in the isolated rabbit vagus nerve. *Anesth Analg* 1987;66:123–126.

65. Datta S, Hurley RJ, Naulty JS, et al. Plasma and cerebrospinal fluid progesterone concentrations in pregnant and nonpregnant women. *Anesth Analg* 1986;65:950–954.

66. Scott DB. Inferior vena cava occlusion in late pregnancy and its importance in anaesthesia. *Br J Anaesth* 1968;40:120–128.

67. Marx GF. Regional analgesia in obstetrics. *Anaesthesist* 1972;20:84–91.

68. McCausland AM, Hyman C, Winsor T, Trotter AD. Venous distensibility during pregnancy. *Am J Obstet Gynecol* 1965;81:472–476.

69. Greiss FC Jr, Crandell DL. Therapy for hypotension induced by spinal anesthesia during pregnancy: Observations on gravid ewes. *JAMA* 1965;191:793–796.

70. Wollman SB, Marx GF. Acute hydration for prevention of hypotension of spinal anesthesia in parturients. *Anesthesiology* 1968;29:374–380.

71. Marx GF, Cosmi EV, Wollman SB. Biochemical status and clinical condition of mother and infant at cesarean section. *Anesth Analg* 1969;48:986–993.

72. Collins KM, Bevan DR, Beard RW. Fluid loading to reduce abnormalities of fetal heart rate and maternal hypotension during epidural analgesia in labour. *Br Med J* 1978;2:1460–1461.

73. Huovinen K, Lehtovirta P, Forrs M, Kivalo I, Teramo K. Changes in placental intervillous blood flow measured by the Xenon method during lumbar epidural block for elective caesarean section. *Acta Anaesthesiol Scand* 1979;23:529–533.

74. Lewis M, Thomas P, Wilkes FG. Hypotension during epidural analgesia for caesarean section: Arterial and central venous pressure changes after acute intravenous loading with two liters of Hartmann's solution. *Anaesthesia* 1983;38:250–253.

75. Rout CC, Rocke DA, Levin J, Gouws E, Reddy D. A re-evaluation of the role of crystalloid preload in the prevention of hypotension associated with spinal anesthesia for elective cesarean section *Anesthesiology* 1993;79:262–269.

76. Ueyama H, Yan-Ling H, Tanigami H, Mashimo T, Yoshiya I. Effects of crystalloid and colloid preload on blood volume in the parturient undergoing spinal anesthesia for elective cesarean section. *Anesthesiology* 1999;91:1571–1576.

77. Marx GF. Bupivacaine cardiotoxicity: Concentration or dose? *Anesthesiology* 1986;65:116.

78. Albright GA. Cardiac arrest following regional anesthesia with etidocaine or bupivacaine. *Anesthesiology* 1979;51:285–287.

79. Marx GF. Maternal complications of regional analgesia. *Reg Anesth* 1981;6:104–107.

80. Guidelines for cardiopulmonary resuscitation and emergency cardiac care: Recommendations of the 1992 National Conference. *JAMA* 1992;268:2249.

81. Marx GF. Cardiopulmonary resuscitation of late-pregnant women. *Anesthesiology* 1982;56:156.

82. Rees GAD, Willis BA. Resuscitation in late pregnancy. *Anaesthesia* 1988;43:347–349.

83. Moore DC, Thompson GE, Crawford RD. Long-acting local anesthetic drugs and convulsions with hypoxia and acidosis. *Anesthesiology* 1982;56:230–232.

84. American Society of Anesthesiologists. Practice Guidelines for Obstetrical Anesthesia: A report by the American Society of Anesthesiologists' task force. *Anesthesiology* 1999;90:600–611.

85. Leighton BL, Norris MC, Sosis M. Limitations of epinephrine as a marker of intravascular injection in laboring women. *Anesthesiology* 1987;66:688–691.

86. Hood DD, Dewan DM, James FM III. Maternal and fetal effects of epinephrine in gravid ewes. *Anesthesiology* 1986;64:610–613.

87. Marx GF, Elstein ID, Schuss M, Anyaegbunam A, Fleischer A. Effects of epidural block with lignocaine and lignocaine-adrenaline

on umbilical artery velocity wave ratios. *Br J Obstet Gynaecol* 1990;97: 517–520.

88. Chadwick HS, Posner K, Caplan RA, Ward RJ, Cheney FW. A comparison of obstetric and nonobstetric anesthesia malpractice claims. *Anesthesiology* 1991;74:242–249.

89. Morgan BM. Maternal death: A review of maternal deaths at one hospital from 1958–1978. *Anaesthesia* 1980;35:334–338.

90. Breheny F, McCarthy J. Maternal mortality: A review of maternal deaths over twenty years at the National Maternity Hospital, Dublin. *Anaesthesia* 1982;37:561–564.

91. Nagaya K, Fetters MD, Ishikawa M, et al. Causes of maternal mortality in Japan. *JAMA* 2000;283:2661–2667.

92. Lee JS, Singh P. Progress in decreasing maternal mortality. *Semin Anesth* 2000;19:46–50.

Shnider and Levinson's Anesthesia for Obstetrics,
edited by Samuel C. Hughes, et al.
Lippincott Williams & Wilkins,
Philadelphia, © 2001.

CHAPTER 25

OBSTETRIC ANESTHESIA AND LAWSUITS

PART I GENERAL CONSIDERATIONS AND RECOMMENDATIONS

RICHARD E. DODGE. ESQ. (DECEASED)

The unfortunate reality facing today's physician is that medical malpractice litigation, like the postoperative wound infection, is a fact of medical life. While the risk of lawsuits can be minimized to a certain extent, it cannot be eliminated. Time and space preclude an exhaustive discussion of the fault system that is the foundation of American jurisprudence as it applies to compensating "victims" of alleged medical malpractice. We will, however, attempt to provide an overview of this subject with special emphasis on obstetric anesthesia.

Every medical specialty has its own subset of diagnostic or treatment decisions that are at least partially unique to that discipline. So, too, are malpractice issues. While many medical-legal issues transcend most or all medical specialties, there are, of necessity, subjects that are totally or in part germane only to a particular specialty or group of closely aligned specialties. In discussing medical-legal concepts as they pertain to medical-malpractice litigation, we will focus whenever possible on anesthesiology and anesthesia for obstetrics.

A MEDICAL MALPRACTICE PERSPECTIVE, PAST AND PRESENT

Medical malpractice lawsuits are not a new phenomenon. Our system has as its genesis English Common Law. Accordingly, the tort system as we know it has been present in one form or another since the U.S. Constitution was implemented. Of course, each state has seen fit to fashion its tort system according to the will of its legislative, executive, and judicial branches. What this means as a practical matter is that, while there are obvious similarities among states, there are also dramatic and sometimes inexplicable differences.

For example, California, for decades a pacesetter in promulgating an ever-widening network of laws that expanded liability in all aspects of human endeavor, enacted the so-called Medical Injury Compensation Reform Act, known as MICRA, in 1975 (1). Among its many features was a provision limiting noneconomic damages to $250,000. Noneconomic damages are those for so-called pain and suffering in personal injury cases. In wrongful death cases, they include such subjective losses as care, comfort, society, love, affection, and sexual relationships. This $250,000 limit remains in effect today; however, it may well be that this limit will be raised in the future. Other states have limitations on noneconomic damages that vary from $250,000 to $1,000,000 (Utah, $250,000 [2]; Oregon, $500,000 [3]; New Mexico, $500,000 [4]; West Virginia, $1,000,000 [5]).

However high the limit is raised, it will never approach the jury awards seen in states such as Ohio, Texas, New York, Pennsylvania, and New Jersey, to name a few, which have no limit on noneconomic damages. Because of the highly subjective nature of this element of damages, it is very difficult from the standpoint of lawyers, doctors, and malpractice insurance carriers to predict with any certainty the amount of a verdict in states having no damage limitation. Multimillion dollar, eight-figure damage awards have been granted in these states. While these numbers do not represent the norm by any means, they are illustrative of the vast differences in substantive law that exist from state to state. An injured patient in California, for example, is limited to $250,000 in general damages for a particular injury, whereas a patient with the exact same injury in a state without general damages limitations might recover literally millions of dollars. The only difference between the two situations is geographic.

Another purely geographic difference pertains to the time in which a disgruntled patient may file a lawsuit. The most common time frame, called the Statute of Limitations, is 1, 2, or 3 years in most states. However, exceptions exist in many states in cases involving birth injuries, minors, and the mentally disabled. There is virtually no uniformity among states insofar as time limitations for filing lawsuits are concerned.

Many other differences exist from jurisdiction to jurisdiction. These include the presence or absence of laws respecting the periodic payment of future economic damages, restrictive caps on attorneys fees earned by plaintiffs' lawyers, and the admissibility of evidence pertaining to insurance and other benefits payable to the plaintiff.

The significance of these many differences will affect physicians practicing the same specialty in different geographic areas. Malpractice insurance premium rates, of course, will vary according to the jury verdict profile and loss ratios that exist in particular states.

Suffice it to say that medical malpractice litigation is alive and well in the United States. There are numerous and complex reasons for the evolution of this system. While its history is of some intellectual interest, other features are of much more importance to the practicing physician. The present state of the law in general and how it affects the obstetric anesthesiologist in particular are significant. Topics ranging from how to reduce the risk of liability exposure of the individual physician to the impact of emotionally and financially draining lawsuits are of paramount importance to the medical community. We will attempt to address these issues and offer an explanation of just what constitutes medical malpractice in the eyes of the law.

MEDICAL MALPRACTICE

Contrary to popular belief, lawsuits against physicians are guided by reasonably well-defined standards. What is less well-defined and much less certain, however, is the application of these standards to a particular case by a jury composed of lay people. Every citizen of the United States, even a physician, is constitutionally guaranteed a trial by a jury of his or her *peers*. However, the argument is frequently heard that a jury whose composition usually includes individuals without a trace of medical knowledge clearly does not provide a doctor with a jury of peers. For a group of lay persons to decide complex and often obscure medical issues that are often poorly understood by even the medical profession is a situation viewed with distrust and skepticism by most physicians.

However, to better understand the system and the way in which the medical profession is ultimately judged, it is helpful to review the actual charge, or instructions, given to a jury by the judge presiding over a trial. These are the actual standards by which a jury is told that they must decide the case brought against the physician accused of medical malpractice. While the language may differ from state to state and from state court to federal court, the general tenor of the instructions is the same.

The jury is first told what the *duty* of the physician is.

A physician, performing professional services for a patient, owes that patient the following duties of care:

1. The duty to have that degree of learning and skill ordinarily possessed by reputable physicians, practicing in the same or a similar locality and under similar circumstances;

2. The duty to use the care and skill ordinarily exercised in like cases by reputable members of the profession practicing in the same or a similar locality under similar circumstances; and

3. The duty to use reasonable diligence and his or her best judgment in the exercise of skill and the application of learning.

A failure to perform any one of these duties is negligence (6).

If the physician is a specialist, the following additional description of the duty is provided:

It is the duty of a physician who holds himself or herself out as a specialist in a particular field of medical, surgical, or other healing science to have the knowledge and skill ordinarily possessed, and to use the care and skill ordinarily used, by reputable specialists practicing in the same field and in the same or a similar locality and under similar circumstances. A failure to fulfill such duty is negligence (7).

The jury may also be told what a breach of that duty *is not*. The following two passages are guidelines that further define the above-quoted standards. These are applicable to all specialties, including that of obstetric anesthesia:

A physician is *not* necessarily negligent because he or she errs in judgment or because his or her efforts prove unsuccessful. The physician is negligent if the error in judgment or lack of success is due to a failure to perform any of the duties as defined in these instructions [emphasis added] (8).

Where there is more than one recognized method of diagnosis or treatment, and no one of them is used exclusively and uniformly by all practitioners of good standing, a physician is *not* negligent if, in exercising his or her best judgment, he or she selects one of the approved methods, which later turns out to be a wrong selection or one not favored by certain other practitioners [emphasis added] (9).

Finally, the jury, having been instructed as to what medical negligence is and is not, receives instructions on the method by which the standard of care required of physicians *must* be proved:

You must determine the standard of professional learning, skill, and care required of the defendant *only* from the opinions of the physicians, including the defendant, who have testified as expert witnesses as to such standard.

You should consider each such opinion and should weigh the qualifications of the witness and the reasons given for his or her opinion. Give each opinion the weight to which you deem it entitled.

You must resolve any conflict in the testimony of the witnesses by weighing each of the opinions expressed against the others,

taking into consideration the reasons given for the opinion; the facts relied upon by the witness; and the relative credibility, special knowledge, skill, experience, training, and education of the witness (10).

One can see that if these guidelines are followed, the jury should arrive at the just and correct verdict. It should be noted here that medical malpractice disputes can be submitted to a judge sitting without a jury or to binding arbitration. The arbitration procedure most commonly involves a single arbitrator or a three-member arbitration panel. Arbitration is ordinarily a matter of contract entered into before treatment by the patient and his or her physician or health maintenance organization (HMO) representative. That a jury is not involved, however, does not change the rules pertaining to the duty of a physician, the breach thereof, and the method of proof. Furthermore, the burden of proof always rests with the plaintiff to prove the charges, regardless of the forum. In most cases, it is not necessary for a defendant to prove or disprove anything from the standpoint of having any burden of proof.

While anecdotal and aberrant jury verdict reports are known to all, the fact is that juries usually do the right thing. Although the current medical-legal, governmental, and managed care environment makes it difficult, the physician should not lose faith in that part of the legal system that is an inseparable component of the practice of medicine. While frustrating, cumbersome, and at times illogical and time-consuming, by and large, the correct result is obtained.

THE MALPRACTICE DILEMMA AND HOW TO AVOID IT
General Considerations

While it may seem like ancient history to many, the advent of intraoperative monitoring is perhaps the single most important breakthrough in terms of patient care for the anesthesiologist in recent decades. That this is true is proven by the most practical of objective tests, the medical malpractice insurance marketplace. For many years, one of the highest-risk medical specialties was anesthesia. This high risk translated to enormous jury verdicts in many cases and a corresponding increase in medical malpractice insurance premiums. The reason for the damage potential is obvious. Injuries related to anesthesia management frequently resulted in catastrophic injuries involving death and brain damage. In the case of obstetric anesthesia, brain-injured mothers and babies were often alleged to have received substandard anesthesia care. With the advent of monitoring devices like the pulse oximeter, and the improved and standardized training of anesthesia specialists, the incidence of this type of injury has declined significantly. That decline has seen a corresponding drop in the incidence of anesthesia-related claims. In 1997, according to statistics compiled by Physician Insurance Association of America (PIAA), anesthesiology claims decreased by almost one third compared with reported claims a decade earlier. Indemnity paid over the same time frame showed an even more dramatic fall of more than 50% (11). While medical malpractice claims remain a significant risk to the anesthesiologist, the risk has decreased. Nevertheless, as will be discussed, obstetric anesthesia claims probably are not decreasing as dramatically as general anesthesia claims.

Despite unimagined technology and gadgetry, however, there is not now nor will there be in the foreseeable future a substitute for the training, experience, background, and care provided by the skilled anesthesiologist. Standardized residency training programs help to ensure this quality of care. It goes without saying that not only is the conscientious pursuit of excellence in this exquisitely sensitive specialty the essence of the obstetric anesthesia professional, but it also is the single best defense against medical malpractice lawsuits.

While there are unquestionably valid malpractice claims that should be fairly compensated, it is likewise true that there are many more unmeritorious claims made against doctors who are entirely undeserving of being a target. Included in the PIAA assessment of the 28 specialty groups database, anesthesiology as a specialty ranked eighth in 1997 in claims reported. There was no breakdown for obstetric anesthesia claims (12).

When sued, the physician often feels as though his or her professional integrity is challenged. It is absolutely essential to understand that the emotional baggage that accompanies a claim by an unhappy patient and her lawyer pales in comparison to the invaluable service provided to a pregnant woman and her fetus by the anesthesiologist. There is infrequently an attitude instilled in the physician that the unpleasantness associated with a medical malpractice lawsuit outweighs the rewards of this profession. Nothing could be further from the truth. To give in to the temptation to change specialties, reduce one's practice, or retire altogether is to surrender to the system that has produced the inconsistent and confusing body of laws governing medical malpractice litigation under which physicians now find themselves practicing. While this system is composed of many fine, dedicated professionals, it also contains the seeds of greed and selfishness that so many in our ever-increasingly litigious society find compelling.

On a practical level, there are some obvious approaches that greatly assist the doctor's case once litigation begins. *It cannot be emphasized too early or too often, however, that training, experience, and the maintenance of ever-expanding technical skills is always the frontline defense against these claims.* The delivery of careful, thoughtful anesthesia care as dictated by the circumstances of a particular case is the principal component of the successful defense of the anesthesiologist.

Documentation

Meticulous documentation of an anesthesia record is essential. Since cases frequently do not come to trial for 2, 3, 4 or more years after the commencement of litigation, the chart will be the primary source of information upon which the doctor's testimony will be based. Missing entries related to, for example, oxygen saturation, tidal volume, medications employed, or other important components of a complete anesthesia record are often difficult to explain and impossible to remember. While habit and custom can be used to recreate a situation, there is no substitute for an accurate record. For example, noting left uterine displacement with a simple "LUD" on the record is far better than later testifying to your habit and custom.

If a complication occurs that is or possibly could be related to anesthesia, the event should be carefully documented. For example, if there is a delay in performing a crash cesarean section and there is the remotest suggestion that part of the delay was due to the anesthesiologist, the circumstances surrounding the case, the time the anesthesiologist was notified, and the times of all significant events must be documented in the chart as soon after the case as time permits. Again, it will be difficult if not impossible to recall exact times involved in the case days or weeks after an event, let alone months or years later.

Preanesthesia evaluations must always be summarized in the chart. While the lack of documentation does not in any way imply that the entirety of the patient's anesthesia treatment was not done perfectly, it necessarily raises an inference that some important part of the evaluation was omitted. As with any missing chart entry, resourceful lawyers challenging a doctor's care and treatment will exploit these omissions in an effort to convince the jury that a particular patient's case was mishandled. An essential part of the preanesthesia interview and examination, of course, includes a review of the pertinent portions of the patient's chart, consultation with the obstetrician and other involved specialists as necessary, and the informed consent discussion to be addressed in the next section.

There are many potential theories of liability, including those pertaining to documentation, that await the unwary physician, and this short chapter is not an exhaustive or comprehensive description of potential problem areas for the anesthesiologist. Some obvious activities to be avoided, however, include any alteration of the medical or anesthesia record after litigation has been threatened or commenced. On the other hand, it is not uncommon to clarify or author a late entry shortly after a case has been concluded simply for the sake of completeness and accuracy. When such a change or augmentation is made, the additions must be dated and initialed by the author. It should be obvious that changes and corrections are made frequently to medical records while medical care continues to be delivered or while a case is fresh in the mind of the nurse or physician. On the other hand, only negative inferences will be drawn when a record is changed months or years after a case is completed and a claim has been made.

Informed Consent

Generally speaking, the law of informed consent requires a physician to inform his or her patient of both the anticipated benefits hoped for by a particular course of treatment as well as any risks that are inherent in such a course of treatment. The law requires this so that the patient may ultimately decide whether to undergo a particular recommended type of treatment. The law extends this requirement to anesthesia as well as to all other aspects of medicine. However, this law has a practical application. It is clearly not necessary for the physician to discuss with the patient all possible complications, the pharmacologic component of anesthesia agents that are going to be administered, or potential negative outcomes that, although possible, are primarily theoretic and very unlikely to occur. It is well recognized that a patient must be advised of the major risks associated with a particular form of treatment, including anesthesia, so that the patient is able to make an informed decision about medical care. However, it is only the major risks that are known to result in serious bodily harm such as death, neurologic damage, infection, hemorrhage, and the like that must be imparted to the patient. Remote risks or risks that can result in only minor complications generally do not require elucidation.

In order to prevail in a case based on a lack of informed consent, it is also not enough for a patient simply to testify that, had she been informed of a particular risk, she would not have consented to the procedure. Obviously, many patients who are motivated to sue their physician for failure to obtain their informed consent are going to so testify. Therefore, the standard required by the law is the so-called "reasonable patient" standard. That is, would a reasonable patient, had she been informed of a particular risk and its incidence, nevertheless have consented to the treatment. By and large, the answer is in the affirmative. That is, a reasonable person in the position of the plaintiff would have so consented. As can be seen, then, if an adverse consequence occurs as a result of anesthesia, an anesthesiologist is not rendered liable simply because the patient was not informed of that risk.

If the complication that occurred was rare or unusual and one commonly recognized as such, the plaintiff/patient has a 3-fold hurdle to overcome. First, the patient must prove that she was not informed of the risk; second, there must be proof that a reasonable patient would not have consented to the treatment had she been informed of the risk; and, third, if the risk is considered to be remote, there is no liability if the standard of care does not require that that remote risk be imparted to a patient. As noted earlier, this standard of care can be determined only by qualified expert witnesses. In this example, the expert would be testifying on the issue of informed consent and what is required in a particular situation of a reputable anesthesiologist practicing under similar circumstances.

Informed consent issues, like every other aspect of the care and treatment delivered to a patient, require documentation.

The major risks of general anesthesia must be discussed and documented. Likewise, the risk of *no* anesthesia must be discussed and memorialized if that is an issue. For example, a mother who has experienced a difficult delivery may well have a recollection different than her anesthesiologist about the conversation covering the risks and benefits of "natural childbirth" as it pertains to anesthesia. By way of illustration, a shoulder dystocia resulting in an Erb's palsy, temporary or permanent, frequently results in a lawsuit. It is not uncommon in these cases for a mother who has requested no analgesia or anesthesia to later recall a distinct conversation with her anesthesiologist in which she allegedly told the doctor that she did not want anesthesia or analgesia *unless* there was a danger to her baby. If the anesthesia record has not been carefully documented, including a summary of the discussions of risks and benefits, the case may well turn on who the jury decides to believe. On the other hand, if the discussion of options, risks, and benefits, including the request for no anesthesia or analgesia, is well documented, the edge clearly shifts to the doctor.

It is not necessary, obviously, to record the entirety of a conversation or author a note that tries to convey a verbatim transcript of the interchange. A note documenting that the usual risks and benefits of anesthesia have been discussed with the patient and that the patient understands and consents to a particular course of action is usually sufficient. If there are unusual aspects of the case, such as a mother requesting no anesthesia or analgesia, the note should be more comprehensive and should detail the fact that the physician has discussed that situation with his or her patient and the patient wishes to proceed as indicated.

Pragmatic Problems

There are problems that frequently occur in ongoing litigation that are largely unrelated to medical treatment. Often, a lawsuit filed against a hospital, obstetrician, delivering physician, or others initially does not involve the anesthesiologist or other members of the team taking care of the mother and child. There may be a request for a deposition of the anesthesiologist, which frequently comes directly from the attorney representing the patient. The usual contact will include assurances that the deposition is only informational and there is no contemplation that the physician to be deposed would ever become involved as a defendant in the case. If such an approach is made, it must never be assumed that the deposition will not have legal consequences for the deponent. While the deposition may, in fact, be strictly designed to discover factual matters, one should also bear in mind that the deposition can be, and frequently is, used to set up the physician by adroit questioning so as to make him or her a viable defendant in the pending litigation.

Likewise, it is not uncommon under these circumstances for an attorney to attempt to use the deposition testimony of a non-defendant as an expert opinion against the involved physicians. It must be kept in mind that deposition testimony has the same force and effect as testimony given in court. The unwary physician who is sent to such a deposition unrepresented and unprepared is in jeopardy of inadvertently becoming involved in the case or providing unintended expert testimony. In cases involving physicians who are in private practice and/or who are independent contractors vis-à-vis a hospital, the malpractice insurance carrier for that physician will not only gladly provide the doctor with legal representation, but it will also undoubtedly insist upon the doctor being represented if informed of the deposition ahead of time. Likewise, in hospital-based practices or with doctors practicing in HMO environments, requests for depositions under these circumstances should be reported to the appropriate administrative personnel so that legal representation can be provided.

It is a fact that a warm and caring attitude adopted by a doctor toward the patient is sometimes the greatest deterrent to litigation, regardless of the outcome that may occur in a particular case. The anesthesiologist is hindered to a certain extent by the lack of any significant or ongoing physician/patient relationship. The anesthesiologist usually has only short-term personal contacts with the patient. Aside from brief conversations in the preanesthesia interview or short encounters during labor or in the recovery room, there is little chance to develop a solid doctor/patient relationship. However, particularly with regard to obstetric anesthesia, the physician involved does have a better chance than perhaps the physician administering general anesthesia to a patient in a nonobstetric situation to develop at least a cordial and pleasant acquaintanceship. The preanesthesia examination and evaluation are not uncommonly conducted by the anesthesiologist who actually administers the obstetric anesthesia. During the course of this contact, it is certainly to be encouraged that the physician commiserate with the patient, encourage the patient, and react to the patient positively. The mental outlook of a mother who is anticipating the birth of a child may ordinarily be considered somewhat more positive than the general anesthesia patient facing gall bladder surgery or some other equally unpleasant operative event. It hopefully goes without saying that the anesthesiologist should use every opportunity of patient contact to establish a friendly, professional working relationship. Furthermore, it is a fact in this age of expanding public awareness and access through the miracle of modern communication and the Internet that patients are generally much better informed and much more inquisitive than the same patient profile of a decade ago. Patients with a little knowledge on a particular subject, even one as involved as anesthesia, may be somewhat trying in their questioning and desire for additional information. It is just this type of patient that the prudent physician will take the time to respond to positively.

TRENDS

An increasing number of situations occur that are largely beyond the control of the anesthesiologist. Nevertheless, it is important to be aware of cases in which the anesthesiologist practicing obstetric anesthesia may become involved in litigation despite a seemingly peripheral role. The bottom line effect of this trend is the proliferation of malpractice actions against obstetric anesthesiologists at a time when general anesthesia claims are declining. These lawsuits have significant consequences for the physician. The trauma associated with being sued; the time taken away from one's practice or family to participate in the defense of the case; the concern that a verdict will exceed the physician's malpractice insurance policy limits; and the financial and professional consequences of reporting requirements imposed by hospitals, insurance companies, preferred provider organizations, HMOs, and others are all factors materially affecting the involved physician, no matter how meritless the suit or claim may be.

Perhaps because of spiraling jury verdicts and the fact that malpractice insurance policy limits do not always provide adequate coverage for these verdicts, there appears to be an increasing tendency to include additional defendants in cases in which traditionally only the obstetrician or the obstetrician and the hospital have been named as defendants. We are now seeing the inclusion of the anesthesiologist as a defendant in an increasing number of cases. In addition to the anesthesiologist, the attending pediatrician and members of the resuscitation team, particularly physicians, may be at risk for inclusion in these cases.

Obviously, there must be a theory proffered other than the lack of insurance coverage. The resourceful plaintiff's bar has sought to expand the potential liability of the anesthesiologist practicing obstetric anesthesia via several scenarios. One theory seeks to include the anesthesiologist as a member of a team jointly responsible for delaying an emergency cesarean section, theoretically resulting in injury to the fetus. Another targets the resuscitation of a depressed infant in cases when some delay has allegedly occurred and caused damage to the newborn.

Still another is predicated on the assertion that **anesthesiologists practicing obstetric anesthesia** frequently have expertise beyond general anesthesiologists in the interpretation of the fetal heart rate monitor tracing. Obstetric anesthesiologists have been sued in cases when they have been in the labor room to check on their patient at a time when a nonreassuring tracing has occurred. Although the obstetricians and nursing staff are primarily responsible for fetal monitoring, the contention is often made that the anesthesiologist, by virtue of his or her expertise, has a duty to inform the obstetrician and make sure the cause of the nonreassuring pattern is evaluated and, if necessary, intervention undertaken.

There are multiple situations that occur in the busy anesthesia practice in the labor and delivery area that can have medical-legal ramifications. The occurrence of these situations cannot be prevented. The skillful, caring physician, however, can react to a particular situation using his or her training and expertise to accomplish the best outcome possible under the circumstances. The obstetric anesthesiologist is not a guarantor of a perfect result in every case–the burden of the obstetric anesthesiologist is to deliver that level of care determined by the situation at hand and in accordance with well-established standards that have stood the test of time.

CONCLUSION

It would be understandable if anesthesiologists, and indeed other medical specialists, were disheartened by the liability risks with which they are confronted each time a patient is anesthetized or treated. The malpractice crisis that swept the United States in the spring of 1975 highlighted the complexity of the professional liability problem. The publicity generated at the time, however, did not accurately reflect the true state of affairs, and it is anticipated that in the future, as in the past, physicians will prevail in the vast majority of lawsuits brought by patients.

It should also be kept in mind that the occurrence of an injury associated with anesthesia or other medical treatment does not in itself establish negligence and, as a consequence, liability. The plaintiff must always prove that the defendant-physician failed to follow standard practice in treating the patient and that it was his or her failure to do so that caused the injury of which the plaintiff complains. Anesthesiologists who understand their relationship to the patient and to other physicians involved in the treatment and who remain vigilant to the standards in the medical community significantly reduce their exposure to malpractice liability.

REFERENCES

1. California Bus. & Prof. Code §6146, subd.(a); Civ. Code, §§3333.1, subd.(a), 3333.2, subd.(a); Code Civ. Proc. §§340.5, 364, subd.(a), 667.7, subds.(a),(e)(4), 1295, subd.(a).
2. Utah Stats. 78-14-7.1.
3. Oregon Revised Stats. 18.560.
4. New Mexico Stats. Annotated 41-5-3.
5. West Virginia Code, ch. 55, art. 7B §8.
6. BAJI (8th ed). California Jury Instructions. BAJI No. 6.00.1.
7. BAJI (8th ed). California Jury Instructions. BAJI No. 6.01.
8. BAJI (8th ed). California Jury Instructions. BAJI No. 6.02.
9. BAJI (8th ed). California Jury Instructions. BAJI No. 6.03.
10. BAJI (8th ed). California Jury Instructions. BAJI No. 6.30.
11. Physician Insurers Association of America. *A Risk Management Review of Anesthesiology Claims (1997)*. VI. Ex 6. Rockville, MD: Physician Insurers Association of America; 1997.
12. Physician Insurers Association of America. *A Risk Management Review of Anesthesiology Claims (1997)*. IV. Ex 2. Rockville, MD: Physician Insurers Association of America; 1997.

PART II REVIEW OF OBSTETRIC ANESTHESIA CLOSED CLAIMS

H. S. CHADWICK, M.D. AND HOLLY C. GUNN, M.D.

In 1985, the Committee on Professional Liability of the American Society of Anesthesiologists (ASA) launched a project to review malpractice claims against anesthesiologists. The goals of the project were to identify patterns of anesthetic-related injury in order to devise strategies to minimize adverse outcomes, improve patient safety, and limit liability risk. That project continues today. Practicing anesthesiologists travel to the offices of professional liability insurance carriers across the nation to review no-longer-active (closed) files of malpractice claims against anesthesiologists. These physician-reviewers complete a data-collection instrument (consisting of a standardized questionnaire and narrative summary) on all claims for which there is enough information to reconstruct the sequence of events and determine the nature of the injury. Data reviewed typically consist of hospital records, including anesthesia records, deposition summaries, expert and peer reviews, legal outcome reports, and information concerning the cost of the settlement or award. Each data collection instrument is reviewed by three physician members of the ASA Closed Claims Committee before being entered into a computer database for future analysis.

The project has yielded a number of studies and publications, including two analyses focusing on claims involving obstetric anesthesia (1, 2). The obstetric-related claims are of particular interest to those who practice obstetric anesthesia. As of June 1998, 4183 files (excluding those for dental injuries) have been reviewed and entered into the ASA Closed Claims Project database. The last comprehensive analysis of the obstetric related-cases was published in 1996, when the database contained 3533 files (434 obstetric anesthesia related) (2). This represents the most recent analysis of the obstetric data and is the primary source of the information presented here.

PROBLEMS AND BENEFITS OF CLOSED CLAIMS ANALYSIS

There are, unfortunately, limitations to closed claims data analysis that must be considered. Most importantly, the true incidence of a specific complication cannot be determined because we do not know, for any given period, the total number of claims filed or the total number of anesthetics given. Additionally, we know that most injuries attributable to medical error do not result in a malpractice claim (3). Conversely, anesthesiologists may be named in a claim in which there was no anesthetic-related injury. Finally, there is a significant delay between the occurrence of the event and the time the insurance file is closed. Because of time lag, critical liability issues that emerge today may be more applicable to anesthesia practice 5 to 10 years ago.

Closed claims analysis, however, provides information on problem areas in obstetric anesthesia that is otherwise difficult to obtain, including what types of injuries result in claims, what anesthetic events lead to such injuries, what proportion of claims result in settlement or awards, and the dollar amount of the payments. Prior to the analysis of closed claims data, maternal mortality statistics were one of the main sources of information on anesthetic complications and liability risk (4–8). Mortality data, however, only consider one of the most adverse outcomes, and miss other causes of significant morbidity. Closed claims analysis includes alleged injuries ranging from fairly minor to very severe. Additionally, unlike other sources of information, identification of these outcomes does not rely on self-reporting by the medical community, but instead highlights problems that

are significant from the consumer's point of view. Finally, these claims are probably very representative of all liability files involving obstetric anesthesia care in the United States, as the 35 participating liability carriers insure more than 50% of anesthesiologists in this country (9). Thus, despite their limitations, data from the ASA Closed Claims Project have much to offer practitioners of obstetric anesthesia regarding areas of potential liability risk and, hopefully, strategies for avoiding adverse anesthetic outcomes.

OBSTETRIC VS. NONOBSTETRIC CLAIMS

Of the 3533 claims recorded in the ASA Closed Claims Project database as of January 1995, 12% (434) involved anesthesia for cesarean section (71%) or vaginal delivery (29%). The mean maternal age was 28 years for patients with obstetric claims vs. 42 years for patients with nonobstetric claims.

Sixty-seven percent (290) of obstetric claims were associated with regional anesthesia, and 31% (133) with general anesthesia. In contrast, only 17% of the nonobstetric claims were associated with regional anesthesia, and 76% with general anesthesia. However, the distribution of regional and general anesthesia for claims involving cesarean section appears similar to the frequency with which these types of anesthetics are used for cesarean delivery throughout the country. The anesthesia work force survey conducted in 1981 (10) and again in 1992 (11) revealed a dramatic increase in the proportion of cesarean sections done by regional anesthesia and a decrease in those done using general anesthesia. A preliminary analysis of the entire ASA database (n = 4183) illustrates a similar trend in the claims for cases involving regional and general anesthesia for cesarean delivery (Fig. 25.1) (9). The similarity in percentages and trends between the anesthesia work force surveys and the closed claims data suggests that anesthetic choice for cesarean section is not inherently more (or less) likely to result in a malpractice suit.

OBSTETRIC ANESTHESIA–RELATED INJURIES

Table 25.1 lists all injuries or complications with a frequency of 5% or greater in the obstetric files, as well as the type of anesthetic and mode of delivery. Maternal death (n = 83) and newborn brain damage (n = 82) continue to be the most common injuries. Maternal death was more commonly associated with general anesthesia and cesarean delivery. Since the 1970s, the proportion of deaths in obstetric closed claims involving regional anesthesia has been declining, while that involving general anesthesia has remained relatively constant (9). It may be that, as the number of women having general anesthetics for cesarean section decreases, the highest-risk patients may be represented to a greater extent in the general anesthesia group.

To better illustrate the obstetric files compared with those of the nonobstetric population, Table 25.2 outlines the most common injuries listed in the obstetric claims, excluding those involving injury to the newborn only. It is noteworthy that, while death is the leading maternal injury resulting in a claim, it constitutes a significantly smaller proportion of total claims compared with the nonobstetric population.

The main reason for this finding appears to be the large proportion of relatively minor injuries—including headache, pain during anesthesia, back pain, and emotional distress—

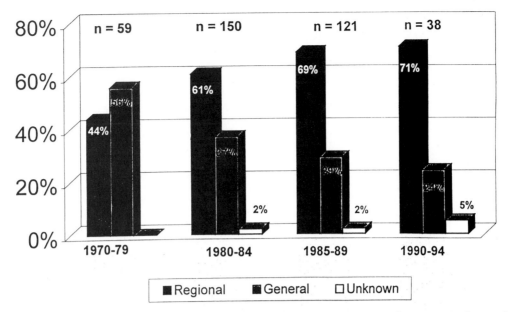

Figure 25.1. Anesthetic technique for C-sections. The proportion of files in which the anesthetic technique for cesarean section was either a regional or general anesthetic is shown as the percentage of the total number of claims for the indicated years. (Data from American Society of Anesthesiologists Closed Claims Project; n = 4183.) (Cheney FW. Personal communication, 1998).

represented in the maternal claims. These four categories total 47% of maternal claims, compared to only 8% of nonobstetric claims. The cause of this disparity is multifactorial. In contrast to claims for maternal death, these minor injuries (with the exception of emotional distress) are more commonly associated with regional anesthesia. The popularity of regional anesthesia techniques in obstetrics, combined with the greater incidence of postlumbar puncture headache in young females, likely accounts for the greater number of headache claims in this population (12, 13). Similarly, claims for back pain may be more likely in a population with a high rate of regional anesthesia and because of the high rate of back pain associated with pregnancy itself (14, 15). The majority of claims for headache and back pain are associated with regional anesthesia for vaginal delivery. This may be due to greater use of regional techniques for vaginal delivery than for cesarean section, or possibly to a

higher incidence of these complications in women who experience labor and periods of bearing down, as some have suggested (16, 17). In contrast, almost all claims for pain during anesthesia are associated with cesarean delivery. Apparently, inadequate analgesia for labor and vaginal delivery is seldom a source of liability risk, but pain during cesarean section is a great concern. Claims for pain during cesarean section almost always are made in the setting of regional anesthesia. Some of these claims may result from a reluctance on the part of anesthesia personnel to convert to general anesthesia during cesarean delivery due to the increased risk of airway difficulties and pulmonary aspiration.

While the high proportion of files with relatively minor maternal injuries may reflect a higher incidence of such problems in this group, other factors, such as unrealistic expectations or general dissatisfaction with the anesthetic care, undoubtedly contribute to the filing of these claims. The higher proportion

Table 25.1. MOST COMMON INJURIES IN THE OBSTETRIC ANESTHESIA FILES*

	OB Files (n = 434)	Regional Anesthesia (n = 290)	General Anesthesia (n = 133)	Cesarean Section (n = 310)	Vaginal Delivery (n = 124)
	% (n)	% (n)	% (n)	% (n)	% (n)
Maternal death	19 (83)	11 (31)[†]	39 (52)	23 (71)[†]	10 (12)
Newborn brain damage	19 (82)	18 (51)	21 (28)	17 (52)	24 (30)
Headache	15 (64)	21 (61)[†]	2 (2)	10 (32)[†]	26 (32)
Maternal nerve damage	10 (43)	13 (38)[†]	4 (5)	10 (30)	10 (13)
Pain during anesthesia	9 (37)	12 (36)[†]	0 (0)	11 (35)[†]	2 (2)
Back pain	8 (36)	12 (36)[†]	0 (0)	6 (18)[‡]	15 (18)
Maternal brain damage	7 (32)	6 (17)	11 (14)	9 (29)[†]	2 (3)
Emotional distress	7 (31)	8 (23)	6 (8)	7 (23)	6 (8)
Newborn death	6 (27)	6 (16)	6 (8)	6 (18)	7 (9)
Aspiration pneumonitis	5 (20)	1 (2)[†]	14 (18)	5 (16)	3 (4)

*Based on American Society of Anesthesiologists Closed Claims Project (n = 3533). The most common injuries in the obstetric group of files are shown in order of decreasing frequency. Percentages are based on the total files in each group. Some files indicated more than one injury and are represented more than once. In some files, the type of anesthetic was not recorded. Files involving "brain damage" only include patients who were alive when the file was closed.
[†] $P \le .01$ for regional vs. general anesthesia, and for cesarean section vs. vaginal delivery.
[‡] $P \le .05$ for cesarean section vs. vaginal delivery.
Data from Chadwick HS. An analysis of obstetric anesthesia cases from the American Society of Anesthesiologists Closed Claims Project database. *Int J Obstet-Anesth* 1996;5:258–263.

Table 25.2. MATERNAL INJURIES COMPARED TO SIMILAR INJURIES IN THE NONOBSTETRIC FILES

	Maternal Injury Files % (No.) (n = 356)	Nonobstetric Files % (No.) (n = 3099)
Maternal/patient death	23 (83)*	36 (1111)
Headache	18 (64)*	2 (50)
Maternal/patient nerve damage	12 (43)†	17 (523)
Pain during anesthesia	10 (37)*	1 (27)
Back pain	10 (34)*	1 (37)
Maternal/patient brain damage	9 (32)†	13 (403)
Emotional distress	9 (31)*	4 (115)
Aspiration pneumonitis	6 (20)†	2 (58)

Based on American Society of Anesthesiologists Closed Claims Project (n = 3533). The most common maternal injuries in the obstetric anesthesia files are shown in order of decreasing frequency. Percentages are based on the total files in each group. Some files, especially those with a fatal outcome, had more than one injury and are represented more than once. Cases involving brain damage only include patients who were alive when the file was closed.
*P ≤ .01
†P ≤ .05
Data from Chadwick HS. An analysis of obstetric anesthesia cases from the American Society of Anesthesiologists Closed Claims Project database. *Int J Obstet Anesth* 1996;5:258–263.

of claims for emotional distress in obstetric vs. nonobstetric groups highlights the value of establishing and maintaining good patient rapport and communication while providing obstetric anesthesia.

NEWBORN BRAIN INJURY

Newborn brain damage accounts for a high proportion (19%) of obstetric anesthesia-related claims, yet it does not show a significant association with type of anesthetic or mode of delivery. Because newborn brain damage may occur as a result of an antepartum, intrapartum, or postpartum event, it is difficult to determine to what degree anesthesia care is causally related to the newborn's injury. The anesthesiologist reviewers felt that only 46% of newborn brain injury claims and 26% of newborn death claims were related to anesthetic care. This is in contrast to the remainder of obstetric claims, 72% of which were determined to be related to anesthetic care. Anesthesiologists are more likely to be unfairly named in a claim for newborn injury, given the often imprecise timing and etiology of the injury and the devastating impact on the family. Reassuringly, however, the payment rate is lower for both newborn brain damage (44%) and death (41%) than for other obstetric claims (52%). This suggests that the insurance industry and legal system are, to some extent, able to recognize and unwilling to compensate a number of these claims against anesthesiologists.

EVENTS LEADING TO INJURIES

In order to use closed claim data to avoid future adverse anesthetic outcomes, we must not only identify what injuries occur, but also understand what critical anesthetic events precipitate these injuries. The most commonly identified damaging events for both obstetric and nonobstetric files in the ASA Closed Claims Project database are listed in Table 25.3. Not surprisingly, critical respiratory events are most common for both groups, constituting 30% of all nonobstetric damaging events and 18% of obstetric damaging events. Of the respiratory events, there is a trend for more problems with difficult intubation or pulmonary aspiration in obstetric files compared with nonobstetric files. The closed claims data, therefore, are consistent with reports that difficult intubation and pulmonary aspiration are the leading causes of anesthetic-related maternal mortality (see Chapter 25, part I), and they support the widely held belief that obstetric patients are at greater risk of having these complications.

The greater proportion of obstetric files in which pulmonary aspiration was identified as the *primary* damaging event is particularly noteworthy because 88% (15/17) of these events occurred

Table 25.3. MOST COMMON DAMAGING EVENTS IN THE OBSTETRIC ANESTHESIA FILES

	Non-OB Files % (No.) (n = 3099)	OB Files % (No.) (n = 434)	OB Regional % (No.) (n = 290)	OB General % (No.) (n = 133)
Respiratory system	30 (914)*	18 (80)	6 (16)*	47 (63)
Difficult intubation	6 (181)	7 (30)	< 0.5 (1)*	22 (29)
Aspiration	2 (52)	4 (17)	1 (2)*	11 (15)
Esophageal intubation	6 (178)*	2 (10)	1 (2)	6 (8)
Inadequate ventilation/oxygenation	9 (266)*	2 (9)	2 (6)	2 (2)
Bronchospasm	1 (43)	2 (7)	1 (2)	4 (5)
Premature extubation	1 (42)	1 (3)	0 (0)	2 (3)
Airway obstruction	3 (82)*	< 0.5 (2)	1 (2)	0 (0)
Inadequate F_{IO_2}	< 0.5 (5)	< 0.5 (2)	< 0.5 (1)	1 (1)
Convulsion	1 (45)*	9 (34)	12 (30)*	3 (4)
Equipment Problems	10 (315)*	6 (27)	8 (23)	3 (4)
Cardiovascular system	9 (287)*	4 (18)	4 (13)	3 (4)
Wrong drug/dose	4 (113)	3 (13)	2 (6)	5 (7)

Based on the American Society of Anesthesiologists Closed Claims Project (n = 3533). The most common damaging events in the obstetric files are shown in order of decreasing frequency. Percentages are based on the total files in each group. Specific damaging events were not identified in all cases. Some files indicated more than one damaging event, although only the most significant is listed. Statistical comparisons are made between obstetric and equivalent nonobstetric files, as well as between obstetric regional and obstetric general anesthetics.
*P ≤ .01
Data from Chadwick HS. An analysis of obstetric anesthesia cases from the American Society of Anesthesiologists Closed Claims Project database. *Int J Obstet Anesth* 1996;5:258–263.

in association with general anesthesia, which represented only 31% of obstetric files. This is in contrast to the nonobstetric files, in which 76% of all claims involved general anesthesia. Pulmonary aspiration was actually noted in 7% (29) of the obstetric files, although it was not necessarily always considered the primary damaging event. In 25 of these cases, the primary anesthetic technique was general anesthesia. In 10 cases, aspiration occurred during difficult intubation or following esophageal intubation, and in seven cases, mask general anesthesia was being used. In three cases, vomiting and aspiration occurred at the time of induction without cricoid pressure. Two cases of aspiration associated with regional anesthesia occurred during resuscitation and intubation efforts following high spinal blocks. In two other cases, aspiration was associated with successful regional anesthesia. In one case, heavy sedation was implicated; in the other, the patient apparently vomited following delivery of the infant.

These data reemphasize the importance of considering every obstetric patient presenting for delivery as having a full stomach. They also suggest that avoidance of mask anesthesia, use of routine antacid prophylaxis, and correct application of cricoid pressure may substantially reduce respiratory critical events and injuries resulting in claims. The frequency with which adverse outcomes are linked with difficult intubation reinforces the need to have appropriate protocols and equipment in place at all times for managing patients in whom tracheal intubation proves difficult.

Obesity has long been considered a risk factor for anesthetic complications, particularly with regard to airway management. The obstetric closed claims files indicate that damaging events related to the respiratory system were significantly more common among obese (32%) than nonobese (7%) parturients ($P \leq .01$). Death also was more common in the obese obstetric patients. Other injuries, however, were not significantly different in obese vs. nonobese obstetric patients, with the exception of a trend toward more airway trauma and back pain among the obese patients. These data underscore the need to be cautious and to have emergency algorithms and equipment prepared at all times when caring for these women.

While respiratory events as a group constitute the largest proportion of damaging events, the single most common damaging event in the obstetric closed claims files was convulsion (Table 25.3). Four cases of convulsion were associated with general anesthesia, and one with spinal anesthesia. These cases are clearly not a result of local anesthetic toxicity. The remaining 29 cases occurred in association with epidural anesthesia, 22 of which appear related to local anesthetic toxicity. In nine of these cases there is no documentation that a test dose of any kind was given. In the remaining 13, test doses were used, but only three were epinephrine-containing test doses. In those files in which convulsion was listed as the primary damaging event, the outcome was neurologic injury or death to the mother, newborn, or both in 74% of the cases.

The problem of local anesthetic toxicity in parturients became apparent in the early 1980s, resulting in strong warnings against the epidural use of 0.75% bupivacaine in obstetrics. Fortunately, since about 1984, the number of claims involving convulsions has decreased substantially. Undoubtedly, the quality of obstetric anesthesia care (including use of appropriate monitoring and resuscitation equipment) has greatly increased in the past 15 years. The current trend of using effective test doses and fractionating epidural local anesthetic injections, as well as not using bupivacaine 0.75%, has undoubtedly contributed to a reduction in the risks of serious adverse outcomes associated with epidural anesthesia in obstetric patients.

Many obstetric patients express concern regarding the risk of nerve injury when they are contemplating regional anesthesia for labor and delivery or cesarean section. Because such injuries are infrequent, most anesthesiologists tend to minimize the risks of such complications. Interestingly, however, nerve damage was

Table 25.4. CAUSES OF BLOCK-RELATED MATERNAL NERVE INJURIES

Likely Etiology	% (No.) (n = 21)
Needle or catheter trauma	52 (11)
Neurotoxicity	19 (4)
Ischemia (e.g., abscess, hematoma, hypotension, vasospasm)	14 (3)
Other identified causes	10 (2)
Undetermined	5 (1)

Based on the American Society of Anesthesiologists Closed Claims Project (n = 3533). A panel of 5 anesthesiologists independently reviewed all maternal nerve injury closed claims files in which peridural or spinal anesthesia was used (n = 38). In 21 (55%) of these cases, the injury was judged to be a result of the regional block procedure. The likely mechanism of injury in these cases is indicated in the table.
Data from Chadwick HS. An analysis of obstetric anesthesia cases from the American Society of Anesthesiologists Closed Claims Project database. *Int J Obstet Anesth* 1996;5:258–263.

the third most common maternal claim (Table 25.2), accounting for 12% of maternal injury files. To better understand the etiologies of these injuries, a panel of anesthesiologists reviewed the closed claims files of each maternal nerve injury case involving epidural or spinal anesthesia (18). Of these claims, the panel judged 55% (21/38) to be a consequence of anesthetic procedures or care. Table 25.4 lists the probable mechanism of injury for these 21 cases. Interestingly, the nerve injury in the majority of these cases appeared to be a result of direct trauma to neural tissue by either needle or catheter. Severe pain or paresthesia during needle or catheter placement or during local anesthetic injection was a prominent feature in these claims. Other mechanisms of injury, such as apparent neurotoxicity and ischemic causes (epidural abscess, hypotension, or vascular insufficiency) were less common. In fact, no cases of epidural hematoma were identified in the maternal injury claims. This analysis suggests that, while nerve injury in obstetrics may be a relatively frequent source of claims against anesthesiologists, often the anesthetic does not appear to be a causative factor.

Careful attention to persistent pain and/or paresthesia during block placement may help to avoid adverse anesthetic outcomes. Additionally, detailed anesthetic documentation and careful neurologic evaluation in the event of injury are critical in defending against an unjust claim (19).

INFORMED CONSENT

Lack of informed consent can be a specific cause of action for bringing suit against a physician. Historically, failure to obtain informed consent has been considered battery (unlawful touching). Informed consent statutes have been adopted in most state legislatures within the past 30 to 40 years, which recognize and protect individual patient's rights of self-determination and autonomy. As such, prior to providing medical care, a physician is obliged to obtain informed consent from the patient or a legally authorized surrogate decision-maker.

In order to defend against a claim of lack of informed consent, it is vital for the health care provider to document the informed consent process in the medical record. A patient signed form is not a necessity but may provide compelling evidence that informed consent was obtained. In some jurisdictions, a form signed by the patient, containing the necessary elements, will shift the burden of proof to the patient claiming that they were not informed of relevant risks *and/or* alternatives (19).

According to a 1986 study, many anesthesiologists were not adequately documenting either general or specific risks of anesthesia (20). A survey of U.S. and United Kingdom (U.K.) obstetric anesthesiologists indicated that 52% of U.S. and only 15% of U.K. anesthesiologists obtained a separate written consent for epidural labor analgesia (21). There has been much concern among anesthesiologists about the adequacy of the informed consent process when women are experiencing severe pain in labor. Ideally, anesthesia options and risks should be discussed before the patient is in severe pain. Unfortunately, often the anesthesiologist first encounters the patient when she is well into the stresses of active labor. Although the consent process can be tailored to the circumstances at hand, maternal pain and distress do not obviate the need for obtaining informed consent for a semi-elective procedure. A recent survey of Canadian women indicated a strong preference to be informed of all possible complications of epidural anesthesia, especially serious ones, even when the risk was quite low (22). This study and others have emphasized the desire among women to have these discussions as early in labor as possible.

Interestingly, the absence of appropriate informed consent has rarely been the *primary* reason for a medical malpractice suit in cases involving labor analgesia. Knapp searched the Lexis database in 1990 and found only three cases that addressed the adequacy of informed consent for anesthesia during labor (23). In each case, the court ruled in favor of the defendant anesthesiologist. The most recent closed claims data (n = 4183, 517 obstetric cases) show that in 24% of the obstetric files informed consent was not documented. However, informed consent issues were mentioned in only six of the narrative statements of these 517 obstetric files. In only one case did the lack of informed consent seem to be the primary focus of the claim (9).

PAYMENTS

Both obstetrics and anesthesiology are considered to be medical specialties with high-risk liability. Well-publicized cases involving huge awards reinforce the idea that obstetric anesthesiology is a particularly high-risk subspecialty. The ASA Closed Claims data, however, provide a somewhat different perspective. The obstetric anesthesia–related files account for 12% of the ASA Closed Claims database. Similarly, the obstetric files constitute 11% of the total number of payments made and 14% of the total dollars expended. Consequently, the obstetric payments, taken as a group, were not disproportionately frequent or large compared with payments in the nonobstetric claims.

Additional payment information is provided in Table 25.5. Payments are considered to be any expenditure by the insurance carrier in the form of settlement or award. General anes-

thesia cases accounted for a significantly higher payment rate and median dollar expenditure. This reflects the higher rate of serious complications (e.g., death, brain injury) in the claims involving general anesthesia. Overall, a lower percentage of claims were paid in the obstetric group. For cases in which payments were made, the median payment was significantly greater in the obstetric claims. The overall dollar difference, however, is not astounding or surprising. The median age of patients (mother and newborn) in obstetric claims is younger than in nonobstetric claims. While the obstetric files contain a smaller proportion of deaths (maternal and newborn), there is a greater proportion of brain injuries (maternal and newborn) compared with the nonobstetric files. Financial compensation for brain injury often exceeds that for death due to the projected need for life-long care.

CONCLUSION

The ASA Closed Claims Project permits a great deal of insight into the nature of insurance claims related to the provision of obstetric anesthesia, and reveals a liability risk profile that differs from nonobstetric claims. Complications involving the respiratory system account for the largest proportion of damaging events in both groups, and problems with difficult intubation and pulmonary aspiration are disproportionately represented in the obstetric files, confirming most anesthesiologists' belief that the pregnant patient's airway demands additional attention and care. As for regional anesthesia–related claims in obstetrics, local anesthetic toxicity remains a concern, although the number of such claims appears to be declining. Nerve damage also constitutes a relatively large percentage of claims, although the cause-and-effect relationship with regional block placement may not always be apparent. Direct trauma to neural tissue appears to be the most common etiology of anesthesia-related damage.

The most surprising difference, however, between obstetric and nonobstetric claims is the large proportion of claims for relatively minor injuries in the obstetric files. While reducing major adverse anesthetic outcomes in obstetrics is important, attention must be paid to limiting liability risk associated with less critical outcomes such as headache, pain during anesthesia, and emotional distress. To some extent, the large proportion of relatively minor injuries in the obstetric files may be due to a greater incidence of such problems in these patients. However, detailed review of these files suggests that, in many cases, patients either were unhappy with the care provided or felt that they were ignored or mistreated. Clearly, factors other than adverse outcome or major injury may be important in motivating

Table 25.5. PAYMENT DATA

	Non-OB Files % (No.) (n = 3099)	OB Files % (No.) (n = 434)	OB Regional % (No.) (n = 290)	OB General % (No.) (n = 133)
No payment	33 (1018)*	39 (171)	44 (129)†	28 (37)
Payments made	59 (1814)*	52 (224)	45 (130)†	66 (88)
Median payment	$100,000†	$200,000	$77,500†	$345,426
Range	$15–$23.2 million	$675–$6.8 million	$675–$6.8 million	$750–$6 million

Based on the American Society of Anesthesiologists Closed Claims Project (n = 3533). Payment frequency and dollar amounts (not adjusted for inflation) are illustrated. Percentages are based on the total number of files in each group and do not total 100% due to missing data. Statistical comparisons are made between payment distributions for obstetric and nonobstetric claims, and for obstetric regional and obstetric general anesthetics. Claims with no payments were excluded from calculations of median payment and range.
*$P \leq .05$
†$P \leq .01$
Data from Chadwick HS. An analysis of obstetric anesthesia cases from the American Society of Anesthesiologists Closed Claims Project database. *Int J Obstet Anesth* 1996;5:258–263.

a patient to bring a claim. It has been suggested that the number of patients harmed by negligent care who actually enter a claim may be less than 2% (3), supporting the idea that patients will not bring a lawsuit unless they feel they or a loved one has been unjustly treated. Malpractice litigation seems to serve the purposes not only of reparation of injury and deterrence of substandard care, but also emotional vindication (24, 25).

One of the benefits of closed claims analysis is that we can gain insight into what is important from the patient's perspective. In obstetric anesthesia, it is clear that relatively minor problems and complications may assume great significance. Therefore, anesthesia care providers should attempt to conduct themselves in a manner such that patients will not be motivated to bring a suit for an unexpected outcome (26). Measures should include establishing and maintaining good rapport throughout the peripartum period, and responding quickly and compassionately when complications do occur. Whenever possible, anesthesiologists should involve themselves in the prenatal education process. A careful preanesthetic evaluation is very important and should occur as early in labor as possible. Special care should be taken to provide patients with realistic expectations and knowledge of the potential major and common minor risks associated with anesthetic procedures, and this should be clearly documented in the medical record.

REFERENCES

1. Chadwick HS, Posner K, Caplan RA, et al. A comparison of obstetric and nonobstetric anesthesia malpractice claims. *Anesthesiology* 1991;74:242–249.
2. Chadwick HS. An analysis of obstetric anesthesia cases from the American Society of Anesthesiologists Closed Claims Project database. *Int J Obstet Anesth* 1996;5:258–263.
3. Localio AR, Lawthers AG, Brennan TA, et al. Relation between malpractice claims and adverse events due to negligence. Results of the Harvard Medical Practice Study III. *N Engl J Med* 1991;325:245–251.
4. Klein MD, Clahr J. Factors in the decline of maternal mortality. *JAMA* 1958;168:237–242.
5. Greiss FC, Anderson SH. Elimination of maternal deaths from anesthesia. *Obstet Gynecol* 1967;29:677–681.
6. Morgan M. Anaesthetic contribution to maternal mortality. *Br J Anaesth* 1987;59:842–855.
7. Bassell GM, Marx GF. Anesthesia-related maternal mortality. In: Shnider SM, Levinson G, eds. *Anesthesia for Obstetrics*. 3rd ed. Baltimore: Williams & Wilkins; 1993:455–466.
8. Turnbull A, Tindall VR, Beard RW, et al. *Report on Confidential Enquiries into Maternal Deaths in England and Wales, 1982–84*. London: HMSO; 1989.
9. Cheney FW. Personal communication, 1998.
10. Gibbs CP, Krischer J, Peckham BM, et al. Obstetric anesthesia: A national survey. *Anesthesiology* 1986;65:298–306.
11. Hawkins JL, Gibbs CP, Orleans M, et al. Obstetric anesthesia work force survey, 1981 versus 1992. *Anesthesiology* 1997;87:135–143.
12. Gielen M. Post dural puncture headache (PDPH): A review. *Reg Anesth* 1989;14:101–106.
13. Lybecker H, Moller JT, May O, Nielsen HK. Incidence and prediction of postdural puncture headache. *Anesth Analg* 1990;70:389–394.
14. Grove LH. Backache, headache, and bladder dysfunction after delivery. *Br J Anaesth* 1973;45:1147–1149.
15. Breen TW, Ransil BJ, Groves PA, Oriol NE. Factors associated with back pain after childbirth. *Anesthesiology* 1994;81:29–34.
16. Okell RW, Sprigge JS. Unintentional dural puncture. A survey of recognition and management. *Anaesthesia* 1987;42:1110–1113.
17. MacArthur C, Lewis M, Knox EC, Crawford JS. Epidural anaesthesia and long term backache after childbirth. *Br Med J* 1990;301:9–12.
18. Chadwick HS, Gunn HC, Ross BK, et al. Nerve injury and regional anesthesia in obstetrics—a review of the ASA Closed Claims Project database [abstract]. *Anesthesiology* 1995;83:A951.
19. Overview of anesthesia liability. *Healthcare Risk Control* 1996;4:2–6.
20. Moore R, DiBlasio W, Amini S. Anesthesia informed consent in New Jersey [abstract]. *Anesthesiology* 1986;65:A468.
21. Bush DJ. A comparison of informed consent for obstetric anaesthesia in the U.S.A. and the U.K. *Int J Obstet Anesth* 1995;4:1–6.
22. Pattee C, Ballantyne M, Milne B. Epidural analgesia for labour and delivery: Informed consent issues. *Can J Anaesth* 1997;44:918–923.
23. Knapp RM. Legal view of informed consent for anesthesia during labor [letter]. *Anesthesiology* 1990;72:211.
24. Hickson GB, Clayton EW, Githens PB, Sloan FA. Factors that prompted families to file medical malpractice claims following perinatal injuries. *JAMA* 1992;267:1359–1363.
25. Meyers AR. "Lumping it": The hidden denominator of the medical malpractice crisis. *Am J Public Health* 1987;77:1544–1548.
26. Palmer SK, Gibbs CP. Risk management in obstetric anesthesia. *Int Anesthesiol Clin* 1989;27:188–199.

FIVE

NONOBSTETRIC DISORDERS DURING PREGNANCY

Shnider and Levinson's Anesthesia for Obstetrics,
edited by Samuel C. Hughes, et al.
Lippincott Williams & Wilkins,
Philadelphia, © 2001.

CHAPTER 26

ANESTHESIA FOR THE PREGNANT CARDIAC PATIENT

DENNIS T. MANGANO, PH.D., M.D.

The pregnant patient with heart disease challenges the anesthesiologist's skills. Pregnancy and labor impose unique demands on the circulation, and anesthesia during delivery may compromise an already stressed cardiovascular system. To avoid such compromise, the anesthesiologist must be aware of the nature and progression of heart disease during pregnancy; the normal physiology of labor, delivery, and the puerperium; the cardiovascular effects of various anesthetic regimens; and the therapies used to manage acute complications. This chapter discusses the clinical manifestations, pathophysiology, and anesthetic management of serious cardiovascular diseases during pregnancy and parturition. The first section reviews the overall incidence, morbidity, and mortality of heart disease. Cardiovascular changes during pregnancy are summarized, and anesthetic guidelines are presented. The second, third, and fourth sections, respectively, discuss rheumatic heart disease, congenital heart disease, and other significant cardiovascular diseases that anesthesiologists managing parturients are likely to encounter. The final section reviews the effects of cardiac therapeutics on the fetus.

GENERAL CONSIDERATIONS

Over a 30 year period, the incidence of heart disease during pregnancy has declined from 3.6% to approximately 1.6% (Fig. 26.1) (1–12). Rheumatic heart disease, despite declining incidence, still accounts for most cases. However, the incidence of congenital heart disease in pregnant patients is steadily increasing, as a greater number of women with congenital heart lesions reach childbearing age due to improved medical and surgical therapies (1, 4, 13). Maternal mortality during pregnancy with rheumatic heart disease varies from less than 1% in asymptomatic patients to 17% in patients with mitral stenosis complicated by atrial fibrillation (Table 26.1) (8). Congenital heart disease is associated with a broad range of maternal and fetal mortality. With specific diseases, including primary pulmonary hypertension, dominant right-to-left shunt (Eisenmenger's syndrome, tetralogy of Fallot), severe aortic stenosis, and coarctation of the aorta, mortality is high regardless of the stage of disease progression (1, 14, 15).

Cardiovascular Changes During Pregnancy and Parturition

The cardiovascular changes associated with pregnancy and parturition that were discussed in Chapter 1 are briefly summarized here (16–21). Pregnancy *per se* exerts a progressive stress on the cardiovascular system that labor and delivery exacerbate (Figs. 26.2 to 26.5) (16–32). During labor, pain and apprehension increase, precipitating a progressive increase in stroke volume and cardiac output to 45% above prelabor values (20, 26–28). Uterine contraction further stresses the system by causing, in effect, an autotransfusion; with each contraction, central blood volume and cardiac output increase further by 10% to 25% (21). After delivery, central blood volume again increases,

and obstruction of the vena cava and aorta is relieved, resulting in a marked increase in stroke volume (up to 80% of prelabor values). Systemic vascular resistance decreases (20). Although well tolerated by the normal heart, the acute preload stress associated with delivery may represent an intolerable physiologic stress to a diseased heart that has become increasingly compromised throughout pregnancy and labor. When combined with postdelivery cardiovascular changes and those induced by hemorrhage or administration of oxytocic drugs, rapid decompensation may occur.

An Overview of Anesthetic Considerations

Anesthesia for the pregnant patient with heart disease requires an understanding of the type, severity, and progression of the disease in the context of normal cardiovascular adaptations to pregnancy. Preanesthetic detection of a symptomatic history either at rest or with exercise is of paramount importance because such a history correlates directly with morbidity and mortality (4, 33, 34). Physical examination plus consultation with the primary physician and cardiologist are necessary to define the severity of the disease.

Choice of Technique

For most cardiac diseases, no one anesthetic approach is exclusively indicated or contraindicated (35). The anesthesiologist's assessment of the patient's ability to tolerate pain during labor and surgery; the autotransfusion of uterine contraction; and the effects of postdelivery changes induced by relief of vena caval obstruction, oxytocic agents, and hemorrhage must each be considered to determine the best technique. The primary concern of the anesthesiologist is to avoid and/or treat specific pathophysiologic changes that can exacerbate the disease process. Cardiac medications required prior to pregnancy usually should be continued throughout pregnancy, labor, and delivery.

Monitoring Concerns

The decision to use invasive techniques (e.g., a radial arterial line or thermodilution pulmonary artery catheter) depends on the severity and progression of the disease. Most asymptomatic patients who show no disease progression and have no signs of impaired right or left ventricular performance will have an uneventful course and do not require invasive monitoring. Exceptions are patients, even if asymptomatic, with primary pulmonary hypertension (36–41), right-to-left shunt (14, 15, 42), dissecting aortic aneurysm (43), severe aortic stenosis (44–49), or coarctation of the aorta (50). Patients with severe heart disease should undergo complete hemodynamic profiling, including measurement of cardiac output, vascular resistance, central venous pressure (CVP), and pulmonary capillary wedge (PCW) pressure. Based on these measurements, a therapeutic plan should be designed for handling each of the acute complications that may occur with the specific disease. Although pulmonary artery catheterization is time-consuming, requires expertise, and may have associated morbidity and mortality, the author believes that

Table 26.1. INCIDENCE AND MORTALITY OF RHEUMATIC AND CONGENITAL HEART DISEASE IN PREGNANCY

	Distribution (%)	Mortality (%) Maternal	Mortality (%) Fetal	References
Rheumatic heart disease (75%)				
Mitral stenosis	90.0	1–17	3.5	1, 3, 4, 86, 107
Mitral insufficiency	6.5			
Aortic insufficiency	2.5			
Aortic stenosis	1.0			
	100.0			
Congenital heart disease (25%)				
Ventricular septal defect	7–26	7–40	2–16	13, 102–105
Atrial septal defect	8–38	1–12	1–12	1, 4, 7, 13, 98, 102
Patent ductus arteriosus	6–20	5–6	17	4, 13, 97, 98
Tetralogy of Fallot	2–15	4–12	36–59	1, 4, 7, 13, 98, 110, 111, 113, 114
Eisenmenger's syndrome	2–4	12–33	30–54	1, 2, 4, 101, 104, 105, 111
Coarctation of the aorta	4–18	3–9	10–20	4, 104, 120, 121
Aortic stenosis	2–10		22	1, 4, 98, 107
Pulmonic stenosis	8–16		4	1, 4, 98, 128
Primary pulmonary hypertension	1–2	53	7	1, 4, 99, 100, 104

the information derived from pulmonary artery monitoring in the presence of severe cardiac disease is worth the imposed risk.

Postoperative Care

Because the hemodynamic aberrations associated with labor and delivery may continue after delivery, patients with symptomatic heart disease who have had a complicated labor and delivery period should be monitored in an intensive care unit.

Management of Complications

Treatment of complications that occur during an anesthetic course may involve the use of electrocardioversion or pharmacologic agents such as digoxin, propranolol, lidocaine, metaraminol, sodium nitroprusside, and phentolamine. These drugs may have untoward fetal effects. Consequently, their use depends on the severity of maternal impairment and consideration of whether the risk of severe fetal morbidity outweighs the maternal morbidity associated with foregoing therapy. The author's philosophy is to correct immediately any severe maternal impairment, even though the therapy may cause fetal morbidity.

Finally, it should be clearly understood that there are few well-controlled studies addressing the effects of anesthetics and

therapeutics on pregnant patients with heart disease. However, the physiologic changes occurring during pregnancy, the pathophysiology of cardiac disease processes, and the effects of anesthetics on pregnant patients without cardiovascular disease are well documented. The anesthetic and therapeutic considerations and recommendations stated in this chapter have been synthesized from these mostly independent bodies of information and represent the opinions of this author.

RHEUMATIC HEART DISEASE

Rheumatic fever is a diffuse inflammatory disease affecting the heart, joints, and subcutaneous tissues following group A β-hemolytic streptococcal infection. Acute rheumatic fever is evidenced by a history of a streptococcal infection and a subsequent clinical picture that usually includes recurrent migratory polyarthritis with or without carditis. Polyarthritis tends to be self-limited, but the carditis can progressively and permanently damage valves or heart muscle. Although the prophylactic administration of antibiotics generally prevents the sequelae of rheumatic fever, rheumatic heart disease continues to be a common cause of death in the United States and in many other countries (33, 34, 51–55). Left or right ventricular failure, atrial dysrhythmias, systemic or pulmonary embolism, and infective endocarditis may complicate rheumatic heart disease during pregnancy (Table 26.2). Although the incidence of these complications during pregnancy has progressively decreased, they still occur in 15% of patients. The most common sequelae encountered in parturients are mitral valve impairments of stenosis, insufficiency, or prolapse, or aortic valve compromise by stenosis or insufficiency.

Mitral Stenosis

Rheumatic fever usually first occurs in 6- to 15-year-old children. If carditis occurs, mitral insufficiency ensues, followed in about 5 years by mitral stenosis. Symptoms usually do not appear for another 15 years. Pulmonary congestion, pulmonary hypertension, and right ventricular failure develop 5 to 10 years after the occurrence of symptoms (56, 57). On average, symptoms appear at 31 years and proceed in 7 years to total incapacity (58). Without surgical correction, 20% of incapacitated patients die in 6 months, 50% in 5 years, 75% in 10 years, and 90% in 15 years (58–63).

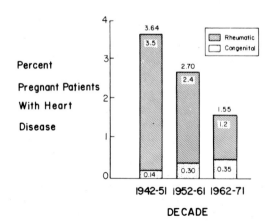

Figure 26.1. Incidence and distribution of heart disease during pregnancy over 3 decades. (Data from a review of more than 50,000 cases reported in Szekely PP, Snaith L, eds. *Heart Disease and Pregnancy.* London: Churchill Livingstone; 1974.)

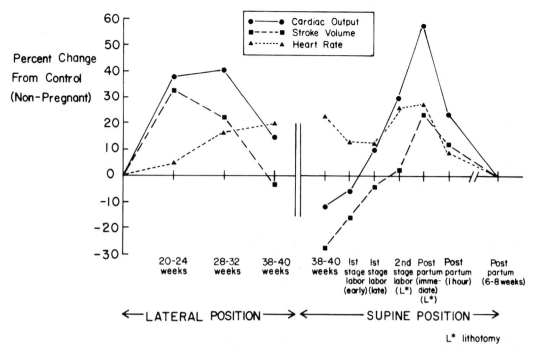

Figure 26.2. Maternal cardiovascular changes during pregnancy and labor from studies on patients in the lateral and supine positions. (Based on data reported by Ueland K, Hansen J. Maternal cardiovascular dynamics. II. Posture and uterine contractions. *Am J Obstet Gynecol* 1969;103:1–7; Ueland K, Hansen J. Maternal cardiovascular dynamics. III. Labor and delivery under local and caudal analgesia. *Am J Obstet Gynecol* 1969;103:8–18; and Ueland K, Novy M, Peterson E, Metcalf J. Maternal cardiovascular dynamics. IV. The influence of gestational age on the maternal cardiovascular response to posture and exercise. *Am J Obstet Gynecol* 1969;104:156–164.)

Clinical Manifestations

Signs and Symptoms. The initial symptoms of mitral stenosis are fatigue and dyspnea on exertion, with progression to paroxysmal nocturnal dyspnea, orthopnea, and dyspnea at rest. Hemoptysis with rupture of bronchopulmonary varices and pulmonary or systemic arterial embolization rarely occur. If mitral stenosis is severe, superimposition of stress such as atrial fibrillation, pulmonary embolism, infection, or pregnancy may precipitate rapid decompensation.

Physical examination may reveal a presystolic or middiastolic murmur that, if faint, will be heard only when the patient lies on her left side. The intensity of the murmur correlates poorly with the degree of stenosis, perhaps because other hemodynamic effects (e.g., depressed cardiac output) reduce flow through the valve. In addition to this murmur, an opening snap may be heard at the base of the heart along the left sternal border. Atrial fibrillation occurs in approximately one third of patients with severe mitral stenosis.

Test Indicators. Radiologic studies yield normal results early in the course of mitral stenosis, but left atrial and right ventricular enlargement occur as the disease progresses. Severe mitral stenosis may produce generalized pulmonary edema.

Electrocardiographic studies show a broadened P wave in lead V_1, signifying left atrial enlargement. Right-axis deviation signifies right ventricular enlargement. Cardiac catheterization commonly shows capillary wedge pressures of 25 to 30 mm Hg (normal is 0 to 12 mm Hg) occurring when the mitral valve orifice area is less than 2 cm². There is an associated increase in pulmonary vascular resistance. Severe mitral stenosis is consistent with valvular diastolic pressure gradients in excess of 25 mm Hg (normal is 5 mm Hg or less) (34, 62, 63).

Pathophysiology

The decrease in mitral valve orifice area impairs left ventricular filling (Fig. 26.6). Initially, the left atrium may overcome this obstruction, but, eventually, ventricular filling will decrease,

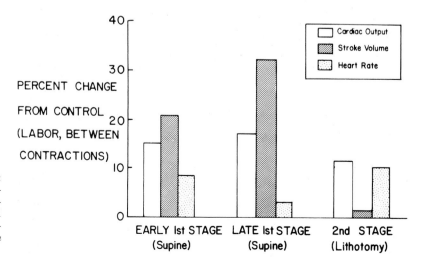

Figure 26.3. Effects of uterine contractions on cardiac output, stroke volume, and heart rate during labor. Values represent percentage increases from control measurements in late pregnancy. (Redrawn from Ueland K, Hansen J. Maternal cardiovascular dynamics. III. Labor and delivery under local and caudal analgesia. *Am J Obstet Gynecol* 1969;103:8–18.)

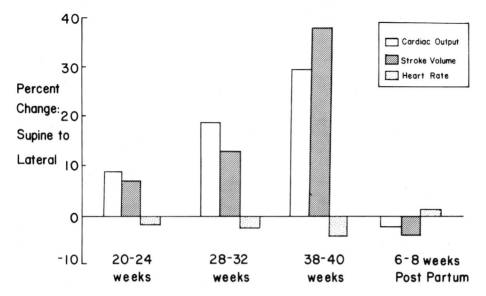

Figure 26.4. Percentage change in cardiac output, stroke volume, and heart rate when the pregnant woman turns from supine to lateral position. (Redrawn from Ueland K, Hansen J. Maternal cardiovascular dynamics. II. Posture and uterine contractions. *Am J Obstet Gynecol* 1969;103:1–7.)

followed by an increase in left atrial volume and pressure, and in pulmonary venous and PCW pressures. Transudation of fluid into the pulmonary interstitial space occurs, pulmonary compliance decreases, and the work of breathing rises, producing progressive dyspnea on exertion. With pulmonary hypertension, pulmonary artery medial thickening and fibrosis result, and pulmonary vascular resistance becomes permanently elevated. Right ventricular hypertrophy, dilation, and failure follow, leading to tricuspid insufficiency with hepatic and peripheral congestion. Atrial fibrillation, tachycardia, or increased metabolic demands (e.g., pregnancy and labor) may exacerbate these processes (31, 32, 64–66).

Pregnancy-Induced Changes. With pregnancy, an anatomically moderate stenosis can become functionally severe (7, 62, 63). Pregnant patients with mitral stenosis have an increased incidence of pulmonary congestion (25%), atrial fibrillation (7%), and paroxysmal atrial tachycardia (3%) (4). Left ventricular dysfunction is uncommon (15%) with pure mitral stenosis (34), and its presence suggests an associated element of mitral or aortic insufficiency.

Table 26.2. PREGNANT PATIENTS WITH RHEUMATIC HEART DISEASE

Major Complications	Incidence (%)
Left or right ventricular failure	8.5
Atrial dysrhythmias	6.5
Systemic or pulmonary embolism	1.6
Infective endocarditis	0.4

Data adapted from Szekely P, Snaith L. *Heart Disease and Pregnancy.* London: Churchill Livingstone; 1974.

Anesthetic Considerations

Asymptomatic parturients without evidence of pulmonary congestion have minimally increased risk; thus, they do not require additional invasive monitoring but should be attended with caution. The presence of marked symptoms significantly

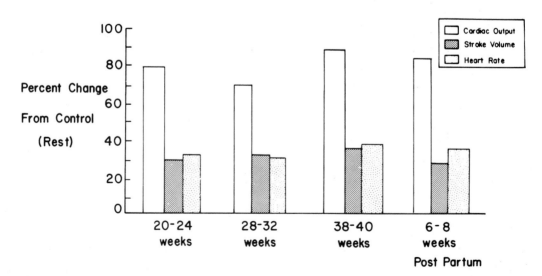

Figure 26.5. Effects of moderate exercise on cardiac output, stroke volume, and heart rate during pregnancy. (Redrawn from Ueland K, Novy M, Peterson E, Metcalf J. Maternal cardiovascular dynamics. IV. The influence of gestational age on the maternal cardiovascular response to posture and exercise. *Am J Obstet Gynecol* 1969;104:856–864.)

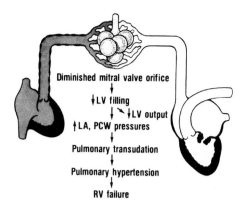

Figure 26.6. Pathophysiology of mitral stenosis. *LV,* left ventricle; *LA,* left atrial; *PCW,* pulmonary capillary wedge; *RV,* right ventricle.

increases parturient risk, warranting radial and pulmonary artery monitoring (Fig. 26.7). Specific factors to consider (Table 26.3) include:

- *Neither sinus tachycardia nor atrial fibrillation with a rapid ventricular response is tolerated well.*

Digoxin therapy used to control atrial fibrillation prior to pregnancy should be continued (with readjustment of dose, if necessary) to maintain ventricular rates below 110 beats per min (bpm). Development of atrial fibrillation with a rapid ventricular response may dramatically decrease cardiac output and produce pulmonary edema (61). The treatment is cardioversion starting with 25 watt-sec energy. The fetal safety of cardioversion has been documented (67–69). If cardioversion is unavailable, or if time (minutes) allows, propranolol (0.2 to 0.5 mg intravenously every 3 minutes) may be used to lower ventricular rate below 110 bpm. Propranolol administration should be discontinued when a total dose of 0.1 mg $\cdot$ kg^{-1} has been given or evidence of heart failure occurs (increasing PCW), and concern regarding side effects should be appreciated (see Therapy section) (70–73). Digitalization is used in stable situations where prolonged but not immediate (seconds to minutes) ventricular rate control is necessary. Digoxin 0.50 mg is given intravenously over 10 minutes followed by 0.25 mg intravenously every 2 hours to achieve a full digitalizing dose. Each dose has an effect in 15 minutes, with full effect in 1 to 2 hours. Potential side effects should be understood by the clinician (32, 74).

Sinus tachycardia in excess of 140 bpm or resulting in decreased cardiac output or increased PCW should be corrected immediately by reversing a precipitating event (pain, light gen-

Table 26.3. MITRAL STENOSIS: ANESTHETIC CONSIDERATIONS

1. Prevent rapid ventricular rates.
2. Minimize increases in central blood volume.
3. Avoid marked decreases in systemic vascular resistance.
4. Prevent increases in pulmonary artery pressure.

eral anesthesia, hypercarbia, acidosis) or by administering propranolol as just described.

- *Marked increases in central blood volume are poorly tolerated.*

Overtransfusion, Trendelenburg position, or autotransfusion via uterine contraction can precipitate right ventricular failure, pulmonary hypertension, pulmonary edema, or atrial fibrillation. Increases in CVP or PCW may be used to assess increases in central blood volume.

- *Marked decreases in systemic vascular resistance may not be tolerated.*

With severe stenosis, decreases in systemic vascular resistance are compensated for by increases in heart rate (stroke volume is fixed). This response is limited and marked increases in heart rate may lead to decompensation. The author recommends that, if necessary, systemic vascular resistance be maintained with an intravenous infusion of metaraminol (10 mg in 250 mL saline). Ephedrine is not recommended because it may increase heart rate.

- *Pulmonary hypertension and right ventricular failure can be exacerbated by multiple factors.*

Any degree of hypercarbia, hypoxia, acidosis, lung hyperinflation, or increased lung water can elevate pulmonary vascular resistance. Prostaglandins used to treat uterine atony should be used with caution since they may have effects on the pulmonary vasculature.

If pulmonary hypertension and right ventricular compromise persist, inotropic support with dopamine (3 to 8 μg $\cdot$ kg^{-1} $\cdot$ min^{-1}) and pulmonary vasodilation with low-dose sodium nitroprusside (0.1 to 0.5 μg $\cdot$ kg $\cdot$ min^{-1}) are recommended. Higher doses of nitroprusside may produce undesirable vasodilation and elevated maternal and fetal cyanide levels (see final section). Prolonged mechanical ventilation may be required if hemodynamic or pulmonary complications occur.

Anesthesia for Vaginal Delivery and Cesarean Section

Vaginal delivery. The author recommends segmental lumbar epidural anesthesia for labor and vaginal delivery (62, 63, 75, 76). This eliminates the pain and tachycardia that attend uterine contractions. Perineal analgesia blocks the urge to push and

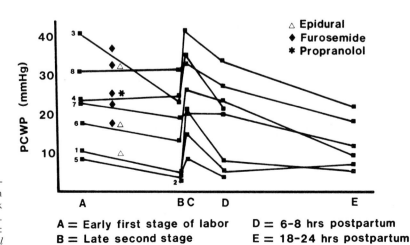

Figure 26.7. Intrapartum alterations in pulmonary capillary wedge pressure (*PCWP*) in eight patients with mitral stenosis. (Reprinted by permission from Clark SL, Phelan JP, Greenspoon J, Aldahl D, Horenstein J. Labor and delivery in the presence of mitral stenosis: Central hemodynamic observations. *Am J Obstet Gynecol* 1985;152:984–988.)

A = Early first stage of labor   D = 6-8 hrs postpartum
B = Late second stage   E = 18-24 hrs postpartum
C = 5-15 min postpartum

thereby prevents exertion, fatigue, and the deleterious effect of a Valsalva maneuver. Fetal descent is accomplished by the uterine contractions per se, and delivery is facilitated with vacuum extraction or outlet forceps. Hypotension may be prevented by continuous left uterine displacement and judicious fluid infusion. Prophylactic ephedrine and rapid hydration should be avoided. If hypotension occurs, metaraminol is the preferred vasopressor.

Cesarean section: regional anesthesia. Either regional or general anesthesia may be used for cesarean section. A continuous lumbar epidural block is preferred to spinal anesthesia because epidural anesthesia produces more controllable hemodynamic changes. The anesthetic level should be established slowly by titrating local anesthetic through the epidural catheter. Epinephrine is omitted from the local anesthetic solution because of the potential for tachycardia and peripheral vasodilation. If hypotension occurs associated with decreased PCW pressure, it may be cautiously treated with fluid infusion to reestablish normal filling pressures. If PCW pressure remains normal or if pulmonary artery monitoring is not possible, hypotension should be corrected by infusion of metaraminol. The combined spinal epidural technique may also be used (see Chapter 9).

Cesarean section: general anesthesia. If general anesthesia is used, drugs that produce tachycardia, such as atropine, pancuronium, meperidine, and ketamine, should be avoided. Parturients with mild stenosis may be managed with an intravenous thiopental induction, intubation, and light general anesthesia. Those with moderate or severe stenosis may be unduly stressed by this regimen, and a slow induction with halothane or intravenous fentanyl is recommended. If significant right or left ventricular compromise exists, fentanyl is preferred over halothane. With either technique, tachycardia may follow endotracheal intubation or surgical incision and should be treated by increasing anesthetic depth or by administration of propranolol. A halothane or fentanyl induction increases the risk of maternal aspiration or neonatal depression, but the author believes that the benefits outweigh these hazards.

Postoperative care. Because mitral stenosis may produce pulmonary dysfunction, respiratory adequacy (arterial blood gases, pulmonary mechanics, chest roentgenogram) must be assessed on weaning from controlled ventilation. Intensive care unit monitoring may be necessary.

Mitral Insufficiency

Mitral insufficiency is the second most common valvular defect in pregnancy (4, 56, 77). Left ventricular volume work is chronically increased. This is usually tolerated well, and patients with insufficiency may remain asymptomatic for 30 to 40 years. However, congestive heart failure follows, and with symptoms, a rapid downhill course occurs with a 5-year mortality of 50%. Other complications occurring during the fourth or fifth decade are atrial fibrillation, systemic embolization, and bacterial endocarditis (56, 78, 79).

Because complications usually occur late in life–after the childbearing age–most patients with mitral regurgitation tolerate pregnancy well. However, Szekely and Snaith (4) reported a 5.5% incidence of pulmonary congestion during pregnancy. In addition, they reported a 4.3% incidence of atrial tachycardia, a 2.8% incidence of pulmonary embolism, and an 8.5% incidence of infective endocarditis.

Clinical Manifestations

Signs and Symptoms. The principal symptoms of advanced mitral insufficiency are those of left ventricular failure. The cardinal sign is a pansystolic murmur of blowing quality, loudest at the cardiac apex, referred to the left axilla or the infrascapular area. Atrial fibrillation occurs in approximately one third

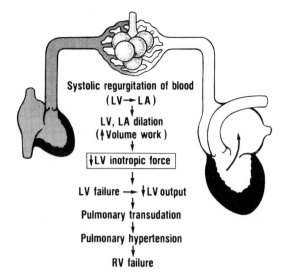

Figure 26.8. Pathophysiology of mitral insufficiency. *LV,* left ventricle; *LA,* left atrium; *RV,* right ventricle.

of patients. Late sequelae associated with mitral insufficiency include pulmonary congestion, pulmonary hypertension, and right ventricular enlargement (33, 52).

Test Indicators. Electrocardiographic results appear normal with mild mitral insufficiency but reveal signs of left ventricular and, at times, right ventricular hypertrophy in the presence of advanced disease. Similarly, roentgenographic results are normal with mild mitral insufficiency but demonstrate left ventricular and, especially, left atrial enlargement in severe cases.

Pathophysiology

Mitral insufficiency causes regurgitation of blood from the left ventricle through the incompetent mitral valve into the left atrium (Fig. 26.8). With chronic mitral insufficiency, the left atrium adapts to the increased blood volume by dilating and increasing compliance. When left atrial pressure rises, pulmonary venous and PCW pressures also rise, causing pulmonary congestion and edema. With progressive left ventricular failure, pulmonary hypertension and right ventricular compromise will occur. Left atrial pressure does not increase until late in the course of the disease; thus, the left atrium protects the pulmonary venous, capillary, and arterial beds from pressure overload. Left ventricular dilation also occurs because of the increase in preload afforded by the hypervolemic left atrium. Forward ejection of blood through the aortic valve can be impaired by as much as 50% to 60% and depends on the ratio of resistance through the aortic valve to resistance through the insufficient mitral valve. Reduction of left ventricular afterload can therefore play an important role in decreasing the amount of regurgitant blood flow and increasing forward cardiac output.

Pregnancy-Induced Changes. With pregnancy comes an increase in intravascular volume that may be intolerable to the chronically compromised left ventricle, resulting in pulmonary congestion (26–28, 80). Changes in systemic resistance may play an important role. The decreased peripheral resistance of pregnancy may improve forward flow at the expense of regurgitant flow (81). In contrast, pain, apprehension, uterine contractions, or surgical stimulation associated with labor and delivery may increase systemic vascular resistance by augmenting sympathetic activity. The resultant decrease in forward flow and increase in regurgitant flow may precipitate acute left ventricular failure and pulmonary congestion (80). It should be noted that the murmurs of mitral and aortic insufficiency may decrease during pregnancy (82).

Table 26.4. MITRAL INSUFFICIENCY: ANESTHETIC CONSIDERATIONS

1. Prevent peripheral vasoconstriction.
2. Avoid myocardial depressants.
3. Treat acute atrial fibrillation immediately.
4. Maintain a normal or slightly elevated heart rate.
5. Monitor pulmonary capillary wedge pressure and intensity of murmur.

Anesthetic Considerations

Asymptomatic patients with mild mitral insufficiency and an unchanging murmur throughout pregnancy may be approached in a routine but cautious fashion. Symptomatic patients typically warrant monitoring by radial and pulmonary artery catheterization. Table 26.4 provides the important anesthetic considerations. Principal among these are:

- *Marked increases in systemic vascular resistance can cause acute decompensation of the left ventricle.*

Treatment consists of left ventricular afterload reduction with low doses of sodium nitroprusside (0.1 to 0.5 $\mu g \cdot kg^{-1} \cdot min^{-1}$) or phentolamine (0.1 to 1 $\mu g \cdot kg^{-1} \cdot min^{-1}$).

- *Atrial fibrillation can cause left ventricular decompensation.*

The preferred treatment is direct current countershock as outlined in the section on mitral stenosis.

- *Myocardial depressants are not well tolerated.*

Because left ventricular impairment usually accompanies mitral insufficiency, even minimal myocardial depression may result in significant compromise.

- *Bradycardia is poorly tolerated.*

Forward stroke volume may be limited, and cardiac output will depend principally on heart rate. Maintenance of normal to slightly elevated heart rates is advocated.

- *The amount of regurgitant flow correlates with the intensity of the insufficiency murmur and the size of the V wave in the PCW pressure tracing.*

Both can be useful parameters in assessing the amount of ventricular failure with chronic insufficiency. PCW pressure is a poor measure of left atrial volume or left ventricular end-diastolic volume since the left atrium is very compliant; however, minor changes in pressure are indicative of changes in left ventricular end-diastolic volume. With acute mitral insufficiency, the left atrium is less compliant, so that changes in PCW pressures correlate with changes in left atrial and left ventricular end-diastolic pressures. The anesthetic considerations for pulmonary hypertension and right ventricular compromise delineated in the section on mitral stenosis also apply here.

- *Afterload reduction may be useful therapy.*

Left ventricular failure may benefit from afterload reduction with small amounts of sodium nitroprusside or phentolamine, combined with dopamine to give left ventricular inotropic support.

Anesthesia for Vaginal Delivery and Cesarean Section

Regional anesthesia. For labor and vaginal delivery, lumbar epidural analgesia is recommended. This technique will prevent the peripheral vasoconstriction associated with the pain of labor and will increase the forward flow of blood. This latter advantage also applies to regional vs. general anesthesia for cesarean section. However, regional anesthesia will increase venous capacitance and may require administration of intravenous fluids to maintain the filling volume of the enlarged left ventricle. Constant left uterine displacement and a 10-degree Trendelenburg position should be used to maintain venous return. The positive inotropic and chronotropic effects of ephedrine are especially useful in preventing and treating hypotension.

Inhalation anesthesia. Nitrous oxide–relaxant anesthesia may be dangerous because of the associated peripheral vasoconstriction. However, when combined with sodium nitroprusside to prevent peripheral vasoconstriction, this approach may be useful in patients with compromised ventricular function because it avoids myocardial depression and maintains an elevated heart rate. In patients without severe ventricular compromise, a halogenated agent may be added to the nitrous oxide.

Mitral Valve Prolapse

Mitral valve prolapse (MVP) is the most common congenital valvular lesion, occurring in 5% to 10% of the general population. Because of the broad spectrum of pathologic changes in the mitral valve apparatus occurring with this syndrome, it is identified by various names, including systolic click-murmur, Barlow's disease, billowing mitral valve, mitral cusp, sloppy mitral valve, and redundant cusp. MVP is most prevalent in younger females, commonly during the childbearing years. In 85% of patients with MVP, the disease is asymptomatic and benign. In the remaining 15%, mitral regurgitation develops over a 10- to 15-year period and requires alteration of medical management.

Parturients with MVP without mitral insufficiency typically tolerate pregnancy and delivery well (83, 84). Complications have been reported only with mitral insufficiency or other coexisting diseases, such as pregnancy-induced hypertension.

Clinical Manifestations

Signs and Symptoms. Although most patients with MVP are asymptomatic, diverse clinical manifestations are associated with the syndrome, including anxiety, palpitations, dyspnea, chest discomfort, light-headedness, emotional disturbance, and signs indicative of autonomic nervous dysfunction, such as orthostatic hypotension. Patients are sometimes marfanoid or have thoracic skeletal abnormalities.

The cardinal sign of MVP is a mid-to-late systolic click, occurring after the beginning of the upstroke of the carotid pulse. Often, the click is accompanied by a mid-to-late crescendo systolic murmur, with murmur duration reflecting the severity of the mitral regurgitation. If MVP is severe, the click occurs early and the murmur becomes holosystolic. The clinical presentation of MVP with mitral insufficiency reflects these same symptoms.

Test Indicators. Electrocardiographic results usually are normal in asymptomatic patients but occasionally may reflect inverted or biphasic T waves and nonspecific ST changes in the inferior leads. Arrhythmias are common, particularly paroxysmal supraventricular tachycardia due to presence of atrioventricular bypass tracts. Other supraventricular and ventricular tachyarrhythmias, bradyarrhythmias, and conduction block have been reported with this condition. Echocardiographic findings are significant and often diagnostic of MVP. M-mode echocardiography demonstrates sudden posterior movement of the posterior leaflet during midsystole, resulting in a "question mark" sign as well as "hammocking" of the posterior leaflet into the left atrium. Two-dimensional echocardiography may be the most definitive test, demonstrating mitral valve leaflets in the left atrium during ventricular systole.

Pathophysiology

With MVP, the cordae tendineae are elongated, causing the mitral leaflets to prolapse into the left atrium when ventricular volume decreases during mid-to-late systole. The systolic click is produced by a sudden tensing of the elongated cordae and the prolapsing leaflets. The crescendo systolic murmur represents retrograde flow during systole from the left ventricle to the left atrium. Conditions that decrease left ventricular volume, such as hypovolemia, venodilation, increased airway pressure, and tachycardia, cause an earlier prolapsing of the mitral leaflets during systole and an earlier and louder crescendo murmur with increased regurgitation. However, conditions that increase ventricular volume, such as bradycardia, afterload augmentation, hypervolemia, and negative inotropic agents, delay the systolic click and murmur and, at times, may mask these signs of MVP.

Generally, when the systolic click and murmur occur earlier in the cycle, the degree of regurgitation is greater. However, certain conditions, such as infusion of venodilators (nitrates) or augmentation of afterload (phenylephrine), cause paradoxical changes. For example, the administration of nitrates decreases ventricular volume, producing an earlier systolic click and murmur, but the associated reduction in left ventricular systolic pressure decreases both the regurgitant fraction and murmur intensity. Similarly, administration of phenylephrine increases systemic vascular resistance, thereby delaying the systolic click and murmur onset, but the associated increase in ventricular volume and systolic pressure increases regurgitation and murmur intensity. When mitral insufficiency occurs with MVP, the anesthetic considerations are therefore similar to those guiding management of parturients with mitral insufficiency alone.

Pregnancy-Induced Changes.   With pregnancy, the normal physiologic changes appear to have little effect on patients with MVP when no other cardiovascular abnormalities are present. Compared with pregnant patients without cardiac disorders, parturients with MVP do not have a higher incidence of antepartum and intrapartum complications or increased signs of fetal distress. However, the co-presence of MVP and a cardiovascular disorder, such as pregnancy-induced hypertension, can result in significant complications such as congestive heart failure.

Anesthetic Considerations

Asymptomatic patients without mitral insufficiency with an unchanging murmur throughout pregnancy should be managed in a routine but cautious manner. However, patients who manifest symptoms of mitral insufficiency or those with crescendo murmurs that increase in intensity during pregnancy warrant special consideration. Table 26.5 provides the principal anesthetic considerations. Of particular concern are the following:

- *Reduction in left ventricular volume generally is not tolerated well and increases the degree of prolapse.*

Treatment consists of reversing these effects (such as decreasing airway pressure) and administration of intravenous fluids. It is essential to maintain intravascular and intraventricular volume and provide acute treatment of blood loss.

- *Antiarrhythmic drugs should be continued pre-, intra-, and post-operatively.*

Treatment of paroxysmal supraventricular tachycardia, especially when decreased peripheral perfusion occurs, should be aggressive (see section on cardiac arrhythmias).

- *With moderate-to-severe mitral insufficiency, steps must be taken to decrease the regurgitant fraction and enhance forward flow.*

In these parturients, it is important to prevent peripheral vasoconstriction, avoid the use of myocardial depressants, and maintain a normal to slightly elevated heart rate.

- *In parturients with mild or no insufficiency, maneuvers or drugs that increase ventricular volume will decrease the degree of prolapse.*

Generally, these patients require no special considerations or treatment modalities. Maintenance of ventricular volume,

---

Table 26.5. MITRAL VALVE PROLAPSE: ANESTHETIC CONSIDERATIONS

1. Avoid decreases in preload.
2. Continue antiarrhythmic therapy.
3. With mitral valve prolapse and moderate-to-severe mitral insufficiency, the same considerations as listed for mitral insufficiency alone apply.

---

afterload, and normal or even depressed contractility should be beneficial.

Anesthesia for Vaginal Delivery and Cesarean Section

Regional anesthesia. Lumbar epidural analgesia is recommended for labor and vaginal delivery in patients with moderate-to-severe mitral insufficiency (85). This technique prevents the peripheral vasoconstriction associated with the pain of labor and will increase the forward flow of blood. This advantage also applies to the use of regional rather than general anesthesia for cesarean section. With regional anesthesia, the increase in venous capacitance will require the administration of intravenous fluid to maintain the filling volume of the enlarged left ventricle and to minimize the degree of prolapse. Left uterine displacement and Trendelenburg positioning should be used to maintain venous return.

Inhalation anesthesia. Nitrous oxide–relaxant anesthesia, when accompanied by tachycardia and peripheral vasoconstriction, may be detrimental in parturients with MVP for several reasons. Tachycardia may reduce intraventricular volume and increase the degree of prolapse. Peripheral vasoconstriction will increase left ventricular systolic pressure and regurgitant flow. However, in parturients without severe ventricular dysfunction, the inhalational agents can be used effectively. And in patients with marked ventricular dysfunction, a nitrous oxide–relaxant technique actually may be beneficial because it will not further compromise myocardial function. In these parturients, normal to low-normal systemic vascular resistance can be maintained by administration of agents such as sodium nitroprusside.

No particular anesthetic technique appears to be superior in MVP patients with mild or no mitral insufficiency.

Aortic Stenosis

Aortic stenosis appears as the dominant valve lesion in 0.5% to 3% of parturients (1, 4, 7, 44–49, 80). This relative rarity results from the 35- to 40-year latent period between acute rheumatic fever and symptoms of severe stenosis: congestive heart failure, syncope, and angina. Most patients become symptomatic in their fifth or sixth decade (86). Progressive decompensation follows the appearance of symptoms, with 50% mortality within 5 years. Sudden death occurs in 3% to 10% of these patients (33, 34, 56, 87). Asymptomatic pregnant patients with aortic stenosis are not at increased risk (4), although they have reduced hemodynamic responses to the demands of pregnancy and exercise (88). Symptomatic aortic stenosis markedly increases maternal and fetal morbidity and mortality (1, 4, 7, 44–49, 89).

Clinical Manifestations

The cross-sectional area of the aortic valve orifice in normal adults is 2.6 to 3.5 cm^2 (90). A 25% to 50% decrease in area results in a loud aortic systolic murmur. Narrowing to less than 1 cm^2 markedly increases left ventricular end-diastolic pressures (Fig. 26.9). Areas below 0.75 cm^2 produce exertional dyspnea, angina pectoris, and syncope (34, 90–92). The principal physical finding is a systolic ejection murmur loudest in the second right intercostal space adjacent to the sternum and radiating into the neck. Intensity of the murmur may not correlate with the degree of stenosis. A low cardiac output or decreased velocity of ejection reduces the intensity of the murmur. The electrocardiogram in severe aortic stenosis shows left ventricular hypertrophy and, occasionally, a left bundle branch block. Radiographs may show left ventricular enlargement, poststenotic dilation of the aorta, and, in older adults, calcification of the aortic valve. Catheterization findings are usually normal when the aortic valve orifice area exceeds 1 cm^2. Smaller areas usually produce a systolic pressure gradient between the aorta and left ventricle. A gradient of 50 mm Hg or more indicates severe stenosis, except in patients with congestive heart failure, where reduced left

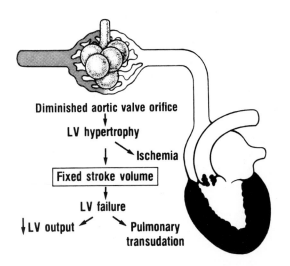

Figure 26.9. Pathophysiology of aortic stenosis. *LV*, left ventricle.

ventricular stroke volume may produce only 30 mm Hg gradients, even with severe aortic stenosis (21, 33, 45).

Anesthetic Considerations

The presence of symptoms, evidence of left ventricular failure, or progression of stenosis suggests a need for radial and pulmonary artery monitoring (46). The following considerations should be noted (Table 26.6):

- *Decreases in systemic vascular resistance are poorly tolerated.*

In healthy parturients, increases in stroke volume and heart rate usually compensate for a decrease in systemic vascular resistance. Aortic stenosis relatively fixes stroke volume, and patients with stenosis must rely on elevation of heart rate to maintain blood pressure. However, elevations of heart rate above 140 bpm will decrease diastolic filling and cardiac output. Vascular resistance should be maintained during anesthesia by using light levels or by administering a vasoconstrictor (e.g., metaraminol).

- *Bradycardia is poorly tolerated for the reasons described earlier for aortic insufficiency.*

Bradycardia increases the duration of ventricular diastole and thus the amount of blood regurgitated across the aortic valve. Heart rates should be maintained between 80 and 100 bpm.

- *Decreases in venous return and left ventricular filling are poorly tolerated.*

Due to the increased and fixed afterload, left ventricular stroke volume will be maintained only if the end-diastolic volume is adequate. Marked decreases in ventricular filling will decrease stroke volume and cardiac output (Fig. 26.10). Additionally, since the ventricle is noncompliant, small changes in fluid loading will result in large changes in filling pressure (Fig. 26.11).

Anesthesia for Vaginal Delivery and Cesarean Section

Parturients with aortic stenosis usually tolerate the hemodynamic effects of pain and stress. When possible, sympathetic blockade should be avoided.

Vaginal delivery. For labor and vaginal delivery, systemic medication, inhalation analgesia, and pudendal nerve block

---

Table 26.6. AORTIC STENOSIS: ANESTHETIC CONSIDERATIONS

1. Avoid decreases in systemic vascular resistance.
2. Avoid bradycardia.
3. Maintain venous return and left ventricular filling.

---

anesthesia have been utilized. If regional analgesia is desired, the use of intrathecal opioids alone, or co-administered with dilute concentrations of epidural local anesthetics, is useful. This can be achieved by use of the combined spinal-epidural techniques discussed in Chapter 9. Because hypotension is poorly tolerated, maternal blood pressure should be sustained with left uterine displacement, fluids, and administration of metaraminol or ephedrine.

Cesarean section. General anesthesia with the standard nitrous oxide—relaxant technique is recommended for cesarean section (93). Halogenated anesthetics, with their potential for undue myocardial depression, should be avoided when evidence exists of severe left ventricular compromise. Signs or symptoms of ventricular ischemia associated with hypotension indicate the need to elevate or maintain systemic vascular resistance with metaraminol.

Aortic Insufficiency

A 7- to 10-year latent period after an acute attack of rheumatic fever usually precedes the development of aortic regurgitation with associated widened pulse pressure, decreased systemic diastolic pressure, and bounding peripheral pulses (34, 56). The disease usually remains asymptomatic for another 7 to 10 years. Patients presenting with (a) left ventricular enlargement, (b) electrocardiographic evidence of ventricular hypertrophy, and (c) a large peripheral pulse pressure have a 33% chance of developing heart failure, angina, or death within 1 year; a 50% chance within 2 years; a 65% chance within 3 years; and an 87% chance within 6 years (56). Patients with one or two of these signs have a 10% chance of developing heart failure, angina, or death over a 10-year period, and patients with none of these signs have uneventful courses over the same period (33, 34, 52).

Because symptoms usually develop during the fourth or fifth decade of life, most patients with dominant aortic insufficiency have uneventful pregnancies. However, heart failure complicates 3% to 9% of such cases during pregnancy (1, 4, 7, 80).

Clinical Manifestations

Signs and Symptoms. The symptoms of aortic insufficiency relate to left ventricular failure. Moderately severe insufficiency produces a widened pulse pressure, with diastolic blood pressures below 60 mm Hg (33, 34, 56) and systolic pressures that are commonly less than 160 mm Hg. An early blowing diastolic murmur usually is heard along the left sternal border in the second, third, or fourth intercostal space. Duration of the diastolic murmur depends on the severity of aortic insufficiency.

Test Indicators. Electrocardiographic evidence of severe insufficiency displays increased QRS amplitude, depressed ST segments, inverted T waves, and a horizontal axis. Atrial fibrillation suggests concomitant mitral valve disease or myocardial failure with moderately severe aortic insufficiency. Chest roentgenography will reveal left ventricular dilation.

Pathophysiology

Left ventricular volume overload occurs with aortic insufficiency (Fig. 26.12). This volume depends on the area of the regurgitation orifice, the diastolic pressure gradient between aorta and left ventricle, and the duration of diastole (94). With chronic volume overload, the left ventricle becomes eccentrically distended and compliance increases. Left ventricular end-diastolic pressure remains normal for several years. The left ventricle usually tolerates this chronic increase in left ventricular volume work and can become markedly distended without evidencing cardiac failure. However, once failure begins, forward stroke volume decreases, end-diastolic volume precipitously increases, and left ventricular end-diastolic pressure rises above normal. Pulmonary capillary congestion and signs of pulmonary edema follow (34, 95).

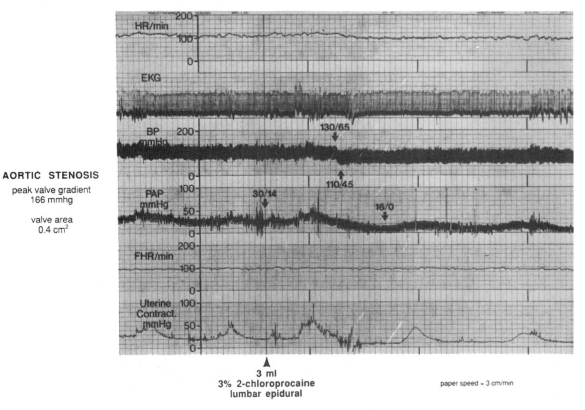

Figure 26.10. Hemodynamic responses to an epidural test dose of a rapid-acting anesthetic in a patient with severe aortic stenosis. *HR*, heart rate; *ECG*, electrocardiogram; *BP*, blood pressure; *PAP*, pulmonary artery pressure; *FHR*, fetal heart rate. Shortly after injection of 3 mL 3% 2-chloroprocaine, there was a dramatic fall in PAP and BP, likely resulting from a small but rapid increase in vascular capacitance. (Reprinted by permission from Easterling TR, Chadwick HS, Otto CM, Benedetti TJ. Aortic stenosis in pregnancy. *Obstet Gynecol* 1988;72:113–118.)

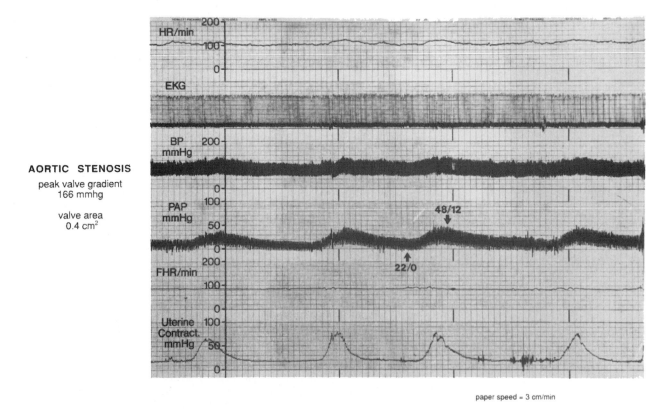

Figure 26.11. Hemodynamic responses of a patient with severe stenosis to increased vascular return associated with uterine contractions. *HR*, heart rate; *ECG*, electrocardiogram; *BP*, blood pressure; *PAP*, pulmonary artery pressure; *FHR* = fetal heart rate. (Reprinted by permission from Easterling TR, Chadwick HS, Otto CM, Benedetti TJ. Aortic stenosis in pregnancy. *Obstet Gynecol* 1988;72:113–118.)

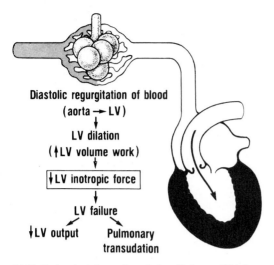

Figure 26.12. Pathophysiology of aortic insufficiency. *LV,* left ventricle.

Pregnancy-Induced Changes. The decrease in systemic vascular resistance and the increase in heart rate during pregnancy may reduce both the regurgitant flow and the intensity of the murmur of insufficiency (82, 96). In contrast, the increase in intravascular volume throughout pregnancy and the increases in systemic vascular resistance with the stress of labor and delivery can lead to left ventricular dysfunction.

Anesthetic Considerations

Asymptomatic patients without signs of pulmonary congestion have minimally increased risk. Symptomatic patients with increased murmur intensity, decreased diastolic blood pressure, increased peripheral pulse pressure, or signs of pulmonary congestion are at increased risk and may benefit from radial artery and pulmonary artery catheterization. Factors to consider (Table 26.7) include the following:

- *Increases in systemic vascular resistance can precipitate left ventricular failure.*

Elevated resistance should be corrected by titration with a low dose of vasodilator such as sodium nitroprusside or phentolamine. Usually, a dose of nitroprusside 0.5 μg · kg^{-1} · min^{-1} or less is all that is needed.

- *Bradycardia is poorly tolerated.*

As with aortic stenosis, bradycardia increases the duration of ventricular diastole and, consequently, the amount of blood regurgitated across the aortic valve. Heart rates should be maintained between 80 and 100 bpm.

- *Myocardial depressants exacerbate left ventricular failure.*

Aortic insufficiency usually produces left ventricular impairment. If myocardial reserve is small, minimal myocardial depression may result in failure.

- *Decreasing diastolic blood pressure, increasing arterial pulse pressure, or increasing intensity or duration of the aortic murmur indicate left ventricular compromise.*

PCW pressure elevation is a late sign, and even small elevations may suggest significant left ventricular failure.

- *Afterload reduction may be useful therapy.*

Table 26.7. AORTIC INSUFFICIENCY: ANESTHETIC CONSIDERATIONS

1. Avoid marked increases in systemic vascular resistance.
2. Maintain a normal or slightly elevated heart rate.
3. Avoid myocardial depressants.
4. Monitor arterial diastolic pressure, pulmonary capillary wedge pressure, and intensity of murmur.

Left ventricular failure may benefit from afterload reduction with small amounts of sodium nitroprusside or phentolamine, combined with dopamine to give left ventricular inotropic support.

Anesthesia for Vaginal Delivery and Cesarean Section

Anesthetic management of parturients with aortic insufficiency is comparable to that for patients with mitral insufficiency (see previous section). Continuous lumbar epidural analgesia will prevent peripheral vasoconstriction and is recommended for vaginal delivery. For cesarean section, regional or general anesthesia, as described in the section on mitral insufficiency, may be used with appropriate monitoring.

CONGENITAL HEART DISEASE

The major categories of congenital heart disease are *left-to-right shunt* (atrial septal defect [ASD], ventricular septal defect [VSD], patent ductus arteriosus [PDA]), *right-to-left shunt* (tetralogy of Fallot, Eisenmenger's syndrome), and *congenital valvular and vascular lesions* (coarctation of the aorta, aortic stenosis, pulmonary stenosis) (1, 4, 7, 8, 14, 15, 42, 50, 97–104).

Pregnancy in women with congenital heart disease may be affected by several factors, including cardiac status, anatomic diagnosis, co-existing pulmonary hypertension, type of surgical repair (if any), and residual postoperative impairment.

Left-to-Right Shunt

Atrial Septal Defect

ASD occurs in 17.5% of adults with congenital heart disease and is the most common congenital heart lesion (4, 13, 97, 98). ASD is consistent with prolonged longevity (8, 99). Cardiac dysrhythmia, pulmonary hypertension, right ventricular failure, and left ventricular failure are commonly not seen until the fourth or fifth decade. Most women with uncorrected ASD tolerate pregnancy well, even when pulmonary blood flow is increased (4, 13). However, the risk of left ventricular failure during pregnancy is increased (1, 7, 100). Maternal and fetal mortality ranges between 1% and 12% (1, 4, 7, 100, 101).

Clinical Manifestations

Signs and Symptoms. Physical examination reveals fixed expiratory splitting of the second heart sound and a systolic ejection murmur at the upper left sternal border, whose intensity varies with the degree of left-to-right shunt (34).

Test Indicators. Electrocardiography usually demonstrates right-axis deviation with an ostium secundum defect. Chest roentgenography may reveal right ventricular enlargement, pulmonary artery prominence, and increased pulmonary vascular markings. Cardiac catheterization of the parturient usually indicates normal pulmonary artery, right ventricular, and right atrial pressures, even with moderate right ventricular dilation.

Pathophysiology. The left-to-right shunting increases right ventricular preload, right ventricular volume work, and pulmonary blood flow. However, a compensatory decrease in pulmonary vascular resistance keeps pulmonary artery pressures normal until the fourth or fifth decade. The increase in right and left atrial blood volume eventually causes right and left atrial distention and associated supraventricular dysrhythmias, particularly atrial fibrillation. The chronically elevated pulmonary blood flow causes pulmonary vascular changes, leading to increased pulmonary vascular resistance, and pulmonary hypertension. Right ventricular failure may occur with a prolonged increase in volume work, particularly when pressure work increases secondary to pulmonary hypertension.

PREGNANCY-INDUCED CHANGES. Pregnancy accelerates these changes by increasing blood volume and cardiac output with consequent increases in left-to-right shunt, right and left

Table 26.8. ATRIAL SEPTAL DEFECT: ANESTHETIC CONSIDERATIONS

1. Prevent or immediately treat supraventricular dysrhythmias.
2. Avoid increases in systemic vascular resistance.
3. Avoid decreases in pulmonary vascular resistance.
4. With pulmonary hypertension, avoid further increases in pulmonary vascular resistance.

ventricular volume work, and pulmonary blood flow. Pulmonary hypertension and right and left ventricular dysfunction may follow. Left atrial distention may precipitate supraventricular dysrhythmias. Supraventricular dysrhythmias are particularly hazardous because incomplete emptying of the left atrium occurs, and left atrial volume and pressure increase and exacerbate the left-to-right shunt.

Anesthetic Considerations. Most asymptomatic patients without evidence of pulmonary hypertension or right ventricular compromise do not require unusual care. Symptoms, pulmonary hypertension, or right ventricular failure indicate radial artery, pulmonary artery, and right atrial pressure monitoring. The following considerations should be noted (Table 26.8):

- *Supraventricular dysrhythmias are poorly tolerated and may increase left-to-right shunt.*

Medications (digoxin, quinidine, etc.) given to control chronic supraventricular dysrhythmias should be continued and adjusted throughout pregnancy and the puerperium. The acute onset of supraventricular dysrhythmias should be treated with direct current cardioversion or propranolol if right ventricular failure or systemic hypotension occurs. Digitalization is recommended if these complications are absent.

- *Increased systemic vascular resistance may not be tolerated.*

Such increase will exacerbate the shunt by increasing aortic-outflow (and therefore mitral-outflow) impedance relative to the impedance of the ASD (fixed).

- *Marked decreases in pulmonary vascular resistance are poorly tolerated.*

An increase in peripheral resistance or a decrease in pulmonary resistance may increase the left-to-right shunt and cause systemic hypotension.

- *Increases in pulmonary vascular resistance exacerbate preexisting pulmonary hypertension, which may precipitate right ventricular failure.*

Anesthesia for Vaginal Delivery and Cesarean Section. For labor, vaginal delivery, and cesarean section, segmental continuous lumbar epidural anesthesia avoids the hazard of increases in systemic vascular resistance. General anesthesia may be used if the above considerations are borne in mind.

Ventricular Septal Defect

VSD occurs in 7% of adults with congenital heart disease. The size of the VSD and the degree of pulmonary hypertension determine the course of patients with VSD (13, 34, 102). In most adult patients, the VSD is small, with a minimal left-to-right shunt, insignificant pulmonary hypertension, and no symptoms. Pregnancy usually is uneventful (13), but rarely may be complicated by bacterial endocarditis or congestive heart failure (13, 86, 99).

The few patients with uncorrected large VSDs usually display growth retardation, recurrent respiratory infection, pulmonary hypertension, and left and right ventricular compromise (97). Their mortality during pregnancy is between 7% and 40% (4, 7, 103–105). Severe right ventricular failure with shunt reversal (Eisenmenger's syndrome) (106) is the major complication. Operative correction of the VSD before pregnancy does not increase maternal or fetal morbidity or mortality during pregnancy (4, 13–15, 107).

Clinical Manifestations. A small VSD produces a mild pansystolic murmur in the fourth or fifth left intercostal space, a nor-

mal chest roentgenogram, and a right bundle branch pattern on the electrocardiogram. Intracardiac pressures are normal, with minimal left-to-right shunting. A moderate-to-large VSD produces loud pansystolic murmurs with expiratory splitting of the second heart sound and evidence of left ventricular enlargement. Eventually, right ventricular enlargement occurs. Right ventricle oxygen saturation is increased as a result of the left-to-right shunt. Right ventricular end-diastolic pressure, pulmonary artery pressure, and left ventricular end-diastolic pressure are increased. A moderate VSD usually decreases pulmonary vascular resistance; a large VSD usually increases it. Prolonged elevation of pulmonary vascular resistance causes bidirectional and, eventually, right-to-left shunting with concomitant cyanosis and clubbing.

Pathophysiology. The left-to-right shunt associated with a small VSD initially increases pulmonary blood flow and secondarily decreases pulmonary vascular resistance, thereby preserving normal pulmonary artery pressures. The increase in left ventricular volume work is well tolerated. With a larger VSD, the greater left-to-right shunt markedly increases pulmonary blood flow, but pulmonary vascular resistance cannot compensate for this increased flow and pulmonary hypertension develops. The increase in left ventricular volume work leads to left ventricular dysfunction, elevation of PCW pressure, and exacerbation of the pulmonary hypertension. Right ventricular failure results, with eventual equalization of right and left ventricular pressures, followed by bidirectional or reverse shunting with peripheral cyanosis (104, 105).

PREGNANCY-INDUCED CHANGES. With pregnancy, elevations in heart rate, cardiac output, and intravascular volume may increase the left-to-right shunt, exacerbate pulmonary hypertension, and cause left and right ventricular failure. Elevation of vascular resistance in response to the stress associated with labor and surgical stimulus increases right and left ventricular dysfunction. Bidirectional shunting or right-to-left shunting may result. If right ventricular afterload increases as much as left afterload, then there may be no increase in shunting.

Anesthetic Considerations. A small VSD in an asymptomatic patient with normal ventricular function does not require specialized monitoring. Symptoms, abnormal ventricular function, or a large VSD indicates monitoring via radial and pulmonary artery catheters. Table 26.9 lists the anesthetic considerations. Chief among these are the following:

- *Increases in systemic vascular resistance may not be tolerated.*

Elevated resistance should be corrected by titration with a low dose of vasodilator such as sodium nitroprusside or phentolamine. Usually, a dose of nitroprusside $0.5 \ \mu g \cdot kg^{-1} \cdot min^{-1}$ or less is all that is needed.

- *Marked increases in heart rate are poorly tolerated.*

An increased systemic vascular resistance or heart rate may increase the left-to-right shunt. Pulmonary hypertension and ventricular failure may follow. Therefore, adequate anesthesia is essential to prevent the sympathetic response that attends pain during labor and delivery, endotracheal intubation, and surgical stimulation. Vasodilation with low doses of sodium nitroprusside or phentolamine (0.1 to $0.5 \ \mu g \cdot kg^{-1} \cdot min^{-1}$) may be needed to reduce shunting and improve cardiac output.

Table 26.9. VENTRICULAR SEPTAL DEFECT: ANESTHETIC CONSIDERATIONS

1. Avoid marked increases in systemic vascular resistance.
2. Avoid marked increases in heart rate.
3. With pulmonary hypertension, avoid marked decreases in systemic vascular resistance.
4. With pulmonary hypertension, avoid marked increases in pulmonary vascular resistance.

• *With pulmonary hypertension and right ventricular compromise, marked decreases in systemic vascular resistance may not be well tolerated.*

With a marked decrease in systemic vascular resistance, a right-to-left shunt and hypoxia will occur. Pressure decreases consequent to regional anesthesia should be corrected.

• *Factors that increase pulmonary vascular resistance should be avoided in patients with pulmonary hypertension and evidence of right ventricular compromise.*

These factors are discussed in the sections on mitral stenosis and primary pulmonary hypertension.

Anesthesia for Vaginal Delivery and Cesarean Section. For labor and vaginal delivery, continuous lumbar epidural anesthesia permits control of systemic resistance and painful stimuli. For cesarean section, either regional or general anesthesia may be used. If regional anesthesia is selected, a continuous lumbar epidural technique will ensure slower changes in systemic resistance and allow more time for correction of pressure changes. General anesthesia that combines inhalation and opioid techniques may best minimize increases in systemic vascular resistance and myocardial depression. Addition of a vasodilator may be necessary.

Potential complications. Peripheral cyanosis in the presence of an elevated cardiac output indicates an imbalance between the pulmonary and systemic resistances with right-to-left shunt as the most probable cause. One hundred percent oxygen should be delivered. Systemic vascular resistance should be increased by decreasing anesthetic depth or by administering small amounts of metaraminol. Peripheral cyanosis associated with a depressed cardiac output indicates right and/or left ventricular failure. Therapy includes an increase in oxygen delivery, withdrawal of anesthesia, and use of an inotrope such as dopamine.

Patent Ductus Arteriosus

PDA constitutes 15% of all congenital heart disease (4). The current practice of early surgical intervention rarely makes this a significant finding during pregnancy. Patients with a small ductus usually have a benign clinical course until the fourth or fifth decade of life, when left or right ventricular failure may occur. However, a ductus of large internal diameter (greater than 1 cm) may produce growth retardation, respiratory infection, congestive heart failure, and pulmonary hypertension during childhood and early adult life. Even without congestive heart failure prior to pregnancy, maternal mortality from ventricular failure is 5% to 6% in untreated pregnant patients (4, 13).

Clinical Manifestations

Signs and Symptoms. A PDA produces a continuous murmur, enveloping the second heart sound with late systolic accentuation, terminating in late or middiastole, and radiating to the first left intercostal space. A large ductus enlarges the left ventricle and widens the arterial pulse pressure.

Test Indicators. Electrocardiographic results can be normal (with a small ductus) or demonstrate left or right ventricular hypertrophy (with a large ductus). Similarly, chest roentgenography data can appear normal (with a small ductus) or can demonstrate left ventricular, left atrial, or pulmonary artery enlargement. Right ventricular enlargement is seen with severe pulmonary hypertension.

Pathophysiology. The left-to-right shunt of aortic blood via the ductus to the pulmonary artery increases central circulatory flow at the expense of peripheral flow. Both length and cross section of the ductus determine resistance to flow and hence the amount of left-to-right shunt. A small internal diameter (less than 1 cm) generally permits a small left-to-right flow. A secondary decrease in pulmonary vascular resistance prevents the increase in pulmonary artery flow from producing pulmonary hypertension. Both the left and right ventricles tolerate this small increase in flow.

Table 26.10. PATENT DUCTUS ARTERIOSIS: ANESTHETIC CONSIDERATIONS

1. Avoid increases in systemic vascular resistance.
2. Avoid marked increases in blood volume.
3. With pulmonary hypertension, avoid marked decreases in systemic vascular resistance or increases in pulmonary vascular resistance.
4. With left ventricular failure, avoid myocardial depressants.

A ductus with a moderate internal diameter (1 to 2 cm) permits a significant increase in pulmonary blood flow. Pulmonary hypertension ultimately results from the inability of the pulmonary vasculature to compensate for the increased flow. Left ventricular volume work is increased, followed eventually by left ventricular failure. With failure, elevation of left ventricular end-diastolic pressure further exacerbates the pulmonary hypertension. Progressive medial hypertrophy and intimal fibrosis increase pulmonary resistance, and right ventricular failure follows.

A large internal diameter (greater than 2 cm) telescopes the temporal development of the above changes. Severe pulmonary hypertension with right ventricular failure may eventually produce a right-to-left shunt and peripheral cyanosis (Eisenmenger's syndrome).

Pregnancy-induced Changes. The increased intravascular volume associated with pregnancy can increase shunting, pulmonary hypertension, and left ventricular volume work. In addition, the increased heart rate and stroke volume will increase myocardial oxygen demand and may compromise left ventricular function during stressful periods, such as uterine contractions. The decrease in systemic vascular resistance, seen throughout pregnancy and particularly during the postpartum period, can lead to shunt reversal and cyanosis, especially in patients with a large ductus.

Anesthetic Considerations. Asymptomatic patients with normal hemodynamics and no evidence of ventricular dysfunction do not require unusual care. Evidence of left ventricular failure, pulmonary hypertension, right ventricular failure, or reversal of the left-to-right shunt indicates monitoring via an arterial line and a pulmonary artery catheter. The following are the important considerations (Table 26.10):

• *Increases in systemic vascular resistance may not be tolerated.*

Proportionate increases in pulmonary vascular resistance may not occur, and left-to-right shunt may increase.

• *Marked increases in blood volume may be poorly tolerated.*

Acute hypervolemia may precipitate failure by increasing left ventricular volume work and oxygen consumption.

• *Marked decreases in systemic vascular resistance or increases in pulmonary resistance may lead to reverse shunting in patients with pre-existing pulmonary hypertension and right ventricular compromise.*

See section on Eisenmenger's syndrome.

• *Patients with left ventricular failure may not tolerate additional myocardial depression.*

Anesthesia for Vaginal Delivery and Cesarean Section.

Choice of technique. Use of a continuous epidural technique for labor, vaginal delivery, and cesarean section prevents increases in systemic vascular resistance associated with pain. In addition, decreases in systemic vascular resistance may reduce a left-to-right shunt. If general anesthesia is selected for cesarean section, increases in systemic vascular resistance should be rapidly treated by deepening anesthesia or administration of a vasodilating agent such as sodium nitroprusside or phentolamine.

Monitoring concerns. The use of simultaneous pulse oximetry of the right hand and foot as a monitor of both pulmonary function and shunt fraction has been shown to be useful (108). Blood flow to the right arm is predominantly preductal; accordingly, Sao_2 in the right arm is determined by Fio_2, pulmonary function, and cardiac output, as well as the degree and direction through the PDA. When the Sao_2 of the right arm is constant, the Sao_2 of the foot changes inversely with the amount of right-to-left shunting through the PDA.

Right-to-Left Shunt

Tetralogy of Fallot

Tetralogy of Fallot constitutes 15% of all congenital heart disease and is the most common cyanotic congenital heart disease (14, 15, 34, 98, 109). This anomaly is characterized by right ventricular outflow obstruction, VSD, right ventricular hypertrophy, and overriding aorta. In the past, few women demonstrated tetralogy of Fallot during pregnancy because most died before the childbearing age. However, antibiotic therapy and palliative or corrective surgery have increased the number of parturients presenting with corrected or uncorrected tetralogy of Fallot (13, 97, 98).

Pregnancy increases the morbidity and mortality of uncorrected tetralogy of Fallot, particularly in patients with a history of syncope, polycythemia, decreased arterial oxygen saturation (less than 80%), and right ventricular hypertension (1, 5, 7, 14, 15, 104, 110–112). Left ventricular failure, bacterial endocarditis, and cerebral thrombosis are increased. Most complications develop immediately postpartum when systemic vascular resistance is lowest, thus exacerbating the right-to-left shunt. With uncorrected tetralogy of Fallot, 40% of parturients sustain heart failure and 12% die (1). The fetal death rate is 36%. Patients undergoing pulmonary valvulotomy during pregnancy are not at increased risk, but fetal mortality approaches 50% (42, 113, 114). Maternal mortality is not increased in patients with a corrected tetralogy of Fallot, but fetal mortality can be as high as 25% (1, 107, 110).

Clinical Manifestations. Uncorrected tetralogy of Fallot causes cyanosis, clubbing, and a systolic thrill at the left sternal border near the second or third intercostal space. The degree of pulmonary hypertension and pulmonary blood flow determine the loudness of the thrill. The electrocardiogram suggests right ventricular hypertrophy. Chest roentgenogram demonstrates an enlarged heart but sparse peripheral pulmonary vasculature. Catheterization reveals decreased pulmonary artery pressure and significant right-to-left shunt.

Pathophysiology. The increased resistance to right ventricular outflow promotes right-to-left shunting via the VSD. Shunting and, therefore, cyanosis depend on the size of the VSD, the obstruction to outflow from the right ventricle, and the ability of the right ventricle to overcome that obstruction. The obstruction may result from a fixed pulmonic stenosis or dynamic infundibular hypertrophy. If infundibular hypertrophy exists, increases in myocardial contractility or decreases in right ventricular volume may increase outflow obstruction (see section on asymmetric septal hypertrophy). If significant hypertrophy does not exist, maintenance of right ventricular contractility is important for preservation of pulmonary blood flow and peripheral oxygenation. Regardless of the type of right ventricular outflow obstruction, decreases in systemic vascular resistance may exacerbate shunting and produce cyanosis.

Pregnancy-induced Changes. Labor and postpartum changes may compromise parturients with tetralogy of Fallot. The stress of labor may increase pulmonary vascular resistance, thereby increasing the right-to-left shunt. Decreases in systemic vascular resistance noted throughout pregnancy and after delivery may increase the right-to-left shunt and produce cyanosis. Finally, patients with infundibular obstruction may be particularly at risk during labor, when increases in contractility may be highest.

Anesthetic Considerations. If the tetralogy has not been corrected, then special considerations are warranted, including radial artery and CVP monitoring. Patients with corrected tetralogy of Fallot may have residual right ventricular failure and re-

Table 26.11. TETRALOGY OF FALLOT: ANESTHETIC CONSIDERATIONS

1. Avoid decreases in systemic vascular resistance.
2. Avoid decreases in blood volume.
3. Avoid decreases in venous return.
4. Avoid myocardial depressants.

quire special considerations (see section on primary pulmonary hypertension). In the absence of symptoms or right ventricular compromise, the usual anesthetic considerations can be applied, but the following factors should be noted (Table 26.11):

- *Decreases in systemic vascular resistance, blood volume, or venous return are not well tolerated.*

A reduction in systemic vascular resistance increases right-to-left shunt, while a decline in blood volume or in venous return compromises right ventricular perfusion of the lungs. High central blood volumes are essential to maintain right ventricular output when this ventricle is compromised.

- *Myocardial depression may not be well tolerated.*

With right ventricular compromise, inotropic support with dopamine may be necessary to offset the effects of even small amounts of myocardial depression.

Anesthesia for Vaginal Delivery and Cesarean Section.
Vaginal delivery. Labor and vaginal delivery in parturients with tetralogy of Fallot are best managed with systemic medication, inhalation analgesia, or paracervical or pudendal block anesthesia. Epidural or spinal anesthesia should be used with extreme caution. To avoid decreases in systemic vascular resistance and venous return, the author recommends volume infusion and continuous left uterine displacement. Ephedrine should be administered cautiously because it may produce a marked increase in pulmonary vascular resistance.

Cesarean section. A general anesthetic technique is preferred for cesarean section. In the absence of infundibular obstruction, a light level of anesthesia should be well tolerated, and nitrous oxide—relaxant anesthesia (with postoperative opioid analgesia) may be most successful. With infundibular stenosis, neither increases in myocardial contractility or heart rate nor decreases in ventricular volume will be well tolerated. The most effective approach in these cases is likely to be a volatile anesthetic such as halothane or isoflurane. Maintaining a normal or slightly elevated right ventricular filling pressure and systemic vascular resistance is important (see section on asymmetric septal hypertrophy).

Complications. The presence of an increasing peripheral cyanosis in patients without infundibular obstruction usually indicates a decrease in systemic vascular resistance or increased right ventricular compromise. Treatment consists of delivering the maximum concentration of oxygen and decreasing the anesthetic depth.

In patients with a history of significant infundibular obstruction, an increase in peripheral cyanosis typically is precipitated by tachycardia, increased myocardial contractility, or decreased right ventricular volume. Treatment consists of increasing the depth of halothane or isoflurane anesthesia, increasing venous return and central blood volume, and decreasing contractility and heart rate by titration of propranolol.

Eisenmenger's Syndrome

Eisenmenger's syndrome consists of pulmonary hypertension and a right-to-left or bidirectional shunt with peripheral cyanosis (13, 34). The shunt may be atrial, ventricular, or aortopulmonary. A left-to-right shunt reversal commonly occurs during the end stages of PDA, VSD, and ASD (98). Approximately 3% of all patients with congenital heart disease are reported to have Eisenmenger's syndrome; prognosis is poor for most of these patients, with survival beyond the age of 40 unlikely. Unfortunately,

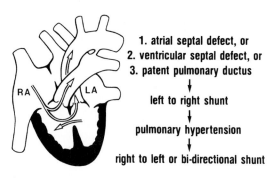

1. atrial septal defect, or
2. ventricular septal defect, or
3. patent pulmonary ductus
↓
left to right shunt
↓
pulmonary hypertension
↓
right to left or bi-directional shunt

Figure 26.13. Pathophysiology of Eisenmenger's syndrome. *RA*, right atrium; *LA*, left atrium.

the condition of high pulmonary artery pressures with a fixed vascular resistance is not reversible by surgical intervention (13, 98, 102).

Maternal and fetal prognoses depend on the severity of the pulmonary hypertension (2, 102): maternal mortality has been reported to be between 12% and 33%, and fetal mortality between 30% and 54%; however, these rates may be low due to underreporting or misdiagnosis (97, 98, 101, 104–108, 110, 111, 115).

Clinical Manifestations

Signs and Symptoms. Clinical manifestations of Eisenmenger's syndrome depend on the degree of pulmonary hypertension and right-to-left shunt (2, 34, 106, 108, 114). The type of murmur detected is a function of the specific right-to-left defect (e.g., a systolic ejection murmur with ASD or a holosystolic murmur with VSD).

Test Indicators. Electrocardiography usually demonstrates right ventricular hypertrophy with right-axis deviation. Chest roentgenography typically reveals increased pulmonary artery markings with a prominent right ventricle.

Pathophysiology. The degree of right-to-left shunt depends on three factors: (a) the severity of the pulmonary hypertension and size of right-to-left circulatory communication (Fig. 26.13); (b) the relationship between the pulmonic and systemic vascular resistance, i.e., increases in pulmonary vascular resistance or decreases in systemic vascular resistance exacerbate the right-to-left shunt, producing peripheral cyanosis; and (c) the contractile state of the right ventricle (progressive right ventricular dysfunction decreases pulmonary blood flow and increases shunt).

Pregnancy-induced Changes. Pregnancy is not well tolerated in patients with Eisenmenger's syndrome. Pulmonary vascular resistance is fixed and therefore unaltered by the physiology of pregnancy. However, the normal decrease in systemic vascular resistance does occur, markedly increasing the right-to-left shunt (7, 104, 116). With elevated shunt, increases in heart rate and stroke volume increase right ventricular oxygen consumption and, in the presence of relatively desaturated blood, may produce right ventricular compromise (34, 116).

Anesthetic Considerations. All patients with Eisenmenger's syndrome are at extremely high risk and should be monitored invasively by radial arterial and central venous catheterization. The chief concerns are (Table 26.12):

Table 26.12. EISENMENGER'S SYNDROME: ANESTHETIC CONSIDERATIONS

1. Avoid decreases in systemic vascular resistance.
2. Avoid decreases in venous return.
3. Avoid increases in pulmonary vascular resistance (e.g., hypercarbia, acidosis, hypoxia).

- *Decreases in systemic vascular resistance or venous return are not well tolerated.* (See section on tetralogy of Fallot.)
- *Elevations in pulmonary vascular resistance are not well tolerated.* Even minimal hypercarbia, acidosis, and hypoxia should be avoided and treated aggressively when they occur (see section on primary pulmonary hypertension).

Anesthesia for Vaginal Delivery and Cesarean Section. Anesthetic management of parturients with Eisenmenger's syndrome is identical to that of patients with tetralogy of Fallot (117–119) (see preceding section on tetralogy of Fallot). However, diuresis usually occurs following delivery, increasing hematocrit and thereby decreasing blood viscosity and pulmonary blood flow. Adequate crystalloid replacement and maintaining hematocrit levels below 55% are recommended.

Other Congenital Heart Diseases

Coarctation of the Aorta

Coarctation of the aorta represents approximately 8% of all cases of congenital heart disease in adults (98). Most cases are surgically corrected in early childhood, decreasing the incidence of coarctation in the pregnant population. Parturients with a corrected lesion do not have a higher than normal risk of maternal and fetal morbidity and mortality (7, 120, 121). However, an uncorrected lesion can result in maternal mortality of 3% to 9% and fetal mortality as high as 20% (4, 7, 50, 120, 121). The principal maternal risks are left ventricular failure, aortic rupture, and infective endocarditis. The offspring of affected women have a higher incidence of congenital heart disease (3% to 5%) than those born of mothers without heart disease (4, 13, 50).

Clinical Manifestations

Signs and Symptoms. Physical examination usually reveals a significant difference in blood pressures in the upper and lower extremities, or in the right and left upper extremities. Other signs include an increase in intensity of the aortic component of the second heart sound, a medium-pitched systolic blowing murmur (heard best between the scapulae), a ventricular heave, and a laterally displaced point of maximal impulse.

Test Indicators. Late in the course of the disease, electrocardiographic evidence will demonstrate signs of left ventricular hypertrophy. Chest roentgenography will demonstrate left ventricular enlargement and a characteristic "three" sign in the aortic knob. Cardiac catheterization is indicated in complicated cases and is useful in assessing the severity of the disease.

Pathophysiology. Coarctation, like aortic stenosis, represents a fixed obstruction to left ventricular ejection. Stroke volume tends to be limited, and increases in cardiac output are achieved primarily through increases in heart rate. Due to increased left ventricular afterload, ventricular pressure work increases and concentric hypertrophy occurs. Patients with mild coarctation tolerate this well, and progression to ventricular dilation and failure occurs late in the course. With severe coarctation, ventricular changes occur earlier, along with pathologic changes in the arterial wall at the site of coarctation that serve as the nidus for dissection and rupture.

Pregnancy-induced Changes. Pregnancy may exacerbate both left ventricular compromise and vascular wall damage. Because stroke volume is limited, the increase in intravascular volume and metabolic demand characteristic of pregnancy can be accommodated only by increases in heart rate. During periods of high demand (labor) or of acute increases in intravascular volume (uterine contraction), even supranormal heart rates may not compensate for the limited stroke volume, resulting in left ventricular failure. Pregnancy also can precipitate anatomic changes in the aortic intima and media that may induce vascular wall damage (120, 121). For example, aortic dissection and rupture may occur due to an increase in the rate of ejection of blood from the left ventricle in response to the increase in heart rate and contractility that occurs with labor and delivery.

Table 26.13. COARCTATION OF THE AORTA: ANESTHETIC CONSIDERATIONS

1. Avoid decreases in systemic vascular resistance.
2. Avoid bradycardia.
3. Maintain left ventricular filling.

Finally, systemic arterial dilation during pregnancy and immediately after delivery may not be tolerated because stroke volume is fixed.

Anesthetic Considerations. Asymptomatic parturients without left ventricular enlargement or dysfunction can be managed like healthy patients. Those at moderate-to-high risk should be monitored by radial and pulmonary artery catheterization. Table 26.13 provides the anesthetic considerations for this population. Chief among these are:

• *Decreases in systemic vascular resistance are not well tolerated.*

Because stroke volume is fixed, compensation for decreases in systemic vascular resistance is limited. Hypotension may result. Maintaining systemic vascular resistance in the normal to slightly elevated range with either metaraminol or "light" anesthesia is recommended. Particular caution should be given to the period immediately after delivery.

• *Decreases in heart rate are not well tolerated.*

With fixed stroke volume, cardiac output is determined primarily by heart rate. Vagal stimulants, medications, or anesthetics that decrease heart rate or depress the sinus node should be avoided. Bradycardia should be treated by removing the precipitant cause and administration, if necessary, of atropine or isoproterenol.

• *Decreases in left ventricular filling are not well tolerated.*

If there is a fixed obstruction to left ventricular emptying, adequate stroke volume will require high end-diastolic volumes. Venous return must be maintained, hypovolemia avoided, and atrial dysrhythmias treated promptly.

Anesthesia for Vaginal Delivery and Cesarean Section. Anesthetic management of patients with coarctation of the aorta is similar to that of patients with rheumatic aortic stenosis (see section on rheumatic heart disease). For vaginal delivery, systemic medication, inhalation analgesia, or pudendal nerve block is recommended. For cesarean section, light general anesthesia using a nitrous oxide—relaxant technique is suggested; this approach can maintain increased levels of heart rate, contractility, and vascular resistance. If the possibility of aortic dissection exists, the anesthetic considerations listed in the section on dissecting aneurysm of the aorta should be noted.

Congenital Aortic Stenosis

Congenital aortic stenosis can be supravalvular, valvular, or subvalvular (122–124). The supravalvular lesion has been described in the maternal rubella syndrome (125), where the narrowing occurs just distal to the coronary artery orifices. The subvalvular lesion may be diaphragmatic or muscular (such as asymmetric septal hypertrophy). The most common valvular lesion, i.e., the most common congenital malformation of the heart, is the bicuspid aortic valve, which occurs in 1% to 2% of the general population (126). Unlike the supravalvular and subvalvular forms, the bicuspid form may not become clinically apparent until late in adult life. Studies by Bacon and Matthews (127) suggested that 20% to 30% of patients with a congenitally bicuspid aortic valve eventually develop aortic stenosis secondary to blood turbulence and fibrin deposition.

Effects on Pregnancy. The literature on parturients with congenital aortic stenosis is limited to a few studies (1, 4, 44, 46, 100). Among 14 such parturients, 10 pregnancies were uncomplicated. Of the remaining four cases, one pregnancy was terminated because of intractable heart failure and three women required aortic valvulotomy during pregnancy. One

of these three patients had an uncomplicated postoperative course and subsequent successful delivery, one had a miscarriage 10 days after surgery, and the third delivered a child with congenital abnormalities who died at the age of 4 months. Maternal morbidity and fetal mortality thus appear to increase with congenital aortic stenosis.

Anesthetic Considerations. Aside from asymmetric septal hypertrophy (which is discussed later in this chapter), the pathophysiology and anesthetic considerations of congenital aortic stenosis are similar to those already described for rheumatic aortic stenosis (Table 26.6).

Congenital Pulmonic Stenosis

Isolated pulmonic stenosis constitutes approximately 13% of all congenital heart disease (98). The lesion may be valvular or subvalvular (infundibular stenosis) (128). The valvular lesion usually is nonprogressive until late in adult life (34). However, the subvalvular lesion, which has a different pathophysiology, can be progressive. The considerations for patients with subvalvular stenosis are discussed in the section on asymmetric septal hypertrophy. Only valvular stenosis is discussed here.

Effects on Pregnancy. Similar to congenital aortic stenosis, the literature on pulmonic stenosis is limited. Reviews of 71 patients with isolated pulmonic stenosis during pregnancy (1, 4) indicate no maternal mortality and three fetal deaths; complications of right ventricular failure occurred in five of 71 pregnancies.

Clinical Manifestations

Signs and Symptoms. Severe right ventricular failure decreases left ventricular output, producing symptoms of fatigue and syncope. Auscultation reveals a pulmonic ejection click following the first heart sound and a systolic ejection murmur in the second left intercostal space. With increasing severity of pulmonic stenosis, the murmur has an increased duration and a late systolic accentuation; the pulmonic component of the second heart sound is delayed, with an expiratory splitting of the second heart sound.

Test Indicators. With mild pulmonic stenosis, electrocardiography usually reveals a right bundle branch block. With severe stenosis, a predominant R wave occurs in lead V_1 that usually exceeds 20 mm in height (129) and correlates with a right ventricular systolic pressure of at least 80 mm Hg (130). Right ventricular strain manifested by negative T waves in the right precordial leads also may occur. The characteristic radiologic finding is prominence of the left pulmonary artery, accompanied by right ventricular and atrial enlargement.

Pathophysiology. With progressive stenosis of the right ventricular outflow tract, pressure work increases and concentric hypertrophy occurs. The right ventricle seems to adapt readily to this situation, maintaining output until late in the course of the disease, when systolic pressure exceeds approximately 80 mm Hg (131). As right ventricular output decreases, so does left ventricular preload and thus cardiac output. Systemic vascular resistance increases in an effort to compensate for decreased left ventricular output. However, as right ventricular failure progresses, further decreases in cardiac output are uncompensated, and symptoms of low cardiac output, such as fatigue and syncope, occur with exercise and later at rest.

Pregnancy-induced Changes. Although patients with isolated pulmonary valvular stenosis have uneventful courses until late in life (34), the extension of the childbearing years due to new reproductive technologies may increase the number of parturients presenting with this disease. The stresses of pregnancy, labor, and delivery are likely to complicate the parturient's course (1, 4). For example, pregnancy-induced increases in intravascular volume (increasing right ventricular preload, stroke work, and oxygen consumption) and in heart rate (increasing oxygen consumption) can precipitate right ventricular failure. Similarly, pregnancy-related decreases in systemic vascular resistance, particularly postdelivery, may counteract

Table 26.14. CONGENITAL PULMONIC STENOSIS: ANESTHETIC CONSIDERATIONS

1. Avoid marked increases in intravascular volume.
2. Avoid marked decreases in venous return.
3. Avoid bradycardia.
4. Avoid marked decreases in systemic vascular resistance.
5. Avoid myocardial depressants.

---

compensatory mechanisms required during low right ventricular output states.

Anesthetic Considerations. Patients who are asymptomatic without progression of right ventricular compromise may be managed in standard fashion. The initial sign of impending right ventricular failure may be a subtle but progressive rise in end-diastolic pressure or CVP. Radial artery and CVP monitoring are advocated. In providing anesthesia, the following considerations should be noted (Table 26.14):

• *Marked increases or decreases in right ventricular filling pressure are not well tolerated.*

Maintaining right ventricular filling pressure in its usual range is necessary for effective ventricular contraction in response to increased pulmonic resistance. Excessive volume transfusion may overdistend the right ventricle, furthering right ventricular failure. A sudden decline in venous return, such as obstruction of the vena cava or acute hemorrhage, will decrease the effectiveness of right ventricular contraction.

• *Decreases in heart rate are not well tolerated.*

Right ventricular output will depend primarily on heart rate because stroke volume is limited. It is important to maintain at least normal (90 to 110 bpm) heart rates by choosing drugs with a positive chronotropic effect and by using light anesthesia.

• *Marked decreases in systemic vascular resistance may not be tolerated.*

With a low output state, systemic pressure is preserved by increases in vascular resistance. Maintaining a normal-to-high systemic vascular resistance using light levels of general anesthesia or a vasoconstrictor such as ephedrine or metaraminol is advocated.

• *Negative inotropes may not be well tolerated.*

The contractile state of the right ventricle may be compromised, and further myocardial depression may result from negative inotropes such as halothane or enflurane. Use of medications or techniques with positive inotropic action is therefore recommended.

Anesthesia for Vaginal Delivery and Cesarean Section.

Vaginal delivery. Techniques that reduce systemic vascular resistance and venous return should be used with extreme caution for labor and vaginal delivery. Better choices are systemic or inhalation analgesics and pudendal blocks. If epidural, caudal, or spinal anesthesia is chosen, prophylactic administration of intravenous fluids and ephedrine is recommended. Maintaining a normal CVP is necessary. Decreases in systemic vascular resistance should be anticipated and immediately corrected with left uterine displacement and administration of ephedrine or metaraminol.

Cesarean section. General anesthesia using a nitrous oxide–relaxant technique is recommended, with a goal of maintaining vascular resistance, heart rate, and myocardial contractility. If signs of right ventricular failure develop (elevation of filling pressure), the level of anesthesia should be decreased and an inotrope such as dopamine administered.

OTHER HEART DISEASES

There are a number of other significant, but relatively rare, cardiac diseases that the anesthesiologist may encounter. Recent case reports suggest that such conditions can be approached safely despite their inherent difficulties (132, 133). The anesthetic considerations will vary depending on the disease itself and its progression.

Primary Pulmonary Hypertension

Primary pulmonary hypertension is a disease that particularly affects young women (134, 135), resulting in maternal mortality of more than 50% (36–41, 104, 107, 129, 136–138). Most deaths occur during the periods of labor and the puerperium, and the pattern is similar to that described in Eisenmenger's syndrome (7, 13, 100, 104, 139). There is speculation that amniotic fluid embolism might be a possible precipitating factor in the fulminant course of this disease during labor and the puerperium (4, 29, 30).

Clinical Manifestations

Signs and Symptoms. The principal symptoms of this disease, exertional dyspnea and fatigue, are due to a low fixed cardiac output, and typically occur late in its natural course (as differentiated from other causes of pulmonary hypertension). The signs of the disease depend on the degree of pulmonary hypertension and right ventricular compromise. Usually, patients are acyanotic, and have cool extremities with poor peripheral pulses and a quiet precordium. Prominent A waves in the deep jugular veins can be noted. Late in the disease, a systolic ejection murmur is heard over the pulmonary valve, and evidence of tricuspid insufficiency also can be detected.

Test Indicators. Electrocardiography typically reveals right ventricular hypertrophy and right atrial enlargement. Chest roentgenography shows a prominent main pulmonary artery and a slightly enlarged heart with a right atrial and right ventricular configuration. Late in the course of the disease, heart size may increase considerably. Cardiac catheterization demonstrates isolated pulmonary hypertension despite normal PCW pressure.

Pathophysiology

Pulmonary hypertension is present when pulmonary artery pressure exceeds 30/15 mm Hg or mean pulmonary artery pressure exceeds 25 mm Hg (124). With elevation of pulmonary pressure, morphologic changes occurring in the pulmonary vasculature produce medial hypertrophy and intimal fibrosis. A large spectrum of changes can occur in this vasculature, and the reactivity of these vessels can be quite variable. With increasing pulmonary hypertension, right ventricular afterload and thus right ventricular pressure work increase. The right ventricle hypertrophies and eventually fails, causing an elevated right ventricular end-diastolic pressure and a decreased cardiac output. This elevation of end-diastolic pressure is reflected in an increase in CVP, which produces passive congestion of the liver and peripheral edema. With progression of the disease, the right ventricle will become dilated, and tricuspid insufficiency will occur. Characteristically, throughout this course, neither PCW nor left ventricular preload is elevated. The left ventricle usually functions well; however, left ventricular output declines because of the failing right ventricle.

Pregnancy-Induced Changes. Pregnancy is accompanied by a broad spectrum of physiologic changes, including sympathetic, thrombogenic, mechanical (pulmonary capacity), and inflammatory changes, all of which can exacerbate substantial changes in pulmonary artery resistance, impedance, and external medicated construction. Both chronic and acute disturbances of these changes occur, especially during labor and delivery, which may readily exacerbate pulmonary hypertension and secondary right ventricular dysfunction.

Anesthetic Considerations

It is imperative that the degree of pulmonary hypertension and right ventricular failure be assessed before proceeding with an anesthetic plan. If possible, the reactivity of the pulmonary vasculature should be determined to assess responsiveness to pharmacologic vasodilation. Monitoring of radial artery and pulmonary artery pressure is recommended in all patients (37, 140). Chief anesthetic considerations (Table 26.15) include:

• *Increases in pulmonary vascular resistance are not well tolerated.*

Hypercarbia, hypoxia, acidosis, lung hyperinflation, pharmacologic vasoconstrictors, and stress can markedly increase pulmonary vascular resistance and should be avoided.

• *Marked decreases in right ventricular volume are not well tolerated.*

Early correction of fluid and blood loss and avoidance of inferior vena caval obstruction are important to maintaining normal to slightly elevated CVP.

• *Marked decreases in systemic vascular resistance may not be well tolerated.*

Cardiac output is limited by a fixed right ventricular output, compromising the ability to compensate for decreases in systemic vascular resistance.

• *Right ventricular contractility may be compromised, and negative inotropes may result in marked depression of ventricular function.*

Anesthesia for Vaginal Delivery and Cesarean Section

In parturients with primary pulmonary hypertension, pain, anxiety, and stress are especially detrimental because pulmonary vascular resistance may increase markedly. Adequate psychologic support and analgesia are mandatory.

Vaginal delivery. Intravenous opioids, inhalation analgesia, intrathecal morphine (141), and paracervical and pudendal nerve blocks are recommended for labor and vaginal delivery. However, neonatal depression may occur in response to the presence of opioids, and the use of neonatal naloxone should be anticipated. Opioids also may cause maternal hypercapnia, potentially increasing pulmonary vascular resistance. Despite these limitations, these techniques are preferred to major conduction anesthesia because they are not associated with marked peripheral vasodilation and decreased venous return. Conduction anesthesia can be performed safely if attention to detail is meticulous, as demonstrated by several recent case reports (37, 140). These parturients are frequently ideal candidates for subarachnoid and/or epidural opioids, as described in Chapters 8 and 9.

If a continuous epidural technique with local anesthetic agents is used, a very cautious and slow titration of local anesthetic is recommended. Meticulous attention must be given to changes in venous capacitance and vascular resistance. Continuous intravenous titration of fluids is necessary. Correction of small decreases in systemic vascular resistance is not advocated, because the treatment might have a marked effect on the pulmonary vascular resistance. Only marked decreases in systemic vascular resistance should be corrected by titration of ephedrine.

Cesarean section. General anesthesia is preferred. However, the conventional rapid induction with thiopental, succinylcholine, and endotracheal intubation may precipitate marked pulmonary hypertension and right ventricular failure. One suggested approach is an inhalation induction with halothane and oxygen. There is some evidence that use of an inhalation agent such as halothane or isoflurane may decrease pulmonary vascular resistance (142). Intubation should not be performed until an adequate depth of anesthesia is achieved. To avoid possible hypoventilation and hypercarbia during induction, it is suggested that the patient be paralyzed immediately after loss of consciousness; ventilation can then be controlled. Hyperinflation of the lungs should be avoided, and a tidal volume of 5 to 10 mL · kg^{-1} is recommended.

Complications. To alleviate the increased risk of aspiration associated with inhalation induction and paralysis, antacids should be administered prior to induction and cricoid pressure should be applied continuously until intubation is performed.

The most serious complication is right ventricular decompensation resulting from increases in pulmonary hypertension. An early sign is a subtle but progressive elevation of CVP even though other parameters are stable and normal. If this should occur, hypercarbia, hypoxia, acidosis, and light anesthesia should be excluded as causal or corrected. If the situation persists, inotropes such as dopamine or isoproterenol should be titrated slowly. If these measures fail, pulmonary vasodilation with low-dose sodium nitroprusside or phentolamine (0.1 to 0.5 μg · kg^{-1} · min^{-1}) should be attempted.

Hypertensive Disorders

The incidence of hypertension during pregnancy from all causes is approximately 6%, with one quarter of these patients having preexisting hypertension (143–146). In addition to essential hypertension, the principal causes of hypertension are toxemia, renal disease, and, more rarely, coarctation of the aorta and pheochromocytoma. Both maternal and fetal morbidity and mortality appear to be affected by the occurrence, degree, pattern, and treatment of hypertension during pregnancy (4, 23, 24, 135, 143–151). With essential hypertension, parturients whose blood pressure does not exceed 160/100 mm Hg before and during the first 20 weeks of pregnancy usually have an excellent prognosis (143). Those who demonstrate the characteristic reduction in systolic blood pressure during the second trimester also seem to have much lower fetal mortality (4.6%) compared with those who show no decrease (16%). Parturients with essential hypertension taking antihypertensive drugs during pregnancy had a lower incidence of toxemia (6% vs. 18%) and fetal mortality (9% vs. 24%) than a similar group of patients managed with rest, sedation, salt restriction, and no pharmacologic therapy (143).

The cardiovascular changes occurring in patients with preeclampsia-eclampsia and essential hypertension have been studied and compared with those changes seen in normal pregnancy. Recent data seem to indicate that parturients with preeclampsia or essential hypertension have a lower cardiac index and smaller increase in blood volume than those with hypertension during pregnancy. Parturients with toxemia have increased sensitivity to the effects of catecholamines (152), vasopressin (153), and angiotensin II (154). As in normal pregnancy, patients with essential hypertension seem to have a marked increase in sensitivity to ganglionic-blocking drugs, which may precipitate severe hypotension. However, patients with pregnancy-induced hypertension do not demonstrate this sensitivity (155, 156). A complete discussion of pregnancy-induced hypertension is found in Chapter 16.

Clinical Manifestations

Signs and Symptoms. The clinical manifestations of hypertension depend on its etiologic factors. In general, symptoms of serious end-organ involvement, such as transient cerebral ischemic attacks, left ventricular failure, angina, and renal insufficiency, are indicative of longstanding or malignant hypertension and warrant special consideration. Especially noteworthy are signs of left ventricular hypertrophy or dilation, which indicate more severe myocardial damage. These signs are a displaced point of maximal impulse, left ventricular heave on physical examination, left ventricular strain pattern (in addition to an excessive left ventricular voltage pattern) demonstrated electrocardiographically, and an enlarged and "boot-shaped" heart visible with chest roentgenography.

Pathophysiology

Hypertension affects nearly all organs of the body. Two pathophysiologic changes are noteworthy: First, long-standing or severe hypertension may cause arterial damage and alter both the distribution of organ blood flow and its autoregulatory processes. There is evidence that these tissues may require perfusion pressures to maintain tissue blood flow (34, 157). Second, with increased systemic pressure, left ventricular pressure work progressively increases, and the ventricle concentrically hypertrophies. Ventricular dilation and cardiomegaly occur later in the disease process when significant myocardial compromise and failure occur (33, 34).

Pregnancy-Induced Changes.   The normal changes associated with pregnancy of increased intravascular volume, increased cardiac demand (heart rate, stroke volume), acute increases in systemic vascular resistance with stress, and altered renal or endocrine function can complicate the course of preexisting hypertension, uncover essential hypertension, or precipitate new forms of hypertension, such as pregnancy-induced hypertension. Both maternal and fetal morbidity and mortality appear to be affected by the occurrence, degree, pattern, and treatment of hypertension during pregnancy (4, 143–150). The final result is left ventricular ischemia and failure, with decreased cardiac output and decreased organ (including uterine) perfusion.

Anesthetic Considerations

The continuation of antihypertensive therapy is recommended. In parturients with severe or malignant hypertension prior to delivery, blood pressure should be reduced to reasonable levels (160 to 180/100 to 110 mm Hg) with intravenous vasodilators, such as labetalol or hydralazine. Slow titration is recommended, as these patients may be very sensitive to vasodilators. When there is left ventricular failure, radial and pulmonary artery monitoring are recommended.

Anesthesia for Vaginal Delivery and Cesarean Section

Vaginal delivery. For labor and vaginal delivery, regional anesthesia is recommended and is discussed fully in Chapter 16. Specifically, a continuous lumbar epidural technique is recommended to ensure that labor pain does not exacerbate hypertension and its sequelae. However, intravascular volume may be relatively decreased and sympathectomy may lead to severe hypotension, indicating hydration prior to administration of block and correction of hypotension with left uterine displacement and small amounts of ephedrine (2.5 mg intravenously).

Cesarean section. Either regional or general anesthesia is appropriate. With regional anesthesia, administration of at least 1000 mL crystalloid prior to blockade is recommended. With general anesthesia, addition of a halogenated agent should prevent the acute increase in blood pressure associated with light levels of anesthesia. The presence of severe or malignant hypertension associated with left ventricular dysfunction warrants radial artery and PCW pressure monitoring. Sodium nitroprusside or phentolamine may be necessary to treat an acute hypertensive crisis.

Cardiomyopathy of Pregnancy

The occurrence of left ventricular failure without known causes late in the course of pregnancy or during the first 6 months of the postpartum period has been called the cardiomyopathy of pregnancy, peripartum cardiomyopathy, puerperal cardiomyopathy, and postpartum heart disease (4, 158–169). It is unclear whether this condition is closely related to pregnancy or whether pregnancy exacerbates a preexisting, latent myocardial disorder. The incidence of this disorder is increased in older multiparous women; in the presence of twins, toxemia, viral infection, poor nutrition, and genetic disorders; and in members of the black race (170). The long-term prognosis is highly variable. Mortality ranges from 15% to 60% (3, 4, 144, 162, 164–169). The occurrence of heart failure during subsequent pregnancies and long-term survival appear to depend on the return of heart size to normal within 6 months after the first episode of cardiomyopathy. A study (160) of the clinical course of this disease in 27 women found that all patients presented with left ventricular failure during the last month of pregnancy or within the first 5 months of the postpartum period. In 14 of 27 patients, heart size returned to normal within 6 months; in the remaining 13 women, cardiomegaly persisted. Eleven of these thirteen patients had chronic congestive heart failure and died after an average of 4.7 years.

Clinical Manifestations

The clinical manifestations associated with this disorder are signs and symptoms of left or right ventricular failure (4, 34). Pulmonary embolism or infarction also may occur (171). Electrocardiography demonstrates left ventricular hypertrophy, diffuse STT wave abnormalities, or left ventricular conduction defects. Chest roentgenographic evidence is consistent with either left, right, or biventricular failure.

Pathophysiology

Patients may remain asymptomatic with significant left or right myocardial damage until a physiologic stress such as pregnancy occurs. With pregnancy, several normal physiologic changes may produce a deleterious effect, for example, the increase in preload associated with uterine contraction or surgery and the increase in cardiac demand (heart rate, stroke volume, contractility) will increase stress on myocardial function. With progressive ventricular failure, end-diastolic volume increases (decreasing subendocardial blood flow), cardiac output decreases (decreasing coronary perfusion), and myocardial oxygen demand increases. The result is a myocardial oxygen supply-demand imbalance, leading to further ventricular compromise.

Anesthetic Considerations

Patients presenting with ventricular failure (left or right) prior to delivery should be treated with bed rest, salt restriction, diuresis, digitalization, and preload-afterload reduction as necessary. If ventricular failure persists at the time of delivery, radial and pulmonary artery monitoring are recommended. Acute increases in afterload occurring with endotracheal intubation or surgical incision can precipitate left ventricular failure and should be anticipated and controlled by administration of a vasodilator.

Anesthesia for Vaginal Delivery and Cesarean Section

Vaginal delivery. Regional anesthesia is recommended for labor and vaginal delivery. A continuous epidural technique is indicated to avoid deleterious increases in afterload secondary to stress. The resulting reduction in preload and afterload may be beneficial in patients with ventricular compromise. A slow titration of the local anesthetic is suggested. Prehydration and prophylactic ephedrine should not be used routinely. Continuous fetal heart rate (FHR) monitoring will help determine when a decrease in blood pressure should be treated.

Cesarean section. Either regional or general anesthesia may be used. If general anesthesia is chosen, a nitrous oxide–relaxant technique is recommended in parturients with marked ventricular failure. Afterload reduction with either sodium nitroprusside or phentolamine may be necessary. If regional anesthesia is chosen, a continuous epidural technique is recommended because significant changes in systemic vascular resistance and venous capacitance will occur more slowly and are more easily corrected. The successful use of the combined spinal-edipural technique has been reported (171a).

Dissecting Aneurysm of the Aorta

Although dissecting aneurysm of the aorta is more commonly found in men over 50 years of age, there is a well-recognized association between pregnancy and this condition (172). Up to 50% of dissecting aneurysms reported in women less than 40 years of age have occurred in association with pregnancy (172–174). Possible etiologic factors are syphilis, sepsis, Erdheim's medial necrosis, arteriosclerosis, and coarctation of the aorta. Pathologic changes occurring with pregnancy, such as hypertension, influence the course of aortic dissection; however, the effect of pregnancy per se on histologic change in the aorta is controversial (7, 173). Maternal mortality ranges from 19% to 91% (2, 167) and depends on the extent of the process and location of the intimal tear, and is similar to that in nonpregnant patients (4).

Clinical Manifestations

Signs and Symptoms. An abrupt, excruciating pain is the most characteristic feature of dissecting aortic aneurysm. Most often, the pain begins in the thorax or abdomen and migrates posteriorly to the interscapular or lumbar areas (33, 34). However, pain also can originate in the neck, extremities, or jaw. Painless dissection is most common in patients with Marfan's syndrome. Physical examination usually demonstrates hypertension and tachycardia, but hypotension also may occur. If the ascending aorta is involved, a murmur of aortic insufficiency may be found; if the abdominal aorta is involved, a palpable tender aneurysm may be detected. Other findings include asymmetric pulses in the major vessels, focal neurologic signs, or evidence of myocardial ischemia.

Pathophysiology

Dissection occurs with aortic degeneration and the hydraulic stresses of pulsatile flow. In approximately 70% of patients, the dissection originates in the ascending aorta, and in the remainder, distal to the left subclavian artery (34). Dissection may be localized or may extend throughout the aorta. Proximal extension may involve the aortic valve (producing aortic insufficiency), the pericardium, or the left pleural space. Distal extension may involve the femoral vessels. In addition, dissection can occur primarily in the anterior or posterior regions of the aorta. With posterior dissection, tamponade may occur and slow the dissection process; with anterior dissection, acute rupture may occur, with hemorrhage into a body cavity.

Anesthetic Considerations for Vaginal Delivery and Cesarean Section

The Nonemergent Situation. Patients having a history of aortic dissection that has been well-controlled medically should continue their medication regimen throughout pregnancy, labor, and delivery. Regional anesthesia for labor and delivery (vaginal or cesarean section) is recommended. Maintaining both a pain-free state and normal to slightly decreased blood pressure (a systolic pressure between 90 and 110 mm Hg) is necessary. FHR should be monitored continuously to determine the acceptable degree of hypotension. If general anesthesia is selected for cesarean section, an inhalation technique with halothane is suggested because this approach will reduce the likelihood of hypertension and tachycardia and may decrease the force of ventricular ejection of blood.

Management of complications. Trimethaphan and propranolol are useful for control of hypertension and tachycardia. These drugs are recommended if hemodynamic control cannot be achieved by a quiet environment, reassurance, pain control with a regional anesthetic, and mild sedation.

Rupture with severe hemorrhage should always be anticipated. Two large-bore intravenous catheters should be placed, at least 8 U whole blood should be available, and preparations should be made for rapid intubation and resuscitation.

The Emergent Situation. All efforts should be made to expedite surgery in parturients presenting with progressive dissection requiring emergency correction. The method of induction of anesthesia is critical.

Inhalation induction with halothane is recommended in patients who are normotensive to hypertensive. Control of blood pressure and minimization of the response to endotracheal intubation will help prevent hemodynamic decompensation prior to surgical control of the aorta. Immediately prior to induction, the surgical field should be prepared and draped, and the surgeon should be ready to make an incision and cross-clamp the aorta should severe hypotension occur with induction or intubation. Patients who are mildly to severely hypotensive may not be able to tolerate an inhalation agent, a barbiturate, or even an opioid prior to intubation. Rapid induction with succinylcholine with or without ketamine is recommended. Even with marked sympathetic stimulation, blood pressure may not increase because of severe intravascular volume depletion. Immediate surgical control of the aorta is the only treatment.

Classic cesarean section should be performed once control of the aortic dissection is achieved.

Asymmetric Septal Hypertrophy

Asymmetric septal hypertrophy (ASH) typically occurs in adults in their third or fourth decade. Also known as idiopathic hypertrophic subvalvular stenosis, ASH is a cardiomyopathy characterized by a marked hypertrophy of the ventricle involving the interventricular septum and the outflow tract (124, 175–179). During ventricular systole, constriction of the outflow tract occurs, producing obstruction to ventricular ejection.

The course of patients with ASH during pregnancy appears to be variable. Increased risk of left ventricular failure and supraventricular dysrhythmias has been reported in one study of 12 patients (180), where one patient developed left ventricular failure during the last month of pregnancy and two developed atrial dysrhythmias in late pregnancy. Three of the 12 patients died during the first postpartum year. Alternatively, studies of 13 patients with ASH during pregnancy (181) report only one complicated pregnancy, marked by episodes of supraventricular tachycardia without evidence of left ventricular failure. All the latter patients had normal deliveries, with no evidence of increased morbidity or mortality during the postpartum period.

Clinical Manifestations

Signs and Symptoms. The most frequent symptoms of patients with ASH are exertional dyspnea, angina pectoris, and syncope (171). Late in the course of the disease, symptoms of left ventricular failure also occur. Physical examination usually reveals an enlarged heart with a left ventricular lift, a double apical impulse, and a systolic murmur commencing late after the first heart sound and best heard at the apex (34).

Test Indicators. Electrocardiography usually demonstrates abnormal results, including evidence of left ventricular hypertrophy, a Wolff-Parkinson-White syndrome, or abnormal Q waves in the inferior or left precordial leads (171). Chest roentgenography usually displays an enlarged left ventricle.

Pathophysiology

Patients with ASH involving the left ventricle exhibit a marked hypertrophy of the entire left ventricle, with bulging of the ventricular myocardium in the septal region several centimeters below the aortic valve. The ventricular cavity is relatively small.

Table 26.16. ASYMMETRIC SEPTAL HYPERTROPHY: ANESTHETIC CONSIDERATIONS

1. Avoid decreases in blood volume and venous return.
2. Avoid or correct supraventricular tachycardia, atrial fibrillation, and atrial flutter.
3. Avoid decreases in systemic vascular resistance.
4. Avoid increases in myocardial contractility.
5. Treat ventricular compromise with phenylephrine, intravenous fluids, and propranolol.

With each systolic contraction, the muscle around the outflow tract constricts and left ventricular ejection is obstructed. Progression of left ventricular hypertrophy eventually leads to ventricular failure.

Agents or events that increase myocardial contractility will exacerbate left ventricular outflow obstruction and precipitate failure (34). Decreases in systemic vascular resistance also may cause an increase in left ventricular ejection force and increase obstruction (33, 34). Decreases in left ventricular preload will reduce the size of the left ventricle cavity during systole and increase obstruction (182). Therefore, neither a rapid atrial rate nor the loss of atrial kick is well tolerated (183).

Pregnancy-Induced Changes. The increase in intravascular volume associated with pregnancy is helpful in patients with ASH because it causes left ventricular distention and decreases the amount of outflow obstruction (182, 183). In contrast, the decrease in systemic vascular resistance and the increase in heart rate and myocardial contractility characteristic of pregnancy may be deleterious and may precipitate left ventricular failure.

Anesthetic Considerations

Symptomatic patients and those with a hemodynamically significant atrial dysrhythmia should have their blood pressure monitored directly using a radial artery catheter and by pulmonary artery cathter. Chief anesthetic considerations (Table 26.16) include:

* *Decreases in preload are not well tolerated.*

Maintaining slight hypervolemia is recommended because the increase in ventricular volume tends to decrease the amount of outflow obstruction.

* *Supraventricular tachycardia, atrial fibrillation, or atrial flutter is not well tolerated.*

These dysrhythmias will decrease ventricular filling. Immediate treatment with direct current cardioversion or propranolol is advocated.

* *Decreases in systemic vascular resistance are not well tolerated.*

Maintaining a normal to a slightly elevated systemic resistance is recommended to minimize the degree of outflow obstruction.

* *Increases in contractility may not be well tolerated.*

Increases in myocardial contractility may markedly increase outflow obstruction.

* *Treatment of ventricular failure with ASH is markedly different from the usual treatment of failure.*

With ASH, increasing afterload (metaraminol) and preload (intravenous fluids), and decreasing heart rate (propranolol) and contractility (propranolol and halothane) are efficacious.

Anesthesia for Vaginal Delivery and Cesarean Section

Vaginal delivery. Anesthesia for labor and vaginal delivery is best provided with systemic or inhalation analgesics and paracervical and pudendal blocks. Major regional anesthetic techniques may reduce systemic vascular resistance and venous return, thereby increasing outflow obstruction, but can be used if the attention to detail is meticulous (184–188). If regional techniques are chosen, prophylactic administration of intravenous fluids, continuous left uterine displacement, and, if necessary, metaraminol infusion may be used to maintain blood pressure.

Cesarean section. General anesthesia with an inhalation agent such as halothane is recommended because the degree of outflow obstruction may be reduced by the negative inotropic and chronotropic effects of halothane (189). Anesthesia for patients with ASH includes significant risk (190, 191); although we advocate general anesthesia, there are case reports of regional anesthesia for cesarean section (192).

Coronary Artery Disease

Coronary artery disease occurring prior to or during pregnancy is uncommon and has been reported in approximately 1 in 10,000 pregnancies (4). Among cases of acute myocardial infarction during pregnancy, maternal and fetal mortality rates are each estimated to be about 35% (4, 7, 193–201). Seventy percent of pregnant patients who succumb had a myocardial infarction during the last trimester. The clinical manifestations and pathophysiology of coronary artery disease are similar to those in the nonpregnant patient (33, 34).

Anesthetic Considerations

Parturients having a history of crescendo angina, recent (6 weeks) myocardial infarction, or congestive heart failure should have their blood pressure monitored directly using a radial artery catheter and a pulmonary artery catheter. Those maintained on nitrates or propranolol for treatment of angina should continue taking these medications throughout pregnancy, labor, delivery, and the puerperium.

A study using continuous Holter monitoring in 25 patients undergoing elective cesarean section under either spinal or epidural anesthesia demonstrated that ST-segment depression is common (202). Specifically, ST-segment depression suggestive of myocardial ischemia was detected in 16 patients, eight of whom had entirely normal regional wall motion on two-dimensional precordial echocardiography. It was interesting that patients in whom ST depression developed had significantly more tachycardia at delivery than those without ST depression. Thus, ST-segment depression may be a nonspecific finding in this population. Although they could not identify the cause of the echocardiographic changes, the relationship between ST depression and heart rate suggests that it may be, at least in part, a rate-related phenomenon. Regarding newer therapeutic approaches in the pregnant patient, fibrinolytics (203, 204), angioplasty (205, 206), and coronary artery bypass grafting have received increased attention over the past decade (133, 207–214). In most cases, these techniques–if meticulously applied–can be used successfully for treatment of acute myocardial infarction in the pregnant patient.

Anesthesia for Vaginal Delivery and Cesarean Section

Vaginal delivery. Regional anesthesia is recommended for labor and vaginal delivery. A regional technique will minimize pain and stress, which could precipitate angina, and may decrease afterload and preload, which will be beneficial. However, a severe decrease in afterload (producing systemic diastolic pressures below 50 mm Hg) or a large increase in heart rate (greater than 120 bpm) can precipitate decreased diastolic filling of the coronary arteries and angina. Correction with metaraminol or propranolol, respectively, is advocated. Administration of nitroglycerin to treat angina in the presence of a sympathetic block may cause a further decrease in preload and cardiac output, potentially producing more ischemia.

Cesarean section. Either regional or general anesthesia is appropriate. The considerations for regional anesthesia are presented above. For general anesthesia, the most important consideration is minimizing the stress of intubation and surgery. If there is no evidence of congestive failure, an inhalation technique is recommended. If congestive failure is present and general anesthesia is selected, a nitrous oxide—relaxant technique with opioid supplementation is suggested. Electrocardiographic evidence of myocardial ischemia (lead V_5 optimally) should be approached by first "normalizing" blood pressure and heart rate, changing the anesthetic level, or administering therapeutic drugs (sodium nitroprusside, propranolol). With normalized vital signs but persistent evidence of ischemia, administration of sublingual nitroglycerin is suggested.

Postoperative care. The rapid hemodynamic changes that occur during the postpartum period can precipitate ischemia. An uneventful delivery does not ensure that the parturient will have an uncomplicated course. The marked changes in systemic vascular resistance and blood volume occurring during the postpartum period warrant close monitoring, preferably in an intensive care unit.

Pericarditis

Pericarditis is an uncommon complication during pregnancy, with few cases reported (215–217). Tamponade is even less common. The anesthetic considerations for pericarditis are similar to those cited for the nonpregnant patient. Most important is a clear understanding of the physiologic significance of the pericarditis. Precordial (or even transesophageal) echocardiography can be performed safely, and will provide invaluable information (216).

Pregnancy After Valvular Surgery

There have been more than 700 cases of pregnancy reported after mitral valvulotomy and more than 150 cases after mitral and aortic valve replacement (4, 218).

Mitral Valvulotomy

Patients with a previous mitral valvulotomy have increased maternal and fetal mortality, pulmonary embolization, and atrial fibrillation (Table 26.17) (4, 219–221). These complications may be related to residual right and left ventricular dysfunction, residual pulmonary hypertension, and a dilated, compliant left atrium. Compared with parturients with prosthetic valves (especially mitral valves), the incidence of these complications is lower, but it is still significantly higher than that in parturients without heart disease, necessitating special anesthetic considerations.

Anesthetic Considerations.
- *Assessment of the status of the valvulotomy should be made throughout pregnancy and prior to delivery.*

Changes in signs or symptoms with pregnancy and exercise are particularly important because they may indicate residual or new mitral stenosis or insufficiency. The previously discussed anesthetic considerations for these lesions should be applied (Tables 26.3 and 26.4).
- *Residual pulmonary hypertension may exist despite correction of the valvular lesion.*

Pulmonary hypertension may be subtle, and symptoms of associated low cardiac output may be precipitated only with exercise or stress. If symptoms or signs exist, the considerations listed for primary pulmonary hypertension also apply here (Table 26.15).

- *Residual right or left ventricular dysfunction may exist.*

Patients with corrected mitral valvular lesions have decreased cardiac output and a decreased response of cardiac output with exercise. The considerations are those described for mitral stenosis and insufficiency (Tables 26.3 and 26.4).
- *Atrial fibrillation is associated with a marked increase in morbidity.*

There is an increased incidence of systemic embolization and left atrial failure (pulmonary edema with a depressed cardiac output). Maintenance and adjustment of medications such as digoxin or quinidine are necessary throughout pregnancy, labor, and delivery. Treatment of acute atrial fibrillation is outlined in the sections on mitral stenosis and dysrhythmias.
- *The choice of anesthetic is dependent on the type and severity of residual disease involving the mitral valve, pulmonary artery, and left and right ventricles.*

For a discussion of these considerations, see the sections on mitral stenosis and insufficiency.

Mitral Valve Replacement

More than 100 cases of pregnancy after mitral valve replacement have been reported (4, 7, 222–226). Although maternal mortality does not differ significantly from that associated with valvulotomy, maternal morbidity, fetal mortality, and fetal malformations are significantly increased (Table 26.17).

In the nonpregnant population, mitral valve replacement is associated with a number of chronic postoperative complications: thromboembolism, paravalvular regurgitation, ball or disk variance, hemolysis, and endocarditis. Typically, these patients also have a low resting cardiac output, a subnormal increase in cardiac output with exercise, residual pulmonary vascular disease, and some degree of right or left ventricular dysfunction (60, 61, 227–229). Pregnancy aggravates these complications further because of increased intravascular volume, increased myocardial oxygen demand, and increased risk of thromboembolism.

Anesthetic Considerations.
- *All patients should be assumed to have some degree of residual myocardial dysfunction and pulmonary hypertension.*

Occurrence or progression of any signs or symptoms of mitral valve disease during pregnancy, especially with exercise or stress, indicates the presence of a considerable amount of residual myocardial damage. The anesthetic considerations listed in the previous section and in the sections on mitral valve disease should be applied.
- *Pulmonary artery monitoring is recommended with symptomatic disease or with evidence of ventricular compromise or pulmonary hypertension.*

Because the risk of endocarditis is increased in parturients with mitral valve disease, a strictly sterile technique must be used in the placement and maintenance of the pulmonary artery catheter.
- *These patients are invariably anticoagulated.*

Usually, coumarin anticoagulants are replaced with heparin during pregnancy (230–237). One anesthetic approach is to continue heparin therapy throughout labor and delivery, avoiding all forms of regional anesthesia, and using systemic medication, inhalation analgesia, and general anesthesia, if necessary. The

---

Table 26.17. MATERNAL AND FETAL COMPLICATIONS IN PATIENTS WITH PREVIOUS VALVULAR SURGERY

Surgical Procedure	Mortality (%)		Maternal Morbidity (Emboli, Hemorrhage) %	Incidence of Fetal Malformations	References
	Maternal	*Fetal*			
Mitral valvulotomy	2.4–5.5	5.5–16.5	6.6–8.0	1	4, 219–221
Mitral valve replacement	1.2	41	36	20	4, 222–226
Mitral and aortic valve replacement	0	87	Unknown	Unknown	4, 222–226
Aortic valve replacement	0	14	21	2	4, 222–226

second approach is to discontinue heparin therapy immediately prior to labor and administer protamine until coagulation normalizes. Regional anesthesia can then be conducted and heparin resumed 24 hours after removal of the epidural catheter (234). Because experience with the latter technique is limited, the morbidity associated with this technique cannot be assessed accurately at this time.

Aortic Valve Replacement

Patients with an aortic valve prosthesis have a lower incidence of complications than those with a mitral prosthesis (Table 26.17) (4, 222–226). The reasons for this difference can be attributed to the difference in myocardial function and the more restricted use of anticoagulants in patients with aortic valve prostheses (235–237). Generally, cardiac output at rest and in response to exercise is normal in patients with aortic valve prostheses, and ventricular function is better (238–240). However, abnormalities do exist and depend principally on preoperative myocardial status and the quality of valve function. Complications in nonpregnant patients include ball and disc variance, paravalvular regurgitation, hemolysis, endocarditis, and thromboembolism. Compared to patients with mitral valve prostheses, however, risk of thromboembolism, residual pulmonary hypertension, or right ventricular compromise is lower. As with mitral valve replacement, pregnancy aggravates these complications further because of increased intravascular volume, increased myocardial oxygen demand, and increased aorta outflow impedance (218, 241, 242).

Anesthetic Considerations
- *All patients should be assumed to have some degree of residual myocardial dysfunction.*

Symptoms or signs of left ventricular compromise, especially with stress or exercise, are indicative of increased risk, and the anesthetic considerations delineated earlier for aortic insufficiency and aortic stenosis should be applied (Tables 26.6 and 26.7).
- *Pulmonary artery monitoring is recommended with symptomatic disease or with evidence of left ventricular compromise.*
- *If the patient is anticoagulated, anesthetic management should be modified as discussed previously.*

Cardiac Transplantation

Cardiac transplantation is now increasingly performed, and a growing number of reports of pregnancy following orthotopic heart transplantation have been published (243–253). These results are encouraging, but further study documenting the safety of this procedure in the pregnant patient is necessary, given the expected increase in this population.

Open-Heart Surgery During Pregnancy

More than 1000 cases of cardiac surgery during pregnancy have been reported (4, 5, 60, 61, 133, 208, 210–214, 242–253). Based on these cases, mortality in parturients undergoing open-heart surgery does not appear to differ from that in nonpregnant patients. In contrast, fetal mortality is very high (33% to 50%), suggesting that less invasive procedures, such as closed valvulotomy, should be considered. The feasibility of closed mitral and aortic valvulotomy (percutaneous balloon techniques) recently has been demonstrated (254, 255).

Anesthetic Considerations

Basic considerations for anesthetic management of pregnant patients undergoing nonobstetric surgeries are discussed in Chapter 13. A detailed delineation of the anesthetic considerations for parturients undergoing open-heart surgery is beyond the scope of this chapter. However, the following recommendations should be noted:

- *The anesthetic considerations previously delineated for the various cardiac lesions are particularly applicable for patients undergoing open-heart surgery.*
- *The fetus should be monitored closely during the intraoperative and postoperative periods (Chapter 36).*
- *Monitoring of systemic vascular resistance and systemic blood pressure is recommended throughout the perioperative period, especially during cardiopulmonary bypass.*

Uterine blood flow depends on both uterine perfusion pressure and vascular resistance. Agents that increase systemic vascular resistance likely also increase uterine vascular resistance, which may precipitate a decrease in uterine blood flow if systemic pressure is elevated. If continuous FHR monitoring indicates fetal distress during cardiopulmonary bypass and arterial pressure is low, perfusion pressure should be increased by increasing flow rate. If fetal distress occurs and vascular resistance is high, small doses of hydralazine are recommended.

CARDIAC DYSRHYTHMIAS

Cardiac dysrhythmias are common during pregnancy, even in patients without detectable organic heart disease. Some type of dysrhythmia, most of which is benign, usually presents during "normal" pregnancy, labor, and delivery (4, 7, 8, 237, 256–259). The more serious dysrhythmias usually are found in association with rheumatic heart disease and are presented below (31).

Atrial Fibrillation

The presence of atrial fibrillation during pregnancy usually is associated with advanced rheumatic mitral valve disease, primarily dominant mitral stenosis (4, 7, 31). Specifically, following mitral valvulotomy, the incidence of atrial fibrillation is higher in pregnant (31%) than in nonpregnant (16.5%) patients (8). A recent onset of atrial fibrillation during pregnancy increases mortality and the incidence of heart failure and embolization. In one study, among 117 parturients in whom atrial fibrillation occurred, maternal mortality was 17%; fetal mortality, 50%; and heart failure developed in 52% of cases (1). Similarly, among patients who developed atrial fibrillation during pregnancy, 62% had associated heart failure, and the incidence of systemic (13%) and pulmonary (18%) embolization was high (4). In approximately half of these cases, heart failure developed before the onset of atrial fibrillation, and in the remaining half, 1 week to 6 months after onset.

Anesthetic Considerations and Management

Parturients with a history of atrial fibrillation who have responded well to treatment should be maintained on their current pharmacologic therapy (such as digitalis, propanolol, verapamil) throughout pregnancy. However, effects on the fetus (as discussed in the following section) should be considered on a case-by-case basis. Therapeutic dosage should be adjusted to achieve ventricular rates between 90 and 110 bpm. The effects of cardiac therapeutics on the fetus will be discussed in the following section. Patients without underlying heart disease who develop new atrial fibrillation during pregnancy, labor, and delivery should be treated immediately if evidence of hypotension, left ventricular failure, or myocardial ischemia exists. With mild-to-moderate changes, rapid digitalization is the appropriate treatment to slow the ventricular response, but requires a minimum of 15 to 30 minutes before significant slowing occurs. When the patient is fully digitalized, restoration of a sinus rhythm can be accomplished with quinidine or procainamide. If the ventricular response is profound, inducing an acute life-threatening situation, direct current cardioversion, starting with 100 watt/sec, should be instituted immediately. If electrocardioversion is unavailable or if more time permits (minutes), propanolol should be administered. In patients with advanced rheumatic heart disease who develop atrial fibrillation, rapid decompensation can occur, warranting immediate direct current cardioversion or propanolol administration. The physiologic changes associated with pregnancy, however, have little effect on the choice of therapy, or its dose or energy level (in the case of cardioversion).

Finally, changes associated with labor and delivery may acutely precipitate a rapid ventricular response, and therefore in these patients the above-listed equipment and pharmacologic therapies should be immediately accessible to the anesthesiologist, by placement at the patient's bedside.

Atrial Flutter

Atrial flutter is rare and less common than atrial fibrillation. The atrial rate is usually between 280 and 320 bpm with a 2:1 block, resulting in a ventricular rate of about 150 bpm.

Anesthetic Considerations and Management

As with atrial fibrillation there are few reports of atrial flutter during pregnancy (1, 4). The clinical implications and general guidelines of therapy are similar to those for atrial fibrillation. However, treatment with direct current cardioversion usually requires less energy, with a rate of 20 watt/sec often successful. Approximately 30% of patients will convert to atrial fibrillation, usually with a slower ventricular response. Atrial fibrillation is then treated as just described.

Finally, changes associated with labor and delivery may acutely precipitate a rapid ventricular response, and therefore in these patients the above-listed equipment and pharmacologic therapies should be immediately accessible to the anesthesiologist, by placement at the patient's bedside.

Paroxysmal Atrial Tachycardia

Paroxysmal atrial tachycardia (PAT) can occur during pregnancy with or without underlying organic heart disease (1, 4). In structurally normal hearts, the presence of PAT does not increase maternal morbidity (256). When associated with mitral stenosis in parturients with rheumatic heart disease, PAT is reportedly associated with a 14% incidence of heart failure and a 5.5% mortality rate (1, 4). Eighty-five percent of PAT cases occurred during pregnancy, labor, and delivery, and 15% postpartum. Peak incidence occurred during the third trimester of pregnancy. Moderate-to-severe mitral stenosis was present in 90% of patients and mitral regurgitation in 10%. All patients manifested cardiac enlargement. Eighty-eight percent of the paroxysms lasting for more than 6 hours were associated with left ventricular failure, whereas paroxysms lasting less than 2 hours were not.

Anesthetic Considerations and Management

The treatment for life-threatening PAT during pregnancy is direct current countershock. If more time permits, any of the following modalities can be instituted: edrophonium (5 to 10 mg intravenously), carotid sinus stimulation, propranolol, or digoxin. Neosynphrine, sometimes used to slow the heart reflex by stimulating baroreceptors (reflex), should be used cautiously in the pregnant patient. As with other dysrhythmias, changes associated with labor and delivery may acutely precipitate a rapid ventricular response, and therefore in these patients the above-listed equipment and pharmacologic therapies should be immediately accessible to the anesthesiologist, by placement at the patient's bedside.

Other Dysrhythmias

Other dysrhythmias occurring during pregnancy, such as heart block, bundle-branch block, Wolff-Parkinson-White syndrome, and ventricular dysrhythmias, are uncommon but can precipitate significant complications, especially in the patient with un-

derlying organic heart disease (1, 4, 88, 256–259). Again, the anesthesiologist should be prepared to treat heart block, Wolff-Parkinson-White syndrome, and ventricular dysrhythmias, and medications should be prepared should they occur during labor.

EFFECTS OF CARDIAC THERAPEUTICS ON THE FETUS

A variety of pharmacologic therapies (antiarrhythmics, vasopressors, and vasodilators), as well as electrocardioversion, are used to treat maternal cardiac disorders (33, 34). The effects of these therapeutics on the fetus and uterine blood flow and contractility must be considered. Many of the drugs are discussed in general below and in more detail in the chapters on obstetrical anesthesia and uterine blood flow (Chapter 2), the effects of anesthesia on uterine activity and labor (Chapter 3), perinatal pharmacology (Chapter 4), and choice of local anesthetics in obstetrics (Chapter 5).

Antiarrhythmics

Lidocaine

High maternal blood levels of lidocaine (greater than $5 \ \mu g \cdot mL^{-1}$) are associated with neonatal depression. The usual therapeutic level for suppression of ventricular dysrhythmias is 2 to $5 \ \mu g \cdot mL^{-1}$ (33), which is comparable to that found with conventional obstetric anesthesia. Very high blood levels of lidocaine, greater than $200 \ \mu g \cdot mL^{-1}$ in pregnant ewes, were found to cause a dose-related, transient (2 to 3 minutes) decrease in uterine blood flow and a simultaneous increase in intrauterine pressure (239). However, constant intravenous infusion (plasma level of 2 to $4 \ \mu g \cdot mL^{-1}$) did not significantly change maternal or fetal hemodynamics or blood gases, or uterine blood flow or tone (260, 261).

Quinidine

Few studies have investigated the safety of quinidine use during pregnancy. However, because pregnancy is associated with a decrease in plasma pseudocholinesterase activity, quinidine may exacerbate the effects of esters such as succinylcholine. In fact, quinidine recently has been shown to have an inhibitory effect on plasma pseudocholinesterase, which may explain the increased effect of the esters (262). It should, therefore, be used cautiously.

Propranolol

Propranolol crosses the placenta (263). Interference with autonomic responses during labor (264) and depressant effects on the neonate have been reported (144). Fetal bradycardia and hypoglycemia resolving over a prolonged period (3 days) have been associated with propranolol (265). Decreased fetal hepatic metabolism may prolong the half-life of propranolol. In pregnant ewes, propranolol impairs the fetal response to anoxia (266, 267).

Esmolol

Esmolol hydrochloride, a β_1-adrenergic selective antagonist with an elimination half-life of 9 minutes, has been increasingly used recently to control perioperative hypertension or tachyarrhythmias because of its ease of titratability. Recent investigations have shown that esmolol crosses the placental membrane of gravid ewes rapidly (268), and production of an equivalent degree of β_1-blockade is slow following prolonged infusion. Another study has demonstrated that the metabolism of esmolol is as rapid in the fetus as it is in the mother (269). FHR and blood pressure decreased 12% and 7%, respectively, but fetal acid-base status remained unaltered. The dosage and safety of this drug in any individual patient should be considered in any elective situation. A number of reports caution against its use in pregnant patients (70–73).

Labetalol

Labetalol hydrochloride, a nonselective β_1-adrenergic and selective α_1-adrenergic blocking agent, is widely used in treating intraoperative and postoperative hypertension. It has been demonstrated to be safe for both the mother and fetus for treatment of both acute and chronic hypertension (270, 271).

Verapamil

Verapamil has been shown to decrease uterine blood flow in awake pregnant ewes (272). These changes may not be physiologically important to the fetus, but may be consequential in patients with cardiovascular dysfunction. Placental transfer of verapamil hydrochloride is limited in the pregnant ewe, but the fetal heart demonstrates a prolonged PR-interval without changes in the acid-base status.

Amiodarone

Amiodarone has been shown to produce both coronary and peripheral vasodilation, probably by interfering with vascular smooth muscle excitation contracture coupling. Successful use during pregnancy has been reported (273–281). However, several case reports described the use of epidural anesthesia in a patient receiving amiodarone therapy for recurrent atrial and ventricular dysrhythmias, as well as interactions between amiodarone and digoxin during pregnancy. Attention to anesthetic interaction was emphasized. Furthermore, several reports highlight fetal and neonatal side effects (280, 281), including neonatal hypothyroidism (280).

Nicardipine

Nifedipine and nicardipine have been shown to have substantial tocolytic effects in vitro and in vivo. However, their safety during pregnancy remains unknown. Recently, in the pregnant rabbit, nicardipine was found to be associated with an increase in heart rate and cardiac output and a fall in uteroplacental blood flow (282). Nifedipine effectively lowers maternal blood pressure and heart rate, but does not decrease uterine blood flow in awake pygmy goats (283). Further studies are required to document the safety of such agents.

Adenosine

A number of more recent reports have emphasized the value of adenosine for treatment of dysrhythmias during pregnancy (284–287) and guidelines have been suggested (288).

Vasopressors and Inotropes

Norepinephrine

In pregnant ewes with sympatholytic hypotension, norepinephrine restores maternal blood pressure to normal without increasing uterine blood flow (289). In normotensive ewes, uterine blood flow decreases despite a marked increase in maternal blood pressure (290). Norepinephrine also produces an increase in uterine tonus and intensity and frequency of contraction (291).

Metaraminol

In pregnant ewes with spinal hypotension, metaraminol will restore maternal blood pressure to normal and, on average, will increase uterine blood flow to 70% to 80% of normal (292). Some reports indicate that maternal blood pressure and uterine blood flow are returned to normal, but fetal acidosis and hypoxia may not be corrected (293).

Phenylephrine, Methoxamine, and Angiotensin II

In pregnant ewes with spinal hypotension, these drugs restore maternal blood pressure to normal but without increasing reduced uterine blood flow (294). In normotensive ewes, these agents produce uterine vasoconstriction and decrease uterine blood flow.

Ephedrine

In hypotensive pregnant ewes, ephedrine restores maternal blood pressure to normal, increases uterine blood flow to 85% of normal, and corrects fetal hypoxia and acidosis (290, 292–294). Comparison with metaraminol revealed that ephedrine caused less maternal bradycardia and a greater increase in uterine blood flow (295).

It has been demonstrated that ephedrine may increase fetal atrial natriuretic peptide (296), likely because it crosses the placenta freely. Although potentially important, this finding presently has unknown implications.

Epinephrine

Despite increases in systemic blood pressure, epinephrine markedly decreases uterine blood flow. In low doses, epinephrine decreases uterine contractility, and in high doses, increases uterine contractility (295).

Isoproterenol

Isoproterenol causes a decrease in mean blood pressure and uterine blood flow. No direct vasodilation of gravid uterine vessels has been demonstrated. Uterine contractions are inhibited by approximately 50% when doses of 2 to 8 $\mu g \cdot kg^{-1} \cdot min^{-1}$ are administered (297).

Dopamine

Differing effects of dopamine on uterine blood flow have been reported (298–303). In normotensive sheep, dopamine increased uterine blood flow despite an increase in uterine vascular resistance (301). However, in pregnant ewes, high does of dopamine increased maternal cardiac output and blood pressure, but decreased uterine blood flow without changing renal blood flow (302). Doses less than 10 $\mu g \cdot kg^{-1} \cdot min^{-1}$ produced no significant change in maternal hemodynamics. In pregnant ewes with spinal hypotension and decreased uterine blood flow, dopamine in doses sufficient to maintain blood pressure at control values (20 to 40 $\mu g \cdot kg^{-1} \cdot min^{-1}$) further decreased uterine blood flow and increased uterine vascular resistance (302). In hypotensive patients undergoing cesarean section, dopamine (2 to 10 $\mu g \cdot kg^{-1} \cdot min^{-1}$) restored systolic pressure to 100 mm Hg without depression of Apgar scores. However, depression of maternal arterial Po_2 was found compared with controls. Infants also had a significantly lower Po_2 in umbilical arterial and venous blood than control (303). Further studies are necessary to resolve the apparently conflicting effects of this drug.

Digoxin

Digoxin crosses the placental barrier in both the exteriorized and the intrauterine fetal lamb preparations, and the half-life is significantly longer in the ewe. The amount that crossed the placenta was found to be small but could preserve cardiac function in these preparations. No toxicity was found. Observations of three women during their 11th and 12th weeks of pregnancy showed that less than 1% of the administered digoxin was detectable in the fetus (304). In contrast, one case report revealed that digoxin may profoundly affect the fetus. A mother who ingested 8.9 mg digoxin during her eighth month of pregnancy gave birth to an infant with digitalis intoxication who died shortly after birth (305). Because of drug distribution, metabolism, and elimination in the neonatal period, the digoxin therapeutic index is narrow in the neonate (306).

Amrinone and Milrinone

Few studies are available on amrinone and milrinone use during pregnancy. Amrinone has a favorable effect on oxygen balance in the failing ventricle (307). However, a report demonstrated that milrinone was associated with maternal tachycardia and an increase in uterine blood flow, but did not appear to affect fetal status (308). In a pregnant ewe study, milrinone had no adverse effects on uterine blood flow and fetal well-being (309).

The transplacental passage of milrinone was documented in the baboon model with a maternal-fetal serum ratio of approximately 4:1 (310). In this model, the FHR and fetal arterial blood gas values were unaltered during continuous milrinone administration. The authors suggested that milrinone's vasodilator effects coupled with its positive cardiac inotropic activity may be of benefit in patients with severe preeclampsia and myocardial failure. The clinical pharmacokinetics of these and other cardiovascular drugs have been recently reviewed, but experience in the parturient remains limited (311).

Vasodilators

Sodium Nitroprusside

In pregnant ewes with phenylephrine-induced hypertension, sodium nitroprusside restores blood pressure to normal values but uterine blood flow remains depressed (312). Prolonged administration in ewes may produce fetal death from cyanide toxicity (313).

Hydralazine

In pregnant ewes, hydralazine decreases blood pressure to control values during phenylephrine-induced hypertension and increases uterine blood flow by 15% (312). Compared with sodium nitroprusside, hydralazine is slower in onset but produces a greater increase in cardiac output and heart rate, and a greater decrease in systemic vascular resistance, at the same systemic pressure (312).

Direct Current Cardioversion

Use of direct current cardioversion during pregnancy has been reported by Vogel et al. (68), Sussman et al. (259), Schroeder and Harrison (69), and Ogburn et al. (314). Energies as high as 100 watt/sec have been used. Gestation and delivery were normal in all cases. Monitoring of FHR revealed no apparent effect on the fetus.

CONCLUSION

The anesthetic considerations for the pregnant patient with cardiac disease naturally vary according to the nature of the disease and its progression. However, some general guidelines can be offered:

- *Continue cardiac medications throughout pregnancy, labor, and delivery.*
- *Avoid marked changes in systemic or pulmonary vascular resistance,* e.g., increased systemic vascular resistance in the presence of mitral or aortic insufficiency, and of VSD, ASD, or PDA without pulmonary compromise; decreased systemic vascular resistance in the presence of stenosis, pulmonary hypertension, and/or ventricular compromise; and increased or decreased pulmonary vascular resistance in the presence of a shunt (VSD, ASD, PDA).
- *Prevent or treat factors that can increase a shunt* (e.g., decreased pulmonary or systemic vascular resistance, supraventricular dysrhythmia) *and those that can precipitate reverse shunting* (e.g., increased pulmonary vascular resistance concurrent with decreased systemic vascular resistance).
- *Avoid the use of myocardial depressants when either ventricle is compromised or at risk.*
- *Avoid any factors that can precipitate ventricular dysfunction or failure,* e.g., marked changes in ventricular volume or filling pressures, such as an increase in right ventricular filling pressure in the presence of pulmonic stenosis.

- *Adapt anesthetic technique to the demands of the parturient's disease,* e.g., regional epidural techniques are applicable in the presence of many cardiac conditions, but not tetralogy of Fallot, aortic or pulmonic stenosis, or pulmonary hypertension, where systemic medication and inhalation analgesia are recommended.
- *Avoid any anesthetic agents or drugs that may contribute to marked changes in heart rate, blood volume, peripheral vasoconstriction, venous return, and ventricular filling volumes.*
- *Apply radial and pulmonary artery monitoring in almost all parturients with cardiac disease, and monitoring of central venous pressure where appropriate,* e.g., in patients with pulmonic stenosis.
- *Know the effects on the fetus of cardiac therapeutics that may be administered intraoperatively,* e.g., lidocaine and propranolol cause neonatal depression, isoproterenol inhibits uterine contractions, and sodium nitroprusside has been implicated in a case of fetal cyanide toxicity.

REFERENCES

1. Mendelson CL, ed. *Cardiac Disease in Pregnancy.* Philadelphia: Davis; 1960.
2. Mendelson CL. Acute cor pulmonale and pregnancy. *Clin Obstet Gynecol* 1968;11:992–1009.
3. Barnes CG, ed. *Medical Disorders in Obstetric Practice.* 3rd ed. Oxford: Blackwell; 1970.
4. Szekely P, Snaith L, eds. *Heart Disease and Pregnancy.* London: Churchill Livingstone; 1974.
5. Ueland K. Cardiovascular diseases complicating pregnancy. *Clin Obstet Gynecol* 1978;21:429–442.
6. Niswander K, Berendes H, Deutschberger J, Lipko N, Westphal MC. Fetal mortality following potentially anoxigenic conditions. *Am J Obstet Gynecol* 1967;98:871–876.
7. Burwell CS, Metcalfe J, eds. *Heart Disease and Pregnancy.* Boston: Little Brown; 1958:210–220.
8. Szekely P, Snaith L. Atrial fibrillation and pregnancy. *Br Med J* 1961;1:1407–1410.
9. Sugrue D, Blake S, MacDonald D. Pregnancy complicated by maternal heart disease at the National Maternity Hospital, Dublin, Ireland 1969–1978. *Am J Obstet Gynecol* 1981;139:1–6.
10. Hess DB, Hess WL. Cardiovascular disease and pregnancy. *Obstet Gynecol Clin North Am* 1992;19:679–692.
11. American College of Obstetricians and Gynecologists. *Cardiac Disease in Pregnancy.* ACOG Technical Bulletin No. 168, 1992.
12. Buehler JW, Kaunitz AM, Hogue CJ, Hughes JM, Smith JC, Rochat RW. Maternal mortality in women aged 35 years or older: United States. *JAMA* 1986;255:53–57.
13. Cannell DE, Vernon CP. Congenital heart disease and pregnancy. *Am J Obstet Gynecol* 1961;85:744–753.
14. McCaffrey FM, Sherman FS. Pregnancy and congenital heart disease: The Magee-Women's Hospital. *J Matern Fetal Med* 1995;4: 152–159.
15. Shime J, Mocarski EJM, Hastings D, et al. Congenital heart disease in pregnancy: Short and long term implications. *Am J Obstet Gynecol* 1989;156:313–322.
16. Kerr M. Cardiovascular dynamics in pregnancy and labor. *Br Med Bull* 1968;24:19–24.
17. Liley AW. Clinical and laboratory significance of variations in maternal and plasma volume in pregnancy. *Int J Gynaecol Obstet* 1970;8:358–362.
18. Metcalfe MJ, Rawles JM, Shirreffs C, Jennings K. Six year follow up of a consecutive series of patients presenting to the coronary care unit with acute chest pain: prognostic importance of the electrocardiogram. *Br Heart J* 1990;63:267–272.
19. Ueland K, Novy M, Peterson E, Metcalfe J. Maternal cardiovascular dynamics. IV. The influence of gestational age on the maternal cardiovascular response to posture and exercise. *Am J Obstet Gynecol* 1969;104:856–864.
20. Ueland K, Hansen J. Maternal cardiovascular dynamics. III. Labor and delivery under local and caudal analgesia. *Am J Obstet Gynecol* 1969;103:8–18.
21. Ueland K, Hansen J. Maternal cardiovascular dynamics. II. Posture and uterine contractions. *Am J Obstet Gynecol* 1969;103:1–7.
22. Adesanya CO, Anjorin FL, Sada IA, Parry EH, Sagnella GA, MacGregor GA. Atrial natriuretic peptide, aldosterone, and plasma

renin activity in peripartum heart failure. *Br Heart J* 1991;65: 152–154.

23. Cunningham FG, Lindheimer MD. Hypertension in pregnancy. *N Engl J Med* 1992;326:927–932.

24. Robson SC, Redfern N, Walkinshaw SA. A protocol for the intrapartum management of severe preeclampsia. *Int J Obstet Anesth.* 1992;1:222–229.

25. Black S, Cucchiara RF, Nishimura RA, Michenfelder JD. Parameters affecting occurrence of paradoxical air embolism. *Anesthesiology* 1989;71:235–241.

26. Sutton MS, Cole P, Plappert M, Saltzman D, Goldhaber S. Effects of subsequent pregnancy on left ventricular function in peripartum cardiomyopathy. *Am Heart J* 1991;121:1776–1778.

27. Lampert MB, Weinert L, Hibbard J, Korcarz C, Lindheimer M, Lang RM. Contractile reserve in patients with peripartum cardiomyopathy and recovered left ventricular function. *Am J Obstet Gynecol* 1997;176:189–195.

28. Witlin AG, Mabie WC, Sibai BM. Peripartum cardiomyopathy: A longitudinal echocardiographic study. *Am J Obstet Gynecol* 1997; 177:1129–1132.

29. Splinter WM, Dwane PD, Wigle RD, McGrath MJ. Anaesthetic management of emergency caesarean section followed by pulmonary embolectomy. *Can J Anaesth* 1989;36:689–692.

30. Esposito RA, Grossi EA, Coppa G, et al. Successful treatment of postpartum shock caused by amniotic fluid embolism with cardiopulmonary bypass and pulmonary artery thromboembolectomy. *Obstet Gynecol* 1990;163:572–574.

31. Rotmensch HH, Rotmensch S, Elkayam U. Management of cardiac arrhythmias during pregnancy: Current concepts. *Drugs* 1987; 33:623–633.

32. Weiner CP, Thompson MI. Direct treatment of fetal supraventricular tachycardia after failed transplacental therapy. *Am J Obstet Gynecol* 1988;158:570–573.

33. Hurst JW, ed. *The Heart.* New York: McGraw-Hill; 1978.

34. Fowler NO, ed. *Cardiac Diagnosis and Treatment.* New York: Harper & Row; 1976.

35. Milsom I, Forssman L, Biber B, Dottori O, Rydgren B, Sivertsson R. Maternal haemodynamic changes during cesarean section: A comparison of epidural and general anaesthesia. *Acta Anaesthesiol Scand* 1985;29:161–167.

36. Slomka F, Salmeron S, Zetlaoui P, Cohen H, Simonneau G, Samii K. Primary pulmonary hypertension and pregnancy: Anesthetic management for delivery. *Anesthesiology* 1988;69:959–961.

37. Robinson DE, Leicht CH. Epidural analgesia with low-dose bupivacaine and fentanyl for labor and delivery in a parturient with severe pulmonary hypertension. *Anesthesiology* 1988;68:285–288.

38. Smedstad KG, Cramb R, Morison DH. Primary pulmonary hypertension: A series of eight cases. *Can J Anesth* 1994;41:502–512.

39. Lawlor MC, Johnson C. Anesthetic management of emergency cesarean delivery in a patient with Noonan and Eisenmenger's syndrome. *Reg Anesth* 1994;19:142–145.

40. Khan MJ, Bhatt SB, Kye JJ. Anesthetic considerations for parturients with primary pulmonary hypertension: Review of the literature and clinical presentation. *Int J Obstet Anesth* 1996;5:36–41.

41. Tampakoudis P, Grimbizis G, Chatzinicolaou K, Mantalenakis S. Successful pregnancy in a patient with severe pulmonary hypertension. *Gynecol Obstet Invest* 1996;42:63–65.

42. Clarkson PM, Wilson NJ, Neutze JM, North RA, Calder AL, Barratt-Boyes BG. Outcome of pregnancy after the Mustard operation for transposition of the great arteries with intact ventricular septum. *J Am Coll Cardiol* 1994;24:190–193.

43. Bevacqua BK. Supraventricular tachycardia associated with postpartum metoclopramide administration. *Anesthesiology* 1988; 68:124–125.

44. Lao TT, Sermer M, MaGee L, Farine D, Colman JM. Congenital aortic stenosis and pregnancy. A reappraisal. *Am J Obstet Gynecol* 1993;169:540–545.

45. Hustead ST, Quick A, Gibbs HR, Werner CA, Manlik D. "Pseudocritical" aortic stenosis during pregnancy: Role for Doppler assessment of aortic valve area. *Am Heart J* 1989;117:1383–1385.

46. Easterling TR, Chadwick HS, Otto CM, Benedetti TJ. Aortic stenosis in pregnancy. *Obstet Gynecol* 1988;72:113–118.

47. Colcough G. Epidural anesthesia for cesarean delivery in a parturient with aortic stenosis. *Reg Anesth* 1990;15:273–274.

48. Brian JE Jr, Seifen AB, Clark RB, Robertson DM, Quirk JG. Aortic stenosis, cesarean delivery, and epidural anesthesia. *J Clin Anesth* 1993;5:154–157.

49. Pittard A, Vucevic M. Regional anaesthesia with a subarachnoid microcatheter for caesarean section in a parturient with aortic stenosis. *Anaesthesia* 1998;53:169–173.

50. Dizon-Townson D, Magee KP, Twickler DM, Cox SM. Coarctation of the abdominal aorta in pregnancy: Diagnosis by magnetic resonance imaging. *Obstet Gynecol* 1995;85:817–819.

51. Sonnenblick E, Lesch M, eds. *Valvular Heart Disease.* New York: Grune & Stratton; 1974.

52. Spagnuolo M, Pasternack B, Taranta A. Risk of rheumatic fever recurrences after streptococcal infections. *N Engl J Med* 1971;285:641–647.

53. Jones TD. The diagnosis of rheumatic fever. *JAMA* 1944;126:481.

54. Seaworth BJ, Durack DT. Infective endocarditis in obstetric and gynecologic practice. *Am J Obstet Gynecol* 1986;154:180–188.

55. Cox SM, Leveno KJ. Pregnancy complicated by bacterial endocarditis. *Clin Obstet Gynecol* 1989;32:48–53.

56. Rappaport E. Natural history of aortic and mitral valve disease. *Am J Cardiol* 1975;35:221–227.

57. Selzer A, Cohn E. Natural history of mitral stenosis: A review. *Circulation* 1972;45:878–980.

58. Wood P. An appreciation of mitral stenosis. *Br Med J* 1954;1:1051–1063.

59. Keith TA, Fowler NO, Helmsworth JA, Gralnick H. The course of surgically modified mitral stenosis. *Am J Med* 1963;34:308–319.

60. Hultgren H, Hubis H, Shumway N. Cardiac function following mitral valve replacement. *Am Heart J* 1968;75:302–312.

61. Braunwald E, Braunwald N, Ross J, Morrow AG. Effects of mitral valve replacement on the pulmonary vascular dynamics of patients with pulmonary hypertension. *N Engl J Med* 1965;273:509–514.

62. Al Kasab SM, Sabag T, al Zaibag M, et al. Beta adrenergic receptor blockade in the management of pregnant women with mitral stenosis. *Am J Obstet Gynecol* 1990;163:37–40.

63. Ziskind Z, Etchin A, Frenkel Y, et al. Epidural anesthesia with the Trendelenburg position for cesarean section with or without a cardiac surgical procedure in patients with severe mitral stenosis: A hemodynamic study. *J Cardiothorac Anesth* 1990;4:354–359.

64. Stott DK, Marpole DGF, Brostow JD, Kloster FE, Griswold HE. The role of left atrial transport in aortic and mitral stenosis. *Circulation* 1970;41:1031–1041.

65. Hildner FJ, Javier RP, Cohen LS, et al. Myocardial dysfunction associated with valvular heart disease. *Am J Cardiol* 1972;30: 319–326.

66. Arani DT, Carleton RA. The deleterious role of tachycardia in mitral stenosis. *Circulation* 1967;36:511–516.

67. Hemmings GT, Whalley DG, O'Connor PJ, Benjamin A, Dunn C. Invasive monitoring and anaesthetic management of a parturient with mitral stenosis. *Can J Anesth* 1987;34:182–185.

68. Vogel JHK, Pryor R, Blount SG Jr. Direct-current defibrillation during pregnancy. *JAMA* 1965;193:970–971.

69. Schroeder JS, Harrison DC. Repeated cardioversion during pregnancy: Treatment of refractory paroxysmal atrial tachycardia during three successive pregnancies. *Am J Cardiol* 1971;27:445–446.

70. Eisenach JC, Castro MI. Maternally administered esmolol produces fetal beta-adrenergic blockade and hypoxemia in sheep. *Anesthesiology* 1989;71:718–722.

71. Larson CP Jr, Shuer LM, Cohen SE. Maternally administered esmolol decreases fetal as well as maternal heart rate. *J Clin Anesth* 1990;2:427–429.

72. Losasso TJ, Muzzi DA, Cucchiara RF. Response of fetal heart rate to maternal administration of esmolol. *Anesthesiology* 1991;74:782–784.

73. Ducey JP, Kanpe KG. Maternal esmolol administration resulting in fetal distress and cesarean section in a term pregnancy. *Anesthesiology* 1992;77:829–832.

74. Lasser DM, Basi L. Fetal response time to transplacental digoxin therapy for supraventricular tachyarrhythmia: A meta-analysis. *J Matern Fetal Med* 1993;2:70–74.

75. Lynch C III, Rizor RF. Anesthetic management and monitoring of a parturient with mitral and aortic valvular disease. *Anesth Analg* 1982;61:788–792.

76. Clark SL, Phelan JP, Greenspoon J, Aldahl D, Horenstein J. Labor and delivery in the presence of mitral stenosis: Central hemodynamic observations. *Am J Obstet Gynecol* 1985;152:984–988.

77. Rokey R, Hsu HW, Moise KJ Jr, Adam K, Wasserstrum N. Inaccurate noninvasive mitral valve area calculation during pregnancy. *Obstet Gynecol* 1994;84:950–955.

78. Perloff JK, Roberts WC. The mitral apparatus: Functional anatomy of mitral regurgitation. *Circulation* 1972;46:227–239.

79. Braunwald E. Mitral regurgitation, physiological, clinical and surgical considerations. *N Engl J Med* 1969;281:425–433.

80. Baxley WA, Kennedy JW, Feild B, Dodge HT. Hemodynamics in ruptured chordae tendineae and chronic rheumatic mitral regurgitation. *Circulation* 1973;48:1288–1294.

81. Goodman DJ, Rossen RM, Holloway EL, Alderman EL, Harrison DC. Effect of nitroprusside on left ventricular dynamics in mitral regurgitation. *Circulation* 1974;50:1025–1032.

82. Marcus FI, Ewy GA, O'Rourke RA, Walsh B, Belich AC. The effect of pregnancy on the murmurs of mitral and aortic regurgitation. *Circulation* 1970;41:795–805.

83. Shapiro EP, Trimble EL, Robinson JC, Estruch MT, Gottlieb SH. Safety of labor and delivery in women with mitral valve prolapse. *Am J Cardiol* 1985;56:806–807.

84. Alcantara LG, Marx GF. Cesarean section under epidural analgesia in a parturient with mitral valve prolapse. *Anesth Analg* 1987;66:902–903.

85. Alderson JD. Cardiovascular collapse following epidural anaesthesia for caesarean section in a patient with aortic incompetence. *Anaesthesia* 1987;42:643–645.

86. Dack S, Bader ME, Bader RA, Gelb IJ. Heart disease. In: Rovinsky J, Guttmacher A, eds. *Medical, Surgical and Gynecologic Complications of Pregnancy*. Baltimore: Williams & Wilkins; 1965:1.

87. Frank S, Johnson A, Ross J Jr. Natural history of aortic valvular stenosis. *Br Heart J* 1973;35:41–46.

88. Ueland K, Novy MJ, Metcalfe J. Hemodynamic responses of patients with heart disease to pregnancy and exercise. *Am J Obstet Gynecol* 1972;113:47–59.

89. Arias F, Pineda J. Aortic stenosis and pregnancy. *J Reprod Med* 1978;20:229–232.

90. Frank S, Ross J Jr. The natural history of severe acquired valvular aortic stenosis. *Am J Cardiol* 1967;19:128–129.

91. Liedtke AJ, Gentzler RD II, Babb JD, Hunter AS, Gault JH. Determinants of cardiac performance in severe aortic stenosis. *Chest* 1976;69:192–200.

92. Lee SJK, Jonsson B, Bevegard S, Karlof I, Astrom H. Hemodynamic changes at rest and during exercise in a patient with aortic stenosis of varying severity. *Am Heart J* 1970;79:318–331.

93. Redfern N, Bower S, Bullock RE, Hull CJ. Alfentanil for caeserean section complicated by severe aortic stenosis. *Br J Anaesth* 1987;59:1309–1312.

94. Brawley RK, Morrow AG. Direct determinations of aortic blood flow in patients with aortic regurgitation. *Circulation* 1967;35:32–45.

95. Schlant RC, Nutter DO. Heart failure in valvular heart disease. *Medicine* 1971;50:421–451.

96. Judge TP, Kennedy JW, Bennett LJ, Wills RE, Murray JA, Blackmon JR. Quantitative hemodynamic effects of heart rate in aortic regurgitation. *Circulation* 1971;44:355–367.

97. Rudolph AM, ed. *Congenital Diseases of the Heart*. Chicago: Year Book Medical Publishers; 1974.

98. Campbell M. The incidence and later distribution of malformations of the heart. In: Watson H, ed. *Paediatric Cardiology*. London: Lloyd-Luke; 1968:71.

99. Snaith L, Szekely P. Cardiovascular surgery in relation to pregnancy. In: Marcus S, Marcus C, eds. *Advances in Obstetrics and Gynecology*. Baltimore: Williams & Wilkins; 1967:220.

100. Jewett JF, Ober WB. Primary pulmonary hypertension as a cause of maternal death. *Am J Obstet Gynecol* 1956;71:1335–1341.

101. Copeland WE, Wooley CF, Ryan JM, Runco V, Levin HS. Pregnancy and congenital heart disease. *Am J Obstet Gynecol* 1963;86:107–110.

102. Bloomfield DK. The natural history of ventricular septal defect in patients surviving infancy. *Circulation* 1964;29:914–955.

103. Ullery JC. The management of pregnancy complicated by heart disease. *Am J Obstet Gynecol* 1954;67:834–866.

104. Jones AM, Howitt G. Eisenmenger's syndrome in pregnancy. *Br Med J* 1965;1:1627–1631.

105. Neilson G, Galea EG, Blunt A. Eisenmenger's syndrome and pregnancy. *Med J Aust* 1971;1:431–434.

106. Eisenmenger V. Die angeborenen defecte der kammerscheidewand des herzens. *Z Klin Med* 1897;32:1–29.

107. Ueland K. Cardiac surgery and pregnancy. *Am J Obstet Gynecol* 1965;92:148–162.

108. Pollack KL, Chestnut DH, Wenstrom KD. Anesthetic management of a parturient with Eisenmenger's syndrome. *Anesth Analg* 1990;70:212–215.

109. Sellers JD, Block FE Jr, McDonald JS. Anesthetic management

110. Meyer EC, Tulsky AS, Sigmann P, Silber EN. Pregnancy in the presence of tetralogy of Fallot. *Am J Cardiol* 1964;14:874–879.

111. Jacoby WJ. Pregnancy with tetralogy and pentalogy of Fallot. *Am J Cardiol* 1964;14:866–873.

112. Kirklin JW, Karp RB (eds.). *The Tetralogy of Fallot*. Philadelphia, W. B. Saunders, 1970.

113. Dunborg G, Broustet P, Bricaud H, Fontan F, Trarieux M, Fontanille P. Correction complete d'une triade de Fallott en Circulation extracorporelle chez une femme enceinte. *Arch Mal Coeur* 1959;52:1389–1391.

114. Baker JL, Russell CS, Grainger RG, Taylor DG, Thornton JA, Verel D. Closed pulmonary valvotomy in the management of Fallot's tetralogy complicated by pregnancy. *J Obstet Gynaecol Br Commonw* 1963;70:154–157.

115. Avila WS, Grinberg M, Snitcowsky R, et al. Maternal and fetal outcome in pregnant women with Eisenmenger's syndrome. *Eur Heart J* 1995;16:460–464.

116. Cutforth R, Catchlove B, Knight LW, Dudgeon G. The Eisenmenger's syndrome and pregnancy. *Aust N Z J Obstet Gynaecol* 1968;8:202–210.

117. Spinnato JA, Kraynack BJ, Cooper MW. Eisenmenger's syndrome in pregnancy: Epidural anesthesia for elective cesarean section. *N Engl J Med* 1981;304:1215–1217.

118. Robinson S. Pulmonary artery catheters in Eisenmenger's syndrome: Many risks, few benefits. *Anesthesiology* 1983;58:588–589.

119. Muller BJ, Steude G. General anesthesia administered to a patient with Eisenmenger's syndrome undergoing cesarean section. *Anesthesiol Rev* 1982;9:32–35.

120. Goodwin JF. Pregnancy and coarctation of the aorta. *Clin Obstet Gynecol* 1961;4:645–664.

121. Deal K, Wooley CF. Coarctation of the aorta and pregnancy. *Ann Intern Med* 1973;78:706–713.

122. Cohen LS, Friedman WF, Braunwald E. Natural history of mild congenital aortic stenosis elucidated by serial hemodynamic studies. *Am J Cardiol* 1972;30:1–5.

123. Pansegrau DG, Kioshos JM, Durnin RE, Kroetz FW. Supravalvular aortic stenosis in adults. *Am J Cardiol* 1973;31:635–641.

124. Parker B. The course in idiopathic hypertrophic muscular subaortic stenosis. *Ann Intern Med* 1969;70:903–911.

125. Varghese PH, Izukawa T, Rowe RD. Supravalvular aortic stenosis as part of rubella syndrome with discussion of pathogenesis. *Br Heart J* 1969;31:59–62.

126. Roberts WC. The congenitally bicuspid aortic valve: A study of 85 autopsy cases. *Am J Cardiol* 1970;26:72–83.

127. Bacon APC, Matthews MB. Congenital bicuspid aortic valves and the etiology of isolated aortic valvular stenosis. *Q J Med* 1959; 28:545–560.

128. Kirklin JW, Connolly DC, Ellis FH Jr, Burchell HB, Edwards JE, Wood EH. Problems in the diagnosis and surgical treatment of pulmonic stenosis with intact ventricular septum. *Circulation* 1953;8:849–863.

129. Bentivoglio LG, Maranhao V, Downing DF. Electrocardiogram in pulmonary stenosis with intact septa. *Am Heart J* 1960;59:347–357.

130. Cayler GG, Ongley P, Nadas AS. Relation of systolic pressure in the right ventricle to the electrocardiogram: A study of patients with pulmonary stenosis and intact ventricular septum. *N Engl J Med* 1958;258:979–982.

131. Moller I, Wennevold A, Lyngborg KE. The natural history of pulmonary stenosis: Long-term follow-up with serial heart catheterizations. *Cardiology* 1973;58:193–202.

132. Wilton NCT, Traber KB, Deschner LS. Anaesthetic management for caesarean section in a patient with uncorrected truncus arteriosus. *Br J Anaesth* 1989;62:434–438.

133. Strickland RA, Oliver WC Jr, Chantigian RC, Ney JA, Danielson GK. Anesthesia, cardiopulmonary bypass and the pregnant patient. *Mayo Clin Proc* 1991;66:411–429.

134. Kaufman JM, Ruble PE. The current status of the pregnant cardiac patient. *Ann Intern Med* 1958;48:1157–1170.

135. Wagenvoort CA, Wagenvoort N, eds. *Pathology of Pulmonary Hypertension*. New York: Wiley & Sons; 1977.

136. Coleman PN, Edmunds AWB, Tregillus J. Primary pulmonary hypertension in three sibs. *Br Heart J* 1959;21:81–88.

137. Breen TW, Janzen JA. Pulmonary hypertension and cardiomyopathy: Anaesthetic management for caesarean section. *Can J Anaesth* 1991;38:895–899.

of labor in a patient with dextrocardia, congenitally corrected transposition, Wolff-Parkinson-White syndrome, and congestive heart failure. *Am J Obstet Gynecol* 1989;161:1001–1003.

138. Roberts NV, Keast PJ. Pulmonary hypertension and pregnancy—a lethal combination. *Anaesth Intensive Care* 1990;18:366–374.

139. Nelson DM, Main E, Crafford W, Ahumada GG. Peripartum heart failure due to primary pulmonary hypertension. *Obstet Gynecol* 1983;62(suppl):58S–63S.

140. Power KJ, Avery AF. Extradural analgesia in the intrapartum management of a patient with pulmonary hypertension. *Br J Anaesth* 1989;63:116–120.

141. Abboud TK, Raya J, Noueihid R, Daniel J. Intrathecal morphine for relief of labor pain in a parturient with severe pulmonary hypertension. *Anesthesiology* 1983;59:477–479.

142. Stoelting RK, Reis RR, Longnecker DE. Hemodynamic responses to nitrous oxide-halothane and halothane in patients with valvular heart disease. *Anesthesiology* 1972;37:430–435.

143. Sullivan JM. Blood pressure elevation in pregnancy. *Prog Cardiovasc Dis* 1974;16:375.

144. Barnes CG, ed. *Medical Disorders in Obstetric Practice.* Oxford: Blackwell; 1970:50–60.

145. Browne FJ. Chronic hypertension and pregnancy. *Br Med J* 1947;2:283.

146. Wallen I. The infant mortality in specific hypertensive disease of pregnancy and in essential hypertension. *Am J Obstet Gynecol* 1953;66:36–45.

147. Kincaid-Smith P, Bullen M, Mills J. Prolonged use of methyldopa in severe hypertension in pregnancy. *Br Med J* 1966;1:274–276.

148. Leather HM, Humphreys DM, Baker P, Chad MA. A controlled trial of hypotensive agents in hypertension in pregnancy. *Lancet* 1968;2:488–490.

149. Ross JH, Wright JA. Successful twin pregnancy after treatment of malignant essential hypertension. *Br Med J* 1958;2:545.

150. Hamilton M. Presymptomatic diagnosis of hypertension. In: *Proceedings of the 5th International Congress of Hygiene and Preventive Medicine.* Vol I. Rome; 1968:132.

151. Smith SL, Douglas BH, Langford HG. A model of preeclampsia. *Johns Hopkins Med J* 1967;120:220–224.

152. Chesley LC, Talledo E, Bohler CS, Zuspan FP. Vascular reactivity to angiotensin II and norepinephrine in pregnant and nonpregnant women. *Am J Obstet Gynecol* 1965;91:837–842.

153. Dieckmann WJ, Michel HL. Vascular effects of posterior pituitary extracts in pregnant women. *Am J Obstet Gynecol* 1937;33:131.

154. Talledo OE, Chesley LC, Zuspan FP. Renin-angiotensin system in normal and toxemic pregnancies. *Am J Obstet Gynecol* 1968;100:218–221.

155. Brust AA, Assali NS, Ferris EB. Evaluation of neurogenic and humoral factors in blood pressure maintenance in normal and toxemic pregnancy using tetraethylammonium chloride. *J Clin Invest* 1948;27:717.

156. Assali NS, Prystowsky H. Studies on autonomic blockade. *J Clin Invest* 1950;29:1354–1366.

157. Koch-Weser J. Correlation of pathophysiology and pharmacotherapy in primary hypertension. *Am J Cardiol* 1973;32:499–510.

158. Walsh JJ, Burch GE. Postpartal heart disease. *Arch Intern Med* 1961;108:817–822.

159. Demakis JG, Rahimtoola SH. Peripartum cardiomyopathy. *Circulation* 1971;44:964–968.

160. Demakis JG, Rahimtoola SH, Sutton GC, et al. Natural course of peripartum cardiomyopathy. *Circulation* 1971;44:1053–1061.

161. Veille JC. Peripartum cardiomyopathies: A review. *Am J Obstet Gynecol* 1984;148:805–818.

162. Homans DC. Peripartum cardiomyopathy. *N Engl J Med* 1985;312:1432–1437.

163. Gambling DR, Flanagan ML, Huckell VF, Lucas SB, Kim JHK. Anaesthetic management and non-invasive monitoring for caesarean section in a patient with cardiomyopathy. *Can J Anesth* 1987;34:505–508.

164. Connelly NR, Chin MT, Parker RK, Moran T, Fitzpatrick T. Pregnancy and delivery in a patient with recent peripartum cardiomyopathy. *Int J Obstet Anesth* 1998;7:38.

165. Ladwig P, Fischer E. Peripartum cardiomyopathy. *Aust N Z J Obstet Gynaecol* 1997;37:156.

166. Witlin AG, Mabie WC, Sibai BM. Peripartum cardiomyopathy: An ominous diagnosis. *Am J Obstet Gynecol* 1997;176:182–188.

167. Brown CS, Bertolet BD. Peripartum cardiomyopathy: A comprehensive review. *Am J Obstet Gynecol* 1998;178:409–414.

168. McIndoe AK, Hammond EJ, Babington R. Peripartum cardiomyopathy presenting as a cardiac arrest at induction of anesthesia for emergency cesarean section. *Br J Anaesth* 1995;75:97–101.

169. George LM, Gatt SP, Lowe S. Peripartum cardiomyopathy: Four case histories and a commentary on anesthetic management. *Anaesth Intensive Care* 1997;25:292–296.

170. Goodwin JF, Oakley CM. The cardiomyopathies. *Br Heart J* 1972;34:545–552.

171. Stuart KL. Cardiomyopathy of pregnancy and the puerperium. *Q J Med* 1968;37:463–478.

171a. Pirlet M, Baird M, Pryn S, et al. Low dose combined Spinal-epidural anaesthesia for caesarean section in a patient with peripartum cardiomyopathy. *Int J Obstet Anesth* 2000;9:189–192.

172. Kitchen DH. Dissecting aneurysm of the aorta in pregnancy. *J Obstet Gynaecol Br Commonw* 1974;81:410–413.

173. Schnitker MA, Bayer CA. Dissecting aneurysm of the aorta in young individuals, particularly in association with pregnancy: With report of a case. *Ann Intern Med* 1944;20:486.

174. McGeachy TE, Paullin JE. Dissecting aneurysm of the aorta. *JAMA* 1937;108:1690.

175. Frank S, Braunwald E. Idiopathic hypertrophic subaortic stenosis: Clinical analysis of 126 patients with emphasis on the natural history. *Circulation* 1968;37:759–788.

176. Powell JW Jr, Whiting RB, Dinsmore RE, Sanders CA. Symptomatic prognosis in patients with idiopathic hypertrophic subaortic stenosis (IHSS). *Am J Med* 1973;55:15–24.

177. Reis RL, Peterson LM, Mason DT, Simon AL, Morrow AG. Congenital fixed subvalvular aortic stenosis: An anatomical classification and correlations with operative results. *Circulation* 1971;43(suppl 1):11–18.

178. Swan DA, Bell B, Oakley CM, Goodwin J. Analysis of symptomatic course and prognosis and treatment of hypertrophic obstructive cardiomyopathy. *Br Heart J* 1971;33:671–685.

179. Braunwald E, Lambrew CT, Rockoff SD, Ross J Jr, Morow AG. Idiopathic hypertrophic subaortic stenosis. I. A description of the disease based upon an analysis of 64 patients. *Circulation* 1964;30(suppl IV):3–213.

180. Brown AK, Doukas N, Riding WD, Jones WE. Cardiomyopathy and pregnancy. *Br Heart J* 1967;29:387–393.

181. Turner GM, Oakley CM, Dixon HG. Management of pregnancy complicated by hypertrophic obstructive cardiomyopathy. *Br Med J* 1968;11:281–284.

182. Mason DT, Braunwald E Jr, Ross J. Effects of changes in body position on the severity of obstruction to left ventricular outflow in idiopathic hypertrophic subaortic stenosis. *Circulation* 1966;33:374–382.

183. Glancy DL, Shepherd RL, Beiser GD, Epstein SE. The dynamic nature of left ventricular outflow obstruction in idiopathic hypertrophic subaortic stenosis. *Ann Intern Med* 1971;75:589–592.

184. Loubser P, Suh K, Cohen S. Adverse effects of spinal anesthesia in a patient with idiopathic hypertrophic subaortic stenosis. *Anesthesiology* 1984;60:228–230.

185. Baraka A, Jabbour S, Itani I. Severe bradycardia following epidural anesthesia in a patient with idiopathic hypertrophic subaortic stenosis. *Anesth Analg* 1987;66:1337–1338.

186. Minnich ME, Quirk JG, Clark RB. Epidural anesthesia for vaginal delivery in a patient with idiopathic hypertrophic subaortic stenosis. *Anesthesiology* 1987;67:590–592.

187. Paix B, Cyna A, Belperio P, Simmons S. Epidural analgesia for labour and delivery in a parturient with congenital hypertrophic obstructive cardiomyopathy. *Anaesth Intensive Care* 1999;27:59–62.

188. Ho KM, Kee WD, Poon MC. Combined spinal and epidural analgesia in a parturient with idiopathic hypertrophic subaortic stenosis. *Anesthesiology* 1997;87:168–169.

189. Boccio RV, Chung JH, Harrison DM. Anesthetic management of cesarean section in a patient with idiopathic hypertrophic subaortic stenosis. *Anesthesiology* 1986;65:663–665.

190. Haering JM, Comunale ME, Parker RA, et al. Cardiac risk of noncardiac surgery in patients with asymmetric septal hypertrophy. *Anesthesiology* 1996;85:254–259.

191. Fairley CJ, Clarke JT. Use of esmolol in a parturient with hypertrophic obstructive cardiomyopathy. *Br J Anaesth* 1995;75:801–804.

192. Autore C, Brauneis S, Apponi F, Commisso C, Pinto G, Fedele F. Epidural anesthesia for cesarean section in patients with hypertrophic cardiomyopathy: A report of three cases. *Anesthesiology* 1999;90:1205–1207.

193. Watson H, Emslie-Smith D, Herring J, Hill IGW. Myocardial infarction during pregnancy and the puerperium. *Lancet* 1960;2:523–525.

194. Fletcher E, Knox EW, Morton P. Acute myocardial infarction in pregnancy. *Br Med J* 1967;11:586–590.

195. Ginz B. Myocardial infarction in pregnancy. *J Obstet Gynaecol Br Commonw* 1970;77:610–615.

196. Husaini MH. Myocardial infarction during pregnancy: Report of two cases with a review of the literature. *Postgrad Med J* 1971;47:660–665.

197. Curry JJ, Quintana FJ. Myocardial infarction with ventricular fibrillation during pregnancy treated by direct current defibrillation with fetal survival. *Chest* 1970;58:82–88.

198. Canning B St J, Green AT, Mulcahy R. Coronary heart disease in the puerperium. *J Obstet Gynaecol Br Commonw* 1969;76:1018–1020.

199. Hankins GD, Wendel GD, Leveno KJ, Stoneham J. Myocardial infarction during pregnancy: A review. *Obstet Gynecol* 1985;65:139–146.

200. Makkonen M, Hietakorpi S, Orden MR, Saarikoski S. Myocardial infarction during pregnancy. *Eur J Obstet Gynecol Reprod Biol* 1995;58:81–83.

201. Trouton TG, Sidhu H, Adgey AA. Myocardial infarction in pregnancy. *Int J Cardiol* 1988;18:35–39.

202. McLintic AJ, Pringle SD, Lilley S, Houston AB, Thorburn J. Electrocardiographic changes during cesarean section under regional anesthesia. *Anesth Analg* 1992;74:26–31.

203. Webber MD, Halligan RE, Schumacher JA. Acute infarction, intracoronary thrombolysis, and primary PTCA in pregnancy. *Cathet Cardiovasc Diagn* 1997;42:38–43.

204. Schumacher B, Belfort MA, Card RJ. Successful treatment of acute myocardial infarction during pregnancy with tissue plasminogen activator. *Am J Obstet Gynecol* 1997;176:716–719.

205. Saxena R, Nolan TE, von Dohlen T, Houghton JL. Postpartum myocardial infarction treated by balloon coronary angioplasty. *Obstet Gynecol* 1992;79:810–812.

206. Sanchez-Ramos L, Chami YG, Bass TA, DelValle GO, Adair CD. Myocardial infarction during pregnancy: Management with transluminal coronary angioplasty and metallic intracoronary stents. *Am J Obstet Gynecol* 1994;171:1392–1393.

207. Farmakides G, Schulman H, Mohtashemi M, Ducey J, Fuss R, Mantell P. Uterine-umbilical velocimetry in open-heart surgery. *Am J Obstet Gynecol* 1987;156:1221–1222.

208. Burke AB, Hur D, Bolan JC, Corso P, Resano FG. Sinusoidal fetal heart rate pattern during cardiopulmonary bypass. *Am J Obstet Gynecol* 1990;163:17–18.

209. Frenkel Y, Barkai G, Reisin L, Rath S, Maschiach S, Battler A. Pregnancy after myocardial infarction: Are we playing safe? *Obstet Gynecol* 1991;77:822–825.

210. Silberman S, Fink D, Berko RS, Mendzelevski B, Bitran D. Coronary artery bypass surgery during pregnancy. *Eur J Cardiothorac Surg* 1996;10:925–926.

211. Khandelwal M, Rasanen J, Ludormirski A, Addonizio P, Reece EA. Evaluation of fetal and uterine hemodynamics during maternal cardiopulmonary bypass. *Obstet Gynecol* 1996;88:667–671.

212. Parry AJ, Westaby S. Cardiopulmonary bypass during pregnancy. *Ann Thorac Surg* 1996;61:1865–1869.

213. Dufour P, Berard J, Vinatier D, et al. Pregnancy after myocardial infarction and a coronary artery bypass graft. *Arch Gynecol Obstet* 1997;259:209–213.

214. Yun EM, Royak A, Liu X, et al. The effects of cardiopulmonary bypass on uterine blood flow [abstract]. *Anesthesiology* 1997;87:A876.

215. Sachs BP, Lorell BH, Mehrez M, Damien N. Constrictive pericarditis and pregnancy. *Am J Obstet Gynecol* 1986;154:156–157.

216. Moustafa E, Zina AA, Kassem M, El-Tabbakh G. Echocardiography of the pericardium in pregnancy. *Obstet Gynecol* 1987;69:851–853.

217. Simpson WG, DePriest PD, Conover WB. Acute pericarditis complicated by cardiac tamponade during pregnancy. *Am J Obstet Gynecol* 1989;160:415–416.

218. Lee CN, Wu CC, Lin PY, Hsieh FJ, Chen HY. Pregnancy following cardiac valve replacement. *Obstet Gynecol* 1994;83:353–356.

219. Schenker JG, Polishuk WZ. Pregnancy following mitral valvotomy: A survey of 182 patients. *Obstet Gynecol* 1968;32:214–220.

220. Wallace WA, Ellis LB. Pregnancy following closed mitral valvuloplasty: Long-term follow-up. *Circulation* 1969;40(suppl III):211.

221. Wallace WA, Harken DE, Ellis LB. Pregnancy following closed mitral valvuloplasty: Long-term study with remarks concerning necessity for cardiac management. *JAMA* 1971;217:297–304.

222. Harrison RC, Roschke EJ. Pregnancy in patients with cardiac prostheses. *Clin Obstet Gynecol* 1975;18:107–123.

223. Villoria FE, Montoya L, Recasens E. Proteis valvulares y'embarazo. *Rev Clin Esp* 1976;140:537.

224. Lutz DJ, Noller KL, Spittell J Jr, Danielson GK, Fish CR. Pregnancy and its complications following cardiac valve prosthesis. *Am J Obstet Gynecol* 1978;131:460–468.

225. Ibera-Perez C, Arevalo-Toledo N, Alvarez-De la Cadena O, Noreiga-Guerra L. The course of pregnancy in patients with artificial heart valves. *Am J Med* 1976;61:504–512.

226. Buxbaum A, Aygen MM, Shahin W, Levy MJ, Ekerling B. Pregnancy in patients with prosthetic heart valves. *Chest* 1971;59:639–642.

227. Kloster F, Bristow D, Starr A, McCord CW, Griswold HE. Serial cardiac output and blood volume studies following cardiac valve replacement. *Circulation* 1966;33:528–539.

228. Austen W, Corning H, Moran J, Sanders CA, Scannel JG. Cardiac hemodynamics immediately following mitral valve surgery. *J Thorac Cardiovasc Surg* 1966;51:468–473.

229. Gilbert CS, Sullivan GJ, McLaughlin JJ. Heart disease in pregnancy: Ten year report from the Lewis Memorial Maternal Hospital. *Obstet Gynecol* 1957;9:58–63.

230. Tejani N. Anticoagulant therapy with cardiac valve prosthesis during pregnancy. *Obstet Gynecol* 1973;42:785–793.

231. Varkey GP, Brindle GF. Peridural anaesthesia and anticoagulant therapy. *Can Anaesth Soc J* 1974;21:106–109.

232. Shaul WL, Hall JG. Multiple congenital anomalies associated with oral anticoagulants. *Am J Obstet Gynecol* 1977;127:191–198.

233. Bloomfield DK. Fetal deaths and malformations associated with the use of coumarin derivatives in pregnancy: A critical review. *Am J Obstet Gynecol* 1970;107:883–888.

234. Saks DM, Marx GF. Management of a parturient with cardiac valve prosthesis. *Anesth Analg* 1976;55:214–216.

235. Stevenson RE, Burton OM, Ferlanto GJ, Taylor HA. Hazards of oral anticoagulants during pregnancy. *JAMA* 1980;243:1549–1551.

236. Hall JG, Pauli RM, Wilson KM. Maternal and fetal sequelae of anticoagulation during pregnancy. *Am J Med* 1980;68:122–140.

237. Nageotte MP, Freeman RK, Garite TJ, Block RA. Anticoagulation in pregnancy. *Am J Obstet Gynecol* 1981;141:472–473.

238. Bristow JD, McCord CW, Starr A, Ritzman LW, Griswold HE. Clinical and hemodynamic results of aortic valvular replacement with a ball-valve prosthesis. *Circulation* 1964;29:I-36–I-46.

239. McHenry MM, Smeloff EA, Davey TB, Kaufman B, Fong WY. Hemodynamic results with full-flow orifice prosthetic valves. *Circulation* 1967;35:I-24–I-37.

240. Ross J Jr, Morrow AG, Mason DT, Braunwald E. Left ventricular function following replacement of the aortic valve: Hemodynamic response to muscular exercise. *Circulation* 1966;33:675–679.

241. Paulus DA, Layon AJ, Mayfield WR, D'Amico R, Taylor WJ, James CF. Intrauterine pregnancy and aortic valve replacement. *J Clin Anesth* 1995;7:338–346.

242. Tzankis G, Morse DS. Cesarean section and reoperative aortic valve replacement in a 38-week old parturient. *J Cardiothorac Vasc Anesth* 1996;10:516–518.

243. Lowenstein BR, Vain NW, Perrone SV, Wright DR, Boullon FJ, Favaloro RG. Successful pregnancy and vaginal delivery after heart transplantation. *Am J Obstet Gynecol* 1988;158:589–590.

244. Kossoy LR, Herbert CM III, Wentz AC. Management of heart transplant recipient: Guidelines for the obstetrician-gynecologist. *Am J Obstet Gynecol* 1988;159:490–499.

245. Key TC, Resnik R, Dittrich HC, Reisner LS. Successful pregnancy after cardiac transplantation. *Am J Obstet Gynecol* 1989;160:367–371.

246. Hedon B, Montoya F, Cabrol A. Twin pregnancy and vaginal birth after heart transplantation. *Lancet* 1990;335:476–477.

247. Camann WR, Goldman GA, Johnson MD, Moore J, Greene M. Cesarean delivery of a patient with a transplanted heart. *Anesthesiology* 1989;71:618.

248. Carvalho AC, Almeida D, Cohen M, et al. Successful pregnancy, delivery and puerperium in a heart transplant patient with previous peripartum cardiomyopathy. *Eur Heart J* 1992;13:1589–1591.

249. Wagoner LE, Taylor DO, Olsen SL, et al. Immunosuppressive therapy, management, and outcome of heart transplant recipients during pregnancy. *J Heart Lung Transplant* 1993;12:993–999.

250. Camann WR, Jarcho JA, Mintz KJ, Greene MF. Uncomplicated vaginal delivery 14 months after cardiac transplantation. *Am Heart J* 1991;121:939–941.

251. Kim KM, Sukhani R, Slogoff S, Tomich PG. Central hemodynamic changes associated with pregnancy in a long-term cardiac transplant recipient. *Am J Obstet Gynecol* 1996;174:1651–1653.

252. Eskander M, Gader S, Ong BY. Two successful vaginal deliveries in a heart transplant recipient. *Obstet Gynecol* 1996;87:880.

253. Scott JR, Wagoner LE, Olsen SL, et al. Pregnancy in heart transplant recipients: Management and outcome. *Obstet Gynecol* 1993;82:324–327.

254. Vosloo S, Reichart B. The feasibility of closed mitral valvotomy in pregnancy. *J Thorac Cardiovasc Surg* 1987;93:675–679.

255. Angel JL, Chapman C, Knuppel RA, Morales WJ, Sims CJ. Percutaneous balloon aortic valvuloplasty in pregnancy. *Obstet Gynecol* 1988;72:438–440.

256. Szekely P, Snaith L. Paroxysmal tachycardia in pregnancy. *Br Heart J* 1953;15:195–198.

257. Mendelson CL. Disorders of the heart beat in pregnancy. *Am J Obstet Gynecol* 1956;72:1268–1299.

258. Mowbray R. Heart block and pregnancy: A review. *J Obstet Gynecol* 1948;72:432.

259. Sussman HF, Duque D, Lesser ME. Atrial flutter with 1:1 AV conduction. *Dis Chest* 1966;49:99–102.

260. Biehl D, Shnider SM, Levinson G, Callender K. The direct effects of circulating lidocaine on uterine blood flow and foetal well being in the pregnant ewe. *Can Anaesth Soc J* 1977;24:445–451.

261. Biehl D, Shnider SM, Levinson G, Callender K. Placental transfer of lidocaine. *Anesthesiology* 1978;8:409–412.

262. Kambam JR, Franks JJ, Smith BE. Inhibitory effect of quinidine on plasma pseudocholinesterase activity in pregnant women. *Am J Obstet Gynecol* 1987;157:897–899.

263. Joelsson I, Barton MD. The response of the unanesthetized sheep fetus to sympathomimetic amines and adrenergic agents. *Am J Obstet Gynecol* 1969;114:43–50.

264. Joelsson I, Barton MD. The effect of blockade on the receptors of the sympathetic nervous system of the fetus. *Acta Obstet Gynecol Scand* 1969;48:75–79.

265. Renou P, Newman W, Wood C. Autonomic control of fetal heart rate. *Am J Obstet Gynecol* 1969;105:949–953.

266. Tunstall ME. The effect of propranolol on the onset of breathing at birth. *Br J Anaesth* 1969;41:792.

267. Reed RL, Cheney CB, Fearon RE, Hook R, Hehre FW. Propranolol therapy throughout pregnancy: A case report. *Anesth Analg* 1974;53:214–218.

268. Ostman PL, Chestnut DH, Robillard JE, Weiner CP, Hdez MJ. Transplacental passage and hemodynamic effects of esmolol in the gravid ewe. *Anesthesiology* 1988;69:738–741.

269. Frishman WH, Chesner M. Beta-adrenergic blockers in pregnancy. *Am Heart J* 1988;115:147–152.

270. MacPherson M, Broughton PF, Rutter N. The effect of maternal labetalol on the newborn infant. *Br J Obstet Gynaecol* 1986;93:539–542.

271. Michael CA. Intravenous labetalol and intravenous diazoxide in severe hypertension complicating pregnancy. *Aust N Z J Obstet Gynaecol* 1986;26:26–29.

272. Murad SH, Tabsh KM, Conklin KA, et al. Verapamil: Placental transfer and effects on maternal and fetal hemodynamics and atrioventricular conduction in the pregnant ewe. *Anesthesiology* 1985;62:49–53.

273. Koblin DD, Romanoff ME, Martin DE, et al. Anesthetic management of the parturient receiving amiodarone. *Anesthesiology* 1987;66:551–553.

274. Dicke JM. Cardiac arrhythmias in pregnant women. *Contemporary OB/GYN* 1983;22:158.

275. Fulgencio JP, Hamza J. Anaesthesia for cesarean section in a patient receiving high dose amiodarone for fetal supraventricular tachycardia. *Anaesthesia* 1994;49:406–408.

276. McKenna WJ, Harris L, Rowland E, Whitelaw A, Storey G, Holt D. Amiodarone therapy during pregnancy. *Am J Cardiol* 1983;51:1231–1233.

277. Rey E, Bachrach LK, Burrow GN. Effects of amiodarone during pregnancy. *Can Med Assoc J* 1987;136:959–960.

278. Foster CJ, Love HG. Amiodarone in pregnancy: Case report and review of the literature. *Int J Cardiol* 1988;20:307–316.

279. Gembruch U, Manz M, Bald R, et al. Repeated intravascular treatment with amiodarone in a fetus with refractory supraventricular tachycardia and hydrops fetalis. *Am Heart J* 1989;118:1335–1338.

280. Laurent M, Betremieux P, Biron Y, LeHelloco A. Neonatal hypothyroidism after treatment with amiodarone during pregnancy. *Am J Cardiol* 1987;60:942.

281. Widerhorn J, Bhandari AK, Bughi S, Rahimtoola SH, Elkayam U. Fetal and neonatal adverse effects profile of amiodarone treatment during pregnancy. *Am Heart J* 1991;122:1162–1166.

282. Lirette M, Holbrook RH, Katz M. Cardiovascular and urine blood flow changes during nicardipine HCl tocolysis in the rabbit. *Obstet Gynecol* 1987;69:79–82.

283. Veille JC, Bissonnette JM, Hohimer AR. The effect of a calcium channel blocker (nifedipine) on uterine blood flow in the pregnant goat. *Am J Obstet Gynecol* 1986;154:1160–1163.

284. Belardinelli L, Linden J, Berne RM. The cardiac effects of adenosine. *Prog Cardiovasc Dis* 198;32:73–97.

285. Mason BA, Ogunyemi D, Punla O, Koos BJ. Maternal and fetal cardiorespiratory responses to adenosine in sheep. *Am J Obstet Gynecol* 1993;168:1558–1561.

286. Mason BA, Ricci-Goodman J, Koos BJ. Adenosine in the treatment of maternal paroxysmal supraventricular tachycardia. *Obstet Gynecol* 1992;80:478–480.

287. Afridi I, Moise KJ Jr, Rokey R. Termination of supraventricular tachycardia with intravenous adenosine in a pregnant woman with Wolff-Parkinson-White syndrome. *Obstet Gynecol* 1992;80:481–483.

288. Dalvi BV, Chaudhuri A, Kulkarni HL, Kale PA. Therapeutic guidelines for congenital complete heart block presenting in pregnancy. *Obstet Gynecol* 1992;79:802–804.

289. Greiss FC Jr, Crandell DL. Therapy for hypotension induced by spinal anesthesia during pregnancy. *JAMA* 1965;191:793–796.

290. Greiss FC Jr, Pick JR. The uterine vascular bed: Adrenergic receptors. *Obstet Gynecol* 1964;23:209–213.

291. Cibils LA, Pose SV, Zuspan FP. Effect of 1-norepinephrine infusion of uterine contractility and the cardiovascular system. *Am J Obstet Gynecol* 1962;84:307–317.

292. James FM III, Greiss FC, Kemp RA. An evaluation of vasopressor therapy for maternal hypotension during spinal anesthesia. *Anesthesiology* 1970;33:25–34.

293. Lucas W, Kirschbaum T, Assali NS. Spinal shock and fetal oxygenation. *Am J Obstet Gynecol* 1965;93:583–587.

294. Levinson G, Shnider SM. Vasopressors in obstetrics. In: Zauder H, ed. *Clinical Anesthesia*. Philadelphia: Davis; 1973:77.

295. Shnider SM, deLorimier AA, Holl JW, Chapler FK, Morishima HO. Vasopressors in obstetrics. I. Correction of fetal acidosis with ephedrine during spinal hypotension. *Am J Obstet Gynecol* 1968;102:911–919.

296. Johnson MD, Datta S, Murphy M, Carr D, Ostheimer GW. Atrial natriuretic peptide in maternal and umbilical cord blood during elective cesarean section [abstract]. *Anesthesiology* 1988;69:A703.

297. Kaiser IH, Harris JS. The effect of adrenaline on the pregnant human uterus. *Am J Obstet Gynecol* 1950;59:775–784.

298. Kresnow N, Rolett EL, Yurchak PM, Hood WB Jr, Gorlin R. Isoproterenol and cardiovascular performance. *Am J Med* 1964;37:514–525.

299. Mahon WA, Reid DWJ, Day RA. The in vivo effects of beta adrenergic stimulation and blockade on the human uterus at term. *J Pharmacol Exp Ther* 1967;156:178–185.

300. Blanchard K, Dandavino A, Nuwayhid B, Brinkman CR III, Assali NS. Systemic and uterine hemodynamic responses to dopamine in pregnant and nonpregnant sheep. *Am J Obstet Gynecol* 1978;130:669–673.

301. Callender K, Levinson G, Shnider SM, Feduska NJ, Biehl DR, Ring G. Dopamine administration in the normotensive pregnant ewe. *Obstet Gynecol* 1978;51:586–589.

302. Rolbin SH, Levinson G, Shnider SM, Biehl DR, Wright RG. Dopamine treatment of spinal hypotension decreases uterine blood flow in the pregnant ewe. *Anesthesiology* 1979;51:36–40.

303. Clark RB, Brunner JA. Dopamine as a vasopressor for the treatment of spinal hypotension during cesarean section. *Anesthesiology* 1980;53:514–517.

304. Okita GT, Plotz EJ, Davis ME. Placental transfer of radioactive digitoxin in pregnant women and its fetal distribution. *Circ Res* 1956;4:376–380.

305. Sherman JL, Locke RV. Transplacental neonatal digitalis intoxication. *Am J Cardiol* 1960;6:834–837.

306. Cambonie G, an Haack K, Guyon G, et al. [Digitalis intoxication during the neonatal period: role of dehydration.] *Arch Pediatr* 2000;7:633–636.

307. Notterman DA. Inotropic agents. Catecholamines, digoxin, amrinone. *Crit Care Clin* 1991;7:583–613.

308. Baumann AL, Santos AC, Wlody D, Pedersen H, Morishima HO, Finster M. Maternal and fetal effects of milrinone and dopamine [abstract]. *Anesthesiology* 1989;71:A855.

309. Santos AC, Baumann AL, Wlody D, Pedersen H, Morishima HO, Finster M. The maternal and fetal effects of milrinone and

dopamine in normotensive pregnant ewes. *Am J Obstet Gynecol* 1992; 166:257–262.

310. Atkinson BD, Fishburne Jr JL, Hales KA, Levy GH, Rayburn WF. Placental transfer of milrinone in the nonhuman primate (baboon). *Am J Obstet Gynecol* 1996;174:895–896.

311. Kirsten R, Nelson K, Kirsten D, Heintz B. Clinical pharmacokinetics of vasodilators. Part II. *Clinical Pharmacokinet* 1998;35: 9–36.

312. Ring G, Krames E, Shnider SM, Wallis KL, Levinson G. Comparison of nitroprusside and hydralazine in hypertensive pregnant ewes. *Obstet Gynecol* 1977;51:598–602.

313. Naulty J, Cefalo RC, Lewis PE. Fetal toxicity of nitroprusside in the pregnant ewe. *Am J Obstet Gynecol* 1981;139:708–711.

314. Ogburn PL Jr, Schmidt G, Linman J, Cefalo RC. Paroxysmal tachycardia and cardioversion during pregnancy. *J Reprod Med* 1982;27:359–362.

Shnider and Levinson's Anesthesia for Obstetrics,
edited by Samuel C. Hughes, et al.
Lippincott Williams & Wilkins,
Philadelphia, © 2001.

CHAPTER 27

PERIOPERATIVE MANAGEMENT OF THE PREGNANT PATIENT WITH ASTHMA

A. SUE CARLISLE, PH.D., M.D.

Asthma is a very common chronic disease that affects approximately 14 to 15 million people in the United States alone and as many as 150 million people worldwide. The incidence in the general population is rising, as is the death rate associated with exacerbation of the disease (1). Asthma is also the most common respiratory disease in women of childbearing age, and it is estimated that 4% of all pregnancies are complicated by asthma (2).

The physiologic changes in the respiratory system that occur during pregnancy have been discussed extensively in Chapter 1. These include changes in minute ventilation and lung volumes, and are normally well tolerated; however, in the asthmatic patient, they represent additional physiologic stress placed on an already-compromised respiratory system. They may also mask symptoms of a worsening disease. It has been stated that asthma may improve, worsen, or remain unchanged during pregnancy (3). This variance undoubtedly is related to the interactions of a disease having multifactorial etiologies with the complex physiologic, immunologic, and hormonal changes of pregnancy. Evidence suggests, moreover, that women with severe asthma tend to have more pronounced exacerbations of the disease during pregnancy. This makes it imperative that careful management of asthma is provided both with prenatal care and during delivery (4).

DEFINITIONS, CLASSIFICATION, AND PATHOPHYSIOLOGY

A consensus definition for asthma (5, 6) states that it is a chronic inflammatory disease of the airways involving multiple components of the immune system, including mast cells, eosinophils, neutrophils, and T lymphocytes. The inflammatory response produces widespread but variable airflow obstruction that reverses either spontaneously or with treatment (Fig. 27.1) Asthma is associated with acute bronchoconstriction, airway edema, mucus plug formation, and airway wall remodeling (7). Exacerbations may be caused by a wide variety of stimuli, including allergens, chemicals, pollutants, tobacco smoke, infections, or exercise. The clinical manifestations are wheezing, shortness of breath, cough, and chest tightness.

The clinical symptoms commonly seen in asthmatic patients are the result of a combination of several factors that interact to produce airway smooth muscle hyperreactivity and hypertrophy, as well as inflammation that produces secretions and edema. In the chronic state, destruction of the airway epithelium also occurs, and this results in the deposition of collagen below the basement membrane, with permanent scarring of the airway.

The improved understanding of the pathophysiology of asthma has led to a reclassification of the condition. The previously used categories of "extrinsic or allergic" and "intrinsic or nonallergic," while useful in describing the extremes of the spectrum of disease, are known to have significant overlap and to manifest as an inflammatory response (8). It is now recognized that there is an important genetic predisposition

to allergic responses resulting in inflammation in most cases of both childhood-onset (previously extrinsic) and adult-onset (previously intrinsic) asthma. The presence of different genetic expressions may help explain the variable degrees of expression of the various components of the disease in different patients (9–11).

Asthma has traditionally been classified as mild, moderate, or severe, based on responses to therapy and the need to intensify therapy (6). Moreover, it has been recognized that the chronicity and the patterns of the disease activity are also important (12, 13). Table 27.1 illustrates the relationship of the frequency and chronicity of the symptoms to the changes in airflow as measured by pulmonary function tests. Recognition of the category into which a parturient falls and any changes that have occurred during the pregnancy will guide the intensity of therapy during the pregnancy and may play an important role in predicting the likelihood of a severe exacerbation during labor and delivery.

Autonomic dysfunction is thought to play a large role in the smooth muscle hyperreactivity in some asthmatics (14–19). Neural control of airway tone involves the autonomic system (15, 20) and cell-derived mediators, which stimulate the smooth muscle (Fig. 27.1) (14, 16, 21, 22). Cysteinyl leukotrienes have been identified as important pro-inflammatory mediators in many patients (23). The sustained release of these and other pro-inflammatory mediators is thought to contribute to the chronic, self-perpetuating injury to the airways (7, 24–26).

PREGNANCY AND ASTHMA
Effects of Asthma on Pregnancy

Outcome studies and epidemiologic studies on the effects of asthma on pregnancy have been recently reviewed by Schatz (27). These studies have shown that the rate of prematurity, pregnancy-induced hypertension, excess perinatal mortality, and low birth weight are all increased in asthmatic women, particularly in those who are severe steroid-dependent asthmatics. Other adverse outcomes that appear to be increased in asthmatics include pre- and postpartum hemorrhage, preterm labor and premature rupture of membranes, neonatal hypoxia, and transient tachypnea of the newborn. The need to induce labor and the rate of cesarean section also appear to be higher in asthmatics.

Schatz (28) points out that the mechanism leading to increased adverse outcome may be related to the disease process itself, to the treatment of the disease, or to some other, as yet undefined, process. It has been suggested that the autonomic abnormalities associated with asthma and bronchial hyperreactivity may also be manifested in other systems, including vascular and uterine smooth muscle hyperreactivity. This could relate to the increased incidence of pregnancy-induced hypertension and preterm labor in this population. Other possible

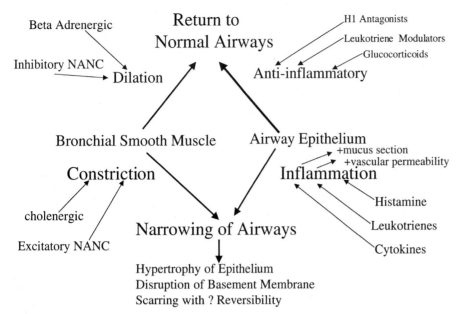

Figure 27.1. **Pathophysiology of Asthma.** The inflammation of the airway leads to airway narrowing via an increase in vascular permeability, mucus secretion, and eventually hypertrophy of the epithelium and disruption of the basement membrane with possible permanent scarring of the airway. The mediators of inflammation are histamine, leukotrienes, and cytokines. The antiinflammatory agents that act on the mediators are H_1-blockers, leukotriene modulators, and glucocorticoids, respectively. The autonomic control of the bronchial smooth muscle is cholinergic and excitatory nonadrenergic-noncholinergic (NANC), which produce constriction, and β-adrenergic and inhibitory NANC, which produce dilation.

contributors to the increase in adverse outcomes may relate to the higher incidence of tobacco abuse by patients who have severe asthma exacerbation during pregnancy. The incidence of asthma is higher in the African-American population (29), as is perinatal morbidity (6). This association may skew outcome data. It is most likely, however, that the majority of adverse outcomes are related to poor asthma control during pregnancy (30–32), independent of genetic background.

The effect of asthma on oxygen delivery to the fetus has also been reviewed (6, 33). The work of breathing is markedly increased during a normal pregnancy as a result of increased oxygen consumption and increased minute ventilation via an increase in tidal volume (see Chapter 1). The increased work of breathing and increased oxygen consumption are further increased during labor. This increased demand requires that peak flows be maintained at a normal level. Even a mild exacerbation of asthma could interfere with the ability of the patient to maintain the normal increased minute ventilation associated with

pregnancy. This would result in both maternal hypoxemia and acute carbon dioxide retention. The maternal carbon dioxide changes would shift the pH acutely and result in decreased fetal oxygenation. Since fetal oxygen extraction occurs on the steep portion of the oxygen-hemoglobin dissociation curve, decreases in maternal arterial oxygen saturation to less than 95% can result in insufficient fetal oxygenation (34). Extreme hyperventilation (alkalosis) can lead to insufficient fetal oxygenation by shifting the affinity of maternal hemoglobin for oxygen (35).

Cardiovascular changes that normally occur during pregnancy also can be adversely affected by exacerbations in asthma. These normal changes include an increase in blood volume and a decrease in systemic and pulmonary vascular resistance. Most asthmatics become dehydrated during exacerbations, and airway obstruction produces an increase in intrathoracic pressure. Both of these changes will decrease cardiac output. The decrease in cardiac output will then compromise the adequacy of uterine blood flow. Since the uterine vessels have little capacity to

---

Table 27.1. CLASSIFICATIONS OF ASTHMA SEVERITY*

	Symptoms[†]	Nighttime Symptoms	Lung Function
STEP 4 Severe persistent	• Continuous symptoms • Limited physical activity • Frequent exacerbations	Frequent	• FEV_1 or PEF ≤60% predicted • PEF variability >30%
STEP 3 Moderate persistent	• Daily symptoms • Daily use of inhaled short-acting β_2-agonist • Exacerbations affect activity • Exacerbations ≥2 times a week; may last days	>1 time a week	• FEV_1 or PEF ≥60%–<80% predicted • PEF variability >30%
STEP 2 Mild persistent	• Symptoms >2 times a week but <1 time a day • Exacerbations may affect activity	>2 times a month	FEV_1 or PEF >80% predicted PEF variability 20%–30%
STEP 1 Mild intermittent	• Symptoms ≤2 times a week • Asymptomatic and normal PEF between exacerbations • Exacerbations brief (from a few hours to a few days); intensity may vary	≤2 times a month	FEV_1 or PEF ≥80% predicted PEF variability <20%

FEV_1 = forced expiratory volume in 1 second; PEF = peak expiratory flow.

*The presence of one of the features of severity in any category is sufficient to place a patient in that category. An individual should be assigned to the most severe grade in which any feature occurs. The characteristics noted in this table are general and may overlap because asthma is highly variable. Furthermore, an individual's classification may change over time.

†Patients at any level of severity can have mild, moderate, or severe exacerbations. Some patients with intermittent asthma experience severe and life-threatening exacerbations separated by long periods of normal lung function and no symptoms.

Reprinted by permission from National Institutes of Health/National Heart, Lung, and Blood Institute. *Expert Panel Report 2. Guidelines for the Diagnosis and Management of Asthma.* Bethesda, MD: National Institutes of Health; 1997.

Table 27.2. PERIOPERATIVE CAUSES OF ASTHMATIC SYMPTOMS

Physiologic
  Exacerbation of chronic asthma
  Acute asthma
  Chronic obstructive pulmonary disease
  Pulmonary embolism (amniotic fluid, thrombus, air)
  Congestive heart failure
  Gastroesophageal reflux disease with chronic aspiration
  Acute lung injury with noncardiac pulmonary edema
  Acute respiratory distress syndrome
  Hypersensitivity (drug or allergy)-induced pulmonary
    infiltrates and/or edema
  Anaphylactic or anaphylactoid reaction
Anatomic
  Pneumothorax
  Laryngeal or vocal cord dysfunction
  Laryngeal edema
  Mucus plugging of airways
Mechanical
  Mechanical obstruction of airway (tumor, foreign body)
  Mechanical obstruction of endotracheal tube
  Endobronchial intubation

autoregulate and the vessels of young healthy people are quite good at autoregulation, a small decrease in cardiac output may not be manifested in the maternal vital signs but may adversely affect the fetus (34).

Treatment of Asthma During Pregnancy

While the anesthesiologist may not routinely have the responsibility for management of asthma during pregnancy, a working knowledge of the currently available modalities for treatment of asthma will improve the care during delivery. Also, more patients are being seen prenatally in early consultation while planning for delivery. It is imperative that the consultant have a good understanding of the importance of the optimal management of asthma, both during the pregnancy and during delivery. The consultant also must be able to distinguish between asthma and other causes of cough, wheezing, and respiratory insufficiency (Table 27.2), and to avoid drugs that exacerbate asthma (Table 27.3).

As previously discussed, epidemiologic and outcome studies suggest that poor treatment of asthma during pregnancy may contribute significantly to adverse outcomes (6, 27, 36). The safety of the use of β_2 agonists has been established by evaluation of available human data (37). Multivariate analysis of outcome data (38, 39) examining the question of the safety of asthma medications suggested that the use of oral corticosteroids may be associated with an increased incidence of pregnancy-induced hypertension. Some evidence suggests that oral corticosteroids may also be weakly associated with low-birth weight and even more weakly associated with cleft palate (40). No other drug associations with adverse outcomes were revealed by this analysis. Recent reports by Luskin (41) and Schatz (30) have further

Table 27.3. DRUGS ASSOCIATED WITH EXACERBATIONS OF ASTHMA

Non-β1 selective antagonists (labetalol, propranolol)
Non-β1 selective ophthalmic preparations (timolol)
Aspirin and tartrazine dyes (in sensitive patients)
Nonsteroidal antiinflammatory drugs (in aspirin-sensitive patients)
Prostaglandin F$_2$-α
Ergot alkaloids
Sulfiting agents (metabisulfite, sodium bisulfite)

substantiated this safety profile, and it is generally agreed that the risk of untreated asthma far exceeds the risk of the medications. The National Institutes of Health Working Group on Asthma and Pregnancy (2) strongly recommends that aggressive management of asthma be instituted before pregnancy if possible, and continued throughout pregnancy, labor, and delivery. The specific drugs recommended by the Working Group are illustrated in Table 27.4. Despite these recommendations, many patients continue to receive inadequate therapy during pregnancy (42).

The Expert Panel of the National Asthma Education and Prevention Program (6) outlines the components of asthma treatment. These include removal of triggers to exacerbations, careful monitoring, patient education, and stepwise use of drugs, with distinction made between acute and chronic treatment (Table 27.1). The initial medications should be inhaled short-acting β_2-agonists (e.g., albuterol) for **mild intermittent asthma** (step 1), and addition of an antiinflammatory such as an inhaled steroid or cromolyn, with possible use of sustained-release theophylline for **mild persistent asthma** (step 2). The treatment of **moderate persistent asthma** (step 3) includes the use of long-acting β_2 agonists (e.g., salmeterol) and intensification of the inhaled steroids. **Severe persistent asthma** (step 4) is treated with the addition of systemic steroid to the previously started medications. Schatz and Zeigler (31) have published a modification of these recommendations, and this simplified step approach is illustrated in Table 27.5. Anticholinergics, such as ipratropium, may also be useful in some patients (2). During labor and delivery, both short-acting, rapid-onset β_2 agonists and steroids should be used for any level of exacerbation of asthma. Additionally, it is obvious that supplemental oxygen should be provided if there is any suggestion of inadequate oxygen delivery to the fetus at any time during the pregnancy or delivery.

The recognition of the role of leukotrienes in the pathophysiology of asthma (43–45) has led to much interest in the use of leukotriene modifiers in the treatment and prevention of asthma. Initial studies of these medications for treatment of mild persistent asthma in adults have been promising; however, insufficient experience with these medications precludes the firm recommendation for their use during pregnancy (6, 46). Animal studies have suggested that two of these leukotriene modifiers, montelukast and zafirlukast, may be safe during pregnancy. A third leukotriene modifier, zileuton, has been shown in animal studies to be associated with poor intrauterine growth, long-bone abnormalities, and cleft-palate. Zileuton therefore may not be safe and should be avoided during pregnancy (47–49).

Status Asthmaticus

Status asthmaticus, or near-fatal asthma, is described as severe bronchospasm unresponsive to intensive β_2 agonists and systemic corticosteroids, and requiring ventilatory support for respiratory failure (50, 51). Some asthmatics will progress to status asthmaticus during pregnancy or delivery, either despite adequate treatment or because of inadequate treatment. Severe respiratory compromise requiring mechanical ventilatory support is a particularly challenging situation in that maintenance of adequate fetal blood flow and oxygenation may be difficult or impossible in these critically ill patients. Adequate ventilation may be hard to achieve, and permissive hypercarbia, frequently used in nonpregnant patients, may adversely affect fetal oxygenation, as previously discussed.

Management of status asthmaticus in the nonpregnant patient usually requires the use of continuous high-flow oxygen delivery systems or mechanical ventilation. Additionally, intensive inhaled β_2 agonists, systemic steroids, methylxanthines, anticholinergics (such as ipratropium), sedation, and sometimes muscle relaxants are needed to achieve adequate ventilation and oxygenation (50, 51). Alternative treatments, including magnesium sulfate (52–57), heliox (58–60), and plasma exchange

Table 27.4. DRUGS AND DOSAGES FOR ASTHMA AND ASSOCIATED CONDITIONS PREFERRED FOR USE DURING PREGNANCY

Drug Class	Specific Drug	Dosage
Antiinflammatory	Cromolyn sodium	2 puffs qid (inhalation) 2 sprays in each nostril bid to qid (intranasal for nasal symptoms)
	Beclomethasone	2–5 puffs bid to qid (inhalation) 2 sprays in each nostril bid (intranasal for allergic rhinitis)
	Prednisone	Burst for active symptoms: 40 mg a day, single or divided dose for 1 week, then taper for 1 week. If prolonged course is required, single a.m. dose on alternate days may minimize adverse effects
Bronchodilator	Inhaled β_2-agonist Theophylline	2 puffs every 4 hours as needed Oral: Dose to reach serum concentration level of 8–12 μg/mL
Antihistamine	Chlorpheniramine	4 mg by mouth up to qid 8–12 mg sustained-release bid
	Tripelennamine	25–50 mg by mouth up to qid 100 mg sustained-release bid
Decongestant	Pseudoephedrine	60 mg by mouth up to qid 120 mg sustained-release bid
Cough	Oxymetazoline Guaifenesin	Intranasal spray or drops up to 5 days for rhinosinusitis 2 tsp by mouth qid
Antibiotics	Dextromethorphan Amoxicillin	— 3 weeks therapy for sinusitis

bid = twice daily; qid = four times daily.
This table presents drugs and suggested dosages for the home management of asthma and associated conditions. Drugs and dosages for the treatment of exacerbations in the emergency department or hospital are presented in the full report of the working group.
Reprinted by permission from the National Asthma Education Program. *Report of the Working Group on Asthma and Pregnancy*. Bethesda, MD: National Institutes of Health; 1992.

(61), have been used with some success. In some instances, the use of volatile anesthetics is also required (51, 62). Volatile anesthetics, such as halothane isoflurane (63–65) and sevoflurane (66, 67), have all been shown to provide some improvement of bronchospasm.

The use of sedatives is vitally important in the treatment of status asthmaticus in that the patient must be able to tolerate intensive ventilatory support and possible hypercapnia. These agents routinely include benzodiazepines and opioids. There is some evidence that propofol, which could be used as an infusion for sedation, may provide some mild bronchodilatory effect; however, the evidence for this action is weak (68–70). There is some speculation that metabisulfite-containing propofol could worsen bronchospasm in patients who are sensitive to

this agent (71). Dexmedetomidine, a potent α_2 agonist, has recently been approved for sedation and analgesia in critically ill patients. This agent appears to cause less respiratory depression (72) and fewer hemodynamic changes than other agents (73), and therefore might be a useful drug in status asthmaticus. No information is yet available, however, regarding the safety of this drug during pregnancy.

In the pregnant patient, choice of treatment must be considered not only with respect to the effect on the maternal pulmonary and cardiovascular systems, but also with respect to the effect on fetal well-being. As discussed previously, severe bronchospasm produces an increase in intrathoracic pressure that may compromise cardiac output. Positive pressure ventilation may make the decrease in cardiac output even more

Table 27.5. PHARMACOLOGICAL STEP THERAPY OF CHRONIC ASTHMA DURING PREGNANCY*

Category	Frequency/Severity of Symptoms	Pulmonary Function (Untreated)*	Step Therapy
Mild	<3 times per week; nocturnal symptoms <2 times per month	1 >80%	Inhaled β_2-agonists, as required
Moderate	≥3 times per week; exacerbations affect sleep or activity	60%–80%	As for "mild," plus inhaled sodium cromoglycate (cromolyn sodium); substitute inhaled beclomethasone dipropionate; add oral theophylline
Severe	Daily; limited activity; frequent nocturnal symptoms; frequent acute exacerbations	<60%	As for "moderate," plus oral corticosteroids (burst for active symptoms, alternate day or daily if necessary)

*Forced expiratory volume in 1 second (FEV$_1$) or peak expiratory flow rate, based on the norm for the patient, which may be the standardized norm or personal best.
Based on the recommendations of the National Asthma Education Program. *Report of the Working Group on Asthma During Pregnancy*. Bethesda, MD: National Institutes of Health; 1997.
Reprinted by permission from Schatz M, Zeigler RS. Asthma and allergy in pregnancy. *Clin Perinatol* 1997;24:407–432.

pronounced. Positioning of the patient to prevent aortocaval compression is important in order to counteract the effects of increased intrathoracic pressure. Vasodilation produced by volatile anesthetics or sedatives may further compromise effective maternal blood volume and therefore fetal circulation. β_2 agonists may cause excessive tachycardia. Theophylline also may cause tachycardia in the mother, as well as producing unwanted effects in the fetus, such as atrial arrhythmias (74). Heliox should be used only when adequate oxygenation can be achieved with an FIO_2 of 0.4 or less, since any mixture with less than 0.6 of heliox is ineffective. Magnesium infusion might be of particular use in the patient with pregnancy-induced hypertension and asthma. Additionally, there is some evidence that epidural anesthesia alone can be efficacious in termination of status asthmaticus in the parturient (75).

All of the interventions discussed for the nonpregnant patient should be used, but special care must be taken in the pregnant patient. Optimum volume status must be maintained and oxygenation maximized during exacerbations of asthma, and the fetus must be monitored carefully in the critically ill patient. Several case reports advise either early termination of the pregnancy or early delivery of the viable fetus (76). In some cases, this may be necessary to ensure the survival of the mother. Some case reports have indicated that delivery has resulted in immediate improvement in the respiratory status of the patient (76, 77).

INDUCTION OF LABOR

The hyperreactivity of the airways of the asthmatic patient has been a source of study for many years (15, 78, 79). It is clear from these studies that asthmatics are particularly sensitive to prostaglandin $F_{2\alpha}$, and this agent has been shown to provoke bronchospasm in induction of labor (80). The effect of prostaglandin E_2 on bronchial smooth muscle is relaxation; however, this agent has been shown to cause bronchospasm when inhaled (81). Oxytocin, which is the usual induction agent, appears not to have adverse effects in asthmatics and should be the agent of choice.

ANESTHESIA FOR LABOR AND DELIVERY IN THE ASTHMATIC PATIENT

The anesthetic management of the nonpregnant asthmatic patient has recently been reviewed by Gal (82). The basic principles outlined in that review also apply to the pregnant patient, and include optimization of pulmonary status prior to initiation of the anesthetic, avoidance of bronchospasm-triggering agents such as histamine releasers, and avoidance of airway irritation by an endotracheal tube whenever possible. The additional considerations required for the pregnant patient include increased risk of aspiration from reflux, risk of a difficult airway, the need to maintain adequate uterine forces, and the need to maintain adequate fetal blood flow and oxygenation (83). The increased work of breathing and increased oxygen use by the parturient are also considerations in the asthmatic patient.

While most asthmatics will deliver without an exacerbation of symptoms (37), the consequences of an exacerbation must be considered in that an asthmatic patient may have little of the respiratory reserve required during normal labor. Some asthmatic patients may deliver with little or no analgesia; however, the need to minimize the increased work of breathing and oxygen use strongly supports the use of effective analgesia in early labor (e.g., systemic medications [Chapter 7] and regional techniques [Chapter 8]), and the use of epidural or subarachnoid block for cesarean section. General anesthesia may be required under some circumstances.

Systemic Analgesics

The use of opioids in asthmatic patients has been controversial in that any respiratory depression may not be tolerated, and

some opioids, particularly high-dose morphine, are associated with histamine release (84). Despite these concerns, the general consensus is that the importance of analgesia in early labor in this patient population greatly outweighs these other considerations. Fentanyl and meperidine are the opioids used most commonly for analgesia. Careful respiratory monitoring should be employed during the use of any respiratory depressants in the asthmatic.

Regional Analgesia

Paracervical or pudendal blocks are sometimes used during labor and delivery (see Chapter 8). These blocks have the advantage of providing some analgesia without sedation or respiratory muscle compromise. The disadvantage of these techniques is that the analgesia is frequently inadequate and this would be a concern in the asthmatic parturient.

Neuraxial Anesthesia for Vaginal Delivery or Cesarean Section

It has long been recognized that use of epidural anesthesia results in decreased catecholamine levels (85) and decreased oxygen consumption (86) during labor. As previously discussed, this may be of vital importance for the asthmatic; therefore, strong consideration should be given to use of neuraxial anesthesia in these patients. This could be provided with spinal, epidural, or combined spinal-epidural technique. There are isolated case reports of bronchospasm associated with spinal anesthesia (87, 88), but the trigger for the bronchospasm was unclear in all of these cases. The majority of patients do not manifest this response. There is also a theoretic concern that patients on steroid therapy may be at greater risk for epidural or intrathecal infections.

Agents for epidural or subarachnoid blocks are discussed in detail elsewhere in this book (Chapters 5, 8, 11), and there are no special considerations regarding choice of local anesthetics for this population. Careful attention must be paid to avoidance of high block, which could be associated with compromise of respiratory muscle function (Fig. 27.2). The importance of maintenance of adequate intravascular volume cannot be overemphasized. If opioids are used either epidurally or intrathecally, the patient must be carefully monitored for respiratory depression.

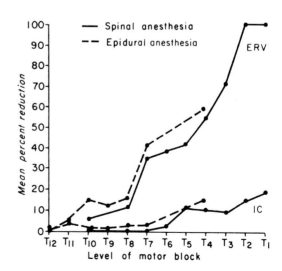

Figure 27.2. Effect of level of motor nerve block during spinal and epidural anesthesia on inspiratory capacity (*IC*) and expiratory reserve volume (*ERV*). Changes in ventilatory parameters are plotted as percentage reduction from control. (Reprinted by permission from Freund FG, Bonica JJ, Ward RJ, Akamatsu TJ, Kennedy WF. Ventilatory reserve and level of motor block during high spinal and epidural anesthesia. *Anesthesiology* 1967;28:834–837.)

General Anesthesia

General anesthesia must be provided if neuraxial anesthesia is contraindicated. The likelihood of exacerbation of bronchospasm is much higher with the placement of an endotracheal tube (89). The need for a rapid sequence induction further increases the possibility of bronchospasm in that the endotracheal tube may be placed with an anesthetic level insufficient to blunt airway reflexes.

The most commonly used agents for induction of anesthesia for cesarean section are thiopental, ketamine, and propofol. Ketamine had been thought to have mild bronchodilatory action related to the release of endogenous catecholamines, but the evidence supporting this effect in humans is poor. Propofol has been shown to be efficacious in blunting airway responsiveness (90) and also may have weak bronchodilating action (68, 91–93). These properties may make it the agent of choice with respect to the airways; however, hemodynamic changes associated with induction with propofol must be managed appropriately and aggressively in the parturient. Thiopental has the disadvantage of causing histamine release in some patients, and theoretically this could be a trigger for bronchospasm in the asthmatic patient. The dose of less than $4 \text{ mg} \cdot \text{kg}^{-1}$, which is the dose some consider safe to avoid fetal depression, may be insufficient as a single agent to blunt airway reflexes in the asthmatic patient. Thiopental has, however, been safely used routinely in asthmatics (89, 94). It is essential that either a dose adequate for blunting airway reflexes (4 to $6 \text{ mg} \cdot \text{kg}^{-1}$) be administered or adjuvant medication be used.

Intravenous lidocaine has been shown to be useful as an adjuvant to the above-mentioned induction (95). The administration of $1 \text{ mg} \cdot \text{kg}^{-1}$ lidocaine will attenuate both airway reflexes and hemodynamic responses associated with endotracheal intubation. Aerosolized lidocaine should not be used since it and many other aerosolized agents have been shown to be airway irritants in the asthmatic (96, 97).

Muscle relaxation must be provided for cesarean section. Succinylcholine is usually employed for initial relaxation for rapid sequence intubation. Newer agents such as rocuronium (98, 99) [100, 101] may be safe alternatives for an asthmatic patient. Some neuromuscular blocking agents (e.g., atracurium and rapacuronium) (see Chapter 11) can potentially worsen bronchospasm, both by histamine release (101) and by alteration of inhibitory pathways that usually block vagally mediated receptors. Vecuronium seems not to exhibit this property (102). Reversal of neuromuscular blockade with neostigmine can also exacerbate airflow obstruction by increasing secretions and bronchospasm; however, the use of glycopyrrolate or atropine can attenuate this response. Edrophonium apparently is less likely than neostigmine to cause bronchospasm (103) and might be a better choice in the asthmatic patient. Alternatively, muscle relaxation could be achieved by continued use of succinylcholine to avoid the need for reversal agents.

Halogenated agents are usually utilized to maintain general anesthesia for cesarean section (Chapter 11). This is particularly appropriate in asthmatic patients since halothane, isoflurane, and sevoflurane all have bronchodilating properties (51, 62–66). Halothane, which was classically used for anesthesia for cesarean sections, has the disadvantage of causing cardiac irritability, particularly in the setting of high catecholamine states or in conjunction with aminophylline use (104). Isoflurane and sevoflurane are now used more commonly in this setting. The disadvantage of using high alveolar concentrations of volatile anesthetics (>1.0 to 1.5 MAC) for control of bronchospasm after delivery is the risk of increased bleeding or frank hemorrhage from uterine relaxation.

Termination of general anesthesia in the nonpregnant asthmatic is usually accomplished with extubation of the trachea during deep anesthesia. This is not possible in the parturient since the risk of aspiration is high. The patient should be treated during surgery with β_2 agonists and steroids, and the trachea extubated with the patient awake. A lidocaine infusion may be useful during emergence in order to decrease airway reactivity. Postoperative mechanical ventilation may be necessary until the airway obstruction is controlled.

POSTPARTUM HEMORRHAGE

It has been shown by review of numerous outcome studies (27) that asthmatics have a higher incidence of significant postpartum hemorrhage than nonasthmatics. The reason for this is unknown but could be related to abnormalities in smooth muscle and the neural regulation of contraction (15). It may also be related to the peripartum use of β_2 agonists.

The management of postpartum hemorrhage is discussed in detail elsewhere in this book (Chapter 20). The recommendations for the use of oxytocin are valid for the asthmatic; however, the use of ergot alkaloids such as methylergonovine (Methergine) and ergonovine (Ergotrate) may be relatively contraindicated in asthmatics in that they can exacerbate bronchospasm (31, 105). Prostaglandin E and prostaglandin $F_{2\alpha}$ both cause uterine contractions. Prostaglandin $F_{2\alpha}$ (Hemabate) is readily available and frequently used to treat uterine atony. This agent has been reported to cause bronchospasm (80) in the asthmatic. Prostaglandin E causes bronchodilation, but the only available formulation is a vaginal suppository or gel, which is not useful in this clinical setting. The risk-benefit ratio for using these agents in this population must be carefully considered, and management of severe bronchospasm might be preferable to cardiovascular collapse from uncontrolled hemorrhage. This is emphasized by the recent analysis of maternal mortality in Japan that cited hemorrhage as the most important cause of preventable deaths (106).

HYPERTENSION, PREECLAMPSIA, AND ASTHMA

Elevated blood pressure during pregnancy may be the result of chronic hypertension or pregnancy-induced hypertension. Review of the literature by Schatz (27) revealed an increased incidence of pregnancy-induced hypertension in the asthmatic population. The treatment of chronic or pregnancy-induced hypertension in the asthmatic patient poses special problems. Additionally, aspirin, which is now controversial in the pregnancy-induced hypertensive patient (107, 108), must be used with caution in the asthmatic population since it is known to be a trigger for bronchospasm in a subset of these patients.

The mainstay of treatment of hypertension in the nonpregnant, nonasthmatic patient is β-blockade, and there is significant experience with use of labetalol for pregnancy-induced hypertension (109, 110). All β-blockers, especially non–β_1-selective agents, should be used with caution in the asthmatic patient. Vasodilators such as hydralazine, calcium-channel blockers, nitroglycerin, and nitroprusside may be better agents for control of hypertension in the asthmatic patient with pregnancy-induced hypertension; however, they can cause hypoxemia in that they adversely affect ventilation-perfusion matching by interfering with hypoxic pulmonary vasoconstriction. Careful attention must be paid to maintaining adequate maternal oxygenation when using these agents. Magnesium infusions are frequently used in these patients for seizure prophylaxis and may have some benefit in treatment of bronchospasm (52–56). Volume expansion is critical in both asthma- and pregnancy-induced hypertension.

Anesthetic considerations for delivery of asthmatic parturients with pregnancy-induced hypertension must include all of the previously discussed airway problems and the possibility of coagulopathy and increased risk of pulmonary edema. Neuraxial anesthesia is the preferred option unless there are clear contraindications.

SUMMARY

Asthma is a chronic inflammatory disease of the airways that leads to airflow limitation by bronchoconstriction, airway edema, mucus secretion with plug formation, and eventually airway remodeling and scarring. The response of this disease to pregnancy is highly varied. The general consensus is that vigorous control of the disease during pregnancy leads to a better outcome.

Anesthetic considerations for the asthmatic parturient must include prevention whenever possible and management of acute exacerbations. Effective analgesia during labor and delivery can be important to ensure adequate fetal oxygen delivery. Neuraxial techniques are usually the preferred modality for analgesia and anesthesia. If necessary, general anesthesia may be safely administered if the previously discussed precautions are followed.

REFERENCES

1. Committee of the Environmental and Occupational Health Assembly of the American Thoracic Society. Health effects of outdoor pollution. *Am J Respir Crit Care Med* 1996;153:3–50.
2. National Asthma Education Program. *Management of Asthma During Pregnancy. Executive Summary: Report of the Working Group on Asthma and Pregnancy.* Bethesda, MD: National Institutes of Health; 1992. NIH publication 93-3279A.
3. Schatz M, Zeiger RS. Asthma and allergy in pregnancy. *Clin Perinatol* 1997;24:407–432.
4. American College of Obstetricians and Gynecologists. Pulmonary disease in pregnancy. ACOG Technical Bulletin No. 224. *Int J Gynaecol Obstet* 1996;54:187–196.
5. Lemanske RF, Busse WW. Primer on allergic and immunologic diseases, 4th edition. *JAMA* 1997;278:1855–1873.
6. National Asthma Education and Prevention Program. *Guidelines for the Diagnosis and Management of Asthma.* Bethesda, MD: National Institutes of Health; 1997.
7. Fahy JV, Corry DB, Boushey HA. Airway inflammation and remodeling in asthma. *Curr Opin Pulm Med* 2000;6:15–20.
8. Walker C, Bode E, Boer L, Hansel TT, Blaser K, Virchow JC. Allergic and nonallergic asthmatics have distinct patterns of T-cell activation and cytokine production in peripheral blood and bronchoalveolar lavage. *Am Rev Respir Dis* 1992;146:109–115.
9. Sanford A, Weir T, Pare P. The genetics of asthma. *Am J Respir Crit Care Med* 1996;153:1749–1765.
10. Reihasaus E, Innis M, MacIntyre N, Liggett SB. Mutations in the gene encoding for the beta 2-adrenergic receptor in normal and asthmatic subjects. *Am J Respir Cell Mol Biol* 1993;8:334–339.
11. Postma DS, Bleecker ER, Amelung PJ, et al. Genetic susceptibility to asthma- bronchial hyper-responsiveness coinherited with a major gene for atopy. *N Engl J Med* 1995;333:894–900.
12. Lenfant C, Khaltaev N. *Global Initiatives for Asthma: Global Strategy for Asthma Management and Prevention.* Bethesda, MD: National Heart, Lung, and Blood Institute/World Health Organization; 1993. NHLBI/WHO Workshop Report; 1–176.
13. Bussee WW, Lemanske RF Jr. Asthma. *N Engl J Med* 2001;344:350–362.
14. Hirshman CA. Airway reactivity in humans. *Anesthesiology* 1983;58:170–177.
15. Bai TR. Beta 2-adrenergic receptors in asthma: A current perspective. *Lung* 1992;170:125–141.
16. Leff AR, Hamann KJ, Wegner DC. Inflammation and cell-cell interactions in airway hyper-responsiveness. *Am J Physiol* 1991;260:L189–L206.
17. Colasurdo GN, Larsen GL, eds. Airway hyperresponsiveness. In: *Asthma and Rhinitis.* Boston: Blackwell Scientific Publications; 1995:1044–1056.
18. Hargreave FE, Dolovich J, O'Byrne PM, et al. The origin of airway hyper-responsiveness. *J Allergy Clin Immunol* 1986;78:825–832.
19. Lemanske RF Jr, MA K. The assessment of autonomic nervous system function. In: Spector, SL. *Provocative Challenge Procedures: Background and Methodology.* Mount Kisco, NY: Futura Publishing Co; 1989:131–166.

20. Reihsaus E, Innis M, MacIntyre N, Liggett SB. Mutations in the gene encoding for the beta 2-adrenergic receptor in normal and asthmatic subjects. *Am J Respir Cell Mol Biol* 1993;8:334–339.
21. Brodie DH, Lotz M, Cuomo AJ, et al. Cytokines in symptomatic asthma airways. *J Allergy Clin Immunol* 1992;89:958–967.
22. Vittori E, Marini M, Fasoli A, et al. Increased expression of endothelin in bronchial epithelial cells of asthmatic patients and effect of corticosteroids. *Am Rev Respir Dis* 1992;146:1320–1325.
23. Lewis RA, Austen KF, Soberman RJ. Leukotrienes and other products of the 5-lipoxygenase pathway. Biochemistry and relation to pathobiology in human diseases. *N Engl J Med* 1990;323:645–655.
24. James DG, Kay AB. Are you TH-1 or TH-2 [editorial]? *Clin Exp Allergy* 1995;25:389–390.
25. Ricci M, Rossi O, Bertoni M, Matucci A. The importance of TH2-like cells in the pathogenesis of airway allergic inflammation. *Clin Exp Allergy* 1993;23:360–369.
26. Horwitz RJ, Busse WW. Inflammation and asthma. *Clin Chest Med* 1995;16:583–602.
27. Schatz M. Interrelationships between asthma and pregnancy: A literature review. *J Allergy Clin Immunol* 1999;103(suppl):S330–S336.
28. Schatz M. Asthma and pregnancy: Background, recommendations, and issues. Introduction to the workshop. *J Allergy Clin Immunol* 1999;103(suppl):S329.
29. Joseph CL, Ownby DR, Peterson EL, Johnson CC. Racial differences in physiologic parameters related to asthma among middle-class children. *Chest* 2000;117:1336–1344.
30. Schatz M. Asthma and pregnancy. *Lancet* 1999;353:1202–1204.
31. Schatz M, Zeigler RS. Asthma and allergy during pregnancy. In: Bierman CW, Pearlman DS, et al., eds. *Allergy, Clinical Immunology and Asthma Management in Infants, Children and Adults.* 3rd ed. Orlando, FL: WB Saunders Co; 1996:729–742.
32. Schatz M, Zeiger RS, Harden K, Hoffman CC, Chilingar L, Petitti D. The safety of asthma and allergy medications during pregnancy. *J Allergy Clin Immunol* 1997;100:301–306.
33. Cousins L. Fetal oxygenation, assessment of fetal well-being and obstetric management of the pregnant patient with asthma. *J Allergy Clin Immunol* 1999;103(suppl):S343–S349.
34. Clark SL. Shock in the pregnant patient. *Semin Perinatol* 1990;14:52–58.
35. Levinson G, Shnider SM, deLorimier AA, Steffenson JL. Effects of maternal hyperventilation on uterine blood flow and fetal oxygenation and acid-base status. *Anesthesiology* 1974;40:340–347.
36. Stenius-Aarniala BC, Hedman J, Teramo KA. Acute asthma during pregnancy. *Thorax* 1996;51:411–414.
37. Schatz M, Zeiger RS, Harden KM. The safety of inhaled beta-agonist bronchodilators during pregnancy. *J Allergy Clin Immunol* 1988;82:686–695.
38. Schatz M. Asthma treatment during pregnancy. What can be safely taken? *Drug Safety* 1997;16:342–350.
39. Schatz M, Zeiger RS. Asthma and allergy in pregnancy. *Clin Perinatol* 1997;24:407–432.
40. Rodriguez-Pinilla E, Martinez-Frias ML. Corticosteroids during pregnancy and oral clefts: A case-control study. *Teratology* 1998;58:2–5.
41. Luskin AT. An overview of the recommendations of the Working Group on Asthma and Pregnancy. National Asthma Education and Prevention Program. *J Allergy Clin Immunol* 1999;103(suppl):S350–S353.
42. Cydulka RK, Emerman CL, Schreiber D, et al. Acute asthma among pregnant women presenting to the emergency department. *Am J Respir Crit Care Med* 1999;160:887–892.
43. Goldstein RA, Paul WE, Metcalfe DD, et al. Asthma. *Ann Intern Med* 1994;121:698–708.
44. Wenzel SE. Antileukotriene drugs in the management of asthma. *JAMA* 1998;280:2068–2069.
45. Malmstrom K, Rodriguez-Gomez G, Guerra J, et al. Oral Montelukast, inhaled beclomethasone, and placebo for chronic asthma. A randomized, controlled trial. *Ann Intern Med* 1999;130:487–495.
46. Edelman JM, Turpin JA, Bronsky EA, et al. Oral montelukast compared with inhaled salmeterol to prevent exercise-induced bronchoconstriction. A randomized, double-blind trial. Exercise Study Group. *Ann Intern Med* 2000;132:97–104.
47. Drugs for asthma. *Med Lett Drugs Ther* 1999;41:5–10.

48. Drugs for asthma. *Med Lett Drugs Ther* 2000;42:19–24.
49. American College of Obstetricians and Gynecologists; American College of Allergy, Asthma and Immunology. The use of newer asthma and allergy medications during pregnancy. *Ann Allergy Asthma Immunol* 2000;84:475–480.
50. Corbridge TC, Thomas C, Hall JB. The assessment and management of adults with status asthmaticus. *Am J Respir Crit Care Med* 1995;151:1296–1316.
51. Cohen NH, Eigen H, Shaughnessy TE. Status asthmaticus. *Crit Care Clin* 1997;13:459–476.
52. Bloch H, Silverman R, Mancherje N, et al. Intravenous magnesium sulfate as an adjunct in the treatment of acute asthma. *Chest* 1995;107:1576–1581.
53. Schiermeyer RP, Finkelstein JA. Rapid infusion of magnesium sulfate obviates need for intubation in status asthmaticus. *Am J Emerg Med* 1994;12:164–166.
54. Skobeloff EM, Kim D, Spivey WH. Magnesium sulfate for the treatment of bronchospasm complicating acute bronchitis in a four-month pregnant woman. *Ann Emerg Med* 1993;22:1365–1367.
55. McLean RM. Magnesium and its therapeutic uses: A review. *Am J Med* 1994;96:63–75.
56. Frakes MA, Richardson LE II. Magnesium sulfate therapy in certain emergency conditions. *Am J Emerg Med* 1997;15:182–187.
57. Swain R, Kaplan-Machlis B. Magnesium for the next millennium. *South Med J* 1999;92:1040–1047.
58. Gluck EH, Onorato DJ, Castriotta R. Helium-oxygen mixtures in intubated patients with status asthmaticus and respiratory acidosis. *Chest* 1990;98:693–698.
59. Manthous CA, Hall JB, Caputo MA, et al. Heliox improves pulse paradoxus and peak expiratory flow in nonintubated patients with severe asthma. *Am J Respir Crit Care Med* 1995;151:310–314.
60. Schaeffer EM, Pohlman A, Morgan S, Hall JB. Oxygenation in status asthmaticus improves during ventilation with helium-oxygen. *Crit Care Med* 1999;27:2666–2670.
61. Frazen D, Gunther H, Borberg H, Wassermann K. Plasma exchange: An option for the treatment of life-threatening status asthmaticus in pregnancy [letter]. *Eur Respir J* 1999;13:938–939.
62. Rook GA, Choi JH, Bishop MJ. The effect of isoflurane, halothane, sevoflurane, and thiopental/nitrous oxide on respiratory system resistance after tracheal intubation. *Anesthesiology* 1997;86:1294–1299.
63. Echeverria M, Gelb AW, Wexler HR, et al. Enflurane and halothane in status asthmaticus. *Chest* 1986;89:152–154.
64. Johnston RG, Noseworthy TW, Friesen EG, et al. Isoflurane therapy for status asthmaticus in children and adults. *Chest* 1990;97:698–701.
65. Saulnier FF, Durocher, AV, Deturek RA, Lefèbvre MC, Wattel FE. Respiratory and hemodynamic effects of halothane in status asthmaticus. *Intensive Care Med* 1990;16:104–107.
66. Green WB Jr. The ventilatory effects of sevoflurane. *Anesth Analg* 1995;81(suppl):S23–S26.
67. Que JC, Lusaya VO. Sevoflurane induction for emergency cesarean section in a parturient in status asthmaticus. *Anesthesiology* 1999;90:1475–1460.
68. Conti G, Dellutri D, Vilardi V, et al. Propofol induces bronchodilation in mechanically ventilated chronic obstructive pulmonary disease (COPD) patients. *Acta Anaesthesiol Scand* 1993;37:105–109.
69. Clarkson K, Power CK, O'Connell F, et al. A comparative evaluation of propofol and midazolam as sedative agents in fiberoptic bronchoscopy. *Chest* 1993;104:1029–1031.
70. Dureuil B. Diprivan and asthma. *Ann Fr Anesth Reanim* 1994;13:620–622.
71. Taylor SL, Bush RK, Selner JC, et al. Sensitivity to sulfited foods among sulfite-sensitive subjects with asthma. *J Allergy Clin Immunol* 1988;81:1159–1167.
72. Bhana N, Goa KL, McClellan KJ. Dexmedetomidine. *Drugs* 2000;59:263–270.
73. Talke P, Chen R, Thomas B, et al. The hemodynamic and adrenergic effects of perioperative dexmedetomidine infusion after vascular surgery. *Anesth Analg* 2000;90:834–839.
74. Ron M, Hochner-Celnikier D, Menczel J, et al. Maternal-fetal transfer of aminophylline. *Acta Obstet Gynecol Scand* 1984;63:217–218.
75. Younker M, Clark T, Tessem J, et al. Bupivacaine-fentanyl epidural analgesia for a parturient in status asthmaticus. *Can J Anaesth* 1987;34:609–612.

76. Shanies HM, Ventakataraman MT, Peter T. Reversal of intractable acute severe asthma by first trimester termination of pregnancy. *J Asthma* 1997;34:169–172.
77. Gelber M, Sidi Y, Gassner S, et al. Uncontrollable life-threatening status asthmaticus–an indicatory for termination of pregnancy by cesarean section. *Respiration* 1984;46:320–322.
78. Boushey HA, Holtzman MJ, Shelley JM, Nadel JA. Bronchial hyperactivity. *Am Rev Respir Dis* 1980;121:389–413.
79. Bai TR. Abnormalities in airway smooth muscle in fatal asthma. *Am Rev Respir Dis* 1990;141:552–557.
80. Fishburne JJ, Brenner WE, Braaksma JT, Hendricks CH. Bronchospasm complicating intravenous prostaglandin F$_2$ alpha for therapeutic abortion. *Obstet Gynecol* 1972;39:892–896.
81. Mathé AA, Hedqvist P. Effect of prostaglandins F$_2$ alpha and E$_2$ on airway conductance in healthy subjects and asthmatic patients. *Am Rev Respir Dis* 1975;111:313–320.
82. Gal TJ. Anesthesia for the patient with reactive airway disease (review course lectures). *Anesth Analg* 2000;13–20.
83. Shnider SM. Choice of anesthesia for labor and delivery. *Obstet Gynecol* 1981;58(suppl):24S–34S.
84. Aviado DM. Regulation of bronchomotor tone during anesthesia. *Anesthesiology* 1975;42:68–80.
85. Shnider SM, Abboud TK, Artal R, et al. Maternal catecholamines decrease during labor after lumbar epidural anesthesia. *Am J Obstet Gynecol* 1983;147:13–15.
86. Húgerdal M, Morgan CW, Sumner AE, Gutsche BB. Minute ventilation and oxygen consumption during labor with epidural analgesia. *Anesthesiology* 1983;59:425–427.
87. Mallampati SR. Bronchospasm during spinal anesthesia. *Anesth Analg* 1981;60:839–840.
88. Kawabata KM. [Two cases of asthmatic attack caused by spinal anesthesia]. *Masui.* 1996;45:102–106.
89. Shnider SM, Papper EM. Anesthesia for the asthmatic patient. *Anesthesiology* 1961;22:886–892.
90. Pizov R, Brown RH, Weiss YS, et al. Wheezing during induction of general anesthesia in patients with and without asthma. A randomized, blinded trial. *Anesthesiology* 1995;82:1111–1116.
91. Eames WO, Rooke GA, Wu RS, Bishop MJ. Comparison of the effects of etomidate, propofol, and thiopental on respiratory resistance after tracheal intubation. *Anesthesiology* 1996;84:1307–1311.
92. Brown RH, Wagner EM. Mechanisms of bronchoprotection by anesthetic induction agents: Propofol versus ketamine. *Anesthesiology* 1999;90:822–828.
93. Kakinohana M, Fujimine T, Kakinohana O. [Propofol anesthesia for an emergent caesarean section in a patient with asthma]. *Masui* 1999;48:900–902.
94. Grunberg G, Cohen JD, Keslin J, Gassner S. Facilitation of mechanical ventilation in status asthmaticus with continuous intravenous thiopental. *Chest* 1991;99:1216–1219.
95. Fung DL. Emergency anesthesia for asthma patients. *Clin Rev Allergy* 1985;3:127–141.
96. Downes H, Hirshman CA. Lidocaine aerosols do not prevent allergic bronchoconstriction. *Anesth Analg* 1981;60:28–32.
97. Downes H, Hirshman CA, Leon DA. Comparison of local anesthetics as bronchodilator aerosols. *Anesthesiology* 1983;58:216–220.
98. Kirkegaard-Nielsen H, Caldwell JE, Berry PD. Rapid tracheal intubation with rocuronium: A probability approach to determining dose. *Anesthesiology* 1999;91:131–136.
99. Heier T, Caldwell JE. Rapid tracheal intubation with large-dose rocuronium: A probability-based approach. *Anesth Analg* 2000;90:175–179.
100. Levy JH, Pitts M, Thanopoulos A, et al. The effect of rapacuronium on histamine release and hemodynamics in adult patients undergoing general anesthesia. *Anesth Analog* 1999;89:290–295.
101. Caldwell JE, Lau M, Fisher DM. Atracurium versus vecuronium in asthmatic patients. A blinded, randomized comparison of adverse events. *Anesthesiology* 1995;83:986–991.
102. Vettermann J, Beck KC, Lindahl SG, Brichant JF, Rehder K. Actions of enflurane, isoflurane, vecuronium, atracurium, and pancuronium on pulmonary resistance in dogs. *Anesthesiology* 1988;69:688–695.
103. Shibata O, Kanairo M, Zhang S, et al. Anticholinesterase drugs stimulate phosphatidylinositol response in rat tracheal slices. *Anesth Analg* 1996;82:1211–1214.

104. Stirt JA, Berger JM, Ricker SM, Sullivan SF. Arrhythmogenic effects of aminophylline during halothane anesthesia in experimental animals. *Anesth Analg* 1980;59:410–416.

105. Crawford JS. Bronchospasm following ergometrine [letter]. *Anaesthesia* 1980;35:397–398.

106. Naagaya K, Fetters MD, Ishikawa M, et al. Causes of maternal mortality in Japan. *JAMA* 2000;283:2661–2667.

107. Collaborative Low-dose Aspirin Study in Pregnancy Collaborative Group (CLASP). A randomised trial of low-dose aspirin for the prevention and treatment of pre-eclampsia among 9,364 pregnant women. *Lancet* 1994;343:619–629.

108. Dumont A, Flahault A, Beaufils M, et al. Effect of aspirin in pregnant women is dependent on increase in bleeding time. *Am J Obstet Gynecol* 1999;180:135–140.

109. Scardo JA, Vermillion ST, Newman RB, et al. A randomized, double-blind, hemodynamic evaluation of nifedipine and labetalol in preeclamptic hypertensive emergencies. *Am J Obstet Gynecol* 1999;181:862–866.

110. Vermillion ST, Scardo JA, Newman RB, Chauhan SP. A randomized, double-blind trial of oral nifedipine and intravenous labetalol in hypertensive emergencies of pregnancy. *Am J Obstet Gynecol* 1999;181:858–861.

Shnider and Levinson's Anesthesia for Obstetrics,
edited by Samuel C. Hughes, et al.
Lippincott Williams & Wilkins,
Philadelphia, © 2001.

CHAPTER 28

ANESTHESIA FOR THE PREGNANT DIABETIC PATIENT

SANJAY DATTA, M.D., F.F.A.R.C.S.

Diabetes mellitus (DM) is extremely common in the general population, occurring with an incidence as high as 4.5% of all pregnancies (1) and a range of 2% to 4% (2, 3). During pregnancy, 90% of DM cases represent gestational diabetes mellitus (GDM) (3). Advances in the obstetric and anesthetic management of diabetic parturients have considerably decreased perinatal mortality for insulin-dependent diabetic mothers (2, 4). With optimal care before and during gestation, women with diabetes should have a perinatal mortality rate roughly equivalent to that observed in normal pregnancies (2). This chapter reviews the metabolic and hormonal adjustments observed in normal and diabetic pregnancies. It also reviews the maternal, fetal, and neonatal complications of diabetes during pregnancy, and modern modes of treatment.

FUEL-HORMONE BALANCE DURING PREGNANCY

Hyperplasia of the beta cells of the maternal islets of Langerhans is associated with pregnancy. Islets from pregnant animals secrete more insulin and are more sensitive to a lower dose of glucose than are islets from nonpregnant animals (5). These morphologic and secretory changes can be induced by treating animals with gestational hormones such as estrogen, progesterone, and human placental lactogen. Compared with nonpregnant controls, humans in the second half of pregnancy have higher basal plasma concentrations of immunoreactive insulin. Therefore, any glucose load produces a faster increase in insulin to higher peak plasma concentrations.

Pregnancy produces major changes in the homeostasis of all metabolic fuels. Plasma concentrations of glucose in the postabsorptive state decline as pregnancy advances, owing to increasing placental uptake of glucose and a probable limitation on hepatic output of glucose. Gluconeogenesis could be limited by a relative lack of the major substrate alanine.

Although fat deposition is accentuated in early pregnancy, later in gestation lipolysis is enhanced, and in the postabsorptive state more glycerol and free fatty acids (FFAs) are released. The lipolytic effects of human placental lactogen override the antilipolytic influence of insulin. Ketogenesis is also accentuated in the postabsorptive state during pregnancy.

During normal pregnancy, the balance of metabolic fuels also differs for the fed state. Despite associated hyperinsulinism, the disposal of glucose is impaired, producing somewhat higher maternal blood levels, perhaps to ensure maximal "feeding" of the conceptus. The antiinsulin effects of gestation have been attributed to interference of human placental lactogen, progesterone, and cortisol (6). The decay of administered insulin in plasma is not greater during pregnancy, despite the presence of placental insulin receptors and degrading enzymes. Glucagon is well suppressed by glucose during pregnancy, and the secretory response of glucagon to amino acids is not higher than levels during nonpregnancy.

METABOLIC DISORDERS IN PARTURIENTS

Deficient secretion of insulin in parturients with Type I DM (insulin-dependent DM, formerly IDDM) increases glucose concentrations in the blood after meals. In the postabsorptive state, the liver manufactures more glucose by breakdown of glycogen secondary to lack of inhibition by insulin. Concentrations of insulin-sensitive branched-chain amino acids such as leucine, isoleucine, and valine are higher in diabetic pregnant women with fasting hyperglycemia (i.e., having glucose levels higher than 105 mg $\cdot$ dL^{-1} during fasting) (3). Criteria for diagnosis of DM and GDM are listed in Table 28.1. The diagnosis of GDM is made when either of the two values are met or exceeded for fasting plasma glucose or 2-hour postprandial glucose.

Gluconeogenesis takes place largely from the mobilization of amino acids and glycerol from the muscle and fat stores, respectively. Some of the FFAs released from adipose cells can be converted in the liver to triglycerides, cholesterol, and phospholipids (7). Knopp et al. (8) found elevated plasma triglyceride levels in obese pregnant women with gestational or adult-onset diabetes. In contrast, when compared with normal parturients, patients with juvenile-onset diabetes did not differ in plasma triglyceride levels. Due to a lack of insulin in diabetic patients, increased amounts of FFAs are converted to ketone bodies, acetoacetate, and β-hydroxybutyric acid. During pregnancy, the physiologic changes of insulin resistance, increased lipolysis, and ketogenesis increase metabolic disturbances in diabetic women.

DIABETIC KETOACIDOSIS

Diabetic ketoacidosis is a major cause of perinatal morbidity. The fetal death rate can be as high as 90%. Without careful and rigorous treatment, diabetic pregnant women are at increased risk of severe hyperglycemia and ketoacidosis (9). Four factors are mainly responsible for ketoacidosis in diabetics: a relative insulin deficiency, an excess of stress hormone, a lack of food, and dehydration. Glucose accumulates in extracellular fluid because of relative insulin deficiency and excessive stress hormone. With a lack of effect of insulin on adipose cells and due to elevated catecholamine and glucagon levels, excessive amounts of FFAs are released. These increased FFAs provide increased substrate for hepatic ketogenesis. Water loss from osmotic diuresis secondary to glucosuria is excessive. Despite dehydration and hyperosmolarity, most patients with ketoacidosis can be hyponatremic. Insulin deficiency and glucagon excess exacerbate the loss of sodium in urine. Another major factor in hyponatremia is the shift of intracellular water to the extracellular space, because without adequate insulin, cells are impermeable to glucose. Urinary and gastrointestinal losses produce a marked deficit in total body potassium. The potential for hyponatremia and hypokalemia must be a major consideration when treatment is formulated.

Table 28.1. CLASSIFICATION OF DIABETES COMPLICATING PREGNANCY

Class	Onset	Fasting Plasma Glucose	2-Hour Postprandial Glucose	Therapy
A_1	Gestational	$<105 \text{ mg} \cdot \text{dL}^{-1}$	$<120 \text{ mg} \cdot \text{dL}^{-1}$	Diet
A_2	Gestational	$>105 \text{ mg} \cdot \text{dL}^{-1}$	$>120 \text{ mg} \cdot \text{dL}^{-1}$	Insulin

Class	Age of Onset	Duration (Years)	Vascular Disease	Therapy
B	>20	<10	None	Insulin
C	10–19	10–19	None	Insulin
D	<10	>20	Benign retinopathy	Insulin
F	Any	Any	Nephropathy*	Insulin
R	Any	Any	Proliferative retinopathy	Insulin
H	Any	Any	Heart	Insulin

*When diagnosed during pregnancy: 500 mg or more proteinuria per 24 hours measured before 20 weeks of gestation.
Table adapted by permission from the American College of Obstetricians and Gynecologists. *Management of Diabetes Mellitus in Pregnancy.* ACOG Technical Bulletin No. 29; May 1986.

Hypertension

The incidence of hypertension and preeclampsia is higher in diabetic parturients than in the normal population (Tables 28.2 and 28.3). Diabetic parturients with associated nephropathy and hypertension may be more prone to pulmonary edema. This is related to both low colloidal oncotic pressure and left ventricular dysfunction (10).

Stiff Joint Syndrome

Stiff joint syndrome (SJS) is a rare condition seen in patients with type I DM of long standing and consists of rapidly progressive microangiopathy; nonfamilial short stature; tight, waxy skin; and limited joint mobility or joint contractures. SJS frequently first involves the small joints of the digits and hands; therefore, the failure to approximate the palmar surfaces of the interphalangeal joints ("prayer sign") is highly correlated with SJS (Fig. 28.1). Involvement of the atlantooccipital joint may prohibit proper extension of the neck, and one might encounter difficult intubation in such a patient (11). While Hogan et al. (11) suggested that 32% of diabetic patients undergoing renal or pancreatic transplants had a difficult intubation, a more recent and much larger review by Warner et al. (12) demonstrated that only 2.1% of the patients had a difficult intubation. None of these patients with severe diabetes undergoing organ transplantation required extraordinary techniques for successful airway management.

WHITE'S CLASSIFICATION OF PREGNANT DIABETIC WOMEN

In 1949, White classified diabetic pregnant women on the basis of the duration and severity of diabetes; the classification is still used in a modified form today (see Table 28.1) (13). This system, which was used worldwide, was originally designed to predict perinatal outcome and define arbitrary management goals. Because perinatal mortality has declined dramatically in all of White's classes, this system is no longer commonly used to describe and compare populations of pregnant diabetic women. However, certain characteristics of patients in the different White classes are still pertinent. The risk of complications is minimal in GDM patients (glucose intolerance of pregnancy) or in patients whose diabetes is well controlled by diet alone. Such patients may otherwise be managed as normal pregnant women. When insulin is required in a gestational diabetic to keep fasting plasma glucose levels below $105 \text{ mg} \cdot \text{dL}^{-1}$ or 2-hour postprandial plasma glucose levels below $120 \text{ mg} \cdot \text{dL}^{-1}$, with appropriate management fetal and neonatal risk are generally equivalent to that of nongestational diabetics requiring insulin (i.e., type B or C). The most complicated and difficult pregnancies occur in women with renal, retinal, or coronary vascular disease.

The White's classification currently is used largely for describing epidemiologic data in clinical trials. Clinically, Pedersen's classification may be important to predict maternal outcome. It suggests the use of four prognostically poor signs of pregnancy related to maternal complications: diabetic ketoacidosis, preeclampsia, pyelonephritis, and maternal neglect are associated with poor outcome in pregnancy. The incidence of complications can be reduced by good metabolic control. Perinatal morbidity and mortality are affected by other maternal complications, both diabetic and nondiabetic (14).

PERINATAL MORBIDITY

Even with substantial advances in the treatment of diabetes, maternal mortality is slightly higher in diabetic parturients

Table 28.2. INCIDENCE OF PREMATURITY, HYPERTENSIVE COMPLICATIONS, AND PREMATURE DELIVERIES CAUSED BY PREECLAMPSIA IN GRAVIDAS WITH INSULIN-REQUIRING DIABETES ANTEDATING PREGNANCY

White's Class*	Prematurity (%) (<37 weeks)	Hypertensive Complications (%)	Premature Deliveries Due to Preeclampsia (%)
B	20.4	17.5	23.8
C	17.4	23.1	28.6
D	25.7	30.7	26.9
F	52.5	66.1	45.2
R	30.5	25.0	36.8
All classes combined	26.2	29.8	32.7

*All subjects grouped in White's classes (N = 420).
Modified from Greene MF, Hare JW, Krache M, et al. Prematurity among insulin-requiring diabetic gravid women. *Am J Obstet Gynecol* 1989;161:106–111.

Table 28.3. OUTCOME OF PREGNANCIES COMPLICATED BY INSULIN-DEPENDENT DIABETES COMPARED WITH NATIONAL DATA IN SWEDEN

	Type 1 Diabetes	National Data	P Value
No. of births	491	279,000	
PIH or preeclampsia (%)	20.6	5.0	<.001
Premature delivery (%)*	24.6	6.0	<.001
Cesarean section (%)	45.2	12.0	<.001
Mean birthweight (g)	3450	3430	NS
Mean gestational age (wk)	38	40	<.0001
LGA (%)	20.0	3.5	<.001
SGA (%)	1.0	2.5	<.05
Perinatal mortality (%)	3.1	0.7	<.0001
Stillbirths (%)	2.1	0.4	<.01

LGA = large for gestational age; NS = not significant; PIH = pregnancy-induced hypertension; SGA = small for gestational age.
*Gestational age less than 259 days.
Reprinted by permission from Hanson U, Pearson B. Outcome of pregnancies complicated by Type I insulin-dependent diabetes in Sweden: Acute pregnancy complications, neonatal mortality, and morbidity. *Am J Perinatol* 1993;10:330–333.

(15). Maternal infection rates are significantly higher in diabetic parturients compared with normal pregnant patients. Peripartum urogenital, respiratory, and endometrial infections occur much more frequently in parturients with type I DM (14). Ramos et al. investigated the risk of group B streptococcus colonization

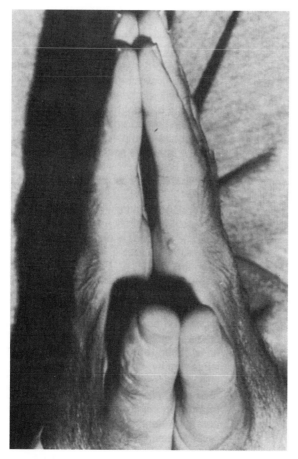

Figure 28.1. The patient is unable to approximate the palmar surfaces of the phalangeal joints, despite maximal effort (a "prayer sign"), because of diabetic stiff joint syndrome, which may also involve the atlantooccipital joint. (Reprinted by permission from Hogan K, Russy D, Springman SR. Difficult laryngoscopy and diabetes mellitus. *Anesth Analg* 1988;67:1162–1165.)

in women with DM during pregnancy (16). Women with DM had higher colonization rates, and the authors concluded that carbohydrate intolerance appeared to be an independent risk factor for group B streptococcus colonization. The authors also suggested the importance of group B streptococcus screening in this group of patients and intrapartum treatment with antibiotics. Incidences of preeclampsia are close to three times higher in type I diabetes compared with normal pregnant patients (13.6% vs. 5%) (17). The rate increases with the severity and duration of diabetes. An imbalance between the thromboxane and prostacyclin ratio has been observed in DM, which might be an important factor related to the higher incidence of preeclampsia in diabetic parturients. Some obstetricians advise the use of prophylactic low-dose aspirin therapy in DM because of the increased incidence of preeclampsia. Diabetic nephropathy can worsen during pregnancy, and long-term maternal mortality and morbidity are high in these patients. Similarly, diabetic retinopathy can deteriorate during pregnancy. Valsalva maneuvers during the second stage of labor may predispose to vitreous hemorrhage.

The leading causes of morbidity among neonates of diabetic mothers are major congenital anomalies, intrauterine fetal distress, prematurity, respiratory distress syndrome (RDS) (18), macrosomia, birth trauma, and neonatal hypoglycemia (19). With normalization of maternal glucose levels and better techniques to assess fetal well-being and maturity, congenital anomalies are the most frequent cause of perinatal mortality and morbidity in diabetic parturients (2). The incidence of congenital anomalies is up to three times higher in infants of diabetic mothers (see Table 28.4). Poor metabolic control during the period from 4 to 8 weeks of pregnancy appears to be related to a higher incidence of such anomalies (20).

Diabetes during pregnancy can affect the fetus in two extreme ways. Macrosomia has been observed to be common in diabetic parturients. The postulated mechanism is the presence of fetal hyperglycemia and hyperinsulinemia in the uncontrolled diabetic mothers. However, even with strict maternal glycemic control, the rate of macrosomia varies between 8% and 43% (21). Although the exact mechanism is not known, some authorities suggest that it may be related to the difficulty in achieving the euglycemia state in long-standing diabetic patients, as well as other factors such as maternal weight and genetic predisposition

Table 28.4. CONGENITAL MALFORMATION IN INFANTS OF DIABETIC MOTHERS

Anomaly	Ratio of Incidences	Gestational Age After Ovulation (wk)
Caudal regression	252	3
Situs invarsus	84	4
Spina bifida, hydrocephalus, or other central nervous system defect	2	4
Anencephalus	3	4
Heart anomalies	4	
Transposition of great vessels		5
Ventricular septal defect		6
Atrial septal defect		6
Anal/rectal atresia	3	6
Renal anomalies	5	
Agenesis	6	5
Cystic kidney	4	5
Ureter duplex	23	5

Adapted from Mills J, Baker L, Goldman AS. Malformations in infants of diabetic mothers occur before the seventh gestational week. Implications for treatment. *Diabetics* 1979;28:292–293; and American College of Obstetricians and Gynecologists. Technical Bulletin No. 200; November/December 1994.

for macrosomia. At the other extreme, diabetic parturients with vascular involvement or superimposed preeclampsia are at increased risk of intrauterine growth–restricted (IUGR) babies with increased rates of fetal morbidity and mortality. In addition to increased perinatal mortality, morbidity is also greater among infants born to diabetic women. Hypoglycemia, hyperbilirubinemia, and hyperglycemia occur much more frequently in infants of diabetic mothers.

MANAGEMENT
Diet and Insulin Therapy

The diet of a diabetic parturient should consist of 30 to 35 cal $\cdot$ kg^{-1} ideal body weight. Carbohydrates should comprise 40% to 50% of the total calories, the remaining calories being divided between fat and protein. Lewis et al. (22) suggested that more protein be included in the diet to keep glucose concentrations at a constant level.

The goal of insulin therapy during pregnancy is avoidance of hyperglycemia and hypoglycemic reactions. The percentage of hemoglobin A$_{1c}$ (HbA$_{1c}$), a minor variant of hemoglobin A, increases with the severity of the disease (Fig. 28.2). HbA$_{1c}$ also correlates well with mean daily capillary blood glucose levels over a few weeks during pregnancy. A sequential measurement of HbA$_{1c}$ (range 5% to 10%) will provide the physician with another indicator of long-term control (Fig. 28.3). However, because insulin dosage must frequently be adjusted during the metabolically dynamic state of pregnancy, glucose levels (in capillary blood or urine) must be ascertained several times each day. Self-monitoring of capillary blood glucose levels at home with glucose oxidase strips and portable reflectance colorimeters has proved reliable in almost all patients and provides excellent end points of therapy (see Table 28.5) (23). At the Brigham and Women's Hospital, the obstetrician's goal is to keep the average capillary blood glucose level at 100 mg $\cdot$ dL^{-1} or less during fasting, and at less than 140 mg $\cdot$ dL^{-1} at 2 hours after eating.

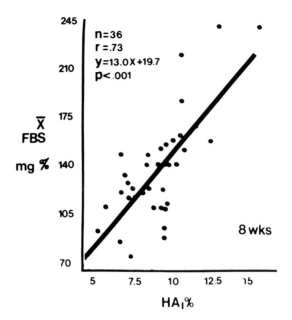

Figure 28.3. Linear regression analysis of hemoglobin A$_1$ (*HA$_1$*) from pregnant diabetic patients on mean of fasting blood sugar (*FBS*) values from prior 8 weeks. Standard error of the estimate = 26.9 mg $\cdot$ 100 mL^{-1}. (Reprinted by permission from O'Shaughnessy R, Russ J, Zuspan FP. Glycosylated hemoglobins and diabetes mellitus in pregnancy. *Am J Obstet Gynecol* 1979;135:783–790.)

Most insulin-dependent parturients require at least two injections of a 1:2 mixture of regular and intermediate-acting insulin each day to prevent fasting and postprandial hyperglycemia. Usually, two thirds of the insulin is given before breakfast, and one third before supper. Occasionally, to manage patients whose blood glucose level is difficult to control, regular insulin is given three or four times each day with one or two injections of intermediate-acting insulin. Small portable pumps for continuous infusions of regular insulin are used at some perinatal centers.

Amino acid composition varies among bovine, porcine, and human insulin. This has been speculated to be the cause of the immunogenicity of animal insulins in humans. Recently, technology has been focused on reshaping the amino acid structure of human insulin to make it more effective when administered subcutaneously, as well as to offer other important pharmacologic profiles. Insulin lispro has been approved for clinical use in the United States. This agent has some distinct clinical advantages. However, insufficient data are available at present regarding its potential teratogenic effect, and it has not been used in pregnant women. Future studies will ultimately dictate the use of this agent in pregnant patients with DM (24).

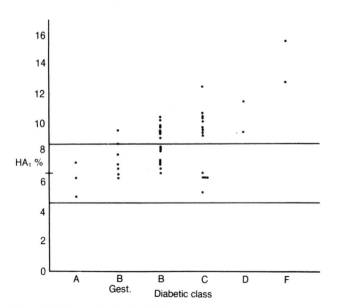

Figure 28.2. Hemoglobin A$_1$ (*HA$_1$*) measurements (n = 43) in 21 pregnant diabetic patients by diabetic class. Gestational class B includes gestational diabetics who require insulin to keep fasting blood sugar less than 100 mg $\cdot$ 100 mL^{-1}. Normal range for pregnancy is indicated (4.7% to 8.7%). Stepwise increase in HA$_1$ by class related to increases in mean blood sugar, which also increased by class. (Reprinted by permission from O'Shaughnessy R, Russ J, Zuspan FP. Glycosylated hemoglobins and diabetes mellitus in pregnancy. *Am J Obstet Gynecol* 1979;135: 783–790.)

Table 28.5. THERAPEUTIC OBJECTIVES FOR PLASMA GLUCOSE LEVELS IN PREGNANCIES COMPLICATED BY DIABETES MELLITUS

	Plasma Glucose Level
Fasting	60–90 mg $\cdot$ dL^{-1}
Before breakfast, dinner, or bedtime snack	60–105 mg $\cdot$ dL^{-1}
After meals:	
1 hour	<130–140 mg $\cdot$ dL^{-1}
2 hours	<120 mg $\cdot$ dL^{-1}
Early morning (0200–0600)	60–90 mg $\cdot$ dL^{-1}

Modified from American College of Obstetricians and Gynecologists. ACOG Technical Bulletin No. 200; November/December 1994.

Monitoring of the Fetus

In the past, the incidence of sudden intrauterine death in the third trimester of pregnancy complicated by DM was as high as 5% to 10%. Poor control of DM accompanied by ketoacidosis, preeclampsia, and diabetes-induced nephropathy were the major causes. Other factors included a combination of relative fetal hypoxia and hyperglycemia, severe hypoglycemia, and fetal myocardial dysfunction.

More recent technologic advances have allowed the early detection of fetal distress, facilitating the prevention of stillbirths. For example, ultrasound quantitates fetal activity patterns. Formerly, measurement of estriol levels in maternal urine and serum was an important diagnostic tool because estriol is produced by the placenta from aromatization of dehydroepiandrosterone sulfate. Currently, ultrasound and other examinations of fetal well-being have replaced estriol determinations.

Ultrasonography to evaluate fetal growth, estimate weight, and detect hydramnios and malformations has proven extremely valuable. Fetal echocardiography at 20 to 22 weeks of gestation may be useful in diagnosing cardiac anomalies. In the third trimester, biophysical surveillance (see Chapter 35) can be used as indicated, and will vary with the extent of the disease and the degree of control.

Timing and Route of Delivery

Unless risks to the mother and fetus make it impossible, delivery should not be induced until the 38th week of gestation to reduce neonatal morbidity from preterm deliveries. Before delivery is induced, fetal lung maturity should be determined by amniotic fluid assay (Fig. 28.4) (see Chapter 35).

The route of delivery is determined by several factors. Bernstein and Catalano examined factors contributing to the risk of cesarean section in parturients with GDM (25). In this study, infant birth weight was not different among the vaginal delivery and cesarean section groups (3374 ± 559 g vs. 3520 ± 456 g).

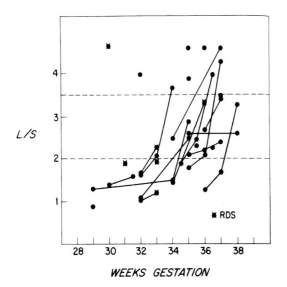

Figure 28.4. Lecithin-sphingomyelin (*L/S*) values obtained at amniocentesis in pregnant women with diabetic nephropathy. Values representing sequential samples in the same patient are connected with *solid lines*. *Dotted line* at 2 indicates usual level of predicted fetal lung maturity for infants of nondiabetic mothers. *Dotted line* at 3.5 indicates levels used to predict low risk of severe respiratory distress syndrome in insulin-dependent diabetes mellitus. Amniotic fluid sample with an L/S value of 4.5 at 30 weeks was obtained after treatment of gravida with dexamethasone. (Reprinted by permission from Kitzmiller JL, Aiello LM, Kaldany A, Younger MD. Diabetic vascular disease complicating pregnancy. *Clin Obstet Gynecol* 1981;24:112.)

However, the factors that were significant for the cesarean section group were (a) nulliparity, (b) maternal pregravid body mass index, (c) fetal position at delivery, and (d) all estimates of neonatal body fat. The authors concluded that increased newborn fat was associated independently with the rate of cesarean section. Of interest, the authors did not observe epidural analgesia as a contributing factor to the need for cesarean section.

Sonographic studies can diagnose macrosomia (if present) and give the obstetrician the choice of elective cesarean section to avoid the chance of a shoulder dystocia with a vaginal delivery, although this is controversial. While Conway and Langer (26) found the rate of shoulder dystocia with elective cesarean delivery was reduced from 2.2% to 0.7%, this has not been a consistent finding (27, 28).

Diabetes and Preterm Labor

Beta-Adrenergic drugs such as salbutamol (29), terbutaline, and ritodrine (30) are used in more routine patients to arrest preterm labor. These drugs can cause hyperglycemia and, subsequently, metabolic acidosis as a result of increased lactate and ketones. Thus, magnesium sulfate is the preferred intravenous tocolytic agent for women with DM. Corticosteroids are also used to accelerate lung maturation in preterm babies. In diabetic subjects, these drugs also possess a potent hyperglycemic effect (31). As a result, severely uncontrolled diabetes can occur within a few hours of starting treatment, leading to a substantial increase in insulin requirement. Therefore, corticosteroids should be used carefully. An increase in serum glucose is best prevented by continuous intravenous infusion of low doses of regular insulin and frequent glucose monitoring.

Glucose and Insulin Therapy During Labor or Before Cesarean Section

Tight control of diabetes in the intrapartum period is essential. Maternal hypoglycemia may interfere with the progress of labor, whereas hyperglycemia may increase fetal distress.

Glucose crosses the placenta by facilitated diffusion. Oakley et al. (32) reported that the difference in maternal and fetal blood glucose levels was approximately 20 mg·dL^{-1} or less when maternal blood glucose levels were within the physiologic range. In one study, when the maternal glucose level exceeded 300 mg·dL^{-1}, the fetal blood glucose level plateaued at 150 to 200 mg·dL^{-1}. In another study, there did not seem to be an upper limit on placental glucose transfer.

Disturbed glucose homeostasis during labor can result in neonatal hypoglycemia. Light et al. (33) observed a direct correlation between the rate of disappearance of glucose in infants of diabetic mothers (and ultimate neonatal hypoglycemia) and the concentration of glucose in umbilical cord blood. This relationship has been attributed to maternal hyperglycemia producing fetal hyperglycemia and consequently fetal hyperinsulinemia.

Lactate concentrations increase in the plasma of the fetus when glucose or fructose levels are high in pregnant women (34) or animals (35). Shelley (36) observed an increased accumulation of lactate in fetal lambs during hyperglycemia and hypoxia, and Bassett and Madill (37) confirmed these results. However, hyperglycemia did not appear to be harmful to well-oxygenated fetuses. Robillard et al. (38) compared fetal blood gases, pH, and plasma lactate concentrations at different levels of hyperglycemia in well-oxygenated sheep fetuses. Plasma lactate concentration increased, pH decreased (from 7.38 to 7.32), and blood gases were stable in the fetus when fetal plasma glucose concentrations were over 150 mg·dL^{-1}. However, severe metabolic acidosis and concomitant decreases in blood gases and pH (from 7.38 to 7.18) occurred when fetal plasma glucose concentrations were over 300 mg·dL^{-1}. Acute hyperglycemia may accentuate metabolic acidosis secondary to acute hypoxia.

During labor and delivery, glucose control is usually managed by intravenous delivery of insulin. West and Lowy (39) described low-dose intravenous infusion of insulin and glucose during labor. Parturients were given a normal dose of insulin the day before delivery, and thereafter food was withheld after 10 P.M. The next morning, the patients were given 1 L 5% dextrose every 6 hours together with Actrapid insulin, usually 1 to 2 $U \cdot h^{-1}$. The insulin infusion was adjusted to keep the blood glucose concentrations between 90 and 125 $mg \cdot dL^{-1}$. None of the neonates became hypoglycemic.

Additionally, Soler and Malins (40) achieved good metabolic control of diabetic mothers and their babies by administering a standard dose of intermediate-acting insulin (i.e., 24 U for those requiring more than 60 $U \cdot h^{-1}$ in the third trimester, and 16 U for those requiring less). During labor, Soler and Malins infused 200 mL 5% dextrose (10 g glucose) hourly. This regimen was very successful if the blood glucose level during fasting on the day of induction of labor was less than 100 mg/dL. If the blood glucose level was higher, they recommended an intravenous infusion of insulin during labor.

Brudenell (41) reported a higher incidence of fetal distress when mothers were given a subcutaneous injection of insulin (21%) instead of an intravenous infusion of insulin (4%). In their technical bulletin, the American College of Obstetricians and Gynecologists describes a recommended technique for low-dose, constant insulin infusion for the intrapartum period (see Table 28.6).

The author's protocol for administering insulin during labor varies according to the fasting blood glucose level. If such levels are less than 120 $mg \cdot dL^{-1}$, intermediate-acting insulin is administered in one third the daily dose given during pregnancy, and capillary blood glucose levels are measured every 1 to 2 hours during labor. If capillary blood glucose levels exceed 120 $mg \cdot dL^{-1}$ during labor, an intravenous infusion of 0.5 to 2 $U \cdot h^{-1}$ regular insulin is added. If the original fasting blood glucose levels are higher than 120 $mg \cdot dL^{-1}$, an intravenous infusion of insulin is used from the very beginning. In diabetic parturients, surprisingly little insulin is required to keep blood glucose levels almost normal during labor. If cesarean section is scheduled early in the morning, no insulin is given until after surgery. However, if abdominal delivery is planned later in the day, this author follows the same protocol as for labor.

Anesthetic Considerations

Optimal anesthetic management of diabetic parturients requires an understanding of specific pathophysiologic changes that occur in such patients.

ALTERED UTEROPLACENTAL BLOOD FLOW

Placental abnormalities are associated with even mild, well-controlled GDM in the mother (42). Nylund et al. (43) compared the uteroplacental blood flow index in the last trimester of pregnancy for 26 women with DM with that for 41 healthy control parturients. After injecting indium-113m intravenously, these investigators recorded the radiation over the placenta with a computer-linked gamma camera. Uteroplacental blood flow was decreased 35% to 45% in diabetic parturients. Also, the index tended to be further impaired in those patients with higher blood glucose values. However, the reduction in the blood flow index in GDM did not differ statistically from that in severe DM. This result substantiated the ultrastructural study of the placenta by Jones and Fox (42), who observed identical placental abnormalities in women with well-controlled diabetes and in parturients with long-standing, moderately controlled disease. Bjork and Persson (44) observed that the placenta of diabetic patients was denser because the villi were enlarged. These enlarged villi can reduce the uteroplacental blood flow by reducing the intervillous space. Such changes in placental perfusion cause the infants of diabetic parturients to be more vulnerable to reduced placental blood flow.

Doppler ultrasonography is used to determine the uteroplacental blood flow. Reece et al. observed the fetal umbilical artery blood flow with Doppler studies in 56 pregnant diabetics; 14 of these patients had associated vascular complications (45). The mean Doppler values decreased uteroplacental blood flow in diabetic patients with vasculopathy compared to nondiabetic control parturients. Systolic/diastolic (S/D) ratio at the third trimester was greater than 30 in about 50% of patients with vasculopathy. The authors observed a tendency toward worse outcomes with S/D ratio approaching 40. There was also a significant increase in Doppler indices in the presence of maternal vasculopathy with associated hypertension and deteriorating renal insufficiency. Intrauterine growth restriction and neonatal metabolic complications were also associated with decreased umbilical artery blood flow. Interestingly, the authors did not observe any correlation between Doppler indices and glucose values. They speculated that Doppler velocity studies may be clinically important to determine the presence of decreased uteroplacental blood flow.

IMPAIRMENT OF OXYGEN TRANSPORT

HbA_{1c} is two to three times higher in insulin-treated diabetics than in patients without diabetes (46). In HbA_{1c}, glucose has entered the internal cavity of hemoglobin, and as glucose becomes covalently bound to two beta-chains, the approximation of the H helices to each other is prevented. This movement is a normal allosteric response of the hemoglobin molecule for oxygen loading. In contrast to hemoglobin A, the oxygen affinity of HbA_{1c} is little affected by the in vitro addition of 2,3-diphosphoglycerate (2,3-DPG). No effect occurs because the binding of 2,3-DPG to hemoglobin is impaired by the presence of a hexose on the NH_2-terminal residues of HbA_{1c} (47). Madsen and Ditzel (48) observed that red blood cell oxygen transport, saturation, and oxygen tension are impaired in patients with Type IDM (Figs. 28.5 and 28.6). In poorly regulated patients in whom

---

Table 28.6. LOW-DOSAGE CONSTANT INSULIN INFUSION FOR INTRAPARTUM MATERNAL GLYCEMIC MANAGEMENT

1. Withhold a.m. insulin injection
2. Start glucose infusion (5% dextrose in water) at 125 $mL \cdot h^{-1}$ (6.25 g glucose/h)
3. Begin infusion of regular insulin at 0.5 $U \cdot h^{-1}$ (Dilution is 25 U regular insulin in 250 mL normal saline with 25 mL flushed through the IV tubing)
4. Monitor maternal glucose levels every 1–2 hours
5. Adjust insulin infusion

Plasma Capillary Glucose ($mg \cdot dL^{-1}$)	Infusion Rate ($U \cdot h^{-1}$)	Fluids (125 $mL \cdot h^{-1}$)
< 80	Insulin off	5% D/LR
80–100	0.5	5% D/LR
101–140	1.0	5% D/LR
141–180	1.5	Normal saline
181–220	2.0	Normal saline
> 220	2.5	Normal saline

Modified from American College of Obstetricians and Gynecologists. ACOG Technical Bulletin No. 200; November/December 1994, and Moore TR. Diabetes in pregnancy. In: Creasy RK, Resnik R, eds. *Maternal-Fetal Medicine*. Philadelphia; WB Saunders; 1999:989.

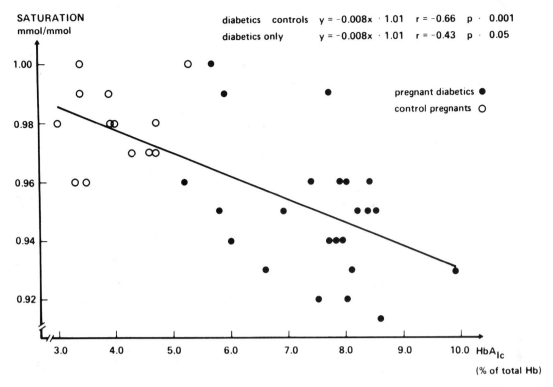

Figure 28.5. Correlation between hemoglobin A_{1c} and arterial oxygen saturation in diabetic women and in the total material. (Reprinted by permission from Madsen H, Ditzel J. Changes in red blood cell oxygen transport in diabetic pregnancy. *Am J Obstet Gynecol* 1982;143:421–424.)

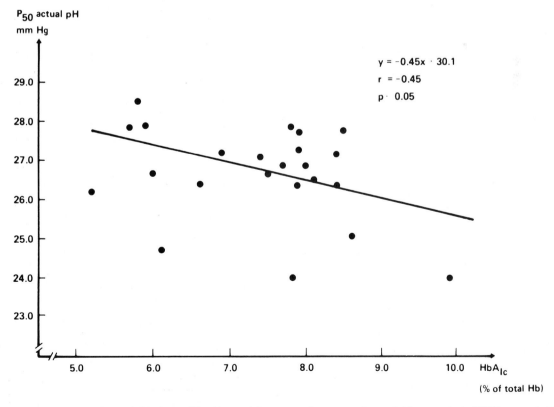

Figure 28.6. Correlation between hemoglobin A_{1c} and P_{50} (the partial pressure of oxygen at a hemoglobin saturation of 50%) at actual pH in diabetic women. (Reprinted by permission from Madsen H, Ditzel J. Changes in red blood cell oxygen transport in diabetic pregnancy. *Am J Obstet Gynecol* 1982;143:421–424.)

concentrations of HbA_{1c} are higher and concentrations of 2,3-DPG tend to be lower, oxygen release at the tissue level may be more impaired.

Another disadvantage of poorly controlled of maternal diabetes is a chronic fluctuation of fetal blood glucose. Maternal hyperglycemia will be associated with fetal hyperglycemia and subsequently may lead to fetal hypoxemia and acidosis (49).

ALTERED BUFFERING CAPACITY IN INFANTS OF DIABETIC MOTHERS

In 1981, Brouillard et al. (50) observed that the infants of diabetic mothers may have a decreased buffering capacity and a different response to an increased acid load. In these infants, the affinity of hemoglobin to oxygen increased. Values for the Po_2 at a hemoglobin saturation of 50% (P_{50}) were significantly lower in infants of diabetic mothers than in infants of nondiabetic mothers (17.9 vs. 22.6 torr). Normally, as CO_2 or fixed acid increases in the blood, oxyhemoglobin affinity decreases and O_2 is released, thereby increasing the amount of reduced hemoglobin. This reduced hemoglobin is thus available for buffering. This principle is the "Bohr effect." When CO_2 or fixed acid is decreased in the blood, oxyhemoglobin affinity increases. Thus, more hemoglobin is available for binding with O_2 because of its release of hydrogen ion. This is called the "Haldane effect." The higher intracellular pH values in infants of diabetic mothers is consistent with the fact that oxyhemoglobin affinity was also higher.

Decreased Epinephrine Responses to Hypoglycemia During Sleep

In an interesting study, Jones et al. observed the counter-regulatory-hormone responses to insulin-induced hypoglycemia in eight adolescent subjects in three sets of conditions: (a) awake during the day, (b) asleep at night, and (c) awake at night (51). They measured plasma-free insulin, epinephrine, norepinephrine, cortisol, and growth hormone during the study period. Sleep was monitored by polysomnography. In diabetics who were insulin dependent, plasma epinephrine responses to hypoglycemia were blunted during sleep (70 ± 14 pg·mL^{-1} vs. 238 ± 39 pg·mL^{-1}) compared with normals. The plasma norepinephrine concentrations also decreased during sleep; however, plasma cortisol concentrations did not increase. In conclusion, Jones et al. suggested that sleep can impair counterregulatory-hormone response to hypoglycemia in diabetic patients requiring insulin. The importance of this finding may be clinically significant while caring for the patient with DM during general anesthesia.

The multiplicity of problems associated with DM makes the infants of diabetic mothers more vulnerable to hypoxia; hence, careful anesthetic management is mandatory.

Anesthetic Management

For labor and vaginal delivery, moderate pain relief can be obtained by administering small doses of opioids in the early part of the first stage of labor. Lumbar epidural block can provide excellent pain relief for both labor and delivery. Pearson (52) noted that the fetus commenced the second stage in a less acidotic state when mothers were given epidural anesthesia than when mothers were given no anesthesia. Acidosis was metabolic in origin and was related to high lactate concentration. In 1983, Shnider et al. (53) showed that epidural anesthesia reduced the maternal endogenous catecholamines during labor, a reduction that might benefit placental perfusion. Such a benefit might be more important in diabetic parturients. Valsalva maneuvers during the second stage of labor may be contraindicated in parturients with diabetic retinopathy, because it might predispose

to vitreous hemorrhage. Epidural analgesia and anesthesia will help to avoid involuntary Valsalva maneuvers and allow for a controlled delivery. Spinal anesthesia also can be used if required at the time of delivery.

If rapid infusion of a crystalloid solution is necessary to treat hypotension, it is important to avoid dextrose-containing solutions for fluid bolus. It is important to consider that the fetus of a diabetic mother may be more susceptible to hypoxia secondary to hypotension than a fetus of a nondiabetic mother. Aggressive treatment with rapid fluid administration and vasopressors is indicated.

Anesthesia for cesarean section requires special attention for diabetic parturients. The incidence of cardiovascular depression is higher during regional anesthesia for cesarean section, and is related to higher sympathetic blockade accentuated by compression of the inferior vena cava and aorta by the uterus. Hypotension may specifically be detrimental in the presence of IUGR babies.

In 1977, Datta and Brown (54) compared spinal and general anesthesia for abdominal delivery in healthy mothers and diabetic parturients. Infants of diabetic mothers receiving spinal anesthesia were more acidotic than infants of diabetic mothers receiving general anesthesia. Acidosis appeared to be related to both maternal diabetes and maternal hypotension. Subsequently, maternal and neonatal acid-base values were also examined after epidural anesthesia was administered in this group of diabetic parturients (55). The incidence of neonatal acidosis (i.e., an umbilical artery pH value of 7.20 or less) during epidural anesthesia was 60%. Fetal acidosis was related to both the degree of maternal diabetes and the presence of maternal hypotension. The umbilical artery pH value was always greater than 7.20 when the mother was not hypotensive.

The genesis of fetal acidosis in diabetic parturients appears to be complex. The human placenta produces lactate in vitro, especially during hypoxia (56) or increased glycogen deposition, as occurs in maternal diabetes (13). The placenta of the ewe can also produce lactic acid (57). In sheep, such lactate accounts for 25% of fetal oxygen consumption, compared with 50% attributable to glucose use. Glycogen-rich placentas of diabetic parturients might contribute lactate to fetal blood during conditions of relative hypoxia, such as decreased uterine blood flow, which may occur during hypotension.

In pregnant women, elevated fetal blood glucose levels have been associated with acidosis at birth. Swanstrom and Bratteby (58) observed a significant correlation between blood glucose concentrations and base deficits in infants with low 1-minute Apgar scores. In a randomized-controlled study of maternal intravenous fluid administration (with or without dextrose) in healthy patients undergoing cesarean delivery, Kenepp et al. (59) found significantly lower umbilical artery pH values in glucose-loaded infants. Fetal lactic acidemia might occur as a result of hypoxia (secondary to maternal hypotension) in the presence of hyperglycemia after acute volume loading with solutions containing dextrose. To test this hypothesis, Kitzmiller et al. (60) noted the effect of acute hyperglycemia in monkey fetuses in response to acute maternal hypoxia. Hyperglycemic fetuses had 1) a greater reduction in arterial oxygen tension and content than did normoglycemic controls, despite similar values for maternal Pao_2 in each group, and 2) severe metabolic acidosis, compared with a modest reduction of arterial pH in normoglycemic fetuses. However, hyperglycemic monkey fetuses exposed to moderate maternal hypoxia did not have greater increases in blood lactate levels than did normoglycemic fetuses. Further investigation is necessary to determine the full nature of the interrelationship between blood glucose levels, oxygen content, and pH in pregnancies complicated by hyperglycemia. A significant risk of neonatal hypoglycemia accompanies the risk of maternal and fetal hyperglycemia when volume expansion with dextrose-containing solutions are used before cesarean section in diabetic parturients. Soler and Malins (40)

Table 28.7. COMPARISON OF ACID-BASE AND BLOOD GAS DATA IN TWO STUDIES ON SPINAL ANESTHESIA FOR CESAREAN SECTION FOR DIABETIC AND NONDIABETIC PATIENTS

	1977		1982*	
	Healthy (n = 15)	*Diabetic (n = 15)*	*Healthy (n = 10)*	*Diabetic (n = 10)*
Maternal artery[†]				
pH	7.43 ± 0.02[‡]	7.43 ± 0.01	7.42 ± 0.01	7.40 ± 0.006
Po_2 (torr)	218 ± 9	209 ± 7	200 ± 9	205 ± 8
Pco_2 (torr)	34 ± 4	33 ± 1	33 ± 2	33 ± 1
BD (mEq/L)	0.67 ± 0.68	0.86 ± 0.56	1.3 ± 0.6	2.7 ± 0.5
Umbilical vein[†]				
pH	7.34 ± 0.01	7.29 ± 0.02	7.35 ± 0.01	7.33 ± 0.01
Po_2 (torr)	37 ± 3	30 ± 2	30 ± 1	32 ± 3
Pco_2 (torr)	48 ± 2	52 ± 2	45 ± 2	48 ± 2
Umbilical artery[†]				
pH	7.28 ± 0.01	7.20 ± 0.02	7.30 ± 0.01	7.27 ± 0.01
Po_2 (torr)	18 ± 1	18 ± 2	22 ± 2	20 ± 2
Pco_2 (torr)	63 ± 2	67 ± 2	50 ± 2.5	56 ± 2
BD (mEq/L)	1.87 ± 0.73	5.67 ± 0.98	3 ± 0.7	4 ± 1
Δ Base deficit[‡]	0.58 ± 0.25	4.14 ± 1.01	1.7 ± 0.3	1.4 ± 1

BD = base deficit; Pco_2 = carbon dioxide partial pressure; Po_2 = oxygen partial pressure.
*Prehydration was accomplished with dextrose-free solution, and developing hypotension was treated immediately with ephedrine.
[†]Values are mean ± SE.
[‡]Maternal artery base deficit–umbilical artery base deficit.
Data from Datta S, Brown WU Jr. Acid-base status in diabetic mothers and their infants following general or spinal anesthesia for cesarean section. *Anesthesiology* 1977 47:272–276; and Datta S, Kitzmiller JL, Naulty JS, Ostheimer GW, Weiss JB. Acid-base status of diabetic mothers and their infants following spinal anesthesia for cesarean section. *Anesth Analg* 1982;61:662–665.

reported an incidence of over 40% in their series when the mean maternal blood glucose level at delivery was more than 130 mg·dL^{-1}.

Finally, Carson et al. (61) observed that chronic infusion of insulin directly into the sheep fetus increased fetal glucose uptake and oxidative use of glucose by the fetus and, surprisingly, reduced fetal arterial oxygen content. They speculated that hyperinsulinemia may increase oxygen consumption and that fetal hyperglycemia and hyperinsulinemia might result in reduced fetal oxygenation in pregnancies complicated by uncontrolled diabetes (61).

This author and colleagues (62) reevaluated acid-base status in 10 rigidly controlled insulin-dependent diabetic mothers and 10 healthy nondiabetic mothers undergoing spinal anesthesia for cesarean section. Dextrose-free intravenous solutions were used for volume expansion before induction of anesthesia, and hypotension was prevented in all cases by prompt treatment with ephedrine. No significant differences occurred in acid-base values between diabetic and nondiabetic mothers, or between infants of diabetic mothers and infants of control patients. Therefore, if maternal diabetes is well controlled, if dextrose-containing solutions are not used for maternal intravascular volume expansion before delivery, and if maternal hypotension is avoided, spinal anesthesia appears to be a safe technique for diabetic mothers undergoing cesarean section (Table 28.7) (62, 63).

In summary, the following criteria should be considered in the administration of anesthesia for cesarean section in diabetic patients:

1. A well-conducted spinal or epidural anesthetic can be safely administered, with particular attention to avoiding hypotension and rapid fluid administration with dextrose solutions.
2. Acute hydration should be provided by administration of a dextrose-free solution before induction of anesthesia.

Solutions containing dextrose should be administered by constant infusion pump at the rate of 5 to 7.5 g·h^{-1}, if needed.
3. Hypotension should be treated promptly with intravenous administration of ephedrine. Minor degrees of hypotension may be less well tolerated in the diabetic parturient.
4. Routine left uterine displacement should be provided from the beginning of induction of anesthesia until delivery. Uterine and placental blood flow may be decreased because of underlying DM.
5. If general anesthesia is to be used, data suggest that good neonatal outcome should be expected. The anesthesiologist should be aware of SJS and consider the possibility of difficult intubation in such patients.
6. During general anesthesia, there is a decreased epinephrine response to hypoglycemia. Maintaining glucose infusions and monitoring glucose concentrations should be considered, especially if an insulin infusion is continued or prolonged in the surgical procedure.
7. After the procedure, regular insulin can be administered as needed in small doses. Lev-Ran (64) noted a decrease in insulin requirement to zero for 1 or 2 days in 11 of 12 patients undergoing cesarean section; in 3 of these 11 patients, hypoglycemia appeared. This temporary decrease in insulin requirement was followed by a steep rise in blood glucose levels. Thus, judicious use of insulin and careful monitoring of glucose levels is essential at this stage.

REFERENCES

1. Rubin R, Altman W, Mendelson D. Health care expenditures for people with diabetes mellitus, 1992. *J Clin Endocrinol Metab* 1994;78:809A–809F.
2. American College of Obstetricians and Gynecologists. *Diabetes and Pregnancy.* ACOG Technical Bulletin No. 200, December 1994.

3. American Diabetes Association. Report of the Expert Committee on the Diagnosis and Classification of Diabetes Mellitus. *Diabetes Care* 1997;20:1183–1197.

4. Kitzmiller JL, Cloherty JP, Younger MD, et al. Diabetic pregnancy and perinatal morbidity. *Am J Obstet Gynecol* 1978;131:560–580.

5. Kitzmiller JL. The endocrine pancreas and maternal metabolism. In: Tulchinski DT, Ryan RJ, eds. *Maternal-Fetal Endocrinology*. Philadelphia: WB Saunders; 1980:58–83.

6. Malaisse WJ, Malaisse-Lagae F, Picard C, Flament-Durand J. Effects of pregnancy and chorionic growth hormone upon insulin secretion. *Endocrinology* 1969;84:41–44.

7. Kalkhoff RK, Jacobson M, Lemper D. Relative effects of progesterone, pregnancy and the augmented insulin response. *J Clin Endocrinol* 1970;31:24–28.

8. Knopp RH, Montes A, Childs M, Li JR, Mabuchi H. Metabolic adjustments in normal and diabetic pregnancy. *Clin Obstet Gynecol* 1981;24:21–49.

9. Kitzmiller JL. Diabetic ketoacidosis. *Contemp Obstet Gynecol* 1982; 20:141–168.

10. Datta S, Greene MF. The diabetic parturient. In: Datta S, ed. *Anesthetic and Obstetric Management of High Risk Pregnancy*. St Louis, Mosby Year Book; 1996:407–422.

11. Hogan K, Rusy D, Springman SR. Difficult laryngoscopy and diabetes mellitus. *Anesth Analg* 1988;67:1162–1165.

12. Warner M, Contreras M, Warner M, et al. Diabetes mellitus and difficult laryngoscopy in renal and pancreatic transplant patients. *Anesth Analg* 1998;86:516–519.

13. White P. Diabetes mellitus in pregnancy. *Clin Perinatol* 1974;1: 331–347.

14. Garner P. Type I diabetes mellitus and pregnancy. *Lancet* 1995; 346:157–161.

15. Gabbe SG, Mestman JG, Freeman RK, et al. Management and outcome of pregnancy in diabetes mellitus, classes B to R. *Am J Obstet Gynecol* 1977;129:723–732.

16. Ramos E, Gaudier FL, Hearing LR, DelValle GO, Jenkins S, Briones D. Group B streptococcus colonization in pregnant diabetic women. *Obstet Gynecol* 1997; 89:257–260.

17. Garner PR, D'Alton ME, Dudley DK, Huard P, Hardie M. Pre-eclampsia in diabetic pregnancies. *Am J Obstet Gynecol* 1990; 163:505–508.

18. Robert MF, Neff NK, Hubbell JP, Taeusch HW, Avery ME. Maternal diabetes and the respiratory distress syndrome. *N Engl J Med* 1976;294:354–360.

19. Datta S, Kitzmiller J. Anesthetic and obstetric management of diabetic pregnant women. *Clin Perinatol* 1982;9:153–166.

20. Gabbe SG. Congenital malformations in infants of diabetic mothers. *Obstet Gynecol Surv* 1977;32:125–132.

21. Campanaro J, Okun N, Stenstrom R, Garner PR. Macrosomia: The relative importance of diabetes as a predisposing factor. *Am J Obstet Gynecol* 1991;164:136–137.

22. Lewis SB, Murray WK, Wallin JD, et al. Improved glucose control in nonhospitalized pregnant diabetic patients. *Obstet Gynecol* 1976; 48:260–267.

23. Counstan DR. Recent advances in the management of diabetic pregnant women. *Clin Perinatol* 1980;7:299–311.

24. Holleman F, Hoekstra JBL. Insulin lispro. *N Engl J Med* 1997;183: 176–183.

25. Bernstein IM, Catalano PM. Examination of factors contributing to the risk of cesarean delivery in women with gestational diabetes. *Obstet Gynecol* 1994; 83:462–465.

26. Conway D, Langer O. Elective delivery for macrosomia in diabetic pregnancy [abstract]. *Am J Obstet Gynecol* 1996;174:A331.

27. Coombs C, Singh N, Khoury J. Elective induction versus spontaneous labor after sonographic diagnosis of fetal macrosomia. *Obstet Gynecol* 1993;81:492–496.

28. Adashek J, Lagrew D, Iriye B, et al. The influence of ultrasound examination at term on the rate of cesarean section. *Am J Obstet Gynecol* 1996;174:328.

29. Fredholm BB, Lunell NO, Persson B, Wager J. Actions of salbutamol in late pregnancy: Plasma cyclic AMP, insulin and C-peptide, carbohydrate and lipid metabolites in diabetic and nondiabetic women. *Diabetologia* 1978;14:235–242.

30. Steel JM, Parboosingh J. Insulin requirements in pregnant diabetics with premature labour controlled by ritodrine. *Br Med J* 1977; 1:880.

31. Watkins PJ. Diabetic control in pregnancy and labour. *J R Soc Med* 1978;71:202–204.

32. Oakley NW, Beard RW, Turner RC. Effect of sustained maternal hyperglycemia in normal and diabetic pregnancies. *Br Med J* 1972; 1:466–469.

33. Light IJ, Keenan WJ, Sutherland J. Maternal intravenous glucose administration as a cause of hypoglycemia in the infant of the diabetic mother. *Am J Obstet Gynecol* 1972;113:345–350.

34. Pearson JF, Shuttleworth R. The metabolic effects of a hypertonic fructose infusion on the mother and fetus during labor. *Am J Obstet Gynecol* 1971;111:259–265.

35. Ames AC, Cobbolds Maddock J. Lactic acidosis complicating treatment of ketosis in labour. *Br Med J* 1975;4:611–613.

36. Shelley HJ. The use of chronically catheterized foetal lambs for the foetal metabolism in combine. In: Gross RS, Dawes KW, Nathanielsz PW, eds. *Foetal and Neonatal Physiology*. St Louis: Cambridge University Press; 1973:360–381.

37. Bassett JM, Madill D. Influence of prolonged glucose infusions on plasma insulin and growth hormone concentrations of foetal lambs. *J Endocrinol* 1974;62:299–309.

38. Robillard JE, Sessions C, Kennedy RL, Smith FG Jr. Metabolic effects of constant hypertonic glucose infusion in well-oxygenated fetuses. *Am J Obstet Gynecol* 1978;130:199–203.

39. West TET, Lowy C. Control of blood glucose during labor in diabetic women with combined glucose and low dose insulin infusion. *Br Med J* 1977;1:1252–1254.

40. Soler NG, Malins JM. Diabetic pregnancy: Management of diabetes on the day of delivery. *Diabetologica* 1978;15:441–446.

41. Brudenell JM. Delivering the baby of the diabetic mother. *J R Soc Med* 1978;71:207–211.

42. Jones CJP, Fox H. Placental changes in gestational diabetes. An ultrastructural study. *Obstet Gynecol* 1976;48:274–280.

43. Nylund L, Lunell N-O, Lewander R, Persson B, Sarby B. Uteroplacental blood flow in diabetic pregnancy: Measurements with indium 113m and a computer-linked gamma camera. *Am J Obstet Gynecol* 1982;144:298–302.

44. Bjork O, Persson B. Placental changes in relation to the degree of metabolic control in diabetes mellitus. *Placenta* 1983;3: 367–378.

45. Reece EA, Hagay Z, Assimakopoulos E, et al. Diabetes mellitus in pregnancy and assessment of umbilical artery waveforms using pulsed Doppler ultrasonography. *J Ultrasound Med* 1994;13:73–80.

46. Trivelli LA, Ranney HM, Lai H-T. Hemoglobin components in patients with diabetes mellitus. *N Engl J Med* 1971;284:353–357.

47. Bunn HF, Briehl RW. The interaction of 2, 3-diphosphoglycerate with various human hemoglobin. *J Clin Invest* 1970;49:1088–1095.

48. Madsen H, Ditzel J. Changes in red blood cell oxygen transport in diabetic pregnancy. *Am J Obstet Gynecol* 1982;143:421–424.

49. Milley JR, Rosenberg AA, Phillipps AF, et al. The effect of insulin on ovine fetal oxygen extraction. *Am J Obstet Gynecol* 1984;149: 673–680.

50. Brouillard RG, Kitzmiller JL, Datta S. Buffering capacity and oxyhemoglobin affinity in infants of diabetic mothers [abstract]. *Anesthesiology* 1981;55:A318.

51. Jones TW, Porter P, Sherwin RS, et al. Decreased epinephrine responses to hypoglycemia during sleep. *N Engl J Med* 1998;338: 1657–1662.

52. Pearson JF. The effect of continuous lumbar epidural block on maternal and fetal acid-base balance during labor and at delivery. In: Doughty A, ed. *Proceedings of the Symposium on Epidural Analgesia in Obstetrics*. London: Lewis; 1972:16–30.

53. Shnider SM, Abboud T, Artal R, Henriksen EH, Stefani SJ, Levinson G. Maternal endogenous catecholamines decrease during labor after lumbar epidural anesthesia. *Am J Obstet Gynecol* 1983;147:13–15.

54. Datta S, Brown WU Jr. Acid-base status in diabetic mothers and their infants following general or spinal anesthesia for cesarean section. *Anesthesiology* 1977;47:272–276.

55. Datta S, Brown WU Jr, Ostheimer GW, Weiss JB, Alper MH. Epidural anesthesia for cesarean section in diabetic parturients: Maternal and neonatal acid base status and bupivacaine concentration. *Anesth Analg* 1981;60:574–580.

56. Gabbe SG, Demer SLM, Greep RO, Villee AC. The effects of hypoxia on placental glycogen metabolism. *Am J Obstet Gynecol* 1972; 114: 540–545.

57. Shelley JH, Bassett JM, Milner RDG. Control of carbohydrate metabolism in the fetus and newborn. *Br Med Bull* 1975;31:37–43.

58. Swanstrom S, Bratteby LE. Metabolic effects of obstetric regional analgesia and of asphyxia in the newborn infant during the first two hours after birth. *Acta Paediatr Scand* 1981;70:791–800.

59. Kenepp NB, Shelley WC, Kuman S, Gutsche BB, Gabbe S, Delivoria-Papadopoulos M. Effects on newborn of hydration with glucose in patients undergoing cesarean section with regional anaesthesia. *Lancet* 1980;1:645.

60. Kitzmiller J, Phillipe M, VonOeyen P, Datta S, Brouillard E. Hyperglycemia, hypoxia and fetal acidosis in rhesus monkeys. In: *Abstracts of Scientific Papers of the Society for Gynecologic Investigation.* St. Louis: 1981:98.

61. Carson BS, Phillips AF, Simmon MA, Battaglia FC, Meschia G. Effects of a sustained insulin infusion upon glucose uptake and oxygenation of the ovine fetus. *Pediatr Res* 1980;13:147–152.

62. Datta S, Kitzmiller JL, Naulty JS, Ostheimer GW, Weiss JB. Acid-base status of diabetic mothers and their infants following spinal anesthesia for cesarean section. *Anesth Analg* 1982;61:662–665.

63. Ramanathan S, Khoo P, Arismendy J. Perioperative maternal and neonatal acid base status and glucose metabolism in patients with insulin diabetes mellitus. *Anesth Analg* 1991;73:105–111.

64. Lev-Ran A. Sharp temporary drop in insulin requirement after cesarean section in diabetic patients. *Am J Obstet Gynecol* 1974;120:905–908.

Shnider and Levinson's Anesthesia for Obstetrics,
edited by Samuel C. Hughes, et al.
Lippincott Williams & Wilkins,
Philadelphia, © 2001.

CHAPTER 29

ANESTHESIA FOR NEUROSURGERY DURING PREGNANCY

BARBARA A. DODSON, M.A., M.D. AND MARK A. ROSEN, M.D.

With improved management of the major obstetric problems of hemorrhage, infection, and pregnancy-induced hypertension, maternal mortality has progressively declined over the past four decades. This has resulted in a relative increase in maternal deaths from nonobstetric causes. Although trauma, particularly motor vehicle accidents, continues to be the leading nonobstetric cause of death (1), neurologic diseases constitute another major source of nonobstetrical mortalities. These neurologic causes include either primary or metastatic brain tumors, acute brain injury and subarachnoid hemorrhage (SAH), either traumatic or nontraumatic in origin. Indeed, nontraumatic SAH accounts for between 5% and 12% of all maternal deaths and is the third most common nonobstetrical cause of maternal mortality (2–5). Nontraumatic causes for SAH include rupture of an intracranial aneurysm or arterioveneous malformation, pregnancy- induced hypertension, and drug abuse (6–8). In addition, other neurologic disorders, such as pseudotumor cerebri, stroke, obstetric nerve palsies, pituitary tumors, cerebral cysts or abscesses, hydrocephalus, epilepsy, or spinal cord diseases, can develop in the pregnant patient (9). This chapter will discuss the neuroanesthetic management of pregnant women. Although not all of the entities listed above will be discussed, the principles of neuroanesthetic management reviewed in this chapter are widely applicable.

INTRACRANIAL TUMORS DURING PREGNANCY

In general, the relationship between pregnancy and intracranial tumors that present with symptoms during pregnancy is probably fortuitous. There appears to be no higher incidence of primary brain tumors in pregnant women as compared to the general age-matched population (9, 10). However, pregnancy may precipitate or exacerbate clinical symptoms. Possible mechanisms for this exacerbation include acceleration of tumor growth, increase of peritumor edema secondary to the generalized water retention associated with pregnancy, engorgement of blood vessels supplying blood flow to the tumor, and the immunotolerance to foreign tissue antigens that occurs during pregnancy (9, 11). A relationship may also exist between pregnancy hormones and the rate of brain tumor growth mediated through specific intracellular receptors (10, 12, 13). Brain tumors in pregnant women have no special clinical features. Pregnancy does not alter the clinical signs, symptoms, indicators for diagnostic testing, use of corticosteroid treatment for cerebral edema or use of radiation treatment for tumors (with appropriate fetal shielding). However, clinical diagnoses of neurological conditions such as brain tumors, are frequency delayed in pregnant women because neurologic symptoms may be mistaken for those secondary to the gravid state. Nausea and vomiting may be interpreted as normal first trimester occurrences or hyperemesis of pregnancy. Headache, and/or visual changes may be mistakenly attributed to pregnancy-induced hypertension and seizures (eclampsia) (9–12, 14).

Histologically, the brain tumor most frequently encountered is glioma, usually diagnosed during the third trimester (11). However, studies suggest a possible relationship between pregnancy and two tumor types, pituitary tumors and meningiomas. Pregnancy-induced hormonal changes include increases in lactotrophs and prolactin production, and decreases in gonadotropins and growth hormone. Although the incidence of pituitary ademonas in the gravid population is similar to the general population, pregnancy-induced hormonal changes can induce an increase in the size of prolactinomas, especially microadenomas (9, 13, 15, 16). This enlargement can disclose a previously undiagnosed tumor, or cause a known pituitary tumor to become symptomatic, producing mass effects and even acute pituitary hemorrhage and infarction (pituitary apoplexy).

Patients may present with signs of a mass lesion (acute headache, nausea or vomiting, acute visual loss, etc.) and/or of hypopituitarism (hypoglycemia, hyponatremia, hypotension, anorexia, fatigue, cold intolerance, diabetes insipitus, etc.). These abnormalities need prompt recognition and treatment to avoid serious morbidity and mortality.

Posterior pituitary problems in pregnancy usually manifest as diabetes insipitus, with a pregnancy-specific variety resulting from excessive degradation of AVP by placental vasopressinase. The condition is treated with the analog desmopressin (DDAVP), which is resistant to vasopressinase (13, 16, 17). Pituitary infarction may also occur in the normal pituitary, often in association with hypovolemic-induced hypotension from peripartum hemorrhage (Sheehan's syndrome) (18). Symptoms include signs of hypopituitarism listed above, postpartum failure to lactate, ammenorrhea, and orthostatic hypotension unresponsive to volume replacement (9, 13, 16, 17). Hypopituitarism during pregnancy may also be the result of lymphocytic adenohypophysitis, an autoimmune endocrine disorder (17, 19, 20).

Meningiomas are a common form of brain tumor, usually well circumscribed, slow growing, and benign. However, tumor recurrence can be clinically significant among patients after incomplete surgical resections. Abundant literature supports a hormonal component in meningiomas. The presence of estrogen and progesterone receptors in a large proportion of human meningioma tissues is well established (12, 21). In addition, many meningiomas have receptors for epidermal growth factor (22). The reported increased growth rates of meningiomas during pregnancy supports a relationship between high progesterone concentrations and the growth of meningiomas (10, 12, 23).

With the exception of choriocarinoma, no extracranial tumors that are likely to metastasize to the brain are uniquely related to pregnancy (9, 10, 24). The incidence of choriocarinoma is one in 50,000 full-term pregnancies but one in 30 molar pregnancies. There is a high incidence of brain metastases with choriocarinomas, approximately 4% to 17% (25, 26). Although, they can occur during pregnancy, such tumors and their metastases usually present in the postpartum period or later (10). Some clinicians have suggested the surgical excision of brain metastases prior to chemotherapy, as these lesions are hemorrhagic and can form neoplastic aneurysms (9, 25–27).

No definitive guidelines presently exist as to the optimal time to perform relatively elective neurosurgery in the pregnant patient. When possible, neurosurgical intervention is usually deferred until after delivery when the maternal physiology returns to nongravid baseline and fetal risks are nonexistent. However, indications for surgery also depend on tumor location and histology. In addition, the clinical course of the tumor may be aggravated by pregnancy, necessitating surgery for improved maternal and fetal outcomes. In most cases, pregnancy may continue under close supervision until the baby is reasonably mature. Labor may be induced in suitable cases. The obstetrical management of patients with brain tumors is discussed later in this chapter.

SEIZURES AND PREGNANCY

A common presentation for neurosurgical lesions including brain tumors and arteriovenous malformations (AVMs) is seizures. The increased estrogens and chorionic gonadotropin levels of pregnancy appear to lower the seizure threshold. Indeed, seizures first appear during pregnancy in 13% of all epileptic women. Pregnant women with epilepsy constitute 0.5% of all pregnancies (28, 29). Although antiepileptic drugs (AEDs) have been implicated as the major cause of teratogenesis in infants born to mothers with epilepsy (28, 30), uncontrolled seizures are also associated with maternal and fetal risk with the attendant potential for maternal and fetal hypoxia and acidosis far outweighs the risks of AED use. Therefore, optimal seizure control during pregnancy remains an important goal (29, 31). To prevent seizures during labor, proper control should be achieved during the third trimester. Benzodiazepines or phenytoin are found to be effective for seizure cessation during labor and delivery. Specific treatment regiments are beyond the scope of this chapter. Neurologic consultation may be useful in the management of the parturient with epilepsy. Practice Parameters developed by the American Academy of Neurology Quality Standards Subcommittee have been published for the neurologic care of pregnant women with epilepsy (31). AEDs can induce both a folate deficiency and vitamin K deficiency. Therefore, all women of childbearing age who take AEDs should take folate supplementation. Vitamin K administration should be maternally administered during the last month of pregnancy and may be required in the newborn at birth to prevent hemorrhagic disease of the newborn (28, 31, 32).

PSEUDOTUMOR CEREBRI

Pseudotumor cerebri or benign intracranial hypertension is a disease in young women of childbearing age characterized by elevated intracranial pressure in the absence of structural intracranial disease, such as intracranial mass lesion or obstructive hydrocephalus. The underlying physiologic factor appears to be decreased absorption of cerebrospinal fluid (CSF). It is associated with a number of conditions including obesity, pregnancy, oral contraceptives and mild closed head injury (9, 33, 34). Symptoms are those of increased intracranial pressure, including headache, nausea and vomiting, and visual changes. Pseudotumor cerebri is generally a benign process with a high remission rate. Therapy is usually symptomatic. However, it can be associated with serious visual complications. Therefore, one of the therapeutic goals is to avoid visual loss. Patients with progressive visual loss resistant to medical therapy may require neurosurgical or ophthalmologic intervention. This includes ventricular or lumboperitoneal shunting or optic nerve sheath decompression.

STROKE AND PREGNANCY

Cerebrovascular events, both ischemic and hemorrhagic, are well-recognized neurologic complications of pregnancy. The incidence of ischemic and hemorrhagic stroke associated with pregnancy or the puerperium varies considerably in the literature with rates quoted from 5 to 210 per 100,000 deliveries and 2 to 70 per 100,000 deliveries, respectively. These stroke rates are approximately 5 to 13 times higher than in a nonpregnant woman of the same age, leading some authors to suggest that pregnancy itself is a risk factor for stroke (9, 35–38). Unfortunately, this is still the case in many medically underdeveloped countries because of higher rates of multiple pregnancies and untreated pregnancy-induced hypertension (39). However, methodological weaknesses in most of the older studies may have resulted in an overestimation of the actual incidence of pregnancy-associated stroke in developed countries. Two recent multicenter studies examining the rates in large, well-defined populations suggest a much lower rate. The first, a combined four year retrospective/prospective study by Sharshar et al., examined the records of women who suffered a cerebrovascular event during pregnancy or the first 2 weeks postpartum in the 63 maternity hospitals (348, 295 deliveries) in the Ile de France region of France, which serves a population base of 10.6 million (36). They identified 31 cases of stroke (15 cerebral infarctions and 16 intracerebral hemorrhages) for an incidence rate of 4.3 per 100,000 deliveries and 4.6 per 100,000 deliveries, respectively. The second, a two year retrospective study by Kittner et al., examined the records for all women between the ages of 15 through 44 discharged from 46 hospitals in the metropolitan Washington D.C. and central Maryland area, which serves a population base of 1.05 million women (38). They identified 32 cases of stroke in women who were pregnant or were up to 6 weeks postpartum (17 cerebral infarctions and 14 intracerebral hemorrhages) for an incidence rate of 11 per 100,000 deliveries and 9 per 100,000 deliveries, respectively. In both these studies the risk of stroke, both ischemic and hemorrhagic, was increased during the puerperium and early (6 weeks) postpartum period but not during pregnancy itself (Fig. 29.1). Physiologic changes occurring during the puerperium that may increase the risk of stroke include large decreases in blood volume, rapid changes in hormonal status, hypercoagulable state or vessel wall changes.

Some authors have suggested a possible correlation between increase rates of restroke and subsequent pregnancies. A recent retrospective study by Lamy et al. investigated the effect of pregnancy on the risk of recurrent stroke in 441 women (age 15 to 40 years) who had suffered an ischemic stroke (373 arterial and 68 venous) (40). The risk of recurrence was 1% within 1 year and 2.3% within 5 years, with the risk greatest among those women with a known cause of the initial stroke. There were 187 pregnancies after stroke in 125 women. Pregnancy did not appear to increase the risk of recurrent stroke and a history of ischemic stroke is not necessarily a contraindication to subsequent pregnancy.

Multiple etiologies have been reported for strokes during pregnancy and the puerperium (Table 29.1) (9, 38, 41). The relative frequency for the multiple causes is not well known because most studies include small patient numbers or did not include detailed etiologic investigation. However, pregnancy-induced hypertension appears to be the most common determinant associated with both nonhemorrhagic stroke and intraparenchymal hemorrhage in the pregnant and postpartum patient. Kittner et al. found pregnancy-induced hypertension was associated with 24% of cerebral infarctions and 14% of intracerebral hemorrhage in their study (Fig. 29.1) (38). The French investigators found an even higher incidence of pregnancy-induced hypertension associated strokes with rates of 47% and 44% for cerebral infarction and intracerebral hemorrhage, respectively (36). Intraparenchymal hemorrhage is a common (>40%) finding at autopsy of women dying from eclampsia (42). Hemorrhage

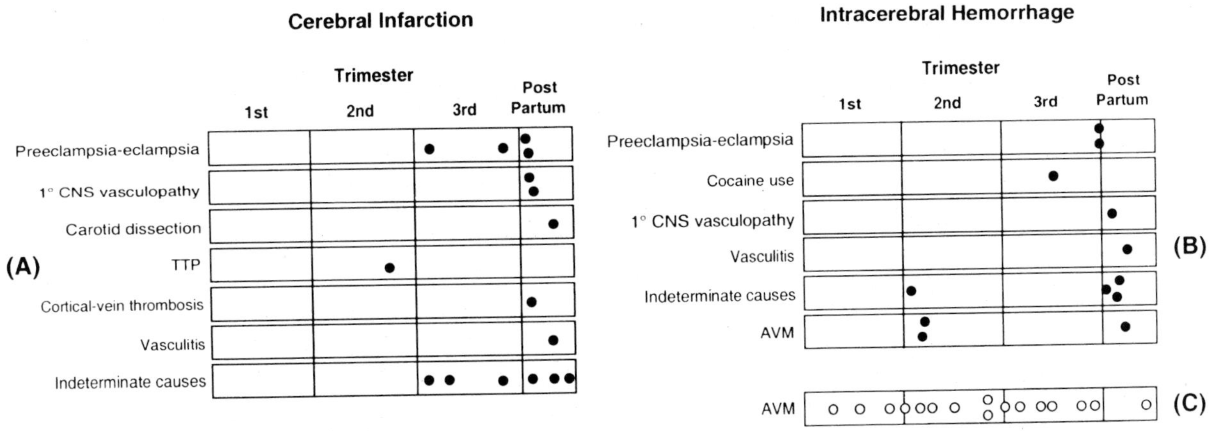

Figure 29.1. **Timing of stroke during pregnancy or postpartum, according to cause.** CNS, central nervous system; TTP, thrombotic thrombocytopenic purpuria. The closed circles represent week of occurrence for cerebral infarcts **(A)** and intracerebral hemorrhages **(B)** as reported by Kittner et al. The open circles represent the week of occurrence for AVM-related hemorrhages **(C)** as reported by Horton et al. (Adapted from Kittner SJ, Stern BJ, Feeser BR, et al. Pregnancy and the risk of stroke. *N Engl J Med* 1996;335:768–774; Horton JC, Chambers WA, Lyons SL, et al. Pregnancy and the risk of hemorrhage from cerebral arteriovenous malformations. *Neurosurgery* 1990;27:867–871, with permission.)

secondary to eclampsia is a consequence of severe hypertension with resultant vasospasm, loss of autoregulatory control and breakdown of the blood brain barrier (9, 41). Pregnancy-induced hypertension related coagulopathies may also play a role (42). Eclampsia-related intracerebral hemorrhage is associated with poor fetal and maternal outcomes (36).

SUBARACHNOID HEMORRHAGE AND PREGNANCY

Maternal intracranial hemorrhage occurs in 0.01% to 0.05% of all pregnancies. Although rare, subarachnoid hemorrhage (SAH) accounts for between 5% and 12% of all maternal deaths and is the third most common nonobstetrical cause of maternal death (2–5). With SAH, the extravasation of blood into the closed intracranial space can increase intracranial pressure (ICP), producing symptoms ranging from headache and drowsiness to coma, rapid brain displacement, and death, depending on the severity of the hemorrhage. The hemorrhage may remain subarachnoid or blood may dissect into brain parenchyma, resulting in focal neurologic deficits. The blood and its breakdown products irritate the meninges, parenchyma, and blood vessels. Meningeal irritation causes headache and sterile meningitis, which can lead to subacute or chronic-communicating hydrocephalus. Brain irritation can evoke adverse descending autonomic discharges, causing hypertension, cardiac arrhythmias, and electrolyte and water disturbances. Delayed cerebral ischemia or vasospasm, caused in part by the breakdown products of extravasated blood, can lead to ischemia or infarction, resulting in neurologic deficits.

There are multiple etiologies for SAH and include trauma, AVMs, intracranial aneurysms, eclampsia, vasculitis, choriocarcinoma and cerebral venous thrombosis (Table 29.1). The most common, nonpregnancy-related causes are ruptured intracranial arterial aneurysms and AVMs (2, 9, 37, 41).

Intracranial Aneurysms

Intracranial aneurysms are congenital or acquired lesions arising from a structural defect in the muscularis and/or media of the arterial wall. They most frequently occur at the apices of bifurcation in the cerebral arterial vessels with approximately 85% occurring in the anterior circulation (Fig. 29.2). The resulting aneurysms are usually less than 1 cm in diameter but can be as large as 5 cm. Autopsy specimens from women of reproductive age reveal a 0.5% to 1.0% incidence of unruptured saccular

aneurysms (43). The most common clinical presentation is that of SAH, including severe headache, nausea, vomiting and/or loss of consciousness. Although rupture can occur at rest, there is frequently a history of elevated blood pressure, either chronic or secondary to physical exertion, valsalva maneuver or drug abuse (44, 45). Despite recent advances in neurosurgical care, aneurysmal rupture still carries a very high morbidity and mortality (44). Approximately 35% to 50% of all patients will die from an initial bleed, 17% prior to reaching neurosurgical care. The natural history of aneurysms is malevolent with >50% incidence of re-rupture within the first 6 months. Approximately 20% of the re-bleeds will occur within the first 2 weeks of the initial bleed, with the overall highest incidence within the first 24 hours. Re-rupture increases mortality by 25% to 60%. Outcome from ruptured intracerebral aneurysm is closely correlated to the initial clinical condition of a patient with the Hunt/Hess classification system, the most commonly used grading system for predictive purposes (Table 29.2) (46, 47).

Although re-bleed is traditionally the most feared complication of aneurysmal rupture, delayed ischemia or vasospasm remains the leading cause of disability and death in the aneurysm patients surviving to reach neurosurgical care (48–50). Approximately 20% to 35% of patients with aneurysmal SAH will develop clinical manifestations of cerebral ischemia or vasospasm, of which half will either die or be left with severe neurological deficits. To improve total outcome, neurosurgical care has become directed towards more aggressive therapy to prevent and/or treat this severe complication. This includes early surgery, the intraoperative use of temporary proximal aneurysm clips instead of induced hypotension and use of the calcium-channel blockers, particularly nimodipine (49, 51). Other post-clipping treatment modalities include hypervolemic, hypertensive therapy and cerebral angioplasty (48, 52, 53).

Arteriovenous Malformations

Cerebral AVMs belong to a group of vascular abnormalities that involve the central nervous system. This group includes capillary telangiectasias, venous malformations, cavernous angiomas and intracranial arteriovenous malformations and fistulae (54). AVMs are generally congenital in origin, arising early in fetal life during the development of primitive vasculature into arteries, veins and capillaries. Changes in arteriovenous architecture may also be induced by trauma and occlusion of branch arteries or venous sinuses (55).

Table 29.1. MAJOR CAUSES OF STROKE DURING PREGNANCY OR THE PUERPERIUM

I. Arterial ischemic strokes

Cardioembolic disorders
  Atrial fibrillation
  Bacterial and nonbacterial endocarditis
  Mital valve prolapse
  Paradoxical embolism
  Peripartum cardiomyopathy
  Prosthetic heart valves
  Rheumatic heart disease

Cerebral angiopathies
  Atherosclerosis
  Arterial dissection erythematosus, Takayasu's disease

Fibromuscular dysplasia
Postpartum cerebral angiopathy

Hematologic disorders
  Antiphospholipid antibodies
  Antithrombin II, protein C, protein S deficiency
  Disseminated intravascular coagulation
  Homocystinuria
  Sickle-cell disease
  Thrombotic thrombocytemic purpura

Other causes
  Choriocarcinoma
  Pregnancy-induced hypertension and/or eclampsia
  Embolism: air, amniotic fluid, fat
  Drug abuse
  Pituitary apoplexy (Sheehan's syndrome)

II. Cerebral venous thrombosis

Antithrombin II, protein C, protein S deficiency
Eclampsia
Homocystinuria
Paroxysmal nocturnal hemoglobinuria
Sickle-cell disease

III. Intracranial hemorrhage

Arterial aneurysm
Arterial hypertension
Arteriovenous malformation
Bacterial endocarditis
Choriocarcinoma
Cerebral venous thrombosis
Disseminated intravascular coagulation
Drug abuse

Pregnancy-induced hypertension
Hematologic disorders
Moyamoya disease

Trauma
Tumor

Causes are listed in alphabetical order.
Adapted from Mas JL, Lamy C. Stroke in pregnancy and the puerperium. *J Neurol* 1998;245:305–313.

There are four anatomical features to an AVM: the nidus, arterial feeders, arterial collaterals, and the venous outflow. The nidus is that portion of the AVM containing the plexus of thin-walled vessels, lacking normal smooth muscle and elastic laminae, which constitutes the abnormal arterial-to-venous connections (54). The vast majority (70% to 90%) of AVMs are supertentorial (Fig. 29.3). However, AVMs can also occur intracerebral, in the posterior fossa, in the dura and in or around the spinal cord. In the past, some AVMs have been referred to as cryptic. This term has been largely replaced by the designation "angiographically occult vascular malformations" (AOVMs). AOVMs constitute a group of low-flow cerebrovascular and spinovascular lesions capable of both hemorrhage and inducing seizure. There is a 4% to 10% incidence of aneurysms associated with AVMs (56–59). Aneurysms associated with AVMs are at risk for rupture before, during, and immediately after AVM treatment, both surgical and endovascular. Therefore, the coexistence of an aneurysm with an AVM should be a consideration when forming an anesthetic plan.

Most AVMs are high-flow, low-resistance shunts with mean transmural pressures 45% to 70% of the systemic mean arterial pressure (MAP). Because AVM transmural pressure is generally less than in aneurysms, rupture is usually less devastating. However, spontaneous hemorrhage still carries a significant morbidity and mortality, with reported rates ranging from 23% to 50%, and 10% to 29%, respectively, for initial hemorrhage and increases with each bleeding episode (59–62). However, these numbers may be high, reflecting combined morbidity and mortality from both AVM-related hemorrhage as well as hemorrhage from coexisting aneurysms (63).

Indications for surgery have traditionally been hemorrhage, intractable epilepsy and progressive neurological deficits. Unruptured AVMs were originally thought to be relatively benign lesions with surgical risks outweighing the natural history of the lesions. However, with an annual hemorrhage rate estimated at 2% to 4% per year, an unruptured AVM represents a cumulative threat for patients <50 years old, with a significant mortality and serious morbidity rate (approximately 0.1% to 0.3% per year and 2% to 3% per year, respectively) over a 15- to 20-year period (56, 61). Therefore, with improved surgical outcomes from the use of microsurgical and endovascular techniques as well as developments in neuroanesthesia, a more aggressive neurosurgical stance has been adopted towards the excision of unruptured AVMs (62, 64).

Interestingly, unlike aneurysms, most studies suggest little correlation between chronic or acute hypertension and spontaneous hemorrhage for AVMs (60, 65). In an analysis of 545 patients, hemorrhage occurred during sleep in 36% of the patients in comparison to <25% incidence during traditional high systemic pressure activities such as heavy lifting, straining while defecating, coitus or "emotional distress" (56, 60, 66). Szabo et al. (66) conducted a combined prospective/retrospective study and found no incidence of hemorrhage in awake patients undergoing radiosurgery for AVM obliteration despite a documented 30% increase in systemic arterial pressure during application of the stereotactic head frame. However, AVM-related hemorrhage has been reported following both amphetamine and cocaine abuse (45, 67). In any case, hypertension is a known risk factor in aneurysmal rupture. Given the high percentage of coexisting aneurysms with AVMs, hemodynamic control should be a high priority in any patient with an AVM.

Pregnancy and Risk of SAH

There is considerable debate as to whether pregnancy increases the risk for aneurysmal or AVM-related SAH. The belief that aneurysms are more prone to rupture during labor has not been confirmed. Indeed, in a retrospective study of 154 cases of verified intracranial hemorrhage during pregnancy, 90% of the ruptures occurred during pregnancy, 8% during the puerperium and only 2% occurred during delivery (Fig. 29.4) (2). As with other studies, 34% of these patients with SAH also had symptoms of pregnancy-induced hypertension. Hunt et al. estimated that with an overall 0.5% to 1% incidence of unruptured aneurysms in the general population, between 20,000 and 40,000 women deliver successfully each year in the United States despite the presence of an intracranial aneurysm (68). Indeed, there appears to be no relationship between parity and aneurysmal rupture (2). Some authors report an increased tendency for aneurysm-related SAH with increasing gestational age, suggesting a possible role for hemodynamic, hormonal or other physiologic changes of pregnancy in aneurysmal rupture (2, 41). However, recent studies have not supported a relationship between gestational age and aneurysmal rupture (36, 38). The relative paucity of first semester hemorrhages as compared to

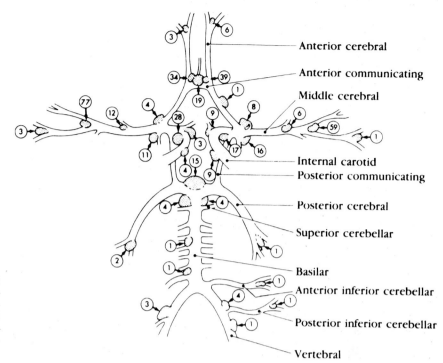

Figure 29.2. **Location of 407 aneurysms in 300 consecutive patients.** Numbers in circles represent the incidence. (From Peerless SJ. Intracranial aneurysms, neurosurgery. In: Newfield P, Cottrell JE, eds. *Handbook of neuroanesthesia: Clinical and Physiologic Essentials,* 2nd ed. Boston: Little, Brown, 1991, with permission.)

the other two trimesters may also represent unrecognized early pregnancy in SAH patients or unrecognized spontaneous abortion after hemorrhage.

The existence of a relationship between pregnancy and increased risk for AVM-related hemorrhage is quite controversial. A report frequently cited as evidence that pregnancy increases the risk of AVM rupture is a 1974 study by Robinson et al. (3). The authors retrospectively examined the records of 1,747 patients admitted with a diagnosis of SAH, aneurysm or AVM to the Regional Neurosurgical Centre in Liverpool, UK, as demonstrated by either angiography or autopsy, between 1954 and 1970. Not all patients had SAH. Of the 164 women less than 45 years old, 67 were defined as having pregnancy-associated lesions; that is, lesions diagnosed either during pregnancy or within 2 years preceding or following pregnancy. AVMs accounted for 36% (24/67) of the lesions in this subgroup, a relative rate of 4 times greater than the total group. The authors then placed the risk for AVM-related hemorrhage at 87%, suggesting an association between pregnancy and hemorrhage from an AVM. These data have been used by some physicians to warn women with AVMs to avoid or terminate pregnancies. This study has been criticized for its methodology, including its rather broad time span (i.e., pregnancy ±2 years) in defining a pregnancy-related lesion. More recent data do not support the conclusions

of Robinson et al. (4, 5, 44, 69). Incidence for first cerebral hemorrhage appears to be identical between pregnant and nonpregnant women (0.035 per person-year). Distribution of AVMs in the pregnant population follows that for the general population, with peak incidence in the 20 to 40 age group (Fig. 29.5). A possible relationship has been suggested between the hemodynamic, coagulation and endocrinological changes that usually occur

Table 29.2. HUNT/ HESS CLASSIFICATION OF ANEURYSMS

Grade 0: Unruptured
Grade 1: +/− mild headache, alert and oriented with no motor deficits
Grade 2: Moderate to severe symptoms, no deficits except cranial nerve III
Grade 3: Confused , drowsy, mild focal deficits
Grade 4: Semicomatose or comatose, with or without lateralizing signs
Grade 5: Deep coma, decerebrate rigidity, moribund

From Hunt WE, Hess RM. Surgical risk as related to time of intervention in the repair of intracranial aneurysms. *J Neurosurg* 1968;28:14–20, with permission.

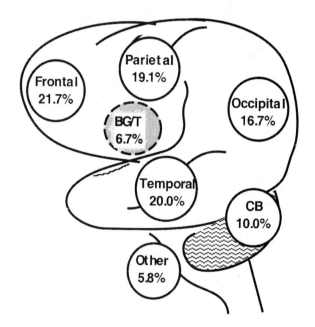

Figure 29.3. **Anatomical location of arteriovenous malformation (AVM).** The figure indicates the primary AVM location from a series of 120 consecutive patients who underwent surgical resection. In some cases, the AVM was located in more than one zone. CB, cerebellum; BG/T, basal ganglia (1.7%)/thalamus (5.0%); other, corpus callosum, intraventricular, brainstem, etc. (Adapted from Hamilton MG, Spetzler RF. The prospective application of a grading system for arteriovenous malformations. *Neurosurgery* 1994;34:2–6, with permission.)

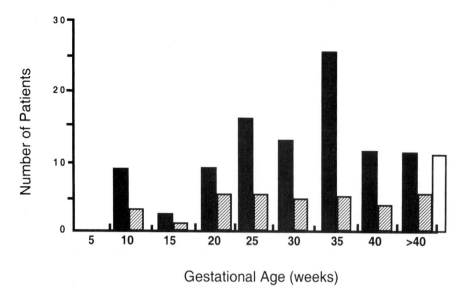

Figure 29.4. **Gestational age at first hemorrhage from aneurysm or arteriovenous malformation (AVM).** The figure shows the distribution of patients in the series report by Dias and Sekhar with respect to gestational age at the time of the initial hemorrhage for aneurysm-related hemorrhages (closed bars, $n = 103$), or an AVM hemorrhage (stippled bars, $n = 36$). The open bars represents patients with postpartum hemorrhages ($n = 11$). (Adapted from Dias MS, Sekhar LN. Intracranial hemorrhage from aneurysms and arteriovenous malformations during pregnancy and the puerperium. *Neurosurgery* 1990;27:855–866, with permission.)

between 20 weeks' gestation and 6 weeks' postpartum and an increased risk for AVM-related hemorrhage (5). However, both Horton et al (Fig. 29.1) and Dias and Sekhat (Fig. 29.4) found the incidence of AVM-related hemorrhage to be relatively-evenly distributed throughout the gestational and postpartum period (2, 4). Robinson reported a 27% risk for AVM-related re-bleed during pregnancy (3). However, this may not be statistically different from the 18% annual rate for re-hemorrhage seen in the general population presenting with an AVM-related bleed (70).

Cerebral Venous Thrombosis

As the name implies, cerebral venous thrombosis is a thrombosis of the cerebral cortical veins and venous sinuses which is frequently associated with pregnancy and the puerperium. The clot may extend into the superior sagittal or lateral sinuses. Symptoms include headache, seizure, abnormal reflexes or neurologic deficits. The incidence rate in North America and Western European ranges from 2 to 60 per 100,000 deliveries (average 10 to 20 per 100,000 deliveries). The vast majority occurs in the puerperium, ranging from 3 days to 4 weeks postpartum with 80% occurring in the second and third week postpartum (37, 41, 71). Possible etiologies include hypercoagulable state, stasis of intracerebral blood flow, and traumatic

damage to the endothelial lining of cerebral veins and sinuses during labor (72). Dehydration and infection contribute to the higher incidence in developing countries. With increasing sophistication in diagnostic techniques and the use of anticoagulation, the current mortality in developed countries is between 6% and 10% (73). The use of anticoagulants is somewhat controversial because of the potential risk of bleeding into an already hemorrhagic infarction. However, most authors believe the risk from a catastrophic intracerebral hemorrhage overcome potential problems from anticoagulation, and suggest its use in pregnancy-related cerebral venous thrombosis. Although still somewhat experimental, intraventional neuroradiology for intracranial fibrinolytic therapy provides another modality for treatment (74, 75).

Diagnosis and Treatment of Subarachnoid Hemorrhage

Neurovascular lesions sometimes can be diagnosed before rupture via a history of headaches, seizures, bruits, cranial nerve palsies, or focal neurologic deficits. However, the most common presentation is SAH. The initial symptoms are the abrupt onset of severe headache ("worst headache of my life"), photophobia, nuchal rigidity, diplopia, nausea, vomiting, vertigo, disturbances of consciousness ranging from drowsiness or confusion

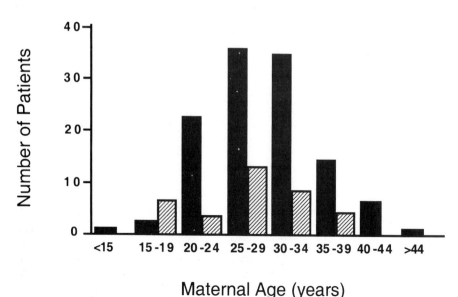

Figure 29.5. **Maternal age at time of intracranial hemorrhage during pregnancy.** The figure demonstrations the age distribution for patients presenting with an intracranial hemorrhage during pregnancy from either an aneurysmal rupture (closed bars, $n = 118$) or an AVM hemorrhage (stippled bars, $n = 36$). This distribution is similar to that for the general population with respect to age at time of initial hemorrhage. (Adapted from Dias MS, Sekhar LN. Intracranial hemorrhage from aneurysms and arteriovenous malformations during pregnancy and the puerperium. *Neurosurgery* 1990;27:855–866, with permission.)

to coma, seizures, migraines, bruits, and possibly focal or lateralizing neurologic deficits. SAH is diagnosed by history and physical examination and confirmed by computerized tomographic (CT) scanning, magnetic resonance imaging (MRI), and the appearance of grossly bloody or xanthochronic CSF obtained by lumbar puncture. Lumbar puncture should be avoided in patients with lateralizing signs or signs of increased intracranial pressure (ICP). Angiography is used to confirm the diagnosis and localize the lesion and its blood supply. Although lesions less than 1 cm may not be visible on radiographic studies, the bleeding site can often be located. Care of the fetus and parturient during radiologic procedures is discussed in more detail below.

The multiple causes for SAH must be considered in the differential diagnosis (Table 29.1). It can be particularly difficult distinguishing between symptoms of SAH and pregnancy-induced hypertension (PIH). Hypertension, proteinuria and convulsions or coma can occur with both conditions. When hypertension and proteinuria are severe and edema generalized, the diagnosis is usually PIH. Although both symptomatologies include headache, the PIH headache is typically frontal and boring (or throbbing), whereas that of SAH is explosive or bursting. In addition, epigastric pain occasionally accompanies pregnancy-induced hypertension, but not SAH. Unusually high blood pressure also occurs more frequently with pregnancy-induced hypertension, but the hemorrhage of a ruptured aneurysm of AVM may raise ICP and cause a reflex increase in blood pressure. Because these profiles are similar, early neurologic consultation is advised whenever the diagnosis is uncertain or pregnancy-induced hypertensive patients present with unusual findings.

Once the diagnosis of SAH is made, the management should be based on neurosurgical rather than obstetric considerations (2, 7, 9, 76, 77). Successful outcome of SAH requires aggressive and prompt investigation and treatment. Treatment goals for pregnant and nonpregnant patients is to preserve life, reduce disability, prevent recurrent hemorrhage, and (for the pregnant patient) preserve fetal life. The initial treatment of SAH is usually conservative including antihypertensives to blunt increases in blood pressure caused by preexisting disease, irritation from subarachnoid blood or mass effect, steroids to reduce cerebral edema and anticonvulsants to treat and/or prevent seizures.

The decision for and timing of surgical treatment for SAH will depend on its underlying cause, the site and accessibility of the lesion and the patient's overall clinical condition, with particular emphasis on neurological status. Surgery in the parturient always has associated risks to both the fetus and the mother. However, because the morbidity and mortality associated with recurrent aneurysmal bleeding is significant, surgical or endovascular management of aneurysms in the gravid patient is recommended (68, 78). Indeed, Dias and Sekhart found that surgical management of aneurysms was associated with lower maternal and fetal mortality than nontreatment (2). Craniotomy for aneurysm clipping has been successfully performed at all stages of pregnancy (68, 77, 79, 80). As with aneurysms, the decision to operate on an AVM after rupture should be neurosurgical rather than obstetrical (76). At present, no definitive guidelines exist as to the optimal time to perform elective surgery. In most neurosurgical practices, pregnant women with an unruptured AVM and those stable posthemorrhage are allowed to reach term gestation, followed by elective postpartum excision of the AVM (2–5, 76).

ANESTHETIC CONSIDERATIONS DURING INTERVENTIONAL NEURORADIOLOGY

Prior to surgery, most patients undergo neurointerventional radiological procedures. These procedure include superselective angiography, endovascular coiling of aneurysms, AVMs, and feeding vessels into tumors, angioplasty or intraarterial placement of papervine for vasospasm (6, 7). In some cases, particularly those involving aneurysms of the posterior circulation, endovascular coiling of the aneurysm may be the preferred treatment (81, 82). Use of endovascular embolization has been one of the major advances in the treatment of AVMs. Anesthetic care is frequently necessary during these procedures (83).

The neuroradiology suite itself can be a difficult environment in which to perform a safe anesthetic. It is frequently an off-site location, far from either obstetrical or anesthetic support if the need should arise. Equipment placement and patient positioning can prevent rapid airway access. Most angiography tables cannot change from the supine position. Intubation and central line placement can be easier to perform while the patient lies on a gurney that can be maneuvered into a head-down position. Also, the inability to place the angiography table into a left or right tilt can complicate initiation of left uterine displacement for a pregnant woman. Lighting levels are often low to facilitate imaging and can interfere with visual assessment of patient color and respiratory effort. These features must be considered in the formulation of any anesthetic plan. Finally, the extensive use of fluoroscopy during these procedures necessitates comprehensive radiation precautions for the mother, fetus and the anesthesiologist.

One concern frequently expressed is for potential risk of radiation-induced fetal abnormalities. Radiation effects are highly dependent upon fetal age at time of exposure (84, 85). Radiation damage can result in embryonic death during embryogenesis (first 2 weeks of pregnancy), congenital abnormalities during organogesis (weeks 2 through 7 of gestation) and growth restriction with microcephaly, restriction secondary to neuronal depletion and increase incidence of childhood cancers (week 8 until birth). Neurons are at particular risks during neuroblast proliferation and cortical migration (weeks 8 through 15) (84). However, the radiation to the abdomen and pelvis from direct cranial radiation is secondary to scatter and extremely limited, generally less than 0.1 millirad. With such an extremely small exposure, the medical benefit of neuroradiographic procedures outweigh maternal and fetal radiation risks. The interventional neuroradiologist can further limit maternal and fetal radiation exposure by abdominal shielding, limiting abdominal fluoroscopy with rapid catheter placement and modern digital imaging systems (82).

As with anesthesia for open neurosurgical procedure, the neurological status, particularly those suggestive compromised cerebral circulation or increased ICP, as well as general physical condition of the patient, must be evaluated prior to interventional neuroradiologic treatment. Endovascular procedures may be performed under monitored anesthetic care (MAC) or general anesthesia. Although the procedures are often long and can be uncomfortable, pain control is usually quite adequate with a MAC technique. The use of a MAC technique can be extremely important during embolization of eloquent (i.e., speech-related) areas, as it permits the continuous evaluation of the patient's higher neurologic functions. However, certain patients are not good candidates for a sedation-based technique. Patients must be able to follow commands since movement artifacts can make superselective angiography difficult if not impossible to perform safely. Movement blurs the fluoroscopic image and increases the risk of vessel perforation. Medical conditions such as severe arthritis, persistent cough or a history of claustrophobia may prevent a patient from lying still for these long periods. General anesthesia with controlled ventilation should be used for patients in whom hypercapnia from sedation may exacerbate ICP.

Many agents have been used for conscious sedation. Modest doses of propofol, midazolam, droperidol, fentanyl, sufentanil and alfentanil have all been used with good effect. However, patients must be closely watched for oversedation. Monitors should include those for BP, ECG, and pulse oximetry. Oxygen via nasal prongs should be administered to all patients. Nasal prongs also provide a useful port for monitoring end-tidal CO_2 via capnography. The choice of agents for the induction and maintenance of general anesthesia, as discussed in detail below, should reflect the need for hemodynamic stability, rapid emergence at the end of the procedure and the medical and neurologic requirements of the patient. Close attention must be given to blood pressure control.

Patients are often anticoagulated, usually with heparin, during endovascular procedures to prevent inappropriate thrombus formation (i.e., in response to the catheters). The goal is to have the activated clotting time (ACT) at approximately $1\frac{1}{2}$ times (normal) baseline levels. The ACT should be checked hourly to determine need for additional heparin. Protamine should be immediately available in case of need for emergent reversal of anticoagulation, such as with inadvertent vessel perforation.

Endovascular embolization procedures themselves have mortality and serious morbidity rates of 2% to 4%, and 1.3% to 22%, respectively (70, 86, 87). The most common endovascular-related complications are hemorrhage and ischemia secondary to occlusion of main-draining veins, inadvertent occlusion of normal vessels, or vessel perforation. New neurologic deficits may manifest as either ischemic deficits, such as aphasia, hemianopsia or hemiplegia, or as seizures. Patients may also exhibit signs of increased ICP secondary to hyperemic complications. Post-treatment seizures may either be new onset or a continuation of a preexisting epileptic state. Pulmonary embolism may also occur for the shunting of particulate material used in the embolization procedure into the system circulation.

The contrast medium can result in a variety of complications, including adverse reactions to the contrast medium itself. The osmotic load from the contrast dye may be sufficient to induce congestive heart failure in some patients. The contrast medium also induces an osmotic diuresis that can result in maternal hypovolemia and electrolyte abnormalities that can affect the fetus. Patients at high risk include those who are fluid restricted (either iatrogenic or from poor intake) or have undergone multiple contrast-using procedures within a short period of time. Contrast dyes can also potentially increase ICP in at-risk patients. Therefore, close attention must be given to the fluid and electrolyte status of patients undergoing embolization procedures. Extravasation of contrast material into brain parenchyma can induce seizure, requiring initiation of anticonvulsant therapy.

Acute, severe intracranial bleeding can occur during embolization procedures as a result of feeding artery perforation by a guidewire or catheter, rupture of a coexisting aneurysm or secondary to hyperemic complications (86, 87). Treatment depends upon the etiology of the bleeding. Small perforations may be treated conservatively without immediate neuroradiological or neurosurgical intervention. In many cases, the catheter itself may be used to occlude the perforation. Radiological intervention may include embolization of the vessel proximal to the site of bleeding. The outcome from emergency surgical intervention to control severe hemorrhage is grim (87). Most of these patients will die intraoperatively from exsanguination or uncontrollable cerebral hypertension. The anesthetic management of patients with vessel perforation depends on their neurologic status. After discussion with the neuroradiologists, systemic anticoagulants should be immediately reversed. Awake patients will complain almost immediately of a severe headache. Many will also have nausea. Therefore, it is important to make a cardiovascularly stable patient comfortable with antiemetics and analgesics. If an emergency craniotomy is deemed necessary, multiple large-bore IVs should be placed and a rapid transfusion device prepared.

ANESTHETIC MANAGEMENT FOR NEUROSURGERY IN THE PREGNANT PATIENT

The particular hazards of anesthesia during pregnancy stem from physiologic changes in the mother and potential adverse effects on the fetus. Hormonal secretions from the corpus luteum and the placenta and the mechanical effects of the gravid uterus induce major changes in practically every organ system. It is important to understand these changes and their implications for anesthetic management to ensure the safest possible administration of anesthesia during pregnancy. These concerns are the subject of Chapters 1 and 13.

The goals of the perioperative management of the pregnant patient with an intracranial lesion include avoiding further neurological injury from re-bleed, delayed cerebral ischemia, increased ICP and/or metabolic complications, such as diabetes insipitus, as well as maintaining overall maternal and fetal well-being. The anesthetic management of these patients requires meticulous attention to hemodynamic control as relatively minor changes could result in devastating consequences. Hypertension could result in a re-bleed in the cases of SAH. In addition, the mass effect of a tumor or SAH as well as disruption of cerebral autoregulation in many of these patients puts them at risk for cerebral ischemia. In addition, the anesthetic management must be designed as to avoid fetal asphyxia, teratogencity and induction of preterm labor.

INTRACRANIAL PRESSURE DILEMMA IN THE PREGNANT PATIENT

A major dilemma in the neuroanesthetic care of pregnant women is how to balance various treatment modalities commonly used during neurosurgery to decrease intracranial pressure or to decrease the risk of aneurysmal rupture against their potential adverse effect on maternal-fetal physiology. The issues surrounding the use of hyperventilation, diuretics and controlled hypertension are discussed in detail below. Other treatments that can help to decrease ICP include maneuvers to improve venous return such as a slight head-up position, decreasing the tidal volume, decompressing the stomach, and checking patient position to ensure adequate drainage of neck veins. Decreasing the concentration of volatile anesthetic used by substituting an agent with less effect on cerebral blood flow (CBF), such as propofol, may also help decrease ICP.

Hypocapnia/Hyperventilation

Hyperventilation is frequently used in neurosurgery to decrease elevated ICP and to facilitate surgical exposure. In patients with intact cerebral autoregulation and normal CO_2 reactivity, CBF varies linearly with $Paco_2$ values from 20 to 80 mm Hg. However, the use of hyperventilation is limited in the pregnant patient. First, pregnancy induces a compensated respiratory alkalosis resulting in a normal maternal $Paco_2$ of 32 mm Hg, with a pH of 7.40 to 7.45. This produces a leftward shift in the cerebral autoregulatory curve, thus reducing the amount of change in CBF possible with hyperventilation. Second, maternal $Paco_2$ directly affects fetal $Paco_2$. Maternal alkalosis constricts pH-sensitive umbilical vessels, decreasing umbilical blood flow. It also induces a leftward shift in the oxyhemoglobin dissociation curve, increasing the affinity of maternal hemoglobin for oxygen, thus decreasing placental transfer of oxygen to the fetal circulation. Third, hypocapnia produced by excessive positive-pressure ventilation may increase mean intrathoracic pressure, decrease venous return, and decrease cardiac output, causing a decrease in uterine blood flow. All of these mechanisms can result in fetal hypoxia and acidosis. Thus, in theory, the use of hyperventilation should be avoided. However, mild hyperventilation that decreases $Paco_2$ by 5 to 10 mm Hg is probably safe, although the fetal heart rate must be monitored for adverse effects. Fetuses with good reserves will not become acidotic in response to moderate maternal hyperventilation, but those in precarious or borderline situations may react adversely to even mild degrees of maternal hyperventilation. The use of hyperventilation should be limited in extent and duration to the minimum required, based on clinical judgment. The pregnant patient is also at increased risk for hypercapnia. In a manner analogous to chronically hyperventilated patients, with the compensated respiratory alkalosis of pregnancy, $Paco_2$ values of 40 to 45 mm Hg actually represent hypercapnia. The resultant increase in CBF can be detrimental to the patient with limited cerebral compliance, producing significant increases in ICP. Maternal hypercapnia also produces respiratory acidosis in the fetus.

Osmotic Diuretics

Mannitol an osmotic diuretic, is frequently used during neurosurgical procedures both to decrease intracranial edema by reducing cerebral intracellular water content. However, it may adversely affect the fetus by inducing maternal dehydration resulting in maternal hypotension, uterine hypoperfusion and fetal injury (88). Mannitol crosses the placenta to a variable extend and can accumulate in the fetus (89). Animal studies have shown a shift in free water from the fetus to the mother following a maternal infusion of mannitol. This can produce increased fetal osmolality and plasma sodium, decreased fetal blood volume, total body water and extracellular fluid volume, resulting in severe fetal dehydration (90–92). However, low doses of osmotic diuretic agents have been used without adverse fetal outcome (9). **Osmotic diuretics should be used with caution and at low doses ($0.25 \text{ g} \cdot \text{kg}^{-1}$) in pregnant women, recognizing potential adverse fetal effects.**

Furosemide is a loop-diuretic that also crosses the placenta and may induce dose-dependent fetal diuresis partially mediated by increases in fetal vascular pressure (93, 94). Although amniotic fluid volume increases and fetal blood volume decreases, the reduction in blood volume is small compared with the urine volume excreted (95). It has been used in the parturient without adverse maternal or fetal effects and may provide an alternate to mannitol in some procedures (96–98). In any case, *diuretics should be used with caution.* Maternal serum osmolality should be followed intraoperatively and maintained at levels less than 300 to 310 $\text{mOsm} \cdot \text{kg}^{-1}$.

Deliberate Hypotension

Deliberate or controlled hypotension has been used during resection of neurovascular lesions to reduce the risk of intraoperative rupture and hemorrhage. Indeed, intraoperative rupture increases operative mortality and serious morbidity by >25%. There are three periods of highest risk: (a) induction of anesthesia; (b) dissection of the aneurysmal sac; and (c) application of the clip. Use of short-acting beta-blockers, such as labetalol and esmolol, are quite useful in maintaining meticulous blood pressure control during the induction period. Traditionally, deliberate hypotension has been used extensively during the other two periods to reduce the pressure in the aneurysmal sac (50, 80). The most commonly used antihypertensive agents are volatile anesthetics, nitroglycerin and sodium nitroprusside.

Low concentrations of halogenated agents, such as **isoflurane** or **desflurane** are not associated with significant reductions in uterine blood flow because of concomitant decreases in uterine vascular resistance. However, high concentrations of these agents can depress myocardial contractility and produce significant hypotension, causing decreased uterine blood flow and consequently fetal asphyxia. In addition, all volatile agents will increase CBF in a dose-dependent fashion with halothane the most potent cerebral vasodilator. Low concentrations

(<0.5 MAC) of isoflurane and desflurane are usually well tolerated by patients with intact cerebral autoregulation with the dose-dependent increase in CBF offset by mild hyperventilation. But, as discussed above, hyperventilation itself may be problematic in the pregnant patient.

Sodium nitroprusside (SNP) is a potent intravenous-antihypertensive agent that rapidly crosses the placenta. Its metabolites are also problematic. SNP is degraded to cyanogen, then transformed to thiocyanate (by the liver enzyme rhodonase). Cyanogen is potentially toxic to the fetus (99). In pregnant animals given SNP, peak arterial cyanide levels appearing in the fetus are significantly higher than those in the mother. This may be due to a more rapid fetal formation of cyanide or to a slower fetal rate of detoxification and excretion. In hypertensive pregnant sheep given SNP, the hemodynamic effects of the drug compromise uterine blood flow (100). It also appears to induce a concentration-dependent reduction in fetal arterial perfusion pressure in the fetal-placental circulation (101). Although SNP has been used in the gravid patient to treat systemic and pulmonary hypertension and to induce intraoperative hypotension without adverse fetal effects (102–104), its administration should be limited to small doses for limited periods of time. If tachyphylaxis or metabolic acidosis develop or if more than $0.5 \text{ mg} \cdot \text{kg}^{-1} \cdot \text{h}^{-1}$ is infused, SNP should be promptly discontinued. Animal data suggest the co-administration of sodium thiosulfate with SNP at doses currently in use for nonpregnant patients may prevent fetal, as well as maternal, cyanide toxicity in cases that may require long-term infusion of SNP (105).

Nitroglycerin (NTG) has been successfully used as an intravenous antihypertensive agent in the parturient without adverse fetal or neonatal effects (106, 107). It is essentially nontoxic and metabolizes to glyceryl dinitrate and nitrite in the presence of glutathione. Furthermore, recent studies suggest that prenatal application of nitroglycerin to facilitate obstetric management results in nitroglycerin levels in umbilical plasma that were two to three orders of magnitude lower than that found in maternal plasma (108). NTG appears to have a relaxant effect on the uterus (109). However, in sheep, nitroglycerin infusion can cause a significant increase in maternal and fetal heart rate and a significant decrease in maternal and fetal mean arterial pressure at a dosage of 10 $\mu g \cdot \text{kg}^{-1} \cdot \text{min}^{-1}$ (110). Onset is slower than that of SNP, and more patients are resistant to its hypotensive effect. Since NTG is absorbed on many plastics, it should be infused using glass bottles and polyethylene tubing.

Potential Complications of Deliberate Hypotension

All three agents have been used successfully. There are, however, significant problems with the use of deliberate hypotension for post-SAH patients. The first problem is in determining a safe lower blood pressure limit. The commonly quoted value of mean arterial pressure (MAP) of approximately 50 mm Hg as the lower limit assumes an intact normal cerebral autoregulation, which rarely exists in post-SAH patients. Usually, there is a loss of autoregulation with cerebral perfusion pressure (CPP) passively dependent on MAP. Therefore, a decrease in MAP can lead to a decrease in CPP with subsequent cerebral ischemia, both acute and delayed (i.e., cerebral vasospasm). Other preexisting conditions, such as hypertension, renal, hepatic and/or cardiac disease, must also be considered in determining a safe lower limit. Additionally, whatever agent is used to induce hypotension, the anesthesiologist should be prepared for exaggerated hypotensive responses in neurosurgical patients receiving calcium-channel blockers and/or made relatively hypovolemic by diuretics or contrast media.

There are additional concerns in the use of deliberate hypotension in the pregnant patient. Maternal blood pressure directly affects uterine arterial blood flow such that deliberate maternal hypotension can decrease uterine blood flow enough to induce fetal asphyxia. The successful use of controlled hypotension has been reported in aneurysmal repair in the pregnant patient (79, 104, 111–113). Minielly et al. reported that transient-controlled hypotension was well tolerated in the fetus and normal fetal heart rate returned with resumption of normal maternal system pressure. They also thought that the fetus tolerated controlled hypotension better than other forms of maternal hypotension, such as hemorrhage. However, risk of fetal bradycardia increases with the institution of controlled hypotension (114, 115), and fetal death or distress (based on fetal heart rate monitoring) has also been reported from its use (99, 116, 117). The "success" reported is often measured by a living fetus or live birth with no assessment of fetal neurologic status or pediatric follow-up.

The hazard to the fetus depends on the severity and duration of the maternal hypotension. Fetal risk is directly related to uterine blood flow, which varies directly with maternal blood pressure. When uterine blood flow is reduced sufficiently, fetal asphyxia results, damaging the fetal central nervous system, heart, and lungs. In fetal monkeys who sustained asphyxia of intermediate severity and duration with consequent acidosis, permanent brain injury occurred, producing lesions similar to those of human cerebral palsy (118). Severe asphyxia produced fetal death from myocardial failure. When it is necessary to induce hypotension in pregnant patients, blood pressure reduction should be limited in depth and duration to the minimum required, based on clinical judgment. The fetal heart rate should be closely monitored because fetal tolerance will depend on fetoplacental reserve. Maternal arterial pH should be measured frequently to avoid risks of severe fetal or maternal compromise.

The trend in neurosurgery has been away from use of deliberate hypotension to the use of temporary proximal clips. As discussed above, delayed ischemia or vasospasm remains the major cause of death and disability in post-SAH patients. Temporary proximal clips reduce aneurysmal pressure and provide hemostatic control during dissection and permanent clip application while permitting normal perfusion in the majority of the cerebral circulation (50, 51, 80, 119). During periods of arterial occlusion, anesthetic techniques should focus on maximizing cerebral perfusion including $Paco_2$ in the low-normal range (30 to 35 mm Hg), and of MAP in the patient's high-normal range. Occasionally, vasopressors may be necessary to maintain adequate CPP. Usually during pregnancy, ephedrine is the vasopressor of choice (see Chapter 11). The safety of phenylephrine, a vasopressor often used during neurosurgical procedures, has not been determined under these circumstances. Modalities for brain protection may also be used during periods of temporary clipping. These include electroencephalography (EEG) burst suppression by barbiturates, propofol or etomidate, and mild intraoperative hypothermia.

BRAIN PROTECTION
Pharmacologic Agents

Barbiturates are the prototype for pharmacological agents used in brain protection. Several authors have advocated their routine, sometimes high dose (up to 2 to 5 g of thiopental) use during periods of increased risks for cerebral ischemia such as temporary aneurysm clipping (120–122). Mechanisms hypothesized for their protective properties include a reduction in cerebral activity by a barbiturate-induced decrease in cerebral metabolic oxygen consumption ($CMRO_2$), free radical scavenging, redistribution of regional cerebral blood flow, membrane stabilization and reduction in intracranial pressure (123). Although evidence has not supported their use in cases of complete global ischemia (124), animal studies and some clinical evidence suggest a protective effect during periods of focal ischemia (120, 121, 125). However, there are few prospective, randomized clinical studies and most reports are either nonrandomized comparisons to historical outcomes or anecdotal. The standard end-

point for barbiturate dosage is titration to EEG burst suppression (50, 80, 126). The use of barbiturates for burst suppression must be made on a patient-by-patient basis with the potential for neuroprotection weighed against possible barbiturate-induced complications such as hypotension and delayed anesthetic emergence. The intravenous anesthetics, etomidate and propofol, have also been proposed as neuroprotective agents during neurosurgery (127–129). Like the barbiturates, etomidate can reduce $CMRO_2$ and produce EEG burst-suppression (119). In general, animal studies have been inconclusive and further animal and clinical studies are necessary to define etomidate's role as a neuroprotective agent. There has been considerable interest in propofol as an anesthetic for neurosurgery (129, 130). Its effects on $CMRO_2$, CBF and EEG activity are similar to those seen with thiopental. In addition, its short duration of action resulting in smooth and rapid emergence makes it an attractive alternative to the barbiturates (130, 131). However, at present, barbiturates continue to be the most popular intravenous agent used in brain protection protocols.

Hypothermia

Mild hypothermia (32°C to 34°C) has become a popular technique for brain protection during craniotomy (132–134). Numerous studies suggest mild hypothermia to be superior to other modalities in decreasing the histological and biochemical sequelae of cerebral ischemic injury (133, 135). Traditionally, hypothermia is thought to provide cerebral protection by lowering $CMRO_2$. Indeed, $CMRO_2$ is decreased by 7% for each 1°C decrease in body temperature. However, more recent studies suggested other mechanisms, such excitatory amino acid antagonism, may also be involved in the protective effects of hypothermia (133, 135). Presently in most neuroanesthesia practices, passive or active intraoperative cooling of patients to 33°C to 34°C is frequently used during at-risk periods for cerebral ischemia. However, the possible benefits of mild hypothermia must be balanced against its potential deleterious effects. Hypothermia produces a temperature-dependent decrease in amplitude and increase in latency in somatosensory-evoked potential (SSEP) waveforms, complicating interpretation of intraoperative waveform changes. Mild hypothermia is also associated with increased incidence of postoperative complications including increased myocardial work from shivering, myocardial ischemia, impaired resistance to surgical wound infections and coagulopathies (132, 136). One possible intraoperative temperature-control strategy is to allow the patient to passively cool to mild hypothermia (33°C to 34°C) during opening and resection with subsequent patient rewarming to normothermia during closure. Rewarming is most easily accomplished by use of force warm air devices. In addition, fluid warmers should be used if large volumes of fluid and/or blood products are infused. Hypothermia does not appear to increase the risk of fetal morbidity (113, 116, 137–139). Although uterine vascular resistance increases and uteroplacental blood flow decreases during hypothermia, oxygen transfer is unaffected. If maternal respiratory acidosis is prevented, the gas and acid-base contents of fetal blood will parallel those of the mother (140). The fetus will also become hypothermic, and its metabolic needs will proportionately decrease (141). For example, the fetal heart rate parallels the decrease in maternal heart rate during cooling, increasing again during rewarming (137).

BLOOD AND FLUID THERAPY

Considerable debate exists over the use of crystalloids versus colloids for fluid replacement during neurosurgery. Both isotonic crystalloids and colloids do not appear to induce edema in the normal brain (142). However, disruption of the blood brain barrier increases its permeability, suggesting a possible preferential use of colloid under conditions of extensive intracranial resection (143). Fluid replacement should be sufficient to provided adequate intravascular volume and peripheral tissue perfusion as monitored by urine output, blood chemistries, central venous and/or pulmonary artery pressures. Large volumes of free water, such as from hypotonic solution, should be avoided to prevent increases in extracellular fluid which can result in cerebral edema.

Blood loss can be rapid and substantial during neurosurgical treatments of neurovascular lesions. Techniques for intraoperative blood salvaging can be useful for these cases, but of limited usefulness in cases involving malignancies (144). Neurosurgical cases require meticulous homeostasis. Even small hematomas can have catastrophic consequences, particularly infratentorial. Therefore, care should be given when using synthetic colloids such as 6% hydroxyethyl starch because of its potential for inducing a von Willebrand-like coagulopathy (maximum dose of $20 \text{ g} \cdot \text{kg}^{-1} \cdot 24 \text{ h}$) (145). Blood transfusions should not be dictated by a single hemoglobin or hematocrit "trigger" value but rather should be based on the patient's risks of developing complications from inadequate oxygenation. In general, a hemoglobin level of $8.0 \text{ g} \cdot \text{dL}^{-1}$ (hematocrit of 24% to 25%) is generally considered an appropriate threshold for transfusion in surgical patients with no risk factors for ischemia, either cerebral or cardiovascular. However, neurosurgical patients are frequently transfused to maintain hemoglobin levels of $9.0 \text{ g} \cdot \text{dL}^{-1}$ (hematocrit of 27% to 28%) to prevent large volumes of crystalloid, which may result in cerebral edema.

ANESTHETIC COURSE FOR NEUROSURGERY

Preoperative Evaluation

The preoperative anesthetic evaluation should also include a detailed neurologic examination both to establish baseline neurologic function and in planning the postoperative management of these patients. The preoperative neurological examination should focus on signs of increased ICP and focal neurological deficits (47). The Glascow Coma Scale is frequently used to quantify neurologic status (Table 29.3) (146). For patients with intracranial aneurysms, their clinical grade should be assessed according to the Hunt/Hess classification system (Table 29.2) (47). Higher grades in this system are often associated with vasospasm, increased ICP and higher surgical morbidity and mortality. Any neurologic deterioration associated with preoperative decreases in blood pressure should be noted to avoid intraoperative systemic blood pressures from falling below critical perfusion levels. Patients should be evaluated for a history of seizures. The fluid and electrolyte status of the patient should be

evaluated and corrected if necessary. Patients who have undergone preoperative angiography are particularly prone to fluid and electrolyte abnormalities secondary to contrast-induced diuresis.

Preoperative diagnostic studies should be examined for other abnormalities, such as a coexistence lesion (multiple aneurysms or AVM with coexisting aneurysm), or a midline shift suggestive of a mass effect. The location of the lesion should be ascertained preoperatively with respect to potential perioperative complications, such as extensive vascularity or cranial nerve involvement. Patients should be examined for signs and symptoms of mass effect and/or lower cranial nerve involvement. Of particular importance are cranial nerve-related symptoms such as dysarthria, dysphagia, dyspnea or history of aspiration pneumonia. Intraoperative surgical manipulation of a tumor or vascular lesion near the brain stem can result in brain stem and/or cranial nerve dysfunction. Surgical stimulation of cranial nerves V and/or X can produce intraoperative hemodynamic changes. Involvement of cranial nerves IX and/or X can result in respiratory compromise and postoperative intubation may be required for airway protection. Previous neurosurgical procedures can produce limitations in mouth opening. In particular, neurosurgical approaches require extensive resection of the temporalis muscle which can produce pseudoankylosis of the temporomanidibular joint mandible. The resulting pseudoankylosis can produce limitations in mandibular opening severe enough as to require fiberoptic intubation, blind nasotracheal intubation or tracheostomy for airway management (147, 148). Particularly at risk are patients undergoing subsequent surgery performed within 1 month of operations involving incision of the temporalis muscle. For patients with suspected airway involvement, indirect laryngoscopy and radiologic head and neck studies can be useful in planning perioperative airway management.

Electrocardiographic changes are frequently noted following SAH, occurring in 25% to 75% of all patients (149). These changes can include T wave inversion or flattening, S-T segment depression or elevation, U waves and prolonged Q-T intervals. Sinus bradycardia, premature ventricular contractions as well as more malignant tachyarryhmias can occur. The clinical significance of ECG changes following SAH is somewhat controversial. Traditionally, they were considered insignificant for patients without previous cardiac disease. However, several recent studies have demonstrated cardiac injury, as measured by echocardiographic changes and elevated cardiac enzymes and tropinin levels following SAH (150–153). It is thought that SAH induces cardiac injury by producing a "stunned myocardium." This is a term first coined by Braumwauld and is thought to represent the effect of intense sympathetic outpouring following hypothalamic stimulation by SAH (154). This outpouring can lead to both vasoconstriction of the coronary arteries and a direct cardiotoxic effect by norepinephrine on the myocardium (myocytolysis). Cardiogenic changes induced by SAH can include pulmonary edema, regional wall motion abnormalities and decrease ejection fractions in the absence of previous cardiovascular disease. The degree of cardiac changes appears to correlate with severity of neurological injuries (151).

Patient positioning during surgery should also be considered during the preoperative assessment. The patient should be questioned about any preexisting conditions, such as arthritis, limitations for neck movement (i.e., cervical radiculopathy, history of carotid bruit, etc.) that may complicate positioning. Ideally, after the beginning of the second trimester, gravid patients should not be placed supine or prone when transported to surgery or positioned on the surgical table. If placed supine, left uterine displacement should be used. Proper positioning will minimize the risk of obstruction of the vena cava by removing the weight of the gravid uterus from the great vessels. The patient's legs should be wrapped in elastic bandages and placed level to her heart to facilitate venous return from the lower extremities and to prevent possible deep vein thrombosis formation.

Table 29.3. GLASGOW COMA SCALE

Category	Response	Score
Eye opening	None	1
	To pain	2
	To voice	3
	Spontaneously	4
Verbal	None	1
	Incomprehensible	2
	Garbled words	3
	Confused speech	4
	Oriented speech	5
Motor	Flaccid	1
	Abnormal extension	2
	Abnormal flexion	3
	Normal flexion	4
	Localizing pain	5
	Follow commands	6

From Teasdale G, Jennett B. Assessment of coma and impaired consciousness. A practical scale. *Lancet* 1974;2:81–84, with permission.

Premedication should be tailored to reflect the patient's medical and neurologic status. Special efforts should be made to decrease the patient's apprehension by providing reassurance and emotional support. Maternal stress and anxiety are associated with an increased release of endogenous catecholamines that decreases uterine blood flow, potentially harming the fetus. Care must be taken to avoid oversedation leading to hypercarbia in patients at-risk for increased ICP. Preoperative sedation may be omitted in many cases, with increased safety for the patient. If possible, patients should be given medication to reduce gastric acidity.

Anesthetic Technique

Maternal and Fetal Monitoring

Appropriate monitors should be placed prior to induction. These monitors include ECG, pulse oximetry, capnography and blood pressure monitoring. Many anesthesiologists prefer to place an intraarterial catheter for arterial blood pressure monitoring prior to induction. Patients can undergo extensive and rapid blood loss during surgical resection of neurovascular lesions. Therefore, venous access must be sufficient to permit rapid transfusion of blood products. A central venous catheter, pulmonary artery catheter and/or transesophageal echocardiography (TEE) may be useful in monitoring fluid replacement therapy, particularly for patients with multiple trauma and/or cardiovascular disease. A precordial Doppler and end-tidal nitrogen monitoring should also be used in cases with potential for venous air embolism, such as those performed in the sitting position.

Whenever possible, fetal and uterine monitors should be used for patients in their second and third trimesters of pregnancy. If the uterine fundus is above the level of the umbilicus, an external tocodynamometer is usually effective for monitoring uterine activity. An external Doppler fetal heart rate monitor will usually detect fetal heart rate after the 16th week of gestation. Doppler monitoring is particularly useful because changes in heart rate may signal an abnormality in maternal ventilation, uterine perfusion, or fetal well-being. For example, anesthetics that readily transverse the placenta diminish the normal beat-to-beat variability of the fetal heart rate. The decrease in fetal heart rate during induced hypothermia parallels a decrease in the maternal heart rate (Fig. 29.6). However, when patterns of bradycardia emerge, they may indicate a fetal response to maternal hypotension or hypoxia. Maternal systolic blood pressure of less than 100 mm Hg may be associated with pathologic fetal bradycardia, which can begin a few minutes after the onset of maternal hypotension and may be preceded by a transient mild tachycardia. Therefore, close observation of maternal blood pressure and prompt treatment of hypotension and hypoxia are essential if the fetus is to have the best chance of surviving with an intact nervous system. If persistent signs of fetal distress occur that are not readily reversed by standard interventions (increased oxygenation, change in maternal position, blood pressure changes, etc.), then the neurosurgical procedure should be temporarily suspended while an emergent cesarean section is performed. Likewise, if labor commences intraoperatively and delivery becomes eminent during a neurosurgical procedure, then the procedure should be temporarily suspended, while the infant is delivered vaginally or by cesarean section, as is obstetrically indicated. Personnel for immediate neonatal resuscitation should be present, as the neonate will be anesthetized.

Induction Dilemma in the Pregnant Woman

One of the major concerns in anesthetizing a pregnant woman for a neurosurgical procedure is how to balance neurosurgical risks with obstetrical risks during the induction period. Neurosurgical concerns dictate that induction must be smooth with impeccable blood pressure control. Decreased blood pressure may produce ischemic changes in hypoperfused areas as well as

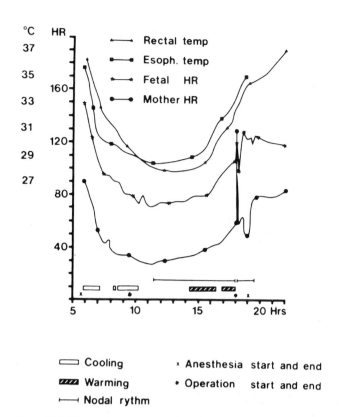

Figure 29.6. Maternal temperature (esophageal and rectal) and heart rate (maternal and fetal) during anesthesia with hypothermia. The times when cooling and warming of the mother were performed and the time during which the mother had modal rhythm are indicated. The hours indicate the time of the day. (From Stange K, Hallidin M. Hypothermia in pregnancy. *Anesthesiology* 1983;58:460–461, with permission.)

compromising uterine blood flow. Hypertension may rupture an aneurysm or worsen cerebral hypertension. However, pregnant women at more than 20 weeks of gestation and women with a history of significant gastric reflux are at-risk for possible regurgitation and aspiration. For these patients, a rapid-sequence technique of intravenous induction and endotracheal intubation should be performed. For patients in whom intubation may be difficult (abnormal airway, morbid obesity, etc.), an awake, fiberoptic intubation with good topicalization of the airway may be the most appropriate method for securing the airway. With respect to a rapid sequence induction, succinylcholine $(1 \text{ mg} \cdot \text{kg}^{-1})$ and higher dose vecuronium $(0.1 \text{ mg} \cdot \text{kg}^{-1}$ 4 minutes after a $0.01 \text{ mg} \cdot \text{kg}^{-1}$ predose) or rocuronium $(1 \text{ mg} \cdot \text{kg}^{-1})$ have all been used with good effect (155, 156). Some clinicians will ask the conscious patient to voluntarily hyperventilate immediately before induction and intubation. There is some concern in the literature over a possible rise in ICP following the use of succinylcholine (157, 158). However, studies suggest that succinylcholine alone causes little if any clinical effects on ICP or CBF (159, 160).

Of more clinical importance is the effect on intracranial dynamics of performing laryngoscopy and intubation under inadequate levels of anesthesia. Indeed, the ability to control hemodynamics and ICP during induction is the most important consideration in choosing an induction drug (50, 80). Thiopental and propofol are both popular induction agents for neurosurgery. Dosage for induction should be decided on a case-to-case basis, with care taken in the hemodynamically compromised patient. Hemodynamic responses to laryngoscopy, intubation, placement of pins for head fixation and incision must be anticipated. Agents used to blunt these responses include additional doses of the induction agent, lidocaine, and beta-blockers, particularly esmolol (50, 80). In some cases, nitroglycerin or nitroprusside may also be necessary.

Maintenance

Inhalational, balanced and total intravenous anesthetic (TIVA) techniques have all been advocated for induction and maintenance of anesthesia for these procedures. Agents frequently used include nitrous oxide/opioids (fentanyl, sufentanil, alfentanil and remifentanil), isoflurane, desflurane and propofol. One must consider surgical requirements, hemodynamic stability, capability for rapid postoperative emergence and the patient's medical and neurologic status in choosing a particular technique (58, 80). Once adequate controlled ventilation has been established, volatile anesthesia can be used to supplement the intravenous agents used for induction. Isoflurane and desflurane may be preferable to halothane because they have less effect on cerebral blood volume and thus helps to maintain cerebral perfusion and because they reduce $CMRO_2$. In addition, the low blood gas solubilities of isoflurane and desflurane permit more rapid anesthetic elimination at the conclusion of the surgical procedure. The dose-dependent increase in CBF by both isoflurane and desflurane is usually not clinically significant at the low (<0.5 MAC) doses utilized during neurosurgical procedures. However, it may be an issue for patients with abnormal cerebral autoregulation. In those individuals, fixed agents, such as propofol, midazolam or thiopental may be more appropriate. Ketamine should be avoided in patients with neurosurgical lesions, because of its ability to markedly increase CBF.

Omission of muscle relaxants may be requested intraoperatively during surgical resection to permit identification of nerves by direct stimulation. Evoked potentials may be used intraoperatively to monitor the functional integrity of specific sensory and/or motor pathways (126). Subcortical, spinal, and peripheral evoked responses as well as direct recordings from cortex or cranial nerves are relatively robust, therefore, either an opioid-based or an inhalational technique should not interfere with interpretation of evoked potential morphology (161). Muscle relaxants have minimal effect on electrocorticography (EEG) and somatosensory evoked potentials (SSEPs) and may indeed improve SSEP recordings by decreasing movement artifacts.

Both EEG and SSEP monitoring are being used with increasing frequency during surgical procedures. Both modalities can be useful in testing the integrity of ascending sensory pathways to detect potentially reversible ischemia-induced functional derangements either from retraction of cerebral tissues or temporary or permanent clipping (119, 126, 162, 163). However, both EEG and SSEP monitoring are quite sensitive to anesthetic effects particularly those secondary to volatile anesthetics and nitrous oxide (161, 164–169). Several authors have advocated use of a TIVA technique whenever intraoperative SSEP monitoring is utilized (166, 167). Rather than any one anesthetic technique, one should remain flexible as choice of agents will also be influenced by patient physiology and disease. Baseline SSEPs should be determined after obtaining an adequate depth of anesthesia for the surgical procedure. In most cases the signal will be sufficient in strength and stability to permit monitoring for changes during surgical manipulation, despite the attenuation induced by a typical balanced anesthetic technique (i.e., nitrous oxide-oxygen, opioid, low concentration of inhalation agent). If not, a systematic approach should be used to improve the signal. The neurophysiologist should attempt to optimize recording techniques and conditions. If these measures do not adequately improve the signal, then, if possible, the anesthesiologist should attempt to decrease the concentration/dose of agents that may decrease the response (e.g., nitrous oxide, inhalational agent), substituting instead agents with less effect on SSEPs (e.g., opioids, propofol). Physiologic factors such as Pao_2, $Paco_2$, systemic blood pressure and temperature can also alter SSEPs and EEGs and should be optimized if possible during intraoperative recordings (165). It is important to maintain stable conditions, both anesthetic and physiologic, during critical neurophysiologic monitoring period to avoid confounding changes to the waveforms (161). If such monitoring is contemplated, a preinduction discussion about anesthetic and monitoring re-

quirements should occur amongst the anesthesiologist, neurosurgeon and electrophysiologist.

Manipulation of the optic nerve, stellate ganglion, carotid sheath and dura can all produce wide blood pressure swings, bradycardia, dysrhythmias, prolonged QT intervals, and sinus arrest. These cardiovascular alterations usually resolve without treatment when manipulation/retraction of these structures is relieved. Infiltration of the area with a local anesthetic such as lidocaine (without epinephrine) can also be useful in ameliorating these responses.

POSTOPERATIVE ANESTHETIC MANAGEMENT

Emergence

In general, the anesthetic technique should be tailored to permit a prompt awakening upon completion of the surgical procedure whenever possible. The ability to neurologically evaluate a patient in the immediate postoperative period can allow for the early diagnosis and treatment of operative complications, such as hematoma formation. Care should be taken to prevent hypertension during surgical closure and postoperatively which can lead to bleeding in the surgical bed as well as possible cardiovascular complications, such as myocardial ischemia. Sympathetic blockers such as esmolol, labetalol and metoprolol and vasodilators such as hydralazine, nitroglycerin and sodium nitroprusside have all been used successfully for blood pressure control.

Airway

The decision to permit resumption of spontaneous respiration or to continue controlled ventilation into the immediate postoperative period should be made on a patient-to-patient basis. Factors influencing the decision include the nature of the procedure, particularly whether or not there was airway involvement, preoperative physical status, the presence of preexisting respiratory disease, duration of the procedure and amount of intravenous fluids given. If ventilation has been via an oral or nasally placed endotracheal tube, extubation must not occur until the patient is fully awake with appropriate intact airway reflexes. The endotracheal tube should not be removed if there is a potential for significant upper airway edema that may compromise the unprotected airway as might be seen in the patient with head and face trauma. Particular attention should be given to the submandibular areas as extensive edema will push the tongue cephalad and posterior, jeopardizing the airway. Care must be taken in determining the degree of cerebral edema as it will continue into the postoperative period with maximum swelling at 12 to 18 hours postprocedure. If substantial edema is present secondary to the surgical procedure and/or fluid replacement, a waiting period of 24 to 36 hours is usually indicated. It is not uncommon for these patients to require reintubation either for airway protection, respiratory insufficiency or upper airway obstruction. Cranial nerve involvement is also a factor in tracheal extubation criteria. A diminished gag reflex either from the disease process or secondary to surgical manipulation will place the patient at risk for aspiration. In addition, the patient should be observed for signs of stridor in the postoperative period. Possible causes for inspiratory stridor include laryngospasm from blood and/or secretions, foreign body aspiration, laryngeal edema or vocal cord dysfunction.

Delayed Awakening

Neurosurgical patients frequently exhibit delayed postoperative awakening. Care should be taken in determining possible causes for this delay as some can represent acute conditions requiring immediate medical and/or surgical attention. The frequent long duration of neurosurgical procedures can result in prolonged sedation and/or hypothermia. Neurologic causes for delayed emergence include intracerebral hematoma, subarachnoid hemorrhage and acute ischemic stroke. Excessive retraction on the frontal lobes can result in "acute brain" or "frontal lobe" syndrome or cerebral ischemic injury with postoperative mental status changes including prolonged emergence. Pneumocephalus can result from air forced from the nasal cavity into the CSF space and can cause meningitis and altered neurologic function.

Hyperemic Complications

Hyperemic complications are defined as perioperative edema or hemorrhage following neurosurgery, particularly after AVM removal. Hemorrhage can be secondary to incomplete removal of a lesion or inadequate hemostasis of the surgical bed. Perioperative edema and hemorrhage may be secondary to venous outflow obstruction by surgical ligation or embolization of draining veins or reduced venous drainage following AVM removal. Several mechanisms, such as the normal perfusion pressure breakthrough (NPPB) theory of Spetzler et al., have been proposed to explain hyperemia following AVM removal (170). Increasing brain size during closure and/or decreasing neurological status in the immediate postoperative period should alert one to the possibility of a hyperemic complication.

Delayed Cerebral Ischemia or Vasospasm

As discussed above, delayed ischemia or vasospasm remains the leading cause of severe morbidity and mortality in aneurysmal patients surviving to hospitalization. However, vasospasm is generally a diagnosis of exclusion and other causes for neurological deterioration (i.e., re-bleed, hydrocephalus, hypoxia, etc.) must be ruled out. The calcium-channel blocker, nimodipine, has been shown to improve SAH-induced vasospasm and has become a standard prophylactic therapy (48, 49, 53, 171). In areas of dysfunctional autoregulation, cerebral perfusion is passively dependent on systemic arterial pressure. Hypertensive/hypervolumic therapy is directed at improving

cerebral perfusion by increasing systemic pressures at least 20% to 30% above baseline using agents such as dopamine and phenylephrine and increasing CVP to 12 to 15 mm Hg with either albumin or sodium-containing isomolar cystalloid. Patients need close monitoring for cardiovascular and/or pulmonary complications of the therapy (53). Furthermore, these maneuvers may have adverse consequences on uterine blood flow, and therefore fetal well-being. The fetus should be monitored and clinical judgement utilized to consider the potential maternal benefit vs. the potential fetal risk. Complications from fluid overloading are common and can be quite severe, particularly for patients with preexisting cardiac disease. For patients with symptomatic vasospasm refractory to medical management, cerebral angioplasty or intracranial intraarterial papaverine may be required to prevent ischemic complications (52).

OBSTETRICAL MANAGEMENT OF PATIENTS WITH NEUROSURGICAL DISEASES

The method of delivery for the parturient with a neurosurgical disease should be based on obstetrical considerations (2, 6, 12, 41, 68, 172). Vaginal deliveries can be safely performed both before and after aneurysm clipping and AVM or tumor removal unless there are obstetrical indications to the contrary (14, 173, 174). Although some obstetricians prefer to perform cesarean sections to avoid Valsalva maneuvers associated with vaginal delivery (3, 175), the method of delivery (vaginal versus cesarean section) appears to have no influence on either fetal or maternal outcome (2, 111, 172, 173, 176). Indeed, Dias and Sekhar found that for patients with either unclipped aneurysms or unresected AVMs, cesarean section afforded no improvement in maternal or fetal outcome than vaginal delivery (Fig. 29.7) (2). Cesarean section may be appropriate for patients with acute bleeding near

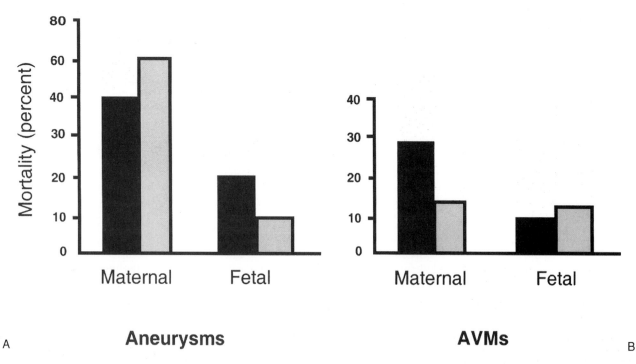

A   **Aneurysms**   **AVMs**   B

Figure 29.7. Effect of obstetrical management on outcome after arteriovenous malformation (AVM) hemorrhage. This figure demonstrates the maternal and fetal mortality (in percent) associated with vaginal delivery (closed bars) or cesarean section (stippled bars) in patients with hemorrhage from aneurysms (**A**) or AVMs (**B**). There were no statistically differences in either fetal or maternal outcomes between the two obstetrical techniques. (Adapted from Dias MS, Sekhar LN. Intracranial hemorrhage from aneurysms and arteriovenous malformations during pregnancy and the puerperium. *Neurosurgery* 1990;27:855–866, with permission.)

term, as part of a combined neurosurgical and obstetrical procedure or for fetal salvage in a moribund parturient (41, 115, 177–180). Therefore, method of delivery and type of anesthesia should be made upon obstetrical and anesthetic rather than neurosurgical considerations.

Preventing hypertension and increased ICP is crucial to managing labor and delivery successfully in women with documented unclipped aneurysms, unexcised AVMs, or intracranial tumors. Several adjunctive maneuvers have been suggested to decrease the hemodynamic changes that occur during labor and delivery. These include shortening the second stage of labor and avoiding maternal straining with the Valsalva maneuver (14, 41, 68, 181, 182). Immediately following the Valsalva maneuver, there is a reduction in CSF pressure accompanied by an increase in cardiac output and blood pressure, which is the result of increased venous return to the heart. The net effect on transmural pressure of cerebral vessels is not precisely known. Until cerebral hemodynamics during labor are better understood, it is best to avoid Valsalva maneuvers in women with cerebrovascular disease, thus reducing the possibility of rupturing tenuous cerebral vessels. Of interest, the risk for intracranial hemorrhage in the presence of an untreated neurovascular lesion does not significantly differ between vaginal delivery and cesarean section (2, 3, 183).

Techniques for shortening the second stage of labor to avoid maternal straining include the administration of epidural or combined spinal epidural (CSE) analgesia for the use of outlet forceps or vacuum extraction. For the first stage of labor, a properly administered epidural or CSE block will decrease pain and the increased blood pressure and cardiac output associated with painful uterine contractions. It can prevent the Valsalva maneuver by blocking the reflex urge to bear down. However, epidural or spinal techniques may have increased risk for patients with increased ICP. For epidurals, increasing ICP by injecting local anesthetic into the epidural space and elevating CSF pressure. Dural puncture may cause a sudden leakage of CSF that decreases CSF pressure and produces cerebellar herniation. Although the likelihood of dural puncture and elevated CSF pressure is somewhat reduced with the caudal approach to the epidural space, caudal anesthesia has been associated with neurologic sequelae among patients with increased ICP. The use of epidural or CSE techniques are not contraindicated, per se, for labor analgesia for parturients with increased ICP, but their benefits must be carefully considered with respect to potential maternal risks.

Alternate forms of analgesia, although less effective than epidural or caudal anesthesia, include paracervical and pudendal blocks, inhalation analgesics, and systemic opioids. Paracervical blocks have been associated with fetal compromise, but they may be a useful alternative for women with increased ICP. Pudendal blocks are safe and useful for the second stage of labor. However, administration of opioids and inhalation agents during spontaneous ventilation may raise $Paco_2$, induce maternal respiratory acidosis, increase cerebral blood flow, and raise ICP. If general anesthesia is necessary for cesarean section, vaginal delivery or manual removal of the placenta, the rapid-sequence intravenous induction technique described earlier should be used. When cesarean delivery is required, epidural anesthesia with a sensory level of T4 is recommended. Low-spinal anesthesia is another alternative. This approach may be contraindicated for patients who have intracranial hypertension in the presence of an aneurysm or AVM. A reduction in CSF pressure may increase aneurysmal transmural pressure, increasing the potential for rupture.

The increased ICP associated with pseudotumor cerebri is *not* a contraindication to labor and delivery. Labor analgesia or cesarean section anesthesia can be provided by an epidural or spinal technique (33, 176, 184). Spinal anesthesia has been advocated as the method of choice for cesarean section for patients with pseudotumor cerebri because of its safety and technical ease and a postdural puncture CSF leak would actually be beneficial

(185). Before performing a regional anesthetic for patients with lumboperitoneal shunts, localization of the site of entry of the shunt into the subarachnoid space is important (176).

If labor supervenes after SAH, a procedure combining cesarean section and neurosurgery may be used, although vaginal and cesarean delivery should be considered before neurosurgical intervention (173). The choice of procedure in this situation is guided by the severity of the maternal clinical condition, the feasibility of treating preterm labor, and the maturity of and potential hazard to the fetus.

After successful surgical occlusion of an aneurysm or AVM, there appears to be no need for specialized management of labor and delivery. Even induction of labor with an oxytocic agent is not contraindicated. Considering that the incidence of unruptured aneurysms in women is reportedly 0.5% to 1%, many pregnant women with this vascular lesion apparently undergo labor and deliver without incident.

Maternal SAH may result in the particularly difficult medical and ethical situation of maternal coma or brain death during pregnancy (177, 178, 186–189). Dillon et al. proposed a management plan for maternal coma and brain death during pregnancy based on fetal gestational age and chance of extrauterine survival (177). Suggested measures for physiologic support in pregnancy complicated by maternal brain death, published by Field et al., are listed in Table 29.4. In general, for patients who fulfill the Harvard Criteria for brain death (unresponsiveness, no movement or breathing, no reflexes and a flat EEG), one can anticipate prolonging somatic life for up to 2 weeks (186). Most authors suggest cesarean section for delivery in cases of maternal coma or brain death. Because two patients (the mother and the

---

Table 29.4. SUGGESTED MEASURES FOR PHYSIOLOGIC SUPPORT IN PREGNANCY COMPLICATED BY MATERNAL BRAIN DEATH

Mechanical ventilation with ventilator with volume present.
Start with a tidal volume of 10 to 15 mL $\cdot$ kg^{-1}, respiratory rate of 10 to 12 breaths per minute and a Flo$_2$ of 1.0. Make subsequent ventilator adjustments to the basis of arterial blood gas determinations.
Decrease the Flo$_2$ to <0.6 while maintaining the Pao$_2$ at ≥90 mm Hg.
Adjust the respiratory rate to maintain Paco$_2$ at 28 to 32 mm Hg. If the Pao$_2$ is <60 mm Hg while the Flo$_2$ >0.5, add positive end-expiratory pressure by starting at 3 to 5 cm of water and titrating upward until the oxygenation improves or the cardiac output declines.

Vasopressors to treat fluid-resistant hypotension.
Start with a continuous intravenous infusion of dopamine (2 to 5 μg $\cdot$ kg^{-1} $\cdot$ min^{-1}), and titrate upward until mean arterial blood pressure of 80 to 100 mm Hg is reached.
If the desired mean arterial pressure is not achieved at dopamine rates of 12 to 15 μg $\cdot$ kg^{-1} $\cdot$ min^{-1}, add dopamine at a continuous infusion rate of 2.5 to 15.0 μg $\cdot$ kg^{-1} $\cdot$ min^{-1}.

Warming or cooling blankets to treat temperature lability. Nutritional support using enteral tube feedings or total parenteral nutrition.
Maintain daily energy intake of 126 to 147 kJ $\cdot$ kg^{-1} for ideal body weight.
Treat hyperglycemia with insulin.

Treat endocrine abnormalities with replacement hormones.
Vasopression.
Thyroxine.
Corticosteroids.

Aggressive surveillance for and treatment of infections.

Heparin prophylaxis.

From Field DR, Gates EA, Creasy RK, et al. Maternal brain death during pregnancy: medical and ethical issues. *JAMA* 1988;260: 816–822, with permission.

fetus), as well as the surviving family members, will be affected by decisions about life support, each case should be assessed individually (186, 189).

REFERENCES

1. Shah KH, Simons RK, Holbrook T, et al. Trauma in pregnancy: maternal and fetal outcomes. *J Trauma* 1998;45:83–86.
2. Dias MS, Sekhar LN. Intracranial hemorrhage from aneurysms and arteriovenous malformations during pregnancy and the puerperium. *Neurosurgery* 1990;27:855–866.
3. Robinson JL, Hall CS, Sedzimir CB. Arteriovenous malformations, aneurysms and pregnancy. *J Neurosurg* 1974;41:63–70.
4. Horton JC, Chambers WA, Lyons SL, et al. Pregnancy and the risk of hemorrhage from cerebral arteriovenous malformations. *Neurosurgery* 1990;27:867–872.
5. Sadasivan B, Malik GM, Lee C, et al. Vascular malformations and prenancy. *Surg Neurol* 1990;33:305–313.
6. Levy DM, Jaspan T. Anaesthesia for caesarean section in a patient with recent subarachnoid haemorrhage and severe pre-eclampsia. *Anaesthesia* 1999;54:994–998.
7. Bendok BR, Getch CC, Malisch TW, et al. Treatment of aneurysmal subarachnoid hemorrhage. *Semin Neurol* 1998;18:521–531.
8. Henderson CE, Torbey M. Rupture of intracranial aneurysm associated with cocaine use during pregnancy. *Am J Perinatol* 1988;5:142–143.
9. Fox MW, Harms RW, Davis DH. Selected neurologic complications of pregnancy. *Mayo Clin Proc* 1990;65:1595–1618.
10. Simon RH. Brain tumors in pregnancy. *Semin Neurol* 1988;8:214–821.
11. Depret-Mosser S, Jomin M, Monnier JC, et al. Cerebral tumors and pregnancy. Apropos of 8 cases. *J Gynecol Obstet Biol Reprod* 1993;22:71–80.
12. Isla A, Alvarez F, Gonzalez A, et al. Brain tumor and pregnancy. *Obstet Gynecol* 1997;89:19–23.
13. Nader S. Pituitary disorders and pregnancy. *Semin Perinatol* 1990;14:24–33.
14. Chaudhuri P, Wallenburg HC. Brain tumors and pregnancy. Presentation of a case and a review of the literature. *Eur J Obstet Gynecol Reprod Biol* 1980;11:109–114.
15. Scheithauer BW, Sano T, Kovacs KT, et al. The pituitary gland in pregnancy: a clinicopathologic and immunohistochemical study of 69 cases. *Mayo Clin Proc* 1990;65:461–474.
16. Prager D, Braunstein GD. Pituitary disorders during pregnancy. *Endocrinol Metab Clin North Am* 1995;24:1–14.
17. Molitch ME. Pituitary diseases in pregnancy. *Semin Perinatol* 1998;22:457–470.
18. Sheenan H. Postpartum necrosis of the anterior pituitary. *J Pathol Bacteriol* 1937;45:189–214.
19. Ishihara T, Hino M, Kurahachi H, et al. Long-term clinical course of two cases of lymphocytic adenohypophysitis. *Endocrinol J* 1996;43:433–840.
20. Patel MC, Guneratne N, Haq N, et al. Peripartum hypopituitarism and lymphocytic hypophysitis. *Q J Med* 1995;88:571–580.
21. Moresco RM, Scheithauer BW, Lucignani G, et al. Oestrogen receptors in meningiomas: a correlative PET and immunohistochemical study. *Nucl Med Commun* 1997;18:606–615.
22. Koper JW, Lamberts SW. Meningiomas, epidermal growth factor and progesterone. *Hum Reprod* 1994;9:190–194.
23. Schlehofer B, Blettner M, Wahrendorf J. Association between brain tumors and menopausal status. *J Natl Cancer Inst* 1992;84:1346–1349.
24. Roelvink NC, Kamphorst W, van Alphen HA, et al. Pregnancy-related primary brain and spinal tumors. *Arch Neurol* 1987;44:209–215.
25. Small W Jr, Lurain JR, Shetty RM, et al. Gestational trophoblastic disease metastatic to the brain. *Radiology* 1996;200:277–280.
26. Bakri Y, Berkowitz RS, Goldstein DP, et al. Brain metastases of gestational trophoblastic tumor. *J Reprod Med* 1994;39:179–184.
27. Flam F. Emergency surgery in gestational trophoblastic tumours. *Eur J Obstet Gynecol Reprod Biol* 1994;55:183–186.
28. Yerby MS. Pregnancy and epilepsy. *Epilepsia* 1991;32:S51–S59.
29. Nulman I, Laslo D, Koren G. Treatment of epilepsy in pregnancy. *Drugs* 1999;57:535–544.
30. Lindhout D, Omtzigt JG. Pregnancy and the risk of teratogenicity. *Epilepsia* 1992;33:S41–S48.
31. Zahn CA, Morrell MJ, Collins SD, et al. Management issues for women with epilepsy: a review of the literature. *Neurology* 1998;51:949–956.
32. Gilmore J, Pennell PB, Stern BJ. Medication use during pregnancy for neurologic conditions. *Neurol Clin* 1998;16:189–206.
33. Peterson CM, Kelly JV. Pseudotumor cerebri in pregnancy. Case reports and review of literature. *Obstet Gynecol Surv* 1985;40:323–329.
34. Digre KB, Varner MW, Corbett JJ. Pseudotumor cerebri and pregnancy. *Neurology* 1984;34:721–729.
35. Wiebers DO, Whisnant JP. The incidence of stroke among pregnant women in Rochester, Minn, 1955 through 1979. *JAMA* 1985;254:3055–3057.
36. Sharshar T, Lamy C, Mas JL. Incidence and causes of strokes associated with pregnancy and puerperium. A study in public hospitals of Ile de France. Stroke in Pregnancy Study Group. *Stroke* 1995;26:930–936.
37. Simolke GA, Cox SM, Cunningham FG. Cerebrovascular accidents complicating pregnancy and the puerperium. *Obstet Gynecol* 1991;78:37–42.
38. Kittner SJ, Stern BJ, Feeser BR, et al. Pregnancy and the risk of stroke. *N Engl J Med* 1996;335:768–774.
39. Qureshi AI, Giles WH, Croft JB, et al. Number of pregnancies and risk for stroke and stroke subtypes. *Arch Neurol* 1997;54:203–206.
40. Lamy C, Hamon J-B, Coste J, et al. Ischemic stroke and subsequent pregnancies: for the French Study Group on stroke in pregnancy. *Neurology* 2000;54:A141–142.
41. Mas JL, Lamy C. Stroke in pregnancy and the puerperium. *J Neurol* 1998;245:305–313.
42. Richards A, Graham D, Bullock R. Clinicopathological study of neurological complications due to hypertensive disorders of pregnancy. *J Neurol Neurosurg Psychiatry* 1988;51:416–421.
43. Rinkel GJ, Djibuti M, van Gijn J. Prevalence and risk of rupture of intracranial aneurysms: a systematic review. *Stroke* 1998;29:251–256.
44. Barrow DL, Reisner A. Natural history of intracranial aneurysms and vascular malformations. *Clin Neurosurg* 1993;40:3–39.
45. Daras M, Tuchman AJ, Koppel BS, et al. Neurovascular complications of cocaine. *Acta Neurol Scand* 1994;90:124–129.
46. Roux PD, Winn HR. Management of the ruptured aneurysm. *Neurosurg Clin North Am* 1998;9:525–540.
47. Hunt WE, Hess RM. Surgical risk as related to time of intervention in the repair of intracranial aneurysms. *J Neurosurg* 1968;28:14–20.
48. Mayberg MR. Cerebral vasospasm. *Neurosurg Clin North Am* 1998;9:615–627.
49. Allen GS, Ahn HS, Preziosi TJ, et al. Cerebral arterial spasm—a controlled trial of nimodipine in patients with subarachnoid hemorrhage. *N Engl J Med* 1983;308:619–624.
50. Young WL. Cerebral aneurysms: current anaesthetic management and future horizons. *Can J Anaesth* 1998;45:R17–R31.
51. Taylor CL, Selman WR, Kiefer SP, et al. Temporary vessel occlusion during intracranial aneurysm repair. *Neurosurgery* 1996;39:893–906.
52. Higashida RT, Halbach VV, Dowd CF, et al. Intravascular balloon dilatation therapy for intracranial arterial vasospasm: patient selection, technique, and clinical results. *Neurosurg Rev* 1992;15:89–95.
53. McGrath BJ, Guy J, Borel CO, et al. Perioperative management of aneurysmal subarachnoid hemorrhage: Part 2. Postoperative management. *Anesth Analg* 1995;81:1295–1302.
54. McCormick WF. Pathology of vascular malformations of the brain. In: Wilson CB, Stein BM, eds. *Intracranial Arteriovenous Malformations*. Baltimore: Williams & Wilkins, 1984:44–63.
55. Ozawa T, Miyasaka Y, Tanaka R, et al. Dural-pial arteriovenous malformation after sinus thrombosis. *Stroke* 1998;29:1721–1724.
56. Brown RD Jr, Wiebers DO, Forbes G, et al. The natural history of unruptured intracranial arteriovenous malformations. *J Neurosurg* 1988;68:352–357.
57. Redekop G, TerBrugge K, Montanera W, et al. Arterial aneurysms associated with cerebral arteriovenous malformations: classification, incidence, and risk of hemorrhage. *J Neurosurg* 1998;89:539–546.
58. Thompson RC, Steinberg GK, Levy RP, et al. The management of patients with arteriovenous malformations and associated intracranial aneurysms. *Neurosurgery* 1998;43:202–212.
59. Brown RD Jr, Wiebers DO, Forbes GS. Unruptured intracranial aneurysms and arteriovenous malformations: frequency of intracranial hemorrhage and relationship of lesions. *J Neurosurg* 1990;73:859–863.
60. Perret G, Grip A. Report on the cooperative study of intracranial aneurysms and subarachnoid hemorrhage. Section VI.

Arteriovenous malformations. An analysis of 545 cases of craino-cerebral arteriovenous malformations and fistulae reported to the Cooperative Study. *J Neurosurg* 1966;25:467–490.

61. Samson DS, Batjer HH. Preoperative evaluation of the risk/benefit ratio for arteriovenous malformations of the brain. In: Wilson CB, Stein BM, ed. *Neurosurgery update II: Vascular, Spinal, Pediatric, and Functional Neurosurgery.* New York: McGraw-Hill, 1991:129–133.

62. Nussbaum ES, Heros RC, Camarata PJ. Surgical treatment of intracranial arteriovenous malformations with an analysis of cost-effectiveness. *Clin Neurosurg* 1995;42:348–369.

63. Hartmann A, Mast H, Mohr JP, et al. Morbidity of intracranial hemorrhage in patients with cerebral arteriovenous malformation. *Stroke* 1998;29:931–934.

64. Pollock BE, Flickinger JC, Lunsford LD, et al. Hemorrhage risk after stereotactic radiosurgery of cerebral arteriovenous malformations. *Neurosurgery* 1996;38:652–661.

65. Witlin AG, Friedman SA, Egerman RS, et al. Cerebrovascular disorders complicating pregnancy—beyond eclampsia. *Am J Obstet Gynecol* 1997;176:1139–1148.

66. Szabo MD, Crosby G, Sundaram P, et al. Hypertension does not cause spontaneous hemorrhage of intracranial arteriovenous malformations. *Anesthesiology* 1989;70:761–763.

67. Selmi F, Davies KG, Sharma RR, et al. Intracerebral haemorrhage due to amphetamine abuse: report of two cases with underlying arteriovenous malformations. *Br J Neurosurg* 1995;9:93–96.

68. Hunt HB, Schifrin BS, Suzuki K. Ruptured berry aneurysms and pregnancy. *Obstet Gynecol* 1974;43:827–837.

69. Moskopp D, Janssen B, Schmidt S, et al. Is there an unusual incidence of the manifestation of intracranial angiomas in pregnancy? Risk assessment based on 17,733 patients over 10 years. *Zentralbl Neurochir* 1992;53:40–46.

70. The Arteriovenous Malformation Study Group. Arteriovenous malformations in the brain of adults. *N Engl J Med* 1999;340:1812–1818.

71. Donaldson JO, Lee NS. Arterial and venous stroke associated with pregnancy. *Neurol Clin* 1994;12:583–599.

72. Dulli DA, Luzzio CC, Williams EC, et al. Cerebral venous thrombosis and activated protein C resistance. *Stroke* 1996;27:1731–1733.

73. Ameri A, Bousser MG. Cerebral venous thrombosis. *Neurol Clin* 1992;10:87–111.

74. Novak Z, Coldwell DM, Brega KE. Selective infusion of urokinase and thrombectomy in the treatment of acute cerebral sinus thrombosis. *Am J Neuroradiol* 2000;21:143–145.

75. Chow K, Gobin YP, Saver J, et al. Endovascular treatment of dural sinus thrombosis with rheolytic thrombectomy and intra-arterial thrombolysis. *Stroke* 2000;31:1420–1425.

76. Lanzino G, Jensen ME, Cappelletto B, et al. Arteriovenous malformations that rupture during pregnancy: a management dilemma. *Acta Neurochir* 1994;126:102–106.

77. Reichman OH, Karlman RL. Berry aneurysm. *Surg Clin North Am* 1995;75:115–121.

78. Stoodley MA, Macdonald RL, Weir BK. Pregnancy and intracranial aneurysms. *Neurosurg Clin North Am* 1998;9:549–556.

79. Dias MS. Neurovascular emergencies in pregnancy. *Clin Obstet Gynecol* 1994;37:337–354.

80. Guy J, McGrath BJ, Borel CO, et al. Perioperative management of aneurysmal subarachnoid hemorrhage: Part 1. Operative management. *Anesth Analg* 1995;81:1060–1072.

81. Vinuela F, Duckwiler G, Mawad M. Guglielmi detachable coil embolization of acute intracranial aneurysm: perioperative anatomical and clinical outcome in 403 patients. *J Neurosurg* 1997;86:475–482.

82. Meyers PM, Halbach VV, Malek AM, et al. Endovascular treatment of cerebral artery aneurysms during pregnancy: report of three cases. *Am J Neuroradiol* 2000;21:1306–1311.

83. Young WL, Pile-Spellman J. Anesthetic considerations for interventional neuroradiology. *Anesthesiology* 1994;80:427–456.

84. Little JB. Low-dose radiation effects: interactions and synergism. *Health Phys* 1990;59:49–55.

85. Brent RL. Radiation teratogenesis. *Teratology* 1980;21:281–298.

86. Valavanis A, Yasargil MG. The endovascular treatment of brain arteriovenous malformations. *Adv Tech Stand Neurosurg* 1998;24:131–2–14.

87. Halbach VV, Higashida RT, Dowd CF, et al. Management of vascular perforations that occur during neurointerventional procedures. *Am J Neuroradiol* 1991;12:319–327.

88. Barno A, Freeman DW. Maternal deaths due to spontaneous subarachnoid hemorrhage. *Am J Obstet Gynecol* 1976;125:384–392.

89. Basso A, Fernandez A, Althabe O, et al. Passage of mannitol from mother to amniotic fluid and fetus. *Obstet Gynecol* 1977;49:628–631.

90. Bruns PD, Linder RO, Drose VE, et al. The placental transfer of water from fetus to mother following the intravenous infusion of hypertonic mannitol to the maternal rabbit. *Am J Obstet Gynecol* 1963;86:160–167.

91. Battaglia F, Prystowsky H, Smisson C, et al. Fetal blood studies. XIII. The effect of the administration of fluids intravenously to mothers upon the concentrations of water and electrolytes in plasma of human fetuses. *Pediatrics* 1960;25:2–10.

92. Ross MG, Ervin MG, Leake RD, et al. Bulk flow of amniotic fluid water in response to maternal osmotic challenge. *Am J Obstet Gynecol* 1983;147:697–701.

93. Kelly TF, Moore TR, Brace RA. Hemodynamic and fluid responses to furosemide infusion in the ovine fetus. *Am J Obstet Gynecol* 1993;168:260–268.

94. Beermann B, Groschinsky-Grind M, Fahraeus L, et al. Placental transfer of furosemide. *Clin Pharmacol Ther* 1978;24:560–562.

95. Wladimiroff JW. Effect of frusemide on fetal urine production. *Br J Obstet Gynaecol* 1975;82:221–224.

96. Katz VL, Peterson R, Cefalo RC. Pseudotumor cerebri and pregnancy. *Am J Perinatol* 1989;6:442–445.

97. Leman RB, Assey ME. Heart disease and pregnancy. *South Med J* 1981;74:944–946.

98. Wilson AL, Matzke GR. The treatment of hypertension in pregnancy. *Drug Intell Clin Pharm* 1981;15:21–26.

99. Naulty J, Cefalo RC, Lewis PE. Fetal toxicity of nitroprusside in the pregnant ewe. *Am J Obstet Gynecol* 1981;139:708–711.

100. Lieb SM, Zugaib M, Nuwayhid B, et al. Nitroprusside-induced hemodynamic alterations in normotensive and hypertensive pregnant sheep. *Am J Obstet Gynecol* 1981;139:925–931.

101. Read MA, Giles WB, Leitch IM, et al. Vascular responses to sodium nitroprusside in the human fetal-placental circulation. *Reprod Fertil Dev* 1995;7:1557–1561.

102. Shoemaker CT, Meyers M. Sodium nitroprusside for control of severe hypertensive disease of pregnancy: a case report and discussion of potential toxicity. *Am J Obstet Gynecol* 1984;149:171–173.

103. Baker AB. Management of severe pregnancy-induced hypertension, or gestosis, with sodium nitroprusside. *Anaesth Intensive Care* 1990;18:361–365.

104. Rigg D, McDonogh A. Use of sodium nitroprusside for deliberate hypotension during pregnancy. *Br J Anaesth* 1981;53:985–987.

105. Curry SC, Carlton MW, Raschke RA. Prevention of fetal and maternal cyanide toxicity from nitroprusside with coinfusion of sodium thiosulfate in gravid ewes. *Anesth Analg* 1997;84:1121–1126.

106. Hood DD, Dewan DM, James FM III, et al. The use of nitroglycerin in preventing the hypertensive response to tracheal intubation on severe preeclamptics. *Anesthesiology* 1985;63:329–332.

107. Silver HM. Acute hypertensive crisis in pregnancy. *Med Clin North Am* 1989;73:623–638.

108. David M, Walka MM, Schmid B, et al. Nitroglycerin application during cesarean delivery: plasma levels, fetal/maternal ratio of nitroglycerin, and effects in newborns. *Am J Obstet Gynecol* 2000;182:955–961.

109. Langevin PB, Katovich MJ, Wood CE, et al. The effect of nitroglycerin on the gravid uterus in sheep and rabbits. *Anesth Analg* 2000;90:337–343.

110. Skarsgard ED, VanderWall KJ, Morris JA, et al. Effects of nitroglycerin and indomethacin on fetal-maternal circulation and on fetal cerebral blood flow and metabolism in sheep. *Am J Obstet Gynecol* 1999;181:440–445.

111. Minielly R, Yuzpe AA, Drake CG. Subarachnoid hemorrhage secondary to ruptured cerebral aneurysm in pregnancy. *Obstet Gynecol* 1979;53:64–70.

112. van Buul BJ, Nijhuis JG, Slappendel R, et al. General anesthesia for surgical repair of intracranial aneurysm in pregnancy: effects on fetal heart rate. *Am J Perinatol* 1993;10:183–186.

113. Wilson F, Sedzimir CB. Hypothermia and hypotension during craniotomy in a pregnant woman. *Lancet* 1959;2:947–949.

114. Katz JD, Hook R, Barash PG. Fetal heart rate monitoring in pregnant patients undergoing surgery. *Am J Obstet Gynecol* 1976;125:267–269.

115. Lennon RL, Sundt TM Jr, Gronert GA. Combined cesarean section and clipping of intracerebral aneurysm. *Anesthesiology* 1984;60:240-242.

116. Robinson JL, Hall CJ, Sedzimir CB. Subarachnoid hemorrhage in pregnancy. *J Neurosurg* 1972;36:27–33.

117. Lewis PE, Cefalo RC, Naulty JS, et al. Placental transfer and fetal toxicity of sodium nitroprusside. *Gynecol Invest* 1977;8:46.

118. Brann AW Jr, Myers RE. Central nervous system findings in the newborn monkey following severe in utero partial asphyxia. *Neurology* 1975;25:327–338.

119. Samson D, Batjer HH, Bowman G, et al. A clinical study of the parameters and effects of temporary arterial occlusion in the management of intracranial aneurysms. *Neurosurgery* 1994;34:22–28.

120. Spetzler RF, Hadley MN. Protection against cerebral ischemia: the role of barbiturates. *Cerebrovasc Brain Metab Rev* 1989;1:212–229.

121. Nussmeier NA, Arlund C, Slogoff S. Neuropsychiatric complications after cardiopulmonary bypass: cerebral protection by a barbiturate. *Anesthesiology* 1986;64:165–170.

122. Lavine SD, Masri LS, Levy ML, et al. Temporary occlusion of the middle cerebral artery in intracranial aneurysm surgery: time limitation and advantage of brain protection. *J Neurosurg* 1997;87:817–824.

123. Sakabe T, Nakakimura K. Effect of anesthetic agents and other drugs on cerebral blood flow, metabolism and intracranial pressure. In: Cottrell JE, Smith DS, eds. *Anesthesia and Neurosurgery.* St. Louis: Mosby, 1994:149–174.

124. Brain Resuscitation Clinical Trial I Study Group. Randomized clinical study of thiopental loading in comatose survivors of cardiac arrest. *N Engl J Med* 1986;314:397–403.

125. Hall R, Murdoch J. Brain protection: physiological and pharmacological considerations. Part II: The pharmacology of brain protection. *Can J Anaesth* 1990;37:762–777.

126. Guerit JM. Neuromonitoring in the operating room: why, when, and how to monitor? *Electroencephalogr Clin Neurophysiol* 1998;106:1–21.

127. Cheng MA, Theard MA, Tempelhoff R. Intravenous agents and intraoperative neuroprotection. Beyond barbiturates. *Crit Care Clin* 1997;13:185–199.

128. Schievink WI, Zabramski JM. Brain protection for cerebral aneurysm surgery. *Neurosurg Clin North Am* 1998;9:661–671.

129. Ravussin P, de Tribolet N. Total intravenous anesthesia with propofol for burst suppression in cerebral aneurysm surgery: preliminary report of 42 patients. *Neurosurgery* 1993;32:236–240.

130. Todd MM, Warner DS, Sokoll MD, et al. A prospective, comparative trial of three anesthetics for elective supratentorial craniotomy. Propofol/fentanyl, isoflurane/nitrous oxide, and fentanyl/nitrous oxide. *Anesthesiology* 1993;78:1005–1020.

131. Weir DL, Goodchild CS, Graham DI. Propofol: Effects on indices of cerebral ischemia. *J Neurosurg Anesthesiol* 1989;1:284–289.

132. Sessler DI. Deliberate mild hypothermia. *J Neurosurg Anesthesiol* 1995;7:38–46.

133. Baker KZ, Young WL, Stone JG, et al. Deliberate mild intraoperative hypothermia for craniotomy. *Anesthesiology* 1994;81:361–367.

134. Ogilvy CS, Carter BS, Kaplan S, et al. Temporary vessel occlusion for aneurysm surgery: risk factors for stroke in patients protected by induced hypothermia and hypertension and intravenous mannitol administration. *J Neurosurg* 1996;84:785–791.

135. Sano T, Drummond JC, Patel PM, et al. A comparison of the cerebral protective effects of isoflurane and mild hypothermia in a model of incomplete forebrain ischemia in the rat. *Anesthesiology* 1992;76:221–228.

136. Watts DD, Trask A, Soeken K, et al. Hypothermic coagulopathy in trauma: effect of varying levels of hypothermia on enzyme speed, platelet function, and fibrinolytic activity. *J Trauma* 1998;44:846–854.

137. Stange K, Halldin M. Hypothermia in pregnancy. *Anesthesiology* 1983;58:460–461.

138. Matsuki A, Oyama T. Operation under hypothermia in a pregnant woman with an intracranial arteriovenous malformation. *Can Anaesth Soc J* 1972;19:184–191.

139. Boba A. Hypothermia: appraisal of risk in 110 consecutive patients. *J Neurosurg* 1962;19:924–933.

140. Vandewater SL, Paul WM. Observations on the foetus during experimental hypothermia. *Can Anaesth Soc J* 1960;7:44–51.

141. Assali NS, Westin B. Effects of hypothermia on uterine circulation and on the fetus. *Proc Soc Exp Biol Med* 1962;109:485–488.

142. Zornow MH, Prough DS. Fluid management in patients with traumatic brain injury. *New Horiz* 1995;3:488–498.

143. Tranmer BI, Iacobacci RI, Kindt GW. Effects of crystalloid and colloid infusions on intracranial pressure and computerized electroencephalographic data in dogs with vasogenic brain edema. *Neurosurgery* 1989;25:173–178.

144. Williamson KR, Taswell HF. Indications for intraoperative blood salvage. *J Clin Apheresis* 1990;5:100–103.

145. Claes Y, Van Hemelrijck J, Van Gerven M, et al. Influence of hydroxyethyl starch on coagulation in patients during the perioperative period. *Anesth Analg* 1992;75:24–30.

146. Teasdale G, Jennett B. Assessment of coma and impaired consciousness. A practical scale. *Lancet* 1974;2:81–84.

147. Kawaguchi M, Sakamoto T, Furuya H, et al. Pseudoankylosis of the mandible after supratentorial craniotomy. *Anesth Analg* 1996;83:731–734.

148. Nitzan DW, Azaz B, Constantini S. Severe limitation in mouth opening following transtemporal neurosurgical procedures: diagnosis, treatment, and prevention. *J Neurosurg* 1992;76:623–625.

149. Davis TP, Alexander J, Lesch M. Electrocardiographic changes associated with acute cerebrovascular disease: a clinical review. *Prog Cardiovasc Dis* 1993;36:245–260.

150. Di Pasquale G, Andreoli A, Lusa AM, et al. Cardiologic complications of subarachnoid hemorrhage. *J Neurosurg Sci* 1998;42:33–36.

151. Zaroff JG, Rordorf GA, Newell JB, et al. Cardiac outcome in patients with subarachnoid hemorrhage and electrocardiographic abnormalities. *Neurosurgery* 1999;44:34–39.

152. Kono T, Morita H, Kuroiwa T, et al. Left ventricular wall motion abnormalities in patients with subarachnoid hemorrhage: neurogenic stunned myocardium. *J Am Coll Cardiol* 1994;24:636–640.

153. Horowitz MB, Willet D, Keffer J. The use of cardiac troponin-I (cTnI) to determine the incidence of myocardial ischemia and injury in patients with aneurysm and presumed aneurysmal subarachnoid hemorrhage. *Acta Neurochir* 1998;140:87–93.

154. Braunwald E, Kloner RA. The stunned myocardium: prolonged, post ischemic ventricular dysfunction. *Circulation* 1982;66:1146–1149.

155. Abouleish EI, Abboud TK, Bikhazi G, et al. Rapacuronium for modified rapid sequence induction in elective caesarean section: neuromuscular blocking effects and safety compared with succinylcholine, and placental transfer. *Br J Anaesth* 1999;83:862–867.

156. Abouleish E, Abboud T, Lechevalier T, et al. Rocuronium (Org 9426) for caesarean section. *Br J Anaesth* 1994;73:336–341.

157. Cottrell JE, Hartung J, Giffin JP, et al. Intracranial and hemodynamic changes after succinylcholine administration in cats. *Anesth Analg* 1983;62:1006–1009.

158. Shapiro HM, Aidinis SJ. Neurosurgical anesthesia. *Surg Clin North Am* 1975;55:913.

159. Brown MM, Parr MJ, Manara AR. The effect of suxamethonium on intracranial pressure and cerebral perfusion pressure in patients with severe head injuries following blunt trauma. *Eur J Anaesthesiol* 1996;13:474–477.

160. Kovarik WD, Mayberg TS, Lam AM, et al. Succinylcholine does not change intracranial pressure, cerebral blood flow velocity, or the electroencephalogram in patients with neurologic injury. *Anesth Analg* 1994;78:469–473.

161. Sloan TB. Anesthetic effects on electrophysiologic recordings. *J Clin Neurophysiol* 1998;15:217–226.

162. Friedman WA, Chadwick GM, Verhoeven FJ, et al. Monitoring of somatosensory evoked potentials during surgery for middle cerebral artery aneurysms. *Neurosurgery* 1991;29:83–88.

163. Lopez JR, Chang SD, Steinberg GK. The use of electrophysiological monitoring in the intraoperative management of intracranial aneurysms. *J Neurol Neurosurg Psychiatry* 1999;66:189–196.

164. Peterson DO, Drummond JC, Todd MM. Effects of halothane, enflurane, isoflurane, and nitrous oxide on somatosensory evoked potentials in humans. *Anesthesiology* 1986;65:35–40.

165. Bendo A, Cass IS, Hartune J, et al. In: Barash PG, ed. *Anesthesia for Neurosurgery, Clinical Anesthesia*, 3rd ed. Philadelphia: Lippincott–Raven Publishers, 1997.

166. Kalkman CJ, Traast H, Zuurmond WW, et al. Differential effects of propofol and nitrous oxide on posterior tibial nerve somatosensory cortical evoked potentials during alfentanil anaesthesia. *Br J Anaesth* 1991;66:483–489.

167. Taniguchi M, Nadstawek J, Pechstein U, et al. Total intravenous anesthesia for improvement of intraoperative monitoring of

somatosensory evoked potentials during aneurysm surgery. *Neurosurgery* 1992;31:891–897.

168. Koht A, Schutz W, Schmidt G, et al. Effects of etomidate, midazolam, and thiopental on median nerve somatosensory evoked potentials and the additive effects of fentanyl and nitrous oxide. *Anesth Analg* 1988;67:435–441.

169. Sloan TB, Koht A. Depression of cortical somatosensory evoked potentials by nitrous oxide. *Br J Anaesth* 1985;57:849–852.

170. Spetzler RF, Wilson CB, Weinstewin P, et al. Normal perfusion pressure breakthrough theory. *Clin Neurosurg* 1978;25:651–672.

171. Feigin VL, Rinkel GJ, Algra A, et al. Calcium antagonists in patients with aneurysmal subarachnoid hemorrhage: a systematic review. *Neurology* 1998;50:876–883.

172. Yih PS, Cheong KF. Anaesthesia for caesarean section in a patient with an intracranial arteriovenous malformation. *Anaesth Intensive Care* 1999;27:66–68.

173. Young DC, Leveno KJ, Whalley PJ. Induced delivery prior to surgery for ruptured cerebral aneurysm. *Obstet Gynecol* 1983;61:749–752.

174. Finfer SR. Management of labour and delivery in patients with intracranial neoplasms. *Br J Anaesth* 1991;67:784–787.

175. Tewari KS, Cappuccini F, Asrat T, et al. Obstetric emergencies precipitated by malignant brain tumors. *Am J Obstet Gynecol* 2000;182:1215–1221.

176. Kassam SH, Hadi HA, Fadel HE, et al. Benign intracranial hypertension in pregnancy: current diagnostic and therapeutic approach. *Obstet Gynecol Surv* 1983;38:314–321.

177. Dillon WP, Lee RV, Tronolone MJ, et al. Life support and maternal death during pregnancy. *JAMA* 1982;248:1089–1091.

178. Catanzarite VA, Willms DC, Holdy KE, et al. Brain death during pregnancy: tocolytic therapy and aggressive maternal support on behalf of the fetus. *Am J Perinatol* 1997;14:431–434.

179. Depret-Mosser S, Monnier JC, Bouthors-Ducloy AS, et al. Cerebral aneurysms and pregnancy: 4 cases. *J Gynecol Obstet Biol Reprod* 1992;21:947–954.

180. Chang L, Looi-Lyons L, Bartosik L, et al. Anesthesia for cesarean section in two patients with brain tumours. *Can J Anaesth* 1999;46:61–65.

181. Daane TA, Tandy RW. Rupture of congenital intracranial aneurysms in pregnancy. *Obstet Gynecol* 1960;15:305–314.

182. Baker JW. Subarachnoid haemorrhage associated with pregnancy. *Aust N Z J Obstet Gynaecol* 1969;9:12–17.

183. Fliegner JR, Hooper RS, Kloss M. Subarachnoid haemorrhage and pregnancy. *J Obstet Gynaecol Br Commonw* 1969;76:912–917.

184. Palop R, Choed-Amphai E, Miller R. Epidural anesthesia for delivery complicated by benign intracranial hypertension. *Anesthesiology* 1979;50:159–160.

185. Abouleish E, Ali V, Tang RA. Benign intracranial hypertension and anesthesia for cesarean section. *Anesthesiology* 1985;63:705–707.

186. Hill LM, Parker D, O'Neill BP. Management of maternal vegetative state during pregnancy. *Mayo Clin Proc* 1985;60:469–472.

187. Field DR, Gates EA, Creasy RK, et al. Maternal brain death during pregnancy: medical and ethical issues. *JAMA* 1988;260:816–822.

188. Vives A, Carmona F, Zabala E, et al. Maternal brain death during pregnancy. *Int J Gynaecol Obstet* 1996;52:67–69.

189. Loewy EH. The pregnant brain dead and the fetus: must we always try to wrest life from death? *Am J Obstet Gynecol* 1987;157:1097–1101.

Shnider and Levinson's Anesthesia for Obstetrics,
edited by Samuel C. Hughes, et al.
Lippincott Williams & Wilkins,
Philadelphia, © 2001.

CHAPTER 30

ANESTHESIA FOR THE PREGNANT PATIENT WITH NEUROMUSCULAR DISORDERS

SAMUEL C. HUGHES, M.D.

Neuromuscular diseases are not common during the childbearing years, but when they occur, have important implications for the obstetrician and the anesthesiologist. This group of diseases may markedly affect the management of a patient and the administration of drugs during labor and delivery (1–4). This chapter reviews the more common anesthetic problems encountered and those that might serve as guides to managing similar or related problems. All of these conditions require highly-individualized care to balance complex medical conditions and their specific presentations during pregnancy. Consultation among the obstetrician, the neurologist and the anesthesiologist may be particularly helpful in this group of patients.

MYOTONIC SYNDROMES

The myotonic syndromes are a group of autosomal dominant degenerative diseases including *myotonia congenita, myotonic dystrophy,* and *paramyotonia congenita.* The latter is the rarest of these syndromes and appears only on exposure to cold (1). A case of cold-induced abortion in a woman with paramyotonia congenita has been reported (5). In all three syndromes, the skeletal muscle is especially affected and generally characterized by weakness and wasting. Smooth muscle can also be affected. Myotonia is characterized by difficulty in initiating muscle movement with delayed muscle relaxation following contraction and is present to some degree in all three manifestations. The basic defect may be in membrane chloride permeability (6).

Myotonia congenita is rare and consists of myotonia and pseudohypertrophy of some voluntary muscles. Dystrophic changes do not occur. The myotonia is said to be most severe following rest but improved with exercise. The disease is most often autosomal dominant, appearing in childhood and rarely progressing in severity. In its purest form, myotonia congenita does not affect the cardiac and smooth muscles. Unlike myotonic dystrophy, there is no mental deterioration, infertility, or decrease in life expectancy. This disease often responds to oral therapy with phenytoin, quinine sulfate, or procainamide, which may diminish muscle stiffness and cramping. In one reported case, the disease increased in severity during pregnancy and improved after delivery with no obstetric complications (7).

Myotonic dystrophy (also called *myotonia atrophica*) is the most common and most severe of these syndromes. Onset is often in the second decade of life, but it may present without myotonia in neonates in a severe form characterized by thin, weak muscles (congenital myotonic dystrophy). When onset is neonatal, death often results within a few months from respiratory weakness (8). Infants who survive have difficulty with swallowing and sucking initially. Children with this congenital form are mentally retarded and eventually display the full syndrome (9). Myotonic dystrophy occurs in three to five in 100,000 (10) and is an autosomal dominant transmitted disease, but has a wide variety of expression. For some individuals bearing the gene, the only manifestation may be cataracts in old age. Electromyographic changes occur early in the disease, before myotonia, and can be demonstrated clinically (11). Death usually occurs during the sixth decade of life from bulbar involvement, cardiac defects, or aspiration pneumonia.

Typically, patients with myotonic dystrophy demonstrate myotonia and wasting of skeletal muscles including facial, cervical, and proximal limb muscles. Often, they exhibit an early frontal baldness, gonadal atrophy, and endocrine failure. Other manifestations of particular importance to the anesthesiologist are cardiac conduction defects with a prolonged P-R interval and heart block that may cause benign arrhythmias or sudden death. Cardiomyopathy and pulmonary complications may be significant. Respiratory involvement is related to impaired mechanical ability. There may be weakness of both the diaphragm and intercostal muscles accompanied by chronic hypoventilation, hypercapnia, and decreased arterial oxygen saturation. During the perioperative period, decreased pharyngeal muscle strength and repeated aspiration can cause further respiratory problems.

Although smooth muscle involvement can occur, there have not been adequate numbers of obstetric cases reported to study the effect of myotonic dystrophy on labor. However, prolonged labor, uterine atony, and hemorrhage have been associated with the syndrome (12–17). The disease has been associated with ovarian insufficiency, amenorrhea, infertility, and, among women who become pregnant, a high incidence of spontaneous abortion (7, 17, 18). However, fertility may not be reduced except in those with severe disease (19). The small number of patients studied makes it unwise to relate the effects of the disease to the course of labor and delivery. Increased muscle weakness during pregnancy has been related to the effects of progesterone (20). Involvement of the adrenal glands may result in adrenocortical insufficiency. Polyhydramnios is reportedly associated with the disease, and may indicate an affected fetus with severe muscular dysfunction and poor swallowing.

In one review of 15 obstetric patients with myotonic dystrophy, eight had spontaneous vaginal deliveries, five required low forceps delivery or vacuum extraction, and two required cesarean delivery (13). Other investigators have reported an increased severity of symptoms at about the seventh month of pregnancy, and the increased muscle weakness may make it difficult for the patient to fully cooperate in the delivery (21). Tocolysis with ritodrine, a beta-mimetic used to delay premature labor, reportedly provoked the symptoms of myotonic dystrophy (22, 23).

Anesthetic Management of Patients with Myotonic Syndromes

The anesthesiologist managing a patient with myotonic dystrophy should evaluate the extent of the disease, the potential for untoward responses to otherwise routine anesthetic agents, and the obstetric course of the patient. The initial evaluation should include an estimation of pulmonary function and an electrocardiogram (ECG) to determine the potential for restrictive lung disease and cardiac arrhythmias (24). Holter monitoring and an echocardiogram may be useful as well as baseline blood gas analysis. If analgesia for labor pain is required, opioids and sedatives should be used with caution. All central nervous system depressants, including thiopental, diazepam, and inhalation agents, have been associated with apnea in these patients (25, 26). Imposing a central respiratory depression on an already atrophic respiratory musculature would most likely cause respiratory difficulty in these patients. Regional anesthesia including epidural, spinal or pudendal block provides satisfactory anesthesia and avoids the risk of respiratory depression. Consequently, the anesthetic technique suggested for patients with myotonic disorders is local or conduction anesthesia (27–35). Warming of fluids, use of warming blankets, and prewarming the labor and delivery rooms will reduce myotonic crisis (generalized contractures) (36).

If general anesthesia is required, a cautious approach is suggested. Patients may be extremely sensitive to intravenous induction agents (37). **The use of depolarizing muscle relaxants in a patient with myotonic dystrophy is considered extremely hazardous and should be avoided.** Marked, generalized skeletal muscle contracture proportional to the dose will develop, leading to difficulty in ventilating the patient (Fig. 30.1) (25). A review of the literature on succinylcholine, however, reveals that both relaxation of the myotonic state and general myotonia have been reported following the use of the drug, suggesting that the response of myotonic patients to this drug is unpredictable (38) (Table 30.1).

The response of these patients to nondepolarizing muscle relaxants appears normal, although a prolonged response to curare has been reported (39). Rapid-sequence endotracheal intubation can be accomplished with a sufficient dose of a nondepolarizing agent. Successful use of a priming dose of atracurium has been reported (16). Propofol has been used successfully (40), but an exaggerated physiologic response has also been reported (41). Anesthesia can be maintained with nitrous oxide, oxygen, and a potent inhalation agent. Opioids should be used sparingly following delivery of the infant. Extubation should be performed only when a patient is fully alert and able to maintain good ventilation. Despite an earlier report of myotonic crisis (generalized contractures) precipitated by the drug (28), reversal of muscle relaxants with neostigmine appears to be safe (25), although this remains controversial (38).

Generalized contractures may result from mechanical, as well as electrical stimulation. Neither regional anesthesia or nondepolarizing muscle relaxants prevent myotonic spasms. The effects of volatile anesthetic agents are uncertain but appear to be minimal. However, muscles in myotonic spasm will become flaccid when injected with a local anesthetic. Uterine myotonia

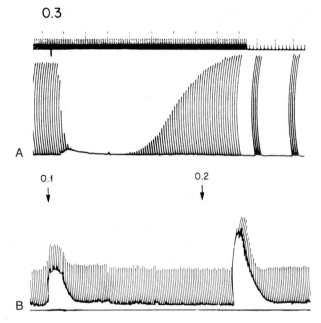

Figure 30.1. The response of a patient with myotonia to succinylcholine, demonstrated by evoked thumb adduction in response to stimulation of the ulnar nerve at 0.15 Hz. Time scale = 1 min. **A:** Normal response. **B:** Abnormal contracture seen when succinylcholine is administered to a patient with myotonia. (Adapted from Mitchell MM, Ali HH, Savarese JJ. Myotonia and neuromuscular blocking agents. *Anesthesiology* 1978;49:44–48.)

at cesarean section requiring topical local anesthetic to relax the uterus and continue surgery has been reported (30). There is no agreement on the treatment of generalized-sustained muscle contraction if it occurs during surgery, but intravenous administration of quinine (300 to 600 mg) has been used, as have large doses of steroids (42). Dantrolene has also been suggested (1).

In summary, patients having myotonic syndromes often present with significant multisystem disease having variable effects on pregnancy. For labor and delivery, regional anesthesia may avoid many of the risks of general anesthesia while providing adequate analgesia or anesthesia. The outcome and potential difficulties will no doubt be related to the severity of the mother's disease.

EPILEPSY

Epilepsy is a chronic seizure disorder affecting approximately 0.4% to 2% of the population (43, 44). Seizures may be caused by

Table 30.1. NEUROMUSCULAR DISORDERS AND THEIR RESPONSE TO MUSCLE RELAXANTS

Neuromuscular Disorders	Response to Succinylcholine	Response to Nondepolarizing Muscle Relaxants
Upper motor neuron lesion	Hyperkalemia, monitor unaffected side	Resistant
Lower motor neuron lesion	Hyperkalemia, monitor unaffected side	Sensitive
Neurofibromatosis	Contractures, resistant to succinylcholine	Sensitive
Myasthenia gravis	Resistant/sensitive if on anticholinesterase	Sensitive
Myasthenia syndrome	Sensitive	Sensitive
Muscular dystrophy	nl/hyperkalemia	nl/sensitive
Myotonia	Contractures/hyperkalemia	Resistant
Peripheral neuropathy	Resistant	sensitive

nl, normal
Adapted from Azar I. The response of patients with neuromuscular disorders to muscle relaxants: a review. Anesthesiology 1984;61:173–187.

Table 30.2. CAUSES OF SEIZURES DURING PREGNANCY

Eclampsia
Idiopathic epilepsy
Head trauma
Metabolic disorders
   Uremia
   Hypoglycemia
   Electrolyte abnormalities
   Hepatic failure
   Subtherapeutic serum levels of anticonvulsants
Meningitis
Encephalitis
Drug or alcohol withdrawal
Drug overdose (e.g., cocaine)
Arteriovenous malformation
Brain tumor

intracranial birth injury, metabolic disturbances, trauma, acute infection, brain tumors, or alcoholism; they may also be of idiopathic origin (Table 30.2). The latter is perhaps the most common and may occur at any age, but usually appears before the age of 20. In obstetric patients, the typical presentation is idiopathic epilepsy with drug therapy in progress.

A review of the Norwegian Medical Birth Registry compared 371 epileptic women with over 100,000 nonepileptic women and found that epileptic women had an increased incidence of hemorrhage, toxemia, and obstetric intervention (including forceps and cesarean delivery) (45). In addition, neonatal mortality was approximately fourfold higher. The authors concluded that women with epilepsy should be considered a high-risk group. Although there is controversy about the extent of the problem (46), these patients deserve careful consideration and monitoring during their pregnancies and deliveries. However, a review of 151 pregnancies in 1998 suggested most women with epilepsy will have an uncomplicated pregnancy and normal, healthy infants (47) (Table 30.3).

Interaction of Pregnancy and Epilepsy

True idiopathic epilepsy may be first diagnosed during pregnancy. The incidence of epilepsy for women in the childbearing years has been reported to be 50 per 100,000 (48). However, there is no evidence that pregnancy causes epilepsy or is in itself epileptogenic. In one review of 59 epileptic mothers studied through 153 pregnancies, 45% had more frequent seizures, 50% showed no change, and 5% had fewer seizures (49). In a prospective study of 154 pregnancies in epileptic women, 32% had more frequent seizures, 23% showed no change in frequency, 14% showed a decrease, while 31% were seizure free during the pregnancy and immediately postpartum (50). Management and control of antiepileptic drugs may explain the variable results reported. A recent retrospective study of 151 pregnancies in 124 epileptic women reported only 21% of women with increased frequency of seizures (47).

Pregnancy produces several physiologic and metabolic changes that may affect the course of epilepsy. Arterial CO_2 tension decreases during pregnancy, but arterial pH usually changes little because of adequate metabolic compensation. During labor, severe pain producing hyperventilation may produce alkalosis and vomiting and potentiate pH changes, thereby inducing seizures. During pregnancy, fluid retention may be epileptogenic and patients should ideally avoid rapid weight gains. In addition, renal plasma flow and glomerular filtration rate increase markedly. In one study phenobarbitone clearance did not show any significant changes, whereas the clearance of phenytoin increased, often by as much as 100% (51). The resulting decrease in serum phenytoin could lead to an increased frequency of seizures; serum levels should therefore be monitored frequently during pregnancy (Fig. 30.2) (52). Because the clearance of phenytoin returns to normal within a few months of delivery, drug dosage must be carefully adjusted postpartum to avoid drug intoxication.

Obstetric patients with epilepsy may also become more complicated because of patients' variable compliance to drug therapy during pregnancy. For example, patients may be more conscientious about taking medication during pregnancy or may decrease medication because of concern for teratogenicity. It has been suggested that in some cases, the emotional factors and stress surrounding pregnancy also may influence epilepsy.

Teratogenic Effects of Anticonvulsant Therapy

The incidence of congenital malformations in the offspring of epileptic women is about two and one-half times that for the general population (53). This may be due to anticonvulsant medication, but a genetic predisposition cannot be ruled out. One of the problems reported is the so called fetal hydantoin syndrome, which presents with altered growth and development

Table 30.3. NEONATAL OUTCOME IN 151 PREGNANCIES OF WOMEN WITH EPILEPSY COMPARED TO A BACKGROUND COHORT OF 38,983 WOMEN

	Women with Epilepsy			Controls	
	n	%	95% CI	*n*	%
Sex distribution					
Girls	72	48	(40.5–57.0)	18,751	48
Boys	79	52	(43.7–60.1)	20,460	52
Birth weight					
<2,500 g	7	5	(1.9–9.4)	2,699	7
2,500–4,500 g	137	90	—	34,483	89
>4,500 g	7	5	(1.9–9.4)	1,458	4
Preterm births	7	5	(1.9–9.4)	2,699	7
Referral to intensive neonatal care unit	30	20	(13.9–27.3)	2,700	7
Perinatal deaths	2	1.3	(0.2–4.7)	181	0.5
Fetal malformations	8	5.3	(2.3–10.3)	585	1.5

Perinatal deaths among newborns of epileptic mothers (1.3%) was more frequent but not significantly increased compared to the background population of 0.5%. While congenital malformations also occurred more frequently (5.3% vs. 1.5%), they were generally mild in nature and there were no neural tube defects.
From Sabers A, a' Rogvi-Hansen B, Dam M, et al. Pregnancy and epilepsy: a retrospective study of 151 pregnancies. *Acta Neurol Scand* 1998;97:164–170, with permission.

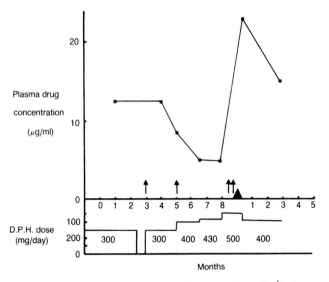

Figure 30.2. Plasma concentration of phenytoin ($\mu g \cdot mL^{-1}$) during pregnancy with the doses administered. The time of childbirth is shown by the *solid triangle*; the *arrows* indicate the occurrence of seizures. Therapeutic range for phenytoin is 10 to 20 mg $\cdot$ mL^{-1}. (Adapted from Lander CM, Edwards VE, Eadie MJ, et al. Plasma anticonvulsant concentrations during pregnancy. *Neurology* 1977;27:128–131.)

and the potential for cleft lip and palate, cardiac lesions, and hypoplasia of nails and digits. However, this has been noted with administration of barbiturates as well. Because treatment of epilepsy often consists of more than one drug, it is difficult to assign blame to a particular drug. Valproic acid therapy in pregnancy may be associated with a 1% risk of neural tube deflects. However, there is conflict in the studies and all of the major antiepileptic drugs (phenobarbital, carbamazepine, phenytoin, and valproic acid) have been identified as being teratogenic. One possible mechanism for teratogenicity is folate deficiency and folate supplementation is recommended. Other drugs in use include primidone, ethosuximide, and clonazepam (54, 55). Thus, if seizure medication is needed, the medication that is most effective should be used. Monotherapy may decrease the chances of teratogenicity (54). Ideally, the epileptic woman contemplating pregnancy should have her anticonvulsant medication tapered to the minimum effective dosage, changed to monotherapy, or discontinued (if possible) before conception. For many women, discontinuing drug therapy is not possible and major manipulation of drug therapy should ideally be avoided during pregnancy. However, most women with epilepsy, even those taking anticonvulsant medications, will have uneventful pregnancies and can expect to deliver healthy babies (47). It must be remembered that seizures put both the mother and fetus at risk and that *status epilepticus* is life threatening with a maternal mortality of 25% reported and a fetal death rate of

50% reported (56). Thus, appropriate anticonvulsant therapy is necessary.

When barbiturates are used to control seizures, the placental transfer of the drug is rapid. The ratio of umbilical cord vein to maternal artery phenobarbital concentration is 0.95 (57). Neonates may suffer from a drug-induced depression of vitamin K-dependent clotting factors (58). Maternal vitamin K supplements are recommended in late pregnancy. Because phenobarbital, primidone, or phenytoin may produce a transient depression of prothrombin and factors V and VII, vitamin K should be administered to neonates of mothers receiving anticonvulsant therapy. In addition, neonates may demonstrate the clinical signs of barbiturate withdrawal, including hyperexcitability, tremulousness, and decreased sucking. The newborn should be carefully observed for these signs for several days in the nursery.

Status Epilepticus During Pregnancy

Status epilepticus can occur with pregnancy, triggered by physiologic changes or alterations in drug level and therapy. It should be treated vigorously with standard anticonvulsant therapy and routine airway management with special attention to the potential for aspiration. Intubation, paralysis with muscle relaxants, and controlled ventilation with oxygen protect the patient from aspirating, decrease respiratory and metabolic acidosis, and ensure adequate oxygenation of mother and fetus. Phenytoin (Dilantin) as a slow intravenous drip (13 to 18 mg $\cdot$ kg^{-1}) is the drug of choice for terminating status epilepticus, although it may cause a drop in blood pressure and mild atrioventricular block. Lorazepam (Ativan®), diazepam (Valium®), or midazolam (Versed®) in incremental doses or phenobarbital (Luminal®) at a dose of 10 to 20 mg $\cdot$ kg^{-1} may be given intravenously but may cause respiratory depression. Even with therapy, the maternal mortality for *status epilepticus* may be as high as 10% to 25% (43, 56). However, if the condition is properly managed in obstetric patients, the outcome has been reported to be good, with the pregnancy continuing to term (49).

Anesthetic Management of Patients with Epilepsy

The anesthesiologist managing a pregnant epileptic patient must consider the cause of the epilepsy and the treatment in progress, as well as the obstetric course. Anticonvulsant drugs being taken should be identified. The availability of drug serum levels, drawn late in the pregnancy or in early labor, would make it possible to optimize dosage. The therapeutic range for phenytoin is 10 to 20 mg $\cdot$ mL^{-1}, which is usually achieved by taking 3 to 5 mg $\cdot$ kg^{-1} per day. The therapeutic range for phenobarbital is 10 to 50 mg $\cdot$ kg^{-1}, achieved with a daily dose of 1 to 5 mg $\cdot$ kg^{-1} per day (Table 30.4).

Table 30.4. COMMONLY USED ANTIEPILEPTIC DRUGS

Generic Name	Trade Name	Dosage (Adult p.o.)	Half-life	Therapeutic Range
Phenytoin	Dilantin	3–5 mg $\cdot$ kg^{-1}/day	24 h (variable)	10–20 μg $\cdot$ mL^{-1}
Phenobarbitol	Luminol	1–5 mg $\cdot$ kg^{-1}/day	90 h	10–50 μg $\cdot$ mL^{-1}
Primidone	Mysoline	10–25 mg $\cdot$ kg^{-1}/day	8 h	2–10 μg $\cdot$ mL^{-1}
Carbamazepine	Tergretol	600–1,200 mg/day	13–17 h	4–12 μg $\cdot$ mL^{-1}
Clonazepam	Clonopine	0.1–0.2 mg $\cdot$ kg^{-1}	24–48 h	5–70 μg $\cdot$ mL^{-1}
Sodium Valproate	Depakene	30–60 mg $\cdot$ kg^{-1}	6–20 h	50–100 μg $\cdot$ mL^{-1}
Ethosuximide	Zarontin	20–40 mg $\cdot$ kg^{-1}	60 h	40–100 μg $\cdot$ mL^{-1}

Drug interactions may be complex with epileptic patients. For example, the addition of phenobarbital to the therapeutic regimen of a patient receiving phenytoin may decrease the phenytoin serum level by enzyme induction. On the other hand, drugs that compete with phenytoin for a common metabolic pathway (e.g., dicumarol, isoniazid, sulfonamides, diazepam, and chloramphenicol) may increase the phenytoin serum levels. Phenobarbital enzyme induction speeds metabolism of methoxyflurane (59), but this agent is of little consequence in modern practice. Hepatic enzyme induction by either phenobarbital or phenytoin may affect drug dosing as well as metabolite production.

Fortunately, local anesthetics do not appear to interact significantly with anticonvulsant medications; in fact, lidocaine has been used to terminate epileptic seizures (60). However, high plasma levels (lidocaine >8 to 10 $\mu g \cdot mL$) achieved with rapid accidental intravenous injection can still cause convulsions. Well-conducted regional anesthesia is therefore a safe and appropriate choice for the typical epileptic patient. During labor and delivery, regional anesthetics prevent the hyperventilation and respiratory alkalosis that could provoke seizure. Well-conducted regional anesthesia for labor and delivery has proved successful and without unique complications.

If general anesthesia is indicated, the routine technique as described elsewhere in this text is satisfactory. In animals, d-tubocurarine interacts with both phenytoin and lidocaine, causing a greater than usual depression of twitch height in epileptic patients, and prolonged neuromuscular blockade (61). Monitoring the neuromuscular function and use of short-acting agents should avoid any potential problems. Some investigators advise against using any drugs with the potential for causing convulsion or seizure-like activity, including ketamine, etomidate, meperidine (metabolite), althesin, and enflurane or sevoflurane (62, 63). However, enflurane does not appear to increase seizure activity in patients with a history of convulsive disorders (64, 65) and inhalation agents have been used to treat *status epilepticus*. A routine inducting agent with thiopental followed by succinylcholine to facilitate intubation and then oxygen, nitrous oxide, and isoflurane to maintain anesthesia are suggested. Routine intravenous opioids such as morphine are suggested for postoperative pain management although some clinicians would avoid meperidine. However, seizures related to meperidine are unlikely unless large total doses of meperidine are administered.

NEUROFIBROMATOSIS

Neurofibromatosis was first described by Von Recklinghausen in 1882. The disease is inherited as an autosomal dominant disorder and occurs in one in 3,000 births (66). The defective gene causing the disorder has now been identified, the NFI gene or chromosome 17J (67). Neurofibromatosis type 1 is the most common form. The classic manifestations include café au lait spots or increased skin pigmentation and neurofibromas involving the skin. Neurofibromas may arise from the neurilemma sheath (Schwann cells), the fibroblasts of peripheral nerves, and melanocytes. The tumors may involve nerve roots or blood vessels and arise in or around most organs and body cavities. They are often totally benign and only a cosmetic problem. Expressivity of the gene is highly variable. Occasionally, they produce serious problems, such as intracranial tumors (in 5% to 10% of patients) or a compromised airway, the latter developing particularly if they occur in the mediastinum or cervical regions (68). In most patients, neurofibromatosis is a multifaceted syndrome associated with some osseous changes and (in rare cases) endocrine disorders such as pheochromocytoma and hyperthyroidism (69). The association with pheochromocytoma is probably overestimated, and some authors indicate that the frequency with which they coincide is only 1% (68). In

5% to 10% of cases of neurofibromatosis, one of the tumors will become sarcomatous (66).

Pregnancy and Neurofibromatosis

The pregnant patient with neurofibromatosis may have particular problems caused by the increase in neurofibroma size associated with pregnancy and the potential for hemorrhaging into the lesions themselves (69). Tumor growth regresses after pregnancy. A predisposition to hypertension related to diffuse vascular changes is suggested (70). It is difficult to judge how common these problems are, but because paravertebral and spinal neurofibromas are often present, the pregnant patient should be observed for any change in neurologic function (Fig. 30.3). Patients with neurofibromatosis should be considered high risk obstetric patients (71). Spontaneous hemothorax has also been reported in the parturient with neurofibromatosis (72) as well as dystosia in labor because of obstruction from pelvic neurofibroma (73).

Vascular changes have also been associated with the disease and, in advanced form, may be characterized by fibrous transformation of the intima (74). Renovascular hypertension associated with neurofibromatosis is often diagnosed before age 20 and may be present in the obstetric patient. Swapp and Main (69) reviewed 11 patients with 24 pregnancies. Ten of these patients were already hypertensive or developed hypertension with pregnancy. While the blood pressure elevations of these patients was mild, renovascular hypertension must be considered in the

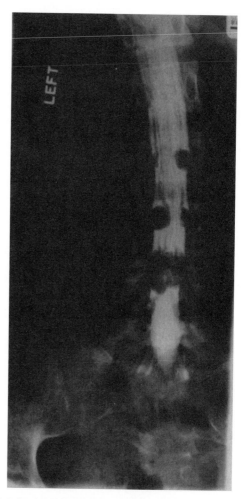

Figure 30.3. Lumbar spine and pelvis showing neurofibromas encroaching on the spine of a 25-year-old woman with neurofibromatosis. This patient had only mild upper extremity symptomatology at the time of this radiographic study.

differential diagnosis of hypertension during pregnancy or at delivery.

Anesthetic Management of Patients with Neurofibromatosis

The initial evaluation of the patient should include a particularly careful history to elicit signs and symptoms indicative of significant disease. That is, simple café au lait spots and cutaneous neurofibromas are probably not cause for alarm. However, intracranial neurofibromas or lesions near the spine might alter the management of pregnancy significantly. A history of labile hypertension might be indicative of pheochromocytoma or of renal vascular disease. Such cardiac lesions as pulmonary stenosis and coarctation of the aorta have also been reported in these patients. Spontaneous hemothorax, rupture of renal artery and other aneurysms have proved fatal in rare case reports (72, 75).

There are several reports of abnormal responses to muscle relaxants in patients with neurofibromatosis (76–78). It is suggested that these patients have a prolonged response to nondepolarizing muscle relaxants. Furthermore, some patients with neurofibromatosis are reported to be resistant to succinylcholine, whereas others have a prolonged response. An abnormal response to muscle relaxants might be attributed to a denervation phenomenon produced by generalized neurofibromatosis, but there is no good evidence that this occurs (1, 78). This author has used both succinylcholine and nondepolarizing agents in these patients with unremarkable results. However, given the diversity of the clinical features of this disease, using the minimal effective dose and monitoring neuromuscular function carefully are recommended when relaxants are required.

In most cases the patient can be managed in a routine manner and according to her wishes, as the obstetric course requires. There are no unique considerations for selecting drugs or techniques unless there is more extensive disease present (as suggested in the preceding section). The possibility of cystic lung lesions leading to pneumothorax should be considered if intubation is required. The anesthesiologist must also examine the airway for evidence of laryngeal or neck involvement, which would make intubation difficult. Muscle relaxants should be carefully monitored. Regional anesthesia is perfectly acceptable, but before administering a conduction block, an attempt should be made to elicit symptomatology and document the presence of paraspinous tumors. Epidural analgesia in labor has been successful but careful selection of patients is suggested, avoiding those with spinal cord neurofibromas (79).

Since one-third of these patients are diagnosed only by chance on routine physical examination and one-third are referred because of cosmetic problems, it is expected that the outcome in most cases of pregnant patients with neurofibromatosis will be good (80).

ACUTE IDIOPATHIC POLYNEURITIS: LANDRY-GUILLAIN-BARRÉ SYNDROME

The Landry-Guillain-Barré-Strohl syndrome (LGBS) was first described by Landry in 1859 as a neurologic disorder with ascending paralysis and later modified by specific cerebrospinal fluid (CSF) findings by Guillain, Barré, and Strohl in 1916 (81). It is an acute inflammatory, demyelinating disease with axonal degeneration of the peripheral nerves. The cause of LGBS remains unknown, but a viral etiology is possible and is linked to an aberrant immune response. The clinical profile has been well documented and the prognosis has improved. The diagnosis is based on typical clinical findings supported by the demonstration of increased protein in the CSF with a normal cell count. The rise in protein probably results from inflammation of nerve roots in the subarachnoid space. There is segmental demyelination throughout the peripheral nervous system.

The syndrome of idiopathic polyneuritis is characterized by the onset of weakness and paralysis that may evolve over days or weeks. It is usually symmetric and ascending in nature, spreading cephalad from simple paresis and impaired tendon reflexes of the lower extremities to possible bulbar symptoms with respiratory depression over a 2-week course. The patient recovers in approximately 6 months, but residual findings occur in perhaps 5% to 10% of these patients. An older review of 10 series including 425 nonobstetric patients with LGBS revealed a 21% mortality (82). While maternal deaths have been reported, improved medical management of the disease during pregnancy should make this uncommon (83, 84).

When considering a diagnosis of LGBS during pregnancy, it is important to rule out disorders with similar symptomatology, such as vitamin B complex deficiency associated with hyperemesis gravidarum, porphyria, or poisoning with lead or other heavy materials. There are no preventive measures for LGBS nor is there any cure, so treatment is symptomatic. The onset of dyspnea, cyanosis, and bronchial congestion is symptomatic of respiratory failure and possible pulmonary infection, both leading causes of maternal death in this syndrome. Improved medical support, including early diagnosis of impending respiratory failure and aggressive intervention in the more serious cases, has undoubtedly improved the outlook for these patients. A case report from UCSF demonstrating the joint efforts of the obstetric and anesthesia-intensive care team is an example of successful patient management in the potentially life-threatening situation (Fig. 30.4). Plasmapheresis may decrease the duration of mechanical ventilation and this technique has been used successfully during pregnancy without complications (85). However, plasmapheresis is not without risks and it should be reserved for more extreme cases.

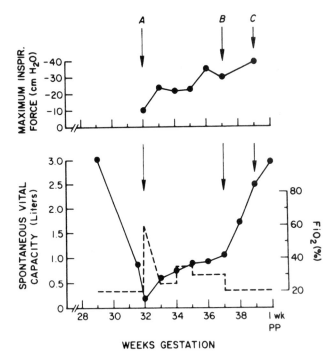

Figure 30.4. Respiratory function during late pregnancy in a patient with LGBS. **Top figure:** Maximum inspiratory force. **Lower figure:** Vital capacity (solid line). The FIo_2 is shown by the broken line. **A:** Initiation of mechanical ventilation. **B:** Cessation of mechanical ventilation. **C:** Delivery. PP, postpartum period. The rapid fall in vital capacity and decreased maximum inspiratory force (normal is 40 cm H_2O or more) necessitated ventilatory support at 32 weeks' gestation. A tracheotomy was performed and the patient was ventilated until 37 weeks' gestation with delivery of a healthy infant 2 weeks later (From Bravo RH, Katz M, Inturrisi M, et al. Obstetric management of Landry-Guillian-Barré syndrome: a case report. *Am J Obstet Gynecol* 1982;142:714–715, with permission.)

Pregnancy and Landry-Guillain-Barré-Strohl Syndrome (LGBS)

The onset of LGBS does not occur at any particular point during the pregnancy. There appears to be no direct relationship between LGBS onset or severity and pregnancy, and there is no reason to terminate a pregnancy because of the disease. The pulmonary changes in pregnancy may increase the need for ventilation. The earlier reports of maternal and perinatal mortality (>10%), indicate that these patients require expert care (86). Infants born to mothers with LGBS are normal, and there is no evidence that the disease is teratogenic. The factors involved in immunopathogenesis appear not to cross the placenta. Infant survival is at least 88% (81). The higher incidence of prematurity is probably related to the severity of the disease and the necessity for respiratory intervention, but with careful support maternal recovery and delivery of a healthy baby can be expected in most cases.

Anesthetic Management of Patients with Landry-Guillain-Barré-Strohl Syndrome

Anesthesia for patients with LGBS is controversial. If general anesthesia is required, these patients are like any patients with generalized weakness and disability. Succinylcholine should not be administered because an excessive release of potassium could result. These patients may also be more sensitive to nondepolarizing muscle relaxants. Controlled ventilation should be used, and the need to support ventilation postoperatively should be anticipated. If intravenous analgesia is considered, opioids should be used with care in LGBS patients with bulbar involvement. Autonomic nervous system dysfunction may occur, with wide fluctuations in blood pressure and heart rate (87). Serial measurements of pulmonary function may be necessary during labor and delivery when a combination of increased respiratory demands, patient position, and poor respiratory function may seriously compromise the patient.

The use of regional anesthesia is controversial. Regional anesthesia is avoided by many in patients with neurologic dysfunction, and psychoprophylaxis and local anesthesia have been recommended (88). However, several anesthesiologists from major centers have stated that regional analgesia exerted no influence on the course of chronic neurologic diseases (89). They reported on two LGBS patients given regional anesthesia without resulting problems. This opinion has been criticized, however, because of the absence of detailed information on agents, dosages, and the length of follow-up (90). Others have reported successful use of epidural analgesia for labor and for cesarean section with no complications (91, 92). The use of epidural anesthesia may be acceptable for analgesia during labor and perhaps delivery (when expulsive forces are decreased and vacuum or forceps extraction may be required), especially because the use of opioids in LGBS patients introduces the potential for respiratory depression. The use of regional anesthesia may also be possible for cesarean delivery in patients with adequate pulmonary function. However, if cesarean delivery is indicated in patients with significant bulbar involvement, a general anesthetic is more appropriate because of the potential for respiratory compromise. Aspiration prophylaxis in these patients is particularly important.

For LGBS patients particularly, pulmonary function should be carefully monitored with respiratory support at hand. The close cooperation of the obstetrician and the anesthesiologist, and appropriate intensive care support as needed, should enable the mother to deliver a healthy baby.

MULTIPLE SCLEROSIS

Multiple sclerosis (MS) is a demyelinating disease of the central nervous system characterized by multiple, random sites of demyelination in the brain and spinal cord. It is a remittent disease of young adults with exacerbation and remissions occurring over the years. The diagnosis depends on physical findings, neurologic history, and the exclusion of other neuromuscular diseases. There is no known cure for the disease; treatment includes physical therapy and symptomatic care. Steroids or other immunosuppressive therapies may shorten the length of an acute attack. It has been suggested that beta interferon may significantly reduce the relapse rate and potential disabilities (93).

MS is not a hereditary disorder, although it is more common in some families. Relatively few cases have been reported among the obstetric population. While the historical literature suggests that women with MS neither married nor had children, more recent analysis indicates otherwise and fails to demonstrate definite adverse effects of pregnancy on the long-term course of the disease. There is a tendency for remission during pregnancy and an increased frequency of multiple sclerosis exacerbation in the first 3 to 6 months after delivery (94).

The etiology of MS is unknown, but it is interesting to note the close relationship between geographic latitude and the risk of developing the disease. There is a lower incidence of the disease at the equator, for example, where the incidence may be one per 100,000 when compared to the northern temperate zones of North America and Europe, where it is one per 1,000. It is generally believed that there is a viral agent that initiates an altered immune reaction in a genetically susceptible individual.

The course of the disease is characterized by exacerbations and remissions with symptoms (depending on site of demyelination) developing over 2 to 3 days, stabilizing for several weeks, then clearing. Common symptoms include general motor weakness, ataxia, blurred vision, and bladder and bowel dysfunction. The interval between exacerbations may be several years but is unpredictable. Eventually, residual symptoms lead to profound disability. However, the young obstetric patient is often without significant permanent disability and may be in a period of remission.

Pregnancy and Multiple Sclerosis (MS)

The effect of pregnancy on the course of multiple sclerosis is ill defined but appears to have no effect on the long-term neurologic disability. Infection, fever, excessive fatigue, and emotional trauma or stress may cause relapses or exacerbations. During pregnancy, all of these conditions may occur and produce a relapse of the disease or an exacerbation in symptomatology. However, it appears that there is a slight decrease in the relapse incidence during pregnancy. In a large, prospective study of 269 pregnancies in 254 women, the rate of relapse of multiple sclerosis declined from 0.7 ± 0.9 per woman per year in the year prior to pregnancy to 0.2 ± 1.0 during the third trimester ($P < 0.001$) (Fig. 30.5). This increased in the three months postpartum to 1.2 ± 2.0 (95,96). Others also reported that the postpartum period was potentially a concern for an increased incidence of relapse (97, 98).

In summary, patients with MS may have a relapse of the disease during pregnancy, but the overall risk may actually decline during pregnancy. The postpartum period (3 to 6 months) shows an increased incidence of relapse. It is unclear whether physical, emotional, or the many physiologic, immunologic, or hormonal changes of pregnancy are responsible for the change in the disease status. Furthermore, one must keep in mind that the incidence of both MS and pregnancy is higher during the third decade of life and it is difficult to make definitive statements about their interactions.

Anesthetic Management of Patients with MS

Although surgery and anesthesia have been implicated in the exacerbation of MS, there is little evidence to support any intrinsic relationship (99). The method of delivery chosen for the preg-

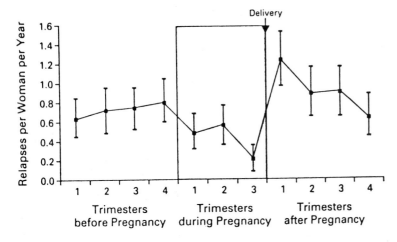

Figure 30.5. Rate of relapse per woman per year for each 3-month period before, during and after pregnancy in 227 pregnancies resulting in a live birth among women with multiple sclerosis. The values shown are means and 95% confidence intervals. The rate of relapse declined during pregnancy and increased during the first 3 months postpartum before returning to the prepregnancy rate. (From Confaveux C, Hutchinson M, Hours M, et al. Rate of pregnancy-related relapse in multiple sclerosis. *N Engl J Med* 1998;339:285–291, with permission.)

nant MS patient should be based on obstetric considerations. General anesthesia using drugs such as succinylcholine, barbiturates, opioids, and various volatile agents has been successful. In one review, in which 42 MS patients were given 88 general anesthetics, only one patient experienced an attack of the disease during the postoperative period. As a result, the rate of relapse was only 0.14 relapse per patient year (100) (Table 30.5). This compared favorably with an expected rate of approximately 0.27 relapse per patient year at that center.

Regional anesthesia has been associated with a relapse of MS, although the evidence is not strong and there are few published data. The study just mentioned reviewed seven patients given nine spinal anesthetics (100). One relapse occurred, and the authors suggested that spinal anesthesia might be best avoided in pregnant MS patients. The same authors concluded that local anesthesia (e.g., peripheral blocks) was completely safe. However, the blood–brain barrier may be impaired in these patients, resulting in a toxic response to local anesthetic at lower than expected doses (101).

There is no strong evidence that spinal or lumbar epidural anesthesia exacerbates MS, and there have been no controlled studies. Most reports are anecdotal in nature because of the small number of patients studied. In one of the few large studies, Schapira demonstrated that spinal puncture alone did not exacerbate the disease (102). In his review of 250 diagnostic spinal taps, 231 patients reported no change in their disease, 14 reported *improvement,* and only five reported deterioration of their condition. Myelography was undertaken in five of these patients with no apparent adverse effects. However, the possibility of a relapse or exacerbated symptoms resulting from the effects of spinal or epidural anesthesia cannot be ignored. The controversy historically with 2-chloroprocaine and more recently with lidocaine suggest that a local anesthetic or their additives can be neurotoxic, particularly in high concentrations (see Chapter 5). This may be a particular concern with demyelinated nerves in an MS patient.

Epidural anesthesia, however, has been used successfully for labor and delivery (89, 96, 103). In one clinical report,

the patient experienced mild MS exacerbations in the form of hypoesthesia on the inner thigh following delivery (103). Although this response lasted for several weeks, the authors concluded that the use of epidural anesthesia should not be prohibited in pregnant MS patients. Warren and Datta suggested that epidural anesthesia might be less risky than spinal anesthesia because the concentration of local anesthetic in the white matter of the spinal cord is lower—1.37 mg · kg^{-1} (spinal) versus 0.4 mg · kg^{-1} (epidural) (103). A clinical review from the same institution and representing 32 pregnancies in 20 women suggested that higher concentrations of local anesthetics may increase the relapse rate (104). The women who received epidural anesthesia for vaginal delivery did not have a higher incidence of relapse than those who received local infiltration. Among the five women who had cesarean section, one had a relapse that led the authors to be cautious concerning concentrated local anesthetics. However, the obstetric course that leads to the need for higher concentrations of local anesthetics seems the most likely cause of any increase in the incidence of relapse. In the largest review to date of 269 pregnancies in 254 women with MS, 42 parturients received epidural analgesia, which had no adverse effect on the rate of relapse or the progression of the disease (96). Although the relationship between the use of regional anesthesia and potential problems for MS patients is not well investigated, using as dilute a solution of local anesthetic as possible for lumbar epidural administration seems prudent. However, when required for cesarean section, either spinal anesthesia or epidural anesthesia may be administered.

When a general anesthetic is required, the routine sequence of thiopental, succinylcholine, N_2O/O_2, and halothane or isoflurane is suggested; opioids, diazepam, and other standard agents have also been used successfully. The earlier suggestion that sodium thiopental may have a deleterious effect on the course of MS or may cause a relapse (105) has not been substantiated (100, 106). The potential of succinylcholine-induced increased release of potassium from muscle tissue is unlikely unless there is severe neurologic deficit with muscle wasting. In the otherwise healthy patient with MS in remission, the use of succinylcholine is acceptable (38). There has been some concern about the effects of the volatile agents on the immune response and postoperative infection, but there is no evidence that immune status following surgery is affected significantly by the choice of anesthetic agent or technique.

Perhaps as important as the choice of anesthetic agent or technique is the practice of dealing openly with the pregnant MS patient, providing choice, support, and as much information as the patient can assimilate. The effects of regional anesthetic, for example, should be explained ahead of time because this resulting muscle weakness could easily be confused with exacerbation of the disease. In our practice at UCSF, a patient with MS would be offered regional anesthesia as indicated by the obstetric plan or the patient's need for analgesia.

Table 30.5. MULTIPLE SCLEROSIS AND ANESTHESIA

Number of Patients	Anesthetics	Number of MS Exacerbations
42	88 general	1
7	9 spinal	1
1	3 caudal	0
98	1,000 local	14

Adapted from Bamford C, Sibley W, Laguna J. Anesthesia in multiple sclerosis. *Can J Neurol Sci* 1978;5:41–44.

Table 30.6. PATHOGENESIS OF MYASTHENIA GRAVIS: AN AUTOIMMUNE DISORDER

A 70–90% decrease in number of acetylcholine receptors
Acetylcholine receptor IgG antibodies in 70% or more of patients
Abnormality in T-cell function responsible for abnormal
   autoimmune response
Postsynaptic membrane abnormalities
Wider clefts between nerve and muscle

MYASTHENIA GRAVIS

First described in 1672, myasthenia gravis is a chronic disease characterized by weakness and easy fatigability. It is a chronic, autoimmune disease involving the neuromuscular junction. Myasthenia gravis most often affects the oculomotor, facial, laryngeal, pharyngeal, and respiratory muscles; and the latter are of particular concern to the anesthesiologist. Patients generally recover somewhat with rest and improve with anticholinesterase therapy. Myasthenia can occur at all ages and is twice as common in females. Onset is usually in the third decade of life for women, with an overall incidence of approximately one in 19,000 to one in 40,000 (107). The disease may be totally benign or life threatening. The pathogenesis includes findings of specific abnormalities at the neuromuscular junction of striated muscle while the myometrium remains unaffected (Table 30.6), and its contractile force is unimpaired. The chief defect is a reduction in the acetylcholine receptors at the postsynaptic neuromuscular junction. The disease may be aggravated to variable extents by several factors, including infection, excitement, fatigue, loss of sleep, diet, and alcohol use. Furthermore, menstruation or pregnancy may cause an exacerbation of myasthenia gravis in many patients.

Pregnancy and Myasthenia Gravis

In a series of 225 myasthenia gravis patients with 322 pregnancies, it was noted that 28.6% experienced remissions, 41% a relapse of their condition, and 29% experienced postpartum exacerbation of the disease (108, 109). Other studies have also reported similar changes in symptomatology (110, 111). In addition, the experience of previous pregnancy was not found to be helpful in predicting the course of subsequent pregnancies. It has been suggested that altered hormonal relationships during pregnancy may cause a relapse of the disease (112). However, neither the administration of birth control pills nor estrogen therapy appears to benefit the myasthenic patient. In addition, the incidence of exacerbations is high (30%) in the postpartum period when hormonal changes are normalizing (108, 109). In summary, the course of the disease during pregnancy, labor, and delivery is highly variable and unpredictable, and requires the careful attention of the obstetric team. A maternal mortality rate of 4% has been reported, however (108). The patient's presentation may vary from benign to full-blown myasthenic crisis (too little anticholinesterase) or cholinergic crisis (too much anticholinesterase). A cholinergic crisis may be associated with excessive tearing, hypersalivation, bradycardia, sweating, abdominal cramping, and diarrhea. A "nonreactive crisis" has been reported and results from the sudden development of refractoriness to antiacetylcholinesterase medications. This may have been related to the administration of betamethasone (113). The correct diagnosis is imperative for acute management.

EDROPHONIUM TEST

Edrophonium chloride (Tensilon) is very similar in action to neostigmine but shorter acting. Both are anticholinesterases and are quaternary ammonium compounds that do not cross the blood–brain barrier. Consequently, there is minimal placental transfer of these compounds (114). When given intravenously, edrophonium chloride can rapidly demonstrate the presence of myasthenia gravis. Even if it exacerbates the condition (cholinergic crisis), this effect is short lasting (115). The patient's muscle strength should first be assessed by vital capacity, grip strength, or other objective methods so that changes may be noted and the patient should be pretreated with atropine 0.6 mg. Next, 1 to 2 mg of edrophonium chloride should be administered intravenously, and if there is no deterioration in symptoms, a further dose of 8 mg may be given (total 10 mg). If inadequately treated, the patient will have a rapid increase in muscle strength (myasthenic crisis) and if there is no improvement or deterioration of muscle strength, the diagnosis of cholinergic crisis is made.

Intravenous neostigmine methylsulfate has also been used as a test, but it is slower in onset and longer in duration. This test must be performed with equipment for respiratory intervention at hand because fatalities have occurred. It has been suggested that uterine cholinergic receptors may be affected by intravenous anticholinesterase therapy, resulting in increased uterine tone and an increased incidence of abortions and possibly premature labor. Although reported results vary, intravenous drug therapy should nevertheless be considered carefully during pregnancy.

Labor and Delivery

The factors previously mentioned that affect the course of myasthenia gravis may be present during labor. They include emotional stress, physical exertion, minor infections, and fatigue. However, the disease does not affect labor itself; the use of outlet forceps may shorten the second stage of labor and avoid fatigue. The first stage of labor is unaffected because the uterus is nonstriated muscle. The cesarean section rate is not increased in these patients. However, problems may result from pharmacologic intervention during labor and delivery. For example, aminoglycosides, kanamycin, and gentamicin reportedly exacerbate the symptoms of myasthenia gravis by presynaptic block (116). Magnesium sulfate, commonly used in the treatment of pregnancy-induced hypertension, may produce a neuromuscular block in the myasthenic patient, resulting in respiratory insufficiency (117). The use of magnesium sulfate is therefore best avoided in these patients.

Anesthetic Management of Patients with Myasthenia Gravis

Preanesthetic assessment of a patient with myasthenia gravis ideally begins with a visit by the anesthesiologist before labor. A formal consultation when the patient is near term might be appropriate to evaluate the patient and the extent of her illness. The laboratory work required to evaluate these patients is more extensive than that usually performed, as is the history taking and physical examination for myasthenic symptoms (Table 30.7). Bulbar weakness, for example, may lead to nutritional

Table 30.7. SUGGESTED PREOPERATIVE ASSESSMENT IN MYASTHENIA GRAVIS

Assess extent of respiratory or bulbar involvement.
Determine frequency and severity of myasthenic attacks.
Note type and dosage of anticholinesterase and other drugs.
Consider pulmonary function test.
Conduct laboratory studies: Complete blood cell count, electrolytes,
   serum protein, electrocardiogram, and chest radiographic series

Table 30.8. TREATMENT OF MYASTHENIA GRAVIS

Anticholinesterase therapy

Thymectomy in younger patients (improvement in 57–86% of patients; drug-free remission in approximately 33%)

Corticosteroids for immunosuppressive actions (improvement in 70–100% of patients)

Azathioprine (improvement in 45% of patients)

Cyclosporine, cyclophosphamide (immunosuppressive)

Plasmapheresis (improvement in 45% of patients but of short duration)

compromise and abnormalities of hemoglobin, serum electrolytes, or protein. Because focal necrosis of the myocardium has been reported, an ECG is recommended (118, 119). Recently performed pulmonary function tests help to determine the extent of the disease and efficacy of therapy and provide information valuable for managing possible respiratory insufficiency. Clearly, the anesthetic management of patients with myasthenia gravis must be based on careful preanesthetic assessment and tailored to the particular obstetric situation.

Anticholinesterase therapy is the mainstay of treatment for myasthenic patients and should be adjusted to provide optimal symptomatic relief before labor. Other therapeutic modalities are often helpful in more difficult cases (Table 30.8). Plasmapheresis may be helpful but the benefits are of short duration (120, 121). Azathioprine may be useful but it is ideally avoided in pregnancy because of possible *teratogenicity*. Anticholinesterase therapy must be maintained during labor and constantly reevaluated. Because gastric uptake is unreliable during labor and delivery, it is recommended that the patient's routine oral dose be converted to the equivalent intramuscular dose (Table 30.9). Physostigmine is not used because it crosses the blood–brain barrier and causes stimulation. Pyridostigmine is preferred since the muscarinic side effects are less.

The postpartum period may also be hazardous. Plausche reported that approximately 30% of pregnant myasthenic patients have exacerbated symptoms during this period (108). Thus, the patient should be monitored postpartum with adjustment of anticholinesterase therapy as needed (122). Breast-feeding is probably not a risk to the mother, provided she is well rested and may be safe for the neonate because anticholinesterase drugs are not transmitted in detectable amounts in breast milk (123).

ANESTHESIA FOR VAGINAL DELIVERY

Traditional intravenous analgesia and sedation with opioids and tranquilizers must be used cautiously in myasthenic patients, particularly if there is respiratory or bulbar involvement. It is recommended that these drugs be administered in less than the usual doses to avoid retention of secretions and respiratory depression. Many clinicians recommend the use of regional anesthesia for vaginal delivery of myasthenic patients (111, 115, 122–125).

Whether administered as a CSE or routine continuous epidural, regional anesthesia provides pain relief with minimal or no systemic medication, prevents fatigue, and allows for the use of

Table 30.9. COMMONLY USED ANTICHOLINESTERASE DRUGS AND EQUIVALENT DOSES

Drug	IV Dose (mg)	IM Dose (mg)	Oral Dose (mg)
Neostigmine (Prostigmine)	0.5	0.7–1.0	15.0
Pyridostigmine (Mestinon)	2.0	3.0–4.0	60.0

outlet forceps (when necessary) to shorten the second stage of labor. Although high blood levels of local anesthetics may interfere with neuromuscular transmission, this is unlikely to be a clinical problem. The levels required to alter neuromuscular transmission (in animal models) are toxic, and despite the pathology of the myasthenic patient's neuromuscular junction, there is no evidence of an altered response to local anesthetics in these patients (126).

2-chloroprocaine, an ester-type local anesthetic metabolized by plasma cholinesterase, is not recommended for epidural anesthesia in a myasthenic patient receiving anticholinesterase therapy (122). For patients receiving anticholinesterase therapy, plasma cholinesterase activity is significantly decreased, which increases the risk of anesthetic overdose or toxicity (127). Amide local anesthetics may be more appropriate because their metabolism is unaltered. There appears to be no contraindication to intraspinal opioids, although particular attention to monitoring of respiratory function in the patient with bulbar involvement is suggested (see Chapter 9). When general anesthesia is required for vaginal delivery, the anesthesiologist must perform a rapid-sequence induction with immediate intubation because of the possibility of a full stomach. In a severely compromised myasthenic patient, intubation may be accomplished with thiopental alone, although a muscle relaxant is often also required. Propofol has been used as an induction agent in obstetric patients with myasthenia gravis (128). Because these patients are especially sensitive to nondepolarizing agents, the onset of muscle relaxation is rapid and can be obtained with 2 to 3 mg of curare (129). Because the redistribution and excretion of curare is unaltered by the disease, the duration of effect is the same as that in normal patients. However, use of small doses of rocuronium, vecuronium, or other muscle relaxants with a short half-life is recommended (130).

Intubation can be equally well accomplished using succinylcholine (30 to 50 mg), but anticholinesterase therapy prolongs the duration of succinylcholine effects for as much as 90 minutes. According to some experts, the response to succinylcholine is unpredictable, and it is claimed that some patients may be resistant to succinylcholine (38). Once intubation is complete, ventilation should be controlled and any of the volatile inhalation agents may be used (if necessary) to relax the uterus or to supplement N_2O and O_2 until delivery is accomplished.

ANESTHESIA FOR CESAREAN DELIVERY

Either regional or general anesthesia can be used for cesarean delivery, provided careful attention is given to the extent of respiratory involvement. If the patient presents with only ocular myasthenia or minimal disease with no anticholinesterase therapy, anesthetic management is relatively routine. However, if there is bulbar or respiratory muscle movement, general anesthesia with endotracheal intubation is more appropriate, unless the disease is well controlled with anticholinesterase therapy. Even then, careful consideration should be given to the combined effects of a high motor block, use of intraspinal opioids, and preexisting respiratory problems in these patients.

During general anesthesia, the use of muscle relaxants in the myasthenic patient is usually unnecessary and best avoided. If a small dose of a short-acting agent is used to facilitate endotracheal intubation, it will probably suffice for the surgery as well. If further relaxation is needed, a small dose of an intermediate or short-acting muscle relaxant in incremental doses is recommended, with careful monitoring of the response (122, 130). In myasthenic patients undergoing thymectomy, Baraka and Dajani (131) used atracurium (0.09 to 0.21 $mg \cdot kg^{-1}$) and achieved 75% to 90% neuromuscular block. The newer nondepolarizing short-acting drugs have proved very useful (130). Reversal of nondepolarizing muscle relaxants can be accomplished with incremental doses of neostigmine (0.5 mg) or pyridostigmine (1 mg) with the response monitored by a nerve stimulator. If the patient's disease was well controlled before surgery, extubation should be expected without complications. However, this is not always possible and pulmonary function tests preoperatively may help predict the success of extubation (132).

In the postoperative period, the patient must be monitored very carefully for 48 hours. The anticholinesterase requirements may vary, and repeated evaluation (including measurements of vital capacity) is suggested. Adequate ventilatory support, endotracheal suctioning, and chest physical therapy must be readily available. If a regional anesthetic has been used, postoperative administration of epidural morphine may provide pain relief uncomplicated by the significant sedation and respiratory depression that might result from larger doses of intramuscular or intravenous opioids. The catheter could be left in place for 24 hours, or longer if needed, to facilitate pain management. Intrathecal morphine (0.1 to 0.25 mg) is also very effective and may provide adequate analgesia for 12 to 24 hours (132).

Neonatal Myasthenia Gravis

Neonatal myasthenia gravis is a transient disease occurring in approximately 12% of the infants born to mothers with myasthenia gravis (133). It usually presents with generalized muscle weakness, weak reflexes, and respiratory distress and is probably caused by placental transfer of maternal antibodies (134). Although 80% of these cases appear within the first 24 hours of life, neonatal myasthenia can occur up to 4 days after birth (2). Placental transfer of maternal anticholinesterases may explain the delayed onset. The infant who has not become symptomatic by the fourth day postpartum may be allowed to leave the hospital. If the condition is suspected, it can be diagnosed by rapid improvement in movement and crying following an intramuscular injection of 0.5 to 1 mg of edrophonium.

The anesthesiologist or an appropriate staff member must be prepared to intervene in the delivery room if the respiratory status of the infant is inadequate. The previous delivery of a healthy infant by a myasthenic mother does not preclude the birth of an infant with neonatal myasthenia gravis on a subsequent delivery. A perinatal mortality of approximately 68 per 1,000 live births has been reported (108). The obstetric team must always be prepared to diagnose and treat the problem. Approximately 80% of infants with neonatal myasthenia gravis require anticholinesterase therapy, but the disease spontaneously clears within 2 to 4 weeks (133, 135) (Table 30.10). The goal in treating these infants is to allow feeding and breathing without producing a vigorous cry or strong, active movement, for fear of invoking cholinergic weakness requiring further inter-

vention with atropine. As the infant's strength improves, anticholinesterase therapy should be tapered off and the length of the interval between treatments increased. Complete recovery can be expected.

SPINAL CORD INJURY: PARAPLEGIA AND QUADRIPLEGIA

Spinal cord transection is most commonly caused by trauma and results in either paralysis of the lower extremities (paraplegia) or of all four extremities (quadriplegia). Extensive cord damage from infection, tumors, or vascular lesions may also cause permanent spinal cord damage and create similar chronic problems (136). In the United States, approximately 11,000 new spinal cord injuries are reported each year and 50% occur in persons between 15 and 25 years of age. Women represent 15% of cases (3). Effective rehabilitation and modern reproductive technology is likely to increase the number of these patients considering pregnancy. Thus, the anesthesiologist will need to consider the specific problems of pregnancy, labor and delivery in these women (137).

Acute transection of the spinal cord produces a flaccid paralysis and loss of sensation below the lesion. The initial phase characterized by hypotension, bradycardia, and the potential ECG abnormalities indicative of myocardial damage, lasts for 2 to 3 weeks and requires careful medical attention. Amenorrhea lasting for 3 to 9 months following spinal cord injury is common (138). The chronic state that follows the injury is characterized by potential muscle rigidity and spasm, as well as anemia and recurrent urinary infections, especially during pregnancy. The risk of a stillbirth or fetal abnormality appears to be increased for the women who suffer spinal cord injury during pregnancy (139).

Autonomic Hyperreflexia: Mass Reflex

This reflex was first described in 1917 by Head and Riddoch and consists of pilomotor erection, excessive sweating, facial flushing, dilated pupils, severe headache, bradycardia, and severe paroxysmal hypertension (140). Increased blood pressure can result in loss of consciousness and convulsions if the stimulus is not removed, and retinal as well as fatal cerebral or subarachnoid hemorrhages have been reported (141). The syndrome appears not to occur if the lesion is below T7 but occurs in over 85% of patients with a cord injury above this level (142, 143).

Autonomic hyperreflexia is the result of afferent impulses entering the isolated cord and initiating focal segmental reflexes that are neither modulated nor inhibited by higher centers (144, 145). Stimulation of the skin below the cord lesion, bladder distension, fecal impaction, rectal examination, genital stimulation, or contraction of a hollow viscus including the gut and uterus may bring about a massive stimulation of the sympathetic nervous system. The isolated adrenal glands receive their sympathetic nerve supply from the greater splanchnic nerve (T5 to T9) and may be partially responsible for the response. However, Debarge and co-workers (146) concluded that the response was more likely caused by norepinephrine from the adrenergic sympathetic nerve endings than by any direct outflow from the adrenal glands. They also suggest that the pressor response to similar doses of catecholamines was greater in quadriplegic patients than in normal control subjects, which helps to explain the severe hypertension resulting from relatively minimal stimulation in some cases. Regardless of the cause, the body's only defense mechanism for uncontrolled paroxysmal hypertension is vagally mediated bradycardia resulting from stimulation of carotid sinus baroreceptors and aortic arch receptors (Fig. 30.6) (147). During uterine contractions, premature ventricular beats, ventricular bigeminy, atrioventricular nodal block, and prominent U waves have been observed (2).

A further concern for the anesthesiologist is the risk of hyperkalemia resulting from the administration of succinylcholine in

Table 30.10. ANTICHOLINESTERASE DRUGS IN NEONATAL MYASTHENIA GRAVIS

Drug	Dosage
Diagnosis	
Edrophonium (Tensilon)—for rapid diagnosis	0.5–1 mg IV
Neostigmine (Prostigmine)	0.1–0.2 mg IM
Treatment	
Pyridostigmine	1 mg · kg^{-1} PO syrup or tablets q 3–4 hr
Neostigmine	0.3 mg · kg^{-1} PO; 0.05–0.25 mg IM q 2–4
Atropine	0.025–0.05 mg sc

Therapy for neonatal myasthenia gravis must be titrated to the symptomatic response of the newborn once the diagnosis is made. Adapted from Rudolph AM, Hoffman JIE, Rudolph CD, eds, *Pediatrics*, 20th ed. Norwalk, CT: Appleton & Lange 1996:1975–1976.

Autonomic Hyperreflexia

uterine contractions
(hollow viscus distension)

⬇

reflex sympathetic discharge
with no supraspinal modification

⬇

autonomic hyperreflexia with hypertension,
and stimulation of aortic arch receptors and
carotid sinus baroreceptors resulting in

⬇

increased vagal discharge to SA node
and bradycardia

Figure 30.6. Etiology and signs of an autonomic hyperreflexic response.

these patients. The hyperkalemic response may occur with many neuromuscular diseases, as well as with massive trauma or crush or burn injuries (148). The risk is not great during the first few hours following cord damage, but the administration of a depolarizing muscle relaxant may be hazardous for up to 6 months or more following the injury, and it is best to avoid succinylcholine if there is any question. The degree of hyperkalemia resulting from the administration of succinylcholine to a patient with recent central nervous system damage can be catastrophic (Table 30.11). The short-acting nondepolarizing agents, vecuronium, atracurium, rocuronium and others obviate this problem.

Labor and Delivery

In 1872, Sir James Simpson demonstrated normal parturition in swine after removal of the thoracic and lumbar cord (149). Cord damage per se is not an indication for cesarean delivery, and a vaginal delivery can be expected unless there is an obstetric reason to indicate otherwise. In a review of 39 deliveries of 26 paraplegic women, 21 had normal vaginal deliveries, 15 forceps deliveries, and only three cesarean deliveries (149). The relatively high rate of forceps deliveries was undoubtedly due to the paralysis of musculature responsible for the expulsive forces. In a more recent review of 52 pregnancies in women with spinal cord injuries, the cesarean section delivery rate was 47% for women with a lesion above T5 and 26% for women with a lesion below that level (150). Preterm labor occurred in 19% of the women. Autonomic hyperreflexia occurred in nine of 12 women with a spinal cord lesion above the T5 level.

With complete cord transection above the T10 level, a painless labor can be expected. However, if cord damage is incomplete or below this level, painful labor may result. If cord damage is above the T10 level, there is also an increased incidence of premature labor that may not be appreciated by the patient. Weekly examination in the third trimester of pregnancy is recommended (es-

Table 30.11. HYPERKALEMIA AFTER ADMINISTRATION OF SUCCINYLCHOLINE (60 MG IV)

Time (min)	K⁺	Electrocardiogram
1	3.88	Normal Sinus rhythm
3	8.93	↑↑T waves and
5	9.05	Wide QRS

Electrocardiographic and plasma potassium changes following 60 mg IV succinylcholine in a patient with recent onset of hemiparesis. Adapted from Cooperman LH, Strobel GE, Kennel EM. Massive hyperkalemia after administration of succinylcholine. *Anesthesiology* 1970;32:161–164.

Table 30.12. MEDICAL COMPLICATIONS OF SPINAL CORD INJURY AGGRAVATED BY PREGNANCY

Pulmonary
  Decreased respiratory reserve
  Atelectasis and pneumonia
  Impaired cough
Hematologic
  Anemia
  Thromboembolic phenomenon
Urogenital
  Chronic urinary tract infection
  Proteinuria
  Renal insufficiency
  Urinary tract calculi
Dermatologic
  Decubitus ulcers
Cardiovascular
  Hypotension
Autonomic hyperreflexia

From Crosby ET, St-Jean B, Reid D, et al. Obstetrical anaesthesia and analgesia in chronic spinal cord–injured women. *Can J Anaesth* 1992; 39:487–494.

pecially in multigravidas) to detect cervical changes indicative of the onset of labor (151). Uterine contractions can stimulate autonomic hyperreflexia and this must be considered in management for labor and delivery. Many of the numerous medical complications of spinal cord injuries are aggravated by pregnancy (Table 30.12).

Anesthetic Management of Patients with Spinal Cord Transection

Depending on the level of the cord lesion, analgesia for labor and delivery per se is probably rarely required for these patients. The general medical condition of the patient and the extent of cord damage must first be evaluated. A history of increased blood pressure with urinary retention, for example, should alert the health care team to the possible presence of autonomic hyperreflexia.

For control of autonomic hyperreflexia in any patient with a T7 level injury or higher, epidural anesthesia should be considered. The ability of epidural analgesia to block autonomic

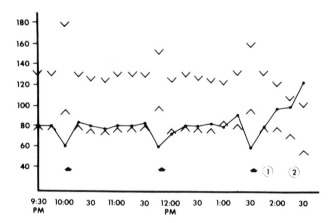

Figure 30.7. Epidural anesthesia and autonomic hyperreflexia: the vital signs of a 24-year-old paraplegic (T4 level) woman in labor showing the response to bupivacaine 0.25% via an epidural catheter. Δ, diastolic pressure; ∇, systolic pressure; ●, pulse rate; ↑, epidural injection of 0.25% bupivacaine; 1, first twin delivered; 2, second twin delivered. (Adapted from Watson DW, Downey GO. Epidural anesthesia for labor and delivery of twins of a paraplegic mother. *Anesthesiology* 1980;52:259–261.)

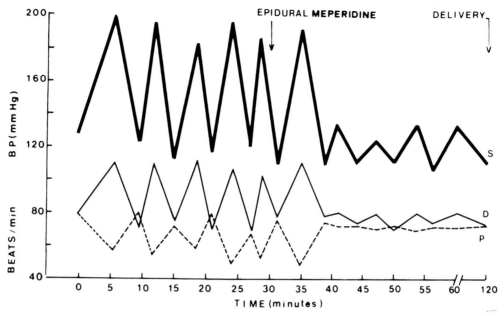

Figure 30.8. Epidural meperidine and autonomic hyperreflexia. A graphic recording of blood pressure and heart rate changes before and after administration of epidural meperidine. S, systolic blood pressure; D, diastolic blood pressure; P, heart rate. (From Baraka A. Epidural meperidine for control of autonomic hyperreflexia in a paraplegic parturient. *Anesthesiology* 1985;62:688–690, with permission.)

hyperreflexia is well established but seems to be regularly overlooked by some (152–155). Although spinal anesthetics provide adequate anesthesia, administering a continuous epidural anesthetic offers more flexibility. Stirt and co-workers (145) reported effective control of autonomic hyperreflexia during labor using epidural anesthesia in a quadriplegic patient. Eight hours after the onset of labor, the patient experienced facial flushing, apprehension, and diaphoresis, and her blood pressure increased to 220/110 with a contraction. An epidural anesthetic was administered to modify or block this response and a healthy newborn was later delivered with forceps.

A similar course was undertaken in the delivery of twins from a paraplegic mother; in this case, 0.25% bupivacaine was effective in blocking autonomic hyperreflexia (Fig. 30.7) (147). In another case, in which the use of sodium nitroprusside to control blood pressure during evacuation of a dead fetus was attempted, it became necessary to administer a continuous epidural block to control wide swings in the patient's blood pressure (155). Clearly, when considering the use of sodium nitroprusside in these patients, placental transfer of the drug, as well as difficulty in titrating the dose and potential toxicity, must be carefully evaluated (156). The success of regional anesthesia in controlling autonomic hyperreflexia and providing extended anesthesia for

pregnant cord-injured patients makes it the clear choice (4, 145, 147, 153, 155, 157, 158). A case report suggested that epidural meperidine may be useful as well (Fig. 30.8) (159). However, epidural fentanyl was not entirely successful in blocking autonomic hyperreflexia in another case report (160). Meperidine's success is related to its local anesthetic properties and this author suggests the use of routine local anesthetics.

A regional anesthetic (either spinal or epidural) is also appropriate for cesarean delivery (158). One author has suggested that general anesthesia can be used to control blood pressure in cord-injured patients during general surgery (161). However, the depth of anesthesia required to achieve this, the uterine atony induced by the use of volatile inhalation agents, and the requisite use of significant intravenous agents that profoundly affect the newborn make general anesthesia a less desirable choice for these patients (Table 30.13). Nevertheless, if general anesthesia is to be used for a cesarean delivery, a rapid-sequence intubation with cricoid pressure can be accomplished using a short-acting nondepolarizing agent to facilitate intubation. The latter is necessary if the cord injury is more recent than 6 months to 1 year. Although the general anesthetic will provide unconsciousness and amnesia, a regional anesthetic should also be used to block autonomic hyperreflexia.

Table 30.13. ANESTHESIA AND THE CONTROL OF BLOOD PRESSURE IN PATIENTS WITH SPINAL CORD INJURY

Group (N)	Anesthetic Technique	Preanesthesia Systolic Blood Pressure (mm Hg)	Intraoperative Systolic Blood Pressure (mm Hg)	Significance (*P*)
A (19)	Topical anesthesia sedation, or no anesthesia	135 ± 20	172 ± 44	<0.005
B (13)	General anesthesia	110 ± 13	107 ± 34	<0.8
C (46)	Spinal anesthesia	117 ± 19	103 ± 21	<0.001

Values are means ± SD. Preanesthetic systolic blood pressure: A vs. B, $P < 0.001$; A vs. C, $P < 0.005$; B vs. C, $P < 0.3$. Intraoperative systolic blood pressure: A vs. B $P < 0.001$; A vs. C, $P < 0.001$; B vs. C, $P < 0.7$. Both general anesthesia and spinal anesthesia effectively controlled blood pressure change in patients at risk for autonomic hyperreflexia. From Lambert DH, Deane RS, Mazuzan JE. Anesthesia and the control of blood pressure in patients with spinal cord injury. *Anesth Analg* 1982;61:344–348.

REFERENCES

1. Abouleish E. Neurologic disease. In: James FM, Wheeler AS, eds. *Obstetric Anesthesia: the Complicated Patient.* Philadelphia: Davis, 1982:57–86.
2. Donaldson JO. *Neurology of Pregnancy.* Philadelphia: Saunders, 1978.
3. American College of Obstetricians & Gynecologists (ACOG). Obstetric management of patients with spinal cord injury (ACOG Committee opinion no. 121). *Int J Obstet Gynecol* 1993; 42:206.
4. Hambly PR, Martin B. Anaesthesia for chronic spinal cord lesions. *Anaesthesia* 1998;53:273–289.
5. Chitayat D, Etchell M, Wilson D. Cold-induced abortion in paramyotonia congenita. *Am J Obstet Gynecol* 1988;158:435–436.
6. Barchi RL. Myotonia. An evaluation of the chloride hypothesis. *Arch Neurol* 1975;32:175–180.
7. Hakim A, Thomlinson J. Myotonia congenita in pregnancy. *J Obstet Gynaecol Br Commonw* 1969;76:561–562.
8. Hageman ATM, Gabréls FJ, Liem KD, et al. Congenital myotonic dystrophy; a report on thirteen cases and a review of the literature. *J Neurosci* 1993;115:95.
9. Harper PS. Myotonic dystrophy in infancy and childhood. In: *Myotonic Dystrophy.* London: WB Saunders, 1989:195.BL
10. Harper PS. The genetic basis of myotonic dystrophy. In: *Myotonic dystrophy.* London: WB Saunders, 1989:318.
11. Chutorian AB, Koenigsberger R. The muscular dystrophies. In: Kelley UC, ed. *Brenneman's Practice of Pediatrics.* Hagerstown, MD: Harper & Row, 1971:6–10.
12. Harvey JC, Sherbourne DH, Siegel CI. Smooth muscle involvement in myotonic dystrophy. *Am J Med* 1965;39:81–90.
13. Sarnat HB, O'Connor T, Byrne PA. Clinical effects of myotonic dystrophy on pregnancy and the neonate. *Arch Neurol* 1976;33:459–465.
14. Jaffe R, Mock M, Abromowicz J, et al. Myotonic dystrophy and pregnancy: a review. *Obstet Gynecol Surv* 1986;41:272.
15. Sun SF, Binder J, Streib E, et al. Myotonic dystrophy: obstetric and neonatal complications. *South Med J* 1985;78:823.
16. Walpole AR, Ross AW. Acute cord prolapse in an obstetric patient with myotonic dystrophica. *Anaesth Intensive Care* 1992;20:526.
17. Russell SH, Hirsch NP. Anaesthesia and myotonia. *Br J Anaesth* 1994; 72:210–216.
18. Gardy HH. Dystrophia myotonica in pregnancy: report of a case. *Obstet Gynecol* 1963;21:441–445.
19. Gilchrist JM. Muscle disease in the pregnant woman. In: Devinsky O, Feldman E, Hainline B, eds. *Neurological Complications of Pregnancy.* New York: Raven Press, 1994:193.
20. Hopkins A, Wray S. The effect of pregnancy on dystrophia myotonica. *Neurology* 1967;17:166–168.
21. Dunn LJ, Dierker LJ. Recurrent hydramnios in association with myotoneia dystrophica. *Obstet Gyencol* 1973;42:104–106.
22. Sholl JS, Hughey MJ, Hirschmann RA. Myotonic muscular dystrophy associated with ritodrine tocolysis. *Am J Obstet Gynecol* 1985; 151:83–86.
23. Streib EW, Sun SF. Myotonic muscular dystrophy associated with ritodrine tocolysis. *Am J Obstet Gynecol* 1985;153:593.
24. Perlof JK, Stevenson WG, Roberts NK, et al. Cardiac involvement in myotonic dystrophy (Steinert's disease): a prospective study of 225 patients. *Am J Cardiol* 1984;54:1074–1081.
25. Mitchell MM, Ali HH, Savarese JJ. Myotonia and neuromuscular blocking agents. *Anesthesiology* 1978;49:44–48.
26. Dundee JW. Thiopentone in dystrophica myotonica. *Anesth Analg* 1952;31:257–262.
27. Wheeler AS, James FM. Local anesthesia for laparoscopy in a case of myotonia dystrophia [Letter]. *Anesthesiology* 1979;50:169.
28. Kaufman L. Anaesthesia in dystrophia myotonica (abridged): a review of the hazards of anaesthesia. *Proc R Soc Med* 1960;53:183–188.
29. Harris MN. Extradural anesthesia and dystrophia myotonia. *Anaesthesia* 1984;39:1032–1033.
30. Cope DK, Miller JN. Local and spinal anesthesia for cesarean section in a patient with myotonic dystrophy. *Anesth Analg* 1986;65:687–690.
31. Patterson RA, Tousignant M, Skene DS. Cesarean section for twins in a patient with myotonic dystrophy. *Can Anaesth Soc J* 1985;32:418–421.
32. Camann WR, Johnson MD. Anesthesia management of a parturient with myotonia dystrophia: a case report. *Reg Anesth* 1990;15:41–43.
33. O'Connor PJ, Caldicott LD, Braithwaite P. Urgent caesarean section with a patient with myotonic dystrophy: A case report and review. *Int J Obstet Anesth* 1996;5:272.
34. Driver IK, Broadway JW. Dystrophia myotonica: Combined spinal-epidural anaesthesia for caesarean section. *Int J Obstet Anesth* 1996;5:275.
35. Campbell AM, Thompson N. Anaesthesia for Caesarean section in a patient with myotonic dystrophy receiving warfarin therapy. *Can J Anaesth* 1995;42:409.
36. Stevens JD, Wauchob TD. Dystrophia myotonica—emergency caesarean section with spinal anesthesia. *Eur J Anaesthesiol* 1991;8:305.
37. Pollard BJ, Young TM. Anaesthesia in myotonia dystrophica. *Anaesthesia* 1989;44:699.
38. Azar I. The response of patients with neuromuscular disorders to the muscle relaxants: a review. *Anesthesiology* 1984;61:173–187.
39. Mudge BJ, Taylor PB, Vanderspek AFL. Perioperative hazards in myotonic dystrophy. *Anaesthesia* 1980;35:492–495.
40. White DA, Smyth DG. Continuous infusion of propofol in dystrophia myotonica. *Can J Anaesth* 1989;36:200.
41. Speedy H. Exaggerated responses to propofol in myotonic dystrophy. *Br J Anaesth* 1990;64:110–112.
42. Hook R, Anderson EF, Noto P. Anesthetic management of a parturient with myotonia atrophica. *Anesthesiology* 1975;43:689–692.
43. Dichter MA. The epilepsies and convulsive disorders. In: Petersdorf RG, Adams RD, Braunwald E, et al., eds. *Harrison's Principles of Internal Medicine,* 10th ed. New York: McGraw-Hill, 1983:2018–2028.
44. Schuster A. Seizures in pregnancy: emergency medicine. *Emerg Med Clin North Am* 1994;12:1013–1015.
45. Bjerkedal T, Bahna SL. The course and outcome of pregnancy in women with epilepsy. *Acta Obstet Gynecol Scand* 1973;52:245–248.
46. Hiilsmaa VK, Bardy A, Teramo K. Obstetric outcome in women with epilepsy. *Am J Obstet Gynecol* 1985;152:499–504.
47. Sabers A, a'Rogvi-Hansen B, Dam M, et al. Pregnancy and epilepsy: a retrospective study of 151 pregnancies. *Acta Neurol Scand* 1998;97:164–170.
48. Hopkins A. Neurological disorders. *Clin Obstet Gynecol* 1977;4:419–433.
49. Knight AH, Rhind EG. Epilepsy and pregnancy: a study of 153 pregnancies in 59 patients. *Epilepsia* 1975;16:99–110.
50. Bardy AH. Incidence of seizures during pregnancy, labor and peurperium in epileptic women: A prospective study. *Acta Neurol Scand* 1987;75:356–363.
51. Mygind KI, Mogens D, Christiansen J. Phenytoin and phenobarbitone plasma clearance during pregnancy. *Acta Neurol Scand* 1976;54:160–166.
52. Lander CM, Edwards VE, Eadie MJ, et al. Plasma anticonvulsant concentrations during pregnancy. *Neurology* 1977;27:128–131.
53. Laidlaw JL, Richens A. *A Textbook of Epilepsy.* London: Churchill Livingstone, 1976.
54. Coleman MT, Rund DA. Nonobstetric conditions causing hypoxia during pregnancy: Asthma and epilepsy. *Am J Obstet Gynecol* 1997;177:1–7.
55. Gilmore J, Pennell PP, Stern BJ. Medication used during pregnancy for neurologic conditions. *Neurol Clin North Am* 1998;16:189–206.
56. Donaldson JO. Neurologic emergencies in pregnancy. *Obstet Gynecol Clin North Am* 1991;18:199–212.
57. Melchior JC, Svensmark O, Trolle D. Placental transfer of phenobarbitone in epileptic women and elimination in newborns. *Lancet* 1967;2:860–861.
58. Solomon GE, Hilgartner MW, Kutt H. Coagulation defects caused by phenobarbitol and primidone. *Neurology* 1973;23:445–451.
59. Van Dyke RA. Metabolism of volatile anesthetics. III. Induction of microsomal dechlorinating and ether-cleaving enzymes. *J Pharmacol Exp Ther* 1966;154:364–369.
60. Bohm E, Flodmark S, Ptersen I. Effect of lidocaine (Xylocaine) on seizure and interseizure electroencephalograms in epileptics. *Arch Neurol Psychiatry* 1959;81:550–556.
61. Harrah HD, Way WL, Katzung BG. The interaction of d-tubocurarine with antiarrhythmic drugs. *Anesthesiology* 1970;33:406–410.
62. Evans DEN. Anesthesia and the epileptic patient: a review. *Anaesthesia* 1975;30:34–45.
63. Komatsu H, Tsaie S, Endo S, et al. Electrical seizures during sevoflorane anesthesia in two pediatric patients with epilepsy. *Anesthesiology* 1994;81:535–537.
64. Roizen MF. Anesthetic implications of concurrent diseases. In: Miller R, ed. *Anesthesia.* New York: Churchill Livingstone, 2000:969–974.

65. Oshima E, Urabe N, Shingu K, et al. Anticonvulsant actions of enflurane on epilepsy models in cats. *Anesthesiology* 1985;63:29–40.

66. Adams RP, DeLong GR. Developmental and other congenital abnormalities of the nervous system. In: Petersdorf RG, Adams RD, Braunwald E, et al., eds. *Harrison's Principles of Internal Medicine,* 10th ed. New York: McGraw-Hill, 1983:2133–2142.

67. Hudson SM. Recent developments in the diagnosis and development of neurofibromatosis. *Arch Dis Child* 1989;64:745.

68. DeFalque RJ, Musunuru VS. Diseases of the nervous system. In: Stoelting AK, Dierdorf SF, eds. *Anesthesia and Co-existing Disease.* New York: Churchill Livingstone, 1983:314–316.

69. Swapp GH, Main RA. Neurofibromatosis in pregnancy. *Br J Dermatol* 1973;88:431–435.

70. Sharma JB, Gulati N, Malik S. Maternal and perinatal complications in neurofibromatosis during pregnancy. *Int J Obstet Anesth* 1991;34:221.

71. Blum K, Kambich M. Maternal genetic disease and pregnancy. *Clin Perinatol* 1997;24:251–265.

72. Brady DB, Bolan JC. Neurofibromatosis and spontaneous hemothorax in pregnancy: two case reports. *Obstet Gynecol* 1984;63:35S.

73. Griffiths ML, Theron EJ. Obstructed labour from pelvic neurofibroma [Letter]. *S Afr Med J* 1978;53:781.

74. Bourke E, Gatenby PBB. Renal artery dysplasia with hypertension in neurofibromatosis. *Br J Med* 1971;3:681–682.

75. Tapp E, Hickling RS. Renal artery rupture in a pregnant woman with neurofibromatosis. *J Pathol* 1962;97:398–399.

76. Manser J. Abnormal responses in Von Recklinghausen's disease [Letter]. *Br J Anaesth* 1970;42:183.

77. Magbagbeola JAO. Abnormal responses to muscle relaxants in a patient with Von Recklinghausen's disease (multiple neurofibromatosis) [Letter]. *Br J Anaesth* 1970;42:710.

78. Baraka A. Myasthenic response to muscle relaxants in Von Recklinghausen's disease. *Br J Anaesth* 1974;46:701–703.

79. Dounas M, Mercier F, Lhuissier C, et al. Epidural analgesia for labour in a parturient with neurofibromatosis. *Can J Anaesth* 1994;42:420–424.

80. Dugoff L, Sujansky E. Neurofibromatosis type 1 and pregnancy. *Am J Med Genet* 1996;66:7–10.

81. Ahlberg G, Ahlmark G. The Landry-Guillain-Barré syndrome and pregnancy. *Acta Obstet Gynecol Scand* 1978;57:377–380.

82. Ravn H. The Landry-Guillain-Barré syndrome: a survey and a clinical report of 127 cases. *Acta Neurol Scand* 1967;43 (Suppl):1–64,.

83. Osler LD, Sidell AD. The Guillain-Barré syndrome: the need for exact diagnosis criteria. *N Engl J Med* 1960;262:964–969.

84. Rudolph JH, Norris FH Jr, Garvey PH, et al. The Landry-Guillain-Barré syndrome in pregnancy: a review. *Obstet Gynecol* 1965;26:265–271.

85. Hurley TJ, Brunson AD, RL A, et al. Landrey-Guillain-Barré Strohl syndrome in pregnancy: report of the cases treated with plasmapheresis. *Obstet Gynecol* 1991;78:482–485.

86. Bravo RH, Katz M, Inturrisi M, et al. Obstetric management of Landry-Guillain-Barré syndrome: a case report. *Am J Obstet Gynecol* 1982;142:714–715.

87. Greenland P, Griggs RC. Arrhythmic complications in Guillain-Barré syndrome. *Arch Intern Med* 1980;140:1053–1055.

88. Elstein M, Legg NJ, Murphy M, et al. Guillain-Barré syndrome in pregnancy. *Anaesthesia* 1971;26:216–224.

89. Crawford JS, James FM III, Nolte H, et al. Regional anesthesia for patients with chronic neurological disease and similar conditions [Letter]. *Anaesthesia* 1981;36:821.

90. Jones RM, Healy TEJ. A reply [Letter]. *Anaesthesia* 1981;36:821–822.

91. McGrady EM. Management of labour and delivery in a patient with Guillain-Barré syndrome [Letter]. *Anaesthesia* 1987;42:894.

92. Hall JK, Straka PE. Successful epidural analgesia in a primagravida after recovery from Guillain-Barré syndrome [Letter]. *Reg Anesth* 1988;13:129.

93. Johnson KP. The historical development of interferons as multiple sclerosis therapies. *J Mol Med* 1997;75:89–94.

94. Abramsky O. Pregnancy and multiple sclerosis. *Ann Neurol* 1994;36:38–46.

95. Whitaker JN. Effects of pregnancy and delivery on disease activity in multiple sclerosis [Editorial]. *N Engl J Med* 1998;339:339–340.

96. Confaureaux C, Hutchinson M, Hours MM, et al. Rate of pregnancy-related relapse in multiple sclerosis. *N Engl J Med* 1998;339:285–291.

97. Muller R. Pregnancy in disseminated sclerosis. *Acta Psychiatr Neurol Scand* 1951;26:397–409.

98. Damek P, Schuster EA. Pregnancy and multiple sclerosis. *Mayo Clin Proc* 1997;72:977–989.

99. Ridley A, Schapira K. Influence of surgical procedures on the course of multiple sclerosis. *Neurology* 1961;11:81–82.

100. Bamford C, Sibley W, Laguna J. Anesthesia in multiple sclerosis. *Can J Neurol Sci* 1978;5:41–44.

101. Eickhoff K, Wikstrom J, Poser S, et al. Protein profile of cerebrospinal fluid in multiple sclerosis with special reference to the function of the blood brain barrier. *J Neurol* 1977;214:207–215.

102. Schapira K. Is lumbar puncture harmful in multiple sclerosis? *J Neurol Neurosurg Psychiatry* 1959;22:238.

103. Warren TM, Datta S, Ostheimer GW. Lumbar epidural anesthesia in a patient with multiple sclerosis. *Anesth Analg* 1982;61:1022–1023.

104. Bader AM, Hunt CO, Datta S, et al. Anesthesia for the obstetric patient with multiple sclerosis. *J Clin Anesth* 1988;1:21–24.

105. Baskett PJF, Armstrong R. Anaesthetic problems in multiple sclerosis. Are certain agents contraindicated? *Anaesthesia* 1976;31:1211–1216.

106. Siemkowicz E. Multiple sclerosis and surgery. *Anaesthesia* 1976;31:1211–1216.

107. Foldes FF, McNall PG. Myasthenia gravis: a guide for anesthesiologists. *Anesthesiology* 1962;23:837–872.

108. Plausche WC. Myasthenia gravis in mothers and their newborn. *Clin Obstet Gynecol* 1991;34:82–87.

109. Plausche WC. Myasthenia gravis in pregnancy. *Am J Obstet Gynecol* 1979;29:691.

110. Osserman KE. Obstetrics. In: Osserman KE, ed. *Myasthenia Gravis.* New York: Grune & Stratton, 1958:239–242.

111. Mitchell PJ, Bebbington M. Myasthenia gravis in pregnancy. *Obstet Gynecol* 1992;80:178–181.

112. Frenkel M, Ehrlich EN. The influence of progesterone and mineralocorticoids upon myasthenia gravis. *Ann Intern Med* 1964;60:971–981.

113. Catanzarite VA, Mittargue AM, Sandberg EC, et al. Respiratory arrest during therapy for premature labor in a patient with myasthenia gravis. *Obstet Gynecol* 1984;64:819–822.

114. Edery H, Porath G, Zahavy J. Passage of 2-hydroxyaminomethyl-N-methylpyridinium methanesulfonate to the fetus and cerebral spaces. *Toxicol Appl Pharmacol* 1966;9:341–346.

115. Foldes FF. Myasthenia gravis. *Monogr Anesthesiol* 1975;3:345–393.

116. Hokkanen E. The aggravating effect of some antibiotics on the neuromuscular blockade in myasthenia gravis. *Acta Neurol Scand* 1964;40:346–352.

117. Cohen BA, London RS, Goldstein PG. Myasthenia gravis and preeclampsia. *Obstet Gynecol* 1976;48:355.

118. Genkins G, Mendelow H, Sobel HJ, et al. Myasthenia gravis: analysis of thirty-one consecutive postmortem examinations. In: Viets H, ed. *Myasthenia Gravis.* Springfield, IL: Charles C Thomas, 1961:519–530.

119. Mendelow H. Pathology. In: Osserman KE, ed. *Myasthenia Gravis.* New York: Grune & Stratton, 1958:10–43.

120. Reimann PM, Mason PD. Plasmapheresis technique and complications. *Intensive Care Med* 1990;16:3–9.

121. Massey JM, Sanders DS. Single fiber electromyography in myasthenia gravis during pregnancy. *Muscle Nerve* 1993;16:458–460.

122. Rolbin SH, Levinson G, Shnider SM, et al. Anesthetic considerations for myasthenia gravis and pregnancy. *Anesth Analg* 1978;57:441–447.

123. McNall PG, Jafarnia MR. Management of myasthenia gravis in the obstetrical patient. *Am J Obstet Gynecol* 1965;92:518–525.

124. Coaldrake LA, Livingstone PA. Myasthenia gravis in pregnancy. *Anaesth Intensive Care* 1983;11:254–257.

125. D'Angelo R, Gerancher JC. Combined spinal and epidural analgesia in a parturient with severe myasthenia gravis. *Reg Anesth* 1998;23:201–203.

126. Usubiaga JE, Wikinski JA, Morales RL, et al. Interaction of intravenously administered procaine, lidocaine and succinylcholine in anesthetized subjects. *Anesth Analg* 1967;46:39–45.

127. Foldes FF, Smith JC. The interaction of human cholinesterases with anticholinesterases used in the therapy of myasthenia gravis. *Ann NY Acad Sci* 1966;135:287–301.

128. O'Flaherty D, Pennant JH, Raok, et al. Total intravenous anesthesia with propofol for transsternal thyomectomy in myasthenia gravis. *J Clin Anesth* 1992;4:241.

129. Mulder DG, Braitman H, Wei-i L, et al. Surgical management in myasthenia gravis. *J Thorac Cardiovasc Surg* 1972;63:105–113.

130. Baraka A. Anaesthesia and myasthenia gravis. *Can J Anaesth* 1992; 39:476–486.

131. Baraka A, Dajani A. Atracurium in myasthenics undergoing thymectomy. *Anesth Analg* 1984;63:1127–1130.

132. Naguib M, Dawlatly A, Ashour M, et al. Multivariate determinants of the need for postoperative ventilation in myasthenia gravis. *Can J Anaesth* 1998;43:1006–1013.

133. Namba T, Brown SB, Grob D. Neonatal myasthenia gravis: report of two cases and review of the literature. *Pediatrics* 1970;45:488–504.

134. Keesey J, Lindstrom J, Cokely H, et al. Antiacetylcholine receptor antibody in neonatal myasthenia gravis [Letter]. *N Engl J Med* 1977;296:55.

135. Penn AS. Diseases of the neuromuscular junction. In: Rudolph AM, Hoffman JIE, Rudolph C, eds. *Pediatrics,* 19th ed. Norwalk, CT: Appleton & Lange, 1991:1801.

136. Guttmann L. *Spinal Cord Injuries: Comprehensive Management and Research.* Oxford: Blackwell Scientific, 1973.

137. Hughes SJ, Short DJ, Usherwood MM, et al. Management of the pregnant woman with spinal cord injuries. *Br J Obstet Gynaecol* 1991;98:513–521.

138. Cross LL, Meythaler JM, Tuel SM, et al. Pregnancy, labor and delivery post spinal cord injury. *Paraplegia* 1992;30:390–396.

139. Goller H, Paeslack V. Our experiences about pregnancy and delivery of the paraplegic women. *Paraplegia* 1970;8:161–166.

140. Head H, Riddoch G. The automatic bladder, excessive sweating and some other reflex conditions in gross injuries of the spinal cord. *Brain* 1917;40:188–263.

141. Kurnick NB. Autonomic hyperreflexia and its control in patients with spinal cord lesions. *Ann Intern Med* 1956;44:678–686.

142. Kendrick WW, Scott JW, Jousse AT, et al. Reflex sweating and hypertension in traumatic transverse myelitis. *Treatment Servs Bull Can (Ottawa)* 1953;8:437–448.

143. Ciliberti BJ, Goldfein J, Rovenstine EA. Hypertension during anesthesia in patients with spinal cord injuries. *Anesthesiology* 1953;15:273–279.

144. Quimby CW Jr, Williams RN, Greifenstein FE. Anesthetic problems of the acute quadriplegic patient. *Anesth Analg* 1973;52:333–340.

145. Stirt JA, Marco A, Conklin KA. Obstetric anesthesia for a quadriplegic patient with autonomic hyperreflexia. *Anesthesiology* 1979;51:560–562.

146. Debarge O, Christensen NJ, Corbett JL, et al. Plasma catecholamines in tetraplegics. *Paraplegia* 1974;12:44–49.

147. Watson DW, Downey GO. Epidural anesthesia for labor and delivery of twins of a paraplegic mother. *Anesthesiology* 1980;52:259–261.

148. Cooperman LH, Strobel GE, Kennell EM. Massive hyperkalemia after administration of succinycholine. *Anesthesiology* 1970;32:161–164.

149. Robertson DNS. Pregnancy and labour in the paraplegic. *Paraplegia* 1972;10:209–212.

150. Westgren W, Hultling C, Levi R, et al. Pregnancy and delivery in women with a traumatic spinal cord injury in Sweden, 1980–1991. *Obstet Gynecol* 1993;81:926–930.

151. Rossier AB, Ruffieux M, Ziegler WH. Pregnancy and labour in high traumatic spinal cord lesions. *Paraplegia* 1969;7:210–216.

152. Young BK, Katz M, Klein SA. Pregnancy after spinal cord injury: altered maternal and fetal response to labor. *Obstet Gynecol* 1983;62:59–63.

153. Marx GF. Editorial comment. *Obstet Anesth Digest* 1984;4:6.

154. Katz VL, Thorp JM, Cefolo RC. Epidural analgesia and autonomic hyperreflexia: a case report. *Am J Obstet Gynecol* 1990;162:471–472.

155. Ravindran RS, Cummins DF, Smith IE. Experience with the use of nitroprusside and subsequent epidural analgesia in a pregnant quadriplegic patient. *Anesth Analg* 1981;60:61–63.

156. Lewis PE, Cefalo RC, Naulty JS, et al. Placental transfer and fetal toxicity of sodium nitroprusside. *Gynecol Invest* 1977;8:46.

157. Kobayashi A, Mizobe T, Tojo H, et al. Autonomic hyperreflexia during labour. *Can J Anaesth* 1995;12:1134–1136.

158. Eldridge J, Kipling M, Smith JW. Anaesthetic management of a woman who became paraplegic at 22 weeks gestation after a spontaneous spinal cord haemorrhage secondary to a presumed arteriovenous malformation. *Br J Anaesth* 1998;81:976–978.

159. Baraka A. Epidural meperidine for control of autonomic hyperreflexia in a paraplegic parturient. *Anesthesiology* 1985;62:688–690.

160. Abouleish E, Hanley ES, Palmer SM. Can epidural fentanyl control autonomic hyperreflexia in a quadriplegic parturient? *Anesth Analg* 1989;68:523–526.

161. Lambert DH, Deane RS, Mazuzan JE. Anesthesia and the control of blood pressure in patients with spinal cord injury. *Anesth Analg* 1982;61:344–348.

Shnider and Levinson's Anesthesia for Obstetrics,
edited by Samuel C. Hughes, et al.
Lippincott Williams & Wilkins,
Philadelphia, © 2001.

CHAPTER 31

ANESTHESIA FOR THE MORBIDLY OBESE PREGNANT PATIENT

SHEILA E. COHEN, M.B., Ch. B., F.F.A.R.S.

DEFINITIONS

Obesity is a disease of modern civilization that afflicts more than 20% of the United States population. It is more than a social or cosmetic problem to the pregnant patient, as evidenced by accumulating data that point to significantly increased maternal and fetal risk with this condition (1–5). In a report of maternal mortality in Michigan, obesity was a risk factor in 80% of anesthetic deaths (2). Because of the prevalence of obesity in our society, the obese parturient may be the most common high-risk patient encountered by the obstetric anesthesiologist. Although obesity usually results from excessive caloric intake and not abnormal metabolism, the cause is often obscure. Hereditary, environmental, social, economic, and psychologic factors all seem to be important (6). The tendency to obesity begins early in life, with an increased number of fat cells being present in the first year. Familial eating patterns tend to result in obese mothers overfeeding their children, so that they similarly become overweight.

Obesity is defined as an excess of body fat. In nonobese young men approximately 15 to 18% of body weight is composed of fat; in females this figure is 20 to 25% (6). In both groups the proportion of body fat tends to increase with age. Although sophisticated measurements of body fat are necessary to accurately define and quantify obesity, in most instances the diagnosis is readily apparent. Obesity can be classified in a variety of ways. Individuals less than 20% in excess of ideal weight have been described as **overweight**, and those more than 20% as **obese**. Morbid obesity is said to be present when body weight is more than twice normal, or when it exceeds by more than 100 lbs. the ideal weight for age and height. Ideal weight can be taken from insurance tables, standard formulas (7) or can be estimated simply using the **Broca Index**:

$$\text{Ideal weight (kg)} = \text{height (cm)} - 100.$$

Techniques used to quantify adiposity more accurately have included complex measurements of body density and determinations of fat or water content by isotopic or chemical dilution. Simple methods include measurement of skinfold thickness, indices such as weight/height, or the **ponderal index** (height/$^3\sqrt{\text{weight}}$). The most useful of these simple measurements of obesity is the **body mass index** (BMI), which affords the best correlation with the degree of adiposity and is least affected by variations in height (8).

$$\text{BMI} = \frac{\text{weight (kg)}}{\text{height (m}^2)}$$

A BMI of less than 25 is normal, 25 to 29.9 is considered overweight, and over 30 frank obesity. A BMI greater than 40 is classified as morbid obesity.

Standard definitions of obesity may be unhelpful in the pregnant patient as *prepregnant* weight may not be known. Also, weight gained in pregnancy results not only from increased adipose tissue but from the expanded blood volume, the uter-ine contents, and edema. Although a variety of definitions for obesity have been used in the parturient (e.g., body weight greater than 80–114 kg or 50–300% greater than ideal weight for height), currently definitions based on BMI are considered most appropriate for clinical and research purposes (9).

Among obese individuals there are two subgroups: those with simple obesity, and a small minority, comprising 5 to 10%, who exhibit the obesity hypoventilation syndrome (OHS), also referred to as the "Pickwickian syndrome" (10). Patients in the latter category are extremely obese and suffer from hypoventilation (hypoxemia and hypercarbia), somnolence, edema, polycythemia, and cardiomegaly. It is fortunate that most obese parturients do not suffer from this syndrome, as it carries with it significant risk of morbidity and mortality.

RISKS OF THE OBESE PARTURIENT

Obesity induces changes in anatomy, physiology, psychopathology, and biotransformation of anesthetic agents. Similarly, pregnancy is associated with significant deviations from the normal state. When these two conditions coexist, the resultant effect is unpredictable and potentially hazardous. In addition, obese individuals frequently suffer from other medical problems, including cardiovascular disease (particularly hypertension and coronary artery disease), diabetes, cirrhosis, and cholelithiasis. Fatty infiltration of the liver can occur, and abnormal liver function tests have been reported (11). These conditions and obstetric factors render the obese parturient and her newborn particularly prone to developing complications during pregnancy (3, 4, 9, 12–20). The complications reported in association with obesity in pregnancy are listed in Table 31.1. A recent study from France found that maternal complications increased markedly in frequency as the degree of maternal obesity increased (Table 31.2) (21). Because the definitions of obesity vary markedly among investigators, comparisons among studies are difficult. Most of the literature is not confined to morbidly obese parturients (who comprise about 6 to 10% of pregnant women in the United States) (16) but includes those with lesser degrees of obesity. Chronic or pregnancy-induced hypertension has been reported in from 23% to 79%, and diabetes in 4% to 46%, of obese parturients (3, 4, 12–14, 16–21). Among morbidly obese gravidas presenting for anesthesia in one institution, 47% had antenatal medical disease (19). These rates, which are 5 to 10 times those in normal weight mothers, explain much of the maternal and fetal morbidity. The newborns of obese parturients are large for gestational age (3, 4, 9, 16, 17), with obesity and diabetes both positively influencing fetal weight. The degree of macrosomia is surprising in view of the lower than normal pregnancy weight gain and the increased incidence of hypertension and multiple gestation (4, 9, 17). Prolonged gestation is common in obesity and results in frequent induction of labor (16, 17, 19). Some studies also have reported increased incidences of dysfunctional labor, failed induction, and prolongation of the second stage (14, 16).

Table 31.1. PREGNANCY-RELATED COMPLICATIONS IN THE OBESE PARTURIENT

Maternal Complications	Obstetric/Neonatal Complications
Gestational diabetes	Increased perinatal mortality[a]
Hypertension (chronic and PIH)	Birth defects
Urinary tract infection	Inadequate weight gain
Increased cesarean section rate	Prolonged gestation
	Macrosomia
Anesthetic complications	Twins/breech/malpresentation
Blood loss > 1,000 mL at cesarean	Dysfunctional labor patterns
	Shoulder dystocia
Prolonged surgery	Birth trauma
Thrombophlebitis	Neonatal hypoglycemia
Wound infections/dehiscence	

[a] Only when antenatal complications present.

The larger babies born to obese mothers may be more at risk for birth trauma and asphyxia, often as a consequence of shoulder dystocia (4, 16). This, along with a higher incidence of malpresentations and twins and a tendency to dysfunctional labors, may explain the high rate of operative delivery quoted in a number of studies. In contrast, Gross et al. (17) found no significant differences in abnormalities of labor or the rate of either operative vaginal or primary cesarean deliveries in a series of moderately overweight women weighing more than 90 kg, although the rate of repeat cesarean sections was increased. In a large study involving 10,000 parturients of various weights, Garbaciak et al. (3) reported an increased incidence of primary cesarean section in obese and morbidly obese parturients. When antepartum complications were present, the incidence increased from 18% in normal weight women to 23% in both obese and morbidly obese mothers. When antepartum complications were absent, the cesarean section rates were 10%, 12%, and 20% in normal weight, obese, and morbidly obese mothers, respectively. The marked increase in the latter group may relate to the more frequent occurrence of fetal umbilical cord accidents, meconium staining, and late decelerations noted in these patients (3). These complications did not affect perinatal mortality, however, which was increased only in the infants of mothers with antepartum complications such as diabetes or hypertension. In an analysis of almost 57,000 pregnancies, Naeye (18) challenged the hypothesis that adverse neonatal

outcome in obesity is related only to maternal complications and fetal macrosomia, providing data demonstrating a progressive increase in perinatal mortality with increasing pregravid maternal weight. Although factors inherently related to obesity, such as maternal diabetes, advanced maternal age, and an increased incidence of dizygous twinning, were associated with greater mortality, acute chorioamnionitis with consequent preterm labor made the biggest contribution to adverse perinatal outcome. It is not known how chorioamnionitis might be related to increased maternal weight. In addition to these problems, there is growing evidence that maternal obesity is associated with an increased risk of congenital abnormalities, particularly neural tube defects (22).

Many of the above complicating conditions necessitate operative vaginal delivery or cesarean section, with a concomitant need for anesthesia. Hood and Dewan (19) reported a 62% cesarean section rate in 117 women weighing over 300 lb, while Wolfe et al. (20) similarly found that 58% of 107 women weighing from 200 to 504 lb required primary cesarean section. Although few studies relate specifically to pregnant patients, anesthesia and surgery in nonpregnant obese patients have been associated with increased morbidity and mortality (23–30). Following surgery for duodenal ulcer, perioperative mortality in obese patients was two and one half to three times that of nonobese patients (23). Sudden death, not apparently due to myocardial infarction, has been reported during anesthesia in these patients. In a critical review of the literature, Pasulka et al. (29) concluded that the risks to the obese patient of *elective* surgery performed in specialized centers by experienced personnel may not be significantly increased. Unfortunately, this is seldom the situation faced by most obstetric patients. Maternal mortality statistics provide convincing evidence that obesity is a significant hazard to the pregnant patient. Obesity was a risk factor in 12 of 15 anesthesia-related maternal deaths in Michigan between 1972 and 1984 (2), with inability to accomplish endotracheal intubation the principal cause of death in recent years. In an earlier report from the Chicago Maternity Center, four of seven maternal deaths occurred in women weighing more than 200 lb (31). Similar data from Minnesota between 1963 and 1972 revealed that 12% of all maternal deaths occurred in obese women; pulmonary embolus was the leading cause of death in this series (15). Mortality data do not classify obesity as a cause of death, however it seems clear that anesthesia, surgery, and pregnancy pose significant risks to the obese woman. Perioperative morbidity also is increased in obese individuals (32). Complications during cesarean section include prolonged surgery

Table 31.2. DEGREE OF OBESITY AND INCIDENCE OF MATERNAL COMPLICATIONS DURING PREGNANCY

	Normal	Overweight	Obese	Morbidly Obese	p value
Number of subjects	54	48	34	30	
Hypertension (%)	9	33[a]	55[a]	79[a]	< 0.0001
Preeclampsia (%)	4	18	30[a]	43[a]	< 0.0001
Gestational diabetes (%)	2	12	39[a]	45[a]	< 0.0001
Insulin (% patients)	0	2	12[a]	21[a]	< 0.001
Insulin (% diabetics)	0	17	31[a]	46[a]	< 0.001
Urinary infection (%)	17	9	29	38	< 0.02
Preterm labor (%)	15	13	23	28	Not significant
Cesarean section (%)	9	17	15	43[a]	< 0.002
Primary cesarean section (%)	7	10	6	33[a]	< 0.006

Normal, BMI 18–24.9; overweight, BMI 25–29.9; obese, BMI 30–34.9; morbidly obese, BMI > 35 a, significantly different from normal weight group.
Adapted from Galtier-Dereure F, Montpeyroux F, Boulot P, et al . Weight excess before pregnancy: complications and cost, *Int J Obesity* 1995;19:443–448.

and excessive blood loss, whereas in the postoperative period, wound infections and thrombophlebitis occur with greatly increased frequency (16, 20, 29, 32).

PHYSIOLOGIC DISTURBANCES

The physiologic changes that accompany both pregnancy (33) (see Chapter 1) and obesity (29, 34) have been extensively studied. However, few data relate specifically to obese parturients. During pregnancy, the most major changes result from hormonal influences and the mechanical effects of the enlarging uterus. The metabolic demands of the fetus, placenta, and breasts also are responsible for some changes, but these exert a relatively minor influence compared with the other causes. In the obese state, most of the deviations from normal result from the added metabolic and mechanical burden of excess fat. Although many of the physiologic changes in obesity and pregnancy are in the same direction, the magnitude of the resultant abnormality frequently is not known. In view of the wide variation in the degree of physiologic derangement that can exist, evaluation of each patient is mandatory.

Respiratory Changes

Lung Volumes

Both pregnancy and obesity result in an exaggerated lumbar lordosis. In very obese patients, a thoracic kyphosis may also be present (28, 33, 34). The normal parturient has a widened transverse diameter of the chest because of cephalad pressure by the gravid uterus. In obesity, the chest wall tends to be splinted in a position of inspiration by abdominal fat, which elevates the ribs. Although diaphragmatic movement again is greater than normal, chest wall adiposity significantly hinders respiratory excursion. Chest wall compliance is decreased in pregnancy and, to a much greater extent, in obesity. In the latter condition, compliance relates directly to the weight of adiposity in this region, rather than to total body weight. Inspiratory capacity is therefore abnormal in obesity, but not in normal pregnancy. In addition, in very obese individuals respiratory muscle efficiency is frequently reduced (34). In a study of healthy young adults with moderate to severe obesity, Ray et al. (35) found that respiratory changes were of two types: those which changed in proportion to the degree of obesity, such as expiratory reserve volume (ERV) and diffusing capacity for carbon monoxide, and those which changed only in extreme obesity, such as vital capacity, total lung capacity, and maximum voluntary ventilation.

Individually, pregnancy and obesity are associated with a decrease in ERV and, hence, functional residual capacity (FRC). This results from cephalad pressure by the gravid uterus in pregnancy, and intraabdominal fat and added weight on the chest wall in obesity (28, 33, 34). In obese nonpregnant individuals, ERV may be reduced to 20% of its predicted value in the sitting position and may be totally obliterated in the Trendelenburg position (Fig. 31.1). The net effect is that FRC may be smaller than closing capacity (the lung volume at which terminal airways close during expiration), leading to closure of dependent airways during tidal ventilation. This results in shunting of deoxygenated blood through nonventilated alveoli, with consequent arterial hypoxemia. Shunt fractions of 10% to 25% of cardiac output have been reported in obesity (36). Although in pregnancy FRC is reduced by 20% to 30%, airway closure in the sitting position has variously been reported not to occur (37) or, conversely, to be present in about 25% of women, the majority of whom, however, were smokers (38). Assumption of the supine, lithotomy, or Trendelenburg position (Fig. 31.1), induction of general anesthesia, and the insertion of abdominal packs during surgery all result in additional decreases in FRC in both preg-

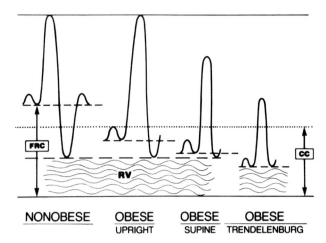

Figure 31.1. Effect of position change on lung volumes in nonobese compared with markedly obese subjects. *FRC,* functional residual capacity; *RV,* residual volume; *CC,* closing capacity. (From Vaughan RW. Pulmonary and cardiovascular derangements in the obese patient. In: Brown BR Jr, ed. *Anesthesia and the Obese Patient.* Philadelphia: Davis, 1982:19–39, with permission.)

nancy and obesity. In these situations there is the potential for significant deterioration in oxygen saturation. Damia et al. (39) demonstrated decreases in FRC of 51% following induction of general anesthesia and muscle paralysis in a group of morbidly obese surgical patients. This decrease, which was considerably greater than that seen in normal weight patients, resulted in lung volumes less than baseline residual volumes. FRC returned toward preanesthesia values after laparotomy incision, only to decrease again with skin closure (39). Extrapolation of these findings to obese parturients undergoing cesarean section suggests that pulmonary function might improve significantly after abdominal incision and delivery of the fetus.

It is fortunate that the effects of obesity and pregnancy on lung volumes do not appear to be additive. When the obese gravida reaches the second half of pregnancy, subdiaphragmatic uterine compression would be expected to lead to further encroachment on FRC, with increased airway closure and ventilation-perfusion mismatching. In one of the few investigations of respiratory function in obese parturients, Eng and associates (40) studied women weighing 50 to 140% above normal (Table 31.3). Measurements were made during the last trimester of pregnancy and 2 months postpartum, when it was assumed that normalcy had resumed. Although the usual respiratory changes of pregnancy occurred, they were not exaggerated and FRC decreased to a lesser extent than normal. Surprisingly, FRC was larger than had previously been reported for both pregnant and obese individuals. The authors postulated that their results were due to measurements having been made with subjects in the sitting rather than the supine position, as was the case in other studies. In spite of FRC being greater than anticipated, moderate hypoxemia was present with mean Pao_2 values of 85 and 86 for pregnant and nonpregnant states, respectively. In this study obesity had a significant deleterious effect on ventilation-perfusion mismatching, but this was not further worsened by the pregnant state. It should be noted that only half of the patients in this study could be classified as morbidly obese. In a study of considerably more obese individuals, Blass (41) similarly concluded that pregnancy did not have a detrimental effect on oxygenation. Arterial Po_2 was higher in 27 gravidas between 250 and 500 lb presenting for cesarean section than it was in women of similar weights who had undergone gastrojejunal bypass. However, these groups are not strictly comparable because patients undergoing remedial surgery may have been more severely incapacitated by their obesity. The authors suggest

Table 31.3. RESPIRATORY FUNCTION DURING PREGNANCY[a]

	Third Trimester (Pregnant)	Postpartum (Nonpregnant)
Lung volumes		
VC(L)	3.76	3.92
ERV	0.79	0.94[b]
FRC	2.06	2.14
FEV 1.0	3.2	3.3
Arterial blood gases		
pH	7.44	7.44
P_{O_2} (mm Hg)	85	86
P_{CO_2} (mm Hg)	30	36[b]
Base excess (mEq/L)	−4.2	+0.03[b]

[a] Respiratory function in 12 obese women during the last trimester of pregnancy and 2 months postpartum (nonpregnant). The change in FRC is not statistically significant and represents a decrease during pregnancy of only 3%. Ventilatory changes are similar to those found in nonobese parturients.
[b] $P < 0.001$ compared to the pregnant state.
VC, vital capacity; ERV, expiratory reserve volume; FRC, functional residual capacity; FEV 1.0, forced expiratory volume in 1 sec.
Data from Eng M, Butler J, Bonica J. Respiratory function in pregnant obese women. *Am J Obstet Gynecol* 1975;123:241–245.

that the hyperventilation and flaring of the chest wall that occur during pregnancy exert a beneficial effect in obese women.

Ventilation

Pregnancy is associated with small (10% to 20%) increases in oxygen consumption and metabolic rate and a large (70%) increase in alveolar ventilation (33). These appear to be hormonally induced (progesterone and estrogen effect) rather than a response to increased metabolism. In obesity, hyperventilation at rest is usual as the excess fat "organ" requires oxygen and generates carbon dioxide; additional cardiorespiratory work is necessary just to mechanically transport the additional weight (28). In patients with simple morbid obesity, the mechanical cost of breathing is increased by 30%, and with OHS, it is increased by as much as 300% above that of normal individuals (42). Eng et al. (40) reported ventilatory changes in obese parturients similar to those in their normal counterparts. Nevertheless, this added burden results in the obese parturient expending significant amounts of energy on ventilatory work, particularly during an unmedicated labor when hyperventilation is often extreme.

Cardiovascular Changes

Similar changes in cardiovascular function are induced by both pregnancy and obesity (28, 33, 34, 36). The increases in cardiac output and blood volume in pregnancy are predominantly a function of hormonal influences, with the added effect of the low-resistance placental circulation acting as an arteriovenous shunt. Whereas in pregnancy cardiac output increases by 35% to 45%, in obesity it may double. In the latter condition, blood volume and cardiac output expand in proportion to the increased mass of fat tissue that must be perfused. Also, the additional work of breathing and hypoxemia (if present) stimulate cardiac output. In obesity, resting left ventricular end-diastolic pressure is at the upper limit of normal, explaining the increase in stroke volume that is present. In contrast to the normal pregnant state in which blood pressure decreases because of lowered vascular resistance, in obesity systolic and diastolic pressures may be elevated with increased systemic vascular resistance. In a study of pregnant women at 36 weeks' gestation, M-mode echocardiography found no difference in left ventricular end-

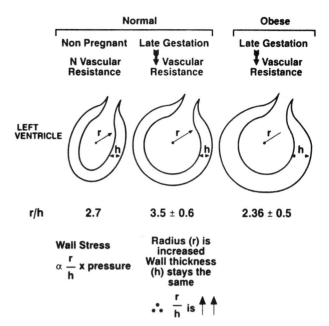

Figure 31.2. Cardiovascular effects of pregnancy. Illustration of radius-to-wall thickness ratio (r/h) in nonpregnant, pregnant, and obese pregnant patients. The ratio in obese pregnant patients was significantly smaller than in pregnant patients but similar to that of nonpregnant patients. (From Veille JC, Hanson R. Obesity, pregnancy and left ventricular functioning during the third trimester. *Am J Obstet Gynecol* 1994;171:980–983, with permission.)

diastolic dimension, fractional shortening and cardiac index between a group of obese parturients (average weight 282 lb) free from cardiac disease, hypertension, or diabetes and a group of nonobese controls (43). However, left ventricular hypertrophy, with a decreased radius-to-wall thickness ratio, was present in the obese parturients (Fig. 31.2), an adaptation that may be important in preserving left ventricular function. As nonpregnant obese patients were not studied, it could not be determined whether these changes were specific to pregnancy or related to maternal obesity. Also, the findings may not be applicable to extremely obese parturients in whom cardiovascular disease is common. Abnormal mean pulmonary artery and pulmonary capillary pressures have been reported in some extremely obese subjects at rest, with excessive increases occurring after exercise (44).

The hemodynamic stresses of pregnancy place the obese woman at significantly increased risk. Cardiac work and myocardial oxygen consumption already are increased during gestation, yet must respond to additional demands imposed by a 45% elevation in cardiac output during labor and an 80% increase in the immediate postpartum period. The peripartum period poses particular risk to mothers with hypertension or coronary artery disease. During the second half of pregnancy, aortocaval compression by the uterus in the supine position can severely reduce cardiac output and placental perfusion. This problem is greatly exacerbated in the obese parturient when a large fat panniculus further compresses the great vessels.

Gastrointestinal Changes

The problems in the normal pregnant woman of delayed gastric emptying, diminished lower esophageal sphincter tone, and hyperacidity are compounded in the obese parturient by a high incidence of hiatus hernia and greatly elevated intragastric pressure. The latter results from compression of intraabdominal structures by omental fat and the weight of the panniculus. Vaughan et al. (45) found 75% of obese surgical patients at risk for developing aspiration pneumonitis, having both a gastric pH

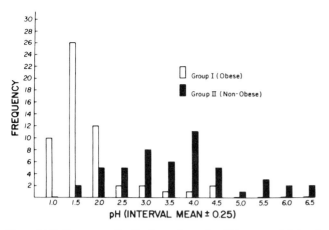

Figure 31.3. Frequency distributions of gastric pH in group I (obese) and group II (nonobese) surgical patients. The distribution curve for group I patients is skewed to the left. (From Vaughan RW, Bauer S, Wise L. Volume and pH of gastric juice in obese patients. *Anesthesiology* 1975;43:686–689, with permission.)

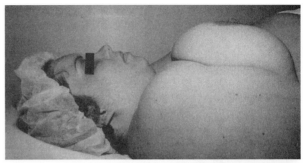

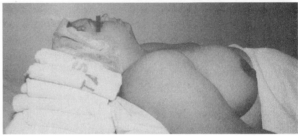

Figure 31.4. A: Obese pregnant woman in the supine position. The atlantooccipital gap is obliterated by fat and access with a laryngoscope is hindered by large breasts. **B:** The same patient positioned with the shoulders elevated and the occiput further elevated so that the head assumes the "sniffing" position. Access to the airway is greatly facilitated.

of less than 2.5 and a volume in excess of 25 mL (Fig. 31.3). In Roberts and Shirley's study of pregnant patients (46), obesity similarly conferred added risk. Among women in labor weighing over 160 lb, mean gastric volume was 131 mL, compared with only 22 mL in women of normal weight.

Pathophysiology of Obesity Hypoventilation Syndrome

In some massively obese patients, hyperventilation gives way to hypoventilation, with consequent hypercapnia, hypoxemia, polycythemia, and somnolence (47). Pulmonary artery pressure is often high and cardiac failure can result. Fortunately, this syndrome usually develops later in life and these patients seldom become pregnant.

EVALUATION OF THE PATIENT

An anesthetic consultation during pregnancy is highly desirable in view of the potential pathophysiologic changes described above. If this has not been accomplished, it should be performed on admission to the labor suite. At this examination the respiratory and cardiovascular systems must be carefully evaluated, inquiring for symptoms of dyspnea, edema, dizziness in the supine position (indicating severe aortocaval compression), and exercise tolerance. The blood pressure should be checked with an adequately sized cuff, bearing in mind that a standard-sized cuff rather than a large cuff will incorrectly classify 37% of women with large upper arms as hypertensive (48). The chest should be examined for signs of left ventricular hypertrophy and pulmonary congestion. Severe "heartburn" indicates that significant gastroesophageal reflux is present.

It is most important at this time to carefully evaluate the airway, because failed intubation, currently the leading cause of maternal anesthetic mortality, is a particular hazard in the obese parturient. Difficulty relates to the degree of adiposity of the face, shoulders, neck, and breasts. The usual atlantooccipital gap is frequently nonexistent in the obese individual (Fig. 31.4), with the result that extension of the head is either impossible or results in bowing of the cervical spine and forward displacement of the larynx (49). Insertion of the laryngoscope may be obstructed by the enlarged breasts (Fig. 31.4), particularly when the patient is in a position of left lateral tilt. A history of easy intubation with prior anesthetics is no guarantee that problems will not be encountered, because weight usually has increased significantly during pregnancy. Inspection of the distribution of body fat, with evaluation of the lumbar area for ease of pal-

pation of bony landmarks and degree of lordosis, is important with respect to performance of regional anesthesia. The arms should be examined to predict potential difficulty with insertion of intravenous and intraarterial catheters.

In addition to the usual laboratory investigations, an electrocardiogram, liver function tests, and a glucose tolerance test may be indicated. Measurement of oxyhemoglobin saturation in the sitting, supine, and Trendelenburg positions using a pulse oximeter provides an easy way to assess the present degree of airway closure and the potential for deterioration with further decreases in FRC. In patients demonstrating desaturation with these maneuvers or in those with extreme obesity, pulmonary function tests and arterial blood gas analysis should be performed. Finally, the predelivery visit affords an ideal opportunity to explain to the patient the problems engendered by her condition and to apprise her of the risks and benefits of alternative analgesic management plans. Although this is not always apparent, many morbidly obese individuals are embarrassed and depressed by their excessive weight. If the anesthesiologist is to secure the patient's cooperation and trust, disparaging remarks about her weight and the difficulties that it will cause must be avoided.

ANESTHETIC CONSIDERATIONS
Drug Metabolism and Toxicity in the Obese Individual

Intravenous Agents

Pharmacokinetics in obese patients differ from those in nonobese individuals because of changes in the volume of distribution, drug clearance, protein binding, and renal and hepatic clearance (28). The interaction of these factors is complex and the effects vary with different drugs. Volume of distribution is increased in obesity for some drugs (e.g., thiopental, sufentanil, lidocaine and benzodiazepines (28, 50), whereas for others it remains unchanged (e.g., propofol, digoxin, cimetidine) (28, 51). An increased volume of distribution of a drug usually prolongs its elimination, even though clearance may be unchanged or increased. The physiologic changes of pregnancy, including

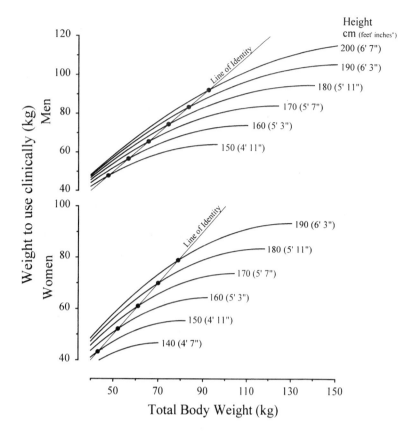

Figure 31.5. A nomogram relating total body weight, height, and gender to the body weight that should be used to calculate dose from recommendations that are scaled to body weight. The dots show ideal body weight. Data are derived from calculations relating total body weight to lean body mass and assume that published dosing recommendations scaled to total body weight are exactly correct for persons of ideal body weight, which accounts for the finding that the dots line up on the line of identity. (From Bouillon T, Shafer SL. Does size matter? [Editorial]. *Anesthesiology* 1998;89:557–560, with permission.)

increased blood volume and cardiac output and decreased protein binding, further complicate prediction of the pharmacokinetics of a particular drug in the parturient. Bouillon and Shafer (52), in a recent editorial, discussed whether dosage in obese patients should be based on total body weight, or scaled to lean body mass or ideal body weight. Because dosing of depressant drugs such as opioids or thiopental based on total body weight may cause profound overdose with serious consequences (53), they advocate scaling doses of intravenous agents to lean body mass. They provide nomograms relating total body weight, height, and gender to the weight that can be used clinically to calculate dose from recommendations based on total body weight (Fig. 31.5). These nomograms are derived from calculations of lean body mass and assume that published dosing recommendations scaled to total body weight are exactly correct for persons of ideal body weight. For patients smaller than ideal body weight, dose can be scaled to total body weight (as this approximates lean body mass); in patients significantly heavier than ideal body weight, dose can be scaled to ideal body weight, or to ideal body weight plus some fraction of the difference between total body weight and ideal weight as shown in Figure 31.5. It can be seen that it is rarely appropriate to scale dose to a weight greater than 80 kg in a woman. An alternative and acceptable strategy is simply to use standard doses without adjustment for weight (52, 54). How can these recommendations be applied to the obese parturient? Although the increased blood volume in pregnancy theoretically could justify an increase in dosage, this might be offset by the decreased anesthetic requirements present during pregnancy. A cautious approach, supported by clinical experience, is to use normal or only moderately increased initial doses of induction agents, opioids, and benzodiazepines, administering additional drug as indicated by the patient's response.

Inhaled Anesthetics

Abnormal biotransformation of volatile anesthetic agents, with increased formation of reactive intermediates or toxic end products, has been reported in morbidly obese patients (55, 56).

Extremely lipid-soluble agents, such as methoxyflurane, are retained in the abnormally large depot of body fat and subsequently undergo prolonged biodegradation. Young et al. (55) reported peak inorganic fluoride levels after methoxyflurane anesthesia that were higher in obese surgical patients than in normal controls. Mean peak serum inorganic fluoride levels of 56 μmol in obese patients were in the range associated with subclinical nephrotoxicity, while four individuals had peak levels in the toxic range. Similarly, fluoride production after enflurane administration to obese patients occurs at a rate twice that in nonobese patients exposed to comparable dosages (56). Maximum serum fluoride levels in obese individuals were 60% higher after enflurane than in normal patients (28 versus 17 μmol) but were insufficiently high to result in abnormal renal function. Isoflurane is metabolized to a much lesser extent than is enflurane and results in considerably lower fluoride levels in obese patients (Fig. 31.6) (57). Unlike enflurane, fluoride levels after isoflurane are similar in obese and normal weight patients. Halothane is not usually metabolized to form inorganic fluoride. However, in morbidly obese patients, elevated inorganic fluoride levels follow halothane administration, indicating that reductive metabolism has taken place (58). This is of concern, because this abnormal metabolic pathway has been associated with halothane hepatotoxicity in animals. To date, there is no evidence that halothane administration to obese individuals routinely results in hepatic dysfunction, although some believe the risk of halothane hepatotoxicity may be increased. Although serum bromide levels following halothane anesthesia are higher in obese patients than in normal individuals, sedative levels are not attained (58).

Among the newer inhalational agents, desflurane does not undergo significant metabolism, whereas sevoflurane is metabolized to inorganic fluoride. However, in contrast to methoxyflurane, sevoflurane is not highly lipid-soluble and is cleared rapidly from the body. Frink et al. (59) found similar biotransformation and inorganic fluoride concentrations in obese and nonobese surgical patients after sevoflurane anesthesia, concluding that this agent posed no increased risk of nephrotoxicity to obese

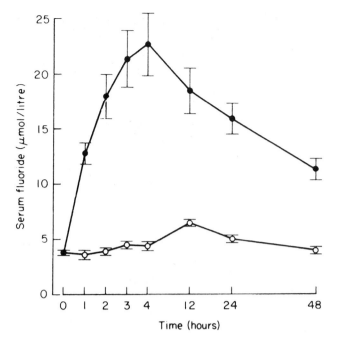

Figure 31.6. Serum inorganic fluoride levels (μmol/L) after enflurane anesthesia (●) and isoflurane anesthesia (○) in obese surgical patients (mean ± SEM). (From Strube PJ, Hulands GH, Halsey MJ. Serum fluoride levels in morbidly obese patients: enflurane compared with isoflurane anaesthesia. *Anaesthesia* 1987;42:685–689, with permission.)

patients. In another study, Higuchi et al. (60) reported higher serum fluoride levels after sevoflurane anesthesia in mildly obese patients than in normal weight controls, although neither group had abnormal renal function. In contrast to Frink's study, anesthetic exposure in Higuchi's patients was prolonged (more than 9 hours), all subjects were male, and most patients had fatty liver infiltration which may have increased hepatic uptake of sevoflurane. Because of the rapid excretion of sevoflurane, total exposure to inorganic fluoride (the "area under the curve") is much less than with methoxyflurane or enflurane. In addition, metabolism of sevoflurane occurs almost exclusively in the liver, in contrast to that of methoxyflurane, which occurs in both the kidneys and the liver. Probably for these reasons, nephrotoxicity after sevoflurane has not been reported in obese individuals.

Although delayed recovery from inhalation anesthesia in obesity might be expected because of retention of volatile agents in body fat, this does not appear to be the case with most modern agents. Cork et al. (61) found no difference between the recovery time of obese individuals who had received fentanyl and those who had received halothane or enflurane.

Muscle Relaxants

Bentley et al. (62) concluded that dose requirements of succinylcholine were increased in obesity in proportion to body weight, BMI, and surface area, rather than relating to lean body mass as might be expected. This was attributed to the increases in blood and extracellular fluid volumes, which are proportionate to the enlarged body surface area (6), as well as to an increase in pseudocholinesterase levels in obesity (62). However, other experts have observed that doses only moderately increased over normal doses produce adequate intubating conditions without the risk of a prolonged duration of effect (28). Studies in which pancuronium was administered to obese patients also have yielded conflicting results. Tsueda et al. (63) found that larger dose requirements for pancuronium in obese patients were related to body surface area, whereas Söderberg et al. (36) suggested that dosage should be based on ideal body weight. Varin and colleagues (64) studied atracurium in obese patients and recommended dosing on the basis of body weight. Although the volume of distribution for atracurium was not increased in these obese patients, a higher drug concentration was required to obtain a degree of blockade comparable to that of nonobese patients (64). The duration of neuromuscular blockade is not prolonged even when large doses of atracurium are given (Fig. 31.7A) (64, 65), probably because drug disposition does not depend on hepatic or renal clearance. In contrast, prolonged recovery from vecuronium has been reported in obesity (Fig. 31.7B) and has been attributed to delayed hepatic elimination, possibly resulting from fatty infiltration of the liver or a relative reduction in hepatic blood flow (65). Overdosage with relaxants other than atracurium can be minimized by reducing maintenance doses and increasing the interval between supplements. Regardless of which drug is used, incremental dosing and intraoperative monitoring of neuromuscular function is essential. Strict postanesthetic surveillance is important to detect residual muscle paralysis and respiratory depression from intravenous or inhalation agents, or from magnesium therapy.

Monitoring

The sophistication of monitoring techniques employed should depend on the degree of obesity (and consequent cardiopulmonary impairment) and whether other conditions such as preeclampsia or diabetes are present. A correctly sized blood

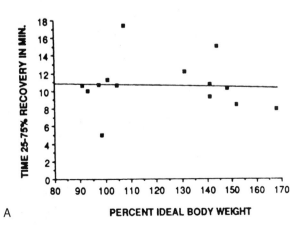

A

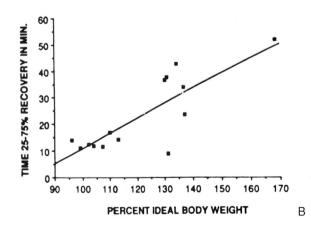

B

Figure 31.7. Regression lines relating time for 25% to 75% recovery of twitch response and body weight in surgical patients following. **A:** Atracurium, 0.5 mg/kg (*r* = 0.06). **B:** Vecuronium, 0.1 mg/kg (*r* = 0.81). (From Weinstein JA, Matteo RS, Ornstein E, et al. Pharmacodynamics of vecuronium and atracurium in the obese surgical patient. *Anesth Analg* 1988;67:1149–1153, with permission.)

pressure cuff is adequate for the moderately obese mother having an uncomplicated labor. In more complex situations an automated device, or an intraarterial catheter that facilitates repeated blood gas analyses, is preferable. Central venous and pulmonary artery catheters may be indicated in special situations such as preeclampsia or cardiac or respiratory failure. Percutaneous placement of these monitors and even an intravenous catheter can prove very difficult, and occasionally a cutdown is necessary. Noninvasive monitoring of oxygenation with pulse oximetry is mandatory during general and regional anesthesia for cesarean section and is helpful during labor in the morbidly obese parturient. End-tidal carbon dioxide monitoring also should be used during general anesthesia to confirm correct placement of the endotracheal tube and permit appropriate adjustment of ventilation. The electrocardiogram must be monitored during major anesthesia and a nerve stimulator used whenever muscle relaxants are employed. During labor, monitoring of contractions and fetal heart rate is often hindered by the thickness of the abdominal wall. Direct internal monitoring of these parameters with a scalp electrode and an intrauterine pressure catheter is usually necessary.

Anesthesia for Vaginal Delivery

During labor the mother should remain in the lateral sitting or semirecumbent position to minimize closure of dependent airways and aortocaval compression. Intravenous access is best secured early in labor. The anesthesiologist should consider administering oxygen throughout labor to prevent hypoxemia, which may result from ventilation perfusion abnormalities and from the enormously increased metabolic and cardiorespiratory activity. The use of pulse oximetry may be particularly helpful for management of these patients. Regional analgesia decreases respiratory work and oxygen consumption, improves oxygenation, and prevents the increase in cardiac output that results from catecholamine secretion during labor. It also is advantageous in view of the frequent need for operative vaginal or cesarean delivery (19). Insertion of an epidural catheter early in labor is recommended by the authors to allow time for placement and confirmation that the block is functional.

Major technical difficulties can present when instituting regional anesthesia in obese parturients, although the distribution of fat is sometimes such that the procedure is easier than would have been predicted from weight alone. As might be expected, the depth at which the epidural space is located correlates strongly with patient weight and the degree of obesity (66, 67). Hood and associates (19) found that, whereas 94% of morbidly obese parturients ultimately obtained successful epidural anesthesia, the catheter had to be replaced once in 46% of patients and two or more times in 21% of patients. Increasing patient weight significantly decreased the likelihood of successful epidural placement by residents, but not by attending anesthesiologists (19). Ranta et al. (68) similarly reported that senior anesthetists were consulted more often to administer the epidural block in obese patients compared with control patients, and that the paramedian approach was used in more cases (25% versus 7%). Also, unintentional intravenous catheter placement occurred in 17% of obese women compared with 3% of controls, resulting in a high incidence of multiple punctures (68). Experienced personnel must be available to perform these challenging procedures and special long needles (15 or 20 cm) are sometimes required. When a normal length needle is used, it may be submerged up the hilt, thereby indenting the subcutaneous tissue. In this circumstance, an assistant may be needed to prevent displacement of the needle by securing it with a hemostat (69). A loss-of-resistance technique is preferable to the "hanging drop" method, because epidural pressure in obesity cannot be relied upon to be subatmospheric. The sitting position is most comfortable for the patient and provides the easiest identification of the midline; elevation of the legs in front of the patient

also helps to flex the back. If no bony landmarks can be located, extensive infiltration of the area with local anesthetic enables exploration with a fine needle to localize a vertebral spinous process or lamina. Wallace et al. (70) performed preliminary studies using indirect sonographic guidance to identify the midline and were able, by measuring the skin-to-lamina distance, to predict the perpendicular depth from the skin to the epidural space. An unintended laterally directed needle (which can result in a unilateral block) thus could be avoided, as this would be associated with a greater than predicted skin-to-epidural space distance. Ultrasonic guidance also may help decide when a longer needle is necessary, and may decrease the risk of dural puncture as the operator can predict the depth of needle insertion at which loss of resistance is expected. However, further experience is needed before this technique can become clinically useful.

Once the epidural space has been located, insertion of the catheter for at least 5 cm is recommended, to prevent displacement of the catheter due to mobility of the layer of subcutaneous fat (3). For the same reason, secure taping of the catheter also is essential. A recent study at the author's institution found that, if the epidural catheter is inserted and securely taped to the skin when the patient is sitting, there is potential for catheter displacement when the patient moves to the lateral decubitus position (72). When the block was performed with the patient sitting and the catheter was not secured at the skin, as the patient assumed the lateral position the catheter moved relative to the skin and appeared to be drawn in towards the epidural space (72). This probably occurs because the distance to the epidural space is greater when the patient is in the lateral position compared with the sitting position (73). The appearance of the unsecured catheter disappearing under the skin results from the tissues expanding as the patient changes position. The catheter in this circumstance is gripped by the ligamentum flavum and should remain at the original distance it was placed in the epidural space. If, however, the catheter is firmly taped to the skin while the patient is still in the sitting position, when she lies on her side the epidural catheter may be pulled out of the epidural space toward the skin by an amount equal to the increased distance to the epidural space in the lateral position. The potential for catheter displacement is considerably greater in obese patients (as tissue depth increases) with catheter movement of 4 to 5 cm occurring in very obese patients (72). This phenomenon may explain the high failure rate after epidural catheter placement in some studies of morbidly obese parturients (19). The problem is best avoided by securing the catheter only after the patient has assumed the lateral position (maintaining sterility of the catheter during the process). The alternatives of performing the block with the patient in the lateral position or inserting the catheter an additional distance into the epidural space may be associated, respectively, with greater technical difficulty and an increased incidence of unilateral blocks. Another cause for block failure reported in obese patients is kinking of the catheter, a problem which has been overcome by placing the operator's hands under the patient's lumbar and thoracic area and pulling the adhesive tape, catheter and subcutaneous tissues in a cephalad direction (74). Maintaining a well-functioning epidural catheter is particularly important in morbidly obese patients because of the high incidence of cesarean section during labor (19).

Some studies have suggested that a lesser volume of local anesthetic is needed to provide adequate epidural analgesia in the obese individual (75, 76), perhaps because adipose tissue and increased venous distension from severe aortocaval compression decrease the capacity of the epidural space. However, one study found that obesity did not influence the height of block achieved after epidural bupivacaine administration during labor (77). A block that is too high or too dense will further weaken respiratory muscle function and impair the ability to push in the second stage of labor. Infusions of dilute solutions of local anesthetics combined with opioids provide excellent analgesia for labor, with minimal motor blockade. Although these mixtures have not specifically been studied in obese parturients, they appear ideal because they allow the patient to move herself and facilitate maternal expulsive efforts during the second stage of labor. Conservative doses of opioids are recommended, as experience with use of intraspinal opioids for postcesarean analgesia suggests that the obese parturient is at greater risk of respiratory depression (78, 79).

When epidural catheter placement for labor analgesia proves technically difficult, a single spinal injection of an opioid can be given [e.g., fentanyl 25 μg, or sufentanil, 7.5 to 10 μg (80)] with or without bupivacaine 1.25 to 2.5 mg, with the goal of establishing analgesia while efforts to insert the epidural catheter at the same or an adjacent interspace proceed. Combined spinal-epidural analgesia (CSE) using a needle-through-needle technique also can be used and may facilitate identification of the epidural space and actually decrease the risk of postdural puncture headache (81). Because fetal bradycardia occasionally follows intrathecal opioid analgesia (80, 82), this technique may be less desirable than epidural analgesia in the obese parturient, in whom injection of a surgical dose of local anesthetic via an untested epidural catheter (or the alternative of emergency general anesthesia) may be hazardous should emergency cesarean section become necessary. Continuous spinal anesthesia using low doses of opioids and local anesthetic also can be considered for labor analgesia, particularly when unintended intrathecal catheter placement occurs during attempted epidural block. Although dural puncture occurs more frequently during attempted epidural block in obese parturients, the incidence of postdural puncture headache appears to be lower in morbidly obese than in normal weight patients (19, 83). Currently, small gauge spinal catheters are not commercially available because of several cases of cauda equina syndrome following administration of large doses of local anesthetics through these devices (84). Single dose spinal block using local anesthetic is appropriate for the second stage of labor, particularly when operative vaginal delivery is planned. Although several investigators have reported higher than expected levels of spinal blockade in obese nonpregnant patients (85–87) (attributing this to increased cerebrospinal fluid pressure caused by epidural venous congestion or excessive extradural fat), a recent study in pregnant patients did not confirm these findings (88). A factor that might increase cephalad spread in obese parturients is the large buttocks that effectively place the patient in a Trendelenburg position relative to the true horizontal of the operating table (89).

If regional analgesia proves technically impossible, first-stage labor pain can be managed with small doses of intravenous opioids via bolus or patient-controlled administration, with careful monitoring of maternal respiration using pulse oximetry. Inhalation analgesia with nitrous oxide can be administered for the latter part of the first and all of the second stage of labor, provided that consciousness and active laryngeal reflexes are maintained and oxygen saturation is closely monitored. Anesthesia can be induced particularly rapidly, because of the degree of hyperventilation present during labor and the decreased FRC of the obese parturient. Methoxyflurane should not be used for reasons already discussed. General anesthesia should rarely be necessary for vaginal delivery, but if unavoidable, it should be performed as described in the following for cesarean section. It must be remembered that the Trendelenburg and lithotomy positions, which often are employed during vaginal delivery, have a deleterious effect on oxygenation. In these situations, positive pressure ventilation should be used to prevent airway closure.

Anesthesia for Cesarean Section

Obese parturients presenting for cesarean section have a high incidence of complications such as diabetes or preeclampsia, with the coexisting medical condition often directly or indirectly being the cause for the procedure. As previously discussed, perioperative morbidity and mortality are high in this group. Reviews of anesthesia for obese patients (1, 16, 25–27, 30, 71, 90–93) describe problems with both regional and general anesthesia. In recent years, general anesthesia has been implicated more often than regional in causing maternal deaths in obese patients (1, 2) and in pregnant women in general (94). For elective cesarean section, regional anesthesia is advantageous because it usually avoids airway difficulties and results in a lower incidence of intraoperative hypertension and postoperative respiratory complications (69, 90–92). The major goals of anesthetic management are prevention of aspiration, careful management of the airway and of ventilation, and avoidance of additional cardiovascular stress and hypotension. Technical difficulties relate to transporting the patient to the operating room, securing her on a narrow operating table, and displacing the uterus adequately to avoid aortocaval compression.

Much discussion has centered on the ideal surgical approach to the uterus (93, 95). Caudad retraction of the panniculus to permit a midline incision traditionally has been favored because abdominal access is facilitated and operating time until delivery minimized. However, Ahern and Goodlin (95) preferred cephalad retraction to enable a Pfannenstiel incision, which has less potential for wound dehiscence and for causing hypoxemia in the postoperative period. In a study of morbidity following cesarean section in obese women, Wolfe et al. (20) found that choice of skin incision did not influence the postoperative course. If a transverse incision is considered desirable, an attempt should be made to retract the panniculus vertically, thus removing its weight from the great vessels (Fig. 31.8). Severe aortocaval compression caused by cephalad retraction of a 70-kg panniculus has resulted in death of the fetus in one extremely obese woman (93). Cephalad retraction of a large panniculus also decreases chest wall compliance, causing dyspnea in patients who are awake and necessitating higher inflation pressures in those undergoing general anesthesia. Whenever possible, fetal heart rate should be monitored during the

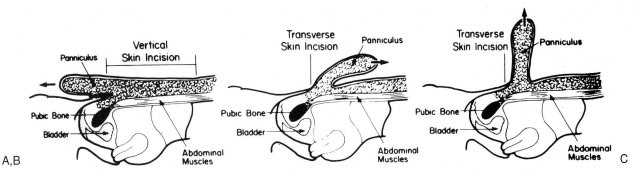

Figure 31.8. The panniculus is shown (**A**) retracted caudad to permit a vertical incision above; (**B**) retracted cephalad to permit a transverse Pfannenstiel incision; and (**C**) retracted vertically. Direction of retraction is shown by arrows. (From Hodgkinson R, Husain FJ. Caesarean section associated with gross obesity. *Br J Anaesth* 1980;52:919–923, with permission.)

surgical procedure. The induction-delivery interval is often prolonged, and fetal deterioration can result from decreases in uterine perfusion due to excessive retraction or abnormalities in maternal ventilation.

General Anesthesia

General endotracheal anesthesia is necessary for some emergency cesarean deliveries or for elective cases when regional anesthesia is contraindicated or not feasible for technical reasons.

Prevention of Aspiration Pneumonitis.   To decrease the risk of pneumonitis should aspiration occur, measures should be taken to increase gastric pH and decrease gastric volume. In elective cases, a histamine H2-receptor antagonist administered the night before and the morning of operation may be useful in reducing gastric pH. In a study in nonpregnant obese surgical patients, only 13% of those who had received cimetidine had a gastric pH of less than 2.5, compared with 65% of patients who had been premedicated with atropine or glycopyrrolate (96). Using the same criteria, Lam et al. (97) found only 10% of morbidly obese patients at risk from aspiration following intravenous injection of 300 mg of cimetidine at least 60 min before induction of anesthesia, compared with 77% in the control group. Some clinicians administer prophylactic oral or intravenous ranitidine for morbidly obese parturients in labor as a precaution should general anesthesia become necessary. Metoclopramide, a dopamine antagonist that increases lower esophageal sphincter tone in gravid patients (98), may be particularly beneficial in obese mothers. A 10- to 20-mg dose administered intravenously 30 min or more before induction of anesthesia may also accelerate gastric motility and, hence, decrease the volume of gastric contents (99). When an obese patient is admitted to the labor ward for urgent cesarean section, an H2 blocker and metoclopramide should be administered immediately to inhibit gastric acid secretion and facilitate emptying of food that may be in the stomach. However, all patients should receive 30 mL of a nonparticulate antacid, such as 0.3 molar sodium citrate, immediately before induction of anesthesia to neutralize gastric pH.

Airway Management.   Endotracheal intubation can present major difficulties in the obese parturient because of fat deposits in the neck, shoulders, and breasts. Failed intubation, often in association with pulmonary aspiration, is one of the most common causes of anesthetic deaths in obese parturients (2). Hood and Dewan (19) encountered difficulty with intubation in almost one third of parturients weighing more than 300 lb who required general anesthesia for cesarean section. Problems should be anticipated beforehand, rather than discovering after induction of anesthesia that the patient can neither be intubated nor ventilated. In obese patients, mask ventilation may be hindered by the fact that mandibular advancement does not improve the retropalatal airway as it does in normal weight patients (100). Careful positioning before induction of anesthesia as shown in Figure 31.4 can greatly facilitate access to the airway. The shoulders are elevated, allowing the breasts to fall away from the neck and chin, while folded towels are used to support the occiput and place the head in the sniffing position. This opens up an area that is often submerged in rolls of fat, allowing insertion of the laryngoscope. The short-handled laryngoscope (101) and the adjustable-angle blade (102) can be helpful in the obese parturient (Fig. 31.9), as well as the intubating laryngeal mask airway (LMA) devices using fiberoptic light sources such as the Billard laryngoscope. An added hazard in obese parturients is laryngeal edema, which can accompany grossly excessive weight gain in pregnancy (103) or generalized edema in preeclampsia (104). A small-diameter endotracheal tube should therefore always be prepared. The anesthesiologist should have difficult intubation equipment immediately available and should be familiar with the American Society of Anesthesiologists Practice Parameter on the Difficult Airway

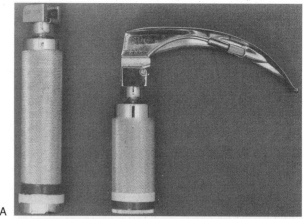

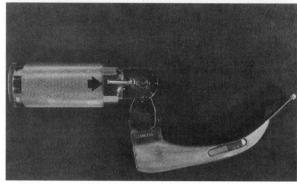

Figure 31.9. **A:** Short handle (right) for laryngoscope compared with conventional length handle (left). **B:** Adjustable-angle laryngoscope. A blade lock (arrow) allows positioning of the blade at 180, 135, 90, or 45 degrees to the handle. The blade can be inserted parallel to the handle and the angle then decreased to 135 or 90 degrees to allow tongue retraction and exposure of the larynx. (From Patil VU, Stehling LC, Zauder HL. An adjustable laryngoscope handle for difficult intubations. *Anesthesiology* 1984;60:609, with permission.)

(105). Equipment should include a LMA and/or a device such as the Combitube ®, to facilitate ventilating the patient should attempts at intubation fail. A 12- or 14-gauge intravenous cannula or a specially designed cricothyrotomy needle with which the anesthesiologist is familiar can be introduced through the cricothyroid membrane into the trachea and connected to a high pressure jet ventilator (106, 107). Technical difficulties should be anticipated because of adiposity of the neck and low compliance of the chest wall. If airway obstruction or failed intubation does occur, hypoxia and acidosis develop with alarming rapidity. The decreased FRC stores less oxygen, while oxygen consumption, carbon dioxide production and the severity of acidosis are greatly increased in the obese parturient. An oximeter and a capnograph are essential when airway complications arise in the obese parturient. If difficulty with the airway is anticipated before induction of anesthesia and time permits, awake fiberoptic intubation can be performed using appropriate sedation and adequate topicalization of the airway. Fiberoptic laryngoscopy is not to be recommended in the emergency situation to practitioners unskilled in this technique. An alternative approach in urgent situations is to perform awake direct laryngoscopy, topicalizing the upper airway if time permits. Most patients will allow the anesthesiologist "one quick look" with a laryngoscope to evaluate the airway with the patient awake. If the epiglottis is visible, intubation with the aid of a flexible Eschmann introducer is often possible after induction of general anesthesia. A recent case report describes use of an LMA to facilitate awake intubation in a morbidly obese parturient undergoing cesarean section (108). Because of the risk associated with general anesthesia, spinal anesthesia is often the best choice for urgent cesarean section when the airway seems certain to present difficulties. If this is not feasible, starting the operation using local anesthesia (while attempts at awake intubation proceed) is preferable to inducing general anesthesia in a patient who cannot be intubated or ventilated.

Anesthetic Technique. Rapid induction of anesthesia with thiopental (e.g., 5 mg · kg^{-1} ideal body weight or a standard dose of 350 to 500 mg) and succinylcholine (1 mg · kg^{-1} total body weight or a standard dose of 120 to 140 mg) is usually performed in the emergency situation, and in elective cases if the airway appears favorable. Concurrent with injection of the induction agents, cricoid pressure should be applied by a skilled assistant. The optimal method of preoxygenation before induction in the obese parturient is controversial. In obese surgical patients (109) and nonobese pregnant patients (110), 3 minutes of preoxygenation and four vital capacity breaths proved equally effective at increasing arterial oxygen tension. However, the former technique resulted in slight retention of carbon dioxide in morbidly obese patients (109). Of most importance in the obese parturient, in whom intubation difficulties are common, is the safe duration of apnea. In a study of normal healthy patients, Gambee et al. (111) demonstrated longer times to desaturation during apnea following 3 min of preoxygenation than following four vital capacity breaths in nonpregnant patients. Because oxygen saturation during apnea decreases much more quickly in both morbidly obese patients (112) and pregnant women (113), a 3- to 5-min period of denitrogenation is recommended in the obese parturient.

Anesthesia can be maintained with nitrous oxide 50% (provided oxygen saturation remains satisfactory) and a low concentration of a volatile anesthetic until delivery, after which the latter may be discontinued and a short-acting opioid administered. Paralysis with a neuromuscular blocking agent is usually necessary to facilitate surgical access. Positive pressure ventilation with relatively large tidal volumes minimizes airway closure (34, 114), although volumes in excess of 13 mL · kg^{-1} ideal body weight did not improve oxygenation in one study of nonpregnant obese patients (115). Positive end-expiratory pressure may not improve oxygenation, because it also decreases cardiac output (114, 116). Catecholamine release during endotracheal intubation can be hazardous in the hypertensive obese gravida, who is particularly prone to developing pulmonary edema because of her expanded blood volume. Treatment of severe hypertension with vasodilators or short-acting beta-adrenergic blockers may be indicated; the choice of drug therapy will depend on the presence or absence of invasive monitoring. The obese mother must be fully awake before extubation, and postoperative ventilation must be continued if adequate arousal and respiratory and neuromuscular function cannot be demonstrated. Because hypoxemia is common in obese patients in the immediate postoperative period, oxygen saturation should be monitored and supplemental oxygen administered in the postanesthetic care unit (117).

Regional Anesthesia

Regional blockade avoids intubation difficulties and, provided hypotension does not develop, is associated with greater cardiovascular stability than is general anesthesia in the hypertensive parturient (118). Also, aspiration should be less of a hazard. However, this risk does exist with regional anesthesia, and the precautions recommended for general anesthesia should be employed. Postoperative respiratory complications have been reported to occur less frequently with regional than with general anesthesia (90).

Epidural anesthesia may be preferable to spinal anesthesia for cesarean section in morbidly obese parturients because of its greater controllability, and the ability to titrate the block to the desired level and extend it for prolonged procedures. However, spinal anesthesia is often technically easier to perform,

provides more dense anesthesia, and is useful in the moderately obese gravida in whom prolonged surgery is not anticipated. Long-acting local anesthetics such as bupivacaine should be used, with the addition of opioids and perhaps epinephrine to ensure a dense block of adequate duration. Combined spinal-epidural anesthesia has the advantage of providing a dense initial block while permitting extension of anesthesia for lengthy procedures. A disadvantage of CSE is that the epidural catheter is not confirmed to be functional until later in the operation, when general anesthesia may be the only alternative if the catheter is misplaced or intravascular and additional anesthesia is needed. Also, if a long epidural needle is required, a needle-through-needle technique may not be feasible unless small-gauge pencil-point spinal needles of adequate length to puncture the dura in this circumstance are available. Continuous spinal anesthesia offers an alternative approach in cases in which the surgical procedure is likely to be long and difficult.

Hypotension with regional anesthesia must be prevented by preloading the circulation with fluids, adequate displacement of the uterus and the panniculus from the inferior vena cava and aorta, and prompt treatment of any decrease in blood pressure with additional fluids and ephedrine. When all these precautions were taken, the incidence of hypotension (<100 mm Hg systolic blood pressure) was only 12% in one series of obese patients receiving epidural anesthesia for cesarean section (75). Several studies have reported higher levels of regional anesthetic block in obese patients (75, 76, 85–87, 90). Hodgkinson and Husain (75) found the extent of epidural block for cesarean section was positively correlated with BMI and body weight. These authors also found that, in obese patients, cephalad spread of epidural block was limited when the patient was in the sitting position, in contrast to patients of normal weight in whom gravity did not affect the block (76). In contrast, other studies have not confirmed decreased epidural dose requirements in obese pregnant patients (77) and have found no influence of the sitting position on the upper level of epidural block (77, 119). Similar controversy exists with spinal anesthesia. Whereas some studies in nonpregnant patients have reported decreased drug requirements with spinal anesthesia, a recent study found that neither body weight nor weight gained during pregnancy influenced the spread of spinal block during cesarean section in the term parturient (88). Decreasing the local anesthetic dosage in obese parturients is not recommended, because of the serious consequences of unsatisfactory anesthesia. An inadequate spinal block may necessitate emergency induction of general anesthesia after the operation has started, presenting a hazardous situation for the obese gravida. Control of the level of spinal blockade can be accomplished by using routine doses of hyperbaric solutions, with careful positioning of the patient in a slight head-up position as soon as an adequate level of anesthesia has been obtained. Regardless of any potential effect on the level of anesthetic block, both spinal and epidural anesthesia are performed most easily with the obese patient in the sitting position, as this facilitates identification of the midline.

Embarrassment of ventilation by large breasts, the fat panniculus, and insertion of packs in the abdomen must be guarded against. Sedation following delivery should be kept to a minimum to avoid hypoventilation. If respiratory inadequacy does occur, general anesthesia with endotracheal intubation and positive pressure ventilation must be undertaken. A major advantage of regional anesthesia is that it permits the use of intraspinal opioid analgesia, postoperatively. Leaving the epidural catheter in situ allows for continuation of analgesia for several days if necessary.

Postoperative Management

The obese parturient continues to be at risk after delivery, particularly if surgical intervention was necessary. Wound dehiscences and infections are more frequent in these individuals,

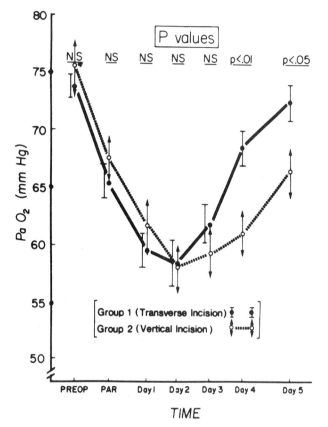

Figure 31.10. Decrease in Pao$_2$ (torr) with time postoperatively in group I (transverse incision) and group II (vertical incision) patients (From Vaughan RW, Wise L. Choice of abdominal operative incision in the obese patient: a study using blood gas measurements. *Ann Surg* 1975;181:829–835, with permission.)

and hospitalization is often prolonged. Postoperative respiratory complications are frequent (29) and hypoxemia can persist for several days (Fig. 31.10) (120, 121). Vertical abdominal incisions result in more severe hypoxemia on the second to fifth postoperative day than do transverse incisions (Fig. 31.10) (121). Supplemental oxygen should be administered and the patient placed in the sitting position, as this minimizes airway closure and improves oxygenation (122). Intensive chest physiotherapy is helpful to aid the clearing of secretions. Severely obese patients in whom cardiac or respiratory dysfunction was present preoperatively should recover in the intensive care unit, at least for the first 24 to 48 hours.

Adequate postoperative analgesia is essential if deep breathing is to be encouraged and atelectasis avoided. Parenteral, epidural, or spinal opioids (123–126) or epidurally administered local anesthetics (90, 92) can be employed, but care must be taken to avoid central respiratory depression or respiratory muscle weakness. The analgesia that results from intraspinal opioids encourages better ventilation, earlier mobility (thus guarding against deep vein thrombosis), and earlier restoration of bowel function, and it facilitates nursing care (123, 124). However, because respiratory depression is a greater risk in the obese parturient (78, 79, 127), particularly those with sleep apnea (128), continuous monitoring of ventilation for the first 24 hours is mandatory either on the postpartum ward or in the intensive care unit. Prophylaxis against deep vein thrombosis with low-dose heparin is advocated by many for obese surgical patients (129, 130) because thrombophlebitis leading to pulmonary embolism is a major cause of mortality, particularly in the postpartum period (15). The issue of heparin prophylaxis in the presence of regional anesthesia is controversial, and is discussed in detail elsewhere (130, 131).

CONCLUSION

In the obese parturient, morbidity and mortality are high because of abnormal anatomy, physiology, and responses to anesthesia. Hypertension, hypotension, hypoxia, and acidosis can develop with great rapidity when complications occur. The margin of safety in these circumstances is very much reduced. The anesthesiologist must be aware of the particular problems of the morbidly obese mother and ensure that an appropriate level of expertise is available for her care. All too often, the attitude of the health care team mirrors the negative view that society holds of these people, with the result that they are not afforded the obese individuals attention warranted by their medical condition.

REFERENCES

1. Endler GC. The risk of anesthesia in obese parturients. *J Perinatol* 1990;10:175–179.
2. Endler GC, Mariona FG, Sokol RJ, et al. Anesthesia-related maternal mortality in Michigan. *Am J Obstet Gynecol* 1988;159:187–193.
3. Garbaciak JA, Richter M, Miller MS, et al. Maternal weight and pregnancy complications. *Am J Obstet Gynecol* 1985;152:238–245.
4. Kliegman RM, Gross T. Perinatal problems of the obese mother and her infant. *Obstet Gynecol* 1985;66:299–306.
5. Bongain A, Isnard V, Gillet JY. Obesity in obstetrics and gynecology. *Eur J Obstet Gynecol Reprod Biol* 1998;77:217–228.
6. Bray GA. *The Obese Patient, vol. 9.* Philadelphia: WB Saunders, 1976:2–93.
7. Abernathy DR, Greenblatt DJ, Divoli M, et al. Alterations in drug distribution and clearance due to obesity. *J Pharmacol Exp Ther* 1981;217:681–685.
8. Executive Summary of the Clinical Guidelines on the Identification, Evaluation and Treatment of Overweight and Obesity in Adults. Expert panel on the identification, evaluation, and treatment of overweight and obesity in adults. *Arch Intern Med* 1998;158:1855–1867.
9. Wolfe HM, Gross TL. Obesity in pregnancy. *Clin Obstet Gynecol* 1994;37:596–604.
10. Burwell CS, Robin ED, Whaley RD, et al. Extreme obesity associated with alveolar hypoventilation: a Pickwickian syndrome. *Am J Med* 1956;21:811–818.
11. Bentley JB. The liver in obesity. In: Brown BR Jr, ed. *Anesthesia and the Obese Patient.* Philadelphia: Davis, 1982:41–53.
12. Roopnarinesingh SS, Pathak UN. Obesity in the Jamaican parturient. *J Obstet Gynaecol Br Commonw* 1970;77:895–899.
13. Tracy TA, Miller GL. Obstetric problems of the massively obese. *Obstet Gynecol* 1969;33:204–208.
14. Freedman MA, Wilds PL, George WM. Grotesque obesity: a serious complication of labor and delivery. *South Med J* 1972;65:732–736.
15. Maeder EC, Barno A, Mecklenburg F. Obesity: a maternal high-risk factor. *Obstet Gynecol* 1975;45:669–671.
16. Johnson SR, Kolberg BH, Varner MW, et al. Maternal obesity and pregnancy. *Surg Gynecol Obstet* 1987;164:431–437.
17. Gross T, Sokol RJ, King KC. Obesity in pregnancy: risks and outcome. *Obstet Gynecol* 1980;56:446–450.
18. Naeye RL. Maternal body weight and pregnancy outcome. *Am J Clin Nutr* 1990;273–299.
19. Hood DD, Dewan DM. Anesthesia outcome in the morbidly obese parturient. *Anesthesiology* 1993;79:1210–1218.
20. Wolfe HM, Gross TL, Sokol RJ, et al. Determinants of morbidity in obese women delivered by cesarean. *Obstet Gynecol* 1988;71:691–696.
21. Galtier Dereure F, Montpeyroux F, Boulot P, et al. Weight excess before pregnancy: complications and cost. *Int J Obesity* 1995;19:443–448.
22. Prentice A, Goldberg G. Maternal obesity increases congenital malformations. *Nutr Rev* 1996;54:146–152.
23. Postlethwait RW, Johnson WD. Complications following surgery for duodenal ulcer in obese patients. *Arch Surg* 1972;105:438–440.
24. Fisher A, Waterhouse TD, Adams AP. Obesity: Its relation to anaesthesia. *Anaesthesia* 1975;30:633–647.
25. Catenacci AJ, Anderson JD, Boersma D. Anesthetic hazards of obesity. *JAMA* 1973;175:657–665.
26. Fox GS. Anesthesia for intestinal short circuiting in the morbidly obese with reference to the pathophysiology of gross obesity. *Can Anaesth Soc J* 1975;22:307–315.

27. Gould AB. Effect of obesity on respiratory complications following general anesthesia. *Anesth Analg* 1962;41:448–452.

28. Shenkman Z, Shir Y, Brodsky JB. Perioperative management of the obese patient. *Br J Anaesth* 1993;70:349–359.

29. Pasulka PS, Bistrian BR, Benotti PN, et al. The risks in obese patients. *Ann Intern Med* 1986;104:540–546.

30. Øberg B, Poulsen TD. Obesity: an anesthetic challenge. *Acta Anaesthesiol Scand* 1996;40:191–200.

31. Benaron HBW, Tucker BE. The effect of obstetric management and factors beyond clinical control on maternal mortality rates at the Chicago Maternity Center from 1959 to 1963. *Am J Obstet Gynecol* 1971;110:1113–1118.

32. Nielsen TK, Hökegård KH. Postoperative cesarean section morbidity: a prospective study. *Am J Obstet Gynecol* 1983;146:911–916.

33. Cohen SE. Why is the pregnant patient different? *Semin Anesth* 1982;1:73–82.

34. Vaughan RW. Pulmonary and cardiovascular derangements in the obese patient. In: Brown BR Jr, ed. *Anesthesia and the Obese Patient.* Philadelphia: Davis, 1982:19–39.

35. Ray CS, Sue DY, Bray G, et al. Effects of obesity on respiratory function. *Am Rev Resp Dis* 1983;128:501–506.

36. Söderberg M, Thomson D, White T. Respiration, circulation and anesthetic management in obesity: Investigation before and after jejunoileal bypass. *Acta Anaesthesiol Scand* 1977;21:55–61.

37. Templeton A, Kelman GR. Maternal blood gases (PAO_2-Pao_2), physiological shunt and VD/VT in normal pregnancy. *Br J Anaesth* 1976;48:1001–1104.

38. Holdcroft A, Bevan DR, O'Sullivan JC, et al. Airway closure and pregnancy. *Anaesthesia* 1977;32:517–523.

39. Damia G, Mascheroni D, Croci M, et al. Perioperative changes in functional residual capacity in morbidly obese patients. *Br J Anaesth* 1988;60:574–578.

40. Eng M, Butler J, Bonica J. Respiratory function in pregnant obese women. *Am J Obstet Gynecol* 1975;123:241–245.

41. Blass NH. Regional anesthesia in the morbidly obese. *Reg Anesth* 1979;4:20–22.

42. Sharp JT, Henry JP, Sweany SK, et al. The total work of breathing in normal and obese men. *J Clin Invest* 1964;43:728–738.

43. Veille JC, Hanson R. Obesity, pregnancy, and left ventricular functioning during the third trimester. *Am J Obstet Gynecol* 1994;171:980–983.

44. Backman L, Freyschuss V, Holbug D, et al. Cardiovascular function in extreme obesity. *Acta Med Scand* 1973;193:437–446.

45. Vaughan RW, Bauer S, Wise L. Volume and pH of gastric juice in obese patients. *Anesthesiology* 1975;43:686–689.

46. Roberts RB, Shirley MA. Reducing the risk of acid aspiration during cesarean section. *Anesth Analg* 1974;53:859–860.

47. Rochester DF, Enson Y. Current concepts in the pathogenesis of the obesity-hypoventilation syndrome. *Am J Med* 1974;57:402–420.

48. Maxwell MH, Schroth PC, Waks AV. Error in blood pressure measurement due to incorrect cuff size in obese patients. *Lancet* 1982;2:33–35.

49. Nichol HC, Zuck D. Difficult laryngoscopy. The "anterior" larynx and the atlantooccipital gap. *Br J Anaesth* 1983;55:141–144.

50. Schwartz AE, Matteo RS, Orstein E, et al. Pharmacokinetics of sufentanil in obese patients. *Anesth Analg* 1991;73:790–793.

51. Servin F, Farinotti R, Haberer JP, et al. Propofol infusion for maintenance of anesthesia in morbidly obese patients receiving nitrous oxide. *Anesthesiology* 1993;78:657–665.

52. Bouillon T, Shafer SL. Does size matter? [Editorial]. *Anesthesiology* 1998;89:557–560.

53. Egan TD, Huizinga B, Gupta SK, et al. Remifentanil pharmacokinetics in obese versus lean elective surgery patients. *Anesthesiology* 1998;89:562–573.

54. Gepts E, Shafer SL, Camu F, et al. Linearity of pharmacokinetics and model estimation of sufentanil. *Anesthesiology* 1995;83:1194–1204.

55. Young SR, Stoelting RK, Peterson C, et al. Anesthetic biotransformation and renal function in obese patients during and after methoxyflurane or halothane anesthesia. *Anesthesiology* 1975;42:451–457.

56. Bentley JB, Vaughan RW, Miller MS, et al. Serum inorganic fluoride levels in obese patients during and after enflurane anesthesia. *Anesth Analg* 1979;58:409–412.

57. Strube PJ, Hulands GH, Halsey MJ. Serum fluoride levels in morbidly obese patients: Enflurane compared with isoflurane anaesthesia. *Anaesthesia* 1987;42:685–689.

58. Bentley JB, Vaughan RM, Gandolfi AJ, et al. Halothane biotransformation in obese and nonobese patients. *Anesthesiology* 1982;57:94–97.

59. Frink EJ, Malan TP, Brown EA, et al. Plasma inorganic fluoride levels with sevoflurane anesthesia in morbidly obese and nonobese patients. *Anesth Analg* 1993;76:1333–1337.

60. Higuchi H, Satoh T, Arimura S, et al. Serum inorganic fluoride levels in mildly obese patients during and after sevoflurane anesthesia. *Anesth Analg* 1993;77:1018–1021.

61. Cork RC, Vaughan RW, Bentley JB. Best general anesthetic agent for the morbidly obese patient. *Anesthesiology* 1980;53:A258.

62. Bentley JB, Borel JD, Vaughan RW, et al. Weight, pseudocholinesterase activity and succinylcholine requirement. *Anesthesiology* 1982;57:48–49.

63. Tsueda K, Warren JE, McCafferty LA, et al. Pancuronium bromide requirements during anesthesia for the morbidly obese. *Anesthesiology* 1978;48:436–439.

64. Varin F, Ducharme J, Théorêt Y, et al. Influence of extreme obesity on the body disposition and neuromuscular blocking effect of atracurium. *Clin Pharmacol Ther* 1990;48:18–25.

65. Weinstein JA, Matteo RS, Ornstein E, et al. Pharmacodynamics of vecuronium and atracurium in the obese surgical patient. *Anesth Analg* 1988;67:1149–1153.

66. Palmer SK, Abram SE, Maitra AM, et al. Distance from the skin to the lumbar epidural space in an obstetric population. *Anesth Analg* 1983;62:944–946.

67. Maiklejohn BH. Distance from the skin to the lumbar epidural space in an obstetric population. *Reg Anesth* 1990;15:134–136.

68. Ranta P, Jouppila P, Spalding M, et al. The effect of maternal obesity on labour and labour pain. *Anaesthesia* 1995;50:322–326.

69. Maitra AM, Palmer SK, Bachhuber SR, et al. Continuous epidural analgesia for cesarean section in a patient with morbid obesity. *Anesth Analg* 1979;58:348–349.

70. Wallace DH, Currie JM, Gilstrap LC. Indirect sonographic guidance for epidural anesthesia in obese pregnant patients. *Reg Anesth* 1992;17:233–236.

71. Dewan DD. Anesthesia for the morbidly obese parturient. In: Hood DD, ed. *Problems in Anesthesia, vol. 3.* Philadelphia: JB Lippincott, 1989:56–68.

72. Hamilton CL, Riley ET, Cohen SE. Changes in the position of epidural catheters associated with patient movement. *Anesthesiology* 1997;86:778–784.

73. Hamza J, Smida M, Benhamou D, et al. Parturients' posture during epidural placement affects the distance from skin to epidural space. *J Clin Anaesth* 1995;7:1–4.

74. Leith P, Sanborn R, Brock-Utne JG. Intraoperative epidural catheter malfunction in two obese patients. *Acta Anaesthesiol Scand* 1997;41:651–653.

75. Hodgkinson R, Husain FJ. Obesity and the cephalad spread of analgesia following epidural administration of bupivacaine for cesarean section. *Anesth Analg* 1980;59:89–92.

76. Hodgkinson R, Husain FJ. Obesity and spread of epidural anesthesia. *Anesth Analg* 1981;60:421–424.

77. Milligan KR, Cramp P, Schatz L, et al. The effect of patient position and obesity on the spread of epidural analgesia. *Int J Obstet Anesth* 1993;2,134–136.

78. Brockway MS, Noble DW, Sharwood-Smith GH, et al. Profound respiratory depression after extradural fentanyl. *Br J Anaesth* 1990;64:243–245.

79. Abouleish E, Rawal N, Rashad MN. The addition of 0.2 mg subarachnoid morphine to hyperbaric bupivacaine for cesarean delivery: a prospective study of 856 cases. *Reg Anesth* 1991;16:137–140.

80. Cohen SE, Cherry CM, Holbrook RH, et al. Intrathecal sufentanil for labor analgesia—sensory changes, side effects, and fetal heart rate changes. *Anesth Analg* 1993;77:1155–1160.

81. Norris MC, Grieco WM, Borkowski M, et al. Complications of labor analgesia: epidural versus combined spinal-epidural techniques. *Anesth Analg* 1995;79:529–537.

82. Clarke VT, Smiley RM, Finster M. Uterine hyperactivity after intrathecal injection of fentanyl for analgesia during labor: a cause of fetal bradycardia? *Anesthesiology* 1994;81:1083.

83. Faure E, Moreno R, Thisted R. Incidence of postdural puncture headache in morbidly obese patients. *Reg Anesth* 1994;19:361–363.

84. Rigler ML, Drasner K, Krejcie TC, et al. Cauda equina syndrome after continuous spinal anesthesia. *Anesth Analg* 1991;72:275–281.

85. Pitkänen MT. Body mass and spread of spinal anesthesia with bupivacaine. *Anesth Analg* 1987;66:127–131.

86. Taivainen T, Tuominen M, Rosenberg PH. Influence of obesity on the spread of spinal analgesia after injection of plain 0.5% bupivacaine at the L3-4 or L4-5 interspace. *Br J Anaesth* 1990;64:542–546.

87. McCulloch WJD, Littlewood DG. Influence of obesity on spinal analgesia with isobaric 0.5% bupivacaine. *Br J Anaesth* 1986;58: 610–614.

88. Ekeløf NP, Jensen J, Poulsen J, et al. Weight gained during pregnancy does not influence the spread of analgesia in the term parturient. *Acta Anaesthesiol Scand* 1997;41:884–887.

89. Greene N. *Physiology of Spinal Anesthesia*, 3rd ed. Baltimore: Williams & Wilkins, 1981:6.

90. Buckley FP, Robinson NB, Simonowitz DA, et al. Anaesthesia in the morbidly obese. *Anaesthesia* 1983;38:840–851.

91. Bromage PR, Fox GS. Obesity: Its relation to anaesthesia. *Anaesthesia* 1976;31:557–558.

92. Gelman S, Laws HL, Potzick J, et al. Thoracic epidural vs. balanced anesthesia in morbid obesity: an intraoperative and postoperative hemodynamic study. *Anesth Analg* 1980;59:902–908.

93. Hodgkinson R, Husain FJ. Caesarean section associated with gross obesity. *Br J Anaesth* 1980;52:919–923.

94. Hawkins JL, Koonin LM, Palmer SK, et al. Anesthesia-related deaths during obstetric delivery in the United States, 1979–1980. *Anesthesiology* 1997;86:277–284.

95. Ahern JK, Goodlin RC. Cesarean section in the massively obese. *Obstet Gynecol* 1978;51:509–510.

96. Wilson SL, Mantena NR, Halverson JD. Effects of atropine, glycopyrrolate, and cimetidine on gastric secretions in morbidly obese patients. *Anesth Analg* 1981;60:37–40.

97. Lam AM, Grace DM, Penny FJ, et al. Prophylactic intravenous cimetidine reduces the risk of acid aspiration in morbidly obese patients. *Anesthesiology* 1986;65:684–687.

98. Brock-Utne JG, Dow TGB, Welman S, et al. The effect of metoclopramide on the lower esophageal spincter in late pregnancy. *Anaesth Intens Care* 1978;6:26–29.

99. Bylsma-Howell M, Riggs KW, McMorland GH, et al. Placental transport of metoclopramide: assessment of maternal and neonatal effects. *Can Anaesth Soc J* 1983;30:487–492.

100. Isono S, Tanaka A, Tagaito Y, et al. Pharyngeal patency in response to advancement of the mandible in obese anesthetized persons. *Anesthesiology* 1997;87:1055–1062.

101. Datta S, Briwa J. Modified laryngoscope for endotracheal intubation of obese patients. *Anesth Analg* 1981;60:120–121.

102. Langeron O, Semjen F, Bourgain J-L, et al. Comparison of the intubating laryngeal mask airway with the fiberoptic intubation in anticipated difficult airway management. *Anesthesiology* 2001;94: 968–972.

103. Spotoft H, Christensen P. Laryngeal oedema accompanying weight gain in pregnancy. *Anaesthesia* 1981;36:71.

104. Seager SJ, Macdonald R. Laryngeal oedema and preeclampsia. *Anaesthesia* 1980;5:360–362.

105. Practice Guidelines for Management of the Difficult Airway. A report by the American Society of Anesthesiologists Task Force on Management of the Difficult Airway. *Anesthesiology* 1993;78; 597–602.

106. Millar WL. Management of a difficult airway in obstetrics. *Anesthesiology* 1980;52:523–524.

107. Benumof JL, Scheller MS. The importance of transtracheal ventilation in the management of the difficult airway. *Anesthesiology* 1989;71:769–778.

108. Godley M, Reddy AR. Use of LMA for awake intubation for caesarean section. *Can J Anaesth* 1996;43:299–302.

109. Goldberg ME, Norris MC, Larijani GE, et al. Preoxygenation in the morbidly obese: a comparison of two techniques. *Anesth Analg* 1989;68:520–522.

110. Norris MC, Dewan DM. Preoxygenation for cesarean section: a comparison of two techniques. *Anesthesiology* 1985;62:827–829.

111. Gambee AM, Hertzka RE, Fisher DM. Preoxygenation techniques: comparison of three minutes and four breaths. *Anesth Analg* 1987;66:468–470.

112. Jense HG, Dubin SA, Silverstein PI, et al. Effect of obesity on safe duration of apnea in anesthetized humans. *Anesth Analg* 1991;72:89–93.

113. Archer GW, Marx GF. Arterial oxygen tension during apnea in parturient women. *Br J Anaesth* 1974;46:358–360.

114. Eriksen J, Anderson J, Rasmussen JP, et al. Effects of ventilation with large tidal volumes or positive end-expiratory pressure on cardiorespiratory function in anaesthetized obese patients. *Acta Anaesthesiol* 1978;22:241–248.

115. Bardoczky GI, Yernault JC, Houben JJ, et al. Large tidal volume ventilation does not improve oxygenation in morbidly obese patients during anesthesia. *Anesth Analg* 1995;81:385–388.

116. Salem MR, Dalal FY, Zygmunt MP, et al. Does PEEP improve intraoperative arterial oxygenation in grossly obese patients? *Anesthesiology* 1978;48:280–281.

117. Morris RW, Buschman A, Warren DL, et al. The prevalence of hypoxemia detected by pulse oximetry during recovery from anesthesia. *J Clin Monit* 1988;4:16–20.

118. Hodgkinson R, Husain FJ, Hayashi RH. Systemic and pulmonary blood pressure during caesarean section in parturients with gestational hypertension. *Can Anaesth Soc J* 1980;27:389–394.

119. Park WY, Hagins FM, Massengale MD, et al. The sitting position and anesthetic spread in the epidural space. *Anesth Analg* 1984;63: 863–864.

120. Vaughan RW, Engelhardt RC, Wise L. Postoperative hypoxemia in obese patients. *Ann Surg* 1974;180:877–882.

121. Vaughan RW, Wise L. Choice of abdominal operative incision in the obese patient: a study using blood gas measurements. *Ann Surg* 1975;181:829–835.

122. Vaughan RW, Wise L. Postoperative arterial blood gas measurements in obese patients: effect of position on gas exchange. *Ann Surg* 1975;182:705–707.

123. Rawal BM, Sjöstrand U, Christoffersson E, et al. Comparison of intramuscular and epidural morphine for postoperative analgesia in the grossly obese: influence on postoperative ambulation and pulmonary function. *Anesth Analg* 1984;63:583–592.

124. Cohen SE, Woods WA. The role of epidural morphine in the postcesarean patient: efficacy and effects of bonding. *Anesthesiology* 1983;58:500–504.

125. Cohen SE, Subak L, Brose WG, et al. Analgesia following cesarean section: patient evaluations and costs of five opioid techniques. *Reg Anesth* 1991;16:141–149.

126. Rosen MA, Hughes SC, Shnider SM, et al. Epidural morphine for the relief of postoperative pain after cesarean delivery. *Anesth Analg* 1983;62:666–672.

127. Fuller JG, McMorland GH, Douglas J, et al. Epidural morphine for analgesia after caesarean section: a report of 4880 patients. *Can J Anaesth* 1990;37:636–640.

128. Ostermeier AM, Roizen MF, Hautkappe M, et al. Three sudden postoperative respiratory arrests associated with epidural opioids in patients with sleep apnea. *Anesth Analg* 1997;85:452–460.

129. Kakkar VV. Prevention of fatal postoperative thromboembolism by low dose heparin: An international multicenter trial. *Lancet* 1975;2:45–51.

130. Odoom JA, Sih IL. Epidural analgesia and anticoagulant therapy. *Anaesthesia* 1983;38:254–259.

131. Neuraxial anesthesia and anticoagulation (a consensus conference). *Reg Anesth Pain Med* 1998:23.

Shnider and Levinson's Anesthesia for Obstetrics,
edited by Samuel C. Hughes, et al.
Lippincott Williams & Wilkins,
Philadelphia, © 2001.

CHAPTER 32

ANESTHESIA FOR THE PREGNANT PATIENT WITH IMMUNOLOGIC DISORDERS

MARGARET SREBRNJAK, B.Sc., M.D., F.R.C.P.C. AND STEPHEN HALPERN, M.D., M.Sc., F.R.C.P.C.

Immunologic mechanisms play a role in a wide variety of pathologic states. These may be acute and life threatening, such as severe anaphylaxis, or they may be subacute or chronic, such as rheumatoid arthritis (RA) and allograft rejection. None of these immunologic diseases preclude pregnancy. Acute events can occur at any time but are most common during labor and delivery, when parenteral drugs are administered most frequently. In addition, acute anaphylactic reactions to such environmental antigens as latex have recently become a major concern both for patients and staff. Chronic diseases may cause a decrease in fertility and an increase in first trimester abortions, but a significant number of these patients can deliver viable fetuses. This chapter reviews the pathophysiology of immune-mediated tissue injury, common syndromes relevant to the parturient and their appropriate anesthetic management.

THE IMMUNE SYSTEM

The immune system is composed of cellular elements (lymphocytes, mast cells, plasma cells, and macrophages), their humoral products (e.g., immunoglobulins and cytokines), and complement. Normally these interact in an organized fashion to rid the body of foreign material (e.g., antigens and haptens) that may cause harm. Inherent in the system is the capacity of the cellular elements to communicate with each other and modulate function both through direct contact and humoral mediators (1). However, in the process, both the cellular and soluble elements may cause inflammation and tissue damage. Destruction of normal tissue may also occur in autoimmune disorders in which the immune response is directed against autoantigens.

There are four classic mechanisms by which the immune system causes injury: immediate hypersensitivity (type 1), cytotoxic reactions (type II), circulating immune complexes (type III), and delayed hypersensitivity reactions (type IV). These are summarized in Table 32.1.

Immediate Hypersensitivity (Type I)

Immediate hypersensitivity or anaphylaxis is a reaction that requires the recognition of antigens by the immunoglobulin type E (IgE). During the initial encounter, B type lymphocytes become sensitized to the foreign antigen. Plasma cells are produced, and specific IgE to that antigen is liberated. The immunoglobulins then bind to circulating mast cells in the tissues, or basophils in the plasma and are ready to participate in an anaphylactic reaction when stimulated on a subsequent exposure. A previous uneventful single or repeated exposures to the same or similar drugs does not exclude the future possibility of severe allergic reactions. With recognition of the allergen and cross-linking of two IgE molecules, there is a conformational change in the cell membrane resulting in the release of mediators (2). These include histamine, serotonin, slow-reacting substance of anaphylaxis (SRS-A), platelet-activating factor

(PAF), and tryptase (1). Together, they cause vasodilation and an increased permeability in capacitance vessels and arteries leading a fall in blood pressure and edema. Smooth muscle contraction in the airways leads to bronchospasm and the irritation of neural elements, results in pruritus and cutaneous erythema (3). Histamine may also predispose the heart to arrhythmias as it can slow atrioventricular conduction but the smooth muscle of the pregnant uterus is unaffected (4). The mediators, in addition to acting as chemotactic factors to inflammatory cells, also activate other pathways (Fig. 32.1).

In general, the clinical manifestations of immediate hypersensitivity depend on the individual's susceptibility to the antigen, the amount of allergen encountered, and the conditions of exposure. Hence, symptoms can be mild or life-threatening (3) (Fig. 32.2).

Anaphylactoid and Anaphylactic Reactions

Pathophysiologically, anaphylactic reactions are distinct from anaphylactoid reactions, however clinically, they may be indistinguishable. For example, the ability of muscle relaxants and opioids to release histamine directly from mast cells is a nonimmune mediated or anaphylactoid reaction (5, 6). Other pharmacological agents such as radiocontrast dye activate complement factors (6). Many anaphylactoid reactions can be attenuated with antihistamines and the slow administration of drugs. In addition, these reactions do not require prior sensitization to an antigen. Most drugs can cause both types of reactions (Fig. 32.1).

Cytotoxic Reactions (Type II)

The cytotoxic immune response is initiated by the combination of circulating IgM or IgG antibodies, with antigens in the cell membrane. These antibodies either act as opsonins and cause cell destruction in the reticuloendothelial system by splenic trapping, or they bind to complement.

When antibodies are directed toward red blood cells, life-threatening hemolysis occurs, as is the case with the transfusion of ABO-incompatible blood. Complement activation, in addition to causing cell lysis, releases activated coagulation enzymes, fibrinolysins, and kinins. These lead to severe hemodynamic and renal compromise, as well as disseminated intravascular coagulation. Other examples of this mechanism of hypersensitivity include autoimmune hemolytic anemia, immune thrombocytopenic purpura, and in pregnancy, erythroblastosis fetalis. The latter will be considered below.

Immune Complex Diseases (Type III)

Immune complex diseases occur when antigen-antibody complexes are deposited in various tissues which cause complement activation and the release of vasoactive and chemotactic factors. Acutely, neutrophils phagocytize the immune complexes and

Table 32.1. IMMUNE MECHANISMS OF TISSUE INJURY

Mechanism	Mediators	Examples
Type I: Immediate hypersensitivity	IgE; histamine, serotonin, SRS-A, PAF, tryptase	Anaphylactic shock Atopy
Type II: Cytotoxic reactions	IgG or IgM; complement	Hemolytic transfusion reactions Autoimmune hemolytic reactions Erythroblastosis fetalis ITP
Type III: Immune complex–mediated	Antigen-antibody complexes; complement, neutrophils	SLE, rheumatoid arthritis Systemic sclerosis
Type IV: Delayed type hypersensitivity	T lymphocytes; lymphokines, macrophages, complement[a], antibodies[a]	Allograft rejection

[a] Not required for the reaction to take place.
IgE, immunoglobulin Type E; SRS-A, slow-reacting substance of anaplylaxia; PAF, platelet activating factor; IgM, Immunoglobulin Type M; ITP, immune thrombocytopenia; SIE, systemic lupus erythematosis.

release lysosomal enzymes. Monocytes and T lymphocytes arrive later and continue the cell destruction. Patients with autoimmune diseases, not only have complement activation from the soluble antigens and antibodies but as the concentration of multimolecular complexes increases, they precipitate and deposit in vascular beds, glomerular basement membranes, and serous cavities resulting in vasculitis, glomerulonephritis, and polyserositis. During normal pregnancies, immune complexes can be detected in the circulation in the third trimester of pregnancy but these are usually removed by the reticuloendothelial system (7). In addition, circulating immune complexes or the antibody component of these, can be detected in cord blood after delivery (7, 8).

Delayed Hypersensitivity Reactions (Type IV)

Delayed hypersensitivity, as exemplified by allograft rejection and by the tuberculin skin test, is mediated by T lymphocytes. Unlike reactions caused by histamine release, which occur immediately, the signs of inflammation occur approximately 12 hours after the antigen is introduced, with a peak severity at 24 to 48 hours. On exposure, previously sensitized T lymphocytes release mediators that attract macrophages and other T lymphocytes to the site of antigen production. In the environment of a number of mediators, these cells then become cytotoxic or "killer" cells. Although antibodies and complement are not necessary for this type of reaction, they are often involved.

TYPE I IMMUNE RESPONSE
Allergy to Anesthetic and Nonanesthetic Agents
Epidemiology

The frequency of allergic reactions during anesthesia ranges from one in 6,000 to one in 25,000 anesthetics (9, 10) with a mortality of 4% to 6% (11). Over 75% of anesthetic allergies occur in women (10). The frequency of anesthetic allergy to

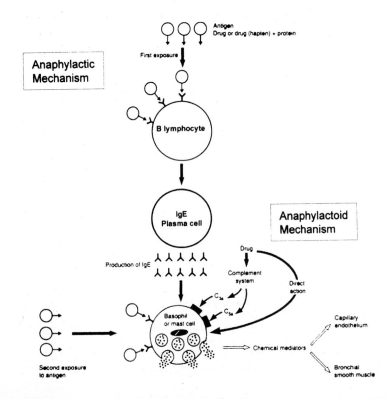

Figure 32.1. Anaphylactic and anaphylactoid mechanisms of drug reactions: C3a and C5a are specific complement factors. (Adapted from Naguib M, Magboul M. Adverse effects of neuromuscular blockers and their antagonists. *Drug Safety* 1998; 18:99–116.)

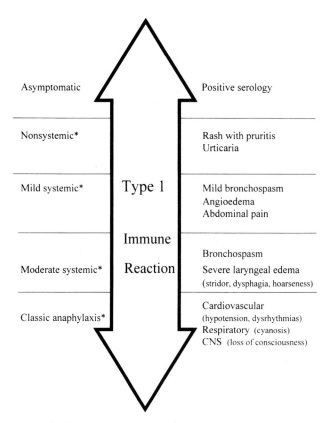

Figure 32.2. *The clinical manifestations of immediate hypersensitivity may also include any of the above signs and symptoms. (Adapted from Kwittken PL, Sweinberg SK, Campbell DE, et al. Latex hypersensitivity in children: clinical presentatiion and detection of latex-specific immunoglobulin E. *Pediatrics* 1995;95:693–699.)

Table 32.2. SIGNS AND SYMPTOMS ASSOCIATED WITH ANAPHYLAXIS

Onset Time	55%, <10 min; 11%, >30 min
Hypotension or circulatory collapse	59–92%
Bronchospasm	36–59%
Tachycardia	94%
Arrhythmias (including bradycardia)	10–18%
Cutaneous flushing/urticaria	45–64%
Angioedema	31–48%

Data from Fisher MM, Baldo BA. The incidence and clinical features of anaphylactic reactions during anaesthesia in Australia. *Ann Fr Anesth Reanim* 1993;12:97–104; Galletly DC, Treuren BC. Anaphylactoid reactions during anaesthesia. *Anaesthesia* 1985;40:329–333; and Laxenaire MC, Moneret-Vautrin DA, Vervloet D. The French experience of anaphylactoid reactions. *Int Anesthesiol Clin* 1985;23:145–160.

that 24% of the patients who reacted to muscle relaxants had a history of allergy to antibiotics (16).

Presentation

In general, agents that have been used for long, continuous periods before the onset of an acute reaction are less likely to be implicated as a cause of hypersensitivity than agents recently introduced (5). The onset of symptoms is often rapid (within minutes), although, the occasional patient may develop signs and symptoms hours later (17).

The awake patient may complain of nonspecific cutaneous burning and pruritus. They may also have nausea, vomiting and abdominal cramps. Angioedema may be centralized about the face and pharyngeal structures or it may be generalized resulting in cardiovascular collapse. Other signs include tachycardia and a falling oxygen saturation. Bronchospasm and increased airway pressures in a patient under general anesthesia are common. Draping may hide early skin manifestations thus extra vigilance is required. Overall, the signs and symptoms of anaphylaxis in any one particular patient can be varied (3, 9) (Table 32.2).

There is a broad differential diagnosis for anaphylaxis in pregnancy and this is presented in Figure 32.4. In addition, the pregnant patient may not present with classical signs such as bronchospasm and skin flushing. Severe hypotension may be all that is evident (18).

Management

Management should start by discontinuing the offending antigen and supporting the airway, breathing and circulation. An intravenous infusion should be started whether or not the reaction

specific agents in one series appears in Figure 32.3. In the pregnant woman, there are the additional concerns of the neonate. Fortunately, there is no genetic basis for anesthetic allergy and there is no passage of maternal IgE across the placenta (12, 13).

The relationship between atopy or multiple allergies and the risk of experiencing severe clinical anaphylaxis during anesthesia is controversial. Neither atopy nor a history of multiple allergies are reliable predictors of anaphylaxis to medications, but atopy may be a risk factor for latex allergy (14). However, patients who have had anaphylaxis in the operating room, will often have positive tests to a number of agents. One center reported a 7.7% prevalence of latex sensitivity in patients allergic to general anesthetic agents (15). Another group found

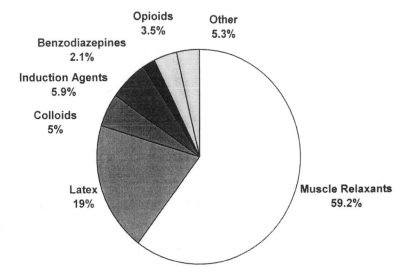

Figure 32.3. Causes of anesthetic-related anaphylaxis. (Adapted from Laxenaire MC, et le. Group d'étude des réactions anaphylactoides peranesthésique: Substances responsables des chocs anaphylactiques peranesthésiques. Troisième enquête multicentrique française (1992–1994). *Ann Fr Anesth Réanim* 1996;15:1211–1218.)

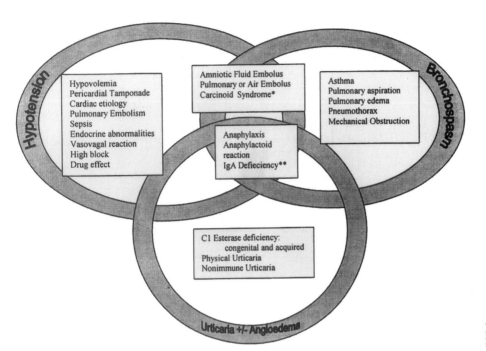

Figure 32.4. Differential diagnosis of anaphylaxis. *Flushing but no edema or urticaria, **with transfusion only.

is mild or severe as reactions may evolve. Biphasic reactions, characterized by a recurrence of symptoms following recovery, have been described in 5% of patients (19).

The airway must be patent and breathing adequate. If severe upper airway obstruction with stridor and cyanosis occurs, endotracheal intubation or cricothyroidotomy should be performed immediately. Artificial ventilation may require a prolonged expiratory time and positive end expiratory pressure in the presence of noncardiogenic pulmonary edema and bronchospasm (19). Overall, the effect of anaphylaxis on the fetus is limited to inadequate placental perfusion and oxygenation. Since, the placenta is metabolically active producing very high levels of diamine oxidase (a histaminase that metabolizes both histamine and other related endogenous mediators) the fetus is not exposed to the inflammatory mediators (13). Severe hypotension and hypoxia leads to fetal asphyxia which may not be severe enough to produce fetal death but can lead to severe central nervous system injury (20). Asphyxia may also occur with the maternal administration of exogenous catecholamines causing maternal uterine vasoconstriction (21). While epinephrine is clearly the drug of choice in the nonpregnant patient, its use in pregnancy is controversial because of its effects on uterine artery resistance (21, 22). Ephedrine is well known to preserve uterine blood flow (23) thus in the absence of cardiovascular collapse and severe bronchospasm, it may be a better alternative (24). When epinephrine is indicated, it should be used in the minimum effective dose in conjunction with left uterine displacement and fluid boluses, to correct hypotension and bronchospasm. Fortunately, even in severe cases of anaphylaxis when large doses of epinephrine are required, prompt delivery of the fetus has limited maternal and fetal morbidity and mortality (13). Thus, if hypotension persists despite initial therapy, immediate delivery could be lifesaving for both (18). If the parturient has no palpable blood pressure then the protocol for cardiac arrest in the pregnant patient should be instituted, including delivery of the fetus after 5 minutes if necessary (25). Aortocaval compression will be relieved, ventilation made easier, CPR more effective and the fetus will be spared the hypoxic and hypotensive environment.

The usual dose of epinephrine is 1 to 2 μg·kg^{-1} or 200 to 500 μg, intramuscularly repeated every 10 to 15 minutes until an intravenous can be obtained. An epinephrine infusion of 1 to 4 μg/min may be required if symptoms persist. Ventricu-

lar arrhythmias are common with intravenous dosing therefore electrocardiographic monitoring is needed (19).

Histamine receptor-blocking drugs and corticosteroids, are useful adjuncts for immediate life-threatening anaphylaxis and may be all that is needed in mild reactions. Antihistamines are particularly effective for angioedema and urticaria, while corticosteroids may reduce the risk of a recurring or protracted anaphylaxis. Salbutamol and aminophylline are indicated for refractory bronchospasm (17, 19).

If an urgent or emergency cesarean section is required, regional anesthesia may be preferred if the patient is hemodynamically stable and the fetus is not in distress. However, the patient may develop severe pharyngeal and laryngeal edema later, which may make general anesthesia problematic. In addition, following intubation, extra caution is warranted on the removal of the endotracheal tube as airway edema may take time to resolve. The management is summarized in Table 32.3.

Assessment of the Event

Once the patient is stabilized attempts should be made to determine the cause of the reaction. The causative agent may not be identified acutely but blood tests can be performed which may suggest that the reaction was either anaphylactic or

---

Table 32.3. MANAGEMENT OF ANAPHYLAXIS IN THE PREGNANT PATIENT

1. Discontinue the suspected offending antigen.
2. Airway and breathing
   a. If necessary, intubate or perform cricothyroidomy.
   b. Supplemental oxygen
3. Circulation of mother and fetus
   a. Position parturient in left lateral position.
   b. Fluid boluses of a balance salt solution
   c. If vasopressors are required consider ephedrine; otherwise, start with epinephrine (subcutaneous dosing is also appropriate).
4. Emergency delivery if the parturient or viable fetus is not responding to therapy
5. Adjuvant therapy
   a. Corticosteroids
   b. Histamine receptor blocking drugs
6. Intensive post reaction monitoring of mother and fetus

anaphylactoid. The tests should be done immediately and at regular intervals as required to determine the nature of the reaction. A complete blood count showing the lack of basophils in the initial reaction sample is highly indicative of an anaphylactic response (6). Histamine levels are generally not useful as they are difficult to measure and return to baseline within 15 to 60 minutes (26). A decrease in C3 and C4 implicate an immune reaction, but not an IgE mediated one and decreases in C3 alone, indicate non-immune mediated reaction. Variations in IgE levels are not sensitive or specific (6). Recently, mast cell tryptase, which is stored in mast cell granules, is being considered as a specific marker for anaphylaxis (27). It is stable in *post mortem* blood and also for prolonged periods and has the advantage of being elevated for several hours (26, 27).

After the acute event, the patient should be referred to an allergy/immunology specialist. However, specific tests must wait at least 6 weeks while the mediators and immunoglobulins return to prereaction levels.

Specific Allergies

Local Anesthetics. Many patients have had adverse reactions to local anesthetics and are subsequently labeled as allergic to the "-caines" (i.e., local anesthetics). While acute hypersensitivity reactions to both ester (28) and amide (29) local anesthetics have been reported, they are extremely rare, comprising only about 1% of all adverse reactions to these drugs (30). Other reactions such as those in Table 32.4 may be misdiagnosed as an allergic response (31). Local anesthetics have been divided into two groups, based on their chemical structure. The benzoic acid (group I) local anesthetics include drugs such as benzocaine, chloroprocaine, procaine and tetracaine. The amide group (group II) includes bupivacaine, etidocaine, lidocaine, mepivacaine, prilocaine, and ropivacaine. There is no evidence that drugs from group I cross-react with drugs in group II. However, drugs within group I may cross-react with each other, particularly on patch testing. There may also be some cross reactivity between drugs in group II diagnosed by patch testing and skin prick tests (32–34).

Some cases of acute hypersensitivity associated with local anesthetics are secondary to other factors such as preservatives (35), other drugs, or environmental (36) and psychological factors (37).

Ideally, the pregnant patient who has experienced an adverse response to local anesthetics should be seen during pregnancy

by an anesthesiologist because these drugs may be vital for the provision of pain relief or anesthesia in the future. Often, the patient's history is not compatible with anaphylaxis and another diagnosis is suggested such as a relative overdose, intravascular injection, or the effect of vasoconstrictors in the solution. However, if the history is suggestive of an acute hypersensitivity reaction, it is best to avoid the offending agent if it is known. A different chemical group may be used. If the offending agent is unknown, intradermal testing and progressive subcutaneous challenge with an amide anesthetic may be useful. The extreme rarity of allergic reactions to local anesthetics and the proven safety of provocative challenge testing makes the risk of a reaction extremely small, even in parturients (38). This approach may also be useful in patients who do not have a classical history of anaphylaxis and require reassurance (39).

Induction Agents. Thiopental allergy has been well documented but both etomidate and ketamine are very rare causes of anaphylaxis (9).

At one time, reactions to propofol were quite common, as the vehicle was cremaphor EL, which has a long history of inducing anaphylactoid reactions. A change to a mixture of soybean oil, egg lecithin (phosphatide) and glycerol was successful in reducing the incidence. The egg lecithin is extracted from egg yolk, which is distinct from egg albumin, the component to which most patients are allergic. In addition, sensitivity to Intralipid in patients with a history of parenteral nutrition or dermatologic products may be an important cross sensitivity to those allergic to the actual propofol molecule (40).

Muscle Relaxants. Fifty-nine percent of the anaphylactic reactions during general anesthesia are due to muscle relaxants (41). Surprisingly, many of the patients who react to relaxants do so on their first intravenous exposure. Ninety percent to 95% of anaphylactic reactions to muscle relaxants occur in women. This may be due to sensitization through exposure to quaternary or tertiary ammonium ions in cosmetics and disinfectants (9). Once a patient becomes sensitized, there is up to a 65% chance of cross-reactivity among muscle relaxants by skin test, especially between pancuronium and vecuronium (42). In addition, all muscle relaxants have the ability to cause direct histamine release (9).

Opioids. Opioids can be classified by their structural derivatives, with morphine, codeine, hydromorphone, and oxycodone in one group and fentanyl, sufentanil, alfentanil and meperidine in another group. Cross-reactivity for anaphylaxis is more likely within each group but, since immune-mediated reactions are so rare, the true prevalence is unknown (43). In addition, most of the reactions to opioids are secondary to direct mast cell mediator release rather than immediate hypersensitivity (9).

Nonanesthetic Drugs. Antibiotics are a common group of drugs implicated in anaphylaxis. The prevalence of penicillin allergy is 2%. Cross-reactivity between penicillins and cephalosporins has been reported to be 10% for first generation cephalosporins and 3% for third generation cephalosporins (44).

Surprisingly, although corticosteroids are a first line medication in the treatment of anaphylaxis, allergy has been reported. Allergic contact dermatitis is seen in up to 4% of patients on patch testing, with anaphylaxis occurring much less frequently. The majority of reactions have occurred with methylprednisolone and hydrocortisone. Prednisone, betamethasone and dexamethasone allergy is uncommon (45).

Among pregnant as well as nonpregnant patients, other proven allergies include chlorhexidine (46), ethylene oxide (47), ranitidine (48), dextran-containing colloids (49), and povidone-iodine (50).

Although there are numerous case reports implicating synthetic oxytocin (51) as a cause of allergy, only a few have been documented by skin test (52). The test itself must be interpreted cautiously, since oxytocin can be irritating to the skin (53, 54) and inactive ingredients may be the source of the anaphylaxis

Table 32.4. DIFFERENTIAL DIAGNOSIS FOR LOCAL ANESTHETIC REACTIONS IN 205 PATIENTS WITH A HISTORY OF ALLERGY

Reaction	Number	Percent
True anaphylaxis	2	1
True anaphylaxis to an additive	2	1
Delayed hypersensitivity	4	2
Vasovagal	82	40
Psychological reactions	10	5
Reactions to other drugs	17	8
Operative dental trauma	21	10
Possible reactions to additives	39	19
Intravascular epinephrine	6	3
Supine hypotension	1	0.5
Hereditary angioedema	2	1
Skin irritation from topical preparations	4	2
Unknown (challenge negative)	6	3
Subarachnoid spread	8	4
Infection	1	0.5

Adapted from Fisher MMD, Bowey CJ. Alleged allergy to local anaesthetics. *Anaesth Intensive Care* 1997;25:611–614.

Table 32.5. DEFINITIONS RELATING TO LATEX ALLERGY

Natural rubber latex: Latex that is derived primarily from the sap of the tree *Hevea braziliensis.*

Natural rubber latex process: Process in which products that are made by converting the concentrated emulsion into finished goods by dipping, i.e., gloves, condoms, and tourniquets.

Dry rubber process: Products that are made from dried or milled sheets that are compression molded or converted back into solution; i.e., syringe plungers, anesthesia masks, vial stoppers, baby nipples.

Synthetic rubber: Products that are derived from synthetic materials and therefore not associated with allergy. Some products contain a mixture of synthetic and natural rubber latex and these are considered natural latex products.

Latex-controlled environment: An environment in which no latex gloves are used and no latex accessories come into contact with the patient.

Latex sensitivity: Refers to a positive result on skin testing or serological tests for latex-specific IgE. This includes symptomatic and asymptomatic patients.

Latex allergy: Allergic symptoms that occur on exposure to latex products or skin test.

Table 32.6. RISK GROUPS FOR LATEX ALLERGY

1. Health care workers
2. Workers with other occupational exposure to latex
3. Patients with a history of multiple surgeries secondary to:
   a. congenital genitourinary tract anomalies
   b. children with spina bifida
4. Individuals with a history of hay fever, rhiinitis, asthma, or eczema (atopy)
5. Individuals with a history of food allergy to tropical fruits (avocado, kiwi, banana), chestnuts, or stone fruits
6. Individuals with severe dermatitis of their hands who also wear latex gloves

(53). Many of the case reports that have implicated oxytocin as the cause of anaphylaxis may more likely be due to latex (55).

Latex Allergy

Latex allergy is a ubiquitous substance in medical devices used for labor and delivery. Clinicians need to be aware of the risks presented by these devices, both to their patients as well as themselves. Therefore, it is imperative that anesthesiologists become familiar with all aspects of the allergy to prevent not only overt reactions but to prevent sensitization (56). Definitions for common terms used with respect to latex allergy appear in Table 32.5.

Background. Universal precautions for viral infections have increased the use of latex containing gloves and medical equipment exponentially since 1985. As a result, there has been an increasing prevalence of latex-related sensitivities with three types of reactions recognized. The most dramatic are the IgE-mediated reactions. The second and third types of reactions are restricted to cutaneous manifestations; namely Type IV allergic contact dermatitis and irritant contact dermatitis (57, 58).

Natural rubber is primarily derived from the milky sap of the rubber tree called *Hevea brasiliensis.* This sap is composed of the cytoplasm of the laticiferous cells and thus contains a number of organic compounds including rubber particles. The particles are surrounded by a layer of proteins and lipids. Although, the proteins only account for 2% of the composition of rubber, they are responsible for the type I reaction (57). Since several proteins may be involved, patients' reactions to different products may vary greatly, depending on the levels of a particular protein. If the specific protein the patient is allergic to is present only in low concentrations, a striking reaction may not occur (59). New protein antigens may also be made during processing which may make testing more difficult (57).

Once the tree is tapped, the sap undergoes one of two processes. The natural rubber latex process refers to products that are made from the concentrated suspension. The fluid mixture is processed with the addition of various accelerators and antioxidants to enhance and speed up the rubber process. Different devices will require different combinations of chemicals to give the product its particular properties. Porcelain molds are then dipped into the resulting mixture and heated. Before gloves are removed from the molds, cornstarch powder is added, as a

lubricant (57). Other devices made from this process include condoms and urinary catheters (60). The *dry natural rubber process* uses coagulated natural latex, which is stored in the form of dried sheets. Products are manufactured either by compression molding or by conversion into solution. Items involved in this process include anesthesia masks, syringe plungers, vial stoppers, injection ports and electrode pads. There may be lower levels of natural latex proteins in this manufacture method (60).

Risk Groups. In the general population the prevalence of positive latex serology has been suggested to be between 0.37% and 6.4% (61, 62). The American Academy of Allergy, Asthma and Immunology identified high-risk groups including health care workers, workers with occupational exposure, and children with spina bifida and genitourinary abnormalities (63) (Table 32.6). Other factors such as food allergy, atopy, and multiple surgeries may increase the risk of latex sensitivity to a lesser extent.

Health Care Workers and Occupational Exposure. Among anesthesia staff the prevalence of latex sensitization ranges from 12.5% to 15.8% (64, 65), which is in keeping with other exposed health care workers (66). In addition, latex sensitization occurs with a yearly incidence of 1% in health care workers (67).

The majority of patients with latex sensitization, diagnosed by serology, are asymptomatic. Brown et al. found that of the 12.5% of anesthesia staff who tested positive, only 2.4% had symptoms. The remaining 10.1% had occult allergy and were at risk for developing symptoms if exposure continued (64).

Latex antigens can be reduced in the labor suite by changing to *low-protein* gloves or powderless gloves (67). The benefits of low-protein gloves are clear. However, gloves with cornstarch powder can carry the latex antigens and aerosolize them (63). Most of the latex allergens become airborne when the gloves are donned or removed but resuspension from clothing or settled dust also contributes (68). The inhalation of powder by sensitive individuals cause symptoms of latex asthma in 2.5% (69). In addition, powder-free gloves also undergo a washing process that extracts or denatures residual rubber proteins (57).

Latex workers not involved in health care are also at risk. One study found that 11% of workers in a glove manufacturing plant were skin test positive to latex with half of them also having occupational asthma (70).

Spina Bifida and Multiple Surgeries. Patients with spina bifida have a high degree of sensitization of 34% to 72% (71, 72). However, Konz et al. showed that only 4% of spinal cord injury patients with a similar number of surgeries to spina bifida patients had latex sensitivity. It is possible that children exposed to latex through surgery during the first days of life may preferentially produce IgE antibody (71).

Food allergy. Foods commonly associated with latex sensitivity include chestnut, banana, and avocado. Other implicated foods include kiwi, tomato, and potato (73). Investigators have shown that over 50% of patients with latex allergy have hypersensitivity to foods both by clinical history as well as by skin prick test (63). There are peptides common to these foods and latex which cross-react immunologically (73). Further testing for possible latex hypersensitivity in these patients should be considered but not all patients with these allergies will require latex avoidance (74).

Atopy and Latex Allergy. The occurrence of atopic diseases increases the risk of latex sensitization, especially if the patients are already in a high-risk category. In a *nonatopic, nonexposed* population of patients, only 0.37% have been found to be skin test positive compared to 9.44% of *atopic* patients. When atopic patients are *exposed* to latex through a variety of means, the prevalence of sensitization increases to 36.4% (61).

Presentation

Patients with a history of sensitivity to rubber give quite clear descriptions of the clinical manifestations of type I reactions. Typical histories include oral itching, facial redness or swelling to latex toy balloons and during dental examinations. Others describe pruritus and swelling following vaginal exams or the use of condoms. Contact urticaria on the hands is commonly described when wearing latex gloves. Bronchospasm and rhinoconjunctivitis have been described on exposure to latex glove powder. More severe reactions such as anaphylaxis have been reported with parenteral or mucosal exposure such as occurs during surgical procedures and barium enemas (72). There are very few cases of serious allergic reactions to latex from unbroken skin exposure (72, 75). In addition, anaphylaxis may not occur with every exposure (74).

In the operating room, the onset can be insidious (76) with the major exposure occurring once the incision is opened which is often 20 to 40 minutes after induction, long after typically responsible anesthetic agents are given.

Management

Preoperative Identification. A specific history of latex allergy should be sought in all patients, although, a negative history is common (64). Patients with a history of spina bifida should have all procedures done in a latex-controlled environment regardless of history (63). With a latex safe protocol in place, latex allergic patients can be expected to experience an allergic reaction 0% to 0.3% of the time in the absence of protocol violation (77). Skin tests should be considered in patients who are members of high risk groups or have a clinical history suggestive of latex allergy (63, 74).

Intraoperative Management. There are no current standards for managing patients with latex allergy or sensitization. Many work sites have formulated policies and procedures on their own. Our recommendations appear in Table 32.7. In addition, each hospital should compile a site-specific list of available latex-free devices.

The use of corticosteroids and histamine receptor blocking drugs have been advocated by some as premedication to minimize the consequences of inadvertent latex exposure (74). However, this strategy is not universal and does not replace the policy of latex avoidance (77).

Ensuring that the latex-sensitive patient is first of the day (74) helps to minimize the exposure to latex laden powder in the air. However, in the obstetrical suite this may not be practical. Fortunately, studies have shown that air-borne latex powder can fall significantly just within 2.5 hours (68).

Low-protein or low-powder gloves are not acceptable in those who are latex sensitized. Alternative materials include styrene, styrene-butadiene, neoprene, and polyvinylchloride. Health care workers, in general, should use nonlatex gloves for activities not likely to involve contact with infectious materials and powder-free low-protein latex gloves for other "at risk" exposures (57). The Centers for Disease Control and Prevention and the Occupational Safety and Health Administration have stated that there are no significant differences in barrier protec-

Table 32.7. RECOMMENDATIONS FOR THE MANAGEMENT OF LATEX-SENSITIVE AND ALLERGIC PATIENTS[a]

1. **Identify:** Identify the latex-sensitive patient and ensure the entire health care team is aware.

2. **Timing:** For operative procedures, arrange the list so that the patient is the first of the day or ensure that greater than 2.5 h has passed since the last case.

3. **Gloves:** Alternatives include styrene, styrene-butadiene, neoprene, and polyvinylchloride, but *not* low-protein or powderless gloves.

4. **Syringes:** Glass or nonnatural latex syringes are preferred. Regular syringes are acceptable, providing that the drugs are freshly drawn and given.

5. **Medications:** Ampules are ideal. Remove natural rubber stoppers from multidose vials.

6. **Intravenous sets:** Tape over injection ports and use stopcocks. Avoid buretrols. Regular intravenous bags or minibags may be used. Add medications through the port to be spiked.

7. **Cotton wrappings** will protect the patient's skin from latex-based blood pressure cuffs or tubing, and esmarch's bandage should be avoided.

8. **Anesthesia equipment:** Manual ventilation bags and ventilator bellows should be nonlatex. Breathing circuit (disposable) of polyvinylchloride should be packaged separately from a latex rebreathing bag.

9. **All products** such as urinary catheters, tapes, tourniquets, and surgical drains should be latex free. If latex devices are imperative, they should be washed thoroughly.

[a] Adapted from American Society of Anesthesiologists. Natural rubber latex allergy: considerations for anesthesiologists. ASA guidelines. American Society of Anesthesiologists, 1999.

tion between intact latex and vinyl gloves although vinyl gloves rip more easily. However, studies have shown that leakage rates may approach 52% in vinyl and latex nonsterile gloves while the mean leakage rates in both sterile latex and vinyl gloves occur in 1% and 9% respectively (78).

The use of syringes with natural rubber plungers in the latex allergic patient is acceptable, providing that the drugs are freshly drawn. By injecting the contents immediately, less protein may be released from the plunger. Natural rubber vial stoppers from multidose vials should be removed (74, 75, 77, 79). Today, however, a large majority of vial stoppers are made from synthetic rubber and therefore do not pose a problem. Although there have been case reports of reactions to natural rubber traced to intravenous fluids and tubing (80), to date, no extractable proteins have been isolated (81).

The internal components of the anesthesia machine may be lined with natural rubber thus it may not be possible to be 100% latex free (72). A filter should be placed in the breathing circuit to deal with this problem (76). Both manual ventilation bags and ventilator bellows should be nonlatex. If there is no choice but to use latex-containing devices they should be washed thoroughly (77).

Postoperative Management. Patients with a history of latex allergy should wear a medical alert bracelet. If life-threatening reactions to latex have occurred the patient should also carry epinephrine and antihistamines in a self-administered form.

Latex Allergy and the Parturient

There are numerous reports in the literature of latex allergy in parturients. In the cases of vaginal delivery, symptoms have developed during examinations of the cervix (82), following delivery of the placenta (83) and with the suturing of episiotomy wounds (84). In cesarean sections, symptoms typically follow the intravenous injection of oxytocin after the delivery of the newborn (54, 55, 85, 86). At that point in the surgery the latex proteins from the surgical gloves become mixed with blood at the placental site during manipulation of the uterus. With oxytocin and the resulting uterine contractions, a bolus of latex proteins is deposited into the circulation leading to symptoms in the subsequent minutes (55, 85). This mechanism may account for a number of patients who were labeled as allergic to oxytocin (51, 87) or other drugs when in fact they were more likely allergic to latex. One case report actually followed with a retraction of suspected fentanyl allergy when latex allergy was confirmed (88). Other case reports where there was no identifiable cause for allergy are probably secondary to latex as well (89–91).

Hand Dermatitis

Hand dermatitis, which includes both allergic contact dermatitis and common irritant dermatitis, occurs in up to 26% of hospital workers (64, 92). Although, neither of them are considered immediate type hypersensitivity, their occurrence is a risk factor for such a reaction. The damaged and abraded skin provide a means by which latex antigen can enter the body and sensitize (64, 92). *Allergic contact dermatitis,* a type IV hypersensitivity, is the predominant immunological response to natural rubber latex outnumbering immediate allergic reactions 4 to1 (57). Generally, these reactions appear over 4 to 6 hours after exposure and peak within 48 hours. It is caused by a hypersensitivity to the accelerators and antioxidants during manufacture, and not the latex proteins (57). Signs and symptoms may include erythematous or scaling patches with vesicles, bullae and erosions (92). *Irritant dermatitis,* a non immune mediated reaction, is characterized by the development of itchy, dry, scaling skin with fissures or erosions (92). It is caused by moisture under the gloves, other workplace chemicals, and repeated hand washing (57). It is best to avoid barrier creams that may enhance skin penetration of the latex allergens. Persons with irritant or allergic contact dermatitis should use nonlatex gloves or cotton liners for protection and should be referred for allergy testing (74).

Food and Drug Administration and Latex-Labeling Regulations

As of September 30, 1998, latex-containing products that are intended for human contact must be labeled as containing natural rubber latex or dry latex. If the devices are solely for export this regulation does not apply. In addition, the term hypoallergenicity will no longer be applied to latex devices. Many health care workers misinterpret this label as making reference to latex content, when it actually refers to the use of minimal chemicals or additives in the manufacture of the gloves (60).

ALLERGY TESTING

Allergy tests fall into two groups: in vivo or in vitro testing. These tests determine if a patient is susceptible to a reaction from a range of drugs by attempting to detect either a reaction by IgE antibodies or by quantitating IgE levels. All in vivo testing should be done in a facility with resuscitation equipment as anaphylaxis may occur.

Skin Testing

The value of skin tests has been well established in the diagnosis of anaphylaxis to anesthetic agents. It is more sensitive than in vitro testing and is the diagnostic procedure of choice (93). However, there is difficulty in studying some anesthetic agents as many cause direct histamine release or simply irritation, which can affect the interpretation of results. Systemic administration of medications such as antihistamines, tricyclic antidepressants,

---

Table 32.8. SKIN TESTS

Skin prick test (SPT)
  Use undiluted drug unless histamine releasing (then dilute 1:10).
  Place one drop of drug on the volar aspect of forearm.
  Prick the skin at a 45 degree angle through the drop with a
    25-gauge needle to a depth where the skin can be lifted.
  Wipe area after 15 min, and measure wheal and flare.
  Positive wheals are measured at 90 degree angles and averaged.
  A positive test is a wheal 2–5 mm greater than control.

Intradermal test
  Start with a 1:100,000 dilution of the drug.
  Increase the concentration by 10 after each injection.
  Inject 0.02–0.05 mL of reagent into the dermis.
  Wait 20–30 min before injecting more concentrated solutions.
  Observe for wheal and flare as above.
  Typically, the severity of the response is correlated to the
    concentration of the reagent.

Adapted from Fisher MM, Bowey CJ. Intradermal compared with prick testing in the diagnosis of anaesthetic allergy. *Br J Anaesth* 1997;79:59–63; and Bousquet J, Michel FB. *In vivo* methods for studying allergy. Skin tests, techniques and interpretation. In: Middleton E, Reed C, Ellis E, et al., eds. *Allergy Principles and Practice,* 4th ed. Toronto: Mosby Press, 1993:573–594.

and sympathomimetic agents can also give false negative results. In addition, appropriate positive (histamine or codeine) and negative (saline) controls should be used (5, 94).

There are two types of skin tests; the skin prick test and the intradermal skin test. The agreement between the two is 93% to 97% (93). Compared to intradermal skin testing, prick tests are less apt to give systemic reactions and they to correlate better with clinical sensitivity. Therefore prick testing is used to *screen* for hypersensitivity and intradermal tests, which are more sensitive but less specific, are performed following negative prick tests (94). Negative skin prick tests and intracutaneous tests are reliable negative predictors of anaphylaxis (9). Case reports of true anaphylaxis during testing are rare, with one review noting 6 fatalities from 1945 to 1987 and none from 1985 to 1989 (95). Testing methods appear in Table 32.8 (9, 93, 94).

When testing for local anesthetic allergy one must ensure that the solution is free from epinephrine, sulfites and parabens. While false positive reactions are relatively common (up to 12%), false negative skin tests and subsequent subcutaneous challenge tests are extremely rare (31, 96).

Standardized, commercial skin test reagents for latex are not yet available in the United States, but many allergy centers prepare their own while still maintaining a high degree of sensitivity and specificity (63). An example of a positive reaction following a skin prick test to latex appears in Figure 32.5.

In Vitro Testing

In vitro testing has the advantage of not placing a patient at risk for a reaction, which is ideal during pregnancy. The US Food and Drug Administration or (FDA) has approved four different serum tests for latex. They utilize the radioallergo absorbant test (RAST) or the enzyme allerg sorbent test (EAST) (56). However, significant levels do not give an indication if a reaction will occur nor will absolute levels indicate the degree of the reaction. It is also less specific and sensitive than skin tests (93). False negatives may occur following the weeks after anaphylaxis as the IgE antibody is temporarily depleted. Currently available test reagents include thiopental, ethylene oxide, protamine, latex as well as a number of muscle relaxants. A negative result may not be useful but a positive test can help identify a patient at risk (57).

When there is disagreement between tests and it is not possible to tell which test is correct, a challenge may be ordered. Often, with general anesthetic agents, antibiotics, and latex, there are

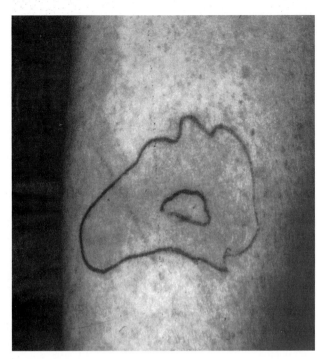

Figure 32.5. Positive skin prick response to latex. (Courtesy of Dr. S.M. Tarlo and Dr. G. Sussman.)

alternatives. In the case of latex allergy, a challenge may consist of a glove use test or an inhalational challenge with latex glove powder. The use test consists of wearing a rubber glove on a wet hand or more commonly just a wet finger. A positive reaction consists of itching and possible urticaria within 30 minutes.

DIFFERENTIAL DIAGNOSIS OF ANAPHYLAXIS

There is a broad differential diagnosis to anaphylaxis because of the numerous conditions that may present with urticaria and angioedema (Fig. 32.4). While urticaria has been defined as well-circumscribed, raised, pruritic, and erythematous lesions caused by edema involving the superficial dermis, angioedema is the extension of the edema to deeper areas of the dermis, subcutaneous tissue or submucosa without the pruritus. Urticaria may be secondary to physical stimuli such as cold, heat, pressure, exercise or secondary to conditions such as systemic mastocytosis. In the vast majority of patients the cause is unknown (97, 98). The following discussion will highlight some of the conditions that can mimic anaphylaxis while others in the differential diagnosis appear in many internal medicine textbooks.

Hereditary Angioedema

Hereditary angioedema is a disorder characterized by deficient or dysfunctional levels of C1 inhibitor. As an uncommon disorder, the interval between the onset of symptoms and diagnosis approaches 20 years. Acquired forms of C1 inhibitor deficiency have been associated with lymphoproliferative disorders and SLE (99).

Clinically, the disorder is characterized by deep swelling of the dermis in the genitalia, face and gastrointestinal tract. The swelling is nonpruritic, nonerythematous and asymmetric. It can be triggered by anxiety, minor trauma or emotional upset, and lasts from 24 hours to several days. Urticaria implicates another diagnosis. The abdominal edema can lead to nau-

sea, vomiting, diarrhea, ascites or the symptoms of an acute abdomen (99).

Angioedema of the pharyngeal and laryngeal structures may lead to life-threatening airway obstruction and is a leading cause of mortality. Signs can occur over minutes to hours with the early signs and symptoms consisting of voice change and dysphagia (99).

Pregnancy may be protective. For prophylaxis against a reaction, parturients have been given fresh frozen plasma for both vaginal and operative deliveries. Danazol which is used commonly in nonpregnant patients, has rarely been used peripartum because it is also an androgen (100). For acute attacks, fresh frozen plasma and more recently, C1 inhibitor concentrate has been administered. Fresh frozen plasma has the disadvantage that it also contains the kinins and substrates involved in the disorder. Unfortunately, the inhibitor concentrate which, can start resolving symptoms within 1 hour and provides protection for 2 to 3 days, is not universally approved for clinical use (99, 101).

Vaginal delivery may be impeded by perineal edema and abdominal pain may obscure obstetric disorders (101). The airway, as described above, may become compromised as a result of straining. Regional analgesia is advised to lessen the pain and the anxiety (101).

General anesthesia for cesarean delivery carries the risk of difficult intubation and extubation since these acts can precipitate extreme pharyngeal edema. Tracheostomy may be necessary but is not always effective (99, 101). It should be noted that although this disorder has features of anaphylaxis, corticosteroids, antifibrinolytics, epinephrine, and antihistamines are not efficacious in the quiescent or acute situation (99).

Laryngopathia Gravidarum

Laryngopathia gravidarum is a rare often acute, noninfectious, inflammatory process of the laryngeal tissues in multigravida patients. The acute form tends to occur just before parturition while the chronic form occurs earlier and can recur in subsequent pregnancies. Both resolve spontaneously postpartum.

Symptoms include progressive dyspnea, hoarseness, sore throat and odynophagia in the absence of fever, lymphadenopathy, or cough. The larynx and frequently the epiglottis demonstrate patchy edema and congestion but the aryepiglottic folds, arytenoids and vestibular regions are smooth and pale. The true vocal cords are unaffected. A tracheostomy may be required in severe cases (102).

Amniotic Fluid Embolus

This topic is discussed more thoroughly in Chapter 19. Some researchers feel that amniotic fluid embolism might be an IgE-mediated anaphylactic reaction with the source of the potential offending antigen resting in the placenta, fetus or amniotic fluid (103). This would explain the varied clinical presentation and the fact that mast cells are involved (104).

Immunoglobulin A Deficiency

This disorder, a deficiency of immunoglobulin A in the serum and mucous secretions, occurs with a frequency of one in 400 to one in 750 individuals. Ten percent to 48% of these individuals will produce IgG antibodies to IgA, and with the transfusion of blood products they are at risk for a severe hypersensitivity reaction (97). Under normal circumstances patients may be asymptomatic but they may also have asthma, atopy and recurrent respiratory infections. Systemic lupus erythematosus (SLE) and rheumatoid arthritis (RA) have been associated with the disease (105).

Systemic Mastocytosis

This disorder is characterized by an abnormal increase in mast cells. The condition consists of urticarial lesions and in 10% of patients, systemic involvement (106). Degranulation of the mast cells can occur with physical and psychological stimuli, alcohol and drugs known to release histamine. Systemic symptoms include pruritus, flushing, palpitations, bronchospasm, lower abdominal pain, gastroesophageal reflux disease and vascular collapse. Patients may also suffer from anemia, thrombocytopenia, osteoporosis, pathological fractures and bleeding diatheses (106).

TYPE II IMMUNE RESPONSE

Type II reactions can occur in pregnancy. Immune thrombocytopenic purpura has been discussed elsewhere, and erythroblastosis fetalis is presented below.

Erythroblastosis Fetalis

Maternal IgG antibodies can be produced against fetal erythrocytes if they contain antigenic material foreign to the mother. The antibody may then cross the placenta and coat fetal red blood cells. This causes destruction of the erythrocytes resulting in anemia, the severity of which depends on the maternal antibody titre and the time of onset. Common antigens involved include those of the Rh, Kell, or Duffy systems (107).

Most affected neonates are either asymptomatic or managed with phototherapy. Others may require blood transfusions for severe anemia or exchange transfusion to prevent brain damage from the hyperbilirubinemia. However, there are a number of severely affected fetuses that must be treated in utero. Evaluations early in gestation require the measurement of bilirubin in the amniotic fluid as well as determining the rate of rise of maternal antibody titres (108). Hydrops fetalis may occur if the fetus is not treated. The clinical manifestations consist of generalized edema, pleural and pericardial effusions, ascites, severe anemia, and hepatosplenomegaly. Hepatosplenomegaly occurs on the basis of extramedulary erythropoiesis in an attempt to increase red cell production. Coagulation may be impaired by the lack of vitamin K-dependent clotting factors from liver involvement, or thrombocytopenia secondary to splenomegaly. Cardiac decompensation and portal hypertension can also occur (109).

The fetal heart rate tracing often reflects the severity of the anemia. Although a sinusoidal pattern has been associated with severe anemia, this pattern can be transient or absent, and is not very specific or sensitive (110). As the fetus' condition worsens, the tracing progresses from nonreactive to a persistent tachycardia or decelerations. However, the fetal heart rate can be normal in spite of increased flow, indicating that other mechanisms such as a decrease in blood viscosity are important in maintaining cardiac output.

Severely affected fetuses are treated with intrauterine transfusions. Rh-negative blood is used to maintain the fetal hematocrit at an acceptable level until fetal lung maturity is achieved. Fetal immobilization may be required to reduce the risk of needle trauma. This may be accomplished indirectly with maternal sedation or, more commonly by injecting a neuromuscular blocking agent, in small doses, directly into the umbilical vein or by fetal intramuscular injection. While many agents have been used for this purpose, vecuronium in doses of $0.1~\text{mg}\cdot\text{kg}^{-1}$ estimated fetal weight, provide immobilization for a short period of time, allowing the obstetrician to evaluate the fetus postoperatively (111).

Despite transfusions, the fetus continues to be at risk. If severely affected, the mother may require a cesarean delivery early. If vaginal delivery is planned, continuous segmental epidural analgesia is safe and effective for the relief of pain in the first stage of labor. Catecholamine release and hyperventilation due to labor pain are diminished. Furthermore, if hypotension is prevented, uterine intervillous blood flow may be increased (112). Organomegaly, especially if associated with tense ascites, can lead to dystocia during delivery. Asphyxia may also occur due to anemia or heart failure.

COLLAGEN VASCULAR DISEASES

Collagen vascular diseases affect women of childbearing years and complicate the management of pregnancy. RA, SLE, and progressive systemic sclerosis are considered below.

Rheumatoid Arthritis

Rheumatoid arthritis is a chronic inflammatory disease of diarthrodial joints that is frequently combined with the dysfunction of other organ systems. It is more common in females and can occur in any age group. The etiologic factors of the disease are unknown, but there is strong evidence that tissue damage is caused by immune complexes, complement, and lysosomal enzymes. Juvenile RA is a similar disease with an onset before age 16 years. This condition can result in crippling sequelae by childbearing age (113).

The severity of joint involvement ranges from mild inflammation and thickened synovium to articular cartilage destruction and ankylosis. The ankylosis can result in a significant restriction of joint movement. Tendons and ligaments may also be weakened, leading to instability and subluxation. The small joints of the hands and feet are usually affected first, but any synovial joint can be involved including the cervical spine, temporomandibular joints, and the cricoarytenoid joints. This latter group may have significant implications for the anesthesiologist and airway management.

The Cervical Spine

The cervical spine is involved in up to 85% of patients with RA. Women with severe involvement of the hands and feet are more likely to have severe cervical disease (114). The cervical spine may become unstable when rheumatoid synovitis causes loss of articular cartilage, bony erosion and laxity of the transverse ligament. Any segment of the cervical spine can be affected but atlantoaxial subluxation, basilar invagination and subaxial subluxation are the more common lesions. Atlantoaxial subluxation can occur in any patient but is more common in those who have had the disease for more than 10 years. Figure 32.6 shows a common configuration of subaxial and vertical subluxation. Patients may be asymptomatic or they may present with neurological symptoms suggestive of cord or nerve root compression. Neck pain from subaxial instability or disk degeneration and headache from compression of the greater occipital nerve are frequently seen. However, patients who are asymptomatic are also at risk for severe neurological complications or sudden death from cord compression (115).

Temporomandibular and Laryngeal Joints

More than 50% of patients with RA have jaw symptoms (114). Ankylosis of the temporomandibular joint may make mouth opening so restricted that oral intubation is difficult. Patients with juvenile RA may also be difficult to intubate due to micrognathia from mandibular disease.

Cricoarytenoid arthritis is present in about 59% of patients with RA. Approximately 14% have constriction of the glottic opening leading to stridor and obstructive sleep apnea (114). They may also complain of hoarseness, wheezing, sore throat and dysphagia. Cricoarytenoiditis may result in reduced vocal cord mobility and recurrent aspiration pneumonitis.

Patient Assessment

Airway and Cervical Spine.   Ideally, the patient should be seen by an anesthesiologist before she is in labor to identify potential airway problems. Observing for at least a 4-cm opening when she opens her mouth can test the temporomandibular joint.

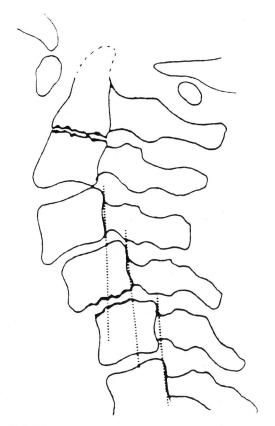

Figure 32.6. Subaxial and vertical subluxation. (From Santaverta S, Kankaanpaa U, Sandelin J, et al. Evaluation of patients with rheumatoid cervical spine. *Scand J Rheumatol* 1987;16:13, with permission.)

The patient should also be viewed from the side to note micrognathia.

The cervical spine must be carefully evaluated both by history and physical examination. X-rays of the cervical spine including anterioposterior, open mouth, and flexion/extension views may show odontoid erosions, subaxial subluxations, apophyseal joint erosions, and disk space narrowing. Whether or not routine cervical radiographs should be obtained in all patients with RA undergoing general anesthesia is controversial (114).

The diagnosis of rheumatoid cricoarytenoid arthritis necessitates a full otolaryngological examination using indirect or direct fiberoptic laryngoscopy.

General Assessment. Other skeletal abnormalities due to rheumatoid or juvenile RA include deformities of the hips, that limit flexion and abduction (116) and bony pelvis abnormalities that may lead to cephalopelvic disproportion. The intervertebral facet joints of the lumbar vertebral column may also be involved. Examination of the back including radiographs (taken before pregnancy) may be helpful in showing which facets are least affected which may facilitate epidural/spinal needle placement.

Visceral involvement is common, especially if the patient has high serum rheumatoid factor (117). Lung manifestations include restrictive lung disease secondary to pleural effusions, kyphosis from spinal disease, and (to a lesser extent) fixation of the ribs by arthritis (114). As the gravid uterus becomes larger, this restriction may become more severe because of impaired diaphragmatic excursion. Heart function may be compromised due to pericardial effusions, conduction defects, valvular heart disease and cardiomyopathies. Cardiac and respiratory reserve may be reduced with the progression of pregnancy as well as with labor and delivery.

Medications are often continued during pregnancy. Corticosteroids and nonsterioidal antiinflammatory drugs (NSAIDS) such as salicylates, indomethacin, naproxen, and diclofenac are not known to be teratogenic. Other, agents such as methotrex-

ate, cyclophosphamide and chlorambucil may be teratogenic and are stopped before conception (118). Large doses of aspirin near the time of delivery predispose patients to delayed and prolonged labor and an increased risk of blood loss during delivery (117). Physiological maternal anemia can be aggravated by iron deficiency secondary to gastrointestinal loss. In a fetus of more than 27 weeks gestation, ibuprofen may cause premature closure of the ductus arteriosis, but this effect resolves within 24 hours of stopping the drug (119). In addition, newborns exposed to high doses of aspirin in utero may have an increased incidence of central nervous system bleeding after delivery. Platelet function may be impaired for days after discontinuing the drug. The risks and benefits of epidural analgesia in patients taking NSAIDS must be weighed against the very slight increased risk of epidural hematoma.

Analgesia and Anesthesia for Labor and Delivery

For patients with mild disease, that is, those with no joint deformities and those who do not require drug therapy, the methods for administering pain relief during labor and delivery are the same as those in normal pregnancy. All patients on NSAIDS should have large bove access and blood available for delivery because of the increased risk of postpartum hemorrhage.

Severe contractures of the large joints may be present. The range of motion of each of these joints should be determined before any neuroaxial blockade so that over extension and dislocation do not occur under anesthesia. It is particularly important to test the hip joints by maximally abducting and flexing them before placing the patient in stirrups. Some patients have osteoporosis secondary to steroid treatment or immobility, and care must be taken with positioning to avoid fractures. Finally, peripheral neuropathy can complicate RA. Although this is not an absolute contraindication to regional anesthesia, it should be documented before commencement of the block.

Anesthesia for vaginal delivery can be managed in the usual fashion with the following in mind. If the patient has severe airway abnormalities, early epidural should be encouraged if coagulation is normal. The use of opioids in these patients should be used with caution, as sedation may lead to the loss of muscle tone resulting in upper airway obstruction. Patients with flexion deformities of the cervical spine and micrognathia are most prone (120). It may not be safely overcome with the usual maneuvers and cervical subluxation and quadriplegia may occur. Care must be taken to avoid local anesthetic toxicity with epidural, pudendal and paracervical blocks for these same reasons. Spinal anesthesia using a small dose of lidocaine, bupivacaine, or tetracaine can be used for a saddle block to facilitate forceps delivery.

Patients with long-standing, crippling RA are likely to require a cesarean section because of hip joint or pelvic bony involvement. For elective cesarean section, lumbar epidural, spinal, or general anesthesia can be used. If there are upper airway deformities or cervical spine abnormalities, conduction anesthesia is preferred if technically possible. If general anesthesia is used in patients with severe airway deformities, the airway must be secured while the patient is awake. Awake intubation with minimal manipulation of the cervical spine is imperative; a fiberoptic technique is recommended (see Chapter 21). Topical anesthesia of the upper airway is required and small doses of an opioid or benzodiazepine is acceptable providing that sedation is minimized. Glycopyrolate, which does not cross the placenta to any great extent, will also decrease airway secretions. In the awake patient, pain or paresthesia during intubation may warn of the limits of the patient's cervical spine before permanent neurologic damage has occurred. A tracheostomy under local anesthesia may be necessary if other options fail. After the procedure, the patient must be fully awake with a return in full muscle function before extubation. If glottic narrowing is severe, she should be observed for several hours postextubation in an area where reintubation or tracheostomy can be performed.

Ideally, the head and neck should be positioned prior to induction to avoid any neurological sequelae. Several pillows can support the head if there is a preexisting severe flexion deformity of the neck. Otherwise the neutral position is ideal. The arms may have to be placed at the sides if there is restriction of shoulder movement. Some patients require hip flexion, which can be accomplished by placing pillows under the knees.

If an emergency cesarean section is required in a patient with a severely deformed upper airway, the experience of the anesthesiologist and the operating team determines the conduct of anesthesia. Extension of an epidural, rapid spinal anesthesia, or awake intubation prior to general anesthesia are options. If the operating team has had experience using local anesthesia, an abdominal wall field block with local infiltration using 1% to 2% 2-chloroprocaine is an alternative. Supplemental sedation is usually required but loss of consciousness should be avoided.

Systemic Lupus Erythematosus

Systemic lupus erythematosus (SLE) is a chronic inflammatory disease thought to be caused by a disturbance in immunoregulatory mechanisms resulting from the interaction of genetic, hormonal, and environmental factors (121). Most patients with the disorder have hypergammaglobulinemia and a reduction in serum complement. In addition, immune deposits have been found in the glomerular basement membrane on renal biopsy and at the dermal-epidermal junction in skin biopsies. However, unlike RA, the joint symptoms are usually mild and severe deformities are rare. There is a high incidence of the disease in females (female/male ratio is 9:1) (122), many of whom are of childbearing age.

Pregnancy and Systemic Lupus Erythematosus

The effect of pregnancy on the progression of SLE is difficult to determine because exacerbations and remissions punctuate the natural history of the disease. A systematic review of the available studies is inconclusive (123). Women with lupus tend to have more complications such as hypertension, bladder infections, diabetes, hyperglycemia and preeclampsia with 7% experiencing a life-threatening complication. The most common in this latter group include arterial or venous thrombosis secondary to antiphospholipid antibodies, renal failure requiring dialysis, and uterine rupture (124). Women with lupus who become pregnant are also at high risk for preterm delivery, preeclampsia and interventions such as induction of labor and cesarean section for fetal reasons (125).

Lupus flares can occur at any time. Later in pregnancy, the signs and symptoms such as arthralgias, anemia, thrombocytopenia, worsening hypertension, proteinuria, and renal dysfunction can be very similar to toxemia. More severe manifestations such as encephalopathy, abdominal pain, and hepatic failure again do not distinguish the two disorders. The treatment for a lupus flare includes high doses of corticosteroids and antihypertensive agents, while preeclampsia is aided by delivery of the infant (125). Laboratory measures such as serum complement are generally not helpful.

Patient Assessment

The signs and symptoms associated with SLE may be mild and confined to one organ system or fulminating, leading rapidly to death. Fever, weight loss, and fatigue may be the first signs of the disease. The skin may be affected, causing the classic malar "butterfly rash." Involvement of mucous membranes with painful ulcerations in the pharynx, mouth, or vagina may also occur (121).

Polyserositis is relatively common, with pleurisy occurring in 50% of cases. If the patient is dyspneic, the respiratory system should be assessed to rule out pulmonary vasculitis, infarction, hemorrhage, or pleural effusions. Hypoxemia should be treated with oxygen both for maternal comfort and fetal well-being.

The heart may be affected in a number of ways. Pericarditis with chest pain occurs in over 50% of patients with SLE but cardiac tamponade is uncommon. Del Rio and co-workers have demonstrated that patients with SLE have a decreased myocardial reserve (125). Coronary arteritis, focal or generalized myocarditis, or focal necrosis and atrophy of the myocardium may cause this. Some patients have cardiac valvular lesions (Libman-Sacks endocarditis) that are usually asymptomatic. However, prophylactic antibiotics against bacterial endocarditis are indicated for labor and delivery. The cardiovascular system is best evaluated by physical examination. An ECG may be useful to assess rhythm abnormalities and ischemic changes.

Lupus nephritis is common and accounts for the majority of fatalities due to SLE. During pregnancy, 43% of women who experience flares have renal involvement (124). A urinalysis, blood urea nitrogen, serum creatinine, serum electrolytes, and blood sugar studies should be performed. Casts in the urine sediment indicate active nephritis. Hypokalemia and glucose intolerance are common in patients receiving corticosteroids.

There may be several coagulation defects in patients with SLE. The platelet count may be low in active disease because of antiplatelet antibodies and splenomegaly. In addition, specific circulating anticoagulants may be present. These are diagnosed by demonstration of factor specificity and are associated with abnormal bleeding. Factor VIII inhibitors are the most common (126). Their presence contraindicates the use of regional block.

The presence of high antiphospholipid antibody titres and a history of recurrent venous or arterial clotting and fetal loss characterize the antiphospholipid antibody syndrome. This antibody is often reported as the "lupus anticoagulant" because in the laboratory causes an elevated activated thromboplastin time (APTT), although clinically, it causes thrombosis. While this syndrome is often treated with immunosuppressants such as corticosteroids, other therapy such as low-molecular-weight heparin and/or aspirin may also be used in an attempt to reduce the incidence of thrombosis. In many cases, heparin may be stopped before labor and delivery, if not, regional anesthesia may be contraindicated despite normal coagulation indices (123). It is best to wait 12 to 24 hours (or longer in patients with renal failure) after the last dose of low-molecular-weight heparin before initiating a neuraxial block, depending on the dose of heparin (127, 128).

Many of the neurological complications of SLE may be due to the vasculitis or to steroid treatment. Up to 25% of deaths in SLE patients occur because of intracerebral bleeding or status epilepticus (120). Other manifestations include psychosis, transverse myelopathy, cranial nerve palsies, and peripheral neuropathy.

The polyarthralgia or arthritis associated with SLE follows the same distribution as RA but is usually milder and not deforming. Avascular necrosis of the head of the femur may result from either chronic steroid therapy or vasculitis.

Approximately 10% of infants have neonatal lupus erythematosis caused by transplacental passage of maternal autoantibodies. Of these, approximately half have skin manifestations that resemble those seen in the adult. Between 1% and 2% of infants are born with complete heart block. This is usually irreversible and may cause neonatal or infant death (129).

Analgesia and Anesthesia for Labor and Delivery

Analgesia for vaginal delivery includes opioids, inhalational analgesia, or if coagulation is normal, continuous lumbar epidural analgesia. Intrathecal or epidural opioids, with or without local anesthetic may be useful. A neurological examination should be done before initiating a conduction block. Although a fixed neurological deficit is not an absolute contraindication to regional block, it should be documented. If raised intracranial pressure is suspected, options other than regional blockade should be considered, such as patient-controlled intravenous opioids. If regional block is contemplated, the risks and benefits of the procedure should be thoroughly discussed with the patient.

Cesarean section may be performed safely under regional or general anesthesia. All patients with SLE should have units of compatible blood prepared in advance because cross-matching problems can arise as the result of irregular antibodies in the serum. If severe renal disease is present, a central venous or pulmonary artery catheter may be required to assess and optimize cardiac output. Hourly urine output using a Foley catheter should be measured. An arterial line may be placed to monitor blood pressure if hypertension is difficult to control. These monitors are especially helpful in preventing pulmonary edema when giving the patient crystalloid and when replacing blood volume after uterine incision. Supplemental oxygen should be given to the patient throughout the procedure.

If general anesthesia is indicated for maternal or fetal reasons, the usual rapid-sequence induction may have to be modified for extremely ill patients with severe cardiac disease. If myocardial function is poor, oxygen is administered, appropriate monitoring is initiated, and anesthesia induced with a reduced dose of thiopental combined with an opioid such as fentanyl. This technique results in less myocardial depression. Succinylcholine is still used as a muscle relaxant to facilitate endotracheal intubation unless the patient has recently suffered paralysis from a cerebrovascular accident. In this situation succinylcholine may cause massive hyperkalemia. A nondepolarizing muscle relaxant such as rocuronium may be used. Agents that require renal excretion to terminate their action should be avoided if renal failure is present. Finally, the delivery should take place in a facility that is prepared to take care of the infant should it be affected with neonatal SLE.

Progressive Systemic Sclerosis (Scleroderma)

Progressive systemic sclerosis (PSS) is a generalized disorder of connective tissue characterized by inflammatory, fibrotic, and vascular lesions in the skin and viscera. The disease is more common in women than men with an average age of onset of 40 years (130). Although the cause is unknown, it has been classified as an autoimmune disorder because autoimmune hemolytic anemia, hypergammaglobulinemia, rheumatoid factor, and numerous autoantibodies have been found in patients with this disease. In addition to skin involvement, PSS causes impairment of kidney, heart, lung, and gastrointestinal tract function (131).

Pregnancy and Progressive Systemic Sclerosis

Pregnancies complicated by PSS put both the mother and fetus at high risk. In one review of 17 case reports, 42% of patients experienced a worsening of their PSS during pregnancy and three women died. There is also an increased incidence of preeclampsia and eclampsia (132). The fetal morbidity is not caused by the maternal auto-antibodies associated with PSS but in the stressed environment caused by maternal organ compromise and hypertension (133). Prematurity and perinatal deaths occur particularly in patients with renal disease (134).

Patient Assessment

The skin becomes sclerosed and thickened from the dermis to the subcutaneous tissue (134). The skin of the extremities is often bound down to the digits and may extend proximally to include the trunk. It may be impossible to clinically assess the position of the fetus if the induration of the skin over the abdomen is severe (136). The skin of the face may become tightly adherent to underlying structures, limiting the ability to open the mouth. Thus orotracheal intubation may be difficult (137).

The kidneys are involved in almost half of patients with PSS. Proteinuria, hypertension, and azotemia are the usual manifestations (137). Renal crisis may be the most significant complication of scleroderma in pregnancy and is a cause of maternal mortality (138). This occurs most often in patients with diffuse,

rapidly progressing skin thickening. The crisis consists of progressive renal failure and malignant hypertension leading to headaches, hypertensive encephalopathy, retinopathy, seizures and left ventricular failure (139). While the condition may respond to a number of antihypertensive agents, angiotensin converting enzyme inhibitors appear to be most effective (138). This class of drugs is not generally recommended in pregnancy because of potential risks to the neonate such as refractory hypotension and oliguria, but it may be life-saving for the mother (140a, 140b). The entire gastrointestinal tract can be involved with PSS, causing malnutrition secondary to malabsorption. This may also cause a prolongation of the prothrombin time due to malabsorption of vitamin K. There is also abnormal esophageal motility, lower esophageal sphincter incompetence, and peptic strictures (140a, 140b). Swallowing may be difficult due to tongue and palate abnormalities. These changes make the aspiration of both lower esophageal and gastric contents a hazard.

Pulmonary function is often impaired. Interstitial fibrosis may lead to pulmonary hypertension, a restrictive lung defect, and a decrease in diffusing capacity (131, 141). In pregnancy, the gravid uterus and an increased metabolic rate may further aggravate hypoxemia. Hypoxia may increase pulmonary artery pressures further, leading to cor pulmonale. Arterial blood gases and chest X-rays may be required.

Similar to both RA and SLE, peripheral joints are often arthritic. This can lead to severe deformities, particularly of the small joints of the hands and feet.

One of the hallmarks of PSS is an increase in vascular reactivity to cold. Raynaud's phenomenon is common and is associated with a decrease in renal blood flow in some patients (142). In addition, coronary vascular spasm may occur, causing arrhythmias and angina in patients with anatomically normal coronary arteries (143). The myocardium may show focal or generalized fibrosis leading to congestive heart failure.

During pregnancy, aspirin and antihypertensive agents are the most frequent drugs prescribed.

Analgesia and Anesthesia for Labor and Delivery

The pregnant patient with severe PSS poses several difficult anesthetic management problems. Often there is a lack of suitable peripheral veins for intravenous therapy. In the patient with Raynaud's phenomena, injection of drugs or the infusion of cold fluids into the small veins may lead to digit necrosis and gangrene. Therefore, it is desirable to use a large forearm or central vein for these purposes. To keep vascular spasms to a minimum, the patient should be kept warm using blankets and fluid warmers. Blood pressure may be difficult to measure but indwelling arterial catheters should be avoided if possible because these may provoke distal vasospasm and gangrene.

Epidural analgesia may be indicated for relief of labor pain or operative delivery. Technically this may be difficult because of changes in the overlying skin or arthritis in the lumbar spine. Vasopressors should be used in small doses intravenously to avoid severe hypertension and vasospasm. For the same reasons, ergot preparations should be used with caution.

General anesthesia may be required for fetal distress. The problems associated with this technique depend on the patient's pathophysiologic condition. Before induction, an attempt should be made to empty the lower esophagus of secretions with an orogastric tube. Next, a nonparticulate antacid should be given. Since the patient often has decreased esophageal motility and distal strictures, oral antacids may not neutralize gastric acid, although it is helpful to neutralize the residual contents in the esophagus. Ranitidine may be useful to reduce gastric acid secretion. Metoclopramide is used to accelerate gastric emptying, but its efficacy in PSS has not been proven. The facial deformities may make tight placement of an anesthetic mask more difficult when preoxygenating. If a difficult intubation is suspected because of restricted mouth opening, awake oral intubation under local anesthesia using a fiberoptic laryngoscope prior to induction may be the safest way to secure the airway. If oral intubation fails, a tracheostomy may be required.

Intraoperative monitoring is often difficult in patients with PSS, and the benefits of using each monitoring device must be weighed against the risks. A Foley catheter should be used and hourly urine output should be recorded. Blood pressure should be monitored noninvasively. Noninvasive measurement of oxygen saturation and end-tidal carbon dioxide reduces the need for obtaining arterial blood. Unfortunately, pulse oximetry may be of limited use in patients with severe vasospastic disease since all sites (fingers, ears, nose) may be affected.

A pulmonary artery catheter is helpful if congestive heart failure or severe pulmonary hypertension is present. Unfortunately, it is technically difficult to correctly position the catheter if the heart is severely dilated and pulmonary artery pressures are high. In addition, cardiac arrhythmias are common.

TRANSPLANTED ORGANS AND PREGNANCY

Transplantation allows women, whose health and fertility have been restored by organ transplants, the ability to conceive (144). Since the first transplant in 1958 (145), hundreds of such women have become pregnant, with the recent majority having healthy newborns and an intact functioning graft. However, there is a consistently high incidence of complications that these patients and their fetuses experience.

To successfully manage the parturient with an allograft, the anesthesiologist must review a number of considerations. These are summarized in Table 32.9 and can be applied to any parturient with a solid organ transplant.

In many transplant patients the primary disease that led to the transplant may continue to require attention. Complications from previous organ failure may also persist or recur. The unique physiology of the donor organ, such as cardiac allografts, may be problematic and acute or chronic rejection may lead to impaired transplant function. The therapies to maintain graft tolerance may have side effects and toxicities especially to the renal system. In addition, immunosuppressants, in being effective pharmacologically, increase the risk of opportunistic and reactivated infections such as cytomegalovirus (in the mother and fetus). It is especially problematic when pregnancy occurs soon after transplantation and higher levels of immunosuppression are used (146). Although, the drugs are not carcinogenic they do impair the ability of the body to deal with abnormal cells should they form. As a result, these patients are 50 to 100 times more likely to develop lymphoproliferative disorders, lymphoma and solid tumors then agematened controls (147).

Pregnancy, labor and delivery are high risk periods for these patients. A significant portion of the morbidity is secondary to the immunosuppressants and associated renal dysfunction (146). Regardless of the solid organ transplanted, hypertension

Table 32.9. ANESTHETIC CONSIDERATIONS FOR THE PREGNANT TRANSPLANT PATIENT

1. **Primary disease**
   a. Other organ systems affected
   b. Residual complications from previous end-organ failure
2. **Organ transplanted**
   a. Current function or residual dysfunction
   b. Physiology of the transplanted organ
   c. Acute and chronic rejection
3. **Treatment**
   a. Side effects and toxicity of immunosuppressants
   b. Risk of malignancy
   c. Risk of infection
4. **Pregnancy**
   a. Physiology of the transplanted organ
   b. Risk of preeclampsia and hypertension
   c. Vaginal or cesarean delivery
      i. Anesthetic options
      ii. Monitoring
      iii. Strict asepsis
      iv. Possible complicated surgical delivery
   d. Fetus
      i. Teratogenesis
      ii. Prematurity
      iii. Intrauterine growth restriction
      iv. Side effects of drugs
      v. Long-term effects

occurs in 21% to 56% of parturients and preeclampsia occurs in up to 29% (148). Women with normal graft and kidney function are less likely to have these complications (146, 148). In addition, 37% to 54% of newborns are premature and 32% to 50% of them are growth restricted (148).

When formulating the anesthetic plan, the history, physical examination and laboratory investigations should reflect the extent of the parturient's systemic disease and obstetrical complications. The complete medical record must be reviewed. Renal dysfunction and hypertension is common in all transplant patients thus a complete evaluation requires that both conditions be clarified. An electrocardiogram should also be performed on all patients taking long-term corticosteroids (147). Complicated labors and deliveries should be anticipated. The past surgery may make cesarean delivery more difficult and current organ dysfunction may necessitate the use of additional monitoring. Regional anesthesia is preferred overall, but contraindications may require one to employ other analgesic techniques or general anesthesia. Strict asepsis during procedures in immunocompromised patients is vital. Table 32.10 outlines some of the pregnancy outcomes and maternal co-morbidities found in transplant patients.

Cardiac Transplants

Cardiac transplantation is indicated for patients with endstage heart disease including idiopathic dilated cardiomyopathy,

Table 32.10. COMPLICATIONS IN 500 PREGNANCIES IN TRANSPLANT RECIPIENTS

	Prematurity	Hypertension	Preeclampsia	Infection	Rejection
Kidney					
noncyclosporin	52%	21%	20%	18%	7%
cyclosporin	54%	56%	29%	22%	11%
Liver	39%	45%	20%	26%	13%
Heart	38%	31%	13%	15%	23%

Data from Radomski JS, Ahlswede BA, Jarrell BE, et al. Outcomes of 500 pregnancies in 335 female kidney, liver, and heart transplant recipients. *Transplant Proc* 1995;27:1089–1090.

obstructive cardiomyopathy, congenital heart disease and ischemic heart disease. These patients do very well, with 1- and 3-year survival rates of 81% and 73%, respectively (149). Pregnancy does not seem to increase the risk of complications (150). In particular, those who have experienced previous peripartum cardiomyopathy have not had a recurrence of their original disease in subsequent pregnancies (151).

During normal pregnancies, cardiac output increases 40%, and during labor and delivery, it increases a further 80% (152). Cardiac transplant patients follow a similar pattern (150). Although, investigators have shown that the exercise capacity in uncomplicated heart transplant recipients only approaches 60% to 70% of predicted, due to the lower contribution from the atria as well as higher filling pressures, it appears to be adequate (153). Thus, if the patient is symptom-free preconception, then pregnancy should be tolerated without significant functional impairment (152).

The Denervated Heart

At the time of transplantation, the heart is fully denervated. Over years, a variable amount of patchy reinnervation may occur (153). The lack of innervation disrupts the normal sympathetic response to exercise or situations of hemodynamic stress such as labor and delivery, intubation and hypoxia (154). In addition, the donor heart loses its parasympathetic or vagal innervation. It beats at an intrinsic rate of 90 to 110 beats per minute and does not respond normally to carotid sinus massage or vagal maneuvers such as valsalva (154). Bradycardias associated with spinal anesthesia or externalization of the uterus will not occur (154–155). The indirect chronotropic response to vagolytic muscle relaxants, anticholinergics, anticholinesterases, phenylephrine or nitroprusside is lost (154, 155). The heart only responds to direct acting agents. Thus, the methods of choice for treatment of bradycardia are isoprenaline, catecholamines or cardiac pacing (154). The lack of direct innervation of the parasympathetic and sympathetic nervous systems means that in stressful situations the transplanted heart must rely on circulating catecholamines for its chronotropic and inotropic effect. This does not occur immediately but gradually over a period of 5 to 6 minutes (154). There may also be an upregulation of receptors, resulting in an increased sensitivity to circulating catecholamines (155).

Patient Assessment

Patients with a cardiac allograft must have a detailed history and assessment of exercise capabilities performed in addition to the usual anesthetic history and physical examination. The risk in these patients of developing premature multivessel coronary stenosis is 18% at 1 year and 44% after 3 years regardless of traditional risk factors. The etiology of the accelerated atherosclerosis is multifactorial, but it may be caused by chronic graft rejection (156). Unfortunately, episodes of myocardial ischemia may be silent due to the lack of innervation of the donor heart, with paroxysmal dyspnea and poor exercise tolerance, being the only symptom (153, 154). Acute graft rejection may be suggested by a history of dysrhythmias and left ventricular dysfunction. With better immunosuppression, rejection is more asymptomatic (154). The presence of right ventricular enlargement and tricuspid regurgitation occurs in two-thirds of patients but by one year this resolves in half of them. Left ventricular size and function remains normal (153). Patients may have a pacemaker as bradyarrhythmias are seen in up to 20% of patients. These devices should be evaluated during pregnancy.

Laboratory investigations are similar to any other solid organ transplant parturient with special emphasis on renal function. The electrocardiogram may include two P waves and some degree of right bundle branch block and dysrhythmias. Other pertinent investigations include those to detect myocardial ischemia and graft rejection. Chest X-rays are performed if indicated.

Analgesia and Anesthesia for Labor and Delivery

Epidural analgesia (or a combined spinal epidural technique), following adequate prehydration, has been tolerated well for labor pain. If hypotension occurs, the heart cannot increase its cardiac output by increasing its heart rate but must rely on an increase in stroke volume from an influx of venous return. Therefore, the transplanted heart is considered preload-dependent and sensitive to hypovolemia (154). For the treatment of hypotension, fluids and phenylephrine are preferred (152). Indirect acting vasopressors such as ephedrine have been used but may be inadequate and unpredictable (155). It may be prudent to institute epidural analgesia early to minimize the hyperdynamic cardiovascular responses to labor and delivery. It can also be extended into the postpartum period to alleviate sympathetic stimulation associated with postoperative pain (152).

Epinephrine in solutions for test dosing or for cesarean section have been used successfully, although some authors raise the concern of exaggerated responses secondary to receptor supersensitivity in the case of intravascular injection (152, 155). Since the response to intravenous epinephrine in a test dose is unreliable, it is not recommended in this context. However, local anesthetics with epinephrine (1:400,000), given in divided doses may enhance the block for cesarean section.

Noninvasive hemodynamic and oxygen saturation monitoring is adequate in most cases. Monitoring for ischemia may be necessary if the history is positive (155). The benefit of hemodynamic monitoring must be balanced against the potential risk of infection. It is generally not required if the patient has a normal exercise tolerance (152).

The mode of delivery is dependent on obstetrical indications and should a cesarean section be required, cautious extension of a labor epidural is safe (152). The precipitous drop in preload associated with spinal anesthesia may not be tolerated (155).

According to the American Heart Association guidelines, there is insufficient data to support specific recommendations regarding endocarditis prophylaxis in those with a previous heart transplant. Since they may have valvular dysfunction or may experience repeated rejection episodes requiring higher doses of immunosuppression, they are classified at moderate risk to develop bacterial endocarditis. Thus according to the guidelines, cesarean section does not require prophylaxis while operative vaginal delivery may warrant antibiotics. Amoxicillin or ampicillin is recommended. Vancomycin can be used for patients allergic to penicillins (157).

Lung Transplants

Lung transplantation is performed for a number of endstage conditions such as alpha-1 antitrypsin deficiency, cystic fibrosis, pulmonary fibrosis and primary pulmonary hypertension. The reported 4-year survival of a single-and double-lung transplant is 53% and 62% respectively (158). The number of lung transplant recipients who become pregnant is extremely small and their outcomes are much less favorable than other solid organ transplants. Many cases are characterized by patients experiencing some degree of decline in lung function in the peripartum period either due to infection or rejection (159). Declining lung function is often attributed to obliterative bronchiolitis, a form of chronic rejection (158). The offspring, on the other hand, do not experience a morbidity or mortality greater than other offspring of transplant patients (159, 160).

The respiratory changes during pregnancy are considerable and have been reviewed in great depth in Chapter 1. As there have been relatively few lung transplant parturients and many suffer a declining forced expiratory reserve volume over one second (FEV_1), it is unclear how donor lung volumes and capacities change in pregnancy in optimal circumstances.

Physiology of the Transplanted Lung

In the past, double-lung transplants were performed en bloc with denervation of the carina and the heart. More recent methods include sequential single-lung transplantation without resection of the carina. In this method the bronchi distal to the anastomosis are not innervated and do not respond to stimuli. However, bronchospasm can still occur due to inhaled metaacholine and histamine. Beta-2 agents will cause bronchodilation.

Early after transplant, the lymphatics are disrupted, making the patient more susceptible to pulmonary edema from fluid overload. In the canine model, lymphatic drainage is reestablished within 2 to 4 weeks (158).

Patient Assessment

From the perspective of the anesthesiologist, the considerations are very similar to transplant patients with other solid organ allografts. Particular attention should be given to current lung function. Shortness of breath, a deteriorating exercise tolerance and a slight fever may signal rejection (158). The history should be reviewed as well as past and recent pulmonary function tests. FEV_1 should be sought as it gives an indication of functional capacity (160).

Chest radiographs and invasive procedures should be performed if clinically indicated (161). Resting arterial blood gases are generally normal (158).

Analgesia and Anesthesia for Labor and Delivery

Since the third trimester is associated with a high incidence of declining lung function, regional anesthesia for labor pain is preferred. Combined spinal epidurals have been successfully performed for cesarean section (161), although we would favor continuous lumbar epidural anesthesia with gradual titration of fluids and block height. In patients dependent on intercostal muscles for respiration, a high block may cause respiratory insufficiency.

In patients with double-lung transplants, sedated patients may be at increased risk of aspiration if the carina is denervated. Fluid boluses should be given judiciously since poor lymphatic drainage may make the patient more prone to pulmonary edema (158). The mode of delivery is dependent on obstetrical indications. Invasive monitoring may be required in severely compromised parturients. If general anesthesia is used, the endotracheal tube must not traumatize the tracheal suture lines (155).

The number of parturients with heart-lung transplants is small and the effects uncertain. Cardiac transplant rejection appears to be less problematic, as lung rejection is more limiting (160).

Liver Transplants

There are many indications for liver transplants including both congenital and acquired diseases. Examples of acquired diseases include chronic active viral hepatitis, alcoholic cirrhosis, sclerosing cholangitis, hepatoma, and primary biliary cirrhosis. Congenital diseases such as alpha-1 antitrypsin deficiency and Wilson's disease may have multisystem involvement which is not completely treated with transplantation. Overall, the 5-year survival of liver transplant patients is 70% to 75% (144, 162).

Pregnancy does not appear to alter hepatic allograft function and there is only a small incidence of graft rejection (163). Liver dysfunction if present, does not appear to have adverse effects on the pregnancy (164).

During normal pregnancies alkaline phosphatase levels (APL) rise in 42% to 77% of parturients. This is secondary to placental ALP. However, the liver transaminases remain normal while other enzymes may increase or decrease (165). As enzymes increase, one of the early signs of rejection, there may be significant confusion to the diagnosis in a parturient with a liver

allograft (166). Repeated liver biopsies and eventual treatment with increasing doses of immunosuppressants may be necessary. However, mild to moderate elevations that antedate conception and remain stable during pregnancies are common and do not require aggressive evaluation (146).

Patient Assessment

Assessment of the parturient with liver transplantation requires the evaluation of the primary disease and the function of the new liver. Evaluation should reflect the considerations outlined earlier (Table 32.9). Co-existing anemia, thrombocytopenia and coagulation abnormalities may contraindicate regional anesthesia. More severe liver dysfunction resulting in encephalopathy, increased intracranial pressure and extensive intrapulmonary shunting (167) are beyond the scope of this chapter. If substance abuse was a factor in the failure of the original liver, then it should be reconsidered in this setting.

Laboratory investigations such as a complete blood count, coagulation profile, biochemistry, renal function and liver biochemical tests need to be performed.

Analgesia and Anesthesia for Labor and Delivery

Regional anesthesia has been used effectively in liver transplant patients with normal liver function and coagulation profile. The mode of delivery is dependent on obstetrical indications and additional monitoring will depend on concurrent medical conditions (146). If general anesthesia is employed for cesarean section, isoflurane may be the vapor of choice, as it increases hepatic artery blood flow (166).

Liver Transplantation in the Parturient

Although there is significant literature regarding pregnancy in the previously transplanted patient, liver transplantation may occur during pregnancy as in the case of hepatic rupture secondary to preeclampsia or hepatic failure due to chronic or fulminant viral hepatic failure (146). It may be associated with immediate delivery of the fetus or with ongoing maturation of the fetus in utero. Considerations include the risk of bleeding or infection with termination versus the possible suboptimal surgical, anesthetic or postoperative management if the pregnancy is continued (146). Neonatal morbidity and mortality relates to prematurity and in utero ischemic insults (168).

Kidney Transplants

Longstanding insulin-dependent diabetes mellitus, hypertension, and collagen vascular disorders are common primary conditions that can lead to chronic renal failure. Despite transplantation these disorders can continue to have significant implications for the anesthesiologist. Patient survival after kidney transplantation at 1 year is 98%, with graft success at 85% (144). Many reports confirm no deleterious effect of pregnancy on a renal graft that was functioning well before pregnancy and 94% of pregnancies that go beyond the first trimester end successfully (169). Surprisingly, hypertension, preeclampsia, diabetes and multiple pregnancies do not increase the risk of graft loss (170). However, rejection is increased in parturients with pre-existing or deteriorating renal function and proteinuria (170).

In normal parturients renal blood flow and glomerular filtration rate increase considerably to a peak at the end of the second trimester of 60% (155). The kidneys enlarge and the ureters and renal pelves dilate (155). In patients with well-functioning renal allografts, the glomerular filtration rate also increases despite being denervated and often derived from a male donor (169). Well-functioning renal allografts mirror these changes. Proteinuria in the third trimester occurs in 40% of patients but in the absence of hypertension it is usually not significant (169).

Table 32.11. COMPLICATIONS ASSOCIATED WITH CHRONIC RENAL FAILURE

Cardiovascular	Increased cardiac output
	Hypertension
	Coronary artery disease
	Uremic pericarditis
Respiratory	Pulmonary edema
	Pleural effusion
	Increased 2,3-diphosphoglycerate
Neurologic	Autonomic dysfunction
	Peripheral neuropathy
Renal	Uremia
	Hyperkalemia
	Hyperparathyroidism
Gastrointestinal	Inadequate gastric emptying
	Nausea and vomiting
Hematologic	Anemia: if transfused risk of HIV,
	Hepatitis B,
	Hepatitis C
	Dysfunctional platelets
Endocrine and metabolic	Metabolic acidosis
Musculoskeletal	Renal osteodystrophy
Other	Infection risk
	Poor skin quality and impaired healing

Patient Assessment

Effects of chronic renal failure are summarized in Table 32.11. Many of the conditions associated with chronic renal failure patients persist despite transplantation. Also a renal allograft does not confer normal kidney function and any impairment should be noted. Chronic renal failure neuropathy is common. Transplantation may improve uremic peripheral neuropathies but is unlikely to improve uremic autonomic dysfunction suggesting that the former is a metabolic problem and the latter is structural (see pancreatic transplants for full description) (171). An evaluation for autonomic and peripheral neuropathies includes an assessment for silent myocardial ischemia, delayed gastric emptying, and lower limb sensory and motor changes.

Physical examination should include a thorough cardiorespiratory and neurological exam. With the extraperitoneal location of the kidney, it is at risk for compression by the enlarging uterus leading to obstruction and pelvic pain (172). The obstruction may become so severe that it may necessitate the placement of nephrotomy tubes (173).

Laboratory investigations include a complete blood count, blood chemistry, renal function, plasma protein, calcium, phosphate, liver function tests and coagulation profile. Serum electrolytes may need to be repeated during labor in patients with unstable kidney function. An electrocardiogram should also be performed.

Analgesia and Anesthesia for Labor and Delivery

Regional techniques are good options for analgesia or anesthesia in the renal transplant patient providing that there is no evidence of coagulopathy. Fluid loading must be done cautiously if there is any underlying kidney dysfunction.

The role of extra monitoring in addition to the standard monitors is dependent on the patient's co-existing conditions. Patients with significant myocardial dysfunction and ischemia that require meticulous fluid management, may need invasive hemodynamic and continuous electrocardiographic monitoring.

A few centers prefer to deliver all newborns by cesarean section but routine vaginal delivery is the preferred mode (172). Cesarean delivery may be prolonged and difficult, secondary to the previous abdominal surgery. Positioning and intravenous

access should take into account the existing arteriovenous fistulas. The choice of general anesthetic agents should be based on current renal function. Inhalational agents such as isoflurane that are free of nephrotoxic metabolites are preferred.

Postoperative pain management may need to be modified in the setting of renal dysfunction. Intramuscular, intravenous and neuroaxial morphine should be given judiciously. Active metabolites of morphine are eliminated slowly in the presence of renal failure. However, fentanyl, alfentanil and sufentanil, appear to act no differently in renal patients (174). Nonsteroidal antiinflammatory medications are not recommended for postoperative pain control because of the high risk of nephrotoxicity (175).

Pancreas Transplantation

Since the late 1970s, pancreatic transplantation have allowed many insulin dependent diabetics the freedom from insulin injections with improved glycemic control. One-year and 5-year graft function approach 75% and 60%, respectively (176). Successful pregnancies and deliveries have been documented.

The surgical procedure itself has gone through a number of revisions. Initially a portion of the intestine along with the pancreas was transplanted to allow for drainage of the exocrine secretions. However due to a number of problems, modifications were required which included ligating the exocrine gland ducts or draining the secretions via the intestine or bladder. This allowed the donor pancreas to be placed in the pelvic area (177).

Normal pregnancies are characterized initially by a brief fall in insulin requirements followed by a gradual increase. There are also lower fasting glucose levels (178). Parturients with functioning pancreatic grafts appear to follow these trends (176, 179).

Patient Evaluation

Ninety-five percent of those who receive a pancreatic transplant have also received a kidney (180). Thus, the anesthesiologist must be aware of the complicated medical history of these patients. Overall, maternal co-morbidities are similar to those with kidney transplants except for a higher risk of infection (173).

Diabetics can develop a wide range of neuropathies from focal neuropathies such as femoral or cranial, to diffuse, such as autonomic dysfunction. Autonomic neuropathies occur in one-sixth of diabetics and are a particular concern to the anesthesiologist (181). It may lead to gastroparesis, diarrhea, postural hypotension and silent myocardial ischemia (182). Silent myocardial ischemia may be suspected with a reduced exercise tolerance. There is controversy whether or not the neuropathies improve following pancreatic transplantation (182, 183). In the presence of a long history of diabetes mellitus, pancreatic allografts may only stabilize or improve marginally nerve function over a number of years (180, 181).

In addition to the usual history with the above considerations in mind, a thorough physical examination should be performed. Extra attention should be paid to the cardiovascular system specifically looking for signs of autonomic neuropathy. Patients exhibit a lack of variability in heart rate during deep breathing and valsalva maneuvers (181). They may also experience a fall in systolic blood pressure on standing. The stiff joint syndrome may be found in 33% of young insulin dependent diabetics. It is characterized by multiple joint contractures (including the laryngeal and cervical areas) that may not be obvious on physical examination. It predisposes patients to difficult laryngoscopy during general anesthesia. It may be alluded to by "the prayer sign" which is defined as the inability of the patient to approximate the palmar surfaces of the phalangeal joints despite maximal effort (178, 184).

Standard laboratory investigations include hematology, biochemistry, renal function and an electrocardiogram. As a result of shortening of the QT interval due to autonomic neuropathy, these parturients are at risk for arrhythmias (181). Rejection episodes may be detected by monitoring serum creatinine (if a kidney from the same donor was also transplanted) or urinary amylase (if a urinary exocrine drainage was attached) (180).

Analgesia and Anesthesia for Labor and Delivery

Management of analgesia and anesthesia is similar to those with kidney transplants. Delivery has been predominately by cesarean delivery because of the fear that vaginal deliveries could be harmful to the grafts (179). Regardless of the anesthetic method, the anesthesiologist must be aware that the autonomic neuropathies may persist. Respiratory arrest following the administration of analgesics in this latter group have occurred, thus opioids should be given judiciously (181). Indications for additional monitoring are dependent on similar criteria to kidney transplant patients. If there is concern about silent myocardial ischemia, a V5 lead should be used in operative procedures.

IMMUNOSUPPRESSANTS DURING PREGNANCY

Immunosuppressants are indicated in patients with a number of underlying conditions including autoimmune diseases and transplantation. The drugs used before pregnancy are often carried through with adjustments in doses to maintain therapeutic levels. As a result, the anesthesiologist must be aware of the pertinent effects of this class of drugs on the mother and fetus. Transplant regimens are also complicated in that they often involve more than one drug. The side effects may act synergistically or may simply become more numerous. Finally, these potent drugs may interact with the parturient's concurrent medical problems.

All immunosuppressants or their active metabolites cross the placenta (185). The major side effects include early delivery and growth-restricted newborns. They have not been shown to be teratogenic in humans at therapeutic doses, but side effects do occur.

Azathioprine

Azathioprine is a purine analogue which interferes with the clonal proliferation of T and B lymphocytes. It is dose limited due to myelosuppression thus raising the concern of thrombocytopenia. In the pregnant patient it can cause neonatal myelosuppression, the effect of which can be reversed by avoiding this problem in the maternal bone marrow (146). Both prematurity and fetal growth impairment occur. Animal studies have shown isolated cases of congenital anomalies but human studies do not confirm this (186). A listing of relevant side effects is in Table 32.12.

Corticosteroids

Corticosteroids have been used for the treatment of a variety of medical problems including transplantation, asthma and autoimmune diseases. It acts by altering lymphocyte function and decreasing the number of circulating lymphocytes (146). In the obstetrical setting it has been associated with premature rupture of membranes, premature delivery and intrauterine growth restriction (187). The high incidence of early ruptured membranes may be related to an altering of vaginal flora and the weakening of membranes (146). Exposure to corticosteroids by the fetus is minimal, since the placenta has an abundance of an enzyme that metabolizes it into inactive forms leaving no more than 10% of the active drug to reach the fetus (186). In animal studies only under the influence of very high doses there has been the suggestion that corticosteroids may increase the incidence of cleft lip and palate. This has not been demonstrated in humans (146). Early case reports have described newborns

with adrenal insufficiency but more recent research finds this unusual (188), especially with doses of less than the equivalent of 15 mg of prednisone (144). "Pulse" dose steroids during labor may not be necessary but increased doses during a cesarean section should be given if the patient has been chronically treated within the year (162). Three doses of 100 mg of hydrocortisone sodium succinate, every eight hours, starting immediately preoperatively is an acceptable regimen (186).

A list of side effects has been summarized in Table 32.12. Osteonecrosis and osteoporosis, especially of the weight-bearing joints should be considered when positioning the patient during the labor and delivery process especially with neuroaxial analgesia (186).

Cyclosporine

Cyclosporine has changed transplantation since its introduction in 1978. It acts by interfering with the production of interleukin-2 and other cytokines. Metabolism involves the cytochrome P-450 system. Levels can vary depending what other drugs the patient is taking (146).

There is a long experience with cyclosporine and pregnancy. In the nonpregnant patient it produces renal dysfunction not only by its nephrotoxic effects, but also by its vasoconstrictive properties. This toxicity is dose related and is usually reversible. However, over the long term cyclosporine may cause persistent renal dysfunction and hypertension (189). Once pregnant, it is this renal dysfunction that predisposes transplant recipients to preeclampsia (164).

There have been multiple studies both in humans and animals examining the effects of cyclosporine and anesthetic agents. Animal studies suggested that cyclosporine could interact with barbiturates and opioids resulting in an increase in their effects but this was not confirmed in humans. However, cyclosporine may increase the depth and duration of action of neuromuscular blockers (189). Other side effects appear in Table 32.12.

Tacrolimas (FK-506) and Sirolimas

Tacrolimas is a new cyclosporine-like immunosuppressant. It acts by inhibiting the production of interleukin 2 and other mediators (190). It has many of the benefits of cyclosporin with less adverse effects. In particular, it causes less arterial hypertension and renal dysfunction (164). The small number of studies suggest that there is a low incidence of hypertension, preeclampsia and abnormalities in allograft function (191). An advantage of tacrolimas is that many patients do not require co-therapy with corticosteroids (146). Tacrolimas has not been found to be teratogenic although there have been a few case reports of reversible cardiomyopathy especially in transplanted children. Recently, a case report of twin newborns with severe cardiomyopathy has appeared with no other definable cause (190). Common adverse effects on the newborn include reduced birth weight and prematurity similar to the other immunosuppressants (191). Of interest has been the observation of transient hyperkalemia in up to 36% of exposed newborns (146).

Sirolimas resembles tacrolimus but acts to block interleukin-2 dependent proliferation. Side effects include hyperlipidemia, thrombocytopenia and increased liver transaminases. There is no impaired glucose metabolism or toxicity of the nervous or renal system (192).

Antimalarial Drugs, Gold Compounds, and Methotrexate

Antimalarial drugs such as chloroquine and hydroxychloroquine have been used for a number of years for the treatment of SLE and RA. They do cross the placenta and early case reports suggested that these drugs caused eye and inner ear damage.

Table 32.12. SIDE EFFECTS OF COMMON IMMUNOSUPPRESSANTS

	Corticosteroids	Azathioprine	Tacrolimus	Cyclosporine
Cardiovascular	Hypertension		Dyspnea Palpitations	Hypertension
Neurological	Psychosis Mood changes		Headache Tremor	Tremors Palmer and plantar parasthesia:
			Parasthesias Seizures Focal neurological deficits	Headache Confusion Seizures
Gastrointestinal	Peptic ulcer disease Pancreatitis	Hepatotoxicity Nausea and vomiting Hypersensitivity Pancreatitis	Nausea and vomiting	Nausea and vomiting Mild hepatic dysfunction
Hematological		Myelosuppression	Thrombocytopenia with sirolimas	
Renal and metabolism	Glucose intolerance Salt and water retention		Nephrotoxicity Hyperkalemia Glucose intolerance	Nephrotoxicity Hyperkalemia Hypomagnesemia Inhibition of insulin secretion
Musculoskeletal	Myopathy Osteoporosis Osteonecrosis	Arthralgias		
Skin	Thin skin/ easy bruising Poor wound healing Acne	Rash Stomatitis		

Other	Weight gain
	Infection risk
	
	Cataracts
		Increased risk of neoplasia
		  and infection
			Increased risk of neoplasia	Parenteral cyclosporin
				  is solubilized in
				  Cremophor which had
				  been associated with
				  allergic reactions.
				Increased risk of
				  malignancy and
				  infection
				Gingival hyperplasia
				Hypertrichosis

Obstetrical	PROM Preterm delivery	Preterm delivery	Preterm delivery	Preeclampsia Preterm delivery

Fetus/newborn	Not a human teratogen
	IUGR
	Adrenal insufficiency
		Not a teratogen
		IUGR
		Neonatal bone marrow
		  suppression (correlates
		  with maternal suppression)
			Transient neonatal
			  hyperkalemia
			Mild reversible renal
			  dysfunction
			Normal growth
				Not a teratogen
				IUGR

PROM, premature rupture of membranes; IUGR, intrauterine growth restriction.

However, more recent reviews and case studies have shown no increase in congenital anomalies (186).

Since gold compounds do cross the placenta readily, it is recommended that patients delay conception for 1-2 month after cessation of therapy. Gold compounds can accumulate in the fetal liver and kidney, although the frequency of congenital anomalies is uncertain (186).

Methotrexate is a folic acid antagonist that prevents the synthesis of purine nucleotides and interferes with DNA synthesis. It has been used in patients with RA, SLE and severe cases of asthma. It is not taken in pregnancy as it is associated with spontaneous abortions and fetal anomalies. Low doses early in pregnancy may be tolerated (186).

Allergy Drugs during Pregnancy

Large studies following asthmatics through pregnancy found no significant relationship between major congenital malformations and exposure to beta agonists, theophylline, corticosteroids, or antihistamines. However, theophylline may increase the risk of preterm delivery. Preferred antihistamines include chlorpheniramine and tripelenanamine (187).

Compared to oral corticosteroids, which are associated with preeclampsia, preterm delivery and low-birth-weight infants, inhaled steroids are not associated with these outcomes (187).

REFERENCES

1. Melvold RW. Review of immunology. In: Patterson R, ed. *Allergic Diseases: Diagnosis and Management,* 5th ed. Philadephia: Lippincott–Raven Publishers, 1995:1–26.
2. Stoelting R. Allergic reactions during anesthesia. *Anesth Analg* 1983;62:341–356.
3. Leynadier F. Pathophysiological and clinical aspects of immediate hypersensitivity to latex. *Clin Rev Allergy* 1993;11:371–380.
4. Garrison GC. Histamine, bradykinin and 5-hydroxytryptamine and their antagonists. In: Gilman AG, Rall TW, Nies AS, et al., eds. *The Pharmacological Basis of Therapeutics,* 8th ed. New York: Pergamon Press, 1990:575–599.
5. Weiss ME, Adkinson NF, Hirshman CA. Evaluation of allergic drug reactions in the perioperative period. *Anesthesiology* 1989;71:483–486.
6. Watkins J. Investigation of allergic and hypersensitivity reactions to anaesthetic agents. *Br J Anaesth* 1987;59:104–111.
7. Gleicher N, Adelsberg BR, Lui TL, et al. Immune complexes in pregnancy. III. Immune complexes in immune-complex associated conditions. *Am J Obstet Gynecol* 1982;142:1011–1015.

8. Eisenberg RA, Cohen PL. The role of immunologic mechanisms in the pathogenesis of rheumatic diseases. In: Schumacher Jr HR, ed. *Primer on Rheumatic Disease*, 9th ed. Atlanta: The Arthritis Foundation, 1988:36–44.

9. Nicklas RA, Bernstein IL, Li JT, et al. Anaphylaxis during general anesthesia, the intraoperative period , and the postoperative period. *J Allergy Clin Immunol* 1998;101(Suppl):S512–S516.

10. Laxenaire MC, Mouton C, Moneret-Vautrin DA, et al. Drugs and other agents involved in anaphylactic shock occurring during anaesthesia. A French multicenter epidemiological inquiry. *Ann Fr Anesth Réanim* 1993;12:91–96.

11. Moscicki RA, Sockin SM, Corsello BF, et al. Anaphylaxis during induction of general anesthesia: subsequent evaluation and management. *J Allergy Clin Immunol* 1990;86:325–332.

12. Fisher MM, Baldo BA. The incidence and clinical features of anaphylactic reactions during anaesthesia in Australia. *Ann Fr Anesth Réanim* 1993;12:97–104.

13. Baraka A, Sfeir S. Anaphylactic cardiac arrest in a parturient. *JAMA* 1980;243:1745–1746.

14. Fisher MM, Outhred A, Bowey CJ. Can clinical anaphylaxis to anaesthetic drugs be predicted from allergic history? *Br J Anaesth* 1987;59:690–692.

15. Tan BB, Lear JT, Watts J, et al. Perioperative collapse: prevalence of latex allergy in patients sensitive to anaesthetic agents. *Contact Dermatitis* 1997;36:47–50.

16. Galletly DC, Treuren BC. Anaphylactoid reactions during anaesthesia. *Anaesthesia* 1985;40:329–333.

17. Nicklas RA, Bernstein IL, Li JT, et al. Algorithm for the treatment of acute anaphylaxis. *J Allergy Clin Immunol* 1998;101(Suppl) :S469–S471.

18. Rosen M, Harmer M. Anaphylactic reactions during anaesthesia in pregnancy: safe in our hands? *Int J Obstet Anesth* 1992;1:183–184.

19. Fisher M. Treatment of acute anaphylaxis. *Br Med J* 1995;311:731–733.

20. Luciano R, Zuppa AA, Maragliano G, et al. Fetal encephalopathy after maternal anaphylaxis. *Biol Neonate* 1997;71:190–193.

21. Myers RE. Two patterns of perinatal brain damage and their conditions of occurrence. *Am J Obstet Gynecol* 1972;112:246–276.

22. Gallagher JS. Anaphylaxis in pregnancy. *Obstet Gynecol* 1988;71:491–493.

23. Ralston DH, Shnider SM, deLorimier AA. Effects of equipotent ephedrine, metaraminol, mephentermine and methoxamine on uterine blood flow in the pregnant ewe. *Anesthesiology* 1974;40:354–370.

24. Entman SS, Moise KJ. Anaphylaxis in pregnancy. *South Med J* 1984;77:402.

25. American Heart Association and the International Liason committe on R esuscitation. Guidelines 2000 for cardiopulmonary resuscitation and emergency cardiovascular care. Cardiac arrest associated with pregnancy. *Circulation* 2000;102:247–249.

26. Clendenen SR, Harper JV, Wharen RE, et al. Anaphylactic reaction after cisatracurium. *Anesthesiology* 1997;87:690–692.

27. Renz CL, Laroche D, Thurn JD, et al. Tryptase levels are not increased during vancomycin-induced anaphylactoid reactions. *Anesthesiology* 1998;89:620–625.

28. Incaudo G, Shatz M, Patterson R, et al. Administration of local anesthetics to patients with prior history of adverse reactions. *J Allergy Clin Immunol* 1978;61:339–345.

29. Brown DT, Beamish D, Wildsmith JAW. Allergic reaction to an amide local anesthetic. *Br J Anaesth* 1981;53:435–437.

30. Fisher MMD, Bowey CJ. Alleged allergy to local anaesthetics. *Anaesth Intensive Care* 1997;25:611–614.

31. Shatz M. Adverse reactions to local anesthetics. *Immunol Allergy Clin North Am* 1992;12:585–609.

32. Curley RK, Macfarlane AW, King CM. Contact sensitivity to the amide local anesthetics lidocaine, prilocaine, and mepivicaine: case report and review of the literature. *Arch Dermatol* 1986;122:924–926.

33. Cuesta-Herranz J, Heras M, Fernández M, et al. Allergic reaction caused by local anesthetic agents belonging to the amide group. *J Allergy Clin Immunol* 1997;99:427–428.

34. Warrington RJ, McPhillips S. Allergic reaction to local anesthetics in the amide group. *J Allergy Clin Immunol* 1997;99:855.

35. Nagel JE, Fuscaldo JT, Fireman P. Paraben allergy. *JAMA* 1977;237:1594–1595.

36. Mehta Y, Luxton MC. A mistaken case of hypersensitivity to local anaesthetic. *Anaesthesia* 1986;41:219–220.

37. Jackson D, Chen AH, Bennett CR. Identifying true lidocaine allergy. *J Am Dent Assoc* 1994;125:1362–1366.

38. Palmer CM, Voulgaropoulos D. Management of the parturient with a history of local anesthetic allergy. *Anesth Analg* 1993;77:625–628.

39. Nicklas RA, Bernstein IL, Li JT, et al. Local anesthetics. *J Allergy Clin Immunol* 1998;101(Suppl) :S510–S511.

40. DeLeon-Casasola OA, Weiss A, Lema MJ. Anaphylaxis due to propofol. *Anesthesiology* 1992;77:384–386.

41. Laxenaire MC. Substances responsables des chocs anaphylactiques peranesthésiques. Troisième enquête multicentrique française (1992–1994). *Ann Fr Anesth Réanim* 1996;15:1211–1218.

42. Leynadier F, Dry J. Anaphylaxis to muscle-relaxant drugs: study of cross- reactivity by skin tests. *Int Arch Allergy Appl Immunol* 1991;94:349–353.

43. Knowles SR. Allergic reactions during general anesthesia. *Can J Clin Pharmacol* 1998;5:33–39.

44. deShazo RD, Kemp SF. Allergic reactions to drugs and biologic agents. *JAMA* 1997;278:1895–1906.

45. Moreno-Ancillo A, Martín-Mu noz F, Martín-Barroso JA, et al. Anaphylaxis to 6-alpha-methylprednisolone in an eight-year-old child. *J Allergy Clin Immunol* 1996;97:1169–1171.

46. Porter BJ, Acharya U, Ormerod AD, et al. Latex/chlorhexidine-induced anaphylaxis in pregnancy. *Allergy* 1998; 53:455–457.

47. Olivieri P, Berchet-Montaut MP, Thomas P. Analgésie obstétricale chez une femme allergique à l'oxyde d'éthylène. *Ann Fr Anesth Réanim* 1988;7:346–348.

48. Powell JA, Maycock EJ. Anaphylactoid reaction to ranitidine in an obstetric patient. *Anaesth Intensive Care* 1993;21:702–703.

49. Paull J. A prospective study of dextran-induced anaphylactoid reactions in 5745 patients. *Anaesth Intensive Care* 1987;15:163–167.

50. Waran KD, Munsick RA. Anaphylaxis from povidone-iodine. *Lancet* 1995;345:1506.

51. Slater RM, Bowles BJ, Pumphrey RS. Anaphylactoid reaction to oxytocin in pregnancy. *Anaesthesia* 1985;40:655–656.

52. Kawarabayashi T, Narisawa Y, Nakamura K, et al. Anaphylactoid reaction to oxytocin during cesarean section. *Gynecol Obstet Invest* 1988;25:277–279.

53. Maycock EJ, Russell WC. Anaphylactoid reaction to Syntocinon. *Anaesth Intensive Care* 1993;21:211–212.

54. Deusch E, Reider N, Marth C. Anaphylactic reaction to latex during cesarean delivery. *Obstet Gynecol* 1996;88:727.

55. Motin J, Guilloux L, Dubost R, et al. Incidents et accidents peropératoires. Analyse de 62 cas en chirurgie et obstétrique. *Soins Chir* 1997;182:25.

56. ASA. *Natural rubber latex allergy: consideration for anesthesiologists. ASA guidelines.* American Society of Anesthesiologists, 1999.

57. Hamann CP. Natural rubber latex protein sensitivity in review. *Am J Contact Derm* 1993;4:4–21.

58. United States Department of Health and Human Services, National Institute for Occupational Safety and Health. *Preventing Allergic Reactions to Natural Rubber Latex in the workplace.* Washington, DC: NIOSH, 1997:97–135.

59. Center for Devices and Radiological Health. Natural rubber-containing medical devices; user labeling. *Federal Register* 1997;62:51021–51030.

60. Moneret-Vautrin DA, Beaudouin E, Widmer S, et al. Prospective study of risk factors in natural rubber latex hypersensitivity. *J Allergy Clin Immunol* 1993;92:668–677.

61. Ownby DR, Ownby HE, McCullough J, et al. The prevalence of anti-latex IgE antibodies in 1000 volunteer blood donors. *J Allergy Clin Immunol* 1996;97:1188–1192

62. Nicklas RA, Bernstein IL, Li JT, et al. Latex. *J Allergy Clin Immunol* 1998;101:S496–S497.

63. Brown RH, Schauble JF, Hamilton RG. Prevalence of latex allergy among anesthesiologists. *Anesthesiology* 1998;89:292–299.

64. Konrad C, Fieber T, Gerber H, et al. The prevalence of latex sensitivity among anesthesiology staff. *Anesth Analg* 1997;84:629–633.

65. Arellano R, Bradley J, Sussman G. Prevalence of latex sensitization among hospital physicians occupationally exposed to latex gloves. *Anesthesiology* 1992;77:905–908.

66. Sussman GL, Liss GM, Deal K, et al. Incidence of latex sensitization among latex glove users. *J Allergy Clin Immunol* 1998;101:171–178.

67. Swanson MC, Bubak ME, Hunt LW, et al. Quantification of occupational latex aeroallergens in a medical center. *J Allergy Clin Immunol* 1994;94:445–451.
68. Vandenplas O, Delwiche JP, Evrard G, et al. Prevalence of occupational asthma due to latex among hospital personnel. *Am J Respir Crit Care Med* 1995;151:54–60.
69. Tarlo SM, Wong L, Roos J, et al. Occupational asthma caused by latex in a surgical glove manufacturing plant. *J Allergy Clin Immunol* 1990;85:626–631.
70. Konz KR, Chia JK, Kurup VP, et al. Comparison of latex hypersensitivity among patients with neurologic defects. *J Allergy Clin Immunol* 1995;95:950–954.
71. Committee Report. Task force on allergic reactions to latex. *J Allergy Clin Immunol* 1993;92:16–18.
72. Beezhold DH, Sussman GL, Liss GM, et al. Latex allergy can induce clinical reactions to specific foods. *Clin Exp Allergy* 1996;26:416–422.
73. Sussman G, Gold M. *Guidelines for the Management of Latex Allergies and Safe Latex Use in Healthcare Facilities.* Ottawa: CHA Press, 1996.
74. Holzman RS. Latex allergy: an emerging operating room problem. *Anesth Analg* 1993;76:635–641.
75. Dakin MJ, Yentis SM. Latex allergy: a strategy for management. *Anaesthesia* 1998;53:774–781.
76. Holzman RS. Clinical management of latex-allergic children. *Anesth Analg* 1997;85:529–533.
77. DeGroot-Kosolcharoen J, Jones JM. Permeability of latex and vinyl gloves to water and blood. *Am J Infect Control* 1989;17:196–201.
78. Yunginger JW, Jones RT, Fransway AF, et al. Latex allergen contents of medical and consumer rubber products. *J Allergy Clin Immunol* 1993;91:A403.
79. Schwartz HA, Zurowski, D. Anaphylaxis to latex in intravenous fluids. *J Allergy Clin Immunol* 1993;92:358–359.
80. Yunginger JW, Jones RT, Fransway AF, et al. Extractable latex allergens and proteins in disposable medical gloves and other rubber products. *J Allergy Clin Immunol* 1994;93:836–842.
81. Santos R, Hernández-Ayup S, Galache P, et al. Severe latex allergy after a vaginal examination during labor: a case report. *Am J Obstet Gynecol* 1997;177:1543–1544.
82. Laurent J, Malet R, Smiejan JM, et al. Latex hypersensitivity after natural delivery. *J Allergy Clin Immunol* 1992;89:779–780.
83. Turjanmaa K, Reunala T, Tuimala R, et al. Allergy to latex gloves: unusual complication during delivery. *Br Med J* 1988;297:1029.
84. Péchinot M. Allergie au latex au décours d'une césarienne. *Ann Fr Anesth Réanim* 1997;16:79–80.
85. Jorrot JC, Mercier F, Pecquet C, et al. Choc anaphylactique peropératoire au latex. *Ann Fr Anesth Réanim* 1989;8:278–279.
86. Morriss WW, Lavies NG, Anderson SK, et al. Acute respiratory distress during caesarean section under spinal anaesthesia. A probable case of anaphylactoid reaction to Syntocinon. *Anaesthesia* 1994;49:41–43.
87. Zucker-Pinchoff B, Chandler MJ. Latex anaphylaxis masquerading as fentanyl anaphylaxis: retraction of a case report. *Anesthesiology* 1993;79:1152–1153.
88. Jackson IJ, Bryson MR, McPhail S, et al. Recurrent anaphylactoid reaction during caesarean section. *Anaesthesia* 1989;44:585–587.
89. Rae SM, Milne MK, Wildsmith JA. Anaphylaxis associated with, but not caused by, extradural bupivicaine. *Br J Anaesth* 1997;78:224–226.
90. Lee J J. Anaphylactoid reaction following epidural block: local anaesthetic or latex? *Anaesthesia* 1994;49:263.
91. Holness DR, Tarlo SM, Sussman G, et al. Exposure characteristics and cutaneous problems in operating room staff. *Contact Dermatitis* 1995;32:352–358.
92. Fisher MM, Bowey CJ. Intradermal compared with prick testing in the diagnosis of anaesthetic allergy. *Br J Anaesth* 1997;79:59–63.
93. Bousquet J, Michel FB. In vivo methods for studying allergy. Skin tests, techniques and interpretation. In: Middleton E, Reed C, Ellis E, et al., eds. *Allergy. Principles and Practice,* 4th ed. Toronto: Mosby Press, 1993:573–594.
94. Reid MJ, Lockey RF, Turkeltaub PC, et al. Survey of fatalities from skin testing and immunotherapy 1985–1989. *J Allergy Clin Immunol* 1993;92:6–15.
95. Shatz M. Skin testing and incremental challenge in the evaluation of adverse reactions to local anesthetics. *J Allergy Clin Immunol* 1984;74:606–616.
96. Austen KF. Disease of Immediate Hypersensitivity. In: Fauci A, Braunwald E, Isselbacher K, et al., eds. *Harrison's Principles of Internal Medicine,* 14th ed. Toronto: McGraw-Hill, 1998:1860–1869.
97. Bolognia JL, Braverman IM. Skin manifestations of internal disease . In: Fauci A, Braunwald E, Isselbacher K, et al., eds. *Harrison's Principles of Internal Medicine,* 14th ed. Toronto: McGraw-Hill, 1998;57:310–328.
98. Jensen NF, Weiler JM. C1 esterase inhibitor deficiency, airway compromise, and anesthesia. *Anesth Analg* 1998;87:480–488.
99. Boulos AN, Brown R, Hukin A, et al. Danazol prophylaxis for delivery in hereditary angioneurotic oedema. *Br J Obstet Gynaecol* 1994;101:1094–1095.
100. Cox M, Holdcroft A. Hereditary angioneurotic oedema: current management in pregnancy. *Anaesthesia* 1995;50:547–549.
101. Bhatia PL, Singh MS, Jha BK. Laryngopathia gravidarum. *Ear Nose Throat J* 1981;60:408–412.
102. Benson MD, Lindberg RE. Amniotic fluid embolism, anaphylaxis, and tryptase. *Am J Obstet Gynecol* 1996;175:737.
103. Fineschi V, Gambassi R, Gherardi M, et al. The diagnosis of amniotic fluid embolism: an immunohistochemical study for the quantification of pulmonary mast cell tryptase. *Int J Legal Med* 1998;111:238–243.
104. Branigan EF, Stevenson MM, Charles D. Blood transfusion reaction in a patient with immunoglobulin A deficiency. *Obstet Gynecol* 1983;61:47S–49S.
105. Borgeat A, Ruetsch YA. Anesthesia in a patient with malignant systemic mastocytosis using a total intravenous anesthetic technique. *Anesth Analg* 1998;86:442–444.
106. Howard H, Martlew V, McFayden I, et al. Consequences for fetal and neonate of maternal red cell alloimmunisation. *Arch Dis Child* 1998;78:F62– F66.
107. Bowman JM. Rherythroblastosis fetalis 1975. *Semin Hematol* 1975;12:189–207.
108. Rote NS. Pathophysiology of Rh immunization. *Clin Obstet Gynecol* 1982;25:243–253.
109. Haines CJ, Read MD. Characteristic fetal heart rate changes in severe rhesus isoimmunization. *Aust N Z J Obstet Gynaecol* 1983;23:114–116.
110. Leveque C, Murat I, Toubas F, et al. Fetal neuromuscular blockade with vecuronium bromide: studies during intravascular intrauterine transfusion in isoimmunized pregnancy. *Anesthesiology* 1992;76:642–644.
111. Hollmén AL, Jouppila R, Jouppila P, et al. Effect of extradural analgesia using bupivacaine and 2-chloroprocaine on intervillous blood flow during normal labor. *Br J Anaesth* 1982;54:837–842.
112. Hess EV. Rheumatoid arthritis: epidemiology, etiology, rheumatoid factor, pathology, pathogenesis. In: Schemacher HR Jr, ed. *Primer on Rheumatic Diseases,* 9th ed. Atlanta: The Arthritis Foundation, 1988:83–96.
113. Matti MV, Sharrock NE. Anesthesia on the rheumatoid patient. *Rheum Dis Clin North Am* 1998;24:19–27.
114. Rawlins BA, Girardi FP, Boachie-Adjei O. Rheumatoid arthritis of the cervical spine. *Rheum Dis Clin North Am* 1998;24:55–65.
115. Hodgekinson R. Anesthetic management of a parturient with severe rheumatoid arthritis. *Anesth Analg* 1981;60:611–612.
116. Bulmash JM. Rheumatoid arthritis in pregnancy. *Obstet Gynecol Ann* 1979;8:223–276.
117. Nelson JL, Østensen M. Pregnancy and rheumatoid arthritis. *Rheum Dis Clin North Am* 1997;23:195–212.
118. Moise KJ Jr, Huhta JC, Sharif DS, et al. Indomethacin in the treatment of premature labor. Effect on the fetal ductus arteriosis. *N Engl J Med* 1988;319:327–331.
119. Edelist G. Principles of anesthetic management in rheumatoid arthritic patients. *Anesth Analg* 1964;43:227–231.
120. Alacorn-Segovia D. Systemic lupus erythematosus: Pathology and pathogenesis. In: Schumacher HR Jr, ed. *Primer on Rheumatic Diseases,* 9th ed. Atlanta: The Arthritis Foundation, 1988:97–110.
121. Scott JS. Systemic lupus erythematosus and allied disorders in pregnancy. *Clin Obstet Gynecol* 1979;6:461–471.
122. Boumpas DT, Fessler BJ, Austin III HA, et al. Systemic Lupus Erythematosis: Emerging Concepts. Part 2: Dermatologic and joint disease, the antiphospolipid antibody syndrome, pregnancy and hormonal therapy, morbidity and mortality, and pathogenesis. *Ann Intern Med* 1995;123:42–52.

123. Petrie M. Hopkins lupus pregnancy center: 1987–1996. *Rheum Dis North Am* 1997;23:1–13.

124. Mascola MA, Repke JT. Obstetric management of the high-risk lupus pregnancy. *Rheum Dis Clin North Am* 1997;23:119–132.

125. del Rio A, Vazquez JJ, Sobrino JA, et al. Myocardial involvement in systemic lupus erythematosus: a non-invasive study of left ventricular function. *Chest* 1978;74:414–417.

126. Reece EA, Romero R, Hobbins J. Coagulopathy associated with Factor VIII Inhibitor: a literature review. *J Reprod Med* 1984;29:53–58.

127. Horlocker T, Wedel D. Spinal and epidural blockade and perioperative low molecular weight heparin: smooth sailing on the Titanic. *Anesth Analg* 1998;86:1153–1156.

128. Neuroaxial anesthesia and anticoagulation (Consensus statement). Anesthesia Society of Regional Anesthesia (ASRA), May 1998.

129. Reichlin M. Systemic lupus erythematosus and pregnancy. *J Reprod Med* 1998;43:355–360.

130. Steen VD. Scleroderma and pregnancy. *Rheum Disease Clin North Am* 1998;23:133–147.

131. Medsger TA. Systemic sclerosis and localized scleroderma. In: Schumacher Jr, HR, ed. *Primer on rheumatic diseases*, 9th ed. Atlanta: The Arthritis Foundation, 1988:111–117.

132. Karlen JR, Cooke WA. Renal scleroderma in pregnancy. *Obstet Gynecol* 1974;44:349–354.

133. Levy DL. Fetal-neonatal involvement in maternal autoimmune disease. *Obstet Gynecol Surv* 1982;37(suppl):122–127.

134. Maymon R, Fegin M. Scleroderma in pregnancy. *Obstet Gynecol Surv* 1989;44:530–534.

135. Johnson TR, Banner EA, Winklemann RK. Scleroderma in pregnancy. *Obstet Gynecol* 1964;23:467–469.

136. Swanesaratnam V, Chong HL. Scleroderma and pregnancy. *Aust N Z J Obstet Gynaecol* 1982;22:123–124.

137. Cannon PJ, Hassar M, Case DB, et al. The relationship between hypertension and renal failure in scleroderma (progressive systemic sclerosis) to structural and functional abnormalities of the renal cortical circulation. *Medicine* 1974;53:1–46.

138. Gilliand BG. Systemic sclerosis. In: Fauci AS, Braunwald E, Isslebacher KJ, et al., eds. *Harrison's Principles of Internal Medicine*, 14th ed. Toronto: McGraw-Hill, 1998:1888–1896.

139. Steen VD, Cosantino JP, Shapiro AP, et al. Outcome of renal crisis in systemic sclerosis: relation to the availability of angiotensin converting enzyme (ACE) inhibitors. *Ann Intern Med* 1990;113:352–357.

140a. Mastrobattista JM. Angiotensin converting enzyme inhibitors in pregnancy. *Semin Perinatol* 1997;21:124–132.

140b. Weisman RA, Calceterra TC. Head and neck manifestations of scleroderma. *Ann Otol Rhinol Laryngol* 1978;87:332–339.

141. Young RH, Mark GJ. Pulmonary vascular changes in scleroderma. *Am J Med* 1978;64:998–1004.

142. Cannon PJ, Hassar M, Case DB, et al. The relationship between hypertension and renal failure in scleroderma (progressive systemic sclerosis) to structural and functional abnormalities of the renal cortical circulation. *Medicine* 1974;53:1–46.

143. Bulkley BH, Ridolfi RL, Salyer WR, et al. Myocardial lesions of progressive systemic sclerosis: a cause of cardiac dysfunction. *Circulation* 1976;53:483–490.

144. Kirk EP. Organ transplantation and pregnancy. A case report and review. *Am J Obstet Gynecol* 1991;164:1629–1634.

145. Murray JE, Reid DE, Harrison JH, et al. Successful pregnancies after human renal transplant. *N Engl J Med* 1963;269:341–343.

146. Casele HL, Laifer SA. Pregnancy after liver transplantation. *Semin Perinatol* 1998;22:149–155.

147. Cardella CJ, Brady HR. Kidney transplantation. *Mod Med Can* 1988;43:824–836.

148. Radomski JS, Ahlswede BA, Jarrell BE, et al. Outcomes of 500 pregnancies in 335 female kidney, liver, and heart transplant recipients. *Transplant Proc* 1995;27:1089–1090.

149. Yuh-Jer Shen A, Mansukhani PW. Is pregnancy contraindicated after cardiac transplantation? A case report and literature review. *Int J Cardiol* 1997;60:151–156.

150. Troché V, Ville Y, Fernandez H. Pregnancy after heart or heart-lung transplantation: a series of 10 pregnancies. *Br J Obstet Gynaecol* 1998;105:454–458.

151. Scott JR, Wagoner LE, Olsen SL, et al. Pregnancy in heart transplant recipients: Management and outcome. *Obstet Gynecol* 1993;82:324–327.

152. Kim KM, Sukhani R, Slogoff S, et al. Central hemodynamic changes associated with pregnancy in a long-term cardiac transplant recipient. *Am J Obstet Gynecol* 1996;174:1651–1653.

153. Taylor AJ, Bergin JD. Cardiac transplantation for the cardiologist not trained in transplantation. *Am Heart J* 1995;129:578–592.

154. Dash, A. Anesthesia for patients with a previous heart transplant. *Int Anesthesiol Clin* 1995;33:1–9.

155. Riley ET. Obstetric management of patients with transplants. *Int Anesthesiol Clin* 1995;33:125–140.

156. Uretsky BF, Murali S, Reddy PS, et al. Development of coronary artery disease in cardiac transplant patients receiving immunosuppressive therapy with cyclosporine and prednisone. *Circulation* 1987;76:827–834.

157. Dajani A, Taubert K, Wilson W, et al. Prevention of bacterial endocarditis: recommendations by the American Heart Association. *Circulation* 1997;96:358–366.

158. Haddow G. Anaesthesia for patients after lung transplantation. *Can J Anaesth* 1997;44:182–197.

159. Armenti VT, Gertner GS, Eisenberg JA, et al. National Transplantation Pregnancy Registry: outcomes of pregnancies in lung recipients. *Transplant Proc* 1998;30:1528–1530.

160. Parry D, Hextall A, Banner N, et al. Pregnancy following lung transplantation. *Transplant Proc* 1997;29:629.

161. Parry D, Hextall A, Robinson VP, et al. Pregnancy following a single lung transplant. *Thorax* 1996;51:1162–1164.

162. Ville Y, Fernandez H, Samuel D, et al. Pregnancy in liver transplant recipients: course and outcome in 19 cases. *Am J Obstet Gynecol* 1993;168:896–902.

163. Pruvot FR, Declerck N, Valat-Rigot AS, et al. Pregnancy after liver transplantation: Focusing on risks to the mother. *Transplant Proc* 1997;29:2470–2471.

164. Casele HL, Laifer SA. Association of pregnancy complications and choice of immunosuppressant in liver transplant patients. *Transplantation* 1998;65:581–583.

165. Van Dyke R. The liver in pregnancy. In: Zakim D, Boyer T, eds. *Hepatology: a Textbook of Liver Disease, vol. II.* 3rd ed. Toronto: WB Saunders, 1996;1734–1759.

166. Avraamides EJ, Craen RA, Gelb AW. Anaesthetic management of a pregnant, post liver transplant patient for dental surgery. *Anaesth Intensive Care* 1997;25:68–70.

167. Kutt JL, Mezon BR. Anesthesia and liver transplantation. *Anesthesiol Clin North Am* 1994;12:717–727.

168. Catnach SM, McCarthy M, Jauniaux E, et al. Liver transplantation during pregnancy complicated by cytomegalovirus infection. *Transplantation* 1995;60:510–511.

169. Davison JM, Milne JEC. Pregnancy and renal transplantation. *Br J Urol* 1997;80(Suppl):29–32.

170. Armenti VT, McGrory CH, Cater JR, et al. Pregnancy outcomes in female renal transplant recipients. *Transplant Proc* 1998;30:1732–1734.

171. Solders G, Persson A, Wilczek H. Autonomic system dysfunction and polyneuropathy in nondiabetic uremia. *Transplantation* 1986;41:616–619.

172. Vennarecci G, Pisani F, Tisone G, et.al. Kidney transplantation and pregnancy. *Transplant Proc* 1997;29:2797–2798.

173. McGrory CH, Groshek MA, Sollinger HW, et al. Pregnancy outcomes in female pancreas-kidney recipients. *Transplant Proc* 1999;31:652–653.

174. Moote CA. Anesthesia for renal transplantation. *Anesthesiol Clin North Am* 1994;12:691–711.

175. Stahl RAK. Non-steroidal anti-inflammatory agents in patients with a renal transplant. *Nephrol Dial Transplant* 1998;13:1119–1121.

176. Moudry-Munns KC, Barrou B, Sutherland DER. Pregnancy after pancreas transplantation: Report from the International Pancreas Transplant Registry. *Transplant Proc* 1996;28:3639.

177. DeWolf AM. Multiviscera and pancreas transplantation. *Int Anesthesiol Clin* 1991;29:111–136.

178. Tarshis J, Datta S. Anesthesia for the pregnant diabetic patient. *Anesthesiol Clin North Am* 1998;16:441–458.

179. Barrou BM, Gruessner AC, Sutherland DER, et al. Pregnancy after pancreas transplantation in the cyclosporine era. *Transplantation* 1998;65:524–527.

180. Sutherland DER, Gruessner AC, Gruessner RWG. Pancreas transplantation: a review. *Transplant Proc* 1998;30:1940–1943.

181. Watkins PJ. Diabetic autonomic neuropathy. *N Engl J Med* 1990; 322:1078–1079.

182. Hathaway DK, Abell T, Cardoso S, et. al. Improvement in autonomic and gastric function following pancreas-kidney versus kidney-alone transplantation and the correlation with quality of life. *Transplantation* 1994;57:816–822.

183. Groth CG, Bolinder J, Solders G, et al. Diabetic patients subjected to combined pancreas and kidney transplantation or kidney transplantation alone: outcome after 5 to 10 years. *Transplant Proc* 1998;30:3413.

184. Ralley FE. The diabetic patient: a challenge or just routine? *Can J Anaesth* 1996;43:R14–R23.

185. Little BB. Immunosuppressant therapy during gestation. *Semin Perinatol* 1997;21:143–148.

186. Esplin MS, Branch DW. Immunosuppressive drugs and pregnancy. *Obstet Gynecol Clin North Am* 1997;24:601–616.

187. Schatz M, Zeiger RS, Harden K, et al. The safety of asthma and allergy medications during pregnancy. *J Allergy Clin Immunol* 1997;100:301–306.

188. Kozlowska-Boszko B, Soluch L, Rybus J, et al. Does chronic glucocorticosteroid therapy in pregnant renal allograft recipients affect cortisol levels in neonates? *Transplant Proc* 1996;28:3490–3491.

189. Payne N. Anesthetic implications of immunosuppressants used for transplantation. *Int Anesthesiol Clin* 1995;33:93–106.

190. Vyas S, Kumar A, Piecuch S, et al. Outcome of twin pregnancy in a renal transplant recipient treated with tacrolimas. *Transplantation* 1999;67:490–492.

191. Jain A, Venkataramanan R, Fung JJ, et al. Pregnancy after liver transplantation under tacrolimus. *Transplantation* 1997;64:559–565.

192. Watson CJE, Friend PJ, Jamieson NV, et al. Sirolimus: a potent new immunosuppressant for liver transplantation. *Transplantation* 1999;67:505–509.

Shnider and Levinson's Anesthesia for Obstetrics,
edited by Samuel C. Hughes, et al.
Lippincott Williams & Wilkins,
Philadelphia, © 2001.

CHAPTER 33

HUMAN IMMUNODEFICIENCY VIRUS IN THE DELIVERY SUITE

SAMUEL C. HUGHES, M.D. AND PATRICIA A. DAILEY, M.D.

The human immunodeficiency virus (HIV) infection is a newly recognized microbe responsible for the pandemic of acquired immunodeficiency syndrome (AIDS) (1). We did not become aware of the virus until 1981, but it is now estimated that on a worldwide basis 2.3 million HIV-infected women give birth each year worldwide (2). Without treatment, 20% to 40% of the infants born to these women will become infected. In the United States, 6,000 to 7,000 HIV-infected women deliver each year (2). To put this into perspective, between 1987 and 1990, there were approximately 363 pregnancy-related deaths per year in the United States (3). AIDS was initially seen as a disease of homosexual men but women represented 23% of newly reported AIDS cases in 1998 (4) (Fig. 33.1). Many patients are unaware of their HIV infection and since the disease is increasingly spread through heterosexual contact, it is the rare labor and delivery ward that will not care for the HIV-infected parturients (5, 6).

EPIDEMIOLOGY AND SCOPE OF THE DISEASE

In the United States, an estimated 650,000 to 900,000 people are infected with HIV (1). Estimates for HIV-infection have run as high as 1.5 million Americans and 200,000 or more are unaware of their infection. On a worldwide basis, more than 33 million people are infected and 43% of them are women (7). There were 5.8 million *new* HIV infections in 1998 or approximately 16,000 each day. HIV/AIDS was the fourth leading cause of death in the world and resulted in 2.3 million deaths in 1998 (1). As we enter a new century, it is estimated that as many as 40 million people are HIV infected and AIDS will remain a tragic, costly presence.

In the United States, 753,907 cases of AIDS were reported by the Centers for Disease Control (CDC) through June 2000 (4) with 438,795 AIDS-related deaths, indicating a case fatality rate of 58%. Deaths from AIDS are now declining in the United States (4) (Fig. 33.2) with a clear link to antiretroviral therapy (8). However, between 1982 and 1994, HIV infection rose from not being mentioned to the leading cause of death among people 25 to 44 years of age (Fig. 33.3). Further, there are still 40,000 new HIV infections per year. Although HIV infection is no longer the leading cause of death in this age group, the CDC has estimated that half of the new infections occur in people less than 25 years of age. The infection among heterosexual men and women has obvious implications for labor and delivery suites and obstetric anesthesia. While the geographic differences are dramatic (4) (Fig. 33.4), most hospitals in the United States will treat HIV-infected women. In large urban centers, this remains a very significant concern (9).

Population at Risk

The transmission of HIV varies greatly in different populations. In the developing world and the United States, treatment of sexually transmitted diseases in women has been shown to sig-

nificantly decrease HIV transmission (10). In Northern Europe and the United Kingdom, HIV infection remains predominately a disease of homosexual men (11). In Spain and Italy and parts of Eastern Europe, HIV infection is closely linked with intravenous drug abuse, not unlike many urban centers in the United States (12). For women in the United States, in 1997, injection-drug use accounted for approximately 38% of the AIDS incidence while heterosexual contact accounted for 58% of the cases (4). In Central Africa where 30% of women delivering in some urban centers are HIV positive, HIV is predominately a heterosexual disease (13) (Fig. 33.5). While sub-Saharan Africa currently has the greatest number of patients with the disease, the growth in developing countries, particularly southeast Asia and the Indian subcontinent is extremely rapid. In Thailand the spread of HIV is linked to both drug abuse and heterosexual spread. In 1987, very little HIV was detected but by 1995, one in 80 people in the population were infected. This rate is three to five times higher then the rate in the United States, and it occurred in a very few years. HIV is a unique virus and is an extremely successful *survivor* in our present environment (14, 15).

The anesthesiologist is now faced with a complex disease that didn't appear in the literature until 1981 and couldn't be definitively diagnosed until 1985 (16). While the death rates are declining because of our better understanding of the disease and aggressive drug therapy, the clinician needs to understand the disease, the unique concerns in pregnancy, therapeutic intervention, opportunistic, and associated infections, and infection control techniques. With this knowledge, the anesthesiologist can plan pain relief for labor and possible anesthetic intervention for surgery. The ever-increasing therapeutic pharmacologic intervention must be taken into particular consideration. Opportunistic infection remains a problem with tuberculosis emerging as a particular concern (17). This chapter will focus on these issues and related concerns as the obstetric suite and operating room are now a common interface with the HIV positive patient.

PATHOGENESIS OF HIV

HIV-I virus is a retrovirus and a single-strand RNA virus. After entering the cell, the virus is copied by a reverse transcriptase enabling it to produce double-strand DNA which then integrates into the host's cells. HIV-2 is an extremely similar virus that produces AIDS as well. This virus is common in western Africa but rarely seen in the United States (in this chapter, HIV refers to HIV-1). The most common mode of infection is sexual transmission through the genital mucosa (18). Within 2 days, the virus can be detected in the internal iliac lymph nodes, and within 5 days (4 to 11 days), the virus can be cultured from the plasma. There is a rapid rise in plasma viremia at this point that spreads to lymphoid organs and the brain (19) (Fig. 33.6). The CD_4+ T-lymphocytes (CD_4+ cells) are infected early in the course of the disease and the remaining cell count per mm^3 helps define the disease progression. The decline of the CD_4+ cell count

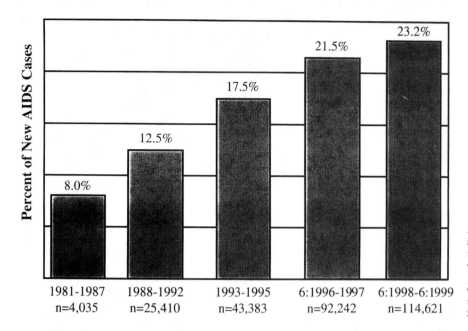

Figure 33.1. Cumulative AIDS cases in women and percent of new U.S. cases. Through 1992, there were only 25,410 cases reported in women, but by June 1999, this total reached 114,621 cumulative AIDS cases. (Data from Centers for Disease Control and Prevention as summarized in successive HIV/AIDS Surveillance Reports.)

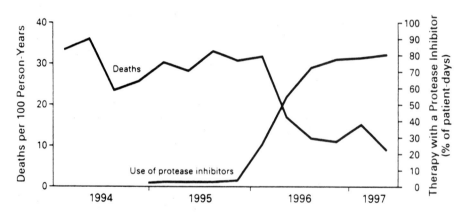

Figure 33.2. Mortality and frequency of use of combination antiretroviral therapy including a protease inhibitor among HIV-infected patients with fewer than 100 CD$_4$+ cells per cubic mm, according to calendar quarter from January 1994 through June 1997. (From Palella FJ, Jr. Delaney KM, Moorman AC, et al. Declining morbidity and mortality among patients with advanced human immunodeficiency virus infection. *N Engl J Med* 1998;338:853–860, with permission.)

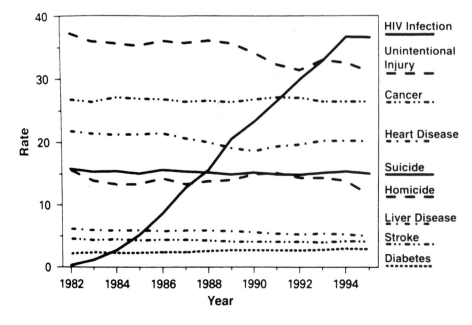

Figure 33.3. Death rates for leading causes of death among persons aged 25–44 years, by year—United States, 1982 to 1995 per 100,000 population. Based on underlying cause of death reported on death certificates using final data for 1982 to 1994 and preliminary data for 1995. While the death rate has now declined slightly, it remains significant. (Data from *MMWR* 1997;4:171. Courtesy of Centers for Disease Control and Prevention.)

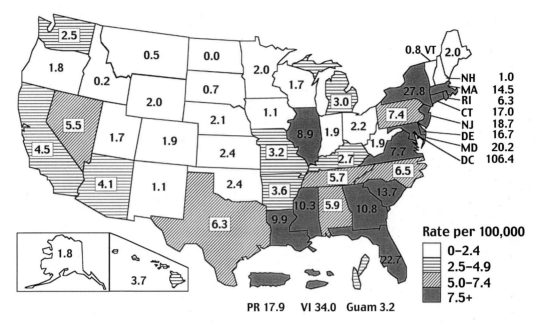

Figure 33.4. Female adult/adolescent annual AIDS rates per 100,000 population for cases reported July 1999 through June 2000, United States. (Data from HIV AIDS Surveillance Report, *MMWR* 2000;12:1. Courtesy of Centers for Disease Control and Prevention.)

marks HIV progression from the initial infection. Plasma viral load (which can be quantitated) is initially extremely high, then declines in the clinical latency period (Fig. 33.7). As constitutional symptoms and opportunistic infections occur (6 to 12 years after infection), viral load again increases in the terminal patient. Because of the high viral load, the patient with an acute

infection is extremely infectious as are those in the late stages of the disease.

Acute infection is a transient, symptomatic illness with symptoms including fever, fatigue, rash, headache, lymphadenopathy, pharyngitis, myalgia or arthralgia and nausea, vomiting and diarrhea. In recent studies, 87% of a group of newly-infected

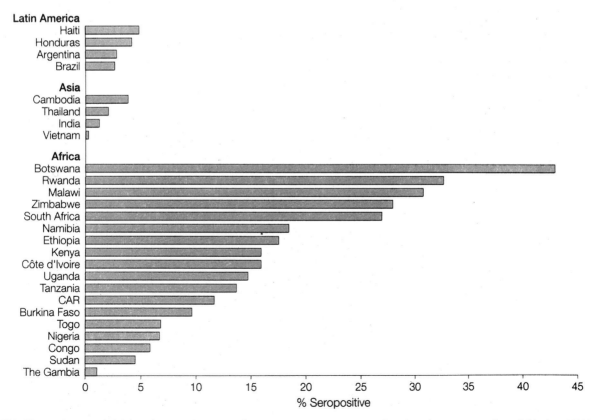

Figure 33.5. Human immunodeficiency virus type 1 seroprevalence among pregnant women. Based on the most recently available data (1996–1998) from the capital cities or major urban centers of selected countries, as compiled by the U.S. Bureau of Census (CAR indicates Central African Republic. (From Cock KM, Fowler MG, Mercier E, et al. Prevention of mother-to-child HIV transmission in resource-poor countries translating research into policy and practice. *JAMA* 2000;283:1175–1182, with permission.)

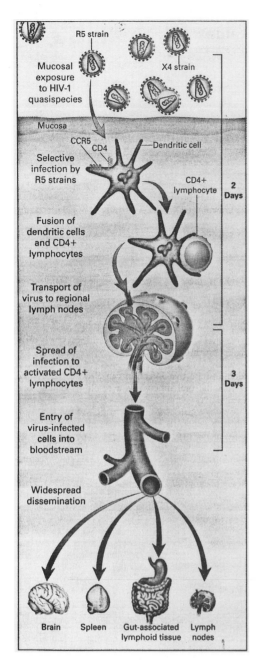

Figure 33.6. Early events in transmucosal HIV-1 infection. The arrows indicate the path of the virus. The viral-envelope protein binds to the CD4 molecule on dendritic cells. Entry into the cells requires the presence of CCR5, a surface chemokine receptor. Dendritic cells, which express the viral coreceptors CD4 and CCR5, are selectively infected by R5 (macrophagetropic) strains. Within 2 days after mucosal exposure, virus can be detected in lymph nodes. Within another 3 days, it can be cultured from plasma. (From Kahn JO, Walker BD. Acute human immunodeficiency virus type 1 infection. *N Engl J Med* 1998;339:33–39, with permission.)

patients had acute symptoms and 95% sought medical evaluation (19, 20). The viral half-life is approximately 6 hours and the turnover may be as high as 1 billion per day. It has been said that HIV is "the fastest genome evolution ever described" (21). While the virus may remain seemingly innocuous for 10 years or more in some individuals, ultimately a rising viral count, extreme compromise of the immune system, and a CD4+ cell count <200 cell/μL, heralds the final stages, the clinical diagnosis of AIDS is made with the occurrence of one of the index conditions (Table 33.1).

HIV Disease: General Considerations

HIV disease is a complex medical disorder that has wide systemic expression and results in multiorgan disease (Table 33.2). These problems are well described, and the management of the HIV-seropositive patient has, in effect, become a medical subspecialty (22). The neurologic, pulmonary, and hematologic changes and abnormalities are of particular concern to the anesthesiologist.

Neurologic involvement begins within days of the initial infection (19) and HIV has been isolated from the cerebrospinal fluid (CSF) during primary infection (23). There are indications of the cellular immune system activation in the central nervous system (CNS) even in the absence of obvious neurologic symptoms or signs. Acute encephalitis has been reported with primary infection but seems uncommon. However, conditions reported with acute infection include: myelopathy, peripheral neuropathy, brachial neuritis, cauda equina syndrome and Guillain-Barré syndrome (24). It is not known what determines the extent of neurologic involvement. However, it is speculated that particular strains of the virus are neurotropic or monocytotropic and thus more likely to cause unique neurologic involvement. The latent phase of the disease appears marked by an autoimmune process triggered by HIV. Demyelinating neuropathies that resemble subacute Guillain-Barré syndrome or chronic inflammatory demyelinating polyneuropathy may be seen. They may respond to corticosteroids, plasmapheresis, or intravenous immunoglobulin (25).

The later stages of the disease lead to severe immune compromise and a wide variety of infectious or opportunistic infections. Meningitis is frequent with cryptococcal infection, a common source, but tuberculosis and syphilitic meningitis are possible. The infectious nature of CSF in the HIV-infected parturient must always be considered. Early in the epidemic, brain biopsies were frequently performed to diagnosis possible tuberculosis lesions versus toxoplasmosis or CNS lymphomas. Currently, these are most often diagnosed without surgery but demonstrate the extent of potential neurologic involvement of the CNS, particularly in the late stages of the disease.

Pulmonary complications are largely related to infectious agents. Indeed, the epidemic began with an obscure report of four homosexual men with *Pneumocystis carini*, which seemed like only a medical curiosity at the time (16). In 1992, *Pneumocystis carinii* pneumonia was the cause of death in 14% of patients while another 18% died of an unspecified pneumonia (26). However, deaths from *Pneumocystis carinii* have declined from the 33% reported in 1987 and may continue to decrease with drug prophylaxis to prevent infection and advance in the management of HIV. However, tuberculosis, aspergillosis and numerous bacterial organisms are frequently causes of pulmonary complications. In 1994, a review of pregnant women with tuberculosis in New York City revealed a rate of active tuberculosis at 12.4 per 100,000 deliveries (1985 to 1990) increasing to 94.8 per 100,000 deliveries (1991 to 1992) (27). Of the 16 patients reviewed, 10 had proven, active pulmonary tuberculosis and two had tuberculosis meningitis. Renal, gastrointestinal and pleural tuberculosis were also diagnosed. Eleven of these women were tested for HIV and seven were seropositive. While this review was limited to two hospitals, it is clear that HIV disease and tuberculosis will remain significantly linked epidemics well into the future (17, 28).

Hematological abnormalities occur with acute HIV infection and are indeed a hallmark of the disease. A lymphocytosis composed of CD8+ T-lymphocytes may appear within two weeks of infection. A mild thrombocytopenia is common but not clinically important (29). However, Kaslow et al. noted that thrombocytopenia occurred in 2.8% of patients with a CD4+ T cell count of >700 cells/mL, but this rate increased to 10.8% when cell counts decreased below 250 (30). Thrombocytopenia may develop as the disease progresses due to a variety of causes such as

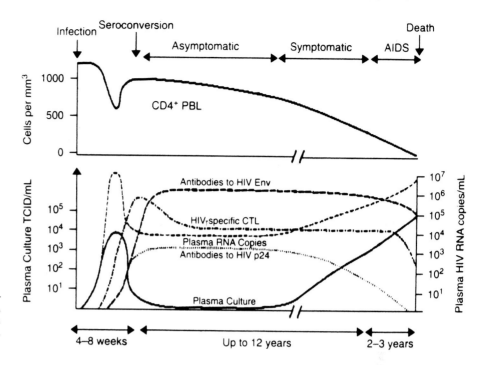

Figure 33.7. Natural history of HIV-1 infection. (From Sande MA, Volberding PA, eds. *The Medical Management of AIDS*, 5th ed. Philadelphia: WB Saunders, 1997:29, with permission.)

HIV-related immune thrombocytopenia (ITP), retroviral infection of megakaryocytes, or drug-induced thrombocytopenia (31).

HIV Disease: Effect of Pregnancy

The possible interaction of pregnancy and HIV disease was initially controversial (32–35). Early reports suggested that the gravidae had a decrease in their CD_4+ T-lymphocyte counts during pregnancy (36, 37) and there were reports of rapid progress to an AIDS diagnosis (38–40). Others have suggested no overall effect on lymphocyte cell parameters or the disease itself (41, 42). This potential interaction is difficult to

Table 33.1. INDEX CONDITIONS FOR THE DIAGNOSIS OF AIDS IN HIV POSITIVE PATIENT

Bacterial infection, multiple or recurrent
Candida of the bronchi, trachea, lungs or esophageal
CD_4+ T-lymphocyte count < 200 cells/μL
Cervical cancer, invasive
Coccidioidomycosis, disseminated or extrapulmonary
Cryptococcosis, extrapulmonary
Cryptosporidiosis, chronic intestinal (>1 month)
Cytomegalovirus other than liver, spleen, lymph nodes
Cytomegalovirus retinitis or CMV (with loss of vision)
Herpes simplex virus with chronic ulcers (>1 month), bronchitis, pneumonitis, esophagitis
HIV-related encephalopathy
Histoplasmosis, disseminated or extrapulmonary
Isophoriasis, chronic intestinal (>1 month)
Kaposi's sarcoma
Burkitt's lymphoma
Immunoblastic lymphoma
Lymphoma of the brain, primary
Mycobacterium avium complex or *kansasii*, disseminated or extrapulmonary
Mycobacterium tuberculosis—any site
Mycobacterium, any other species, pulmonary or extrapulmonary
Pneumocystis carinii pneumonia
Pneumonia, recurrent
Progressive multifocal leukoencephalopathy (PML)
Recurrent *Salmonella* septicemia
Toxoplasmosis of the brain
Wasting syndrome due to HIV

Data from the CDC 1993 revised classification system for HIV infection (definition became effective January, 1993): *MMWR* 1992;41:RR-17. Index clinical conditions remain as listed, December 1999

Table 33.2. HIV-MULTIORGAN DISEASE

Respiratory complications
 Pneumocystis carinii
 Bacterial pneumonia
 Tuberculosis
 Aspergillosis
 Cytomegalovirus
 Oral/pharyngeal candidiasis, herpetic infections

Hematologic
 Leukopenia
 Thrombocytopenia
 Anemia
 Drug toxicity

Cardiac
 Endocarditis (IV drug abuse)
 Pericarditis
 Focal myocarditis

Gastrointestinal
 Infectious diarrhea, proctitis
 Acalculous cholecystitis
 Vomiting, loss of appetite, cachexia
 Dysphagia (*Candida albicans*, cytomegalovirus), esophagitis
 Liver disease, hepatitis B and C, other infections

Neurologic problems in AIDS patients
 Distal, symmetrical sensory neuropathy: numbness; tingling, painful dysesthesias and paresthesias
 Chronic, inflammatory demyelinating polyneuropathy
 AIDS encephalopathy or AIDS dementia complex: cognitive, motor and behavioral changes
 Vacuolar myelopathy: sensory disturbance, spasticity and hyperreflexia (acute or chronic progression)
 Segmental (focal) myelopathy, acute or subacute (less common)
 Opportunistic infections or malignancies to include: toxoplasmosis, cryptococcal meningitis, progressive multifocal leukoencephalopathy, cytomegalovirus infection, herpes simplex virus, brain lymphomas or tuberculous lesions

evaluate because of the many obstetric variables, possible effect of drug use, nutritional factors and social factors. However, a large study in HIV-infected and uninfected Malawian gravidae suggested no difference in lymphocyte subsets (13). A recent study of 226 HIV-infected women during pregnancy in the United States was supportive of this conclusion (43).

More recently, measurement of direct viral load by measuring HIV ribonucleic acid (RNA) levels during pregnancy and postpartum has been used to evaluate the influence of pregnancy on HIV infection. Pregnancy had little immediate effect on HIV viral load in HIV-seropositive women (44). Thus, data suggest pregnancy has no acute effect on the course of HIV disease. Tragically, in large urban centers patients with significant, untreated HIV disease complicated by opportunistic infections may first come to medical attention during their pregnancy. These patients require the attention of medical specialists to manage their disease during pregnancy and prevent vertical transmission to the fetus.

Even with early HIV disease, careful medical evaluation during pregnancy is required. However, despite the many potential medical concerns, pregnancy and delivery may be very uneventful and the primary concern is to prevent vertical transmission (mother to fetus and newborn) of HIV.

Vertical Transmission: HIV Infection from Mother to Infant

In the United States, HIV infection in newborns has undergone a dramatic decline of more than 60% (45) (Fig. 33.8). On a worldwide basis, however, as many as 600,000 infants may be infected with HIV each year during the perinatal period (13, 46). Maternal-infant or vertical transmission is the primary means by which children become infected with HIV. If untreated, 15% to 40% of infants born to HIV-seropositive mothers will become infected in utero during labor, delivery or by breast-feeding (47). The risk of intrauterine infection is 4.4% and may not be affected by maternal zidovudine (AZT) therapy (48). The intrapartum time period accounts for 60% of the risk of perinatal HIV transmission and the remainder is via breast-feeding (49, 49a).

It has now been demonstrated that the maternal plasma HIV-1 RNA level is the best predictor of the risk of perinatal HIV-1 transmission and that reducing this level below 500 viral copies per mL will minimize this risk (50, 51). Breaks in placental barrier, prolonged rupture of membranes (>4 h), high cervicoaginal viral load (may not correlate with systemic viral load), lack of zidovudine treatment and vaginal delivery lead to increased rates of vertical transmission (49–53). The AIDS Clinical Trial Group (ACTG) Study 076 demonstrated a reduction in vertical transmission of HIV from 25.5% to 8.3% with maternal zidovudine therapy (47, 54). The U.S. Public Health Service Task Force has issued new recommendations including the use of zidovudine chemoprophylaxis to prevent perinatal transmission and offering the parturient antiretroviral therapy during pregnancy to treat the primary infection (52). Combination antiretroviral therapy (for example, zidovudine, lamivudine and nelfinavir or indinavir) during pregnancy has been successfully used and leads to a decreased viral load, increased CD$_4$+ T-lymphocyte cell count and lack of HIV vertical transmission (53). This study was particularly noteworthy because the women had advanced disease, prior histories of vertical transmission and/or substance abuse. Shorter courses of zidovudine and nevirapine have been successfully tried and may prove effective and more affordable in the developing world (55, 56).

Elective Cesarean Delivery

Management of HIV-seropositive women includes attempts to minimize the infant's exposure to maternal blood and genital secretions to decrease perinatal HIV transmission. This involves avoiding percutaneous umbilical cord sampling, fetal scalp clips (when possible), fetal scalp sampling, delivery techniques that could produce abrasions in the infant's skin (i.e., vacuum or

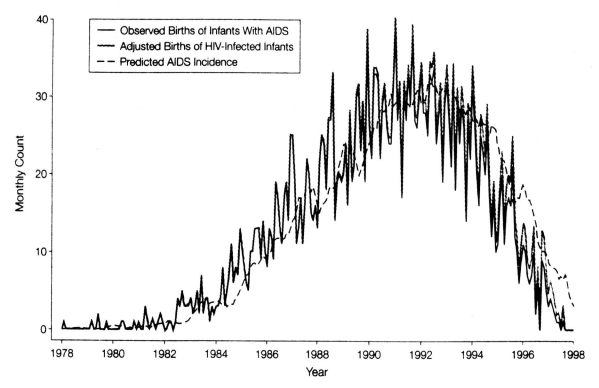

Figure 33.8. AIDS diagnoses reported through June 1998 for children diagnosed as having AIDS in the first year of life. AIDS, acquired immunodeficiency syndrome; HIV, human immunodeficiency virus. (From Lindegren ML, Byers RH, Thomas P, et al. Trends in perinatal transmission of HIV/AIDS in the United States. *JAMA* 1999;282:531–538, with permission.)

Table 33.3. ELECTIVE CESAREAN DELIVERY TO REDUCE THE TRANSMISSION OF HIV: RATES OF VERTICAL TRANSMISSION

	Elective Cesarean Delivery	Other Mode of Delivery
No antiretroviral therapy	10.4%	19.0%
Antiretroviral therapy	2.0%	7.3%

These data demonstrate the strong correlation between elective cesarean delivery and a lower risk of vertical HIV transmission (odds ratio 0.73).
Data from the International Perinatal HIV Group. The mode of delivery and the risk of vertical transmission of human immunodeficiency virus type 1–a meta-analysis of 15 prospective cohort studies. *N Engl J Med* 1999;340:977–987.

forceps), and immediate removal of maternal blood and fluids from the infant. However, numerous studies began to suggest a relationship between the mode of delivery and the vertical transmission rate (57–60). More recently, two large studies have demonstrated a significant decrease in the risk of vertical transmission with elective cesarean delivery (61, 62) (Table 33.3). It must be kept in mind that a parturient with a viral load below the limits of detection and/or one of several combination drug therapies may also have an extremely low HIV vertical transmission rate with a vaginal delivery. Further, cesarean sections are associated with higher maternal mortality rates, increases in postoperative morbidity and increased uterine rupture in subsequent pregnancies and these risks may be magnified in the developing world (63, 64). However, the American College of Obstetricians and Gynecologists (ACOG) has stated HIV-infected women should be offered a scheduled cesarean delivery to further reduce the risk of vertical transmission beyond that achievable with drug prophylaxis alone (115).

The available data indicate no reduction in the transmission rate if the cesarean delivery is performed after the onset of labor or rupture of membranes. Delivery at 38 completed weeks' gestation is recommended to reduce the likelihood of the onset of labor or rupture of membranes before delivery (65). Pregnant patients should also receive antiretroviral therapy according to currently accepted guidelines for nonpregnant adults (66). It is further noted that no combination of therapies can absolutely guarantee the lack of newborn transmission. The patient's autonomy in making this decision must be respected. The risk factors for perinatal HIV transmission continue to be evaluated (67). Discussion and controversy will continue around the issue of testing for HIV and management of the disease (68, 69). However, more aggressive medical and surgical management of the HIV-seropositive parturient will have benefits for both the mother and the newborn.

Drug Therapy: Side Effects and Drug Interaction

The routine use of new, increasingly intensive antiretroviral therapies has led to significant declines in morbidity and mortality in HIV disease (8, 70). Data suggesting intensive combination drug therapy, including a protease inhibitor, should be routine for patients with advanced disease.

There is an ever-increasing list of antiretroviral drugs available for the management of HIV disease, each with unique side effects (Table 33.4). The protease inhibitors have proven highly effective but also have wide-ranging side effects. Hyperlipidemia, glucose intolerance, abnormal fat distribution and high serum aminotransferase concentrations have been reported, (71) but rarely hepatitis. The manufacturers' drug inserts for the protease inhibitors report hemorrhage in patients with hemophilia

and drug therapy but there is little documented in the literature. While there are numerous other side effects, the most important concern may be the inhibition of cytochrome P-450 (CYP) 3A4 which is important for the metabolism of many drugs. It has recently been demonstrated that ritonavir significantly inhibits the metabolism of fentanyl among volunteers receiving a brief course of ritonavir (72) (Fig. 33.9). Ritonavir reduced the clearance of fentanyl by 67%, from 15.6 ± 8.2 to 5.2 ± 2 mL . min^{-1}kg^{-1} ($P < 0.01$). The results suggest a strong interaction between ritonavir and fentanyl and indicate the need to modify fentanyl dosing in these patients, at least when ritonavir is initially used. The risk of respiratory depression over a longer time period after fentanyl administration than would be otherwise be expected, seems likely, particularly with higher fentanyl doses. When smaller bolus doses of fentanyl are used, it is advisable to maintain respiratory monitoring for a longer period of time than usual. Caution is urged when administering benzodiazepines and opioids to patients receiving protease inhibitors but there is little clinical data upon which to base firm recommendations. The author's clinical experience (SCH), however, suggests that with careful titration, routine drugs, such as midazolam, fentanyl and morphine can be safely used. Conversely, the FDA approval of the protease inhibitors was very rapid and based upon very little clinical experience (largely in men). Further, the use of protease inhibitors in the parturient is extremely new (53, 73), and the clinician must be alert to possible unreported side effects, direct drug interactions and other drug toxicity.

The HIV-seropositive parturient may be taking numerous other drugs for prophylaxis or treatment of *pneumocystis carinii*, tuberculosis, toxoplasmosis, mycobacterium avium, fungal infection or herpes simplex (74) (Table 33.5). These drugs, as well as the use of antiviral therapy, has led to a decrease in deaths from opportunistic infections (Fig. 33.2). All of the drugs listed may have considerable side effects and the potential of unique drug interactions. A careful review of the drugs currently in use by the patient, updated laboratory analysis (Hct, liver enzymes, CD_4+ cell count), direct questioning of the patient for drug side effects and consultation with the primary care physician or HIV specialist will be extremely useful, when possible, given the lack of experience with these drugs in the parturient.

Neonatal and Fetal Effects

The administration of antiretroviral drugs will benefit the parturient by treating the underlying HIV disease and decrease vertical transmission even with the abbreviated maternal regimens that are begun intrapartum or in the first 48 hours of the newborn's life (75). However, despite the current recommendations and ongoing treatment of parturients with numerous antiretroviral agents, there is insufficient information to address the effect of exposure on the newborn. This is true even with zidovudine exposure, the drug with the greatest clinical experience. The long-term risks for neoplasia or organ-system toxicity in children is unknown (52). However, recent reports are encouraging. In one report with over 700 children with known zidovudine exposure in utero, there was no evidence of tumors with short-term (19–38 months) follow-up (76).

In a further prospective study of 234 HIV-uninfected children born to 230 HIV-infected women, slightly more than half were exposed to zidovudine in utero while the rest received a placebo (77). The median age at follow-up was 4.2 years (3.2 to 5.6 years). There were no significant differences in weight, height, head circumference or cognitive development function. There were also no deaths or malignancies. While there were no observed adverse effects observed in the HIV-uninfected children with in utero and neonatal exposure to zidovudine, extensive, continued evaluation is necessary to assess the long-term safety of intervention and this is ongoing. As new

Table 33.4. ANTIRETROVIRAL DRUGS FOR MANAGEMENT OF HIV INFECTION[a]

Drug	Dose	Side Effects
Nucleoside reverse transcriptase inhibitors		
Zidovudine (ZDV, AZT, Retrovir®)[b]	100 mg, 6×/day	Marrow suppression, anemia, hepatic steatosis, myopathy, lactic acidosis, headache, gastrointestinal disturbances; inhibits cytochrome P-450
Lamivudine (3TC, Epivir®)[b]	300 mg, b.i.d—commonly used with ZDV	Generally benign, often second drug of choice for triple therapy; may have diarrhea, headache, nausea, but is well tolerated.
Didanosine (DDI, Videx®)	200 mg, b.i.d.	Pancreatitis (fatalities reported), peripheral neuropathy, diarrhea
Zalcitabine (ddC, HIVID®)	0.75 mg, t.i.d.	Peripheral neuropathy, pancreatitis, stomatitis
Stavudine (d4T, Zerit®)	40 mg, b.i.d.	Peripheral neuropathy (may be severe), pancreatitis
Abacavir (Ziagen®)	300 mg, t.i.d.	Mild nausea, headache; hypersensitivity
Protease inhibitors		
Saquinavir mesylate (Invirase or Fortoase®)	600 mg, t.i.d.	Nausea, diarrhea, abdominal discomfort (improved with Fortoase®); inhibits cytochrome P-450
Indinavir sulfate (Crixivan®)	800 mg, t.i.d.	Nephrolithiasis (increased H_2O intake recommended), abdominal discomfort, hyperbilirubinemia; may increase levels of midazolam, triazolam; appears to inhibit cytochrome P-450
Nelfinavir mesylate (Viracept®)	750 mg, t.i.d.	Diarrhea; well tolerated; appears to inhibit cytochrome P-450
Ritonavir (Norvir®)	600 mg, b.i.d.	Nausea, vomiting, diarrhea, anorexia; elevated triglycerides, creatine kinase, transaminases; inhibits cytochrome P-450 (potent); not recommended with antiarrhythmics or sedative/hypnotics
Amprenavir (Agenerase®)	1,200 mg, b.i.d.	Rash, limited data; inhibits cytochrome P-450
Nonnucleoside reverse transcriptase inhibitors		
Nevirapine (Viramune®)	200 mg q.d., increasing to b.i.d. over 2 weeks	Skin rash, severe in some cases requiring hospitalzation; recommend caution with oral contraceptives; activates cytochrome P-450.
Delavirdine (Rescriptor®)	400 mg, t.i.d.	May increase concentrations of some antiarrhythmic drugs, plasma level of sedative hypnotics, calcium-channel blockers, and warfarin; rash, headache, nausea; inhibits cytochrome P-450
Efavirenz (Sustiva®)	600 mg/day in p.m.	Dizziness, light-headedness; may be teratogenic, not recommended in Pregnancy.

[a] This is a list of drugs commonly used or disused as of December 1999. There are currently numerous other drugs being investigated. The rapid approval by the Food and Drug Administration of most of the drugs in this table means that there is often minimal clinical experience. This is particularly true with regards to the parturient. The clinician should be alert to unusual or unexpected side effects or drug interactions. Updated information can be obtained from http://HIV on Site.ucsf.edu. This UCSF website by Dr. S. Deeks and Dr. P. Volberding (AIDS Knowledge Base-4) is updated regularly.

[b] Zidovudine (300 mg) and lamivudine (150 mg) are now combined into one tablet and marketed as Combivir and administered b.i.d. Other drugs are increasingly available in single tablet preparations for patient convenience.

antiretroviral drugs are used as well as prophylactic drug therapy for opportunistic diseases, possible toxic effects upon the neonate or later in the child's life must be carefully considered.

Anesthesia for Labor and Delivery

When planning an anesthetic for any patient with a major medical disease, a careful review of the disease process itself, the current status of the patient's disease and any therapy administered is necessary. As noted earlier in this chapter, HIV/AIDS is a multiorgan disease and drug therapy is complex and continues to change and evolve (Table 33.2). Further, in the patient with advanced disease (CD^4+ T-lymphocytes <200 cells/μL) numerous opportunistic infections and possible malignancies may complicate the anesthetic management along with pulmonary and hematologic problems. For exam-

ple, a prolonged, partial thromboplastin time (PTT) in a HIV-infected parturient may be secondary to the presence of a so-called lupus anticoagulant that is an in vitro abnormality This results in an artificially prolonged PTT that has little clinical significance. The presence of a lupus anticoagulant is confirmed by a prolonged Russell viper venom test (78).

The wide range of neurologic complications associated with the disease must also be considered. In 1985, in the early phase of the epidemic, it was said that approximately 10% of patients with AIDS first presented with neurologic signs and symptoms (79). While this is no longer true, the early involvement of the CNS with viral infection and the potentially catastrophic neurologic involvement of the CNS in the terminal phases of the disease, is well documented (25).

A large number of HIV-infected pregnant women are also at risk for the many potential problems associated with drug

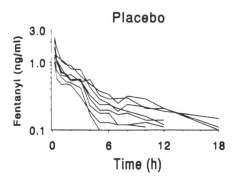
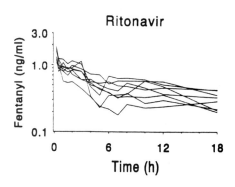

Figure 33.9. Plasma concentrations of fentanyl after an intravenous dose of 5 $\mu g \cdot kg^{-1}$ fentanyl following pretreatment with oral placebo (left) or ritonavir (right) in 11 healthy volunteers. (From Olkkola KT, Palkama VJ, Neuvonen PJ. Ritonavir's role in reducing fentanyl clearance and prolonging its half-life. *Anesthesiology* 1999;91:681–685, with permission.)

abuse. In a review of 96 HIV-infected parturients who delivered in a two year period (1990 to 1992), approximately 45% were noted to be intravenous drug users, nearly 50% had a history of veneral disease, approximately 25% were anemic (Hct <30%), and 12% had hepatitis (80).

Despite the many potential complications in the HIV-positive parturient, it has been this author's experience that these patients have few problems related to their anesthetic management, particularly in the earlier stages of infection. The underlying HIV disease and obstetric considerations will dictate the course of management and the anesthetic requirements.

Regional anesthesia is the most common technique in obstetric anesthesia. However, early in the HIV epidemic, many clinicians were hesitant to perform regional anesthesia in the HIV-seropositive patient (81). It was feared that the HIV infection could be "spread" to the CNS by epidural or spinal anesthesia.We now realize that the virus finds its way to the CNS quite early in the course of the infection (Fig. 33.6). Failure to be able to culture the virus from the CSF probably results from sampling error, not the absence of the virus in the fluid (82). Safety of regional anesthesia and exten-

sive clinical experience in the parturient has now been addressed in at least two studies as well as a case report (80, 83, 84). There is no information to suggest that subarachnoid or epidural anesthesia is contraindicated in HIV-infected patients.

In a prospective study of the immunologic function and clinical course of 30 HIV- infected parturients at San Francisco General Hospital, we demonstrated that regional anesthesia could be performed without adverse sequelae (83). The patients had extensive laboratory and medical evaluation before delivery and were followed for at least 4 to 6 months postpartum. There were no neurologic or infectious problems related to the regional anesthetics administered ($n = 18$) or the obstetric course. The immune function of the parturients remained stable in the peripartum period (CD$_4$+ T-lymphocytes, CD$_8$+ T-lymphocytes and serum p24 antigen). Another review of 96 HIV-positive parturients confirmed these findings (80). Regional anesthesia for cesarean section and other surgical procedures in the parturient may be particularly beneficial in that limited parenteral opioids are usually needed and the possible side effects that may occur with delayed metabolism caused by protease inhibitors can be avoided (71). We have had extensive clinical experience with various regional anesthetic techniques (primarily with male patients in the general operating room) from the beginning of the epidemic over 20 years ago. Spinal and epidural anesthesia have been used extensively with no adverse sequelae. Thus, when regional anesthesia is indicated in the HIV-positive parturient and there are no obvious contraindications (coagulopathy, infection at the site of block placement, for example) it can be used in a routine manner.

The use of an **epidural blood patch** (EBP) is appropriate when indicated to treat a postdural puncture headache (PDPH). Despite the theoretic risks, there are no serious complications related to this technique in the HIV-seropositive patient (85–89). The report by Tom et al., although a study of men, was quite careful in the acute and long-term follow-up of HIV-positive patients who received an EBP (86). Thus, while conservative management of a PDPH may be considered initially, there is no evidence to suggest that there are any unique risks of an EBP in the HIV-seropositive patient.

Finally, the use of combined spinal epidural (CSE) analgesia is increasing in obstetric anesthesia. However, there are scattered reports of meningitis among non-HIV infected patients associated with the CSE technique generating some controversy about the safety of routinely breaching the dural barrier (90–92). Is the HIV-seropositive parturient at increased risk for this potential complication? Is the possibility of some unrecognized or undiagnosed systemic infection greater in these patients so that routinely entering the dura might increase the risk of infection? While this remains open to speculation, the current evidence and clinical experience suggests that this is unlikely. However, as increasing numbers of HIV- seropositive parturients are being managed (Fig. 33.1), the clinician should consider this potential risk. Despite these threatening concerns, the author uses CSE when it appears beneficial and has routinely used spinal anesthesia in patients with HIV disease.

Table 33.5. PROPHYLAXIS FOR OPPORTUNISTIC INFECTIONS: DRUGS AND TOXICITY

Indication	Drug	Possible Toxicity
Pneumocysstis carinii + toxoplasmosis	Trimethoprim sulfamethoxazole	Severe rash may occur, fever, marrow suppression
Pneumocystis carinii [a]	Pentamidine	Nephrotoxicity, ↑ K$^+$, ↓ Ca^{++}, ↑amylase
Mycobacterium avium complex	Azithromycin Clarithromycin Rifabutin	Gastrointestinal Gastrointestinal Rash, neutropenia, gastrointestinal intolerance
Fungal infection	Fluconazole	Nausea, skin rash, gastrointestinal disturbances (↓ metabolism of warfarin), neutropenia, thrombocytopenia, hypotension, renal failure, ↑ liver enzymes
Herpes simplex	Acyclovir	Marrow suppression, renal failure, ↑ liver enzymes

[a] Other drugs in use for *Pneumocystis carinii* prophylasis or treatment include clindamycin, primaquine, atovaquone, and dapsone.
From Hughes SC. Human immunodeficiency virus and obstetric anesthesia. *Anesthesiol Clin North Am* 1998;16:397–418, with permission.

When **general anesthesia is** indicated, it can be safely performed in the routine manner. While there are data documenting transient immunologic changes secondary to anesthesia and surgery, it has not been linked to adverse clinical outcome and remains largely a theoretical concern (93–97). Thus, while an earlier report cautioned against the use of inhalation anesthetics (97), this seems overly speculative and runs counter to the extensive clinical experience in the intervening years. There is no known unique contraindication to a routine general anesthetic in a HIV-infected parturient.

When general anesthesia is indicated for the parturient because of emergency surgery, the patient's preference, or for other clinical reasons, it can be administered safely. If the patient is receiving protease inhibitors, use of benzodiazepines and opioids should be limited to small bolus doses as indicated. Routine monitoring in the usual post-anesthesia recovery area may need to be extended if larger doses of opioids are used because their metabolism is inhibited due to protease inhibitors (72). At San Francisco General Hospital, we recover parturients in the usual manner on the labor and delivery unit with particular focus on continuous pulse oximetry and close observation of respiratory function is recommended.

Prevention of HIV Transmission by Health Care Workers

The HIV epidemic has made all health care workers (HCW) more aware of the infectious risks to themselves and their patients in the hospital setting. There are documented cases of HIV, hepatitis B (HBV) and hepatitis C (HCV) transmission from patient to HCW and from HCW to patient, although the greatest risk is to the HCW (98). The Occupational Safety and Health Administration (OSHA) Bloodborne Pathogens Standard mandated "universal precautions" or universal blood and body fluid precautions (99, 100). These directives are meant to protect both the patient and the HCW. Through June 1999 in the United States, there were 55 documented cases and 136 possible cases of occupationally- acquired HIV infections in HCW (4). Infection of a patient with HIV by a HCW is *extremely* rare by comparison and easily avoided with universal precautions.

A review of all data on a worldwide basis, including the United States, noted only 94 cases of occupationally-acquired HIV with 190 possible cases reported (101). In another review of infection control practices in an obstetric suite of a large urban hospital, it was found that there was contact with blood or amniotic fluid in 39% of vaginal deliveries and 50% of the cesarean de-

liveries, and that the majority of the contacts were preventable with barrier precautions, i.e., gloves, mask and eye shields (102). In a separate study of anesthesia personnel performing a variety of routine procedures, there was contact with blood or body fluids 18% to 87% of the time, varying with the procedure including 34% with catheterization of the epidural space (103). The authors noted that 98% of the contact with blood could be prevented by using gloves routinely. The use of barrier precautions to include gloves, mask and eye shields is vital. Gowns should be worn if gross contamination is likely. These guidelines will decrease the risk of transmission of HCV as well, which is four times as prevalent in the population than HIV and thus an even greater risk (104). Immunization is the primary strategy for prevention of HBV infection in anesthesiologists.

Percutaneous Injury: Risk of Occupational Infection

The greatest risk to HCW for infection with HBV, HCV or HIV is through percutaneous injury. The Centers for Disease Control (CDC) noted that 79% of HCW who seroconverted to HIV positive were exposed by hollow-bore needles (104). In a multicenter review of anesthesia personnel, 138 contaminated percutaneous injuries occurred and 74% of these were with contaminated hollow-bore needles (105). When the individual injuries were studied, 74% were judged to be preventable. Use of universal precautions and engineered safety devices, particularly use of non-needle systems and "safer" intravenous catheters, can greatly reduce our risks.

The risks of exposure to blood-borne pathogens have been carefully reviewed and estimates of possible disease transmission calculated (106) (Table 33.6). This risk will vary according to several factors (Table 33.7). This information should be used to consider post exposure prophylaxis (PEP) after a needlestick or other exposure to blood or body fluids.

Postexposure Prophylaxis (PEP)

If exposure to potentially infectious blood or body fluids occurs, immediate cleaning of the wound and risk assessment are vital. Use of multidrug prophylactic antiviral therapy for HIV exposure is now recommended (107). The effective management of PEP is supported by the current favorable results of antiviral therapy in the parturient to prevent vertical transmission (discussed earlier in this chapter) (46, 51). Current therapy recommendations for PEP would include at

Table 33.6. RISK ASSESSMENT AFTER OCCUPATIONAL EXPOSURE TO BLOOD-BORNE PATHOGENS

Virus	Risk of Transmission		Infectious Material	
	Percutaneous Injury [a]	*Mucosal/Broken Skin*	*Documented*	*Unlikely*
HBV	20–40% (30%)	Not quantified, > HCV and HIV	Blood, blood products	Urine, feces
HCV	3–10% (2–4%)	Not quantified, plausible if undocumented	Blood, blood products	Saliva, urine, feces
HIV	0.2–0.5% (0.3%)	Not quantified, documented	Blood, blood products, bodily fluids	Saliva, urine, feces

[a] Percentages are those often quoted for risk of transmission as compared to wide-ranging figures. This data not only compares the relative risk but points out that the risk to health care workers is percutaneous injury, i.e, needlestick.
From Gerberding JL. Management of occupational exposure to blood-borne viruses. *N Engl J Med* 1997;332:444–451, with permission.

Table 33.7. FACTORS INDEPENDENTLY ASSOCIATED WITH PERCUTANEOUS INJURY TRANSMISSION RISK

Risk Factor	Odds Ratio
Deep (intramuscular) Injury	16.1
Visible blood on sharp device	5.2
Device used to enter artery or vein	5.1
Source patient with terminal AIDS	6.4
ZDV prophylaxis used	0.2

$p < 0.05$ by logistic regression analysis in a case-control study. Data from CDC. Case control study of HIV seroconversion in health-care workers after percutaneous exposure to HIV-infected blood—from United Kingdom and United States, January 1988 to August 1994. *MMWR* 1995;44:929.

least zidovudine and lamivudine for four weeks and possibly the addition of a protease inhibitor such as nelfinavir or indinavir. Consultation with local experts and current CDC recommendations are suggested. The CDC home page at http://www.cdc.gov is regularly updated and a valuable resource. There is no recommended postexposure prophylaxis for HCV currently. HBV is transmitted at an extremely high rate (20% to 40%) with percutaneous injury and the HCW is advised to determine their antibody status to HBV after parenteral exposure with risk of infection. Antibody titers <10 mIU/mL in the previously vaccinated HCW require a vaccine booster and hepatitis B immune globulin (HBIG) to protect against HBV infection until antibody response develops. It is not known how long protection is incurred after the initial series of HBV vaccination but it appears extremely effective. There is now a lower incidence of HBV infection in the health care worker community than the population at large.

CONCLUSION

HIV disease is well established on a worldwide basis and until a vaccine is developed, it appears likely to be an increasing concern to women of childbearing age. It will be the rare obstetric suite that does not manage the HIV-seropositive patients, knowingly or unknowingly. These patients require access to increasingly effective antiretroviral therapy, careful evaluation for other infections, malignancies, or opportunistic diseases and anesthetic management as indicated by the obstetric requirements. While the patient must be evaluated for the numerous potential complications of the disease, there are no unique contraindications to regional or general anesthesia. Universal precautions must be observed in these and all patients. The increasing use of multiple antiretroviral therapies in the parturient will lead to better maternal outcome, increased lifespan and decreased vertical transmission.

REFERENCES

1. Fauci A. The AIDS epidemic: considerations for the 21st century. *N Engl J Med* 1999;341:1046–1050.
2. Riley LE, Greene MF. Elective cesarean delivery to reduce the transmission of HIV [Editorial]. *N Engl J Med* 1999;340:1032–1033.
3. Berg CJ, Atrash HK, Koonin LM, et al. Pregnancy-related mortality in the United States, 1987–1990. *Obstet Gynecol* 1996;88:161–167.
4. Centers for Disease Control and Prevention. *HIV/AIDS surveillance report*. Atlanta: CDC, 2000:1–43.
5. Rosenberg PS, Biggar RJ. Trends in HIV incidence among young adults in the United States. *JAMA* 1998;279:1894–1899.
6. Chirgwin KD, Feldman J, Dehovitz JA, et al. Incidence and risk factors for heterosexually acquired HIV in an inner-city cohort of women: temporal association with pregnancy. *J Acquir Immune Defic Syndr* 1999;20:295–299.
7. WHO. *AIDS Epidemic Update: December, 1998.* Geneva: Joint United Nation Programme on HIV/AIDS (UNAIDS), World Health Organization, 1998.
8. Palella Jr FJ, Delaney KM, Moorman AC, et al. Declining morbidity and mortality among patients with advanced human immunodeficiency virus infection. *N Engl J Med* 1998;338:853–886.
9. Hughes S. AIDS: the focus turns to women [Editorial]. *Int J Obstet Anesth* 1993;2:1–2.
10. Grosskurth H, Mosha F, Todd J, et al. Impact of improved treatment of sexually transmitted diseases on HIV infection in rural Tanzania. Randomized, controlled trial. *Lancet* 1995;346:530–536.
11. Piatak M Jr, Saag LC, Yang SJ, et al. High levels of HIV-1 in plasma during all stages of infection determined by competitive PCR. *Science* 1993;259:1749–1754.
12. Karon JM, Rosenberg PS, McQuillan G, et al. Prevalence of HIV infection in the United States, 1984–1992. *JAMA* 1996;276:126–131.
13. Cock KM, Fowler MG, Mercier E, et al. Prevention of mother-to-child HIV transmission in resource-poor countries translating research into policy and practice. *JAMA* 2000;283:1175–1182.
14. Rosenberg PS. Scope of the AIDS epidemic in the United States. *Science* 1995;270:1372–1375.
15. Rotello G. Sexual ecology. In: *AIDS and the destiny of gay men.* New York, Penguin Group, 1997.
16. Gottlieb M. *Pneumocystis carinii* pneumonia and mucosal candidiasis in previously healthy homosexual men: evidence of a new acquired cellular immunodeficiency. *N Engl J Med* 1981;305:1425–1430.
17. Dye C, Schule S, Colin P, et al. Global burden of tuberculosis—estimated incidence, prevalence, and mortality by country. *JAMA* 1999;282:677–686.
18. Royce RA, Sè na A, Cates W Jr., et al. Sexual transmission of HIV. *N Engl J Med* 1997;336:1072–1078.
19. Kahn J, Walker B. Acute human immunodeficiency virus type 1 infection. *N Engl J Med* 1998;339:33–39.
20. Schaker T, Collier AC, Hughes J, et al. Clinical and epidemiologic features of primary HIV infection. *Ann Intern Med* 1996;125:257–264.
21. Johnstone FD. HIV and pregnancy. *Br J Obstet Gynaecol* 1996;103:1184–1190.
22. Sande MA, Volberding PA, eds. *The Medical Management of AIDS*, 5th ed. Philadelphia: WB Saunders, 1997.
23. Dennings DW, Anderson J, Rudge P, et al. Acute myelopathy associated with primary infections with human immunodeficiency virus. *Br Med J* 1987;294: 143–144.
24. Cari A, Cooper D. Primary HIV infection. In: Sande MA, Voldberding PA, eds. *The Medical Management of AIDS*, 5th ed. Philadelphia: WB Saunders, 1997:91.
25. Price RW. Management of the neurologic complications of HIV-1 infection and AIDS. In: Sande MA, Volberding PA, eds. *The Medical Management of AIDS*, 5th ed. Philadelphia: WB Saunders, 1997:197–199.
26. Selik RM, Chu SY, Ward JW. Trends in infectious diseases and cancers among persons dying of HIV infection in the United States from 1987 to 1992. *Ann Intern Med* 1995;123:933–936.
27. Margono F, Mroueh J, Garely A, et al. Resurgence of active tuberculosis among pregnant women. *Obstet Gynecol* 1994;83:911–914.
28. Starke JR. Tuberculosis: An old disease but a new threat to the mother, fetus and neonate. Clin Perinatol 1997;24:107-127.
29. Ho D, Sarngadharan M, Resnick L, et al. Primary human T-lymphotropic virus type III infection. *Ann Intern Med* 1985;103:880–883.
30. Kaslow, RA, Phair JP, Friedman HB, et al. Infection with the human immunodeficiency virus: clinical manifestations and their relationship to immune deficiency. A report of the Multicenter AIDS Cohort Study. *Ann Intern Med* 1987;107: 474–480.
31. Hambleton J. Complications of HIV infection. In: Sande M, Volberding P, eds. *The Medical Management of AIDS*, 5th ed. Philadelphia: WB Saunders, 1997: 242–244.
32. Coyne BA, Landers DV. The immunology of HIV disease and pregnancy and possible interactions. *Obstet Gynecol Clin North Am* 1990;17:595–606.
33. Clark SJ, Saag MS, Decker WD, et al. High titers of cytopathic virus in plasma of patients with symptomatic primary HIV-1 infection. *N Engl J Med* 1991;324: 954–960.

34. Dinsmoor MJ, Christmas JT. Changes in T-lymphocyte subpopulations during pregnancy complicated by human immunodeficiency virus infection. *Am J Obstet Gynecol* 1992;167:1575–1579.

35. Selik RM, Chu Sy, Buehler JW. HIV infection as a leading cause of death among young adults in U.S. cities and states. *JAMA* 1993;269:2991–2994.

36. Biggar RJ, Pahwa S, Minkoff H, et al. Immunosuppression in pregnant women infected with human immunodeficiency virus. *Am J Obstet Gynecol* 1989;161: 1239–1244.

37. Scott GB, Fischl MA, Klimas N, et al. Mothers of infants with acquired immunodeficiency syndrome: evidence of both symptomatic and asymptomatic carriers. *JAMA* 1985;253:363–366.

38. Minkoff H, de Regt RH, Landesman S, et al. *Pneumocystis carinii* pneumonia associated with acquired immunodeficiency syndrome in pregnancy: a report of three maternal deaths. *Obstet Gynecol* 1986;67:284–287.

39. Koonin LM, Ellerbrock TV, Atrash HK, et al. Pregnancy-associated deaths due to AIDS in the United States. *JAMA* 1989;261:1306–1309.

40. Nightingale SD, Jockusch JD, Haslund I, et al. Logarithmic relationship of CD4 count to survival in patients with human immunodeficiency virus infection. *Arch Intern Med* 1993;153:1313–1318.

41. Coulam CB, Silverfield JC, Kazmar RE, et al. T-lymphocyte subsets during pregnancy and the menstrual cycle. *Am J Reprod Immunol* 1983;4:88–90.

42. Glassman AB, Bennett CE, Christopher JB, et al. Immunity during pregnancy: lymphocyte subpopulations and mitogen responsiveness. *Ann Clin Lab Sci* 1985;15:357–362.

43. Tuomala RE, Kalish LA, Zorilla C, et al. Changes in total CD_4+ and CD_8+ T-lymphocytes during pregnancy and 1 year postpartum in human immunodeficiency virus-infected women. *Obstet Gynecol* 1997;89:967–974.

44. Burns D, Landesman S, Minkoff H, et al. The influence of pregnancy on human immunodeficiency virus type 1 infection: antepartum and postpartum changes in human immunodeficiency virus type 1 viral load. *Am J Obstet Gynecol* 1998;178:355–359.

45. Lindegren ML, Byers RJ Jr, Thomas P, et al. Trends in perinatal transmission of HIV/AIDS in the United States. *JAMA* 1999;282:531–538

46. World Health Organization (WHO). Global AIDS surveillance—part 1. *Wkly Epidemiol Rec* 1997;72:357–360.

47. Connor EM, Sperling RS, Gelber R, et al. Reduction of maternal-infant transmission of human immunodeficiency virus type 1 with zidovudine treatment. *N Engl J Med* 1994;331:1175–1180.

48. Kuhn L, Stekett R, Weedom J, et al. Distinct risk factors for intrauterine and intrapartum immunodeficiency virus transmission and consequences for disease progression in infected children. *J Infect Dis* 1999;179:52–58.

49. Mofenson LM. Mother-child HIV-1 transmission: timing and determinants. *Obstet Gynecol Clin North Am* 1997;24:759–781.

49a. Nduati R, John G, Mbori-Ngacha D, et al. Effect of breast-feeding and formula feeding on transmission of HIV-1. *JAMA* 2000;283:1167–1174.

50. Mofenson LM, Lamhert J, Stiehm ER, et al. Risk factors for perinatal transmission of HIV type 1 in women treated with zidovudine. *N Engl J Med* 1999;341:385–393.

51. Garcia PM, Kalish LA, Pitt J, et al. Maternal levels of plasma human immunodeficiency virus type 1 RNA and the risk of perinatal transmission. *N Engl J Med* 1999;341:394–402.

52. Centers for Disease Control and Prevention. Public Health Service Task Force recommendations for the use of antiretroviral drugs in pregnant women infected with HIV-1 for maternal health, and for reducing perinatal HIV-1 transmission in the United States. *MMWR* 1998;47(RR-2):1–30.

53. McGowan JP, Crane M, Wiznia AA, et al. Combination antiretroviral therapy in human immunodeficiency virus-infected pregnant women. *Obstet Gynecol* 1999;94:641–646.

54. Centers of Disease Control and Prevention. Update: perinatally acquired HIV/AIDS—United States, 1997. *MMWR* 1997;46:1086–1092.

55. Guay LA, Musoke P, Fleming T, et al. Intrapartum and neonatal single-dose nevirapine compared with zidovudine for prevention of mother-to-child transmission of HIV- 1 in Kampala, Uganda: HIVNET 012 randomised trial. *Lancet* 1999;354:795–802.

56. Marseille E, Kahn JG, Mmiro F, et al. Cost effectiveness of single-dose nevirapine regimen for mothers and babies to decrease vertical HIV -1 transmission in sub-Saharan Africa. *Lancet* 1999;354:803–809.

57. European Collaborative Study. Caesarean section and risk of vertical transmission of HIV-1 infection. *Lancet* 1994;343:1464–1467.

58. Maguire A, Sanchez E, Fortuny C, et al. Potential risk factors for vertical HIV-1 transmission in Catalonia, Spain: the protective role of cesarean section. *AIDS* 1997;11:1851–1857.

59. Kind C, Rudin C, Siegrist C-A, et al. Prevention of vertical HIV transmission: additive protective effect of elective cesarean section and zidovudine prophylaxia. *AIDS* 1998;12:205–210.

60. Mandelbrot L, Le Chenadec J, Berrebi A, et al. Perinatal HIV-1 transmission: interaction between zidovudine prophylaxia and mode of delivery in the French Perinatal Cohort. *JAMA* 1998;280:55–60.

61. European Mode of Delivery Collaboration. Elective caesarean section versus vaginal delivery in prevention of vertical HIV-1 transmission: a randomized clinical trial. *Lancet* 1999;353:1035–1039.

62. International Perinatal HIV Group. The mode of delivery and the risk of vertical transmission of human immunodeficiency virus type 1: a meta-analysis of 15 prospective cohort studies. *N Engl J Med* 1999;340:977–987.

63. Kuhn L, Abobat R, Coutsoudis A, et al. Cesarean deliveries and maternal-infant HIV transmission: results from a prospective study in South Africa. *J Acquir Immune Defic Syndr* 1996;11:478–483.

64. Semprini AE, Castagna C, Ravizza M, et al. The incidence of complications after caesarean section in 156 HIV -positive women. *AIDS* 1995;9:913–917.

65. ACOG Committee Opinion. Scheduled cesarean delivery and the prevention of vertical transmission of HIV infection. *Int J Gynaceol Obstet* 1999;66:305–306.

66. Centers for Disease Control and Prevention. Report of the NIH Panel to define principles of therapy of HIV infection and guidelines for the use of antiretroviral agents in HIV-infected adults and adolescents. *MMWR* 1998;47 (RR-5):1–82.

67. Shapiro DE, Sperling RS, Mandelbrot L, et al. Risk factors for perinatal human immunodeficiency virus transmission in patients receiving zidovudine prophylaxis. *Obstet Gynecol* 1999;94:897–908.

68. Grimes RM, Richards EP, Helfgott AW, et al. Legal considerations in screening pregnant women for human immunodeficiency virus. *Am J Obstet Gynecol* 1999;180:259–264.

69. Minkoff H, O'Sullivan MJ. The case for rapid HIV testing during labor. *JAMA* 1998;279:1743–1744.

70. Carpenter CCJ, Fischl MA, Hammer SM, et al. Antiretroviral therapy for HIV infection in 1997: updated recommendations of the International AIDS Society—USA panel. *JAMA* 1997;277:1962–1969.

71. Flexner C. HIV-protease inhibitors [Review]. *N Engl J Med* 1998;338:1281–1292.

72. Olkkola KT, Palkama VJ, Neuvonen PJ. Ritonavir's role in reducing fentanyl clearance and prolonging its half-life. *Anesthesiology* 1999;91:681–685.

73. Mandelbrot L, Landreau-Mascaro A, Rekacewica C, et al. Lamivudine-Zidovudine combination for prevention of maternal-infant transmission of HIV-1. *JAMA* 2001;285:2083–2093.

74. Hughes SC. Human immunodeficiency virus and obstetric anesthesia. *Anesthesiol Clin North Am* 1998;16:397–418.

75. Wade NA, Birkhead GS, Warren BL, et al. Abbreviated regimens of zidovudine prophylaxis and perinatal transmission of the human immunodeficiency virus. *N Engl J Med* 1998;339:1409–1414.

76. Hanson IC, Antonelli TA, Sperling RS, et al. Lack of tumors in infants with perinatal HIV-1 exposure and fetal/neonatal exposure to zidovudine. *J Acquir Immune Defic Syndr* 1999;20:463–467.

77. Culnane M, Fowler MG, Lee SS, et al. Lack of long-term effects of in utero exposure to zidovudine among uninfected children born to HIV-infected women. *JAMA* 1999;281:151–157.

78. Bloom E, Abrahms DI, Rodgers G. Lupus anticoagulant in the acquired immunodeficiency syndrome. *JAMA* 1986;256:491–493.

79. Levy RM, Bredesen DE, Rosenblum ML. Neurological manifestations of the acquired immunodeficiency syndrome (AIDS): experience at UCSF and review of the literature. *J Neurosurg* 1985;62:475–495.

80. Gershon RY, Manning-Williams D. Anesthesia and the HIV-infected parturient: a retrospective study. *Int J Obstet Anesth* 1997;6:76–81.

81. Greene ER. Spinal and epidural anesthesia in patients with the acquired immunodeficiency syndrome. *Anesth Analg* 1986;65:1090–1091.

82. Spector SA, Hsia K, Pratt D, et al. Virologic markers of human immunodeficiency virus type 1 in cerebrospinal fluid. *J Infect Dis* 1993;168:68–74.

83. Hughes SC, Dailey PA, Landers D, et al. Parturients infected with human immunodeficiency virus and regional anesthesia: clinical and immunologic response. *Anesthesiology* 1995;82:32–37.

84. Birnback DJ, Bourlier RA, Choi R, et al. Anaesthetic management of caesarean section in a patient with active recurrent genital herpes and AIDS-related dementia. *Br J Anaesth* 1995;75:639–641.

85. Frame WA, Lichtmann MW. Blood patch in the HIV-positive patient [Letter]. *Anesthesiology* 1990;73:1297.

86. Tom DJ, Gulevich SJ, Shapiro HM, et al. Epidural blood patch in the HIV-1 positive patient. *Anesthesiology* 1992;76:943–947.

87. Bevacqua BK, Sluck AV. Epidural blood patch in a patient with HIV infection. *Anesthesiology* 1991;74:952–953.

88. Gibbons JJ. Postdural puncture headache in the HIV-positive patient [Letter]. *Anesthesiology* 1991;74:953.

89. Newman P, Carrington D, Clarke J. Epidural blood patch is contraindicated in HIV-positive patients. *Int J Obstet Anesth* 1999;7:167–169.

90. Stalard B. Another complication of combined extradural- subarachnoid technique [Letter]. *Br J Anaesth* 1994;73:426.

91. Harding SA, Collis RE, Morgan BM. Meningitis after combined spinal-extradural anesthesia in obstetrics. *Br J Anaesth* 1994;73:545–547.

92. Russell R, Plaat F. The dura is too vulnerable to be breached routinely in labour. *Int J Anesth* 1999;8:56–61.

93. Clark W. Prevention of anesthesia-induced immunosuppression: a novel strategy involving interferons [Editorial]. *Anesthesiology* 1993;78:627–628.

94. Dailey PA. Human immunodeficiency virus in the delivery suite. In: Shnider SM, Levinson G, eds. *Anesthesia for Obstetrics,* 3rd ed. Baltimore: Williams & Wilkins, 1993:617–632.

95. Scannell KA. Surgery and human immunodeficiency virus disease. *J Acquir Immune Defic Syndr* 1984;2:43–53.

96. Markovic SN, Knight PR, Murasko DM. Inhibition of interferon stimulation of natural killer cell activity in mice anesthetized with halothane or isoflurane. *Anesthesiology* 1993;78:700–706.

97. Thomson DA. Anesthesia and the immune system. *J Burn Care Rehabil* 1987;8:483–487.

98. Hughes SC. *HIV and other occupational exposures: risk management (review course).* Dallas: American Society of Anesthesiology, 1999.

99. Department of Labor, Occupational Safety and Health Administration. Occupational exposure to bloodborne pathogens. Final rule (29 CFR part 1910.1030). *Federal Register* 1991;56:64004–64182.

100. Centers for Disease Control. Recommendations for follow-up of health-care-workers after occupational exposure to hepatitis C virus. *MMWR* 1997;46:603–606.

101. Ippolito G, Puro V, Heptonstall J, et al. Occupational human immunodeficiency virus infection in health care workers: worldwide cases through September 1997. *Clin Infect Dis* 1999;28:365–383.

102. Panlilio AL, Welch BA, Bell DM, et al. Blood and amniotic fluid contact sustained by obstetric personnel during deliveries. *Am J Obstet Gynecol* 1992;167:703–708.

103. Kristensen M, Sloth E, Jensen TK. Relationship between anesthetic procedure and contact of anesthesia personnel with patient body fluids. *Anesthesiology* 1990;73:619–624.

104. Centers for Disease Control and Prevention. Public health service guidelines for management of health-care worker exposure to HIV and recommendations for post exposure prophylaxis. *MMWR* 1998;47:1–33.

105. Greene E, Berry A, Jagger J, et al. Multicenter study of contaminated percutaneous injuries in anesthesia personnel. *Anesthesiology* 1998;89:1362–1372.

106. Gerberding JL. Management of occupational exposure to bloodborne viruses. *N Engl J Med* 1995;332:444–451.

107. Gerberding JL Prophylaxis for occupational exposure to HIV. *Ann Intern Med* 1996;125:497-501.

108. Hader SL, Smith DK, Moore JS, et al. HIV infection in women in the United States: status at the millennium. *JAMA* 2001;1184–1192.

SIX

FETUS AND NEWBORN

Shnider and Levinson's Anesthesia for Obstetrics,
edited by Samuel C. Hughes, et al.
Lippincott Williams & Wilkins,
Philadelphia, © 2001.

CHAPTER 34

ANESTHESIA AND THE DRUG-ADDICTED MOTHER

SAMUEL C. HUGHES, M.D. AND CHARLIZE KESSIN, M.D.

Anesthesiologists are confronted with the problems of maternal drug addiction when drug-addicted or drug-intoxicated patients request analgesia for labor or require anesthesia for elective or emergency cesarean section, and when a drug-affected neonate requires resuscitation or suffers from withdrawal symptoms. Illicit drugs can have acute effects on the mother and fetus, which lead to emergency intervention. Thus, it is important for the anesthesiologist to be familiar with the consequences of the drugs most commonly abused by pregnant women. This chapter reviews the effects of the most common illicit drugs among pregnant women and the repercussions on the fetus and/or neonate. In addition, the effects of other non-illicit substances, including alcohol, tobacco, and caffeine, will be discussed. Finally, some guidelines for the management of anesthesia in drug-addicted mothers are provided.

CURRENT TRENDS

Illicit drug use during pregnancy is unfortunately far from a rare event. In the United States, the National Institute on Drug Abuse (NIDA) estimated in 1990 that 5.5% of pregnant women, or nearly 250,000 women, had used illicit drugs during pregnancy (1). In an earlier report by the NIDA, it was estimated that, of 56 million women in the United States of childbearing age, 15%, or 8 million women, were substance abusers (2). In addition, a much larger number of women, 18.8%, or 757,000, used alcohol during their pregnancy, and there were even more who smoked cigarettes (1) (Table 34.1). Comby and Shiono had even higher estimates of maternal exposure rates to illicit drugs during pregnancy: cocaine 4% to 5%; marijuana 17%; cigarettes 38%; and alcohol 73% (3). Newborn exposure to drugs in utero continues to be a national concern, with an unknown hundreds of thousands affected each year. It is estimated that 5% of women of childbearing age can be considered "heavy" drinkers. Many women take multiple drugs such as the combination of cocaine, alcohol, and marijuana (2). In a study of cocaine-abusing parturients undergoing cesarean section by Kain et al. (4), it was noted that 44% to 55% also used alcohol and cigarettes. Of those who were positive for cocaine by urine analysis at the prenatal visit and on admission to labor and delivery, many had a history of opioid (27%), marijuana (15%), sedative (33%), or stimulant (18%) use during pregnancy.

The simultaneous abuse of several substances makes it difficult to determine the effects of a particular drug. In addition, malnutrition, inadequate medical care, and infectious diseases can also be responsible for some of the adverse effects observed in drug addicts. Delayed diagnosis of pregnancy among drug-addicted women results in continued drug exposure in the fetus during the most vulnerable stage (5). Most drugs that are abused readily cross the placenta and are often not only directly fetotoxic but have indirect effects on the fetus. They disrupt normal maternal nutrition and may have maternal cardiovascular effects that interfere with normal placental blood supply.

Both cocaine use and cigarette smoking have been associated with placenta previa. Catecholamine-mediated vasospasm leads

to decreased placental perfusion and a secondary hypertrophy of the placenta. This results in implantation over a larger area, including the lower uterine segment and cervical os, which may be the mechanism in common. While the exact mechanism is unclear, the fourfold risk of placenta previa with cocaine use is significant for the practice of obstetric anesthesia (6, 7).

The effects of illicit drugs on the newborn are varied and in some cases controversial, but may include acute drug effects in the delivery room, drug withdrawal later in the nursery, or long-term consequences from congenital anatomic malformations or behavioral teratology. A comprehensive, geographically based study (California) on substance abuse by pregnant women collected urine from 30,000 women at delivery in 1992 and screened for illicit substances (tobacco use was self-reported) (8). If this study is extrapolated to the United States at large, an estimated 440,000 infants per year, or approximately 11% of 4 million births, are exposed to alcohol or drugs in the days before delivery. Illicit drug use during pregnancy is also part of the duel epidemic—human immunodeficiency virus (HIV) and drug abuse. In the Women and Infant Transmission Study (WITS), which followed 530 HIV-infected women and their infants, 42% of the women used "hard drugs," e.g., cocaine, heroin/opioids, methadone, or used other injection drugs (9). Of these patients, 44% used multiple drugs. Both illicit drug abuse and HIV infection (see Chapter 33) in pregnant women will continue to be significant concerns, particularly in large urban centers. However, alcohol and cigarette abuse are far more common and, thus, may do the most harm (1).

ALCOHOL

It is estimated that there are 15.1 million alcohol-abusing individuals in the United States, and approximately 4.6 million are women (10). At least 1 million of these women are of childbearing age, and alcohol abuse often involves other drug abuse (tobacco or possibly illegal drugs). A recent survey documented that alcohol use by pregnant women is increasing after a decline in the early 1990s (9). In 1995, it was found that 15.3% of women consumed alcohol during their pregnancy and 3.5% were frequent users (11).

The chief abnormality associated with the abuse of alcohol during pregnancy is the "fetal alcohol syndrome" (FAS) (12). This syndrome includes a characteristic facies, prenatal and postnatal growth deficiency, microcephaly, and mental retardation (Fig. 34.1). FAS occurs in about one-third of the infants born to mothers who drink three or more ounces of absolute alcohol per day during pregnancy. However, a safe level of maternal alcohol consumption during pregnancy has never been defined (13). Children with FAS are almost always born to those women who consume "large" amounts of alcohol during pregnancy, but studies have reported neurobehavioral deficits, intrauterine growth restriction, and head and facial abnormalities in infants of "moderate" alcohol consumers (12–18). Most likely, heavy alcohol consumption throughout pregnancy produces the wide variety of effects characteristic of FAS, whereas episodic drinking

Table 34.1. DRUG USE DURING PREGNANCY IN WOMEN DELIVERING IN THE UNITED STATES

Illict drug use	**5.5%**	
Marijuana	2.9%	(119,000)
Cocaine	1.1%	(45,000)
Heroin	0.1%	(3,600)
Psychotherapeutic drugs (without prescription)	1.5%	(61,000)
Other drug use	**39.2%**	
Cigarettes	20.4%	(820,000)
Alcohol(during pregnancy)	18.8%	(757,000)

Data from National Institute on Drug Abuse (NIDA), National Pregnancy and Health Survey: drug use among women deliverying live births, 1992. Marwick C. Challenging report on pregnancy and drug abuse. *JAMA* 1998;280:1039–1040.

or drinking lesser amounts produces the incomplete pattern of anomalies according to the period of exposure.

FAS has recently been labeled the "fetal alcohol abuse syndrome" (FAAS) by one clinician (19, 20). This designation implies that very low levels of alcohol consumption do not lead to the syndrome and may result in inappropriate diagnosis in children. Studies in animals support the conclusion that alcohol-related birth effects occur only at blood-alcohol levels above 0.1% (100 mg · dL^{-1}), which is legal intoxication, a level consistent with heavy drinking (20).

When there is a history of alcohol abuse and not all the characteristics of FAS are present, the term "fetal alcohol effects" (fae) has been used. this has also been labeled "alcohol abuse–related birth defects" (20). The use of the term FAE has been questioned, but it still is used by some clinicians (21). Mental retardation in later life has been one of the most common problems of alcohol exposure in utero and can be present in one-third of the infants without the more obvious signs of FAS. Ethanol appears to be responsible for FAS and FAE (17).

Multiple mechanisms have been proposed for the fetal effects of maternal alcohol ingestion. First, ethanol can disrupt normal maternal nutrition by impairing intestinal absorption of nutrients and by disturbing liver function. Second, ethanol crosses the placenta, and the primary metabolite of ethanol, acetaldehyde, is believed to have direct toxicity on the fetus. Third, ethanol (and/or acetaldehyde) may also be toxic to the pla-

centa. Ethanol is teratogenic in a variety of animals, and the same anomalies are found in humans (18). Acute alcohol intoxication can also have distressing effects on the fetus, causing tachycardia, decreased heart rate variability, and late and variable decelerations (22). Studies in the rhesus monkey have shown that maternal ethanol levels of 200 to 300 mg · dL^{-1} reduce umbilical blood flow and fetal oxygenation (Fig. 34.2) (23). However, this would represent an extremely high blood alcohol level in humans. The effects of low levels of alcohol on the fetus are controversial (22, 23). Chronic alcoholic women may have a greater risk for abruptio placentae, spontaneous abortions, and stillbirth (24).

Anesthetic Considerations

Many problems face the anesthesiologist when taking care of an alcoholic because nearly all systems in the body are affected (25). The main problems include hemodynamic instability and increased resistance to neuroleptics and analgesics (26). Cardiovascular disease is the leading cause of death in alcoholics, and cardiomyopathy should be considered in all cases of heavy alcohol abuse (27). The induction of general anesthesia should be by a "rapid-sequence" technique, which is routine for pregnant woman.

However, there is cross-tolerance of alcohol with barbiturates, minor tranquilizers, and the usual anesthetic doses of inhalation agents; therefore, induction doses of thiopental should be increased to a maximum of 6 mg · kg^{-1}. Most alcoholics require a larger induction dose of thiopental due to tolerance and to an expanded plasma volume. However, routinely doubling the induction dose for alcoholics may be dangerous for those with hypoalbuminemia and cardiomyopathy (28). Similar findings of increased tolerance in the *chronic* alcoholic and the additive effect during *acute* intoxication have been described for propofol (29). Particular attention should be directed at the state of hydration and prevention of hypoglycemia.

During *acute* intoxication, ethanol and barbiturates produce a supra-additive effect. Even in *chronic* alcoholics, acute intoxication causes an increase in the half-life of barbiturates, and under this circumstance induction doses should also be decreased.

Other factors can complicate rapid sequence induction of anesthesia. Cerebral tolerance to hypoxia is decreased significantly in the presence of only mild intoxication. Pregnant women pose a greater risk for acid aspiration syndrome than nonpregnant patients (see Chapter 22). When acutely intoxicated

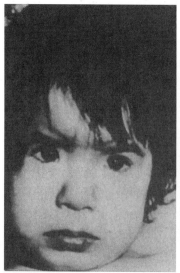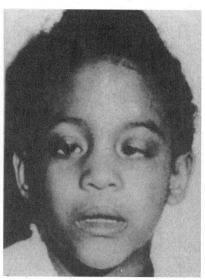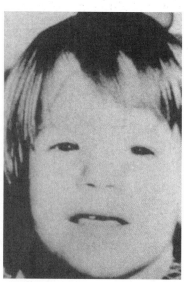

A,B   C

Figure 34.1. Fetal alcohol effects. Affected children of chronic alcoholic women at 1 year, 3 years and 9 months, and 2 1/2 years. Note the short palpebral fissures for all children and strabismus and ptosis of the eyelid. (From James KL. *Smith's Recognizable Patterns of Human Malformation,* 4th ed. Philadelphia: WB Saunders, 1988:492, with permission.)

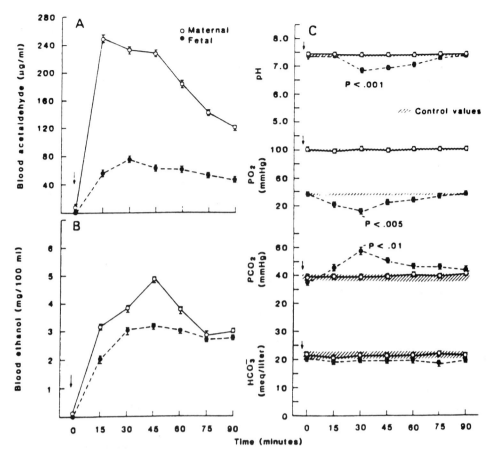

Figure 34.2. Ethanol (**A**) and acetaldehyde (**B**) in maternal ($\circ$) and fetal ($\sum$) blood ($n = 5$). **C:** Maternal and fetal blood gas values ($n = 5$) and of the control group ($n = 4$). Results are means $\pm$ SD. The shaded areas represent normal control values. (From Mukherjee AB, Hodgen GD. Maternal ethanol exposure induces transient impairment of umbilical circulation and fetal hypoxia in monkeys. *Science* 1982;218:700–702, with permission.)

with alcohol, this risk is increased because alcohol is a potent stimulus to gastric acid secretion. In addition, there is a significant delay in gastric emptying caused by alcohol. Maintenance of anesthesia is rarely a problem; however, anesthetic requirements are usually increased unless acute intoxication is present. However, the postoperative period may be complicated by alcohol withdrawal.

When the patient is not intoxicated, as for elective procedures, a withdrawal syndrome may occur. A minor withdrawal syndrome occurs in the majority of alcoholics within 6 to 8 hours of abstinence, and this is often the moment that elective interventions are started (30). This stage of the withdrawal syndrome is characterized by tremor, sweating, anorexia, vomiting, muscle weakness, and cramps. Autonomic imbalance also produces tachycardia, systolic hypertension, and dysrhythmias. Propranolol may control some of these symptoms, but pure beta-blocking agents may adversely affect the neonate's ability to adapt to the stress of delivery. Sedation is usually unnecessary, but small IV doses of diazepam (2.5 to 5 mg) or midazolam (1 to 3 mg) can reduce autonomic hyperactivity without resulting in neonatal depression.

Pulmonary and liver disease are frequent among alcoholics. As many as 66% may have abnormal chest x-ray findings (31). Succinylcholine activity may be prolonged by liver disease due to diminished cholinesterase activity. The action of nondepolarizing neuromuscular blocking agents may be prolonged because of abnormal potassium or magnesium levels or, in fact, may be shortened in liver disease or malnutrition due to altered protein binding. Use of a neuromuscular twitch monitor is recommended. Esophageal varices may make the insertion of nasogastric tubes, esophageal stethoscopes, and temperature probes hazardous, and extreme care must be exercised.

Regional anesthesia is successful in alcoholics, but additional sedation may be required in the agitated alcoholic. Liver disease may produce coagulation defects, which may exclude the use of epidural and intrathecal techniques. Alcoholic neuropathy is not aggravated by or a medical contraindication to regional anesthesia, but it is prudent to document any signs or symptoms of peripheral neuropathy. Severe hypotension may result from dehydration, cardiomyopathy, or autonomic neuropathy preoperatively. However, many of these problems are not manifested in the younger alcoholic patient most likely to present for delivery.

TOBACCO

There is no doubt concerning the adverse effects of tobacco on health to include that of the pregnant patient. Cigarettes are the most commonly used drug during pregnancy. Nearly 2,000 compounds have been identified in cigarette smoke. In addition to nicotine, other toxic components include carbon monoxide and cyanide, which have been implicated in observed fetal effects (31). Nicotine causes an increase in maternal heart rate (MHR), systolic and diastolic blood pressure, and peripheral vasoconstriction (32). Infants born to mothers who smoke during pregnancy tend to be lighter in weight than infants born to nonsmokers. This and other fetal concerns may be related to vitamin B_{12} depletion caused by cyanide. Fetal problems also can be explained by the vasoconstrictive effects of nicotine and the reduction of uteroplacental blood flow (33). Fetal hypoxia by decreased uterine blood flow (UBF) or carbon monoxide is also felt to be causative. There are strong associations between cigarette smoking and low birth weight (34), abruptio placentae (35), and impaired respiratory function in newborns (36).

A recent study of 400 adolescents and women, age 14 to 40 years, suggests that cigarette smoking and cocaine use are independently associated with an increased risk of spontaneous abortions (37). The Centers for Disease Control and Prevention (CDC) reported in 1999 that 11% to 23% of pregnant women continued to smoke in the last 3 months of pregnancy (38). A large meta-analysis supports a casual role for smoking in preterm delivery (39).

The incidence of prematurity may double from 6% to 12% when the mother smokes at least 20 cigarettes per day. At birth, these infants often have a higher hematocrit because carbon monoxide is fixed to the hemoglobin of the fetus and the relative hypoxemia causes an increase in the erythropoiesis. A syndrome with hyperexcitability, crying, and feeding difficulties has been observed, without need of treatment with sedatives. Sleep disturbances and learning difficulties have also been reported. Some studies suggest that the deleterious effects of nicotine on brain development extend for a period sufficient to cause long-lasting alterations that are eventually expressed as neurobehavioral teratogenic effects (40). Cigarette smoking causes a reduction in fetal breathing movements. Sudden infant death syndrome (SIDS) occurs twice as frequently in infants of mothers who smoke than of those who do not. Neonatal tolerance to hypoxia after prenatal nicotine exposure may also play a role in SIDS (41). The known effects of nicotine on fetal breathing may extend into the neonatal period. Perinatal mortality is also higher among infants born to smokers. A Swedish study noted a 50% increased risk of cancer among infants of mothers who smoked at least 10 cigarettes per day (42). Since many parturients who abuse drugs are multidrug users, the effects of cigarette smoking may be compounded by other substances.

Anesthetic Considerations

The longer a patient stops smoking before anesthesia, the greater the benefits. A period of 48 hours should be sufficient for carboxyhemoglobin of all smokers to fall to a nonsmoker's level and to produce a rise in oxygen content and availability. This has been demonstrated in pregnant women, in whom smoking abstinence for 48 hours produced an 8% increase in available oxygen (43). To facilitate a decrease in maternal smoking, it has been suggested that nicotine replacement therapy during pregnancy may be beneficial (44, 45). Intraoperative and postoperative respiratory morbidity in smokers is increased by mucus hypersecretion, impairment of tracheobronchial clearance, and small airway narrowing. Acute bronchoconstriction is often treated with halogenated hydrocarbons or with beta-mimetics such as terbutaline or other bronchodilators. Fewer cardiovascular problems are to be expected after 12 to 24 hours of abstinence from carbon monoxide and nicotine elimination. Several days are required to improve ciliary function and 1 to 2 weeks to reduce the sputum volume. However, 4 to 6 weeks of abstinence are necessary to greatly decrease postoperative respiratory morbidity (46). Smoking has also been suggested to be responsible for increased gastric fluid volume, placing smokers at a higher risk for pulmonary aspiration (47). In an otherwise healthy parturient, the anesthetic concerns for those who abuse tobacco are limited to pulmonary function; many potential problems may be avoided with regional anesthesia.

CAFFEINE

Caffeine is the most widely consumed behaviorally active substance in the world. The per capita consumption of coffee in the United States is nearly 3.5 kg per year (48, 49). Caffeine is also contained in tea, colas, and chocolate (50). This translates to 150 mg of caffeine, which is the equivalent of one to two cups per day and 80% of pregnant women ingest caffeine daily. Caffeine acts on the dopaminergic system in a similar manner as amphetamines and cocaine (51). Caffeine readily crosses the placenta and can have a half-life of 100 hours in the infant because of their inability to metabolize caffeine (52). Caffeine is a known teratogen in animals (53) and causes a wide variety of other potential concerns (54–56). Caffeine has been loosely linked to birth defects in humans while other researchers did not find any adverse maternal or newborn effects (50, 57, 58). Still further studies demonstrated an association between caffeine with spontaneous abortion, stillbirth, preterm delivery and low-birth weight (59, 60). A recent meta-analysis demonstrated a small increase in the risk of spontaneous abortion and low-birth weight (61). This is supported by an excellent study that linked extremely high serum paraxanthine plasma levels, the chief metabolite of caffeine, to women who had spontaneous abortions (62). The serum plasma levels achieved equate to a 60 kg women who has 6 cups (nonsmokers) to 11 cups (smokers) of coffee per day.

This evidence supports the advice from the Food and Drug Administration (FDA) for pregnant women to "avoid caffeine-containing food and drugs if possible or consume them only sparingly" (63). Consumption of numerous cups of coffee or tea each day has risk. Three cases of fetal arrhythmia resulting from excessive intake of caffeine by mothers during pregnancy have been reported (64). In two cases, the arrhythmia resolved gradually over three days after birth without medical intervention. They were not associated with maternal arrhythmia or hemodynamic instability.

Anesthetic Considerations

A significant problem encountered in a patient with substantial coffee use is caffeine withdrawal in the postoperative period. The most consistent feature of caffeine withdrawal is headache (65, 66), fatigue, and anxiety. Headache is an important potential side-effect of general and spinal anesthesia or may occur after an inadvertent dural puncture during epidural anesthesia. Before performing a blood patch to relieve symptoms of a postdural puncture headache (PDPH), caffeine withdrawal should be considered. However, the postural nature of a PDPH is unique. The administration of oral caffeine (300 mg) or intravenous caffeine (500 mg) have been administered to treat PDPH and may be beneficial with postoperative caffeine withdrawal (see Chapter 23, page 414). However, seizures have been reported in an obstetric patient who had received oral caffeine (1,000 mg during a 23-hour period) for a PDPH (67). Limiting oral intake to 600 mg/24 hr for medical management of headaches is recommended. Intravenous caffeine therapy for a PDPH in a 71-year-old man resulted in a transient atrial fibrillation that underscores the potential risk and obvious anesthetic concerns with intravenous administration or perhaps even high oral intake of caffeine in some patients (68).

OPIOIDS

Opioid abuse is widespread but estimates vary significantly. The true incidence is difficult to evaluate and certainly varies by geographic location and within populations. A recent report of heroin use during pregnancy suggested a 0.1% incidence (1), while opioid use was estimated by others to range from less than 1% to 2% (8, 69) to as high as 21% in specific populations (70). NIDA reported that 88,000 women were using heroin regularly, and 650,000 had used it at least once, (71) while another review suggested 300,000 infants are exposed to opioids in utero (72). The NIDA report also noted that 5 million women of childbearing age use illicit substances.

A report by the California Department of Health Services in 1997 noted that a higher incidence of drug-related deaths in urban areas continues to be a problem. In San Francisco, deaths from illicit drug use (non-obstetric) directly related to heroin (153 persons) were significantly greater than deaths from

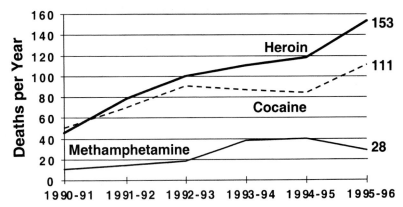

Figure 34.3. Death in San Francisco caused by drugs from 1990 through 1996 (fiscal year). The numbers represent deaths caused specifically by heroin, cocaine, or methamphetamines, not including drug-related deaths. The increasing availability of potent, inexpensive heroin has led to increased deaths. None of these deaths were known to be in pregnant women, but they point to the increasing use of street drugs in the culture. (Data is from the California State Department of Health Services, April 1997.)

cocaine (111 persons) (Fig. 34.3). The purity and declining price of heroin on the street seems linked to these findings. While these deaths were not in pregnant women, it is an indication of the increasing availability and abuse of heroin and cocaine in larger urban centers. By comparison, it was reported that 144 deaths resulted from heroin abuse in Seattle in 1998; one of the highest per capita rates in the United States (73). This compares with 147 heroin-related deaths in Frankfurt, Germany in 1992 which was reduced to 26 in 1999 by use of safe-injection rooms provided by a social program. While the latter is extremely controversial, it indicates the extent of the problem and risks to the pregnant women in many urban areas. Heroin is the most common opioid abused during pregnancy. It may be consumed by smoking, intranasal inhalation or intravenous injection. The medical complications of injection drug use are listed in Table 34.2. An increasing number of women are also on methadone maintenance and the number of pregnant women in these programs has increased (74).

Exposure during pregnancy to opioids has been reported to produce intrauterine growth restriction, preterm labor, abruptio placentae, chorioamnionitis, and an increased risk of cesarean section for fetal distress (24). There is an increased risk for fetal loss and low-birth weight as well, but all of these concerns are multifactorial in origin (4). As noted earlier, polysubstance abuse is common and it is difficult to separate individual effects. Maternal life-style also puts the infant at risk. Infants of women enrolled in methadone maintenance programs have been reported to have an overall better perinatal outcome by some (75, 76), but there are conflicting reports (77, 78). Withdrawal from opioids in the third trimester can result in meconium staining, perinatal asphyxia and neonatal death. However, success with methadone weaning has been reported without detrimental effects on the fetus or neonate (79). Neonates of women addicted to opioids exhibit withdrawal after delivery and can have an increased likelihood of respiratory distress, seizures, hyperthermia, an increased incidence of SIDS and other serious consequences (Table 34.3). Neonatal withdrawal has been reported in infants born of mothers receiving less than 10 mg of methadone per day (80). Neonatal withdrawal may last for several months and has a mortality rate of 1%, usually associated with infection, prematurity and other consequences of opioid abuse. Substance abuse during pregnancy continues to be costly to the infant and society at large (81).

Anesthetic Considerations

Cesarean section is required more often in drug-dependent women. The most common reason is fetal distress. Intravenous induction of general anesthesia, using the usual rapid-sequence technique, is effective for opioid addicts although some authors have reported an increased incidence of hypotension (82). Provided that the patient's normal opioid requirements

Table 34.2. MEDICAL COMPLICATIONS OF INJECTION DRUG USE

Infectious
  HIV
  Hepatitis
  Tuberculosis
  Tetanus
  "Cotton fever"
  Malaria
Soft tissue
  Abscess
  Necrotizing fasciitis
  Tetanus
  Rhabdomyolysis
  Retained needle fragments
Cardiovascular
  Endocarditis
  Thrombophlebitis
  Venosclerosis
  Mycotic aneurysm
  Embolic occlusion
Pulmonary
  Pulmonary edema
  Septic pulmonary emboli
  Interstitial damage
  Pneumonia
  Pneumothorax
  Angiothrombotic pulmonary
  Hypertension
Neurologic
  Cerebral infarction
  Intracranial hemmorrhage
  CNS abscess
  Meningitis
  Parkinsonian syndrome
Bone and joint
  Septic arthritis
  Osteomyelitis
Gastrointestinal
  Pseudo–obstruction
  Hypoglycemia
Ocular
  Endophthalmitis
  Central retinal artery occlusion
  Granulomas
Other
  Renal
  Endocrine
  Immunologic
  Traumatic

This table summarizes the potential complications related to intravenous drug abuse. From Stackhouse RA, Hughes SC. Drug Abuse and HIV Disease in the obstetric patient: clinical issues in obstetric anesthesia. *Current Anaesth and Critical Care* 2000; 11:97–103, with permission.

Table 34.3. CLINICAL SIGNS OF NEONATAL WITHDRAWAL SYNDROME

Control nervous system dysfunction
Irritable, excessive crying
Jittery, tremulous
Hyperactive reflexes
Increased tone
Sleep disturbance
Seizures
Autonomic dysfunction
Excessive sweating
Mottling
Hyperthermia
Hypertension
Respiratory symptoms
Tachypnea
Nasal stuffiness
Gastrointestinal and feeding disturbances
Diarrhea
Excessive sucking
Hyperphagia

From Martinez A, Partridge JC, Bean X, et al. Perinatal substance abuse. In Taeusch HW, Ballard RA, eds. *Avery's Diseases of the Newborn*. Philadelphia, WB Saunders,1998.

are met, cross-tolerance is not a major problem during the maintenance phase of anesthesia.

Methadone may have an influence on the reactivity of the nonstress test and lead to unnecessary interventions (83). Fetal distress can originate from withdrawal resulting in sympathetic hyperactivity and leading to fetal hypoxia (84). The symptoms of opioid withdrawal appear 8 to 12 hours after the last dose. Symptoms of withdrawal may begin mildly with yawning, rhinorrhea and a generalized irritability and progress to diarrhea, dehydration, tachycardia, hypertension and fever. Meconium accumulation on the placenta has been found in heroin-addicted women and thought to be caused by the stress of fetal withdrawal. To avoid withdrawal, it is important for an opioid addict to receive her regular daily dose of opioid (85). This dose must be considered as a physiologic requirement and should not be omitted if regional techniques are employed for labor analgesia or cesarean section. However, the administration of opioid agonist-antagonists, such as nalbuphine or butorphanol, to patients addicted to opioids should be avoided because they may result in withdrawal (86). There is a higher incidence of infectious disease in heroin-abusing patients, including endocarditis and infectious arthritis, which some consider a relative contraindication to the use of regional techniques (87), but this author and colleagues at San Francisco General Hospital have frequently used regional anesthesia in this patient group. Because opioid addicts and women receiving methadone maintenance have a 25% incidence of chronic anemia, replacement of blood loss must be considered (88). Establishing intravenous access can create major difficulties in the opioid addict, and often central venous access (CVP) is the only possibility. Placement of a CVP catheter will often involve the anesthesiologist or a surgical specialist.

Maternal health concerns beyond the obvious direct effects related to opioid or other illicit drug use include numerous infectious diseases and medical problems related to intravenous drug abuse. These include HIV infection, hepatitis B and C, endocarditis and numerous neurologic and pulmonary complications (Table 34.2). A recent report of 33 pregnant women with extra-pulmonary tuberculosis highlighted the potential catastrophic consequences if this diagnosis is missed or not treated (89). In this review, the absence of systemic symptoms and the reluctance to perform appropriate radiographic studies during pregnancy resulted in early onset of paraplegia in two women from spinal tuberculosis. The condition of the women improved with anti-tuberculosis drug therapy. This group

of patients require careful multispecialty medical evaluation during their pregnancy.

A unique, potential problem facing the anesthesiologist is the concern when an addict takes an additional dose of opioids before coming to the hospital or before a surgical procedure. This frequently results from patient anxiety or an attempt to provide self-administered analgesia. This may result in unexpected maternal sequelae and potential neonatal respiratory depression. Naloxone, which is usually the drug of choice when respiration is depressed from opioid abuse (90), should not be used in the pregnant woman or in the depressed newborn of a opioid-addicted woman, except in very small, titrated doses. Ventilation is the therapy of choice because naloxone can result in acute withdrawal symptoms in the newborn. Postoperative analgesia may be a problem. Intermittent injections of opioids are likely to result in insufficient pain relief, and continuous infusions may be more successful because they produce a more constant blood level of opioid. The use of spinal and epidural opiates has not been sufficiently studied in this group of patients, but the authors' experience indicate it is safe and effective at the usual doses. At San Francisco General Hospital, intrathecal epidural morphine and fentanyl have been used effectively and safely in patients receiving methadone maintenance. Patients who abuse opioids and have surgery need acute pain relief as well as chronic opioid maintenance. Opioid tolerance may be extreme with use of 1 to 2 grams of heroin per day. While the purity of street drugs vary widely, this can be equivalent to 1,000 to 2,000 mg of morphine per day. Correlation of "street use" of opioids with actual opioid or methadone requirements is difficult and is best achieved by titrating the opioid to physiologic responses. However, with IV drug users (IVDU), tolerance decreases rapidly with complete withdrawal and more routine doses of opioids must be used.

The early use of regional anesthesia during labor in IVDU parturients is helpful. Anxiety and fear of pain are common and the establishment of an effective regional blockade helps build a rapport with the patient and provides a route of anesthesia for cesarean section if needed. If the patient is on methadone maintenance, this should be continued during labor and postoperatively.

COCAINE

Cocaine was the first local anesthetic and is derived from the *Erythroxylon coca* plant. It is used less frequently today in clinical practice, but the abuse of cocaine has become a public health concern. In a report published in 1995, it was noted that cocaine was responsible for 42.6% of drug-related deaths (91). At that time, it was estimated that 15% of the U.S. population had used cocaine at least once, as many as 8 million used it regularly, and 5,000 Americans tried cocaine for the first time each day. Unfortunately, cocaine abuse in pregnant women paralleled the increase in the general population at that time (8). Prevalence of substance abuse in the parturient measured by anonymous toxicology screens have ranged from 0.4% to 40%, (92) with marijuana and cocaine being commonly detected. In the early 1990s, approximately 10% of the newborns at San Francisco General Hospital were positive for benzoylegonine, a metabolite of cocaine, indicating maternal use within the last week. While this number has declined more recently, cocaine abuse in the pregnant patient remains a significant concern.

A rapid assay for cocaine metabolites has been developed and screening of patients at risk for multiple drugs is common (93). The problems related to the abuse of cocaine are more obvious in larger urban centers. However, a survey of college students in the United States in 1997 noted that 14.4% of students had tried cocaine. Among students who were at least 25 years old, this increased to 28.1% (94). Cocaine use during pregnancy has potential serious medical and obstetrical complications and the obstetric anesthesiologist must be aware of these concerns (95–98).

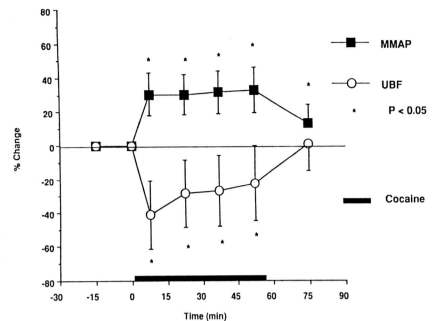

Figure 34.4. Percentage of change in maternal mean arterial pressure (MMAP) and uterine blood flow (UBF) during cocaine administration to pregnant ewes (*n* = 10). Values are expressed as mean ± SD. Changes are compared to baseline values with significance noted (*P < 0.05). (From Vertommen JD, Hughes SC, Rosen MA, et al. Hydralazine does not restore uterine blood flow during cocaine-induced hypertension in the pregnant ewe. *Anesthesiology* 1992;76:580–587, with permission.)

Pharmacology and Physiologic Response

Cocaine acts as a local anesthetic at sodium and potassium channels but also blocks the re-uptake of catecholamines and neurotransmitters at nerve terminals, including norepinephrine, dopamine, epinephrine, and serotonin. Increased levels of catecholamines lead to tachycardia, vasoconstriction, hypertension and decreased UBF. Studies in animal models have shown a decrease in uterine and placental perfusion and an increase in uterine contractility after cocaine (Fig. 34.4) (99–101). Cocaine has been shown to augment contractility of pregnant human myometrium in vitro by both adrenergic and nonadrenergic mechanisms (102).

Cocaine readily crosses the placenta and may constrict vessels in the placenta and umbilical cord. Women who used cocaine in the third trimester reported feeling contractions and increased fetal activity within minutes of cocaine use (103). There is a link to spontaneous abortions and cocaine use (38). There is also an increased rate of abruptio placenta which may be related to the vasoconstrictive effects of cocaine (104–106). Fetal distress and abruptio placenta are common causes of emergent cesarean section among cocaine abusers (107). The cocaine epidemic led to a statement by the American College of Obstetricians and Gynecologists in the form of a committee opinion that recommended frequent testing and counseling for women at risk (108). Fetal and maternal clinical concerns are summarized in Table 34.4.

Maternal Complications

Many of the medical complications of cocaine are related to its blockade of catecholamine reuptake with significant

consequences (109–111). However, there are unique concerns for the parturient that may lead to emergency anesthetic intervention for maternal or fetal safety (Table 34.4). Maternal complications have included abruptio placenta (104–106, 112), uterine rupture (114), fetal demise in utero (115, 116), and premature labor and delivery (106, 116). There is an increased incidence of fetal distress and it is a common cause for cesarean section in these patients (107). Pulmonary complications of smoking cocaine may be significant (Table 34.5). In the postpartum period, a case of maternal hypertension and seizure that resulted in an intracerebral hemorrhage has been reported. The initial diagnosis was pregnancy-induced hypertension (PIH) but proved to be the result of postpartum cocaine abuse (117). Maternal hypertension, hyperreflexia and convulsions from cocaine abuse can mimic PIH and cocaine abuse must be included in the differential diagnosis of hypertension in pregnancy.

Neonatal Complications

Neonates born to cocaine-abusing mothers show transient signs of CNS irritability (118). Some infants have abnormal

Table 34.4. COCAINE AND OBSTETRIC ANESTHESIA: CAUSES OF EMERGENCY INTERVENTION

Abruptio placentae
Acute fetal distress
Premature rupture of membranes
Uterine rupture
Maternal seizure, coma
Severe maternal hypertension
Myocardial or neurologic complications

Table 34.5. PULMONARY COMPLICATIONS OF SMOKED COCAINE[a]

Acute respiratory symptoms
Exacerbation of asthma
Thermal airway injury
Deterioration in lung function
Pneumothorax and pneumomediastinum
Bronchiolitis obliterans with organizing pneumonia
Pulmonary hemorrhage
Noncardiogenic pulmonary edema
Pulmonary infiltrates with eosinophilia/interstitial pneumonitis
pulmonary vascular disease/pulmonary infarction

[a] Smoked cocaine is cocaine in freebase form (vs. cocaine hydrochloride) and is also referred to as "crack cocaine" or "freebase." Cocaine hydrochloride decomposes if burned but the base from can be smoked. From Haim DY, Lippmann ML, Golaberg SK, et al. The pulmonary complications of crack cocaine, a comprehensive review. Chest 1995; 107:233–240,with permission.

Table 34.6. ASSOCIATED CLINICAL FEATURES IN THE MOTHER AND INFANT WITH COCAINE USE DURING PREGNANCY

Pregnancy
Spontaneous abortions
Abruptio placentae
Stillbirths
Premature delivery
Growth
Low birth weight
Intrauterine growth restriction
Small head size
Infections
Perinatal HIV
Congenital syphilis
Malformations
Urogenital
Brain
Midline defects (agenesis of the corpus callosum, septo-optic dysplasia)
Skull defects, encephaloceles
Ocular
Vascular disruption (limb reduction, intestinal atresia)
Cardiac
Neurodevelopmental Findings
Neonates
Impaired organizational state
Hypertonia,tremor
Seizures
Brainstem conduction delays
SIDS
Infants and children
Hypertonia in infancy
Abnormal behaviors (?)

HIV, human immunodeficiency virus; SIDS, sudden infant death syndrome. From Chiriboga CA. Cocaine and the fetus: methodological issues and neurologic correlates. In: Konkol RJ, Olsen GD, eds. *Prenatal Cocaine Exposure.* Boca Raton, FL, CRC Press 1996, with permission.

electroencephalograms during the first week of life. Signs of withdrawal after prenatal cocaine exposure occur in a significant number of infants (119). Cerebral infarction has been reported in the infants of mothers who used cocaine just before labor and delivery (120). While still controversial, a recent study demonstrated that cocaine use is associated with low-birth weight and fetal growth restriction (121). Spontaneous neonatal intestinal perforation in a preterm infant exposed to cocaine in utero has been reported (122). While other causes of neonatal intestinal perforation and necrotizing enterocolitis were considered, the authors concluded that the perforation was linked to cocaine. Cocaine-exposed infants have congenital defects, more medical complications, longer hospital stays and may suffer from long-term developmental deficits (Table 34.6) (95, 123, 124). Characteristic facies have been described but this may relate to alcohol or other drug abuse (Figs. 34.5 and 34.6). The neurobehavioral effects on newborns from prenatal cocaine exposure are controversial. The findings range from demonstrating no abnormalities to finding impairments in arousal, neurological function, neurophysiological function, and state regulation (125).

While stroke, seizures and congenital anomalies (fourfold increase in genitourinary anomalies) have been reported , most cocaine associations appear to be transient and resolve in infancy and early childhood. One study in children between 4 and 6 years of age noted that prenatal cocaine exposure predicted poor visual motor performance (126). However, these children did not differ from controls on gross neurological motor and expressive language measures. The conflicting reports may re-

late to the inability to detect subtle neurobehavioral differences or cognitive deficits or to better quantitate prenatal cocaine exposure. Persistent neurobehavioral effects, for example, were demonstrated in a group of infants (tested at 6.5 to 13 months of age) with heavy prenatal cocaine exposure (127). Recently, evaluation of 386 mother—infant pairs using the Brazelton Neonatal Behavioral Assessment Scale and Neonatal Stress Scale noted that the single, most-important predictor of neonatal outcome is the frequency, quantity , and method of cocaine delivery (128). Further long-term studies will be needed to fully evaluate the specific, long-term effects of maternal cocaine abuse on the children and young adults who were exposed in utero. The anesthetic concerns in this group of patients will be discussed in conjunction with amphetamine abuse because of the similarities in issues for the anesthesiologist.

AMPHETAMINES

Amphetamines and methamphetamines are sympathomimetic amines. Their stimulatory effect on the sympathetic nervous system is caused by an increase in neurotransmitters released from presynaptic terminals. Amphetamines (methylphenethylamine) and methamphetamines (*N*-methylated form) have been used orally and intravenously as well as inhaled or "snorted." Crystal methamphetamine ("ice") is a smokable form of the drug that is not unlike "crack" cocaine regarding the potential adverse maternal and neonatal outcome (129).

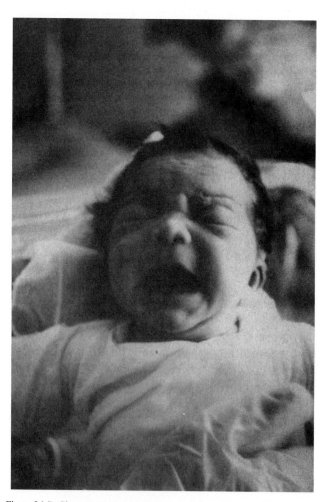

Figure 34.5. Characteristic facies of infant exposed prenatally to cocaine only. Note marked periorbital and eyelid edema and "double eyebrow" crease. These babies often appear irritable, but this is not a consistent finding.

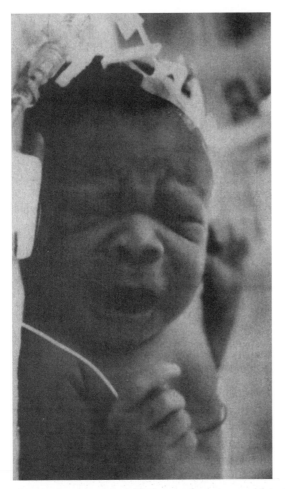

Figure 34.6. Facies of infant exposed prenatally to cocaine and alcohol. Note severe periorbital and eyelid edema "double eyebrow" crease. Features consistent with fetal alcohol exposure (long smooth philtrum, thin upper lip, bitemporal narrowing) are also recognizable.

The clinical effects of amphetamines are often indistinguishable from those of cocaine. In the pregnant ewe model, methamphetamine administration resulted in decreased UBF and caused fetal hypoxia (130). Fetal lactic acidemia, hyperglycemia, and increased catecholamines have been reported in the animal model as well. In women, amphetamine abuse appears to be popular in part because of appetite suppression and weight loss. The pregnant patient may continue taking the drug while unknowingly being pregnant. The d,L-isomer of amphetamine was first marketed in 1931 as Benzedrine. In the 1950s, obstetricians prescribed low-dose oral amphetamines to reduce weight gain during pregnancy. There are conflicting reports regarding the potential of congenital abnormalities or neurologic sequelae in the newborn (131, 132). In a study from Sweden, however, there was an increase in the incidence of preterm labor, placental abruption, fetal distress, and postpartum hemorrhage (133). Thus, both cocaine and amphetamine abuse seem to result in an increase in the incidence of placental abruption, intrauterine growth restriction and preterm delivery with fetal distress but this is not a consistent finding (132).

As with cocaine, infants born to mothers who abused amphetamines during pregnancy may have a variety of symptoms including abnormal sleep pattern, tremors, hypertonia, high-pitched cry, poor or frantic sucking, vomiting, sneezing, and tachypnea (131). Some infants who were studied using ultrasonographic examination of the brain and who were otherwise entirely well, had evidence of brain lesions. Amphetamine-exposed infants exhibit lethargy, poor feeding, decreased alertness, and severe lassitude, and some infants have minor neurologic abnormalities.

The maternal response to acute amphetamine administration may be prolonged hypertension, tachycardia, arrhythmias, hyperreflexia, and fever, which appears to be very similar to cocaine intoxication and mimic PIH or malignant hyperthermia. Chronic use may lead to psychosis and to significant management concerns during pregnancy and delivery. This group of patients frequently abuse multiple drugs, further clouding the specific effects of amphetamines.

Anesthetic Considerations

Identification of the parturient at risk for problems related to cocaine and amphetamine abuse is often difficult. While a positive history and dramatic cardiovascular physiologic response is seen with acute drug intoxication, the patient will often deny drug abuse and the physical findings will be less obvious at delivery. In several studies, 35% to 55% of pregnant women with a positive urine test for cocaine denied drug use (134). The absence of prenatal care was found to be an important predictor of cocaine abuse.

Both cocaine and amphetamine abuse result in catecholamine excess during acute intoxication and catecholamine depletion in the chronic addict. The anesthesiologist can help minimize potential increases in uterine vascular resistance caused by an excess of catecholamines by reducing pain and anxiety during labor (135). Early placement of an epidural will decrease pain, lower maternal catecholamines and may benefit a potentially compromised fetus. However, as discussed later in this chapter, both regional and general anesthesia may result in adverse effects in this patient group.

Control of Maternal Cardiovascular Response

Drug-addicted mothers often arrive at the hospital because labor has been induced by drugs, including cocaine and amphetamines. Severe hypertension and/or abruptio placentae may be present in these patients and require immediate intervention. Pregnancy enhances the action of cocaine on the cardiovascular system and puts the parturients at increased risk (136). The best drugs to treat the hypertension resulting from cocaine abuse is poorly defined. **Hydralazine** had been the drug of choice by many obstetricians to treat hypertension in the pregnant patient but can lead to tachycardia which may be unacceptable in a patient who is already tachycardic from cocaine or amphetamine abuse (137). Other choices of treatment to consider include **labetalol** (138, 139), **esmolol** (140), and **nitroglycerin** (NTG) (141). However, beta-blocking agents are avoided in the pregnant patient by some. In addition, propranolol has been reported to result in severe hypertension when used to treat cocaine intoxication (142). **Calcium channel-blocking** agents (143) and **neuroleptics** (144) also have been advocated for treatment of cocaine intoxication and small doses of **benzodiazepines** have proven helpful (diazepam 2.5 to 10 mg IV). NTG may be beneficial in cocaine-intoxicated patients for whom coronary artery vasoconstriction is an additional concern.

We investigated hydralazine for control of cocaine-induced hypertension at UCSF in the gravid ewe (97). The intravenous administration of cocaine increased maternal mean arterial blood pressure (MABP) by approximately 30% and decreased UBF by 25% to 45% (see Fig. 34.4). While hydralazine successfully controlled MABP, UBF remained significantly decreased and MHR increased by approximately 120% (Fig. 34.7). Labetalol was investigated in a similar protocol in the gravid ewe and effectively controlled maternal MABP and MHR. While UBF remained decreased, we concluded that labetalol may be preferable to hydralazine for treatment of the acutely cocaine-intoxicated parturient (138). While this was a study in

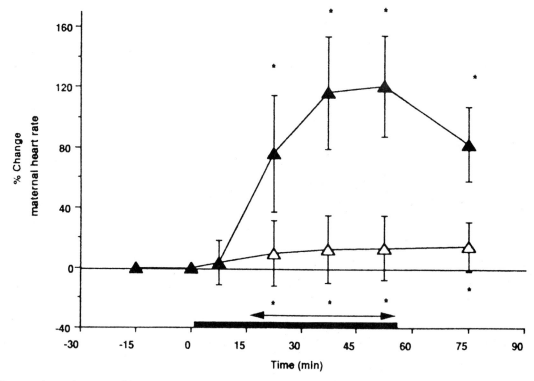

Figure 34.7. Percent change in maternal heart rate during cocaine administration with hydralazine ($n = 10$; filled triangles) and without (open triangles) hydralazine therapy (control $n = 10$). Hydralazine treatment began at 16 min and was discontinued at 55 min and is represent by the arrow. The heavy bar represents the time of cocaine administration. Values are expressed as mean ± SD. Changes are compared to baseline values with significance noted (*$P < 0.05$). (From Vertommen JD, Hughes SC, Rosen MA, et al. Hydralazine does not restore uterine blood flow during cocaine-induced hypertension in the pregnant ewe. *Anesthesiology* 1992;76:580–587, with permission.)

the ewe, labetalol is now commonly used in this clinical setting in labor and delivery in parturients.

Two animal models (145, 146) and clinical use in the pregnant patient (147, 148) suggested that NTG would be particularly beneficial in the management of cocaine-induced hypertension during pregnancy. In an attempt to decrease maternal MABP and improve UBF, NTG was also investigated using the

gravid ewe in our laboratory (141). Kessin et al. demonstrated that NTG administration in the gravid ewe effectively treated cocaine-induced maternal hypertension but it had no significant effect upon UBF (Fig. 34.8) (141). NTG also increased MHR by approximately 75%. It was concluded that single-drug therapy for acute cocaine intoxication with NTG is not ideal and the increase in MHR may lead to further adverse sequelae.

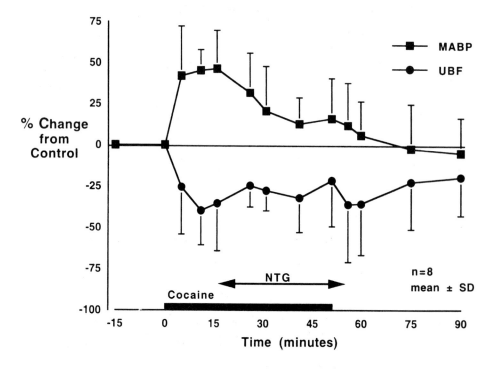

Figure 34.8. Percentage change in maternal mean arterial pressure (MABP) and uterine blood flow (UBF) during cocaine administration to pregnant ewe and treatment with nitroglycerine (NTG). Values are expressed as mean ± SD, and changes are compared to baseline values. While NTG effectively controlled the MABP of the ewe, the UBF remained decreased. (Data from Kessin C, Hughes SC, Rosen MA, et al. Cocaine-induced hypertension and response to treatment with nitroglycerin in the pregnant ewe. *Anesthesiology* 1995;83:A937.)

Labetalol has become the drug of choice to manage the acute cocaine crises (140, 149). However, the nonselective beta-blocking effects of labetalol are much more potent than its alpha-blocking effects, and the potential consequences of relatively unopposed alpha effects must be considered (140). This has been reported with propranolol (142, 150), but labetalol remains the most effective drug to manage acute hypertension *caused by cocaine* in the parturient. It may be used in combination with NTG if necessary. However, acute management of maternal cardiovascular response to cocaine remains controversial and consideration must be given to other maternal risks, the clinical setting, and fetal status (116, 147, 148, 151–154).

Regional anesthesia remains an effective choice if not otherwise contraindicated. While thrombocytopenia has been reported in association with cocaine abuse (155), more recent investigations have not found this to be true (156). An increased incidence of hypotension has been associated with epidural anesthesia for cesarean section in parturients who were cocaine abusers (4, 157). Kain et al. reported that hypotension occurred significantly more often in cocaine abusers than in the control group (44% vs. 10%, $P = 0.04$) with epidural anesthesia for cesarean section in cocaine-abusing parturients. Further, Birnbach et al. reported that ephedrine may not be an effective vasopressor in these patients due to depleted catecholamines and recommended that phenylephrine should be used if ephedrine is not effective in treating maternal hypotension with regional anesthesia (158). It has been suggested that the segmental level of the epidural for cesarean section might be raised gradually to decrease the incidence of hypotension (95). However, there are no contraindications to spinal anesthesia for cesarean section for these patients but adequate fluid hydration, careful positioning and immediate availability of ephedrine and phenylephrine must be provided.

General anesthesia may be indicated for emergency cesarean section particularly for acute fetal distress or maternal abruptio placenta. In the cohort study by Kain et al., the most frequent reasons for cesarean section in cocaine-abusing parturients were fetal distress (48%) and abruptio placentae (21%). With endotracheal intubation, diastolic blood pressure was significantly higher among parturients who used cocaine (99 ± 13 mm Hg vs. 87 ± 18 mm Hg), while they found no ventricular dysrhythmias or coronary ischemic episodes. However, clinical experience and studies in animal models require that the anesthesiologist be prepared to treat an increased incidence of hypertension, arrhythmias, myocardial ischemia and severe maternal tachycardia (97, 147, 148, 152, 154, 159).

Volatile anesthetic agents may sensitize the myocardium to dysrhythmias induced by catecholamines and halothane is not recommended in the parturient suspected of cocaine abuse. Ketamine is a potent sympathomimetic drug and is either best avoided or titrated with caution. It has been reported to cause hypertension and pulmonary edema in a patient with substance abuse (154). The minimum alveolar concentration (MAC) is decreased with chronic cocaine or amphetamine abuse but may be increased with acute drug use. Careful titration of isoflurane for general anesthesia has proven effective but there are no controlled studies (160).

MARIJUANA

Marijuana is a common drug of abuse. A nationwide survey of college students found that nearly 50% of students had at least tried marijuana (161). Use during pregnancy ranges from less than 5% (self reporting) to 35% (maternal urine testing). In a prospective-multicenter cohort study, it was found that 11% of pregnant women used marijuana, 2.3% used cocaine and 35% smoked cigarettes (162). The active ingredient is delta-9-tetrahydrocannabinol (THC), which can cause a mild tachycardia and an increase in arterial blood pressure along with a generalized euphoria.

The onset is 10 to 15 minutes, and the effects may persist for 3 to 5 hours.

THC rapidly crosses the placenta and accumulation of the drug in fatty tissue makes elimination very slow which results in prolonged exposure (up to 30 days) in the fetus (163). There are little convincing data to link marijuana to congenital anomalies (163, 164). Earlier reports suggested an association between marijuana and decreased birth weight and preterm delivery but this has not been substantiated (162). These patients often abuse numerous drugs and have less prenatal care and thus, studies that do not carefully control for other factors may have misleading results.

Marijuana is smoked, and as with cigarette smoking, it elevates the carbon monoxide levels in the blood, resulting in less oxygen available for the fetus. Newborns exposed to prenatal marijuana have been found to have changes on the Brazelton Neonatal Behavioral Assessment Scores (165), but other investigators have not confirmed this finding (166).

Anesthetic Considerations

There is little evidence of significant problems related to anesthesia with marijuana use in most patients. Like smoking cigarettes, there may be pulmonary concerns such as respiratory tract infections (167). A mild maternal tachycardia is possible (168), but with significant tachycardia or elevation in arterial blood pressure, other routine obstetric diagnoses (as well as cocaine or amphetamine use) should be suspected. Potentiation of the pharmacodynamic effects of epinephrine added to local anesthetics has been reported (168). The duration of action of both ketamine and thiopental is prolonged and in an animal model, there is an additive effect with volatile agents (169, 170). Recent use of marijuana may lead to additive effects with concomitantly administered sedatives (88). In addition, marijuana inhibits cholinesterase activity and may prolong the action of succinylcholine (171). While the acutely intoxicated patient is potentially at risk for adverse interaction with anesthetic drugs, this has not been reported in obstetric anesthesia despite the widespread use of marijuana. There are no contraindications to either regional or general anesthesia, as indicated.

CONCLUSION

Drug use in the parturient can lead to catastrophic results for the mother, the fetus, or the newborn. The risk varies widely with the drugs considered in this chapter. Although cigarettes and alcohol are the most widely abused drugs, these drugs are usually of less concern to the anesthesiologist when compared to cocaine or heroin. Women who abuse drugs often use multiple drugs and fail to report their use when questioned. Neonatal outcome studies are often poorly controlled or plagued by numerous confounding factors and their results often conflict. However, significant sequelae from both illicit and legal drug use is well documented. The anesthesiologist should remain alert to possible maternal drug abuse and potential interaction with the obstetric course and anesthetic implications, and the potential impact on the fetus and newborn.

REFERENCES

1. Marwick C. Challenging report on pregnancy and drug abuse. *JAMA* 1998;280:1039–1040.
2. Silverman S. Scope, specifics of maternal drug use, and effects on fetus are beginning to emerge from studies. *JAMA* 1989;261:1688–1689.
3. Comby DS, Shiono PH. Estimating the number of substance-exposed infants. In: Behrman RE, ed. *Drug-Exposed Infants.* Los Altos, CA: David and Lucile Packard Foundation, Center for the Future of Children, 1991.

4. Kain ZM, Mayers LC, Ferris CA, et al. Cocaine-abusing parturients undergoing cesarean section, a cohort study. *Anesthesiology* 1996;85:1028–1035.

5. Silverman S. Combinations of drugs taken by pregnant women add to problems in determining fetal damage. *JAMA* 1989;261:1694.

6. Macones GA, Sehdev HM, Parry S, et al. The association between cocaine use and placental previa. *Am J Obstet Gynecol* 1997; 1097–1100.

7. Handler AS, Mason ED, Rosenberg DL, et al. The relationship between exposure during pregnancy to cigarette smoking and cocaine use and placenta previa. *Am J Obstet Gynecol* 1994;170:884–889.

8. Vega WA, Kolody B, Hwang J, et al. Prevalence and magnitude of perinatal substance exposures in California. *N Engl J Med* 1993;329:850–854.

9. Rodriquez EM, Mofsen LM, Chang B-H, et al. Association of maternal drug use during pregnancy with maternal HIV culture positivity and perinatal transmission. *AIDS* 1996;10:273–282.

10. Williams GD, Grant BF, Harford TC, et al. Population projections using DSM-III criteria: alcohol abuse and dependence, 1990–2000. *Alcohol Health Res World* 1989;13:366–370.

11. Ebrahim SH, Luman ET, Floyd RL, et al. Alcohol consumption by pregnant women in the United States during 1988–1995. *Obstet Gynecol* 1998;92:187–192.

12. Little RE, Asker RL, Sampson PD, et al. Fetal growth and moderate drinking in early pregnancy. *Am J Epidemiol* 1986;123:270–278.

13. Becker CE. Alcohol and drug use: is there a "safe" amount? *West J Med* 1984;141:884–890.

14. Coles CD, Smith IE, Lancaster JS, et al. Persistence over the first month of neurobehavioral differences in infants exposed to alcohol prenatally. *Infant Behav Dev* 1987;10:23–27.

15. Russell M. Clinical implications of recent research on the fetal alcohol syndrome. *Bull NY Acad Med* 1991;67:207–222.

16. Emhart CB, Sokol RJ, Martier S, et al. Alcohol teratogenicity in the human: a detailed assessment of specificity, critical period and threshold. *Am J Obstet Gynecol* 1987;156:33–39.

17. Fisher SE, Karl PI. Maternal ethanol use and selective fetal malnutrition. *Recent Dev Alcohol* 1988;6:277–289.

18. Clarren SK, Smith DW. The fetal alcohol syndrome. *N Engl J Med* 1978;298:1063–1067.

19. Abel EL. *Fetal Alcohol Abuse Syndrome Revisited.* New York: Plenum Press, 1998.

20. Abel EL. Prevention of alcohol abuse-related birth effects: 1. Public education efforts. *Alcohol Alcohol* 1998;4:411–416.

21. Aose JM, Jones KL, Clauen SK. Do we need the term "FAE"? *Pediatrics* 1995;95:428

22. Silva PD, Miller KD, Madden J, et al. Abnormal fetal heart rate pattern associated with severe intrapartum ethanol intoxication. *J Reprod Med* 1987;32:144–146.

23. Mukherjee AB, Hodgen GD. Maternal ethanol exposure induces transient impairment of umbilical circulation and fetal hypoxia in monkeys. *Science* 1982;218:700–702.

24. Martinez AM, Partridge JC, Bean X, et al. Perinatal substance abuse. In: Taeusch HW, Ballard RA, eds. *Avery's Disorders of the Newborn.* Philadelphia: WB Saunders, 1998.

25. O'Daniel L. Anesthetic management of the alcoholic patient. *AANAJ* 1980;48:445–451.

26. St. Haxholdt O, Krintel JJ, Johannson G. Pre-operative alcohol infusion. *Anaesthesia* 1984;39:240–245.

27. Edwards R, Mosher VB. Alcohol abuse, anaesthesia and intensive care. *Anaesthesia* 1980;35:474–489.

28. Klatsky AL. Cardiovascular effects of alcohol. *Am J Med Sci* 1995;37:28–37.

29. Du Cailar J, d'Athis F, Eledjam JJ, et al. Propofol et éthylisme. *Ann Fr Anesth Reanim* 1987;6:332–333.

30. Edwards R. Anaesthesia and alcohol. *BMJ* 1985;291:423–424.

31. Fried PA, O'Connell CM. A comparison of the effects of prenatal exposure to tobacco, alcohol, cannabis and caffeine on birth size and subsequent growth. *Neurotoxicol Teratol* 1987;9:79–85.

32. Vert P, Lebrun F. Les nuissances toxiques pour le foetus: L'alcohol, les drogues psychoactives et le tabac. *Rev Prat* 1998;38:825–831.

33. Walsh RA. Effects of maternal smoking on adverse pregnancy outcomes: examination of the criteria of causation. *Hum Biol* 1994;66:1059–1092.

34. Secker-Walker RH, Vacek PM, Flynn BS, et al. Smoking in pregnancy, exhaled carbon monoxide, and birth weight. *Obstet Gynecol* 1997;89:648–653.

35. Ananth CV, Smulian JC, Vintzileos AM. Incidence of placental abruption in relation to cigarette smoking and hypertensive disorders during pregnancy: a meta-analysis of observational studies. *Obstet Gynecol* 1999;93:622–628.

36. Hoo AF, Henschen M, Dezateux C, et al. Respiratory function among preterm infants whose mothers smoked during pregnancy. *Am J Respir Crit Care Med* 1998;158:700–705.

37. Ness RB, Brisse JA, Hirschinger N, et al. Cocaine and tobacco use and the risks of spontaneous abortion. *N Engl J Med* 1999;340:333–339.

38. Centers for Disease Control and Prevention. Prevalence of selected maternal and infant characteristics, pregnancy risk assessment monitoring system. *MMWR* 1999;48(SS-5):6.

39. Shah NR, Bracken MB. Asystemic review and meta-analysis of prospective studies on the association between maternal cigarette smoking and preterm delivery. *Am J Obstet Gynecol* 2000;182:465–472.

40. Slotkin TA, Cho H, Whitmore WL. Effects of prenatal nicotine exposure on neuronatal development. Selective actions on central and peripheral catecholaminergic pathways. *Brain Res Bull* 1987;18:601–611.

41. Slotkin TA, Lappi SE, McCook EC, et al. Loss of neonatal hypoxia tolerance after prenatal nicotine exposure: implications for sudden infant death syndrome. *Brain Res Bull* 1995;38:69.

42. Stjerfeldt M, Berglund K, Lindsten J, et al. Maternal smoking during pregnancy and risk of childhood cancer. *Lancet* 1986;1:1350–1352.

43. Davies JM, Latto IP, Jones JG, et al. Effects of stopping smoking for 48 hours on oxygen availability from the blood: a study on pregnant women. *BMJ* 1979;2:355–356.

44. American College of Obstetricians and Gynecologists. *Smoking and reproductive health. ACOG Technical Bulletin No. 180.* Washington, DC: ACOG, 1993.

45. Benowitz NL. Nicotine replacement therapy during pregnancy. *JAMA* 1991;266:3174–3177.

46. Pearse AC, Jones RM. Smoking and anesthesia: preoperative abstinence and perioperative morbidity. *Anesthesiology* 1984;61:576–584.

47. Wright DJ, Pandya A. Smoking and gastric juice volume in outpatients. *Can Anaesth Soc J* 1979;26:328.

48. Fredholm BB, Bättig K, Holmén J, et al. Actions of caffeine in the brain with special reference to factors that contribute to its widespread use. *Pharmacol Rev* 1999;51:83–133.

49. Eskenazi B. Caffeine: filtering the facts [Editorial]. *N Engl J Med* 1999;341:1688–1699.

50. Armstrong BG, McDonald AD, Sloan M. Cigarettes, alcohol and coffee consumption and spontaneous abortion. *Am J Public Health* 1992;82:85.

51. Nehlig A. Are we dependent upon coffee and caffeine: a review on human and animal data. *Neurosci Biobehav Rev* 1999;23:563–576.

52. Eskenazi B. Caffeine during pregnancy: grounds for concern? *JAMA* 1993;270:2973–2974.

53. Smith SE, McElhatton PR, Sullivan FM. Effects of administering caffeine to pregnant rats either as a single daily dose or as divided doses four times a day. *Food Chem Toxicol* 1987;25:125.

54. Nehlig A, Debry G. Potential teratogenic and neurodevelopmental consequences of coffee and caffeine exposure: a review on human and animal data. *Neurotoxicol Teratol* 1994;16:531–543.

55. Tye K, Pollard I, Karlsson L, et al. Caffeine exposure in utero increases the incidence of apnea in adult rats. *Reprod Toxicol* 1993;7:449–452.

56. Fisher S, Guillet R. Neonatal caffeine alters passive avoidance retention in rats in an age- and gender-related manner. *Brain Res Dev Brain Res* 1997;98:145–149.

57. Linn S, Schoenbaum SC, Monson RR, et al. No association between coffee consumption and adverse outcomes of pregnancy. *N Engl J Med* 1982;360:141–145.

58. Mills JL, Holmes LB, Aarons JH, et al. Moderate caffeine use and the risk of spontaneous abortion and intrauterine growth retardation. *JAMA* 1993;269:593–597.

59. Heller J. What do we know about the risks of caffeine consumption in pregnancy? *Br J Addict* 1987;82:885–889.

60. Srisuphan W, Bracken MB. Caffeine consumption during pregnancy and association with late spontaneous abortion. *Am J Obstet Gynecol* 1986;154:14–20.

61. Fernandes O, Sabharwal M, Smiley T, et al. Moderate to heavy caffeine consumption during pregnancy and relationship to

spontaneous abortion and abnormal fetal growth: a meta analysis. *Reprod Toxicol* 1998;12:435–444.

62. Klebanoff MA, Levine RJ, Der Somonian R, et al. Maternal serum paraxanthine, a caffeine metabolite, and the risk of spontaneous abortion. *N Engl J Med* 1999;341:1639–1644.

63. Food and Drug Administration. *Caffeine in Pregnancy*. Rockville, MD: FDA, 1981;81:1081.

64. Oei SG, Vosters RPK, van der Hagen NLG. Fetal arrhythmia caused by excessive intake of caffeine by pregnant women. *BMJ* 1989;298:568.

65. Galletly DC, Fennelly M, Whitwam JG. Does caffeine withdrawal contribute to postanesthetic morbidity? *Lancet* 1989;1:1335.

66. Fennely M, Galletly DC, Purdie GL. Is caffeine withdrawal the mechanism of postoperative headache? *Anesth Analg* 1991;72:449–453.

67. Paech M. Unexpected postpartum seizures associated with post dural puncture headache treated with caffeine. *Int J Obstet Anesth* 1996;5:43–46.

68. McSwiney M, Phillips J. Post dural puncture headache. *Acta Anaesthesiol Scand* 1995;39:990–995.

69. Chasnoff IJ, Landress HJ, Barrett ME. The prevalence of illicit drug and alcohol use during pregnancy and discrepancies in mandatory reporting in Pinellas County, Florida. *N Engl J Med* 1990;322:1202–1206.

70. Ostrea EM, Brady M, Gause S, et al. Drug screening of newborns by meconium analysis: a large-scale, prospective, epidemiologic study. *Pediatrics* 1992;89:107–113.

71. National Institute on Drug Abuse. *National household survey on drug abuse: main findings*. DHHS publication no. 94-3012. Rockville, MD: U.S. Department of Health and Human Services, 1992.

72. Sprauve ME. Substance abuse and HIV in pregnancy. *Clin Obstet Gynecol* 1996;39:316–332.

73. Verhovek SH. Conference seeks ways to reduce heroin deaths. *New York Times* 2000 Jan 16:13.

74. Brown HL, Britton KA, Mahoffey D, et al. Methadone maintenance in pregnancy: a reappraisal. *Am J Obstet Gynecol* 1998;179:459–463.

75. Harper RG, Solish GI, Purow HM, et al. The effect of a methadone treatment program on heroin addicts and their newborn infants. *Pediatrics* 1974;54:300–305.

76. Hamid MA. Methadone maintenance in pregnancy: consequences to care and outcome. *Obstet Gynecol* 1988;71:399–404.

77. Lipschitz MH, Wilson GS. Patterns of growth and development in narcotic-exposed children: methodological issues in controlled studies on effects of prenatal exposure to drug abuse. *NIDA Res Monogr* 1991;114:323–329.

78. Zuckerman B, Bresnahan K. Developmental and behavioral consequences of prenatal drug and alcohol exposure. *Pediatr Clin North Am* 1991;38:1387–1406.

79. Mass U, Kattner E, Weingart-Jesse B, et al. Infrequent neonate opiate withdrawal following maternal detoxification during pregnancy. *J Perinat Med* 1990;18:111–118.

80. Malpas TJ, Darlow BA, Lennox R, et al. Maternal methadone dosage and neonatal withdrawal. *Aust N Z J Obstet Gynaecol* 1995;35:175–177.

81. Stichler JF, Weiss M, Wright NE. Examining the "cost" of substance abuse in pregnancy: patient outcome and resource utilization. *J Perinatol* 1998;18:384–388.

82. Boyle RK. Intra- and postoperative anaesthetic management of an opioid addict undergoing caesarean section. *Anaesth Intensive Care* 1991;19:276–279.

83. Archie CL, Lee MI, Sokol RJ, et al. The effects of methadone treatment on the reactivity of the nonstress test. *Obstet Gynecol* 1989;74:254–255.

84. Naeye RL, Blanc W, LeBlanc W, et al. Fetal complications of maternal heroin addiction: abnormal growth, infections and episodes of stress. *J Pediatr* 1973;83:1055–1061.

85. Jage J. Anaesthesia und analgesie bei opiatabhängigen. *Anaesthesist* 1988;37:470–482.

86. Weintrauab SJ, Naulty JS. Acute abstinence syndrome after epidural injection of butorphanol. *Anesth Analg* 1985;64:452–453.

87. Gomar C, Luis M, Nalda MA. Sacro-illitis in a heroin addict. *Anaesthesia* 1984;39:167–170.

88. Wood PR, Soni N. Anaesthesia and substance abuse. *Anaesthesia* 1989;44:672–680.

89. Jana N, Vasishta K, Saha SC, et al. Obstetrical outcomes among women with extra pulmonary tuberculosis. *N Engl J Med* 1999;341:645–649.

90. Bradberry JC, Raebel MA. Continuous infusion of naloxone in the treatment of narcotic overdose. *Drug Intell Clin Pharm* 1981;15:945–949.

91. Harwood HJ. Inhalants: a policy analysis of the problem in the United States. In Kozel N, Sloboda Z, De La Rosa N (eds). Epidemiology of Inhalant Abuse: An International Perspective, Rockvile, MD. *NIDA Res Monogr* 1995:274–303.

92. Hanlon-Lundberg KM, Williams M, Rhim T. Accelerated fetal lung maturity profiles and maternal cocaine exposure. *Obstet Gynecol* 1996;87:128–132.

93. Birnbach DJ, Stein DJ, Grunebaum A, et al. Cocaine screening of parturients without prenatal care: an evaluation of a rapid screening assay. *Anesth Analg* 1997;84:76–79.

94. Centers for Disease Control and Prevention. CDC surveillance summaries, November 14, 1997. *MMWR* 1997;46:10.

95. Kain ZN, Rimar S, Barash PG. Cocaine abuse in the parturient and effects on the fetus and neonate. *Anesth Analg* 1993;77:835–845.

96. Rozenak D, Diamant YZ, Yaffe H, et al. Cocaine: maternal use during pregnancy and its effect on the mother, the fetus and the infant. *Obstet Gynecol Surv* 1990;45:348–359.

97. Vertommen JD, Hughes SC, Rosen MA, et al. Hydralazine does not restore uterine blood flow in cocaine-induced hypertension in the pregnant ewe. *Anesthesiology* 1992;76:580–597.

98. Haim DY, Lippmann ML, Goldberg SK, et al. The pulmonary complications of crack cocaine: a comprehensive review. *Chest* 1995;107:233–240.

99. Woods JR, Plessinger MA, Clark KE. Effect of cocaine on uterine blood flow and fetal oxygenation. *JAMA* 1987;257:957–961.

100. Moore TR, Sorg J, Miller L. Hemodynamic effects of intravenous cocaine on the pregnant ewe and fetus. *Am J Obstet Gynecol* 1986;155:883–888.

101. Foutz SE, Kotelko DM, Shnider SM, et al. Placental transfer and effects of cocaine on uterine blood flow and the fetus. *Anesthesiology* 1983;59:A442.

102. Hurd WW, Betz AL, Dombrowski MP, et al. Cocaine augments contractility of pregnant human uterus by both adrenergic and nonadrenergic mechanisms. *Am J Obstet Gynecol* 1998;178:1077–1081.

103. Smith CG, Asch RH. Drug abuse and reproduction. *Fertil Steril* 1987;48:355–373.

104. Burkett G, Yasin SY, Palow D, et al. Patterns of cocaine binging: effect on pregnancy. *Am J Obstet Gynecol* 1994;171:372–379.

105. Wehbeh H, Matthews RP, McCalla S, et al. The effect of recent cocaine use on the progress of labor. *Am J Obstet Gynecol* 1995;172:1014–1018.

106. Plessinger MA, Woods JR. Maternal, placental and fetal pathophysiology of cocaine exposure during pregnancy. *Clin Obstet Gynecol* 1993;36:267–278.

107. Zain ZN, Mayers LC, Ferris CA, et al. Cocaine-abusing parturients undergoing cesarean section. *Anesthesiology* 1996;85:1026–1035.

108. American College of Obstetrics and Gynecology: Committee on Obstetrics, Maternal and Fetal Medicine. *Cocaine in pregnancy*. Committee Opinion no. 114. Washington, DC: ACOG, 1992.

109. Cregler K, Mark H. Medical complications of cocaine abuse. *N Engl J Med* 1986;315:1495–1500.

110. Levine SR, Brust JCM, Futrell N, et al. Cerebrovascular complications of the use of the "crack" form of alkaloidal cocaine. *N Engl J Med* 1990;323:699–704.

111. Lampley EC, Williams S, Myers SA. Cocaine-associated rhabdomyolysis causing renal failure in pregnancy. *Obstet Gynecol* 1996;87:804–806.

112. Mooney EE, Boggess KA, Herbert WN, et al. Placental pathology in patients using cocaine: An observational study. *Obstet Gynecol* 1998;91:925–929.

113. Mishra A, Landzberg BR, Parente JT. Uterine rupture in association with alkaloidal ("crack") abuse. *Am J Obstet Gynecol* 1995;173:243–244.

114. Martinez A, Larabee K, Monga M. Cocaine is associated with intrauterine fetal death in women with suspected preterm labor. *Am J Perinatol* 1996;13:164–166.

115. Collins KA, Davis GJ, Lantz PE. An unusual case of maternal-fetal death due to vaginal insufflation of cocaine. *Am J Forensic Med Pathol* 1994;15:335–339.

116. Dinsmoor MJ, Irons SJ, Christmas JT. Preterm rupture of membranes associated with recent cocaine use. *Am J Obstet Gynecol* 1994;171:305–309.

117. Mercado A, Johnson G, Calver D, et al. Cocaine, pregnancy and postpartum intracerebral hemorrhage. *Obstet Gynecol* 1989;73:467–468.

118. Dixon SD. Effects of transplacental exposure to cocaine and methamphetamine on the neonate. *West J Med* 1989;150:436–442.

119. Fulroth R, Phillips B, Durand DJ. Perinatal outcome of infants exposed to cocaine and/or heroin in utero. *Am J Dis Child* 1989;143:905–910.

120. Tenorio GM, Nazvi M, Bickers GH, et al. Intrauterine stroke and maternal polydrug use. *Clin Pediatr* 1988;27:565–567.

121. Spraure ME, Lindsay MK, Herbert S, et al. Adverse perinatal outcome in parturients who use crack cocaine. *Obstet Gynecol* 1997;89:674–678.

122. Thé TG, Young M, Rosser S. In-utero cocaine exposure and neonatal intestinal perforation: a case report. *JAMA* 1995;87:889–891.

123. Holzman C, Paneth N. Maternal cocaine use during pregnancy and perinatal outcomes. *Epidemiol Rev* 1994;16:315–334.

124. Finnegan LP, Mellot JM, Williams LR, et al. Perinatal exposure to cocaine: human studies. *NIDA Res Monogr* 1992;391–409.

125. Chiriboga CA. Neurological correlates of fetal cocaine exposure. *Ann N Y Acad Sci* 1998;846:109–125.

126. Bender SL, Word CO, DiClemente RJ, et al. The developmental implications of prenatal and/or postnatal crack cocaine exposure in preschool children: a preliminary report. *J Dev Behav Pediatr* 1995;16:418–430.

127. Jacobson SW, Jacobson JL, Sokol RJ, et al. New evidence for neurobehavioral effects of in utero cocaine exposure. *J Pediatr* 1996;129:581–590.

128. Datta-Bhutada S, Johnson HL, Rosen TS. Intrauterine cocaine and crack exposure: neonatal outcome. *J Perinatol* 1998;18:183–188.

129. Cho AK. Ice: a new dosage of an old drug. *Science* 1990;249:631

130. Stek AM, Baker RE, Fisher BA. Fetal responses to maternal methamphetamine administration in sheep. *Am J Obstet Gynecol* 1995;173:1592–1598.

131. Oro AS, Dixon DS. Perinatal cocaine and methamphetamine exposure: maternal and neonatal correlates. *J Pediatr* 1987;11:571–578.

132. Little BB, Snell LM, Gilstrap LC. Methamphetamine abuse during pregnancy: outcome and fetal effects. *Obstet Gynecol* 1988;72:541–544.

133. Erickson M, Larsson C, Windbladh B, et al. The influence of amphetamine addiction on pregnancy and the newborn infants. *Acta Paediatr Scand* 1978;67:95–99.

134. Akin ZEN, Rim S, Barite PG. Cocaine abuse in the parturient and effects on the fetus and neonate. *Anesth Analg* 1993;77:835–845.

135. Hollmén A, Jouppila R, Jouppila P, et al. Effect of extradural analgesia using bupivacaine and 2-chloroprocaine on intervillous blood flow during normal labour. *Br J Anaesth* 1982;54:837–842.

136. Woods JR Jr, Scott KJ, Plessinger MA. Pregnancy enhances cocaine's actions on the heart and within the peripheral circulation. *Am J Obstet Gynecol* 1994;170:1027–1035.

137. Jouppila P, Kirkinen P, Koivula A, et al. Effects of dihydralazine infusion on the fetoplacental blood flow and maternal prostanoids. *Obstet Gynecol* 1985;65:115–118.

138. Hughes SC, Vertommen JD, Rosen MA, et al. Cocaine-induced hypertension in the ewe and response to treatment with labetalol. *Anesthesiology* 1991;75:A1075.

139. Gay RG, Loper KA. Control of cocaine-induced hypertension with labetalol. *Anesth Analg* 1988;67:91–94

140. Pollan S, Tadjziechy M. Esmolol in the management of epinephrine- and cocaine-induced cardiovascular toxicity. *Anesth Analg* 1989;69:663–664.

141. Kessin C, Hughes SC, Rosen MA, et al. Cocaine-induced hypertension and response to treatment with nitroglycerine in the pregnant ewe. *Anesthesiology* 1995;83:A937.

142. Ramoska E, Sacchetti AD. Propranolol-induced hypertension in treatment of cocaine intoxication. *Ann Emerg Med* 1985;14:1112–1113.

143. Nahas G, Trouvé R, Demus JF, et al. A calcium channel blocker as antidote to the cardiac effects of cocaine intoxication. *N Engl J Med* 1985;313:519–520.

144. Catravas JD, Waters IW. Acute cocaine intoxication in the conscious dog: studies on the mechanism of lethality. *J Pharmacol Exp Ther* 1981;217:350–356.

145. Wheeler AS, James III FM, Meis PJ, et al. Effects of nitroglycer-ine and nitroprusside on the uterine vasculature of gravid ewes. *Anesthesiology* 1980;52:390–394.

146. Craft Jr JB, Co EG, Yonekura ML, et al. Nitroglycerin therapy for phenylephrine- induced hypertension in pregnant ewes. *Anesth Analg* 1980;59:494–499.

147. Liu SS, Forrester RM, Murphy GS, et al. Anaesthetic management of a parturient with myocardial infarction related to cocaine use. *Can J Anaesth* 1992;39:858–861.

148. Bulbul ZP, Rosenthal DN, Kleinman CS. Myocardial infarction in the perinatal period secondary to maternal cocaine abuse. *Arch Pediatr Adolesc Med* 1994;148:1092–1096.

149. Lobl JK, Carbone LD. Emergency management of cocaine intoxication: counteracting the effects of today's "favorite drug." *Postgrad Med* 1992;91:161–166.

150. Goehrer JD, Moliteruo DJ, Willard JE, et al. Influence of labetalol on cocaine-induced coronary vasoconstriction in humans. *Am J Med* 1993;94:608–610.

151. Thatcher SS, Corfman R, Grosso J, et al. Cocaine use and acute rupture of ectopic pregnancies. *Obstet Gynecol* 1989;74:478–479.

152. Towers CV, Pircon RA, Nageotte MP, et al. Cocaine intoxication presenting as preeclampsia and eclampsia. *Obstet Gynecol* 1993;81:545–547.

153. Moens MD, Caliendo MJ, Marshall W, et al. Hepatic rupture in pregnancy associated with cocaine use. *Am J Obstet Gynecol* 1993;82:687–689.

154. Murphy Jr JL. Hypertension and pulmonary oedema associated with ketamine administration in a patient with a history of substance abuse. *Can J Anaesth* 1993;40:160–164.

155. Lessinger CA. Severe thrombocytopenia associated with cocaine abuse. *Am Intern Med* 1990;112:708–710.

156. Gershon RY, Fisher AJ, Graves WL. The cocaine-abusing parturient is not at an increased risk for thrombocytopenia. *Anesth Analg* 1996;82:865–866.

157. Birnbach D, Grunebaum A, Collins E, et al. The effect of cocaine on epidural anesthesia. *Am J Obstet Gynecol* 1991;164:400S.

158. Birnbach DJ, Stein DJ, Danzer BI, et al. Ephedrine resistance in the cocaine-positive parturient. Prevalence and treatment. *Anesthesiology* 1996;85:A892.

159. Boylan JF, Cheng DC, Sandler AW, et al. Cocaine toxicity and isoflurane anesthesia: hemodynamic, myocardial, metabolic and regional blood flow effects in swine. *J Cardiothorac Vasc Anesth* 1996;10:772–777.

160. Fleming JA, Byck R, Barash PG. Pharmacology and therapeutic applications of cocaine. *Anesthesiology* 1990;73:518–531.

161. Centers for Disease Control and Prevention (CDC). Youth Risk Behavior Surveillance: National College Health Risk Behavior Survey, United States, 1995. *MMWR* 1997;46:11.

162. Shiono PH, Klebanoff MA, Nugent RP, et al. The impact of cocaine and marijuana use on low-birth weight and preterm birth: a multicenter study. *Am J Obstet Gynecol* 1995;172:19–27.

163. Zuckerman B, Frank DA, Hingson R, et al. Effects of maternal marijuana and cocaine use on fetal growth. *N Engl J Med* 1989;320:762–768.

164. Fried PA, Watkinson B, Willan A. Marijuana use during pregnancy and decreased length of gestation. *Am J Obstet Gynecol* 1984;150:23–27.

165. Fried PA, Makin JE. Neonatal behavioral correlates of prenatal exposure to marijuana in a low risk population. *Neurotoxicol Teratol* 1987;9:1

166. Dreher MC, Nugent K, Hudgins R. Prenatal marijuana exposure and neonatal outcomes in Jamaica: an ethnographic study. *Pediatrics* 1994;93:254.

167. Wheeler SF. Substance abuse during pregnancy. *Prim Care* 1993;20:191–207.

168. Beaconsfield P, Ginsburg J, Rainsbury R. Marijuana smoking: cardiovascular effects in man and possible mechanisms. *N Engl J Med* 1972;287:209–212.

169. Stoelting RK, Martz RC, Gartner J, et al. Effects of delta 9-tetra-break hydrocannabinol on halothane MAC in dogs. *Anesthesiology* 1973;38:521–524.

170. Vitez TS, Way WL, Miller RD, et al. Effects of delta 9-tetrahydrocannabinol on cyclopropane MAC in the rat. *Anesthesiology* 1973;38:525–527.

171. Ltasch L, Christ R. Probleme der anaesthesie bei Drogen-abhängigen. *Anaesthesist* 1988;37:123–139.

Shnider and Levinson's Anesthesia for Obstetrics,
edited by Samuel C. Hughes, et al.
Lippincott Williams & Wilkins,
Philadelphia, © 2001.

CHAPTER 35

FETAL EVALUATION: ROUTINE AND INDICATED TESTS

SARAH J. KILPATRICK, M.D., Ph.D. AND
RUSSELL K. LAROS, JR., M.D.

A variety of tests are currently available to aid the clinician in fetal evaluation. These tests generally fall into two categories: those offered as a part of routine prenatal care and those utilized when indicated by a specific risk factor. The anesthesiologist should be aware of the fetal status before undertaking care of the mother. Problems such as intrauterine growth restriction, prematurity, or the presence of fetal anomalies may influence the choice of anesthesia. All available tests are not reviewed in this chapter; rather, discussion is limited to routine and indicated tests that have found the widest clinical acceptance. In each instance, the physiologic basis for the particular study is briefly reviewed, and those clinical situations where it is of greatest value are discussed. For a glossary of abbreviations used throughout this chapter, see Table 35.1.

FIRST AND SECOND TRIMESTER FETAL EVALUATION

Aneuploidy and Neural Tube Defect Screening

The risk of aneuploidy, numeric chromosome abnormalities, increases with maternal age. At age 35, the risk is approximately 0.5% at term and 0.8% in the second trimester. Traditionally, women 35 years old and older have been offered invasive tests (discussed below) to determine fetal chromosomes. However, there is a 0.5% risk of miscarriage with these tests (1). Because of this risk there has been much interest in developing noninvasive tools to better predict risk of aneuploidy and thus reduce the number of women who choose an invasive test. Since most fetuses with aneuploidy are actually born to women under 35 (only 20% of trisomy 21 occurs in women over age 34 because more women under 35 are having babies), the screening tests are offered to all women. Another group of anomalies, neural tube defects such as anencephaly and meningomyelecele, can be detected with a serum screen as well. The incidence of neural tube defects is not increased with maternal age. Early identification of these defects can allow termination if desired.

Maternal Serum Triple Marker Screening

As implied in the name, three maternal serum analytes are used currently as markers for elevated risk of aneuploidy or neural tube defects. These are alpha-fetoprotein (AFP), estriol, and beta-human chorionic gonadotropin (hCG). Because all three markers are gestational age–dependent, the test is useful only when performed between 15 and 20 weeks' gestation, and the gestational age of the pregnancy is known (2). The purpose of triple marker screening is to provide an individual patient with her specific risk for trisomy 18, trisomy 21, and neural tube defect.

AFP is produced primarily in the fetal liver with lesser amounts coming from the yolk sac and the gastrointestinal tract. The fetal serum level reaches a maximum at 13 weeks' gestation and declines thereafter, becoming virtually absent after the age of

2 years. Amniotic fluid levels parallel the fetal serum levels at a ratio of about 1:150, with the maximum levels occurring at 12 to 14 weeks' gestation. The maternal serum levels are lower than the fetal levels by a factor of 10,000. However, maternal serum levels increase progressively until the 32nd week of pregnancy and then decline modestly to term. Normal values are usually defined at a given gestational age based on multiples of the median (MOM). Values greater than 2.5 MOM are considered abnormally high, and those less than 0.4 MOM are considered low (3, 4). Trisomy 21 and trisomy 18 are associated with a lower maternal serum alpha-fetoprotein (MSAFP), and utilizing AFP alone 25% of trisomy 21 fetuses will be detected (5).

In the majority of fetuses with an open neural tube defect, the amniotic fluid AFP and consequently the maternal serum AFP will be elevated. In fact, 80% of fetal neural tube defects, including anencephaly and meningomyelecele, can be identified by a maternal serum AFP greater than 2.0 MOM if screened between 15 and 20 weeks' gestation (6, 7). Abnormally high or low MSAFP values must be appropriately evaluated to rule in or out the various conditions listed in Table 35.2. The standard evaluation includes a level 2 ultrasound and possibly an amniocentesis for fetal chromosome and amniotic fluid AFP evaluation. Cases of unexplained, high MSAFP should have antepartum fetal surveillance in the third trimester because of the association of intrauterine growth restriction (IUGR), fetal demise and oligohydramnios in these women (8, 9). Unexplained elevated MSAFP may be a marker for a placental abnormality resulting in too much AFP leaking into the maternal serum as well as a later poor outcome (10).

Soon after the implementation of routine AFP screening, data became available that incorporating estriol and hCG levels added sensitivity to the screening tool for identifying fetuses at increased risk for trisomy 21 and 18 defects (11). Triple marker screening will detect 60% of fetal trisomy 21 in women under age 35 and 90% in women older than 35 (2, 12, 13). In addition, triple marker screening will detect 60% of trisomy 18 fetuses (14).

During the first few weeks of pregnancy the corpus luteum produces most of the circulating estrogens. With regression of the corpus luteum, maternal estrogens do not decrease, but rather there is a sharp rise in maternal plasma estrone (E_1), estradiol (E_2), and estriol (E_3). This rise is due to increased placental production of estrogens from conversion of fetal 16 alpha-DHEA-S. The 16 alpha-DHEA-S in turn comes from conversion of diethylstilboestrol (DES) produced by fetal adrenal and liver (15). Before estriol was used as a second trimester screening test, urinary estriol was followed in the third trimester as a marker of fetal well-being in high-risk pregnancies because normal levels were dependent on normal fetal adrenal function (16). Urinary estriol surveillance for fetal well-being has been replaced by more sensitive and specific tests of antepartum fetal testing. However, second trimester maternal serum estriol has proven to be important for aneuploidy screening (2). HCG is also produced by the trophoblastic tissue and is highest in the

Table 35.1. GLOSSARY OF TERMS USED WITH ABBREVIATIONS

Alpha-fetoprotein (AFP)
Amniotic fluid index (AFI)
Beta-human chorionic gonadotropin (hCG)
Biparietal diameter (BPD)
Biophysical profile (BPP)
Chorionic villus sampling (CVS)
Contraction stress test (CST)
Estrone (E$_1$)
Estradiol (E$_2$)
Estriol (E$_3$)
Fetal lung maturity index (FLM)
Intrauterine growth restriction (IUGR)
Lecithin/spingomyelin (L/S ratio)
Maternal serum alpha-fetoprotein (MSAFP)
Multiples of the median (MOM)
Nonstress test (NST)
Oxytocin challenge test (OCT)
Phosphatidylglycerol (PG)
Respiratory distress syndrome (RDS)
Surfactant/albumin (SA ratio)
Systolic/diastolic (SD ratio)
Vibroacoustic stimulation (VAS)

first 12 weeks. It was noted that estriol is decreased in fetuses with trisomy 21 and trisomy 18, and hCG is increased in those with trisomy 21 but decreased in those with trisomy 18 (17–19). Based on these associations, curves incorporating maternal serum AFP, estriol, and hCG values between 15 and 20 weeks with gestational age, maternal age, weight, race and smoking history were computer generated to produce a specific risk of the mother having a fetus with trisomy 21 or 18. The patient may use this information to decide if she wants an amniocentesis to evaluate chromosomes. In general, since the risk of miscarriage from an amniocentesis is 0.5%, unless the risk for aneuploidy is higher, amniocentesis is not offered. Second trimester maternal serum marker screening is now a part of routine prenatal care throughout the United States. New analytes including serum inhibin A, urinary hCG and total estrogens are currently being investigated for use as aneuploidy screening tools (20–22).

Nuchal Translucency Screening

Nuchal translucency (NT) screening is a new technique to assess aneuploidy risk (23). An ultrasound of the fetus is done at 10 to 14 weeks' gestation and the nuchal fold is measured. The measurement is recorded into a computer program, that af-

Table 35.2. CONDITIONS ASSOCIATED WITH ABNORMAL MATERNAL α-FETOPROTEIN LEVELS

Elevated
Neural tube defects
Multiple gestations
Fetal death
Abdominal wall defects: omphalocele and gastroschisis
Esophageal and duodenal atresia
Congenital nephrosis
Cystic hygroma
Subsequent intrauterine growth restriction and poor fetal outcome
Renal anomalies
Sacrococcygeal teratoma
Underestimation of fetal age

Low
Chromosomal abnormalities (especially trisomies)
Fetal death
Overestimation of gestational age

ter recording maternal and gestational age, calculates a specific aneuploidy risk. In a study of 96,000 women, 82% of aneuploidies were diagnosed by NT screening (23). The wider the nuchal translucency the higher the risk for aneuploidy.

Aneuploidy Determination

Invasive tests including chorionic villus sampling (CVS) and amniocentesis are offered routinely to women at age 35 and older, and to women who have had a screening test indicating an increased risk for aneuploidy (24). Both tests have a 0.5% risk of miscarriage. CVS is performed usually at 12 weeks' gestation and is a placental biopsy obtained by aspiration with a small catheter (25). The procedure is performed with ultrasound guidance either transcervically or transabdominally for easiest access to the placenta. The chorionic villi obtained are then cultured and fetal chromosomes determined. Results are generally available in 7 to 10 days. The advantage of this procedure is that the patient will know the chromosomes by about 14 weeks.

Amniocentesis is done between 16 and 18 weeks' gestation. Ultrasound guidance is used to obtain 20 mL of amniotic fluid from which fetal lymphocytes are cultured to determine chromosomes. Since they are harder to culture than villi, the results take longer: 10 to 14 days. The patient will have results back by 17 to 20 weeks' gestation. A final procedure to determine fetal chromosomes is to obtain fetal blood by percutaneous umbilical blood sampling or cordocentesis. With ultrasound guidance a needle is placed directly into the fetal umbilical vein or artery for blood sampling. This procedure has a much higher fetal loss risk of approximately 1% to 2% and is reserved for rare instances in the third trimester when knowledge of fetal chromosomes may affect delivery management (26). Fetal cells obtained by CVS, amniocentesis or cordocentesis may be used for DNA analysis to determine various genetic diseases. Essentially any genetic disease for which there has been a gene identified can be diagnosed in the fetus.

Ultrasonography

Prenatal ultrasound is virtually ubiquitous today even appearing in television advertisements for health insurance. Despite its patient appeal, it remains controversial whether routine antenatal ultrasound alters pregnancy outcome or is cost effective (27). There are two levels of ultrasound examination: basic and directed, sometimes referred to as level 1 and level 2. Another name for the directed ultrasound exam is a fetal survey. The difference in these examinations is the level of detail used. There are strict guidelines developed by the American Institute for Ultrasound in Medicine for level 1 ultrasound (28). In a level 1 ultrasound, fetal anatomy, age, weight, growth, placental location, amniotic fluid, cervix, adnexa, and uterus are assessed (Fig. 35.1). This is the standard ultrasound unless there is a specific concern for a fetal anomaly. A directed ultrasound is ordered when there is an increased risk for a specific fetal anomaly, e.g., an abnormal triple screen, a history of maternal anti-seizure medication use, or polyhydramnios (Fig. 35.2). A directed ultrasound examination includes the basic portion and a more detailed evaluation of the anatomic area of concern. For example, for the patient with an elevated MSAFP (neural tube defect risk) then the brain and spinal cord would be the anatomic areas closely examined. In general, directed ultrasounds are done in tertiary care centers or by physicians with particular training in prenatal ultrasonography. The most common indications for prenatal ultrasonography are determination of fetal dating, fetal growth, placental location, and examination for fetal anomalies.

Fetal Dating

Fetal age can be determined quite accurately with ultrasound. Because all fetuses start at about the same size but vary widely in

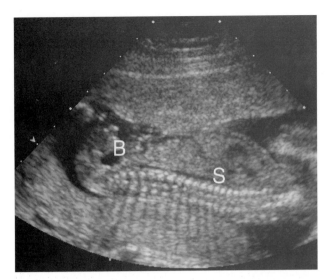

Figure 35.1. Level 1 sonogram performed at 18 weeks' gestation showing fetal spine and urinary bladder. S, spine; B, bladder. (Courtesy of Dr. R. Filly, University of California San Francisco.)

size as they approach term, the accuracy of an ultrasonic determination of age varies inversely with the age. Although a variety of structures can be measured and have been found to correlate well with fetal age, those most widely used are the biparietal diameter (BPD), gestational sac diameter, crown-rump length, abdominal circumference, and femur length. The use of a combination of measurements will usually give a more reliable estimate of fetal age. Crown rump length is the most accurate for dating and between 7 and 13 weeks the error in dating is no greater than 3 to 5 days (29). From 14 to 20 weeks' gestation, the error of an ultrasonically determined gestational age utilizing regression equations incorporating multiple measurements such as head circumference and femur length is plus or minus 8% or approximately 1 week (30). Dating in the third trimester is not accurate because the error is plus or minus 2 weeks and should not be used to change fetal dates. Thus, if dating is a concern then the ultrasound should be done in the first or second trimester if possible. In addition, there are now a number of reports presenting nomograms for estimation of fetal weight. The most common one is derived from Hadlock data and uses biparietal diameter, abdominal circumference, femur length and

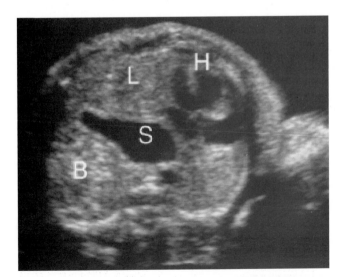

Figure 35.2. Level 2 sonogram at 22 weeks' gestation showing congenital diaphragmatic hernia. L, liver; H, heart; B, bowel; S, stomach. (Courtesy of Dr. R. Filly, University of California San Francisco.)

head circumference (29–30). Unfortunately, all current methods have a large margin of error particularly at the larger weights where the error may be as high as 15% (31).

Fetal Growth

As part of the basic ultrasound both an estimated fetal weight and percentile is usually reported. Percentiles between 10% and 90% are considered normal. A percentile of less than 10% is used as the definition of IUGR. Serial sonography can be used to follow percentiles. Campbell and Wilkin (32), using a second-degree polynomial regression formula, were able to identify infants weighing less than 5% below their expected weight for gestational age with a 95% confidence at 32 weeks' gestation; this accuracy decreased to 63% at 38 weeks. Their false-positive rate was just over 1% at all gestational ages. Unfortunately, other studies have not been nearly as successful at defining IUGR and suggest a specificity and sensitivity of ultrasonic diagnoses of only 70% (33, 34).

Another indication to perform ultrasound is to rule out fetal macrosomia. Macrosomia is characterized either as a fetal weight above the 90th percentile or greater than 4,000 or 4,500 g. The absolute weight definition is used because of the increased incidence of birth trauma experienced by these very large infants. Macrosomia may be constitutional but also may be secondary to maternal glucose intolerance. The highest incidence of birth injury is in macrosomic neonates of mothers with diabetes (35, 36). However, because of the high error in large fetuses, the utility of a macrosomia diagnosis is controversial (37–39). For example, one study suggested that, to prevent one permanent brachial plexus injury in fetuses with estimated weights of 4,500 grams or more, 3,695 cesarean sections would need to be performed for a cost of $8.7 million (39).

Placental Localization

Ultrasound can be used very effectively to locate the placenta. Such localization can be accomplished with 95% accuracy during the latter part of gestation and thus is very useful in the management of patients with antepartum hemorrhage. The diagnosis of placenta previa is made by ultrasound. However, the diagnosis of placental abruption is made clinically because there is a high false negative rate with ultrasound (40, 41).

Determination of Fetal Anomalies

A directed or level 2 fetal ultrasound is done when there is a suspicion of a fetal anomaly. The suspicion may be from the patient's history, an abnormal serum marker result, or an abnormality observed on a basic ultrasound. The accuracy in predicting fetal anomalies is best after 18 weeks gestation and thus directed scans generally are not done prior to that time. The importance of fetal anomaly determination is that it will give the patient and her physician the choices of termination, where to delivery her baby, and the possibility of fetal surgery. For example, if it is known that the fetus has an operable lesion such as a gastroschisis, then the patient should be delivered in a center that has pediatric surgery and a level 3 intensive care nursery. If there is concern for a fetal cardiac anomaly, then in addition to a level 2 scan a fetal echocardiogram should also be performed. The diagnostic accuracy of ultrasound is limited for cardiac anomalies and that accuracy is markedly improved with fetal echocardiography. The most common indications for fetal echocardiography are a prior baby with a cardiac anomaly, maternal or paternal congenital cardiac disease, and pregestational diabetes.

Limited Ultrasound

Finally, there are many times when ultrasound is used in a limited fashion. This terminology is used to indicate that the entire basic scan will not be done, but rather only a limited view will be taken. Limited use includes determination of fetal lie, use during a procedure such as an amniocentesis or fetal version, and evaluation of amniotic fluid volume during antepartum fetal testing.

THIRD TRIMESTER FETAL EVALUATION

The third trimester is generally defined as greater than 23 weeks and corresponds to fetal viability. In the past it was defined as greater than 27 weeks. Most of the tests to be described in this section are used to influence delivery timing and are used only if indicated. Thus, there are no routine third trimester tests for fetal evaluation. Ultrasound is often used in the third trimester and will only be mentioned briefly.

Determination of Lung Maturity

Determination of fetal lung maturity may be important to avoid delivering a baby at risk for respiratory distress syndrome (RDS) which is associated with significant morbidity and mortality. The clinical circumstances when determining fetal lung maturity are important and include preterm rupture of membranes, preterm labor, planning an elective cesarean section or induction before 39 weeks, and planning an elective cesarean section or induction in a pregestational diabetic patient.

Amniotic fluid can be obtained by transabdominal amniocentesis or collected transvaginally in the patient with ruptured membranes and analyzed by various tests for fetal lung maturity. The rational for the tests and the common tests available will be discussed below. Each test has a specific result associated with low risk of RDS, referred to as "mature." If the test result is less than the mature value it is referred to as "immature." If the result is immature then the physician has the option to delay delivery if possible or to give the mother corticosteroids to reduce the risk of RDS.

Amniotic Fluid Surfactant Determination

The pathophysiology of RDS and the measurement of amniotic fluid surfactant activity has been reviewed in detail (42). The surfactant complex is made up primarily of phospholipids, the most abundant of which is lecithin. Lecithin is secreted by type II alveolar cells and is excreted into the fetal trachea and thence into the amniotic fluid. During early gestation only a small amount of surfactant activity is present. However, with maturation of the appropriate enzyme system between 34 and 36 weeks' gestation, there is an abrupt rise in amniotic fluid surfactant activity (Fig. 35.3). This rise in activity above a critical level is accompanied by a virtual absence of RDS in the neonate. With any of the tests described below the risk of RDS with a mature lung index is < 2% (43, 44).

There are now multiple tests available to measure surfactant activity as markers for a low risk of RDS including the ratio of the major phospholipids lecithin and sphingomyelin (L/S ratio) as described by Gluck (45), and the fetal lung maturity index (FLM) or surfactant/albumin (SA) ratio (44, 46) and others (47). The L/S ratio is measured using thin-layer chromatography; a positive ratio is generally considered to be greater than 2 and assures a low risk that the fetus will develop RDS. The SA ratio is measured by fluorescence polarization and greater than or equal to 50 is considered mature. Phosphatidylglycerol (PG), the unique phospholipid of lung surfactant, first appears when the L/S ratio exceeds 2 and indicates secretion of mature lung surfactant. Analysis of PG in amniotic fluid serves as an additional index of lung maturity and may be less prone to error when the specimen is contaminated by blood (43, 47). Presence of PG is considered the most conservative measure of lung maturity because it has the fewest false positives that is the lowest risk of RDS. However, using the presence of PG as an indicator for lung immaturity will result in many false negatives. In other words, there will be mature L/S ratios before PG is present. Presence of PG is still considered the best test of fetal lung maturity in pregestational diabetics because of data

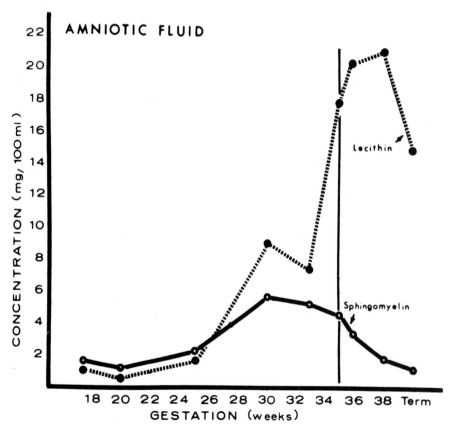

Figure 35.3. Levels of lecithin and sphingomyelin in amniotic fluid at increasing gestational ages. An acute rise in lecithin at 35 weeks marks pulmonary maturity. (From Gluck L, Kulovich MV, Borer RC Jr, et al. The diagnosis of the respiratory distress syndrome (RDS) by amniocentesis. *Am J Obstet Gynecol* 1971;109:440–445, with permission.)

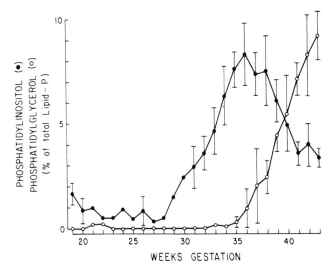

Figure 35.4. The content of PI (*solid circles*) and PG (*open circles*) in amniotic fluid during normal gestation. The phospholipids were quantified by measuring the phosphorus (P) content and expressed as percentages of total lipid phosphorus. Mean ± SD of three to five samples are shown for each point. (From Hallman M, Kulovich M, Kirkpatrick E, et al. Phosphatidylinositol and phosphatidylglycerol in amniotic fluid: indices of lung maturity. *Am J Obstet Gynecol* 1976;125:613–623, with permission.)

suggesting delayed lung maturity in fetuses of diabetic mothers (48–50). The relative percentage of phospholipid represented by phosphatidylinositol and PG in amniotic fluid at varying gestational ages is depicted in Figure 35.4. Measuring surfactant activity will aid the clinician in timing deliveries in a variety of situations. Hack and associates (51) found that 12% of all infants admitted to the intensive care nursery with RDS were the products of elective interventions (cesarean sections or inductions). These findings suggest that some study of lung maturity should be used before elective repeat cesarean section or induction of labor in almost every case. The American College of Obstetricians and Gynecologists (ACOG) has recommended that an amniocentesis for lung maturity should be performed in any pregnancy when an elective induction or cesarean section is planned before 39 weeks' gestation (52).

Fetal Therapy

In addition to rapid karyotyping, cordocentesis may be used to obtain a sample of fetal blood for other indications. The most common indications for this procedure are determination of fetal hemoglobin and fetal transfusion in suspected fetal anemia, such as fetal hydrops or isoimmunization with Rh or atypical red cell antigens. Rarer indications are evaluation of fetal platelet count in alloimmune thrombocytopenia and suspected intrauterine infection (53, 54). There are significant risks to cordocentesis including fetal bradycardia, fetal loss, amnionitis and rupture of membranes (26).

Fetal Anemia

The most common cause of fetal anemia is isoimmunization from atypical red cell antibodies such as anti-Kell, anti-Kidd, and Rh antibodies such as anti-c, C, D, e, and E. If the maternal antibody screen is positive and the titer is greater than $\frac{1}{8}$ or rising, then amniocentesis is offered to determine amniotic fluid bilirubin as a marker of fetal hemolysis. Bilirubin is found in the amniotic fluid of normal pregnancies between the 12th and 36th week of gestation. The analysis for bilirubin is done spectrophotometrically by scanning the absorbance of amniotic fluid at wave lengths at 450 nm (Fig. 35.5). The delta OD 450, as a marker of bilirubin concentration in amniotic fluid, is then

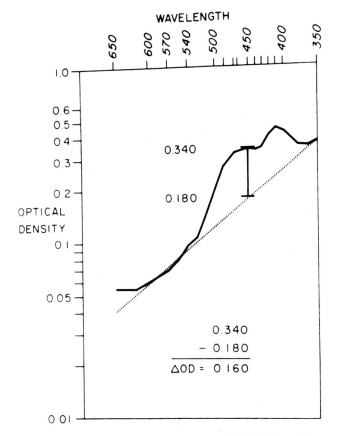

Figure 35.5. Determination of ΔOD 450 in amniotic fluid. An arbitrary *broken line* has been drawn connecting the spectrophotometric readings obtained at 375 and 600 nm. The *solid vertical line* represents the ΔOD at 450 nm. (From Merkatz IR, Aladjem S, Little B. The value of biochemical estimations on amniotic fluid in management of the high-risk pregnancy. *Clin Perinatol* 1974;1:301–319, with permission.)

plotted by gestational age on a Liley graph to determine severity of the disease (55–57). Appropriate management, including intrauterine fetal transfusion, early delivery, subsequent amniocentesis or no therapeutic intervention, is determined from where on the Liley graph the OD 450 falls (Fig. 35.6) (55, 58, 59). If the result is in high zone 2 or zone 3, then delivery or fetal transfusion is warranted because there is a high likelihood of severe fetal anemia and death if nothing is done. If the result is in zone 1 observation is appropriate.

Direct intravascular transfusion via cordocentesis is the usual route of transfusion for the anemic fetus. This approach allows a pre-transfusion and post-transfusion measurement of the fetal hematocrit. Occasionally if it is difficult to perform an intravascular transfusion, a fetal intraperitoneal transfusion can be done. The current approach to diagnosis and treatment should allow a woman with severe isoimmunization an 80% to 90% chance of a successful fetal outcome (60–62). Long-term outcome in these fetuses is excellent (63). The same technique of fetal blood sampling and possible fetal platelet transfusion is used in the management of fetuses with alloimmune thrombocytopenia (64).

ANTEPARTUM FETAL SURVEILLANCE

Antepartum fetal surveillance includes a number of tests designed to assess fetal well-being. These tests should only be used if indicated because like all screening tests there is a significant risk of false positives in a low prevalence population. The purpose of antepartum surveillance is to identify the fetus at risk for stillbirth or significant morbidity. The tests most commonly used

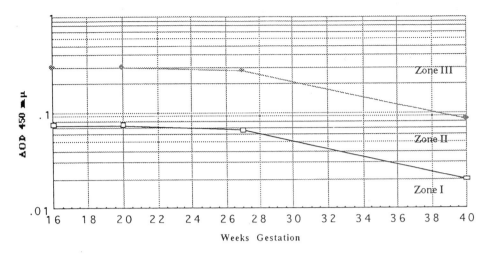

Figure 35.6. An example of the Liley curve used to assess severity of isoimmunization by plotting ΔOD 450 by gestational age. (Adapted from Merkatz IR, Aladjem S, Little B. The value of biochemical estimations on amniotic fluid in management of the high-risk pregnancy. *Clin Perinatol* 1974;1:301–319.)

today depend on the underlying concept that fetal well-being can be accurately predicted by a combination of events including accelerations of the fetal heart rate, normal fetal movement, lack of fetal heart rate decelerations with contractions, and normal volume of amniotic fluid. The three most common testing schemes used are nonstress test (NST) and amniotic fluid assessment; contraction stress test (CST); and biophysical profile (BPP). As described below, the sensitivity and specificity of these three tests for predicting fetal demise are similar with a false negative rate of ≤ 0.8/1000 or less, so the choice of which test to use is up to the provider (65–67).

Nonstress Test and Amniotic Fluid Assessment

The NST is so named because it does not require contractions (stress) to assess the fetus. The normal response is a reactive NST defined as the presence of at least two heart rate accelerations 15 beats above the fetal heart rate baseline lasting 15 seconds in 20 minutes. The presence of a reactive NST is associated with a false negative rate of 3% (65). That is, there is a 3% likelihood that the fetus will not be alive in one week after a reactive NST. If after 20 minutes the NST is nonreactive there are several methods to stimulate the fetus including giving the mother oral fluids or IV fluids and using vibroacoustic stimulation (VAS). VAS evolved from observations of fetal heart rate change in response to

various stimuli, including sound. The sound stimulus most commonly used is an electronic artificial larynx, which generates sound levels averaging 82 dB. A stimulus is applied for 1 second with repeated applications at 1 minute intervals for a maximum of three times if no accelerations are noted after the initial application. Two or more accelerations of at least 15 bpm lasting 15 seconds in a 10 minute period constitutes a reactive test. Reactivity after VAS has the same predictive value as spontaneous reactivity (68). VAS has also recently been used during labor to evaluate a nonreactive strip with reduced variability (69). Persistent nonreactive NSTs require further evaluation such as a CST or BPP. When amniotic fluid volume is also assessed and found to be in the normal range, the false negative rate of the NST and AF assessment is 0.8/1,000 (67). The most commonly used technique of amniotic fluid assessment is the amniotic fluid index (AFI) (71). The normal range of AFI is 8.1 to 24 cm. An AFI of less than 5.1 is oligohydramnios and 5.1 to 8.0 is considered low normal (71). The combination of NST and AFI is the most often used scheme for antenatal testing and is also called the modified BPP (67).

Contraction Stress Test

The Contraction Stress Test (CST) is considered a stress test because it evaluates the fetal heart rate response to repeated

Table 35.3. SCORING SYSTEM FOR THE BIOPHYSICAL PROFILE

Biophysical Variable	Normal (Score = 2)	Abnormal (Score = 0)
1. Fetal breathing movements	At least one episode of at least 30 sec duration in 30-min observation	Absent or no episode of ≥30 sec in 30 min
2. Gross body movement	At least three discrete body/limb movements in 30 min (episodes of active continuous movement considered as a single movement)	Two or fewer episodes of body/limb movements in 30 min
3. Fetal tone	At least one episode of active extension with return to flexion of fetal limb (s) or trunk. Opening and closing of hand considered normal tone	Either slow extension with return to partial flexion or movement of limb in full extension or absent fetal movement
4. Reactive fetal heart rate	At least two episodes of acceleration of ≥15 bpm and at least 15-sec duration associated with fetal movement in 30 min	Less than two accelerations or acceleration < 15 bpm in 30 min
5. Qualitative amniotic fluid volume	At least one pocket of amniotic fluid that measures at least 1 cm in two perpendicular planes	Either no amniotic fluid pockets or a pocket < 1 cm in two perpendicular planes

From Manning FA, Morrison I, Lang IR, et al. Antepartum determination of fetal health: composite biophysical profile scoring. *Clin Perinatol* 1982;9:285–296, with permission.

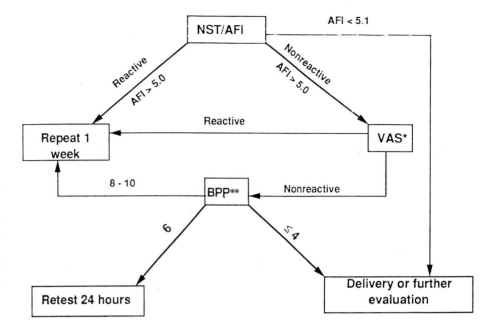

Figure 35.7. A schema for antepartum fetal heart rate testing using the modified biophysical profile. NST, nonstress test; AFI, amniotic fluid index; VAS, vibroacoustic stimulation; BPP, biophysical profile. **If NST has decelerations, consider CST rather than BPP. If CST is negative, retest in 1 week. If CST is positive, deliver or hospitalize. (Adapted from Everston LR, Gauathier RJ, Schifrin BS, et al. Antepartum fetal heart rate testing. *Am J Obstet Gynecol* 1979;133:29–33.)

contractions. During a uterine contraction there is a significant fall in uteroplacental blood flow and thus, a decrease in the amount of oxygen delivered to the fetus. The normal fetoplacental unit has sufficient respiratory reserve to withstand uterine contractions without production of transient episodes of fetal hypoxia and hypercarbia. However, in situations of placental insufficiency, the added stress of contractions may cause transient hypoxia and hypercarbia that is reflected by changes in the fetal heart rate pattern (see Chapter 36). The normal response is either accelerations or no decelerations and is referred to as a negative CST which is associated with continued fetal well-being for at least 7 days (65). An abnormal or non- reassuring response is repetitive late decelerations associated with the majority of contractions and is called a positive CST (72, 73). A positive CST warrants delivery or continuous monitoring. A positive CST does not necessarily require a cesarean section for delivery because many patients with a positive CST will tolerate labor. To be adequate a CST must have three uterine contractions felt by the mother in ten minutes. A suspicious CST is one that does not meet criteria for either negative or positive and warrants additional testing. The false negative rate of a negative CST is 0.1% for fetal death in one week (74). Contractions for a CST may be generated spontaneously with oxytocin (oxytocin challenge test: OCT) or by breast stimulation. Uterine contractions and fetal heart rate are monitored with an external recording device. The method of performing an oxytocin challenge test has been detailed elsewhere (75).

Biophysical Profile

The biophysical profile (BPP) was developed because it was hoped that the assessment of multiple variables would better define fetal status (76, 77). Five variables: fetal breathing movements, fetal movements, fetal tone, amniotic fluid volume, and the nonstress test, are measured in the same observation period. The scoring system devised by Manning and associates (78) is shown in Table 35.3. A score of 8 to 10 is normal, 4 to 6 is suspect and should be repeated within 24 hours, and 0 to 2 indicates a very sick fetus that should be delivered immediately. The false negative rate of a BPP score of 8 to 10 is 0.1% (66, 77). The likelihood of stillbirth or neonatal demise increases significantly with falling BPP scores with the perinatal mortality risk of 8%, 15%, and 50% with BPP of 4, 2, and 0, respectively (79).

As noted above, the likelihood of a false negative result or stillbirth, is similar for all three of these testing schemes. Therefore, any of them may be used. Because the false positive rate

will increase in low-risk populations, resulting in inappropriate inductions, antenatal testing should be used only in high-risk pregnancies. Common indications for antepartum testing include postdates (beyond 41.5 weeks), hypertensive disease, diabetes mellitus, IUGR, history of previous stillbirth, unexplained elevated maternal serum AFP, twins with discordant growth or IUGR, cyanotic heart disease, hyperthyroidism and decreased fetal movement. Usually testing is performed weekly unless otherwise indicated. One schema for antepartum testing is shown in Figure 35.7.

DOPPLER VELOCIMETRY

Doppler velocimetry utilizes ultrasound to measure maternal and fetal blood flow. Figure 35.8 depicts flow as a function of time and is the type of waveform seen in the umbilical artery. The systolic/diastolic (S/D) ratio, Pourcelot ratio and pulsatility index have all been evaluated in a variety of clinical conditions. Data have been accumulated on umbilical, uterine, and

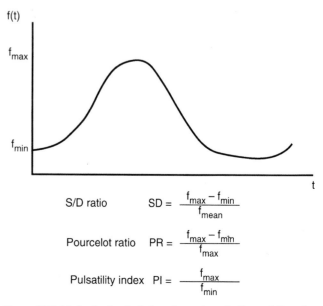

$$\text{S/D ratio} \quad SD = \frac{f_{max} - f_{min}}{f_{mean}}$$

$$\text{Pourcelot ratio} \quad PR = \frac{f_{max} - f_{min}}{f_{max}}$$

$$\text{Pulsatility index} \quad PI = \frac{f_{max}}{f_{min}}$$

Figure 35.8. Method of calculating the various indices of Doppler velocimetry.

fetal carotid artery blood flow with the hope that they may provide a better physiologic understanding of the cause of abnormal growth in both singleton and multiple pregnancies (80–82). Devoe and colleagues examined the diagnostic value of NST, amniotic fluid volume, and umbilical artery velocimetry in 1,000 high-risk patients (83). Unfortunately, Doppler velocimetry had the poorest sensitivity and the lowest positive predictive value. The role of Doppler velocimetry in routine antepartum testing is not yet clear because it has not been shown to provide better information than that provided by the standard tests: NST, AFI, BPP, or CST. However, in fetuses with IUGR Doppler assessment of umbilical blood flow may be helpful. If there is absent or reversed diastolic flow, suggesting high placental resistance, there is a high likelihood of fetal distress and perinatal mortality and delivery should be strongly considered (84).

CONCLUSION

There are now available a number of studies that aid the clinician in management of both normal and abnormal pregnancies. Thoughtful use of these studies does improve perinatal outcome. As new studies are developed and those presently available become better defined, even more accurate fetal surveillance and lower fetal morbidity and mortality can be anticipated.

REFERENCES

1. *NICHD Consensus Conference on Antenatal Diagnosis. NIH publication no. 80–1973.* Washington, DC: NIH, 1979.
2. Phillips OP, Elias S, Shulman LP, et al. Maternal serum screening for fetal Down syndrome in women less than 35 years of age using alpha-fetoprotein, hCG, and unconjugated estriol: a prospective 2-year study. *Obstet Gynecol* 1992;80:353–358.
3. Milunsky A, Flyate E. Prenatal diagnosis of neural tube defects: problems and pitfalls—analysis of 2495 cases using the fetoprotein assay. *Obstet Gynecol* 1976;48:1–5.
4. Richard DS, Seeds JW, Katz VL, et al. Elevated maternal-fetoprotein with normal ultrasound: Is amniocentesis always appropriate? A review of 20,069 screened patients. *Obstet Gynecol* 1988;71:203–207.
5. DiMaio MS, Baumgarten A, Greenstein RM, et al. Screening for fetal Down's syndrome in pregnancy by measuring maternal serum alpha-fetoprotein levels. *N Engl J Med* 1987;317:342–346.
6. Report of U.K. Collaborative Study on Alpha-fetoprotein in Relation to Neural-tube Defects. Maternal serum alpha-fetoprotein measurement in antenatal screening for anencephaly and spina bifida in early pregnancy. *Lancet* 1977;2:1323–1332.
7. American College of Obstetricians and Gynecologists. Maternal serum screening. *ACOG Educ Bull* 1996;228:1–9.
8. Simpson JL, Elias S, Morgan CD, et al. Does unexplained second-trimester (15 to 20 weeks' gestation) maternal serum alpha-fetoprotein elevation presage adverse perinatal outcome? *Am J Obstet Gynecol* 1991;164:829–836.
9. Wenstrom KD, Owen J, Davis RO, et al. Prognostic significance of unexplained elevated amniotic fluid alpha-fetoprotein. *Obstet Gynecol* 1996;87:213–216.
10. Katz VL, Chescheir NC, Cefalo RC. Unexplained elevations of maternal serum alpha-fetoprotein. *Obstet Gynecol Surv* 1990;45:719–726.
11. MacDonald ML, Wagner RM, Slotnick RN. Sensitivity and specificity of screening for Down syndrome with alpha-fetoprotein, hCG, unconjugated estriol, and maternal age. *Obstet Gynecol* 1991;77:63–68.
12. Haddow JE, Palomaki GE, Knight GJ, et al. Prenatal screening for Down's syndrome with use of maternal serum markers. *N Engl J Med* 1992;327:588–593.
13. Haddow JE, Palomaki GE, Knight GJ, et al. Reducing the need for amniocentesis in women 35 years of age or older with serum markers for screening. *N Engl J Med* 1994;330:1114–1118.
14. Canick JA, Palomaki GE, Osathanondh R. Prenatal screening for trisomy 18 in the second trimester. *Prenat Diagn* 1990;10:546–548.
15. Siiteri PK, MacDonald PC. Placental estrogen biosynthesis during human pregnancy. *J Clin Endocrinol Metab* 1966;26:751–761.

16. Distler W, Gabbe SG, Freeman RK, et al. Estriol in pregnancy. V. Unconjugated and total plasma estriol in management of pregnant diabetic patients. *Am J Obstet Gynecol* 1978;130:424–431.
17. Bogart MH, Pandian MR, Jones OW. Abnormal maternal serum chorionic gonadotropin levels in pregnancies with fetal chromosome abnormalities. *Prenat Diagn* 1987;7:623.
18. Canick JA, Knight GJ, Palomaki GE, et al. Low second trimester maternal serum unconjugated oestriol in pregnancies with Down's syndrome. *Br J Obstet Gynaecol* 1988;95:330.
19. Merkatz IR, Nitowsky HM, Macri JN, et al. An association between low maternal serum alpha-fetoprotein and fetal chromosomal abnormalities. *Am J Obstet Gynecol* 1984;148:886–889.
20. Casals E, Fortuny A, Grudzinskas JG, et al. First-trimester biochemical screening for Down syndrome with the use of PAPP-A, AFP, and beta-hCG. *Prenat Diagn* 1996;16:405–410.
21. Cuckle HS, Iles RK, Sehmi IK, et al. Urinary multiple marker screening for Down's syndrome. *Prenat Diagn* 1995;15:745–751.
22. Wenstrom KD, Chu DC, Owen J, et al. Maternal serum alpha-fetoprotein and dimeric inhibin A detect aneuploidies other than Down syndrome. *Am J Obstet Gynecol* 1998;179:966–970.
23. Snijders RJ, Noble P, Sebire N, et al. UK multicentre project on assessment of risk of trisomy 21 by maternal age and fetal nuchal-translucency thickness at 10 - 14 weeks of gestation. Fetal Medicine Foundation First Trimester Screening Group. *Lancet* 1998;352:343–346.
24. Golbus MS, Conte FA, Schneider EL, et al. Intrauterine diagnosis of genetic defects, results, problems, and follow-up of 100 cases in a prenatal genetic detection center. *Am J Obstet Gynecol* 1974;118:897–905.
25. Rhoads GG, Jackson LG, Schlesselman SE, et al. The safety and efficacy of chorionic villus sampling for early prenatal diagnosis of cytogenetic abnormalities. *N Engl J Med* 1989;320:609–617.
26. Weiner CP, Wenstrom KD, Sipes SL, et al. Risk factors for cordocentesis and fetal intravascular transfusion. *Am J Obstet Gynecol* 1991;165:1020–1025.
27. Ewigman BG, Crane JP, Frigoletto FD, et al. Effect of prenatal ultrasound screening on perinatal outcome. *N Engl J Med* 1993;329:821–827.
28. Callen PW, ed. The obstetric ultrasound examination. In: *Ultrasonography in Obstetrics and Gynecology.* Philadelphia: WB Saunders, 1994:1–14.
29. Hadlock FP. Ultrasound determination of menstrual age. In: Callen PW, ed. *Ultrasonography in Obstetrics and Gynecology.* Philadelphia: WB Saunders, 1994:86–101.
30. Hadlock FP, Deter LR, Harrist RB, et al. Estimating fetal age: computer assisted analysis of multiple fetal growth parameters. *Radiology* 1984;152:497.
31. Hadlock FP, Harrist RB, Fearneyhough TC, et al. Use of femur length/abdominal circumference ratio in detecting the macrosomic fetus. *Radiology* 1984;154:503–505.
32. Campbell S, Wilkin D. Ultrasonic measurement of fetal abdominal circumference in the estimation of fetal weight. *Br J Obstet Gynaecol* 1975;82:689–697.
33. Gross BH, Callen PW, Filly RA. The relationship of fetal transverse body diameter and biparietal diameter in the diagnosis of intrauterine growth retardation. *J Ultrasound Med* 1982;1:361–365.
34. Manning FA, Hill LM, Platt LD. Qualitative amniotic fluid volume determination by ultrasound: antepartum detection of intrauterine growth retardation. *Am J Obstet Gynecol* 1981;139:254–258.
35. Acker DB, Sachs BP, Friedman EA. Risk factors for shoulder dystocia. *Obstet Gynecol* 1985;66:762–768.
36. Modanlou HD, Komatsu G, Dorchester W, et al. Large-for-gestational age neonates: anthropometric reasons for shoulder dystocia. *Obstet Gynecol* 1982;60:417–423.
37. Gonen O, Rosen DJD, Dolfin Z, et al. Induction of labor versus expectant management in macrosomia: a randomized study. *Obstet Gynecol* 1997;89:913–917.
38. Kolderup LB, Laros RK, Musci TJ. Incidence of persistent birth injury in macrosomic infants: association with mode of delivery. *Am J Obstet Gynecol* 1997;177:37–41.
39. Rouse DJ, Owen J, Goldenberg RL, et al. The effectiveness and costs of elective cesarean delivery for fetal macrosomia diagnosed by ultrasound. *JAMA* 1996;276:1480–1486.
40. Kobayashi M, Hillman LM, Fillsti L. Placental localization. *Am J Obstet Gynecol* 1970;106:279–285.
41. Kuhlmann RS, Warsof S. Ultrasound of the placenta. *Clin Obstet Gynecol* 1996;39:519–534.

42. Gluck L. Fetal maturity and amniotic fluid surfactant determinants. In: Spellacy WN, ed. *Management of the High-risk Pregnancy*. Baltimore: University Park Press, 1976:189.

43. Kulovich MV, Hallman MB, Gluck L. The lung profile. I. Normal lung. *Am J Obstet Gynecol* 1979;135:57–63.

44. Russell JC, Cooper CM, Ketchum CH, et al. Multicenter evaluation of TDx test for assessing fetal lung maturity. *Clin Chem* 1989;35:1005–1010.

45. Gluck L, Kulovich MV, Borer RC, et al. Diagnosis of respiratory distress by amniocentesis. *Am J Obstet Gynecol* 1971;109:440–445.

46. Hagen E, Link JC, Arias F. A comparison of the accuracy of the TDx-FLM assay, lecithin-sphingomyelin ratio, and phosphatidylglycerol in the prediction of neonatal respiratory distress syndrome. *Obstet Gynecol* 1993;82:1004–1008.

47. Hallman M, Kulovich M, Kirkpatrick E, et al. Phosphatidylinositol and phosphatidylglycerol in amniotic fluid: indices of lung maturity. *Am J Obstet Gynecol* 1976;125:613–623.

48. Kulovich MV, Gluck L. The lung profile: II. Complicated pregnancies. *Am J Obstet Gynecol* 1979;136:64.

49. Ylinen K. High maternal levels of hemoglobin A1c associated with delayed fetal lung maturation in insulin-dependent diabetic pregnancies. *Acta Obstet Gynecol Scand* 1987;66:263–266.

50. Landon MB, Gabbe SG. Fetal surveillance in the pregnancy complicated by diabetes mellitus. *Clin Obstet Gynecol* 1991;34:535–543.

51. Hack M, Fanaroff AA, Klaus M, et al. Neonatal respiratory distress following elective delivery: a preventable disease? *Am J Obstet Gynecol* 1976;126:43–47.

52. American College of Obstetricians and Gynecologists. Assessment of fetal lung maturity. *ACOG Educ Bull* 1996;230:1–7.

53. Ryan G, Morrow RJ. Fetal blood transfusion. *Fetal Drug Ther* 1994;21:573–587.

54. Weiner CP. Cordocentesis for diagnostic indications: two years' experience. *Obstet Gynecol* 1987;70:664–668.

55. Duerbeck NB, Seeds JW. Rhesus immunization in pregnancy: a review. *Obstet Gynecol Surv* 1993;48:801–810.

56. Bevis DCA. Blood pigment in haemolytic disease of the newborn. *J Obstet Gynaecol Br Commonw* 1956;63:68–75.

57. Liley AW. Liquor amnii analysis in management of pregnancy complicated by Rhesus sensitization. *Am J Obstet Gynecol* 1961;82:1359–1370.

58. Bowman JM. Management of Rh-isoimmunization. *Obstet Gynecol* 1978;52:1–9.

59. Whitfield CR. A three-year assessment of an action line method of timing intervention in rhesus isoimmunization. *Am J Obstet Gynecol* 1970;108:1239–1244.

60. Rodeck CH, Letsky E. How the management of erythroblastosis fetalis has changed. *Br J Obstet Gynaecol* 1989;96:759–763.

61. Harman CR, Bowman JM, Manning FA, et al. Intraperitoneal versus intravascular approach: a case-control comparison. *Am J Obstet Gynecol* 1990;162:1053–1059.

62. Parer JT. Severe Rh isoimmunization: current methods of in utero diagnosis and treatment. *Am J Obstet Gynecol* 1988;158:1323–1329.

63. Hudon L, Moise KJ, Hegemier SE, et al. Long-term neurodevelopmental outcome after intrauterine transfusion for treatment of fetal hemolytic disease. *Am J Obstet Gynecol* 1998;179:858–863.

64. Bussel JB, Berkowitz RL, Lynch L, et al. Antenatal management of alloimmune thrombocytopenia with IV IgG: a randomized trial of the addition of low-dose steroids to IV IgG. *Am J Obstet Gynecol* 1996;174:1414–1423.

65. Freeman RK, Anderson G, Dorchester W. A prospective multi-institutional study of antepartum fetal heart rate monitoring. II. Contraction stress test versus nonstress test for primary surveillance. *Am J Obstet Gynecol* 1982;143:778–781.

66. Manning FA, Morrison I, Harman CR, et al. Fetal assessment based on fetal biophysical profile scoring: experience in 19,221 referred high-risk pregnancies. II. An analysis of false-negative fetal deaths. *Am J Obstet Gynecol* 1987;157:880–884.

67. Miller DA, Rabello YA, Paul RH. The modified biophysical profile: antepartum testing in the 1990s. *Am J Obstet Gynecol* 1996;174:812–817.

68. Smith CV, Phelan JP, Platt LD, et al. Fetal acoustic stimulation testing. II. A randomized clinical comparision with the nonstress test. *Am J Obstet Gynecol* 1986;155:131–134.

69. Zimmer EZ, Divon MY. Fetal vibroacoustic stimulation. *Obstet Gynecol* 1993;81:451–457.

70. Phelan JP, Ohn MO, Smith CV, et al. Amniotic fluid index measurements during pregnancy. *J Reprod Med* 1987;32:603–604.

71. Moore TR, Cayle JE. The amniotic fluid index in normal human pregnancy. *Am J Obstet Gynecol* 1990;162:1168–1173.

72. Farahani G, Vasudeva K, Petric RH, et al. Oxytocin challenge test in high-risk pregnancy. *Obstet Gynecol* 1976;47:159–168.

73. Freeman RK. The use of the oxytocin challenge test for antepartum clinical evaluation of respiratory function. *Am J Obstet Gynecol* 1975;121:481–489.

74. Nageotte MP, Towers CV, Asrat T, et al. The value of a negative antepartum test: contraction stress test and modified biophysical profile. *Obstet Gynecol* 1994;84:231–234.

75. Ray M, Freeman R, Pine S, et al. Clinical experience with the oxytocin challenge test. *Am J Obstet Gynecol* 1972;114:1–9.

76. Manning FA, Platt L, Sipos L. Antepartum fetal evaluation: development of a fetal biophysical profile. *Am J Obstet Gynecol* 1980;136:787–795.

77. Manning FA, Morrison I, Lange IR, et al. Fetal assessment based on fetal biophysical profile scoring: experience in 12,620 referred high risk pregnancies. I. Perinatal mortality by frequency and etiology. *Am J Obstet Gynecol* 1985;151:343–350.

78. Manning FA, Morrison I, Lange IR, et al. Antepartum determination of fetal health: composite biophysical profile screening. *Clin Perinatol* 1982;9:285–296.

79. Manning FA, Morrison I, Harmon CR, et al. The abnormal fetal biophysical profile score. *Am J Obstet Gynecol* 1990;162:918–927.

80. Schulman H, Winter D, Farmakides G, et al. Pregnancy surveillance with Doppler velocimetry of uterine and umbilical arteries. *Am J Obstet Gynecol* 1989;160:192–199.

81. Wladimiroff J, Wijngaard J, Degani S, et al. Cerebral and umbilical artery blood velocity waveforms in normal and growth-retarded pregnancies. *Obstet Gynecol* 1987;69:705–710.

82. Giles W, Trudinger B, Cook C, et al. Umbilical artery blood flow velocity waveforms and twin pregnancy outcome. *Obstet Gynecol* 1988;72:894–899.

83. Devoe L, Gardner P, Dear C, et al. The diagnostic values of concurrent nonstress testing, amniotic fluid measurement, and Doppler velocimetry in screening a general high-risk population. *Am J Obstet Gynecol* 1990;163:1040–1050.

84. Karsdorp VH, van Vugt JM, van Geijn HP, et al. Clinical significance of absent or reversed end diastolic velocity waveforms in umbilical artery. *Lancet* 1994;344:1664.

Shnider and Levinson's Anesthesia for Obstetrics,
edited by Samuel C. Hughes, et al.
Lippincott Williams & Wilkins,
Philadelphia, © 2001.

CHAPTER 36

ELECTRONIC FETAL MONITORING AND DIAGNOSIS OF FETAL ASPHYXIA

JULIAN T. PARER, M.D., PH.D. AND TEKOA L. KING, CNM, MPH

The purpose of electronic fetal heart rate (FHR) monitoring during labor is assessment of fetal oxygenation. Heart rate interpretation is one of the few tools available for assessing fetal status during labor and is the most commonly used method for fetal surveillance during labor in hospitals in the United States (1, 2). However, electronic fetal monitoring (EFM) is an imperfect tool. It has excellent sensitivity for identifying a non-hypoxic fetus but poor predictive value for accurately identifying a hypoxic fetus (3, 4). This is in part because the use of EFM mushroomed into clinical practice before the underlying physiology was well understood.

Intrauterine asphyxia is an uncommon cause of newborn depression but remains the primary adverse outcome one hopes to detect and avoid by EFM (4). The pathologic consequence of asphyxia in the fetus is injury to the developing fetal tissues, primarily the brain, with subsequent neurologic impairment. Historically, birth trauma and/or birth asphyxia were thought to be the origin of most congenital neurologic disorders. Although intrapartum asphyxia is one cause of neurologic disability in children, the majority of these disabilities remain unexplained (5). Evidence suggests that approximately 8% to 15% of cerebral palsy is secondary to intrapartum events (6). Review of the factors affecting the fetal response to asphyxia, the FHR patterns that reflect fetal hypoxemia and the pathophysiologic consequences of intrapartum asphyxia can explain this paradox.

HISTORY OF FETAL HEART RATE MONITORING

EFM was introduced into clinical practice in the early 1960s. Initially, the interpretation of FHR patterns was purely empirical, with a pattern being described as abnormal when a depressed fetus resulted. Transient decelerations of FHR were noted in some cases with a depressed fetus (7, 8). Others noted that variability of the FHR seemed to be a positive sign of fetal health (9). A major source of confusion in interpretation has been that so-called ominous patterns are actually associated with a healthy fetus in a significant number of cases (10, 11).

The first randomized-controlled trial of continuous electronic FHR monitoring compared to intermittent auscultation was published in 1976, and found a several-fold increase in cesarean sections in the groups monitored but no improvement in newborn outcome (12). Several randomized-controlled trials and a meta-analysis followed, with similar findings (13–21). Problems with these trials include inadequate patient numbers to show mortality rate differences compared with a very low intrinsic rate, poorly established and non-standardized criteria for diagnosis of fetal asphyxia (loosely called fetal distress), and differing criteria of fetal hazard for the monitored and unmonitored patient groups (3, 22). The reliability, validity and the relationship between FHR patterns, adverse outcome and ability of obstetric intervention to modify these outcomes had not been established when the randomized-control trails were performed. Overall, FHR interpretation has had a tendency to diagnose asphyxia too frequently, leading to an increased incidence of cesarean delivery.

Despite the limitations of the controlled trials and their findings, electronic FHR monitoring remains very popular and widely used in North America. Clinicians continue to rely heavily on intrapartum EFM for many reasons. The concept of using heart rate changes for the purpose of assessing oxygenation is based on known physiologic mechanisms, has strong biologic plausibility and is a reasonable hypothesis. Resolution of this dilemma necessitates a review of what is known to date about the physiology of the FHR and the factors that influence it.

ETIOLOGIES OF FETAL ASPHYXIA

There are four major mechanisms by which the fetus can experience intrapartum asphyxial stress: (a) decreased maternal arterial oxygen tension, (b) inadequate uterine blood flow to the intervillous space, (c) interruption of umbilical blood flow and rarely, (d) fetal pathology.

Decreased Maternal Arterial Oxygen Tension

A significant decrease in maternal oxygen tension is a relatively rare cause of fetal asphyxia in the intrapartum period. Maternal apnea, pulmonary edema, amniotic fluid embolus, or severe asthma are examples of clinical situations that can result in both maternal and fetal hypoxia.

Inadequate Uterine Blood Flow

Uterine blood flow is one of the major determinants of oxygen exchange across the placenta. Reduction below a certain level will result in inadequate fetal oxygen uptake. This may occur acutely (e.g., abruptio placentae or maternal hypotension with spinal anesthesia), chronically (e.g., severe pregnancy-induced hypertension), or intermittently and/or transiently (e.g., maternal hypotension secondary to supine positioning). Initiation of epidural anesthesia with a resultant sympathectomy can be followed by a brief deceleration that is generally clinically benign if maternal hypotension is promptly corrected.

Interruption of Umbilical Blood Flow

Oxygen delivery from the fetal side of the placenta to the fetal body depends on adequate blood flow in the umbilical cord. When the umbilical cord is occluded fetal hypertension results, which initiates a vagal response that stimulates fetal bradycardia. If the occlusion is intermittent in an otherwise healthy fetus, the FHR will intermittently decrease as evidenced by variable decelerations.

Fetal Pathology

Rarely, the fetus with a co-existing problem may be at increased risk for asphyxia. For example, a fetus with an increased metabolic rate (e.g., pyrexia) or decreased oxygen carrying capacity (e.g., anemia from Rh sensitization) may be less tolerant of the intermittent decreases in oxygen delivery that occur during uterine contractions. In addition, the premature fetus may develop metabolic acidosis sooner than the full term infant under similar conditions.

FETAL RESPONSE TO ASPHYXIA

Asphyxia is a continuum of oxygen deficit that includes hypoxemia, hypercarbia, acidemia, and, ultimately, acidosis. In turn, the fetal response to different degrees of asphyxial insults ranges from a series of physiologic compensatory mechanisms to asphyxial damage.

Transient fetal hypoxemia secondary to cord occlusion or brief decreases in intervillous blood flow during uterine contractions is common during labor. The most important physiologic fetal response is hyperemia-induced redistribution of blood flow, which favors the heart, brain and adrenal glands (23, 24). During fetal hypoxemia, the arterial venous oxygen concentration difference across the myocardial and cerebral circulation decreases and the respective blood flows increase; therefore oxygen consumption of the heart and brain remain constant (23, 25, 26). In other organs and areas of the body, there is reduced blood flow and anaerobic metabolism. If the hypoxemic insult persists or reoccurs too frequently, lactic acid accumulation will result in metabolic acidosis.

When asphyxia becomes severe, these protective mechanisms are overwhelmed, and there is more intense and extensive vasoconstriction. At such degrees of hypoxia, oxygen consumption by all organs, including those previously favored decreases. This precedes a final bradycardia, hypotension, and death by a relatively short-time period. It is thought that hypoxic organ damage occurs during this phase when physiologic decompensation occurs (27).

CLINICAL FETAL HEART RATE MONITORING

Fetal Heart Rate Monitor

Commercial FHR monitors have two major components: a device for detecting each fetal cardiac cycle for processing of the beat-to-beat FHR and a second component for detecting uterine activity. Each of these is displayed on a two-channel strip chart recorder. Both FHR and uterine contractions can be monitored invasively or noninvasively.

Fetal Heart Rate Monitoring

The FHR can be monitored with a Doppler ultrasound transducer or fetal electrode applied directly to the fetal scalp. The most commonly used device is the noninvasive Doppler transducer, which is applied to the maternal abdomen over the fetal back or chest. It uses the frequency shift of an ultrasound wave directed toward the moving fetal heart for detection of cardiac cycles. The monitor counts the time interval between each heart

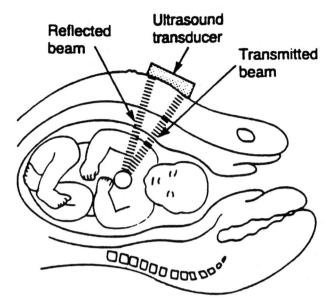

Figure 36.1. The Doppler ultrasound device for detecting cardiac activity. The frequency of the reflected beam is changed when it is reflected from a moving structure. (From Parer JT. *Handbook of Fetal Heart Rate Monitoring*, 2nd ed. Philadelphia: WB Saunders, 1997:104, with permission.)

beat detected, calculates heart rate based on each interval and displays the results every one to two beats. The data are also plotted on paper moving at a rate of 3 cm/min. Because there is variability in the time interval between each beat in a normally oxygenated fetus, the displayed and plotted line typically has a jagged, not smooth or straight appearance. Early Doppler technology tended to exaggerate the FHR variability but improvements in technology have resulted in Doppler recordings that sufficiently reflect actual FHR variability. Although the Doppler transducer is easy to apply, maternal or fetal movement, uterine contractions or maternal positions can interrupt a continuous recording. Another disadvantage is that certain data may be lost in processing of the signal. For example, several machines use a running average of adjacent or several beats to compensate for the lack of discreteness of the signal or for missing data. This tends to disguise some of the beat-to-beat variability (Fig. 36.1).

The direct fetal scalp electrode (FSE) is the most accurate way to assess the FHR but cannot be used unless the cervix is at least 1 to 3 centimeters dilated and the membranes have ruptured. In the invasive mode, an electrode is placed directly to the fetal scalp. A cardiotachometer uses the peak or a threshold voltage of the fetal R wave to measure the interval between each fetal cardiac cycle. The data are processed and displayed and plotted in the same fashion described for the Doppler (Fig. 36.2).

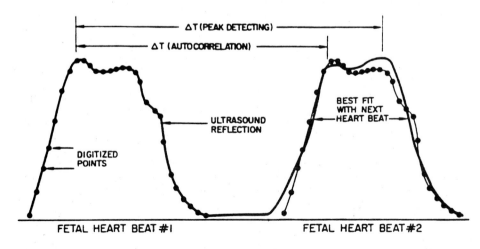

Figure 36.2. Waveforms of two ultrasound cardiac signals compare integration (peak-to-peak) of the first-generation electronic fetal monitor with autocorrelation of the second-generation electronic fetal monitor. (From Hewlett Packard Company, Palo Alto, CA, with permission.)

Uterine Activity Monitoring

During the intrapartum period, the FHR is interpreted relative to uterine activity. Therefore, interpretation of FHR patterns includes assessment of (a) frequency, (b) duration, (c) intensity, and (d) the uterine resting tone between contractions. Uterine activity can be determined by palpation, external tocodynamometer (*tokos* is Greek for childbirth), or the use of an intrauterine pressure catheter. The noninvasive devise for detecting uterine activity is called the tocodynamometer. This is placed on the mother's abdomen over the uterus and detects the tightening that occurs with uterine contractions. Tocodynamometers do not measure resting uterine tone or intensity of uterine contractions but depict the frequency and duration of uterine contractions.

In the invasive mode for detection of uterine activity, a transducer-tipped catheter is placed transvaginally within the amniotic cavity. Intra-amniotic pressure is detected and processed by a strain gauge transducer and displayed on a second channel of the strip chart recorder. This pressure can be directly quantified in mm Hg.

Adequate uterine activity is described clinically as that which achieves acceptable cervical dilation per unit time, generally at least 1 cm/hr dilation in the active phase of labor (28). When cervical dilation proceeds at a slower rate, uterine activity measurements can be used to determine whether such activity is adequate. Adequate uterine activity is generally described as contractions occurring every 2 or 3 minutes of about 50- to 70-mm Hg peak height intensity (about 250 to 300 Montevideo units).

In the United States, accepted standards for scaling of the strip chart recorder for the above devices is paper speed at 3 cm/min on the horizontal scale and FHR displayed on a vertical scale of 30 beats/min/cm. This scaling can be important for interpretation. Beat-to-beat variability, which is recognized as fluctuations of the recorder pen between adjacent or several beats, can be appreciated at the speed noted above. However, if a substantially slower speed is used (1 cm/min) the beat-to-beat variability is obscured. The use of a slow paper speed tends to exaggerate the appearance of heart rate variability. Interpretation of FHR patterns described below also depends on scaling. Thus, familiarity with patterns at one scale can pose difficulties "translating" pattern recognition to a different scale.

Characteristics of the Fetal Heart Rate

Characteristics of FHR patterns are classified as baseline or periodic/episodic (29, 30). The baseline features, rate and variability, are those recorded between uterine contractions. Periodic changes, which occur in association with uterine contractions, and episodic changes, which are those not associated with uterine contractions, will be discussed below (Table 36.1).

Baseline features of the heart rate are those predominant characteristics which can be recognized between uterine contractions. These consist of the following:

Baseline Rate

Baseline FHR is the approximate mean FHR rounded to 5 beats/min during a 10-minute segment, excluding (a) periodic or episodic changes, (b) periods of marked FHR variability, and (c) segments of the baseline which differ by more than 25 beats/min. Currently the **normal baseline FHR** is conventionally considered to be between 110 and 160 beats per minute. Values below 110 are termed bradycardia and those above 160 tachycardia.

Table 36.1. FETAL HEART RATE (FHR) CHARACTERISTICS AND PATTERNS: NOMENCLATURE

Term	Definition
Baseline rate	Mean FHR rounded to increments of 5 bpm during a 10-min segment excluding periodic or episodic changes, periods of marked variability, and segments of baseline that differ by >25 bpm. Duration must be ≥2 min.
Bradycardia	Baseline rate of <110 bpm.
Tachycardia	Baseline rate of >160 bpm.
Variability	Fluctuations in the baseline FHR of 2 cycles/min or greater.
Absent variability	Amplitude from peak to trough undetectable.
Minimal variability	Amplitude from peak to trough > undetectable and ≤5 bpm.
Moderate variability	Amplitude from peak to trough 6–25 bpm.
Marked variability	Amplitude from peak to trough >25 bpm.
Acceleration	Visually apparent abrupt increase (onset to peak is <30 sec) of FHR above baseline. Peak is ≥15 bpm. Duration is ≥15 sec and <2 min. In gestations <32 weeks, Peak of 10 bpm and duration of 10 sec is an acceleration.
Prolonged acceleration	Acceleration >2 min and <10 min duration.
Early deceleration	Visually apparent gradual decrease (onset to nadir is ≥30 sec) of FHR below baseline. Return to baseline associated with a uterine contraction. Nadir of deceleration occurs at the same time as the peak of the contraction Generally, the onset, nadir and recovery of the deceleration occur at the same time as the onset, peak, and recovery of the contraction.
Late deceleration	Visually apparent gradual decrease (onset to nadir is ≥30 sec) of FHR below baseline. Return to baseline associated with a uterine contraction. Nadir of deceleration occurs after the peak of the contraction. Generally, the onset, nadir, and recovery of the deceleration occur after the onset, peak, and recovery of the contraction
Variable deceleration	Visually apparent abrupt decrease (onset to nadir is <30 sec) in FHR below baseline. Decrease is ≥15 bpm. Duration is ≥15 sec and <2 min.
Prolonged deceleration	Visually apparent abrupt decrease (onset to nadir is <30 sec) in FHR below baseline. Decrease is ≥15 bpm. Duration is >2 min. but <10 min.

Adapted from National Institute of Child Health and Human Development Research Planning Workshop. Electronic fetal heart rate monitoring: research guidelines for interpretation. *Am J Obstet Gynecol* 1997;177:1385–1390; and *J Obstet Gynecol Neonat Nurse* 1997;26:635–640.

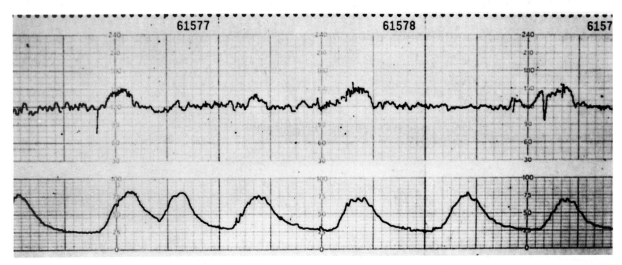

Figure 36.3. Accelerations with contractions. (From Parer JT. *Handbook of Fetal Heart Rate Monitoring*, 2nd ed. Philadelphia: WB Saunders, 1997:150, with permission.)

Fetal Heart Rate Variability

In examining an FHR monitor tracing, in most cases one notes an irregular line. These irregularities demonstrate the FHR variability and represent a slight difference in time interval between each beat, and therefore in calculated FHR that is plotted on the paper. Baseline FHR variability is defined as fluctuations in the baseline FHR of 2 cycles per minute or greater. These fluctuations are somewhat akin to sine waves, but they are irregular in amplitude and frequency. The normal fetus has at least "minimal" variability. Clinically, one recognizes variability visually. There are four basic classes of heart rate variability. They are visually quantified as the amplitude of the peak-to-trough in beats/min as follows:

1. Absent FHR variability, amplitude range undetectable
2. Minimal FHR variability, amplitude range undetectable to 5 beats/min
3. Moderate FHR variability, amplitude range 6 to 25 beats/min
4. Marked FHR variability, amplitude range greater than 25 beats/min

Accelerations

Accelerations are a visually apparent abrupt increase (defined as onset of acceleration to peak in less than 30 seconds) in FHR above the baseline. The increase is calculated from the recently determined portion of the baseline. The acme is 15 beats/min above the baseline, the acceleration lasts at least 15 seconds and less than 2 minutes from the onset to return to baseline. Before

32 weeks of gestation, accelerations are defined as having an acme 10 beats/min above the baseline and duration of 10 seconds (Fig. 36.3). Accelerations are commonly found on tracings from normal fetuses and are associated with a normal well-oxygenated fetus.

VARIANT FETAL HEART RATE PATTERNS

A number of FHR patterns are seen that differ from the "normal" pattern described above but may not be "abnormal." The vast majority of babies born after displaying these patterns has no detectable asphyxial abnormality or sequelae and the pattern is therefore termed "variant." Variant patterns can be modifications in the baseline rate, variability or inclusion of periodic changes described below. Conversely, a few variant FHR patterns discussed below are consistently associated with a significant risk for neonatal acidemia. When placed in the context of the clinical setting, reasonable judgments can be made about the likelihood of fetal acidemia when one assesses progressive change or evolution of patterns and the duration of the variant patterns relative to the presence or absence of variability (Tables 36.2 through 36.4).

Fetal Heart Rate Changes

Bradycardia

Bradycardia is defined as a FHR below 110 beats/min for 10 minutes or longer. Bradycardia in the fetus represents a prolonged

Table 36.2. BRADYCARDIA AND RISK OF FETAL ACIDEMIA

Nonacidemic	Possibly Acidemic	Presumed Acidemia
1. Bradycardia <110 bpm and >80 bpm with minimal or moderate variability	1. Bradycardia < bpm and >60 bpm with moderate or minimal variability	1. Bradycardia <60 bpm
		2. Second stage Bradycardia that loses variability within first 3 min from onset or loses variability for >4 min
Causes include idiopathic bradycardia, congenital heart block	May develop metabolic acidemia if persists	Causes include prolapsed cord, uterine rupture, placental abruption, unexplained

Table 36.3. TACHYCARDIA AND RISK OF FETAL ACIDEMIA

Nonacidemic	Possibly Acidemic	Presumed Acidemia
Tachycardia with moderate or minimal variability; no decelerations	Tachycardia with moderate or minimal variability; mild variable or late decelerations. May develop metabolic acidemia if persists	Tachycardia with absent variability; variable or late decelerations
Causes include elevated maternal temperature, fetal dysrhythmia, medications, prematurity	Causes include fetal sepsis	

stepwise decrease in fetal oxygenation (Fig. 36.4) (31). Fetal bradycardias may be a consequence of vagal activity or the result of fetal hypoxia resulting from fetal inability to maintain a compensatory increase in stroke volume. The hypoxic fetus can increase stroke volume in response to bradycardia but these abilities are limited and insufficient at heart rates below 60 beats/min. Under these conditions, fetal cardiac output cannot be maintained, and umbilical blood flow decreases. This results in insufficient oxygen transport from the fetal placenta to the fetal body and therefore in fetal decompensation (hypoxia). In other words, bradycardia can cause hypoxia or it can result from hypoxia. The depth, duration and presence or absence of variability are critical components for assessment of bradycardia and the likelihood of fetal hypoxemia.

There are a number of non-asphyxial causes of bradycardia. These include the bradyarrhythmias (e.g., complete heart block), certain drugs (e.g., the beta-blockers), or hypothermia. Other fetuses have a heart rate below 110 beats/min but are otherwise totally normal and simply represent a normal variation outside arbitrarily set limits of normal heart rate (Table 36.2).

Terminal Bradycardia

A sudden profound bradycardia is a medical emergency that may signal uterine rupture or placental abruption. This pattern called "terminal" may precede death in utero if birth does not occur rapidly. Studies that have compared the decision to incision times for emergency cesarean section have shown that there is a time-dependent relationship between the onset of

the bradycardia, the depth of the bradycardia, the presence or absence of variability and the development of metabolic acidosis (32). If the bradycardia is between 80 to 100 beats/min and variability is maintained, the fetus will generally stay well oxygenated centrally and can tolerate these rates for an indefinite time (33). Bradycardia with rates of less than 60 beats/minutes, those associated with late or variable decelerations, and those with minimal or absent variability are most often associated with adverse outcome (11, 34–36).

Terminal bradycardias are the most common fetal heart pattern associated with uterine rupture (37, 38). Leung et al. evaluated the fetal consequences of catastrophic uterine rupture when the diagnosis was made at the onset of a fetal bradycardia. All infants with a previously normal FHR pattern born within 17 minutes following the onset of a prolonged deceleration survived without significant perinatal morbidity. If severe late and variable decelerations were present prior to the onset of bradycardia, the fetus tolerated a shorter period of prolonged FHR deceleration and there was a significantly increased risk for metabolic acidosis. In this case, perinatal asphyxia occurred as early as 10 minutes after the onset of the terminal bradycardia.

Second Stage Bradycardia

Bradycardia that occurs during the second stage of labor following a previously normal FHR pattern is much more benign. These may be due to increased vagal tone (e.g., head compression) or occasionally umbilical cord occlusion (4). If the

Table 36.4. VARIABILITY AND RISK OF FETAL ACIDOSIS

Nonacidemic	Possibly Acidemic	Presumed Acidemia
Minimal variability		
Minimal variability: Normal baseline rate No decelerations	Minimal variability with nonrecurrent or mild: Tachycardia Bradycardia Late decelerations Variable decelerations	Minimal variability with persistent or severe: Tachycardia Bradycardia Late decelerations Variable decelerations
Causes include opioids, tranquilizers, MgSO$_4$, barbiturates, anesthetic agents, prematurity, fetal sleep	May develop metabolic acidemia if persistent and/or variability decreases	Causes include metabolic acidemia
Absent variability		
Intermittent absent variability, normal rate without deceleration; preceded by periods of moderate variability	Progressive decrease in variability with decelerations	Absent variability with: Tachycardia Bradycardia Late decelerations Variable decelerations
Causes include idopathic response	May develop metabolic acidemia if persistent and/or variability decreases	Causes include metabolic acidemia

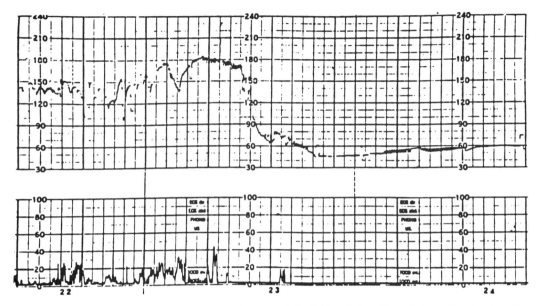

Figure 36.4. Sudden prolonged fetal bradycardia in a woman with an amniotic fluid embolus. There is immediate bradycardia to less than 60 beats/min with the onset of maternal cyanosis and pulmonary edema. There is also loss of fetal heart rate variability. Lower trace is the uterine activity.

variability remains moderate or minimal and the FHR does not decrease below 80 to 90 beats/min, expediting birth is not necessary (33).

Paracervical Block Bradycardia

Post paracervical block bradycardia occurs on the average of 7 minutes after the paracervical block is administered and lasts an average of 8 minutes. The range in both of these values, the decrease in FHR, and associated FHR abnormalities are quite variable. Its incidence varies from 0 to 56% depending on the drug dosage and definition. An average incidence is 15%. Some fetal deaths have been associated with paracervical block bradycardia (39). The etiologic factors are controversial. One theory suggests the most likely cause of the bradycardia is direct fetal toxicity by the local anesthetic drug, not necessarily by direct fetal injection but by rapid uptake by the fetus, possibly via the uterine arteries. The fetal level of the drugs can be quite high, although rarely higher than that of the mother. More probably, local anesthetic agents cause spasm of the uterine arteries, resulting in decreased uterine blood flow and hence fetal asphyxia. Acidosis has been demonstrated in these fetuses by blood sampling during the bradycardia (39). Using minimal quantities and volumes of drug assists minimization of this undesirable side effect of paracervical block. Careful technique to ensure that the drug is placed just submucosally will avoid accidental fetal injection. Paracervical block is contraindicated in the case of a fetus that already has an abnormal FHR pattern.

If bradycardia develops following initiation of a paracervical block, supportive management is recommended. If the pattern resolves and FHR returns to normal, no further evaluation is needed, but repeat paracervical injection should be avoided. Except in rare and profoundly abnormal cases, delivery should be avoided because the bradycardia is typically not severe or long lasting, and the fetus will recover.

Finally, it should also be kept in mind that in the case of a fetal demise, both the external ultrasound transducer and the direct fetal electrode can record maternal heart rate, which will appear the same as a bradycardic FHR. The external transducer can record maternal heart rate from the aorta and the direct lead will record maternal heart rate that is conducted through the dead fetal tissue.

Immediately upon recognition of a bradycardia, attempts should be made to improve fetal oxygenation (Table 36.5).

There is rarely a need for grave concern if a moderate bradycardia with minimal or moderate variability persists. However, if the bradycardia is below 100 beats/min, then more vigorous efforts should be made to alleviate it even in the presence of good FHR variability. A bradycardia below 60 beats/min will almost invariably result in fetal decompensation shortly, and becomes an obstetric emergency to abolish it or deliver the baby before severe central asphyxia occurs.

Tachycardia

A baseline tachycardia (FHR of greater than 160 bpm for 10 minutes or more) may be caused by fetal conditions such as infection, hypoxemia, anemia, prematurity (less than 26 to 28 weeks' gestation), cardiac dysrhythmias, and congenital anomalies or by maternal conditions such as fever, dehydration, infection, or medical problems as in thyroid disease. Beta sympathomimetic drugs, such as terbutaline and ritodrine, may also cause both maternal and fetal tachycardia. Tachycardia represents increased sympathetic and/or decreased parasympathetic autonomic tone. There are a number of causes of tachycardia that do not reflect a risk of fetal acidemia. The most common of these is maternal temperature elevation (Table 36.3).

Fetal tachycardia in the presence of chorioamnionitis may be secondary to the maternal fever or it may be an indication of fetal infection, or both. Thus, the determination of risk for acidemia in a fetus with tachycardia is especially difficult. Tachycardia with moderate variability in the absence of FHR decelerations rarely represents fetal acidemia (10, 35, 40). In the presence of normal FHR variability and no periodic changes, the tachycardia must be assumed to be due to some cause other than oxygen deprivation in the fetus. Tachycardia is sometimes seen during recovery from asphyxia and as discussed above, probably represents catecholamine activity following sympathetic nervous or adrenal medullar activity in response to an acute non-repetitive asphyxial stress. Fetal tachycardia without FHR variability signifies a significant risk for fetal acidemia.

Changes in Fetal Heart Rate Variability

FHR variability is believed to represent an intact neurologic pathway that includes the fetal cerebral cortex, midbrain, vagus nerve, and cardiac conduction system (28). Fetuses with unexplained minimal or absent of FHR variability (Fig. 36.5) and no

Table 36.5. INTRAUTERINE TREATMENT OF VARIANT FETAL HEART RATE (FHR) PATTERNS

FHR Patterns	Causes	Corrective Maneuver	Mechanism
Bradycardia, late decelerations	Hypotension (e.g., supine hypotension, conduction anesthesia)	Intravenous fluids Position change Ephedrine	Increase in UBF
Bradycardia, late decelerations	Excessive uterine activity	Decrease in oxytocin Lateral position	Same as above
Variable decelerations	Transient umbilical cord compression	Position change Amnioinfusion	Return of umbilical blood flow toward normal by decreasing cord compression "Pads" the cord, protecting it from compression
Variable decelerations	Head compression, usually second stage	Push only with alternate contractions	Return of umbilical blood flow toward normal
Late decelerations	Decreased UBF during uterine contraction below limits of usual fetal O$_2$ level	Position change Maternal hyperoxia Tocolytic agents (e.g., terbutaline)	Increase in UBF Increase in maternal-fetal O$_2$ gradient Decrease uterine tonus and/or contractions thus reducing decrease in UBF
Decreasing FHR variability after FHR patterns signifying hypoxia, viz, late or variable decelerations or bradycardia	Prolonged hypoxia/asphyxia	Position change Maternal hyperoxia Tocolytic agents (e.g., terbutaline)	Optimize uterine UBF Increase in maternal-fetal O$_2$ gradient Decrease in uterine tonus and/or contractions, thus reducing associated decrease in UBF

UBF, uterine blood flow.

periodic changes fall into several categories: (a) quiet sleep state; (b) idiopathic reduced FHR variability with no obvious explanation, but without evidence of asphyxia or CNS compromise; (c) centrally acting drugs, e.g., opioids; (d) congenital neurologic abnormality due to either a developmental CNS defect or acquired from an in utero infection or asphyxial event (41, 42); (e) abnormal cardiac conduction system (e.g., complete heart block); and (f) deep asphyxia with inability of the heart to manifest periodic changes. Clinical observations also suggest that some severely growth restricted fetuses may have reduced or even absent FHR variability, even in the absence of demonstrable asphyxia. The mechanism of this depressed variability is not known.

If the FHR variability is reduced or absent on initial placement of the monitor, the clinician's ability to determine if pro-

gressive asphyxia is occurring is more difficult or even impossible without ancillary testing. Delivery is sometimes expedited to give the fetus the benefit of uncertainty, although there is not consensus that this is the correct approach.

Minimal variability without concomitant decelerations is almost always unrelated to fetal acidemia (43). However, a fetus with an abnormal cardiac conduction system, anencephaly or congenital neurologic deficit may present with minimal or absent variability and in the case of congenital neurologic impairment, this FHR pattern may actually represent an asphyxial insult that occurred during the antepartum period (44).

The most important concept is that decreased FHR variability that does result from asphyxia and CNS depression during the intrapartum period follows asphyxial stress patterns such as bradycardia, late decelerations, or variable decelerations. Loss

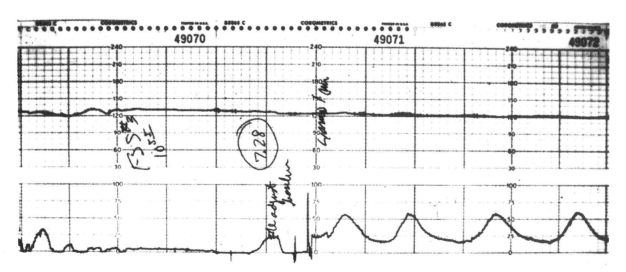

Figure 36.5. No variability of FHR. Patient had severe preeclampsia and received magnesium sulfate and opioids. Normal scalp blood pH (7.28) assures one that absence of variability is not a result of asphyxia. Fetus is not chronically asphyxiated or decompensating. Uterine activity channel has inaccurate trace in first half. (From Parer JT, King TL. Whither fetal heart rate monitoring. *Obstet Gynecol Fertil* 1999;22:149–192, with permission.)

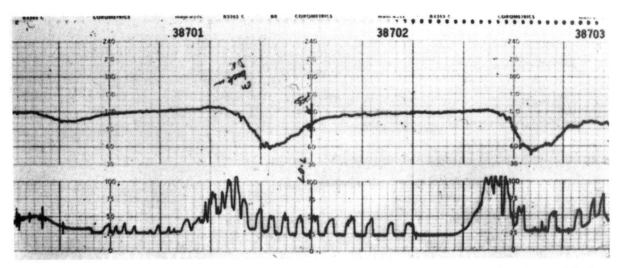

Figure 36.6. Nonreflex late decelerations with virtual absence of FHR variability. Decelerations represent transient asphyxial myocardial failure as well as intermittent vagal decreases in heart rate. Lack of FHR variability also signifies decreased cerebral oxygenation. Note acidemia in fetal scalp blood (7.07). The baby, a 3,340-g girl with Apgar scores of 3 (1 min) and 4 (5 min), was delivered soon after this tracing. Cesarean delivery was considered contraindicated because of severe preeclamptic coagulopathy. (From Parer JT, King TL. Whither fetal heart rate monitoring. *Obstet Gynecol Fertil* 1999;22:149–192, with permission.)

of variability associated with the presence of these periodic patterns during labor is the most sensitive indicator of metabolic acidemia in a fetus (34, 35, 45).

Periodic Changes

Periodic patterns are episodic or periodic changes in FHR. These consist of early decelerations, late decelerations, variable decelerations and/or prolonged decelerations.

Early and Late Decelerations

Early and late decelerations have the following characteristics (29) (Fig. 36.6):

1. They are smooth and rounded in configuration and the mirror image of the contraction.
2. They are persistent, often occurring with each contraction.
3. Their onset, nadir and recovery are generally delayed 10 to 30 seconds after the onset, apex and resolution of the contraction.
4. The depth of the dip can be related to the intensity of the contraction.

Late decelerations are of two varieties (28, 46–48). The first type is sometimes seen when an acute insult (e.g., reduced uter-

ine blood flow due to maternal hypotension) is superimposed on a previously normally oxygenated fetus in the presence of uterine contractions. These late decelerations are caused by a decrease in uterine blood flow (with the uterine contraction) that places the fetus beyond the capacity to extract oxygen. The relatively deoxygenated blood transported from the placenta during the contraction causes fetal hyperemia. Hyperemia results in chemoreceptor-mediated vagal discharge, which causes the transient deceleration. The deceleration is presumed to start "late" relative to the contraction because of the added circulation time from the fetal placental site to the chemoreceptors and also because the progressively decreasing oxygen tension must reach a certain threshold before vagal activity occurs. There may also be baroreceptor activity causing the vagal discharge (46). Between contractions, oxygen delivery is adequate and there is no additional vagal activity, so the baseline heart rate and variability are normal. Because these late decelerations are accompanied by normal FHR variability that signifies normal CNS integrity, the fetus is physiologically "compensated" in the vital organs (Fig. 36.7).

The periodic change historically called "early deceleration" appears to be a variant of the above-described late deceleration. It is not clear why the deceleration is not late, but early decelerations have been noted to evolve into late decelerations.

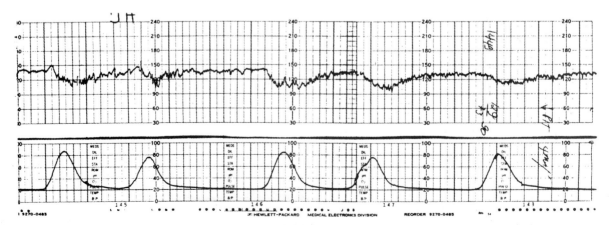

Figure 36.7. Reflex late decelerations. Note retention of moderate (normal) FHR variability. (From Parer JT, King TL. Whither fetal heart rate monitoring. *Obstet Gynecol Fertil* 1999;22:149–192, with permission.)

The second type of late deceleration is a result of the same initial mechanism except that the deoxygenated bolus of blood from the placenta is presumed to be insufficient to support myocardial action. Therefore, for the period of the contraction, there is direct myocardial hypoxic depression (or failure) as well as vagal activity (46, 48). This second variety is seen without variability (Fig. 36.6). It signifies fetal "decompensation" (e.g., inadequate fetal cerebral and myocardial oxygenation). This type of late deceleration is seen most commonly in states of decreased placental reserve, (e.g., pregnancy-induced hypertension or intrauterine growth restriction) or following prolonged asphyxial stresses (e.g., a long period of severe late or variable decelerations). The distinguishing feature between the type of late deceleration caused by chemoreceptor-reflex activity and non-reflex myocardial depression is the presence of FHR variability in the former.

When late decelerations with or without variability occur, efforts should be made to eliminate them by improving maternal and fetal placental blood flows and instituting maternal hyperoxia. Vagal-mediated late decelerations, typically resulting from an acute transient hypoxic episode, generally can be abolished. If not, the fetus may accumulate oxygen debt, though usually not before 30 minutes in a normally grown term fetus who was previously normoxic. When late decelerations persist and variability is lost, the presumption is that the fetus is at risk for myocardial failure and decreased cerebral oxygenation. In this situation, the intermittent decreases in uterine blood flow with each contraction can no longer be tolerated. In utero treatments designed to increase uterine blood flow and oxygenation will be less likely to abolish these late decelerations.

Variable Decelerations

Variable decelerations (Fig. 36.8) have the following characteristics:

1. The appearance of the decrease in FHR is variable in duration, profundity, and shape from uterine contraction to contraction.
2. They are abrupt in onset and cessation, sometimes decreasing 60 beats/min in one or several beats. Therefore, they are neurogenic (vagal) in origin.

Variable decelerations are termed severe when the FHR decreases below 60 beats/min (or 60 beats/min below baseline FHR) and persist longer than 60 seconds in duration. Although other criteria have been proposed this is the one most commonly used. There is no accepted terminology for classifying variable decelerations into mild or moderate categories but in practice most institutions have some commonly agreed upon terms for describing the less severe forms of this periodic pattern.

Variable decelerations represent the firing of the vagus nerve in response to certain stimuli, either umbilical cord compression (generally in the first stage of labor) or possibly substantial head compression (e.g., during maternal voluntary expulsive efforts late in the second stage of labor). Whether the fetus is still normoxic in the central tissues (i.e., physiologically compensated) can be determined by observation of the maintenance of FHR variability.

When severe variable decelerations develop, vigorous efforts should be made to abolish them because it is likely that even the previously normal fetus with normal placental function will eventually decompensate, although not usually before 30 minutes. The term fetus with a normal FHR tracing prior to the onset of variable decelerations usually can tolerate "mild" or "moderate" variable decelerations for a prolonged period.

Significance of Pattern Evolution

During labor, a FHR pattern with decreasing variability due to asphyxia is virtually always preceded by a heart rate pattern signifying potentially hypoxic events, e.g., late decelerations, variable decelerations (usually severe), or a prolonged bradycardia. The normal evolution to decreased or absent variability can also occur with relatively minor decelerations in cases of chorioamnionitis or dysmaturity. If the FHR patterns cannot be improved, i.e., if the patterns indicative of tissue hypoxia persist for a significant period, further diagnosis or delivery may be indicated.

Some patterns are so severe that they must be considered to represent asphyxia unless it can be rapidly ruled out, for example, absent FHR variability associated with profound decelerations (Fig. 36.9), which at times are difficult to distinguish

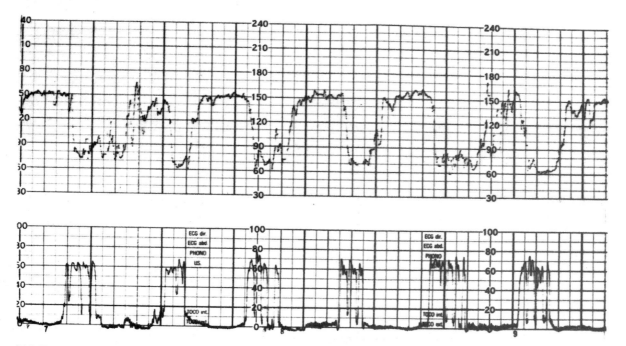

Figure 36.8. Variable decelerations: intrapartum recording using fetal scalp electrode and tocodynamometer. The spikes on the uterine activity channel represent maternal pushing efforts in the second stage of labor. Note normal baseline variability between contractions. Paper speed was 3 cm/min.

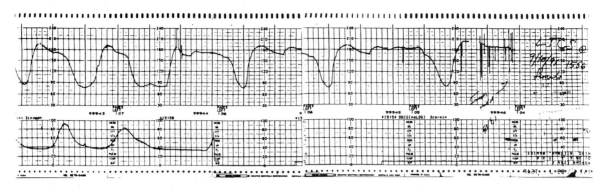

Figure 36.9. This fetal heart rate pattern of profound decelerations and absent fetal heart rate variability must be considered to represent serious asphyxia unless it can be ruled out by ancillary testing, such as fetal scalp sampling. Because the majority of such fetuses are, in fact, deeply asphyxiated, emergent delivery is recommended.

as late or variable. One cannot be certain whether such fetuses have already suffered cerebral damage. Rapid delivery is recommended.

Unusual Fetal Heart Rate Patterns

Sinusoidal Pattern

Sinusoidal pattern is a regular, smooth, sine wavelike baseline with a frequency of approximately 3 to 6/min and an amplitude range of up to 30 beats/min. The regularity of waves and lack of short-term variability distinguish the pattern from long-term variability complexes, which are crudely shaped and irregular.

The pattern was first described in a group of severely affected Rh-isoimmunized fetuses, but has subsequently been noted in association with fetuses that are anemic for other reasons and in asphyxiated infants. It has also been described in cases of normal infants born without depression or acid-base abnormalities, although in the latter cases there is dispute about whether the patterns are truly sinusoidal or whether, because of the moderately irregular pattern, they are variants of long-term variability. Such patterns are also sometimes seen after administration of butorphanol or nalbuphine to the mother. The authors believe an essential characteristic of the sinusoidal pattern is extreme regularity and smoothness.

If the sinusoidal pattern is seen in an Rh-sensitized patient with substantial hemolysis (as noted by the value of the change in optical density at 450 nm in amniotic fluid), this signifies a need for rapid intervention. This may take the form of delivery, or possibly intrauterine transfusion, depending on the gestational age and the preceding Rh data, treatment, and workup.

Management in the absence of Rh disease is somewhat more difficult to recommend. If the pattern is persistent, monotonously regular, and unaccompanied by short-term variability, and cannot be abolished by maneuvers as outlined above, fetal blood sampling is indicated. If fetal blood sampling is not available, delivery is recommended.

However, if the pattern is irregularly sinusoidal or "pseudosinusoidal," intermittently present, and not associated with intervening periodic decelerations, then it is very unlikely to indicate fetal compromise. Hence, immediate delivery is not warranted. Fetal blood sampling may assist in confirming normality in such cases.

Saltatory Pattern

The term "saltatory pattern" is applied when one sees rapid variations in FHR with a frequency of 3 to 6 beats/min, and amplitude range greater than 25 beats/min. It is qualitatively described as marked or excessive variability, and the swings have a strikingly bizarre appearance.

The saltatory pattern was associated with low Apgar scores in early discussions of FHR variability, but it was not possible to relate the time course of the pattern to the fetal depression (9). That is, fetuses with the pattern in the intrapartum period tended to have low Apgar scores, but it was not clear whether the pattern was present immediately before delivery or it preceded an evolution to a more serious FHR pattern.

Saltatory pattern is almost invariably seen during labor rather than in the antepartum period. Because the authors believe the fetus with this pattern is not hemodynamically compensated (although it may suffer from slight asphyxia), it is recommended that attempts be made to abolish it by maneuvers such as maternal positioning, avoidance of hypotension, avoidance of excessive uterine activity, and possibly maternal hyperoxia. The authors do not know of such a pattern that has evolved into fetal decompensation; it probably has similar significance to mild or moderate variable decelerations.

Dysrhythmias

A number of case reports have described numerous fetal dysrhythmias that have been diagnosed in utero. These include complete heart block, premature atrial contractions, premature ventricular contractions, bigeminy, supraventricular tachycardia, paroxysmal atrial tachycardia, blocked atrial premature beats, atrial flutter, and asystole of variable duration.

A great deal of concern was experienced in the past over the fetus with a dysrhythmia. It has become obvious that only rarely are early interventions required and most of these infants can tolerate labor well. The authors have investigated such cases with an attempted fetal ECG using external abdominal electrodes, sonography, and echocardiography. The latter has been most helpful in diagnosing the condition and determining whether there are any obvious structural abnormalities before birth. The authors have used internal fetal monitoring during labor with supplemental fetal blood sampling for the fetus with bizarre FHR patterns. The FHR monitor detects and depicts the interval between beats and is thus a very sensitive dysrhythmia detector. Bradyarrhythmias are the most commonly reported. These appear as FHR tracings of approximately 50 to 60 beats/min with virtually absent FHR variability. Bradycardias and tachycardias may be doubled or halved by the cardiotachometer, particularly in the Doppler mode. This artifact can almost always be ruled out by brief auscultation.

These dysrhythmias generally represent cardiac conduction defects that have an anatomic or functional basis. The persistent types appear to have a worse prognosis than the intermittent ones, the latter often resolving in the newborn.

Complete heart block has an incidence of about one in 20,000 births, and approximately 30% of cases are associated with heart disease, often a cardiac structural abnormality. About 10% of newborns with congenital heart block die in early infancy. Infants with heart block often have mothers with collagen vascular disease, particularly systemic lupus erythematosus, so such women should be screened appropriately.

The extreme tachycardias, generally above 240 beats/min, sometimes have been associated with hydrops, apparently because of intrauterine cardiac failure. There are case reports of in utero treatments with digoxin, adrenergic blocking agents, procainamide, or calcium-channel blockers. In some cases, there has been resolution of the hydrops.

The major problem in the fetus with dysrhythmia is generally in the newborn period. The authors recommend that such infants be delivered in a tertiary care center with immediate access to pediatric cardiology care. Those with heart block may need cardiac pacing and those with a tachycardia may need medication to prevent cardiac failure.

Preterm Fetus

Several investigators have examined both the antepartum and intrapartum FHR patterns of premature fetuses, and their relationship to fetal blood acid-base status (49). There now seems little doubt that the same criteria used in the term fetus can be used for the premature. An important difference, however, is that premature fetuses can quickly develop abnormal patterns, and that these patterns tend to progress much more rapidly in their severity than those in the term fetus.

There are some commonly held beliefs with regard to premature fetuses that are in error. The first is that the premature fetus normally has a tachycardia. The second is that the premature fetus has a "flat baseline." In fact, the average FHR of the 28-week-old fetus is about 150 beats/min with a range of about 130 to 170—that is, only slightly above that of the term fetus. On the second point, most premature fetuses have normal FHR variability, and with its disappearance or absence the management should be the same as that for a term fetus, even in the presence of a tachycardia. However, there is a tendency for premature fetuses to have a smaller amplitude of variability.

Congenital Anomalies

Except as described for the dysrhythmias, the vast majority of fetuses with congenital anomalies have normal FHR patterns and a response to asphyxia similar to that of the normal fetus (50). There are several exceptions, for example complete heart block and anencephaly. Fetuses such as those with Down's syndrome and Trisomy 18, and those with aplastic lungs, meningomyelocele, hydrocephalus, and many others, may have no FHR warning of their defects. However, in one series it was noted that although there was no pathognomonic pattern in such fetuses, the rate of cesarean section for fetal distress was significantly increased (48).

An important exception is seen with Potter's syndrome. Such fetuses are generally recognized as growth restricted because of the oligohydramnios, and in addition may have substantial variable decelerations, presumably for the same reason. That is, umbilical cord compression is more likely without the "padding" of adequate amniotic fluid. A number of such fetuses have been delivered by cesarean section for "fetal distress" with the tragic outcome of rapid neonatal death due to hypoplastic lungs.

There is no simple solution to the problem of emergency intervention (generally cesarean section) for the fetus that is destined to be severely defective or die in the neonatal period. Genetic evaluation in certain high-risk groups may decrease the incidence of such problems.

INTERPRETATION OF FETAL HEART RATE PATTERNS
Prognostic Value of Accelerations and Variability

The two most sensitive indicators of adequate cerebral oxygenation are variability and/or accelerations. A normal baseline rate with moderate variability, accelerations and no periodic changes is highly predictive of a well-oxygenated fetus (10, 11, 35, 51).

In addition, there is a close association between the presence of accelerations and normal FHR variability. It has been well established that the greatest contribution of EFM to fetal healthcare is the ability to predict normal outcomes. A reassuring fetal tracing virtually assures the perinatal team that, barring unforeseen acute insults such as abruptio placentae or prolapsed cord, a well-oxygenated neonate will be born.

Patterns Associated With Risk for Acidemia

The evolution of intrapartum FHR patterns during asphyxia is established, and it is known that FHR variability decreases and then disappears before substantial fetal depression or fetal death occurs in utero. This decrease in FHR variability is considered to correlate clinically with decreased CNS function, which is presumed to precede CNS damage.

From the clinical management perspective, the approach above is important. It suggests that when variability is maintained, there is time for in utero treatment to alleviate the stress patterns before operative delivery is warranted. Conversely, absent FHR variability in the presence of persistent asphyxial stress patterns should indicate immediate delivery. There is some evidence that neurologic damage may begin at 10 minutes in such cases. It is our current belief that a sustained FHR less than 80 beats/min also should be managed by immediate preparation for delivery, whereas rates of 80 to 100 beats/min can be managed more conservatively. In all of these cases, the presence of FHR variability persistently has been the most important prognostic sign of continued fetal CNS compensation. The five FHR patterns that are clearly associated with a risk for newborn acidemia are listed in Table 36.6.

TREATMENT OF THE FETUS IN UTERO

It is now well recognized that fetal oxygenation can be improved, acidosis relieved, and abnormal FHR patterns abolished by certain non-invasive modes of treatment. The FHR patterns that can result in potential fetal hypoxia are presented in Table 36.5, together with the recommended treatment maneuvers and presumed mechanisms for improving fetal oxygenation. These should be the first maneuvers carried out. If the asphyxial insult is acute and the fetus was previously normoxic, there is an excellent chance that the variant FHR pattern will be abolished with in utero treatment.

ANCILLARY METHODS OF DIAGNOSIS

Because EFM has a high false positive rate for determination of fetal hypoxemia, ancillary tests of fetal well being are used when the FHR pattern is indeterminate. Fetal blood sampling, fetal scalp stimulation, and pulse oximetry are discussed.

Fetal Blood Sampling

Fetal blood sampling was introduced initially as an independent means of fetal surveillance during labor (52). The extensive list

---

Table 36.6. FETAL HEART RATE PATTERNS ASSOCIATED WITH RISK FOR ACIDEMIA

Absent variability and:
   Persistent tachycardia
   Bradycardia (<80 bpm)
Absent or minimal variability and:
   Recurrent late decelerations
   Recurrent moderate or severe variable decelerations
   Sinusoidal pattern

of indications for fetal blood sampling originally proposed has shortened in recent years, with the realization of the favorable prognostic significance of FHR variability and development of fetal scalp stimulation (10, 53, 54). Scalp sampling is carried out by placing an endoscope against the fetal presenting part and puncturing the fetal skin using a small blade device, until a droplet of blood wells up. This is collected anaerobically and analyzed for pH and PCO_2 (and other factors if necessary). The bicarbonate or base excess can be calculated by means of the Henderson-Hasselbalch equation. It has been noted that, at pH values above 7.2 to 7.25, the fetus is generally vigorous at birth, whereas a pH below 7.15 is associated with a 2-minute Apgar score of less than 6 in 80% of cases (55). However, there is a considerable overlap in the groups, and a single value such as 7.2 cannot be relied on entirely. Numerous other factors must be taken into account, such as the maternal acid-base status, the relationship of the sampling to uterine contractions, the permanence of the placental insult, the influence of in utero treatment, the type of acidosis, (i.e., respiratory versus metabolic), the stage of labor, and the various other clinical aspects of the particular case.

Fetal scalp sampling has not been widely adopted. It is technically difficult to accomplish and many community hospitals do not have the equipment or lab personnel available as needed.

Fetal Scalp Stimulation

Interestingly, studies involving fetal blood sampling noted a high correlation between the occurrence of accelerations of the FHR during scalp puncture for obtaining a blood sample, and a "normal" pH value, i.e., above 7.20. In a subsequent prospective trial, this observation was validated (45). The technique for eliciting accelerations via scalp stimulation is simple. The fetal scalp is digitally stimulated during a vaginal examination and the FHR monitor observed for an acceleration of 15 seconds duration, peaking at 15 beats/min above the baseline FHR. Because the presence of accelerations is highly predictive of a pH >7.2, scalp stimulation has largely replaced scalp blood sampling in most obstetric units.

Fetal Pulse Oximetry

Fetal pulse oximetry has been introduced as another method to monitor the fetus and to help clarify fetal status in the presence of a non-reassuring FHR pattern. It is hoped that this will reduce the incidence of unnecessary cesarean sections. Although recently approved for use in the United States, this technology has been commercially available in Europe and elsewhere for several years, but has not yet gained widespread acceptance (56).

The fetus has fetal hemoglobin, lower oxygen saturation and a much smaller pulse than adults, resulting in lower signal amplitudes (57). New oximeters have been developed with these factors in mind, using different light wavelengths and a reflectance (rather than transmission) probe, which is placed along the fetal temple, cheek or forehead. The probe is held in place by being wedged between the fetal head and the uterine wall. The technique had limitations that include decreased saturation readings that are artifacts due to venous stasis and frequent technical difficulties that result in an inability to achieve sensor contact. Newer designs have resolved many of these problems.

Studies correlating fetal pulse oximetry with fetal scalp pH and subsequent umbilical artery pH and PO_2 reveal that fetal saturation between 30% to 70% is normal. Values less than 30% saturation for greater than 10 to 15 minutes are concerning for fetal acidosis (58). A recent randomized-controlled trial resulted in a significant decrease in cesarean deliveries for fetal indications (10% control, 5% with oximeter), but a doubling of

cesarean deliveries for dystocia, so the overall cesarean rate was not changed by use of the oximeter (56).

Still other methods of fetal monitoring have included continuous scalp tissue pH, transcutaneous fetal scalp oxygen, and carbon dioxide electrodes; however, these devices never became commercially available because of technical problems (particularly with application to the fetal head), lack of reliability, and expense. Some European investigators have used the fetal ST waveform for analysis, but results are very preliminary.

ROLE OF FETAL HEART RATE MONITORING IN THE DIAGNOSIS OF FETAL ASPHYXIA

Thirty-nine percent of the intrapartum FHR tracings obtained via EFM display periodic FHR patterns, yet only 2% of all newborns have evidence of metabolic acidosis (pH of less than 7.1, with base excess of less than 12) (10, 59). The published studies comparing the incidence of periodic FHR patterns to newborn acidemia have been retrospective case control studies of asphyxiated newborns (35, 41, 60, 61) or prospective studies comparing specific FHR patterns to fetal scalp sample pH or umbilical cord blood pH values at birth (11, 34, 40, 62, 63). It is important to remember that case control and prospective observational designs can demonstrate a statistically significant association but cannot prove that the association elucidated is actually a cause and effect relationship.

Clinical Indicators of Asphyxia

The term "perinatal asphyxia" has been used in the obstetric literature to refer to various degrees of acidosis and/or hypercarbia in the newborn, which makes the use of the term as a diagnosis imprecise (64). The question relevant to clinicians is as follows: What level of perinatal asphyxia is associated with poor newborn outcomes?

There is no precise clinical or biochemical indicator that has a high positive predictive value for perinatal asphyxia. The original outcome measures used in early studies of EFM were cerebral palsy and intrapartum stillbirth. Other outcome measures of potential significance are Apgar scores, newborn seizures, and acidemia at birth. The purpose of this section is to review how well EFM predicts neonatal morbidity.

Cerebral Palsy

At the time FHR monitoring was introduced it was felt that virtually all intrapartum deaths and neonatal cerebral palsy were due to intrapartum asphyxia, yet the prevalence of cerebral palsy has not decreased since the advent of EFM (65). The majority of cases of cerebral palsy appear to be due to developmental defects, neuronal migrational defects, infections, toxins, antepartum ischemic or asphyxial episodes in the fetus, and other causes. The problem with regard to cerebral palsy is that although it is indeed a morbid neonatal outcome, most cases cannot be avoided via the use of EFM. This was summarized succinctly by Ellison, "A technology that defines more than 40% of FHR patterns as deviant cannot possibly be accurate in predicting a very low frequency outcome such as neurologic abnormality." (61) In fact, the incidence of cerebral palsy due to intrapartum asphyxia is of the order of 0.025%, i.e., more than 1,000-fold less than the incidence of variant FHR patterns during labor.

FHR monitoring has decreased the incidence of intrapartum stillbirth. Prior to the introduction of FHR monitoring, approximately one third of all stillbirths or three per 1000 births occurred in the intrapartum period (66). Currently, the overall incidence of intrapartum stillbirth is at most 0.5 of 1,000 births.

Apgar Scores

The Apgar score was designed as a screen for neonatal adaptation to extrauterine life (67). Since its introduction in 1952, this delivery room assessment has assumed a broad role in the prediction of neurologic outcome despite the fact that there is little evidence supporting this use. Normal FHR tracings predict normal Apgar scores 96% of the time and 83% of newborns with low 5 minute Apgar scores are presaged by variant FHR patterns (68). However, despite this concordance, Apgar scores do not predict neonatal morbidity well. Prematurity, neonatal infection or neonatal procedures such as intubation can affect various components of the composite Apgar score for example. Apgar scores are poorly associated with umbilical arterial pH values, which do reflect respiratory and/or metabolic acidosis present at birth (69).

Newborn Seizures

A National Institute of Health review of perinatal causes of neurologic abnormality concluded "neonatal seizures appear to be the best evidence of asphyxia and the best predictor of later damage" (70). Seizures that first occur in the newborn period are predictive of long-term neurologic abnormality (71), and neonatal seizures that are secondary to perinatal asphyxia occur within the first day or so of life (72).

Despite the clear relationship between seizures and long-term outcome, the predictive value of FHR patterns associated with neonatal seizures is poor. Using data from the meta-analysis of FHR monitoring (21), it is estimated that seizures during the newborn period are secondary to intrapartum asphyxia in approximately 2.5 per 1,000 births. Infants who seize have longer hospital stays, and undergo numerous medical procedures and evaluation, but most babies who experience seizures in the newborn period have no residual deficits.

Fetal Acidemia

Fetal acidemia is considered the precursor to more permanent morbidity and therefore is the clinical indicator of value when assessing the risk for adverse neonatal outcome. An umbilical arterial blood acidosis of pH 7.0 or less occurs in about three per 1,000 births (73). A pH value of less than 7.0 is associated with (but not predictive of) neurologic and other organ damage (73–76). Some morbidity is seen in fetuses with an umbilical arterial pH between 7.0 and 7.1. While morbidity seen after pH values in this range are generally not catastrophic or permanent, it can be costly and distressing. A pH of less than 7.1 is at approximately the 2.5th percentile (59), so this gives us a reasonable target population of fetuses which could benefit from FHR monitoring, i.e., 25% of births.

The incidence of umbilical cord pH values needs to be compared to FHR patterns. If we consider variant patterns with reduced or absent FHR variability, the prevalence decreases to 3%. Even this is 100-fold greater than the incidence of intrapartum-induced cerebral palsy, and 10-fold greater than an umbilical arterial pH of less than 7.0, although it is similar to the incidence of pH of less than 7.1.

Healing ability of the brain and the effect of asphyxial events experienced by an ill neonate confound the sensitivity of intrapartum predictors (77). In addition, although the degree of asphyxia can be determined via assessment of acidemia in umbilical cord gases, this does not necessarily reflect the duration of the insult (71). Thus, the detection of acidemia is at best an indirect measure of asphyxia because umbilical cord gases measure the degree of asphyxia but do not directly measure either the fetal response to asphyxia or its duration.

Studies evaluating the intrapartum course of infants with an abnormal newborn course have elucidated those intrapartum factors that both reliably reflect asphyxia and can be attributed to the intrapartum period (75, 78, 79):

Table 36.7. CRITERIA TO DEFINE AN ACUTE INTRAPARTUM HYPOXIC EVENT

Essential criteria:[a]
1. Evidence of a metabolic acidosis in intrapartum fetal, umbilical arterial cord or very early neonatal blood samples. pH <7.00 and base deficit >12 mMol/L.
2. Early onset of severe or moderate neonatal encephalopathy in infants >34 weeks gestation.
3. Cerebral palsy of the spastic quadriplegic or dyskinetic type.

Criteria that together suggest an intrapartum timing but by themselves are nonspecific:[b]
4. A sentinel (signal) hypoxic event occurring immediately before or during labor.
5. A sudden, rapid, and sustained deterioration of the fetal heart rate pattern usually following the hypoxic sentinel event.
6. Apgar score of 0–6 for >5 minutes
7. Early evidence of multisystem involvement.
8. Early imaging evidence of acute cerebral abnormality.

[a] All three of the essential criteria are necessary before an intrapartum hypoxia can be considered the etiology of the cerebral palsy.
[b] If evidence for some of the four to eight criteria is missing or contradictory, the timing of the neuropathology becomes increasingly in doubt.
Adapted from MacLenan A. A template for defining a causal relation between intrapartum events and cerebral palsy: international consensus statement. *BMJ* 1999;319:1054–1059, with permission.

---

1. Umbilical artery metabolic or mixed acidemia with pH of 7.00 or less
2. Five-minute Apgar score of 0 to 3
3. Neonatal neurological sequelae
4. Multi-organ dysfunction

Between 1997 and 1998, an international Task Force composed of specialists and researchers in perinatology, neonatology, midwifery, science and epidemiology reviewed the literature on the causation of cerebral palsy (44). The International Consensus Statement published by this group lists clinical and biochemical criteria that define an acute intrapartum event (Table 36.7).

To date, attempts to compare FHR patterns to subsequent neonatal morbidity have been imprecise. Cerebral palsy and neonatal seizures are extremely rare events and variant heart rate patterns are common. Apgar scores correlate well with FHR patterns but they do not correlate well with long-term outcome or with concomitant newborn acidemia. Although there are no specific FHR patterns or group of patterns that reliably predict brain damage, there is an increase in the literature that suggests there is a correlation between absent variability with severe periodic decelerations or bradycardia, and progressive metabolic acidemia in the fetus. The degree of acidemia that reliably predicts newborn complications is as yet undetermined.

CONCLUSION

The physiologic mechanisms that enhance oxygen delivery to fetal tissue are able to accommodate varying degrees of lower Po_2 without pathologic sequelae. The biochemical events that herald irreversible asphyxial injury have not been determined in terms of acid-base indices and, owing to the wide variability from fetus to fetus, acid-base status at birth may never be a perfect predictor. To date, there are no clinical markers or specific FHR patterns that reliably predict intrapartum asphyxia. Neither are there single neonatal indices (such as Apgar scores, umbilical cord gases, or neonatal seizures) that reliably correlate with intrapartum asphyxia severe enough to cause brain injury. The combination of a mixed acidemia, 5-minute Apgar score of less than 3, seizures within 24 hours of birth, and multi-organ dysfunction as a constellation is the indicator most closely associated with intrapartum asphyxia.

Given the above complexities, the goal of clinical EFM is the detection of those patterns that herald a significant risk of acidemia at a value well before the above described irreversible damage occurs. Absent or minimal variability, especially in the presence of late or variable decelerations, severe variable decelerations, and bradycardias are the patterns most closely associated with fetal acidemia.

REFERENCES

1. Albers LL, Krulewitch CJ. Electronic fetal monitoring in the United States in the 1980s. *Obstet Gynecol* 1993;82:8–10.
2. Ventura SJ, Martin JA, Curtin SC, et al. Report of the final natality statistics. *Mon Vital Stat Rep NCHS* 1996;46:1–11.
3. Martin CB. Electronic fetal monitoring: A brief summary of its development, problems and prospects. *Eur J Obstet Gynaecol Reprod Biol* 1998;78:133–140.
4. Parer JT, King TL. Whither fetal heart rate monitoring. *Obstet Gynecol Fertil* 1999;22:149–192.
5. Nelson KB. The neurologically impaired child and alleged malpractice at birth. *Neurol Clin* 1999;17:283–293.
6. Nelson KB. What proportion of cerebral palsy is related to birth asphyxia? *J Pediatr* 1988;112:572–574.
7. Hon EH. *An Atlas of Fetal Heart Rate Patterns.* New Haven, CT: Harty Press, 1968.
8. Caldeyro-Barcia R, Mendez-Bauer C, Poseiro JJ, et al. Control of human fetal heart rate during labor. In: Cassels D, ed. *The Heart and Circulation in the Newborn and Infant.* New York: Grune & Stratton, 1966:7.
9. Hammacher K, Huter KA, Bokelmann J, et al. Foetal heart frequency and perinatal condition of the foetus and newborn. *Gynaecologia* 1968;166:349–360.
10. Krebs HB, Petres RE, Dunn LE, et al. Intrapartum fetal heart rate monitoring. I. Classification and prognosis of fetal heart rate patterns. *Am J Obstet Gynecol* 1979;133:762–772.
11. Berkus MD, Langer O, Samueloff A, et al. Electronic fetal monitoring: what's reassuring? *Acta Obstet Gynecol Scand* 1999;78:15–21.
12. Havercamp AD, Thompson HE, McFee JG, et al. The evaluation of continuous fetal heart rate monitoring in high-risk pregnancy. *Am J Obstet Gynecol* 1976;125:310–320.
13. Renou P, Chang A, Anderson I, et al. Controlled trial of fetal intensive care. *Am J Obstet Gynecol* 1976;126:470–475.
14. Kelso IM, Parsons RJ, Lawrence GF, et al. An assessment of continuous fetal heart rate monitoring in labor. *Am J Obstet Gynecol* 1978;131:526–532.
15. Havercamp AD, Orleans M, Langerdoerfer S, et al. A controlled trial of differential effects of intrapartum fetal monitoring. *Am J Obstet Gynecol* 1979;134:399–408.
16. Wood C, Renou P, Oats J, et al. A controlled trial of fetal heart rate monitoring in a low risk obstetric population. *Am J Obstet Gynecol* 1981;141:527–534.
17. Neldam S, Osler M, Hansen PK, et al. Intrapartum fetal heart rate monitoring in a combined low-and high-risk population: a controlled trial. *Eur J Obstet Gynecol Reprod Biol* 1986;23:1–11.
18. MacDonald D, Grant A, Sheridan-Pereira M, et al. The Dublin randomized controlled trial of intrapartum fetal heart rate monitoring. *Am J Obstet Gynecol* 1985;152:524–539.
19. Leveno J, Cunningham FG, Nelson S, et al. A prospective comparison of selective and universal electronic fetal monitoring in 34,995 pregnancies. *N Engl J Med* 1986;315:615–641.
20. Luthy DA, Shy KK, van Belle G, et al. A randomized trial of electronic monitoring in labor. *Obstet Gynecol* 1987;69:687–695.
21. Thacker SB, Stroup DF, Peterson HB. Efficacy and safety of intrapartum electronic fetal monitoring: an update. *Obstet Gynecol* 1995;86:613–620.
22. Parer JT, King T. Fetal heart rate monitoring: is it salvageable? *Am J Obstet Gynecol* 2000;182:982–987.
23. Cohn HE, Sacks EJ, Heymann MA, et al. Cardiovascular responses to hypoxemia and acidemia in fetal lambs. *Am J Obstet Gynecol* 1974;120:817–824.
24. Jensen A, Garnier Y, Berger R. Dynamics of fetal circulatory responses to hypoxia and asphyxia. *Eur J Obstet Gynecol Reprod Biol* 1999;84:155–172.
25. Fisher DJ, Heymann MA, Rudolph AM. Fetal myocardial and carbohydrate consumption during acutely induced hypoxia. *Am J Physiol* 1982;242:H657–H661.
26. Jones MD, Sheldon RE, Peeters LL, et al. Fetal cerebral oxygen consumption at different levels of oxygenation. *J Appl Physiol* 1977;43:1080–1084.
27. Yaffe H, Parer JT, Block BS, et al. Cardiorespiratory responses to graded reductions of uterine blood flow in the sheep fetus. *J Dev Physiol* 1987;9:325–336.
28. Parer JT. *Handbook of Fetal Heart Rate Monitoring,* 2nd ed. Philadelphia: Saunders, 1997.
29. Hon EH, Quilligan EJ. The classification of fetal heart rate. II. A revised working classification. *Conn Med* 1967;31:779–784.
30. National Institute of Child Health and Human Development Research Planning Workshop. Electronic fetal heart rate monitoring: research guidelines for interpretation. *Am J Obstet Gynecol* 1997;17:1385–1390.
31. Court DJ, Parer JT. Experimental studies of fetal asphyxia and fetal heart rate interpretation. In: Nathanielsz PW, Parer JT, eds. *Research in Perinatal Medicine.* New York: Perinatology Press, 1984:113–169.
32. Korhonen J, Kariniemi V. Emergency cesarean section: the effect of delay on umbilical arterial gas balance and Apgar scores. *Acta Obstet Gynecol Scand* 1994;73:782–786.
33. Gull H, Jaffa AJ, Oren M, et al. Acid accumulation during end stage bradycardia in term fetuses: how long is too long? *Br J Obstet Gynaecol* 1996;103:1096–1101.
34. Beard RW, Filshie GM, Knight CA, et al. The significance of the changes in the continuous fetal heart rate in the first stage of labour. *J Obstet Gynaecol Br Commonw* 1971;78:865–881.
35. Low JA, Victory R, Derrick EJ. Predictive value of electronic fetal monitoring for intrapartum fetal asphyxia with metabolic acidosis. *Obstet Gynecol* 1999;93:285–291.
36. Dellinger EH, Boehm FH, Crane MM. Electronic fetal heart rate monitoring: early neonatal outcomes associated with normal rate, fetal stress and fetal distress. *Am J Obstet Gynecol* 2000;182:14–20.
37. Menihan CA. Uterine rupture in women attempting a vaginal birth following prior cesarean birth. *J Perinatol* 1998;18:440–443.
38. Leung AS, Leung EK, Paul RH. Uterine rupture after previous cesarean delivery: maternal and fetal consequences. *Am J Obstet Gynecol* 1993;169:945–950.
39. Ralston DH, Shnider SM. The fetal and neonatal effects of regional anesthesia in obstetrics. *Anesthesiology* 1978;48:34–64.
40. Tejani N, Mann LI, Bhakthavathsalan C, et al. Correlation of fetal heart rate–uterine contraction patterns with fetal scalp blood pH. *Obstet Gynecol* 1975;46:392–396.
41. Phelan JP, Ahn MO. Perinatal observations of forty-eight neurologically impaired term infants. *Am J Obstet Gynecol* 1994;171:424–431.
42. Schifrin BS, Hamilton-Rubinstein T, Shields JR. Fetal heart rate patterns and the timing of fetal injury. *J Perinatol* 1994;14:174–181.
43. Parer JT, Livingston EG. What is fetal distress? *Am J Obstet Gynecol* 1990;162:1421–1427.
44. MacLennan AH. A template for defining a causal relationship between acute intrapartum events and cerebral palsy: International Consensus Statement. *BMJ* 1999;319:1016–1017.
45. Clark SL, Gimovsky ML, Miller FC. The scalp stimulation test: a clinical alternative to fetal scalp blood sampling. *Am J Obstet Gynecol* 1984;148:274–277.
46. Martin CB Jr, DeHann J, van der Wildt B, et al. Mechanisms of late decelerations in the fetal heart rate: a study with autonomic blocking agents in fetal lambs. *Eur J Obstet Gynaecol Reprod Biol* 1979;9:361–373.
47. Parer JT, Krueger TR, Harris JL. Fetal oxygen consumption and mechanisms of heart rate response during artificially produced late deceleration of fetal heart rate in sheep. *Am J Obstet Gynecol* 1980;136:478–482.
48. Harris JL, Krueger TR, Parer JT. Mechanisms of late decelerations of the fetal heart rate during hypoxia. *Am J Obstet Gynecol* 1982;144:491–496.
49. Bowes WA, Gabbe SG, Bowes C. Fetal heart rate monitoring in premature infants weighing 1500 grams or less. *Am J Obstet Gynecol* 1980;137:791–796.
50. Garite TJ, Linzey EM, Freeman RK, et al. Fetal heart rate patterns and fetal distress in fetuses with congenital anomalies. *Obstet Gynecol* 1979;53:716–720.
51. Krebs HB, Petres RE, Dunn LJ. Intrapartum fetal heart rate monitoring. V. Fetal heart rate patterns in the second stage of labor. *Am J Obstet Gynecol* 1981;140:435–439.

52. Saling E, Scheider D. Biochemical supervision of the foetus during labour. *J Obstet Gynaecol Br Commonw* 1967;74:799–811.

53. Paul RH, Suidan AK, Yeh SY, et al. Clinical fetal monitoring. VIII. The evaluation and significance of intrapartum baseline FHR variability. *Am J Obstet Gynecol* 1975;123:206–210.

54. Ecker JL, Parer JT. Obstetric evaluation of fetal acid-base balance. *Crit Rev Clin Lab Sci* 1999;36:407–451.

55. Beard RW, Morris ED, Clayton SG. pH of foetal capillary blood as an indicator of the condition of the foetus. *J Obstet Gynaecol Br Commonw* 1967;74:812–822.

56. Garite TJ, Dildy G, McNamara H, et al. A multicenter randomized trial of fetal pulse oximetry. *Am J Obstet Gynecol* 2000;182:S12.

57. Seeds J, Cefalo R, Proctor H, et al. The relationship of intracranial infrared light absorbance to fetal oxygenation. *Am J Obstet Gynecol* 1984;149:679–684.

58. Dildy GA, Clark SL, Loucks CA. Preliminary experience with intrapartum fetal pulse oximetry in humans. *Obstet Gynecol* 1993;81:630–635.

59. Helwig JT, Parer JT, Kilpatrick SJ, et al. Umbilical cord blood acid base state: what is normal? *Am J Obstet Gynecol* 1996;174:1807–1814.

60. Low JA, Cox MJ, Karchmar EJ, et al. The prediction of intrapartum fetal metabolic acidosis by fetal heart rate monitoring. *Am J Obstet Gynecol* 1981;139:229–305.

61. Ellison PH, Foster M, Sheridan-Pereira M, et al. Electronic fetal monitoring, auscultation and neonatal outcome. *Am J Obstet Gynecol* 1991;164:1281–1289.

62. Kubli FW, Hon EH, Khazin AF, et al. Observations on heart rate and pH in the human fetus during labor. *Am J Obstet Gynecol* 1969;104:1190–1206.

63. Fleischer A, Schulman H, Jagani N, et al. The development of fetal acidosis in the presence of an abnormal fetal heart tracing. *Am J Obstet Gynecol* 1982;142:55–60.

64. American College of Obstetricians and Gynecologists. *Inappropriate use of the terms fetal distress and birth asphyxia.* ACOG Committee Opinion. Washington, DC: ACOG, 1998 no. 197.

65. Paneth N, Kiely J. The frequency of cerebral palsy: a review of population studies in industrial nations since 1950. In: Stanley FJ, Alberman E, eds. *The Epidemiology of the Cerebral Palsies.* Philadelphia: JB Lippincott, 1984:46–56.

66. Lilien AA. Term intrapartum fetal death. *Am J Obstet Gynecol* 1970;107:595–603.

67. Apgar V. A proposal for a new method of evaluation of the newborn infant. *Anesth Analg* 1953;32:260–267.

68. Schifrin BS, Dame L. Fetal heart rate patterns: prediction of Apgar score. *JAMA* 1972;219:1322–1325.

69. Sykes GS, Johnson P, Ashworth F, et al. Do Apgar scores indicate asphyxia? *Lancet* 1982;27:494–496.

70. Freeman JM. *Prenatal and perinatal factors associated with brain disorders.* Washington, DC: National Institute of Child Health and Human Development, 1985.

71. Low JA, Galbraith RS, Muir DW, et al. Motor and cognitive deficits after intrapartum asphyxia in the mature fetus. *Am J Obstet Gynecol* 1988;158:356–361.

72. Minchom P, Niswander K, Chalmers I, et al. Antecedents and outcome of very early neonatal seizures in infants born at or after term. *Br J Obstet Gynaecol* 1987;94:431–439.

73. Goldaber KG, Gilstrap LC, Leveno KJ, et al. Pathologic fetal acidemia. *Obstet Gynecol* 1991;78:1103–1108.

74. Low JA, Panagiotopoulos C, Derrick EJ. Newborn complications after intrapartum asphyxia with metabolic acidosis in the term fetus. *Am J Obstet Gynecol* 1994;170:1081–1087.

75. Gilstrap LC, Leveno KJ, Burris J, et al. Diagnosis of birth asphyxia on the basis of fetal pH, Apgar score, and newborn cerebral dysfunction. *Am J Obstet Gynecol* 1989;161:825–830.

76. Winkler CL, Hauth JC, Tucker MJ, et al. Neonatal complications at term as related to the degree of umbilical artery acidemia. *Am J Obstet Gynecol* 1991;164:637–641.

77. Nelson KB, Ellenberg JH. Children who "outgrew" cerebral palsy. *Pediatrics* 1982;69:529–536.

78. American College of Obstetricians and Gynecologists. *Umbilical cord blood acid-base analysis.* ACOG Committee Opinion 91. Washington, DC: ACOG, 1991.

79. Gilstrap LC, Cunningham G. Umbilical cord blood acid-base analysis. In: *Williams Obstetrics,* 19th ed. Ortho Pharmaceutical Corp., Rariton, NJ, 1994.

Shnider and Levinson's Anesthesia for Obstetrics,
edited by Samuel C. Hughes, et al.
Lippincott Williams & Wilkins,
Philadelphia, © 2001.

CHAPTER 37

EVALUATION OF
THE NEONATE

GERSHON LEVINSON, M.D., SAMUEL C. HUGHES, M.D.,
AND MARK A. ROSEN, M.D.

Evaluation of the fetus and neonate is important to detect and treat problems that result in increased perinatal morbidity and mortality. Factors that may modify infant outcome and survival include complications that occur during pregnancy or labor, perinatal asphyxia, anesthetic medications, and the presence of congenital abnormalities. Evaluation prior to delivery is primarily aimed at determining optimal obstetric management, whereas the importance of assessment immediately after birth lies in promptly identifying severely depressed infants who require active resuscitation. In the first hours of life it is imperative that infants who need special observation and therapy are identified and placed in intensive care nurseries. Such management has considerably reduced neonatal mortality, particularly with regard to premature infants. Further evaluation over the early days and months of life enables a prognosis to be formulated as to the long-term physical, neurologic, and psychologic well-being of the infant. In addition, some of these methods of evaluation are utilized to assess outcome in obstetric and anesthetic research.

EVALUATION OF THE NEONATE IN THE DELIVERY ROOM

After delivery, the infant's condition must be rapidly assessed to determine the need for immediate resuscitation. Before the introduction of the Apgar score, the time interval between delivery and the "first gasp" (breathing time) or "first cry" (crying time) was used to identify asphyxiated infants. The underlying hypothesis was that infants who breathed very shortly after birth (i.e., in the first 60 to 90 seconds) were healthy and did not require resuscitation, whereas infants in whom ventilation was delayed were asphyxiated. It was demonstrated subsequently by James et al. (1) that the mere onset of ventilation did not bear a constant relationship to oxygenation.

In 1953, Dr. Virginia Apgar developed her now universally accepted scoring system (2), that evaluation of the newborn immediately after birth was standardized into a simple, reproducible form that all personnel could easily be trained to perform. To ensure objectivity, it was intended that the score be performed by a pediatrician or some other individual not directly involved in care of the mother. The score was designed to clearly identify depressed infants requiring resuscitation and thereafter to follow their progress over the first minutes of life. The score directs the attendant's attention to five vital signs: heart rate, respiratory effort, muscle tone, reflex irritability, and color. Each sign is given a numeric value, as shown in Figure 37.1.

Heart Rate

Heart rate is determined by auscultation of the chest, or less commonly, by observation of the epigastrium or precordium for visible heart beat or by palpation of the cord at the umbilicus. As with the fetus, the neonate at birth usually has a heart rate of over 100 beats/min. A heart rate less than this usually signifies hypoxia. However, an otherwise healthy baby can have a reflex bradycardia from zealous efforts to aspirate the pharynx or empty the stomach. Rarely, bradycardia is due to congenital

heart block or maternal beta-adrenergic blockade therapy (e.g., esmolol) (3). An infant with a heart rate over 100 beats/minute receives a 2, less than 100 beats/minute is scored 1 and absent heart rate is 0.

Respiratory Effort

An infant who is breathing and crying lustily receives a 2 rating, whereas an apneic infant receives a score of 0. All other types of respiratory effort—such as irregular, shallow respiration or weak cry—are scored 1. The respiratory rate, per se, is not considered, only the quality of the respiratory efforts.

Muscle Tone

A baby with active movement or spontaneously flexed arms and legs that resist extension is rated 2, whereas a completely flaccid infant receives a 0 score. Anything in between receives a value of 1. Some maternally administered drugs such as benzodiazepines or magnesium may depress muscle tone without affecting circulation or ventilation (4), whereas others, such as ketamine in large doses ($>2\,\mathrm{mg}\cdot\mathrm{kg}^{-1}$), may increase tone while depressing ventilation (5).

Reflex Irritability

This is tested by either inserting a nasal catheter, flicking the soles of the feet, or drying the baby vigorously. A sneeze or lusty cry is scored 2, a grimace or weak cry 1, and no response 0.

Color

All infants are cyanotic at birth because of their high hemoglobin concentrations and low PaO_2. The disappearance of cyanosis is usually rapid when ventilation and circulation are normal. Many healthy, vigorous infants still have generalized or acrocyanosis at 1 minute due in part to peripheral vasoconstriction in response to the cold delivery room. A completely pink baby receives a score of 2, a pale or blue baby a score of 0, and a neonate with acrocyanosis a score of 1. If an infant seems to be breathing well but remains completely cyanotic despite administration of 100% oxygen, the most common cause is acidosis and pulmonary vasoconstriction. Other causes include cyanotic congenital heart disease, methemoglobinemia, polycythemia, or pulmonary disease such as hypoplastic lungs. The very pale infant may be hypovolemic and hypotensive. Some maternally administered drugs such as magnesium can cause peripheral vasodilation and a pink color in a hypotonic lethargic baby. Normally, babies will have acrocyanosis for more than 10 minutes after birth.

EVALUATION OF THE APGAR SCORE

Of the five criteria in the Apgar score, heart rate and respiratory effort are most important in identifying a distressed newborn, and color is of least value. Modifications of this scoring system with relative weight values for each sign or elimination of the color evaluation have been suggested (6). However, the

Score	A Appearance Color	P Pulse Heart Rate	G Grimace Reflex Irritability	A Activity Muscle Tone	R Respiration Respiratory Effort
0	Blue, pale	Absent	No response	Limp	Absent
1	Body pink, Extremities blue	Below 100	Grimace	Some flexion of extremities	Slow, irregular
2	Completely pink	Over 100	Cough, sneeze, or cry	Active motion	Good, crying

Figure 37.1. Apgar score is based on five signs, each scored 0, 1, or 2.

Apgar score as originally described has achieved its universal acceptance and popularity due in large part to its simplicity and reproducibility. The Apgar score has been claimed to have prognostic significance in regard to development of respiratory distress syndrome (7), neurologic abnormalities (8), and indeed death (9). It quickly identifies those infants requiring active resuscitation, which, by its early initiation, will reduce neonatal morbidity and mortality.

The Apgar score is usually measured at 1 and 5 minutes after birth. If the infant's condition continues to change in response to resuscitative efforts, the score should be repeated at 10 and 20 minutes of life. In addition to its simplicity, this measure has the effect of forcing the birth attendants to focus attention on the neonate at a time when care of the mother may also be demanding their attention. Although it has been used for almost 50 years as an evaluative and prognostic tool, it is useful to review its value and limitations in light of knowledge acquired since its inception.

Apgar Score and Resuscitation

On the basis of 1-minute scores, neonates may be divided into three groups that relate to the degree of depression and thus, to the need for active resuscitation. Several groups (10, 11) have found the Apgar score to correlate well with acid-base measurements performed immediately after birth: infants with scores greater than 7 had either normal values or, more commonly, a mild respiratory acidosis; infants with scores of 4 to 6 were moderately depressed, having a respiratory acidosis with some slight depression of buffer base; and those with low scores (0 to 3) usually had a combined metabolic and respiratory acidosis. This last group frequently had experienced a period of prolonged or severe asphyxia. This is similar to the relationship of fetal scalp samples taken just before delivery and Apgar scores at birth (12) (Fig. 37.2).

This relationship between Apgar score and the acid-base status has been challenged. In a prospective study of 1,210 infants, Sykes et al. (13) found that among babies with Apgar scores less than 7 at 1 and 5 minutes, only 21% and 19%, respectively, were severely acidotic (umbilical artery pH of less than 7.1 and base deficit of more than 13 mmol/liter). Conversely, of the babies with severe acidosis, 73% had Apgar scores over 7 at 1 minute, and 86% had such scores at 5 minutes. The authors caution that the Apgar score should not be considered predictive of neonatal asphyxial damage.

Other investigators have also found a poor correlation between Apgar scores and acid-base status (14–20). Lauener et al.

(14) found that the sensitivity of a 1-minute Apgar score of less than 4 for an umbilical arterial pH of less than 7.15 was 10.7%, whereas the specificity was 98.7%. This indicates that the score was very good at ruling out acidosis but could not be used to predict a low pH. In their study, of all infants with Apgar scores less than 4, only 37% had an umbilical cord arterial pH of less than 7.15. Similar results (i.e., poor positive predictive value but good negative-predictive value) was also found in the

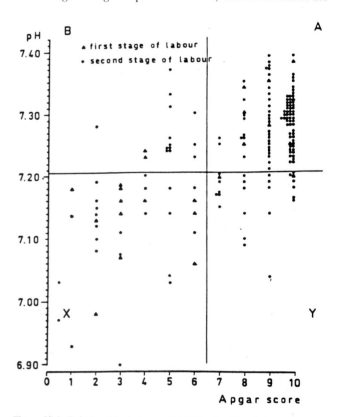

Figure 37.2. Relationship between fetal blood pH and Apgar score at 2 minutes. All samples were taken shortly before delivery. The diagram is arbitrarily divided, separating fetuses regarded as vigorous (Apgar score 7 or above) and those with "normal" pH (above 7.2). Note that there is a general relationship between the two variables (segments *A* and *X*) and also approximately 30% spillover into the false-normal and false-abnormal groups (*B* and *Y*). (From Beard RW, Morris ED, Clayton SG. pH of foetal capillary blood as an indicator of the condition of the foetus. *J Obstet Gynaecol Br Commonw* 1967;74:812–822, with permission.)

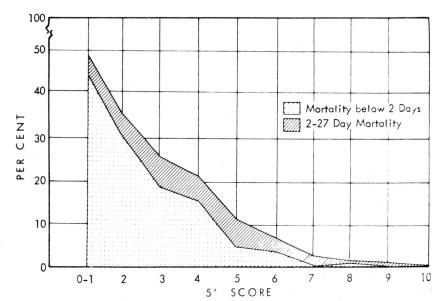

Figure 37.3. Percentage of neonatal mortality within each 5-min Apgar score. (From Drage JS, Berendes H. Apgar scores. and outcome of the newborn. *Pediatr Clin North Am* 1966;13:635–643, with permission.)

relationship between lactic acidemia and Apgar scores (16) and Apgar scores less than 3 and umbilical cord arterial pH of less than 7.21 in preterm infants (19).

As others (21, 22) have pointed out, newborn depression can result from a variety of factors, including maternally administered CNS depressants, birth trauma, or reflex bradycardia from excessively vigorous suctioning of the airway. Severe asphyxia can occur long before delivery, causing permanent damage in a baby whose acid-base status has completely recovered by birth (23). Alternatively, it can occur acutely, shortly before delivery in an otherwise healthy infant; such a baby may be born severely acidotic, but cries immediately, quickly restoring normal acid-base status. Some studies indicate that the combination of either fetal heart rate monitoring or biophysical profile, cord blood pH, and Apgar score is better than any one parameter alone as an evaluation of neonatal status at delivery (see Chapters 35 and 36) (24, 25).

Regardless of the cause of neonatal depression, the degree of intervention required during resuscitation relates to the extent to which the score is lowered. For example, essentially healthy neonates scoring 8 to 10 need no ventilatory assistance, and mild-to-moderately depressed infants (scores 3 to 7) frequently improve rapidly in response to oxygen administered by mask (with positive pressure when necessary), whereas those who are severely depressed (scores 0 to 2) merit immediate active intervention, including endotracheal intubation and perhaps cardiac massage. A detailed description of resuscitation of the newborn based on the Apgar score is described in Chapter 38. A second evaluation of the score at 5 minutes (and subsequently at 5-minute intervals until the score is greater than 7) forces the resuscitation team to assess their progress and better enables them to decide whether to continue their attempts. As a guide to identifying and treating the depressed neonate, the Apgar score has not yet been surpassed by any other index.

Prognostic Value of the Apgar Score

Apgar and James (26) and the Collaborative Study of Cerebral Palsy (27) investigated the correlation between neonatal mortality and Apgar score. In Apgar's study, the mortality in the first 28 days of life, in both full-term and premature infants, was inversely related to the score at 1 minute.

In very low-birth-weight infants, mortality tended to be high at all scores, although in all birth weight groups considered, there was a significant difference in survival in infants whose scores were poor (0 to 3), fair (4 to 6), or good (7 to 10) (26). In an

attempt to establish a more accurate predictive index, the Collaborative Study evaluated scores at both 1 and 5 minutes. They confirmed Apgar results for 1-minute scores, finding mortality in the first 27 days to be 23% for infants having scores of 0 or 1, decreasing to 0.1% for infants with 1-minute scores of 10. The 27-day mortality of infants with 5-minute scores of 0 or 1 was 49%; it decreased with increasing scores. The Collaborative Study also demonstrated that Apgar scores more accurately predicted mortality during the first 2 days of life, rather than the period from 2 to 27 days, and that the 5-minute score was more useful in this respect (Fig. 37.3). In spite of a smaller incidence of low scores at 5 minutes, such scores were much more likely to be associated with increased mortality. When birth weight was considered in conjunction with Apgar score, the highest mortality occurred in infants with both low birth weight and low Apgar scores. There was also a trend to increased mortality in infants weighing over 4000 g, perhaps because these infants were the offspring of diabetic mothers or because they had sustained birth trauma during a difficult delivery.

In a continuation of these studies, the Collaborative Perinatal Project of the National Institute of Neurological and Communicative Disorders and Stroke (NCPP) reported data on 49,000 infants born between 1959 and 1966, further exploring the relationship between mortality and Apgar score (28). While low (0 to 3) 5-minute Apgar scores were associated with a 10- to 15-fold greater mortality in the first year than were high scores (7 to 10), the persistence of a low score was the most significant factor. Among babies who still had a low score 20 minutes after birth, 59% of term infants and 96% of low birth weight (less than 2500 g) infants had died by the end of the first year.

Limitations of the Apgar Score

The Apgar score remains a useful general prognostic tool in predicting short-term mortality for *groups* of infants, particularly those of low birth weight. It has little value, however, when attempting to predict the likelihood of survival in any individual case.

Several problems become apparent when the Apgar score is critically examined as an evaluative index. The intended objectivity of the score may be threatened by lack of personnel available to measure it who are not involved with care of the patient. However, this criticism of subjectivity can be leveled equally and justifiably at most other indices used to assess neonatal condition. Perhaps a more important limitation is the relative crudeness of the measurement, which looks only at the vital functions necessary to sustain life and continues observation for only a very brief period. Many serious neonatal problems do not present until after the infant has left the delivery room, and Apgar herself commented that the score "is no substitute for a careful physical examination and careful observation over the first few hours of life." Because the infant has to be considerably affected to significantly lower the score, subtle effects of perinatal asphyxia or maternal medication may be missed entirely. Newer and more sophisticated techniques of examining the neurologic and behavioral aspects of the newborn have repeatedly demonstrated profound and sometimes prolonged depression in infants who have perfectly normal Apgar scores. Thus, studies using this index as an outcome measure that have judged drug regimens as "safe" must be reinterpreted in the light of more recent data. The Apgar score remains a simple method of assessing the status of the newborn, and determining the necessity for and the effectiveness of resuscitation (29).

NEWBORN ASSESSMENT AND NEONATAL NEUROLOGIC INJURY

In addition to studying mortality, the same groups (8, 28) investigated the value of the Apgar score as a predictor of neonatal morbidity. Neurologic examinations were performed at 1 year of age and were related to 1- and 5-minute Apgar scores and to birth weight (8). Of the 14,115 infants examined, 1.9% were discovered to have definite neurologic abnormalities. When considered in conjunction with Apgar scores at 1 minute, an incidence of 3.6% of neurologically abnormal infants was found in the group who had scores of 0 to 3, whereas the incidence was only 1.6% in infants who had scored 7 to 10. When grouped according to 5-minute score, the disparity was even greater; the incidence of abnormal infants in the "low score" group was four times as high as in the "high score" group. Again, birth weight was an extremely significant factor, with a more than 6-fold increase in neurologic abnormalities in infants weighing 1,001 to 2,000 g at birth compared with those weighing over 2500 g (Figs. 37.4 and 37.5).

The Collaborative Project of the NCPP carefully screened children up to 7 years of age for cerebral palsy (CP), mental retardation, and more minor handicaps (28). Although the incidence of low Apgar scores was higher among infants with CP than among normal children, 73% of CP victims were born with Apgar scores above 7 (Fig. 37.6). Even a 5-minute Apgar score of 0 to 3 correlates poorly with future neurologic outcome. Term infants with Apgar scores of 0 to 3 at 5 minutes have an increased risk of CP,

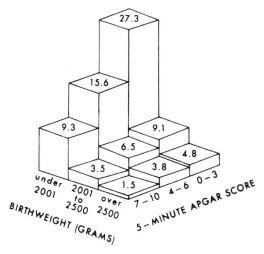

Figure 37.5. Percentage of neurologic abnormality at 1 year of age, by 5-min Apgar score and birth weight groups. (Adapted from Drage JS, Kennedy C, Berendes H, et al. The Apgar score as an index of infant morbidity. *Dev Med Child Neurol* 1966;8:141–148.)

but this increase is only 0.3% to 1% (28, 30). This suggests that factors arising before or after birth are more significant with respect to the etiology of CP than those surrounding the birth process itself. In children free from CP, mental retardation and other disorders were not more commonly associated with low Apgar scores.

The association between perinatal asphyxia and cerebral palsy is weak (31), and the causes of most cases are unknown. Factors found more frequently than expected in babies with cerebral palsy were maternal proteinuria or mental retardation, breech presentation, major congenital malformation in the neonate not involving the CNS, and neonatal seizures. Most children (about 90%) with cerebral palsy are not asphyxiated at birth (32). In the approximately 10% of infants with cerebral palsy who were asphyxiated at birth, it is uncertain if the perinatal asphyxia caused the cerebral palsy or if the asphyxia was incidental or caused by a preexisting fetal abnormality. Similar to the poor correlation of a low Apgar score and cerebral palsy, numerous recent studies have shown no close association between umbilical cord metabolic acidosis and cerebral palsy (33–35).

The current consensus of opinion (36–39) is that to postulate a relationship between perinatal asphyxia and cerebral palsy in an individual patient, the following criteria must be present:

1. Profound umbilical artery metabolic or mixed acidemia (pH of less than 7)
2. Persistence of an Apgar score of 0 to 3 for longer than 5 minutes
3. Evidence of neonatal neurologic sequelae (e.g., seizures, coma, hypotonia and one or more of the following: cardiovascular, gastrointestinal, hematologic, pulmonary, or renal system dysfunction).

Unless these characteristics are all present and other potential causes such as preexisting brain lesions eliminated, a link between the birth asphyxia and subsequent cerebral palsy is unlikely. It is noteworthy that the incidence of cerebral palsy in term infants (one to two out of 1,000) has not changed despite the widespread use of fetal monitoring, the decreased use of forceps, the increased rate of cesarean sections for fetal indications, and improved neonatal resuscitation. The perception that hypoxia at birth accounts for a significant portion of infants with cerebral palsy is clearly unwarranted.

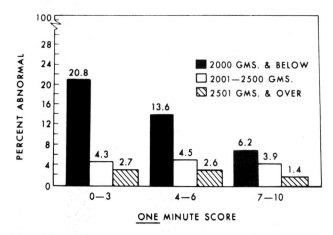

Figure 37.4. Percentage of neurologic abnormality at 1 year of age, by 1-min Apgar score and birth weight groups. (Adapted from Drage JS, Kennedy C, Berendes H, et al. The Apgar score as an index of infant morbidity. *Dev Med Child Neurol* 1966;8:141–148.)

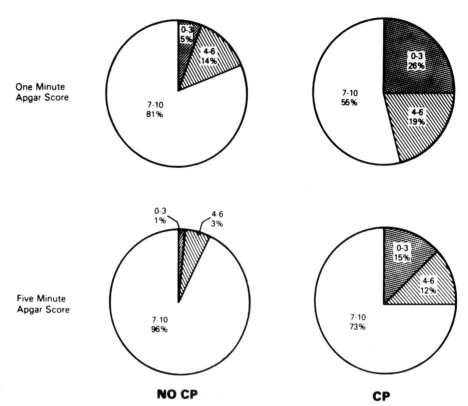

One Minute
Apgar Score

Five Minute
Apgar Score

NO CP   **CP**

Figure 37.6. Distribution of Apgar scores at 1 and 5 min in children with no later cerebral palsy (CP; left), and in those with cerebral palsy (right). (From Nelson KB, Ellenberg JG. Apgar scores as predictors of chronic neurologic disability. *Pediatrics* 1981;68:36–44, with permission.)

LATER EVALUATION OF THE NEONATE
General Examination of the Newborn

As soon as the infant's condition has stabilized after delivery, a careful and thorough examination must be performed to look for abnormalities that may require special management. Developmental anomalies of the nervous system, such as spina bifida or myelomeningocele, are usually obvious, but congenital cardiac disease may be asymptomatic at this stage. An infant who remains cyanotic or whose lungs are difficult to inflate should immediately arouse suspicion of a diagnosis of diaphragmatic hernia, whereas the presence of bubbling secretions would suggest tracheoesophageal fistula. If either of the latter conditions is suspected, further diagnostic measures must be undertaken immediately. Examination of the mouth may reveal cleft lip or palate, a large tongue as in cretinism, or micrognathia as in the Pierre Robin syndrome. It is especially important to recognize these abnormalities because dangerous respiratory obstruction may develop, particularly during feeding.

Continued Observation of the Neonate

In most centers, for the first few hours of life the infant is intensively observed, regardless of whether it is "rooming in" or in a special nursery. During the first 24 hours, the infant undergoes massive physiologic adjustments from intrauterine to extrauterine life. Desmond and associates (40) observed a number of physical signs during the first 10 hours of life in essentially healthy neonates (Fig. 37.7). A period of great activity is seen immediately after birth, which subsides after the first 30 minutes, giving way to sleep for subsequent hours. The infant then once more becomes active and aroused and may pass meconium and cry. Respiratory difficulties such as grunting or intercostal retraction, signifying the presence of respiratory distress syndrome, may not become obvious until this time. CNS damage may manifest itself by irritability, "jitteriness," or seizures; in such cases, a full neurologic examination is indicated.

The biochemical status of the infant is also changing during this period. In normal infants the respiratory acidosis that is usu-

ally present at birth is rapidly corrected during the first hours of life, and by 24 hours, blood gases are similar to those found in utero (41). In sick neonates, serial evaluation of acid-base status using an umbilical arterial catheter may reveal abnormalities that point to the need for oxygen or bicarbonate therapy or ventilatory support. Asphyxiated infants or those severely depressed by anesthetic medication frequently demonstrate a prolonged respiratory acidosis in addition to a metabolic acidosis. The metabolic derangements in these and in premature infants resolve much more slowly than in healthy infants.

Assessment of Weight and Gestational Age

Morbidity and mortality are high in low-birth-weight infants. It is important to recognize that this group comprises two distinct subgroups: (a) infants who are small because they have been born prematurely and (b) infants who are of lower birth weight than would be expected from knowledge of their gestational age. Intrauterine growth standards have been constructed that permit classification of an infant as small, appropriate, or large for gestational-age (42) (Fig. 37.8). Deviation from normal growth occurs in a variety of pathologic conditions. Intrauterine growth restriction may occur in conjunction with chronic maternal hypertension, toxemia, placental insufficiency, cigarette smoking, alcoholism, drug abuse, or severe malnutrition. Frequently, the etiologic factor is unknown. The distinction between premature but appropriate-for-gestational-age infants and full-term infants of similar weight who are small for gestational age is important because different problems may be anticipated in each group. Premature infants are susceptible to respiratory distress, jaundice, hypothermia, intracranial hemorrhage, and retrolental fibroplasia. Small-for-gestational-age infants are more likely to suffer from hypoglycemia and infection, as well as requiring a greater caloric intake that is associated with a higher oxygen consumption (43). Congenital and chromosomal abnormalities occur more frequently in small-for-gestational-age infants.

The prognosis of small-for-gestational-age infants is generally poorer then premature appropriate-for-gestational-age infants of the same weight, as judged by the results of developmental

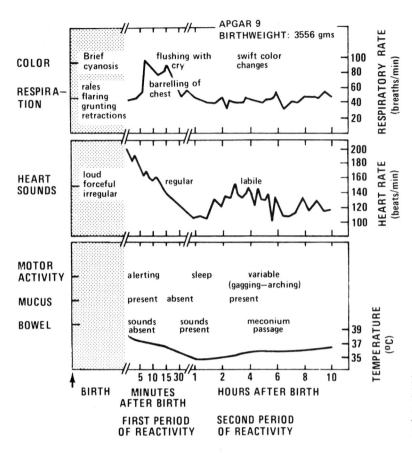

Figure 37.7. Physical findings noted during the first 10 hours of life in a high Apgar score infant delivered under spinal anesthesia without prior premedication. (Adapted from Desmond MM, Rudolph AJ, Phitaksphrai-wan P. The transitional care nursery. *Pediatr Clin North Am* 1966;13:651–668.)

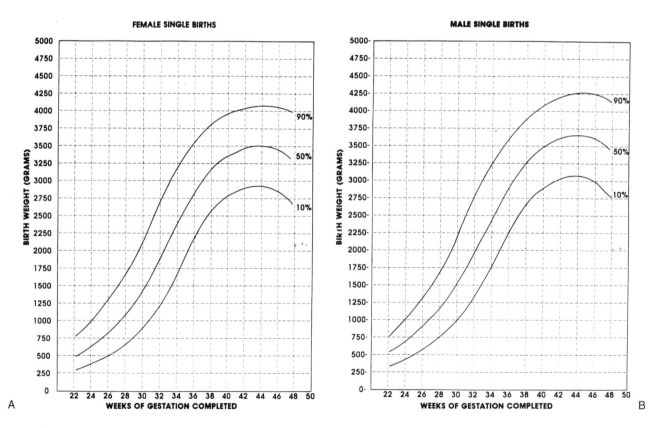

Figure 37.8. University of California San Francisco Perinatal Access System of classification of newborns by birth weight and gestational age: female (**a**) and male (**b**). (From North Coast Perinatal Access System, 1982, with permission.)

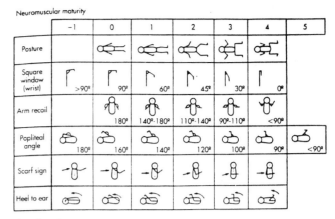

Figure 37.9. New Ballard scoring system for clinical assessment of maturation in newborns. This scoring system has been expanded to include extremely preterm infants and it has been refined to improve the accuracy of assessment of more mature infants. (Adapted from Ballard JL, Khoury JC, Wedig K, et al. New Ballard score, expanded to include extremely premature infants. *J Pediatr* 1991;119:418.)

testing. It can be postulated that the nutritional deficiency or chronic hypoxia that results in low birth weight is also responsible for poor neurologic development. Both morbidity and mortality in the newborn are related to gestational age, following a pattern similar to the relationship with birth weight, that is, rates are highest in infants of lowest birth weight and earliest gestational age and diminish as normal values are approached. Morbidity and mortality are also increased when excessive birth weight or postmaturity is present; large birth weight is often associated with maternal diabetes or difficult deliveries, and in postmaturity the fetus tends to have outgrown its placental supply. Consideration of gestational age with respect to birth weight is, of course, only possible if the former can be accurately determined. Although the date of the last menstrual period provides valuable information, bleeding early in pregnancy frequently cannot be distinguished from a normal period and, thus, the date of conception is unknown. Several schemes have been developed for assessing gestational age that relate development to either the appearance of certain neurologic signs or to external characteristics in the newborn. Although either of these parameters gives a fair estimate of gestational age, the best approximation is provided by the Dubowitz score (44), which uses both sets of criteria. As modified by Ballard (45) (Fig. 37.9), a graded score is awarded for the presence of six neurologic signs that predominantly reflect muscle tone and that are related to maturation of the nervous system. The signs selected are those least affected by the state of arousal of the infant or the presence of neurologic abnormality. Both of these factors had affected previous assessments based on neurologic criteria. Seven external characteristics (including skin texture, color and opacity, nipple formation, and ear form) are similarly considered, and a composite score is obtained. Dubowitz found that different observers could reliably reproduce the total score, be

performed at any time during the first 5 days of life, and be able to accurately assess gestational age to within 1 week.

Neurobehavioral Testing

The inability of the Apgar score to detect subtle or delayed effects of perinatal events led pediatricians, psychologists, and more recently, anesthesiologists to seek more sensitive methods of evaluating the neonate. Although traditional neurologic examination is undoubtedly of diagnostic value in infants with frank neurologic problems, it is of limited value for recognizing the sequelae of lesser perinatal insults and for predicting their influence on future development. For a complete description of the neurologic examination of the neonate and the abnormalities associated with neurologic disorders, the reader is referred to a review of the subject (46).

Dissatisfaction with existing techniques has caused attention to be directed toward other aspects of newborn behavior. As far back as 1957, Graham and co-workers (47) correlated decreased performance in a series of neonatal behavior tests with the severity of perinatal hypoxia. Infants with a history of hypoxia could clearly be distinguished from a control group of "normal" infants. Drugs administered to the mother also may result in subtle and prolonged effects on the newborn, in spite of normal Apgar scores at birth.

Various neurobehavioral tests have been developed that have modified and extended the classic newborn neurologic examination. For many years the infant had been regarded as functioning only reflexively at a spinal or brain stem level. When subjected to closer scrutiny it was appreciated that the newborn is capable of quite organized behavior in the first days of life.

Brazelton (48) observed that maternal medication exaggerated and prolonged the period of relative disorganization that occurs for some period following "normal" delivery. This led him

Name _____ Unit Number _____
Time _____ Blood Gases Po$_2$ _____ Pco$_2$ _____ pH _____
Anesthetic Level _____Type _____ Body Temp _____
Apgar   HR ____ Resp Eff ____ Tone ____ Irrit ____ Color ____Total ____

                    NEURO EXAM:

STATE _____ 1. Response to pinprick   0 1 2 3
                    Habituation no. _____
         _____ 2. Resistance against passive motion
                    A. Pull to sitting   0 1 2 3
                    B. Arm recoil   0 1 2 3
                    C. Truncal tone   0 1 2 3
                    D. General body tone 0 1 2 3
         _____ 3. Rooting   0 1 2 3
         _____ 4. Sucking   0 1 2 3
         _____ 5. Moro response   0 1 2 3
                    Threshold (# of attempts)
                    Extinguishment
         _____ 6. Habituation to light in eyes   No. _____
         _____ 7. Response to sound   0 1 2 3
                    Habituation no. _____
         _____ 8. Placing   0 1 2 3
                 9. Alertness   0 1 2 3
                 10. General assessment   A   B   N   S†
                    (circle)
                    Reasons
                    State _____
                    Lability of state _____

COMMENTS:

Figure 37.10. Protocol for Early Neonatal Neurobehavioral Scale (ENNS) or Scanlon Score. A, abnormal; B, borderline; N, normal; S, superior. (From Scanlon JW, Brown WU Jr, Weiss JB, et al. Neurobehavioral responses of newborn infants after maternal epidural anesthesia. *Anesthesiology* 1974;40:121–128, with permission.)

to develop a more exact way of quantitating the psychophysiologic adaptive changes occurring during the first week after birth. The Brazelton Neonatal Behavioral Assessment Scale (NBAS) (49) has formed the basis of many other such scales and examines various aspects of newborn behavior that are thought to involve the CNS at a cortical level. Such functions include the newborn's ability to alter its state of arousal, suppress meaningless or intrusive stimuli, and respond appropriately to a spectrum of external events in its environment. CNS integrity is also evidenced by the newborn's motor behavior, both in initiating complex motor acts and in reflex motor responses. In the normal infant, smooth arcs of limb movements are present, whereas jerky, hypertonic activity signifies imbalance between flexor and extensor muscle groups and reflects a poorly organized CNS. The NBAS is a comprehensive evaluation of newborn behavior, but it is time consuming and must be performed by a trained observer.

Neonatal behavioral tests have proved sensitive in demonstrating depression of the neonate after perinatal asphyxia, illness, maternal medication, and a variety of other influences. Repeated assessments are most valuable because they allow recovery from such effects to be monitored and permit formulation of a long-term prognosis. The NBAS proved superior to routine neurologic examinations in predicting which infants would be neurologically abnormal at 7 years of age (50). Although both tests succeeded in identifying most of the infants who were ultimately considered to be impaired, the neurologic examination had a higher "false alarm" rate and mislabeled more normal children than the NBAS.

The obstetric anesthesiologist is, of course, most interested in the effects on the neonate of maternally administered drugs. Conway and Brackbill (51) claimed that both maternal analgesia and anesthesia could affect newborn behavior for as long as 4 weeks after birth, although it was difficult in their study to separate the effects of individual drugs, dosages, and anesthetic techniques. Behavioral effects have been correlated with electroencephalographic records of newborns and have confirmed that heavy maternal medication may cause transient CNS depression until the third day of life (52).

With the intention of studying primarily the effects on the neonate of maternal medication and anesthetic techniques, Scanlon and associates (53) devised a neurobehavioral test, the Early Neonatal Neurobehavioral Scale (ENNS), based on the Prechtl and Beintema Neurological Examination (54) and the NBAS (Fig. 37.10). This examination has proved to be relatively simple and rapid to perform, with a high degree of reproducibility between observers. It was initially designed to assess infants during the first 8 to 12 hours of life, this period of time corresponding with the half-life of local anesthetics used for epidural anesthesia. The test must be conducted when the infant is awake but resting quietly in a room without other distracting influences. The observer assesses the infant's state of wakefulness on several occasions, reflex responses (rooting, sucking, Moro's maneuver), muscle tone and power, and responses to light, pinprick, and sound. Decrement behavior or "habituation" after repetition of these stimuli is also recorded. The ability of the infant to decrease and eventually abolish its response to stimuli that are meaningless to it seems to represent the earliest example of processing of information by the cerebral cortex, memory, and perhaps even learning. This property, commonly referred to as habituation, seems to be particularly sensitive to the effects of anesthetic drugs. Even small amounts of maternal systemic medication, such as meperidine (50 mg), have been shown to depress such "higher" CNS functions, as reflected by a slower rate of habituation to a redundant sound stimulus. This parameter and responsiveness to external stimuli were found by Brackbill et al. (55) to be the most sensitive elements of a variety of evaluative tests.

Other investigators (56) consider alterations in motor tone to be more significant than habituation as indicators of neonatal CNS depression. With this in mind, Amiel-Tison, Barrier, and

NEUROLOGICAL AND ADAPTIVE CAPACITY SCORES

			0	1	2
Adaptive Capacity	1	Response to Sound	absent:	mild:	vigorous:
	2	Habituation to Sound	absent:	7-12 stimuli:	< 6 stimuli:
	3	Response to Light	absent:	mild:	brisk blink or startle:
	4	Habituation to Light	absent:	7-12 stimuli:	< 6 stimuli:
	5	Consolability	absent:	difficult:	easy:

TOTAL		ADAPTIVE CAPACITY

			0	1	2
Passive Tone	6	Scarf Sign	encircles the neck:	elbow slightly passes midline:	elbow does not reach midline:
	7	Recoil of Elbows	absent:	slow: weak:	brisk: reproducible:
	8	Popliteal Angle	>110°	100°-110°	< 90°
	9	Recoil of Lower Limbs	absent:	slow: weak:	brisk: reproducible:
Active Tone	10	Active Contraction of Neck Flexors	absent or abnormal:	difficult:	good; head is maintained in the axis of the body:
	11	Active Contraction of Neck Extensors (from leaning forward position)	absent or abnormal:	difficult:	good; head is maintained in the axis of the body:
	12	Palmar Grasp*	absent:	weak:	excellent; reproducible:
	13	Response to Traction (following palmar grasp)	absent:	Lifts part of the body weight:	lifts all of the body weight:
	14	Supporting Reaction (upright position)	absent:	incomplete; transitory:	Strong; supports all body weight:
*Primary Reflexes	15	Automatic Walking*	absent:	difficult to obtain:	perfect; reproducible:
	16	Moro Reflex*	absent:	weak; incomplete:	perfect; complete:
	17	Sucking*	absent:	weak:	perfect; synchronous with swallowing:
General Assessment	18	Alertness	coma:	lethargy:	normal:
	19	Crying	absent:	weak; high pitched; excessive:	normal:
	20	Motor Activity	absent or grossly excessive:	diminished or mildly excessive:	normal:

TOTAL		NEUROLOGICAL

TOTAL SCORE		AT_____	MINUTES OF LIFE

Figure 37.11. Neurologic and Adaptive Capacity Scores (NACS). Asterisks signify primary reflexes. (From Amiel-Tison C, Barrier G, Shnider SM, et al. A new neurologic and adaptive capacity scoring system for evaluating obstetric medications in full-term newborns. *Anesthesiology* 1982;56:340–350, with permission.)

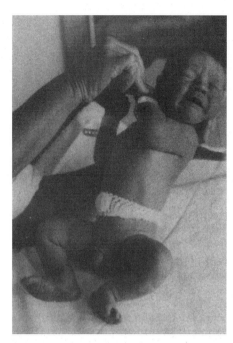

Figure 37.12. Scar sign. The elbow does not reach midline. (From Amiel-Tison C, Barrier G, Shnider SM, et al. A new neurologic and adaptive capacity scoring system for evaluating obstetric medications in full-term newborns. *Anesthesiology* 1982;56:340–350, with permission.)

Shnider designed a neurobehavioral examination, the Neurologic and Adaptive Capacity Score (NACS) (54). This combines elements of the Amiel-Tison neurologic examination (57), the ENNS (53), and the NBAS (49). The NACS was specifically designed as a screening test to detect CNS depression caused by drugs and to distinguish it from that caused by perinatal asphyxia or birth trauma. Twenty criteria are tested and scored as 0, 1, or 2, encompassing five general areas: adaptive capacity, passive tone, active tone, primary reflexes, and alertness (Fig. 37.11). Tests of passive tone include the scarf sign (Fig. 37.12), recoil of elbows and lower limbs (Fig. 37. 13), and measurement of the popliteal angle (Fig. 37.14). Tests of active tone include an assessment of the extensor and flexor muscles of the neck (Fig. 37.15), the response to traction (Fig. 37.16), and the supporting reaction (Fig. 37.17). Primary reflexes include the palmar grasp (Fig. 37.18), automatic walking (Fig. 37.19), the Moro reflex (Fig. 37.20), and the sucking reflex.

The emphasis on motor tone allows unilateral or upper body hypotonus, which sometimes is indicative of mild birth trauma or asphyxia, to be distinguished from global motor depression, which is more likely to result from anesthetic depression. Hypertonus of neck extensors, which can accompany intracranial hypertension, merits a low score on the NACS, whereas it would be scored as 3, an optimal score, in the ENNS. In comparison with that score, less emphasis is placed on reflex activity, and habituation to noxious stimuli such as pinprick and repeated Moro maneuvers are avoided. The latter frequently prove distressing to the mother, who may be observing the examination. In the NACS, as in the NBAS, an optimal response is sought by encouraging the examiner to alter the sequence of the test

according to the state of arousal of the infant, and by retesting items to ensure the best response. The NACS has high interobserver reliability, requires no special equipment, and takes only 3 to 4 minutes to perform (compared with 6 to 10 minutes for the ENNS and 45 minutes for the NBAS). A particular advantage of the NACS is that, as each item is progressively scored from 0 for a poor response to 2 for an optimal response, a total score can be compiled for each infant. This enables easier statistical comparison of different treatment regimens than do other scales, which permit only comparison of numbers of infants with "high" or "low" scores for each specific variable. Arbitrarily, a score of 35 to 40 in the NACS has been designated as representing a neurologically vigorous neonate. When a group of newborns were examined with both the ENNS and NACS, 92% scored equally well on both examinations (56); this is hardly surprising given the similarity of the tests. Valid criticisms of both these scales relate to their subjective nature and the inability in any rapid

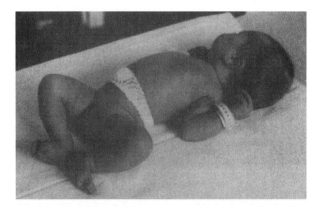

Figure 37.13. Posture and recoil. The infant is in a spontaneously flexed posture. Forearms and lower limbs return briskly to a position of flexion when extended. (From Amiel-Tison C, Barrier G, Shnider SM, et al. A new neurologic and adaptive capacity scoring system for evaluating obstetric medications in full-term newborns. *Anesthesiology* 1982;56:340–350, with permission.)

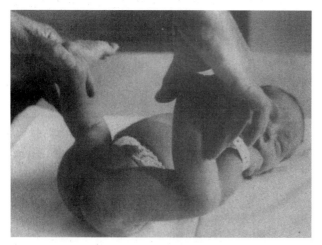

Figure 37.14. Popliteal angle. The angle between the leg and the thigh is the popliteal angle. (From Amiel-Tison C, Barrier G, Shnider SM, et al. A new neurologic and adaptive capacity scoring system for evaluating obstetric medications in full-term newborns. *Anesthesiology* 1982;56:340–350, with permission.)

simple test to evaluate all aspects of newborn behavior (58). Brockhurst et al. reviewed 71 articles that reported studies that used the NACS to correlate neonatal outcome with maternal medication during labor and delivery. They found that few studies reported statistically significant differences in the total NACS, and they speculated that this could be due to lack of actual differences, design limitations due to inadequate number of patients or other serious methodological faults, or lack of sensitivity in the NACS to detect small effects or deviations from normal (59). In fact, in their review, they found that (a) most studies did not follow the recommended NACS assessment protocol by deviating from the recommended assessment times, (b) did not use a controlled environment thereby allowing high levels of ambient light and noise to interfere, and (c) included infants of less than 38 weeks' gestation. In addition, many studies included inappropriate neonates such as preterm and breech deliveries, failed to consider obstetric variables such as length of labor and delivery method, and drug kinetics such as interval between drug administration and delivery. Standardization of the NACS with normal neonates not exposed to medication in utero has not been achieved and a normal range has not been determined. The ability of the NACS to differentiate between drug-induced depression and asphyxia still has not been proven. The NACS has differentiated between the neurobehavioral effects of general and regional anesthesia (60–62), which supports the merits of the scale.

A recent attempt to assess the reliability of the NACS suggested that the test had poor reliability (59%). However, this study of NACS reliability had significant methodological problems. While the validity of the NACS is still not proven, nevertheless it remains one of the most commonly used neurobehavioral tests for assessment of neonatal drug effects.

NEUROBEHAVIORAL EFFECTS OF ANESTHESIA

An increasing mass of information is accumulating that relates newborn behavior to the effects of anesthesia. This has been encouraged by the Food and Drug Administration's requirement that new drugs for use in the parturient be subjected to neurobehavioral testing in the neonate. Most of the studies that are discussed below have used either the ENNS, or more recently, the NACS.

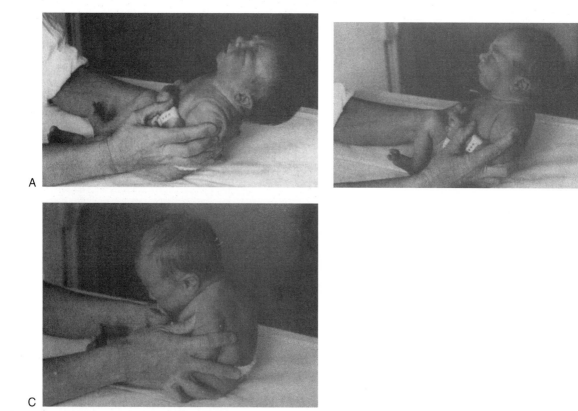

Figure 37.15. **A:** Note position of head in relation to trunk when infant is pulled from supine into sitting position. **B:** Extensor and flexor tone is balanced in the full-term infant. **C:** The head is maintained for a few seconds along the axis of the trunk before dropping forward. (From Amiel-Tison C, Barrier G, Shnider SM, et al. A new neurologic and adaptive capacity scoring system for evaluating obstetric medications in full-term newborns. *Anesthesiology* 1982;56:340–350, with permission.)

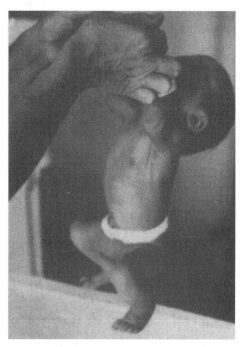

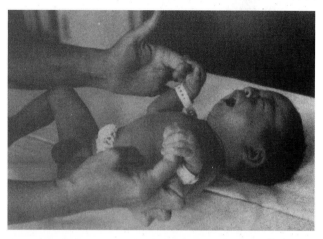

Figure 37.18. Palmar grasp. Flexion of the infant's fingers onto the examiner's index fingers. (From Amiel-Tison C, Barrier G, Shnider SM, et al. A new neurologic and adaptive capacity scoring system for evaluating obstetric medications in full-term newborns. *Anesthesiology* 1982;56:340–350, with permission.)

Figure 37.16. Response to traction. The contraction is spreading to flexor muscles of the upper limbs so that the infant can lift himself or herself completely. (From Amiel-Tison C, Barrier G, Shnider SM, et al. A new neurologic and adaptive capacity scoring system for evaluating obstetric medications in full-term newborns. *Anesthesiology* 1982;56:340–350, with permission.)

Systemic Medications

In general, maternal administration of CNS depressants causes a transient depression of newborn behavior that appears to be related to the presence and quantity of drug in the neonatal circulation. Kron et al. (63) demonstrated that a single injection of 200 mg of secobarbital given to the mother immediately before delivery was associated with poorer sucking responses in the infant for as long as 4 days after birth. Brazelton (48) similarly found a lag of 2 days in the establishment of breast-feeding and 1 day in weight gain in babies of mothers who were heavily medicated in labor, as compared with those whose mothers were not. Visual attentiveness of the newborn also was depressed for as long as 4 days after the administration of opioids or barbiturates to the mother within $1\frac{1}{2}$ hours of delivery (64). Rolbin and co-workers (65) reported that diazepam, in doses of 2.5 to 10 mg, administered 30 to 55 minutes before cesarean section resulted in decreased muscle tone as detected by the ENNS at 4 hours of age. Other aspects of the test were normal, and tone had improved by 24 hours of age.

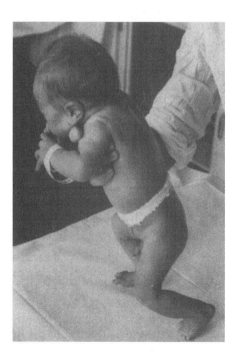

Figure 37.17. Supporting reaction. In the standing position, the legs straighten and the spinal muscles contract. (From Amiel-Tison C, Barrier G, Shnider SM, et al. A new neurologic and adaptive capacity scoring system for evaluating obstetric medications in full-term newborns. *Anesthesiology* 1982;56:340–350, with permission.)

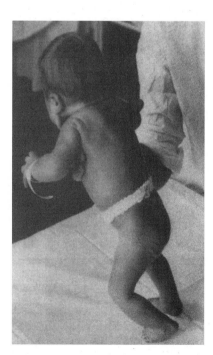

Figure 37.19. Automatic walking. Walking occurs when the supporting reaction is obtained. (From Amiel-Tison C, Barrier G, Shnider SM, et al. A new neurologic and adaptive capacity scoring system for evaluating obstetric medications in full-term newborns. *Anesthesiology* 1982;56:340–350, with permission.)

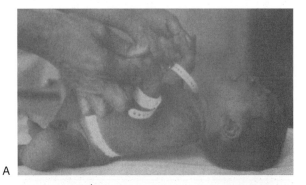

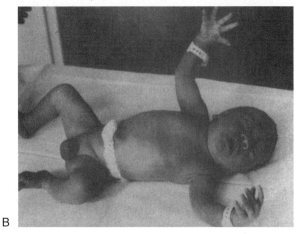

Figure 37.20. Moro reflex. **A:** To achieve neck and trunk angulation, the infant's shoulders are lifted a few centimeters off the table. **B:** The first part of the Moro reflex consists of a brisk abduction and extension of the arms and complete opening of the hands. (From Amiel-Tison C, Barrier G, Shnider SM, et al. A new neurologic and adaptive capacity scoring system for evaluating obstetric medications in full-term newborns. *Anesthesiology* 1982;56:340–350, with permission.)

Numerous studies (66) have evaluated the neonatal effects of meperidine. Fifty to 100 mg of this agent, administered 1 to 3 hours before delivery, does not usually lower Apgar scores, although it does adversely affect newborn behavior. In a large study of 920 term infants, Hodgkinson et al. (67) found that meperidine (50 to 150 mg) administered within 4 hours of delivery globally depressed the ENNS for the first 2 days of life; the degree of depression was dose related. Brackbill and co-workers, (55), using the NBAS and a modification of the habituation test for an auditory stimulus, also reported lower scores in general, and delayed habituation in particular, following similar doses of meperidine. Brower et al. (68) studied neonatal electroencephalogram patterns following maternal meperidine administration and discovered that only the response to auditory stimuli was affected. Perhaps of more importance with respect to adverse effects is the finding by Kron et al. (63) of poorer sucking in infants exposed to moderate doses of this opioid. Unfortunately, in most of the above investigations subjects were selected retrospectively, control groups were lacking, and patients were not differentiated according to socioeconomic status or obstetric complexity. In addition, many patients received a number of analgesic drugs. Leiberman and co-workers (69), in a well-controlled prospective study, compared 145 term infants whose mothers had received 100 to 150 mg doses of meperidine on demand with infants whose mothers had received epidural anesthesia with bupivacaine 0.375%. The only abnormality detected by repeated examinations (NBAS and Prechtl neonatal assessment) up to 42 days of age was decreased habituation to sound on day 3 in the meperidine group.

Fentanyl, a very popular opioid in labor, appears to have little neurobehavioral effects when used in routine clinical doses in labor. Two studies (70, 71) indicate that intravenous fentanyl administration (mean dose 140 ± 32 µg) has a minimal effect on the NACS. However, using patient-controlled intravenous analgesia for labor, it was found that nalbuphine in doses up to 42 mg produced lower NACS scores than did meperidine in doses up to 210 mg (72). Butorphanol, a synthetic opioid agonist/antagonist, has proved to be similar to meperidine with respect to neurobehavioral effects (73).

Several investigators (74, 75) have administered naloxone shortly before delivery to mothers who had received opioids, in an attempt to prevent newborn depression. Disappointingly, benefit was either absent (74) or transient (75) in nature. Administration of naloxone directly to the neonate has proved more effective (76, 77). However, administration of naloxone to infants whose mothers have received opioids cannot be advocated, except when respiratory or CNS depression is present. The naturally occurring endogenous opioids that are present in the neonate may be integral to the newborn's capacity for coping with stress.

Epidural Anesthesia

Scanlon et al. (53) reported that infants of mothers who received epidural anesthesia with either lidocaine or mepivacaine had significantly lower scores than "non-epidural" infants on tests of muscle strength and tone, but behaved normally with respect to habituation to repetitive stimuli. They concluded that these infants were "floppy but alert," and that higher CNS functions had not been depressed by the medication. These effects were present only in the first 8 hours of life, which corresponds with the period during which significant concentrations of local anesthetics were found in the newborn circulation; lidocaine was detected in the neonatal bloodstream for 8 hours and mepivacaine for as long as 24 hours after birth (78). Subsequently, in two separate studies, the same authors found epidural anesthesia using bupivacaine (79) and chloroprocaine (80) to be free from the motor depression seen with lidocaine and mepivacaine. Bupivacaine is present only in very small amounts in the newborn circulation after epidural anesthesia and disappears much more rapidly from the fetal circulation than the other agents; chloroprocaine is rapidly metabolized by plasma cholinesterase. The mechanism by which local anesthetics might affect the newborn is unknown, although an effect on the neuromuscular junction has been postulated.

These studies have been criticized on several grounds: (a) the initial epidural group consisted of a mixture of patients, two-thirds of whom had received mepivacaine and only one-third lidocaine; (b) the number of infants exposed to lidocaine (i.e., 9) is too small to allow firm conclusions to be drawn; (c) the controls for the second and third studies were the same "non-epidural" babies that had formed the controls in the first study several years previously; and (d) approximately one-third of patients in the first study had received opioids or barbiturates in the hours prior to delivery in addition to epidural anesthesia.

A number of studies have indicated that continuous epidural anesthesia with small *intermittent bolus injections* of all commonly used local anesthetics for labor and delivery, including lidocaine, bupivacaine, and chloroprocaine, have no adverse effects on the NACS. These studies with the NACS corroborated previous studies (81, 82) in which the Scanlon ENNS was used to study neurobehavior and did not agree with Scanlon's original report that lidocaine did indeed compromise neurobehavioral function in the neonate (53). Continuous infusion of local anesthetics, frequently employed for labor epidural analgesia, theoretically creates a risk for local anesthetic accumulation in the fetus. Using the NACS, no adverse affects of this continuous administration were found with bupivacaine, chloroprocaine, or lidocaine (83). One would expect that if local anesthetics adversely affected neonatal neurobehavior, the larger doses used for cesarean section would demonstrate these effects in both the NACS or ENNS.

Palahniuk et al. (84), in accordance with Scanlon's group, found transient neonatal hypotonia following epidural lidocaine administered for cesarean section. However, Abboud et al. (81, 85) administered lidocaine, chloroprocaine, and bupivacaine epidurally for labor or cesarean section and found that neonatal neurobehavioral depression was not present in any of the groups. Corroborating these findings, Kileff et al. (86), using the ENNS, compared infants of mothers having cesarean sections with epidural anesthesia using 2% lidocaine or 0.5% bupivacaine. Neonates in the lidocaine group scored as well as those in the bupivacaine group on all items of the ENNS. Kuhnert et al. (87), using the Brazelton Neonatal Behavioral Assessment Scale, compared neonates of mothers given chloroprocaine or lidocaine for vaginal delivery or cesarean section. Only very subtle changes were attributable to lidocaine. No babies had significant hypotonia. Although the differences in effects between the two drug groups were statistically significant, they were so small as to be clinically insignificant. Other investigators (88–90) have confirmed that lidocaine, bupivacaine, chloroprocaine, and etidocaine, even when administered in high dosage for cesarean section, are free from adverse neurobehavioral effects. Similarly, ropivacaine when used for either labor epidurals (91, 92) or for cesarean section (93, 94), has been shown to not decrease the NACS score. Likewise, epidural anesthesia with levobupivacaine 0.5% compared to bupivacaine 0.5% for cesarean section produced equally efficacious anesthesia with no significant differences in Apgar scores or NACS (95).

Epinephrine is commonly added to local anesthetics in epidural anesthesia in concentrations of 1:200,000 to 1:400,000 to decrease systemic absorption and peak blood levels of anesthetic, to provide a longer duration of action, and to intensify motor blockade (96–99). The use of epinephrine in obstetrics is controversial because of possible detrimental effects on uterine blood flow (100–102) and activity (103–107). Epinephrine that is slowly absorbed from the epidural space probably would not have clinically significant effects on uterine blood flow (108–111) and fetal well-being. These assumptions have been corroborated by the findings of no differences in the NACS whether or not epinephrine is added to 1.5% lidocaine (112), 0.5% bupivacaine (113), 2% 2-chloroprocaine (114), or a mixture of bupivacaine 0.25%, butorphanol (1 mg), and epinephrine (115). Thus, for cesarean section in which larger doses of local anesthetic are used and more profound motor blockade is desired, the addition of epinephrine 1:200,000 to the local anesthetic solution may be advantageous and has no detrimental effects on the NACS.

In the United States, 2-chloroprocaine (Nesacaine) has undergone a change in formulation. The sodium bisulfite has been removed as the antioxidant. Studies of bisulfite-free 2-chloroprocaine with and without 1:300,000 epinephrine has shown no detrimental effects on the NACS (116). These findings are similar to those using the old chloroprocaine formulation (114). Lidocaine, bupivacaine, ropivacaine, levobupivacaine and 2-chloroprocaine are widely used in obstetric anesthesia and, in view of the above studies using the NACS and other neurobehavioral tests, appear to be safe drugs for the neonate when administered epidurally to the mother.

Spinal Anesthesia

McGuinness et al. (90) and Hodgkinson et al. (117) compared spinal anesthesia using tetracaine with epidural bupivacaine and with general anesthesia, respectively. Spinal anesthesia produced ENNS scores similar to those with bupivacaine, and significantly better scores than were associated with general anesthesia. The absence of neurobehavioral depression with spinal anesthesia is not surprising, given the extremely low dose of local anesthetic required to provide neural blockade.

Spinal and Epidural Opioids

In general, there has long been concern about maternally administered opioids for potential depressant effects on the newborn. Concern for the newborn, in part, stimulated the initial interest in the use of *intraspinal opioids*; it was thought that low-dose effective analgesia would pose less risk to the neonate. Hughes and co-workers (118) found that newborns delivered of mothers who were given 2, 5, and 7.5 mg of epidural morphine had high Apgar and NACS scores and normal values for umbilical arterial and venous blood gas tension.

Abboud documented the safe use of intrathecal morphine (0.5 to 1 mg) with similar clinical data (119). Intrathecal meperidine also does not depress the NACS (120). Combined spinal epidural anesthesia with fentanyl and bupivacaine has also been shown to have no effect on the newborn (121). Dailey and co-workers (122) found that a continuous maternal intravenous infusion of naloxone to decrease side effects, such as severe itching, did not adversely affect the infant's NACS. We have also found that epidural fentanyl ($1 \mu g \cdot kg^{-1}$) administered with local anesthetics for cesarean section has no adverse effects on the NACS (123), nor is the NACS adversely affected by the addition of fentanyl (50 to 100 μg), either administered in saline or mixed with bupivacaine for labor (124, 125). Use of epidural butorphanol with either bupivacaine (126) or lidocaine (127) for labor does not adversely affect the NACS. Epidural sufentanil for labor analgesia in doses as high as 30 μg does not depress the NACS (128).

Paracervical and Pudendal Block

Data relating neurobehavioral effects of paracervical block are conflicting and difficult to interpret (66). This technique currently is infrequently used in the United States because of the relatively high incidence of fetal bradycardia. Merkow et al. (129) reported that pudendal block with lidocaine, mepivacaine, and 2-chloroprocaine did not result in neurobehavioral depression. In contrast to the neurobehavioral abnormalities found with epidurally administered mepivacaine (53), the habituation response was actually better in the infants who had been exposed to this agent via pudendal block. This difference probably relates to the significantly lower levels of mepivacaine identified following pudendal block, as compared with epidural block ($0.1 \mu g \cdot mL^{-1}$ at 4 hours [129] versus $0.82 \mu g \cdot mL^{-1}$ at 8 hours [53]).

General Anesthesia

The effects of general anesthesia for elective cesarean section or vaginal delivery in normal pregnancies also have been studied. Infants whose mothers had undergone general rather than spinal anesthesia exhibited global depression of neurobehavioral performance, in spite of there being no difference in Apgar scores between the groups (117, 130). Palahniuk et al. (84) compared three anesthetic techniques for cesarean section: (a) methoxyflurane with high-inspired oxygen, (b) nitrous oxide with low-inspired oxygen, and (c) lumbar epidural anesthesia. Although all infants appeared clinically normal, those in the nitrous oxide group were less alert and had lower scores on neurobehavioral testing (ENNS) than the other groups for a period of 24 hours. A different study compared the results of the ENNS in infants whose mothers had received ketamine-nitrous oxide or thiopental-nitrous oxide general anesthesia or 2-chloroprocaine epidural anesthesia for vaginal delivery (131). Epidural anesthesia was associated with the greatest percentage of high scores on the first and second days of life. The infants performed least well after thiopental, with ketamine producing an intermediate effect.

Halogenated anesthetics (halothane, enflurane, and isoflurane) administered at cesarean section in low concentrations to supplement nitrous oxide anesthesia and permit use of a high-inspired oxygen concentration do not adversely affect acid-base status or Apgar scores (84), although some transient depression of the NACS has been noted (132) when the infants are compared to those born with spinal or epidural anesthesia. This was confirmed by other investigators (133). Analgesic concentrations of inhalation agents have been administered for labor and there have been no adverse behavioral effects (134, 135).

SIGNIFICANCE OF NEUROBEHAVIORAL EFFECTS

It is appropriate at this juncture to question the significance, as regards well-being and future development of abnormalities revealed by neurobehavioral testing. Tronick et al. (136) studied the effects of different analgesic regimens for labor on the behavior of normal neonates, attempting to control for other stress factors. Techniques included maternal local and regional anesthesia, and in some cases additional light systemic medication was administered. Only minimal effects were found in all groups. These proved to be transient, and all effects progressively improved over the first 10 days of life.

Similarly, most of the studies discussed in this chapter have found the effects of obstetric analgesia, as currently practiced, to either be absent or of short duration. In contrast, Standley et al. (137) claimed that infants whose mothers had received either systemic analgesia or regional anesthetic blocks performed significantly less well in neurobehavioral examinations on the third day of life than infants whose mothers had no anesthesia. Infants exposed to local anesthetics were said to be most affected. However, this study can be faulted because of the multiplicity of drugs used and the inappropriate grouping together of different anesthetic techniques. Also, complicating obstetric factors were not adequately considered. Friedman et al. (138) have clearly demonstrated the correlation between dysfunctional labor or prolongation of the second stage and adverse neurobehavior. Forceps delivery and anesthesia are associated secondarily with these problems and can be mistakenly considered responsible for their consequences.

In a report that achieved great publicity (139), Brackbill and Broman claimed that poorer physical and intellectual development persisted for up to 7 years in children of mothers who had received medication during childbirth. Although patients (who formed part of the Collaborative Perinatal Project in the 1950s) were claimed to be healthy, women with pregnancy-induced hypertension, difficult deliveries, and other obstetric complications were included. A panel of experts including statisticians, obstetricians, perinatologists, and anesthesiologists, and the Anesthetic and Life Support Committee of the Food and Drug Administration, carefully reviewed their data. Brackbill and Broman's conclusions subsequently were rejected on the grounds that their groups were not homogeneous, statistical analyses were poor, there was no control group, and the postpartum course of the children had not been taken into account (140). In two well-designed, controlled studies that carefully evaluated motor and cognitive abilities of children up to 4 (141, 142) and 5 (143) years of age using a number of tests, no correlation was found between maternal anesthetic technique and later development. As might have been anticipated, emergency cesarean section and peripartum asphyxia adversely affected subsequent development.

There is no evidence that prolonged adverse effects are associated with transient neurobehavioral depression caused by maternal medication. Neurobehavioral assessment techniques have been used predominantly for research and are probably too cumbersome to be applied routinely as a clinical screening tool. At present, neurobehavioral testing is only one method of evaluating the newborn and should not be used in isolation. It should be used in conjunction with the clinical history, Apgar score, physical examination, biochemical, radiologic, and neurologic evaluation.

REFERENCES

1. James LS, Weisbrot IM, Prince CE, et al. The acid-base status of human infants in relation to birth asphyxia and the onset of respiration. *J Pediatr* 1958;52:379–394.
2. Apgar V. A proposal for a new method of evaluation of the newborn infant. *Anesth Analg* 1953;32:260–267.
3. Gladstone GR, Hordof A, Gersony WM. Propranolol administration during pregnancy: effects on the fetus. *J Pediatr* 1975;86:962–964.
4. Flowers CE, Rudolph AJ, Desmond MM. Diazepam (Valium) as an adjunct in obstetric analgesia. *Obstet Gynecol* 1969;34:68–81.
5. Little B, Chang T, Chucot L, et al. Study of ketamine as an obstetric anesthetic agent. *Am J Obstet Gynecol* 1972;113:247–260.
6. Crawford JS. Anaesthesia for caesarean section: A proposal for evaluation with analysis of a method. *Br J Anaesth* 1962;34:179–195.
7. Rudolph AJ, Desmond MM, Pineda RG. Clinical diagnosis of respiratory difficulty in the newborn. *Pediatr Clin North Am* 1966;13:669–692.
8. Drage JS, Kennedy C, Berendes H, et al. The Apgar score as an index of infant morbidity. *Dev Med Child Neurol* 1966;8:141–148.
9. Drage JS, Berendes H. Apgar scores and outcome of the newborn. *Pediatr Clin North Am* 1966;13:635–643.
10. Crawford JS, Davies P, Pearson JE. Significance of the individual components of the Apgar score. *Br J Anaesth* 1973;45:148–158.
11. Marx GF, Mahajan S, Miclat MN. Correlation of biochemical data with Apgar scores at birth and at one minute. *Br J Anaesth* 1977;49:831–833.
12. Beard RW, Morris ED, Clayton SG. pH of foetal capillary blood as an indicator of the condition of the foetus. *Obstet Gynaecol Br Commonw* 1967;74:812–822.
13. Sykes GS, Molloy PM, Johnson P, et al. Do Apgar scores indicate asphyxia? *Lancet* 1982;1:494–496.
14. Lauener PA, Calame A, Janecek P, et al. Systematic pH-measurements in the umbilical artery: causes and predictive value of neonatal acidosis. *J Perinat Med* 1983;11:278–285.
15. Fields LM, Entman SS, Boehm FH. Correlation of the one-minute Apgar score and the pH value of umbilical arterial blood. *South Med J* 1983;76:1477–1479.
16. Suidan JS, Young BK. Outcome of fetuses with lactic acidemia. *Am J Obstet Gynecol* 1984;150:33–37.
17. Boehm FH, Fields L, Entman SS, et al. Correlation of the one minute Apgar score and umbilical cord acid-base status. *South Med J* 1986;79:429–431.
18. Page PO, Martin J, Palmer S, et al. Correlation of neonatal acid-base status with Apgar scores and fetal heart rate tracings. *Am J Obstet Gynecol* 1986;154:1306–1311.
19. Luthy DA, Kirkwood KS, Strickland D, et al. Status of infants at birth and risk for adverse neonatal events and long-term sequelae: a study in low birth weight infants. *Am J Obstet Gynecol* 1987;157:676–679.
20. Marrin M, Paes BA. Birth asphyxia: does the Apgar score have diagnostic value? *Obstet Gynecol* 1988;72:120–123.
21. Crawford JS. Apgar score and neonatal asphyxia. *Lancet* 1982;1:684–685.
22. Hughes-Davies TH. Apgar score and neonatal asphyxia. *Lancet* 1982;1:685.
23. Paul RH, Yonekura L, Cantrell CJ, et al. Fetal injury prior to labor: does it happen? *Am J Obstet Gynecol* 1986;154:1187–1193.
24. Page FO, Martin JN, Palmer SM, et al. Correlation of neonatal acid-base status with Apgar scores and fetal heart rate tracings. *Am J Obstet Gynecol* 1986;154:1306–1311.
25. Vintzileos AM, Gaffney SE, Salinger LM, et al. The relationships among the fetal biophysical profile, umbilical cord pH, and Apgar scores. *Am J Obstet Gynecol* 1987;157:627–631.
26. Apgar V, James LS. Further observations on the newborn scoring system. *Am J Dis Child* 1962;104:419–427.
27. Drage JS, Kennedy C, Schwarz BK. The Apgar score as an index of neonatal mortality: a report from the Collaborative Study on Cerebral Palsy. *Obstet Gynecol* 1964;24:222–230.
28. Nelson KB, Ellenberg JH. Apgar scores as predictors of chronic neurologic disabilities. *Pediatrics* 1981;68:36–44.
29. American College of Obstetricians and Gynecologists: Committee on Obstetric Practice and American Academy of Pediatrics:

Committee on Fetus and Newborn. *Use and abuse of the Apgar score.* ACOG Technical Bulletin 174. Washington, DC: ACOG, 1996.

30. Stanley FJ. Cerebral palsy trends: implications for perinatal care. *Acta Obstet Gynecol Scand* 1994;73:5–9.

31. Nelson KB, Ellenberg JH. Antecedents of cerebral palsy: multivariate analysis of risk. *N Engl J Med* 1986;315:81–86.

32. Blair E, Stanley FJ. Intrapartum asphyxia: a rare cause of cerebral palsy. *J Pediatr* 1988;112:515–519.

33. Ruth VJ, Raivio KO. Perinatal brain damage: predictive value of metabolic acidosis and the Apgar score. *BMJ* 1988;297:24–27.

34. Fee S, Malee K, Deddish R, et al. Severe acidosis and subsequent neurologic status. *Am J Obstet Gynecol* 1990;162:802–806.

35. Dennis J, Johnson A, Mutch L, et al. Acid-base status at birth and neurodevelopmental outcome at four and one-half years. *Am J Obstet Gynecol* 1989;161:213–220.

36. Nelson KB. Perspective on the role of perinatal asphyxia in neurologic outcome: its role in developmental deficits in children. *Can Med Assoc J* 1989;141(suppl):3–10.

37. American College of Obstetricians and Gynecologists. *Fetal and neonatal neurologic injury.* ACOG Technical Bulletin 163. Washington, DC: ACOG, 1992.

38. American College of Obstetricians and Gynecologists. *Utility of umbilical cord blood acid-base assessment.* ACOG Committee Opinion 138. Washington, DC: ACOG, 1994.

39. American College of Obstetricians and Gynecologists. *Inappropriate use of the terms fetal distress and birth asphyxia.* ACOG Committee Opinion 197. Washington, DC: ACOG, 1998.

40. Desmond MM, Rudolph AJ, Phitaksphraiwan P. The transitional care nursery. *Pediatr Clin North Am* 1966;13:651–668.

41. Weisbrot IM, James LS, Prince CE, et al. Acid-base homeostasis of the newborn infant during the first 24 hours of life. *J Pediatr* 1958;52:395–403.

42. Lubchenco LO, Koops BL. Assessment of weight and gestational age. In: Avery GB, ed. *Neonatology: Pathophysiology and Management of the Newborn,* 3rd ed. Philadelphia: JB Lippincott, 1987:235–257.

43. Brazelton TB, Paraker WB, Zuckerman B. Importance of behavioral assessment of the neonate. *Curr Probl Pediatr* 1976;7:34–36.

44. Dubowitz LM, Dubowitz V, Goldberg C. Clinical assessment of gestational age in the newborn infant. *J Pediatr* 1970;77:1–10.

45. Ballard JL, Khoury JC, Wedig K, et al. New Ballard Score, expanded to include extremely premature infants. *J Pediatr* 1991;119:417–423.

46. Volpe JJ. Neurological disorders. In: Avery GB, ed. *Neonatology: Pathophysiology and Management of the Newborn,* 4th ed. Philadelphia: JB Lippincott, 1994:1117–1138.

47. Graham FK, Pennoyer MM, Caldwell BM, et al. Relationship between clinical status and behavior test performance in a newborn group with histories suggesting anoxia. *J Pediatr* 1957;50:177–189.

48. Brazelton TB. Psychophysiologic reactions in the neonate. II. Effect of maternal medication on the neonate and his behavior. *J Pediatr* 1961;58:513–518.

49. Brazelton TB. *Neonatal Behavioral Assessment Scale.* Philadelphia: Lippincott, 1973.

50. Brazelton TB, Parker WB, Zuckerman B. Importance of behavioral assessment of the neonate. *Curr Probl Pediatr* 1976;7:70–75.

51. Conway E, Brackbill Y. Delivery medication and infant outcome: an empirical study. *Monogr Soc Res Child Dev* 1970;35:24–34.

52. Borgstedt AD, Rosen MG. Medication during labor correlated with behavior and EEG of the newborn. *Am J Dis Child* 1968;115:21–24.

53. Scanlon JW, Brown WU Jr, Weiss JB, et al. Neurobehavioral responses of newborn infants after maternal epidural anesthesia. *Anesthesiology* 1974;40:121–128.

54. Prechtl H, Bientema D. *The Neurological Examination of the Full-Term Newborn Infant.* London: Spastics International Medical Publications, 1964.

55. Brackbill Y, Kane J, Manniello RL, et al. Obstetric meperidine usage and assessment of neonatal status. *Anesthesiology* 1974;40:116–120.

56. Amiel-Tison C, Barrier G, Shnider SM, et al. A new neurologic and adaptive capacity scoring system for evaluating obstetric medications in full-term newborns. *Anesthesiology* 1982;56:340–350.

57. Amiel-Tison C. A method for neurological evaluation within the first year of life. Experience with full-term newborns. *Ciba Found Symp* 1978;59:107–126.

58. Tronick E. A critique of the Neonatal Neurologic Adaptive Capacity Score (NASC). *Anesthesiology* 1982;56:338–339.

59. Brockhurst NJ, Littleford JA, Halpern SH. The neurologic and adaptive capacity score: a systematic review of its use in obstetric anesthesia research. *Anesthesiology* 2000;92:237–246.

59a. Halpern SH, Littleford JA, Brockhurst NJ. The neurologic and adaptive capacity score is not a reliable method of newborn evaluation. *Anesthesiology* 2001;94:958–962.

60. Gin T, Yau G, Chan K, et al. Disposition of propofol infusions for caesarean section. *Can J Anaesth* 1991;38:31–36.

61. Mahajan J, Mahajan RP, Singh MM, et al. Anaesthetic technique for elective caesarean section and neurobehavioural status of newborns. *Int J Obstet Anesth* 1992;1:89–93.

62. Abboud TK, Nagappala S, Murakawa K, et al. Comparison of the effects of general and regional anesthesia for cesarean section on neonatal neurologic and adaptive capacity scores. *Anesth Analg* 1985;64:996–1000.

63. Kron RE, Stein M, Goddard KE. Newborn sucking behavior affected by obstetric sedation. *Pediatrics* 1966;37:1012–1016.

64. Stechler G. Newborn attention as affected by medication during labor. *Science* 1964;144:315–317.

65. Rolbin SH, Wright RG, Shnider SM, et al. Diazepam during cesarean section–effects on neonatal Apgar scores, acid-base status, neurobehavioral assessment and maternal and fetal plasma norepinephrine levels. In: *Abstracts of Scientific Papers.* New Orleans: American Society of Anesthesiologists, 1977:449.

66. Dailey PA, Baysinger CL, Levinson G, et al. Neurobehavioral testing of the newborn infant—Effects of obstetric anesthesia. *Clin Perinatol* 1982;9:191–214.

67. Hodgkinson R, Bhatt M, Wang CN. Double-blind comparison of the neurobehavior of neonates following administration of different doses of meperidine to the mother. *Can Anaesth Soc J* 1978;25:405–411.

68. Brower KR, Crowell DH, Leung P, et al. Neonatal electroencephalographic patterns as affected by maternal drugs administered during labor and delivery. *Anesth Analg* 1978;57:303–306.

69. Lieberman BA, Rosenblatt DB, Belsey E, et al. The effects of maternally administered pethidine or epidural bupivacaine on the fetus and newborn. *Br J Obstet Gynaecol* 1979;86:598–606.

70. Rayburn WF, Rathke A, Leuschen MP, et al. Fentanyl citrate during labor. *Am J Obstet Gynecol* 1989;161:202–206.

71. Rayburn WF, Smith CV, Leuschen MP, et al. Comparison of patient-controlled and nurse-administered analgesia using intravenous fentanyl during labor. *Anesth Rev* 1991;18:31–33.

72. Frank M, McAteer EJ, Cattermole R, et al. Nalbuphine for obstetric analgesia. *Anaesthesia* 1987;42:697–703.

73. Hodgkinson R, Hugg RW, Hayashi RH, et al. Double-blind comparison of maternal analgesia and neonatal neurobehavior following intravenous butorphanol and meperidine. *J Int Med Res* 1979;7:224–230.

74. Clark RB, Beard AG, Greifenstein FE, et al. Naloxone in the parturient and her infant. *South Med J* 1976;69:570–575.

75. Hodgkinson R, Bhatt M, Grewal G, et al. Neonatal neurobehavior in the first 48 hours of life: effect of the administration of meperidine with and without naloxone in the mother. *Pediatrics* 1978;62:294–298.

76. Bonta BW, Gagliardi JO, Williams V, et al. Naloxone reversal of mild neurobehavioral depression in normal newborn infants after routine obstetric analgesia. *J Pediatr* 1979;94:102–105.

77. Weiner PC, Hogg MI, Rosen M. Neonatal respiration, feeding and neurobehavioral state: effects of intrapartum bupivacaine, pethidine and pethidine reversal by naloxone. *Anaesthesia* 1979;34:996–1004.

78. Brown WU Jr, Bell GC, Lurie AO, et al. Newborn blood levels of lidocaine and mepivacaine in the first postnatal day following maternal epidural anesthesia. *Anesthesiology* 1975;42:698–706.

79. Scanlon JW, Ostheimer GW, Lurie AO, et al. Neurobehavioral responses and drug concentrations in newborns after maternal epidural anesthesia with bupivacaine. *Anesthesiology* 1976;45:400–405.

80. Brown WU Jr. Neonatal neurobehavioral tests following vaginal delivery under ketamine, thiopental and extradural anesthesia. *Anesth Analg* 1977;56:552–553.

81. Abboud TK, Khoo SS, Miller F, et al. Maternal, fetal, and neonatal responses after epidural anesthesia with bupivacaine, 2-chloroprocaine, or lidocaine. *Anesth Analg* 1982;61:638–644.

82. Abboud TK, Sarkis F, Blikian A, et al. Lack of adverse neurobehavioral effects of lidocaine. *Anesthesiology* 1982;57:A404.

83. Abboud TK, Afrasiabi A, Sarkis F, et al. Continuous infusion epidural analgesia in parturients receiving bupivacaine, chloroprocaine, or lidocaine: maternal, fetal and neonatal effects. *Anesth Analg* 1984;63:421–428.

84. Palahniuk RJ, Scatliff J, Biehl D, et al. Maternal and neonatal effects of methoxyflurane, nitrous oxide and lumbar epidural anaesthesia for caesarean section. *Can J Anaesth* 1977;24:586–596.

85. Abboud TK, Kyung CK, Noueihid R, et al. Epidural bupivacaine, chloroprocaine or lidocaine for cesarean section: maternal and neonatal effects. *Anesth Analg* 1983;62:914–919.

86. Kileff ME, James FM, Dewan DM, et al. Neonatal neurobehavioral responses after epidural anesthesia for cesarean section using lidocaine and bupivacaine. *Anesth Analg* 1984;63:413–417.

87. Kuhnert BR, Harrison MJ, Linn PL, et al. Effect of maternal epidural anesthesia on neonatal behavior. *Anesth Analg* 1984;63:301–308.

88. Datta S, Corke BC, Alper MH, et al. Epidural anesthesia for cesarean section: a comparison of bupivacaine, chloroprocaine, and etidocaine. *Anesthesiology* 1980;52:48–51.

89. Lund PC, Cwik JC, Gannon RT, et al. Etidocaine for caesarean section: effects on mother and baby. *Br J Anaesth* 4 1977;9:457–460.

90. McGuinness GA, Merkow AJ, Kennedy RL, et al. Epidural anesthesia with bupivacaine for cesarean section: neonatal blood levels and neurobehavioral responses. *Anesthesiology* 1978;49:270–273.

91. Eddleston JM, Holland JJ, Griffin RP, et al. A double-blind comparison of 0.25% ropivacaine and 0.25% bupivacaine for extradural analgesia in labour. *Br J Anaesth* 1996;76:66–71.

92. Stienstra R, Jonker TA, Bourdrez P, et al. Ropivacaine 0.25% versus bupivacaine 0.25% for continuous epidural analgesia in labor: a double-blind comparison. *Anesth Analg* 1995;80:285–289.

93. Griffin RP, Reynolds F. Extradural anaesthesia for caesarean section: a double-blind comparison of 0.5% ropivacaine with 0.5% bupivacaine. *Br J Anaesth* 1995;74:512–516.

94. Irestedt L, Emanuelsson B-M, Ekblom A, et al. Ropivacaine 7.5 mg/ml for elective caesarean section: a clinical and pharmacokinetic comparison of 150 mg and 187.5 mg. *Acta Anaesthesiol Scand* 1997;41:1149–1156.

95. Bader AN, Tseng L, Camman WR, et al. Clinical effects and maternal and fetal plasma concentrations of 0.5% epidural levobupivacaine versus bupivacaine for cesarean delivery. *Anesthesiology* 1999;90:1596–1601.

96. Bromage PR, Robson JG. Concentrations of lignocaine in the blood after intravenous, intramuscular, epidural and endotracheal administration. *Anaesthesia* 1961;16:461.

97. Mather LE, Tucker GT, Murphy TM, et al. The effects of adding adrenaline to etidocaine and lignocaine in extradural anaesthesia. II. Pharmacokinetics. *Br J Anaesth* 1976;48:989–994.

98. Scott DB, Jebson PRG, Braid DP, et al. Factors affecting plasma levels of lignocaine and prilocaine. *Br J Anaesth* 1972;44:1040–1049.

99. Bromage PR. Physiology. In: *Epidural Analgesia.* Philadelphia: WB Saunders, 1978:357–360.

100. Rosenfeld CR, Barton MD, Meschia G. Effects of epinephrine on distribution of blood flow in the pregnant ewe. *Am J Obstet Gynecol* 1976;124:156–163.

101. Wallis KL, Shnider SM, Hicks JS, et al. Epidural anesthesia in the normotensive pregnant ewe: effects on uterine blood flow and fetal acid-base status. *Anesthesiology* 1976;44:481–487.

102. Hood DD, Dewan DM, Rose JC, et al. Maternal and fetal effects of intravenous epinephrine containing solutions in gravid ewes. *Anesthesiology* 1983;59:A393.

103. Rucker MP. The action of adrenalin on the pregnant uterus. *South Med J* 1925;18:412.

104. Gunther RE, Bauman J. Obstetrical caudal anesthesia. I. A randomized study comparing 1% mepivacaine with 1% lidocaine plus epinephrine. *Anesthesiology* 1969;31:5–19.

105. Gunther RE, Bellville JW. Obstetrical anesthesia. II. A randomized study comparing 1% mepivacaine with 1% mepivacaine plus epinephrine. *Anesthesiology* 1972;37:288–298.

106. Matadial L, Cibils LA. The effect of epidural anesthesia on uterine activity and blood pressure. *Am J Obstet Gynecol* 1976;125:846–854.

107. Zador G, Nilsson BA. Low-dose intermittent epidural anaesthesia with lidocaine for vaginal delivery. II. Influence on labour and foetal acid-base status. *Acta Obstet Gynecol* 1974;34(suppl):17–30.

108. Levinson G, Shnider SM, Krames E, et al. Epidural anesthesia for cesarean section: effects of epinephrine in the local anesthetic solution. In: *Abstracts of Scientific Papers.* Chicago: American Society of Anesthesiologists, 1975:285–286.

109. deRosayro AM, Hahrwold ML, Hill AB. Cardiovascular effects of epidural epinephrine in the pregnant sheep. *Reg Anesth* 1981;6:4–7.

110. Albright GA, Jouppila R, Hollmén AL, et al. Epinephrine does not alter human intervillous blood flow during epidural anesthesia. *Anesthesiology* 1981;54:131–135.

111. Craft JB Jr, Epstein BS, Coakley CS. Effect of lidocaine with epinephrine versus lidocaine (plain) on induced labor. *Anesth Analg* 1972;51:243–246.

112. Abboud TK, David S, Nagappala S, et al. Maternal, fetal and neonatal effects of lidocaine with and without epinephrine for epidural anesthesia in obstetrics. *Anesth Analg* 1984;63:973–979.

113. Abboud TK, Sheik-Ol-Eslam A, Yanagi T, et al. Safety and efficacy of epinephrine added to bupivacaine for lumbar epidural analgesia in obstetrics. *Anesth Analg* 1985;64:585–591.

114. Abboud TK, DerSarkissian L, Terrasi J, et al. Comparative maternal, fetal and neonatal effects of chloroprocaine with and without epinephrine for epidural anesthesia in obstetrics. *Anesth Analg* 1987;66:71–75.

115. Abboud TK, Afrasiabi A, Zhu J, et al. Bupivacaine/butorphanol/epinephrine for epidural anesthesia in obstetrics: Maternal and neonatal effects. *Reg Anesth* 1989;14:219–224.

116. Abboud TK, Mosaad P, Maker A, et al. Comparative maternal and neonatal effects of the new and the old formulations of 2-chloroprocaine. *Reg Anesth* 1988;13:101–106.

117. Hodgkinson R, Bhatt M, Kim SS, et al. Neonatal neurobehavioral tests following cesarean section under general and spinal anesthesia. *Am J Obstet Gynecol* 1978;132:670–674.

118. Hughes SC, Rosen MA, Shnider SM, et al. Maternal and neonatal effects of epidural morphine for labor and delivery. *Anesth Analg* 1984;63:319–324.

119. Abboud TK, Shnider SM, Dailey PA, et al. Intrathecal administration of hyperbaric morphine for the relief of pain in labour. *Br J Anaesth* 1984;56:1351–1359.

120. Talafre ML, Jacquinot P, Legagneux F, et al. Intrathecal administration of meperidine versus tetracaine for elective cesarean section. *Anesthesiology* 1987;67:A620.

121. Fernando R, Bonello E, Gill P, et al. Neonatal welfare and placental transfer of fentanyl and bupivacaine during ambulatory combined spinal epidural analgesia for labour. *Anaesthesia* 1997; 52:517–524.

122. Dailey PA, Brookshire GL, Shnider SM, et al. The effects of naloxone associated with the intrathecal use of morphine in labor. *Anesth Analg* 1985;64:658–666.

123. Preston P, Rosen M, Hughes SC, et al. Epidural anesthesia with fentanyl and lidocaine for cesarean section: maternal effects and neonatal outcome. *Anesthesiology* 1988;68:938–943.

124. Murakawa K, Abboud TK, Yanagi T, et al. Clinical experience of epidural fentanyl for labor pain. *J Anesthesia (Jpn)* 1987;1:93–95.

125. Cohen SE, Tan S, Albright GA, et al. Epidural fentanyl/bupivacaine mixtures for obstetric analgesia. *Anesthesiology* 1987;67:403–407.

126. Abboud TK, Afrasiabi A, Zhu J, et al. Epidural morphine or butorphanol augments bupivacaine analgesia during labor. *Reg Anesth* 1989;14:115–120.

127. Zhu J, Abboud TK, Afrasiabi A, et al. Epidural butorphanol augments lidocaine analgesia during labor. *Anesthesiology* 1990; 73:A979.

128. Little MS, McNitt JD, Choi HJ, et al. A pilot study of low dose epidural sufentanil and bupivacaine for labor anesthesia. *Anesthesiology* 1987;67:A444.

129. Merkow AJ, McGuinness GA, Erenberg A, et al. The neonatal neurobehavioral effects of bupivacaine, mepivacaine, and 2-chloroprocaine used for pudendal block. *Anesthesiology* 1980;52:309–312.

130. Scanlon JW, Shea E, Alper MH. Neurobehavioral responses of newborn infants following general or spinal anesthesia for cesarean section. In: *Abstracts of Scientific Papers.* Chicago: American Society of Anesthesiologists, 1975:91.

131. Hodgkinson R, Marx GF, Kim SS, et al. Neonatal neurobehavioral tests following vaginal delivery under ketamine, thiopental and extradural anesthesia. *Anesth Analg* 1977;56:548–552.

132. Abboud TK, Nagappala S, Murakawa K, et al. Comparison of the effects of general and regional anesthesia for cesarean section on neonatal neurologic and adaptive capacity scores. *Anesth Analg* 1985;64:996–1000.

133. Mahajan J, Mahajan RP, Singh MM, et al. Anaesthetic technique for elective caesarean section and neurobehavioural status of newborns. *Int J Obstet Anesth* 1992;1:89–93.

134. Stefani SJ, Hughes SC, Shnider SM, et al. Neonatal neurobehavioral effects of inhalation analgesia for delivery. Anesthesiology 1982;56:351–355.

135. Abboud TK, Gangolly J, Mossaad P, et al. Isoflurane in obstetrics. *Anesth Analg* 1989;68:388–391.

136. Tronick E, Wise S, Als H, et al. Regional obstetric anesthesia and newborn behavior: Effects over the first ten days of life. *Pediatrics* 1976;58:95–100.

137. Standley K, Soule AB, Duchowny MS. Local-regional anesthesia during childbirth: effect on newborn behaviors. *Science* 1974;186:634–635.

138. Friedman EA, Sachtleben MR, Bresky PA. Dysfunctional labor. XII. Long-term effects on infants. *Am J Obstet Gynecol* 1977;127:779–783.

139. Kolata GB. Behavioral teratology: birth defects of the mind. *Science* 1978;202:732–734.

140. Kolata GB. Scientists attack report that obstetrical medications endanger children: but natural childbirth advocates rally to its defense. *Science* 1979;204:391–392.

141. Ounsted M, Scott A, Moar V. Delivery and development: to what extent can one associate cause and effect? *J R Soc Med* 1980;73:789–792.

142. Ounsted M. Pain relief during childbirth and development at 4 years. *J R Soc Med* 1981;74:629–630.

143. Van den Berg BJ, Levinson G, Shnider SM, et al. Evaluation of long-term effects of obstetric medication on clinical development. In: *Abstracts of Scientific Papers.* Boston: Society for Obstetric Anesthesia and Perinatology, 1980:52.

Shnider and Levinson's Anesthesia for Obstetrics,
edited by Samuel C. Hughes, et al.
Lippincott Williams & Wilkins,
Philadelphia, © 2001.

CHAPTER 38

RESUSCITATION OF THE NEWBORN

SUSAN H. SNIDERMAN, M.D., GERSHON LEVINSON, M.D., AND
GEORGE A. GREGORY, M.D.

Delivery room resuscitation of the neonate requires an understanding of the physiology of asphyxia and of the changes that occur during the transition from the fetal to the adult circulation.

Immediately after delivery, as the fetus becomes a neonate, major changes in the pulmonary and circulatory systems must occur. The lungs must now assume the role of the placenta in the exchange of oxygen and carbon dioxide. This requires pulmonary expansion, aeration, and pulmonary perfusion. In the vast majority of instances, these changes occur spontaneously. Some infants, however, require resuscitation to make the transition from dependent fetal to independent neonatal existence. This chapter discusses the normal changes at birth, the pathophysiology of asphyxia, and recommended techniques for resuscitation of the newborn.

CHANGES IN THE CIRCULATION AT BIRTH

In utero, blood is oxygenated in the placenta and returns to the fetal heart via the umbilical vein, to the left portal vein, the ductus venosus, and the inferior vena cava (1, 2) (Fig. 38.1). At the junction of the inferior vena cava and right atrium the caval blood divides into two streams. Approximately 40% enters the right heart, where it mixes with venous blood returning via the superior vena cava from the upper part of the body. This blood is ejected by the right ventricle into the pulmonary arteries. However, because the pulmonary vascular resistance is so high, only 7% actually perfuses the fetal lungs; the remainder is shunted across the ductus arteriosus into the descending thoracic aorta. About 60% of the well-oxygenated blood returning via the inferior vena cava is deflected by the crista dividens in the right atrium through the foramen ovale into the left atrium. Although this blood undergoes admixture with the small amount of venous blood returning to the left atrium from the lungs, it is relatively well oxygenated. Thus, the blood perfusing the brain and the coronary arteries has a higher oxygen content than the blood perfusing the lower half of the body, which has been mixed with a large amount of less well-oxygenated blood entering the descending aorta from the ductus arteriosus.

With clamping of the cord and removal of the low-resistance placenta from the systemic circulation at birth, systemic vascular resistance increases, left atrial pressure increases, and flow through the foramen ovale decreases. When the lungs expand with the first breaths, pulmonary vascular resistance decreases, and 90% to 100% of right ventricular output now perfuses the lungs (3, 4). The increased pulmonary venous return to the left atrium forces physiologic closure of the foramen ovale flap. Anatomic closure of the foramen takes several months so that in the newborn, any circulatory disturbance that elevates right as compared to left atrial pressure will cause the foramen to open and venous blood to flow from right to left leading to cyanosis.

As arterial oxygen tension and pH rise, the pulmonary vessels dilate, pulmonary vascular resistance decreases further, pulmonary blood pressure falls below systemic and right-to-left shunting of blood through the ductus arteriosus ceases. In the normal newborn, the rise in arterial oxygen to above 60 mm Hg will cause vasoconstriction of the ductus arteriosus and aid in functional closure (5, 6).

ESTABLISHMENT OF VENTILATION

In utero, the fetal lung is filled with an ultrafiltrate of plasma, approximately 30 $mL \cdot kg^{-1}$ of body weight (7, 8). This fluid produced in the lungs must be removed prior to, during and immediately after birth. Reabsorption of fetal lung fluid begins even prior to the onset of contractions and continues throughout labor. During a vaginal delivery the thorax of the fetus is squeezed while passing through the birth canal. This helps push out approximately two-thirds of the fluid left in the lungs at the end of labor, and the remainder is removed after birth by capillaries and lymphatics (9). Infants delivered by cesarean section do not benefit from the vaginal squeeze and may not have the benefit of labor, which may account for their increased difficulty in establishing normal ventilation (10).

Normal infants make their first respiratory movements within seconds of delivery of the thorax. This is due in part to the elastic recoil of the chest wall following expulsion. During the first breath, a negative pressure of 60 to 100 cm H_2O is generated and up to 80 mL of air inspired (11) (Fig. 38.2). The breath is generally held for about 2 seconds and then only partly exhaled. Approximately 75% of the first breath is retained in the lung as part of the developing functional residual capacity. The next few breaths are similar to the first, with lesser amounts of air retained each time. Once ventilation is established, the normal mature infant has a tidal volume of 5 to 7 $mL \cdot kg^{-1}$, a vital capacity of over 100 mL, a breathing frequency of 30 to 60 times/minute, a minute ventilation of over 500 mL, and a lung compliance of 5 mL/cm H_2O (11).

By 90 seconds after delivery, most infants have begun rhythmic ventilation. Initiation of breathing depends on the condition of the respiratory center, including peripheral chemoreceptors responsive to low pH and low Po_2.

ASPHYXIA

Immediately after birth, if adequate ventilation is not established the ensuing hypoxemia and respiratory and metabolic acidosis will prevent establishment of a normal adult circulation. Pulmonary vascular resistance will remain high and pulmonary blood flow low, and the ductus arteriosus and foramen ovale will remain widely patent with a large right-to-left shunt through both. With progressive hypoxemia and acidosis, myocardial failure and brain damage will occur.

In the extreme case when no pulmonary ventilation occurs in a newborn mammal, by 5 minutes the PaO_2 will fall to under 2 mm Hg, the $PaCO_2$ will rise to 100 mm Hg, and the pH will fall to 7.0 or below (1) (Fig. 38.3). Heart rate and blood pressure will decrease and after a period of gasping, apnea will occur. In the monkey, after 7 minutes of complete asphyxia, there will be irreversible brain damage. After the cessation of gasping, nothing will reinitiate breathing other than artificial ventilation.

CAUSES OF NEONATAL DEPRESSION

A number of factors may depress the respiratory center of the neonate, including drugs administered to the mother (e.g., anesthetics, opioids, sedatives, barbiturates, and magnesium), severe

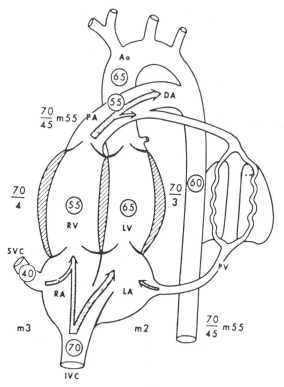

Figure 38.1. The course of the circulation in the heart and great vessels in the late-gestation fetus. (From Rudolph AM. *Congenital Diseases of the Heart.* Chicago: Year Book Medical Publishers, 1974:3, with permission.)

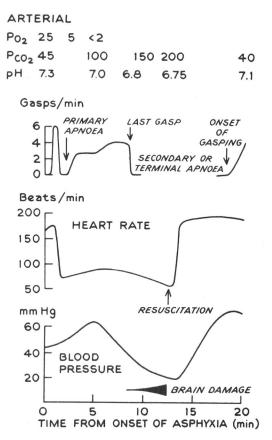

Figure 38.3. Schematic diagram of changes in Rhesus monkeys during asphyxia and resuscitation by positive pressure ventilation. Brain damage was assessed by histologic examination some weeks or months later. (From Dawes GS. *Foetal and Neonatal Physiology.* Chicago: Year Book Medical Publishers, 1968:141–157, with permission.)

intrauterine fetal hypoxia and acidosis, high or low environmental temperature, or CNS trauma associated with the birth process. There is evidence to support less respiratory depression at birth, higher Apgar scores, and more vigorous babies when spinal rather than general anesthesia is used for Cesarean section delivery (12, 13). In addition, certain congenital anomalies may make adaptation to extrauterine life difficult or impossible. Some of these are listed in Table 38.1.

There are also various situations in which serious neonatal morbidity may occur. Identifying these high-risk fetuses prior to birth allows the anesthesiologist, obstetrician, and neonatologist to prepare for immediate resuscitation of the newborn. Some of the factors that should alert the anesthesiologist that the fetus is at high risk are listed in Table 38.2.

The mechanism for the adverse effect on the neonate is obvious in conditions like preeclampsia and anemia, which are asso-

ciated with decreased uteroplacental blood flow or oxygenation. In conditions such as diabetes mellitus, neonatal morbidity and mortality are very high but the precise etiologic factors are not known. Nevertheless, in all these conditions aggressive management of the newborn is indicated.

GOALS OF RESUSCITATION

Neonatal resuscitation should not only save life but also ideally prevent the sequelae of acute asphyxia whenever possible. These sequelae may include hypoxic-ischemic encephalopathy

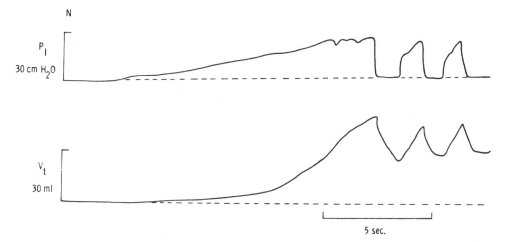

Figure 38.2. Initial lung inflation during resuscitation. (From Jacobs MM, Phibbs RH. Prevention, recognition and treatment of perinatal asphyxia. *J Pediatr* 1981;99:935, with permission.)

Table 38.1. OTHER CAUSES OF NEONATAL DEPRESSION IN THE DELIVERY ROOM

Congenital defects of the respiratory system
Nose: choanal stenosis and atresia
Upper airway: micrognathia (Pierre Robin syndrome)
Larynx
    Webs
    Fusions
    Atresia
    Vocal cord paralysis
    Subglottic stenosis
Trachea
    Tracheal agenesis
    Tracheal rings
    Cartilage
Vascular
    Hemangiomas
    Webs
    Tumors
Bronchi
    Congenital bronchial stenosis
Diaphragmatic hernia
Esophageal atresia and tracheoesophageal fistula
Congenital heart disease
Central nervous system dysfunction (congenital/acquired)
Fetal sepsis

Table 38.2. FACTORS THAT MAY HELP TO IDENTIFY HIGH-RISK FETUSES

Maternal conditions
Preeclampsia-eclampsia
Chronic hypertension
Diabetes mellitus
Chronic renal disease
Maternal malnutrition or severe obesity
Sickle cell disease
Anemia (<9 g hemoglobin)
Rh or ABO incompatibility
Heart disease
Pulmonary disease
Third-trimester bleeding
Drug therapy (e.g., lithium carbonate, magnesium,
    adrenergic-blocking drugs)
Drug or ethanol abuse
Maternal infection
Uterine or pelvic anatomic abnormalities
Prolonged rupture of membranes
Previous fetal or neonatal deaths
Fetal conditions: antepartum
Premature delivery
Postmaturity (>43 weeks)
Intrauterine growth restriction
Multiple births
Oligo- or polyhydramnios
Labor and delivery conditions
Breech or other abnormal presentations
Forceps delivery (other than low elective)
Cesarean section
Prolapsed umbilical cord
Nuchal cord
Prolonged general anesthesia
Excessive sedation or analgesia
Anesthetic complications (such as untreated hypotension
    or hypoxia)
Prolonged or precipitous labor
Uterine hypertonus (spontaneous/oxytocin induced)
Abnormal fetal heart rate or rhythm
Meconium-stained amniotic fluid

with resultant cerebral palsy, cognitive impairment or global developmental delay, multi-organ failure, bone marrow depression, disseminated intravascular coagulation, and asphyxial cardiomyopathy. The degree of organ damage and potential for full recovery depends not only on the severity of the asphyxial event, but its duration as well as the speed and success of resuscitative efforts in restoring oxygen delivery to the tissues.

THE APGAR SCORE

The most widely used method for evaluating the condition of the infant in the delivery room is a score devised by the anesthesiologist Virginia Apgar in 1953 (14, 15). It is fully described in Chapter 37. This easily performed assessment is usually made 1 and 5 minutes after birth. There are five signs: heart rate, respiratory effort, muscle tone, response to stimulation, and skin color. A score of 0, 1, or 2 is assigned according to the presence or absence of each of the signs. Apgar scoring should continue every 5 minutes until the scoring is greater than 7.

UMBILICAL CORD BLOOD SAMPLING

At delivery, the acid-base status and oxygenation of the fetus may be easily ascertained by sampling from a doubly-clamped segment of umbilical cord. This is indicated for babies who have demonstrated fetal distress in utero or who are clinically depressed at 1 minute of age. Some favor routinely measuring umbilical cord blood acid-base status at all deliveries (16). This approach has been discussed fully in Chapter 37. Blood is drawn separately with heparinized syringes from both an umbilical artery and the umbilical vein. It should be recalled that the umbilical vein blood is the best-oxygenated blood. The normal blood gas values are shown in Table 38.3 (17). If both umbilical venous and umbilical artery blood gases show low Po_2 and high Pco_2, then uteroplacental insufficiency was present. If umbilical artery blood shows signs of asphyxia but umbilical venous blood is relatively normal, i.e., a wide venous-arterial difference exists, then umbilical cord compression has likely occurred during labor or the infant is hypovolemic. With partial compression of the umbilical cord or in conditions with low fetal cardiac output, the transit time of fetal blood through the placenta is slowed, thus allowing more time for equilibration with the maternal blood. The umbilical venous blood becomes well oxygenated, but due to hypovolemia or obstruction of blood flow from the placenta to the fetus, an inadequate amount of oxygen is delivered to the fetal tissues and the umbilical arterial blood will demonstrate a low Po_2 and pH with a large base deficit. A depressed neonate with normal umbilical venous oxygen and acid-base values may, in fact, be asphyxiated. It is obvious, therefore, that both the umbilical vein and artery blood should be analyzed for correct assessment of the etiology and significance of neonatal

Table 38.3. NORMAL VALUES FOR UMBILICAL CORD BLOOD[a]

Cord Blood	pH	PCO$_2$ (mm Hg)	PO$_2$ (mm Hg)	Bicarbonate (mEq/L)
Arterial	7.28 ± 0.05 (7.15–7.43)	49.2 ± 8.4 (31.1–74.3)	18.0 ± 6.2 (3.8–33.8)	22.3 ± 2.5 (13.3–27.5)
Venous	7.35 ± 0.05 (7.24–7.49)	38.2 ± 5.6 (23.2–49.2)	29.2 ± 5.9 (15.4–48.2)	20.4 ± 2.1 (15.9–24.7)

[a] Results are for 146 newborns after uncomplicated labor and vaginal delivery at 37 to 42 weeks of gestation. Values are mean ± SD; ranges are given in parentheses.
From Yeomans ER, Hauth JC, Gilstrap LC III, et al. Umbilical cord pH, Pco$_2$, and bicarbonate following uncomplicated term vaginal deliveries. *Am J Obstet Gynecol* 1985;151:798–800, with permission.

depression. If umbilical cord blood gases are normal but the neonate is depressed at birth, common causes include drug depression, sepsis, acute birth trauma, or other factors listed in Table 38.1.

STEPS IN INITIAL RESUSCITATION
Personnel

Every labor and delivery faculty should have a list of both fetal and maternal conditions that require the presence of a resuscitation team at delivery (Table 38.2). The basic team should include at least one physician and one nurse both certified in neonatal resuscitation. For known high-risk deliveries such as extreme prematurity, congenital diaphragmatic hernia, hydrops fetalis, complete placental abruption, a neonatal team should be present at the delivery and should include one neonatologist, another physician and two experienced nursery nurses. Additional personnel such as a respiratory therapist with resuscitation experience may be helpful. An anesthesiologist may be invaluable in managing difficult intubations and ventilation. The most experienced person in attendance should take charge and lead the resuscitation team. While awaiting the birth, tasks should be assigned to each member of the team including management of the airway, placement of ECG monitor leads and the pulse oximeter, insertion of the umbilical catheter, drawing up medications, and charting (18).

Equipment

Each delivery room should contain the basic equipment for resuscitating the depressed newborn (Table 38.4). This includes infant laryngoscopes, supply of batteries and bulbs, various sizes of endotracheal tubes, infant face masks, resuscitation bags, suction bulbs and catheters. In addition, each room should have a mobile or portable (delivery room to nursery) resuscitation bed that provides easy access to the infant for all the personnel involved in the resuscitation. Suction, oxygen and compressed air as well as a blender should be immediately adjacent or physically attached to the resuscitation bed. A source of radiant heat should be mounted above each resuscitation unit. The energy output should be servo-controlled by a sensor taped to the infant's abdomen.

Prior to every delivery, the overhead heater should be turned on to warm the bed and the oxygen and suction should be turned on and tested. The resuscitation bag should fill well and the pop-off pressure should be set at 30 to 50 cm of water and checked. For resuscitation of infants equal to or greater than 37 weeks' gestation, 100% oxygen should be used.

In addition, a special neonatal resuscitation room located immediately adjacent to the delivery room suites is desirable for intensive care of the immature or severely asphyxiated newborn in need of prolonged resuscitation. More sophisticated ventilatory and monitoring equipment and a variety of emergency drugs should be immediately available, as well as umbilical vessel catheter insertion trays and equipment for thoracentesis, paracentesis and fluid resuscitation. This room should be accessible for portable X-ray and ultrasound machines, and should have its own thermostat so that the ambient temperature can be increased above that in the delivery suites.

THERMAL MANAGEMENT

Immediately after birth, particular attention must be given to the prevention of heat loss by the infant. A naked, wet baby delivered into a room at 25°C will rapidly lose heat by conduction, convection, evaporation, and radiation. Catecholamine-mediated, non-shivering thermogenesis by metabolism of brown fat is the principal mechanism utilized by the term neonate in his or her usually futile attempt to maintain normal body temperature.

Table 38.4. EQUIPMENT FOR NEONATAL RESUSCITATION

Basic equipment
Radiantly heated, mobile resuscitation crib
Suction devices: sterile bulb suction *or* DeLee suction trap, meconium aspirator and vacuum suction with sterile catheters (6, 8, 10 French)
Stethoscope
Oxygen source with flowmeter and tubing
Infant resuscitation bag with a pressure-release valve or pressure gauge. The bag must be capable of delivering 90% to 100% oxygen
Infant face masks (newborn and premature sizes)
Infant oropharyngeal airways (newborn and premature sizes)
Laryngoscope with straight blades (no. 0 and 1) (extra bulbs and batteries for laryngoscope)
Sterile endotracheal tubes sizes (2, 2.5, 3, 3.5, and 4 mm) with stylets
Sterile umbilical vessel catheterization tray including 3.5 and 5 French umbilical vessel catheters
Drug tray including:
  Epinephrine 1:10,000
  Naloxone 0.4 $mg \cdot mL^{-1}$ or 0.1 $mg \cdot mL^{-1}$
  Sodium bicarbonate 4.2%
  Dextrose 10%
  Sterile water
  Normal saline
  Volume expanders: either albumin 5% solution, normal saline or Ringer's lactate solution
  Dopamine
Syringes: 1, 3, 5, 10, 20, and 50 mL
Needles: 18, 21, and 25 gauge
Sterile gloves, scissors, adhesive tape, alcohol sponges, and three-way stopcocks
For special neonatal treatment room: All of the above plus:
Oscillometric or Doppler device for neonatal blood pressure
Source of oxygen *and* air with oxygen-air blender
Heated nebulizer
Anaeroid manometer for observing airway pressures during controlled ventilation
Oxygen analyzer
Pulse oximeter
Pressure transducers and monitor for intraarterial and venous pressures
Electrocardiogram and heart rate monitor
Blood gas machine readily available
Thoracocentesis tray including size 10 to 16 French catheters for treatment of pneumothorax

---

This leads to a dramatic increase in oxygen consumption, calorie utilization, and metabolic rate (19–22).

All newborns should be quickly dried with a warm blanket or towel to decrease evaporative heat loss. Newborn infants have a very large surface area to body mass making them especially vulnerable to rate of cold stress. This can lead to respiratory distress, hypoxemia, and hypoglycemia. Therefore, the newborn should be placed underneath a radiant warmer, preferably servo-controlled by a sensor placed on the baby's abdomen or thigh.

ESTABLISHMENT OF THE AIRWAY

As the infant's head is delivered, the mouth and nose are gently suctioned to remove the lung fluid as well as amniotic fluid, blood, mucus, and meconium that might be in the pharynx (Fig. 38.4). Babies born through meconium require more extensive airway management as will be described subsequently. The infant is placed in the head-down position to allow gravity drainage of the pharyngeal fluid. Suctioning of the pharynx and nose should be brief and gentle, because prolonged or too vigorous suctioning may produce breath holding, laryngospasm, profound bradycardia or another arrhythmia.

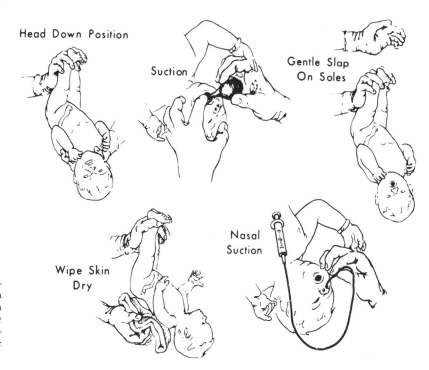

Head Down Position

Suction

Gentle Slap
On Soles

Nasal
Suction

Wipe Skin
Dry

Figure 38.4. Establishment of patency of upper airway by gravity drainage, suctioning, and stimulation
to cry by rubbing the infant with a towel. (From
Gregory GA. Cardiopulmonary resuscitation of the
newborn. In: Shnider SM, Moya F, eds. *The anesthesiologist, Mother and Newborn.* Baltimore: Williams &
Wilkins, 1974:20, with permission.)

In addition to removing debris from the airway with nasal suctioning, anatomic abnormalities such as choanal atresia may be
noted. Babies are nasal breathers and will often develop severe
hypoxia if unable to breathe through their noses.

ESTABLISHMENT OF VENTILATION

The current recommendation of the American Academy of Pediatrics and the American Heart Association is to institute resuscitation prior to the assignment of the 1-minute Apgar score (23).

The vast majority of newborns require only upper airway suctioning, drying of the skin, and a warm ambient environment.
If the infant is not breathing, a brief period of tactile stimulation, including rubbing the infant's back or flicking the soles
of the feet, may be enough to initiate a regular respiratory pattern. If the infant is breathing, color and heart rate should be
assessed. If the pulse is greater than 100, blow-by oxygen should
be provided until the infant's chest, abdomen and mucous membranes are pink. Acrocyanosis is common in the first day of life
in full-term babies who are nonetheless well oxygenated. Occasionally a baby who is vigorous at 1 minute of age will deteriorate shortly thereafter. Possible causes are drug depression
secondary to maternal opioid analgesia in labor, reflex bradycardia or laryngospasm resulting from overly vigorous nasopharyngeal suctioning, hypoxia due to spontaneous pneumothorax,
or a congenital anomaly such as a diaphragmatic hernia, which
can interfere with adaptation to extrauterine life difficult. During this brief observation period, a cursory physical examination
for obvious congenital anomalies should be performed on every
newborn. This will often include aspiration and measurement of
gastric contents. A soft plastic catheter (8 French) is passed into
the stomach. If large amounts of fluid are obtained, i.e., more
than 25 mL, a high bowel obstruction should be suspected; if the
tube curls up in the esophagus or pharynx, esophageal atresia
with or without tracheoesophageal fistula is likely.

BAG AND MASK VENTILATION

Infants who remain apneic after an initial brief period (15 to
30 seconds) of tactile stimulation and infants with ineffective or
gasping ventilation and/or a heart rate of less than 100 beats per
minute require positive-pressure ventilation, typically administered initially with bag and face mask and 100% O_2 (Fig. 38.5).

The upper airway should be cleared and an appropriately
sized face mask should be selected. The mask should just cover
the nose and mouth and should not extend over the eyes or
beyond the chin. The infant's head should be in a neutral position, and care must be taken not to occlude the trachea by
over extending or over flexing the neck. The little finger of the
hand holding the mask can be used to support the mandible.
Pressures of 25 to 30 cm H_2O administered for the first 5 to 10
breaths are usually necessary. Higher pressures up to 50 cm of
water are occasionally required but as pressures increase, the
risk of an iatrogenic pneumothorax increases. Once the lungs
have been inflated, pressures of 12 to 20 cm H_2O are usually

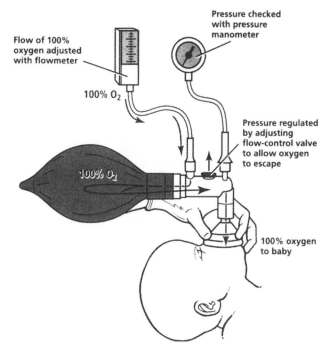

Flow of 100%
oxygen adjusted
with flowmeter

Pressure checked
with pressure
manometer

100% O_2

100% O_2

Pressure regulated
by adjusting
flow-control valve
to allow oxygen
to escape

100% oxygen
to baby

Figure 38.5. Bag and mask ventilation. (From Kattwinkel J, et al. (eds)
Neonatal Resuscitation Textbook, 4th ed. Dallas: American Heart Association
and American Academy of Pediatrics, 2000;3–11, with permission.)

sufficient to deliver an adequate volume. Positive pressure ventilation via a face mask may result in gaseous distension of the stomach, ocular damage due to pressure applied to the eyes, or abrasions of the face. If bag and mask ventilation is continued for more than 2 minutes, an oral or nasogastric catheter (8 French) should be inserted into the stomach with the upper end open to the atmosphere. In addition to correcting hypoxia, positive-pressure ventilation may stimulate sensitive stretch receptors in the pulmonary tree and initiate gasping and then regular ventilation (24). Most infants with respiratory depression secondary to maternal medications during labor or secondary to mild hypoxia during labor may be easily ventilated using this technique and will not require endotracheal intubation. To assess the adequacy of bag and mask ventilation, the chest should be observed for expansion of the lungs with each breath and the heart rate should be monitored.

The use of a laryngeal mask airway has been described in the neonate and may be useful in situations when positive-pressure ventilation with a face mask is ineffective but endotracheal intubation is difficult (25, 26). It is a simpler technique than intubation but has the disadvantage of not allowing for direct endotracheal suctioning of meconium or other particulate matter, and it cannot be used for endotracheal medication administration.

ENDOTRACHEAL INTUBATION

If there is no immediate (in less than 30 seconds) improvement in the clinical condition of the neonate with positive-pressure ventilation with the face mask, prompt endotracheal intubation for ventilation is indicated. **Immediate** endotracheal intubation should be considered for situations in which bag and mask ventilation is likely to be ineffective, such as extreme prematurity with low pulmonary compliance secondary to surfactant deficiency, and in conditions diagnosed by antenatal ultrasound, such as large bilateral pleural effusions and congenital diaphragmatic hernia.

The infant's head should be placed in a neutral "sniffing position" rather than hyperextended. The larynx of the neonate is more anterior than in the adult and at the level of the third cervical vertebra rather than at the sixth. Thus, a small straight blade, such as a Miller 0 to 1, provides the best visualization of the larynx. As the laryngoscope is introduced into the right-hand corner of the mouth, the tongue is moved toward the left and the epiglottis is located (Fig. 38.6). Gentle pressure over the hyoid

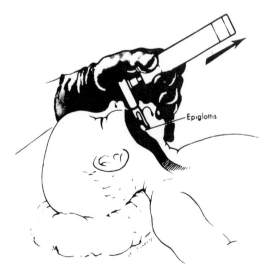

Figure 38.6. Technique for laryngoscopy. Left hand holds the laryngoscope and steadies the head and the little finger depresses the hyoid bone to help bring the larynx into view. (From Gregory GA. Resuscitation of the newborn. *Anesthesiology* 1975;43:225–237, with permission.)

Table 38.5. RECOMMENDATION OF ENDOTRACHEAL TUBE SIZE

Weight	Tube Size	Distance from Lip
<1,000 g	2.5	7 cm
1,000–2,000 g	3.0	8 cm
2,000–3,000 g	3.5	9 cm
>3,500 g	4.0	10 cm

bone with the little finger of the hand holding the laryngoscope will move the larynx posteriorly to help expose the epiglottis. The tip of the laryngoscope blade can be either placed in the vallecula or posterior to the epiglottis, and with gentle upward pressure the cords are visualized. If unable to visualize the larynx or to insert the endotracheal tube after two to three attempts (or about 20 seconds), the neonate should be ventilated with a bag and mask before further attempts are made.

A sterile uncuffed endotracheal tube should be used, a size such that there is a small air leak with positive-pressure ventilation. Too large a tube may cause subglottic stenosis, and too small a tube will not permit adequate ventilation and may become plugged easily. Depending on the weight of the neonate, a size 2.5-mm to 4.0-mm endotracheal tube is chosen (Table 38.5). The tube should be inserted about 2 cm past the cords, and ventilation with 100% oxygen should commence. Although a pressure of 25 to 30 cm H_2O is usually sufficient to ventilate most asphyxiated infants, those with low compliance, as found in erythroblastosis or pulmonary hypoplasia, may require higher pressures.

The correct placement of the endotracheal tube and the adequacy of ventilation must be ascertained immediately (Fig. 38.7). Both sides of the chest should rise equally, breath sounds auscultated in the midaxillary line should be equal bilaterally and louder over the chest than the stomach, and the heart rate, color, and body tone should improve. Inadvertent esophageal or main stem bronchial intubations may occur and must be immediately recognized. Esophageal ventilation will also produce chest movement and sounds. However, the sounds will be louder over the abdomen than the chest, and no chest movement will occur at the apices. Clinically, the infant will continue to deteriorate. A mainstem bronchial intubation may be recognized by asymmetric movement of the chest and absent or decreased breath sounds over the unventilated lung. Breath sounds may be misleading even to the experienced resuscitator, because sound is transmitted well in these small infants with thin chest walls. Thus, relying on this sign alone for diagnosis of correct placement of the endotracheal tube is dangerous. Other evidence that the tube is well positioned includes condensation of water vapor on the inside of the tube during exhalation and improvement in heart rate and color. Capnography, the technique of measuring end-tidal partial pressure of carbon dioxide, is currently being utilized in some resuscitation units to quickly confirm endotracheal as opposed to esophageal intubation.

In the severely asphyxiated infant, there is currently some controversy about whether resuscitation should proceed using 100% FIO_2 versus room air. Accumulation of free oxygen radicals produced during cerebral reperfusion, perhaps facilitated by hyperoxemia, may cause neuronal injury and add significantly to the hypoxic-ischemic insult (27).

CHEST COMPRESSIONS

If after 15 to 30 seconds of positive-pressure ventilation, the heartbeat is absent or barely detectable with a rate less than 80 beats/minute, closed-chest cardiac massage should be initiated (23). Both thumbs are placed on the sternum at the junction of the lower and middle thirds, and the back is supported

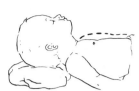

See chest expand

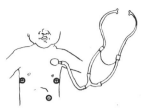

Hear bilateral breath sounds

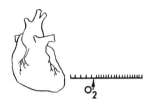

Hear pulse rate increase

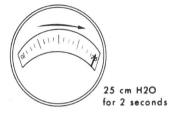

25 cm H2O
for 2 seconds

Avoid excessive pressures

Figure 38.7. Means of determining adequacy of ventilation clinically. (From Shnider SM, ed. *Obstetrical Anesthesia: Current Concepts and Practice.* Baltimore: Williams & Wilkins, 1970:225, with permission.)

with the fingers (Fig. 38.8). The sternum should be compressed to a depth of about one third of the anterior-posterior chest diameter at a rate of 90/minutes. Ventilation should occur at a rate of 30/minute. Within each two-second window, there should be three chest compressions and then a pause in compressions for a breath (23).

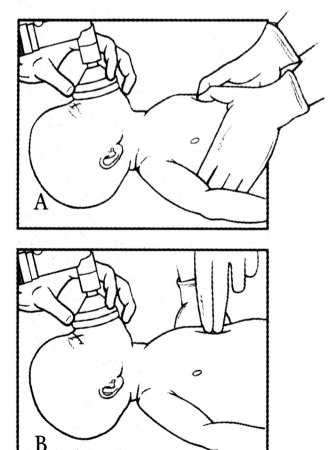

Figure 38.8. **A:** Chest compressions carried out by the preferred thumb compression technique. **B:** Two-finger method. (From Kattwinkel J, et al. (eds). Neonatal Resuscitation Textbook, 4th ed. Dallas: American Heart Association American Academy of Pediatrics, 1990, with permission.)

An alternate technique is shown in Figure 38.8. The tips of the middle finger and either the index or ring finger of one hand are used for compression. The two fingers should be positioned perpendicular to the chest and only the two fingertips should rest on the chest. The other hand can be used to support the infant's back so that the heart is more effectively compressed.

An adequate cardiac output with massage can be ascertained by an improvement in the neonate's color, constriction of the pupils, and palpable arterial pulses. Every two minutes, chest compressions and ventilation should pause so that endogenous heart rate can be measured. Chest compressions may be stopped when the infant's heart rate is greater than 80 beats/minute and peripheral pulses are palpable (28). If cardiac compressions are required for more than 30 to 60 seconds, electrocardiographic leads should be attached to monitor heart rate and rhythm.

EPINEPHRINE

Epinephrine should be given if there is no heart rate or if the heart rate is less than 60 beats/minute and is not increasing in response to ventilation. It may be given via the endotracheal tube (Fig. 38.9) and ventilated into the alveoli or it may be given intravenously once access has been obtained. The response appears to be more rapid when given intravenously (29). Low-dose epinephrine is preferred, i.e. 0.1 to 0.3 mL·kg^{-1} of 1:10,000 epinephrine solution. If there is no response, the dose may be repeated every 3 to 5 minutes and, on occasion, high-dose epinephrine may be given, i.e., 1 to 3 mL·kg^{-1} of 1:10,000. However, the high dose has been associated with severe and possibly organ-damaging vasoconstriction. The most common cause of persistent bradycardia in an asphyxiated neonate is inadequate ventilation secondary to inadequate seal with the mask or improper placement of the endotracheal tube.

UMBILICAL VESSEL CATHETERIZATION

The umbilical vein is larger and much easier to cannulate in an emergency than the umbilical artery. Using sterile technique, a 3.5- or 5-French catheter is inserted into the umbilical vein at the stump of the umbilical cord (30). The catheter is advanced 2 to 3 cm until the point at which blood can first be aspirated. This should place the tip of the catheter just below the intrahepatic

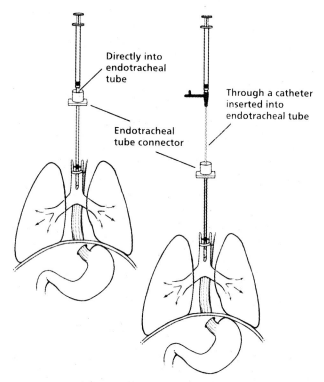

Figure 38.9. Endotracheal instillation of medication. **A:** Direct injection via the endotracheal tube followed by immediate positive pressure ventilation. **B:** Insertion via a feeding tube through the endotracheal tube with subsequent flush of normal saline followed by positive pressure ventilation. (From Kattwinkel J, et al. (eds). *Neonatel Resuscitation Textbook,* 4th ed. Dallas: American Heart Association and American Academy of Pediatrics, 2000;6–5, with permission.)

portion of the umbilical vein (Fig. 38.10). The location of the catheter tip is important because administration of drugs or hypertonic solutions through this catheter may be hazardous if the catheter tip is wedged in a portal venous radicle and may lead to hepatic necrosis or portal vein thrombosis (31). Using the umbilical vein will not permit assessment of oxygenation or systemic blood pressure.

The umbilical artery may be cannulated in situations where monitoring arterial blood gases and/or systemic blood pressure is indicated. This procedure is more difficult and requires more skill than umbilical venous catheterization. In a term infant, the catheter should be advanced to between 9 and 12 cm, depending on the infant's size, which should place the tip above the bifurcation of the aorta and below the celiac, renal, and mesenteric arteries (i.e., ideally between L3 and L4). Blood can be drawn immediately for arterial blood gases and for a spun hematocrit and a transducer can be attached for direct and continuous monitoring of blood pressure. If the catheter is to remain in place, radiographic verification of tip position is indicated.

CORRECTION OF ACIDOSIS

Severe metabolic acidosis or base deficit of 15 mEq/liter or more, should be promptly corrected by alkali administration to assist in achieving normal pulmonary perfusion and oxygenation (3). If the base deficit is known, then the dose of sodium bicarbonate needed may be calculated by the formula:

mEq of base required $=$ base deficit $\times$ 0.3 $\times$ body weight in kg

Usually, one-half the calculated dose is administered and blood gases are then re-evaluated. Subsequent doses are given as necessary. The rate of bicarbonate administration should be slow and the neonatal concentration of bicarbonate should be used. A 4.2% solution (0.5 mEq/mL) is given at a rate no faster than 1 mEq/kg/min. If blood gas analysis is not readily available and the neonate is severely depressed with an Apgar score of five or less at 5 minutes despite adequate ventilation, then a dose of bicarbonate of 2 to 3 mEq/kg may be given at the rate described above.

It has been suggested that there is an association between intracranial hemorrhage and sodium bicarbonate administration (32). Because intraventricular hemorrhage is a common finding in very small, premature infants, particularly those with asphyxia, it is not clear whether the high incidence of hemorrhage reported following *rapid* bicarbonate administration was due to an acute increase in osmolarity, a rise in arterial P_{CO_2}, or the asphyxia for which the bicarbonate was given. Others have reported that if bicarbonate administration is slow and ventilation is controlled, a rapid improvement in neonatal oxygenation can be expected to occur with no increased risk of intraventricular hemorrhage (33).

Sodium bicarbonate should not be infused unless metabolic acidosis or neonatal depression is severe and then only if the bicarbonate is slowly administered and the infant is being effectively ventilated. Mild or moderate metabolic and respiratory acidosis, that is, a pH between 7.05 and 7.3 and a base deficit

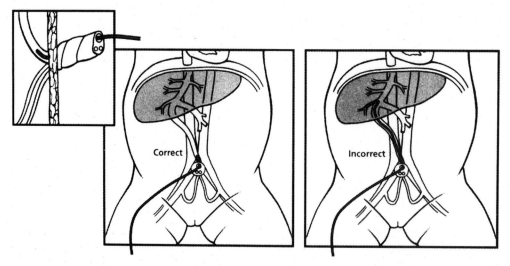

Figure 38.10. Proper placement of umbilical venous catheter for emergency medications. (From Kattwinkel J, et al. (eds). *Neonatal Resuscitation Textbook,* 4th ed. Dallas: American Heart Association and American Academy of Pediatrics, 2000;6–6, with permission.)

of 5 to 15 mEq/liter, usually will be corrected spontaneously or by assisted ventilation and volume expansion when indicated.

If the infant cannot be easily ventilated and has a combined severe respiratory and metabolic acidosis, Tris buffer (THAM), a sodium-free organic buffer that does not raise carbon dioxide levels, may be used instead of sodium bicarbonate to correct the metabolic component of the acidosis.

TREATMENT OF SHOCK

The most common cause of shock in the newborn is hypovolemia. It frequently follows severe intrapartum asphyxia during which a greater than normal portion of fetal blood is shunted to the placenta where it remains after cord clamping and delivery (34). Hypovolemia is also commonly associated with umbilical cord compression in vertex and especially breech vaginal deliveries. Acute compression of the umbilical cord during delivery may result in trapping of fetal blood in the placenta due to occlusion of the compliant umbilical vein while flow continues through the more rigid and muscular umbilical arteries. Ruptured placental or umbilical vessels and feto-maternal transfusion, although occurring far less frequently than intrapartum asphyxia and cord compression, can result in severe hypovolemic shock.

Hypovolemia should be suspected if the neonate is pale and has poor capillary refill, tachycardia, and tachypnea. Precise diagnosis and treatment require constant monitoring of arterial and central venous pressures and heart rate and repeated measurements of PaO_2, $PaCO_2$, pH, and hematocrit. Normal aortic blood pressure measured with the umbilical artery catheter varies with birth weight (28). Figure 38.11 shows the normal mean arterial blood pressure for each birth weight and the 95% confidence limits of this relationship. Newborns with blood pressures below the lower confidence line are hypotensive and most likely hypovolemic. Intrathoracic venous pressures measured with the umbilical venous catheter tip in the right atrium are normally 5 to 12 cm H_2O when measured at end expiration (28). If pressure is less than 5 cm H_2O, hypovolemia is likely.

Hypovolemic shock requires immediate therapy. An infusion of normal saline or Ringer's lactate solution (10 mL·kg^{-1} body weight over a 5- to 10-minute period) should be given until blood

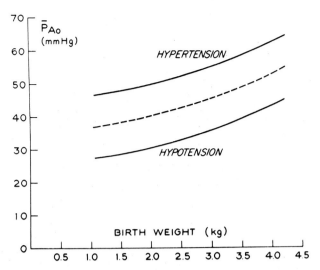

Figure 38.11. Mean aortic blood pressure obtained from an umbilical artery catheter. The dashed line is the average blood pressure at each birth weight, and the solid lines represent the 95% confidence limits. (From Kitterman JA, Phibbs RH, Tooley WH. Aortic blood pressure in normal newborn infants during the first 12 hours of life. *Pediatrics* 1969;44:959–968, with permission.)

is available and the response evaluated to determine whether the dose should be repeated immediately. A 5% albumin/saline solution (or other plasma substitute) can also be used. However, as soon as blood is available, 10 to 20 mL·kg^{-1} of O-negative irradiated packed cells should be given. Repeated infusions of fluid or blood should be given as needed to establish and maintain adequate intravascular pressure.

Frequently a hypovolemic, asphyxiated neonate will have a relatively normal arterial blood pressure and hematocrit due to intense peripheral vasoconstriction. When the acidosis is corrected with bicarbonate and/or hyperventilation, the blood vessels dilate and hypotension occurs, unmasking the presence of hypovolemia (Fig. 38.12). When severe hypovolemia is corrected, a marked metabolic acidemia may reappear after systemic circulatory status and peripheral perfusion improve.

Figure 38.12. Heart rate, hematocrit, and mean aortic pressure in a 1,370 g, 30 weeks' gestation infant with asphyxia at birth and respiratory distress. At 12 min of age, severe metabolic acidosis was treated with NaHCO₃. Hypovolemia then became apparent by the progressive fall in blood pressure. Albumin administration restored blood pressure and alleviated tachycardia. (From Phibbs RH: What is the evidence that blood pressure monitoring is useful? In: Lucey JF, ed. *Problems of Neonatal Intensive Care Units. Report of the 59th Ross Conference on Pediatric Research.* Columbus: Ross Laboratories, 1969:81, with permission.)

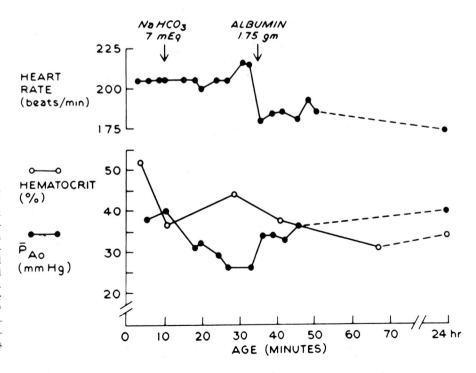

Table 38.6. MEDICATIONS FOR RESUSCITATION OF THE NEWBORN

Medication	Concentration to Administer	Preparation	Dosage/Route	Indications for Use	Rate/Precautions
Epinephrine	1:10,000	1 mL	0.1–0.3 mL·kg^{-1} IV or ET	1. No detectable heart beat 2. Heart rate <80/min despite 30 sec of ventilation and chest compression	Give rapidly
Volume expanders	Whole blood 5% Albumin Normal saline Ringer's lactate solution	40 mL	10 mL·kg^{-1} IV	1. Evidence of acute bleeding 2. Signs of hypovolemia	Give over 5–10 min
Sodium bicarbonate	0.5 mEq/mL (4.2% solution)	20 mL or two 10-mL prefilled syringes	2 mEq/kg IV	Documented or assumed metabolic acidosis	Give *slowly*, over at least 2 min Give only if infant being effectively ventilated
Naloxone	0.4 mg·mL^{-1} 1.0 mg·mL^{-1}	1 mL 1 mL	0.1 mg·kg^{-1} (0.25 mL·kg^{-1}) IV, ET, IM, SQ 0.1 mg·kg^{-1} (0.1 mL·kg^{-1}) IV, ET, IM, SQ	Severe respiratory depression *and* maternal narcotic administration within the past 4 hr	Give rapidly IV, ET preferred IM, SQ acceptable
Dopamine	$\dfrac{6 \times \dfrac{\text{weight}}{\text{(kg)}} \times \dfrac{\text{desired dose}}{(\mu g \cdot kg^{-1} \cdot min)}}{\text{desired fluid (mL} \cdot hr^{-1})}$ =	mg of dopamine per 100 mL of solution	Begin at 5 $\mu g \cdot kg^{-1} \cdot min$ (may increase to 20 $\mu g \cdot kg^{-1} \cdot$ min if necessary) IV	Infant shows evidence of shock and poor peripheral perfusion after giving epinephrine, volume expander, and sodium bicarbonate	Give as a continuous infusion using an infusion pump Monitor HR and BP closely Seek consultation

IV, intravenous; ET, endotracheal; IM, intramuscular; SQ, subcutaneous.
Adapted from Bloom RS, Cropley C. *Textbook of Neonatal Resuscitation.* American Heart Association, 1990.

It should also be noted that hypocapnia due to hyperventilation and hypocapnia can cause vasodilatation and hypotension in the absence of hypovolemia. When the alkalosis is recognized, ventilation should be decreased to see if blood pressure returns to the normal range before giving volume replacement.

With persistent signs of hypovolemia, the presence of metabolic acidosis and the need for sodium bicarbonate should be considered. With persistent hypotension, the administration of dopamine should also be considered (Table 38.6).

WHEN TO STOP RESUSCITATIVE EFFORTS

Resuscitation attempts may be terminated when the Apgar is truly 0 at 1, 5, and 10 minutes indicating no heartbeat despite appropriate resuscitative measures. Most infants who have been resuscitated after 10 to 15 minutes of 0 Apgar score will expire during the immediate neonatal period from multi-organ failure or will survive with severe hypoxic-ischemic encephalopathy and devastating neurologic sequelae. Consideration should also be given to terminating resuscitative efforts in extremely immature infants in whom adequate oxygenation cannot be obtained after 20 to 30 minutes of resuscitation including exogenous surfactant administration.

SPECIAL PROBLEMS IN RESUSCITATION
Routine Tracheal Suctioning for Meconium

Meconium aspiration pneumonitis is the leading respiratory cause of death in the full-term newborn. Treatment of

meconium aspiration should begin in the delivery room. With suctioning of the airways, there is a significant reduction in morbidity and mortality rates (35–38) (Fig. 38.13). Infants who aspirate blood, mucus, meconium, or amniotic fluid in utero often have lower airway obstruction and severe asphyxia after birth. The best-studied and most common example is the meconium aspiration syndrome.

Meconium is the breakdown product of swallowed amniotic fluid, gastrointestinal cells, and intestinal secretions. Aspiration of meconium is uncommon in fetuses of less than 34 weeks of gestation, but increasingly common after 40 weeks of gestation. Mature fetuses respond to stress (hypoxia) with increased gut motility, relaxation of the anal sphincters, defecation (1, 2), and deep, agonal gasping. Normal fetal breathing results in inhalation of about 1 mL of fluid; gasping leads to as much as 60 mL of amniotic fluid and debris being inhaled into the more distal airway. Much of the aspirated material is in the mouth, trachea, and mainstem bronchi. If birth is delayed for more than 24 hours after the in utero passage of meconium, the aspirated material is broken down by the lung fluid and expelled from the lungs by the continuous production of lung fluid. If birth occurs within 12 to 24 hours of aspiration, the meconium in the major airways will move progressively into the periphery of the lung with initiation and maintenance of air breathing. This causes obstruction of small airways, which leads to mismatching of ventilation and perfusion as well as a chemical pneumonitis and the release of vasoactive substances that may initiate pulmonary vasoconstriction and persistent fetal circulation. Ventilation becomes rapid (100 to 150 breaths/min) and shallow and lung compliance decreases to levels seen in infants with hyaline membrane disease (0.8 mL/cm H_2O).

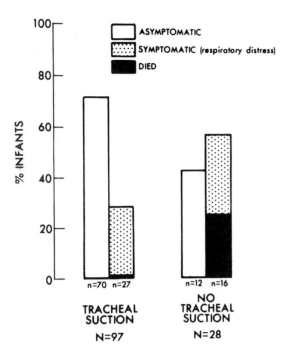

Figure 38.13. Comparison of percentage of incidence of respiratory distress and percentage of mortality in 97 infants who received tracheal suction in the delivery room and 28 infants who did not (numbers of infants below columns); note that one infant died in the tracheal suction group and seven died in the no tracheal suction group. (From Ting P, Brady JP. Tracheal suction in meconium aspiration. *Am J Obstet Gynecol* 1975;122:767–771, with permission.)

The precise management of neonates born through meconium is currently undergoing reevaluation. All agree that the mouth and nose of all these neonates should be suctioned by the obstetrician as soon as the head is out but before the shoulders are delivered and the infant starts breathing. Subsequent endotracheal intubation and suctioning is controversial and is discussed extensively in a review (38). The procedure does have occasional minor risks of hoarseness, sore throat leading to poor feeding and traumatic bleeding, and rarely, more serious injuries such as pneumothorax or esophageal or tracheal perforation (39). A recent very large multicenter prospective-randomized trial was unable to document any significant benefit intubation with endotracheal suctioning in the extremely vigorous neonate (40). Other neonatology neonatologists continue to recommend endotracheal intubation and suctioning of all meconium-stained neonates. Other neonatologists suggest that intubation is only necessary if thick, particulate, "pea-soup" meconium is present. In the presence of thin, watery, yellow-tinged meconium-stained amniotic fluid with no visible particles, they believe no special management is required. Others examine the oropharynx with a laryngoscope and only intubate if meconium is present in the oropharynx or at the vocal cords. Finally, there is now some evidence that, regardless of the nature of the meconium, if the infant is vigorous (Apgar score of 8 or more at 15 to 30 seconds after delivery), intubation is not necessary.

We believe that the respiratory failure induced by meconium aspiration can be prevented in many cases by removing the meconium from the lung and large airways before it can obstruct small airways. All infants born through thick or particulate meconium who are not completely vigorous at birth definitely should undergo endotracheal suction. We also recommend endotracheal suctioning of vigorous infants covered with thick meconium. We do not believe examination of the oropharynx is reliable, as it is difficult to visualize meconium below the cords. Babies born through thin meconium probably do not require special management, but the clinical judgment of the

resuscitator in evaluating the nature of the meconium is crucial. If uncertain, intubation is advised. Similarly, the depressed neonate born through thin meconium may benefit from endotracheal intubation and suction (41, 42). It must be emphasized that despite appropriate management, some infants will still develop meconium aspiration syndrome, respiratory failure, and death, presumably from in utero aspiration.

To remove thick meconium, a 3-mm endotracheal tube is inserted, and suction is applied to the tube by a suction device specially designed for this purpose (Fig. 38.14). After suction is applied, the tube is withdrawn from the trachea. Meconium withdrawn into the tube is immediately expelled from the tube and the trachea is re-intubated to repeat the procedure. If meconium is not recovered, the trachea is not re-intubated. In either case the infant is then allowed to breathe or is ventilated with oxygen as required. The trachea can then be re-intubated if meconium was obtained during the second period of suctioning. Excessive airway pressure must be avoided because pulmonary gas leaks are common following meconium aspiration (35) and can occur any time during the first 3 days of life. In situations where it is likely that the infant has in fact aspirated meconium, 100% oxygen should be provided until oxygen saturation can be monitored to prevent hypoxic pulmonary vasoconstriction. If the above procedure is followed, the mortality from meconium aspiration is only 0.06 per 1,000 live births, compared to 2.2 per 1,000 live births when no suctioning is applied. Infants whose tracheas are suctioned seldom require assisted ventilation following meconium aspiration. However, some infants will develop

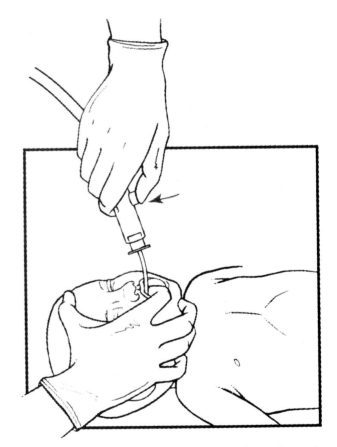

Figure 38.14. An example of a disposable mechanical meconium aspirator. Wall suction is connected to the smaller end with the barbed fitting. Wall suction is set at 80 mm Hg. After the patient is intubated, the larger end (15 mm ID) of the meconium aspirator is connected to the endotracheal tube adapter. The suction control port on top of the aspirator is occluded to regulate suction and remove meconium. (From Kattwinkel J, et al. (eds). *Neonatal Resuscitation Textbook*, 4th ed. Dallas: American Heart Association and American Academy of Pediatrics, 2000;5–15, with permission.)

respiratory failure despite suctioning, probably secondary to an intrauterine aspiration event.

Opioid Depression

When opioids are administered for pain relief during labor and delivery, the infant may be born mildly to moderately depressed. The incidence of respiratory depression secondary to maternal opioid administration increases with the cumulative dosage that a mother received as well as the timing of delivery after the last dose. As in the adult, the usual signs of opioid depression in a neonate are hypoventilation and poor response to stimuli. If respiratory depression is thought to be due to opioid overdose, the infant should receive bag and mask ventilation and then treatment with an opioid antagonist. Naloxone, $0.1 \ mg \cdot kg^{-1}$, is the antagonist of choice. If the mother abuses opioids or is in a methadone maintenance program, the use of naloxone is contraindicated in the neonate because acute withdrawal symptoms including seizures may be precipitated.

Magnesium Intoxication

Babies born to mothers treated with large doses of magnesium for toxemia of pregnancy may display signs of hypermagnesemia. These infants are hypotensive, hypotonic, peripherally vasodilated and often bright red. Because of poor ventilatory effort, they may require intubation and mechanical ventilation until the magnesium level decreases, which may take 24 to 72 hours. Calcium is an effective antidote.

Local Anesthetic Toxicity

Fetal intoxication with local anesthetics can occasionally occur inadvertently during the maternal administration of caudal or paracervical blocks (43, 44). The infants are severely depressed with bradycardia, hypotension, apnea, hypotonia, and convulsions. Careful examination of the baby's head often discloses the needle puncture site. In addition to the usual resuscitation of a severely depressed neonate, these babies may require detoxification using gastric lavage with isotonic saline and exchange transfusion. Rarely cardiac arrhythmias may occur and may require cardioversion during resuscitation (45).

Pneumothorax

Pneumothorax in the delivery room can occur spontaneously, often associated with meconium aspiration (in which ball-valve air trapping occurs) or with other diseases associated with poor lung compliance (such as diaphragmatic hernia and pulmonary hypoplasia). When a pneumothorax occurs in normal lungs, it is usually caused by excessive airway pressures administered in the resuscitation of a depressed newborn. Tension pneumothorax, in which high intrathoracic pressure prevents venous return to the heart, is catastrophic and life-threatening. When the diagnosis of tension pneumothorax is suspected, transillumination of the chest may be very helpful in confirming the presence and the side of the pneumothorax. Immediate management consists of inserting a 25-gauge needle connected to a three-way stopcock and 20-mL syringe into the thoracic cavity in the second intercostal space in the midclavicular line. If air is continuously aspirated, then the needle should be replaced by an adequately sized catheter (10 to 16 French) placed in the intercostal space between the 6th and 7th rib in the mid-axillary line and directed anteriorly. The catheter should be connected to underwater seal continuous suction through an underwater seal.

Resuscitation of the Premature Infant

A resuscitation team should be present for the delivery of a known preterm infant of less than 34 weeks' gestation. The resuscitation room should be kept warm and, for the extremely immature infant, a warming pad can be placed under the infant on the radiant warmer bed. An oxygen-air blender should be used so that the FIO_2 can be lowered in order to maintain the infant's arterial PO_2 between 50 and 70 mm Hg. Care should be taken to avoid any prolonged period of hyperoxemia that may contribute to the development of retinopathy of prematurity. The inhaled gas should be warmed and humidified. Skin and axillary temperatures should be monitored frequently during resuscitation. Most infants of less than 1,000 grams in birth weight (extremely low-birth weight) will require immediate endotracheal intubation for initial stabilization because of decreased lung compliance and decreased chest wall stability. An umbilical arterial catheter should be inserted routinely in the extremely low-birth weight infant for direct monitoring of arterial blood pressure as well as arterial blood gases. Hyperventilation and alkalosis should be avoided to prevent cerebral vasoconstriction with resultant ischemic injury to the periventricular white matter. Hypoglycemia should be anticipated and intravenous access obtained. Consideration should be given to the administration of exogenous surfactant prophylactically in infants of less than 28 weeks of gestation within the first 10 minutes of life. Rescue treatment with surfactant in infants of more than 28 weeks of gestation with evidence of respiratory distress syndrome also should be considered as soon as the infant has been stabilized while still in the resuscitation area. There is evidence to suggest that rescue surfactant is more effective when given within the first hour of life (46).

Major Anomalies and Hydrops Fetalis

Delivery of infants with known severe congenital anomalies or hydrops fetalis should occur in a high-risk center where a full resuscitation team is prepared to emergently deal with problems such as severe anemia, massive pleural and pericardial effusions, massive ascites and airway obstruction. Infants with hydrops may present with pleural effusions and/or ascites severe enough to interfere with lung expansion. Sometimes these large fluid collections can be evacuated prior to delivery under ultrasound needle guidance to facilitate a smoother resuscitation. Otherwise the resuscitation team needs to be prepared to perform bilateral thoracenteses and an abdominal paracentesis if necessary to allow for adequate ventilation and oxygenation.

A recent technique called the "EXIT procedure" was described initially in infants undergoing fetal tracheal occlusion procedures for hypoplastic lungs secondary to congenital diaphragmatic hernia (see Chapter 14) (47). This technique uses high-dose halogenated agents for general anesthesia during Cesarean section delivery to maintain uterine relaxation so that the infant can be maintained on the placental circulation while procedures are performed to provide an adequate airway (see Chapter 21). Bronchoscopy, intubation, and/or tracheostomy may be performed while maintaining adequate gas exchange via the placenta. This technique has already been used in CHAOS syndrome and in providing an immediate airway in infants with large cervical tumors compressing the airway diagnosed prior to delivery (48, 49).

It is our practice to resuscitate infants who present with multiple severe congenital anomalies unless these abnormalities were detected during the pregnancy and a decision was made with the family not to resuscitate the infant at birth. Once the infant has been stabilized, a complete assessment of the abnormalities should be undertaken and the family should participate in decisions about further interventions.

CONCLUSION

Rapid, organized, and skillful resuscitation of the depressed newborn is mandatory. The obstetrician, anesthesiologist, and neonatologist must work as a team in evaluating the newborn, establishing a patent airway, providing adequate ventilation, and

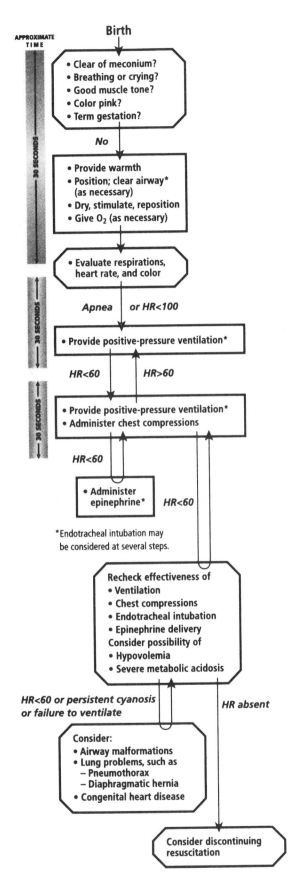

Figure 38.15. Overview of resuscitation of the newborn. (From Kattwinkel J, et al. (eds). *Neonatal Resuscitation Textbook*, 4th ed. Dallas: American Heart Association and American Academy of Pediatrics, 1987:1–5, with permission.)

restoring normal blood volume, cardiac output, and acid-base status. An overview of resuscitation of the newborn in the delivery room, as recommended by the American Heart Association and the American Academy of Pediatrics, is shown in Figure 38.15.

REFERENCES

1. Dawes GS. *Foetal and Neonatal Physiology.* Chicago: Year Book Medical Publishers, 1968:91–105.
2. Rudolph AM, Heymann MA. Fetal and neonatal circulation and respiration. *Ann Rev Physiol* 1974;36:187–207.
3. Rudolph AM, Yuen S. Response of the pulmonary vasculature to hypoxia and H^+ ion concentration changes. *J Clin Invest* 1966;45:399–411.
4. Cassen S, Dawes GS, Mott JC, et al. The vascular resistance of the foetal and newly ventilated lung of the lamb. *J Physiol* 1964;171:61–79.
5. Assali NS, Morris JA, Smith EW, et al. Studies on ductus arteriosus circulation. *Circ Res* 1963;13:478–489.
6. Boreus LO, Malmfors T, McMurphy DM, et al. Demonstration of adrenergic receptor function and innervation in the ductus arteriosus of the human fetus. *Acta Physiol Scand* 1969;77:316–321.
7. Adams FH, Moss AJ, Fagan L. The tracheal fluid of the foetal lamb. *Biol Neonate* 1963;5:151–158.
8. Ross BB. Comparison of foetal pulmonary fluid with foetal plasma and amniotic fluid. *Nature* 1963;199:1100.
9. Karlberg P. The adaptive changes in the immediate postnatal period, with particular reference to respiration. *J Pediatr* 1960;56:585–604.
10. Usher RH, Allen AC, McLean FH. Risk of respiratory distress syndrome related to gestational age, role of delivery and maternal diabetes. *Am J Obstet Gynecol* 1971;111:826–832.
11. Karlberg P. The breaths of life. In: Gluck L. ed. *Modern Perinatal Medicine.* Chicago: Year Book Medical Publishers, 1974:391–408.
12. Hodgson CA, Wauchob, TD. A comparison of spinal and general anaesthesia for elective caesarean section: affect on neonatal condition at birth. *Int J Obstet Anesth* 1994;3:25–30.
13. Mahajan J, Mahajan RP, Singh MM, et al. Anaesthetic technique for elective caesarean section and neurobehavioral status of newborns. *Int J Obstet Anesth* 1992;2:89–93.
14. Apgar V. A proposal for a new method of evaluation of the newborn infant. *Anesth Analg* 1953;32:260–267.
15. Apgar V, James LS. Further observations on the newborn scoring system. *Am J Dis Child* 1962;104:419–428.
16. Johnson JWC, Richards DS, Wagaman RA. The case for routine umbilical blood acid-base studies at delivery. *Am J Obstet Gynecol* 1990;162:621–625.
17. Yeomans ER, Hauth JC, Gilstrap LC III, et al. Umbilical cord pH, Pco_2 and bicarbonate following uncomplicated term vaginal deliveries. *Am J Obstet Gynecol* 1985;151:798–800.
18. Taeusch, HW, Sniderman, S. Neonatal resuscitation. In: Taeusch HW, Christiansen RO, Buescher ES, eds. *Pediatric and Neonatal Tests and Procedures.* Philadelphia: WB Saunders Company, 1996.
19. Aherne W, Hull D. The site of heat production in the newborn infant. *Proc R Soc Med* 1964; 57:1172–1173.
20. Karlberg P, Moore RE, Oliver TK. The thermogenic response of the newborn infant to noradrenaline. *Acta Paediatr Scand* 1962;51:284–292.
21. Dawkins MJR, Scopes JW. Non-shivering thermogenesis and brown adipose tissue in the human newborn infant. *Nature* 1965;206:201–202.
22. Adamsons K Jr, Gandy GM, James LS. The influence of thermal factors upon oxygen consumption of the newborn infant. *J Pediatr* 1965;66:495–508.
23. Kattwinkel J, et al. (eds). *Neonatal Resuscitation Textbook*, 4th ed. Dallas: American Academy of Pediatrics and American Heart Association, 2000.
24. Cross K, Klaus M, Tooley WH, et al. The response of the newborn baby to inflation of the lungs. *J Physiol* 1960;151:551–565.
25. Brimacombe J, Berry A. The laryngeal mask airway for obstetric anesthesia and neonatal resuscitation. *Int J Obstet Anesth* 1994;3:211–218.
26. Paterson SJ, Byrne PJ, Molesky MG, et al. Neonatal resuscitation using the laryngeal mask airway. *Anesthesiology* 1994;80:1248–1253.

27. Kattwinkle J, Niermeyer S, Nadkarni V, et al. Resuscitation of the newly born infant: an advisory statement from the Pediatric Working Group of the International Liaison Committee on Resuscitation. *Resuscitation* 1999;40:71–88.
28. Kitterman JA, Phibbs RH, Tooley WH. Aortic blood pressure in normal newborn infants during the first 12 hours of life. *Pediatrics* 1969;44:959–968.
29. Burchfield DJ. Medication use in neonatal resuscitation. *Clin Perinatol* 1999;26:683–691.
30. Kitterman JA, Phibbs RH, Tooley WH. Catheterization of umbilical vessels in newborn infants. *Pediatr Clin North Am* 1970;17:895–912.
31. Erkan V, Blankenship W, Stahlman MT. The complications of chronic umbilical vessel catheterization. *Pediatr Res* 1968;2:317.
32. Simmons MA, Adcock EW, Bard H, et al. Hypernatremia and intracranial hemorrhage in neonates. *N Engl J Med* 1974;291:6–10.
33. Tooley WH. Alkali therapy in the asphyxiated newborn infant. In: Shnider SM, ed. *Obstetrical Anesthesia.* Baltimore: Williams & Wilkins, 1970:230.
34. Ballard R, Kitterman JR, Phibbs RH, et al. Observations on hypovolemia in the newborn. *Clin Res* 1972;20:278.
35. Gregory GA, Gooding C, Phibbs RH, et al. Meconium aspiration: a prospective study. *J Pediatr* 1974;85:848–852.
36. Ting P, Brady JP. Tracheal suction in meconium aspiration. *Am J Obstet Gynecol* 1975;122:767–771.
37. Carson BS, Losey RW, Bowes WA Jr, et al. Combined obstetric and pediatric approach to prevent meconium aspiration syndrome. *Am J Obstet Gynecol* 1976;126:712–715.
38. Wiswell TE, Tuggle JM, Turner BS. Meconium aspiration syndrome: have we made a difference? *Pediatrics* 1990;85:715–721.
39. Linder N, Aranda JV, Tsur M, et al. Need for endotracheal intubation and suction in meconium-stained neonates. *J Pediatr* 1998;112:613–615.
40. Wiswell TE, Gannon CM, Jacob J, et al. Delivery room management of the apparently vigorous meconium-stained neonate: results of the multicenter, international collaborative trial. *Pediatrics* 2000;105:1–7.
41. Hagerman JR, Conley M, Francis K, et al. Delivery room management of meconium staining of the amniotic fluid and the development of meconium aspiration syndrome. *J Perinatol* 1988;8:127–131.
42. Yeh TF, Harris V, Srinivasan G, et al. Roentgenographic findings in infants with meconium aspiration syndrome. *JAMA* 1979;242:60–63.
43. Finster M, Poppers PJ, Sinclair JC, et al. Accidental intoxication of the fetus with local anesthetic drug during caudal anesthesia. *Am J Obstet Gynecol* 1965;92:922–924.
44. Dodson WE, Hillman RE, Hillman LS. Brain tissue levels in a fatal case of neonatal mepivacaine poisoning. *J Pediatr* 1975;86:624–627.
45. Heinonen KM. Rare procedures during delivery room resuscitation-cardioversion of ventricular tachycardia in an asphytic neonate. *Intensive Care Med* 1992;18:491–492.
46. The OSIRIS Collaborative Group. Early verus delayed neonatal administration of synthetic surfactant—the judgement of OSIRIS. *Lancet* 1992;340:1363.
47. Mychaliska GB, Bealer JF, Graf JL, et al. Operating on placental support: the ex utero intrapartum treatment procedure. *J Pediatr Surg* 1997;32:227–230.
48. Larsen ME, Larsen JW, Hamersley SL, et al. Successful management of fetal cervical teratoma using the EXIT procedure. *J Matern Fetal Med* 1999;8:295–297.
49. DeCou JM, Jones DC, Jacobs HD, et al. Successful ex utero intrapartum treatment (EXIT) procedure for congenital high airway obstruction syndrome (CHAOS) owing to laryngeal atresia. *J Pediatr Surg* 1998;33:1563–1565.

Shnider and Levinson's Anesthesia for Obstetrics,
edited by Samuel C. Hughes, et al.
Lippincott Williams & Wilkins,
Philadelphia, © 2001.

APPENDIX A

GUIDELINES FOR REGIONAL ANESTHESIA IN OBSTETRICS

These guidelines apply to the use of regional anesthesia or analgesia in which local anesthetics are administered to the parturient during labor and delivery. They are intended to encourage quality patient care but cannot guarantee any specific patient outcome. Because the availability of anesthesia resources may vary, members are responsible for interpreting and establishing the guidelines for their own institutions and practices. These guidelines are subject to revision from time to time as warranted by the evolution of technology and practice.

Guideline I: Regional anesthesia should be initiated and maintained only in locations in which appropriate resuscitation equipment and drugs are immediately available to manage procedurally related problems.

Resuscitation equipment should include, but is not limited to: sources of oxygen and suction, equipment to maintain an airway and perform endotracheal intubation, a means to provide positive pressure ventilation, and drugs and equipment for cardiopulmonary resuscitation.

Guideline II: Regional anesthesia should be initiated by a physician with appropriate privileges and maintained by or under the medical direction (1) of such an individual.

Physicians should be approved through the institutional credentialing process to initiate and direct the maintenance of obstetric anesthesia and to manage procedurally related complications.

Guideline III: Regional anesthesia should not be administered until: 1. the patient has been examined by a qualified individual (2); and 2. a physician with obstetrical privileges to perform operative vaginal or cesarean delivery, who has knowledge of the maternal and fetal status and the progress of labor and who approves the initiation of labor anesthesia, is readily available to supervise the labor and manage any obstetric complications that may arise.

Under circumstances defined by department protocol, qualified personnel may perform the initial pelvic examination. The physician responsible for the patient's obstetrical care should be informed of her status so that a decision can be made regarding present risk and further management (2).

Guideline IV: An intravenous infusion should be established before the initiation of regional anesthesia and maintained throughout the duration of the regional anesthetic.

Guideline V: Regional anesthesia for labor and/or vaginal delivery requires that the parturient's vital signs and the fetal heart rate be monitored and documented by a qualified individual. Additional monitoring appropriate to the clinical condition of the parturient and the fetus should be employed when indicated. when extensive regional blockade is administered for complicated vaginal delivery, the standards for basic anesthetic monitoring (3) should be applied.

Guideline VI: Regional anesthesia for cesarean delivery requires that the standards for basic anesthetic monitoring (3) be applied and that a physician with privileges in obstetrics be immediately available.

Guideline VII: Qualified personnel, other than the anesthesiologist attending the mother, should be immediately available to assume responsibility for resuscitation of the newborn (3).

The primary responsibility of the anesthesiologist is to provide care to the mother. If the anesthesiologist is also requested to provide brief assistance in the care of the newborn, the benefit to the child must be compared to the risk to the mother.

Guideline VIII: A physician with appropriate privileges should remain readily available during the regional anesthetic to manage anesthetic complications until the patient's postanesthesia condition is satisfactory and stable.

Guideline IX: All patients recovering from regional anesthesia should receive appropriate postanesthesia care. following cesarean delivery and/or extensive regional blockade, the standards for post-anesthesia care (4) should be applied.

1. A postanesthesia care unit (PACU) should be available to receive patients. The design, equipment and staffing should meet requirements of the facility's accrediting and licensing bodies.
2. When a site other than the PACU is used, equivalent postanesthesia care should be provided.

Guideline X: There should be a policy to assure the availability in the facility of a physician to manage complications and to provide cardiopulmonary resuscitation for patients receiving postanesthesia care.

REFERENCES

1. The Anesthesia Care Team. Approved by ASA House of Delegates October 26, 1982 and last amended October 25, 1995.
2. Guidelines for Perinatal Care. American Academy of Pediatrics and American College of Obstetricians and Gynecologists, 1988.
3. Standards for Basic Anesthetic Monitoring. Approved by ASA House of Delegates October 21, 1986 and last amended October 21, 1998.
4. Standards for Postanesthesia Care. Approved by ASA House of Delegates October 12, 1988 and last amended October 19, 1994.

Shnider and Levinson's Anesthesia for Obstetrics, edited by Samuel C. Hughes, et al. Lippincott Williams & Wilkins, Philadelphia, © 2001.

APPENDIX B

PRACTICE GUIDELINES FOR OBSTETRICAL ANESTHESIA

REPORT BY THE AMERICAN SOCIETY OF ANESTHESIOLOGISTS
TASK FORCE ON OBSTETRICAL ANESTHESIA

Practice guidelines are systematically developed recommendations that assist the practitioner and patient in making decisions about health care. These recommendations may be adopted, modified, or rejected according to clinical needs and constraints.

Practice guidelines are not intended as standards or absolute requirements. The use of practice guidelines cannot guarantee any specific outcome. Practice guidelines are subject to periodic revision as warranted by the evolution of medical knowledge, technology, and practice. The guidelines provide basic recommendations that are supported by analysis of the current literature and by a synthesis of expert opinion, open forum commentary, and clinical feasibility data.

PURPOSES OF THE GUIDELINES FOR OBSTETRICAL ANESTHESIA

The purposes of these Guidelines are to enhance the quality of anesthesia care for obstetric patients, reduce the incidence and severity of anesthesia-related complications, and increase patient satisfaction.

FOCUS OF THE GUIDELINES

The Guidelines focus on the anesthetic management of pregnant patients during labor, non-operative delivery, operative delivery, and selected aspects of postpartum care. The intended patient population includes, but is not limited to intrapartum and postpartum patients with uncomplicated pregnancies or with common obstetric problems. The Guidelines do not apply to patients undergoing surgery during pregnancy, gynecological patients or parturients with chronic medical disease (e.g., severe heart, renal, or neurological disease).

APPLICATION OF THE GUIDELINES

The Guidelines are intended for use by anesthesiologists. They also may serve as a resource for other anesthesia providers and health care professionals who advise or care for patients who will receive anesthesia care during labor, delivery and the immediate postpartum period.

TASK FORCE MEMBERS AND CONSULTANTS

The ASA appointed a Task Force of 11 members to review the published evidence and obtain consultant opinion from a representative body of anesthesiologists and obstetricians. The Task Force members consisted of anesthesiologists in both private and academic practices from various geographic areas of the United States.

The Task Force met its objective in a five-step process. First, original published research studies relevant to these issues were reviewed and analyzed. Second, Consultants from various geographic areas of the United States who practice or work in various settings (e.g., academic and private practice) were asked to participate in opinion surveys and review and comment on drafts of the Guidelines. Third, the Task Force held two open forums

at major national meetings to solicit input from attendees on its draft recommendations. Fourth, all available information was used by the Task Force in developing the Guideline recommendations. Finally, the Consultants were surveyed to assess their opinions on the feasibility of implementing the Guidelines.

AVAILABILITY AND STRENGTH OF EVIDENCE

Evidence-based guidelines are developed by a rigorous analytic process. To assist the reader, the Guidelines make use of several descriptive terms that are easier to understand than the technical terms and data that are used in the actual analyses. These descriptive terms are defined below:

The following terms describe the availability of scientific evidence in the literature.

Insufficient: There are too few published studies to investigate a relationship between a clinical intervention and clinical outcome.

Inconclusive: Published studies are available, but they cannot be used to assess the relationship between a clinical intervention and a clinical outcome because the studies either do not meet predefined criteria for content as defined in the "Focus of the Guidelines," or do not meet research design or analytic standards.

Silent: There are no available studies in the literature that address a relationship of interest.

The following terms describe the strength of scientific data.

Supportive: There is sufficient quantitative information from adequately designed studies to describe a statistically significant relationship ($P < 0.01$) between a clinical intervention and a clinical outcome, using the technique of meta-analysis.

Suggestive: There is enough information from case reports and descriptive studies to provide a directional assessment of the relationship between a clinical intervention and a clinical outcome. This type of qualitative information does not permit a statistical assessment of significance.

Equivocal: Qualitative data have not provided a clear direction for clinical outcomes related to a clinical intervention and (1) there is insufficient quantitative information or (2) aggregated comparative studies have found no quantitatively significant differences among groups or conditions.

The following terms describe survey responses from Consultants for any specified issue. Responses are weighted as agree = +1, undecided = 0, or disagree = −1.

Agree: The average weighted responses must be equal to or greater than +0.30 (on a scale of −1 to 1) to indicate agreement.

Equivocal: The average weighted responses must be between −0.30 and +0.30 (on a scale of −1 to 1) to indicate an equivocal response.

Disagree: The average weighted responses must be equal to or less than −0.30 (on a scale of −1 to 1) to indicate disagreement.

GUIDELINES

I. Perianesthetic evaluation.

1. History and physical examination. The literature is silent regarding the relationship between anesthesia-related obstetric outcomes and the performance of a focused history

and physical examination. However, there is suggestive data that a patient's medical history and/or findings from a physical exam may be related to anesthetic outcomes. The Consultants and Task Force agree that a focused history and physical examination may be associated with reduced maternal, fetal and neonatal complications. The Task Force agrees that the obstetric patient benefits from communication between the anesthesiologist and the obstetrician.

> **Recommendations:** The anesthesiologist should do a focused history and physical examination when consulted to deliver anesthesia care. This should include a maternal health history, an anesthesia-related obstetric history, an airway examination, and a baseline blood pressure measurement. When a regional anesthetic is planned, the back should be examined. Recognition of significant anesthetic risk factors should encourage consultation with the obstetrician.

2. Intrapartum Platelet Count. A platelet count may indicate the severity of a patient's pregnancy-induced hypertension. However, the literature is insufficient to assess the predictive value of a platelet count for anesthesia-related complications in either uncomplicated parturients or those with pregnancy-induced hypertension. The Consultants and Task Force both agree that a routine platelet count in the healthy parturient is not necessary. However, in the patient with pregnancy-induced hypertension, the Consultants and Task Force both agree that the use of a platelet count may reduce the risk of anesthesia-related complications.

> **Recommendations:** A specific platelet count predictive of regional anesthetic complications has not been determined. The anesthesiologist's decision to order or require a platelet count should be individualized and based upon a patient's history, physical examination and clinical signs of a coagulopathy.

3. Blood Type and Screen. The literature is silent regarding whether obtaining a blood type and screen is associated with fewer maternal anesthetic complications. The Consultants and Task Force are equivocal regarding the routine use of a blood type and screen to reduce the risk of anesthesia-related complications.

> Recommendations: The anesthesiologist's decision to order or require a blood type and screen or crossmatch should be individualized and based on anticipated hemorrhagic complications (e.g., placenta previa in a patient with previous uterine surgery).

4. Perianesthetic Recording of the Fetal Heart Rate. The literature suggests that analgesic/anesthetic agents may influence the fetal heart rate pattern. There is insufficient literature to demonstrate that perianesthetic recording of the fetal heart rate prevents fetal complications. However, both the Task Force and Consultants agree that perianesthetic recording of the fetal heart rate reduces fetal and neonatal complications.

> **Recommendations:** The fetal heart rate should be monitored by a qualified individual before and after administration of regional analgesia for labor. The Task Force recognizes that continuous electronic recording of the fetal heart rate may not be necessary in every clinical setting (1) and may not be possible during placement of a regional anesthetic.

II. Fasting in the obstetric patient.
1. Clear Liquids. Published evidence is insufficient regarding the relationship between fasting times for clear liquids and the risk of emesis/reflux or pulmonary aspiration during labor. The Task Force and Consultants agree that oral intake of clear liquids during labor improves maternal comfort and satisfaction. The Task Force and Consultants are equivocal whether oral intake of clear liquids increases maternal risk of pulmonary aspiration.

> **Recommendations:** The oral intake of modest amounts of clear liquids may be allowed for uncomplicated laboring patients. Examples of clear liquids include, but are not limited to, water, fruit juices without pulp, carbonated beverages, clear tea, and black coffee. The volume of liquid ingested is less important than the type of liquid ingested. However, patients with additional risk factors of aspiration (e.g., morbidly obese, diabetic, difficult airway), or patients at increased risk for operative delivery (e.g., non-reassuring fetal heart rate pattern) may have further restrictions of oral intake, determined on a case-by-case basis.

2. **Solids.** A specific fasting time for solids that is predictive of maternal anesthetic complications has not been determined. There is insufficient published evidence to address the safety of *any* particular fasting period for solids for obstetric patients. The Consultants agree that a fasting period for solids of 8 hours or more is preferable for uncomplicated parturients undergoing *elective* cesarean delivery. The Task Force recognizes that in laboring patients the timing of delivery is uncertain; therefore compliance with a predetermined fasting period is not always possible. The Task Force supports a fasting period of at least 6 hours before to elective cesarean delivery.

> **Recommendations:** Solid foods should be avoided in laboring patients. The patient undergoing elective cesarean delivery should have a fasting period for solids consistent with the hospital's policy for non-obstetric patients undergoing elective surgery. Both the amount and type of food ingested must be considered when determining the timing of surgery.

III. Anesthesia Care for Labor and Vaginal Delivery.
A. Overview of Recommendations. Anesthesia care is not necessary for all women for labor and/or delivery. For women who request pain relief for labor and/or delivery, there are many effective analgesic techniques available. Maternal request represents sufficient justification for pain relief, but the selected analgesia technique depends on the medical status of the patient, the progress of the labor, and the resources of the facility. When sufficient resources (e.g., anesthesia and nursing staff) are available, epidural catheter techniques should be one of the analgesic options offered. The primary goal is to provide adequate maternal analgesia with as little motor block as possible when regional analgesia is used for uncomplicated labor and/or vaginal delivery. This can be achieved by the administration of local anesthetic at low concentrations. The concentration of the local anesthetic may be further reduced by the addition of narcotics and still provide adequate analgesia.
B. Specific Recommendations.
1. Epidural Anesthetics.
   a. **Epidural local anesthetics.** The literature supports the use of single-bolus epidural local anesthetics for providing greater quality of analgesia compared to parenteral opioids. However, the literature indicates a reduced incidence of spontaneous vaginal delivery associated with single-bolus epidural local anesthetics. The literature is insufficient to indicate causation. Compared to *single-injection spinal opioids* the literature is equivocal regarding the analgesic efficacy of single-bolus epidural local anesthetics. The literature suggests that epidural local anesthetics compared to spinal opioids are associated with a lower incidence of pruritus. The literature is insufficient to compare the incidence of other side-effects.

b. **The addition of opioids to epidural local anesthetics.** The literature supports that the use of epidural local anesthetics with opioids, when compared with *equal* concentrations of epidural local anesthetics without opioids, provides greater quality and duration of analgesia. The former is associated with reduced motor block and an increased likelihood of spontaneous delivery, possibly as a result of a reduced total dose of local anesthetic administered over time.##

The literature is equivocal regarding the analgesic efficacy of *low* concentrations of epidural local anesthetics with opioids compared to higher concentrations of epidural local anesthetics without opioids. The literature indicates that low concentrations of epidural local anesthetics with opioids compared to *higher* concentrations of epidural local anesthetics are associated with reduced motor block.

No differences in the incidence of nausea, hypotension, duration of labor, or neonatal outcomes are found when epidural local anesthetics with opioids were compared to epidural local anesthetics without opioids. However, the literature indicates that the addition of opioids to epidural local anesthetics results in a higher incidence of pruritus. The literature is insufficient to determine the effects of epidural local anesthetics with opioids on other maternal outcomes (e.g., respiratory depression, urinary retention).

The Task Force and majority of Consultants are supportive of the case-by-case selection of an analgesic technique for labor. The subgroup of Consultants reporting a preferred technique, when all choices are available, selected an epidural local anesthetic technique. When a low concentration of epidural local anesthetic is used, the Consultants and Task Force agree that the addition of an opioid(s) improves analgesia and maternal satisfaction without increasing maternal, fetal or neonatal complications.

Recommendations: The selected analgesic/anesthetic technique should reflect patient needs and preferences, practitioner preferences or skills, and available resources. When an epidural local anesthetic is selected for labor and delivery, the addition of an opioid may allow the use of a lower concentration of local anesthetic and prolong the duration of analgesia. Appropriate resources for the treatment of complications related to epidural local anesthetics (e.g., hypotension, systemic toxicity, high spinal anesthesia) should be available. If opioids are added, treatments for related complications (e.g., pruritus, nausea, respiratory depression) should be available.

c. **Continuous infusion epidural techniques (CIE).** The literature indicates that effective analgesia can be maintained with a low concentration of local anesthetic with an epidural infusion technique. In addition, when an opioid is added to a local anesthetic infusion, an even lower concentration of local anesthetic provides effective analgesia. For example, comparable analgesia is found, with a reduced incidence of motor block, using bupivacaine infusion concentrations of *less than* 0.125% with an opioid compared to bupivacaine concentrations

equal to 0.125% without an opioid.*** No comparative differences are noted for incidence of instrumental delivery.

The literature is equivocal regarding the relationship between different local anesthetic infusion regimens and the incidence of nausea or neonatal outcome. However, the literature suggests that local anesthetic infusions with opioids are associated with a higher incidence of pruritus.

The Task Force and Consultants agree that infusions using low concentrations of local anesthetics with or without opioids provide equivalent analgesia, reduced motor block, and improved maternal satisfaction when compared to higher concentrations of local anesthetic.

Recommendations: Adequate analgesia for uncomplicated labor and delivery should be provided with the secondary goal of producing as little motor block as possible. The lowest concentration of local anesthetic infusion that provides adequate maternal analgesia and satisfaction should be used. For example, an infusion concentration of bupivacaine equal to or greater than 0.25% is unnecessary for labor analgesia for most patients. The addition of an opioid(s) to a low concentration of local anesthetic may improve analgesia and minimize motor block. Resources for the treatment of potential complications should be available.

2. **Spinal Opioids with or without Local Anesthetics.** The literature suggests that spinal opioids with or without local anesthetics provide effective labor analgesia without significantly altering the incidence of neonatal complications. There is insufficient literature to compare spinal opioids with parenteral opioids. However, the Consultants and Task Force agree that spinal opioids provide improved maternal analgesia compared to parenteral opioids.

The literature is equivocal regarding analgesic efficacy of spinal opioids compared to epidural local anesthetics. The Consultants and Task Force agree that spinal opioids provide equivalent analgesia compared to epidural local anesthetics. The Task Force agrees that the rapid onset of analgesia provided by single-injection spinal techniques may be advantageous for selected patients (e.g., advanced labor).

Recommendations: Spinal opioids with or without local anesthetics may be used to provide effective, though time-limited, analgesia for labor. Resources for the treatment of potential complications (e.g., pruritus, nausea, hypotension, respiratory depression) should be available.

3. **Combined Spinal-Epidural Techniques.** Although the literature suggests that combined spinal-epidural techniques (CSE) provide effective analgesia, the literature is insufficient to evaluate the analgesic efficacy of CSE compared to epidural local anesthetics. The literature indicates that use of CSE techniques with opioids when compared to epidural local anesthetics with or without opioids results in a higher incidence of pruritus and nausea. The Task Force and Consultants are equivocal regarding improved analgesia or maternal benefit of CSE versus epidural techniques. Although the literature is insufficient to evaluate fetal and neonatal

---

##No meta analytic differences in the likelihood of spontaneous delivery were found when studies using morphine or meperidine were added to studies using only fentanyl or sufentanil.

***References to pupivacaine are included for illustrative purposes only, and because bupivacaine is the most extensively studied local anesthetic for CIE. The Task Force recognizes that other local anesthestic agents are equally appropriate for CIE.

outcomes of CSE techniques, the Task Force and Consultants agree that CSE does not increase the risk of fetal or neonatal complications.

> **Recommendations:** Combined spinal-epidural techniques may be used to provide rapid and effective analgesia for labor. Resources for the treatment of potential complications (e.g., pruritus, nausea, hypotension, respiratory depression) should be available.

4. **Regional Analgesia and Progress of Labor.** There is insufficient literature to indicate whether timing of analgesia related to cervical dilation affects labor and delivery outcomes. Both the Task Force and Consultants agree that cervical dilation at the time of epidural analgesia administration does not impact the outcome of labor.

The literature indicates that epidural anesthesia may be used in a trial of labor for previous cesarean section patients without adversely affecting the incidence of vaginal delivery. However, randomized comparisons of epidural versus other specific anesthetic techniques were not found, and comparison groups were often confounded.

> **Recommendations:** Cervical dilation is not a reliable means of determining when regional analgesia should be initiated. Regional analgesia should be administered on an individualized basis.

5. **Monitored or Stand-by Anesthesia Care for Complicated Vaginal Delivery.** Monitored anesthesia care refers to instances in which an anesthesiologist has been called upon to provide specific anesthesia services to a particular patient undergoing a planned procedure (2). For these Guidelines, stand-by anesthesia care refers to the availability of the anesthesiologist in the facility, in the event of obstetric complications. The literature is silent regarding the subject of monitored or stand-by anesthesia care in obstetrics. However, the Task Force and Consultants agree that monitored or stand-by anesthesia care for complicated vaginal delivery reduces maternal, fetal, and neonatal complications.

> **Recommendations:** Either monitored or stand-by anesthesia care, determined on a case-by-case basis for complicated vaginal delivery (e.g., breech presentation, twins, and trial of instrumental delivery), should be made available when requested by the obstetrician.

IV. Removal of Retained Placenta.

1. **Anesthetic Choices.** The literature is insufficient to indicate whether a particular type of anesthetic is more effective than another for removal of retained placenta. The literature is also insufficient to assess the relationship between a particular type of anesthetic and maternal complications. The Task Force and Consultants agree that spinal or epidural anesthesia (i.e., regional anesthesia) is associated with reduced maternal complications and improved satisfaction when compared to general anesthesia or sedation/analgesia. The Task Force recognizes that circumstances may occur when general anesthesia or sedation/analgesia may be the more appropriate anesthetic choice (e.g., significant hemorrhage).

> **Recommendations:** Regional anesthesia, general endotracheal anesthesia, or sedation/analgesia may be used for removal of retained placenta. Hemodynamic status should be assessed before giving regional anesthesia to a parturient who has experienced significant bleeding. In cases involving significant maternal hemorrhage, a general anesthetic may be preferable to initiating regional anesthesia. Sedation/analgesia

should be titrated carefully due to the potential risk of pulmonary aspiration in the recently delivered parturient with an unprotected airway.

2. **Nitroglycerin for Uterine Relaxation.** The literature suggests and the Task Force and Consultants agree that the administration of nitroglycerin is effective for uterine relaxation during removal of retained placental tissue.

> **Recommendations:** Nitroglycerin is an alternative to terbutaline sulfate or general endotracheal anesthesia with halogenated agents for uterine relaxation during removal of retained placental tissue. Initiating treatment with a low dose of nitroglycerin may relax the uterus sufficiently while minimizing potential complications (e.g., hypotension).

V. Anesthetic Choices for Cesarean Delivery. The literature suggests that spinal, epidural or CSE anesthetic techniques can be used effectively for cesarean delivery. When compared to regional techniques, the literature indicates that general anesthetics can be administered with shorter induction-to-delivery times. The literature is insufficient to determine the relative risk of maternal death associated with general anesthesia compared to other anesthetic techniques. However, the literature suggests that a greater number of maternal deaths occur when general anesthesia is administered. The literature indicates that a larger proportion of neonates in the general anesthesia groups, compared to those in the regional anesthesia groups, are assigned Apgar scores of less than 7 at 1 and 5 minutes. However, few studies have utilized randomized comparisons of general versus regional anesthesia, resulting in potential selection bias in the reporting of outcomes.

The literature suggests that maternal side effects associated with regional techniques may include hypotension, nausea, vomiting, pruritus and postdural puncture headache. The literature is insufficient to examine the comparative merits of various regional anesthetic techniques. The Consultants agree that regional anesthesia can be administered with fewer maternal and neonatal complications and improved maternal satisfaction when compared to general anesthesia.

The consultants are equivocal about the possibility of increased maternal complications when comparing spinal or epidural anesthesia with CSE techniques. They agree that neonatal complications are not increased.

> **Recommendations:** The decision to use a particular anesthetic technique should be individualized based on several factors. These include anesthetic, obstetric and/or fetal risk factors (e.g., elective versus emergency) and the preferences of the patient and anesthesiologist. Resources for the treatment of potential complications (e.g., airway management, inadequate analgesia, hypotension, pruritus, nausea) should be available

VI. Postpartum Tubal Ligation. There is insufficient literature to evaluate the comparative benefits of local, spinal, epidural or general anesthesia for postpartum tubal ligation. Both the Task Force and Consultants agree that epidural, spinal and general anesthesia can be effectively provided without affecting maternal complications. Neither the Task Force nor the Consultants agree that local techniques provide effective anesthesia, and they are equivocal regarding the impact of local anesthesia on maternal complications. Although the literature is insufficient, the Task Force and Consultants agree that a postpartum tubal ligation can be performed safely within eight hours of delivery in many patients.

> **Recommendations:** Evaluation of the patient for postpartum tubal ligation should include assessment of hemodynamic status (e.g., blood loss) and consideration of anesthetic risks. The patient planning to have an elective

Table 1. SUGGESTED RESOURCES FOR OBSTETRIC HEMORRHAGIC EMERGENCIES[a]

1. Large-bore IV catheters.
2. Fluid warmer.
3. Forced air body warmer.
4. Availability of blood bank resources.
5. Equipment for infusing IV fluids and/or blood products rapidly. Examples include (but are not limited to) hand squeezed fluid chambers, hand inflated pressure bags, and automatic infusion devices.

[a] Important: The items listed in this table represent suggestions. The items should be customized to meet the specific needs, preferences, and skills of the practitioner and health-care facility.

postpartum tubal ligation within 8 hours of delivery should have no oral intake of solid foods during labor and postpartum until the time of surgery. Both the timing of the procedure and the decision to use a particular anesthetic technique (i.e., regional versus general) should be individualized, based on anesthetic and/or obstetric risk factors and patient preferences. The anesthesiologist should be aware that an epidural catheter placed for labor may be more likely to fail with longer post-delivery time intervals. If a postpartum tubal ligation is to be done before the patient is discharged from the hospital, the procedure should not be attempted at a time when it might compromise other aspects of patient care in the labor and delivery area.

VII. Management of Complications.

1. **Resources for Management of Hemorrhagic Emergencies.** The literature suggests that the availability of resources for hemorrhagic emergencies is associated with reduced maternal complications. The Task Force and Consultants agree that the availability of resources for managing hemorrhagic emergencies is associated with reduced maternal, fetal and neonatal complications.

   Recommendations: Institutions providing obstetric care should have resources available to manage hemorrhagic emergencies (Table 1). In an emergency, the use of type-specific or O negative blood is acceptable in the parturient.

2. **Equipment for Management of Airway Emergencies.** The literature suggests, and the Task Force and Consultants agree that the availability of equipment for the management of airway emergencies is associated with reduced maternal complications.

   Recommendations: Labor and delivery units should have equipment and personnel readily available to manage airway emergencies. Basic airway management equipment should be immediately available during the initial provision of regional analgesia (Table 2). In ad-

Table 2. SUGGESTED RESOURCES FOR AIRWAY MANAGEMENT DURING INITIAL PROVISION OF REGIONAL ANESTHESIA[a]

1. Laryngoscope and assorted blades.
2. Endotracheal tubes, with stylets.
3. Oxygen source.
4. Suction source with tubing and catheters.
5. Self-inflating bag and mask for positive pressure ventilation.
6. Medications for blood pressure support, muscle relaxation, and hypnosis.

[a] Important: The items listed in this table represent suggestions. The items should be customized to meet the specific needs, preferences, and skills of the practitioner and health-care facility.

Table 3. SUGGESTED CONTENTS OF A PORTABLE UNIT FOR DIFFICULT AIRWAY MANAGEMENT FOR CESAREAN SECTION ROOMS[a,b]

1. Rigid laryngoscope blades and handles of alternate design and size from those routinely used.[c]
2. Endotracheal tubes of assorted size.
3. Laryngeal mask airways of assorted sizes.
4. At least one device suitable for emergency nonsurgical airway ventilation. Examples include (but are not limited to), retrograde intubation equipment, a hollow jet ventilation stylet or cricothyrotomy kit with or without a transtracheal jet ventilator, and the esophageal-tracheal combitube.
5. Endrotracheal tube guides. Examples include (but are not limited to) semirigid stylets with or without a hollow core for jet ventilation, light wands, and forceps designed to manipulate the distal portion of the endotracheal tube.
6. Equipment suitable for emergency surgical airway access.
7. Topical anesthetics and vasoconstrictors.

[a] Important: The items listed in this table represent suggestions. The items should be customized to meet the specific needs, preferences, and skills of the practitioner and health-care facility.
[b] The Task force believes fiberoptic intubation equipment should be readily available.
Adapted from "Practice guidelines for management of the difficult airway: a report by the American Society of Anesthesiologists Task Force on Management of the Difficult Airway." *Anesthesiology* 1993;78:597–602.

dition, portable equipment for difficult airway management should be readily available in the operative area of labor and delivery units (Table 3).

3. **Central Invasive Hemodynamic Monitoring.** There is insufficient literature to indicate whether pulmonary artery catheterization is associated with improved maternal, fetal or neonatal outcomes in patients with pregnancy-related hypertensive disorders. The literature is silent regarding the management of obstetric patients with central venous catheterization alone. The literature suggests that pulmonary artery catheterization has been used safely in obstetric patients; however, the literature is insufficient to examine specific obstetric outcomes. The Task Force and Consultants agree that it is not necessary to routinely use central invasive hemodynamic monitoring for severe preeclamptic parturients.

   Recommendations: The decision to perform invasive hemodynamic monitoring should be individualized and based on clinical indications that include the patient's medical history and cardiovascular risk factors. The Task Force recognizes that not all practitioners have access to resources for utilization of central venous or pulmonary artery catheters in obstetric units.

4. **Cardiopulmonary Resuscitation.** The literature is insufficient to evaluate the efficacy of CPR in the obstetric patient during labor and delivery. The Task Force is supportive of the immediate availability of basic and advanced life-support equipment in the operative area of labor and delivery units.

   Recommendations: Basic and advanced life-support equipment should be immediately available in the operative area of labor and delivery units. If cardiac arrest occurs during labor and delivery, standard resuscitative measures and procedures, including left uterine displacement, should be taken. In cases of cardiac arrest, the American Heart Association has stated the following: "Several authors now recommend that the decision to perform a perimortem cesarean section should be made rapidly, with delivery effected within 4 to 5 minutes of the arrest" (3).

REFERENCES

1. *Guidelines for Perinatal Care,* 4th ed. Washington, DC: American Academy of Pediatrics and American College of Obstetricians and Gynecologists, 1997:100–102.
2. Position on monitored anesthesia care. In: *ASA Standards, Guidelines and Statements.* American Society of Anesthesiologists, Park Ridge, IL. 1997.
3. Guidelines for Cardiopulmonary Resuscitation and Emergency Cardiac Care: Recommendations of the 1992 national conference. *JAMA* 1992;268:2249.

Developed by the Task Force on Obstetrical Anesthesia: Joy L. Hawkins, M.D. (Chair), Denver, Colorado; James F. Arens, M.D., Galveston, Texas; Brenda A. Bucklin, M.D., Omaha, Nebraska; Robert A. Caplan, M.D., Seattle, Washington; David H. Chestnut, M.D., Birmingham, Alabama; Richard T. Connis, Ph.D., Woodinville, Washington; Patricia A. Dailey, M.D., Hillsborough, California; Larry C. Gilstrap, M.D., Houston, Texas; Stephen C. Grice, M.D., Alpharetta, Georgia; Nancy E. Oriol, M.D., Boston, Masachusetts; Kathryn J. Zuspan, M.D., Edina, Minnesota.

Supported by the American Society of Anesthesiologists, under the direction of James F. Arens, M.D., Chairman of the Ad Hoc Committee on Practice Parameters. Approved by the House of Delegates, October 21, 1998. Effective date January 1, 1999. The methods and analyses used to develop these guidelines are described in *Anesthesiology* 1999;60:600–611. A list of the articles used to describe the guidelines is available by writing to the American Society of Anesthesiologists.

Reprinted with permission from *Anesthesiology* 1999;90:600–611. © 1999 American Society of Anesthesiologists, 520 N. Northwest Highway, Park Ridge, IL 60068-2573.

Shnider and Levinson's Anesthesia for Obstetrics,
edited by Samuel C. Hughes, et al.
Lippincott Williams & Wilkins,
Philadelphia, © 2001.

APPENDIX C

OPTIMAL GOALS FOR ANESTHESIA CARE IN OBSTETRICS

This joint statement from the American Society of Anesthesiologists (ASA) and the American College of Obstetricians and Gynecologists (ACOG) has been designed to address issues of concern to both specialties. Good obstetric care requires the availability of qualified personnel and equipment to administer general or regional anesthesia both electively and emergently. The extent and degree to which anesthesia services are available varies widely among hospitals. However, for any hospital providing obstetric care, certain optimal anesthesia goals should be sought. These include the following:

I. Availability of a licensed practitioner who is credentialed to administer an appropriate anesthetic whenever necessary. For many women, regional anesthesia (spinal, epidural, or combined spinal epidural will be the most appropriate anesthetic.

II. Availability of a licensed practitioner who is credentialed to maintain support of vital functions in any obstetric emergency.

III. Availability of anesthesia and surgical personnel to permit the start of a cesarean delivery within 30 minutes of the decision to perform the procedure; in cases of VBAC, appropriate facilities and personnel, including obstetric anesthesia, nursing personnel, and a physician capable of monitoring labor and performing cesarean delivery, immediately available during active labor to perform emergency cesarean delivery (1). The definition of immediate availability of personnel and facilities remains a local decision, based on each institution's available resources and geographic location.

IV. Appointment of a qualified anesthesiologist to be responsible for all anesthetics administered.

There are obstetric units where obstetricians or obstetrician-supervised nurse anesthetists administer anesthetics. The administration of general or regional anesthesia requires both medical judgment and technical skills. Thus, a physician with privileges in anesthesiology should be readily available.

Persons administering or supervising obstetric anesthesia should be qualified to manage the infrequent but occasionally life-threatening complications of major regional anesthesia such as respiratory and cardiovascular failure, toxic local anesthetic convulsions, or vomiting and aspiration. Mastering and retaining the skills and knowledge necessary to manage these complications require adequate training and frequent application.

To ensure the safest and most effective anesthesia for obstetric patients, the director of anesthesia services, with the approval of the medical staff, should develop and enforce written policies regarding provision of obstetric anesthesia. These include:

I. Availability of a qualified physician with obstetrical privileges to perform operative vaginal or cesarean delivery during administration of anesthesia.

Regional and/or general anesthesia should not be administered until the patient has been examined and the fetal status and progress of labor evaluated by a qualified individual. A physician with obstetrical privileges who has knowledge of the maternal and fetal status and the progress of labor, and who approves the initiation of labor anesthesia, should be readily available to deal with any obstetric complications that may arise.

II. Availability of equipment, facilities and support personnel equal to that provided in the surgical suite.

This should include the availability of a properly equipped and staffed recovery room capable of receiving and caring for all patients recovering from major regional or general anesthesia. Birthing facilities, when used for analgesia or anesthesia, must be appropriately equipped to provide safe anesthetic care during labor and delivery or postanesthesia recovery care.

Personnel other than the surgical team immediately available to assume responsibility for resuscitation of the depressed newborn.

The surgeon and anesthesiologist are responsible for the mother and may not be able to leave her care for the newborn even when a regional anesthetic is functioning adequately. Individuals qualified to perform neonatal resuscitation should demonstrate:

A. Proficiency in rapid and accurate evaluation of the newborn condition, including Apgar scoring.

B. Knowledge of the pathogenesis of depression in a newborn (acidosis, drugs, hypovolemia, trauma, anomalies, and infection) as well as specific indications for resuscitation.

C. Proficiency in newborn airway management, laryngoscopy, endotracheal intubations, suctioning of airways, artificial ventilation, cardiac massage, and maintenance of thermal stability.

In larger maternity units and those functioning as high-risk centers, 24-hour in-house anesthesia, obstetric and neonatal specialists are usually necessary. Preferably, the obstetric anesthesia services should be directed by an anesthesiologist with special training or experience in obstetric anesthesia. These units will also frequently require the availability of more sophisticated monitoring equipment and specially trained nursing personnel.

A survey jointly sponsored by ASA and ACOG found that many hospitals in the United States have not yet achieved the above goals. Deficiencies were most evident in smaller delivery units. Some small delivery units are necessary because of geographic considerations. Currently, approximately 50 percent of hospitals providing obstetric care have fewer than 500 deliveries per year. Providing comprehensive care for obstetric patients in these small units is extremely inefficient, not cost-effective and frequently impossible. Thus, the following recommendations are made:

1. Whenever possible, small units should consolidate.

2. When geographic factors require the existence of smaller units, these units should be part of a well-established regional perinatal system.

The availability of the appropriate personnel to assist in the management of a variety of obstetric problems is a necessary feature of good obstetric care. The presence of a pediatrician or other trained physician at a high-risk cesarean delivery to care for the newborn or the availability of an anesthesiologist during active labor and delivery when vaginal birth after cesarean delivery (VBAC) is attempted, and at a breech or twin delivery are examples. Frequently, these professionals spend a considerable amount of time standing by for the possibility that their services may be needed emergently but may ultimately not be required to perform the tasks for which they are present. Reasonable compensation for these standby services is justifiable and necessary.

A variety of other mechanisms have been suggested to increase the availability and quality of anesthesia services in obstetrics. Improved hospital design to place labor and delivery suites closer to the operating room would allow for more efficient supervision of nurse anesthetists. Anesthesia equipment in the labor and delivery area must be comparable to that in the operating room.

Finally, good interpersonal relations between obstetricians and anesthesiologists are important. Joint meetings between the two departments should be encouraged. Anesthesiologists should recognize the special needs and concerns of the obstetrician, and obstetricians should recognize the anesthesiologist as a consultant in the management of pain and life-support measures. Both should recognize the need to provide high-quality care for all patients.

REFERENCE

1. American College of Obstetricians and Gynecologists. *Vaginal birth after previous Cesarean delivery.* ACOG Practice Bulletin. Washington, DC: ACOG, 1999.

BIBLIOGRAPHY

Committee on Perinatal Health. *Toward improving the outcome of pregnancy: the 1990s and beyond.* White Plains, NY: March of Dimes Birth Defects Foundation, 1993.

Shnider and Levinson's Anesthesia for Obstetrics,
edited by Samuel C. Hughes, et al.
Lippincott Williams & Wilkins,
Philadelphia, © 2001.

APPENDIX D

FETAL AND NEONATAL EFFECTS OF MATERNALLY ADMINISTERED DRUGS

RHONDA K. ARNETTE, M.D.

It is reported that 0.3% to 2.2% of women have surgery during their pregnancy (see Chapter 13) and are thus exposed to anesthetics as well as other drugs. Many more women, unfortunately, are exposed to illicit drugs during pregnancy, with some estimates as high as 5.5% (see Chapter 34). Additionally, four of every five women take medication during their pregnancy, largely as prescribed drugs, and many parturients receive medication during labor and delivery for obstetric considerations or analgesia. When obstetric complications arise, patients may require substantial doses of several drugs to ensure a safe outcome. Thus, the fetal and neonatal effects of many maternally administered drugs are important and are summarized here for quick reference.

It is probable that all maternally administered drugs cross the placenta to some extent. Movement is primarily by passive diffusion. Both a large transplacental drug gradient and a high diffusion constant facilitate movement across the placental membrane. Drugs with a high diffusion constant are those of low molecular weight and high lipid solubility which exist primarily in the nonionized unbound form.

When administered during the first trimester, the period of organogenesis, certain drugs may modify development of fetal tissues with resultant congenital anomalies. However, drugs are not the sole factor which may have an adverse effect on fetal tissue organization and development. In fact, the cause of most malformations is not known. Only a small percentage are directly attributable to known hereditary and environmental factors (the latter including infection, irradiation, and drug use). Organogenesis is complete by the end of the first trimester, with important exceptions being the teeth, genital system, and central nervous system. The vast majority of congenital malformations arise during the first trimester of pregnancy when organ systems are developing and embryonic cells are rapidly dividing. The teratogenic effects of a drug are both dose and time related. The timing of a teratogenic influence is crucial in determining the system affected. In humans, for example, the period of greatest development and organization of the cardiovascular system is between 20 and 40 days after conception, that of the limbs is from 24 to 46 days, and that of the central nervous system is from 15 to 25 days. Exposure to an appropriate teratogen between 15 and 25 days after conception may, for example, result in nervous system but not skeletal anomalies. It is possible that teratogenic drugs exert their effects on development within the first 2 weeks of conception—before the woman knows that she is pregnant. However, from the time of fertilization until implantation of the blastocyst, most deleterious drugs abort the conception rather that deform it.

Only three types of drugs are definitely know to be teratogenic in humans: certain antimetabolites, thalidomide, and steroid hormones with androgenic activity. Epidemiologic surveys have been undertaken to examine the possible association between maternal drug ingestion and congenital defects in the infant. Most studies are difficult to interpret. Associations are loose, and it is impossible to differentiate the effects of a drug from those of the maternal disease for which the medication was prescribed. From these studies, many drugs are highly suspect for inducing fetal abnormalities but the risk is often relatively low. Although considerable work has been done on teratogenicity in animals, it should be stressed that little, if any, parallel exists between the ability to induce abnormalities in a particular species of animal and that in humans.

Drugs administered at any time during pregnancy or labor may modify fetal and newborn physiology. Such changes are usually of no clinical relevance, but, on occasion, they may be either detrimental or beneficial.

Analgesic or anesthetic drugs administered to the mother prior to delivery may depress the fetus and lessen the reserve of the newborn for adapting to extrauterine life. The most widely used method for evaluating the condition of the infant in the delivery room is the Apgar score. There are five signs: heart rate, respiratory effect, muscle tone, response to stimulation, and skin color. A score of 0, 1, or 2 is assigned to the presence or absence of each sign. Apgar scoring quickly identifies those infants with significant depression of vital function. Maternally administered drugs may reduce neonatal vigor and subsequently result in lower Apgar scores. Such drug-induced depression is infrequent in uncomplicated well-conducted obstetrics but may occur, for instance, with general anesthesia for cesarean section. When drug depression does occur, it is in the form of respiratory depression, and ventilation may require support for a short period of time. Neurobehavioral changes have also been described, and this topic is discussed in detail in Chapter 37.

The following table lists some of the more frequently used drugs with their possible effects on the fetus and newborn. Comments and references are included where appropriate.

Drug	Use in Pregnancy	Use in Lactation: American Academy of Pediatrics (AAP) Recommendations Documented when Available	References
Analgesics (opioids)	Small for gestational age and neonatal withdrawal syndrome with chronic use Accelerated appearance of mature L/S ratios in heroin addicts Increased incidence of neonatal jaundice with methadone only Decreased incidence of neonatal jaundice with heroin Neonatal withdrawal syndrome with chronic abuse Intrauterine death associated with maternal opioid withdrawal Neonatal depression with inappropriate doses during labor; morphine most depressant	AAP: Compatible No adverse effects with methadone dose of 20 mg/24 h Morphine: infant may have significant blood levels	(11, 46, 65, 113, 114, 115, 141, 169, 170, 179, 236, 251, 275, 287, 318, 378)
Analgesics (nonopioid)			
Acetaminophen	Appears to be safe in therapeutic doses for short term Case report of severe maternal anemia and fetal kidney disease with continuous high daily doses Fetal liver toxicity with toxic maternal doses	AAP: Compatible	(17, 34, 47, 64, 124, 138, 160, 184, 279)
Aspirin	No evidence of increased risk of congenital anomalies Intrauterine growth restriction and increased incidence of stillbirths Use of full doses near term may be related to increased maternal and neonatal hemorrhagic phenomenon as well as premature ductus arteriosus closure and pulmonary hypertension in the neonate Possibly increased incidence of prolonged gestation and labor with use near term	AAP: Use with caution One case report of metabolic acidosis	(12, 34, 64, 65, 159, 160, 293, 314, 321, 332, 341)
Ibuprofen, Indomethacin, Naproxen, Ketoprofen, Ketorolac	Third trimester use may be associated with increased maternal and hemorrhagic phenomenon, premature ductus closure and pulmonary hypertension in the neonate, oligohydramnios, and prolongation of gestation and labor	AAP: Compatible	(34, 65, 82, 104, 117, 142, 198, 229, 291, 343, 348)
Anticoagulants			
Coumadin	Embryopathy characterized by stippled epiphyses and nasal and limb hypoplasia with first trimester use Risk of fetal hemorrhage with use at any time during gestation CNS abnormalities, including dorsal midline dysplasia, midline cerebellar atrophy, and ventral midline dysplasia, mental restriction and optic atrophy Increased incidence of stillbirths, spontaneous abortions, and fetal death	AAP: Compatible	(20, 21, 32, 34, 51, 65, 84, 102, 125, 156, 194, 253, 301, 330, 350, 371)
Heparin	Does not cross the placenta Maternal heparin-induced thrombocytopenia and osteoporosis	Not excreted in breast milk	(34, 100, 110, 132, 149, 174, 329, 368, 379)
Low molecular weight heparin (LMWH)	Does not cross the placenta Conflicting data on maternal osteoporosis	Excretion in breast milk is unlikely	(34, 109, 151, 221, 239, 240, 261)
Anticholinergics			
Atropine	Decreased fetal breathing but no fetal hypoxia or effect on fetal heart or variability with modest doses	AAP: Compatible	(2, 3, 34, 64, 145, 220)
Glycopyrrolate	No effect on fetal heart rate Does not readily cross the placenta	Limited human data	(2, 3, 34)

(continued)

(continued)

Drug	Use in Pregnancy	Use in Lactation: American Academy of Pediatrics (AAP) Recommendations Documented when Available	References
Anticonvulsants			
Carbamazepine	Pattern of congenital malformations characterized by craniofacial defects, developmental delay, fingernail hypoplasia Neural tube defects	AAP: Compatible	(8, 34, 64, 65, 93, 165, 233, 280, 298, 376, 377)
Phenobarbital	Neonatal withdrawal Neonatal coagulopathy	AAP: Use with caution due to sedative and withdrawal effects One case report of methemaglobinemia	(8, 34, 64, 65, 81, 93, 234)
Phenytoin	Fetal hydantoin syndrome characterized by growth and performance delays, craniofacial abnormalities, limb abnormalities Neonatal coagulapathy	AAP: Compatible One case of methemaglobinemia	(8, 34, 64, 93, 105, 129, 130, 377)
Valproic acid	Neural tube defects Facial defects	AAP: Compatible	(8, 13, 34, 64, 83, 93, 157, 202, 359)
Antidepressants			
Lithium	Possible association with congenital heart defects, particularly Epstein's anomaly Signs of lithium toxicity in the neonate have been reported Possible fetal hypothyroidism and goiter	AAP: Contraindicated due to potential for lithium toxicity	(15, 34, 64, 65, 91, 102, 227, 233, 305, 357)
SSRIs			
Fluoxetine	Studies suggest no increased risk of major congenital malformations; however, higher rates of minor malformations and perinatal complications (prematurity, lower birth weights, poor neonatal adaptation, increased ICU admissions, pulmonary hypertension) have been described Possible increased rate of spontaneous abortions	AAP: Unknown but may be of concern	(34, 44, 60, 64, 65, 181, 252, 369)
Sertraline, Paroxetine	Limited human data	AAP: Unknown but may be of concern	(34, 65)
SNRIs, SARIs, NDRIs, NASAs	Limited human data	AAP: Unknown but may be of concern	(34, 65)
Tricyclics	Studies do not consistently suggest an increased risk of congenital malformations, although case reports have suggested a possible association with limb malformations Neonatal withdrawal symptoms	AAP: Unknown but may be of concern	(7, 34, 64, 65, 89, 152, 180, 217, 267, 316, 320, 358, 369)
Antiemetics			
Diphenhydramine	Studies suggest no increase in fetal anomalies or adverse effects	Limited data	(17, 34, 102, 138, 160, 216, 303, 312)
Droperidol	Limited human data although no adverse effects have been reported	Limited data	(34, 102, 216, 235, 256, 323)
Metoclopramide	Studies suggest no increased risk of fetal anomalies	AAP: Use with caution due to potential CNS effects	(34, 64, 102, 207, 209, 216, 225, 235, 246)
Ondansetron	Limited human data although no adverse effects have been reported	Limited data	(34, 102, 122, 216, 334, 374)
Prochlorperazine	Studies suggest no increased incidence in fetal anomalies Potential for extrapyramidal effects in the neonate	Limited data	(19, 34, 102, 116, 160, 182, 216, 225, 268, 322)
Promethazine	Studies suggest no increased incidence in fetal anomalies Possible impairment of platelet aggregation in the neonate (of questionable clinical significance)	Limited data	(17, 34, 69, 102, 138, 160, 216, 238, 294, 312, 361)

(continued)

(continued)

Drug	Use in Pregnancy	Use in Lactation: American Academy of Pediatrics (AAP) Recommendations Documented when Available	References
Antihypertensives			
ACE inhibitors	Associated with intrauterine growth retardation, oligohydramnios, neonatal renal failure, and neonatal death	AAP: Captopril and enalapril listed as compatible Limited human data with other ACE inhibitors	(24, 33, 34, 64, 102, 121, 131, 172, 241, 265, 282, 286, 307, 308)
Alpha 2 Agonists			
Methyldopa	No apparent adverse effects on the fetus (stable uteroplacental perfusion and fetal hemodynamics)	AAP: Compatible	(14, 34, 64, 98, 102, 106, 127, 173, 230, 271)
Clonidine	Limited human data, but no adverse effects reported	Limited data	(34, 102, 139, 147, 148, 162, 172, 269)
Beta blockers	Possibly associated with intrauterine growth restriction Fetal or neonatal bradycardia Delayed spontaneous breathing in the newborn (more common with intravenous beta blocker) Neonatal hypoglycemia Premature or prolonged labor	AAP: Compatible, although potential for beta blockade exists in the neonate	(34, 39, 40, 64, 92, 102, 103, 112, 154, 199, 200, 203, 204, 208, 212, 231, 264, 289, 290, 299, 336, 347)
Calcium channel blockers	Limited human data (particularly during first trimester), but no adverse affects reported Report of potentiation of muscle weakness when magnesium sulfate is used concurrently	AAP: Captopril and nifedipine listed as compatible Limited human data on other calcium channel blockers	(34, 42, 50, 64, 68, 102, 125, 158, 197, 213, 270, 325, 342)
Diuretics			
Thiazides	May aggravate maternal hypovolemia and reduce placental perfusion Neonatal adverse effects include hypoglycemia, thrombocytopenia, electrolyte imbalance, and intrauterine growth restriction	AAP: Compatible May suppress lactation	(6, 34, 64, 102, 118, 134, 172, 188, 196, 223, 260, 278, 311)
Furosemide	May aggravate maternal hypovolemia and reduce placental perfusion May increase risk of neonatal hyperbilirubinemia Potential neonatal electrolyte imbalance	No adverse effects reported	(34, 52, 102, 107, 201, 339, 349)
Vasodilators			
Hydralazine	Studies suggest no increased incidence of fetal anomalies No adverse effects on uterine blood flow Report of transient neonatal thrombocytopenia with daily third trimester use Report of lupus-like syndrome in neonate	AAP: Compatible	(34, 45, 64, 172, 186, 210, 284, 319, 366, 375)
Antimicrobials			
Antibiotics			
Aminoglycosides	Reports of ototoxicity with streptomycin and kanamycin, although no reports with use of gentamicin Potentiation of neuromuscular blockade with concurrent magnesium sulfate use	AAP: Streptomycin and kanamycin listed as compatible Limited human data with gentamicin	(34, 64, 87, 88, 102, 150, 164, 187, 324, 356, 367)
Cephalosporins	Adverse effects have not been demonstrated, although there are no large studies	AAP: Compatible	(34, 64, 78, 102, 281)
Fluoroquinolones	Limited human data, but reports of arthropathy in immature animals	Limited data	(23, 27, 30, 34, 102, 205, 243, 277)
Macrolides	No adverse effects reported with erythromycin and clindamycin Limited human data with clarithromycin and azithromycin	AAP: Erythromycin and clindamycin listed as compatible Limited data on clarithromycin and azithromycin	(4, 17, 34, 58, 64, 95, 102, 138, 160, 218, 219, 224, 304, 365)

(continued)

(continued)

Drug	Use in Pregnancy	Use in Lactation: American Academy of Pediatrics (AAP) Recommendations Documented when Available	References
Penicillins	Adverse effects have not been demonstrated	AAP: Compatible	(17, 34, 64, 102, 138, 160, 183)
Sulfonamides	Reports of neonatal hyperbilirubinemia when used near delivery Report of hemolytic anemia in a fetus of a mother with G6PD deficiency	AAP: Compatible Use with caution in infant with jaundice or G6PD deficiency and ill, stressed, and premature infants	(34, 62, 64, 75, 102, 111, 135, 137, 171, 206, 244, 254)
Tetracyclines	Fetal risk of teeth discoloration and hypoplasia Skeletal growth restriction	AAP: Compatible	(34, 43, 61, 64, 102, 133, 175, 185, 222, 276, 335)
Antifungals			
Fluconazole	Four neonates with similar pattern of anomalies (craniofacial defects, congenital heart disease, skeletal deformities) with continuous, high-dose therapy in the first trimester No adverse effects with low-dose, short-term therapy, although human data is limited	Limited data	(5, 34, 102, 155, 161, 195, 215, 266)
Antiretrovirals (see Chapter 33) Nucleoside reverse transcriptase inhibitors	—	—	(380, 381)
AZT or ZDV (Zidovudine)	Readily crosses the placenta Studies do not suggest an increased incidence of congenital abnormalities Potential for mitochondrial dysfunction in the fetus	Is excreted in breast milk Limited data	(18, 29, 67, 72, 77, 226, 228, 245, 331, 328, 363)
DDI (Didanosine)	Limited placental transfer Limited human data	Unknown if excreted in breast milk	(18, 226)
ddc (Zalcitabine)	Limited human data	Unknown if excreted in breast milk	—
d4t (Stavudine)	Limited human data Phase I/II study (ACTG 332) underway	Unknown if excreted in breast milk	—
3TC (Epivir, Lamivudine)	Limited human data Readily crosses the placenta	Is excreted in breast milk Limited data	(18, 226)
Protease inhibitors	—	—	(380, 381)
Saquinavir (Invirase)	Limited human data Phase I/II study (ACTG 386) underway	Limited data	—
Ritonavir (Norvir)	Limited human data Phase I/II study (ACTG 354) underway	Limited data	—
Indinavir (Crixivan)	May be associated with hyperbilirubinemia and nephrolithiasis in neonates Phase I/II study (ACTG 358) underway	Limited data	(18, 226)
Nelfinavir (Viracept)	Limited human data Phase I/II study (ACTG 353) underway	Limited data	—
Nonnucleoside reverse transcriptase inhibitors Nevirapine, Efavirenz, Delavirdine, Abacavir	Limited human data	Limited data	—
Antivirals			
Acyclovir	Limited human data but no adverse fetal effects reported	AAP: Compatible	(34, 35, 64, 101, 102, 310)
Anxiolytics			
Benzodiazepines	Earlier studies reported a possible link between diazepam use to oral clefts, while subsequent studies have not shown an association Neonatal withdrawal with chronic use "Floppy infant syndrome" characterized by hypotonia, lethargy, cyanosis, hypothermia, and sucking difficulties with chronic use Decreased fetal variability and fetal movement Altered neonatal thermogenesis	AAP: Unknown but may be of concern	(1, 17, 28, 34, 64, 70, 71, 73, 74, 76, 85, 102, 108, 160, 189, 190, 192, 250, 283, 296, 297, 300, 317, 327, 344)

(continued)

(continued)

Drug	Use in Pregnancy	Use in Lactation: American Academy of Pediatrics (AAP) Recommendations Documented when Available	References
Bronchodilators			
Theophylline	No increased risk of fetal anomalies reported Neonatal and maternal tachycardia, jitteriness, vomiting with high doses	AAP: Compatible but may cause irritability in the newborn	(16, 34, 64, 102, 146, 326, 340)
Albuterol	No increased risk of fetal anomalies reported but little first trimester data Neonatal/fetal and maternal tachycardia Neonatal hypoglycemia	Limited data	(34, 90, 102, 136, 176, 263, 333, 352, 353)
Terbutaline	No increased risk of fetal anomalies reported but little first trimester data Neonatal hypoglycemia Neonatal/fetal and maternal tachycardia	AAP: Compatible	(34, 64, 94, 102, 153, 255, 285, 315, 354)
Corticosteroids			
	Associated with oral clefts in animals, although human data do not support an increased risk of anomalies May be associated with low birth weight One case report of congenital cataracts Prednisone, methyprednisone, hydrocortisone, and prednisolone are converted into relatively inactive forms by an abundance of 11 beta dehydrogenase in the placenta so little active drug reaches the fetus; in contrast, dexamethasone and betamethasone are considerably less well metabolized by the placenta	AAP: Prednisone listed as compatible Limited data on other corticosteroids	(22, 31, 34, 64, 76, 94, 102, 138, 159, 166, 168, 193, 237, 249, 258, 259, 273, 302, 309, 370)
Histamine H$_2$ receptor antagonists			
Omeprazole	One case report of anencephaly Other studies suggest no increased risk of anomalies or adverse fetal/neonatal effects	Limited data	(34, 102, 167, 191, 292, 331, 338)
Cimetidine	Studies suggest no increased risk of anomalies or adverse fetal/neonatal effects	AAP: Compatible	(34, 64, 102, 144, 163, 167, 177, 211)
Hypoglycemics			
Oral hypoglycemics	Conflicting data: some studies have shown an increase in anomalies, while others have not	Unknown effects but potential for hypoglycemia exists	(34, 64, 54, 55, 56, 57, 102, 257, 272)
Insulin	Risk of anomalies is unlikely to be increased as insulin minimally crosses the placenta during the first trimester	Not excreted in breast milk	(34)
Thyroid agents			
Antithyroid			
Propylthiouracil	Mild or transient fetal hypothyroidism and goiter Treatment of choice during pregnancy	AAP: Compatible	(26, 34, 37, 38, 49, 64, 80, 102, 346, 360)
Sodium iodine–131	Fetal hypothyroidism and goiter	AAP: Requires temporary cessation of breast feeding due to the presence of radioactivity in milk	(34, 64, 99, 102, 119, 126, 295)
Thyroid replacement			
Levothyroxine	No increase in anomalies reported	Effect controversial: some suggest sufficient quantities excreted to protect against hypothyroidism, while others do not	(34, 36, 79, 123, 138, 242, 345, 360)

REFERENCES

1. Aarskog D. *Lancet* 1975;2:921.
2. Abboud TK, et al. *Anesth Analg* 1983;62:426–430.
3. Abboud TK, Read J, Miller F, et al. *Obstet Gynecol* 1981;57:224–227.
4. Adair CD, Gunter M, Stovall TG, et al. *Obstet Gynecol* 1998;91:165–168.
5. Aleck KA, Bertley DL. *Am J Med Genet* 1997;72:253–256.
6. Alstatt LB. *J Pediatr* 1965;66:985–988.
7. Altshuler L, Cohen L, Szuba MP, et al. *Am J Psychiatry* 1996;153:592–606.
8. ACOG. *Int J Gynecol Obstet* 1996;56:279–286.
9. Ananth J. *Compr Psychiatry* 1975;16:437–445.
10. Ananth J. *Pharmacopsychiatry* 1976;11:246–260.
11. Annunziato D. *Pediatrics* 1971;47:787.
12. Arcilla RA, Thilenius OG, Ranniger K. *J Pediatr* 1969;75:74–78.
13. Ardinger HH, Atkin JF, Blackston RD, et al. *Am J Med Genet* 1988;29:171–185.
14. Arias F, Zamora J. *Obstet Gynecol* 1979;53:489–494.
15. Arnom RG, Marin-Garcia J, Peeden JN. *Am J Dis Child* 1981;135:941–943.
16. Arwood LL, Dasta JF, Friedman C. *Pediatrics* 1979;63:844–846.
17. Aselton P, Jick H, Milunsky A, et al. *Obstet Gynecol* 1985; 65:451–455.
18. Augenbraun M, Minkoff H. *Obstet Gynecol Clin North Am* 1997;24:833–854.
19. Ayd FJ Jr. *Clin Med* 1964;71:1758–1763.
20. Ayhan A, Yapar EG, Yuce K, et al. *Int J Gynecol Obstet* 1991;35:117–122.
21. Baillie M, Allen ED, Elkington AR. *Br J Ophthalmol* 1980;64:633–635.
22. Ballard PD, Hearney EF, Smith MB. *Teratology* 1977;16:175–180.
23. Baroncini A, Calzolari E, Calabrese O, et al. *Teratology* 1996;53:24A.
24. Barr M Jr, Cotien MM Jr. *Teratology* 1991;44:485–495.
25. Becerra JE, Khourg MJ, Cordero JF, et al. *Pediatrics* 1990;85:1–9.
26. Becks GP, Burrow GN. *Med Clin North Am* 1991;75:121–150.
27. Berkovitch M, Pastuszak A, Gazarian M, et al. *Obstet Gynecol* 1994;84:535–538.
28. Birger M, Homberg R, Insler V. *Int J Gynaecol Obstet* 1980;18:377–382.
29. Blanche S, Tardieu M, Rustin R, et al. *Lancet* 1999;354:1084–1089.
30. Bomford JAL, Ledger JC, O'Keefe BJ, et al. *Drugs* 1993;45 (Suppl 3):461–462.
31. Bongiovanni AM, McPadden AJ. *Fertil Steril* 1960;11:181–186.
32. Born D, Martinez EE, Almeida PAM, et al. *Am Heart J* 1992;124:413–417.
33. Brent RL, Beckman DA. *Teratology* 1991;43:543–546.
34. Briggs GG, Freeman RK, Yaffe SJ, eds. *Drugs in Pregnancy and Lactation: a Reference Guide to Fetal and Neonatal Risk*, 5th ed. Baltimore: Williams and Wilkins, 1998.
35. Brown ZA, Baker DA. *Obstet Gynecol* 1989;73:526–531.
36. Bruner JP, Dellinger EH. *Fetal Diagn Ther* 1997;12:200–204.
37. Burrow GN. *Endocrinol Rev* 1993;14:194–202.
38. Burrow GN. *N Engl J Med* 1978;298:150–153.
39. Butters L, Kennedy S, Rubin PC. *BMJ* 1990;301:587–589.
40. Caldroney RD. *N Engl J Med* 1982;306:810.
41. Campomori A, Bonati M. *Ann Pharmacother* 1997;31:118–119.
42. Carbonne B, Jannet D, Touboul C, et al. *Obstet Gynecol* 1993;81:908–914.
43. Carter MP, Wilson F. *BMJ* 1962;2:407–408.
44. Chambers CD, Johnson KA, Dick LN, et al. *N Engl J Med* 1996;335:1010–1015.
45. Chapman ER, Stovier WE, Magee RA. *Am J Obstet Gynecol* 1954;68:1109–1117.
46. Chappel JN. *JAMA* 1972;221:1516.
47. Char VC, Chandra R, Fletcher AB, et al. *J Pediatr* 1975;86:638–639.
48. Chari RS, Friedman SA, Sibai BM. *Fetal Matern Med Rev.*
49. Cheron RG, Kaplan MM, Larsen PR, et al. *N Engl J Med* 1981;304:525–528.
50. Childress CH, Katz VF. *Obstet Gynecol* 1994;83:616–624.
51. Chong MKB, Harveey D, deSwiet M. *Br J Obstet Gynaecol* 1984;91:1070–1073.
52. Christianson R, Page EW. *Obstet Gynecol* 1976;48:647–652.
53. Clarke CF, Welch CR, Pigo H. *J Obstet Gynecol* 1989;9:301–302.
54. Coetzee EJ, Jackson WPU. *Diabet Res Clin Pract* 1986;1:281–287.
55. Coetzee EJ, Jackson WPU. *S Afr Med J* 1980;58:795–802.
56. Coetzee EJ, Jackson WPU. *S Afr Med J* 1984;65:635–637.
57. Coetzee EJ, Jackson WPU. *S Afr Med J* 1986;5:281–287.
58. Cohen I, Veille J-C, Calkins BM. *JAMA* 1990;263:3160–3163.
59. Cohen LS, Friedman JM, Jefferson JW, et al. *JAMA* 1994;271:146–150.
60. Cohen LS, Rosenbaum JF. *J Clin Psychiatr* 1998;59(Suppl 2):18–28.
61. Cohlan SQ, Bevelander G, Tiamsic T. *Am J Dis Child* 1963;105:453.
62. Colley DP, Kay J, Gibson GT. *Aust J Pharm* 1982;63:570–575.
63. Collins E, Turner G. *Lancet* 1975;2:335–338.
64. Collins R, Yusuf S, Peto R. *BMJ* 1985;290:17–23.
65. Committee on Drugs, AAP. *Pediatrics* 1994;93:137–150.
66. Committee on Drugs, AAP. *Pediatrics* 2000;105:880–887.
67. Conner EM, Sperling RS, Gelber R, et al. *N Engl J Med* 1994;331:1173–1180.
68. Constantine G, Beevers DG, Reynolds AL, et al. *Br J Obstet Gynaecol* 1987;94:1136–1142.
69. Corby DG, Shulman I. *J Pediatr* 1971;79:307–313.
70. Cree JE, Meyer J, Hailey DM. *BMJ* 1973;4:251–255.
71. Crombie DL, Pinsent RJ, Fleming DM. *N Engl J Med* 1975;293:198–199.
72. Culnane M, Fowler MG, Lee SS, et al. *JAMA* 1999;281:151–157.
73. Czeizel A. *Lancet* 1976;13:198–200.
74. Czeizel A. *Reprod Toxicol* 1988;1:183–188.
75. Czeizel A. *Reprod Toxicol* 1990;4:305–313.
76. Czeizel A, Rockenbaur M. *Teratology* 1997;56:335–340.
77. Dabis F, Msellati P, Meda N, et al. *Lancet* 1999;353:786–797.
78. Dashe JS, Gilstrap LC. *Obstet Gynecol Clin North Am* 1997;24:617–629.
79. Davidson KM, Richards DS, Schatz DA, et al. *N Engl J Med* 1991;324:543–546.
80. Davis LE, Lucas MJ, Hankins GDV, et al. *Am J Obstet Gynecol* 1989;160:63–70.
81. Desmond MM, Schwanecke RP, Wilson GS, et al. *J Pediatr* 1972;80:190–197.
82. DeWit W, Van Mourik I, Wiesenhaan PF. *Br J Obstet Gynaecol* 1988;95:303–305.
83. DiLiberti JH, Farndon PA, Dennis NR, et al. *Am J Med Genet* 1984;19:473–481.
84. DiSaia PJ. *Obstet Gynecol* 1966;28:469–471.
85. Dixon JC, Speidel BD, Dixon JJ. *Acta Pediatr* 1998;87:225–226.
86. Dombrowski MP, Brown CL, Berry SM. *J Matern Fetal Med* 1996;5:310–313.
87. Donald PR, Doherty E, Van Zyl FJ. *Cent Afr J Med* 1991;37:268–271.
88. Donald PR, Sellars SL. *S Afr Med J* 1981;60:316–318.
89. Eggermont E, Raveschot J, Deneve V, et al. *Acta Paediatr Belg* 1972;26:197–204.
90. Eggers TR, Doyle LW, Pepperol RJ. *Med J Aust* 1979;1:213–216.
91. Elia J, Katz IR, Simpson GM. *Psychopharmacol Bull* 1987;23:531–586.
92. Eliahou HE, Silverberg DS, Reisin E, et al. *Br J Obstet Gynaecol* 1978;85:431–436.
93. Eller DP, Patterson A, Webb GW. *Obstet Gynecol Clin North Am* 1997;24:523–533.
94. Epstein MF, Nicholls E, Stubblefield PG. *J Pediatr* 1979;94:449–453.
95. Eschenbach DA, Nugent RP, Rao AV, et al. *Am J Obstet Gynecol* 1991;164:734–742.
96. Esplin MS, Branch DW. *Obstet Gynecol Clin North Am* 1997;24:601–615.
97. Farkas VG, Farkas G Jr, et al. *Teratology* 1977;15:57–64.
98. Fidler J, Smith V, Fayers P, et al. *BMJ* 1983;286:1927–1930.
99. Fisher WD, Vooheess ML, Gardner L. *J Pediatr* 1963;62:132–146.
100. Flessa HC, Kapstrom AB, Glueck HI, et al. *Am J Obstet Gynecol* 1965;93:570–573.
101. Frenkel LM, Brown ZA, Bryson YL, et al. *Am J Obstet Gynecol* 1991;164:568–576.
102. Friedman JM, Polifka JE. *Teratogenic Effects of Drugs: a Resource for Clinicians*, 2nd ed. Baltimore: Johns Hopkins University Press, 2000.
103. Frishman WH, Chesner M. *Am Heart J* 1988;115:147–152.
104. Fuchs F. *Am J Obstet Gynecol* 1976;126:809–820.
105. Gaily E, Granstrom M-L, Hiilesmaa V, et al. *J Pediatr* 1988;112:520–529.
106. Gallery EDM, Sounders DM, Hunyor SN, et al. *BMJ* 1979;1:1591–1594.
107. Gant NF, Madden JD, Shteri PK, et al. *Am J Obstet Gynecol* 1976;124:143–148.
108. Gillberg C. *Lancet* 1977;2:244.
109. Gillis S, Shusan A, Eldor A. *Int J Gynecol Obstet* 1993;39:297–301.
110. Ginsberg JS, Kowalchuk G, Hirsh J, et al. *Arch Intern Med* 1989;1449:2233–2236.
111. Ginzler AM, Cherner C. *Am J Obstet Gynecol* 1942;44:46–55.
112. Gladstone GR, Hordof A, Gersony WM. *J Pediatr* 1975;86:962–964.
113. Glass L, Rajegowda BK, Evans HE. *Lancet* 1971;2:685.
114. Glass L, Rajegowda BK, Kahn EJ, et al. *N Engl J Med* 1972;286:746.

115. Gluck L, Kuovich MV. *Am J Obstet Gynecol* 1973;115:539.
116. Godet PF, Marie-Cardine M. *Encephale* 1991;17:534–547.
117. Goldenberg RL, Davis RO, Baker RC. *Am J Obstet Gynecol* 1989;160:1196–1197.
118. Goldman JA, Neri A, Ovadia J, et al. *Am J Obstet Gynecol* 1969;105:556–560.
119. Green HG, Gareis FJ, Shepard TH, et al. *Am J Dis Child* 1971;122:247–249.
120. Greenberger PA, Patterson R. *Ann Inetrn Med* 1983;98:478–480.
121. Guignard JP, Burgener F, Calame A. *Int J Pediatr Nephrol* 1981;2:133.
122. Guikontes E, Spantideas A, Diakakia J. *Lancet* 1992;340:1223.
123. Hadi HA, Strickland D. *Am J Perinatol* 1995;12:455–458.
124. Haibach H, Akhter JE, Muscato MS, et al. *Am J Clin Pathol* 1984;82:240–242.
125. Hall JG, Pauli RM, Wilson KM. *Am J Med* 1980;68:122–140.
126. Hamill GC, Jarmen JA, Wynne MD. *Am J Obstet Gynecol* 1961;81:1018–1023.
127. Hamilton H. *Postgrad Med J* 1968;44:66–69.
128. Hamilton M, Kopelman H. *BMJ* 1963;1:151–155.
129. Hanson JW, Myrianthopoulos NC, Harvey MAS, et al. *J Pediatr* 1976;89:662–668.
130. Hanson JW, Smith DW. *J Pediatr* 1975;87:285–290.
131. Hanssens M, Keirse MJ, Vankelcon F, et al. *Obstet Gynecol* 1991;78:128–135.
132. Haram K, Hervig T, Thordason H, et al. *Acta Obstet Gynecol Scand* 1993;72:674–675.
133. Harcourt JK, Johnson NW, Storey E. *Arch Oral Biol* 1962;7:431.
134. Harley JD, Robin H, Robertson SEJ. *BMJ* 1964;1:696–697.
135. Harris RC, Lucey JF, Maclean JR. *J Pediatr* 1950;23:878.
136. Hastwell G. *Lancet* 1975;2:1212–1213.
137. Heckel GP. *JAMA* 1941;117:1314–1316.
138. Heinonen OP, Slone D, Shapiro S. *Birth Defects and Drugs in Pregnancy.* Littleton, MA: Publishing Sciences Group, 1977.
139. Henderson-Smart DJ, Horvath JS, Phippard AF. *Clin Exp Pharmacol Physiol* 1984;11:351–354.
140. Hertz-Picciotto I, Hopenhayn-Rich C, Golub M, et al. *Epidemiol Rev* 1990;12:108–148.
141. Herzlinder RA, Kandall SR, Vaughan HG. *J Pediatr* 1977;91:638.
142. Hickok DE, Hollenbach KA, Reilley SF, et al. *Am J Obstet Gynecol* 1989;160:1525–1531.
143. Hill WC. *Clin Obstet Gynecol* 1995;38:725–745.
144. Hodgkinson R, Glassenberg R, Joyce TH III, et al. *Anesthesiology* 1982:57:A408.
145. Hon EH, et al. *Am J Obstet Gynecol* 1961;82:291.
146. Horowitz DA, Jablonski WJ, Mehta KA. *Am J Dis Child* 1982;136:73–74.
147. Horvath JS, Korda A, Child A, et al. *Med J Aust* 1985;143:19–21.
148. Horvath JS, Phippand A, Korda A, et al. *Obstet Gynecol* 1985;66:634–638.
149. Howell R, Fidler J, Letsky E, et al. *Br J Obstet Gynaecol* 1983;90:1124–1128.
150. Hulton S-A, Kaplan BS. *Am J Med Genet* 1995;58:91–93.
151. Hunt PJ, Doughty HA, Majumdar G, et al. *Thromb Haemost* 1997;77:39–43.
152. Idanpaan-Heikkila J, Saxen L. *Lancet* 1973;2:282–284.
153. Ingemarrson I, Arulkumaran S, Ratnam SS. *Am J Obstet Gynecol* 1985;153:859–865.
154. Ingemarrson I, Liedholm H, Monton S, et al. *Acta Obstet Gynecol Scand* 1984;118(Suppl):95–97.
155. Inman W, Pearce G, Wilton L. *Eur J Clin Pharmacol* 1994;46:115–118.
156. Iturbe-Alesio I, del Carmen Fonseca M, Mutchinik O, et al. *N Engl J Med* 1986;22:1390–1393.
157. Jager-Roman E, Deichl A, Jakob S, et al. *J Pediatr* 1986;108:997–1004.
158. Jannet D, Carbonne B, Sebban E, et al. *Obstet Gynecol* 1994;84:354–359.
159. Janssen NM, Genta MS. *Arch Intern Med* 2000;160:610–619.
160. Jick H, Holmes LB, Hunter JR, et al. *JAMA* 1981;246:343–346.
161. Jick SS. *Pharmacotherapy* 1999;19:221–222.
162. Johnston CI, Aickin DR. *Med J Aust* 1971;2:132–135.
163. Johnston JR, Moore J, McCaughey W, et al. *Anesth Analg* 1983;62:720–726.
164. Jones HC. *J Natl Med Assoc* 1973;65:201–203.
165. Jones KL, Larco RV, Johnson KA, et al. *N Engl J Med* 1989;320:1661–1666.
166. Julkunen T, Jouhikainen T, Kaaja R. *Lupus* 1993;2:125–131.
167. Kallen B. *Br J Obstet Gynaecol* 1998;105:877–881.
168. Kallen B. Scand J Rheumatol 1998;27(Suppl):119–124.
169. Kandall SR, Albin S, Lowinson J, et al. *Pediatrics* 1976;58:681–685.
170. Kandall SR, Gartner LM. *Pediatr Res* 1973;7:92.
171. Kantor HI, Sutherland DA, Leonard JT, et al. *Obstet Gynecol* 1961;17:494–500.
172. Kheddun SM, Moodley J, Naicker T, et al. *Pharmacol Ther* 1997;74:221–258.
173. Kincaid-Smith P, Bullen M. *BMJ* 1966;1:274–276.
174. King DJ, Delton JG. *Ann Intern Med* 1984;100:535–540.
175. Kline AH, Blattner RJ, Lunin M. *JAMA* 1964;118:178.
176. Korda AR, Lynerum RC, Jones WR. *Med J Aust* 1974;1:744–746.
177. Koren G, Zemlickis DM. *Am J Perinatol* 1991;8:37–38.
178. Kraus AM. *J Pediatr Ophthalmol Strabismus* 1975;12:107–108.
179. Kron RF, Litt M, Finnegan LP. *Pediatr Res* 1973;7:64.
180. Kuenssberg EV, Knox JD. *BMJ* 1972;2:292.
181. Kulin NA, Pastuszak A, Sage SR, et al. *JAMA* 1998;279:609–610.
182. Kullander S, Kallen B. *Acta Obstet Gynecol Scand* 1976;55:105–111.
183. Kullander S, Kallen B. *Acta Obstet Gynecol Scand* 1976;55:287–295.
184. Kurzel RB. *South Med J* 1990;83:953.
185. Kutscher AH, Zegarelli EV, Torvell HM, et al. *Am J Obstet Gynecol* 1986;96:291.
186. Kuzniar J, Skret A, Piela A, et al. *Obstet Gynecol* 1985;66:453–458.
187. L'Hommedieu CS, Nicholas D, Armes DA, et al. *J Pediatr* 1983;102:629–631.
188. Ladner CN, Pearson JW, Herrick CN, et al. *Obstet Gynecol* 1964;23:555–560.
189. Laegreid L, Hayberg G, Lundberg A. *Neuropediatrics* 1992;23:18–23.
190. Laegreid L, Olegard R, Walstrom J, et al. *J Pediatr* 1989;114:126–131.
191. Lalkin A, Loebstein R, Addis A, et al. *Am J Obstet Gynecol* 1998;179:727–730.
192. Lary JM, Khoury MJ, Erickson JD. *Teratology* 1995;51:175.
193. Laskin CA, Bombardier C, Hannah ME, et al. *N Engl J Med* 1997;337:148–153.
194. Lecura F, Desnos M, Taurelle R. *Acta Obstet Gynecol Scand* 1996;75:217–221.
195. Lee BE, Feinberg M, Abraham JJ, et al. *Pediatr Infect Dis J* 1992;11:1062–1064.
196. Leikin SL. *N Engl J Med* 1964;271:161.
197. Levin AC, Doering PL, Hatton RC. *Ann Pharmacother* 1994;28:1371–1378.
198. Levin DL. *Semin Perinatol* 1980;4:35–44.
199. Levitan AA, Manion JC. *Am J Cardiol* 1973;32:247.
200. Lieberman BA, Stirrat GM, Cohen SL, et al. *Br J Obstet Gynaecol* 1978;85:678–683.
201. Lindheimer MD, Katz AL. *N Engl J Med* 1973;288:891–894.
202. Lindhout D, Schmidt D. *Lancet* 1986;2:1392–1393.
203. Lip GY, Beevers M, Churchill D, et al. *Am J Cardiol* 1997;79:1436–1438.
204. Livingstone I, Craswell PW, Beran EB, et al. *Clin Exp Hypertens* 1983;2:341–350.
205. Loebstein R, Addis A, Ho E, et al. *Antimicrob Agents Chemother* 1998;42:1336–1339.
206. Lucey JF, Driscoll TJ Jr. *Pediatrics* 1959:24:498–499.
207. Lussos SA, Bader AM, Thornhill ML, et al. *Reg Anesth* 17:126–130.
208. Lydakis C, Lip GY, Beevers M, et al. *Am J Hypertens* 1999;12:541–547.
209. Lyonnet R, Lucchini G. *J Med Chir Prat* 1967;138:352–355.
210. Mabie WC, Gonzalez AR, Sibia BM, et al. *Obstet Gynecol* 1987;70:328–333.
211. Magee LA, Inocencion G, Kamboj L, et al. *Dig Dis Sci* 1996;41:1145–1149.
212. Magee LA, Ornstein MP, von Dadelszen P. *BMJ* 1999;318:1332–1336.
213. Magee LA, Schick B, Donnenfeld AE, et al. *Am J Obstet Gynecol* 1996;174:823–828.
214. Mandel SJ, Brent GA, Larsen PR. *Thyroid* 1994;4:129–133.
215. Mastroiacovo P, Mazzone T, Botto LD, et al. *Am J Obstet Gynecol* 1996;175:1645–1650.
216. Mazzotta P, Magee LA. *Drugs* 2000;59:781–800.
217. McBride WG. *Med J Aust* 1972;1:492.
218. McCormack WM, Rosner B, Lee Y-H, et al. *Obstet Gynecol* 1987;69:202–207.
219. McGregor JA, French JI, Richter R, et al. *Am J Obstet Gynecol* 1990;163:1580–1591.
220. Meadows SR, et al. *Proc R Soc Med* 1970;63:48.

221. Melissari E, Parker CJ, Wilson NV, et al. *Thromb Haemost* 1992; 68:652–656.
222. Mennie AT. *BMJ* 1962;2:480.
223. Menzies DW. *BMJ.* 1964;1:739–742.
224. Mercer BM, Miodovnik M, Thurnau GR, et al. *JAMA* 1997;278: 989–995.
225. Milkovich L, Van den Berg BJ. *Am J Obstet Gynecol* 1976;125:244–248.
226. Minkoff H, Augenbaum. *Am J Obstet Gynecol* 1997;176:478–489.
227. Mizrahi EM, Hobbs JF, Goldsmith DI. *J Pediatr* 1979;94:493–495.
228. Mofenson LM. *N Engl J Med* 2000;343:803–805.
229. Moise KJ Jr, Huhta JC, Sharif DS, et al. *N Engl J Med* 1988;319:327–331.
230. Montan S, Anandakumar C, Arulkumaran S, et al. *Am J Obstet Gynecol* 1993;168:152–156.
231. Montan S, Ingemarrson I, Marsal K, et al. *BMJ* 1992;304:946–949.
232. Morrell MJ. *Int Pediatr* 1995;10(Suppl):58–65.
233. Morrell P, Sutherland GR, Buamah PK, et al. *Arch Dis Child* 1983;58:539–541.
234. Mountain KR, Hirsh J, Gallus AS. *Lancet* 1970;1:265–268.
235. Nageotte MP, Briggs GG, Towers CV, et al. *Am J Obstet Gynecol* 1996;174:1801–1806.
236. Nathenson G, Cohen MI, Litt IF. *J Pediatr* 1972;81:899–903.
237. Nelson JL, Ostenson M. *Rheum Dis Clin North Am* 1997;23:195–212.
238. Nelson MM, Forfar JO. *BMJ* 1971;1:523–527.
239. Nelson-Piercy C. *Br J Obstet Gynecol* 1994;101:6–8.
240. Nelson-Piercy C, Letsky EA, deSwiet M. *Am J Obstet Gynecol* 1997; 176:1062–1068.
241. Nightingale SL. *JAMA* 1992;267:2445.
242. Noia G, De Santis M, Tocci A, et al. *Fetal Diagn Ther* 1992;7:138–143.
243. Nordy SR, Lietman PS. *Drugs* 1993;45(Suppl 3):59–64.
244. Nyhan WL. *J Pediatr* 1961;59:1.
245. O'Sullivan MJ, Boyer PJJ, Scott GB, et al. *Am J Obstet Gynecol* 1993;168:1510–1516.
246. Orr DA, Bill KM, Gillion KRW, et al. *Anaesthesia* 1993;48:114–119.
247. Ostenson M. *Immunopharmacology* 1996;93:137–150.
248. Ostenson M, Ostenson H. *J Rheumatol* 1996;23:1045–49.
249. Ostenson M, Ramsey-Goldman R. *Drug Safety* 1998;19:389–410.
250. Owen JR, Irani SF, Blair AW. *Arch Dis Child* 1972;47:107–110.
251. Palmer RH, Ouellette EM, Warner L, et al. *Pediatrics* 1974;53:490–494.
252. Pastuszak A, Schick-Boschetto B, Zuber C, et al. *JAMA* 1993;269: 2246–2248.
253. Pavankumar P, Venugopal P, Kaul U, et al. *Scand J Thorac Cardiovasc Surg* 1988;22:19–22.
254. Perkins RP. *Am J Obstet Gynecol* 1971;111:379–381.
255. Peterson A, Peterson K, Tongen S, et al. *J Fam Pract* 1993;36:25–31.
256. Pettit GP, Smith GA, McIlroy WL. *Milit Med* 1976;141:316–317.
257. Piacquadio K, Hollinsworth DR, Murphy H. *Lancet* 1991;338:866–869.
258. Pinsky L, DiGeorge AM. *Science* 1965;147:402–403.
259. Pirson Y, Van Lierde M, Ghysen J, et al. *N Engl J Med* 1985;313:328.
260. Prescott LF. *BMJ* 1964;1:1438.
261. Priollet P, Roncato M, Aiach M, et al. *Br J Haematol* 1986;63:605–606.
262. Pritchard JA, Walley PJ. *Am J Obstet Gynecol* 1961;81:1241–1244.
263. Prociancy RS, Pinheiro CEA. *J Pediatr* 1982;101:612–614.
264. Pruyn SC, Phelan JP, Buchanan GC. *Am J Obstet Gynecol* 1979; 135:485–489.
265. Pryde PG, Sedman AB, Nugent CE, et al. *J Am Soc Nephrol* 1993;3: 1575–1582.
266. Pursley TJ, Blomquist IK, Abraham J, et al. *Clin Infect Dis* 1996; 22:336–340.
267. Rachelefsky G, Flynt J, Ebbin A. *Lancet* 1972;1:838.
268. Rafla N. *Am J Obstet Gynecol* 1987;156:1557.
269. Raftos J, Bauer GE, Lewis RG, et al. *Med J Aust* 1973;1:786–793.
270. Ray D, Dynson D. *Clin Obstet Gynecol* 1995;38:713–721.
271. Redman CWG, Beillin LJ, Bonnar, et al. *Lancet* 1976;2:753.
272. Reece AE, Homko. *Drug Safety* 1998;18:209–220.
273. Reinisch JM. *Science* 1978;202:436–439.
274. Rementeria JL, Bhatt K. *J Pediatr* 1977;90:123–126.
275. Rementeria JL, Nunag NN. *Am J Obstet Gynecol* 1973;116:1152–1156.
276. Rendle-Short TJ. *Lancet* 1962;1:1188.
277. Rodondi LC. *Pharm Ther Forum* 1987;35:4.
278. Rodriquez SU, Leikin SL, Hiller MC. *N Engl J Med* 1964;270:881–884.
279. Rollins DE, Von Bahr C, Glaumann H, et al. *Science* 1979;205:1414–1416.
280. Rosa FW. *N Engl J Med* 1991;324:674–677.
281. Rosa FW. *Reprod Toxicol* 1995;9:583.
282. Rosa FW, Bosco LA, Graham CF, et al. *Obstet Gynecol* 1989;74:371–374.
283. Rosenberg L, Mitchell AA, Parsells JL, et al. *N Engl J Med* 1983; 309:1282–1285.
284. Rosenfeld J, Bott-Kanner G, Boner G, et al. *Eur J Obstet Gynecol* 1986;22:197–204.
285. Roth AC, Milsom I, Forssman L, et al. *Acta Obstet Gynecol Scand* 1990;69:223–228.
286. Rothberg AD, Lorenz R. *Pediatr Pharmacol* 1984;4:189–92.
287. Rothstein P, Gould JB. *Pediatr Clin North Am* 1974;21:307–321.
288. Roubenoff R, Hoyt J, Petri M, et al. *Semin Arthritis Rheum* 1988;18:88–110.
289. Rubin PC. *N Engl J Med* 1981;305:1323–1326.
290. Rubin PC, Butters L, Clark DM, et al. *Lancet* 1983;1:431–434.
291. Rudolph AM. *Obstet Gynecol* 1981;58 (Suppl):63S–67S.
292. Ruigomez A, Rodriguez LAG, Cattaruzzi C, et al. *Am J Epidemiol* 1999;150:476–481.
293. Rumack CM, Guggenheim MA, Rumack BH, et al. *Obstet Gynecol* 1981;58(Suppl):52S–56S.
294. Rumeau-Roquette C, Goujard J, Huel G. *Teratology* 1977;15:57–64.
295. Russel KP, Rose H, Starr P. *Surg Gynecol Obstet* 1957;104:560–564.
296. Safra MJ, Oakley GP Jr. *Lancet* 1975;2:478–480.
297. Safra MJ, Oakley GP Jr. *Lancet* 1976;1:810.
298. Samren EB, van Duijn CM, Koch S, et al. *Epilepsia* 1997;38:981–990.
299. Sandstrom B. *Clin Exp Hypertens* 1982;1:127–141.
300. Saxen I. *Int J Prev Soc Med* 1975;29:103–110.
301. Sbarouni E, Oakley C. *Br Heart J* 1994;71:196–201.
302. Schatz M, Patterson R, et al. *JAMA* 1975;233:804–807.
303. Schatz M, Petitti D. *Asthma Immunol* 1997;78:157–159.
304. Schick B, Hom M, Librizzi R, et al. *Reprod Toxicol* 1996;10:162.
305. Schou M, Amdisen A. *Am J Obstet Gynecol* 1975;122:541.
306. Schou M, Goldfield MD, Weinstein MR, et al. *BMJ* 1973;2:135–136.
307. Schubiger G, Flury G, Nussberger J. *Ann Intern Med* 1988;108:215–216.
308. Scott AA, Purohit DM. *Am J Obstet Gynecol* 1989;160:1223–1224.
309. Scott JR. *Am J Obstet Gynecol* 1977;128:668–676.
310. Scott LL, Sanchez PJ, Jackson GL, et al. *Obstet Gynecol* 1996;69–73.
311. Senior B, Slone D, Shapiro S, et al. *Lancet* 1976;2:377.
312. Seto A, Einarson T, Koren G. *Am J Perinatol* 1997;14:119–124.
313. Shaffer N, Chuachoowong R, Mock PA, et al. *Lancet* 1999;353: 773–780.
314. Shapiro S, Monson RR, Kaufman DW, et al. *Lancet* 1976;1:1375–1376.
315. Sharif DS, Huhta JC, Moise KJ Jr, et al. *J Clin Ultrasound* 1990;18: 85–89.
316. Shearer WT, Schreiner RJ, Marshall RE. *J Pediatr* 1972;81:570–572.
317. Shiono PH, Mills JL. *N Engl J Med* 1984;311:919–920.
318. Shnider SM, Moya F. *Am J Obstet Gynecol* 1964;89:1009.
319. Sibai BM, Anderson GD. *Obstet Gynecol* 1986;67:517–522.
320. Sim M. *BMJ* 1972;2:45.
321. Slone D, Heinonen OP, Kaufman D, et al. *Lancet* 1976:1:1373–1375.
322. Slone D, Siskind V, Heinonen OP, et al. *Am J Obstet Gynecol* 1977; 128:486–488.
323. Smith AM, McNeil WT. *BMJ* 1969;1:572–573.
324. Snider DE Jr, Layde PM, Johnson MW, et al. *Am Rev Respir Dis* 1980;122:65–79.
325. Snyder SW, Cardwell MS. *Am J Obstet Gynecol* 1989; 161:35–36.
326. Spector SL. *Chest* 1984;86(Suppl):1S–5S.
327. Speight AN. *Lancet* 1971;1:878.
328. Sperling RS, Stratton PO, et al. *N Engl J Med* 1992;326:857–861.
329. Squires JW, Pinch LW. *JAMA* 1979;241:2417–2418.
330. Stevenson RE, Burton OM, Ferlanto GJ, et al. *JAMA* 1980;243: 1549–1551.
331. Stuart JC, Kan AF, Rowbottom SJ, et al. *Anaesthesia* 1996;51:415–421.
332. Stuart MJ, Gross SJ, Elrad H, et al. *N Engl J Med* 1982;307:909–913.
333. Thomas DJB, Dove AF, Alberti KGMM. *Br J Obstet Gynaecol* 1977; 84:497–499.
334. Tincello DG, Johnstone MJ. *Postgrad Med J* 1996;72:688–689.
335. Toaff R, Ravid R. *Lancet* 1966;2:281–282.
336. Tonstall ME. *Br J Anaesth* 1969;41:792.
337. Towner D, Kjos SL, Leung B, et al. *Diabetes Care* 1995;18:1446–1451.
338. Tsirigotis M, Yazdani N, Craft I. *Hum Reprod* 1995;10:2177–2178.
339. Turmen T, Thom P, Louidas AT, et al. *J Clin Pharmacol* 1982;22:551–556.

340. Turner ES, Greenberger PA, Patterson R. *Ann Intern Med* 1980; 6:905–918.
341. Turner G, Collins E. *Lancet* 1975;3:338–339.
342. Ulmsten U, Andersson K-E, Wingerup L. *Arch Gynecol* 1980;229: 1–5.
343. Van Den Veyver IB, Moise KJ Jr, Ou C-N, et al. *Obstet Gynecol* 1993;82:500–503.
344. Van Geijn HP, Jongsma HW, Doesburg WH, et al. *Eur J Obstet Gynecol Reprod Biol* 1980;10:187–201.
345. Van Herle AJ, Young RT, Fisher DA, et al. *J Clin Endocrinol Metab* 1975;40:474–477.
346. Van Loon AJ, Derksen JTM, et al. *Prenat Diagn* 1995;15:599–604.
347. Van Zwieten PA, Timmermans PB. J *Cardiovasc Pharmacol* 1985; 5(Suppl 1):S11–S17.
348. Vanhaesebrouck P, Thiery M, Leroy JG, et al. *J Pediatr* 1988;113: 738–743.
349. Vert P, Broquaire M, Legagneur M, et al. *Eur J Clin Pharmocol* 1982; 22:39–45.
350. Vitali E, Donateli F, Quain E, et al. *J Cardiovasc Surg* 1986;27:221– 227.
351. Wager J, Fredholm B, Lunell NO, et al. *Acta Obstet Gyncol Scand* 1982;108(Suppl):41–46.
352. Wager J, Lunell NO, Joelsson I, et al. *Acta Obstet Gynecol Scand* 1977;56:475–478.
353. Wagner CL, Katikaneni LD, Cox TH, et al. *Obstet Gynecol Clin North Am* 1998;25:169–194.
354. Wallace RL, Caldwell DL, Ansbacher R, et al. *Obstet Gynecol* 1978; 51:387–392.
355. Walters BNJ, Redman CWG. *Br J Obstet Gynaecol* 1984;91:330–336.
356. Warkany J. *Teratology* 1979;20:133–138.
357. Warkany J. *Teratology* 1988;38:593–596.
358. Webster PA. *Lancet* 1973;2:318–319.
359. Wegner C, Nau H. *Neurology* 1992;42(Suppl):17–24.
360. Weiner S, Scharf JI, Bolognese RJ, et al. *J Reprod Med* 1980;24: 39–42.
361. Whaun JM, Smith GR, Sochor VA. *Haemostasis* 1980;9:226–237.
362. White A, Andrews E, Eldridge R, et al. *MMWR* 1994;43:409– 416.
363. Wiktor SZ, Ekpini E, Karon JM, et al. *Lancet* 1999;353:781– 785.
364. Wilbanks GD, Bressler B, Peete CH Jr, et al. *JAMA* 1970;213:865– 867.
365. Wilton LV, Pearce GL, Martin RM, et al. *Br J Obstet Gynaecol* 1998; 105:882–889.
366. Winderlov E, Karlamn I, Storsater J. *N Engl J Med* 1980;303:1235.
367. Wing DA, Hendershott CM, Debuque L, et al. *Obstet Gynecol* 1998;92:249–253.
368. Wise PH, Hall AJ. *BMJ* 1980;3:110–111.
369. Wisner KL, Gelenberg AJ, Leonard H, et al. *JAMA* 1999;282:1264– 1269.
370. Wong KL, Chan FY, Lee CP. *J Rheumatol* 1986;13:732–739.
371. Wong V, Chen CH, Chan KC. *Am J Med Genet* 1993;45:17–21.
372. Woods DL, Morrell DF. *BMJ* 1982;285:691–692.
373. Woody J, London W, Wilbanks G. *Pediatrics* 1971;47:94–96.
374. World MJ. *Lancet* 1993;341:185.
375. Yemini M, Shoham Z, Dgoani R, et al. *Eur J Obstet Gynecol Reprod Biol* 1989;30:193–197.
376. Yerby MS, Leavitt A, Erickson DM, et al. *Neurology* 1992;42(Suppl) 132–140.
377. Zahn CA, Morrel MJ, Collins SD, et al. *Neurology* 1998;51:949–956.
378. Zelson C. *N Engl J Med* 1973;288:1393.
379. Zimran A, Shilo S, Fisher D, et al. *Arch Intern Med* 1986;46:386–388.
380. CDC. *MMWR* 1998;47(RR-5):1–82.
381. ACOG. *ACOG Committee Opin* 2000;234:1–3.

INDEX

Note: Page numbers followed by f indicate figures; those followed by t indicate tables.

A

A-a (alveolar-arterial) gradient, during pregnancy, 4
Abacavir (Ziagen), for HIV, 590t
Abortion, fetal malformations managed by, 267, 268t
Abruptio placentae, 364–365, 364f
Abscess, epidural, 422, 423t
Accelerations, 625t, 626, 626f
  prognostic value of, 633
  prolonged, 625t
ACE (angiotensin-converting enzyme) inhibitors, fetal and
    neonatal effects of, 684t
Acetaminophen
  in breast milk, 243
  fetal and neonatal effects of, 682t
Acid aspiration, 395, 397f, 433
Acid-base balance
  Apgar score and, 640–641, 640f
  fetal, with cesarean section, 225
  in infants of diabetic mothers, 504–505, 505t
  of placenta, 25–26
Acid-base imbalance, during labor, 3
Acidemia, fetal, 635
  bradycardia and, 626, 626t
  fetal heart rate patterns at risk for, 633, 633t
  tachycardia and, 627t
Acidosis, fetal, fetal heart rate variability and, 627t
Acquired immunodeficiency syndrome (AIDS). See Human
    immunodeficiency virus (HIV)
Acrocyanosis, in newborn, 639
Activated partial thromboplastin time (aPTT), 303t, 346,
    347t
Active Management of Labor (AML), 41
Active transport, placental transport via, 19–20, 20f
Acupuncture, 97, 97f
Acute idiopathic polyneuritis, 534–535, 534f
Acute intrapartum event, 635, 635t
Acute normovolemic hemodilution (ANH), during cesarean
    section, 369
Acyclovir, fetal and neonatal effects of, 685t
Adenosine, fetal effect of, 479
Adenosine receptors, 150–151, 151f
Adrenocorticotropic hormone, for postdural puncture
    headache, 416
AEDs (antiepileptic drugs), 510, 531–532, 532t
  fetal and neonatal effects of, 683t
AFE See Amniotic fluid embolism
AFI (amniotic fluid index), 618
AFP (alpha-fetoprotein), 613, 614t
Age
  fetal, 614–615
  gestational, 643–645, 644f, 645f
  small for, 323, 643–645, 644f, 645f
Agenerase (amprenavir), for HIV, 590t
Agonist-antagonist agents, systemic, 115–116, 115f
AIDS. See Human immunodeficiency virus (HIV)
Airway
  anatomic examination of, 375–377, 376f–378f, 379f
  assessment of, 375–377, 376f–378f
  difficult
    and aspiration, 399, 399t
    prevention of complications of, 399–400, 399f, 400f
  esophageal gastric tube, 300f, 399
  establishment in newborn of, 660–661, 661f
  laryngeal mask, 384–386, 385f, 385t
  neuroanatomy of, 381–382, 381f, 382f
    after neurosurgery, 521
  pregnancy effect on, 375
  suctioning of, 660–661, 661f, 666–668, 667f
  topical anesthesia/nerve blocks of, 382–384, 383f, 384f
Airway management
  for allergic reactions, 562
  aspiration prophylaxis in, 377–378, 379f
  for cesarean section, 677, 677t
  cricothyrotomy for, 386–387
  emergency, 677, 677t
  equipment for, 379t
  esophageal tracheal combitube for, 386
  extubation in, 387
  with failed tracheal intubation, 379–381, 380f
  fiberoptic intubation in, 381
  for general anesthesia, 377–381, 379f, 379t, 380f
  with obesity, 549, 549f, 554–555, 554f
  positioning for, 379, 379f
  during pregnancy, 6t
  preoxygenation in, 379, 380f
  with regional anesthesia, 677, 677t
  with rheumatoid arthritis, 568–569
  transtracheal insufflation or jet ventilation for, 387
Airway resistance, during pregnancy, 4t
Albumin, for pregnancy-induced hypertension, 308
Albumin concentration, effect on placental drug transfer of,
    62, 63t
Albuterol, fetal and neonatal effects of, 686t
Alcohol abuse, 599–601, 600f, 601f

Alfentanil
  in breast milk, 243
  with bupivacaine, 166
  epidural, 163
  intrathecal, for postoperative pain, 173, 173f
  pharmacokinetics of, 153t
  with pregnancy-induced hypertension, 313
  systemic, 112
Alkalinization, of local anesthetics, 210, 210f
Alkali reserve, during pregnancy, 250t
Allergic contact dermatitis, due to latex allergy, 566
Allergic reactions, 559, 560–566, 560t
  anesthetic causes of, 561f
  assessment of, 562–563
  differential diagnosis of, 561, 562f, 567–568
  epidemiology of, 560–561, 561f
  fetal effects of, 562
  to general anesthetic agents, 563
  to latex, 564–566, 564t, 565t
  to local anesthetics, 563, 563t
  management of, 561–562, 562t
  mechanisms of, 559, 560f, 560t
  to nonanesthetic drugs, 563–564
  to opioids, 563
  presentation of, 561, 561f, 561t
Allergy drugs, during pregnancy, 577
Allergy testing, 566–567, 566t, 567f
α_2-adrenergic agonists, 150, 151f
  fetal and neonatal effects of, 684t
α_2-adrenoreceptors, 150, 151f, 152f
Alpha-fetoprotein (AFP), 613, 614t
Alphaprodine (Nisentil), fetal heart rate with, 107f
Alveolar-arterial (A-a) gradient, during pregnancy, 4
Alveolar dead space, during pregnancy, 4t
Alveolar ventilation, during pregnancy, 3, 4t, 249, 250f
Amide-linked agents, 74f, 77–84
  bupivacaine, 74f, 81–84, 82t, 83f
  chiral compounds, 84–87
  levobupivacaine, 86–87
  lidocaine, 74f, 77–81, 77f, 78f, 78t–80t
    carbonated, 81, 87
  mepivacaine, 74f, 81
  prilocaine, 74f, 81
  ropivacaine, 74f, 84–86, 85f
Amino acids, placental transport of, 19–20
Aminoglycosides, fetal and neonatal effects of, 684t
Amiodarone, fetal effects of, 479
AML (Active Management of Labor), 41
Amnesia, anterograde, from midazolam, 115
Amnestic drugs, systemic, 116–117
Amniocentesis, 614
Amniotic fluid embolism (AFE), 355–359
  vs. anaphylaxis, 567
  clinical presentation and diagnosis of, 355–356, 356t
  incidence of, 355
  mortality from, 355, 356t
  pathogenesis of, 357–358, 358f
  pathophysiology of, 356–357, 356t, 357t
  predisposing conditions for, 355
  treatment of, 358, 358t
Amniotic fluid index (AFI), 618
Amniotic fluid surfactant determination, 616–617, 616f, 617f
Amniotic fluid volume, quantitative, 618t
Amoxicillin, for asthma, 490t
Amphetamines
  abuse of, 603f, 606–607
  teratogenicity of, 252
Amprenavir (Agenerase), for HIV, 590t
Amrinone, effect on fetus of, 479–480
Analgesics, fetal and neonatal effects of, 682t
Anaphylactic reactions, 559, 560f, 563
Anaphylactoid reactions, 559, 560f, 563
Anaphylaxis, 560–568
  anesthetic causes of, 561f
  assessment of, 562–563
  atopy and, 561
  clinical presentation of, 561, 561t
  differential diagnosis of, 561, 562f, 567–568
  fetal effects of, 562
  due to general anesthetic agents, 563
  due to latex, 564–566, 564t, 565t
  due to local anesthetics, 563, 563t
  management of, 561–562, 562t
  mechanisms of, 559, 560f, 560t
  due to nonanesthetic drugs, 563–564
  due to opioids, 563
Anemia
  Cooley's, 350
  fetal, 617, 617f, 618f
  of pregnancy, 7
  sickle-cell, 350t, 351
"Anesthesia and You," 103–104
Anesthesia care, goals of, 679–680
Anesthesia equipment, with latex allergy, 565, 565t

Anesthesia record, 443
Anesthetic machine, 191, 192t
Aneuploidy, 613–614
Aneurysms
  dissecting aortic, 474
  intracranial, 511, 512–513, 513f, 513t, 514f
Angioedema, hereditary, 567
Angiographically occult vascular malformations (AOVMs),
    512
Angiotensin, during pregnancy, 13
Angiotensin-converting enzyme (ACE) inhibitors, fetal and
    neonatal effects of, 684t
Angiotensin II, effect on fetus of, 479
ANH (acute normovolemic hemodilution), during cesarean
    section, 369
Anomalies
  congenital. See Congenital anomalies
  fetal, 615
ANP (atrial natriuretic peptide), during pregnancy, 14
Antacids
  aspiration of, 395–396, 401
  for prevention of aspiration, 401, 433–434
    with cesarean section, 203–204, 215
    with general anesthesia, 378
    with surgery during pregnancy, 251
Antagonists, systemic, 117–118
Antepartum fetal surveillance, 617–619, 618t, 619f
Antepartum risk assessment, 390
Anterior spinal artery syndrome, 419
Antianxiety medication, for cesarean section, 203, 214
Antiarrhythmics, effect on fetus of, 478–479
Antibiotics
  allergic reactions to, 563
  for aspiration, 397
  for asthma, 490t
  fetal and neonatal effects of, 684t–685t
Antibodies, 559
Anticholinergic therapy
  for aspiration prophylaxis, 402
  fetal and neonatal effects of, 682t
Anticoagulants, 349
  fetal and neonatal effects of, 682t
Anticonvulsant therapy, 510, 531–532, 532t
  fetal and neonatal effects of, 683t
Antidepressants, fetal and neonatal effects of, 683t
Antiemetics
  for aspiration prophylaxis, 402
  fetal and neonatal effects of, 683t
Antiepileptic drugs (AEDs), 510, 531–532, 532t
  fetal and neonatal effects of, 683t
Antifactor Xa, during pregnancy, 11t
Antifungals, fetal and neonatal effects of, 685t
Antigens, 559
Antihistamines
  for allergic reactions, 562
  for amniotic fluid embolism, 358
  for asthma, 490t
Antihypertensive agents
  effect on uteroplacental blood flow of, 27t, 33–34, 34f, 35f
  fetal and neonatal effects of, 684t
  for pregnancy-induced hypertension, 306–307
Antiinflammatory drugs, for asthma, 490t
Antilirium (physostigmine), 117
Antimalarial drugs, for immunosuppression, 576–577
Antimicrobials, fetal and neonatal effects of, 684t–685t
Antiphospholipid antibody syndrome, 570
Antiphospholipid-anticardiolipin antibody syndrome, 346
Antiretroviral drugs, 584f, 589, 590t, 591f
  fetal and neonatal effects of, 685t
Antithrombin III (ATIII), 346
  during pregnancy, 11t
Antithyroid medications, fetal and neonatal effects of, 686t
Antivirals, fetal and neonatal effects of, 685t
Anxiety
  with cesarean section, 203, 214
  effect on uteroplacental blood flow of, 27t, 32
Anxiolytics, fetal and neonatal effects of, 685t
A-O (atlanto-occipital) extension, 376, 377f
A-O (atlanto-occipital) gap, with obesity, 549, 549f
Aorta, coarctation of, 456t, 469–470, 470t
Aortic aneurysm, dissecting, 474
Aortic blood pressure, in newborn, 665, 665f
Aortic insufficiency, 456t, 463–465, 465f, 465t
Aortic stenosis
  congenital, 470
  due to rheumatic heart disease, 456t, 462–463, 463f, 463t,
    464f
Aortic valve replacement, pregnancy after, 476t, 477
Aortocaval compression
  decreased uterine activity with, 46
  during pregnancy, 8–10, 9f, 10f
  prevention of, 138
  regional anesthesia and, 136, 137f–139f

AOVMs (angiographically occult vascular malformations), 512
Apgar score, 639–642
  after cesarean section, 223–225, 224t, 225t
  components of, 639, 640f
  evaluation of, 639–642
  fetal heart rate monitoring and, 635
  limitations of, 641–642
  and neonatal neurological injury, 642, 642f, 643f
  prognostic value of, 641, 641f
  and resuscitation, 640–641, 640f, 659
  timing of, 640
aPTT (activated partial thromboplastin time), 303t, 346, 347t
Arachnoid membrane, 125f, 152
  drug transfer across, 152, 152f
Arnold-Chiari syndrome, maternal, 413, 415
Arrhythmias
  with bupivacaine, 82–84, 82t, 83f
  fetal, 632–633
  during pregnancy, 477–478
Arterial blood gases
  with obesity, 548t
  during pregnancy, 3, 4t
Arterial PCO$_2$, during pregnancy, 4t
Arterial PO$_2$, during pregnancy, 4t
Arteriovenous malformations (AVMs)
  cerebral, 511–512, 511f, 513–514, 513f, 514f
  of spine, 412–413
Artery of Adamkiewicz, 410f, 411
Arthritis, rheumatoid, 568–570, 569f
ASD (atrial septal defect), 456t, 465–466, 466t
Asepsis, 422
ASH (asymmetric septal hypertrophy), 474–475, 475t
Asphyxia
  fetal
    clinical indicators of, 634
    etiologies of, 623
    fetal heart rate monitoring in diagnosis of, 634–635, 635t
    fetal heart rate patterns with, 631–632, 632f
    fetal response to, 624
    during surgery on fetus, 274
    during surgery on mother, 259–260, 259f, 260f
  perinatal, 657, 658f
    and cerebral palsy, 642, 643f
Aspirate, volume and pH of, 392–393, 395f, 396f
Aspiration, 391–404
  of acid gastric material, 395, 397f, 433
  with alcohol abuse, 600–601
  of antacids, 395–396, 401
  antibiotic therapy for, 397
  cricoid pressure for, 398–399, 398f, 399f
  with difficult airway, 399–400, 399f, 399t, 400f
  emergent treatment of, 393–394
  epidemiology of, 391, 392t, 393f, 393t
  events surrounding, 398, 398t
  gastric acidity and, 392
  gastric emptying and, 391, 394t
    drugs and, 391–392
  gastroesophageal tone and reflux and gastric pressure and, 392, 394f
  with general anesthesia, 398, 398t
  with laryngeal mask airway, 385
  lawsuits on, 448–449, 448t
  maternal mortality due to, 433–434, 433f
  meconium, 666–668, 667f
  muscle fasciculations and, 398
  of particulate matter, 395–396, 433
  in parturients, 238
  patient education on, 433
  position during induction and, 398
  during pregnancy, 249–251, 433
  prevention of, 215, 377–378, 397–400, 433–434
    antacids for, 203–204, 215, 251, 378, 401
    anticholinergic therapy for, 402
    antiemetics for, 402
    bicarbonate for, 401
    cimetidine for, 239, 401–402, 434
    combination antacid prophylaxis for, 402, 403t
    cricoid pressure for, 378, 379f, 398–399, 398f, 399f, 433, 433f
    emptying of stomach pharmacologically for, 402
    famotidine for, 402
    fasting for, 400–401, 401t
    H$_2$-receptor antagonists for, 239, 378, 401–402, 434
    lansoprazole for, 402
    metoclopramide for, 239, 378, 402, 434
    nizatidine for, 402
    omeprazole for, 239, 402
    ranitidine for, 239, 401–402, 434
  risk factors for, 377–378, 391–393, 394t–396f, 394t
  signs and symptoms of, 393, 397t
  steroid therapy for, 397
  volume and pH and, 392–393, 395f, 396f
Aspiration pneumonitis
  experimental treatment of, 397
  with obesity, 548–549, 549f, 554
  prophylaxis for, 400–403, 401t, 403t
  volume and pH of aspirate in, 392–393, 395f, 396f
Aspirin
  for preeclampsia, 299
  for preterm labor, 336
Asthma, 487–493
  anesthesia with, 491–492, 491f
  classification of, 487, 488t
  defined, 487
  drugs associated with exacerbations of, 489t
  effect on pregnancy of, 487–489
  hypertension and preeclampsia with, 492
  incidence of, 487

induction of labor with, 491
  pathophysiology of, 487, 488f
  perioperative causes of, 489t
  postpartum hemorrhage with, 492
  severity of, 487, 488t
  status asthmaticus in, 489–491
  treatment of, 489, 490t
Asymmetric septal hypertrophy (ASH), 474–475, 475t
ATIII (antithrombin III), 346
  during pregnancy, 11t
Atlanto-occipital (A-O) extension, 376, 377f
Atlanto-occipital (A-O) gap, with obesity, 549, 549f
Atopy, 561
  and latex allergy, 565
Atracurium, with obesity, 551, 551f
Atrial fibrillation
  due to mitral stenosis, 459
  after mitral valvulotomy, 476
  during pregnancy, 477–478
Atrial flutter, during pregnancy, 478
Atrial natriuretic peptide (ANP), during pregnancy, 14
Atrial septal defect (ASD), 456t, 465–466, 466t
Atropine
  in breast milk, 244
  fetal and neonatal effects of, 682t
  for myasthenia gravis, 539t
Autoimmune diseases, 560
Autologous donation, during cesarean section, 369
Automatic walking, 647, 647f, 649f
Autonomic hyperreflexia, 539–541, 540f, 540t, 541f
AVMs (arteriovenous malformations)
  cerebral, 511–512, 511f, 513–514, 513f, 514f
  of spine, 412–413
Awake extubation, 400
Awakening, delayed, after neurosurgery, 521–522
Awards, for malpractice, 441, 450, 450t
Awareness, during general anesthesia, 223, 224t
Azathioprine, for immunosuppression, 576
AZT (zidovudine)
  fetal and neonatal effects of, 685t
  for HIV, 590t

B
Back pain
  with chloroprocaine, 75–76, 76t, 414
  due to regional anesthesia, 143, 413–414
    lawsuits on, 447, 447t, 448t
Bag and mask ventilation, of newborn, 661–662, 661f
Ballard scoring system, 645, 645f
Barbiturates
  with alcohol abuse, 600
  effect on uterine activity and labor of, 43
  effect on uteroplacental blood flow of, 26, 27t, 28f
  neonatal effect of, 649
  as neuroprotective agents, 518
  for seizures, 532
  systemic, 113–114, 113f
Base excess (BE)
  with obesity, 548t
  during pregnancy, 4t
Basal metabolism, during pregnancy, 251f
Bearing-down reflex, epidural analgesia and, 47
Beclomethasone, for asthma, 490t
Bed rest
  for postdural puncture headache, 213, 213f, 415, 415f
  for pregnancy-induced hypertension, 304
Bedsores, 413
Behavioral teratology, 258–259
Benzodiazepines
  in breast milk, 244
  fetal and neonatal effects of, 685t
  systemic, 114–115, 114f
β_2-agonist, for asthma, 490t
β-adrenergic agents
  anesthetic considerations with, 329–331, 330f–333f
  cardiovascular effects of, 326, 327f
  mechanism of action of, 326
  metabolic effects of, 327f, 329, 329f
  myocardial effects of, 328–329
  for preterm labor, 325t, 326–331, 326t, 327f–333f
  pulmonary edema due to, 327–328, 328f
Beta-blockers
  fetal and neonatal effects of, 684t
  for pregnancy-induced hypertension, 306
Beta-human chorionic gonadotropin (hCG), 614
Bicarbonate (HCO$_3$)
  for aspiration prophylaxis, 401
  for cesarean section, 205t
    emergency, 227t
  hypotension with, 136
  with local anesthetics, 87
  for neonatal metabolic acidosis, 664–665, 666t
  placental transfer of, 25
  during pregnancy, 4t
Bicuspid aortic valve, 470
Biophysical profile (BPP), 618t, 619
Birth, circulatory changes at, 657, 658f
Birth weight, 643–645, 644f, 645f
Bleeding. See Hemorrhage
Bleeding time, 346, 347
  in preeclampsia and eclampsia, 303t
Blood flow (Q), studies of, 23–24, 24f
Blood gases
  with obesity, 548t
  during pregnancy, 3, 4t
Blood loss
  during delivery, 7, 11t

with halogenated agents, 222–223, 223t, 224t
  during neurosurgery, 519
Blood patch epidural, for postdural puncture headache, 214, 214t, 416–417
  with HIV, 591
Blood pressure (BP), during pregnancy, 6t, 8, 9t, 11t
Blood salvage, during cesarean section, 369
Blood type and screen, guidelines for, 674
Blood urea nitrogen (BUN), during pregnancy, 13
Blood volume
  with obesity, 548
  postpartum, 238
  in preeclampsia, 299–300, 303t
  during pregnancy, 6t, 7, 7f, 249
Body habitus, 376
Body mass index (BMI), 545
Bohr effect, 504
BP (blood pressure), during pregnancy, 6t, 8, 9t, 11t
BPP (biophysical profile), 618t, 619
Bradycardia
  fetal, 625t, 626–628, 626t, 628f, 629t
  paracervical block, 628
  second stage, 627–628
  terminal, 627
Brain death, maternal, 523–524, 523t
Brain protection, during neurosurgery, 518
Brain tumors, 509–510
Brazelton Neonatal Behavioral Assessment Scale (NBAS), 646
Breach of duty, 442
Breast-feeding
  after meperidine, 110
  after postpartum sterilization, 243–244, 244t
Breech presentation, 288–291
  anesthetic consideration in, 290–291, 291t
  cesarean delivery of, 290–291
  complete (single or double footling), 288, 289t
  etiology of, 288–289
  external cephalic version for, 289
  frank, 288, 289t
  incomplete, 288, 289t
  maternal, fetal, and neonatal hazards of, 290, 290f
  obstetric management of, 289–290, 289t
  partial breech extraction (assisted breech delivery) of, 290
  spontaneous delivery of, 289–290
  total breech extraction of, 290
  types of, 288, 289t
  vaginal delivery of, 289–290, 289t, 290f
Broca Index, 545
Bronchodilators
  for asthma, 490t
  fetal and neonatal effects of, 686t
Brow position, 288, 288f
Buffering capacity, in infants of diabetic mothers, 504–505, 505t
Bulk flow, placental transport via, 20–21, 20f
BUN (blood urea nitrogen), during pregnancy, 13
Bupivacaine (Marcaine, Sensorcaine), 81–84
  and autonomic hyperreflexia, 540f, 541
  in breast milk, 243
  cardiotoxicity of, 82–84, 82t, 83f, 213, 436–437
  for cesarean section, 205t, 208–209, 209, 209f
    emergency, 227t
  cesarean section rate with, 49, 50
  chemical structure of, 74f, 81
  for combined spinal-epidural analgesia, 129, 158, 158f, 159, 159f, 159t
  concentrations of, 82
  current usage of, 84
  effect on first stage of labor of, 45, 46t
  effect on preterm fetus of, 340
  effect on second stage of labor of, 46t, 47, 48, 49, 50–51
  effect on uterine activity of, 44f
  effect on uteroplacental blood flow of, 27t, 31, 31f
  epidural, 82, 84
  fetal distribution of, 67f, 68
  fetal uptake of, 65, 66
  gastric emptying with, 239
  intrathecal, 52, 53, 84
  for lumbar epidural anesthesia, 127t
  minimum local analgesic concentration of, 85, 85f, 86
  neonatal effect of, 650, 651
  opioids with
    for cesarean section, 208–209, 209f, 210–211
    for vaginal delivery, 163–167, 164f–166f, 166t, 167–168, 167t
  pharmacokinetics of, 153t
  placental transfer of, 61, 62, 63, 63f, 63t, 64f, 77
  seizures due to, 436
  for spinal anesthesia, 128, 128t
  test dose of, 134, 135f
BURP maneuver, 379
Butorphanol
  with bupivacaine, 166
  effect on uterine activity and labor of, 45, 46t, 49
  neurotoxicity of, 180, 181f
  systemic, 116, 116f, 116t

C
CABA (chloroaminobenzoic acid), plasma concentration of, 75f
Caffeine
  maternal use of, 602
  for postdural puncture headache, 214, 416, 602
Calcium
  as coagulation factor, 345, 346t
  for magnesium toxicity, 306

Calcium channel blockers
 effect on uteroplacental blood flow of, 27t, 34
 fetal and neonatal effects of, 684t
 for pregnancy-induced hypertension, 306–307
 for preterm labor, 325t, 336
"Cannot intubate, cannot ventilate" (CI/CV) situation, 385–386
Carbamazepine (Tegretol)
 fetal and neonatal effects of, 683t
 for seizures, 532t
Carbocaine. *See* Mepivacaine (Carbocaine)
Carbonated lidocaine, 81, 87
Carbon dioxide (CO_2)
 for laparoscopic sterilization, 239–240
 for laparoscopic surgery, 261
Carbon dioxide (CO_2) transfer, across placenta, 25
Carcinogenesis, transplacental, 259
Cardiac abnormalities, with HIV, 587t
Cardiac arrest
 due to regional anesthesia, 142, 436
 due to total spinal anesthesia, 143, 143f
Cardiac disease. *See also* Cardiac patient(s)
 congenital, 465–471
 incidence of, 455, 455f, 455t
 rheumatic, 456–465, 458t
Cardiac dysrhythmias
 with bupivacaine, 82–84, 82t, 83f
 fetal, 632–633
 during pregnancy, 477–478
Cardiac index, in preeclampsia, 299
Cardiac output
 effect of exercise on, 458f
 effect of positioning on, 458f
 effect of uterine contractions on, 457f
 fetal, 24, 275
 with obesity, 548
 postpartum, 238
 in preeclampsia, 299, 300t, 301f
 during pregnancy, 6t, 7–8, 8f, 11t, 249, 253f, 457f
Cardiac patient(s), 455–480
 anesthetic considerations in, 455–456
 antiarrhythmics for, 478–479
 aortic insufficiency, 456t, 463–465, 465f, 465t
 aortic stenosis, 456t, 462–463, 463f, 463t, 464f, 470
 asymmetric septal hypertrophy, 474–475, 475t
 atrial septal defect, 456t, 465–466, 466t
 cardiac transplantation, 477
 cardiomyopathy of pregnancy, 473–474
 choice of anesthetic technique for, 455
 coarctation of the aorta, 456t, 469–470, 470t
 complications in, 456
 congenital heart disease, 465–471
 coronary artery disease, 475–476
 current cardioversion for, 480
 dissecting aneurysm of the aorta, 474
 dysrhythmias, 477–478
 Eisenmenger's syndrome, 456t, 468–469, 469f, 469t
 general considerations with, 455–456
 with hypertension, 472–473
  primary pulmonary, 456t, 471–472, 472t
 inotropes for, 479–480
 intrathecal morphine for, 156, 157f
 left-to-right shunt, 465–468
 mitral insufficiency, 456t, 460–461, 460f, 461t
 mitral stenosis, 456–460, 456t, 459f, 459t
 mitral valve prolapse, 461–462, 462t
 monitoring of, 455–456
 open-heart surgery for, 477
 patent ductus arteriosus, 456t, 467–468, 467t
 pericarditis, 476
 postoperative care for, 456
 pulmonic stenosis, 417t, 456t, 470–471
 rheumatic heart disease, 456–465, 458t
 right-to-left shunt, 468–469
 tetralogy of Fallot, 456t, 468, 468t
 after valvular surgery, 476–477, 476t
 vasodilators for, 480
 vasopressors for, 479–480
 ventricular septal defect, 456t, 466–467, 466t
Cardiac surgery, during pregnancy, 477
Cardiac transplantation, pregnancy after, 477, 572–573
Cardiff methoxyflurane inhaler, 193
Cardiomyopathy of pregnancy, 473–474
Cardiopulmonary resuscitation (CPR), 436, 677
Cardiotoxicity, of bupivacaine, 82–84, 82t, 83f, 213
Cardiovascular changes
 asthma, 488–489
 hypertension, 472
 obesity, 548, 548f
 during pregnancy, 6–11, 6f–10f, 6t, 7t, 9t, 11t, 238, 455, 457f, 458f
 in puerperium, 238
 systemic lupus erythematosus, 570
Cardiovascular circulation, fetal, 66, 66f, 275–276, 275f, 276f
 effects of anesthesia on, 276–277, 276f–278f, 276t
Cardiovascular collapse, maternal mortality due to, 435–436
Cardiovascular effects
 β-adrenergic agonists, 326, 327f, 328f
 cocaine abuse, 607–609, 608f
 exercise, 458f
 inhalation agents, 195
 positioning, 458f
 uterine contractions, 457f
Cardioversion, 480
 for atrial fibrillation, 459
Carotid dissection, stroke due to, 511f

Catecholamines, effect on uteroplacental blood flow of, 27t, 31–32, 33
Catheter, trauma due to, 419
Cauda equina syndrome, from lidocaine, 77–79, 77f, 78f, 78t, 79t
Caudal anesthesia
 contraindications to, 134
 needle placement for, 125f
 technique of, 131–132, 131f, 131t, 132f
CC (closing capacity)
 with obesity, 547f
 during pregnancy, 4
CDH (congenital diaphragmatic hernia), 269–270, 270f, 615f
Central nervous system (CNS) depressants, neonatal effect of, 649–650
Central nervous system (CNS) effects, of pregnancy-induced hypertension, 302–303
Central nervous system (CNS) toxicity, of regional anesthesia, 140–142, 142t
Central nervous system (CNS) vasculopathy, stroke due to, 511f
Central venous pressure (CVP)
 in preeclampsia, 299, 300, 300t, 302f
 during pregnancy, 6t
 in pregnancy-induced hypertension, 307–308, 311
Cephalosporins
 allergic reactions to, 563
 fetal and neonatal effects of, 684t
Cerebral blood flow, fetal, 276
Cerebral ischemia, after neurosurgery, 522
Cerebral metabolic oxygen consumption ($CMRO_2$), 518
Cerebral oxygenation, during pregnancy, 9, 10f
Cerebral palsy (CP), 634
 Apgar score and, 642, 643f
Cerebral venous thrombosis, 512t, 514
Cerebrospinal fluid (CSF)
 during pregnancy, 12
 transfer of drugs to, 152, 152f
Cerebrovascular events, during pregnancy, 510–511, 511f, 512t, 513f, 513t
Cervical blocks, with combined spinal-epidural anesthesia, 160
Cervical dilation
 epidural analgesia, 45
 measurement of, 41, 42f
Cervical lacerations, 369
Cervical spine, rheumatoid arthritis of, 568, 569f
Cesarean section, 201–228
 airway management for, 677, 677t
 allergic reaction, 562
 aortic stenosis, 463
 asymmetric septal hypertrophy, 475
 blood loss from, 369
 breech presentation, 290–291, 291t
 cardiomyopathy of pregnancy, 473–474
 coronary artery disease, 475–476
 diabetes mellitus, 501
 emergency, 225–228, 227t
 epidural analgesia and, 46t, 47, 48, 49–50, 49t, 50f, 51f
 fetal malformations, 269f
 after fetal surgery, 272
 general anesthesia for, 214–223
  choice of, 201–202, 227–228
  condition of newborn with, 223–225, 224t, 225t
  emergency, 226
  etomidate, 220
  failed intubation with, 215–216, 216f, 217f
  halogenated agents, 221–223, 222f, 222t–224t
  ketamine, 219–220
  maternal and fetal effects of, 217–223
  maternal awareness during, 223, 224t
  maternal ventilation during, 217, 218f, 219f
  muscle relaxants, 220–221, 221t
  nitrous oxide, 221
  premedication for, 214
  preoxygenation for, 216, 217t
  preparation and equipment for, 214–215, 215t
  prevention of aspiration with, 215
  propofol, 220
  reduced requirements for, 214, 214t, 217
  thiopental, 217–219, 219f
 guidelines for, 676
 HIV, 588–589, 589t
 hypertension, 473
 idiopathic thrombocytopenic purpura, 348
 indications for, 201, 203t
 insulin therapy before, 501–502
 levobupivacaine for, 87
 lidocaine for, 80–81
 local anesthesia for, 73–74
 mitral stenosis, 460
 for multiple gestations, 294
 myasthenia gravis, 538–539
 for neurosurgical patients, 522–523, 522f
 newborn status after, 223–225, 224t, 225t
 obesity, 546, 553–556, 553f, 554f, 556f
 patient information on, 104
 for placenta previa, 361–363
 for pregnancy-induced hypertension, 311–314, 312f–314f, 315f
 of preterm infant, 337–340
 primary pulmonary hypertension, 472
 pulmonic stenosis, 471
 rates for, 201, 202f
 regional anesthesia for, 73–74, 201–214
  anesthetic solutions for, 208–213
  antacid administration with, 203–204
  antianxiety medication with, 203

 choice of, 201–202, 227–228
 combined spinal-epidural, 212–213, 212t
 complications of, 204–207, 205t, 206f, 208f, 213–214, 213f, 214t
 condition of newborn with, 223–225, 224t, 225t
 emergency, 226
 epidural, 209–212, 209t–212f
 failed, 213
 high or total spinal or epidural with, 213, 437
 hypotension due to, 204–207, 206f
 postdural puncture headache due to, 207–208, 208f, 213–214, 213f, 214t
 preparation for, 202–204, 204t
 reduced requirements for, 201, 204f, 204t
 supplemental oxygen with, 204, 205f
 technique of, 201–202, 205t
 toxicity of, 213
 via subarachnoid block, 208–209
 with rheumatoid arthritis, 569–570
 ropivacaine for, 86
 with systemic lupus erythematosus, 571
 with tetralogy of Fallot, 468
 trial of labor following, 366
 vaginal birth after, 366
  uterine rupture during, 365–366, 366t
Chemical contaminants, of subarachnoid and epidural spaces, 420–422, 422t
Chest compressions, for newborn, 662–663, 663f
Chest wall compliance
 with obesity, 547
 during pregnancy, 4t
Chiral compounds, 84–87
Chirocaine. *See* Levobupivacaine
Chlordiazepoxide (Librium), teratogenicity of, 253
Chloroaminobenzoic acid (CABA), plasma concentration of, 75f
2-Chloroprocaine (2CP). *See* Chloroprocaine (Nesacaine)
Chloroprocaine (Nesacaine), 75–76
 back pain due to, 75–76, 76t, 414
 for cesarean section, 209, 209t
  emergency, 227, 227t
 chemical structure of, 74f
 current usage of, 76
 effect on other epidural agents of, 75
 effect on preterm fetus of, 340
 effect on second stage of labor of, 50
 effect on uteroplacental blood flow of, 27t, 30, 31, 31f
 with epidural morphine, 173–174
 fetal tachycardia with, 138, 139f
 half-life of, 75, 75t
 for lumbar epidural anesthesia, 126
 neonatal effect of, 650, 651
 pharmacokinetics of, 75, 75f, 75t
 plasma concentration of, 75, 75f
 for pudendal block, 133
 test dose of, 136
 toxicity of, 75–76, 76t
Chlorpheniramine, for asthma, 490t
Chlorpromazine, teratogenicity of, 252
Cholinergic receptors, 150, 152f
Cholinesterase, during pregnancy, 13
Choriocarcinoma, 509–510
Chorionic villus sampling (CVS), 614
CI/CV ("cannot intubate, cannot ventilate") situation, 385–386
Cigarette smoking, 601–602
Cimetidine
 for aspiration prevention, 239, 401–402, 434
 effect on placental drug transfer of, 62
 fetal and neonatal effects of, 686t
 with general anesthesia, 215
 with obesity, 554
Circulation, fetal, 66, 66f, 275–276, 275f, 276f
 effects of anesthesia on, 276–277, 276f–278f, 276t
Citanest (prilocaine), 81
 chemical structure of, 74f
Clonazepam (Klonopin), for seizures, 532t
Clonidine
 effect on second stage of labor of, 51–52
 effect on uteroplacental blood flow of, 27t, 35
 epidural and intrathecal, 174
 fetal and neonatal effects of, 684t
 in patient-controlled epidural analgesia, 167
 placental transfer of, 64, 65f
Closed claims analysis, 446–451, 447f, 447t–450t
Closing capacity (CC)
 with obesity, 547f
 during pregnancy, 4
Closing volume, during pregnancy, 4t
Clotting factors. *See* Coagulation factors
$CMRO_2$ (cerebral metabolic oxygen consumption), 518
CNS (central nervous system) effects, of pregnancy-induced hypertension, 302–303
CNS (central nervous system) toxicity, of regional anesthesia, 140–142, 142t
CNS (central nervous system) vasculopathy, stroke due to, 511f
CO_2 (carbon dioxide)
 for laparoscopic sterilization, 239–240
 for laparoscopic surgery, 261
CO_2 (carbon dioxide) transfer, across placenta, 25
Coagulation
 laboratory methods for study of, 346–347, 347t
 mechanism of, 345–346, 346t
Coagulation abnormalities
 with abruptio placentae, 364–365
 with preeclampsia and eclampsia, 300, 303t

Coagulation abnormalities (*cont.*)
  with systemic lupus erythematosus, 570
  treatment of, 347–349, 347t
Coagulation factors, 345–346, 346t
  acquired or congenital disorders of, 348–349
  during pregnancy, 11, 11t
Coarctation of the aorta, 456t, 469–470, 470t
Cocaine
  abuse of, 604–606
    anesthetic considerations with, 607, 609
    assay for, 604
    epidemiology of, 604
    hypertension due to, 607–609, 608f
    maternal complications of, 605, 605t
    maternal deaths due to, 603f
    neonatal complications of, 605–606, 606f, 606t, 607f
    pharmacology and physiologic response to, 605, 605f
  chemical structure of, 74f
  effect on uteroplacental blood flow of, 27t, 31, 31f
  pharmacology and physiologic response to, 605
  stroke due to, 511f
  teratogenicity of, 256
  for topical anesthesia of nose, 382
Codeine, in breast milk, 243
Coffee, 602
Collagen vascular diseases, 559–560, 560t, 568–572
Colloid oncotic pressure (COP)
  in preeclampsia, 300
  during pregnancy, 8f, 11
Color, in Apgar score, 639, 640f
Coma, 519, 519t
Combined spinal-epidural (CSE) analgesia
  advantages and disadvantages of, 129, 129f
  for cesarean section, 212–213, 212t
  effect on uterine activity and labor of, 52–53, 52t, 53f, 162, 162t
  failure of, 160–161, 161f
  guidelines for, 675
  with obesity, 553, 555
  opioids in, 158–162, 158f–161f, 159t, 161t
  patient information on, 103
  postdural puncture headache due to, 129, 130t, 160, 212, 212f
  side effects of, 129–130, 130f, 130t, 159–161, 160f, 161f
  technique of, 129, 158–159
  for walking epidurals, 129, 161–162, 161t
Concentration gradient, 21, 21f
Conditioned reflexes, 96–97
C1 inhibitor, 346
Congenital anomalies
  with anesthesia during pregnancy, 253–258
    animal studies of, 253–256, 255f
    human studies of, 256–258, 257t, 258f
  with diabetes mellitus, 500, 500t
  fetal heart rate patterns with, 633
  resuscitation with, 668
  of spine, maternal, 412–413
Congenital bilateral hydronephrosis, 271–272, 272f
Congenital diaphragmatic hernia (CDH), 269–270, 270f, 615f
Congenital heart disease, 465–471
  aortic stenosis, 470
  atrial septal defect, 456t, 465–466, 466t
  coarctation of the aorta, 456t, 469–470, 470t
  Eisenmenger's syndrome, 456t, 468–469, 469f, 469t
  incidence of, 455, 456f, 456t
  left-to-right shunt, 465–468
  patent ductus arteriosus, 456t, 467–468, 467t
  pulmonic stenosis, 417t, 456t, 470–471
  right-to-left shunt, 468–469
  tetralogy of Fallot, 456t, 468, 468t
  ventricular septal defect, 456t, 466–467, 466t
Connective tissue disorders, 559–560, 560t, 568–572
Consciousness, with inhalation agents, 194–195
Conscious sedation, for interventional neuroradiology, 515–516
Consent, informed, 443–444, 449–450
Contact dermatitis, due to latex allergy, 566
Continuous infusion lumbar epidural anesthesia, 126–128, 127t
Continuous spinal anesthesia (CSA), 128, 128t, 167
  catheter size for, 78, 167
  for cesarean section, 74
  guidelines for, 78, 78t
  neurotoxicity of, 77
  opioids in, 167
Continuous spinal-epidural (CSE) anesthesia, infection due to, 422–423
Contraction(s)
  cardiovascular effects of, 457f
  hemodynamic effects of, 8, 9f
  physiology of, 325, 326f
Contraction stress test (CST), 618–619
Contrast medium, 516
Conus medullaris
  innervation of, 410–412
  lumbar puncture hazards to, 419f
Convulsions. *See* Seizures
Cooley's anemia, 350
COP (colloid oncotic pressure)
  in preeclampsia, 300
  during pregnancy, 8f, 11
Cordocentesis, for fetal anemia, 617
Coronary artery disease, 475–476
Cortical vein thrombosis
  due to regional anesthesia, 414–415
  stroke due to, 511f
Corticospinal fibers, 124f

Corticosteroids
  for allergic reactions, 562
  allergic reactions to, 563
  for aspiration, 397
  fetal and neonatal effects of, 489, 686t
  for immunosuppression, 576
Cough medications, for asthma, 490t
Coumadin (warfarin), fetal and neonatal effects of, 682t
Coumarin, 349
2-CP. *See* Chloroprocaine (Nesacaine)
CP (cerebral palsy), 634
  Apgar score and, 642, 643f
CPR (cardiopulmonary resuscitation), 436, 677
Cranial nerves, in neurosurgery evaluation, 519
Creatinine, during pregnancy, 13
Cricoarytenoiditis, 568
Cricoid pressure (CP), 378
  for aspiration prevention, 398–399, 398f, 399f, 433, 433f
  with laryngeal mask airway, 384–385, 385f, 385t
Cricothyroid membrane, 376
Cricothyrotomy, 381, 386–387, 434
Crixivan (indinavir sulfate)
  fetal and neonatal effects of, 685t
  for HIV, 590t
Cromolyn sodium, for asthma, 490t
Crown-rump length, 615
Cryoprecipitate, for amniotic fluid embolism, 358
Crystalloid administration, for hypotension, 206–207
CSA. *See* Continuous spinal anesthesia
CSE analgesia. *See* Combined spinal-epidural (CSE) analgesia
CSF (cerebrospinal fluid)
  during pregnancy, 12
  transfer of drugs to, 152, 152f
CST (contraction stress test), 618–619
Curare
  magnesium with, 305, 305f
  for prevention of aspiration, 398
CVP (central venous pressure)
  in preeclampsia, 299, 300, 300t, 302f
  during pregnancy, 6t
  in pregnancy-induced hypertension, 307–308, 311
CVS (chorionic villus sampling), 614
Cyanosis, in newborn, 639
Cyclopropane
  effect on uterine activity and labor of, 43f
  teratogenicity of, 256
Cyclosporine, for immunosuppression, 576
Cytotoxic reactions, 559, 560t, 568
Cytotrophoblast, 19, 20f

D
Damages, for malpractice, 441, 450, 450t
Dantrolene, effect on uteroplacental blood flow of, 27t, 35–36
ddC (zalcitabine)
  fetal and neonatal effects of, 685t
  for HIV, 590t
DDI (didanosine)
  fetal and neonatal effects of, 685t
  for HIV, 590t
DDI (drug-delivery interval), for meperidine, 106–109, 109f, 110, 110f
Dead space, during pregnancy, 4t
Dead space–to–tidal volume ratio, during pregnancy, 4
Decelerations
  early, 625t, 630
  late, 625t, 629t, 630–631, 630f
  prolonged, 625t
  variable, 625t, 629t, 631, 631f
Decongestants, for asthma, 490t
Decubitus ulcers, 413
Deep vein thrombosis
  from laparoscopic surgery, 261
  during pregnancy, 11
Delavirdine (Rescriptor), for HIV, 590t
Delayed awakening, after neurosurgery, 521–522
Delayed hypersensitivity reactions, 560, 560t
Delivery mode
  effect of epidural analgesia on, 46t, 47–52, 49t, 50f, 51t
  effect of intrathecal and combined spinal-epidural analgesia on, 52–53, 52t, 53f
Delivery room, neonatal evaluation in, 639–642, 640f–643f
Demerol. *See* Meperidine
Deposition, 444
Depakene (sodium valproate), for seizures, 532t
Dermatitis, due to latex allergy, 566
Desflurane, 193, 194
  in breast milk, 244
  effect on uterine activity and labor of, 41
  effect on uteroplacental blood flow of, 27t, 29
  maternal and fetal effects of, 221
  during neurosurgery, 517
  in obese patients, 550
  for postpartum sterilization, 243
Desmethyldiazepam, plasma concentration of, 114f
Dexamethasone, for eclampsia, 307
Dexmedetomidine, placental transfer of, 64, 65f
Dextran, for postdural puncture headache, 416
Dextromethorphan, for asthma, 490t
Dextrorotatory enantiomers, 84
d4T (stavudine)
  fetal and neonatal effects of, 685t
  for HIV, 590t
Diabetes mellitus (DM), 497–505
  anesthetic management of, 504–505, 505t
  cesarean section in, 501–502, 502t
  classification of, 497, 498, 498t
  diabetic ketoacidosis in, 497

  diet for, 500
  fetal monitoring with, 501
  gestational, 497
  hemoglobin A_1 in, 500, 500f
  incidence of, 497
  insulin therapy for, 500, 500f, 500t
  labor with, 501–502, 502t
  management of, 500–502, 500f, 500t, 501f, 502t
  outcome of pregnancy with, 498, 499t
  oxygen transport with, 502–504, 503f
  pancreas transplantation for, 575–576
  perinatal morbidity with, 498–500, 499t
  plasma epinephrine response to hypoglycemia in, 504
  plasma glucose levels in, 500, 500t, 501–502, 504
  preeclampsia with, 297–298, 498, 498t
  and preterm labor, 498t, 501
  shoulder dystocia with, 292
  stiff joint syndrome in, 498, 499f
  timing and route of delivery with, 501, 501f
  uteroplacental blood flow with, 502
Diabetic ketoacidosis, 497
Diabetic mothers, infants of
  buffering capacity in, 504–505, 505t
  congenital anomalies in, 499, 499t
"Diabetogenic" profile of pregnancy, 14
Diaphragmatic hernia, congenital, 269–270, 270f, 615f
Diastolic blood pressure, during pregnancy, 6t
Diazepam
  adverse effects of, 115
  with cesarean section, 203, 214
  chemical structure of, 114t
  for eclampsia, 307
  effect on uterine activity and labor of, 43
  effect on uteroplacental blood flow of, 26, 27t
  neonatal effect of, 649
  pharmacokinetics of, 114–115
  plasma concentration of, 114–115, 114f
  systemic, 114–115, 114t
  teratogenicity of, 253
Diazoxide, for pregnancy-induced hypertension, 307
DIC (disseminated intravascular coagulation), 349, 357, 357t
Didanosine (DDI, Videx)
  fetal and neonatal effects of, 685t
  for HIV, 590t
Diet, with diabetes mellitus, 500
Diethyl ether, teratogenicity of, 256
Difficult airway management. *See* Airway, difficult; Airway management
Diffusing capacity, during pregnancy, 4t
Diffusion, placental transport via, 19, 20f, 21–22, 21f
Diffusion distance, 22
Digoxin
  for atrial fibrillation, 459
  effect on fetus of, 479
Dilantin. *See* Phenytoin (Dilantin)
Dinoprostone (prostaglandin E_2)
  with asthma, 491, 492
  gastric emptying of, 392
  for uterine atony, 367, 368t
Diphenhydramine
  fetal and neonatal effects of, 683t
  for nausea, vomiting, or itching, 171t, 176
Direct current cardioversion, 480
Disinfectants, skin, 422
Disodium ethylenediaminetetraacetic acid (EDTA), chloroprocaine with, 75–76, 76t, 209, 209t
Dissecting aneurysm of the aorta, 474
Disseminated intravascular coagulation (DIC), 349, 357, 357t
Dissociative drugs, systemic, 116–117
Diuretics
  fetal and neonatal effects of, 684t
  during neurosurgery, 517
Dizziness, naloxone for, 178t
DM. *See* Diabetes mellitus (DM)
Dobutamine, for amniotic fluid embolism, 358t
Documentation, 443
Dopamine
  for amniotic fluid embolism, 358t
  effect on uteroplacental blood flow of, 27t, 32
  fetal effect of, 479
  for mitral stenosis, 459
  in neonatal resuscitation, 666t
Doppler transducer, fetal heart rate monitoring with, 624, 624f
Doppler velocimetry, 619–620, 619f
Dorsal columns, 124f
Dorsal root, 124f
Dorsal root ganglion, 124f
Double set-up, for antepartum hemorrhage, 361, 362t
Draw-over inhalation analgesia, 193
Droperidol
  fetal and neonatal effects of, 683t
  for nausea, vomiting, or itching, 171t
  neurotoxicity of, 179
  with pregnancy-induced hypertension, 313
Drowsiness, naloxone for, 178t
Drug(s)
  in breast milk, 243–244, 244t
  effect on uterine activity and labor of, 41–54
  effect on uteroplacental circulation of, 26–36, 27t
  fetal and neonatal effects of, 681–686
  fetal distribution of, 66–68, 66f–68f, 66t
  fetal metabolism and excretion of, 68, 68t
  fetal uptake of, 64–66, 65f, 66f
  free, 61, 62f
  half-life of, 61
  pK_a of, 63, 64

Drug(s) (*cont.*)
    placental transfer of, 61–64, 62f–65f, 62t–64t
    protein binding of, 62–63, 63f, 63t, 64f
Drug addiction, 599–609
    alcohol, 599–601, 600f, 601f
    amphetamines, 603f, 606–607
    caffeine, 602
    cocaine, 604–606
        anesthetic considerations with, 607, 609
        assay for, 604
        epidemiology of, 604
        hypertension due to, 607–609, 608f
        maternal complications of, 605, 605t
        maternal deaths due to, 603f
        neonatal complications of, 605–606, 606f, 606t, 607f
        pharmacology and physiologic response to, 605, 605f
    current trends in, 599, 600t
    marijuana, 609
    opioids, 602–604, 603f, 603t, 604t
    tobacco, 601–602
Drug-delivery interval (DDI), for meperidine, 106–109, 109f,
    110, 110f
Ductus arteriosus, 275
    closure of, 657
    patent, 456t, 467–468, 467t
Dural puncture
    headache after. *See* Postdural puncture headache (PDPH)
    unintentional, 420–422, 422t
Dura mater, 125f, 152
Duties of care, 442
Dysrhythmias
    with bupivacaine, 82–84, 82t, 83f
    fetal, 632–633
    during pregnancy, 477–478
Dystocia, 41, 42t
    shoulder, 291–293, 292f, 293t

E
Early decelerations, 625t, 630
Early Neonatal Neurobehavioral Scale (ENNS), 646, 646f
EBP (epidural blood patch), for postdural puncture
    headache, 214, 214t, 416–417
    with HIV, 591
ECG. *See* Electrocardiogram (ECG)
Eclampsia. *See* Pregnancy-induced hypertension (PIH)
    cardiovascular changes with, 472
    convulsions due to, 307
    defined, 297, 298t
    incidence of, 297
    monitoring of, 307–308, 308t
    stroke due to, 510–511, 511f
ECV (external cephalic version), 289
Edema
    after neurosurgery, 522
    in preeclampsia, 299, 301
Edrophonium chloride (Tensilon) test, for myasthenia gravis,
    537, 539t
EDTA (ethylenediaminetetraacetic acid), chloroprocaine
    with, 75–76, 76t, 209, 209t
EEG (electroencephalogram), for neurosurgery, 521
Efavirenz (Sustiva), for HIV, 590t
EFM (electronic fetal monitoring). *See* Fetal heart rate (FHR)
    monitoring
Eisenmenger's syndrome, 456t, 468–469, 469f, 469t
Electrocardiogram (ECG)
    of aortic insufficiency, 463
    of aortic stenosis, 463, 464f
    during fetal surgery, 277, 279f
    of mitral stenosis, 457
    of mitral valve prolapse, 461
    with subarachnoid hemorrhage, 519
Electroencephalogram (EEG), for neurosurgery, 521
Electronic fetal monitoring (EFM). *See* Fetal heart rate (FHR)
    monitoring
Embolism, amniotic fluid. *See* Amniotic fluid embolism (AFE)
Emergency cesarean section, 225–228, 227t
Emergency deliveries, anesthesia for, 390
Emotional distress, lawsuits on, 447–448, 447t, 448t
Emotional stress, teratogenicity of, 258
Emotril trichloroethylene vaporizer, 193
Enantiomers, 84
Endocrine changes, during pregnancy, 13–14
Endocytosis, 21
Endogenous opiates, 149, 150t
β-Endorphin, 150t
Endorphin(s), during pregnancy, 12
Endothelia, in preeclampsia, 298
Endothelin, in amniotic fluid embolism, 357
Endotracheal intubation
    failed, 215–216, 216f, 217f, 379–381, 380f
        maternal mortality due to, 434, 434t
    fiberoptic, 381, 383–384, 384f
    for meconium suctioning, 667–668, 667f
    of newborn, 662, 662f, 662f, 663f
    with obesity, 554, 554f
    during pregnancy, 3
    with pregnancy-induced hypertension, 312–314, 313f, 314f,
        315f
Endotracheal tube (ETT), 383
Endovascular embolization, 516
End-tidal PCO₂, during pregnancy, 249, 250f
Enflurane
    in breast milk, 244
    effect on uterine activity and labor of, 41, 43f
    effect on uteroplacental blood flow of, 29
    efficacy of, 194
    maternal and fetal effects of, 221, 222, 222f, 224t

minimum alveolar concentration for, 249, 251f
    in obese patients, 550, 551f
    teratogenicity of, 256
Enkephalins, 150t
ENNS (Early Neonatal Neurobehavioral Scale), 646, 646f
Entonox, 191–192, 192f, 192t, 193, 193f
Environmental considerations, with inhalation agents, 196
Ephedrine
    for allergic reactions, 562
    effect on uteroplacental blood flow of, 27t, 32, 33f
    fetal effect of, 479
    for hypotension, 138, 139f, 140, 141f, 205–206, 206f, 207
        in preterm labor and delivery, 330, 331f–333f
    for vasoconstriction of nose, 382
Epidural abscess, 422, 423t
Epidural analgesia/anesthesia. *See also* Regional anesthesia
    with asthma, 491, 491f
    and autonomic hyperreflexia, 540–541, 540f, 541f
    bearing-down reflex with, 47
    for breech presentation, 291
    bupivacaine for, 82, 84
    cardiovascular effects of, 11t
    for cesarean section, 74, 201–208
        anesthetic solutions for, 209–213, 209t, 210f, 211f, 212f
        antacid administration with, 203–204
        antianxiety medication with, 203
        choice of, 201–202
        complications of, 204–207, 205t, 206f, 208f, 213–214,
            213f, 214t
        condition of newborn with, 223–225, 224t, 225t
        emergency, 226–227, 227f
        failed, 213
        high or total, 213, 437
        hypotension due to, 204–207, 206f
        postdural puncture headache due to, 207–208, 208f,
            213–214, 213f, 214t
        preparation for, 202–204, 204t
        reduced requirements for, 201, 204f, 204t, 211–212, 241,
            241t
        supplemental oxygen with, 204, 205f
        technique for, 201–202, 205t
    and cesarean section rate, 46t, 47, 49–50, 49t, 50f, 51t
    chloroprocaine for, 76
    contraindications to, 134
    dense or prolonged, 143–144
    effect on uterine activity and labor of, 44–52, 44f
    effect on uteroplacental blood flow of, 27t, 31, 31f
    epinephrine with, 87
    fetal malposition with, 47–48
    fluid bolus with, 46
    forceps deliveries with, 48
    guidelines for, 674–675
    after heart transplantation, 573
    and hyperventilation during labor, 3, 5f
    inadequate or failed, 144
    inadvertent intrathecal injection in, 79
    infusion *vs.* intermittent bolus of, 50–51
    levobupivacaine for, 87
    lidocaine for, 80–81
    lumbar
        continuous infusion, 126–128, 127t
        drug regimens for, 127t
        movement of drug after injection in, 152–153, 152f
        needle placement for, 125f
        positioning for, 125f, 126f
        with pregnancy-induced hypertension, 309–310, 309t,
            310f
        technique of, 123–126, 125f, 126f, 127t
        timing of, 123–124
    for multiple gestations, 294
    with multiple sclerosis, 536
    neonatal effect of, 650–651
    with obesity, 144, 552–553, 555
    opioids in. *See* Epidural opioids
    and oxytocin release, 47
    patient-controlled
        drug regimens for, 127t
        efficacy of, 167
        outcome of labor with, 51
        ropivacaine in, 85, 86
        technique of, 167
    patient information on, 103–104
    "perineal dose" of, 48
    for postpartum sterilization, 240–242, 241f, 241t, 242t, 403
    with pregnancy-induced hypertension, 311
    for preterm labor and delivery, 330
    with progressive systemic sclerosis, 571
    prolonged neural blockade with, 417
    reduced requirements for, 201, 204f, 204t, 211–212, 241,
        241t, 249, 254f, 435
    ropivacaine for, 85–86, 85f
    rostral spread of, 417
    test dose for, 209–210
    timing of, 44, 50
    total, 213
    unilateral, 144
    walking, 129
        efficacy of, 161
        maternal safety of, 161–162, 161t
        neuromuscular coordination with, 413
Epidural blood patch (EBP), for postdural puncture
    headache, 214, 214t, 416–417
    with HIV, 591
Epidural opioids, 162–163
    additives with, 167–168
    complications of, 174–180
    epinephrine with, 174

local anesthetics with, 173–174
    monitoring of, 179
    neonatal effects of, 651
    for postoperative pain management, 168–170, 168f, 169f,
        169t–171t, 173–174, 173t
    progress in labor with, 162–163, 162t, 163f, 163t, 164f
Epidural space, 125f
    chemical contaminants of, 420–422, 422t
    transfer of drugs from, 152, 152f
Epidural veins, engorgement of, 12, 249, 435
Epilepsy, 530–533, 531t, 532f, 532t. *See also* Seizures
Epinephrine
    for allergic reactions, 562
    for amniotic fluid embolism, 358t
    for cesarean section, 210
        emergency, 227t
    in combined spinal-epidural anesthesia, 158–159, 159f
    effect on first stage of labor of, 46
    effect on placental drug transfer of, 61, 63f
    effect on second stage of labor of, 51
    effect on uteroplacental blood flow of, 27t, 32
    epidural, 87
        with epidural opioids, 174
            side effects of, 174
    fetal effect of, 479
    after heart transplantation, 573
    for hypotension, in preterm labor and delivery, 332f
    intrathecal, 52, 87–88, 88f
        side effects of, 174
    with local anesthetics, 87–88, 88f
    for lumbar epidural anesthesia, 127t
    neonatal effect of, 651
    in newborn resuscitation, 663, 664f, 666t
    test dose of, 134–136, 135f, 136f, 436
Episiotomy, for preterm delivery, 340
Epivir (lamivudine)
    fetal and neonatal effects of, 685t
    for HIV, 590t
Equanil (meprobamate), teratogenicity of, 253
Ergonovine (Ergotrate, Ergometrine), for uterine atony, 367,
    368t
Ergot alkaloids
    for abruptio placentae, 365
    for uterine atony, 367, 368t
ERV (expiratory reserve volume)
    with obesity, 547, 548t
    during pregnancy, 3, 4t, 5f, 251f
Erythroblastosis fetalis, 568
Esmolol hydrochloride, effect on fetus of, 478
Esophageal gastric tube airway, 300f, 399
Esophageal tracheal combitube (ETC), 381, 386
Esophagitis, during pregnancy, 12
Ester-linked agents, 74–77, 74f
Estriol, 613–614
Ethanol abuse, 599–601, 600f, 601f
Ether, effect on uterine activity and labor of, 43f
Ethosuximide (Zarontin), for seizures, 533t
Ethylenediaminetetraacetic acid (EDTA), chloroprocaine
    with, 75–76, 76t, 209, 209t
Etidocaine
    chemical structure of, 74f
    neonatal effect of, 651
    placental transfer of, 77
Etomidate
    maternal and fetal effects of, 220
    as neuroprotective agent, 518
ETT (endotracheal tube), 383
EXIT (ex utero intrapartum treatment) procedure, 270–271,
    668
Exocytosis, 21
Expiratory reserve volume (ERV)
    with obesity, 547, 548t
    during pregnancy, 3, 4t, 5f, 251f
External cardiac compression, 436
External cephalic version (ECV), 289
Extradural pressure, during pregnancy, 12
Extubation, 387
    awake, 400
Ex utero intrapartum treatment (EXIT) procedure, 270–271,
    668

F
FAAS (fetal alcohol abuse syndrome), 600
Face mask (FM)
    aspiration risk with, 385
    for newborn ventilation, 661–662, 661f
Face position, 288, 288f
Facilitated diffusion, placental transport via, 19, 20f
FAE (fetal alcohol effects), 600
Famotidine, for aspiration prophylaxis, 402
FAS (fetal alcohol syndrome), 599–600, 600f
Fasting
    for aspiration prophylaxis, 400–401, 401t
    guidelines for, 674
Femoral venous pressure, during pregnancy, 6t, 254f
Fentanyl
    for anxiety with cesarean section, 203, 214
    in breast milk, 243
    with bupivacaine, 163–166, 164f–166f, 166t, 167–168, 167t
    for cesarean section, 209, 208–209, 210–211
    cesarean section rate with, 49, 50
    for combined spinal-epidural analgesia, 129, 158, 158f, 159,
        159f, 159t
    dosage of, 110, 111f
    effect on first stage of labor of, 45, 46t
    effect on second stage labor of, 46t, 48, 49, 50, 51

Fentanyl (*cont.*)
  effect on uterine activity of, 43
  effect on uteroplacental blood flow of, 27t, 35
  epidural
    for cesarean section, 210–211
    for labor and delivery, 163
    neonatal effects of, 179
    neurotoxicity of, 179
    for postoperative pain, 168, 169f
    respiratory depression due to, 175
  for fetal surgery, 273
  gastric emptying with, 239, 391–392
  for inadequate or failed epidural analgesia, 144
  intrathecal, 52, 53, 155, 157f
    neurotoxicity of, 179
    for postoperative pain, 172, 173, 173f, 173t
    progress in labor with, 162
    side effects of, 160
  for lumbar epidural anesthesia, 127t
  neonatal effect of, 110–112, 111f, 112t, 179, 650, 651
  with obesity, 553
  patient-controlled IV, 110, 112
  pharmacokinetics of, 110, 152, 153, 153t
  placental transfer of, 110
  with pregnancy-induced hypertension, 309, 313
  pruritus due to, 174
  ritonavir and, 589, 591f
  with ropivacaine, 86
  systemic, 110–112, 111f, 112t
  transfer across arachnoid membrane of, 152
Ferguson reflex, epidural analgesia and, 47
Fetal acidemia, 635
  bradycardia and, 626, 626t
  fetal heart rate patterns at risk for, 633, 633t
  tachycardia and, 627t
Fetal acidosis, fetal heart rate variability and, 627t
Fetal age, 614–615
Fetal alcohol abuse syndrome (FAAS), 600
Fetal alcohol effects (FAE), 600
Fetal alcohol syndrome (FAS), 599–600, 600f
Fetal anemia, 617, 617f, 618f
Fetal anomalies, 615
  therapeutic alternatives for, 267–269, 268t, 269t
Fetal asphyxia
  clinical indicators of, 634
  etiologies of, 623
  fetal heart rate monitoring in diagnosis of, 634–635, 635t
  fetal heart rate patterns with, 631–632, 632f
  fetal response to, 624
  during surgery on fetus, 274
  during surgery on mother, 259–260, 259f, 260f
Fetal blood sampling, 633–634
Fetal breathing movements, 618t
Fetal dating, 614–615
Fetal distress, emergency cesarean section for, 226, 390
Fetal effects
  of ACE inhibitors, 684t
  of acetaminophen, 682t
  of acyclovir, 685t
  of adenosine, 479
  of allergic reactions, 562
  of α_2-adrenergic agonists, 684t
  of aminoglycosides, 684t
  of amiodarone, 479
  of amphetamine abuse, 607
  of amrinone, 479–480
  of analgesics, 682t
  of angiotensin II, 479
  of antiarrhythmics, 478–479
  of antibiotics, 684t–685t
  of anticholinergic therapy, 682t
  of anticoagulants, 682t
  of anticonvulsant therapy, 683t
  of antidepressants, 683t
  of antiemetics, 683t
  of antiepileptic drugs, 683t
  of antifungals, 685t
  of antihypertensive agents, 684t
  of antimicrobials, 684t–685t
  of antiretroviral drugs, 589–590, 685t
  of antivirals, 685t
  of anxiolytics, 685t
  of atropine, 682t
  of benzodiazepines, 685t
  of beta-blockers, 684t
  of bronchodilators, 686t
  of caffeine, 602
  of calcium channel blockers, 684t
  of carbamazepine, 683t
  of cephalosporins, 684t
  of cigarette smoking, 601–602
  of cimetidine, 686t
  of clonidine, 684t
  of cocaine abuse, 606, 606t
  of corticosteroids, 489, 686t
  of Coumadin, 682t
  of desflurane, 221
  of digoxin, 479
  of diphenhydramine, 683t
  of diuretics, 684t
  of dopamine, 479
  of droperidol, 683t
  of enflurane, 221, 222, 222f, 224t
  of ephedrine, 479
  of epinephrine, 479
  of esmolol hydrochloride, 478
  of etomidate, 220

  of fluconazole, 685t
  of fluoroquinolones, 684t
  of furosemide, 684t
  of general anesthesia, 217–223
  of glycopyrrolate, 682t
  of halothane, 221, 222, 222f, 223t, 224t
  of heparin, 682t
  of histamine-2 (H_2) receptor antagonists, 686t
  of human immunodeficiency virus, 589–590
  of hydralazine, 480, 684t
  of hypoglycemics, 686t
  of hypotension, 137, 139f
  of ibuprofen, 682t
  of indomethacin, 682t
  of inhalation agents, 191, 195–196, 195f
  of inotropes, 479–480
  of insulin, 686t
  of isoflurane, 221, 222, 224t
  of isoproterenol, 479
  of ketoprofen, 682t
  of ketorolac, 682t
  of labetalol hydrochloride, 479
  of lidocaine, 478
  of lithium, 683t
  of macrolides, 684t
  of maternally administered drugs, 681–686
  of metaraminol, 479
  of methoxamine, 479
  of methyldopa, 684t
  of metoclopramide, 683t
  of milrinone, 479–480
  of muscle relaxants, 220–221, 221t
  of naproxen, 682t
  of nicardipine, 479
  of nitrous oxide, 221
  of norepinephrine, 479
  of omeprazole, 686t
  of ondansetron, 683t
  of opioids, 603, 682t
  of penicillins, 685t
  of phenobarbital, 683t
  of phenylephrine, 479
  of phenytoin, 683t
  of pregnancy-induced hypertension, 303
  of prochlorperazine, 683t
  of promethazine, 683t
  of propranolol, 478
  of quinidine, 478
  of rocuronium, 221
  of sevoflurane, 221
  of sodium nitroprusside, 480
  of succinylcholine, 220–221, 221t
  of sulfonamides, 685t
  of tetracyclines, 685t
  of thyroid agents, 686t
  of valproic acid, 683t
  of vasodilators, 480, 684t
  of vasopressors, 479–480
  of vecuronium, 221
  of verapamil, 479
Fetal evaluation, 613–620
  amniotic fluid index in, 618
  of amniotic fluid surfactant, 616–617, 616f, 617f
  of anemia, 617, 617f, 618f
  of aneuploidy, 613–614
  antepartum, 617–619, 618t, 619f
  biophysical profile in, 618f, 619
  contraction stress test in, 618–619
  Doppler velocimetry in, 619–620, 619f
  for fetal anomalies, 615
  for fetal dating, 614–615
  of fetal growth, 615
  first and second trimester, 613–616
  of lung maturity, 616
  maternal serum triple marker screening in, 613–614, 614t
  neural tube defect screening in, 613
  nonstress test in, 618
  nuchal translucency screening in, 614
  for placental localization, 615
  third trimester, 616–617
  ultrasonography in, 614–616, 615f
Fetal growth, evaluation of, 615
Fetal head
  diameter of, 288, 288f
  pressure on neural structures or spinal nutrient arteries by, 410–412
Fetal heart rate (FHR)
  accelerations in, 625t, 626, 626f
    prognostic value of, 633
    prolonged, 625t
  baseline, 625, 625t
  characteristics of, 625–626, 625t
  with congenital anomalies, 533
  decelerations in
    early, 625t, 630
    late, 625t, 629t, 630–631, 630f
    prolonged, 625t
    variable, 625t, 629t, 631, 631f
  dysrhythmias of, 632–633
  periodic changes in, 630–631, 630f, 631f
  of preterm fetus, 633
  reactive, 618t
  saltatory pattern of, 632
  sinusoidal pattern of, 632
  and uterine activity, 625
  variability in, 626
    absent, 625t, 626, 627t, 629–630, 629f

    changes in, 625t, 627t, 628–630, 629f
    decreasing, 629t
    marked, 625t, 626
    minimal, 625t, 626, 627t, 629–630
    moderate, 625t, 626
    prognostic value of, 633
  variant patterns of, 626–633
    bradycardia, 625t, 626–628, 626t, 628f, 629f
    interpretation of, 633, 633t
    intrauterine treatment of, 629f
    significance of, 631–632, 632t
    tachycardia, 625t, 627t, 628
    unusual, 632–633
Fetal heart rate (FHR) abnormalities
  due to combined spinal-epidural analgesia, 129–130, 130t, 160, 160f
  due to magnesium, 305
  due to opioids, 105, 106, 107t, 108f, 149
  due to paracervical block, 132, 132f, 133f
  in utero treatment of, 633
Fetal heart rate (FHR) monitor, 624–625
Fetal heart rate (FHR) monitoring, 623–636
  alternatives to, 633–634
  with diabetes mellitus, 501
  in diagnosis of fetal asphyxia, 634–635, 635t
  during fetal surgery, 277–278, 279f–281f
  guidelines for, 674
  history of, 623
  during maternal surgery, 262, 262f
  during neurosurgery, 520, 520f
  of preterm fetus, 337–338
  technique of, 624–625, 624f
Fetal hydantoin syndrome, 531–532
Fetal lung maturity (FLM), 616–617
  with diabetes mellitus, 501, 501f
Fetal lung maturity (FLM) index, 616
Fetal malposition, with epidural analgesia, 47–48
Fetal oxygenation, with asthma, 488
Fetal pulse oximetry, 634
Fetal scalp electrode (FSE), 624, 624f
Fetal scalp sampling, 634
  and Apgar score, 640, 640f
Fetal scalp stimulation, 634
Fetal surgery, 267–282
  alternatives to, 267–269, 268t, 269t
  anesthetic considerations for, 272–275, 272t, 273f, 274f
  background of, 267, 268t
  cardiovascular considerations in, 275–277, 275f–278f, 276t
  for congenital diaphragmatic hernia, 269–270, 270f
  fetal monitoring for, 277–278, 279f–281f
  future of, 280–282
  indications for, 267, 268t, 269–272, 269t
  prevention of preterm labor during, 278–280
  rationale for, 269, 269t
  risks of, 272
  for teratoma, 268f
  for tracheal occlusion, 270–271, 271f
  for urinary tract obstruction, 271–272, 272f, 273f
Fetal surveillance, 617–619, 618t, 619f
Fetal survey, 614, 615f
Fetal therapy, 617
Fetal tone, 618t
Fetal weight, evaluation of, 615
Fetoscopy, 273
Fetus
  circulation of, 66, 66f, 275–276, 275f, 276f, 657, 658f
    effects of anesthesia on, 276–277, 276f–278f, 276t
  drug distribution in, 66–68, 66f–68f, 66t
  drug metabolism and excretion in, 68, 68t
  drug uptake in, 64–66, 65f, 66f
  effect of cardiac therapeutics on, 478–480
  high-risk, 658, 659t
  oxygen transfer to, 24–25, 24t, 25f
FEV 1.0 (forced expiratory volume in 1 sec)
  with obesity, 548t
  during pregnancy, 4t
FHR. *See* Fetal heart rate
Fiberoptic blades, 384, 384f
Fiberoptic laryngoscopy, 381, 383–384, 384f
Fibrin degradation products, 347t
Fibrinogen
  in coagulation, 345, 346t
  in preeclampsia and eclampsia, 303t
  during pregnancy, 11, 11t
  screening for, 347t
Fibrinolysis, 345–346
  screening for, 347
Fibrin split products, during pregnancy, 11t
Fibronectin
  in amniotic fluid embolism, 358
  in preeclampsia, 298, 299
  and preterm labor, 323
Fick's equation, 21, 63
Filum terminale, 125f
FK-506 (tacrolimus), for immunosuppression, 576
FLM (fetal lung maturity), 616–617
  with diabetes mellitus, 501, 501f
FLM (fetal lung maturity) index, 616
Fluconazole, fetal and neonatal effects of, 685t
Fluid preload, and hypotension, 137, 434–435
Fluid replacement, during neurosurgery, 518–519
Fluid restriction, for pregnancy-induced hypertension, 304
Flumazenil, 118
Fluoroquinolones, fetal and neonatal effects of, 684t
Fluoxetine, fetal and neonatal effects of, 683t
Fluroxene, teratogenicity of, 256

FM (face mask)
  aspiration risk with, 385
  for newborn ventilation, 661–662, 661f
Food allergy, and latex sensitivity, 564–565
Foramen ovale, closure of, 657
Forced expiratory volume in 1 sec (FEV 1.0)
  with obesity, 548t
  during pregnancy, 4t
Forceps deliveries
  with epidural analgesia, 48
  for multiple gestations, 294
Forceps rotation, 287–288
Fortovase (saquinavir mesylate)
  fetal and neonatal effects of, 685t
  for HIV, 590t
Fraction of inspired oxygen, during labor, 5
Frankenhauser's ganglion, 132
FSE (fetal scalp electrode), 624, 624f
Fuel-hormone balance, during pregnancy, 497
Functional residual capacity (FRC)
  with obesity, 547, 547f, 548t
  during pregnancy, 3, 4t, 5, 5f, 249, 251f
Fungal infection, with HIV, 591t
Furosemide
  fetal and neonatal effects of, 684t
  during neurosurgery, 517

G
Gastric acid, during pregnancy, 13, 13f, 392
Gastric contents, pulmonary aspiration of. *See* Aspiration
Gastric emptying
  opioids and, 237, 239, 239t, 391–392
  during pregnancy, 12–13, 238–239, 239t, 249–250, 391, 394f
  and risk of aspiration, 391
Gastric motility, during pregnancy, 12–13
Gastric pressure, during pregnancy, 392, 394f
Gastroesophageal reflux
  barrier pressure to, 378
  during pregnancy, 12, 238–239, 239t, 392
Gastroesophageal tone, and aspiration, 392
Gastrointestinal changes
  with obesity, 548–549, 549f
  during pregnancy, 12–13, 13f, 238–239, 239t, 375
Gastrointestinal complications, of HIV, 587t
Gastrointestinal system, in progressive systemic sclerosis, 571
Gate theory of pain, 97–98
GDM (gestational diabetes mellitus), 497
General anesthesia
  airway management for, 377–381
  allergic reactions to, 563
  aspiration with, 398, 398t
  with asthma, 492
  for breech presentation, 291
  for cesarean section, 214–223
    choice of, 201–202, 227–228
    condition of newborn with, 223–225, 224t, 225t
    emergency, 226
    with etomidate, 220
    failed intubation with, 215–216, 216f, 217f
    with halogenated agents, 221–223, 222f, 222t–224t
    with ketamine, 219–220
    maternal and fetal effects of, 217–223
    maternal awareness during, 223, 224t
    maternal ventilation during, 217, 218f, 219f
    with muscle relaxants, 220–221, 221t
    with nitrous oxide, 221
    premedication for, 214
    preoxygenation for, 216, 217t
    preparation and equipment for, 214–215, 215f
    prevention of aspiration with, 215
    with propofol, 220
    reduced requirements for, 214, 214t, 217
    technique for, 214–215, 215t
    with thiopental, 217–219, 219f
  with cocaine abuse, 609
  with epilepsy, 533
  for fetal surgery, 273, 274
  with HIV, 592
  maternal mortality with, 431–432, 431f, 432t, 433–434, 433f, 434t
  with mitral stenosis, 460
  with multiple sclerosis, 536
  with myasthenia gravis, 538–539
  neonatal effect of, 651–652
  with obesity, 554–555, 554f
  for postpartum sterilization, 242–243, 242t, 243t, 403
  with pregnancy-induced hypertension, 312
  for preterm labor and delivery, 330–331
  with progressive systemic sclerosis, 571–572
  with rheumatoid arthritis, 569
  with spinal cord injury, 541, 541t
  with systemic lupus erythematosus, 571
  for vaginal delivery, 189, 191t
Gestational age, 643–645, 644f, 645f
  small for, 323, 643–645, 644f, 645f
Gestational diabetes mellitus (GDM), 497. *See also* Diabetes mellitus (DM)
Glasgow Coma Scale, 519, 519t
Gliomas, 509
Glomerular filtration rate (GFR), during pregnancy, 13
Glossopharyngeal nerve, 381, 382f
Glove(s), with latex allergy, 565, 565t
Glove anesthesia, 95
Glucose
  placental transport of, 19
  plasma levels of, in diabetes mellitus, 500, 500t, 501–502, 504

Glucose metabolism, during pregnancy, 497
Glucose therapy, during labor or before cesarean section, 501–502
Glucosuria, during pregnancy, 13
Glycopyrrolate, fetal and neonatal effects of, 682t
Gold compounds, for immunosuppression, 577
Gross body movement, fetal, 618t
Guaifenesin, for asthma, 490t

H
Half-life, 61
Halogenated inhalation agents
  with asthma, 492
  effect on uteroplacental blood flow of, 27t, 29–30
  maternal and fetal effects of, 221–223, 222f, 222t–224t
  neonatal effect of, 651–652
Halothane
  effect on uterine activity and labor of, 41, 43f
  effect on uteroplacental blood flow of, 27t, 29
  efficacy of, 194
  for fetal surgery, 276–277, 276f–278f, 276t
  hypotension due to, 260
  maternal and fetal effects of, 221, 222, 222f, 223t, 224t
  minimum alveolar concentration for, 249, 251f
    for fetal surgery, 276, 276t
  in obese patients, 550
  teratogenicity of, 256, 258–259
Hand dermatitis, due to latex allergy, 566
Hb SCD (hemoglobin SC disease), 350t, 351–352
HBV (hepatitis B virus), occupational exposure to, 592t, 593
hCG (human chorionic gonadotropin), 614
HCV (hepatitis C virus), occupational exposure to, 592t, 593
Headache, postdural puncture. *See* Postdural puncture headache (PDPH)
Head-down tilt, for hypotension, 206
Head entrapment, in breech presentation, 290
Health care workers (HCWs)
  HIV in, 592–593, 592t, 593t
  latex allergy in, 564
Heart block, in fetus, 632
Heartburn, during pregnancy, 12, 392
Heart disease. *See also* Cardiac patient(s)
  congenital, 465–471
  incidence of, 455, 455f, 455t
  rheumatic, 456–465, 458t
Heart murmur, during pregnancy, 6
Heart rate
  in Apgar score, 639, 640f
  effect of exercise on, 458t
  effect of positioning on, 458f
  effect of uterine contractions on, 457f
  fetal. *See* Fetal heart rate (FHR)
  during pregnancy, 6t, 8f, 457f
Heart size, during pregnancy, 6, 6f
Heart sounds, during pregnancy, 6
Heart transplantation, pregnancy after, 477, 572–573
Heat loss, in neonate, 660
HELLP syndrome
  defined, 298t
  delivery in, 304
  pathophysiology of, 300–301, 302
Hemabate (prostaglandin $F_{2\alpha}$)
  with asthma, 491, 492
  for uterine atony, 367–369, 368t
Hematocrit
  after cesarean section, 222–223, 223t, 224t
  in preeclampsia, 299–300, 303t
  during pregnancy, 7
Hematologic abnormalities, with HIV, 586–587, 587t
Hematoma
  intraspinal, 420, 421t
  subdural, 413, 415
Hemodilution, during cesarean section, 369
Hemodynamic effects
  of β-adrenergic agonists, 326, 327f, 328f
  of laparoscopic sterilization, 240
  of magnesium sulfate, 333, 334, 334f, 335f
  of obesity, 548, 548f
  of preeclampsia, 299, 300t, 301f, 302f
  of pregnancy, 7f
Hemoglobin, during pregnancy, 7, 11t
Hemoglobin A_1, in diabetes mellitus, 500, 500f, 502, 503f
Hemoglobin C disease, 350t, 352
Hemoglobin concentration, of fetal blood, 24
Hemoglobin C trait, 350t, 352
Hemoglobin E disease, 352, 352t
Hemoglobin H disease, 349, 350t
Hemoglobinopathies, 349–352
  structural, 350–352, 350t
Hemoglobin SC disease (Hb SCD), 350t, 351–352
Hemoglobin S-high F, 350t
Hemoglobin S-β-thalassemia, 350t, 352
Hemorrhage
  due to abruptio placentae, 364–365, 364f
  antepartum, 361–366
  due to cervical and vaginal lacerations, 369
  due to cesarean section, 369
  effects of, 361, 363f
  guidelines for management of, 676, 677t
  mortality due to, 361, 362f
  after neurosurgery, 522
  due to placenta accreta, 363–364, 363f
  due to placenta previa, 361–364, 362f–364f, 362t
  postpartum, 366–370
    with asthma, 492
  due to retained placenta, 367

subarachnoid. *See* Subarachnoid hemorrhage (SAH)
  thromboelastography for, 369–370
  due to uterine atony, 367–369, 368t
  due to uterine rupture, 365–366, 366t
Heparin, 349
  fetal and neonatal effects of, 682t
  after mitral valve replacement, 476–477
  regional anesthesia with, 134
Hepatic changes, during pregnancy, 13–14
Hepatic disease, coagulation factor abnormalities in, 348–349
Hepatic function tests, during pregnancy, 13
Hepatic involvement, in pregnancy-induced hypertension, 302
Hepatic transplantation, 574
Hepatitis B virus (HBV), occupational exposure to, 592t, 593
Hepatitis C virus (HCV), occupational exposure to, 592t, 593
Hereditary angioedema, 567
Hernia, congenital diaphragmatic, 269–270, 270f, 615f
Heroin use, 602–603, 603f
Herpes simplex virus (HSV)
  with epidural morphine, 176
  with HIV, 591t
Hiatal hernias, 392
Histamine, 559
Histamine-2 (H_2) receptor antagonists
  for allergic reactions, 562
  for aspiration prevention, 239, 378, 401–402, 434
    with obesity, 553
  effect on placental drug transfer of, 62
  fetal and neonatal effects of, 686t
History, guidelines for, 673–674
HIV. *See* Human immunodeficiency virus
Hivid (zalcitabine)
  fetal and neonatal effects of, 685t
  for HIV, 590t
Horner's syndrome, 417
Hospitalization, for pregnancy-induced hypertension, 304
HSV (herpes simplex virus)
  with epidural morphine, 176
  with HIV, 591t
H_2 receptor antagonists. *See* Histamine-2 receptor antagonists
Human chorionic gonadotropin (hCG), 614
Human immunodeficiency virus (HIV), 583–593
  anesthesia with, 590–592
  cesarean section for, 588–589, 589t
  clinical diagnosis of AIDS with, 586, 587t
  drug therapy for, 584f, 589, 590t, 591f, 591t
  effect of pregnancy on, 587–588
  epidemiology and scope of, 583, 584f, 585f
  mortality from, 583, 584f
  multiorgan disease in, 586–587, 587t
  natural history of, 585–586, 587f
  neonatal and fetal effects of, 589–590
  occupational exposure to, 592–593, 592t, 593t
  opportunistic infections with, 589, 591t
  pathogenesis of, 583–586, 586f, 587f
  population at risk for, 583, 585f
  transmission by health care workers of, 592
  vertical transmission of, 588, 588f
Hunt/Hess classification, of aneurysms, 513t, 519
Hydralazine
  effect on uteroplacental blood flow of, 27t, 33, 34f, 35f
  fetal and neonatal effects of, 480, 684t
  for hypertension
    cocaine-induced, 607–609, 608f
    pregnancy-induced, 306, 313, 315t
    vasopressor-induced, 143
Hydration
  during labor, 433
  for postdural puncture headache, 213–214, 415–416
Hydronephrosis, congenital bilateral, 271–272, 272f
Hydrops fetalis, resuscitation with, 668
Hydrotherapy, 100
Hydroxyzine
  effect on uterine activity and labor of, 43
  systemic, 114
Hyoscine (scopolamine), systemic, 117
Hypercapnia
  effect on uteroplacental blood flow of, 36
  during surgery, 260
Hypercarbia, teratogenicity of, 258
Hyperemia
  after neurosurgery, 522
  transient fetal, 624
Hyperglycemia, 501–502, 504–505
Hyperkalemia, due to succinylcholine, with spinal cord injury, 539–540, 540t
Hyperreflexia, in pregnancy-induced hypertension, 302
Hypersensitivity
  delayed, 560, 560t
  immediate, 559, 560–568, 560f, 560t, 561f
Hypertension
  anesthetic considerations with, 473
  with asthma, 492
  benign intracranial, 510
  cardiovascular changes with, 472
  cesarean section with, 473
  chronic, 297, 298t
  clinical manifestations of, 472–473
  cocaine-induced, 607–609, 608f
  with diabetes mellitus, 297–298, 498, 498t
  essential, 472–473
  incidence of, 472
  with obesity, 545
  pathophysiology of, 473
  in preeclampsia, 299
  pregnancy-aggravated, 298t

Hypertension (*cont.*)
  pregnancy-induced. *See* Pregnancy-induced hypertension (PIH)
  pregnancy-induced changes in, 473
  primary pulmonary, 456t, 471–472, 472t
  transient, 298t
  vaginal delivery with, 473
  vasopressor-induced, 143
Hypertonus, uterine, 260, 260f
Hypertrophic subvalvular stenosis, idiopathic, 474–475, 475t
Hyperventilation
  effect on uteroplacental blood flow of, 36, 36f
  during labor, 3, 4f, 5f
  during neurosurgery, 516–517
  with obesity, 548
Hypnosis, 95–96
Hypocapnia
  effect on uteroplacental blood flow of, 27t, 36
  during labor, 3, 4f
  during neurosurgery, 516–517
Hypoglycemics, fetal and neonatal effects of, 686t
Hypokalemia, due to β-adrenergic agonists, 329
Hypotension
  due to combined spinal-epidural analgesia, 129, 130f, 130t, 160
  fetal effects of, 137, 139f
  due to halothane, 260
  incidence of, 205, 206f
  with multiple gestations, 294
  during neurosurgery, 517–518
  orthostatic, from opioids, 105
  physiology of, 204–205, 206f
  with preterm labor and delivery, 330, 331f–333f
  prophylactic treatment for, 205–207
  due to regional anesthesia
    for cesarean section, 204–207, 206f
      with obesity, 555
    for vaginal delivery, 136–140, 137f–141f
  supine, 8–10, 9f, 10f, 136, 137f–139f
  during surgery, 260
  volume preloading for, 137, 435–436
Hypothermia, during neurosurgery, 518
Hypoventilation
  during labor, 3, 4f, 5f
  due to obesity, 545, 546
Hypovolemic shock, in newborn, 665–666, 665f, 666t
Hypoxemia, during pregnancy, 6t
Hypoxia
  acute intrapartum, 635, 635t
  during anesthesia, 259, 259f
  effect on uteroplacental blood flow of, 36
  during labor, 3, 4f, 5
  during pregnancy, 5
  teratogenicity of, 258
Hysterotomy, 274–275, 279

I
Ibuprofen, fetal and neonatal effects of, 682t
ICP (intracranial pressure)
  increased, 415
  during neurosurgery, 516–518, 523
Idiopathic hypertrophic subvalvular stenosis, 474–475, 475t
Idiopathic polyneuritis, 534–535, 534f
Idiopathic thrombocytopenic purpura (ITP), 347–348
IgA (immunoglobulin A) deficiency, 567
IgE (immunoglobulin E), 559
IgG (immunoglobulin G), 559
IgM (immunoglobulin M), 559
Imipramine, teratogenicity of, 252
Imitrex (sumatriptan succinate), for postdural puncture headache, 416
Immediate hypersensitivity, 559, 560–568, 560f, 560t, 561f
Immune complex diseases, 559–560, 560t, 568–572
Immune globulins, placental transport of, 21
Immune mechanisms, of tissue injury, 559–560, 560t
Immune response
  type I, 559, 560–568, 560t
  type II, 559, 560t, 568
  type III, 559–560, 560t
  type IV, 560, 560t
Immune system, 559–560, 560f, 560t, 561f
Immunoglobulin A (IgA) deficiency, 567
Immunoglobulin E (IgE), 559
Immunoglobulin G (IgG), 559
Immunoglobulin M (IgM), 559
Immunosuppressants, 576–577, 577t
IM (intramuscular) sedation, maternal mortality with, 431f
Indinavir sulfate (Crixivan)
  fetal and neonatal effects of, 685t
  for HIV, 590t
Indomethacin
  fetal and neonatal effects of, 682t
  after fetal surgery, 280
  for preterm labor, 335–336
Induction agents
  allergic reactions to, 563
  effect on uteroplacental blood flow of, 26–29, 27t, 28f, 29f
  for postpartum sterilization, 242
Infection(s)
  with diabetes mellitus, 499
  due to regional anesthesia, 414, 422–424, 423t
Inferior vena cava occlusion
  during pregnancy, 8–10, 9f, 10f, 249, 254f
  prevention of, 138
  regional anesthesia and, 136, 137f–139f
Informed consent, 443–444, 449–450

Inhalation analgesia/anesthesia, 189–196
  with anesthetic machine, 191, 192t
  cardiovascular effects of, 195
  consciousness with, 194–195
  current use of, 189, 191t
  draw-over, 193
  effect on uterine activity and labor of, 41, 43f, 46t
  effect on uteroplacental blood flow of, 27t, 29–30, 30f
  with Entonox, 191–192, 192f, 192t, 193, 193f
  environmental considerations with, 196
  equipment and methods of administration for, 191, 192f, 192t, 193f
  history of, 189, 190f
  indications for, 189
  intermittent, 192–193, 192f, 192t, 193f
  maternal effects of, 190–191, 193–195, 194f
  with mitral insufficiency, 461
  with mitral valve prolapse, 462
  neonatal effects of, 191, 195–196, 195f
  nitrous oxide for
    efficacy of, 193–194, 194f
    reported use of, 189, 191t
    technique of, 191–192, 192f
  with obesity, 550–551, 551f
  oxygenation with, 195
  for postpartum sterilization, 243
  principles of, 189–191, 191f
  uterine relaxation with, 195
  for vaginal delivery, 189, 191t
  volatile agents for, 193, 193f, 194
Injuries
  events leading to, 448–449, 448t, 449t
  newborn brain, 448
  obstetric anesthesia-related, 446–448, 447t, 448t
Inotropes, fetal effect of, 479–480
Inspiratory capacity
  with obesity, 547
  during pregnancy, 4t, 5f, 251f
Inspiratory reserve volume, during pregnancy, 5f
Insulin, fetal and neonatal effects of, 686t
Insulin sensitivity, during pregnancy, 14
Insulin therapy
  for diabetes mellitus, 500, 500f, 500t
  during labor or before cesarean section, 501–502
Intercristal line, 418–419, 419f
Interlocking twins, 293, 294f
Internal podalic version, 288, 288f, 294
Interspinous ligament, 125f
Intervillous space, circulatory pathways at, 65, 66f
Intraabdominal pressure, during pregnancy, 392, 394f
Intracranial aneurysms, 511, 512–513, 513f, 513t, 514f
Intracranial hypertension, benign, 510
Intracranial pressure (ICP)
  increased, 415
  during neurosurgery, 516–518, 523
Intracranial tumors, 509–510
Intradermal test, 566, 566t
Intragastric pressure, during pregnancy, 392, 394f
Intramuscular (IM) sedation, maternal mortality with, 431f
Intraspinal anesthesia. *See* Spinal anesthesia
Intraspinal opioids, 155–180
  complications of, 174–180
  effect on uteroplacental blood flow of, 27t, 35
  guidelines for, 675
  for labor and delivery, 155–162
  local anesthetics with, 163–168
  neonatal effects of, 178–179, 651
  pharmacology of, 149–153
  for postoperative pain management, 168–174
  progress in labor with, 162–163, 162t, 163f, 164f
Intrathecal anesthesia
  bupivacaine for, 52, 53, 84
  for cesarean section, 74
  effect on uterine activity and labor of, 52–53, 52t, 53f
  epinephrine with, 52, 87–88, 88f
  ropivacaine for, 86
Intrathecal injection, inadvertent, 79
Intrathecal opioids
  complications of, 174–180
  for labor and delivery, 155–157, 156f, 157f, 157t
  monitoring of, 179
  for postoperative pain management, 170–173, 172f, 173f, 173t
  progress in labor with, 162
Intrathecal space, transfer of drugs to, 152, 152f
Intrauterine growth restriction (IUGR)
  with diabetes mellitus, 500
  evaluation of, 615
Intrauterine intervention. *See* Fetal surgery
Intrauterine pressure catheter (IUPC), 41, 42f
Intravascular injection, accidental, 418
Intravenous analgesics. *See* Systemic medication(s)
Intravenous drug users (IVDUs), 603–604, 603t
Intravenous fluid preload, and hypotension, 137, 434–435
Intravenous fluids, for pregnancy-induced hypertension, 308
Intravenous injection, toxic, 418
Intravenous sedation, maternal mortality with, 431f
Intravenous sets, with latex allergy, 565t
Intrinsic maternal obstetric palsy, 410–413, 411f, 412f
Intubation, failed, 215–216, 216f, 217f
  maternal mortality due to, 434, 434t
Invirase (saquinavir mesylate)
  fetal and neonatal effects of, 685t
  for HIV, 590t
In vitro testing, for allergies, 566–567
"Ion trapping," 64, 65f
Iron, placental transport of, 21

Irritant dermatitis, due to latex allergy, 566
Isoflurane
  in breast milk, 244
  effect on uterine activity and labor of, 41, 43f
  effect on uteroplacental blood flow of, 27t, 29, 30f
  efficacy of, 194
  with Entonox, 193, 193f
  for fetal surgery, 276, 277f
  maternal and fetal effects of, 221, 222, 224t
  during neurosurgery, 517
  in obese patients, 550, 551f
  teratogenicity of, 256
Isomers, 84
Isoproterenol
  for amniotic fluid embolism, 358t
  effect on uteroplacental blood flow of, 27t
  fetal effects of, 479
  test dose of, 136
Isoxsuprine, effect on uteroplacental blood flow of, 32
ITP (idiopathic thrombocytopenic purpura), 347–348
IUGR (intrauterine growth restriction)
  with diabetes mellitus, 500
  evaluation of, 615
IUPC (intrauterine pressure catheter), 41, 42f
IV. *See* Intravenous
IVDUs (intravenous drug users), 603–604, 603t

K
Kallikrein, 346
Ketamine
  with asthma, 492
  effect on uterine activity and labor of, 43
  effect on uteroplacental blood flow of, 27t, 29
  for failed regional block, 213
  for inadequate or failed epidural analgesia, 144
  maternal and fetal effects of, 219–220
  neonatal effect of, 651
  with placenta previa, 361
  with pregnancy-induced hypertension, 314
  systemic, 116–117, 117f, 117t
  uterine hypertonus due to, 260, 260f
Ketoacidosis, diabetic, 497
Ketoprofen, fetal and neonatal effects of, 682t
Ketorolac, fetal and neonatal effects of, 682t
Kidney failure, complications with, 575, 575t
Kidney function, in pregnancy-induced hypertension, 301–302
Kidneys, in progressive systemic sclerosis, 571
Kidney transplantation, 574–575, 575t
Klikovich, Stanisav, 189, 190f
Klonopin (clonazepam), for seizures, 532t

L
Labetalol hydrochloride
  effect on uteroplacental blood flow of, 27t, 34
  fetal effects of, 479
  for hypertension
    pregnancy-induced, 306, 313, 314f, 315t
    vasopressor-induced, 143
Labor
  Active Management of, 41
  combined spinal-epidural analgesia for, 158–162, 158f–161f, 159t, 161t, 162, 162t
  drug effects on, 41–54
    with inhalation agents, 41, 43f
    with intrathecal and combined spinal-epidural analgesia, 52–53, 52t, 53f
    with parenteral agents, 43–44, 43f
    with regional anesthesia, 44–52, 44f, 45t, 46t, 47f, 48t
  epidural opioids for, 162–163, 162t, 163f, 163t, 164f
  first stage of, 41
    effect of regional anesthesia on, 44–47, 45t, 46t, 47f
  intrathecal opioids for, 155–156, 156f, 157f, 157t, 162
  maternal position during, 100
  progress of, 41, 42f
  prolonged, 41, 42t
  second stage of, 41
    effect of regional anesthesia on, 45t, 46t, 47–52, 48t, 49t, 50f, 51t
    prolonged, 48t
  third stage of, 41
Lactate
  in hyperglycemia, 501–502
  placental transfer of, 26
Lamaze method, 96–97
Lamivudine (3TC, Epivir)
  fetal and neonatal effects of, 685t
  for HIV, 590t
Landry-Guillain-Barré syndrome (LGBS), 534–535, 534f
Lansoprazole, for aspiration prophylaxis, 402
Laparoscopic sterilization
  breast-feeding after, 243–244, 244t
  complications of, 240
  general anesthesia for, 242–243, 242t, 243t
  local anesthesia for, 240, 240f
  physiologic changes induced by, 239–240
  regional anesthesia for, 240–242, 241f, 241t, 242t
  tubal ligation *vs.*, 237–238
Laparoscopic surgery, during pregnancy, 261
Laryngeal edema, in preeclampsia, 301
Laryngeal joint, rheumatoid arthritis of, 568
Laryngeal mask airway (LMA), 384
  and aspiration, 399–400, 400f
  and cricoid pressure, 384–385, 385f, 385t
  for failed intubation, 216, 381
  for newborn, 662
  with obesity, 554
  ProSeal, 381, 386

Laryngopathia gravidarum, 567
Laryngoscopic line of vision, 376, 377f
Laryngoscopic view classification, 376, 376f
Laryngoscopy
  best attempt at, 379–381
  failed, 215–216, 216f, 217f, 379–381, 380f, 434
  fiberoptic, 381, 383–384, 384f
  of newborn, 662, 662f
  in obese patient, 549, 549f, 554, 554f
Larynx, topical anesthesia/nerve blocks of, 383, 383f
Late decelerations, 625t, 629t, 630–631, 630f
Latex allergy, 564–566, 564t, 565t
Lawsuits
  closed claims analysis of, 446–451, 447f, 447t–450t
  general considerations and recommendations on, 441–445
Lecithin/sphingomyelin (L/S) ratio, 616
  with diabetes mellitus, 501f
Left-to-right shunt, 465–468
Left uterine displacement (LUD), for aortocaval compression, 10, 139
Left ventricular change, during pregnancy, 7f
Left ventricular failure
  due to aortic insufficiency, 463
  in cardiomyopathy of pregnancy, 473–474
  due to mitral insufficiency, 460
Left ventricular stroke work index, in preeclampsia, 300t, 302f
Legal issues. See Lawsuits
Leg wrapping, for hypotension, 207
LESP (lower esophageal sphincter pressure), 378
LES (lower esophageal sphincter) tone
  with laryngeal mask or face mask, 385
  and risk of aspiration, 392
Leukocyte levels, during pregnancy, 11
Leukotriene(s), in amniotic fluid embolism, 357
Leukotriene modifiers, for asthma, 489
Levobupivacaine (Chirocaine), 86–87
  vs. bupivacaine, 86–87
  for combined spinal-epidural analgesia, 129
  current usage of, 87
  fetal distribution of, 67f, 68
Levorotatory enantiomers, 84
Levothyroxine, fetal and neonatal effects of, 686t
LGBS (Landry-Guillain-Barré syndrome), 534–535, 534f
LHR (lung-to-head ratio), 270
Librium (chlordiazepoxide), teratogenicity of, 253
Lidocaine (Xylocaine), 77–81
  alkalinization of, 210, 210f
  with asthma, 492
  background of, 77
  carbonated, 81, 87
  for cesarean section, 205t, 208, 209
    emergency, 227, 227t
  chemical structure of, 74f
  current usage of, 80–81
  effect on first stage of labor of, 45
  effect on preterm fetus of, 338–339, 338f, 339f
  effect on second stage of labor of, 48, 50
  effect on uteroplacental blood flow of, 27t, 30
  with epilepsy, 533
  epinephrine with, 87–88, 88f
  fetal effects of, 478
  fetal uptake of, 64, 65, 65f, 66
  for lumbar epidural anesthesia, 126, 127t
  neonatal effects of, 650, 651
  pharmacokinetics of, 68, 68t, 153t
  placental transfer of, 61–62, 63, 63f, 64f, 77
  for postpartum sterilization, 241, 242
  for pudendal block, 133
  reduced requirement for, 435
  for spinal anesthesia, 128, 128t
  teratogenicity of, 256, 259
  test dose of, 134, 136
  for topical anesthesia
    of larynx and trachea, 383
    of mouth, 382
    of nose, 382
  toxicity of
    major, 77–79, 77f, 78f, 78t, 79t
    minor, 79–80, 79t, 80t, 242
Lie, defined, 287
Ligamentum flavum, 125f
Line of vision (LOV), 376, 377f
Lipophilicity, and rate of transfer across arachnoid membrane, 152, 152f
β-Lipotropin, 150t
Lithium, fetal and neonatal effects of, 683t
Litigation. See Lawsuits
Liver disease, coagulation factor abnormalities in, 348–349
Liver function tests, during pregnancy, 13
Liver transplantation, 574
LMA. See Laryngeal mask airway (LMA)
LMWH (low-molecular weight heparin)
  fetal and neonatal effects of, 682t
  regional anesthesia with, 134
Local anesthetics, 73–88
  adjuvants to, 87–88
  alkalinization of, 210, 210f
  allergic reactions to, 563, 563t
  amide-linked agents, 74f, 77–84
  bupivacaine, 74f, 81–84, 82t, 83f
  chiral compounds, 84–87
  chloroprocaine, 74f, 75–76, 75f, 75t, 76t
  cocaine, 74f
  for continuous spinal anesthesia, 74
  effect on first stage of labor of, 45
  effect on second stage of labor of, 50
  effect on uteroplacental blood flow of, 27t, 30–31, 30f, 31f

enhanced action of, 417–418
for epidural analgesia, 74
with epidural morphine, 173–174
epinephrine with, 87–88, 88f
ester-linked agents, 74–77, 74f
etidocaine, 74f
for intrathecal analgesia, 73
for labor analgesia, 73, 74t
levobupivacaine, 86–87
lidocaine, 74f, 77–81, 77f, 78f, 78t–80t
  carbonated, 81, 87
and lipid-soluble opioids, 163–168, 164f–166f, 166t, 167t
maternal mortality due to, 436–437
meperidine with, 88
mepivacaine, 74f, 81
with obesity, 552–553
for operative delivery, 73
piperocaine, 76
for postpartum sterilization, 240, 240f
prilocaine, 74f, 81
procaine, 74f, 76
requirements of, 73, 74t
ropivacaine, 74f, 84–86, 85f
sodium bicarbonate with, 87
for subarachnoid block, 73–74
tetracaine, 74f, 76–77
toxicity of, 436–437, 449
  in neonate, 668
Lorazepam
  in breast milk, 244
  chemical structure of, 114t
  systemic, 115
Loss-of-resistance test (LORT), 420
LOV (line of vision), 376, 377f
Low-birth-weight infants, 323, 643–645, 644f, 645f
Lower esophageal sphincter pressure (LESP), 378
Lower esophageal sphincter (LES) tone
  with laryngeal mask or face mask, 385
  and risk of aspiration, 392
Low-molecular weight heparin (LMWH)
  fetal and neonatal effects of, 682t
  regional anesthesia with, 134
L/S (lecithin/sphingomyelin) ratio, 616
  with diabetes mellitus, 501f
LUD (left uterine displacement), for aortocaval compression, 10, 139
Lumbar epidural anesthesia/analgesia
  continuous infusion, 126–128, 127t
  drug regimens for, 127t
  movement of drug after injection in, 152–153, 152f
  needle placement for, 125f
  positioning for, 125f, 126f
  with pregnancy-induced hypertension, 309–310, 309f, 310f
  technique of, 123–126, 125f, 126f, 127f
  timing of, 123–124
Lumbar lordosis, 435
Lumbar sympathetic block, 133
Lumbosacral cord, innervation of, 411f
Lumbosacral spine, schematic diagram of, 125f
Luminal (phenobarbital)
  fetal and neonatal effects of, 683t
  for seizures, 532, 532t, 533
  teratogenicity of, 252
Lung capacities, during pregnancy, 3, 5f
Lung compliance, during pregnancy, 4t
Lung inflation, during resuscitation, 657, 658f
Lung maturity, 616–617
Lung-to-head ratio (LHR), 270
Lung transplantation, 573–574
Lung volumes
  with obesity, 547–548, 547f, 548f
  during pregnancy, 3, 5f, 251f
Lupus erythematosus, 570–571

M
MAC (minimum alveolar concentration)
  for fetal surgery, 276, 276f
  during pregnancy, 5, 11, 243, 249f, 251f
MAC (monitored anesthetic care)
  for complicated vaginal delivery, 676
  for interventional neuroradiology, 515–516
Macrolides, fetal and neonatal effects of, 684t
Macrosomia, 499–500, 501
  evaluation of, 615
  with obesity, 545–546
Magnesium sulfate
  anesthetic considerations with, 333–334, 334f
  for closure of hysterotomy, 274, 279–280
  for eclampsia, 307
  effect on uterine activity and labor of, 43f
  effect on uteroplacental blood flow of, 27t, 34–35
  gastric emptying with, 392
  mechanism of action of, 331
  newborn intoxication with, 668
  for pregnancy-induced hypertension, 304–306, 304t, 305f
  for preterm labor, 325t, 331–334, 333t, 334f, 335f
  side effects of, 332–333, 334f
Mallampati classification, 375–376, 376f
Malpractice
  amount of damages/awards for, 441, 450, 450t
  avoidance of, 442–444
  closed claims analysis of, 446–451, 447f, 447t–450t
  filing limit for, 441
  general considerations and recommendations on, 441–445
  standards for, 441–442
  trends in, 444–445

Mandibular space, examination of, 376, 377f
Mannitol, during neurosurgery, 517
MAP (mean arterial pressure)
  in preeclampsia, 300t
  during pregnancy, 6t
Marcaine. See Bupivacaine (Sensorcaine)
Marijuana, 609
Mask ventilation. See also Laryngeal mask airway (LMA)
  "best attempt," 381
  of newborn, 661–662, 661f
Mastocytosis, systemic, 568
Maternal awareness, during general anesthesia, 223, 224t
Maternal effects
  of etomidate, 220
  of general anesthesia, 217–223
  of halogenated inhalation agents, 221–223, 222f, 222t–224t
  of inhalation analgesia/anesthesia, 190–191, 193–195, 194f
  of muscle relaxants, 220–221, 221t
  of nitrous oxide, 193–195, 221
Maternal mortality, 429–437
  from cardiovascular collapse, 435–436
  causes of, 430–431, 430f, 431t, 432, 432t, 433–437
  classification of, 429, 430t
  with diabetes mellitus, 498
  epidemiology of, 429–432, 430f, 430t–432t, 431f, 446, 447t
  with general anesthesia, 431–432, 431f, 432t, 433–434, 433f, 434f
  from inability to intubate trachea, 434, 434t
  lawsuits on, 446, 447f, 448t
  from local anesthetic toxicity, 436–437
  with obesity, 546–547
  from pulmonary aspiration of gastric contents, 433–434, 433f
  with regional anesthesia, 431–432, 431f, 432t, 435–436
  from unrecognized events, 437
Maternal mortality rate, 429
Maternal serum alpha-fetoprotein (MSAFP), 613, 614t
Maternal serum triple marker screening, 613–614, 614t
Maximum breathing capacity, during pregnancy, 4t
McGill Pain Questionnaire, 96f
McRobert's maneuver, 292, 292f
Mean arterial pressure (MAP)
  in preeclampsia, 300t
  during pregnancy, 6t
Meconium, suctioning of, 666–668, 667f
Medical Injury Compensation Reform Act (MICRA), 441
Medications. See Drug(s)
Mendelson's syndrome, 395, 397f, 433
Meningiomas, 509
Meningitis, due to regional anesthesia, 414, 422, 423t
Meperidine (Demerol), 88
  and autonomic hyperreflexia, 541, 541f
  and breast-feeding, 110, 243
  with bupivacaine, 166
  cesarean section rate with, 49, 49t, 50
  dosage of, 105
  drug-delivery interval for, 106–109, 109f
  effect on fetal heart rate of, 106, 108f
  effect on first stage of labor of, 45, 46t
  effect on second stage of labor of, 46t, 49, 49t, 50
  effect on uterine activity of, 43, 43f, 106, 108f
  epidural, 163
    for postoperative pain, 169–170
  gastric emptying with, 239, 391
  half-life of, 106
  intramuscular vs. intravenous, 105, 107f
  intrathecal, for postoperative pain, 173, 173t
  neonatal effects of, 106–110, 108f–110f, 650, 651
  pharmacokinetics of, 105–106, 107f, 153t
  plasma levels of, 106, 107f
  with pregnancy-induced hypertension, 309
  systemic, 105–110, 106f–110f, 106t, 113f
  teratogenicity of, 253
  toxicity of, 88
Mephentermine
  effect on uteroplacental blood flow of, 33f
  for hypotension, in preterm labor and delivery, 332f
Mepivacaine (Carbocaine), 81
  chemical structure of, 74f
  effect on uteroplacental blood flow of, 30, 30f
  fetal uptake of, 64
  neonatal effects of, 650
  pharmacokinetics of, 81
  placental transfer of, 61, 63, 63f, 77
  for pudendal block, 133
  transient neurologic symptoms with, 81
Meprobamate (Equanil, Miltown), teratogenicity of, 253
Metabolic acidosis, in newborn, 664–665
Metabolic alkalosis, effect on uteroplacental blood flow of, 36
Metabolic effects, of β-adrenergic agonists, 327f, 329, 329f
Metaraminol
  effect on fetus of, 479
  effect on uteroplacental blood flow of, 33f
  for mitral stenosis, 459
Methadone, 604
  pharmacokinetics of, 153t
  teratogenicity of, 252
Methamphetamine abuse, 603f, 606–607
Methergine (methylergonovine)
  for abruptio placentae, 365
  for uterine atony, 367, 368f
Methotrexate, for immunosuppression, 577
Methoxamine (Vasoxyl)
  effect on fetus of, 479
  effect on first stage of labor of, 47, 47f
Methoxyflurane (Penthrane)
  Cardiff inhaler for, 193

Methoxyflurane (Penthrane) (*cont.*)
 effect on uterine activity and labor of, 43f
 efficacy of, 194
 in obese patients, 550
 teratogenicity of, 256
Methyldopa, fetal and neonatal effects of, 684t
Methylergonovine (Methergine)
 for abruptio placentae, 365
 for uterine atony, 367, 368t
Methylxanthines, for postdural puncture headache, 416
Metoclopramide
 for aspiration prevention, 239, 378, 402, 434
 fetal and neonatal effects of, 683t
 with general anesthesia, 215
 for nausea and vomiting, 177
 with obesity, 554
Metoprolol, for pregnancy-induced hypertension, 306
Metycaine (piperocaine), 76
MICRA (Medical Injury Compensation Reform Act), 441
Midazolam
 in breast milk, 244
 with cesarean section, 203, 214
 chemical structure of, 114t
 for eclampsia, 307
 for fetal surgery, 273
 systemic, 115
Milrinone, effect on fetus of, 479–480
Miltown (meprobamate), teratogenicity of, 253
Minimum alveolar concentration (MAC)
 for fetal surgery, 276, 276f
 during pregnancy, 5, 11, 243, 249f, 251f
Minimum local analgesic concentration (MLAC), of
 ropivacaine *vs.* bupivacaine, 85, 85f, 86
Minute ventilation, during pregnancy, 3, 4t, 249, 250f, 251f
Mitral insufficiency, 456t, 460–461, 460f, 461t
Mitral stenosis, 456–460
 anesthetic considerations with, 458–460, 459f, 459t
 clinical manifestations of, 457
 pathophysiology of, 457–458, 459f
 pregnancy-induced changes in, 458
 pulmonary capillary wedge pressure in, 459f
Mitral valve prolapse (MVP), 461–462, 462t
Mitral valve replacement, pregnancy after, 476–477, 476t
Mitral valvulotomy, pregnancy after, 476, 476t
Mivacurium, for postpartum sterilization, 242
MLAC (minimum local analgesic concentration), of
 ropivacaine *vs.* bupivacaine, 85, 85f, 86
Monitored anesthetic care
 for complicated vaginal delivery, 676
 for interventional neuroradiology, 515–516
Monitoring
 cardiac patient, 455–456
 epidural and intrathecal opioids, 179
 fetal. *See* Fetal heart rate (FHR) monitoring
 during neurosurgery, 520, 520f
 obese patient, 551–552
 patent ductus arteriosus, 467–468
 pregnancy-induced hypertension, 307–308, 308t, 310–311
 with progressive systemic sclerosis, 572
Montevideo units, 41
Moro reflex, 647, 647f, 650f
Morphine
 in breast milk, 243
 with bupivacaine, 166
 for cesarean section, 205t, 209, 211, 211f
 for continuous spinal anesthesia, 128t
 effect on uterine activity and labor of, 43
 effect on uteroplacental blood flow of, 35
 epidural
  for cesarean section, 211, 211f
  herpes simplex virus with, 176
  for labor and delivery, 162–163, 163f, 163t
  local anesthetic with, 173–174
  for postoperative pain, 168–169, 168f, 169t, 170, 170t
  respiratory depression due to, 175–176, 176f
 intrathecal, 52
  for labor and delivery, 155–156, 156f, 157f, 157t
  neonatal effects of, 179
  for postoperative pain, 171–172, 172f, 173, 173f, 173t
  progress in labor with, 162
  respiratory depression due to, 175, 175f
 neonatal effects of, 651
 pharmacokinetics of, 152, 153, 153t
 systemic, 106f, 113, 113f
 teratogenicity of, 253
 transfer across arachnoid membrane of, 152
Motor tracts, 124f
Mouth, topical anesthesia/nerve blocks of, 382–383
MSAFP (maternal serum alpha-fetoprotein), 613, 614t
Multiple gestations, 293–294, 294f, 294t
Multiple sclerosis (MS), 535–536, 536f, 536t
Muscarinic receptors, 150
Muscle fasciculations, and aspiration, 398
Muscle relaxants
 allergic reactions to, 563
 magnesium sulfate and, 305, 305f, 334
 maternal and fetal effects of, 220–221, 221t
 with obesity, 551, 551f
 for postpartum sterilization, 242–243, 243t
 teratogenicity of, 256
Muscle tone, in Apgar score, 639, 640f
MVP (mitral valve prolapse), 461–462, 462t
Myasthenia gravis, 537–539, 537t–539t
Mycobacterium avium complex, with HIV, 591t
Myocardial effects, of β-adrenergic agonists, 328–329
Myocardial thickness, during pregnancy, 7f
Myotonia atrophica, 529

Myotonia congenita, 529
Myotonic dystrophy, 529
Myotonic syndromes, 529–530, 530f, 530t
Mysoline (primidone), for seizures, 532t

N
N$_2$O. *See* Nitrous oxide
NACS (Neurologic and Adaptive Capacity Score), 647–648,
 647f–650f
NAIT (neonatal alloimmune thrombocytopenia), 348
Nalbuphine
 for pruritus, 176
 systemic, 115–116, 115f
Naloxone
 before delivery, 117–118
 for drowsiness/dizziness, 178t
 for high cervical blocks with CSE anesthesia, 160
 for nausea and vomiting, 171t, 178t
 in neonatal resuscitation, 112, 112t, 650, 651, 666t, 668
 with opiate addiction, 604
 for pruritus, 156, 171t, 176, 178t
 for respiratory depression, 171t
 side effects and use of, 177–178, 178f, 178t
Naltrexone, for pruritus, 178
Naproxen, fetal and neonatal effects of, 682t
Naropin. *See* Ropivacaine
NASAs, fetal and neonatal effects of, 683t
Nasopharynx, topical anesthesia/nerve blocks of, 382
National Pregnancy Mortality Surveillance System, 429, 430
Natural childbirth, 96
Nausea and vomiting
 due to combined spinal-epidural analgesia, 129, 130t, 174f
 due to epidural analgesia, 171t, 174f
 naloxone for, 171t, 178t
 from opioids, 105, 177
 prevention of, 433
NBAS (Neonatal Behavioral Assessment Scale), 646
NDRIs, fetal and neonatal effects of, 683t
Neck mobility, 376, 377f
Neck muscles, in newborn, 647, 647f, 648f
Needle(s), trauma due to, 418–419
Needle size, and postdural puncture headache, 207–208, 208f,
 242, 242t, 415
Negligence, 442
Nelfinavir mesylate (Viracept)
 fetal and neonatal effects of, 685t
 for HIV, 590t
Neonatal alloimmune thrombocytopenia (NAIT), 348
Neonatal Behavioral Assessment Scale (NBAS), 646
Neonatal depression
 Apgar score and, 640–641, 640f
 causes of, 657–658, 659t
 with halogenated agents, 223
 with magnesium, 305
 with meperidine, 106–110, 108f–110f
Neonatal effects
 of ACE inhibitors, 684t
 of acetaminophen, 682t
 of acyclovir, 685t
 of α$_2$-adrenergic agonists, 684t
 of aminoglycosides, 684t
 of amphetamine abuse, 607
 of analgesics, 682t
 of antibiotics, 684t–685t
 of anticholinergic therapy, 682t
 of anticoagulants, 682t
 of anticonvulsant therapy, 683t
 of antidepressants, 683t
 of antiemetics, 683t
 of antifungals, 685t
 of antihypertensive agents, 684t
 of antimicrobials, 684t–685t
 of antiretroviral drugs, 589–590, 685t
 of antivirals, 685t
 of anxiolytics, 685t
 of aspirin, 682t
 of atropine, 682t
 of benzodiazepines, 685t
 of beta-blockers, 684t
 of bronchodilators, 686t
 of bupivacaine, 650, 651
 of calcium channel blockers, 684t
 of carbamazepine, 683t
 of cephalosporins, 684t
 of chloroprocaine, 650, 651
 of cimetidine, 686t
 of clonidine, 684t
 of CNS depressants, 649–650
 of cocaine abuse, 605–606, 606f, 606t, 607f
 of corticosteroids, 489, 686t
 of Coumadin, 682t
 of diphenhydramine, 683t
 of diuretics, 684t
 of droperidol, 683t
 of drugs used in postpartum sterilization, 243–244, 244t
 of epidural analgesia/anesthesia, 650–651
 of epinephrine, 651
 of etidocaine, 651
 of fentanyl, 110–112, 111f, 112t, 179, 650, 651
 of fluconazole, 685t
 of fluoroquinolones, 684t
 of furosemide, 684t
 of general anesthesia, 651–652
 of glycopyrrolate, 682t
 of halogenated inhalation agents, 651–652
 of heparin, 682t
 of histamine-2 (H$_2$) receptor antagonists, 686t

 of hydralazine, 480, 684t
 of hypoglycemics, 686t
 of ibuprofen, 682t
 of indomethacin, 682t
 of inhalation agents, 191, 195–196, 195f
 of insulin, 686t
 of ketamine, 651
 of ketoprofen, 682t
 of ketorolac, 682t
 of levobupivacaine, 651
 of lidocaine, 650, 651
 of lithium, 683t
 of macrolides, 684t
 of maternally administered drugs, 681–686
 of meperidine, 650, 651
 of mepivacaine, 650
 of methyldopa, 684t
 of metoclopramide, 683t
 of morphine, 179, 651
 of naproxen, 682t
 of nitrous oxide, 195, 195f, 651
 of omeprazole, 686t
 of ondansetron, 683t
 of opioids, 668, 682t
  in drug abuse, 603, 604t
  intraspinal, 178–179, 651
  systemic, 649–650
 of paracervical block, 651
 of penicillins, 685t
 of phenobarbital, 683t
 of phenytoin, 683t
 of pregnancy-induced hypertension, 314
 of prochlorperazine, 683t
 of promethazine, 683t
 of pudendal block, 651
 of spinal anesthesia, 178–180, 651
 of sufentanil, 179
 of sulfonamides, 685t
 of systemic medication, 649–650
 of tetracyclines, 685t
 of thiopental, 651
 of thyroid agents, 686t
 of valproic acid, 683t
 of vasodilators, 684t
Neonatal evaluation, 639–652
 Apgar score in, 639–642, 640f, 641f
 after cesarean section, 223–225, 224t, 225t
 continued observation in, 643, 644f
 in delivery room, 639–642, 640f–643f
 general examination in, 643
 at later point, 643–648
 of neurobehavioral abnormalities
  due to anesthesia, 648–652
  significance of, 652
  testing for, 645–648, 646f–650f
 for neurological injury, 642, 642f, 643f
 of weight and gestational age, 643–645, 644f, 645f
Neonatal mortality, Apgar score and, 641, 641f
Neonatal myasthenia gravis, 539, 539t
Neonatal resuscitation, 657–669
 airway in, 660–661, 661f
 Apgar score and, 640–641, 640f, 659
 bag and mask ventilation in, 661–662, 661f
 chest compressions in, 662–663, 663f
 correction of acidosis in, 664–665
 endotracheal intubation in, 662, 662f, 662t, 663f
 epinephrine in, 663, 664f
 equipment for, 660, 660t
 goals of, 658–659
 with hydrops fetalis, 668
 for local anesthetic toxicity, 668
 lung inflation during, 657, 658f
 for magnesium intoxication, 668
 with major anomalies, 668
 medications for, 666t
 for opioid depression, 668
 overview of, 669t
 personnel for, 660
 with placenta previa, 362
 for pneumothorax, 668
 of premature infant, 668
 respiration in, 657, 658f, 661–662, 661f–663f, 662t
 special problems in, 666–668
 thermal management in, 660
 tracheal suctioning in, 660–661, 661f, 666–668, 667f
 treatment of shock in, 665–666, 665f, 666t
 umbilical vessel catheterization in, 663–664, 664f
 when to stop efforts at, 666
Neonate
 brain injury of, lawsuits on, 447t, 448, 448t
 circulatory changes in, 657, 658f
 continued observation of, 643, 644f
 general examination of, 643
 neurobehavioral abnormalities in
  due to anesthesia, 648–652
  significance of, 652
  testing for, 645–648, 646f–650f
 neurological injury in, 642, 642f, 643f
 thermal management of, 660
 weight and gestational age of, 643–645, 644f, 645f
Neostigmine methylsulfate (Prostigmin), 150
 for myasthenia gravis, 539t
Neostigmine methylsulfate (Prostigmin) test, for myasthenia
 gravis, 537, 539t
Neo-Synephrine
 effect on first stage of labor of, 47
 for topical anesthesia of nose, 382

Nephritis, lupus, 570
Nerve injuries
    central vs. peripheral, 412f
    lawsuits on, 447t–449t, 449
Nervous system, during pregnancy, 11–12, 11f
Nesacaine. See Chloroprocaine
Neural blockade, prolonged, 417
Neural compression injury, preexisting, 410
Neural tube defect screening, 613, 614t
Neuraxial anesthesia, with asthma, 491, 941f
Neurobehavioral abnormalities, neonatal
    due to anesthesia, 648–652
    significance of, 652
    testing for, 645–648, 646f–650f
Neurobehavioral examination, after cesarean section, 225
Neurofibromatosis, 533–534, 533f
Neurological injury, neonatal, 642, 642f, 643f
Neurologic and Adaptive Capacity Score (NACS), 647–648,
    647f–650f
Neurologic complications
    of HIV, 586, 587t
    of regional anesthesia, 409–424, 410f, 411t
        due to chemical contaminants, 420–422, 422t
        chronic, 418–422
        cortical vein thrombosis, 414–415
        enhanced local anesthetic action, 417–418
        iatrogenic trauma, 418–419, 419f, 420
        incidence of, 410, 411t
        increased intracranial pressure, 415
        infection, 414, 422–424, 423t
        intrinsic maternal obstetric palsy, 410–413, 411f, 412f
        postdural puncture headache, 414, 414t, 415–417, 416f
        postpartum backache, 413–414
        pressure sores, 413
        shivering, 417
        subarachnoid hemorrhage, 415
        subdural hematoma, 415
        trends in practice and, 423–424
        vascular, 415, 419–420, 421f, 421t
Neuromuscular disorders, 529–541
    epilepsy, 530–533, 531t, 532f, 532t
    Landry-Guillain-Barré syndrome, 534–535, 534f
    multiple sclerosis, 535–536, 536f, 536t
    myasthenia gravis, 537–539, 537t–539t
    myotonic syndromes, 529–530, 530f, 530t
    neurofibromatosis, 533–534, 533f
    spinal cord injury, 539–541, 540f, 540t, 541f, 541t
Neuroradiology, interventional, 515–516
Neurosurgery, 509–524
    anesthetic management for, 516, 519–522
    for arteriovenous malformations, 511–512, 511f, 513–514,
        513f, 514f
    blood and fluid therapy during, 518–519
    brain protection during, 518
    for central venous thrombosis, 512t, 514
    interventional neuroradiology for, 515–516
    for intracranial aneurysms, 511, 512–513, 513f, 513t, 514f
    intracranial pressure during, 516–518
    for intracranial tumors, 509–510
    monitoring during, 520, 520f
    postoperative management after, 521–522
    preoperative evaluation for, 519–520, 519t
    for pseudotumor cerebri, 510
    for seizures, 510
    for stroke, 510–511, 511f, 512t, 513f, 513t
    for subarachnoid hemorrhage, 511–515, 514f
Neurosurgical diseases, obstetrical management with,
    522–524, 522f, 523t
Neurotoxicity
    chloroprocaine, 75–76, 76t
    intraspinal opioids, 179, 180t, 181f
    lidocaine
        major, 77–79, 77f, 78t, 79t
        minor, 79–80, 79t, 80t
Nevirapine (Viramune), for HIV, 590t
Newborn. See Neonate
Nicardipine
    effect on uteroplacental blood flow of, 27t, 34
    fetal effects of, 479
Nicotine, 601–602
Nicotinic receptors, 150
Nifedipine
    effect on uteroplacental blood flow of, 27t, 34
    fetal effects of, 479
    for pregnancy-induced hypertension, 306–307
    for preterm labor, 336
Nipride. See Sodium nitroprusside (Nipride)
Nisentil (alphaprodine), fetal heart rate with, 107f
Nitric oxide synthase, during pregnancy, 14
Nitroglycerin (NTG)
    effect on uteroplacental blood flow of, 27t, 34
    for EXIT procedure, 271
    for fetal heart rate abnormalities, 130, 160
    for fetal surgery, 271, 279
    for hypertension
        cocaine-induced, 608, 608f
        pregnancy-induced, 313, 315t
        vasopressor-induced, 143
    during neurosurgery, 517
    for preterm labor, 336–337
    for retained placenta, 367, 676
Nitroprusside. See Sodium nitroprusside (Nipride)
Nitrous oxide (N$_2$O)
    effect on uteroplacental blood flow of, 29, 30f
    efficacy of, 193–194, 194f
    fetal effects of, 221
    for inadequate or failed epidural analgesia, 144

with inhalation agents, 196
for laparoscopic sterilization, 240–241
maternal awareness with, 223, 224t
maternal effects of, 193–195, 221
neonatal effects of, 195, 195f, 651
reported use of, 189, 191t
technique for, 191–192, 192f
teratogenicity of, 253–256, 255f
Nizatidine, for aspiration prophylaxis, 402
Nondepolarizing muscle relaxants
    with Landry-Guillain-Barré syndrome, 535
    maternal and fetal effects of, 221
    with myotonia, 530, 530t
    with neurofibromatosis, 534
Nonnucleoside reverse transcriptase inhibitors, for HIV, 590t
Nonpharmacologic pain relief, 95–100
    acupuncture for, 97, 97f
    hydrotherapy for, 100
    hypnosis for, 95–96
    maternal position for, 100
    natural childbirth for, 96
    prenatal anesthesia visits for, 100, 103–104
    psychoprophylaxis for, 96–97
    social and professional support for, 99–100, 99f
    sterile water blocks for, 98–99, 99f
    transcutaneous electrical nerve stimulation for, 97–98, 98f
Nonreassuring fetal status, emergency cesarean section for,
    226
Nonsteroidal anti-inflammatory analgesics, for preterm labor,
    335
Nonstress test (NST), 618
Norepinephrine
    for amniotic fluid embolism, 358t
    fetal effects of, 479
Normoperidine, 109, 109f
Norvir (ritonavir)
    fetal and neonatal effects of, 685t
    for HIV, 589, 590t, 591f
Nose, topical anesthesia/nerve blocks of, 382
NST (nonstress test), 618
NTG. See Nitroglycerin
Nuchal translucency (NT) screening, 614
Nucleoside reverse transcriptase inhibitors
    fetal and neonatal effects of, 685t
    for HIV, 590t

O
Obesity, 545–556
    airway management with, 549, 549f, 554–555, 554f
    aspiration pneumonitis with, 548–549, 549f, 554
    cesarean section with, 546, 553–556, 553f, 554f, 556f
    defined, 545
    drug metabolism and toxicity with, 549–551, 550f, 551f
    evaluation of patient with, 549, 549f
    general anesthesia with, 554–555, 554f
    inhaled anesthetics with, 550–551, 551f
    intravenous agents with, 549–550, 550f
    monitoring with, 551–552
    muscle relaxants with, 551, 551f
    physiologic disturbances with, 547–549, 547f–549f, 548t
    postoperative management with, 555–556, 556f
    regional anesthesia with, 552–553, 555
    as risk factor for complications, 449, 545–547, 546t
    vaginal delivery with, 552–553
Obesity hyperventilation syndrome (OHS), 545, 549
Occiput posterior (OP) position, persistent, 287–288
Occupational exposure
    HIV, 592–593, 592t, 593t
    latex, 564
Oliguria, in pregnancy-induced hypertension, 308t
Omeprazole
    for aspiration prevention, 239, 402
    fetal and neonatal effects of, 686t
    with general anesthesia, 215
Ondansetron, fetal and neonatal effects of, 683t
Open-heart surgery, during pregnancy, 477
Opiate(s), endogenous, 149, 150t
Opiate receptors, 149, 150t, 151t
Opioids
    abuse of, 602–604, 603f, 603t, 604t
    allergic reactions to, 563
    in combined spinal-epidural analgesia, 158–162, 158f–161f,
        159t, 161t
        progress in labor with, 162, 162t
    in continuous spinal analgesia, 167
    epidural, 162–163
        additives with, 167–168
        for cesarean section, 210–211, 211f
        complications of, 174–180
        epinephrine with, 174
        local anesthetics with, 173–174
        monitoring of, 179
        neonatal effects of, 651
        patient-controlled, 167
        for postoperative pain management, 168–170, 168f, 169f,
            169t–171t, 173–174, 173t
        progress in labor with, 162–163, 162t, 163t, 164f
    fetal and neonatal effects of, 682t
    and gastric emptying, 237, 239, 239t, 391–392
    intraspinal, 155–180
        complications of, 174–180
        effect on uteroplacental blood flow of, 27t, 35
        for labor and delivery, 155–162
        local anesthetics with, 163–168
        neonatal effects of, 178–179, 651
        for postoperative pain management, 168–174
        progress in labor with, 162–163, 162t, 163f, 164f

intrathecal
    complications of, 174–180
    for labor and delivery, 155–157, 156f, 157f, 157t
    monitoring of, 179
    for postoperative pain management, 170–173, 172f, 173f,
        173t
    progress in labor with, 162
    neonatal effects of, 178–179, 651, 668
    with obesity, 553
    pharmacokinetics and pharmacodynamics of, 152–153,
        152f, 153t
    with ropivacaine, 86
    systemic
        effect on uterine activity and labor of, 43–44, 43f, 45, 46t
        fentanyl, 110–112, 111f, 112t
        inadequacy of, 105, 106f
        intramuscular vs. intravenous, 105, 107f
        meperidine, 105–110, 106f–110f, 106t
        morphine, 106f, 113, 113f
        neonatal effects of, 649–650
        side effects of, 105, 106f, 106t, 107f
        sufentanil, alfentanil, and remifentanil, 112–113, 112f
    teratogenicity of, 253
Opportunistic infections, with HIV, 589, 591t
OP (occiput posterior) position, persistent, 287–288
Organ transplantation, 572–576, 572t
Oropharynx
    examination of, 375–376, 376f
    topical anesthesia/nerve blocks of, 382–383
Orthostatic hypotension, from opioids, 105
Osmotic diuretics, during neurosurgery, 517
Overweight, defined, 545
Oxygen affinity, of fetal blood, 24–25, 25f
Oxygenation
    for cesarean section, 204, 205f
    with inhalation agents, 195, 221–222, 222f
    during labor, 5
    for surgery during pregnancy, 259, 259f
Oxygen capacity, of fetus, 24–25
Oxygen consumption
    during labor, 5
    during pregnancy, 4t, 5, 249, 251f
Oxygen desaturation, from opioids, 105, 106f
Oxygen dissociation curve, of fetus, 24, 25f
Oxygen reserve, during pregnancy, 5
Oxygen tension
    decreased, 623
    fetal, 24
    maternal, 259, 259f
Oxygen transfer, to fetus, 24–25, 24t, 25f
Oxygen transport
    with diabetes mellitus, 502–504, 503f
    during pregnancy, 11
Oxygen uptake, during pregnancy, 4–5
Oxyhemoglobin dissociation curve
    during labor, 3
    during pregnancy, 11
Oxymetazoline, for asthma, 490t
Oxytocin
    for abruptio placentae, 365
    allergic reactions to, 563–564
    epidural analgesia and, 47
    for uterine atony, 367, 368t
    and uterine rupture, 365–366

P
PaCO$_2$
    during pregnancy, 3, 4t
    during surgery, 259–260
Pain
    during anesthesia, lawsuits on, 447, 447t, 448t
    fetal response to, 273–274, 274f
    gate theory of, 97–98
    postoperative
        epidural opioids for, 168–170, 168f, 169f, 169t–171t,
            173–174, 173t
        intrathecal opioids for, 170–173, 172f, 173f, 173t
Pain pathways, 123, 124f, 125f, 149, 150f
    in fetus, 274, 274f
Pain Rating Index (PRI), 96f
Pain relief, nonpharmacologic. See Nonpharmacologic pain
    relief
Pain scores, 95, 96f
Pain threshold, in pregnancy, 249, 252f
Palmar grasp, 647, 647f, 649f
Palsy
    cerebral, 634
        Apgar score and, 642, 643f
    intrinsic maternal obstetric, 410–413, 411f, 412f
Pancreas transplantation, 575–576
Pancuronium
    for fetal surgery, 273
    with obesity, 551
PaO$_2$, during pregnancy, 4t, 5, 6f
Paraaminobenzoic acid, 75
Paracervical block anesthesia, 132–133, 132f, 133f
    bradycardia due to, 628
    neonatal effect of, 651
Paramyotonia congenita, 529
Paranasal sinusitis, due to regional anesthesia, 414
Paraplegia, 539–541, 540f, 540t, 541f, 541t
Parenteral agents, effect on uterine activity and labor of,
    43–44, 43f, 45, 46t
Paroxetine, fetal and neonatal effects of, 683t
Paroxysmal atrial tachycardia (PAT), during pregnancy, 478
Partial exchange transfusion, for sickle-cell anemia,
    351, 351t

Partial thromboplastin time (PTT), 346, 347t
  in preeclampsia and eclampsia, 303t
  during pregnancy, 11t
Particulate aspiration, 395–396, 433
PAT (paroxysmal atrial tachycardia), during pregnancy, 478
Patent ductus arteriosus (PDA), 456t, 467–468, 467f
Patient-controlled analgesia (PCA)
  effect on uterine activity and labor of, 45, 46t
  with pregnancy-induced hypertension, 309
Patient-controlled epidural analgesia (PCEA)
  drug regimens for, 127t
  efficacy of, 167
  outcome of labor with, 51
  ropivacaine in, 85, 86
  technique of, 167
Patient-controlled IV analgesia (PCIA), cesarean section rate with, 49
Patient information, on anesthesia, 103–104
PCA (patient-controlled analgesia)
  effect on uterine activity and labor of, 45, 46t
  with pregnancy-induced hypertension, 309
PCEA. See Patient-controlled epidural analgesia (PCEA)
PCO$_2$
  arterial, during pregnancy, 4t
  end-tidal, during pregnancy, 249, 250f
  with obesity, 548t
PCOP (pulmonary capillary occlusion pressure), in preeclampsia, 299, 300
PCWP (pulmonary capillary wedge pressure)
  in mitral stenosis, 459f
  in preeclampsia, 300t, 302f
  during pregnancy, 7f
PDA (patent ductus arteriosus), 456t, 467–468, 467f
PDPH. See Postdural puncture headache
Peak expiratory flow (PEF), during pregnancy, 4t
"Pencil-point" needles, 208, 208f
Penicillins
  allergic reactions to, 563
  fetal and neonatal effects of, 685t
Penthrane. See Methoxyflurane
Pentobarbital
  systemic, 113
  teratogenicity of, 252
PEP (postexposure prophylaxis), for HIV, 592–593
Perianesthetic evaluation, guidelines for, 673–674
Pericardial effusion, during pregnancy, 6
Pericarditis, 476
Perinatal morbidity, with diabetes mellitus, 498–500, 499t
"Perineal dose," of epidural analgesia, 48
Perineal infiltration, 133
Perphenazine, effect on uterine activity and labor of, 46t
Personnel, for anesthesia care, 679–680
PG (phosphatidylglycerol), in amniotic fluid, 616–617, 617f
PGSIs (prostaglandin synthetase inhibitors), for preterm labor, 325t, 334–336
pH
  of aspirated fluid, 392–393, 395f, 396f
  with obesity, 548t
  during pregnancy, 4t, 250f
Pharmacology. See Drug(s)
Pharyngeal structures, classification of, 215–216, 216f, 375–376, 376f
Phenobarbital (Luminal)
  fetal and neonatal effects of, 683t
  for seizures, 532, 532t, 533
  teratogenicity of, 252
Phenothiazine derivatives, systemic, 114
Phentolamine, for mitral insufficiency, 461
Phenylephrine
  effect on uteroplacental blood flow of, 27t, 32
  fetal effects of, 479
  for hypotension, 140, 141f, 207
  in preterm labor and delivery, 330, 332f, 333f
Phenytoin (Dilantin)
  drug interactions with, 533
  fetal and neonatal effects of, 683t
  for seizures, 531, 532t
  for status epilepticus, 532
Phosphatidylglycerol (PG), in amniotic fluid, 616–617, 617f
Phosphatidylinositol (PI), in amniotic fluid, 617, 617f
Physical examination, guidelines for, 673–674
Physiologic changes, 3–14, 238
  cardiovascular, 6–11, 6f–10f, 6t, 7t, 9t, 11t, 238
  endocrine, 13–14
  gastrointestinal, 12–13, 13f, 238–239, 239t
  hepatic, 13
  neurologic, 11–12, 11f
  renal, 13
  respiratory, 3–6, 4f–6f, 4t, 6t
  in uterine blood flow, 14
Physostigmine (Antilirium), 117
PI (pulsatility index), 23
PI (phosphatidylinositol), in amniotic fluid, 617, 617f
Pickwickian syndrome, 545, 549
PIH. See Pregnancy-induced hypertension
Pinocytosis, placental transport via, 20f, 21
Piperocaine (Metycaine), 76
Pituitary tumors, 509
pK$_a$, of drug, 63, 64
Placenta
  acid-base balance of, 25–26
  anatomy and circulation of, 19, 20f
  area of, 21–22
  carbon dioxide transfer across, 25

localization of, 615
marginal separation of, 364
respiratory gas exchange in, 19–22, 20f, 21f
retained, 367, 676
Placenta accreta, 363–364, 363f
Placenta increta, 363–364, 363f
Placental membrane, permeability of, 22
Placental transfer
  amide-linked agents, 77
  barbiturates, 113, 113f
  drugs, 61–64, 62f–65f, 62t–64t
  inhalation agents, 195
  magnesium, 305–306
  rate of, 21
Placenta percreta, 363–364, 363f
Placenta previa, 361–364, 362f–364f, 362t
Plasma colloid oncotic pressure, during pregnancy, 11
Plasma thromboplastin antecedent deficiency, 349
Plasma volume
  in preeclampsia, 299–300, 303t
  during pregnancy, 6t, 7, 7f
Plasminogen, 346
Platelet(s), aggregation of, 345
Platelet count, 346, 347t
  guidelines for, 674
  during pregnancy, 11, 11t, 420, 420f
Platelet disorders, 347–348
Platelet transfusions, 347
Plethysmography, during fetal surgery, 277
PLMA (ProSeal laryngeal mask airway), 381, 386
Pneumatic compression devices, for hypotension, 207
Pneumatic trauma, 420
Pneumocystis carinii pneumonia, 586, 591f
Pneumonitis, aspiration. See Aspiration pneumonitis
Pneumothorax, in neonate, 668
PO$_2$
  arterial, during pregnancy, 4t
  with obesity, 548t
  transcutaneous, during labor, 9, 9f
Polyneuritis, acute idiopathic, 534–535, 534f
Pontocaine. See tetracaine
Popliteal angle, 647f, 648f
Position
  defined, 287–291
  face or brow, 288, 288f
  persistent occiput posterior, 287–288
Positioning
  for airway management, 379, 379f
  aortocaval compression due to, 8–10, 9f, 10f
  and aspiration, 398
  cardiovascular effects of, 458f
  for hypotension, 206
  during labor, 100
  for postdural puncture headache, 213, 213f, 415, 416f
  with subarachnoid hemorrhage, 519
Positive-pressure ventilation, 217, 218f
Postdural puncture headache (PDPH)
  due to combined spinal-epidural analgesia, 129, 130t, 160, 212, 212f
  differential diagnosis of, 414, 414t
  due to epidural anesthesia, 213–214, 213f, 214t
  due to intrathecal morphine, 156, 157f
  lawsuits on, 447, 447t, 448t
  needle size and, 207–208, 208f, 242, 242t
  prevention of, 207–208, 208f, 213–214, 213f
  risk factors for, 414, 415
  treatment of, 213–214, 213f, 415–417, 416f
    with caffeine, 214, 416, 602
    with epidural blood patch, 214, 214t, 416–417
    with HIV, 591
Postexposure prophylaxis (PEP), for HIV, 592–593
Posthypnotic suggestion, 95
Postoperative pain management
  epidural opioids for, 168–170, 168f, 169f, 169t–171t, 173–174, 173t
  intrathecal opioids for, 170–173, 172f, 173f, 173t
Postpartum care, with pregnancy-induced hypertension, 314
Postpartum hemorrhage, 366–370
  with asthma, 492
Postpartum management, of neurosurgery, 521–522
Postpartum tubal ligation (PPTL). See Tubal ligation
Potter's syndrome, 633
Pourcelot Ratio (PR), 23
Practice guidelines, for obstetrical anesthesia, 673–677
"Prayer sign," 498, 499f
Prednisone, for asthma, 490t
Preeclampsia. See also Pregnancy-induced hypertension (PIH)
  anesthesia and analgesia with, 308–311, 309f, 310f
  with asthma, 492
  cardiovascular changes with, 472
  cesarean section for, 311–314, 312f–314f, 315t
  defined, 297, 298t
  delivery with, 303–304, 308
  with diabetes mellitus, 297–298, 498, 498t
  effect on placental drug transfer of, 61–62
  etiology of, 298–299, 298f, 299t
  incidence of, 297–298
  monitoring of, 307–308, 308t
  pathophysiology of, 299–303, 300t, 301f, 302f, 303t
  postpartum care of mother and neonate with, 314
  severe, 299, 299t
  stroke due to, 510–511, 511f
  therapy for, 303–307, 304t, 305f

maternal safety in, 249–251, 250f–254f
  prevention of preterm labor due to, 260–261
  teratogenicity in, 251–259, 254f, 255f, 257f, 258f
Pregnancy-induced hypertension (PIH), 297–314
  anesthesia and analgesia with, 308–311, 309f, 310f
  cesarean section for, 311–314, 312f–314f, 315t
  convulsions due to, 307
  defined, 297, 298t
  delivery with, 303–304, 308
  etiology of, 298–299, 298f, 299t
  incidence of, 297–298, 298t
  monitoring of, 307–308, 308t
  with obesity, 545
  pathophysiology of, 299–303, 300t, 301f, 302f, 303t
  postpartum care of mother and neonate with, 314
  severe, 299, 299t
  stroke due to, 510–511, 511f
  vs. subarachnoid hemorrhage, 515
  therapy for, 303–307, 304t, 305f
Prehydration
  for hypotension, 206–207
  for pregnancy-induced hypertension, 311
Prematurity. See Preterm labor and delivery
Prenatal visits, to anesthesia clinic, 100, 103–104
Preoxygenation
  in airway management, 379, 380f
  for general anesthesia, 216, 217t
Presentation
  breech, 288–291, 289f, 289t, 290f, 291t
  defined, 287
Pressure sores, 413
Preterm labor and delivery, 323–340
  anesthesia for, 338–340, 338f, 339f
  cesarean section or vaginal delivery in, 337–340
  with cigarette smoking, 602
  defined, 323
  with diabetes mellitus, 498t, 501
  epidemiology of, 323, 324f
  fetal heart rate monitoring in, 633
  induced, for fetal malformations, 267–269, 268t
  prevention of, during fetal surgery, 278–280
  resuscitation after, 668
  risk factors for, 323, 324f
  screening for, 323
  due to surgery, 260–261
  survival rate with, 323, 324f
  tocolytic therapy for, 325–337
    β-adrenergic agents in, 325t, 326–331, 326t, 327f–333f
    calcium entry-blocking drugs in, 325t, 336
    efficacy of, 325–326
    indications for, 323–325, 325t, 326f
    magnesium sulfate in, 325t, 331–334, 333t, 334f, 335f
    nitroglycerin in, 336–337
    prostaglandin synthetase inhibitors in, 325t, 334–336
PRI (Pain Rating Index), 96f
Prilocaine (Citanest), 81
  chemical structure of, 74f
Primary active transport, placental transport via, 19, 20f
Primary pulmonary hypertension, 456t, 471–472, 472t
Primidone (Mysoline), for seizures, 532t
Procaine, 76
  chemical structure of, 74f
  fetal uptake of, 64
  reduced requirement for, 435
Prochlorperazine
  fetal and neonatal effects of, 683t
  teratogenicity of, 252
Progesterone, during pregnancy, 11–12, 435
Progressive systemic sclerosis (PSS), 571–572
Prolonged gestation, with obesity, 545
Prolonged neural blockade, 417
Promethazine
  effect on uterine activity and labor of, 43, 45, 46t, 49
  fetal and neonatal effects of, 683t
  gastric emptying with, 239
  systemic, 114
Propiomazine, systemic, 114
Propofol
  allergic reactions to, 563
  with asthma, 492
  effect on uteroplacental blood flow of, 26, 27t, 29f
  for fetal surgery, 273
  maternal and fetal effects of, 220
  as neuroprotective agent, 518
  for neurosurgery, 520
  with placenta previa, 361
  for postpartum sterilization, 242, 243
  with succinylcholine, 220
Propranolol
  for atrial fibrillation, 459
  fetal effects of, 478
  for pregnancy-induced hypertension, 306
Propylthiouracil, fetal and neonatal effects of, 686t
ProSeal laryngeal mask airway (PLMA), 381, 386
Prostacyclin, in preeclampsia, 299, 301f
Prostaglandin(s)
  for abruptio placentae, 365
  for uterine atony, 367–369, 368t
Prostaglandin E$_2$ (Dinoprostone)
  with asthma, 491, 492
  gastric emptying with, 392
  for uterine atony, 367, 368t
Prostaglandin F$_{2\alpha}$ (Hemabate)
  with asthma, 491, 492
  for uterine atony, 367–369, 368t
Prostaglandin synthetase inhibitors (PGSIs), for preterm labor, 325t, 334–336

Prostigmin (neostigmine methylsulfate), 150
  for myasthenia gravis, 539t
Prostigmin (neostigmine methylsulfate) test, for myasthenia
    gravis, 537, 539t
Protease inhibitors
  fetal and neonatal effects of, 685t
  for HIV, 589, 590t
Protein binding
  effect on fetal drug distribution of, 68, 68f
  effect on placental drug transfer of, 62–63, 63f, 63t, 64f
Protein C, 346
Proteinuria
  in preeclampsia, 299
  during pregnancy, 13
Prothrombin, 345, 346t
  during pregnancy, 11t
Prothrombin time (PT), 346, 347t
  in preeclampsia and eclampsia, 303t
  during pregnancy, 11t
Pruritus
  due to combined spinal-epidural analgesia, 129, 130t, 158,
    160, 174f
  naloxone for, 156, 171t, 176, 178t
  naltrexone for, 178
  due to opioids
    epidural, 171t, 174f
    intraspinal, 176
    intrathecal, 156, 157t, 174f
Pseudoephedrine, for asthma, 490t
Pseudotumor cerebri, 510
Psoas major muscle, lumbosacral cord and, 411f
PSS (progressive systemic sclerosis), 571–572
Psychoprophylaxis, 96–97
PT (prothrombin time), 346, 347t
  in preeclampsia and eclampsia, 303t
  during pregnancy, 11t
PTT (partial thromboplastin time), 346, 347t
  in preeclampsia and eclampsia, 303t
  during pregnancy, 11t
Pudendal block, 133
  neonatal effect of, 651
Pulmonary acid aspiration syndrome, 395, 397f, 433
Pulmonary artery catheter
  guidelines of, 677
  in pregnancy-induced hypertension, 308, 308t
Pulmonary aspiration. See Aspiration
Pulmonary capillary occlusion pressure (PCOP), in
    preeclampsia, 299, 300
Pulmonary capillary wedge pressure (PCWP)
  in mitral stenosis, 459f
  in preeclampsia, 300t, 302f
  during pregnancy, 7f
Pulmonary edema
  due to β-adrenergic agonists, 327–328
  in preeclampsia and eclampsia, 300, 308t, 314
Pulmonary hypertension, primary, 456t, 471–472, 472t
Pulmonary shunt (Qs/Qt), during pregnancy, 3–4
Pulmonary vascular resistance
  in preeclampsia, 299, 300t
  during pregnancy, 7f, 8
Pulmonic stenosis, 417t, 456t, 470–471
Pulsatility index (PI), 23
Pulse oximetry
  fetal, 634
  during fetal surgery, 277–278, 279f–281f
Pyridostigmine, for myasthenia gravis, 539t

Q
Q (blood flow), studies of, 23–24, 24f
Qs/Qt (pulmonary shunt), during pregnancy, 3–4
Quadriplegia, 539–541, 540t, 540t, 541f, 541t
Quincke needle, 208, 208f
Quinidine, effect on fetus of, 478

R
RA (rheumatoid arthritis), 568–570, 569f
Racemic mixtures, 84
Radiation-induced fetal abnormalities, 515
Radicularis magna, 410f, 411
Ranitidine
  for aspiration prevention, 239, 401–402, 434
  effect on placental drug transfer of, 62
  with general anesthesia, 215
  with obesity, 554
Rapacuronium, for neurosurgery, 520
RDS (respiratory distress syndrome), 616–617
"Reasonable patient" standard, 443
Recoil, of elbows, 647, 647f
Recurrent laryngeal nerve (RLN), 381–382
Red blood cell volume, during pregnancy, 6t, 7, 7f
Reflex irritability, in Apgar score, 639, 640f
Regional anesthesia, 123–144. See also Combined
    spinal-epidural (CSE) anesthesia; Epidural
    analgesia/anesthesia; Spinal anesthesia
  agents for. See Local anesthetics
  of airway, 382–384, 383f, 384f
  airway management for, 677, 677t
  with alcohol abuse, 601
  with Arnold-Chiari syndrome, 413
  with arteriovenous malformations, 412–413
  with asthma, 491
  and autonomic hyperreflexia, 540–541, 540f, 541f
  backaches due to, 143, 413–414
  for breech presentation, 291
  caudal, 131–132, 131f, 131t, 132f
  for cesarean section, 73–74, 201–214
    anesthetic solutions for, 208–212

antacid administration with, 203–204
antianxiety medication with, 203
choice of, 201–202, 227–228
combined spinal-epidural, 212–213, 212t
complications of, 204–207, 205t, 206f, 208f, 213–214,
    213f, 214t
condition of newborn with, 223–225, 224t, 225t
emergency, 226
epidural, 209–212, 209t–212f
failed, 213
high or total spinal or epidural with, 213, 437
hypotension due to, 204–207, 206f
postdural puncture headache due to, 207–208, 208f,
    213–214, 213f, 214t
preparation for, 202–204, 204t
reduced requirements for, 201, 204f, 204t, 211–212
supplemental oxygen with, 204, 205f
technique for, 201–202, 205t
toxicity of, 213
via subarachnoid block, 208–209
with cocaine abuse, 609
contraindications to, 134
convulsions due to, 140–142, 142t
dense or prolonged epidural block due to, 143–144
effect on uterine activity and labor of, 44–52, 44f
effect on uteroplacental blood flow of, 27t, 31, 31f
with epilepsy, 533
failed, 213
guidelines for, 671
with HIV, 591
hypotension due to, 136–140, 137f–141f
inadequate or failed, 144
with Landry-Guillain-Barré syndrome, 535
lumbar epidural, 123–126, 125f, 126f, 127f
  continuous infusion, 126–128, 127t
lumbar sympathetic block, 133
magnesium sulfate and, 333–334
with maternal congenital anomalies of the spine, 412–413
maternal mortality with, 431–432, 431f, 432t, 435–436
with mitral insufficiency, 461
with mitral stenosis, 459–460
with mitral valve prolapse, 462
with multiple sclerosis, 536
neurologic complications of, 409–424, 410f, 411t
  due to chemical contaminants, 420–422, 422t
  chronic, 418–422
  cortical vein thrombosis, 414–415
  enhanced local anesthetic action, 417–418
  iatrogenic trauma, 418–419, 419f, 420
  incidence of, 410, 411t
  increased intracranial pressure, 415
  infection, 414, 422–424, 423t
  intrinsic maternal obstetric palsy, 410–413, 411f, 412f
  postdural puncture headache, 414, 414t, 415–417, 416f
  postpartum backache, 413–414
  pressure sores, 413
  shivering, 417
  subarachnoid hemorrhage, 415
  subdural hematoma, 415
  trends in practice and, 423–424
  vascular, 415, 419–420, 421f, 421t
with obesity, 552–553, 555
pain pathways and, 123, 124f, 125f
paracervical block, 132–133, 132f, 133f
patient information on, 103–104
for postpartum sterilization, 240–242, 241f, 241t, 242t, 403
with pregnancy-induced hypertension, 311–312, 312f
  preparation for, 123, 125t
  progress in labor with, 675–676
pudendal block and local perineal infiltration, 133
resuscitation equipment for, 123, 125t
spinal, 128, 128t
  continuous, 128, 128t
test dose regimens for, 134–136, 135f, 136f
total spinal anesthesia due to, 142–143, 143f
unrecognized events during, 437
urinary retention due to, 144
vasopressor-induced hypertension due to, 143
Regurgitation
  aspiration due to, 433
  during pregnancy, 249–251
  prevention of, 433
Remifentanil
  placental transfer of, 64, 64t
  systemic, 112–113
Renal changes, during pregnancy, 13
Renal failure, complications with, 575, 575t
Renal function, in pregnancy-induced hypertension,
    301–302
Renal plasma flow (RPF), during pregnancy, 13
Renal transplantation, 574–575, 575t
Renin, during pregnancy, 13
Rescriptor (delavirdine), for HIV, 590t
Residual volume (RV)
  with obesity, 547f
  during pregnancy, 4t, 5f, 251f
Respiration, establishment of neonatal, 657, 658f, 661–662,
    661f–663f, 662t
Respiratory acidosis, Apgar score and, 640–641, 640f
Respiratory alkalosis, during labor, 3
Respiratory changes
  during laparoscopic sterilization, 240
  with obesity, 547–548, 547f, 548t
  during pregnancy, 3–6, 4f–6f, 4t, 6t, 249, 250f, 251f, 375
Respiratory complications
  of cocaine abuse, 605t
  of HIV, 586, 587t

Respiratory depression
  due to combined spinal-epidural analgesia, 129, 130t, 160
  due to epidural opioids, 171t, 175–176
  due to intrathecal opioids, 175–176
Respiratory distress syndrome (RDS), 616–617
Respiratory effort, in Apgar score, 639, 640f
Respiratory events, leading to injuries, 448, 448t
Respiratory function, in progressive systemic sclerosis, 571
Respiratory gases, effect on uteroplacental blood flow of, 27t,
    36, 36f
Respiratory gas exchange, in placenta, 19–22, 20f, 21f
Respiratory rate, during pregnancy, 4t, 249, 250f
Resuscitation
  cardiopulmonary, 436, 677
  neonatal. See Neonatal resuscitation
Resuscitation equipment, 660, 660t
  for regional anesthesia, 123, 125t
Resuscitation team, 660
Reticulospinal fibers, 124f
Retrovir (zidovudine)
  fetal and neonatal effects of, 685t
  for HIV, 590t
Reverse transcriptase inhibitors
  fetal and neonatal effects of, 685t
  for HIV, 590t
Rh disease, sinusoidal pattern with, 632
Rheumatic heart disease, 456t, 458f
  aortic insufficiency due to, 456t, 463–465, 465f, 465t
  aortic stenosis due to, 456t, 462–463, 463f, 463t, 464f
  incidence of, 455, 456f, 456t
  mitral insufficiency due to, 456t, 460–461, 460f, 461f
  mitral stenosis due to, 456–460, 456t, 459f, 459t
  mitral valve prolapse due to, 461–462, 462t
Rheumatoid arthritis (RA), 568–570, 569f
Right-to-left shunt, 468–469
Ritodrine
  effect on uteroplacental blood flow of, 27t, 32
  epidural anesthesia with, 329, 330f, 332f, 333f
  gastric emptying with, 392
  general anesthesia with, 330–331
  for preterm labor, 326
  side effects of, 327, 328, 329
Ritonavir (Norvir)
  fetal and neonatal effects of, 685t
  for HIV, 589, 590t, 591f
RLN (recurrent laryngeal nerve), 381–382
Rocuronium
  maternal and fetal effects of, 221
  for postpartum sterilization, 243, 243t
Ropivacaine (Naropin), 84–86
  for cesarean section, 86
  chemical structure of, 74f, 84
  clinical potency of, 84–85, 85f, 86
  for combined spinal-epidural analgesia, 129
  current usage of, 85–86, 85f
  effect on first stage of labor of, 45
  effect on second stage of labor of, 50
  effect on uteroplacental blood flow of, 27t, 30–31
  epidural, 85–86, 85f
  fetal distribution of, 67f, 68
  intrathecal, 86
  minimum local analgesic concentration of, 85, 85f, 86
  opioids with, 86
  placental transfer of, 62, 63, 63f, 63t, 77, 85
Rostral spread, of blockade, 417
RPF (renal plasma flow), during pregnancy, 13
Rubber allergy, 564–566, 564t, 565t
RV (residual volume)
  with obesity, 547f
  during pregnancy, 4t, 5f, 251f

S
Sacrococcygeal ligament, 125f
Saddle block. See Spinal anesthesia
SAH. See Subarachnoid hemorrhage
Salicylates, teratogenicity of, 253
Saline instillation, for postdural puncture headache, 213, 416
Saltatory pattern, of fetal heart rate, 632
Saquinavir mesylate (Invirase, Fortovase)
  fetal and neonatal effects of, 685t
  for HIV, 590t
S/A (surfactant/albumin) ratio, 616
SARIs, fetal and neonatal effects of, 683t
SCA (sickle-cell anemia), 350t, 351
Scalp sampling, 634
  and Apgar score, 640, 640f
Scarf sign, 647, 647f
Scleroderma, 571–572
Scopolamine (Hyoscine), systemic, 117
Scopolamine transdermal patches, for nausea and vomiting,
    177
S/D (systolic-to-diastolic) ratio, 23, 24
Secobarbital
  neonatal effect of, 649
  systemic, 113f
Secondary active transport, placental transport via, 19, 20f
Second stage bradycardia, 627–628
Sedation, from opioids, 105, 106f
Sedative-tranquilizers, systemic, 113–115
Seizures
  anesthesia with, 530–533, 531t, 532f, 532t
  causes of, 530–531, 531t
  due to eclampsia, 307
  neonatal outcome with, 531, 531t
  newborn, 635
  during pregnancy, 510, 530–531, 531t
  due to regional anesthesia, 140–142, 142t, 436

Selective serotonin reuptake inhibitors (SSRIs), fetal and neonatal effects of, 683t
Self-hypnosis, 95
Sellick's maneuver, 398–399, 398f, 399f, 433, 433f
Sensorcaine. *See* Bupivacaine (Marcaine, Sensorcaine)
Sepsis, spinal, 422
Sertraline, fetal and neonatal effects of, 683t
Sevoflurane, 193, 194
  in breast milk, 244
  effect on uterine activity and labor of, 41
  effect on uteroplacental blood flow of, 27t, 29
  maternal and fetal effects of, 221
  in obese patients, 550–551
  for postpartum sterilization, 243
SGA (small for gestational age), 323, 643–645, 644f, 645f
Sheehan's syndrome, 509
Shivering, 417
Shock, in newborn, 665–666, 665f, 666t
Shoulder dystocia, 291–293, 292f, 293t
Shunt
  left-to-right, 465–468
  right-to-left, 468–469
Sickle-cell anemia (SCA), 350t, 351
Sickle-cell hemoglobin SC disease, 350t, 351–352
Sickle-cell trait, 350t, 351
SIDS (sudden infant death syndrome), with cigarette smoking, 602
Simpson, James Young, 189, 190f
Sinusitis, due to regional anesthesia, 414
Sinusoidal pattern, of fetal heart rate, 632
Sinus tachycardia, due to mitral stenosis, 459
Sirolimus, for immunosuppression, 576
SJS (stiff joint syndrome), 498, 499f
Skin, in progressive systemic sclerosis, 571
Skin disinfectants, 422
Skin prick test (SPT), 566, 566t, 567f
Skin testing, for allergies, 566, 566t, 567f
SLE (systemic lupus erythematosus), 570–571
SLN (superior laryngeal nerve), 381–382, 383f
SLN (superior laryngeal nerve) block, 383, 383f
Small for gestational age (SGA), 323, 643–645, 644f, 645f
Smoking, 601–602
Snow, John, 189, 190f
SNP. *See* Sodium nitroprusside (SNP, Nipride)
SNRIs, fetal and neonatal effects of, 683t
Social support, during labor, 99–100, 99f
Sodium bicarbonate
  for aspiration prophylaxis, 401
  for cesarean section, 205t
    emergency, 227t
  hypotension with, 136
  with local anesthetics, 87
  for neonatal metabolic acidosis, 664–665, 666t
Sodium citrate
  for aspiration prophylaxis, 401, 434
  with general anesthesia, 215
Sodium iodine-131, fetal and neonatal effects of, 686t
Sodium nitroprusside (SNP, Nipride)
  effect on fetus of, 480
  effect on uteroplacental blood flow of, 27t, 34, 34f
  for hypertension
    pregnancy-induced, 313, 315t
    vasopressor-induced, 143
  for mitral insufficiency, 461
  for mitral stenosis, 459
  during neurosurgery, 517
  for pregnancy-induced hypertension, 307
Sodium restriction, for pregnancy-induced hypertension, 304
Sodium valproate (Depakene), for seizures, 532t
Somatosensory evoked potentials (SSEPs), for neurosurgery, 521
Spina bifida, latex allergy with, 564
Spina bifida occulta, maternal, 412
Spinal anesthesia. *See also* Regional anesthesia
  adenosine agents for, 150–151, 150t
  α_2-adrenergic agents for, 150, 151f, 152f
  with asthma, 491, 491f
  bupivacaine for, 52, 53, 84
  for cesarean section, 73–74, 201–209
    anesthetic solutions for, 208–209
    antacid administration with, 203–204
    antianxiety medication with, 203
    choice of, 201–202
    complications of, 204–207, 205t, 206f, 208f, 213–214, 213f, 214t
    condition of newborn with, 223–225, 224t, 225t
    failed, 213
    high or total, 213, 437
    hypotension due to, 204–207, 206f
    postdural puncture headache due to, 207–208, 208f, 213–214, 213f, 214t
    preparation for, 202–204, 204t
    reduced requirements for, 201, 204f, 204t
    supplemental oxygen with, 204, 205f
    technique for, 201–202, 205t
  cholinergic agents for, 150, 152f
  complications of, 174–177, 174f–177f, 176t
  continuous, 128, 128t, 167
    catheter size for, 78, 167
    for cesarean section, 74
    guidelines for, 78, 78t
    neurotoxicity of, 77
  contraindications to, 134
  effect on uterine activity and labor of, 52–53, 52t, 53f
  effect on uteroplacental blood flow of, 27t, 31, 31f
  epinephrine with, 52, 87–88, 88f
  after "failed spinal," 78–79, 79t, 213

for labor and delivery, 155–162
  levobupivacaine for, 87
  lidocaine for, 81
  local anesthetics with opioids in, 163–168
  neonatal effects of, 178–180, 651
  nonopiate agents in, 150–151, 151f, 151t, 152f
  with obesity, 553, 555
  opioids in, 155–180
    complications of, 174–180
    effect on uteroplacental blood flow of, 27t, 35
    guidelines for, 675
    for labor and delivery, 155–162
    local anesthetics with, 163–168
    neonatal effects of, 178–179, 651
    pharmacology of, 149–153
    for postoperative pain management, 168–174
    progress in labor with, 162–163, 162t, 163f, 164f
  for postoperative pain management, 168–174
  for postpartum sterilization, 240–242, 241f, 241t, 242t, 403
  and progress in labor, 162–163
  ropivacaine for, 86
  with spinal cord injury, 541t
  suggested guidelines for, 79, 79t
  technique of, 128, 128t
  total, 142–143, 143f, 213
  transient neurologic symptoms after, 79–80, 79t, 80t
Spinal cord
  anatomy of, 124f, 125f
  blood supply of, 410f
  synaptic connections in, 124f
Spinal cord injury, 539–541, 540f, 540t, 541f, 541t
Spinal dysraphism, maternal, 412
Spinal nutrient arteries, 410–412
Spinal sepsis, 423
Spinal space, transfer of drugs to, 152, 152f
Spine, maternal congenital anomalies of, 412–413
SpO$_2$, during pregnancy, 5
Sprotte needle, 208, 208f
SPT (skin prick test), 566, 566t, 567f
SSEPs (somatosensory evoked potentials), for neurosurgery, 521
SSRIs (selective serotonin reuptake inhibitors), fetal and neonatal effects of, 683t
Stand-by anesthesia, for complicated vaginal delivery, 676
Status asthmaticus, 489–491
Status epilepticus, 532
Stavudine (d4T, Zerit)
  fetal and neonatal effects of, 685t
  for HIV, 590t
Stereoisomers, 84
Sterile water blocks, 98–99, 99f
Sterilization
  "interval," 237
  postpartum, 237–244, 402–403
    advantage of, 237
    breast-feeding after, 243–244, 244t
    general anesthesia for, 242–243, 242t, 243t, 403
    local anesthesia for, 240, 240f
    physiologic changes induced by laparoscopy during, 239–240
    physiologic changes of pregnancy and puerperium and, 238–239, 239t
    regional anesthesia for, 240–242, 241f, 241t, 242t, 403
    timing of, 237
    tubal ligation *vs.* laparoscopic approach to, 237–238
  prevalence of, 237
Sternomental distance, 376
Steroids. *See* Corticosteroids
Stiff joint syndrome (SJS), 498, 499f
Stomach, pharmacologic emptying of, 402, 434
Stress
  effect on uteroplacental blood flow of, 27t, 32
  teratogenicity of, 258
Stroke, during pregnancy, 510–511, 511f, 512t, 513t, 513f
Stroke volume
  effect of exercise on, 458f
  effect of positioning on, 458f
  effect of uterine contractions on, 457f
  during pregnancy, 6t, 8f, 249, 253f, 457f
ST-segment depression, in coronary artery disease, 475
Subarachnoid block
  with asthma, 491, 491f
  for cesarean section, 73–74, 208–209, 209f
  in combined spinal-epidural anesthesia, 158, 158f
  needle placement for, 125f
  with pregnancy-induced hypertension, 311, 312
  rostral spread of, 417
Subarachnoid hemorrhage (SAH)
  due to arteriovenous malformations, 511–512, 511f, 513–514, 513f, 514f
  diagnosis and treatment of, 514–515
  electrocardiogram with, 519
  due to intracranial aneurysms, 511, 512–513, 513f, 513t, 514f
  during pregnancy, 511–515, 514f
  vs. pregnancy-induced hypertension, 515
  due to regional anesthesia, 415
  risk of, 512–514, 514f
Subarachnoid injection, massive, 418
Subarachnoid space, chemical contaminants of, 420–422, 422t
Subdural block, 142–143, 143f
Subdural hematoma, due to regional anesthesia, 413, 415
Subdural space, 125f
  accidental entry into, 417–418
Submandibular compliance, 376
Substance abuse, 599–609
  alcohol, 599–601, 600f, 601f

amphetamines, 603f, 606–607
  caffeine, 602
  cocaine, 604–606
    anesthetic considerations with, 607, 609
    assay for, 604
    epidemiology of, 604
    hypertension due to, 607–609, 608f
    maternal complications of, 605, 605f
    maternal deaths due to, 603f
    neonatal complications of, 605–606, 606f, 606t, 607f
    pharmacology and physiologic response to, 605, 605f
  current trends in, 599, 600t
  marijuana, 609
  opioids, 602–604, 603f, 603t, 604t
  tobacco, 601–602
Subvalvular stenosis, idiopathic hypertrophic, 474–475, 475t
Succinylcholine
  aspiration with, 398
  with asthma, 492
  effect on uteroplacental blood flow of, 26, 28f–30f
  hyperkalemic response to, with spinal cord injury, 539–540, 540t
  magnesium with, 305, 305f
  maternal and fetal effects of, 220–221, 221t
  with myotonia, 530, 530f, 530t
  for neurosurgery, 520
  with obesity, 551, 555
  with placenta previa, 361
  for postpartum sterilization, 242
  with propofol, 220
Sucking reflex, 647, 647f
Suctioning, of newborn, 660–661, 661f, 666–668, 667f
Sudden infant death syndrome (SIDS), with cigarette smoking, 602
Sufentanil
  in breast milk, 243
  with bupivacaine, 165–166, 166t, 167–168, 167t
  for cesarean section, 209, 211
  for combined spinal-epidural analgesia, 129, 158, 159, 159f, 159t
  for continuous spinal anesthesia, 128t
  effect on labor of, 51, 52
  effect on uteroplacental blood flow of, 27t
  epidural, 163, 164f
    for cesarean section, 211
    neonatal effects of, 179
    for postoperative pain, 169, 169t
  intrathecal, 52, 53
    for postoperative pain, 172, 173, 173f, 173t
    progress in labor with, 162
    side effects of, 160
  for lumbar epidural anesthesia, 127t
  with obesity, 553
  pharmacokinetics of, 152, 153, 153t
  pruritus due to, 174
  with ropivacaine, 86
  systemic, 112, 112t
  transfer across arachnoid membrane of, 152
Suggestibility, 95
Sulfonamides, fetal and neonatal effects of, 685t
Sulindac, for preterm labor, 335
Sumatriptan succinate (Imitrex), for postdural puncture headache, 416
Superior laryngeal nerve (SLN), 381–382, 383f
Superior laryngeal nerve (SLN) block, 383, 383f
Supine-hypotension syndrome, 8–10, 9f, 10f, 136, 137f–139f, 206
Supporting reaction, 647, 647f, 649f
Supportive companion, during labor, 99–100, 99f
Supraspinous ligament, 125f
Surfactant/albumin (S/A) ratio, 616
Surfactant determination, 616–617, 616f, 617f
Surgery, during pregnancy, 249–262
  anesthetic management for, 261–262, 261f, 262f
  avoidance of fetal asphyxia in, 259–260, 259f, 260f
  maternal safety in, 249–251, 250f–254f
  prevention of preterm labor due to, 260–261
  teratogenicity in, 251–259, 254f, 255f, 257f, 258f
"Surgical tocolysis," 278–280
Sustiva (efavirenz), for HIV, 590t
Synaptic connections, in spinal cord, 124f
Syncytiotrophoblast, 19, 20f
Syringe, with latex allergy, 565, 565t
Syringomyelia, 413, 415
Systemic lupus erythematosus (SLE), 570–571
Systemic mastocytosis, 568
Systemic medication(s), 105–118
  with agonist-antagonist agents, 115–116, 115f
  with antagonists, 117–118
  with asthma, 491
  with barbiturates, 113–114, 113f
  with benzodiazepines, 114–115, 114f
  with dissociative or amnestic drugs, 116–117
  effect on uteroplacental blood flow of, 26–29, 27t, 28f, 29f
  neonatal effect of, 649–650
  with obesity, 549–550, 550f
  with opioids, 105–113
    fentanyl, 110–112, 111f, 112t
    inadequacy of, 105, 106f
    meperidine, 105–110, 106f–110f, 106t, 113f
    morphine, 113, 113f
    side effects of, 105, 106f, 106t, 107f
    sufentanil, alfentanil, and remifentanil, 112–113, 112f
  with phenothiazine derivatives and hydroxyzine, 114
  with sedative-tranquilizers, 113–115
  teratogenicity of, 252–253

Systemic vascular resistance
   in mitral stenosis, 459
   in preeclampsia, 300t
   during pregnancy, 7f, 8
Systolic blood pressure, during pregnancy, 6t
Systolic click, due to mitral valve prolapse, 461–462
Systolic ejection murmur, due to aortic stenosis, 462
Systolic-to-diastolic (S/D) ratio, 23, 24

T
Tachycardia, fetal, 625t, 627t, 628, 633
Tacrolimus (FK-506), for immunosuppression, 576
Tamponade, 476
Tecota trichloroethylene vaporizer, 193
TEG (thromboelastography), 369–370
Tegretol (carbamazepine)
   fetal and neonatal effects of, 683t
   for seizures, 532t
Temporary proximal clips, during neurosurgery, 518
Temporomandibular joint, rheumatoid arthritis of, 568
TENS (transcutaneous electrical nerve stimulation), 97–98, 98f
Tensilon (edrophonium chloride) test, for myasthenia gravis, 537, 539t
Teratogenicity, 251–259, 681
   of anesthetics, 253–258
      animal studies of, 253–256, 255f
      human studies of, 256–258, 257f, 258f
   of anticonvulsant therapy, 531–532
   behavioral, 258–259
   carcinogenesis, 259
   of hypoxia and hypercarbia, 258
   of maternal emotional stress and trauma, 258
   susceptibility to, 251–252, 254f, 255f
   of systemic medications, 252–253
Terbutaline
   effect on uteroplacental blood flow of, 27t, 32
   fetal and neonatal effects of, 686t
   for fetal heart rate abnormalities, 130
   for preterm labor, 326, 329, 329f, 331f
Terminal bradycardia, 627
Test dose regimens, for regional anesthesia, 134–136, 135f, 136f
Tetracaine (Pontocaine), 76–77
   for cesarean section, 205t
   chemical structure of, 74f
   for postpartum sterilization, 241
   reduced requirement for, 435
   for spinal anesthesia, 128, 128t
Tetracyclines, fetal and neonatal effects of, 685t
Tetrahydrocannabinol (THC), 609
Tetralogy of Fallot, 456t, 468, 468t
α-Thalassemia, 349–350, 350t
β-Thalassemia, 350, 350t
Thalassemia major, 350
THC (tetrahydrocannabinol), 609
Theophylline
   for asthma, 490t
   fetal and neonatal effects of, 686t
   for postdural puncture headache, 416
Thermal management, of neonate, 660
Thiamylal, teratogenicity of, 252
Thiazide diuretics, fetal and neonatal effects of, 684t
Thiopental
   with alcohol abuse, 600
   allergic reactions to, 563
   with asthma, 492
   in breast milk, 243
   decreased requirements in pregnancy for, 249, 252f
   for eclampsia, 307
   effect on uteroplacental blood flow of, 26, 27t, 28f, 30f
   fetal distribution of, 67f
   maternal and fetal effects of, 217–219, 219f
   neonatal effect of, 651
   as neuroprotective agent, 518
   for neurosurgery, 520
   with obesity, 555
   with placenta previa, 361
   for postpartum sterilization, 242
Thoracic kyphosis, with obesity, 547
3TC (lamivudine)
   fetal and neonatal effects of, 685t
   for HIV, 590t
Thrombin, 345
Thrombin time, 346, 347t
Thrombocytopenia, 347
   with HIV, 586–587
   neonatal alloimmune, 348
   in preeclampsia and eclampsia, 300, 303t
   during pregnancy, 420, 421f
Thromboelastography (TEG), 369–370
Thromboembolism, from laparoscopic surgery, 261
Thrombotic thrombocytopenic purpura (TTP), stroke due to, 511f
Thromboxane, in preeclampsia, 299, 301f, 303t
Thyroid agents, fetal and neonatal effects of, 686t
Thyroid function, during pregnancy, 14
Thyroid replacement therapy, fetal and neonatal effects of, 686t
Thyromental distance, 215, 216f, 376
Tidal volume, during pregnancy, 3, 4t, 5f, 249, 250f
TLC (total lung capacity), during pregnancy, 3, 4t, 5f
TNG (trinitroglycerin), for pregnancy-induced hypertension, 307
TNS (transient neurologic symptoms), after spinal anesthesia, 79–80, 79t, 80t
Tobacco, 601–602

Tocolytic therapy, 325–337
   β-adrenergic agents in, 325t, 326–331, 326t, 327f–333f
   calcium entry-blocking drugs in, 325t, 336
   efficacy of, 325–326
   during fetal surgery, 278–280
   indications for, 323–325, 325t, 326f
   magnesium sulfate in, 325t, 331–334, 333t, 334f, 335f
   nitroglycerin in, 336–337
   prostaglandin synthetase inhibitors in, 325t, 334–336
Tongue, size of, 215–216, 216f
Topical anesthesia, with spinal cord injury, 541t
Total compliance, during pregnancy, 4t
Total lung capacity (TLC), during pregnancy, 3, 4t, 5f
Total peripheral resistance, during pregnancy, 6t
Total pulmonary resistance, during pregnancy, 4t
Total spinal anesthesia, 142–143, 143f
Toxemia of pregnancy. *See* Pregnancy-induced hypertension (PIH)
Toxic intravenous injection, 418
Toxicity
   bupivacaine, 82–84, 82t, 83f, 213
   chloroprocaine, 75–76, 76t
   intraspinal opioids, 179–180, 180t, 181f
   levobupivacaine, 86–87
   lidocaine
      major, 77–79, 77f, 78f, 78t, 79t
      minor, 79–80, 79t, 80t
   local anesthetics, 436–437, 449
      in neonate, 668
   meperidine, 88
   regional anesthesia, 140–142, 142t
Toxoplasmosis, with HIV, 591t
Trachea, topical anesthesia/nerve blocks of, 383
Tracheal intubation. *See* Endotracheal intubation
Tracheal occlusion, 270–271, 271f
Tracheal suctioning, of newborn, 660–661, 661f, 666–668, 667f
Tracheostomy, 381, 434
Traction, newborn response to, 647, 647f, 649f
Tramadol, systemic, 116
Tranquilizers, teratogenicity of, 253
Transcutaneous electrical nerve stimulation (TENS), 97–98, 98f
Transcutaneous PO$_2$, during labor, 9, 9f
Transfusion therapy
   for abruptio placentae, 365
   for fetal anemia, 617
   during neurosurgery, 519
   for sickle-cell anemia, 351, 351t
Transient neurologic symptoms (TNS), after spinal anesthesia, 79–80, 79t, 80t
Transient radicular irritation (TRI), due to lidocaine, 242
Transplacental carcinogenesis, 259
Transplantation, 572–576, 572t
   cardiac, 572–573
   kidney, 574–575, 575t
   liver, 574
   lung, 573–574
   pancreas, 575–576
Transtracheal block, 383
Transtracheal jet ventilation (TTJV), 381, 387
Trauma
   due to regional anesthesia, 418–419, 419f, 420
   teratogenicity of, 258
Trendelenburg position, for hypotension, 206
TRI (transient radicular irritation), due to lidocaine, 242
Trichloroethylene (Trilene), 193, 194
Trickle-down anesthesia, 383
Tricyclic antidepressants, fetal and neonatal effects of, 683t
Trigeminal nerve, 381, 381f
Trimethaphan, for pregnancy-induced hypertension, 307, 315t
Trinitroglycerin (TNG), for pregnancy-induced hypertension, 307
Tripelennamine, for asthma, 490t
Triple marker screening, 613–614, 614t
Trisomy 18, 21, 613–614
Trophoblast, 19, 20f
TTJV (transtracheal jet ventilation), 381, 387
TTP (thrombotic thrombocytopenic purpura), stroke due to, 511f
Tubal ligation, 237–244, 402–403
   breast-feeding after, 243–244, 244t
   general anesthesia for, 242–243, 242t, 243t, 403
   guidelines for, 676
   vs. laparoscopic sterilization, 237–238
   local anesthesia for, 240, 240f
   mortality from, 237
   preparation for, 239
   regional anesthesia for, 240–242, 241f, 241t, 242t, 403
   timing of, 237
Tuberculosis
   with HIV, 586
   with opioid abuse, 604
D-Tubocurarine, magnesium with, 305, 305f
Tubular reabsorption, during pregnancy, 13
Tuffier's line, 418–419, 419f
"Turtle sign," 292
Twin(s), 293–294, 294f, 294t
   abnormal, 271
Twin-to-twin transfusion syndrome, 271

U
UESP (upper esophageal sphincter pressure), 378
Ulcers, decubitus, 413
Ultrasonography, prenatal, 614–616, 615f
Umbilical arterial blood, free drug in, 66–68, 66t

Umbilical artery(ies), 19
   in fetal drug uptake, 65, 66, 66f
Umbilical artery catheterization, 664
Umbilical blood flow, 23–24, 24f
   in fetal drug uptake, 65, 66, 66f
   interruption of, 623
Umbilical cord, prolapsed, in breech presentation, 290
Umbilical cord blood sampling, 659–660, 659t
Umbilical vein, 19
Umbilical vein catheterization, 663–664, 664f
Upper airway edema, in preeclampsia, 301
Upper esophageal sphincter pressure (UESP), 378
Urinary output, with pregnancy-induced hypertension, 308, 308t
Urinary retention
   due to combined spinal-epidural analgesia, 130t
   due to intraspinal morphine, 176–177, 177f
   due to regional anesthesia, 144
Urinary stasis, during pregnancy, 13
Urinary tract obstruction, fetal, 271–272, 272f, 273f
Uterine activity
   defined, 41
   drug effects on, 41–54
      with inhalation agents, 41, 43f
      with intrathecal and combined spinal-epidural analgesia, 52–53, 52t, 53f
      with parenteral agents, 43–44, 43f
      with regional anesthesia, 44–52, 44f
      with test dose of epinephrine, 135, 135f
   fetal heart rate and, 625
   measurement of, 41, 42f
   monitoring of, 625
   in pregnancy-induced hypertension, 303
Uterine arterial blood, concentration of free drug in, 61, 62t
Uterine atony, 367–369, 368t
Uterine bleeding, with halogenated agents, 222–223, 223t, 224t
Uterine blood flow. *See also* Uteroplacental circulation
   distribution of, 61, 62f
   with halogenated agents, 222, 222f
   inadequate, 623
   during pregnancy, 14, 22–23, 22f, 23t, 26
Uterine contractions
   cardiovascular effects of, 457f
   hemodynamic effects of, 8, 9f
   physiology of, 325, 326f
Uterine displacement, for aortocaval compression, 10
Uterine hyperstimulation, due to combined spinal-epidural analgesia, 130
Uterine hypertonus, 260, 260f
Uterine inversion, 367
Uterine relaxation, 41
   during fetal surgery, 278–280
   with inhalation agents, 195
Uterine rupture, 365–366, 366t
   fetal bradycardia due to, 627
Uterine vasoconstriction, 260, 260f
Uteroplacental circulation, 19, 20f. *See also* Uterine blood flow
   animal models of, 26, 28f
   assessment of, 26, 28f
   with diabetes mellitus, 502
   drug effects on, 26–36, 27t
      antihypertensive agents, 27t, 33–34, 34f, 35f
      calcium channel blockers, 27t, 34
      catecholamines, 27t, 31–32, 33f
      clonidine, 27t, 35
      dantrolene, 27t, 35–36
      induction agents, 26–29, 27t, 28f, 29f
      inhalation agents, 27t, 29–30, 30f
      intraspinal opioids, 27t, 35
      local anesthetics, 27t, 30–31, 30f, 31f
      magnesium sulfate, 27t, 34–35
      regional anesthesia, 27t, 31, 31f
      vasopressors, 27t, 32, 33f
   respiratory gases and, 27t, 36, 36f
   stress effects on, 27t, 32

V
Vaginal birth after cesarean (VBAC), 366
   uterine rupture during, 365–366, 366t
Vaginal delivery
   with aortic stenosis, 463
   with asymmetric septal hypertrophy, 475
   of breech presentation, 289–290, 289t, 290f
   with cardiomyopathy of pregnancy, 473
   with coronary artery disease, 475
   general anesthesia for, 189, 191t
   guidelines for, 674–676
   with hypertension, 473
   with idiopathic thrombocytopenic purpura, 348
   with mitral stenosis, 459–460
   of multiple gestations, 294
   with myasthenia gravis, 538
   for neurosurgical patients, 522–523, 522f
   with obesity, 552–553
   with pregnancy-induced hypertension, 303–304, 308
   of preterm infant, 337–340
   primary pulmonary hypertension, 472
   pulmonic stenosis, 471
   rheumatoid arthritis, 569
   systemic lupus erythematosus, 570–571
   tetralogy of Fallot, 468
Vaginal lacerations, 369
Vagus nerve, 381, 382f
Valproic acid, fetal and neonatal effects of, 683t
Valvular surgery, pregnancy after, 476–477, 476t
Variable decelerations, 625t, 629t, 631, 631f

VAS (vibroacoustic stimulation), 618
Vascular malformations, angiographically occult, 512
Vascular resistance, with obesity, 548f
Vasculitis, stroke due to, 511f
Vasculosyncytial membrane, 21
Vasoconstriction, uterine, 260, 260f
Vasodilators, fetal and neonatal effects of, 480, 684t
Vasopressors
    effect on first stage of labor of, 46–47, 47f
    effect on uteroplacental blood flow of, 27t, 32, 33f
    fetal effects of, 479–480
    hypertension induced by, 143
    for hypotension, 138, 139–140, 140f, 141f, 207
Vasospasm, after neurosurgery, 522
Vasoxyl (methoxamine)
    effect on fetus of, 479
    effect on first stage of labor of, 47, 47f
VBAC (vaginal birth after cesarean), 366
    uterine rupture during, 365–366, 366t
VC (vital capacity)
    with obesity, 548t
    during pregnancy, 3, 4t, 5f, 251f
Vecuronium
    for fetal surgery, 273
    maternal and fetal effects of, 221
    for neurosurgery, 520
    with obesity, 551, 551f
    for postpartum sterilization, 243
Ventilation
    establishment in newborn of, 657, 658f
    with general anesthesia, 217, 218f, 219f
    with obesity, 548
    positive-pressure, 217, 218f
    during pregnancy, 3

Ventilation equivalent, during pregnancy, 251f
Ventilatory effort, in Apgar score, 639, 640f
Ventricular outputs, fetal, 24
Ventricular septal defect (VSD), 456t, 466–467, 466t
Ventrolateral column, 124f
Verapamil
    effect on uteroplacental blood flow of, 27t, 34
    fetal effects of, 479
Very low-birth-weight infant, 323
Vesicostomy, fetal, 272
Vibroacoustic stimulation (VAS), 618
Videx (didanosine)
    fetal and neonatal effects of, 685t
    for HIV, 590t
Viracept (nelfinavir mesylate)
    fetal and neonatal effects of, 685t
    for HIV, 590t
Viral infections, due to regional anesthesia, 414
Viramune (nevirapine), for HIV, 590t
Vital capacity (VC)
    with obesity, 548t
    during pregnancy, 3, 4t, 5f, 251f
Vitamin K, for liver disease, 349
Volatile agents
    administration of, 193, 193f
    efficacy of, 194
    neonatal effects of, 195–196
Volume expanders, in neonatal resuscitation, 666t
Volume preload, and hypotension, 137, 434–435
Volume replacement, for hypotension, 206–207
Vomiting. See Nausea and vomiting
von Willebrand factor, 345, 346t
von Willebrand's disease (vWD), 348
VSD (ventricular septal defect), 456t, 466–467, 466t

W
Walking, automatic, 647, 647f, 649f
Walking epidurals, 129
    efficacy of, 161
    maternal safety of, 161–162, 161t
    neuromuscular coordination with, 413
Warfarin (Coumadin), fetal and neonatal effects of, 682t
Waste anesthetic gases, teratogenicity of, 256, 257t
Water, placental transport of, 20–21
Weight, of newborn, 643–645, 644f, 645f
Weight gain, during pregnancy, 7, 7t
Whitacre needle, 208, 208f
Withdrawal
    alcohol, 601
    caffeine, 602
    cocaine, 606
    opioid, 603, 604, 604t

X
Xylocaine. See Lidocaine

Z
Zalcitabine (ddC, Hivid)
    fetal and neonatal effects of, 685t
    for HIV, 590t
Zarontin (ethosuximide), for seizures, 532t
Zavanelli maneuver, 292, 293
Zerit (stavudine)
    fetal and neonatal effects of, 685t
    for HIV, 590t
Ziagen (abacavir), for HIV, 590t
Zidovudine (ZDV, AZT, Retrovir)
    fetal and neonatal effects of, 685t
    for HIV, 590t